a LANGE medical book

CURRENT
Pediatric Diagnosis & Treatment

13th Edition

Edited by

William W. Hay, Jr., MD
Professor, Department of Pediatrics
Director, Training Program in Neonatal-Perinatal Medicine
Director, Neonatal Clinical Research Center
Section of Neonatology and the Division of Perinatal Medicine and Research
University of Colorado School of Medicine and The Children's Hospital, Denver

Jessie R. Groothuis, MD
Professor, Department of Pediatrics
Director, Neonatal High Risk Followup Program
Section of Neonatology
University of Colorado School of Medicine and The Children's Hospital, Denver

Anthony R. Hayward, MD, PhD
Professor, Departments of Pediatrics and Immunology
Head, Section of Pediatric Allergy and Immunology
University of Colorado School of Medicine and The Children's Hospital, Denver

Myron J. Levin, MD
Professor, Departments of Pediatrics and Medicine
Head, Section of Pediatric Infectious Diseases
University of Colorado School of Medicine and The Children's Hospital, Denver

and Associate Authors

The Department of Pediatrics at the University of Colorado School of Medicine is affiliated with
The Children's Hospital of Denver, Colorado

Appleton & Lange
Stamford, Connecticut

Copyright © 1997 by Appleton & Lange
A Simon & Schuster Company

Editors: Add © history of previous editions here; include list of
chapters
not copyrighted by A&L here.

97 98 99 00 01 / 10 9 8 7 6 5 4 3 2 1

Prentice Hall International (UK) Limited, *London*
Prentice Hall of Australia Pty. Limited, *Sydney*
Prentice Hall Canada, Inc. *Toronto*
Prentice Hall Hispanoamericana, S.A., *Mexico*
Prentice Hall of India Private Limited, *New Delhi*
Prentice Hall of Japan, Inc., *Tokyo*
Simon & Schuster Asia Pte. Ltd., *Singapore*
Editora Prentice Hall do Brasil Ltda., *Rio de Janeiro*
Prentice Hall Upper Saddle River, New Jersey

ISBN 0-8385-1400-6
ISSN 0093-8556

Acquisitions Editor: Shelley Reinhardt
Production Editor: Chris Langan
Designer: Mary Skudlarek

Table of Contents

Contributors

Steven H. Abman, MD
Professor, Department of Pediatrics, Section of Pediatric Pulmonary Medicine, University of Colorado School of Medicine and The Children's Hospital, Denver.
Respiratory Tract & Mediastinum

R.B. Abrams, DDS
Assistant Clinical Professor, Department of Growth and Development, University of Colorado School of Dentistry; Director of Dental Education, The Children's Hospital, Denver.
Oral Medicine & Dentistry

Frank J. Accurso, MD
Professor, Department of Pediatrics, Section of Pediatric Pulmonary Medicine, University of Colorado School of Medicine and The Children's Hospital, Denver.
Respiratory Tract & Mediastinum

Edythe A. Albano, MD
Assistant Professor, Department of Pediatrics, Section of Hematology and Oncology, University of Colorado School of Medicine and The Children's Hospital, Denver.
Neoplastic Diseases

Daniel R. Ambruso, MD
Professor, Department of Pediatrics, Section of Pediatric Hematology and Oncology, University of Colorado School of Medicine; Associate Medical Director, Belle Bonfils Blood Center, Denver.
Hematologic Disorders

Trina Menden Anglin, MD, PhD
Medical Officer, Office of Adolescent Health, Maternal & Child Health Bureau, Health Resources & Services Administration, United States Public Health Service, Department of Health & Human Services, Rockville, Maryland.
Adolescent Substance Abuse

F. Keith Battan, MD
Assistant Professor, Department of Pediatrics, Section of Emergency and General Pediatrics, University of Colorado School of Medicine; Associate Director, Emergency Department, The Children's Hospital, Denver.
Emergencies & Injuries

Stephen Berman, MD
Professor, Department of Pediatrics, Section of General Academic Pediatrics University of Colorado School of Medicine and The Children's Hospital; Director of Health Policy, University of Colorado Health Sciences Center, Denver.
Ear, Nose, & Throat

Mark M. Boucek, MD
Professor, Department of Pediatrics, Section of Cardiology; Head, Section of Pediatric Cardiology, University of Colorado School of Medicine and The Children's Hospital, Denver.
Cardiovascular Diseases

Bonnie W. Camp, MD, PhD
Professor Emerita, Departments of Pediatrics and Psychiatry, University of Colorado School of Medicine, Denver.
Developmental Disorders

Kenneth H. Chan, MD
Associate Professor, Department of Pediatric Otolaryngology, University of Colorado School of Medicine; Chairman, Department of Pediatric Otolaryngology, The Children's Hospital, Denver.
Ear, Nose, & Throat

H. Peter Chase, MD
Professor, Department of Pediatrics; Clinical Director, Barbara Davis Center for Childhood Diabetes, University of Colorado School of Medicine, Denver.
Diabetes Mellitus

R. Barkley Clark, MD
Associate Clinical Professor, Department of Psychiatry, Division of Child Psychiatry, University of Colorado Health Sciences Center, Denver.
Psychosocial Aspects of Pediatric & Psychiatric Disorders

Richard C. Dart, MD, PhD
Director, Rocky Mountain Poison and Drug Cen-

ter; Associate Professor of Surgery, Medicine & Pharmacy, University of Colorado School of Medicine, Denver.
Emergencies & Injuries

Emily L. Dobyns, MD
Assistant Professor, Department of Pediatrics, Section of Pediatric Critical Care Medicine, University of Colorado School of Medicine and The Children's Hospital, Denver.
Critical Care

Anthony G. Durmowicz, MD
Assistant Professor, Department of Pediatrics, Section of Pediatric Critical Care Medicine, University of Colorado School of Medicine and The Children's Hospital, Denver.
Critical Care

Robert E. Eilert, MD
Clinical Professor, Department of Orthopedic Surgery, University of Colorado School of Medicine; Chairman, Department of Orthopedic Surgery, The Children's Hospital, Denver.
Orthopedics

George S. Eisenbarth, MD, PhD
Professor of Medicine, Pediatrics, & Immunology, University of Colorado Health Sciences Center; Executive Director, Barbara Davis Center for Childhood Diabetes, Denver.
Diabetes Mellitus

Allan M. Eisenbaum, MD, FAAO, FAAP
Associate Clinical Professor, Department of Ophthalmology, University of Colorado School of Medicine and The Children's Hospital, Denver.
Eye

Leland L. Fan, MD
Professor, Department of Pediatrics, Section of Pediatric Pulmonary Medicine, University of Colorado School of Medicine and The Children's Hospital, Denver.
Respiratory Tract & Mediastinum

Nicholas K. Foreman, MD
Associate Professor, Department of Pediatrics, University of Colorado School of Medicine; Director of Neuro-Oncology, The Children's Hospital, Denver.
Neoplastic Diseases

Erwin W. Gelfand, MD
Professor, Department of Pediatrics and Microbiology/Immunology, University of Colorado School of Medicine; Chairman, Department of

Pediatrics, National Jewish Center for Immunology and Respiratory Medicine, Denver.
Immunodeficiency

Gaia Georgopoulos, MD
Assistant Clinical Professor, Department of Orthopedics, University of Colorado School of Medicine and The Children's Hospital, Denver.
Orthopedics

Edward Goldson, MD
Professor, Department of Pediatrics, Section of Developmental and Behavioral Medicine, University of Colorado School of Medicine and The Children's Hospital, Denver.
Behavioral Disorders & Developmental Variations

Stephen I. Goodman, MD
Professor, Department of Pediatrics, Head, Section of Genetics, Metabolism and Birth Defects, University of Colorado School of Medicine and The Children's Hospital, Denver.
Inborn Errors of Metabolism

Ronald W. Gotlin, MD
Professor, Department of Pediatrics, Section of Pediatric Endocrinology; Director of Medical Student Education, University of Colorado School of Medicine and The Children's Hospital, Denver.
Endocrine Disorders

Carol L. Greene, MD
Associate Professor, Department of Pediatrics, Section of Genetics, Metabolism and Birth Defects, University of Colorado School of Medicine and The Children's Hospital, Denver.
Inborn Errors of Metabolism

Brian S. Greffe, MD, CM
Assistant Professor, Department of Pediatrics, Section of Hematology and Oncology, University of Colorado School of Medicine and The Children's Hospital, Denver.
Neoplastic Diseases

Leon Greos, MD
Clinician and Practicing Allergist, Colorado Allergy and Asthma Clinic, PC, Aurora.
Allergic Disorders

Jessie R. Groothuis, MD
Professor, Department of Pediatrics; Director, Neonatal High Risk Followup Program, Section of Neonatology, University of Colorado School of Medicine and The Children's Hospital, Denver.
Immunization

Randi Jenssen Hagerman, MD
Professor, Department of Pediatrics, Head, Section of Developmental and Behavioral Medicine, University of Colorado School of Medicine and The Children's Hospital, Denver.
Growth & Development

K. Michael Hambidge, MD, BChir, ScD
Professor, Department of Pediatrics; Director, University of Colorado Center for Human Nutrition, University of Colorado Health Sciences Center and The Children's Hospital, Denver.
Normal Childhood Nutrition & Its Disorders

Keith B. Hammond, MS, FIMLS
Senior Instructor, Departments of Pediatrics and Pathology; Director, Pediatric Clinical Research Center Laboratory, University of Colorado School of Medicine and The Children's Hospital, Denver.
Normal Biochemical & Hematologic Values

William W. Hay, Jr., MD
Professor, Department of Pediatrics; Director, Training Program in Neonatal-Perinatal Medicine; Director, Neonatal Clinical Research Center, Section of Neonatology, Division of Perinatal Medicine and Research, University of Colorado School of Medicine and The Children's Hospital, Denver.

Anthony R. Hayward, MD, PhD
Professor, Departments of Pediatrics and Immunology; Head, Section of Pediatric Allergy and Immunology, University of Colorado School of Medicine and The Children's Hospital, Denver.
Immunodeficiency

Roxann M. Headley, MD
Assistant Professor, Department of Pediatrics, Section of General Academic Pediatrics, University of Colorado School of Medicine; Medical Director, Child Health Clinic, The Children's Hospital, Denver.
Ambulatory Pediatrics

Desmond B. Henry, Jr., MD
Clinical Instructor, Departments of Anesthesiology and Pediatrics, University of Colorado School of Medicine; Medical Director, Pediatric Care Unit; Director of Children's Emergency Transport Services, Inc., The Children's Hospital, Denver.
Critical Care

J. Roger Hollister, MD
Professor, Department of Pediatrics, University of Colorado Health Sciences Center; Head, Section of Pediatric Rheumatology, University of Col-

orado School of Medicine and The Children's Hospital, Denver.
Rheumatic Diseases

David W. Kaplan, MD, MPH
Professor, Department of Pediatrics; Head, Section of Adolescent Medicine, University of Colorado School of Medicine and The Children's Hospital, Denver.
Adolescence

Michael S. Kappy, MD, PhD
Professor, Department of Pediatrics, Head, Section of Pediatric Endocrinology, University of Colorado School of Medicine and The Children's Hospital, Denver.
Endocrine Disorders

Elizabeth B. Kozleski, EdD
Assistant Professor, School of Education, Division of Educational Psychology and Special Education, University of Colorado; Associate Professor, Department of Psychiatry, University of Colorado Health Sciences Center, Denver.
Developmental Disorders

Nancy F. Krebs, MD, MS
Assistant Professor, Department of Pediatrics, Section of Nutrition; Associate Director, University of Colorado Center for Human Nutrition, University of Colorado School of Medicine and The Children's Hospital, Denver.
Normal Childhood Nutrition & Its Disorders

Richard D. Krugman, MD
Professor, Department of Pediatrics; Dean, University of Colorado School of Medicine, Denver.
Child Abuse & Neglect

Peter A. Lane, MD
Associate Professor, Department of Pediatrics, Section of Pediatric Hematology and Oncology; Director, Colorado Sickle Cell Treatment and Research Center, University of Colorado School of Medicine and The Children's Hospital, Denver.
Hematologic Disorders

Gary L. Larsen, MD
Professor, Department of Pediatrics; Head, Section of Pediatric Pulmonary Medicine, University of Colorado School of Medicine; Senior Faculty Member, National Jewish Center for Immunology and Respiratory Medicine, Denver.
Respiratory Tract & Mediastinum

Myron J. Levin, MD
Professor, Departments of Pediatrics and Medi-

cine; Head, Section of Pediatric Infectious Diseases, University of Colorado School of Medicine and The Children's Hospital, Denver.
Infections: Viral & Rickettsial
Infections: Parasitic & Mycotic

Stanley L. Loftness, MD, FAAP
Assistant Clinical Professor, Departments of Pediatrics and Anesthesiology, University of Colorado Health Sciences Center; School of Medicine and The Children's Hospital, Denver.
Critical Care

Gary M. Lum, MD
Professor, Departments of Pediatrics and Medicine; Head, Section of Pediatric Renal Medicine, University of Colorado School of Medicine and The Children's Hospital, Denver.
Kidney & Urinary Tract

James V. Lustig, MD
Director, Children's Medical Center of Northwest Ohio, Medical College of Ohio, Toledo.
Ambulatory Pediatrics

Kathleen A. Mammel, MD
Director, Adolescent Pediatrics, William Beaumont Hospital, University of Michigan Medical School, Royal Oak.
Adolescence
Fluid & Electrolyte Therapy

David K. Manchester, MD
Associate Professor, Departments of Pediatrics and Pharmacology, University of Colorado School of Medicine; Co-Director, Division of Genetic Services, The Children's Hospital, Denver.
Genetics & Dysmorphology

Elizabeth J. McFarland, MD
Assistant Professor, Department of Pediatrics, University of Colorado Health Sciences Center; Associate Director, HIV Program, The Children's Hospital, Denver.
Human Immunodeficiency Virus (HIV) Infections:
Acquired Immunodeficiency Syndrome (AIDS)

Paul G. Moe, MD, MS
Professor, Departments of Pediatrics and Neurology, University of Colorado School of Medicine and The Children's Hospital, Denver.
Neurologic & Muscular Disorders

Joseph G. Morelli, MD
Associate Professor, Departments of Pediatrics and Dermatology, University of Colorado School of Medicine and The Children's Hospital, Denver.
Skin

William A. Mueller, DMD
Clinical Associate Professor, Department of Growth & Development, University of Colorado School of Dentistry; Chief of Dentistry, The Children's Hospital, Denver.
Oral Medicine & Dentistry

Michael R. Narkewicz, MD
Associate Professor, Department of Pediatrics, Section of Pediatric Gastroenterology, Hepatology, and Nutrition, and The Pediatric Liver Center, University of Colorado School of Medicine and The Children's Hospital, Denver.
Liver & Pancreas

Rachelle Nuss, MD
Associate Professor, Department of Pediatrics, Section of Pediatric Hematology and Oncology, University of Colorado School of Medicine and The Children's Hospital, Denver.
Hematologic Disorders

Lorrie F. Odom, MD
Professor, Department of Pediatrics, Section of Pediatric Hematology and Oncology, University of Colorado School of Medicine; Clinical Director of Oncology, The Children's Hospital, Denver.
Neoplastic Diseases

John W. Ogle, MD
Associate Professor and Vice Chairman, Department of Pediatrics, University of Colorado School of Medicine; Director, Department of Pediatrics, Denver General Hospital, Denver.
Infections: Bacterial & Spirochetal
Antimicrobial Therapy of Pediatric Infections

Christopher M. Paap, PharmD, BCPS
Assistant Professor, University of Colorado School of Pharmacy; Clinical Specialist, The Children's Hospital, Denver.
Drug Therapy

David S. Pearlman, MD
Clinical Professor, Department of Pediatrics, University of Colorado School of Medicine, Denver.
Allergic Disorders

Adam A. Rosenberg, MD
Professor, Department of Pediatrics, Section of Neonatology, University of Coloraldo School of Medicine and The Children's Hospital, Denver; Medical Director of the Newborn Service, University Hospital, University of Colorado Health Sciences Center, Denver.
The Newborn Infant

Barry H. Rumack, MD
Clinical Professor, Department of Pediatrics, University of Colorado School of Medicine; President and Chief Executive Officer, Micromedex, Inc., Denver.
Emergencies, Injuries, & Poisoning

Michael S. Schaffer, MD
Associate Professor, Department of Pediatrics, Section of Pediatric Cardiology; Director, Department of Electrophysiology, University of Colorado School of Medicine and The Children's Hospital, Denver.
Cardiovascular Diseases

Alan R. Seay, MD
Professor, Departments of Pediatrics and Neurology; and Head, Division of Child Neurology, University of Colorado School of Medicine and The Children's Hospital, Denver.
Neurologic & Muscular Disorders

Eric J. Sigel, MD
Assistant Professor, Department of Pediatrics; Clinical Director, Adolescent Clinic, University of Colorado School of Medicine and The Children's Hospital, Denver.
Sexually Transmitted Disease

Eric A.F. Simoes, MD, DCH
Associate Professor, Department of Pediatrics, Section of Pediatric Infectious Diseases, University of Colorado School of Medicine and The Children's Hospital, Denver.
Immunization

Robert H. Slover, MD
Assistant Professor, Department of Pediatrics, Section of Pediatric Endocrinology, University of Colorado School of Medicine and The Children's Hospital, Denver.
Endocrine Disorders

Ronald J. Sokol, MD
Professor, Department of Pediatrics, Section of Pediatric Gastroenterology, Hepatology, and Nutrition; Medical Director, Pediatric Liver Center, University of Colorado School of Medicine and The Children's Hospital, Denver.
Liver & Pancreas

Judith M. Sondheimer, MD
Professor, Department of Pediatrics; Chief, Section of Pediatric Gastroenterology, Hepatology, and Nutrition, University of Colorado Health Sciences Center and The Children's Hospital, Denver.
Gastrointestinal Tract

Kurt R. Stenmark, MD
Professor, Department of Pediatrics; Head, Section

of Pediatric Critical Care Medicine, University of Colorado School of Medicine and The Children's Hospital, Denver.
Critical Care

Janet M. Stewart, MD
Associate Professor, Department of Pediatrics, Section of Genetics, Metabolism, and Birth Defects, University of Colorado School of Medicine and The Children's Hospital, Denver.
Genetics & Dysmorphology

Linda C. Stork, MD
Associate Professor, Department of Pediatrics, Section of Hematology and Oncology, University of Colorado Health Sciences Center, Denver.
Neoplastic Diseases

Eva Sujansky, MD
Associate Professor, Departments of Pediatrics and Biophysics, Biochemistry and Genetics, University of Colorado School of Medicine; Co-Director, Division of Genetic Services, The Children's Hospital, Denver.
Genetics & Dysmorphology

Elizabeth H. Thilo, MD
Associate Professor, Department of Pediatrics, Section of Neonatology, University of Colorado Health Sciences Center, Denver.
The Newborn Infant

Joanne M. Vitanza, MD
Clinician and Practicing Allergist, Colorado Allergy and Asthma Clinic, PC, Aurora.
Allergic Disorders

Jeffrey S. Wagener, MD
Associate Professor, Department of Pediatrics, Section of Pulmonary Medicine, University of Colorado School of Medicine and The Children's Hospital, Denver.
Respiratory Tract & Mediastinum

Adriana Weinberg, MD
Assistant Professor, Departments of Pediatrics and Medicine, University of Colorado Health Sciences Center, Denver.
Infections: Parasitic & Mycotic

William L. Weston, MD
Professor and Chairman, Department of Dermatology; Professor, Department of Pediatrics, University of Colorado School of Medicine, Denver.
Skin

Carl W. White, MD
Professor, Department of Pediatrics, Section of

Pediatric Pulmonary Medicine, University of Colorado Health Sciences Center; Senior Staff Physician, National Jewish Center for Immunology and Respiratory Medicine, Denver.
Respiratory Tract & Mediastinum

James W. Wiggins, Jr., MD
Professor, Department of Pediatrics, Section of Pediatric Cardiology, University of Colorado School of Medicine and The Children's Hospital, Denver.
Cardiovascular Diseases

Robert R. Wolfe, MD
Professor, Department of Pediatrics, Section of Pediatric Cardiology, University of Colorado School of Medicine and The Children's Hospital, Denver.
Cardiovascular Diseases

Preface

The 13th edition of *Current Pediatric Diagnosis & Treatment* features practical, up-to-date, well-referenced information on the care of children from birth through infancy and adolescence. *CPDT* emphasizes the clinical aspects of pediatric care while also covering the important underlying principles. Its goal is to provide a guide to diagnosis, understanding, and treatment of the medical problems of all pediatric patients in an easy to use and readable format.

INTENDED AUDIENCE

Like all Lange medical books, *CPDT* provides a concise yet comprehensive source of current information. Students will find *CPDT* an authoritative introduction to pediatrics and an excellent source for reference and review. Residents in pediatrics (and other specialties) will appreciate the detailed descriptions of diseases and diagnostic and therapeutic procedures. Pediatricians, family practitioners, nurses, and other health-care providers who work with infants and children also will find *CPDT* a useful reference on management aspects of pediatric medicine.

COVERAGE

Forty-two chapters cover a wide range of topics, including normal growth and development, neonatal medicine, emergency and critical care medicine, and diagnosis and treatment of specific disorders according to major problems and organ systems. A wealth of tables and figures summarize such important information as acute and critical care procedures in the delivery room, the office, the emergency room, and the critical care unit; anti-infective agents; drug dosages; immunization schedules; differential diagnosis; and the development screening tests. The final chapter is a handy guide to normal laboratory values.

NEW TO THE EDITION

The 13th edition of *CPDT* remains an up-to-date, comprehensive pediatric treatise, but this edition is *the most comprehensive revision to date* and significantly improves this classic book. The editors and contributing authors have continued to substantially revise the book, providing recent medical advances and increasing the book's emphasis on ambulatory care, acute critical care, and the practical approach to pediatric disorders. As editors and practicing pediatricians, we have tried to ensure that each chapter reflects the needs and realities of day-to-day practice.

New Chapters: The *two new chapters* deal with two of the most important and timely subjects in pediatric medicine today:

30. Diabetes Mellitus

36. Human Immunodeficiency Virus (HIV) Infections: Acquired Immunodeficiency Syndrome (AIDS)

Chapter Revisions: Nine chapters have been extensively revised, with new authors added in several cases, reflecting substantial new information in each of their areas of pediatric medicine:

9. Ambulatory Pediatrics
10. Immunization
17. Ear, Nose, & Throat
18. Respiratory Tract & Mediastinum
27. Neoplastic Disease
29. Endocrine Disorders
33. Allergic Disorders
35. Infections: Viral & Rickettsial
38. Infections: Parasitic & Mycotic

All other chapters are substantially revised and references have been updated.

ACKNOWLEDGMENTS

The editors and contributing authors wish to thank Karen Goselin, Administrative Assistant, Section of Neonatology and the Department of Pediatrics, for organizational support and secretarial assistance.

William W. Hay, Jr., MD
Jessie R. Groothuis, MD
Anthony R. Hayward, MD, PhD
Myron J. Levin, MD

Denver
November 1996

Growth & Development

1

Randi Jenssen Hagerman, MD

This chapter outlines the continuous and dynamic process of growth and development in children. It emphasizes the interactive aspects of physical, cognitive, social, and emotional development so that the reader can appreciate the impact of each of these domains throughout the span of development.

Our understanding of development has undergone major shifts in this century as we have assimilated new information. Freud emphasized how early emotional experiences determined by the environment shape personality and psychopathology. Piaget focused on the predetermined unfolding of cognitive abilities over time in a specific progression that is innate to the child and relatively independent of the environment. In past decades, however, the influence of the environment has assumed an all-powerful role as people have appreciated how greatly the trauma of dysfunctional families and socioeconomic status affect optimal developmental outcomes. We have now reached a stage of regarding the environmental influences in a context that also takes into account the genetic components of temperament and cognitive abilities in a neurobiologic format. We can now understand development through the interaction of these forces so that the relative importance of any single factor is not inflated unless significant trauma or pathologic circumstances exist.

This chapter is divided into sections according to age so that the interactions of central nervous system maturation; physical, cognitive, and emotional growth; genetic variation; and environmental influences can be discussed at critical age levels. Major development theories are reviewed, and longitudinal changes are summarized in charts and tables to give readers an organizational framework by which to remember trends in development. Development occurs at a variable pace in each child. The developmental milestones cited refer to an average child or to group means, and the variability from child to child must be remembered.

THE NEWBORN

Normal newborns are endowed with a set of reflexes to facilitate survival, including rooting and sucking reflexes, and remarkable sensory abilities. The newborn is no longer considered a blank slate— a totally unformed being who gradually gains abilities according to environmental influences. Instead, the newborn is seen as having genetic strengths and weaknesses in neurocognitive organization that are reflected in temperament, adaptability, responsiveness, and general interaction with the environment. These responses should in turn prompt reciprocal interactions from the parents, which further shape development. The Neonatal Behavioral Assessment scale by Brazelton was developed to measure many of the newborn's characteristics of temperament, including social behavior, orienting responses to stimuli, ability to deal with disturbing stimuli, state of arousal, and motor skills. When these abilities are described to the mother, this assessment can further sensitize her to the unique aspects of her child's behavior and responsiveness. This knowledge may in turn improve their interactions.

The newborn has significant sensory abilities, which have been better identified in the last decade. Hearing is well developed at birth, and speech sounds are preferred. The infant becomes alert and oriented to a female voice with high-pitched tones more readily than to a low-pitched male voice. The lower frequency tones of a male voice are more likely to soothe an infant. High-pitched crying is distressing not only to the newborn but also to adults. Infants can shut out loud or aversive stimuli and simply not respond. Within the first few weeks of life, they learn to recognize the mother's voice and differentiate it from other female voices.

Smell is well developed at birth and plays a significant role in how infants orient themselves to the environment. Infants turn away from aversive smells and respond positively to pleasant ones. By 1 week of age, breast-fed infants recognize and discriminate the smell of their mother's breast pads. They recognize the smell of their mother, not the smell of milk alone. The infant has definite taste preferences at birth, preferring sweet tastes. Infants have more taste buds than adults do and avoid bitter or aversive tastes.

At birth, the retina is well developed, but the lens is rather immobile. Fixation and tracking through the visual field are well developed by 2 months of age. Infants prefer to gaze at a human face rather than geometric designs, and they also prefer curved lines, bright colors, and high contrast. The length of time that an infant fixates on a paired visual stimulus has been interpreted as visual preference and has also been correlated with later cognitive development. Visual fixation tasks are the basis of the "infant IQ" tests marketed recently. Although visual acuity is poor at birth (approximately 20/400), it improves rapidly in the first 6 months of life to 20/40. Strabismus is common after birth but usually resolves by 3 months of age. If it persists, referral to an ophthalmologist is appropriate at 6 months of age.

Brazelton TB: *Neonatal Behavioral Assessment Scale,* 2nd ed. Lippincott, 1984.

Dixon SD, Stein MT: *Encounters With Children: Pediatric Behavior and Development,* 2nd ed. Mosby–Year Book, 1992. (An exceptional review of development with an emphasis on incorporating development issues into general pediatric care.)

Yogman MW, Cook KV, Gersten M: Infant and toddler development: Active organization of the social world. Curr Probl Pediatr 1988 (May);18:259. (A detailed assessment of early cognitive and emotional development.)

THE FIRST YEAR

One of the most distressing features of infants is the amount of time they spend crying in the first few weeks of life. Crying gradually increases during the first 6–12 weeks of age because it is the main modality by which infants express responses to stimuli, both aversive and nonaversive. Crying can be a response to a variety of stimuli, including hunger, a wet diaper, fear, fatigue, and overstimulation. Crying gradually decreases after 12 weeks of age, as the infant develops other responses, such as smiling or reaching, or becomes more adept at self-soothing, such as by sucking the fingers or thumb. In the first weeks of life, however, crying can become a distressing problem for the parents, and crying associated with irritability is often labeled as colic. Particularly sensitive infants with a low tolerance for stimuli can be irritable and difficult to deal with at home. It is useful to help parents understand their infant's temperament and to teach them techniques for avoiding excessive stimuli (because parents often respond to excessive crying by creating excessive stimuli). Parents should be taught ways to calm the child, such as offering nonnutritive sucking, rocking the child, singing to the child, and walking while holding the

child. Perhaps most important for the parents is an understanding of the developmental aspects of crying and the emergence of improved coping skills in the baby after 12 weeks of age.

Piaget describes the first 2 years of life as the sensorimotor period, during which infants learn with increasing sophistication how to link the sensory input from the environment with a motor response. Infants build on primitive reflex patterns of behavior (termed *schema*; sucking is an example) and constantly incorporate or assimilate new experiences to further elaborate their schema. The schema evolve over time as infants accommodate new experiences and as new levels of cognitive ability unfold in a rather orderly sequence. In the first year of life, infants' perception of reality revolves around themselves and what they can see or touch. They follow the trajectory of an object through the field of vision, but prior to 6 months, the object does not exist for them once it leaves the field of vision. At 9–12 months, infants gradually develop the concept of object permanence, or the understanding that objects exist even when they are not seen. They first apply the concept of object permanence to the image of the mother because of her emotional importance; this realization is a critical part of attachment behavior, discussed below. In the second year, children extend their ability to manipulate objects by using instruments, first by imitation and later by trial and error (Table 1–1).

Freud describes the first year of life as the oral stage because so many of the infant's needs are fulfilled by oral means. Nutrition is obtained through sucking on the breast or bottle, and self-soothing also occurs through sucking on fingers or a pacifier. As Mahler emphasizes, this is a stage of symbiosis with the mother, during which the boundaries between mother and infant are blurred. The baby's needs are totally met by the mother, and the mother has been described as manifesting "narcissistic possessiveness" of the infant. This is a very positive and critical interaction in the bidirectional attachment process known as bonding. The parents learn to be aware of and read their infant's cues, which reflect needs. A more sensitive emotional interaction process develops, which can be seen in the mirroring of facial expressions by mother and infant and in their mutual engagement in cycles of attention and inattention, which further develops into social play. A mother who is depressed or cannot respond to the baby's expressions and cues has a profound effect on the infant's future development and attachment. Erickson's terms of basic trust versus mistrust are another way of describing the reciprocal interaction that characterizes this stage (see Table 1–1).

Turn-taking games, which occur between 3 and 6 months of age, are a pleasure for both the parents and the infant and are an extension of mirroring behavior. They also represent an early form of imitative behavior, which is important in later social and cognitive

Table 1–1. Perspectives of human behavior.[1]

Age	Theories of Development			Skill Areas		Psychopathology
	Freud	Erikson	Piaget	Language	Motor	
Birth–18 mo	Oral	Basic trust vs mistrust	Sensorimotor	Body actions; crying; naming; pointing	Reflex sitting, reaching, grasping, walking	Autism; anaclitic depression, colic; disorders of attachment; feeding, sleeping problems
18 mo–3 y	Anal	Autonomy vs shame, doubt	Symbolic (preoperational)	Sentences; telegraph jargon	Climbing, running	Separation issues; negativism; fearfulness; constipation; shyness, withdrawal
3–6 y	Oedipal	Initiative vs guilt	Intuition (preoperational)	Connective words; can be readily understood	Increased coordination; tricycle; jumping	Enuresis; encopresis; anxiety; aggressive acting out; phobias; nightmares
6–11 y	Latency	Industry vs inferiority	Concrete operational	Subordinate sentences; reading and writing; language reasoning	Increased skills; sports, recreational cooperative games	School phobias; obsessive reactions; conversion reactions; depressive equivalents
12–17 y	Adolescence (genital)	Identity vs role confusion	Formal operational	Reason abstract; using language; abstract manipulation	Refinement of skills	Delinquency; promiscuity; schizophrenia; anorexia nervosa; suicide
17–30 y	Young adulthood	Intimacy vs isolation	Formal operational	Reason abstract; using language; abstract manipulation	Refinement of skills	Schizophrenia; borderline personality; adjustment disorders; development of intimate relationship and difficulties with relationships
30–60 y	Adulthood	Generativity vs stagnation	Formal operational	Reason abstract; using language; abstract manipulation	Refinement of skills	Depression; self-doubts; career development issues; family, social network; neuroses
60 y and over	Old age	Ego integration vs despair	Formal operational		Loss of functions (?)	Involutional depression; anxiety; anger; increased dependency

[1]Adapted and reproduced, with permission, from Dixon S: Setting the stage: Theories and concepts of child development. In: *Encounters With Children.* Dixon S, Stein M (editors). Year Book, 1987.

development. More sophisticated games, such as peek-a-boo, occur at approximately 9 months. The infant's thrill at the reappearance of the face that vanished momentarily demonstrates the emerging understanding of object permanence.

Eight to nine months is also a critical time in the attachment process because separation anxiety and stranger anxiety become marked. Kagan describes the infant at this stage as able to appreciate discrepant events that match previously known schema only partially. These new events cause uncertainty and subsequently fear and anxiety. Cognitively, the

infant must be able to retrieve the memory of previous schema and integrate the new information to previous knowledge over an extended time. These abilities are developed by 8 months of age and lead to the fears that subsequently develop: stranger anxiety and separation anxiety. In stranger anxiety, the infant analyzes the face of a stranger, detects the mismatch with previous schema, and may subsequently respond with fear or anxiety, leading to crying. In separation anxiety, the child perceives the difference between the mother's presence and absence by remembering the schema of her presence. Perceiving the inconsistency, the child becomes uncertain and subsequently anxious and fearful. This begins at 8 months, reaches a peak at 15 months, and disappears by the end of 2 years in a relatively orderly progression because central nervous system maturation facilitates the development of new skills. A parent can put the child's understanding of object permanence to good use by placing a picture of the mother near the child or by leaving an object where the child can see it during her absence. A visual substitute for her actual presence may comfort the child.

Bayley N (editor): *Bayley Scales of Infant Development,* 2nd ed. Psychological Corp, 1993.

Dixon SD, Stein MT: *Encounters With Children: Pediatric Behavior and Development,* 2nd ed. Mosby–Year Book, 1992.

Freud A: *Normality and Pathology in Childhood: Assessments of Development.* International Universities Press, 1965.

Ginsberg H, Opper S: *Piaget's Theory of Intellectual Development.* Prentice-Hall, 1969. (A readable review of Piaget's work.)

Kagan J: Canalization of early psychological development. Pediatrics 1982;70:474.

Levine MD, Carey WB, Crocker AC (editors): *Developmental-Behavioral Pediatrics,* 2nd ed. Saunders, 1992.

Piaget J: *The Origins of Intelligence in Children.* Norton, 1952.

Yogman MW, Cook KV, Gersten M: Infant and toddler development: Active organization of the social world. Curr Probl Pediatr 1988 (May);18:259.

GROWTH IN THE FIRST 3 YEARS

Fetal growth in length is most rapid at 4–6 months' gestation. However, adipose tissue begins to develop at 7 months, and weight gain accelerates, causing fetal weight to double during the last 2 months in utero. The rate of growth of males in late fetal development and during the first 6 months postnatally is more rapid than the growth rate of females because of a higher level of testosterone. The birth weight of the newborn correlates with the size, nutritional state, and general health of the mother and represents the influence of uterine constraints on ultimate size. Newborns may lose up to 10% of their birth weight in the first few days of life, but with normal nutrition birth weight is regained in approximately 10 days. The infant subsequently gains approximately 30 g/d for the first several months.

After the first 6 months of life, genetic factors influencing ultimate height begin to exert their effect. The growth percentile, therefore, may shift significantly in the first 4–18 months of life. This shift can be either up or down. An infant who is small for gestational age and has a genetic predisposition to larger stature usually experiences accelerated growth in the first 6 months, and by 18 months a relatively stable new growth percentile is established. The downward shift is seen in large infants who have a genetic predisposition to short stature. A fall-off in their growth percentiles may often be misconstrued as failure to thrive, although a stable growth percentile should be achieved by 18 months of age.

By 1 year of age, infants weigh three times as much as they did at birth and are 1½ times as long. By 2 years of age, the growth velocity curve has stabilized into the rate for mid childhood, which is a weight gain of 2–3 kg/y and a height gain of 5–7.5 cm/y (Figures 1–1 to 1–6). At the second birthday, a child attains approximately 50% of adult height.

The energy requirement during growth also changes dramatically in the first few years of life. Approximately 110 kcal/kg/d is necessary in early infancy because up to 40% of this total energy requirement is used for growth. The percentage used for growth gradually decreases to 3% at 2 years of age and remains at this level even during adolescence. After 2 years of age, the overall energy requirement gradually decreases from 90 kcal/kg/d to 60 kcal/kg/d during middle childhood, and the majority of the energy expenditure is accounted for by activity and basal metabolic rate of the tissues. The gradual decrease is secondary to a decline in the relative mass of organs, such as the brain and the liver, that have a high requirement for energy compared to resting muscle. The relative energy expended during activity increases in adolescence, particularly for males. The percentage of body weight that is muscle increases from 22% at 3 months to 35% at 5 years and 40% at maturity in males. In contrast, organ weight is 17% of body weight in the infant, with 75% of organ weight accounted for by the brain. By maturity, only 5.1% of body weight is organ weight. Fat increases during the first year of life from 12% of body weight at birth. After the infant begins to walk and explore, however, the proportion of fat decreases and remains stable throughout childhood. In adolescence, the proportion of body weight that is fat increases with sexual maturation in girls but not in boys. For further information, see Chapter 11.

Falkner F, Tanner JM (editors): *Developmental Biology: Prenatal Growth.* Vol 1 of: *Human Growth: A Comprehensive Treatise,* 2nd ed. Plenum, 1986.

Falkner F, Tanner JM (editors): *Postnatal Growth Neurobiology.* Vol 2 of: *Human Growth: A Comprehensive Treatise,* 2nd ed. Plenum, 1986. (A detailed analysis of current research in physical growth and brain development.)

Jelliffe DB, Jelliffe EF: *Growth Monitoring and Promotion in Young Children.* Oxford Univ Press, 1990. (A review of growth monitoring methods.)

Lowrey GH: *Growth and Development of Children,* 8th ed. Year Book, 1986. (A detailed analysis of physical growth and development in children.)

Smith DW: *Growth and Its Disorders: Major Problems in Clinical Pediatrics,* Vol 25. Saunders, 1977. (A classic

**GIRLS: BIRTH TO 36 MONTHS
PHYSICAL GROWTH NCHS PERCENTILES***

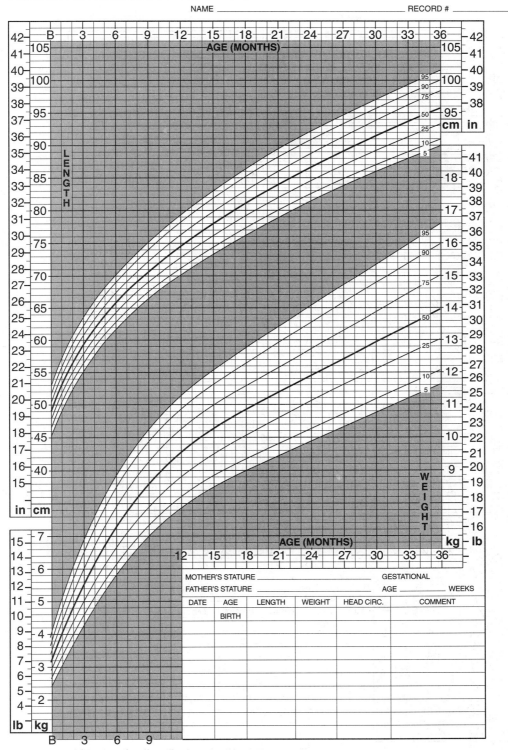

Figure 1–1. Percentile standards for weight and height in girls birth–3 years. (Reproduced, with permission, from Ross Laboratories, Columbus, OH. © 1982 Ross Laboratories.)

BOYS: BIRTH TO 36 MONTHS
PHYSICAL GROWTH NCHS PERCENTILES*

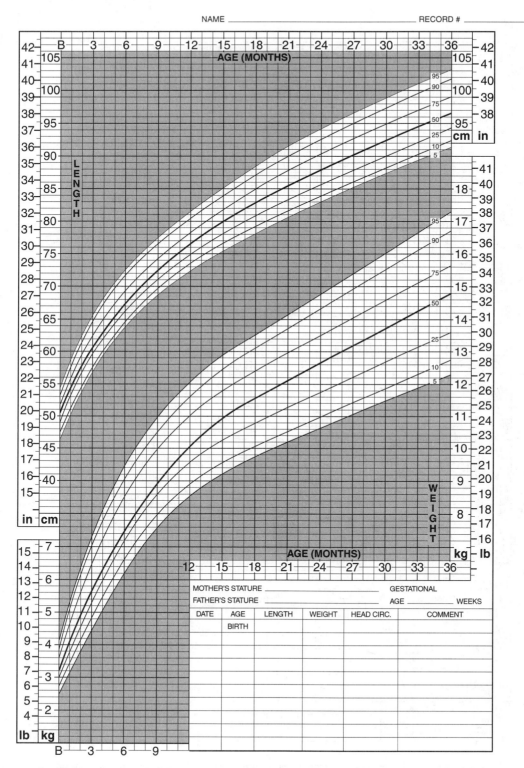

Figure 1–2. Percentile standards for weight and height in boys birth–3 years. (Reproduced, with permission, from Ross Laboratories, Columbus, OH. © 1982 Ross Laboratories.)

GIRLS: 2 TO 18 YEARS
PHYSICAL GROWTH
NCHS PERCENTILES*

Figure 1–3. Percentile standards for weight and height in girls 2–18 years. (Reproduced, with permission, from Ross Laboratories, Columbus, OH. © 1982 Ross Laboratories.)

BOYS: 2 TO 18 YEARS
PHYSICAL GROWTH
NCHS PERCENTILES*

Figure 1–4. Percentile standards for weight and height in boys 2–18 years. (Reproduced, with permission, from Ross Laboratories, Columbus, OH. © 1982 Ross Laboratories.)

Figure 1–5. Head circumference of girls. (Modified and reproduced, with permission, from Nellhaus G: Pediatrics 1968;41:106.)

review of linear growth through childhood and adolescence.)

Tanner JM, Whitehouse RH, Takaishi M: Standards from birth to maturity for height, weight, height velocity: British children. Arch Dis Child 1965;41:454.

Brain Growth

About 100 billion neurons are present in the fully developed brain, and replication of neurons is completed before birth. Most of this growth occurs in the first 3 months of gestation. Cell density subsequently

Figure 1–6. Head circumference of boys. (Modified and reproduced, with permission, from Nellhaus G: Pediatrics 1968;41:106.)

decreases rapidly until birth. After birth, the decrease is slower and ceases at 15 months. At birth, the head is 75% of its adult size and makes up 25% of the baby's length. This ratio changes dramatically in time so that by 25 years of age, the head measures one-eighth of the body length. Postnatally, the brain continues to grow rapidly, completing half of its lifetime growth by the end of the first year. The postnatal growth is the result of an increase in white matter and a proliferation of synaptic connections. After 2 years of age, the head circumference increases only 2 cm/y during middle childhood (see Figures 1–5 and 1–6). By 7 years of age, 90% of brain growth is completed, and many 10-year-olds have the brain weight of an adult.

The cerebellum is the area of the gray matter that develops last. It begins its growth at 30 weeks of gestation and ends at approximately 1 year of age. It is, therefore, particularly vulnerable to trauma, which may occur in late gestation or at birth. The spinal cord extends through the length of the neural canal until the third month of gestation. After this time, the torso of the fetus grows faster than the spinal cord, which is fixed in position superiorly by the brain. The lower end of the spinal cord subsequently rests at a gradually higher vertebral level through later fetal life and, by birth, is located at the third lumbar vertebra. The spinal cord doubles its weight in the first year of life and has increased eightfold by adulthood.

Myelinization begins in the spinal cord by the fourth month of gestation and begins in the brain during the last trimester. At birth, the autonomic system is matured and myelinated. The cranial nerves, except for the optic and olfactory nerves, are also myelinated. The cortex and most of its connection to the thalamus and basal ganglia are incompletely myelinated. It takes at least 2 years for myelinization of these areas and the spinal cord to be complete.

Newborn Reflexes

Reflex movement begins in fetal development as early as 9 weeks' gestation. However, most of the reflexes associated with the newborn develop between 20 and 38 weeks' gestation. Sucking, a basic reflex critical to survival, can first be seen in utero as early as 14 weeks' gestation. The rooting reflex begins by 28 weeks' gestation and is evidenced by the infant's pursing the lips and sucking after turning toward a touch to the cheek. The tonic neck reflex is elicited by forcibly turning the infant's head. In response, the infant extends the arm and leg on the side toward which the head is turned and flexes the opposite side (fencing position stance). This reflex disappears by 8 months of age unless myelinization or brain development is pathologic. The Moro embrace reflex (an embracing movement as a startle response), palmar grasp, and trunk incurving in response to a tactile stimulus to the side of the trunk all develop by 28 weeks' gestation but disappear by 3, 4, and 5 months of age, respectively. Babinski's reflex, which develops just prior to birth in a full-term infant, does not normally disappear until 12–16 months of age, when adequate myelinization has occurred.

EEG & Sleep

The brain also undergoes rapid maturation in the first 2 years of life. Prior to 26 weeks' gestation, the EEG is disorganized and without periodicity. By 8 months' gestation, however, low-amplitude fast waves occur at 16–18 cycles per second. At birth, the waking and sleeping cycles can be differentiated, and by 4 months, sleep spindles appear. During this period, the proportion of total sleep time occupied by active or rapid eye movement (REM) sleep decreases from 50% to 20%. The infant's sleep pattern at the onset of sleep also shifts from REM sleep to quiet sleep. The amount of quiet sleep also gradually increases to a maximum of 70–80% of total sleep time. These changes are a reflection of significant brain maturation, which has occurred by 4 months. Infantile reflexes, as previously mentioned, are disappearing, and the infant is becoming more alert and interactive with the environment. The infant is now reaching for and grasping objects, smiling and laughing out loud, anticipating food on sight, and sitting with support.

Motor Dexterity

The developmental progression of the grasp through the first year illustrates the gradual improvement in motor dexterity. The grasp begins as a raking motion involving mainly the ulnar aspect of the hand at 3–4 months. The thumb is used in the grasp just before 5 months, as the focus shifts to the radial side of the hand. The thumb opposes the finger for picking up a cube just before 7 months, but the neat pincer grasp used for smaller objects, such as a pellet, does not develop until approximately 9 months.

The changes in gross motor skills have a significant impact on the child's exploration of the environment. Sitting alone occurs at 6 months of age, but the onset of walking at 12 months (with a range of 9–17 months in the normal child) introduces the major theme of the second year of life, autonomy.

THE SECOND YEAR

Once children can walk independently, they can move away from the mother and explore the environment on their own. Although they use the mother as a home base and return to her frequently to reassure themselves that she is still there and available for them, they have definitely taken a quantum jump in independence and autonomy. These new themes are closely tied to the child's beginning sense of mastery over the environment and an emerging sense of self.

These issues lead to the "terrible twos" and the frequent verbalizations "no" as children struggle to develop a better idea of what is under their control. This is a fragile time of ego development. Parents should not crush emerging autonomy but develop appropriate limits that foster independent exploration.

As children develop a sense of self, they begin to understand the feelings of others and develop empathy. They hug another who is in distress or become concerned when another is hurt. They begin to understand how another child feels when he or she is hit or hurt, and this realization helps them to inhibit their own aggressive behavior. They also begin to understand right and wrong and parental expectations. They realize when they have done something "bad" and may signify that awareness with "uh oh!" or distress. They also take pleasure in their accomplishments and become more aware of their bodies.

The development of these cognitive, emotional, and physical abilities is related to significant brain maturation, which occurs by 2 years of age. These changes set the stage for toilet training after 18 months of age. Toddlers have developed the sensory abilities to be aware of a full rectum or bladder and are physically able to control their rectal sphincter. They also take great pleasure in their accomplishments, particularly in appropriate elimination, if it is positively reinforced. Children must be given some control over when elimination occurs. If severe restrictions are imposed, the accomplishment of this developmental milestone can become a battle between parent and child, and long- term struggles of control predisposing to encopresis may develop later. Freud terms this period the anal stage because the development issue of bowel control is the major task requiring mastery. It basically represents a more generalized theme of socialized behavior and overall body cleanliness, which is begun to be taught or imposed on the child at this age. The child is encouraged to control impulsive and aggressive behavior by acting in socially appropriate ways. Although Freud describes the by-products of anal regularity on personality development, including punctuality, reliability, cleanliness, and conscientiousness, these themes simply represent abilities emerging at the time that toilet training is also being mastered. (See Chapter 7.)

Cech D, Martin ST: Functional movement development across the life span. Saunders, 1995. (A review of motor development and motor abilities throughout childhood and adulthood.)

Dixon SD, Stein MT: *Encounters With Children: Pediatric Behavior and Development,* 2nd ed. Mosby–Year Book, 1992.

Egan DF: *Developmental Examination of Infants and Preschool Children,* Clinics in Developmental Medicine No. 112. MacKeith, 1990.

Yogman MW, Cook KV, Gersten M: Infant and toddler development: Active organization of the social world. Curr Probl Pediatr 1988 (May);18:259.

Zeitlin S, Williamson GG: Coping in young children: Early intervention practices to enhance adaptive behavior & resilience. Brooks, 1994. (A review of adaptation and coping in young children.)

LANGUAGE DEVELOPMENT: 1–4 YEARS

Communication is important from birth, particularly the nonverbal reciprocal interactions between the infant and caretaker, which have already been described. By 2 months of age, these interactions begin to include vocalizations that involve cooing and reciprocal vocal play between the mother and child. Babbling begins by 6–10 months of age, and the repetition of sounds, such as "da-da-da-da," is facilitated by increasing oral muscular control. Babbling reaches a peak at 12 months. The child then moves into a stage of having needs met by using individual words to represent objects or actions. It is common for children of this age to express wants and needs by pointing to objects. There is significant variability in the number of words acquired by 18 months, with an average of 20–50 words. The failure of parents or siblings to encourage vocalization and their overuse of nonverbal communication, such as pointing, slows the development of expressive vocabulary. Recurrent otitis media, which causes a fluctuating conductive hearing loss, may also have a significant impact on the achievement of early language milestones.

Receptive language usually develops more rapidly than expressive language. Word comprehension begins at 9 months; by 13 months, the receptive vocabulary may be as high as 20–100 words. After 18 months, there is a dramatic increase in expressive and receptive vocabulary, and by the end of the second year, a quantum leap occurs in language development. This leap represents a major change in cognitive development. The child begins to put words and phrases together and begins to use language to represent a new world, the symbolic world. Although the infant begins to use single words to represent objects or people in the latter part of the first year, it is not until the end of the second year that language ability begins to blossom. Children now begin to put verbs into their phrases and focus much of their language on describing their new abilities, often while they are doing them, such as "I go out." They incorporate prepositions into speech and ask why and what questions more frequently. They also begin to appreciate time factors and to understand and use this concept in their speech (Table 1–2).

The Early Language Milestones Scale (ELM) is a simple tool for assessing early language development in the pediatric office setting (Figure 1–7). It is scored in the same fashion as the Denver II (Figure

Table 1–2. Normal speech and language development.

Age	Speech	Language	Articulation[1]
1 mo	Throaty sounds		Vowels: \ah\, \uh\, \ee\
2 mo	Vowel sounds ("eh"), coos		
2½ mo	Squeals		
3 mo	Babbles, initial vowels		
4 mo	Gutteral sounds ("ah," "go")		Consonants, m, p, b
5 mo			Vowels: \o\, \u\
7 mo	Imitates speech sounds		
8 mo			Syllables: da, ba, ka
10 mo		"Dada" or "mama" nonspecifically	Approximates names: baba/bottle
12 mo	Jargon begins (own language)	One word other than "mama" or "dada"	Understandable: 2–3 words
13 mo		Three words	
16 mo		Six words	Consonants: t, d, w, n, h
18–24 mo		Two-word phrases	Understandable 2-word phrases
24–30 mo		Three-word phrases	Understandable 3-word phrases
2 y	Vowels uttered correctly	Approximately 270 words; uses pronouns	Approximately 270 words; uses phrases
3 y	Some degree of hesitancy and uncertainty common	Approximately 900 words; intelligible 4-word phrases	Approximately 900 words; intelligible 4-word phrases
4 y		Approximately 1540 words; intelligible 5-word phrases or sentences	Approximately 1540 words; intelligible 5-word phrases
6 y		Approximately 2560 words; intelligible 6- or 7-word sentences	Approximately 2560 words; intelligible 6- or 7-word sentences
7–8 y	Adult proficiency		

[1]Data on articulation from Berry MF: *Language Disorders of Children.* Appleton-Century-Crofts, 1969; and from Bzoch K, League R: *Receptive-Expressive Emergent Language Scale.* University Park Press, 1970.

1–8) but tests both receptive and expressive language areas in greater depth.

Piaget describes the 2- to 6-year-old stage as preoperational. This stage begins when language has facilitated the creation of mental images in the symbolic sense. The child begins to learn to manipulate the symbolic world. The child sorts out reality from fantasy imperfectly and may be terrified of dreams, wishes, and foolish threats. Most of the child's perception of the world is egocentric or interpreted in reference to wants, needs, or influence. Cause-and-effect relationships are confused with temporal relationships or interpreted egocentrically. For instance, children often focus their understanding of divorce on themselves; for example, "My father left because I was bad" or "My father left because he didn't love me." Illness and the need for medical care are also commonly misinterpreted at this age. The child may make a mental connection between a sibling's illness and a recent argument, a negative comment, or a wish that the sibling be ill. The child may experience significant guilt unless the parents are aware of these misperceptions and take time to sort them out.

At this age, children also endow inanimate objects with human feelings. They also assume that humans cause or create all natural events. For instance, when asked why the sun sets, they may respond that "the sun goes to his house" or "it is pushed down by someone else."

Magical thinking blossoms during the ages of 3–5 as symbolic thinking incorporates more elaborate fantasy. Fantasy facilitates development of role playing, sexual identity, and emotional growth. Children test new experiences in fantasy, both in their imagination and in play. In their play, children often create magical stories and novel situations that reflect issues they are dealing with, such as aggression, relationships, fears, and control issues. Children often invent imaginary friends at this time, and nightmares or fears of monsters are common. At this stage, other

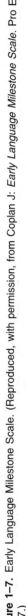

Figure 1–7. Early Language Milestone Scale. (Reproduced, with permission, from Coplan J: *Early Language Milestone Scale*. Pro Ed, 1987.)

13

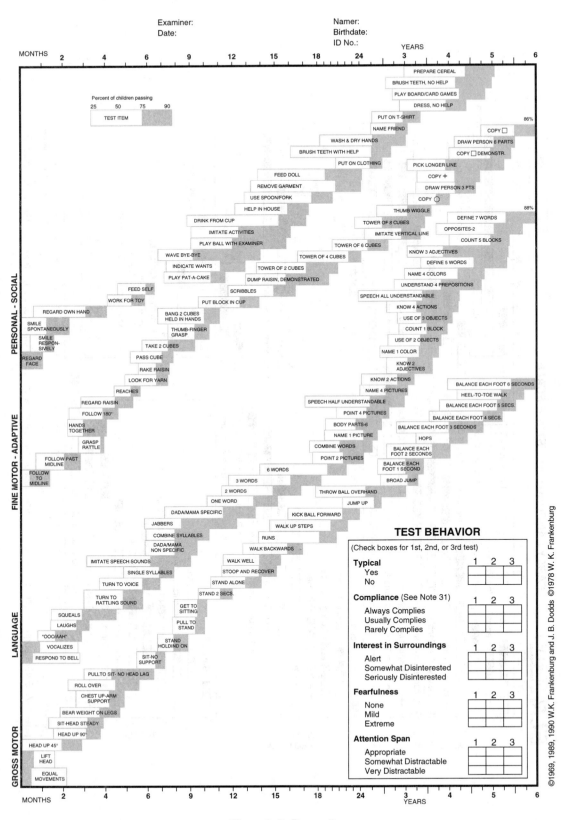

Figure 1–8. Denver II.

children become important in facilitating play, such as in a preschool group. Play gradually becomes more cooperative; shared fantasy leads to game playing. Freud describes the Oedipal phase between the ages of 3 and 6, when there is strong attachment to the parent of the opposite sex. The child's fantasies may focus on play acting the adult role with that parent, although by 6 years of age Oedipal issues are usually resolved, and attachment is redirected to the parent of the same sex.

Bayley N (editor): *Bayley Scales of Infant Development,* 2nd ed. Psychological Corp, 1993.

Billeaud FP: *Communication Disorders in Infants and Toddlers.* Andover Medical, 1993. (This text reviews normal language development and assessment techniques and measures as well as intervention strategies in communication disorders.)

Coplan J: *Early Language Milestone Scale,* Pro Ed, 1987.

Dixon SD, Stein MT: *Encounters With Children: Pediatric Behavior and Development,* 2nd ed. Mosby–Year Book, 1992.

Erikson EH: *Childhood and Society,* 2nd ed. Norton, 1963.

Fraiberg S: *The Magic Years.* Scribner, 1959.

Frankenberg WK et al: The Denver II: A major revision and restandardization of the Denver Developmental Screening Test. Pediatrics 1991;89:91.

Glascoe FP, Dvorkin PH: The role of parents in the detection of developmental and behavioral problems. Pediatrics 1995;95:829.

Levine MD, Carey WB, Crocker AC (editors): *Developmental-Behavioral Pediatrics,* 2nd ed. Saunders, 1992.

Piaget J, Inyhelder B: *The Psychology of the Child.* Basic Books, 1969.

Walker D et al: Early Language Milestone Scale and language screening of young children. Pediatrics 1989; 83:284.

Yogman MW, Cook KV, Gersten M: Infant and toddler development: Active organization of the social world. Curr Probl Pediatr 1988 (May);18:259.

THE EARLY SCHOOL YEARS: 5–7

Attendance in kindergarten at 5 years marks an acceleration in the separation/individuation theme initiated in the preschool years. The child is ready to relate to peers in a more interactive manner than demonstrated by previous parallel play. The brain has reached 90% of its adult weight. At approximately 6 years, a remodeling of the cortex occurs. The Betz cells decrease in length and increase in width. The cortex, in general, shows a decrease in total thickness, with an increase in the number of nerve cells in the different layers. Sensorimotor coordination abilities are maturing and facilitating pencil-and-paper tasks and sports, both part of the school experience.

Cognitive abilities are still at the preoperational stage, and children focus on one variable in a problem at a time. However, by 5½ years, most children

have mastered conservation of length; by 6½ years, conservation of mass and weight; and by 8 years, conservation of volume.

By first grade, there is more pressure on the child to master academic tasks, including the recognition of numbers, letters, and words, and the ability to write. Piaget describes the stage of concrete operations beginning after age 6, when the child is able to perform mental operations concerning concrete objects that involve the manipulation of more than one variable. The child is able to order, number, and classify because these activities are related to concrete objects in the environment and because these activities are stressed in early schooling. Magical thinking diminishes greatly at this time, and the reality of cause-and-effect relationships is better understood. Fantasy and imagination are still strong and are reflected in the themes of play. Table 1–3 lists specific developmental abilities through middle childhood and adolescence.

THE MIDDLE CHILDHOOD YEARS: 7–11

Freud terms these the latency years, during which children are not bothered by significant aggressive or sexual drives but instead devote most of their energies to school and peer group interactions. In reality, throughout this period there is a gradual increase in sexual drives, which is manifested by increasingly aggressive play and interactions with the opposite sex. Fantasy still has an active role in dealing with sexuality before adolescence, and fantasies often focus on movie stars and rock heroes. Organized sports, clubs, and other activities are other modalities that permit preadolescent children to display socially acceptable forms of aggression and sexual interest.

For the 7-year-old, the major developmental task focuses on achievement in school and acceptance by peers. Academic expectations have intensified and require the child to concentrate, attend, and process increasingly complex auditory and visual information. Children with significant learning disabilities or problems of attention may have difficulty in these tasks and subsequently may receive significant negative reinforcement from teachers and even parents. Such children may develop a poor self-image, which may be manifested as behavioral difficulties. The pediatrician must evaluate potential learning disabilities in any child who is not developing adequately at this stage or who presents with emotional or behavioral problems. Their abilities are not as easily documented as milestones in early development. In the school-age child, the quality of the response, the attentional abilities, and the child's emotional approach to the task can make a dramatic difference in how successful the child is at school. The clinician must

Table 1–3. Developmental charts.[1]

1–2 months

Activities to be observed:
Holds head erect and lifts head.
Turns from side to back.
Regards faces and follows objects through visual field.
Drops toys.
Becomes alert in response to voice.

Activities related by parent:
Recognizes parents.
Engages in vocalizations.
Smiles spontaneously.

3–5 months

Activities to be observed:
Grasps cube—first ulnar then later thumb opposition.
Reaches for and brings objects to mouth.
Makes "raspberry" sound.
Sits with support.

Activities related by parent:
Laughs.
Anticipates food on sight.
Turns from back to side.

6–8 months

Activities to be observed:
Sits alone for a short period.
Reaches with one hand.
First scoops up a pellet then grasps it using thumb
    opposition.
Imitates "bye-bye."
Passes object from hand to hand in midline.
Babbles.

Activities related by parent:
Rolls from back to stomach.
Is inhibited by the word *no.*

9–11 months

Activities to be observed:
Stands alone.
Imitates pat-a-cake and peek-a-boo.
Uses thumb and index finger to pick up pellet.

Activities related by parent:
Walks by supporting self on furniture.
Follows one-step verbal commands, eg,
    "Come here," "Give it to me."

1 year

Activities to be observed:
Walks independently.
Says "mama" and "dada" with meaning.
Can use a neat pincer grasp to pick up a pellet.
Releases cube into cup after demonstration.
Gives toys on request.
Tries to build a tower of 2 cubes.

Activities related by parent:
Points to desired objects.
Says 1 or 2 other words.

18 months

Activities to be observed:
Builds tower of 3–4 cubes.
Throws ball.
Scribbles spontaneously.
Seats self in chair.
Dumps pellet from bottle.

Activities related by parent:
Walks up and down stairs with help.
Says 4–20 words.
Understands a 2-step command.
Carries and hugs doll.
Feeds self.

24 months

Activities to be observed:
Speaks short phrases, 2 words or more.
Kicks ball on request.
Builds tower of 6–7 cubes.
Points to named objects or pictures.
Jumps off floor with both feet.
Stands on either foot alone.
Uses pronouns.

Activities related by parent:
Verbalizes toilet needs.
Pulls on simple garment.
Turns pages of book singly.
Plays with domestic mimicry.

30 months

Activities to be observed:
Walks backward.
Begins to hop on one foot.
Uses prepositions.
Copies a crude circle.
Points to objects described by use.
Refers to self as I.
Holds crayon in fist.

Activities related by parent:
Helps put things away.
Carries on a conversation.

3 years

Activities to be observed:
Holds crayon with fingers.
Builds tower of 9–10 cubes.
Imitates 3-cube bridge.
Copies circle.
Gives first and last name.

Activities related by parent:
Rides tricycle using pedals.
Dresses with supervision.

3–4 years

Activities to be observed:
Climbs stairs with alternating feet.
Begins to button and unbutton.
"What do you like to do that's fun?" (Answers using
    plurals, personal pronoun, and verbs.)
Responds to command to place toy *in, on* or *under* table.
Draws a circle when asked to draw a man (girl, boy).
Knows own sex. ("Are you a boy or a girl?")
Gives full name.
Copies a circle already drawn. ("Can you make one like
    this?")

Activities related by parent:
Feeds self at mealtime.
Takes off shoes and jacket.

4–5 years

Activities to be observed:
Runs and turns without losing balance.
May stand on one leg for at least 10 seconds.

(continued)

Table 1–3. Developmental charts. (continued)

Buttons clothes and laces shoes. (Does not tie.)
Counts to 4 by rote.
"Give me 2 sticks." (Able to do so from pile of 4 tongue depressors.)
Draws a man. (Head, 2 appendages, and possibly 2 eyes. No torso yet.)
Knows the days of the week. ("What day comes after Tuesday?")
Gives appropriate answers to: "What must you do if you are sleepy? Hungry? Cold?"
Copies + in imitation.

Activities related by parent:
Self care at toilet. (May need help with wiping.)
Plays outside for at least 30 minutes.
Dresses self except for tying.

5–6 years

Activities to be observed:
Can catch ball.
Skips smoothly.
Copies a + already drawn.
Tells age.
Concept of 10 (eg, counts 10 tongue depressors). May recite to higher number by rote.
Knows right and left hand.
Draws recognizable man with at least 8 details.
Can describe favorite television program in some detail.

Activities related by parent:
Does simple chores at home (eg, taking out garbage, drying silverware).
Goes to school unattended or meets school bus.
Good motor ability but little awareness of dangers.

6–7 years

Activities to be observed:
Copies a △.
Defines words by use. ("What is an orange?" "To eat.")
Knows if morning or afternoon.
Draws a man with 12 details.
Reads several one-syllable printed words. (My, dog, see, boy.)
Uses pencil for printing name.

7–8 years

Activities to be observed:
Counts by 2s and 5s.
Ties shoes.
Copies a ◊.
Knows what day of the week it is. (Not date or year.)
Reads paragraph #1 Durrell:

Reading:
Muff is a little yellow kitten. She drinks milk. she sleeps on a chair. She does not like to get wet.

Corresponding arithmetic:

$$\begin{array}{cccc} 7 & 6 & 6 & 8 \\ +4 & +7 & -4 & -3 \end{array}$$

No evidence of sound substitution in speech (eg, *fr* for *thr*).
Adds and subtracts one-digit numbers.
Draws a man with 16 details.

8–9 years

Activities to be observed:
Defines words better than by use. ("What is an orange?" "A fruit.")
Can give an appropriate answer to the following:

"What is the thing for you to do if . . .
—you've broken something that belongs to someone else?"
—a playmate hits you without meaning to do so?"
Reads paragraph #2 Durrell:

Reading:
A little black dog ran away from home. He played with two big dogs. They ran away from him. It began to rain. He went under a tree. He wanted to go home, but he did not know the way. He saw a boy he knew. The boy took him home.

Corresponding arithmetic:

$$\begin{array}{cccc} & 45 & & \\ 67 & 16 & 14 & 84 \\ + 4 & +27 & - 8 & -36 \end{array}$$

Is learning borrowing and carrying processes in addition and subtraction.

9–10 years

Activities to be observed:
Knows the month, day, and year.
Names the months in order. (15 seconds, 1 error.)
Makes a sentence with these 3 words in it: (One or 2. Can use words orally in proper context.)
   1. work . . . money . . . men
   2. boy . . . river . . . ball
Reads paragraph #3 Durrell:

Reading:
Six boys put up a tent by the side of a river. They took things to eat with them. When the sun went down, they went into the tent to sleep. In the night, a cow came and began to eat grass around the tent. The boys were afraid. They thought it was a bear.

Corresponding arithmetic:

$$\begin{array}{ccc} 5204 & 23 & 837 \\ - 530 & \times 3 & \times 7 \end{array}$$

Should comprehend and answer the question: "What was the cow doing?"
Learning simple multiplication.

10–12 years

Activities to be observed:
Should read and comprehend paragraph #5 Durrell:

Reading:
In 1807, Robert Fulton took the first long trip in a steamboat. He went one hundred and fifty miles up the Hudson River. The boat went five miles an hour. This was faster than a steamboat had ever gone before. Crowds gathered on both banks of the river to see this new kind of boat. They were afraid that its noise and splashing would drive away all the fish.

Corresponding arithmetic:

$$\begin{array}{ccc} 420 & & \\ \times 29 & 9)\overline{72} & 31)\overline{62} \end{array}$$

Answer: "What river was the trip made on?"
Ask to write the sentence: "The fishermen did not like the boat."
Should do multiplication and simple division.

12–15 years

Activities to be observed:
Reads paragraph #7 Durrell:

(continued)

Table 1–3. Developmental charts. (continued)

Reading:	*Corresponding arithmetic:*

Reading:

Golf originated in Holland as a game played on ice. The game in its present form first appeared in Scotland. It became unusually popular and kings found it so enjoyable that it was known as "the royal game." James IV, however, thought that people neglected their work to indulge in this fascinating sport so that it was forbidden in 1457. James relented when he found how attractive the game was, and it immediately regained its former popularity. Golf spread gradually to other countries, being introduced in America in 1890. It has grown in favor until there is hardly a town that does not boast of a private or public course.

Corresponding arithmetic:

$$536)\overline{4762} \qquad \frac{1}{3} \qquad \qquad 7\frac{1}{6}$$
$$+\frac{1}{3} \qquad \qquad - \quad \frac{3}{4}$$

Reduce fractions to lowest forms.

Ask to write a sentence: "Golf originated in Holland as a game played on ice."
Answers questions:
"Why was golf forbidden by James IV?"
"Why did he change his mind?"
Does long division, adds and subtracts fractions.

[1]Modified from Leavitt SR, Goodman H, Harvin D: Pediatrics 1963;31:499.

---

consider all of these aspects to appropriately diagnose learning disabilities. (See Chapter 4.)

Levine MD, Carey WB, Crocker AC (editors): *Developmental-Behavioral Pediatrics,* 2nd ed. Saunders, 1992.

Parker S, Zuckerman B (editors): *Behavioral & Developmental Pediatrics: A Handbook for Primary Care.* Little, Brown, 1995. (A brief survey of evaluation issues, screening instruments in addition to specific management strategies for a large number of developmental & behavioral problems.)

Piaget J, Inyhelder B: *The Psychology of the Child.* Basic Books, 1969.

Vaughan VC, Litt IF: *Child and Adolescent Development: Clinical Implications.* Saunders, 1990. (A thorough review of physical, cognitive, and behavioral development from infancy through adolescence.)

PREPUBERTAL & PUBERTAL GROWTH

The pubertal growth spurt occurs at about 10 years in females and 12½ years in males. The speed of growth increases, reaching a peak of approximately 9 cm/y in females and 10.3 cm/y in males. Different areas of the skeleton attain their peak growth at different times. This is seen most dramatically in the feet, which first experience a growth spurt. This is followed by a rapid increase in leg length and subsequently by trunk growth. Facial growth occurs after peak height velocity. The mandible changes most remarkably, demonstrating a 25% increase in height between 12 and 20 years of age, compared to only a 6–7% increase in the size of the cranial base.

Boys have just over 2 more years of preadolescent growth than girls do; during this time, leg growth increases more dramatically than trunk growth. Girls have a greater spurt in hip width, related to stature, than boys do, although boys exceed girls in most other areas of bone growth.

The Hypothalamic-Pituitary-Gonadal Axis & Puberty

Gonadal development is initiated in the fetus by 10 weeks' gestation, and it is almost complete by age 3 months in the male. This process occurs without significant input from gonadotropins, although placental human chorionic gonadotropin (hCG) plays a significant role in migration of germ cells and differentiation of Leydig's cells. By the 21st week of gestation, the hypothalamus secretes gonadotropin-releasing hormone (GnRH), and the anterior pituitary releases follicle-stimulating hormone (FSH) and luteinizing hormone (LH). Their levels reach a peak by the 23rd to 24th weeks of gestation, which coincides with oocyte maturation in utero, including the development of primary follicles.

In the newborn period, GnRH is secreted in a pulsatile fashion, causing episodic elevations of both FSH and LH. In females, FSH predominates, and in males LH predominates; they stimulate elevations in testosterone and estrogen in the first few months of life. After this period of significant neuroendocrine activity, a quiescent period, with almost undetectable levels of gonadotropins, sets in and lasts through childhood. Hypothalamic secretion of GnRH is suppressed until puberty.

The large fetal adrenal gland regresses significantly after birth until adrenarche at 6–9 years of age. Adrenarche refers to the regrowth of the zona reticularis and the activation of its enzyme systems to produce adrenal steroids such as dehydroepiandrosterone sulfate and 17-ketosteroids. These steroids are partially responsible for body odor, the development of pubic and axillary hair, and stimulation of linear growth. Adrenarche occurs before gonadarche and is probably under the control of adrenocorticotropic hormone (ACTH).

Gonadarche is initiated by the pulsatile secretion of GnRH from the hypothalamus, which in turn stimulates the release of gonadotropins. In early puberty, FSH and LH are secreted during sleep, and there is an increasing amplitude in its pulses as puberty progresses. The efficacy of FSH and LH also changes in that biopotency of these hormones improves as puberty progresses. For additional information on puberty, see Chapter 5.

Falkner F, Tanner JM (editors): *Postnatal Growth Neurobiology.* Vol 2 of: *Human Growth: A Comprehensive Treatise,* 2nd ed. Plenum, 1986.

Lowrey GH: *Growth and Development of Children,* 8th ed. Year Book, 1986.

Vaughan VC, Litt IF: *Child and Adolescent Development: Clinical Implications.* Saunders, 1990.

2

The Newborn Infant

Adam A. Rosenberg, MD, & Elizabeth H. Thilo, MD

Neonatology is a discipline that encompasses all aspects of care for newborn infants. By tradition, the first 28 days of life has been considered the newborn period. Practically, however, neonatal care includes all of the care provided until discharge from the nursery, ranging from a 24-hour stay for term, healthy infants to many months of care for sick, very immature infants. Follow-up care for most newborn infants is usually provided by family physicians and pediatricians. Neonatologists or other physicians skilled in developmental pediatrics, however, may provide special follow-up services for infants discharged from intensive care nurseries. Table 2–1 summarizes the levels of nursery care commonly encountered.

NEONATAL BIRTH WEIGHT & GESTATIONAL AGE DISTRIBUTION

Mortality rates have decreased steadily for infants in all birth weight and gestational age groups with improved neonatal stabilization and intensive care technology. Table 2–2 presents neonatal survival rates by birth weight and gestational age for infants cared for at Maine Medical Center, 1982–1991. These mortality rates are representative of other centers in the United States over the same period. Note that there is an approximately 60% survival rate for infants weighing 600–700 g and that survival rates are over 90% for infants weighing over 1000 g. There is no difference between survival rates for term infants who are large for gestational age (LGA) and those who are appropriate for gestational age (AGA), in large part as a result of better obstetric management of gestational and insulin-dependent diabetic patients. Furthermore, the use of ultrasound allows obstetricians to anticipate delivery of an LGA infant and, if necessary, perform cesarean section, thus avoiding much of the birth trauma associated with LGA infants in the past. The small–for–gesta-

tional age (SGA) infant born very prematurely has a mortality rate comparable to those of premature babies of the same size, whereas the larger and more mature SGA infant has a better survival rate than those of preterm infants of comparable size.

The birth weight and gestational age of all infants must be plotted on some appropriate standard. Birth weight–gestational age distributions vary from one population to the next. Table 2–3 lists some of the factors that affect these distributions. For these reasons, the standards should be prepared from data collected on the local population. When these are not available, any regional standard may be used. The birth weight–gestational age distribution of an infant is simply a screening tool that should always be supplemented by clinical data confirming a tentative diagnosis of intrauterine growth retardation or excessive fetal growth. These clinical data include not only the clinical features of the infant determined during the physical examination but also such factors as the size of each parent and the birth weight–gestational age distribution of infants previously born to the parents.

Table 2–4 lists causes of variations in neonatal size in relation to gestational age. An important distinction to be made, particularly in SGA infants, is whether the growth disorder is symmetric (weight, height, and occipitofrontal circumference [OFC ≤10%]) or asymmetric (sparing of growth in length and OFC). Asymmetric growth retardation implies a problem late in the pregnancy, such as pregnancy-induced hypertension or placental insufficiency. Symmetric growth retardation implies an event of early pregnancy: chromosomal abnormality, drug or alcohol use, congenital viral infections. In general, the outlook for normal growth and development is better in the asymmetrically growth-retarded infant whose intrauterine brain growth has been spared.

Knowledge of a baby's birth weight in relation to gestational age is also helpful in anticipating neonatal problems. LGA babies are at risk for birth trauma, hypoglycemia, polycythemia, congenital anomalies, cardiomyopathy, hyperbilirubinemia, and hypocalcemia. SGA babies are at risk for fetal distress during

Table 2–1. Levels of nursery care.

Level 1 nurseries:
These nurseries care for infants presumed healthy. In such units, screening and surveillance are primary responsibilities. "Rooming-in" units are encouraged, with emphasis support of breast-feeding and assessment of parenting skills.

Level 2 nurseries:
These nurseries care for infants >30 weeks of gestation and ≥1200 g who require special attention short of the need for circulatory or prolonged ventilator support and major surgical procedures. Because they address the greatest diversity of neonatal disorders, these nurseries present perhaps the greatest challenge to health care providers. A high percentage of the problems in such nurseries relates to obstetric complication (eg, birth trauma, fetal distress, obstetric anesthesia).

Level 3 nurseries:
These nurseries are staffed and equipped to care for all newborn infants who are critically ill, regardless of the level of support required. They are regional institutions serving as referral centers for other nurseries and for this reason are often linked with transport services. Optimally, these nurseries should be part of a perinatal center.

Perinatal center:
A perinatal center provides services both to high-risk mothers and to infants requiring level 3 nursery care. Ample data now clearly demonstrate a higher neonatal survival rate for high-risk pregnancies cared for in such centers. The transport of high-risk mothers to perinatal centers is preferred, therefore, to the transport of a critically ill infant following delivery.

Table 2–3. Factors affecting birth weight–gestational age distributions.

1. Socioeconomic factors that affect nutritional level and access to health care
2. Altitude
3. Incidence of environmental factors that affect birth weight (eg, smoking)
4. Racial distribution

labor and delivery, polycythemia, hypoglycemia, and hypocalcemia.

American Academy of Pediatrics: *Guidelines for Perinatal Care,* 3rd ed. American Academy of Pediatrics, 1992.

Hack M et al: Very low birth weight outcomes of the National Institute of Child Health and Human Development Neonatal Network. Pediatrics 1991;87:587.

Hack M et al: Very-low-birth-weight outcomes of the National Institute of Child Health and Human Development Neonatal Network, November 1989 to October 1990. Am J Obstet Gynecol 1995;172:457.

Kempe A et al: Clinical determinants of the racial disparity in very low birth weight. N Engl J Med 1992;327:969.

Phelps DL et al: 28-day survival rates of 6676 neonates with birth weights of 1250 grams or less. Pediatrics 1991;87:7.

Philip AGS: Neonatal mortality rate: Is further improvement possible? J Pediatr 1995;126:427.

Whyte HE et al: Extreme immaturity: Outcome of 568 pregnancies of 23–26 weeks gestation. Obstet Gynecol 1993;82:1.

Wright K et al: New postnatal growth grids for very low birth weight infants. Pediatrics 1993;91:922.

Table 2–2. Comparison of birth weight–specific and gestational age–specific mortality rates for low birth weight infants by time interval at Maine Medical Center neonatal intensive care unit.[1]

	1982–1985		1986–1989		1990–1991	
	No.	**% (corrected)**	**No.**	**% (corrected)**	**No.**	**% (corrected)**
Birth weight (g)						
500–749	45/70	64 (64)[2]	47/71	66 (66)	14/35	40 (38)
750–999	37/97	38 (37)	27/80	34 (31)	6/57	11 (9)
1000–1249	12/99	12 (11)	15/121	12 (12)	4/62	6 (3)
1250–1499	8/106	8 (7)	7/113	6 (5)	1/54	2 (2)
1500–1749[3]	8/121	7 (4)	6/144	4 (2)	3/67	4 (2)
1750–1999[3]	6/107	6 (4)	4/140	3 (1)	3/97	3 (2)
2000–2249[3]	5/91	5 (2)	6/163	4 (1)	2/62	3 (2)
2250–2499[3]	8/106	8 (4)	8/148	5 (1)	4/59	8 (4)
Gestational age (week)						
≤25	51/66	77	53/82	65	17/56	30
26–27	32/87	37	26/93	28	2/44	5
28–29	12/112	11	13/122	11	2/60	3
30–31	9/128	7	7/143	5	6/75	8
32–33	15/193	8	6/255	2	4/140	3
34–35	4/139	3	6/178	3	3/84	4

[1]Reproduced, with permission, from Philip AGS: Neonatal, morality rate: Is further improvement possible? J Pediatr 1995; 126:427.
[2]Figures in parentheses indicate corrected mortality rates after exclusion of deaths from congenital anomaly.
[3]Denominators for these categories are much larger than stated, since many (or most) do not go to the neonatal intensive care unit.

Table 2–4. Etiology of variations in neonatal size in relation to gestational age.

Infants large for gestational age
  Infant of a diabetic mother

Infants small for gestational age
  Asymmetric
    Placental insufficiency secondary to pregnancy-induced
        hypertension or other maternal vascular disease
    Maternal age >35 y
    Poor weight gain during pregnancy
    Multiple gestation
  Symmetric
    Maternal drug use
      Narcotics
      Cocaine
      Alcohol
    Chromosomal abnormalities
    Intrauterine viral infection (eg, cytomegalovirus)

EVALUATION OF THE NEWBORN INFANT

HISTORY

Taking the history in newborn medicine involves three key areas: (1) the medical history of the mother and father, including a relevant genetic history; (2) the previous obstetric history of the mother; and (3) the history of the current pregnancy.

Maternal age, gravidity/parity, and blood type as well as the results of antenatal serologic testing and prior pregnancy outcomes are standard historical questions. Illnesses with genetic implications and all chronic illness in the mother known to affect intrauterine development are of particular importance. The past and current obstetric history must be as detailed as possible, including documentation of any procedures such as ultrasound examinations, amniocentesis, screening tests, and biophysical profiles. The biophysical profile is the prenatal equivalent of an Apgar score, in which five or six indices of fetal well-being are assessed. If chorionic villus biopsy or cordocentesis (umbilical cord blood sampling) has been done, it should be documented together with the information obtained. Any unusual dietary history, drug intake, smoking history, or potential exposure to infectious agents associated with congenital infection should be noted, as well as weight gain during pregnancy, the workplace of the mother, and exercise level. The social history may assist the clinician in assessing parenting skills and the risks of child abuse. Acute problems in the mother, such as urinary tract infection, pregnancy-induced hypertension, bleeding, fetal distress, and meconium in the amniotic fluid should be noted. Duration of ruptured membranes and presence of signs of chorioamnionitis should be elicited. In high-risk groups, the presence of HIV (human immunodeficiency virus) and HBsAg (hepatitis B surface antigen) must be determined.

PHYSICAL EXAMINATION

The extent of the physical examination of a newborn infant depends on the condition of the infant and the environment in which it is being performed. If the pediatrician is in attendance in the delivery room for a normal delivery, a physical examination is largely based on observation coupled with auscultation of the chest and examination for congenital anomalies. Because the infant is recovering from "birth shock," the examination should not be extensive. The examination should include collecting sufficient information for an Apgar score (see Table 2–5) at 1 and 5 minutes of age. In the case of severely depressed infants, a 10-minute score should also be recorded. Serial Apgar scores provide a shorthand description of the severity of intrauterine distress or the quality of the resuscitative efforts made.

The color of the neonate's skin is a very useful indicator. Because there is normally a high blood flow to the skin, any stress that triggers a catecholamine response produces fairly dramatic changes in skin color secondary to changes in the distribution of cardiac output and perfusion of the skin. Cyanosis and pallor are two signs that are evaluated both as an index of oxygenation and as a reflection of changes in skin blood flow. In infants of very low birth weight,

Table 2–5. Infant evaluation at birth (Apgar score).[1,2]

	Score		
	0	**1**	**2**
Heart rate	Absent	Slow (<100)	>100
Respiratory effort	Absent	Slow, irregular	Good, crying
Muscle tone	Limp	Some flexion	Active motion
Response to catheter in nostril[3]	No response	Grimace	Cough or sneeze
Color	Blue or pale	Body pink; extremities blue	Completely pink

[1]Reproduced, with permission, from Apgar V et al: Evaluation of the newborn infant—Second report. JAMA 1958;168:1985. © 1958 American Medical Association.
[2]One minute and 5 minutes after complete birth of the infant (disregarding the cord and the placenta), the following objective signs should be observed and recorded.
[3]Tested after oropharynx is clear.

tissues are fragile and easily bruised. Thus, bruised areas should be considered an indication of deep tissue bleeding that may involve fairly extensive hemorrhage. The bruising not only produces problems with hyperbilirubinemia over the next few days but also can represent acute, significant blood loss that must be treated with volume expansion.

The skeletal examination immediately after delivery serves two purposes: (1) to detect any obvious congenital anomalies, and (2) to detect signs of birth trauma, particularly in LGA infants or infants in whom there has been a prolonged second stage of labor, such as in those with a fractured clavicle or humerus.

The umbilical cord and the placenta should also be examined. The principal feature noted in the cord is the number of vessels. Normally, there are two arteries and one vein. In 1% of deliveries (5–6% of twin deliveries), the cord has only two vessels: an artery and a vein. The latter may be considered a vascular anomaly and, as is the case with other minor anomalies, carries with it a slightly increased risk of associated anomalies. The placenta is usually examined by the physician delivering it. Small placentas are always associated with small infants. The placental examination centers around the identification of membranes and vessels, particularly in multiple gestations. A single chorion always represents monozygotic twinning, whereas a full set of double membranes, amnion and chorion, can be either monozygotic or dizygotic. The placenta is also examined for the frequency and severity of placental infarcts and for evidence of clot (placental abruption) on the maternal side.

General Examination

Heart rate should range from 120 to 160 beats/min, and the respiratory rate is 30–60; blood pressure norms are unrelated to gestational age or birth weight, but are affected by perinatal asphyxia and the need for mechanical ventilation (Table 2–6). *Note:* An irregularly irregular heart rate, usually caused by premature atrial contractions, is a common finding. This irregularity should resolve in the first days of life and is not of pathologic significance.

Length, weight, and head circumference should be plotted on appropriate growth curves to establish percentile and whether the baby is AGA, LGA, or SGA (Figure 2–1).

Gestational Age Estimation

Accurate maternal dates remain the best indicator of gestational age. Other obstetric observations, such as fundal height, time of auscultation of fetal heartbeat with a stethoscope, and early ultrasound examination, provide supporting information. A postnatal examination (Table 2–7) can also be used, because fetal physical characteristics and neurologic development progress in predictable fashion. Table 2–7 item-

Table 2–6. Blood pressure ranges in different groups of the healthy population.[1]

Birth Weight (g)	n	Systolic (mm Hg)	Diastolic (mm Hg)
501–750	18	50–62	26–36
751–1000	39	48–59	23–36
1001–1250	30	49–61	26–35
1251–1500	45	46–56	23–33
1501–1750	51	46–58	23–33
1751–2000	61	48–61	24–35
Gestational Age (weeks)	**n**	**Systolic (mm Hg)**	**Diastolic (mm Hg)**
<24	11	48–63	24–39
24–28	55	48–58	25–36
29–32	110	47–59	24–34
>32	68	48–60	24–34

[1]Reproduced, with permission, from Hegyi T et al: Blood pressure ranges in premature infants. I. The first hours of life. J Pediatr 1994;124:627.

izes the physical and neurologic criteria to be examined. The upper panel is the neuromuscular examination assessing primarily muscle tone and strength. The lower panel catalogs a variety of physical characteristics.

Disappearance of the anterior vascular capsule of the lens is also helpful in determining gestational age. At 27–28 weeks of gestation, the lens capsule is covered by vessels; by 34 weeks, this vasculature is completely atrophied.

Foot length, measured carefully from the heel to the tip of the longest toe, also correlates with gestational age in AGA infants. The foot measures 4.5 cm at 25 weeks' gestation, and increases by 0.25 cm/wk until term.

Skin

Check for bruising, petechiae (common over the presenting part), meconium staining, and jaundice. Peripheral cyanosis is commonly present when the extremities are cool or the infant is polycythemic. Generalized cyanosis merits immediate evaluation. Pallor may be caused by acute or chronic blood loss. Plethora suggests polycythemia. Note vernix caseosa (a whitish, greasy material covering the body that decreases as term approaches) and lanugo (the fine hair covering the preterm infant's skin). Dry skin with cracking and peeling of the superficial layers is common in postterm infants. Edema may be generalized (hydrops) or localized (eg, on the dorsum of the foot in Turner's syndrome). Check for birthmarks, such as capillary hemangiomas (lower occiput, eyelids, forehead) and mongolian spot (bluish-black pigmentation over the back and buttocks). Milia (small white papules over the nose and face) are the result of blocked ducts of sebaceous glands. Miliaria (pustules without a red base) result from blocked ducts of

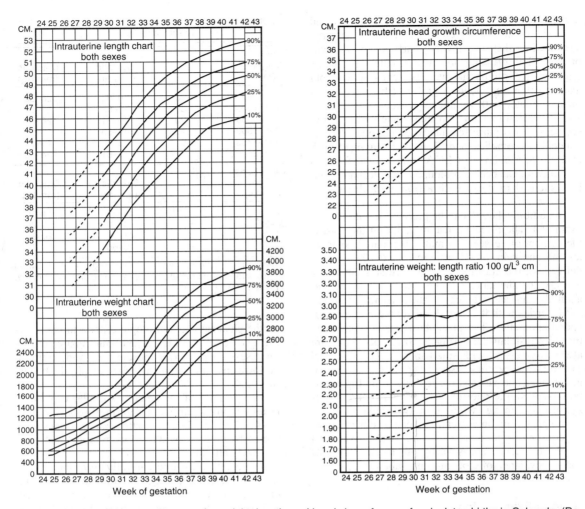

Figure 2–1. Intrauterine growth curves for weight, length, and head circumference for singleton births in Colorado. (Reproduced, with permission, from Lubchenco LO et al: Intrauterine growth in length and head circumference as estimated from live births at gestational ages from 26–42 weeks. Pediatrics 1996;37:403.)

sweat glands. Erythema toxicum is characterized by erythematous raised areas with pustules filled with eosinophils. Pustular melanosis is a pustular rash that leaves a pigmented base when the pustule ruptures. The pustules are noninfectious but contain neutrophils. Jaundice presenting in the first 24 hours of life should be considered abnormal.

Head

Check for cephalohematoma (contained within suture lines) and caput succedaneum (edema over the presenting part that crosses suture lines). Subgaleal (beneath the scalp) hemorrhages are seen infrequently but are not limited by sutures, so that blood loss can be extensive. Skull fractures may be linear or depressed and may be associated with a cephalohematoma. Check the size and presence of the

fontanelles. The anterior fontanelle varies from 1 to 4 cm in any direction, whereas the posterior fontanelle should be less than 1 cm. The third fontanelle is a bony defect along the sagittal suture in the parietal bones. Sutures should be freely mobile. Craniosynostosis is a prematurely fused suture.

Face

Odd facies may be associated with a specific syndrome. Bruising from birth trauma (especially with face presentation) and forceps marks should be identified. Facial nerve palsy is observed when the infant cries; the unaffected side of the mouth moves normally, giving a distorted facial grimace. Face presentations may have considerable soft tissue swelling around the nose and mouth, causing transient airway obstruction.

Table 2–7. New Ballard Score for assessment of fetal maturation of newly born infants.[1,2]

Neuromuscular Maturity

Neuromuscular Maturity Sign	Score							Record Score Here
	−1	0	1	2	3	4	5	
Posture								
Square Window (wrist)	>90°	90°	60°	45°	30°	0°		
Arm Recoil	180°	180°	140°–180°	110°–140°	90°–110°	<90°		
Popliteal Angle		160°	140°	120°	100°	90°	<90°	
Scarf Sign								
Heel to Ear								

Total Neuromuscular Maturity Score

Physical Maturity

Physical Maturity Sign	Score							Record Score Here
	−1	0	1	2	3	4	5	
Skin	Sticky, friable, transparent	Gelatinous, red, translucent	Smooth, pink, visible veins	Superficial peeling &/or rash; few veins	Cracking pale areas rare veins	Parchment, deep cracking; no vessels	Leathery, cracked, wrinkled	
Lanugo	None	Sparse	Abundant	Thinning	Bald areas	Mostly bald		
Plantar Surface	Heel-toe 40–50 mm: −1 <40 mm: −2	>50 mm: no crease	Faint red marks	Anterior transverse crease only	Creases anterior ⅔	Creases over entire sole		
Breast	Imperceptible	Barely perceptible	Flat areola; no bud	Stippled areola; 1- to 2-mm bud	Raised areola; 3- to 4-mm bud	Full areola; 5- to 10-mm bud		
Eye/Ear	Lids fused loosely: −1 tightly: −2	Lids open; pinna flat; stays folded	Slightly curved pinna; soft; slow recoil	Well-curved pinna; soft but ready recoil	Formed & firm instant recoil	Thick cartilage; ear stiff		
Genitals (male)	Scrotum flat, smooth	Scrotum empty; faint rugae	Testes in upper canal; rare rugae	Testes descending; few rugae	Testes down; good rugae	Testes pendulous; deep rugae		
Genitals (female)	Clitoris prominent & labia flat	Prominent clitoris & small labia minora	Prominent clitoris & enlarging minora	Majora & minora equally prominent	Majora large; minora small	Majora cover clitoris & minora		

Total Physical Maturity Score

Maturity	Score	−10	−5	0	5	10	15	20	25	30	35	40	45	50
Rating	Weeks	20	22	24	26	28	30	32	34	36	38	40	42	44

[1]Reproduced, with permission, from Ballard JL et al: New Ballard Score, expanded to include extremely premature infants. J Pediatr 1991;119:417.
[2]See text for a description of the clinical gestational age examination.

Eyes

Subconjunctival hemorrhages are seen frequently as a result of the birth process. Extraocular movements should be assessed. Occasional uncoordinated eye movements are common, but persistent irregular movements are abnormal. The iris should be inspected for abnormalities such as Brushfield's spots (trisomy 21) and colobomas. Examine for the red reflex of the retina. Leukocoria can be caused by glaucoma (cloudy cornea), cataract, or tumor (retinoblastoma). Infants at risk for chorioretinitis (congenital viral infection) should undergo a retinal examination while the pupil is dilated.

Nose

Examine the nose for size and shape. In utero compression can cause deformities. Babies are obligate nose breathers; any nasal obstruction (eg, bilateral choanal atresia) can cause respiratory distress. Unilateral choanal atresia can be checked for by occluding each naris. Purulent nasal discharge suggests congenital syphilis.

Ears

Malformed or malpositioned (low-set or posteriorly rotated) ears are often associated with other congenital anomalies. The tympanic membranes should be visualized.

Mouth

Epithelial (Epstein's) pearls are retention cysts along the gum margins and at the junction of hard and soft palates. Natal teeth may be present and sometimes need to be removed to avoid the risk of aspiration. Check the integrity and shape of the palate; rule out cleft lip and/or palate. A small mandible may be seen with Pierre Robin syndrome and can result in respiratory difficulty as the tongue occludes the airway. A prominent tongue can be seen in trisomy 21 and Beckwith-Wiedemann syndrome. Excessive drooling suggests esophageal atresia.

Neck

Webbing is seen in Turner's syndrome. Sinus tracts may be seen as remnants of branchial clefts. Check for masses: midline (thyroid), anterior to the sternocleidomastoids (branchial cleft cysts), within the sternocleidomastoid (hematoma, torticollis), and posterior to the sternocleidomastoid (cystic hygroma).

Chest & Lungs

Check for fractured clavicles (crepitus, bruising). Increased anteroposterior diameter (barrel chest) can be seen with aspiration syndromes. Check air entry bilaterally. Diminished breath sounds suggest pneumothorax or a space-occupying lesion (eg, diaphragmatic hernia). Check the position of the mediastinum. A shift is seen with pneumothorax (tension) or with a space-occupying lesion. With pneumomediastinum, heart sounds are usually muffled. Expiratory grunting and decreased air entry are seen with hyaline membrane disease. Rales are not diagnostic of disease.

Heart

Examination of the heart is described in detail in Chapter 19. *Note:* Murmurs are most often benign and are not necessarily present in serious congenital heart disease in the newborn. The two most common presentations of heart disease in the newborn are cyanosis and congestive heart failure with abnormalities of pulses. In hypoplastic left heart and critical aortic stenosis, pulses are diminished throughout. In coarctation, pulses are diminished in the lower extremities.

Abdomen

Check for softness, absence of distention, and good bowel sounds. Palpate for kidneys—most abdominal masses in the newborn are associated with the kidneys (multicystic/dysplastic, hydronephrosis, etc). When the abdomen is relaxed, normal-sized kidneys can be appreciated. A markedly scaphoid abdomen plus respiratory distress suggests diaphragmatic hernia. Absence of abdominal musculature (prune-belly syndrome) may occur in association with renal abnormalities. Check the size of the liver and the spleen. These organs are superficial and require only light palpation to discern them in the newborn. The outline of a distended bladder may be seen and palpated above the symphysis pubica.

Genitalia & Anus

Male and female genitals show characteristics according to gestational age (Table 2–7). In the female, an imperforate hymen may be visible. During the first few days, a whitish discharge with or without blood is normal. Rule out ambiguous genitals and abnormal anal openings or fissures. Check the patency and location of the anus.

Skeleton

Check for obvious anomalies, for example, the absence of a bone, clubfoot, and fusion or webbing of digits. Check for extra digits. Examine for hip dislocation by attempting to dislocate the femur posteriorly and then abducting the legs to relocate the femur. Examine for extremity fractures and for palsies (especially brachial plexus injuries). Rule out myelomeningoceles and other spinal deformities (eg, scoliosis). Arthrogryposis (limited joint movement) is seen with in utero limitation of movement because of lack of amniotic fluid or from a congenital muscle disease.

Neurologic Examination

Observe resting tone (normal, term newborns should exhibit flexion of the upper and lower extremities) and spontaneous movements. Look for asymmetry of movements. Extension of extremities should result in spontaneous recoil to the flexed position. Assess the character of the cry; a highpitched cry may be indicative of disease of the central nervous system (eg, hemorrhage). Hypotonia and a weak cry are indicative of systemic disease or a congenital muscle disorder. Check for newborn reflexes:

(1) **Rooting reflex**—Head turns to the side of a facial stimulus.

(2) **Sucking reflex.**

(3) **Traction response**—The infant is pulled by the arms to sitting. Initially, the head lags, then with active flexion comes to midline for a few seconds before falling forward.

(4) **Palmar grasp.**

(5) **Deep tendon reflexes.**

(6) **Placing**—Rub the dorsum of one foot on the underside of a surface. Then the infant will flex the knee and bring the foot up.

(7) **Moro (startle) reflex**—Hold the infant, and support the head. Allow the head to drop 1–2 cm suddenly. The arms will abduct at the shoulder and extend at the elbow. Adduction will follow. The hands show a prominent spreading or extension of the fingers. *Note:* Several beats of ankle clonus and an upgoing Babinski reflex are normal.

American Academy of Pediatrics: *Guidelines for Perinatal Care,* 3rd ed. American Academy of Pediatrics, 1992.

Ballard JL et al: New Ballard Score, expanded to include extremely premature infants. J Pediatr 1991;119:417.

Hegy T et al: Blood pressure ranges in premature infants: II. The first weeks of life. Pediatrics 1996;97:336.

CARE OF THE NORMAL NEWBORN

CARE IMMEDIATELY AFTER DELIVERY

Gently suction the oropharynx. Support body temperature by drying the skin, then swaddle or place the infant beneath a radiant heat source. Assign Apgar scores. If polyhydramnios is present at delivery or if excessive oral secretions are noted, pass a soft catheter into the stomach to rule out esophageal atresia. Routine eye prophylaxis must be done as defined by local health codes (eg, silver nitrate, 1%, or erythromycin ointment) to prevent gonorrheal conjunctivitis. Place identification bands, and obtain footprints.

CORD BLOOD

Cord blood is used for blood typing, Coombs' testing, and serology. Another tube is saved. Cord blood is also useful for other tests, such as electrolytes, glucose, total protein, and toxicology screen. Blood from doubly clamped cord can also be used in testing for pH, base deficit, and lactate concentrations, if needed.

CARE IN THE TRANSITIONAL NURSERY

Check temperature stabilization. Give vitamin K, 1 mg intramuscularly, to prevent hemorrhagic disease of the newborn. Review pertinent history. Plot birth weight and gestational age to assess risk for certain problems, such as hypoglycemia. Indications that the baby is ready for feeding include the following: (1) alertness and vigor, (2) absence of abdominal distention, (3) good bowel sounds, and (4) normal hunger cry. All of these usually occur 2–6 hours after birth, but fetal distress or traumatic delivery may prolong this period.

CONTINUED CARE IN LEVEL 1

The primary responsibilities of the level 1 nursery are care of the well infant, enhancing successful mother-infant bonding, feeding, and teaching the techniques of newborn care. However, surveillance is a key function of the staff; they must be alert for signs and symptoms of illness.

Admission

The prenatal history and immediate postnatal events should be reviewed so that as many problems as possible are anticipated. The determination of birth weight for gestational age is very helpful in this regard. The baby's initial physical examination should be performed within the first 12 hours of life.

Temperature Control

After delivery, body temperature may be labile until the infant has stabilized. Cooling should be avoided, because it can delay normal cardiovascular adjustments and predispose the infant to persistent pulmonary hypertension. Drying the skin is absolutely essential, and radiant heating devices are excellent adjuncts, allowing both warming of the infant and adequate observation.

Observation

The infant should be observed for signs of illness, including temperature instability, change in activity, refusal to feed, pallor, cyanosis, jaundice, tachypnea and respiratory distress, delayed (beyond 24 hours) passage of first stool or void, and bilious vomiting.

Screening Laboratory

Infants born to mothers with type O or Rh-negative blood should have a blood type and direct and indirect Coombs' tests performed on cord blood. The indirect Coombs' test is particularly important in the diagnosis of ABO incompatibility. Chemstrip testing should be performed in infants at risk for hypoglycemia (SGA, preterm, LGA, infant of a diabetic mother [IDM], stressed infant). Values of less than 40 mg/dL should be confirmed with a blood glucose. Hematocrit should be measured at 3–6 hours of age in infants at risk for or with symptoms of polycythemia or anemia. Other tests include the serologic test for syphilis and state- sponsored screens for inborn errors of metabolism, such as phenylketonuria (PKU), galactosemia, sickle cell disease, hypothyroidism, and cystic fibrosis. In well newborns, these metabolic screens are performed just prior to discharge, after 24–48 hours if possible. In some states, a repeat test is required at 8–14 days of age. In infants with prolonged hospital stays, the test should be performed at 1 week of age.

Duration of Stay

The trend over the last several years has been toward shorter hospital stays for well mothers and infants. Criteria for early discharge (<24 hours) at the University of Colorado are presented in Table 2–8. These criteria have been adapted from those suggested by the American Academy of Pediatrics (AAP). Of considerable importance is the fact that most infants who manifest serious cardiorespiratory and infectious

problems do so in the first 6 hours of life. Other problems, such as jaundice and difficulties in breast-feeding, typically occur after 48 hours and can usually be handled on an outpatient basis provided that good follow-up has been arranged. The AAP recommends a follow-up visit within 48–72 hours for any newborn discharged before 48 hours of age. Infants who are small, slightly premature, and breast-feeding are at particular risk for inadequate intake. Suggested guidelines for the follow-up interview and physical examination are shown in Table 2–9. The timing of discharge must be determined in each case based on medical, social, and financial factors.

Adapting Nursery Care to Meet the Needs of the Mother

The life situation of the mother and family is important in their adaptation to the newly born infant. The caretaker needs to be aware of emotional support available to the mother (spouse or other family members), financial security, maturity of the mother, and past psychiatric, drug, or alcohol problems. The family should receive instruction about basic care skills such as feeding, bathing, and cord and circumcision care and information on common newborn problems. One-on-one teaching is preferred, supplemented on a busy service with videotapes and printed material. The baby should room-in with the mother whenever possible. The mother and infant are then supervised by the nursery staff, and individual needs become more quickly apparent.

Circumcision

Circumcision is an elective procedure to be performed only in healthy, stable infants. The procedure has potential medical benefits, including prevention of phimosis, paraphimosis, and balanoposthitis. In addition, circumcision has been shown to decrease the incidence of cancer of the penis and may result in a de-

---

Table 2–8. Criteria for early discharge.[1]

1. Delivery is vertex, single, sterile, and vaginal.
2. Apgar scores of >7 at 1 and 5 min.
3. Gestational age of 38–42 weeks and weight of 2700–4000 g.
4. Minimum length of stay of 20 h; a transition to normal thermoregulation in an open crib, completion of 2 successful feedings, evidence of stool and void, completion of neonatal screening for metabolic disease and blood type and Coombs' test (Rh-negative and O mothers) prior to discharge.
5. Vital signs within normal ranges at discharge:
   Axillary temperature 36.1–37.2 °C
   Heart rate 110–150/min
   Respiratory rate 30–60/min
6. A normal neonatal hospital course with no signs or symptoms that require continuous observation:
   Blood dextrose maintained >45 mg/dL
   Hematocrit 45–65%
   ABO-incompatible infants must be free of clinical jaundice.
7. Physical examination completed by the physician or a trained assistant.
8. Demonstration of mother's understanding and ability to provide adequate care for her newborn; infant care education provided on a one-to-one or classroom basis by the nursing staff prior to discharge.
9. Signed documentation by mother that states her obligation to participate in follow-up care.

[1]Adapted, with permission, from Conrad PD, Wilkening RB, Rosenberg AA: Safety of newborn discharge in less than 36 hours in an indigent population. Am J Dis Child 1989;143:98. Copyright © 1989 American Medical Association.

Table 2–9. Guidelines for the follow-up evaluation.

History
Rhythmic sucking and audible swallowing for at least 10 min total per feeding?
Baby wakes and demands to feed every 2–3 h (at least 8–10 feedings per 24 h)?
Do breasts feel full before feedings, and softer after?
Are there at least 6 noticeably wet diapers per 24 h?
Are there yellow bowel movements (no longer meconium), at least 4 per 24 h?
Is baby still acting hungry after nursing (needs frequent pacifier, sucks hands, rooting)?

Physical assessment
Weight, unclothed: should not be more than 8–10% below birth weight at lowest
Extent of jaundice
Assessment of hydration, alertness, general well-being
Cardiovascular examination: murmur, brachial and femoral pulses, respirations

creased incidence of urinary tract infection. The risks of the procedure include local infection, bleeding, removal of too much skin, and urethral injury. Local anesthesia (dorsal penile nerve block) or topical application of an anesthetic cream reduces the physiologic and behavioral responses of the infant to the procedure. Circumcision is contraindicated in infants with genital abnormalities (eg, hypospadias). Appropriate laboratory evaluation should be performed prior to the procedure in infants with a family history of bleeding.

Discharge Preparation

1. Perform a physical examination.
2. Discuss cord and circumcision care.
3. Make sure the mother has mastered the essentials of newborn care.
4. Review signs and symptoms that cause concern:
   a. Jaundice
   b. Poor feeding
   c. Lethargy: increased sleeping
   d. Vomiting
   e. Fever
5. Review feeding instructions.
6. Arrange follow-up.
7. Verify the identification of the infant and the person accepting the infant at discharge.
8. Check on all screening procedures.

American Academy of Pediatrics: *Guidelines for Perinatal Care,* 3rd ed. American Academy of Pediatrics, 1992.

American Academy of Pediatrics Committee on Fetus and Newborn: Routine evaluation of blood pressure, hematocrit and glucose in newborns. Pediatrics 1993;92:474.

American Academy of Pediatrics Committee on Genetics: Issues in newborn screening. Pediatrics 1992;89:345.

American Academy of Pediatrics Section on Endocrinology and Committee on Genetics, and American Thyroid Association Committee on Public Health: Newborn screening for congenital hypothyroidism: Recommended guidelines. Pediatrics 1993;91:1203.

American Academy of Pediatrics Task Force on Circumcision: Report of the Task Force on Circumcision. Pediatrics 1989;84:388.

American Academy of Pediatrics Vitamin K Ad Hoc Task Force: Controversies concerning vitamin K and the newborn. Pediatrics 1993;91:1001.

Braveman P et al: Early discharge of newborns and mothers: A critical review of the literature. Pediatrics 1995; 96:716.

Britton JR et al: Early discharge of the term newborn: A continued dilemma. Pediatrics 1994;94:291.

Craig JC et al: Effect of circumcision on incidence of urinary tract infection in preschool boys. J Pediatr 1996;128:23.

Report of the 100th Ross Conference on Pediatric Research: *The Term Newborn Infant: A Current Outlook.* Ross Laboratories, 1991.

Snellman LW et al: Prospective evaluation of complications of dorsal penile nerve block for neonatal circumcision. Pediatrics 1995;95:705.

Weatherstone KB et al: Safety and efficacy of a topical anesthetic for neonatal circumcision. Pediatrics 1993;92:710.

PARENT-INFANT RELATIONSHIP

DEVELOPMENT OF PARENT-INFANT BONDING

The steps in maternal attachment can be outlined as follows: (1) planning the pregnancy, (2) confirming the pregnancy, (3) accepting the pregnancy, (4) feeling fetal movement, (5) accepting the fetus as an individual, (6) experiencing birth, (7) hearing and seeing the baby, (8) touching and holding the baby, and (9) caretaking.

The first 1½ hours of life are an important time in the process of mother-infant bonding. The infant is alert and able to follow with the eyes, a response prompting meaningful interaction with the mother. Whether a critical time period for these initial interactions exists is not clear, but increased contact with the infant over the first 3 postpartum days is associated with improved parenting behavior.

THE SICK INFANT

Mothers with high-risk pregnancies are at increased risk for subsequent parenting problems. The involvement of both obstetrician and pediatrician alike before the child's birth enables the family to prepare for anticipated aspects of the baby's care and provides reassurance that the odds are heavily in favor of a live baby who will ultimately be healthy. If the need for neonatal intensive care is anticipated before birth (known congenital anomaly, refractory premature labor), *maternal* transport to the proper facility should be planned. In this way, a mother can be with her baby during critical care. It is also very helpful to allow the parents to tour the unit their baby will occupy before delivery.

The single basic principle in dealing with parents of a sick infant is to provide essential information clearly and accurately to both parents, preferably when they are together. In most circumstances, one can be reasonably positive about the outcome. There is also no reason to emphasize problems that might occur in the future or to deal with individual worries of the physician.

CONGENITAL MALFORMATIONS

The birth of an infant with a congenital malformation is another situation in which staff support is essential. Parental reactions to the birth of a malformed infant follow a predictable course. For most parents, initial shock and denial are followed by a period of sadness and anger, gradual adaptation, and, finally, an increased satisfaction with and ability to care for the baby. The parents must be allowed to pass through these stages and, in effect, mourn the loss of the anticipated normal child. Again, information, including the prognosis for the particular problem, must be provided clearly and accurately to both parents in words they can understand, and with compassion.

DEATH OF AN INFANT

A stillbirth or the death of an infant is a highly stressful family event; there is a significant incidence of psychiatric disorders within 2 years of the death of a neonate. One of the major predispositions is a breakdown of communication between parents. The health care staff needs to encourage the parents to talk with each other, discuss their feelings, and display emotion. The staff should talk with the parents at the time of death and then several months later review the findings of the autopsy, answer questions, and see how the family is doing.

Klaus MH, Kennell JH: Care of the parents. In: *Care of the High-Risk Neonate,* 4th ed. Klaus MH, Fanaroff AA (editors). Saunders, 1993.

Klein M et al: Low birth weight and the battered child syndrome. Am J Dis Child 1971;122:15.

Mahowald MB: Baby Doe committees: A critical evaluation. Clin Perinatol 1988;15:789.

FEEDING OF THE NEWBORN INFANT

WHAT, WHEN, & HOW MUCH TO FEED

The healthy, term infant should be allowed to feed every 2–5 hours on demand. The first feeding usually occurs at 2–6 hours of life. Breast-feeding can start as early as in the delivery room. Although there is a trend toward earlier institution of feedings, evidence that the infant is prepared for feedings should always be present—soft, nondistended abdomen, good bowel sounds, and a strong, rhythmic suck. Breast milk or formula (20 kcal/oz) can be given. Generally, the volume increases from 0.5–1 oz per feeding initially up to above 1.5–2 oz per feeding on day 3. By day 3, the average term newborn takes in about 100 mL/kg/d of milk.

METHODS OF FEEDING

Bottle Feeding

Most commercial bottles and nipples are satisfactory. The preterm infant usually requires a softer nipple with a larger hole.

Breast-feeding

Although a wide range of infant formulas satisfy the nutritional needs of most neonates, breast milk is the standard on which formulas are based. The distribution of calories in human milk is 7% protein, 55% fat, and 38% carbohydrate. The ratio of whey to casein is 60:40. This allows ease of protein digestion, while fat digestion is aided by lipase in the milk. Despite low levels of several vitamins and minerals, bioavailability is high. Infants of mothers who are strict vegetarians should receive supplemental iron, folate, and vitamin B_{12}. Along with nutritional features, other advantages of breast milk include the following: (1) the presence of host resistance factors, including IgA and cellular components thought to decrease the incidence of upper respiratory and gastrointestinal infections in infancy; (2) the possibility that breast-feeding may decrease the frequency and severity of childhood eczema and asthma; (3) promotion of mother-infant bonding; and (4) recent evidence that breast milk as a nutritional source enhances neurodevelopmental outcome.

The nursery staff must be cognizant of problems associated with breast-feeding and be able to provide help and support for mothers in the hospital. Feeding should be fairly frequent in early stages (every 2–3 hours) so that production of milk is stimulated. Initially, nursing time is limited to 5 minutes on each side, then increased to 10 minutes on each side. Care of the nipples should also be reviewed in the hospital.

Gavage Feeding

Intermittent gavage feeding can be used for infants with a weak suck and swallow or for infants who tire easily, including preterm infants and those with medical conditions (eg, respiratory distress or congenital heart disease) precluding nipple feedings. An orogastric tube can be inserted for each feeding, or a soft, indwelling orogastric or nasogastric tube can be used. The position of the tube in the stomach should be checked prior to each feeding. The infant should be fed every 2–3 hours, depending on the age and size of the patient. Generally, infants weighing less than 1200 g require 2-hour feedings, whereas larger infants are fed at 3-hour intervals. Feedings are started at 10–25% of the child's nutritional needs and advanced to full requirements (100–120 kcal/kg/d) over 3–7 days. The more rapid advancement is used in infants weighing more than 1500 g and the slowest in infants weighing less than 1000 g.

Gastrostomy

Gastrostomy feedings are indicated for infants requiring indefinite tube feedings (eg, those with neurologic disease) and for those with certain surgical conditions (eg, some cases of esophageal atresia).

Parenteral Alimentation

Nutrition can effectively be provided with hyperalimentation solutions given through either peripheral or central venous lines. Table 2–10 illustrates the use of hyperalimentation in newborns. Parenteral nutrition is indicated for infants with gastrointestinal anomalies after surgical correction, for preterm infants with necrotizing enterocolitis and other forms of feeding intolerance, and for infants too sick, for any reason, to tolerate enteral feedings. Central hyperalimentation has now been facilitated by Silastic lines that can be placed in the nursery under local anesthesia percutaneously or through a basilic vein cutdown. An umbilical venous line with its tip located at the diaphragm can also be used for central access.

Barness LA (editor): *Pediatric Nutrition Handbook.* American Academy of Pediatrics, 1993.

Beaudry M et al: Relation between infant feeding and infections during the first six months of life. J Pediatr 1995;126:191.

Dewey KG et al: Differences in morbidity between breast-fed and formula-fed infants. J Pediatr 1995;126:696.

Greene HL et al: Guidelines for the use of vitamins, trace elements, calcium, magnesium and phosphorus in infants and children receiving total parenteral nutrition. Am J Clin Nutr 1988;48:1324.

Heird WC, Kashyap S, Gomez MR: Parenteral alimentation of the neonate. Semin Perinatol 1991;15:493.

Lawrence PB: Breast milk: Best source of nutrition for term and preterm infants. Pediatr Clin North Am 1994;41:925.

Lucas A et al: Breast milk and subsequent intelligence quotient in children born preterm. Lancet 1992;339:261.

Lucas A et al: A randomized multicenter study of human milk versus formula and later development in preterm infants. Arch Dis Child 1994;70:F141.

Neuzil J et al: Oxidation of parenteral lipid emulsion by ambient and phototherapy lights: Potential toxicity of routine parenteral feeding. J Pediatr 1995;126:785.

Tsang RC et al (editors): *Nutritional Needs of the Preterm Infant.* Williams & Wilkins, 1993.

NEONATAL INTENSIVE CARE

GENERAL APPROACH

Neonatal intensive care should always have an anticipatory component; that is, obstetricians managing high-risk pregnancies should anticipate delivery as often as possible and discuss specific features of the pregnancy likely to affect the infant immediately after birth. In this way, the course of the labor and the condition of the infant during delivery are known to the baby's caregiver. A pediatrician or neonatologist should be in attendance at high-risk deliveries to provide prompt resuscitation of the infant, when needed.

Table 2–10. Use of parenteral alimentation solutions.

	Volume (mL/kg/d)	Carbohydrate (g/dL)	Protein (g/kg)	Lipid (g/kg)	Calories (kcal/kg)
Peripheral: Short-term (7–10 d)					
Starting solution	100–150	$D_{10}W$	1	1	46–64
Target solution	150	$D_{12.5}W$	2.5	3	102
Central: Long-term (>10 d)					
Starting solution	100–150	$D_{10}W$	1	1	46–64
Target solution	130	$D_{20}W$	3–3.5	3	123

Notes:
1. Protein calories should be no more than 10% of total calories.
2. Advance dextrose in central hyperalimentation as tolerated by 2.5% per day as long as blood glucose remains normal.
3. Advance lipids by 0.5 g/kg/d as long as triglycerides are normal. Use 20% concentration.
4. Total water should be 100–150 mL/kg/d, depending on the child's fluid tolerance.

Monitoring:
1. Chemstrips or blood glucose two or three times a day when changing dextrose concentration, then daily.
2. Electrolytes daily, then twice a week when the child is receiving a stable solution.
3. Weekly blood urea nitrogen and serum creatinine; total protein and serum albumin; serum calcium, phosphate, magnesium, direct bilirubin, and alkaline phosphatase; and CBC with platelet counts.

TRANSPORTATION

Whenever possible, high-risk mothers should be delivered at perinatal centers so that transport of the infant after delivery can be avoided, and mother and baby can remain together after delivery. In such circumstances, the infant is simply moved from the delivery room to the level 2 or 3 nursery. The transport unit should be easily movable and be equipped to provide ventilatory assistance and oxygen therapy to the infant and to maintain body temperature. In transports from one hospital to another, equipment for intravenous infusions should be available, together with appropriate solutions to support circulating blood volume and extracellular fluid volume. Equipment should be on hand to monitor the infant (heart rate, respirations, blood pressure, oxygen saturation). All emergency equipment necessary to resuscitate an infant should be available. The infant should be stabilized prior to transport.

PERINATAL RESUSCITATION

Perinatal resuscitation involves the steps taken by the obstetrician during labor and delivery to support the infant, as well as the traditional resuscitative steps taken by the pediatrician after delivery of the infant. Intrapartum steps to support the infant include the following: maintaining maternal blood pressure with volume expanders if needed, administering maternal oxygen therapy, positioning the mother to improve placental perfusion, readjusting oxytocin infusions or administering a tocolytic if appropriate, minimizing trauma to the infant (particularly important in infants of very low birth weight), suctioning the nasopharynx at delivery of the head if meconium is present in amniotic fluid, obtaining all necessary cord blood samples, and completing an examination of the placenta.

Steps taken by the pediatrician or neonatologist center around support of the following physiologic areas: temperature support, initiation and maintenance of effective ventilation, maintenance of perfusion and hydration, and glucose regulation. These are generally accomplished as discussed in the following paragraphs.

Resuscitation of the Newborn Infant

A number of conditions of pregnancy, labor, and delivery place the infant at risk for birth asphyxia: (1) maternal diseases such as diabetes, pregnancy-induced hypertension, heart and renal disease, and collagen-vascular disease; (2) fetal conditions such as prematurity, multiple births, growth retardation, and fetal anomalies; and (3) labor and delivery conditions, including fetal distress with or without meconium in the amniotic fluid and administration of anesthetics and narcotic analgesics.

Physiology of Birth Asphyxia

Birth asphyxia can be the result of several mechanisms: (1) acute interruption of umbilical blood flow (eg, prolapsed cord with cord compression), (2) premature placental separation, (3) maternal hypotension or hypoxia, (4) chronic placental insufficiency, and (5) failure to execute a proper newborn resuscitation.

The neonatal response to asphyxia follows a predictable pattern that has been demonstrated in a variety of species (Figure 2–2). The initial response to hypoxia is an increase in frequency of respiration and a rise in heart rate and blood pressure. Respirations then cease (primary apnea) as heart rate and blood pressure begin to fall. This initial period of apnea lasts 30–60 seconds. Gasping respirations (3–6/min) then begin, while heart rate and blood pressure gradually decline. Secondary or terminal apnea then ensues, with further decline in heart rate and blood

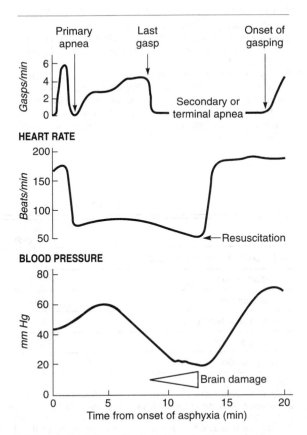

Figure 2–2. Schematic depiction of changes in rhesus monkeys during asphyxia and on resuscitation by positive-pressure ventilation. (Adapted and reproduced, with permission, from Dawes GS: *Fetal and Neonatal Physiology.* Year Book, 1968.)

pressure. The longer the duration of secondary apnea, the greater the risk for hypoxic organ injury. A cardinal feature of the defense against hypoxia is the sacrifice, that is, underperfusion, of certain tissue beds (eg, skin, muscle, gastrointestinal tract), which allows the perfusion of core organs (ie, heart, brain) to be maintained.

The response to resuscitation also follows a predictable pattern. During the period of primary apnea, almost any physical stimulus causes the baby to initiate respirations. Infants in secondary apnea require positive-pressure ventilation. The first sign of recovery is an increase in heart rate, followed by an increase in blood pressure with improved perfusion. The period required for rhythmic, spontaneous respirations to occur is related to the duration of the secondary apnea. As a rough rule, for each 1 minute past the last gasp, 2 minutes of positive-pressure breathing is required before gasping begins, and 4 minutes is required to reach rhythmic breathing. However, these periods can vary, depending on the degree and duration of intrauterine asphyxia. Not until sometime later do spinal and corneal reflexes return. Muscle tone gradually improves over the course of several hours.

Delivery Room Management

When asphyxia is anticipated, a resuscitation team of two persons, one to manage the airway and one to monitor heartbeat and provide assistance, should be present. The necessary equipment and drugs are listed in Table 2–11.

A. Steps in the Resuscitation: See Figure 2–3.

1. Dry the infant well, and place the baby under the radiant heat source.

2. Gently suction the mouth, then the nose.

3. Quickly assess the infant's condition. The best criteria are the infant's respiratory effort (apneic, gasping, regular) and heart rate (>100 or <100). A depressed heart rate indicative of hypoxic myocardial depression is the single most reliable indicator of the need for resuscitation.

4. Generally, infants with heart rates over 100 beats/min require no further intervention. Infants with heart rates less than 100/min and apnea or irregular respiratory efforts should be vigorously stimulated. The baby's back should be rubbed with a towel while oxygen is blown over the baby's face.

5. If the baby fails to respond to tactile stimulation within a few seconds, begin bag and mask ventilation, using a soft mask that seals well around the mouth and nose. For the initial inflations, pressures of 30–40 cm H_2O may be necessary to overcome surface-active forces in the lungs. Adequacy of ventilation is assessed by observing expansion of the infant's chest accompanied by an improvement in heart rate, perfusion, and color. After the first few breaths,

Table 2–11. Equipment for neonatal resuscitation.[1]

Clinical Needs	Equipment
Thermoregulation	Radiant heat source with platform, mattress covered with warm sterile blankets, servo control heating, temperature probe
Airway management	**Suction:** Bulb suction, DeLee suction apparatus, wall vacuum suction with sterile catheters **Ventilation:** Manual infant resuscitation bag connected to manometer capable of delivering 100% oxygen, appropriate masks for term and preterm infants **Intubation:** Neonatal laryngoscope with No. 0 and No. 1 blades; endotracheal tubes (2.5-, 3.0-, 3.5-mm OD with stylet)
Gastric decompression	Nasogastric tubes: 5F and 8F
Administration of drugs and volume replacement	Sterile umbilical catheterization tray, umbilical catheters (3.5F and 5F), volume expanders (Ringer's lactate, 5% albumin), drug box with appropriate neonatal vials and dilutions, sterile syringes, and needles
Transport	Warmed transport isolette with oxygen source

[1]Modified, with permission, from Rosenberg AA: Neonatal adaptation. In *Obstetrics: Normal and Problem Pregnancies.* Gabbe SG, Niebyl JR, Simpson JL (editors). Churchill Livingston, 1996.

lower the peak pressure to 15–20 cm H_2O. The baby's chest movement should resemble that of an easy breath rather than a deep sigh. The rate of bagging should be 40–60 breaths per minute.

6. Most neonates can be effectively resuscitated with a bag and mask. If the infant does not respond to bag and mask ventilation, try to reposition the head (slight extension), reapply the mask to achieve a good seal, consider suctioning the mouth and the oropharynx, and try ventilating with the mouth open. If the infant does not respond favorably within 30 seconds, intubation is appropriate.

Failure to respond to intubation and ventilation can result from (1) mechanical difficulties (Table 2–12), (2) profound asphyxia with myocardial depression, and (3) inadequate circulating blood volume.

Quickly rule out the mechanical causes in Table 2–12. Check to be sure the endotracheal tube passes through the vocal cords. Occlusion of the tube should be suspected when there is resistance to bagging and no chest wall movement. Very few neonates (approximately 0.1%) require either cardiac massage or drugs during resuscitation. Almost all newborns respond to ventilation with 100% oxygen if done effectively.

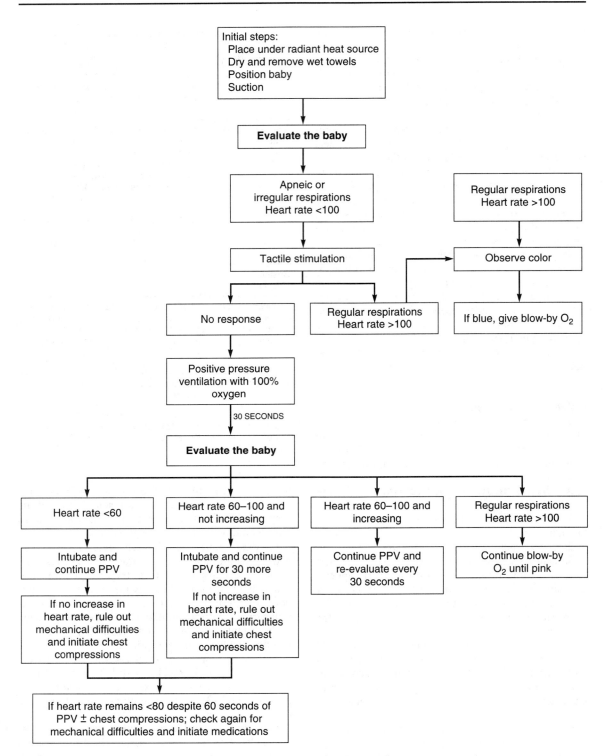

Figure 2–3. Delivery room management.

Table 2–12. Mechanical causes of failed resuscitation.[1]

Etiology	Examples
Equipment failure	Malfunctioning bag, oxygen not connected or running
Endotracheal tube malposition	Esophagus, right main stem bronchus
Occluded endotracheal tube	
Insufficient inflation pressure to expand lungs	
Space-occupying lesions in the thorax	Pneumothorax, pleural effusions, diaphragmatic hernia
Pulmonary hypoplasia	Extreme prematurity, oligohydramnios

[1]Reproduced, with permission, from Rosenberg AA: Neonatal adaptation. In: *Obstetrics: Normal and Problem Pregnancies*. Gabbe SG, Niebyl JR, Simpson JL (editors). Churchill Livingston, 1996.

7. If mechanical causes are ruled out, and the heart rate remains below 80 and is not increasing after intubation and positive-pressure ventilation for 30 seconds, cardiac compression should be initiated. Simultaneous delivery of chest compressions and positive-pressure ventilation is likely to decrease the efficiency of ventilation. Therefore, chest compressions should be interspersed with ventilation at a 3:1 ratio (90 compressions and 30 breaths per minute).

8. If drugs are needed (rarely), the drug of choice is 0.1–0.3 mL/kg of epinephrine, 1:10,000 solution (0.01–0.03 mg/kg), given via the endotracheal tube or an umbilical venous line. Some children and adults who do not respond to standard doses will respond to 0.2 mg/kg, but the safety and efficacy of such a dose have not been adequately evaluated in the newborn. Sodium bicarbonate, 1–2 meq/kg of the neonatal dilution (0.5 meq/mL), can be used for an infant with *documented* metabolic acidosis. If volume loss is suspected, 10 mL/kg of a volume expander (5% albumin, normal saline) should be administered through an umbilical venous line.

B. Continued Resuscitative Measures: The appropriateness of continued resuscitative efforts should be reevaluated in an infant who fails to respond to the above efforts. Today, resuscitative efforts are made even in "apparent stillbirths," that is, infants whose Apgar score at 1 minute is 0–1. Modern resuscitative techniques have led to an increasing survival rate for these infants, with 60% of survivors showing normal development. It is clear from a number of studies that initial resuscitation of these infants should proceed; however, subsequent continued support must depend on response to resuscitation. All studies emphasize that if the Apgar score is not improving markedly over the first 10–15 minutes of life, the mortality rates and the incidence of severe developmental handicap among survivors are high.

C. Special Considerations:

1. Preterm infants—

a. Minimizing heat loss improves survival, so prewarmed towels should be available, and the environmental temperature of the delivery suite should be raised (especially for infants weighing <1500 g).

b. In the extremely low birth weight infant (<1000 g), proceed quickly to intubation.

c. Volume expanders and sodium bicarbonate (if needed) should be infused slowly to avoid rapid swings in blood pressure and serum osmolality.

2. In the case of narcotic administration to the mother during labor, perform the resuscitation as described above. When the baby is stable with good heart rate, color, and perfusion but still has poor respiratory effort, a trial of naloxone hydrochloride (0.1 mg/kg given intramuscularly, subcutaneously, intravenously, or intratracheally) is indicated. Naloxone should not be administered in place of positive-pressure ventilation.

3. Meconium-stained amniotic fluid—

a. The obstetrician carefully suctions the oropharynx and the nasopharynx after delivery of the head with a suction apparatus attached to wall suction.

b. The delivery is then completed, and the baby is given to the resuscitator.

c. If the baby is active and breathing, requiring no resuscitation, and if effective obstetric suctioning has been performed, the airway need not be inspected. Only further suctioning of the mouth and nasopharynx need be performed.

d. The airway of any depressed infant requiring ventilation must be checked and cleared (by passage of a tube below the vocal cords) before positive-pressure ventilation is instituted. Special adapters are available for use with regulated wall suction to allow suction to be applied to the endotracheal tube.

4. Universal precautions should always be observed in the delivery room.

American Heart Association and American Academy of Pediatrics: *Textbook of Neonatal Resuscitation.* American Heart Association/American Academy of Pediatrics, 1994.

Apgar V: A proposal for a new method of evaluation of the newborn infant. Anesth Analg 1953;32:260.

Greenough A: Meconium aspiration syndrome—Prevention and treatment. Early Hum Dev 1995;41:183.

Gupta JM et al: The sequence of events in neonatal apnea. Lancet 1967;2:55.

Jain L et al: Cardiopulmonary resuscitation of apparently stillborn infants: Survival and long-term outcome. J Pediatr 1991;118:778.

Katz VL, Bowes WA: Meconium aspiration syndrome; reflections on a murky subject. Am J Obstet Gynecol 1992;166:171.

Perlman JM, Risser R: Cardiopulmonary resuscitation in the delivery room: Associated clinical events. Arch Pediatr Adolesc Med 1995;149:20.

Wiswell TE, Bent RC: Meconium staining and the meconium aspiration syndrome: Unresolved issues. Pediatr Clin North Am 1993;40:955.

Yoder BA: Meconium-stained amniotic fluid and respiratory complications: Impact of selective tracheal suction. Obstet Gynecol 1994;83:77.

THE PRETERM INFANT

Premature infants account for the majority of high-risk newborns. The preterm infant faces a variety of physiologic handicaps:

(1) The ability to suck, swallow, and breathe in a coordinated fashion is not in place until 34–36 weeks of gestation. Therefore, enteral feedings must be provided by gavage. Furthermore, preterm infants frequently have gastroesophageal influx and an immature gag reflex, which increase the risk of aspiration of feedings.

(2) Decreased ability to maintain body temperature (see below).

(3) Pulmonary immaturity—surfactant deficiency, often with structural immaturity in those infants of less than 26 weeks of gestation. Their condition is complicated by the combination of noncompliant lungs and a compliant chest wall.

(4) Immature control of respiration, leading to apnea and bradycardia.

(5) Persistent patency of the ductus arteriosus, leading to further compromise of pulmonary gas exchange because of overperfusion of the lungs.

(6) Immature cerebral vasculature, predisposing the infant to subependymal/intraventricular hemorrhage.

(7) Impaired substrate absorption by the gastrointestinal tract, compromising nutritional management.

(8) Immature renal function (including both filtration and tubular functions), complicating fluid and electrolyte management.

(9) Increased susceptibility to infection.

(10) Immaturity of metabolic processes, predisposing the infant to hypoglycemia and hypocalcemia.

CARE OF THE PRETERM INFANT

Delivery Room

See Perinatal Resuscitation.

Care in the Nursery

Some general principles, for example, thermoregulation, monitoring, and fluid and electrolyte management, are covered here. Other conditions unique to the preterm infant are discussed under specific headings in the chapter.

A. Thermoregulation: Maintaining a stable body temperature is a function of heat production and conservation balanced against heat loss. Heat is produced at the rate of 4.8 kcal/L of O_2 consumed. Heat production in response to cold stress can occur through voluntary muscle activity, involuntary muscle activity (shivering), and thermogenesis not caused by shivering. Newborns produce heat mainly through the last of these three mechanisms. This metabolic heat production depends on the quantity of brown fat present, which is very limited in the preterm infant. Heat loss to the environment can occur through the following mechanisms: (1) Radiation—transfer of heat from a warmer to a cooler object not in contact. (2) Convection—transfer of heat to the surrounding gaseous environment. This is influenced by air movement and temperature. (3) Conduction—transfer of heat to a cooler object in contact. (4) Evaporation—cooling secondary to water loss through the skin.

Heat loss in the preterm newborn is accelerated because of a large ratio of surface area to body mass and reduced insulation of subcutaneous tissue. Furthermore, water loss through the skin is accelerated because of the immaturity of the skin (especially in infants <27–28 weeks' gestation) and because of the limited ability of skin blood vessels to constrict in response to cold.

For these reasons, the thermal environment of the preterm neonate must be carefully regulated. The infant can be kept warm in an isolette in which the air is heated and convective heat loss is minimized. Alternatively, the infant can be kept warm on an open bed with a radiant heat source. Although evaporative and convective heat losses are greater when the radiant warmer is used, this system allows easy access to a critically ill neonate. Ideally, the infant should be kept in a neutral thermal environment (Figure 2–4). The neutral thermal environment allows the infant to maintain a stable core body temperature with a minimum of metabolic heat production through oxygen consumption. In other words, heat losses have been minimized. This is a desirable goal in an infant who may be at risk for hypoxia as a result of cardiorespiratory disease. Furthermore, the infant is able to utilize calories for growth instead of heat production. The neutral thermal environment for a given infant depends on size, gestational age, and postnatal age. The neutral thermal environment (for either isolette or radiant warmer care) can be obtained by maintaining an abdominal skin temperature of 36.5 °C.

Temperature can be regulated in either isolettes or radiant warmers by manual or servo control adjustments. In manual control, skin temperature is regulated by manually adjusting the environmental temperature of an isolette or the heat output from a radiant warmer so that the infant maintains the desired skin temperature. In servo control, the heating equipment is adjusted automatically to maintain the

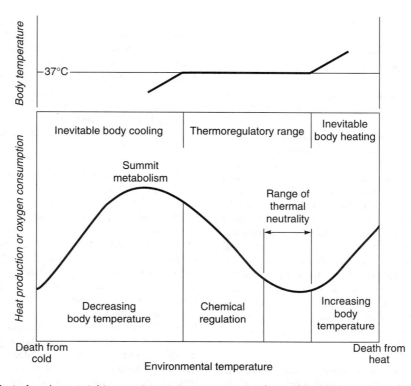

Figure 2–4. Effect of environmental temperature on oxygen consumption and body temperature. (Adapted and reproduced, with permission, from Klaus MH, Fanaroff AA, Martin RJ: The physical environment. In: *Care of the High-Risk Neonate,* 3rd ed. Klaus MH, Fanaroff AA [editors]. Saunders, 1986.)

desired skin temperature. The core temperature of the infant can be estimated from axillary temperatures. Although rectal temperatures provide a slightly better estimation of core temperature, they are discouraged because of the risk of rectal perforation. In infants weighing more than 1200 g, skin temperature is less than core temperature; however, in infants of very low birth weight, core temperature is lower than skin temperature and invariably below normal in the first few hours of life. Generally, when infants reach 1800–2000 g, they can maintain temperature while bundled in a bassinet.

B. Monitoring the High-Risk Infant: Care of the high- risk preterm infant requires sophisticated monitoring techniques. At a minimum, equipment to monitor heart rate, respirations, and blood pressure should be available. Oxygen saturation can be assessed continuously using pulse oximetry. This determination can be correlated with arterial oxygen tension (PaO_2) as needed. Transcutaneous PO_2 and PCO_2 can also be utilized to assess oxygenation and ventilation. Finally, arterial blood gases, electrolytes, glucose, calcium, bilirubin, and other chemistries must be measured on small volumes of blood. Early in the care of a sick preterm infant, the most efficient way to sample blood for tests as well as provide fluids

and monitor blood pressure is through an umbilical arterial line. Once the infant is stable and the need for frequent blood samples is reduced (usually 4–7 days), the umbilical line should be removed. All indwelling lines are associated with morbidity from thrombosis/embolus, infection, and bleeding.

C. Fluid and Electrolyte Therapy: Fluid requirements in preterm infants are a function of (1) insensible losses (skin and respiratory), (2) urine output, (3) stool output (<5% of total), and (4) others, such as nasogastric losses.

In most circumstances, the majority of the fluid requirement is determined by insensible losses and urine losses. The major contribution to insensible water loss is evaporative skin loss. The rate of water loss is a function of gestational age (body weight), environment (losses are greater under a radiant warmer than in an isolette), and the use of phototherapy. Respiratory losses are minimal when infants are breathing humidified oxygen. The renal contribution to water requirement is influenced by the decreased ability of the preterm neonate to concentrate the urine and conserve water.

Electrolyte requirements are minimal for the initial 24–48 hours until there is excretion in the urine. Basal requirements are as follows:

Sodium	3 meq/kg/d
Potassium	2 meq/kg/d
Chloride	2–3 meq/kg/d
Bicarbonate	2–3 meq/kg/d

In the infant of gestational age less than 30 weeks, sodium and bicarbonate losses in the urine are frequently higher.

Initial fluid management after birth is determined by the infant's size. Infants weighing more than 1500 g should start at 80–100 mL/kg/d of 10% dextrose in water ($D_{10}W$), whereas those weighing less should start at 100–120 mL/kg/d of either $D_{10}W$ or 5% dextrose in water (D_5W) (infants <800 g and <26 weeks often become hyperglycemic on $D_{10}W$). The most critical issue in fluid management is monitoring. Measurements of body weight, urine output, fluid and electrolyte intake, serum and urine electrolytes, and glucose (using Chemstrips) allow fairly precise determinations of the infant's water, glucose, and electrolyte needs. Once an infant has stabilized (usually by day 2 or 3), hyperalimentation solutions can be started to meet nutritional as well as water and electrolyte requirements.

Bell EF, Oh W: Fluid and electrolyte management. In: *Neonatology: Pathophysiology and Management of the Newborn,* 4th ed. Avery GB et al (editors). Lippincott, 1994.

Gunn TR, Gluckman PD: Perinatal thermogenesis. Early Hum Dev 1995;42:169.

Hay WW Jr, Thilo E, Curlander JB: Pulse oximetry in neonatal medicine. Clin Perinatol 1991;18:441.

Kjartansson S et al: Water loss from the skin of term and preterm infants nursed under a radiant heater. Pediatr Res 1995;37:233.

Klaus MH, Fanaroff AA, Martin RJ: The physical environment. In: *Care of the High-Risk Neonate,* 4th ed. Klaus MH, Fanaroff AA (editors). Saunders, 1993.

LeBlanc MH: Thermoregulation: Incubators, radiant warmers, artificial skins, and body hoods. Clin Perinatol 1991;18:403.

Mancini AJ et al: Semipermeable dressings improve epidermal barrier function in premature infants. Pediatr Res 1994;36:306.

Scopes JW: Metabolic rate and temperature control in the human body. Br Med Bull 1966;22:88.

Shaffer SG, Weismann DN: Fluid requirements in the preterm infant. Clin Perinatol 1992;19:233.

NUTRITION OF THE HIGH-RISK INFANT

This section addresses a nutritional approach to the very immature infant, for whom nutritional problems are most difficult. The end result of good nutrition is a steady weight gain. The growth of an infant should therefore be charted weekly against one of the standard postnatal growth curves. The average caloric requirement for the growing premature infant is 120 kcal/kg/d. Expected weight gain for the adequately nourished preterm infant is 10–30 g per day.

Infants initially require intravenous glucose infusions to maintain blood glucose concentration in the range of 60–100 mg/dL. Infusions of 5–7 mg/kg/min (approximately 80–100 mL/kg/d of a 10% dextrose solution) are usually needed. Nutritional support in the very low birth weight infant generally is started at 24–48 hours of age with parenteral alimentation solutions given either peripherally or centrally (see Table 2–10). Small-volume trophic feeds with breast milk or 20-cal/oz premature formula should be started as soon as possible and slowly advanced once the infant is stable. Intermittent bolus feedings are preferred, because these appear to stimulate the release of gut-related hormones and may speed the maturation of the gastrointestinal tract. A suggested schedule for feedings is presented in Table 2–13. *Note:* In the extremely low birth weight infant (<1000 g) or the postsurgical neonate, continuous-drip feeds are sometimes better tolerated.

In general, the long-term nutritional support for infants of very low birth weight consists of either breast milk supplemented to increase protein, caloric density, and mineral content or infant formulas modified for preterm infants. In all of these formulas, protein concentrations (approximately 2 g/dL) and caloric concentrations (approximately 24 kcal/oz) are relatively high. In addition, premature formulas contain some of the fat as medium-chain triglycerides, which do not require bile for emulsification, as an energy source. These feedings should not be started immediately. The infant should be gradually advanced to feedings of higher caloric density after the full volume of either breast milk or formula (20 kcal/oz) is tolerated. Success of feedings is assessed by:

- passage of feeds out of the stomach
- abdominal examination free of distention
- normal stool pattern

Carbohydrates

Glucose is the only carbohydrate provided initially; once milk feedings are begun, however, the lactose in the milk provides galactose, an important carbohydrate for the newborn. It is important to monitor blood glucose levels during the transition from intravenous to milk feedings (decreasing the reliance on intravenous glucose infusions), because infants fed intermittently cannot sustain blood glucose concentrations unless gluconeogenesis is well established.

Amino Acids

The amino acid composition of solutions available for intravenous use has been altered to provide a more readily usable form of nitrogen. TrophAmine is the preferred mixture for neonates since its amino

Table 2–13. Suggested feeding regimen for preterm infants.

| Weight (g) | Initial | | | Time to Full Feedings (d) |
	Feeding (mL)	Frequency (hourly)	Advancement (mL/feeding)	
500–800	1	2[1]	1 every 12–24 h	6
800–1000	2	2[1]	1 every 12 h	4–6
1000–1200	2–3	2	1 every 12 h	4
1200–1500	4	2–3	1 every 6–8 h	4
>1500	5–10	3	1 every other feeding	3–4

[1]Second and subsequent feedings offered only after examination of the infant shows the following:
   (1) No distention
   (2) Normal bowel sounds
   (3) No residuals or vomiting

acid profiles are most similar to those seen in infants on breast milk. The same principle—breast milk as the gold standard—has been applied to the design of formulas for premature infants. The increase in protein concentration in these formulas can lead to nitrogen intakes of 3–3.5 g/kg/d. These high intakes can be well utilized if caloric intake is also high.

Fats

Milk, whether breast milk or formula, constitutes a high-fat diet. A relatively high fat intake is important in establishing normal postnatal liver and gastrointestinal function. Deficiencies in essential fatty acids can develop quickly in the infant of very low birth weight, who has little body stores of essential fatty acids at the time of birth. Thus, it is important to make sure these babies receive an adequate amount of essential fatty acids, provided either intravenously or through milk feedings.

Vitamins

Vitamins are initially provided intravenously and later through milk feedings. Fortified breast milk and the formulas for premature infants provide adequate amounts of vitamins. Vitamin K, 1 mg intramuscularly, is given once to all newborns immediately after delivery.

Minerals

Formulas for premature infants contain increased concentrations of calcium and phosphorus. Any premature infant receiving an adequate intake of either fortified breast milk or one of these formulas receives adequate amounts of calcium and phosphorus for bone mineralization. Osteopenia and occasionally rickets are still seen in infants receiving long-term parenteral nutrition or the calciuric diuretic furosemide. Iron supplementation (2 mg/kg/d) is recommended for premature infants, beginning at about

2 months of life. This can be provided by iron-supplemented formulas. In some infants, iron supplementation may be indicated earlier. In particular, infants treated with erythropoietin for prevention of anemia of prematurity require supplemental iron at a dose of 4–8 mg/kg/d. Trace elements are discussed in Chapter 11.

DISCHARGE

Discharge policies are more flexible today. Term, healthy newborns may be discharged in 24 hours or less. Very immature infants are usually ready for discharge when they reach 2000–2500 g, but weight or postconceptual age alone no longer determines the time of discharge; a careful assessment of the infant's progress and the home environment also influences the decision. Factors such as the support for the mother at home and the stability of the family situation play a part in timing of discharge. The infant must at the very least be stable, eating well, and showing steady weight gain at the time of discharge. In addition, staff should observe the parents caring for the infant to confirm that the parents are capable of managing whatever special care the infant requires. Infants with special requirements, for example, oxygen therapy, may be discharged if the family clearly can manage to provide the additional support to the infant at home. The availability of a social worker or visiting nurse makes such discharge decisions easier.

FOLLOW-UP CARE

This term refers to follow-up visits to an ambulatory setting, for the purpose of tracking the achievement of behavioral and developmental landmarks in infants who have received neonatal intensive care.

For infants discharged from level 2 nurseries, follow-up care can be provided by the pediatrician, with consultative visits at special care facilities as required. Infants discharged from level 3 nurseries require specialized follow-up care, because many families need help with physical or neurologic problems and management of home oxygen therapy. In addition, the family needs ongoing support during the first few years of the child's life. The frequency of repeated hospitalizations in many infants who have experienced complications (eg, chronic lung disease and the attendant growth disturbances) after neonatal intensive care underscores the need for such support.

Als H et al: Individualized developmental care for the very low–birth–weight infant. JAMA 1994;272:853.

Ballard RA (editor): *Pediatric Care of the ICN Graduate.* Saunders, 1988.

Barness LA (editor): *Pediatric Nutrition Handbook.* American Academy of Pediatrics, 1993.

Berseth CL: Minimal enteral feedings. Clin Perinatol 1995;22:195.

Bregman J, Kimberlin LVS: Developmental outcome in extremely premature infants. Impact of surfactant. Pediatr Clin North Am 1993;40:937.

Gross SJ, Slagle TA: Feeding the low birthweight infant. Clin Perinatol 1993;20:193.

Hack M et al: School-age outcomes in children with birth weights under 750g. N Engl J Med 1994;331:753.

Hack M et al: Very-low-birth-weight outcomes of the National Institute of Child Health and Human Development Neonatal Network, November 1989 to October 1990. Am J Obstet Gynecol 1995;172:457.

Halsey CL, Collin MF, Anderson CL: Extremely low birth weight children and their peers: A comparison of preschool performance. Pediatrics 1993;91:807.

Kotagal UR et al: Description and evaluation of a program for early discharge of infants from a neonatal intensive care unit. J Pediatr 1995;127:285.

Pereira GR: Nutritional care of the extremely premature infant. Clin Perinatol 1995;22:61.

Rivera A et al: Effect of intravenous amino acids on protein metabolism of preterm infants during the first three days of life. Pediatr Res 1993;33:106.

Saigal S et al: Comprehensive assessment of the health status of extremely low birth weight children at eight years of age: Comparison with a reference group. J Pediatr 1994;125:411.

Schanler RJ: Suitability of human milk for the low-birth-weight infant. Clin Perinatol 1995;22:207.

Schanler RJ, Abrams SA: Postnatal attainment of intrauterine macromineral accretion rates in low birth weight infants fed fortified human milk. J Pediatr 1995;126:441.

Troche B et al: Early minimal feeds promote growth in critically ill premature infants. Biol Neonate 1995;67:172.

Tsang RC et al (editors): *Nutritional Needs of the Preterm Infant.* Williams & Wilkins, 1993.

Victorian Infant Collaborative Study Group: Eight-year outcome in infants with birth weight of 500 to 999 grams: Continuing regional study of 1979 and 1980 births. J Pediatr 1991;118:761.

Victorian Infant Collaborative Study Group: Improvement of outcome for infants of birth weight under 1000 g. Arch Dis Child 1991;66:765.

MULTIPLE BIRTHS

Multiple births represent an important area in perinatal medicine. Twinning occurs in one of every 80 pregnancies. A clear distinction should be made between dizygotic (fraternal) and monozygotic (identical) twins. Race, maternal parity, and maternal age affect only the incidence of dizygotic twinning. Drugs that induce ovulation, such as clomiphene citrate or gonadotropin therapy, increase the incidence of dizygotic twinning quite strikingly.

Examination of the placenta can help establish the type of twinning: two amnionic membranes and two chorionic membranes are found in all cases of dizygotic twins and in one-third of cases of monozygotic twins; one chorionic membrane always indicates monozygotic twins.

COMPLICATIONS OF MULTIPLE BIRTHS

Intrauterine Growth Retardation

There is some degree of intrauterine growth retardation in most multiple pregnancies after 34 weeks. If prenatal care is good, however, the growth retardation is rarely clinically significant. There are two exceptions; the first is the monochorial twin pregnancy in which there is an arteriovenous shunt from one twin's circulation to that of the other (twin-twin transfusion syndrome). The infant on the venous side becomes plethoric and considerably larger than the other, smaller, anemic twin. Morbidity and mortality are considerable in twin-twin transfusion syndrome. Discordance in size, that is, birth weights that are significantly different, can also occur when there are separate placentas; one placenta develops poorly, presumably because of a poor implantation site. In this instance, there is no fetal exchange of blood, but there is a striking difference in the growth rate of the two infants.

Preterm Delivery

Gestation length tends to be inversely related to the number of fetuses. It is the prematurity that tends to increase the mortality or morbidity of twin pregnancies.

OBSTETRIC COMPLICATIONS

Obstetric complications, including polyhydramnios, pregnancy-induced hypertension, premature rupture of membranes, abnormal fetal presentations, and prolapsed umbilical cord, occur more frequently in women with multiple fetuses. In general, most of the complications can be avoided or minimized in terms of their impact on the infant by good obstetric management. Multiple pregnancy should always be identified prenatally with ultrasound examinations; doing so allows the obstetrician and pediatrician or neonatologist to plan their management jointly. The neonatal complications are usually related to prematurity. Prolongation of pregnancy, therefore, leads to a significant reduction in neonatal morbidity.

Follow-up studies of twin pregnancies have yielded conflicting results. In general, the studies do not suggest that twinning has a significant effect on the child's later development, especially if prematurity is excluded as a separate risk factor.

Cheung VYT et al: Preterm discordant twins: What birth weight difference is significant? Am J Obstet Gynecol 1995;172:955.

D'Alton ME, Simpson LL: Syndromes in twins. Semin Perinatol 1995;19:375.

Grether JK et al: Twinning and cerebral palsy: Experience in four northern California counties, births 1983 through 1985. Pediatrics 1993;92:854.

Lopriore E et al: Twin-to-twin transfusion syndrome: New perspectives. J Pediatr 1995;127:675.

Powers WF, Kiely JL: The risks confronting twins: A national perspective. Am J Obstet Gynecol 1994;170:456.

SPECIFIC DISEASES OF THE NEWBORN INFANT

RESPIRATORY DISEASES

1. APNEA

Diagnosis

In preterm infants, recurrent apneic episodes are a common clinical problem. *Apnea* is defined as a respiratory pause lasting more than 20 seconds, or any pause which is accompanied by cyanosis and bradycardia. Shorter respiratory pauses associated with cyanosis or bradycardia also qualify as significant apnea but must be differentiated from periodic breathing, which is common in term as well as preterm infants. *Periodic breathing* is defined as regularly recurring ventilatory cycles interrupted by short pauses not associated with bradycardia or color change. Although apnea in premature infants is often not associated with a predisposing factor, there are a variety of processes that may precipitate apnea (Table 2–14). These processes should at least be con-

Table 2–14. Causes of apnea in the preterm infant.

Temperature instability—both cold and heat stress
Response to passage of a feeding tube
Gastroesophageal reflux
Hypoxemia
Pulmonary parenchymal disease
Patent ductus arteriosus
?Anemia
Infection
Sepsis (viral or bacterial)
Necrotizing enterocolitis
Metabolic causes
Hypoglycemia
Hyponatremia
Intracranial hemorrhage
Posthemorrhagic hydrocephalus
Seizures
Drugs (eg, morphine)
Apnea of prematurity

sidered prior to settling on a diagnosis of apnea of prematurity.

Apnea of prematurity is the most frequent cause of apnea. Most apnea of prematurity is mixed apnea characterized by a centrally (brain stem) mediated respiratory pause preceded or followed by airway obstruction. Less common is pure central or pure obstructive apnea. Apnea of prematurity is the result of immaturity of both the central respiratory regulatory centers and protective mechanisms that aid in maintaining airway patency. Onset, typically during the first 2 weeks of life, is gradual, with the frequency of spells increasing over time. Pathologic apnea can be suspected in an infant with a sudden onset of frequent apneic spells or a sudden onset of very severe spells. Apnea presenting from birth or on the first day of life is unusual, but can occur in the preterm infant who does not require mechanical ventilation for respiratory distress syndrome. In the term or near-term infant, this presentation can suggest the presence of an acute (asphyxia or birth trauma) or chronic (congenital hypotonia, structural central nervous system lesion, etc) neuromuscular abnormality.

The workup is directed by the clinical presentation of the apnea. All infants, regardless of severity and frequency of apnea, require a minimum screening evaluation, including a general assessment of the infant's well-being (eg, tolerance of feedings, stable temperature, normal physical examination), a check of the association of spells to feeding, hematocrit, measurement of Pao_2 or Sao_2, blood glucose, and a review of drug history. Infants with sudden onset of severe apnea may require a more extensive evaluation, including a workup for infection. Other specific tests are dictated by signs in the infant, for example, evaluation for necrotizing enterocolitis in an infant with apnea and abdominal distention.

Treatment

The physician treating apnea should first address

any underlying cause. If the apnea is due simply to prematurity, treatment is dictated by the frequency and severity of apneic spells. Apneic spells frequent enough to interfere with other aspects of care (eg, feeding) or severe enough to necessitate bag and mask ventilation to relieve cyanosis and bradycardia require treatment. Nasal CPAP (continuous positive airway pressure), by treating the obstructive component of apnea, can be an effective treatment for some infants. Intubation and ventilation can eliminate apneic spells but carry the attendant risks of long-term endotracheal intubation. Conclusive evidence that methylxanthines (theophylline and caffeine) are effective in the treatment of apnea have led to their widespread use as first-line therapy. Theophylline can be used, with a loading dose of 5 mg/kg and maintenance dose of 1–2 mg/kg every 6–12 hours. The loading dose of caffeine is 20 mg/kg (caffeine citrate); the maintenance dose is 5–10 mg/kg every 24 hours. Theophylline has a more narrow therapeutic index than caffeine. These agents appear to work as central stimulants. Side effects include tachycardia, feeding intolerance, and (with overdosing) seizures. The minimum dose necessary to decrease the frequency of apnea and eliminate severe spells should be used. Desired drug levels are usually in the range of 5–10 μg/mL for both drugs. Intravenous doxapram infused at a dose of 1 mg/kg/h for 48 hours is effective in some cases of methylxanthine-refractory apnea.

Prognosis

In the majority of premature infants, apneic and bradycardiac spells cease by 34–36 weeks postconception. Occasionally the episodes last longer, and outpatient therapy with methylxanthines may be indicated. Whether to provide home monitoring for such infants is controversial. Apneic and bradycardiac episodes in the nursery are not predictors of later sudden infant death syndrome (SIDS). However, home monitoring in infants still experiencing apnea and bradycardia at the time of hospital discharge is probably a prudent measure. The incidence of SIDS is slightly increased in the preterm infant. Recent work in term infants has shown an increased incidence of SIDS in infants who sleep in the prone position. Whether or not this can be extrapolated to the preterm infant (in particular those with gastroesophageal reflux or persistent respiratory symptoms) is unclear. When possible, a sleeping position on the side with the right side down or supine seems prudent unless contraindicated by reflux or respiratory symptoms.

American Academy of Pediatrics Task Force on Infant Positioning and SIDS: Positioning and SIDS. Pediatrics 1992;89:1120.

Baitram A et al: Doxapram for the initial treatment of idiopathic apnea of prematurity. Biol Neonate 1992;61:209.

Dwyer T et al: The contribution of changes in the prevalence of prone sleeping position to the decline in sudden infant death syndrome in Tasmania. JAMA 1995;273:783.

Kemp JS, Thach BT: A sleep position–dependent mechanism for infant death on sheepskins. Am J Dis Child 1993;147:642.

Kemp JS et al: Physical properties of bedding that may increase risk of sudden infant death syndrome in prone-sleeping infants. Pediatr Res 1994;36:7.

Klonoff-Cohen HS, Edelstein SL: A case-control study of routine and death scene sleep position and sudden infant death syndrome in southern California. JAMA 1995;273:790.

Krongrad E: Infants at high risk for sudden infant death syndrome: Have they been identified? A commentary. Pediatrics 1991;88:1274.

Larsen PB et al: Aminophylline versus caffeine citrate for apnea and bradycardia prophylaxis in premature neonates. Acta Paediatr 1995;84:360.

Miller MJ, Martin RJ: Apnea of prematurity. Clin Perinatol 1992;19:789.

National Institutes of Health Consensus Development Conference on Infantile Apnea and Home Monitoring. Pediatrics 1987;79:292.

Ponsonby A-L et al: Factors potentiating the risk of sudden infant death syndrome associated with the prone position. N Engl J Med 1993;329:377.

Ruggins NR: Pathophysiology of apnea in preterm infants. Arch Dis Child 1991;66:70.

Ruggins NR et al: Site of upper airway obstruction in preterm infants with problematical apnea. Arch Dis Child 1991;66:787.

Willinger M et al: Infant sleep position and risk for sudden infant death syndrome: Report of a meeting held January 13 and 14, 1994, National Institutes of Health, Bethesda, MD. Pediatrics 1994;93:814.

2. RESPIRATORY DISTRESS IN THE NEWBORN

Diagnosis

Respiratory distress is among the most common symptom complexes seen in the newborn. Respiratory distress may result from both noncardiopulmonary and cardiopulmonary causes (Table 2–15). The cardinal clinical features include a respiratory rate of more than 60 per minute with or without associated cyanosis, nasal flaring, intercostal and sternal retractions, and expiratory grunting. It is important to consider the noncardiopulmonary causes listed in Table 2–15, because the natural tendency is to focus on the heart and lungs. Most of the noncardiopulmonary causes can be ruled out by the history, physical examination, and a few simple laboratory tests. The evaluation of cardiovascular disorders is discussed in the next section.

The physician attempting diagnosis of pulmonary disorders must consider the following major concerns in the term infant: transient tachypnea, aspiration syndromes, and congenital pneumonia.

Table 2–15. Causes of respiratory distress in the newborn.[1]

Noncardiopulmonary	Cardiovascular	Pulmonary
Hypothermia or hyperthermia	Left-sided outflow tract obstruction	Upper airway obstruction
Hypoglycemia	Hypoplastic left heart	Choanal atresia
Polycythemia	Aortic stenosis	Vocal cord paralysis
Metabolic acidosis	Coarticulation of the aorta	Lingual thyroid
Drug intoxications or withdrawal	Cyanotic lesions	Meconium aspiration
Insult to the central nervous system	Transposition of the great vessels	Clear fluid aspiration
Asphyxia	Total anomalous pulmonary venous	Transient tachypnea
Hemorrhage	return	Pneumonia
Neuromuscular disease	Tricuspid atresia	Pulmonary hypoplasia
Phrenic nerve injury	Right-sided outflow obstruction	Hyaline membrane disease
Asphyxiating thoracic dystrophy		Pneumothorax
		Pleural effusions
		Mass lesions
		Lobar emphysema
		Cystic adenomatoid malformation

[1]Reproduced, with permission, from Rosenberg AA: Neonatal adaptation. In *Obstetrics: Normal and Problem Pregnancies.* Gabbe SG, Niebyl JR, Simpson JL (editors). Churchill Livingstone, 1996.

A. Transient Tachypnea: The syndrome of transient tachypnea or retained lung fluid presents as respiratory distress in nonasphyxiated term infants (often delivered by cesarean section) or slightly preterm infants. The clinical features include tachypnea, cyanosis, grunting, flaring, and retractions usually present from birth. The chest x-ray film indicating prominent perihilar streaking and fluid in the interlobar fissures is the key to diagnosis. The symptoms generally abate within 12–24 hours, although they can persist longer.

B. Clear Fluid Aspiration: At or before delivery, the infant can aspirate clear amniotic fluid or fluid mixed with blood. The clinical presentation is much like that of transient tachypnea, with the following differences: these infants usually require higher FiO_2 (30–60% versus 25–40% in infants with transient tachypnea), and the course is more protracted (4–7 days). The chest x-ray film reveals hyperexpansion with a more patchy infiltrate pattern than that seen with transient tachypnea.

C. Meconium Aspiration Syndrome: The perinatal course in these infants is often marked by fetal distress, low Apgar scores, and meconium in the amniotic fluid. These infants exhibit tachypnea, retractions, cyanosis, an overdistended, barrel-shaped chest, and coarse breath sounds. The chest x-ray film reveals coarse, irregular infiltrates and hyperexpansion. There is a high incidence of air leaks and, in severe cases, a high rate of persistent pulmonary hypertension (see Cardiovascular Diseases).

D. Congenital Pneumonia: The lungs are the most common site of infection in the neonate. Both bacterial and viral infections can be acquired before, during, or after birth. Most commonly, infections ascend from the genital tract before or during labor. The rupture of membranes more than 12–18 hours prior to delivery is a predisposing factor. The presence of chorioamnionitis in the mother further in-

creases the risk. Infants with congenital pneumonia present with respiratory symptoms as early as in the delivery room, with the majority symptomatic by 6–12 hours of age. The chest x-ray is not helpful in distinguishing congenital pneumonia from other forms of neonatal lung disease. The presence of shock, poor perfusion, and absolute neutropenia on blood count provide corroborating evidence for pneumonia. Tracheal aspirate Gram's stain may be helpful.

E. Spontaneous Pneumothorax: This entity occurs in 1% of all deliveries. Risk is increased by manipulations such as bag and mask ventilation in the delivery room. Clinically, the infants are tachypneic with a small oxygen requirement (25–40% FiO_2). Breath sounds may be asymmetric, and if the pneumothorax is under tension, the mediastinum may be shifted. The diagnosis can be confirmed on x-ray studies. There is a small increased risk of renal abnormalities associated with spontaneous pneumothorax. Therefore, a careful physical examination of the kidneys and observation of urine output are indicated.

F. Other Pulmonary Causes: The other pulmonary causes of respiratory distress are fairly rare. Bilateral choanal atresia should be suspected if there is no air movement when the infant breathes through the nose. These infants present in the delivery room with good color and heart rate while crying. When they quiet down and resume normal breathing, they become cyanotic and bradycardic. Other causes of airway obstruction are usually characterized by some degree of stridor or poor air movement despite good respiratory effort. Pleural effusions can be suspected in hydropic infants (eg, those with erythroblastosis fetalis). Space-occupying lesions cause a shift of the mediastinum and asymmetric breath sounds.

G. Hyaline Membrane Disease: The most common cause of respiratory distress in the preterm infant is hyaline membrane disease. The incidence of this disorder increases from 5% at 35–36 weeks to more than 50% of infants of 26–28 weeks' gestation. This condition is caused by a deficiency of surfactant. Surfactant decreases surface tension in the alveolus during expiration, allowing the alveolus to remain partly expanded, thereby maintaining a functional residual capacity. The absence of surfactant results in poor lung compliance and atelectasis. The infant must expend a great deal of effort to expand the lungs with each breath, and respiratory failure ensues (see Figure 2–5). Infants with hyaline membrane disease demonstrate all the clinical signs of respiratory distress. On auscultation, air movement is diminished despite vigorous respiratory effort. The chest x-ray film demonstrates diffuse bilateral atelectasis causing a "ground-glass" appearance. Major airways are highlighted by the atelectatic air sacs creating air bronchograms. In the unintubated child, there is doming of the diaphragms and hypoexpansion.

Treatment

The cornerstone of treatment of neonatal respiratory distress is the provision of adequate supplemental oxygen to maintain a PaO_2 of 60–70 mm Hg and an arterial saturation of 92–96%. PaO_2 levels less than 50 mm Hg are associated with pulmonary vascular vasoconstriction which can exacerbate hypoxemia, while those greater than 100 mm Hg may increase the risk of retinopathy of prematurity. Oxygen should be warmed, humidified, and given through an air blender. Concentration should be measured with a calibrated oxygen analyzer. An umbilical or peripheral arterial line should be placed in any infant requiring more than 45% FiO_2 by 4–6 hours of life to allow frequent blood gas determinations. Noninva-

sive monitoring with a transcutaneous O_2 monitor or pulse oximeter can provide continuous information.

Other supportive treatment includes intravenous provision of glucose and water. Unless infection can be absolutely ruled out, blood cultures should be obtained and broad-spectrum antibiotics started. Colloid solutions (eg, 5% albumin) can be given in infusions of 10 mL/kg over 30 minutes for low blood pressure, poor perfusion, and metabolic acidosis. Sodium bicarbonate (1–2 meq/kg) is indicated for treatment of a documented metabolic acidosis that has not responded to oxygen, ventilation, and volume. While therapy is instituted, specific workup should be pursued as indicated by history and physical findings. In most cases, a chest x-ray study, blood gas, complete blood count, and blood glucose allow a diagnosis.

Intubation and ventilation should be undertaken for signs of respiratory failure (PaO_2 <60 mm Hg in 70–80% FiO_2 or $PaCO_2$ >50 mm Hg). These guidelines, however, do not apply to infants with hyaline membrane disease. Indication for further respiratory support in these infants is a need for 50% FiO_2 to keep PaO_2 greater than 60 mm Hg. Peak pressures should be adequate to produce chest wall expansion (usually 18–24 cm H_2O). Positive end-expiratory pressure (4–6 cm H_2O) should also be used. Ventilation rates of 20–50 are usually required. The goal is to maintain PaO_2 of 60–70 mm Hg and $PaCO_2$ of 40–50 mm Hg.

Two exogenous surfactants (colfosceril palmitate [Exosurf Neonatal] and beractant [Survanta]) have been approved in the United States by the Food and Drug Administration for use in infants with hyaline membrane disease. Surfactant replacement therapy, used both in the delivery room as prophylaxis and with established hyaline membrane disease as rescue, has been shown to decrease the mortality rate in preterm infants and to decrease air leak complications of the disease. Ventilator settings and oxygen requirements are significantly less in surfactant-treated infants than in controls during the acute course. Although the acute course of respiratory disease is improved, the incidence of other complications of prematurity, such as intracranial hemorrhage, patent ductus arteriosus, and necrotizing enterocolitis, has not been altered by surfactant replacement therapy. In addition, the incidence of chronic lung disease among survivors has not decreased. However, the severity of chronic lung disease is less in surfactant-treated newborns because of the lower inspired oxygen concentrations and ventilator settings made possible during the acute stages of respiratory distress syndrome. The dose of the artificial surfactant Exosurf is 5 mL/kg intratracheally, while that of the bovine-derived Survanta is 4 mL/kg. The usual dosing schedule when the first dose is given in the delivery room to prevent hyaline membrane disease is a total of two or three doses given 8–12 hours apart as long as the infant re-

Figure 2–5. Pressure-volume relationships for the inflation and deflation of surfactant-deficient and surfactant-treated preterm rabbit lungs. (Reproduced, with permission, from Jobe AH: The developmental biology of the lung. In: *Neonatal-Perinatal Medicine: Diseases of the Fetus and Infant,* 5th ed. Fanaroff AA, Martin RJ [editors]. Mosby, 1992.)

mains ventilated on greater than 30–40% inspired oxygen concentration. Rescue surfactant is given as two to four doses 8–12 hours apart. The first dose is optimally administered as soon as possible after birth, preferably prior to 2–4 hours of age. As the disease process evolves, proteins that inhibit surfactant function leak into the air spaces, making surfactant replacement less effective. The second dose should be administered to infants who continue to require ventilation and more than 30% inspired oxygen concentration. A prophylactic strategy may offer some advantage in those infants of 26 weeks' gestation or less. For infants over 26 weeks, early rescue therapy (as soon as possible after birth that a diagnosis of surfactant deficiency can be made) is the strategy of choice. The availability of surfactant replacement therapy has encouraged earlier intubation of infants with hyaline membrane disease. Surfactant replacement has also been used with some success in term infants with secondary surfactant deficiency resulting from pneumonia or meconium aspiration.

Antenatal administration of corticosteroids to the mother is an important strategy utilized by obstetricians to accelerate lung maturation. Infants whose mothers were given corticosteroids more than 24 hours prior to preterm birth have less respiratory distress syndrome and a lower mortality rate than those in untreated pregnancies. Antenatal corticosteroids and exogenous surfactant administration after birth appear to have a synergistic effect on outcome.

The approach to infants who go on to develop chronic lung disease has been aided by the use of dexamethasone (0.5 mg/kg) to decrease lung inflammation. Dexamethasone is most effective when started in chronically ventilated infants at 10 days to 3 weeks of age. Dosing schedules used have varied from a 5-day course to intermittent 3- to 5-day bursts to an initial 3–5 days at full dose followed by a gradual wean in dosage over 4–6 weeks.

Prognosis

Most of the conditions described in the term infant are acute and resolve in the first several days of life. Meconium aspiration syndrome and congenital pneumonia do have a significant rate of associated pulmonary morbidity (chronic lung disease) and mortality (approximately 10–20%). Mortality rates in these disorders have been reduced by use of high-frequency ventilation, inhaled nitric oxide (NO), and extracorporeal membrane oxygenation (ECMO). Mortality rates have decreased dramatically in infants with hyaline membrane disease through the use of continuous positive airway pressure, positive-pressure ventilation, and surfactant replacement therapy. Mortality rates associated with hyaline membrane disease are less than 10% for infants of greater than 28 weeks' gestation. The major long-term sequela is the development of chronic lung disease (defined as the need for oxygen or ventilation after 1 month of age), which occurs in 20% of the survivors of hyaline membrane disease. The incidence is highest at lower gestational ages. The development of chronic lung disease is a function of lung immaturity at birth and exposure to high oxygen concentrations and ventilator barotrauma. Although the use of exogenous surfactants has not decreased the incidence of chronic lung disease, the condition is not as severe in surfactant-treated infants. Up to 10% of infants who develop severe chronic lung disease will die in the first 2 years of life because of respiratory failure, pulmonary infection, or sudden death. Most infants with chronic lung disease do well clinically, despite abnormalities in pulmonary function testing. Some infants with chronic lung disease require home oxygen therapy. This can be monitored with pulse oximetry, with SaO_2 kept at 92–96%. Systemic hypertension can be seen in these patients; frequent blood pressure determinations, therefore, are indicated, as are ECGs and echocardiograms to monitor for left and right ventricular hypertrophy.

Avery ME et al: Transient tachypnea of the newborn. Am J Dis Child 1966;111:380.

Avery ME, Mead J: Surface properties in relation to atelectasis and hyaline membrane disease. Am J Dis Child 1959;97:517.

Blayney M et al: Bronchopulmonary dysplasia: Improvement in lung function between 7 and 10 years of age. J Pediatr 1991;118:201.

Brozanski BS et al: Effect of pulse dexamethasone therapy on the incidence of chronic lung disease in the very low birth weight infant. J Pediatr 1995;126:769.

Clark RH: High-frequency ventilation. J Pediatr 1994;124:661.

Cleary JP et al: Improved oxygenation during synchronized intermittent mandatory ventilation in neonates with respiratory distress syndrome: A randomized crossover study. J Pediatr 1995;126:407.

Collaborative Dexamethasone Trial Group: Dexamethasone therapy in neonatal chronic lung disease: An international placebo-controlled trial. Pediatrics 1991;88:421.

Dunn MS: Surfactant replacement therapy: Prophylaxis or treatment? Pediatrics 1993;92:148.

Durand M et al: Effects of early dexamethasone therapy on pulmonary mechanics and chronic lung disease in very low birth weight infants: A randomized controlled trial. Pediatrics 1995;95:584.

Ferrara TB et al: Survival and follow-up of infants born at 23 to 26 weeks of gestational age: Effects of surfactant therapy. J Pediatr 1994;124:119.

Halliday HL: Overview of clinical trials comparing natural and synthetic surfactants. Biol Neonate 1995;67(Suppl 1):32.

Holtzman RB, Frank L (editors): Bronchopulmonary dysplasia. Clin Perinatol 1992;19:3.

Horbar JD et al: A multicenter randomized trial comparing two surfactants for the treatment of neonatal respiratory distress syndrome. J Pediatr 1993;123:757.

HiFO Study Group: Randomized study of high-frequency oscillatory ventilation in infants with severe respiratory distress syndrome. J Pediatr 1993;122:609.

Jobe AH: Pulmonary surfactant therapy. N Engl J Med 1993;328:861.

Kattwinkel J et al: Prophylactic administration of calf lung surfactant extract is more effective than early treatment of respiratory distress syndrome in neonates of 29 through 32 weeks' gestation. Pediatrics 1993;92:90.

Kendig JW et al: A comparison of surfactant as immediate prophylaxis and as rescue therapy in newborns of less than 30 weeks gestation. N Engl J Med 1991;324:864.

Khammash H et al: Surfactant therapy in full-term neonates with severe respiratory failure. Pediatrics 1993;92:135.

Long W: Synthetic surfactant. Semin Perinatol 1993;17:275.

Long W (editor): Surfactant replacement therapy. Clin Perinatol 1993;20(4).

Long W et al (editors): Symposium on Synthetic Surfactant II: Health and developmental outcomes at one year. J Pediatr 1995;126(5-2).

Merritt TA et al: Overview of exogenous surfactant replacement therapy. J Intens Care Med 1993;8:205.

National Institutes of Health Consensus Development Conference Statement: Effect of corticosteroids on perinatal outcomes, February 28–March 2, 1994. Am J Obstet Gynecol 1995;173:246.

Northway WH et al: Late pulmonary sequelae of bronchopulmonary dysplasia. N Engl J Med 1990;323:1793.

Northway WH Jr et al: Pulmonary disease following respirator therapy of hyaline membrane disease. N Engl J Med 1967;276:357.

Pramanik AK et al: Surfactant replacement therapy for pulmonary diseases. Pediatr Clin North Am 1993;40:913.

Spafford PS et al: Use of natural surfactants to prevent and treat respiratory distress syndrome. Semin Perinatol 1993;17:285.

Wright L (editor): Effect of corticosteroids for fetal maturation on perinatal outcomes. Am J Obstet Gynecol 1995;173(Suppl):253.

CARDIOVASCULAR DISEASES
(See also Chapter 19.)

Diagnosis

Cardiovascular causes of respiratory distress in the neonatal period can be divided into two major groups—structural heart disease and a structurally normal heart with shunting through fetal pathways.

A. Structural Heart Disease: The central presenting features of symptomatic congenital heart disease in the first week of life include cyanosis and congestive heart failure. Cyanotic heart disease can be caused by:

- transposition of the great vessels
- total anomalous pulmonary venous return
- truncus arteriosus (some types)
- tricuspid atresia
- pulmonary atresia/stenosis

Infants with these disorders present with early cyanosis. The hallmark of many of these lesions is cyanosis in an infant without associated respiratory distress. Although early cyanosis is the central feature in these disorders, tachypnea develops over time in many infants either because of increased pulmonary blood flow or secondary to metabolic acidosis from hypoxia. Infants with total anomalous venous return below the diaphragm present early with tachypnea, because the pulmonary venous return is obstructed and pulmonary edema develops. Diagnostic aids include comparing a blood gas or oxygen saturation obtained while the infant breathes 100% oxygen to one obtained while the child breathes room air. Failure of the PaO_2 or SaO_2 to increase when 100% oxygen is breathed suggests cyanotic congenital heart disease. A chest x-ray film with decreased pulmonary markings is consistent with right heart obstruction, and an ECG with left-sided predominance suggests the small right heart seen with tricuspid atresia and other forms of right heart obstruction. Infants with total anomalous pulmonary venous return with obstructed venous return have a small or normal heart size and marked pulmonary edema on chest x-ray. Diagnosis can be confirmed with echocardiography.

Infants with congestive heart failure generally have some form of left-sided outflow tract obstruction. Infants with left-to-right shunt lesions, such as ventricular septal defect, may have murmurs in the newborn period, but clinical symptoms do not occur until pulmonary vascular resistance drops enough to cause significant shunting and subsequent failure (usually 3–4 weeks of age). Infants with left-sided outflow obstruction generally do well the first day or two until the source of all or some of the systemic flow, the ductus arteriosus, narrows. Tachypnea, tachycardia, congestive heart failure, and metabolic acidosis develop. On examination, all of these infants have abnormalities of the pulses. In aortic atresia and stenosis, pulses are all diminished, whereas in coarctation syndromes, differential pulses (diminished in the lower extremities) are evident. Chest x-ray films in these infants show a large heart and pulmonary edema. Arterial blood gases are remarkable for profound metabolic acidosis.

B. Shunting Through Fetal Pathways: The syndrome of persistent pulmonary hypertension occurs when the normal decrease in pulmonary vascular resistance after birth does not occur. Most infants with persistent pulmonary hypertension are full term or postterm and have experienced perinatal asphyxia. Other clinical associations include hypothermia, meconium aspiration syndrome, hyaline membrane disease, polycythemia, neonatal sepsis, chronic intrauterine hypoxia, and pulmonary hypoplasia.

There are three causes of persistent pulmonary hypertension: (1) acute vasoconstriction resulting from perinatal hypoxia, (2) prenatal increase in pulmonary vascular smooth muscle development, and (3) decreased cross-sectional area of the pulmonary vascular bed because of inadequate vessel number. In the first, an acute perinatal event leads to hypoxia and failure of the pulmonary vascular resistance to drop. In the second, abnormal muscularization of the pulmonary resistance vessels results in persistent hypertension after birth. Finally, the third includes infants with pulmonary hypoplasia (eg, diaphragmatic hernia).

Clinically, the syndrome is characterized by onset on the first day of life, usually from birth. Respiratory distress is prominent, and PaO_2 is usually poorly responsive to high concentrations of inspired oxygen. Many of the infants have associated myocardial depression with resulting systemic hypotension. Echocardiography reveals right-to-left shunting at the level of the ductus arteriosus or foramen ovale (or both).

C. Patent Ductus Arteriosus: Patent ductus arteriosus is the most common cardiovascular disorder seen in the preterm infant. Clinically, significant patent ductus arteriosus usually presents on days 3–7 of life as the respiratory distress from hyaline membrane disease is improving. Presentation can be on day 1 or 2, especially in those infants of less than 28 weeks' gestation and in infants treated with surfactant replacement therapy. The signs include a hyperdynamic precordium, increased peripheral pulses, and a widened pulse pressure, with or without a systolic heart murmur. Early presentations are not uncommonly manifested by systemic hypotension without a murmur or hyperdynamic circulation. These signs are often accompanied by an increase in respiratory support. The presence of significant patent ductus arteriosus can be confirmed by echocardiography. Before undertaking medical or surgical ligation, other structural heart disease must be ruled out.

Treatment

For congenital heart disease, early stabilization includes supportive therapy as needed (eg, intravenous glucose, oxygen, ventilation for respiratory failure). Specific therapy includes infusions of prostaglandin E_1, 0.025–0.1 $\mu g/kg/min$, to maintain ductal patency. In some cyanotic lesions (eg, pulmonary atresia), this improves pulmonary blood flow and PaO_2 by allowing shunting through the ductus to the pulmonary artery. In left-sided outflow tract obstruction, systemic blood flow is ductal dependent; prostaglandins improve systemic perfusion and resolve the baby's acidosis. Further specific management, including palliative surgical and cardiac catheterization procedures, is discussed in Chapter 19.

Therapy for persistent pulmonary hypertension involves supportive therapy for other postasphyxia problems (eg, anticonvulsants for seizures, careful fluid and electrolyte management for renal failure). Intravenous glucose should be provided to maintain normal blood sugar, and antibiotics should be administered for possible infection. Specific therapy is aimed at both increasing systemic arterial pressure and decreasing pulmonary arterial pressure to reverse the right-to-left shunting through fetal pathways. First-line therapy includes oxygen and ventilation (to lower pulmonary vascular resistance) and colloid infusions (10 mL/kg, up to 30 mL/kg) to improve systemic pressure. Ideally, systolic pressure should be greater than 60 mm Hg. With compromised cardiac function, systemic pressors can be used as second-line therapy (eg, dopamine, 5–20 $\mu g/kg/min$; dobutamine, 5–20 $\mu g/kg/min$; or both). If oxygenation is still not adequate (PaO_2 <55 mm Hg), a trial of alkalosis by hyperventilation is indicated. Many babies improve as the pH rises above 7.55–7.6. Since alkalosis seems to be helpful, any base deficit should be corrected with sodium bicarbonate to allow less vigorous hyperventilation. Recent studies using the inhaled gas nitric oxide (NO), which is identical or very similar to endogenous endothelium-derived relaxing factor, have shown it to be a very promising and specific pulmonary vasodilator. In addition, use of high-frequency oscillatory ventilation has proved effective in many of these infants, particularly those with severe associated lung disease.

Infants for whom conventional therapy is failing (poor oxygenation despite maximum support) may require extracorporeal membrane oxygenation (ECMO). The infants are placed on bypass with blood exiting the baby from the right atrium and returning to the aortic arch after passing through a membrane oxygenator. The lungs are essentially at rest during the procedure, and with resolution of the pulmonary hypertension, the infants are weaned from ECMO back to conventional ventilator therapy. This therapy can save infants who might otherwise die but has major side effects that must be considered prior to its institution. Neurodevelopmental outcome among survivors of ECMO is similar to that of infants with persistent pulmonary hypertension managed without the procedure.

The ductus arteriosus is managed by medical or surgical ligation. A clinically significant ductus causing compromise in the infant can be closed with indomethacin (0.1–0.2 mg/kg per dose) given intravenously every 12–24 hours for three doses. In about two-thirds of the cases, indomethacin is successful in closing the ductus. If the ductus reopens, a second course of drug may be utilized. If indomethacin fails to close the ductus or if a ductus reopens a second time, surgical ligation should be pursued. In some cases, a more prolonged course of indomethacin is being utilized to prevent recurrences. The major side effect of indomethacin is a transient oliguria, which can be treated by fluid restriction until urine output improves. The drug should not be used if the infant is hyperkalemic, if the creatinine is greater than 2 mg/dL, or if the platelet count is less than 50,000/μL.

Prognosis

The prognosis for the congenital heart lesions,

which depends on the type of lesion, is reviewed in Chapter 19. With persistent pulmonary hypertension, the mortality rate remains approximately 10–15%. Long-term neurologic morbidity occurs in approximately 10% of survivors. An increased incidence of hearing loss has been identified following hyperventilation and alkalosis in this group of infants. The other major long-term morbidity is chronic lung disease secondary to the extensive ventilator support that many of these infants require.

Clark RH: High-frequency ventilation. J Pediatr 1994; 124:661.

Clyman RI: Recommendations for the postnatal use of indomethacin: An analysis of four separate treatment strategies. J Pediatr 1996;128:601.

Finer NN et al: Inhaled nitric oxide in infants referred for extracorporeal membrane oxygenation: Dose response. J Pediatr 1994;124:302.

Glass P et al: Neurodevelopmental status at age five years of neonates treated with extracorporeal membrane oxygenation. J Pediatr 1995;127:447.

Hammerman C, Aramburo MJ: Prolonged indomethacin treatment for the prevention of recurrences of patent ductus arteriosus. J Pediatr 1990;117:771.

Hammerman C et al: Continuous versus multiple rapid infusions of indomethacin: Effects on cerebral blood flow velocity. Pediatrics 1995;95:244.

Henricks-Munoz KD, Walton JP: Hearing loss in infants with persistent fetal circulation. Pediatrics 1988;81:650.

HiFO Study Group: Randomized study of high-frequency oscillatory ventilation in infants with severe respiratory distress syndrome. J Pediatr 1993;122:609.

Kanto WP: A decade of experience with neonatal extracorporeal membrane oxygenation. J Pediatr 1994;124:335.

Kinsella JP, Abman SH: Recent developments in the pathophysiology and treatment of persistent pulmonary hypertension of the newborn. J Pediatr 1995;126:853.

Kinsella JP et al: Clinical responses to prolonged treatment of persistent pulmonary hypertension of the newborn with low doses of inhaled nitric oxide. J Pediatr 1993;123:103.

Roberts JD et al: Inhaled nitric oxide in persistent pulmonary hypertension of the newborn. Lancet 1992;340:818.

Schumacher RE et al: Follow-up of infants treated with extracorporeal membrane oxygenation for newborn respiratory failure. Pediatrics 1991;87:451.

Walsh-Sukys MC: Persistent pulmonary hypertension of the newborn: The black box revisited. Clin Perinatol 1993;20:127.

Wilden SR et al: Prospective, controlled study of developmental outcome in survivors of extracorporeal membrane oxygenation: The first 24 months. Pediatrics 1994;93:404.

Zahka KG, Spector M, Hanisch D: Hypoplastic left-heart syndrome: Norwood operation, transplantation, or compassionate care. Clin Perinatol 1993;20:145.

NEONATAL JAUNDICE

Jaundice is a common neonatal problem. Nearly all newborns develop a serum bilirubin above 2 mg/dL, and 65% of them develop a bilirubin level above 5 mg/dL during the first week of life. Anthropologically speaking, hyperbilirubinemia is likely to confer some biologic advantage if it occurs so often. Bilirubin is a potent antioxidant and peroxyl scavenger which may help the newborn, who is deficient in most antioxidant substances, such as vitamin E, catalase, and superoxide dismutase, to avoid oxygen toxicity in the days after birth. The reason to worry about hyperbilirubinemia is that it can also be toxic, with high levels resulting in an encephalopathy known as kernicterus.

Metabolism of Bilirubin

Heme (iron protoporphyrin) is broken down by heme oxygenase to iron, which is conserved; carbon monoxide, which is exhaled; and biliverdin, which is then further metabolized to bilirubin by the enzyme bilirubin reductase. Each 1 g of hemoglobin breakdown results in the production of 34 mg of bilirubin (1 mg/dL = 17.2 μmol/mL of bilirubin). Bilirubin is carried bound to albumin to the liver, where, in the presence of the enzyme uridyldiphosphoglucuronyl transferase (UDPGT, "glucuronyl transferase"), it is taken up by the hepatocyte and conjugated with two glucuronide molecules. The conjugated bilirubin is then excreted through the bile to the intestine. In the presence of normal gut flora, the conjugated bilirubin is further metabolized to stercobilins and excreted in the stool. In the absence of gut flora, and with slow intestinal motility, as in the first few days of life, the conjugated bilirubin remains in the intestinal lumen, where a mucosal enzyme, β-glucuronidase, can cleave off the glucuronide molecules, leaving unconjugated bilirubin to be reabsorbed (the enterohepatic circulation of bilirubin).

Bilirubin Toxicity

The exact mechanism by which bilirubin is toxic to cells is not known. It is assumed that if the amount of lipid-soluble unconjugated bilirubin exceeds the available binding sites on albumin, there will then be "free" bilirubin which can enter neurons and damage them. The blood-brain barrier probably plays an important role in protecting an individual from brain damage, but its integrity is impossible to measure clinically. It is unknown whether there is a level of bilirubin above which brain damage would always occur, even in a healthy individual.

The syndrome of bilirubin encephalopathy was well described in the era before exchange transfusion as treatment for Rh isoimmunization (see below). The pathologic correlate is known as kernicterus, named for the yellow staining of the subthalamic nuclei ("kerns") seen at autopsy. Clinically, early bilirubin encephalopathy consists of lethargy, hypotonia, and poor sucking, progressing to hypertonia, opisthotonos, and a high-pitched cry. Long-term sequelae include athetoid cerebral palsy, sensorineural deafness, limitation of upward gaze, and dental dysplasia. Whether or not bilirubin causes more subtle neurologic abnormalities remains debatable.

Bilirubin encephalopathy is very rare with current neonatal management. The only infant in which a specific bilirubin level (20 mg/dL [344 μmol/mL] and above) has been associated with an increased risk of kernicterus is the Rh-isoimmunized infant. This observation and management strategy has been extended to other neonates with hemolytic disease, despite a lack of data on the risk in these infants. The risk is likely very small for term infants without hemolysis, even at bilirubin levels of 25 mg/dL (430 μmol/mL) and above. Premature infants are likely at some increased risk because of associated illnesses that may affect the integrity of the blood-brain barrier, and lower albumin levels. For this reason, a lower level of bilirubin is generally assumed to represent the "exchange level" in these infants, and is usually chosen arbitrarily based on the size and gestational age of the infant. One common approach is to use 1% of the birth weight in grams as the "exchange level" in milligrams per deciliter (ie, 12 mg/dL for a 1200-g infant), down to a low of 10 mg/dL, but many other approaches exist.

Causes of Unconjugated Hyperbilirubinemia

The causes of unconjugated hyperbilirubinemia can be grouped into two main categories: overproduction of bilirubin and decreased conjugation of bilirubin (Table 2–16).

A. Increased Bilirubin Production:

Increased production of bilirubin can result from hemolysis and an increased rate of red blood cell destruction, related to the presence of maternal antibodies against fetal cells (Coombs' test–positive), to abnormal red cell membrane shape (ie, spherocytosis), or to abnormal red cell enzymes (ie, glucose-6-phosphate dehydrogenase [G6PD] deficiency). The antibodies can be directed against the major blood group antigens (the type A or B infant of a type O mother), or the minor antigens (the Rh system: D, E, C, d, e, c, Kell, Duffy, etc).

1. Antibody-mediated hemolysis (Coombs' test–positive)—*ABO incompatibility* is common, generally is not severe, and can accompany any pregnancy in a type O mother. The severity is not predictable because of the variability in the amount of naturally occurring anti-A or anti-B IgG antibodies in the mother. Although 20% of pregnancies are the appropriate "set-up" for ABO incompatibility (mother O, baby A or B), only about 33% of such infants are Coombs' test–positive, and only about 20% of these develop pathologic jaundice. In addition to hyperbilirubinemia in the first days of life, these infants may develop a significant anemia over the first several weeks, and may need to be transfused on occasion.

Table 2–16. Etiology of jaundice secondary to unconjugated hyperbilirubemia.

Overproduction of Bilirubin
1. Increased rate of hemolysis
   a. Patients with a positive Coombs' test
      Rh incompatibility
      ABO incompatibility
      Other blood group sensitizations
   b. Patients with a negative Coombs' test
      Abnormal red cell shapes
         Spherocytosis
         Elliptocytosis
         Pyknocytosis
         Stomatocytosis
      Red cell enzyme abnormalities
         Glucose-6-phosphate dehydrogenase deficiency
         Pyruvate kinase deficiency
         Hexokinase deficiency
         Other metabolic defects
   c. Patients with bacterial or viral sepsis
2. Nonhemolytic causes of increased bilirubin load: Unconjugated bilirubin elevated, reticulocyte count normal.
   a. Extravascular hemorrhage
      Cephalohematoma
      Extensive bruising
      Central nervous system hemorrhage
   b. Polycythemia
   c. Exaggerated enterohepatic circulation of bilirubin
      Gastrointestinal tract obstruction
      Functional ileus

Decreased Rate of Conjugation
   (Unconjugated bilirubin elevated, reticulocyte count normal)
"Physiologic" jaundice
Crigler-Najjar syndrome (type I glucuronyl transferase deficiency, autosomal recessive)
Type II glucuronyl transferase deficiency, autosomal dominant
Gilbert's syndrome
?Galactosemia
?Hypothyroidism

Rh isoimmunization is much less common, tends not to be clinically severe with the first pregnancy, and tends to become more severe with each succeeding sensitized pregnancy because of an increased maternal antibody production each time. Most Rh disease can be prevented by administering high-titer RhO(D) immune globulin to an Rh-negative woman after any invasive procedure during pregnancy, as well as after any miscarriage, abortion, or delivery of an Rh-positive infant. In severe cases, erythroblastosis fetalis (hydrops or generalized edema and heart failure related to severe anemia in the fetus) occurs, often resulting in fetal or neonatal death without appropriate antenatal intervention. In less severe cases, hemolysis is the main problem, with resultant hyperbilirubinemia and anemia. The cornerstone of antenatal management once isoimmunization has been diagnosed is transfusion of the fetus with Rh-negative cells, either directly into the umbilical vein via percutaneous cordocentesis or into the fetal abdominal cavity. Following delivery, phototherapy is usually started immediately, with exchange transfusion (see below) as needed. Recently, a dose of intravenous immunoglobulin (IVIG), 500 mg/kg, given to the infant as soon after delivery as the diagosis is made has been shown to decrease the need for exchange transfusion. Ongoing hemolysis will still occur until all maternal antibody is gone; therefore, all these infants need to be followed up carefully over the first 2 months for anemia severe enough to require transfusion.

2. Nonimmune hemolysis (Coombs' test–negative)—*Hereditary spherocytosis* is the most common red cell membrane defect, resulting in hemolysis because of decreased red cell deformability. These infants may present with hyperbilirubinemia severe enough to require exchange transfusion. Mild to moderate splenomegaly may be present. Diagnosis is suspected by peripheral blood smear and confirmed by red cell osmotic fragility study. Family history of anemia, jaundice, and gallstones may be elicited.

G6PD deficiency is the most common red cell enzyme defect resulting in hemolysis, and should be suspected in a male (it is sex-linked) of Mediterranean or Asian descent, particularly when jaundice is of later onset than usual.

3. Nonhemolytic increased bilirubin production—*Enclosed hemorrhage,* such as cephalohematoma, intracranial hemorrhage, or extensive bruising in the skin, can lead to excessive jaundice as the red blood cells are broken down and removed. *Polycythemia* leads to excessive jaundice by increased red cell mass, with increased numbers of cells reaching senescence daily. *Ileus,* either paralytic or mechanical related to a *bowel obstruction,* leads to excessive hyperbilirubinemia secondary to an increased enterohepatic circulation.

B. Decreased Rate of Conjugation:
1. UDPGT deficiency—*Crigler-Najjar syndrome* type I (complete deficiency, autosomal recessive) and type II (partial deficiency, autosomal dominant) will present as excessive and prolonged neonatal jaundice, but both forms are very rare.

Gilbert's syndrome is a mild autosomal dominant disorder affecting 3–6% of the population and characterized by decreased hepatic UDPGT levels. Mild unconjugated hyperbilirubinemia without other liver function abnormalities occurs after puberty. The relationship of this disorder, if any, to neonatal jaundice, is under investigation.

Prolonged Hyperbilirubinemia

Causes of prolonged hyperbilirubinemia include hemolytic disease, breast milk jaundice, Crigler-Najjar syndrome, bowel obstruction, congenital hypothyroidism, and galactosemia. Galactosemia generally presents with hepatomegaly in an ill-appearing, often septic, infant, and the hyperbilirubinemia is usually mixed.

A. Hyperbilirubinemia Caused by Unknown or Multiple Factors:
1. Physiologic jaundice—The contributing factors to physiologic jaundice include UDPGT inactivity at birth, a relatively high red cell mass even in the nonpolycythemic neonate, and an absence of intestinal flora with initially slow intestinal motility leading to an active enterohepatic circulation of bilirubin. To be "physiologic" rather than pathologic, the following criteria apply: (1) clinical jaundice appears after 24 hours of age, (2) total bilirubin rises by less than 5 mg/dL (86 μmol/mL) per day, (3) peak bilirubin occurs at 3–5 days of age with a total bilirubin of no more than 15 mg/dL (258 μmol/mL), and (4) clinical jaundice is resolved by 1 week in the term infant and by 2 weeks in the preterm infant. Hyperbilirubinemia outside of these parameters, or jaundice that requires treatment, is not physiologic and must be evaluated (see below).

2. High altitude—Infants at 3100 m (10,000 ft) have twice the incidence of bilirubin of at least 12 mg/dL (206 μmol/mL) than infants at 1600 m (5200 ft) and four times the incidence of infants at sea level: 39% versus 16% versus 8%, respectively. Possible mechanisms include increased bilirubin production secondary to increased hematocrit and decreased clearance caused by hypoxemia.

3. Racial differences—Asians are more likely than whites or blacks to have a bilirubin of or exceeding 12 mg/dL (206 μmol/mL): 23% versus 10–13% versus 4%, respectively.

4. Prematurity—Premature infants frequently have poor enteral intake, delayed stooling, and increased enterohepatic circulation. Even at 37 weeks' gestation, they are four times more likely to have bilirubin of 13 mg/dL (224 μmol/mL) or more than at 40 weeks.

5. Breast-feeding and jaundice—There are two syndromes of jaundice associated with breast-feeding: breast milk jaundice and breast-feeding–associated jaundice ("lack–of–breast milk" jaundice).

Breast milk jaundice is a syndrome of prolonged unconjugated hyperbilirubinemia believed to be caused by an inhibitor to conjugation in the breast milk of some mothers. Suggested substances have included pregnanediol, free fatty acids, steroids, and β-glucuronidase. The hyperbilirubinemia peaks at 10–15 days of age, with a maximal level of 10–30 mg/dL (172–516 μmol/mL), and declines slowly by 3–12 weeks of age. If nursing is interrupted for 24–48 hours, the bilirubin level falls precipitously and will not rebound to the same level when nursing is resumed.

Breast-feeding–associated jaundice, also known as lack–of–breast milk jaundice, is a common entity. Breast-fed infants have a higher incidence (9%) of bilirubin of or exceeding 13 mg/dL (223 μmol/mL) than formula-fed infants (2%), and are nearly 10 times more likely to have bilirubin of 15 mg/dL (258 μmol/mL) or more than formula-fed infants: 2% versus 0.3%. The pathogenesis appears to be decreased enteral intake and increased enterohepatic circulation. No increase in bilirubin production is seen as measured by carbon monoxide exhalation. Although rarely associated with bilirubin encephalopathy, this type of jaundice should be considered a sign of failure to establish an adequate milk supply and should prompt specific inquiries into this possibility (see Table 2–17). If inadequate intake is present, the infant should receive supplementation with formula if needed, and the mother should be instructed to nurse more frequently and to pump her breasts with an electric breast pump every 2 hours to enhance milk production. A consultation with a certified lactation specialist should be considered, since many physicians feel inadequately prepared to handle these situations. As normal newborn hospital discharge occurs before the milk supply is established, the importance of a follow-up visit 2–3 days after discharge becomes obvious.

These two entities may sometimes overlap in the same infant, as prolonged jaundice is common in breast-fed infants (20–30%), and many of those with high bilirubins in the first days also persist longest.

Evaluation of Hyperbilirubinemia

Clinical jaundice appears at a bilirubin level of 5 mg/dL (86 μmol/mL) and appears first on the head, progressing down the chest and abdomen as the level increases. By the time jaundice is noted on the distal extremities, the level is likely to be at least 15 mg/dL (258 μmol/mL). Infants who develop clinical jaundice on the first day of life, or who appear excessively jaundiced, require evaluation. The minimal evaluation consists of feeding and elimination history, weight (with comparison to birth weight), physical examination for any source of excessive heme breakdown, and laboratory evaluation for blood type, Coombs' test, CBC with smear, and total bilirubin level. A G6PD test should be considered if the infant is an Asian or Mediterranean male, particularly if the jaundice presents later than usual. A fractionated bilirubin level should be obtained if the infant appears acutely ill, if the jaundice is prolonged, or if there is dark urine with light stools.

Because of large interlaboratory variability, serial bilirubin levels should be obtained from a single laboratory whenever possible to make interpretation of levels more meaningful.

A. Treatment of Hyperbilirubinemia Protoporphyrins: Tin-protoporphyrin (Sn-PP) and tin-mesoporphyrin (Sn-MP) are inhibitors of heme oxygenase, the enzyme that begins the catabolism of heme (Fe-protoporphyrin). Studies involving the use of a single injection of these substances given shortly after birth to prevent the formation of bilirubin are ongoing. Although very promising, these drugs are still considered experimental.

B. Phototherapy: Phototherapy is used most commonly, since it is relatively noninvasive and safe. Light at a wavelength absorbed by bilirubin (blue or white spectrum) is used. The unconjugated bilirubin in the skin is converted by such light to a stereoisomer compound which is water-soluble and able to be excreted in the bile without conjugation. A minimum of 10–12 $\mu W/cm^2$ irradiance is required, and efficacy is dose-dependent. The dose can be raised by increasing the body surface area exposed to the light and by moving the lights closer to the baby. The newer bili-blankets (fiberoptic blankets to wrap around the baby) are effective and less disruptive to normal baby handling. When under phototherapy lamps, the infant's eyes should be shielded from the light to prevent possible damage to retinal cells. A frequent side effect of phototherapy is diarrhea, the pathogenesis of which is not clear, but which is symptomatically improved by feeding a non–lactose-containing formula for the duration of the treatment.

Phototherapy is started when the bilirubin level is approximately 5 mg/dL (86 μmol/mL) lower than the "exchange level" for that infant (ie, at levels of 15–18 mg/dL [258–310 μmol/mL] for a term infant). Guidelines for the use of phototherapy in the term infant with and without ABO incompatibility are shown in Tables 2–18 and 2–19. Although phototherapy has been shown to decrease the likelihood of exchange transfusion, the long-term benefits of its use in infants not requiring exchange transfusion are unknown.

C. Exchange Transfusion: Double-volume exchange transfusion (approximately 160–200 mL/kg body weight) remains necessary in the rare case of hemolysis resulting from Rh isoimmunization, ABO incompatibility, or hereditary spherocytosis. In addition to decreasing the bilirubin level by approximately 50% acutely, the exchange also serves to re-

Table 2–17. Signs of inadequate breast milk intake.

Weight loss of >8–10% from birth
Fewer than 6 noticeable wet diapers per day
Fewer than 4 sizable stools per day
Nursing fewer than 8–10 times per 24 h for at least 10 min each feed

Table 2–18. Guidelines for use of phototherapy in the term infant without hemolysis.

Bilirubin ≥15 mg/dL, age <2 d: Evaluation, phototherapy
Bilirubin ≥18 mg/dL, age >2–3 d: Evaluation, phototherapy
Bilirubin ≥20–22 mg/dL, age >3–4 d: Evaluation, phototherapy, consider interruption of nursing and formula supplementation; have mother use electric breast pump to get or keep milk in.
Bilirubin ≥25 mg/dL: As above, plus consider exchange transfusion

Table 2–19. Guidelines for treatment of the term infant with ABO incompatibility.

Phototherapy if:
Bilirubin ≥10 mg/dL at <12 h
Bilirubin ≥12–14 mg/dL at <18 h
Bilirubin ≥15 mg/dL at >24 h

move nearly 80% of the sensitized or abnormal red blood cells and any offending antibody so that ongoing hemolysis will be decreased. The procedure is invasive and is not without risk. The risk of mortality is greatest in the smallest, most immature, and otherwise unstable infants, but sudden death during the procedure can occur in any infant. Because of the rarity of the procedure and its inherent risk, it should be carried out very cautiously, preferably at a referral center.

For the typical exchange transfusion, the umbilical vein is catheterized and reconstituted whole blood with a hematocrit of approximately 50% is used, in aliquots of 8–10 mL per pass. Hypocalcemia occurs during the procedure because of binding to the citrate-phosphate-dextrose anticoagulant and needs to be corrected periodically. Hypoglycemia is common following the procedure and requires close monitoring. Thrombocytopenia occurs because of the removal of platelets. The entire procedure should take 1–2 hours and should be performed using aseptic technique.

American Academy of Pediatrics Provisional Committee for Quality Improvement and Subcommittee on Hyperbilirubinemia: Practice parameter: Management of hyperbilirubinemia in the healthy term newborn. Pediatrics 1994;94:558.

Kappas A et al: Direct comparison of Sn-mesoporphyrin, an inhibitor of bilirubin production, and phototherapy controlling hyperbilirubinemia in term and near-term newborns. Pediatrics 1995;95:468.

Martinez JC et al: Hyperbilirubinemia in the breast-fed newborn: A controlled trial of four interventions. Pediatrics 1993;91:470.

McDonagh AF: Is bilirubin good for you? Clin Perinatol 1990;17:359.

National Institute of Child Health and Human Development: Randomized, controlled trial of phototherapy for neonatal hyperbilirubinemia. Pediatrics 1985;75 (Suppl):381.

Newman TB, Maisels MJ: Evaluation and treatment of jaundice in the term newborn: A kinder, gentler approach. Pediatrics 1992;89:809.

Peterec SM: Management of neonatal Rh disease. Clin Perinatol 1995;22:561.

Rubo J et al: High-dose intravenous immune globulin therapy for hyperbilirubinemia caused by Rh hemolytic disease. J Pediatr 1992;121:93.

Scheidt PC et al: Intelligence at 6 years in relation to neonatal bilirubin level: Follow-up of the National Institute of Child Health and Human Development trial of phototherapy. Pediatrics 1991;87:797.

Scheidt PC et al: Phototherapy for neonatal hyperbilirubinemia: Six-year follow-up of the National Institute of Child Health and Human Development trial. Pediatrics 1990;85:455.

Schreiner RL, Gluck MR: Interlaboratory bilirubin variability. Pediatrics 1982;69:277.

Seidman DS et al: Neonatal hyperbilirubinemia and physical and cognitive performance at 17 years of age. Pediatrics 1991;88:828.

Tan KL: Phototherapy for neonatal jaundice. Clin Perinatol 1991;18:423.

Valaes T et al: Control of jaundice in preterm newborns by an inhibitor of bilirubin production: Studies with tin-mesoporphyrin. Pediatrics 1994;93:1.

Watchko JF, Oski FA: Bilirubin 20 mg/dL = vigintiphobia. Pediatrics 1983;71:660.

Watchko JF, Oski FA: Kernicterus in preterm newborns: Past, present, and future. Pediatrics 1992;90:707.

INFECTIONS OF THE NEWBORN

GENERAL APPROACH

The fetus and the newborn infant are very susceptible to infections. There are three major routes of perinatal infection:

(1) Blood-borne transplacental infection of the fetus (eg, cytomegalovirus, rubella, syphilis).

(2) Ascending infection with a disruption of the barrier provided by the amniotic membranes (eg, bacterial infections after 12–18 hours of ruptured membranes).

(3) Infection upon passage through an infected birth canal or exposure to infected blood at delivery (eg, herpes simplex, hepatitis B, bacterial infections).

The susceptibility of the newborn is related to immaturity of both the cellular and humoral immune systems at birth. This feature is particularly evident in the preterm neonate. Passive protection against some organisms is provided by transfer of IgG across the placenta during the third trimester of pregnancy. Preterm infants, especially those born at less than 30 weeks, do not have the benefit of the full amount of this passively acquired antibody.

Diagnosis

A. History: Maternal and obstetric histories are important in the diagnosis of neonatal infections. The incidence of early-onset (<5 days) neonatal bacterial infection is 4–5:1000 live births. Rupture of membranes more than 24 hours prior to delivery is associated with an infection rate of 1:100, and rupture of membranes with chorioamnionitis with a rate of neonatal infection of 10:100. Irrespective of rupture of membranes, infection rates are five times higher in preterm infants. Other important historical points include immunization of the mother against rubella, a prior history of genital herpes, or viral illness around the time of delivery.

B. Symptoms and Signs: Early-onset bacterial infection is related to perinatal risk factors and presents most commonly on day 1 of life, with the majority of cases at less than 12 hours. Respiratory distress is the most common presenting sign. Other features include low Apgar scores without fetal distress, poor perfusion, and hypotension. Late-onset (presentation at >5 days of age) bacterial infection presents in a more subtle manner, with poor feeding, lethargy, hypotonia, temperature instability, altered perfusion, new or increased oxygen requirement, and apnea. Signs suggestive of congenital viral infections include small size for gestational age, microcephaly, petechiae, jaundice, and hepatosplenomegaly.

C. Laboratory Findings: Low total white counts, absolute neutropenia ($<1000/\mu L$), and elevated ratios of immature to mature neutrophils are suggestive of neonatal bacterial infection. Thrombocytopenia is also a common feature. Other laboratory aids are hypoglycemia or hyperglycemia with no change in glucose administration and unexplained metabolic acidosis. In early-onset bacterial infection, pneumonia is invariably present; chest x-ray films show infiltrates, but these infiltrates cannot be distinguished from infiltrates resulting from other causes of neonatal lung disease. Antigen detection in urine or other body fluids has been helpful in the rapid identification of some bacteria (especially group B streptococcus). Definitive diagnosis is made by positive cultures from blood, cerebrospinal fluid, and so on. Serologies and cultures are useful in the diagnosis of congenital viral infections.

Treatment

A high index of suspicion is important in the diagnosis and treatment of neonatal infection. Table 2–20 presents guidelines for the evaluation and management of *term* infants with risk factors or clinical signs of infection. Because the risk of infection is greater in the preterm infant and because respiratory disease is a common sign of infection, any preterm infant with respiratory disease requires blood cultures and broad-spectrum therapy for 48–72 hours pending the results of cultures. An examination of cerebrospinal fluid should be performed in those infants in whom infection is highly suspected on a clinical basis (eg, associated hypotension, persistent metabolic acidosis, neutropenia). Other specific therapy includes the administration of intravenous gamma globulin (500–750 mg/kg) to infants with known infection or clinical signs very suggestive of true infection. In sick infants, the essentials of good supportive therapy should be provided: intravenous glucose and water, colloid volume support, use of pressors as needed, and oxygen and ventilator support.

Table 2–20. Guidelines for evaluation of neonatal bacterial infection in the term infant.

Risk Factor	Clinical Signs[1]	Evaluation and Treatment
12–18 h after rupture of membranes	None	Observation
>12–18 h after rupture of membranes, chorioamnionitis	None	CBC, blood cultures, broad-spectrum antibiotics for 48–72 h
>12–18 h after rupture of membranes, chorioamnionitis, maternal antibiotics	None	CBC, blood cultures, urine antigen test for group B streptococci, broad-spectrum antibiotics for 48–72 h
None or present	Present	CBC, blood and CSF culture, perhaps urine culture (see below); broad-spectrum antibiotics[2]

[1]If clinical signs consistent with infection are absent, close observation without treatment may be sufficient.
[2]Irrespective of age at presentation, any infant who appears infected by clinical criteria should undergo cerebrospinal fluid (CSF) examination. Urine culture is indicated in the evaluation of infants who were initially well but have developed symptoms after 2–3 days of age.

Prognosis

The prognosis for neonatal infection depends on the specific agent and type of infection. This issue is addressed in the discussion of specific infections.

SPECIFIC INFECTIONS

1. BACTERIAL SEPSIS

The most common organisms causing bacterial sepsis in the newborn are group B β-hemolytic streptococcus (GBS) and gram-negative enterics (especially *Escherichia coli*). Other organisms to consider are *Staphylococcus aureus, Listeria monocytogenes, Enterococcus,* and *Staphylococcus epidermidis* (most common in infants with indwelling central venous lines). Early-onset bacterial sepsis is usually acquired in utero (ascending) or by passage through an infected birth canal. Late-onset bacterial sepsis is more often associated with infection of cerebrospinal fluid or other local infections (eg, osteomyelitis). Clinical signs, laboratory aids, and evaluation have been noted (see above and Table 2–20).

Antibiotic coverage should be directed initially toward suspected organisms. Early-onset sepsis is usually caused by GBS or gram-negative enterics; broad-spectrum coverage, therefore, should include ampicillin plus an aminoglycoside or third-generation cephalosporin. Specific doses and schedules are given in Chapter 34. Late-onset infections can also be caused by the same organisms, but coverage may need to be expanded to include staphylococci. In particular, the preterm infant with indwelling lines is at risk for *S epidermidis,* for which vancomycin is the drug of choice.

Selective intrapartum treatement with ampicillin or penicillin for maternal GBS carriers identified antepartum or intrapartum with associated risk factors (preterm labor, premature rupture of the membranes before 37 weeks, rupture of the membranes beyond 18 hours at any gestational age, multiple births, maternal fever) has proven effective in preventing neonatal GBS infection. If maternal GBS status is unknown, chemoprophylaxis may be indicated for one or more of the risk factors listed above.

2. FUNGAL SEPSIS

With more aggressive neonatal care associated with the survival of smaller infants, infection with *Candida* species has become more common. Infants of low birth weight with central lines who have had repeated exposures to broad-spectrum antibiotics are at highest risk. For infants less than 1500 g, colonization rates of 27% have been demonstrated, with many of these infants developing cutaneous lesions. A much smaller percentage (2–5%) develops systemic disease. Clinical features at presentation are indistinguishable from those of bacterial sepsis. Deep organ involvement (renal tract, endophthalmitis, endocarditis) is commonly associated with systemic candidiasis. Treatment is with the antifungal amphotericin B. In severe infections, flucytosine can be added for synergistic coverage (see Chapter 38). In addition, *Malassezia furfur* is also seen in infants with central lines receiving intravenous fat emulsion. To clear this organism, it is necessary to remove the inciting indwelling line.

3. MENINGITIS

Any newborn with bacterial sepsis is also at risk for meningitis. The incidence is low in infants with early-onset sepsis but is much higher in infants with late-onset infection. The workup for any infant with signs consistent with infection should include a spinal tap. Diagnosis is suggested by a protein greater than 250 mg/dL, glucose less than 30 mg/dL, more than 25 WBCs/μL, and a positive Gram's stain. The diagnosis is confirmed by culture. Most common organisms are GBS and gram-negative enterics. While sepsis can be treated with 10–14 days of antibiotics, meningitis should be treated for 21 days with appropriate antibiotics. The mortality rate for neonatal meningitis is approximately 25%, with significant neurologic morbidity present in one-third of

the survivors. Use of dexamethasone has not been studied in neonates.

4. PNEUMONIA

The respiratory system can be infected in utero or upon passage through the birth canal. Early-onset neonatal infection is usually associated with pneumonia. Pneumonia should also be suspected in older neonates with a recent onset of tachypnea, retractions, and cyanosis. In infants already receiving respiratory support, an increase in oxygen requirement or ventilator settings may indicate pneumonia. Not only bacteria but also viruses (cytomegalovirus, respiratory syncytial virus, adenovirus, influenza, herpes simplex, parainfluenza) and *Chlamydia* can cause the disease. In infants with pre-existing respiratory disease, intercurrent pulmonary infections may contribute to the ultimate severity of chronic lung disease.

5. URINARY TRACT INFECTION

Infection of the urine is uncommon with early-onset infection. Urinary tract infection in the newborn is seen most commonly in association with genitourinary anomalies and is caused by gram-negative enterics. Urine should be evaluated as part of the workup for late-onset infection. Culture should be obtained either by suprapubic aspiration or bladder catheterization. Antibiotic therapy is continued for 10–14 days intravenously. Subsequently, evaluation for genitourinary anomalies, starting with an ultrasound examination and a voiding cystourethrogram, should be undertaken.

6. OSTEOMYELITIS

Osteomyelitis is an uncommon infection in the newborn. It is seen in association with late-onset septicemia, usually with *S aureus* or GBS. More detailed discussion of osteomyelitis can be found in Chapter 24.

7. OTITIS MEDIA

Otitis media may be present in a significant number of long-term nursery residents. It is particularly common in infants who have had prolonged endotracheal intubation or an indwelling nasogastric feeding tube. An evaluation for infection in such an infant is not complete without an ear examination. Gram-negative enterics are more common infecting agents in nursery residents than in outpatients.

8. OMPHALITIS

A normal umbilical cord stump will atrophy and separate at the skin level. A small amount of purulent material at the base of the cord is common but can be minimized by keeping the cord open to air and cleaning the base with alcohol several times each day. The cord can become colonized with streptococci, staphylococci, or gram-negative organisms that can cause local infection. Infections are more common in cords manipulated for venous or arterial lines. Omphalitis is diagnosed when redness and edema are evident in the soft tissues around the stump. Local and systemic cultures should be obtained. Treatment is with broad-spectrum intravenous antibiotics. Complications are determined by the degree of infection of the cord vessels and include septic thrombophlebitis, hepatic abscess, necrotizing fasciitis, and portal vein thrombosis.

9. CONGENITAL VIRAL & PARASITIC INFECTIONS
(See also Chapters 35 and 38.)

Cytomegalovirus

Cytomegalovirus (CMV) is the most common virus known to be transmitted in utero. The incidence of congenital infection ranges from 0.2% to 2.2% among live births. Transmission of CMV can take place as a consequence of either primary or reactivated infection in the mother. An important source of infection is children (especially those in a day care setting), who transmit the virus to parents and workers. The incidence of primary infection in pregnancy is 1–4%, with a 40% transmission rate to the fetus. Of these infants, 85–90% are asymptomatic at birth, whereas 10–15% have clinically apparent disease—hepatosplenomegaly, petechiae, small size for gestational age, direct hyperbilirubinemia, or thrombocytopenia. The risk of neonatal disease is higher when the mother acquires the infection in the first half of pregnancy. The incidence of reactivated infection in pregnancy is less than 1%, with a 0–1% incidence of clinically apparent disease. Diagnosis in a suspected infant should be confirmed with culture of the virus (blood, cerebrospinal fluid, urine, throat, placenta, amniotic fluid). Although experimental, ganciclovir has been used in some severely ill neonates.

The mortality rate in patients with symptomatic congenital CMV may be as high as 20%. Sequelae, including hearing loss, mental retardation, delayed motor development, chorioretinitis and optic atrophy, seizures, language delays, and learning disability, occur in 90% of symptomatic survivors. The incidence is 5–15% in asymptomatic infants; the most frequent finding is hearing loss.

Perinatal infection can also occur with acquisition of virus around the time of delivery. These infections are generally asymptomatic and without sequelae. Postnatal infection is usually asymptomatic but can cause hepatitis, pneumonitis, and neurologic illness in compromised seronegative prematures. The virus can be acquired through transfusions or ingestion of CMV-infected breast milk. Transfusion risk can be minimized by using frozen, washed red blood cells or CMV antibody–negative donors.

Rubella

Congenital rubella infection occurs as a result of rubella infection in the mother during pregnancy. The frequency of infection in the infant is as high as 80% in mothers infected during the first trimester. Infection rates then decline. A high incidence of defects can be attributed to infection acquired during the first trimester but declines with later infection. Clinical features of congenital rubella include adenopathy, bone radiolucencies, encephalitis, cardiac defects (pulmonary arterial hypoplasia and patent ductus arteriosus), cataracts, retinopathy, growth retardation, hepatosplenomegaly, thrombocytopenia, and purpura. The diagnosis should be suspected in cases of a characteristic clinical illness in the mother (rash, adenopathy, arthritis). Maternal illness can be confirmed with serologies. IgG titers in the infant can be compared to those in the mother, and specific IgM may be looked for in the baby. Diagnosis can be confirmed by culture of pharyngeal secretions.

There is no treatment for congenital rubella. Prevention, however, is possible with immunization. Nonimmune patients of childbearing age should be immunized prior to conception. Congenital rubella does cause significant, long-term sequelae, including mental retardation and hearing loss. Sequelae are most severe in infections acquired during the first trimester. Infants infected late in gestation do not suffer long-term sequelae.

Varicella

Congenital varicella is rare (<5% after infection acquired during the first or second trimester) but does cause a recognizable constellation of findings, including limb hypoplasia, cutaneous scars, microcephaly, cortical atrophy, chorioretinitis, and cataracts. Perinatal exposure (5 days before to 2 days after delivery) can cause severe to fatal disseminated varicella. Prophylaxis and therapy are available for perinatal varicella. If maternal varicella develops within the perinatal risk period, 1.25 mL of varicella immune globulin should be given. If this has not been done, the illness can be treated with intravenous acyclovir. (See Chapter 35.)

Hospitalized premature infants of at least 28 weeks' gestation whose mothers have no history of chickenpox and all infants of less than 28 weeks' gestational age should receive varicella immune globulin for postnatal exposure.

Toxoplasmosis

Toxoplasmosis is caused by the parasite *Toxoplasma gondii*. When infection occurs during pregnancy, up to 40% of the children become infected, of whom 15% have severe clinical damage. The means of acquisition include exposure to cat feces and ingestion of raw meat. Fetal damage is most likely to occur when the infection occurs in the second to sixth month of gestation. Clinical findings include growth retardation, chorioretinitis, seizures, jaundice, hydrocephalus, microcephaly, hepatosplenomegaly, adenopathy, cataracts, maculopapular rash, thrombocytopenia, and pneumonia. The majority of affected infants are asymptomatic at birth but show evidence of damage (chorioretinitis, blindness, low IQ) at a later time. Serologies, first for IgG and then the specific IgM antibody, make the diagnosis. Treatment of the acutely infected pregnant woman may prevent transmission to the fetus. Neonatal treatment using pyrimethamine and sulfadiazine with folinic acid can improve long-term outcome (see Chapter 38).

10. PERINATALLY ACQUIRED VIRAL INFECTIONS

Herpes Simplex
(See also Chapter 35.)

Herpes simplex infection is most commonly acquired at the time of birth with passage through an infected birth canal. A mother can have either a primary or a reactivated secondary infection. Primary maternal infection, because of both high titer of organism and no maternal antibodies, poses the greatest risk to the infant. The risk of neonatal infection with vaginal delivery in this setting is 33–50%. Seventy percent of mothers with primary herpes at the time of delivery are asymptomatic. The risk to an infant born to a mother with recurrent herpes simplex virus (HSV) is much lower: less than 3–5%. Time of presentation of localized (skin, eye, mouth) or disseminated disease (pneumonia, shock, hepatitis) in the infant is usually 5–14 days of age. Central nervous system disease usually presents at 14–28 days of age with lethargy and seizures. In about one-third of patients, localized skin, eye, and mouth disease is the first indication of infection. In another third, disseminated or central nervous system disease precedes skin, eye, and mouth findings, while the remaining third have disseminated or central nervous system disease in the absence of skin, eye, and mouth disease. Preliminary diagnosis can be made by scraping the base of a vesicle and finding multinucleated giant cells. Viral culture, usually positive in 24–72 hours, makes the definitive diagnosis. In some cases, newer polymerase chain reaction DNA technology may assist in diagnosis.

Therapy for neonatal herpes is available with adenosine arabinoside or acyclovir. Acyclovir has fewer side effects and is the drug of choice. Both agents are effective in improving survival with central nervous system and disseminated disease and in preventing the spread of localized disease. Prevention is possible by not allowing delivery through an infected birth canal (eg, by cesarean section). However, antepartum cervical cultures are poor predictors of the presence of virus at the time of delivery. Furthermore, given the low incidence of infection in the newborn in secondary maternal infection, cesarean section is not indicated for asymptomatic mothers with a history of herpes. In most settings, cesarean sections are still performed in mothers with active lesions (either primary or secondary) at the time of delivery. Infants born to mothers with a history of HSV infection but no active lesions can be observed closely after birth. Infants born to mothers with active lesions, irrespective of the route of delivery, should be cultured (eye, oropharynx, umbilicus, rectum) 24 hours after delivery. If the infant is colonized (positive cultures), treatment with acyclovir should be considered. In cases of documented primary infection at the time of delivery, the infant should be cultured and started on acyclovir pending the results of cultures. Neonates with documented herpes infection or a likely exposure should be managed with contact isolation. The major problem facing perinatologists is the high percentage of asymptomatic primary maternal infection. In these cases, infection in the neonate is currently not preventable. Therefore, any infant who presents at the right age with symptoms consistent with neonatal herpes should be cultured and started on acyclovir pending the results of those cultures.

Prognosis is good for localized skin and mucosal disease that does not progress. The mortality rate for both disseminated and central nervous system herpes is high, with significant rates of morbidity among survivors despite treatment.

Hepatitis B
(See also Chapter 21.)

Infants can be infected with hepatitis B at the time of birth. Clinical illness is rare in the neonatal period, but exposed infants are at risk to become chronic HBsAg carriers and to develop chronic active hepatitis and are at increased risk for hepatic carcinoma. The presence of HBsAg should be determined in all pregnant women. If the result is positive, the infant should receive hepatitis B immunoglobulin (HBIG) and hepatitis B vaccine as soon as possible after birth, followed by two subsequent vaccine doses at 1 and 6 months of age. If an HBsAg has not been tested prior to birth in a mother at risk, the test should be run after delivery, and hepatitis B vaccine should be given within 12 hours of birth. If the mother is subsequently found to be positive, HBIG should be given as soon as possible (preferably within 48 hours, but not later than 1 week after birth). Subsequent vaccine doses should be given at 1 and 6 months of age. The Centers for Disease Control and Prevention and the American Academy of Pediatrics recommend universal immunization of all newborns with hepatitis B vaccine at birth, at 1–2 months, and at 6–18 months. *Note:* In low birth weight infants, the initial vaccine should be given when the infant reaches a weight of 2000 g.

Enteroviral Infection

Enteroviral infections occur with greatest frequency in the late summer and early fall. Infection is usually acquired in the perinatal period. There is often a history of a maternal illness (fever, diarrhea, rash) in the week prior to delivery. The illness presents in the infant in the first 2 weeks of life. Most commonly, the illness is characterized by fevers, lethargy, irritability, diarrhea, and rash but is not severe. Other symptom complexes include meningoencephalitis and myocarditis, as well as a severe disseminated illness with hepatitis, pneumonia, shock, and disseminated intravascular coagulation. Diagnosis can be confirmed by culture (rectum, cerebrospinal fluid, blood). There is no therapy of proved efficacy. Prognosis is good for all symptom complexes except severe disseminated disease, which carries a high mortality rate.

HIV Infection
(See also Chapter 36.)

Human immunodeficiency virus (HIV) can pass transplacentally, be acquired at the time of delivery, or be transmitted postpartum via breast milk. The prevalence of HIV infection among women of childbearing age is 1.5:1000. Transmission of virus occurs in about 30% of births. Use of zidovudine during pregnancy, intrapartum, and for 6 weeks in the newborn decreases vertical transmission to 8%. The risk of transmission is increased in mothers with advanced disease, low CD4 counts, and p24 antigenemia. Diagnosis is based on clinical, immunologic, and serologic findings. The presence of maternal antibody acquired transplacentally confuses diagnosis in the neonate. An infant who is not infected should remain healthy, and the titer of antibody should decline during the first year of life. Diagnosis can be made in infants in the first few months of life by culture, detection of HIV DNA sequences by polymerase chain reaction, and HIV p24 antigen assay.

Protection of health care workers is also an important issue to consider. Testing should be performed in all pregnant women. Because such testing will still fail to identify some infected patients, however, universal precautions should be used. Gloves should be worn during all procedures involving blood and blood-contaminated fluids, intubation, and any invasive procedures using needles. When a splash exposure is possible (eg, in the delivery room), a mask and eye covers should be used.

11. OTHER INFECTIONS

Congenital Syphilis

The infant is usually infected in utero by transplacental passage of *Treponema pallidum*. Findings consistent with congenital syphilis include mucocutaneous lesions, lymphadenopathy, hepatitis, bony changes, and hydrops. However, in the newborn period, infants are often asymptomatic, so that diagnosis is based on maternal and infant serologic testing and is only presumptive. An infant should be evaluated for congenital syphilis if he or she is born to a mother with positive nontreponemal tests confirmed by a positive treponemal test without documented adequate treatment. Evaluation should include a physical examination, quantitative nontreponemal serologic test for syphilis, cerebrospinal fluid examination, long-bone x-rays, and antitreponemal IgM. A definitive diagnosis can be made on those rare occasions when the organism is identified by dark-field or pathologic examination. Guidelines for therapy are presented in Table 2–21.

Tuberculosis
(See also Chapter 37.)

Congenital tuberculosis is rare (seen in the infant of a mother with hematogenously spread tuberculosis). Women with pulmonary tuberculosis are not likely to infect the fetus until after delivery. Management is based on the mother's situation:

(1) Mother with a positive skin test and negative chest x-ray—Investigate family contacts, treat the mother with isoniazid (INH), and follow up the infant with skin tests.

(2) Mother with newly diagnosed disease or disease treated for 2 or more weeks judged to be noncontagious at delivery—Investigate family contacts, have a chest x-ray and skin test done on the infant at 3–4 months, and treat the infant with INH until testing is done and negative.

(3) Mother with active contagious disease—The mother should be separated from the infant until adequate treatment has been administered to render the mother noncontagious. The infant should be followed up with skin tests, or therapy has been started in the infant as under (2).

(4) Mother with hematogenously spread disease—The infant should be evaluated for congenital tuberculosis, separated from the mother until she is noncontagious, and treated with INH as under (3).

Conjunctivitis

Neisseria gonorrhoeae may colonize an infant during passage through an infected birth canal. Gonococcal ophthalmitis presents at 3–7 days with very purulent conjunctivitis. Diagnosis can be suspected when gram-negative intracellular diplococci are seen on Gram's strain and confirmed by culture. Treatment is with ceftriaxone of cefotaxime (in premature or hyperbilirubinemic infants). Prophylaxis at

Table 2–21. Recommended treatment of neonates (≤4 weeks of age) with proven or possible congenital syphilis.[1]

Clinical Status	Antimicrobial Therapy
Proven or highly probable disease[2]	Aqueous crystalline penicillin G, IV, for 10–14 d[3]
Asymptomatic, normal CSF and radiographic examination—maternal treatment:	
None, inadequate,[4] undocumented, failed, or reinfected	Aqueous crystalline penicillin G, IV, for 10–14 d[3]
Erythromycin	Clinical, serologic follow-up, and benzathine penicillin G, IM, single dose[5]
Adequate therapy but given less than 1 mo before delivery, or mother's response to treatment is not demonstrated by a fourfold decrease in titer of a nontreponemal serologic test	Clinical, serologic follow-up, and benzathine penicillin G, IM, single dose[5]

[1]Reproduced, with permission, from the American Academy of Pediatrics: *Report of the Committee on Infectious Diseases,* 23rd ed. American Academy of Pediatrics. 1994.
[2](1) Physical or x-ray evidence of active disease, (2) serum quantitative nontreponemal titer is at least four times the mother's titer, (3) cerebospinal fluid (CSF) VDRL is reactive or CSF cell count and/or protein is abnormal, or (4) positive antitreponemal IgM antibody test.
[3]100,000–150,000 IU/kg/d given every 8–12 hours. Some experts recommend aqueous procaine penicillin G, 50,000 U/kg IM for 10–14 days.
[4]The mother's penicillin dose is unknown, inadequate, or undocumented.
[5]Some experts recommend aqueous crystalline or procaine penicillin G as for proven or highly probable disease. Others would follow up the infant without therapy if close clinical and serologic follow-up can be assured. The dose of benzathine penicillin G is 50,000 U/kg.

birth is given with 1% silver nitrate or 0.5% erythromycin ointment. Infants born to mothers with known gonococcal disease should also receive a single dose of ceftriaxone.

Chlamydia trachomatis is another important cause of conjunctivitis, presenting at 5 days to several weeks of age with congestion, edema, and minimal discharge. The organism is acquired at birth after passage through an infected birth canal. Acquisition occurs in 50% of infants born to infected women, with a 25–50% risk of conjunctivitis. Prevalence in pregnancy is over 10% in some populations. Diagnosis is by isolation of the organism or by rapid antigen detection tests. Treatment is with oral erythromycin. Topical treatment alone will not eradicate nasopharyngeal carriage, leaving the infant at risk for the development of pneumonitis. Diagnosis in the infant requires therapy of the mother and her sexual partners.

INFECTION CONTROL

The single most important principle in nursery infection control is good hand washing. Hands should be washed with a germicidal soap for 3 minutes prior to entering the nursery to handle patients. This procedure should be repeated between patient visits. Personnel with upper respiratory tract infections should wear masks; those with gastrointestinal tract infections must be rigorous about hand washing. Wounds or herpetic lesions should be covered.

An infected infant with a communicable disease (eg, viral respiratory infection, necrotizing enterocolitis) should be isolated. Ideally, the infant should be placed in a separate room, but if one is not available, a remote site in the nursery and perhaps an isolette should be used. The number of staff caring for the infant and their exposure to other infants should be limited. Gown, gloves, and mask should be worn as indicated for type of infection, and exposed materials should be disposed of separately.

Nursery staff should also take precautions against acquiring HIV infection. Newborns should be handled with gloves prior to initial bathing to remove blood. Gloves should be worn when drawing blood and starting intravenous therapy. Aspiration of meconium from an infant's airway should be performed with wall suction.

American Academy of Pediatrics: *Guidelines for Perinatal Care.* American Academy of Pediatrics, 1992.

American Academy of Pediatrics: *Report of the Committee on Infectious Diseases.* American Academy of Pediatrics, 1994.

American Academy of Pediatrics Committee on Infectious Diseases and Committee on Fetus and Newborn: Guidelines for prevention of group B streptococcal (GBS) infection by chemoprophylaxis. Pediatrics 1992;90:775.

American Academy of Pediatrics Committee on Infectious Diseases: Universal hepatitis B immunization. Pediatrics 1992;89:795.

Beeram MR et al: Lumbar puncture in the evaluation of possible asymptomatic congenital syphilis in neonates. J Pediatr 1996;128:125.

Blanche S et al: Relation of the course of HIV infection in children to the severity of the disease in their mothers at delivery. N Engl J Med 1994;330:308.

Brown ZA et al: Neonatal herpes simplex virus infection in relation to asymptomatic maternal infection at the time of labor. N Engl J Med 1991;324:1247.

Burgard M et al: The use of viral culture and p24 antigen testing to diagnose human immunodeficiency virus infection in neonates. N Engl J Med 1992;327:1192.

Connor EM et al: Reduction of maternal-infant transmission of human immunodeficiency virus type 1 with zidovudine treatment. N Engl J Med 1994;331:1173.

Enders G et al: Consequences of varicella and herpes zoster in pregnancy: Prospective study of 1739 cases. Lancet 1994;343:1548.

Evans HE (editor): Perinatal AIDS. Clin Perinatol 1994;21(1).

Fowler KB et al: The outcome of congenital cytomegalovirus infection in relation to maternal antibody status. N Engl J Med 1992;326:663.

Gibbs RS, Amstey MS, Lezotte DC: Role of cesarean delivery in preventing neonatal herpes virus infection. JAMA 1993;270:94.

Guerina NG et al: Neonatal serologic screening and early treatment for congenital *Toxoplasma gondii* infection. N Engl J Med 1994;330:1858.

Heggie AD et al: Frequency and significance of isolation of *Ureaplasma urealyticum* and *Mycoplasma hominis* from cerebrospinal fluid and tracheal aspirate specimens from low birth weight infants. J Pediatr 1994;124:956.

Ikeda MK, Jenson HB: Evaluation and treatment of congenital syphilis. J Pediatr 1990;117:843.

Kliegman RM, Clapp DW: Rational principles for immunoglobulin prophylaxis and therapy of neonatal infections. Clin Perinatol 1991;18:303.

Kulhanjian JA et al: Identification of women at unsuspected risk of primary infection with HSV type 2 during pregnancy. N Engl J Med 1992;326:916.

McFarlin BL et al: Epidemic syphilis: Maternal factors associated with congenital infection. Am J Obstet Gynecol 1994;170:535.

Miles SA et al: Rapid serologic testing with immune-complex–dissociated HIV p24 antigen for early detection in neonates. N Engl J Med 1993;328:297.

Nataro JP et al: Prospective analysis of coagulase-negative staphylococcal infection in hospitalized infants. J Pediatr 1994;125:798.

Ng PC: Systemic fungal infections in neonates. Arch Dis Child 1994;71:F130.

Nigro G et al: Ganciclovir therapy for symptomatic congenital cytomegalovirus infection in infants: A two-regimen experience. J Pediatr 1994;124:318.

Ohlsson A, Myhr TL: Intrapartum chemoprophylaxis of perinatal group B streptococcal infections: A critical review of randomized controlled trials. Am J Obstet Gynecol 1994;170:910.

Pastuszak AL et al: Outcome after maternal varicella infection in the first 20 weeks of pregnancy. N Engl J Med 1994;330:901.

Peckham C, Gibb D: Mother-to-child transmission of the human immunodeficiency virus. N Engl J Med 1995;333:298.

Pelke S et al: Gowning does not affect colonization or infection rates in a neonatal intensive care unit. Arch Pediatr Adolesc Med 1994;148:1016.

Prober CG et al: Low risk of herpes simplex infections in neonates exposed to the virus at the time of vaginal delivery to mothers with recurrent genital herpes simplex virus infection. N Engl J Med 1987;316:240.

Pylipow M et al: Selective intrapartum prophylaxis for group B streptococcus colonization: Management and outcome of newborns. Pediatrics 1994;93:631.

Remington JS, Klein JO (editors): *Infectious Diseases of the Fetus and Newborn Infant,* 4th ed. Saunders, 1995.

Risk factors for mother-to-child transmission of HIV-1. European Collaborative Study. Lancet 1992;339:1007.

Roizen N et al: Neurologic and developmental outcome in treated congenital toxoplasmosis. Pediatrics 1995;95:11.

Rouse DJ et al: Strategies for the prevention of early-onset group B streptococcal sepsis: A decision analysis. Obstet Gynecol 1994;83:483.

Stamos JK, Rowley AH: Timely diagnosis of congenital infections. Pediatr Clin North Am 1994;41:1017.

St. Louis ME et al: Risk for perinatal HIV-1 transmission according to maternal immunologic, virologic, and placental factors. JAMA 1993;269:2853.

Task Force on Pediatric AIDS: Perinatal human immunodeficiency virus (HIV) testing. Pediatrics 1992;89:791.

Toltzis P: Current issues in neonatal herpes simplex virus infection. Clin Perinatol 1991;18:193.

Weisman LE et al: Early onset group B streptococcal sepsis: A current assessment. J Pediatr 1992;121:428.

Weisman LE et al: Intravenous immune globulin prophylaxis of late- onset sepsis in premature neonates. J Pediatr 1994;125:922.

Whitley R et al: A controlled trial comparing vidarabine with acyclovir in neonatal herpes simplex virus infection. N Engl J Med 1991;324:444.

Wiswell TE et al: No lumbar puncture in the evaluation for early neonatal sepsis: Will meningitis be missed? Pediatrics 1995;95:803.

GASTROINTESTINAL & ABDOMINAL SURGICAL CONDITIONS (See also Chapter 20.)

CONGENITAL CONDITIONS

1. TRACHEOESOPHAGEAL FISTULA & ESOPHAGEAL ATRESIA

Diagnosis

These associated conditions are characterized by a blind esophageal pouch and a fistulous connection between either the proximal or distal esophagus and the airway. In 85% of infants with this condition, the fistula is between the distal esophagus and the airway. Polyhydramnios is common because of the high level of gastrointestinal obstruction. Infants present in the first hours of life with copious secretions, choking, cyanosis, and respiratory distress. Diagnosis can be confirmed with chest x-ray after careful placement of a nasogastric tube to the point at which resistance is met. On chest x-ray, the tube will be seen in the blind pouch. If a tracheoesophageal fistula is present to the distal esophagus, gas will be present in the abdomen.

Treatment

The tube in the proximal pouch should be placed on continuous suction to drain secretions and prevent aspiration. The head of the bed should be elevated to prevent reflux of gastric contents through the distal fistula into the lungs. Intravenous glucose and fluids should be provided and oxygen administered as needed. Definitive treatment is surgical and depends on the distance between the segments of esophagus. If the distance is not too great, the fistula can be ligated and the ends of the esophagus anastomosed. In instances in which the end of the esophagus cannot be anastomosed, the initial surgery entails fistula ligation and a gastrostomy. Antibiotics are usually used postoperatively.

Prognosis

Prognosis is determined primarily by the presence or absence of associated anomalies. Vertebral, cardiac, renal, limb, and anal anomalies are also seen (VACTERL association). Evaluation for other anomalies should be done early in the infant's course.

2. HIGH INTESTINAL OBSTRUCTION

Diagnosis

Infants with high intestinal obstruction present early with vomiting. A history of polyhydramnios is also common. In cases of duodenal atresia, vomitus may or may not contain bile; in cases of malrotation and midgut volvulus and high jejunal atresia, vomitus is bilious. Midgut volvulus may occur with malrotation and involves torsion of the intestine around the superior mesenteric artery that causes occlusion of the vascular supply of most of the small intestine. If not treated promptly, the infant can lose most of the small bowel to ischemic injury. Therefore, *bilious vomiting* in the neonate demands immediate attention and evaluation. Diagnosis of high intestinal obstruction can be confirmed with x-rays. Duodenal atresia is characterized by a double bubble sign (stomach and dilated duodenum). In cases of midgut volvulus, the plain abdominal x-ray may not be definitive. Occasionally, air stops at the level of the ligament of Treitz (level of obstruction). However, air can also be present beyond this point, precluding accurate diagnosis on plain film. Diagnosis can be confirmed with an upper gastrointestinal series to determine whether contrast material passes the ligament of Treitz.

Treatment

A nasogastric tube should be placed to suction for decompression, an intravenous infusion should be started for administering glucose and fluids, and supportive respiratory treatment should be given. The definitive treatment is surgery. Midgut volvulus is an indication for emergency surgery. Other conditions can be handled promptly but need not be done in an emergency fashion. Antibiotics are usually used for these conditions.

Prognosis

Duodenal atresia is associated with trisomy 21. Prognosis in that circumstance is related to other associated conditions (eg, cardiac). Infants with other high intestinal obstructions do well after surgical correction, except those with midgut volvulus who suffer loss of considerable amounts of ischemic small bowel.

3. DISTAL INTESTINAL OBSTRUCTION

Diagnosis

Low intestinal obstruction presents with an increasing intolerance of feedings (spitting progressing to vomiting), abdominal distention, and decreased or absent stooling. Imperforate anus should be diagnosed on initial physical examination prior to onset of symptoms. In the case of a high rectal atresia, however, the obstruction can be missed on the initial examination. Other diagnostic clues to imperforate anus include the presence of perineal fistulas with meconium or the presence of meconium in the urine (rectovesical fistula). Other causes of distal intestinal obstruction include meconium ileus, Hirschsprung's disease, meconium plug syndrome, small left colon syndrome, ileal atresia, and colonic atresia. Plain film of the abdomen shows gaseous distention with multiple air through a considerable portion of the bowel and air-fluid levels. Diagnosis of meconium ileus, meconium plug, and small left colon syndrome can be made by appearance on contrast enema. In cases of meconium plug syndrome, osmotic contrast material (eg, meglumine diatrizoate [Gastrografin]) has a therapeutic as well as a diagnostic use: it induces passage of the plug. Rectal biopsy showing absence of ganglion cells confirms the diagnosis of Hirschsprung's disease.

Treatment

Nasogastric suction to decompress the abdomen, intravenous glucose, fluid and electrolyte replacement, and respiratory support as necessary should be instituted. Antibiotics are usually indicated. The definitive treatment for all these conditions (with the exception of meconium plug syndrome and small left colon syndrome) is surgery.

Prognosis

Up to 10% of infants with meconium plug syndrome are found to have cystic fibrosis, whereas all infants with meconium ileus have cystic fibrosis. In addition, meconium plug syndrome is associated with Hirschsprung's disease. Small left colon syndrome is seen in infants of diabetic mothers. Once the child develops a normal stooling pattern, feedings will usually be tolerated and no further problems noted. Imperforate anus is associated (like tracheoesophageal fistula) with other anomalies—vertebral, renal, cardiac, limb. The other conditions usually carry an excellent prognosis after surgical repair.

4. ABDOMINAL WALL DEFECTS

Omphalocele

Omphaloceles are formed by the incomplete closure of the anterior abdominal wall after return of the midgut to the abdominal cavity. The size of the defect is variable, but usually the omphalocele sac contains some intestine, stomach, liver, and spleen. The abdominal cavity is small and underdeveloped. The umbilical cord can be seen to insert onto the center of the omphalocele sac. There is a high incidence of associated anomalies, including cardiac and other gastrointestinal anomalies, and chromosomal syndromes (trisomy 13). Acute treatment involves covering the defect with a sterile warm saline–soaked dressing to prevent fluid loss, nasogastric tube decompression, intravenous fluids and glucose, and antibiotics. If the abdominal contents will fit, a primary surgical closure is done. If not, a staged closure is performed, with gradual reduction of the omphalocele into the abdominal cavity and a secondary closure. Postoperatively, third-space fluid losses may be extensive; fluid and electrolyte therapy, therefore, must be carefully monitored.

Gastroschisis

Gastroschisis is a defect in the anterior abdominal wall *lateral* to the umbilicus; there is no covering sac, and the herniated viscera is usually limited to intestine. Furthermore, the intestine has been exposed to amniotic fluid and has a thickened, beefy-red appearance. The herniation is thought to occur as a rupture through an ischemic portion of the abdominal wall. Other than intestinal atresia, associated anomalies are uncommon. Therapy is as described for omphalocele; however, primary closures can be successfully performed more frequently.

Diaphragmatic Hernia

This congenital malformation consists of herniation of abdominal organs into the hemithorax (usually left) resulting from a posterolateral defect in the diaphragm. Infants usually present in the delivery room with respiratory distress, cyanosis, decreased breath sounds on the side of the hernia, and shift of the mediastinum to the side opposite the hernia. The infants are often difficult to resuscitate and require early intubation and placement of a nasogastric tube. The rapidity and severity of presentation with respiratory distress are dependent on the degree of pulmonary hypoplasia. The ipsilateral and, to some extent, the contralateral lung are compressed in utero because of the hernia. Treatment is to intubate and ventilate and to decompress the gastrointestinal tract with a nasogastric tube. An intravenous infusion of glucose and fluid should be started. A chest x-ray confirms the diagnosis. Surgery is performed after the infant is stabilized to remove abdominal contents from the thorax and to close the diaphragmatic defect. The postoperative course is often complicated by severe pulmonary hypertension. Therapy with high-frequency ventilation, inhaled NO, and ECMO is often needed in these infants. The mortality rate for this condition is 50%, with survival dependent on the degree of pulmonary hypoplasia in the contralateral lung.

NECROTIZING ENTEROCOLITIS

Necrotizing enterocolitis (NEC) is the most common acquired gastrointestinal emergency in the newborn; it most often affects preterm infants, with an incidence of 10% in infants less than 1500 g. In term infants, it is seen in association with polycythemia, congenital heart disease, and birth asphyxia. The pathogenesis of the disease is a multifactorial interaction between an immature gastrointestinal tract, mucosal injury, and potentially injurious factors in the lumen. Previous intestinal ischemia, bacterial or viral infection, and immunologic immaturity of the gut are felt to play a role in the genesis of NEC. In up to 20% of affected infants, the only risk factor present is prematurity.

Diagnosis

The most common presenting sign is abdominal distention. Other signs include vomiting or increased gastric residuals, heme-positive stools, abdominal tenderness, temperature instability, increased apnea and bradycardia, decreased urine output, and poor perfusion. The complete blood count may show increased white blood cell count with an increased band count or, as the disease progresses, an absolute neutropenia. Thrombocytopenia is often seen along with stress-induced hyperglycemia and metabolic acidosis. Diagnosis is confirmed by the presence of pneumatosis intestinalis (air in the bowel wall) on x-ray. There is a spectrum of disease, and milder cases may exhibit only distention of bowel loops with bowel wall edema (thickened-appearing walls on x-ray).

Prevention

Induction of intestinal maturation with antenatal steroids appears to decrease the incidence of NEC. Use of human milk feeds, early trophic feeds, and a slow advancement of feeding volume may serve to decrease the incidence of NEC, but these issues remain controversial. Immunologic modulation through feeding oral immunoglobulins has also shown some promise, but this requires further study. Epidemics can be interrupted by careful measures to control infection.

Treatment

A. Medical Treatment:

1. Decompression of gut by nasogastric tube.

2. Maintenance of oxygenation; ventilation if necessary.
3. Intravenous fluids (colloid and normal saline) to replace third-space gastrointestinal losses. Enough fluid should be given to restore a good urine output.
4. Broad-spectrum antibiotics, including anaerobic coverage.
5. Close monitoring of vital signs, physical examination, laboratory data (blood gases, white blood cell count, platelet count, x-rays).

B. Surgical Treatment: Indications for surgery are evidence of perforation (free air present on a left lateral decubitus film), a fixed dilated loop of bowel on serial x-rays, abdominal wall cellulitis, and progressive deterioration despite maximal medical support. All these signs are indicative of necrotic bowel. In surgery, necrotic bowel is removed and ostomies are created. Reanastomosis is performed after the disease is resolved and the infant is bigger (usually >2 kg). Infants managed either medically or surgically should not be refed until the disease is resolved—normal abdominal examination, resolution of pneumatosis on x-ray—usually a period of 10–14 days. Nutritional support during this time should be provided by total parenteral nutrition.

Prognosis

Death occurs in 10% of cases. Surgery is needed in less than 25% of cases. Long-term prognosis is determined by the amount of intestine lost. Infants with short bowel require long-term support with intravenous nutrition and therefore have very long hospitalizations. Even for those infants, however, the outcome is favorable because of improved parenteral nutrition formulations. Late strictures occur in 8% of patients whether treated medically or surgically about 3–6 weeks after initial diagnosis. Some of these strictures are severe enough to require surgical intervention.

PERFORATIONS OF THE GASTROINTESTINAL TRACT

Prenatal intestinal perforation causes sterile meconium peritonitis. The perforation most often occurs as a result of meconium ileus, but it can occur with intestinal atresia, volvulus, internal hernias, congenital peritoneal bands, intussception, and gastroschisis. Abdominal x-ray films reveal intraperitoneal calcifications. In most cases, surgical exploration is necessary.

Postnatal intestinal perforation most often occurs in association with necrotizing enterocolitis and causes bacterial peritonitis. Other causes include perforated peptic ulcers (associated with chronic steroid administration), Hirschsprung's disease, intestinal atresia, gastroschisis, and malrotation with volvulus.

Left lateral decubitus abdominal plain films will demonstrate free air over the liver.

Gastric perforation in the newborn occurs most often during the first 5 days of life and is associated with perinatal stress. Perforation is associated with marked abdominal distention and massive pneumoperitoneum on abdominal x-ray.

Postnatal gastrointestinal perforation is a surgical emergency. Vigorous fluid and electrolyte resuscitation, nasogastric suction, and antibiotic coverage are necessary supportive measures.

Adra AM et al: The fetus with gastroschisis: Impact of route of delivery and prenatal ultrasonography. Am J Obstet Gynecol 1996;174:540.

Dillon PW, Cilley RE: Newborn surgical emergencies: Gastrointestinal anomalies, abdominal wall defects. Pediatr Clin North Am 1993;40:1289.

Eibl MM et al: Prevention of necrotizing enterocolitis in low-birth-weight infants by IgA-IgG feeding. N Engl J Med 1988;319:1.

Harrison MR et al: A prospective study of the outcome for fetuses with diaphragmatic hernia. JAMA 1994;271:382.

Kanto WP et al: Recognition and medical management of necrotizing enterocolitis. Clin Perinatol 1994;21:335.

Kays DW: Surgical conditions of the neonatal intestinal tract. Clin Perinatol 1996;23:353.

MacKendrick W, Caplan M: Necrotizing enterocolitis: New thoughts about pathogenesis and potential treatments. Pediatr Clin North Am 1993;40:1047.

Major CA et al: Tocolysis with indomethacin increases the incidence of necrotizing enterocolitis in the low-birth-weight neonate. Am J Obstet Gynecol 1994;170:102.

McClead RE Jr (editor): Neonatal necrotizing enterocolitis: Current concepts and controversies. J Pediatr 1990; 117:S1.

McKeown RE: Role of delayed feeding and of feeding increments in necrotizing enterocolitis. J Pediatr 1992; 121:764.

Stoll BJ: Epidemiology of necrotizing enterocolitis. Clin Perinatol 1994;21:205.

Torfs C, Curry C, Roeper P: Gastroschisis. J Pediatr 1990;116:1.

Vidyasagar D, Reyes H: Neonatal surgery. Clin Perinatol 1989;16:1.

HEMATOLOGIC DISORDERS (See also Chapter 26.)

BLEEDING DISORDERS

Neonatal coagulation is discussed in detail elsewhere in the text. Bleeding in the newborn may result from inherited clotting deficiencies (eg, factor VIII deficiency) or acquired disorders—hemorrhagic disease of the newborn, disseminated intravascular coagulation (DIC), liver failure, and thrombocytopenia.

Hemorrhagic Disease of the Newborn

This disorder is caused by the deficiency of the vitamin K-dependent clotting factors (II, VII, IX, X). Bleeding occurs in 0.25–1.7% of newborns who do not receive vitamin K prophylaxis after birth, generally in the first 2–5 days of age in an otherwise well infant. Sites of bleeding include the gastrointestinal tract, umbilical cord, circumcision site, and nose. Bleeding from vitamin K deficiency is more likely to occur in infants of mothers taking anticonvulsants or sodium warfarin. It is also more common in breast-fed than in formula-fed infants, because of very low amounts of vitamin K in breast milk and slower and more restricted intestinal colonization. Table 2–22 distinguishes clinical and laboratory features of hemorrhagic disease, DIC, and bleeding resulting from hepatic failure. Hemorrhagic disease of the newborn is treated by administering 1 mg of vitamin K. DIC and liver failure are treated by addressing the underlying condition and replacing clotting factors.

Thrombocytopenia

Neonatal thrombocytopenia can be isolated or occur in association with a deficiency of clotting factors (see Table 2–22). The differential diagnosis for thrombocytopenia with distinguishing clinical features is presented in Table 2–23. Treatment of neonatal thrombocytopenia is transfusion of platelets (10 mL/kg of platelets increases the platelet count by approximately 70,000/μL). Indication for transfusion in the term infant is clinical bleeding or a total count less than 10,000–20,000/μL. In the preterm infant at risk for intraventricular hemorrhage, transfusion is indicated for counts less than 40,000–50,000/μL.

Isoimmune thrombocytopenia requires transfusion of maternal platelets, since 98% of the random population will also be platelet antigen–positive. The mother would be the most readily available platelet antigen–negative donor. Treatment with steroids has been disappointing. Treatment with intravenous immunoglobulin (IVIG) infusion (1 g/d) daily for 3 days or until the platelet count has doubled or is over 50,000/μL is recommended. Antenatal therapy of the mother with IVIG with or without steroids is also beneficial, since 20–30% of infants with isoimmune thrombocytopenia will suffer from intracranial hemorrhage, 50% before birth. In infants born to mothers with idiopathic thrombocytopenic purpura, both corticosteroids and IVIG infusion have improved platelet counts. Although some centers obtain a fetal platelet count by cordocentesis at 36–38 weeks with elective cesarean delivery if the platelet count is be-

Table 2–22. Features of infants bleeding from hemorrhagic disease of the newborn (HDN), disseminated intravascular coagulation (DIC), or liver failures.

	HDN	DIC	Liver Failure
Clinical	Well infant; no prophylactic vitamin K	Sick infant; hypoxia, sepsis, etc	Sick infant; hepatitis, inborn errors of metabolism, shock liver
Bleeding	Gastrointestinal tract, umbilical cord, circumcision, nose	Generalized	Generalized
Onset	2–3 d	Any time	Any time
Platelet count	Normal	Decreased	Normal or decreased
Prothrombin time (PT)	Prolonged	Prolonged	Prolonged
Partial thromboplastin time (PTT)	Prolonged	Prolonged	Prolonged
Fibrinogen	Normal	Decreased	Decreased
Factor V	Normal	Decreased	Decreased

Table 2–23. Differential diagnosis of neonatal thrombocytopenia.

Disorder	Clinical Tips
Immune Passively acquired antibody; idiopathic thrombocytopenic purpura, systemic lupus erythematosus, drug-induced	Proper history, maternal thrombocytopenia
Isoimmune sensation to PLA-1 antigen	Positive antiplatelet antibodies in baby's serum, sustained rise in platelets by transfusion of mother's platelets
Infections Bacterial Congenital viral infections	Sick infants with other signs consistent with infections
Syndromes Absent radii Fanconi's anemia	Congenital anomalies, associated pancytopenia
Disseminated intravascular coagulation (DIC)	Sick infants, abnormalities of clotting factors
Giant hemangioma	
Thrombosis	Hyperviscous infants, vascular catheters
High-risk with respiratory distress syndrome, pulmonary hypertension, etc	Isolated decrease in platelets is not uncommon in sick infants even in the absence of DIC

low 50,000/μL, the risk of intracranial bleeding in these infants (in contrast to isoimmune cases) appears to be low. For this reason, other centers advocate no ascertainment of the fetal platelet count and vaginal birth.

Anemia

Anemia can be caused by hemorrhage, hemolysis, or failure to produce red blood cells. Anemia presenting in the first 24–48 hours of life is the result of hemorrhage or hemolysis. Hemorrhage can occur in utero (fetoplacental, fetomaternal, or twin-to-twin), perinatally (cord rupture, placenta previa, incision through placenta at cesarean section), or internally (intracranial hemorrhage, cephalohematoma, ruptured liver or spleen). When the bleeding has been of a chronic nature in utero (eg, slow fetomaternal), infants are pale at birth but well compensated, without signs of volume loss. The initial hematocrit is low. Acute bleeding presents with signs of hypovolemia (tachycardia, poor perfusion, hypotension). The hematocrit initially may be normal or decreased but after several hours of equilibration will be decreased. Hemolysis is caused by blood group incompatibilities, enzyme/membrane abnormalities, infection, and DIC. Initial evaluation should include a review of the perinatal history, a determination of the infant's volume status, and a complete physical examination. A Kleihaur Betke test for fetal cells in the mother's circulation should be done on maternal blood. A complete blood count, blood smear, reticulocyte count, and a direct and indirect Coombs' test should be performed. This simple evaluation should suggest a diagnosis in most infants.

ANEMIA IN THE PREMATURE INFANT

In the premature infant, the hemoglobin reaches its nadir at approximately 8–12 weeks and is 2–3 g/dL lower than that in the term infant. The lower nadir in the premature appears to be the result of a decreased erythropoietin response to the low red cell mass. Symptoms of anemia include poor feeding, lethargy, increased heart rate, poor weight gain, and possibly apnea. The decision to transfuse is based on the presence of clinical symptoms. Transfusion is not indicated in an asymptomatic infant simply because of an arbitrary hematocrit number. Most infants become symptomatic if the hematocrit drops below 20%. With risks to transfusion, alternative therapies have been explored. Erythropoietin alfa (150–250 IU given subcutaneously three times per week) has been shown to increase hematocrit and reticulocyte count and to decrease the frequency and volume of transfused blood. This treatment should be reserved for the highest-risk infants (those less than 28–30 weeks' gestational age and below 1000–1200 g). For optimal effect, supplemental iron at a dose of 4–8 mg/kg/d

should be given along with 15 IU of vitamin E daily. Treatment should start when infants are taking at least two-thirds of their nutrition enterally and should continue through 34–36 weeks postconception.

Supplemental iron should be started in all preterm infants at 2 months after birth to prevent iron deficiency anemia.

POLYCYTHEMIA

Elevated hematocrits occur in 2–5% of live births. Although 50% of polycythemic infants are appropriate for gestational age, the proportion of polycythemic infants is greater in the SGA and LGA populations. Causes of increased hematocrit include (1) twin-twin transfusion, (2) maternal-fetal transfusion, (3) intrapartum transfusion from the placenta, associated with fetal distress, and (4) chronic intrauterine hypoxia (SGA infants, LGA infants of diabetic mothers).

The consequence of polycythemia is hyperviscosity, since the major factor influencing blood viscosity in infants is red cell mass. Hyperviscosity decreases effective perfusion of the capillary beds of the microcirculation. Clinical symptomatology can be related to any organ system (Table 2–24). Diagnostic screening can be done by measuring a capillary (heel stick) hematocrit. If the value is greater than 70%, a peripheral venous hematocrit should be measured. Values greater than 68% at less than 12 hours of age should be considered consistent with hyperviscosity. After 12 hours of age, values greater than 65% should be considered diagnostic.

Treatment for the acute symptoms is recommended for symptomatic infants. Treatment for asymptomatic infants based strictly on hematocrit is controversial. Definitive treatment is accomplished by an isovolemic partial exchange with 5% albumin.

Table 2–24. Organ-related symptoms of hyperviscosity.

Central nervous system	Irritability, jitteriness, seizures, lethargy
Cardiopulmonary	Respiratory distress, secondary to congestive heart failure, or persistent pulmonary hypertension
Gastrointestinal	Vomiting, heme-positive stools, distention, necrotizing enterocolitis
Renal	Decreased urinary output, renal vein thrombosis
Metabolic	Hypoglycemia
Hematologic	Hyperbilirubinemia, thrombocytopenia

The amount to exchange (in milliliters) is calculated using the following formula:

$$\frac{[\text{PVH (\%)} - \text{DH (\%)}] \times \text{BV (mL/kg)} \times \text{Wt (kg)}}{\text{PVH (\%)}}$$

where PVH = peripheral venous hematocrit, DH = desired hematocrit, BV = blood volume, and Wt = weight.

Blood is withdrawn at a steady rate from an umbilical venous line while the replacement solution is infused at the same rate through a peripheral intravenous line over 15–30 minutes. Desired hematocrit value is 50–55%; assumed blood volume is 80 mL/kg.

American Academy of Pediatrics Vitamin K Ad Hoc Task Force: Controversies concerning vitamin K and the newborn. Pediatrics 1993;91:1001.

Black VD et al: Neonatal hyperviscosity: Association with lower achievement and IQ scores at school age. Pediatrics 1989;83:662.

Burrows RF, Kelton JG: Perinatal thrombocytopenia. Clin Perinatol 1995;22:779.

Erslev AJ: Erythropoietin. N Engl J Med 1991;324:1339.

Gallagher PG, Ehrenkranz RA: Erythropoietin therapy for anemia of prematurity. Clin Perinatol 1993;20:167.

Greer FR: Vitamin K deficiency and hemorrhage in infancy. Clin Perinatol 1995;22:759.

Keyes WG et al: Assessing the need for transfusion of premature infants and role of hematocrit, clinical signs, and erythropoietin level. Pediatrics 1989;84:808.

Klebanoff MA et al: The risk of childhood cancer after neonatal exposure to vitamin K. N Engl J Med 1993;329:905.

Lane PA, Hathaway WE: Vitamin K in infancy. J Pediatr 1985;106:351.

Maier RF et al: The effect of epoietin beta (recombinant human erythropoietin) on the need for transfusion in very-low-birth-weight infants. N Engl J Med 1994; 330:1173.

Matsunaga AT, Lubin BH: Hemolytic anemia in the newborn. Clin Perinatol 1995;22:803.

Menell JS, Bussel JB: Antenatal management of the thrombocytopenias. Clin Perinatol 1994;21:591.

Pearson HA: Anemia in the newborn: A diagnostic approach and challenge. Semin Perinatol 1991;15(Suppl 2):2.

Shannon KM et al: Recombinant human erythropoietin stimulates erythropoiesis and reduces erythrocyte transfusions in very low birth weight preterm infants. Pediatrics 1995;95:1.

Soubasi V et al: Follow-up of very low birth weight infants after erythropoietin treatment to prevent anemia of prematurity. J Pediatr 1995;127:291.

Werner EJ: Neonatal polycythemia and hyperviscosity. Clin Perinatol 1995;22:561.

METABOLIC DISORDERS

HYPOGLYCEMIA

Glucose concentration in the fetus is approximately 15 mg/dL less than the maternal glucose concentration. Glucose concentration normally decreases in the immediate postnatal period, with concentrations below 35–40 mg/dL being considered indicative of hypoglycemia. By 3 hours of age, the glucose concentration in normal, term babies stabilizes between 50 and 80 mg/dL. After the first few hours of life, concentrations below 40 mg/dL should be considered abnormal.

The two most commonly encountered groups of newborn infants at high risk for neonatal hypoglycemia are infants of diabetic mothers (IDM) and infants with intrauterine growth retardation (IUGR).

Infant of a Diabetic Mother

The IDM baby represents an example of an infant with abundant glucose stores in the form of glycogen and fat who develops hypoglycemia because of an imbalance in insulin-glucagon secretion resulting from hyperinsulinemia from islet cell hyperplasia. In addition, there are other tissue sites that grow abnormally in utero, probably as a consequence of increased flow of nutrients (carbohydrates, amino acids, and fats) from the maternal circulation. The result is a macrosomic infant who is at increased risk for trauma (bruising, fractures, nerve root injuries, etc) during delivery. Other problems related to the in utero metabolic environment include a cardiomyopathy (asymmetric septal hypertrophy), which can present either as cardiac failure or as respiratory distress, and, more rarely, microcolon, which presents as a low intestinal obstruction. IDMs are also at increased risk for congenital anomalies likely related to first-trimester glucose control. Other neonatal problems include a hypercoagulable state and an increased risk for polycythemia, a combination that predisposes the infant to large venous thromboses (eg, renal vein thrombosis). Finally, these infants are somewhat immature for their gestational age and are at increased risk for hyaline membrane disease, hypocalcemia, and hyperbilirubinemia.

Intrauterine Growth Retardation

The infant with IUGR has very little carbon stores in the form of glycogen and body fat and therefore is prone to hypoglycemia despite relatively appropriate endocrine adjustments to birth. In addition to problems with hypoglycemia, marked hyperglycemia and a transient diabetes mellitus–like syndrome occasionally may develop, particularly in the very preterm

SGA infant. These problems can usually be handled by adjusting glucose intake, although insulin is sometimes needed transiently.

Other Causes of Hypoglycemia

Hypoglycemia can be found with other disorders associated with islet cell hyperplasia (Beckwith's syndrome [macroglossia, omphalocele, macrosomia], erythroblastosis fetalis, nesidioblastosis), inborn errors of metabolism (leucine sensitivity, glycogen storage disease, galactosemia), and endocrine disorders (panhypopituitarism, other deficiencies of counterregulatory hormones). It may also occur as a complication of birth asphyxia, hypoxia secondary to cardiorespiratory disease, or other stresses, including bacterial and viral sepsis.

Diagnosis

The signs of hypoglycemia in the newborn are relatively nonspecific and are usually quite mild, including lethargy, irritability, poor feeding, regurgitation, and jitteriness or tremulousness. More severe symptoms are cardiorespiratory distress, apnea, and seizures. One may find signs associated with catecholamine release, including pallor, sweating, cool extremities, and an increased heart rate. Cardiac failure has been found when hypoglycemia has been severe, particularly in IDM babies with a cardiomyopathy. Infants with hyperinsulinemic states can also experience the onset of hypoglycemia very early (within the first 30–60 minutes of life).

Glucose concentration can be measured by one of the commercially available screening techniques that rely on a test strip method done on a drop of peripheral blood obtained by heel stick. All infants at risk should be screened, including IDMs, SGA infants, premature infants, and any infant with symptoms that could be caused by hypoglycemia. All low or borderline values should be supplemented by direct measurement of blood glucose concentration determined with a glucose analyzer. There is far too great a variance in results obtained by the test strip methods to rely on these alone in following the high-risk groups. It is important to continue surveillance of glucose concentration until the baby has been on full milk feedings for a 24-hour period. Relapse of hypoglycemia thereafter is unlikely but possible, as milk feedings constitute a low-glucose, high-fat intake.

Infants with persistent hypoglycemia requiring intravenous glucose infusions for more than 5 days should be evaluated for less common causes of hypoglycemia. This workup should include evaluation for inborn errors of metabolism, hyperinsulinemic states, and deficiencies of counterregulatory hormones.

Treatment

Therapy is based on provision of glucose either enterally or intravenously. Suggested guidelines for treatment are presented in Table 2–25. It is important

Table 2–25. Hypoglycemia: suggested therapeutic regimens.

Screening Test	Presence of Symptoms	Action
Test strip 20–40 mg/dL	None	Draw blood glucose; if the infant is alert and vigorous, feed; follow with frequent test strips. If the baby continues to have test strips <40 mg/dL, provide IV glucose at 6 mg/kg/min (3.6 mL/kg/h).
Test strip <40 mg/dL	Present	Draw blood glucose; provide bolus of $D_{10}W$ (2 mL/kg) followed by an infusion of 6 mg/kg/min (3.6 mL/kg/h).
Test strip <20 mg/dL	None or present	Draw blood glucose; provide bolus of $D_{10}W$ followed by an infusion of 6 mg/kg/min. If IV access cannot be obtained immediately, an umbilical venous line should be utilized.

to note that in hyperinsulinemic states rapid boluses of glucose are to be avoided. After initial correction with a bolus of $D_{10}W$, 2 mL/kg, glucose infusion should be gradually increased as needed from a starting rate of 6 mg/kg/min. Finally, in both IDM and SGA babies, those with high hematocrits and hypoglycemia are most likely to show clinical signs of hypoglycemia. In such infants, both the hypoglycemia and polycythemia should be treated.

Prognosis

Prognosis of hypoglycemia is good if therapy is prompt. Central nervous system sequelae are seen in infants with neonatal seizures resulting from hypoglycemia.

HYPERGLYCEMIA

Hyperglycemia may develop in preterm infants, particularly those of very low birth weight who are also SGA. Glucose concentrations may exceed 200–250 mg/dL, particularly in the first few days of life. This transient diabetes-like syndrome usually lasts approximately 1–2 weeks. Management may include simply reducing glucose intake while continuing to provide supplemental calories with intravenous amino acids and lipids, coupled with small milk feedings by gavage. Insulin infusions intravenously have also been used to permit a larger intravenous glucose intake without hyperglycemia. This is usually reserved for those infants in whom it has not been possible to begin any gavage milk feedings and in whom caloric intake in the form of amino acids and lipids is small. However, this approach requires careful monitoring of blood glucose concentrations directly. The errors in estimation of blood sugar using screening techniques are far too large to avoid significant hypoglycemic episodes. Since the problem is a transient one, it is usually possible to maintain adequate intake with intermittent gavage feedings plus peripheral alimentation without resorting to intravenous insulin administration.

Hawdon JM et al: Prevention and management of neonatal hypoglycemia. Arch Dis Child 1994;70:F60.

Lucas A et al: Adverse neurodevelopmental outcome of moderate neonatal hypoglycemia. Br Med J 1988; 297:1304.

Ogata ES: Carbohydrate homeostasis. In: *Neonatology: Pathophsiology and Management of the Newborn,* 4th ed. Avery GB, Flatcher MR, MacDonald MG (editors). Lippincott, 1994.

Reece EA, Homko CJ: Infant of the diabetic mother. Semin Perinatol 1994;18:459.

Srinivasan G et al: Plasma glucose values in normal neonates: A new look. J Pediatr 1986;109:114.

HYPOCALCEMIA

Calcium concentration in the immediate newborn period decreases in all newborn infants. The concentration in fetal plasma is higher than that of the neonate or adult. *Hypocalcemia* is usually defined as a total serum concentration less than 7 mg/dL (equivalent to a calcium activity of 3.5 meq/L), although the physiologically active fraction, ionized calcium, should be measured whenever possible. Ionized calcium is usually normal even when total calcium is as low as 6–7 mg/dL. An ionized calcium of greater than 0.9 mmol/L (1.8 meq/L; 3.6 mg/dL) is not likely to be detrimental.

Diagnosis

The clinical signs of hypocalcemia and hypocalcemic tetany include a high-pitched cry, jitteriness, tremulousness, and seizures.

Hypocalcemia tends to occur at two different times in the neonatal period. Early-onset hypocalcemia occurs in the first 2 days of life and has been associated with prematurity, maternal diabetes, asphyxia, and, rarely, maternal hypoparathyroidism. Late-onset hypocalcemia occurs at approximately 7–10 days of age and is seen in infants receiving modified cow's milk rather than infant formula (high phosphorus intake) or in infants with hypoparathyroidism or hypomagnesemia. Mothers in third-world countries often suffer from vitamin D deficiency, which can also contribute to late-onset hypocalcemia.

Treatment

A. Oral Calcium Therapy: The oral administration of calcium salts is a preferred method of treatment for chronic forms of hypocalcemia resulting from hypoparathyroidism, but is rarely used in early-onset hypocalcemia. Calcium in the form of calcium gluconate can be either given as a dilute solution or added to formula feedings several times a day. A dose of 0.5–1 g/kg/d provides approximately 45–90 mg of elemental calcium per kilogram per day. If a 10% solution of calcium gluconate is used, the dose is 5–10 mL/kg/d given in divided doses every 4 or every 6 hours.

B. Intravenous Calcium Therapy: Intravenous calcium therapy is usually needed for infants with symptomatic hypocalcemia or an ionized calcium less than 0.9 mmol/L. A number of precautions must be observed when calcium gluconate is given intravenously. The infusion must be given slowly, so that there is no sudden increase in calcium concentration in blood entering the right atrium, which could cause severe bradycardia and even cardiac arrest. Furthermore, the infusion must be carefully observed, as an IV infiltrate containing calcium can cause full-thickness skin necrosis requiring grafting. For these reasons, IV calcium therapy should be given judiciously and through a central venous line if possible. Intravenous administration of 10% calcium gluconate is usually given as a bolus of 100–200 mg/kg over approximately 10–20 minutes, followed by a continuous infusion (0.5–1 g/kg/d) over 1–2 days. Ten percent calcium chloride (35–70 mg/kg per dose) may result in a larger increment in ionized calcium and greater improvement in mean arterial blood pressure in sick hypocalcemic infants and thus may have a role in the newborn. *Note:* Calcium salts cannot be added to intravenous solutions that contain sodium bicarbonate because they precipitate as calcium carbonate.

Prognosis

The prognosis is good for neonatal seizures entirely caused by hypocalcemia that is promptly treated.

Itani O, Tsang RC: Calcium, phosphorus, and magnesium in the newborn: Pathophysiology and management. In: *Neonatal Nutrition and Metabolism.* Hay WW (editor). Mosby, 1991.

Lynch RE: Ionized calcium: Pediatric perspective. Pediatr Clin North Am 1990;37:373.

Suleimam MY, Zaloga GP: How and when to manage ionized hypocalcemia in critically ill patients. J Crit Illness 1993;8:372.

INFANTS OF MOTHERS WHO ABUSE DRUGS

The problem of newborn infants born to mothers abusing drugs is increasing in all parts of the country. The most common forms of abuse include smoking, alcohol, marihuana, narcotic, and cocaine abuse. Because these mothers frequently abuse many drugs and the history of drug abuse is often unreliable, it is often difficult to pinpoint which drug may be causing the morbidity seen in a newborn infant. Finally, increasingly early hospital discharge makes discovery of these infants based on physical findings and behavior much more difficult.

NARCOTICS

Diagnosis

The withdrawal signs in infants born to mothers who are addicted to heroin or who have been on maintenance methadone programs are similar. The clinical findings in infants born to methadone-maintained mothers seem to be, if anything, more severe and prolonged. Clinical manifestations begin early, usually within the first day or two of life. Symptoms are quite characteristic: irritability and hyperactivity, increased tremors, a high-pitched cry, excessive hunger and salivation, sweating, yawning, sneezing, nasal stuffiness, fist sucking, temperature instability, and regurgitation. More severely affected infants may have seizures, vomiting, and diarrhea, as well as tachypnea. The infants are often small for gestational age. The clinical picture is typical enough to suggest a diagnosis even if a maternal history of drug abuse has not been obtained. Confirmation should be attempted with urine toxicology, but results will be negative unless the last drug dose was within a few days of delivery. Meconium can also be tested for illicit drugs. Since the substances accumulate throughout pregnancy, the number of positives is higher compared to urine testing. However, one cannot determine the timing or duration of exposure through meconium testing.

Treatment

Careful observation of the infant is a requirement. Supportive treatment includes swaddling the infant and providing a quiet, low-light environment. In general, specific treatment should be avoided unless the symptoms and morbidity in the infant warrant it. There is no single drug that has been uniformly effective, and the first choice varies among nurseries. The drugs that have been used include phenobarbital at an initial loading dose of 15–20 mg/kg intramus-

cularly, followed by a maintenance dose of 5 mg/kg/d in two divided doses usually given orally. Paregoric and diazepam have also been used, although these authors prefer phenobarbital because of its safety and predictability of effect. Phenobarbital blood levels should be obtained in the more severely affected infants to ensure that the concentration of the drug remains within the therapeutic range. The treatment can then be tapered over some days, although some treatment may be necessary for weeks following delivery. Both handling and procedures in the nursery should be kept to a minimum. As an alternative, methadone has been used, particularly in the babies born to methadone-maintained mothers.

Prognosis

These infants demonstrate long-term neurobehavioral handicaps. However, it is difficult to separate with certainty the effects of in utero drug exposure from environmental influences during upbringing. Infants of narcotic abusers have an increased risk of sudden infant death syndrome.

ALCOHOL

Diagnosis

The effects of alcohol on the fetus and the newborn are roughly proportionate to the degree of ethanol abuse. Fetal growth and development are adversely affected, and infants can suffer withdrawal similar to that caused by narcotic abuse. Features observed are shown in Table 2–26.

Prognosis

Children with full-blown fetal alcohol syndrome demonstrate postnatal growth deficiency and mild to moderate mental retardation. Those with lesser effects are at increased risk for attention-deficit disorder and subtle developmental delays.

TOBACCO SMOKING

Smoking has been shown to have an impact on the growth rate of the fetus. The more the mother smokes, the greater the degree of intrauterine growth retardation. More recently, smoking during pregnancy has been associated with mild neurodevelopmental handicap. However, it is important to recognize that multiple drug abuse applies to this category as well, and the potential interaction of multiple factors on fetal growth and development must be considered. It is important to recognize that multiple drug abuse applies to this category as well, and the potential interaction of multiple factors on fetal growth and development must be considered.

Table 2–26. Features observed in fetal alcohol syndrome and fetal alcohol effects.[1]

Growth
  Prenatal and postnatal growth deficiency[2]
  Decreased adipose tissue[3]

Performance
  Mental retardation[2]
  Developmental delay
  Fine-motor dysfunction
  Infant irritability,[2] child hyperactivity,[3] and poor attention span
  Speech problems
  Poor coordination, hypotonia[3]
  Cognitive, behavioral, and psychosocial problems

Craniofacial
  Microcephaly[2]
  Short palpebral fissures[2]
  Ptosis[4]
  Retrognathia in infancy[2]
  Maxillary hypoplasia[3]
  Hypoplastic long or smooth philtrum[2]
  Thin vermillion of upper lip[2]
  Short, upturned nose[3]
  Micrognathia in adolescence[3]

Skeletal
  Joint alterations, including camptodactyly, flexion contractures at elbows, congenital hip dislocations
  Foot position defects
  Radioulnar synostosis
  Tapering terminal phalanges, hypoplastic fingernails and toenails[5]
  Cervical spine abnormalities
  Altered palm crease patterns[4]
  Pectus excavatum[4]

Cardiac
  Ventricular septal defect[5]
  Atrial septal defect[4]
  Tetralogy of Fallot, great vessel anomalies[5]

Other
  Cleft lip and/or cleft palate[5]
  Myopia,[5] strabismus[4]
  Epicanthal folds[4]
  Dental malocclusion
  Hearing loss, protuberant ears
  Abnormal thoracic cage
  Strawberry hemangiomata[4]
  Hypoplastic labia majora[4]
  Micro-ophthalmia, blepharophimosis[5]
  Small teeth with faulty enamel[5]
  Hypospadias; small, rotated kidneys; hydronephrosis[5]
  Hirsutism in infancy[5]
  Hernias of diaphragm, umbilicus or groin, diastasis recti[5]

[1]Principal[2,3] and associated[4,5] features observed in 245 affected individuals. (Reproduced, with permission, from the American Academy of Pediatrics Committee on Substance Abuse: Fetal alcohol syndrome and fetal alcohol effects. Pediatrics 1993;91:1004.)
[2] >80% of patients.
[3] >50% of patients.
[4] 26–50% of patients.
[5] 1–25% of patients.

COCAINE

Cocaine abuse is a growing problem in medicine. Its use has increased greatly (10–20% on urban delivery services); moreover, cocaine is often used in association with other drugs. Prenatal cocaine exposure appears to be related to abruptio placenta, birth of small infants because of growth retardation and/or prematurity, and genitourinary malformations. Less certain associations include intestinal atresias, intraventricular hemorrhage, and cerebral infarcts. In high-risk populations, urine toxicology should be performed in mothers and infants. Analysis of meconium allows increased ascertainment by indicating drug use well prior to delivery.

As with other illegal drugs, cocaine seems to have long-term neurobehavioral effects, but multiple drug use and environmental factors preclude assigning specific effects to cocaine with certainty.

TOLUENE EMBRYOPATHY

Solvent abuse (via paint, lacquer, or glue sniffing) is a relatively common form of substance abuse. The active organic solvent in these agents is toluene. Features attributable to in utero toluene exposure include prematurity, intrauterine growth retardation, microcephaly, craniofacial abnormalities similar to that seen with in utero alcohol exposure, nail hypoplasia, and renal anomalies. Long-term effects include postnatal growth deficiency and developmental delay.

OTHER DRUGS

There are two categories under which drugs and their effects on the newborn should be considered. In the first category are drugs to which the fetus is exposed because of exposure to the mother. Many times, these are drugs prescribed for therapy of maternal conditions. The human placenta is relatively permeable, particularly to lipophilic solutes. Whenever possible, therapy should be postponed until after the first trimester. Drugs with potential fetal toxicity include antineoplastics, antithyroid agents, benzodiazepines, Coumadin, lithium, and immunosuppressants.

In the second category are drugs that the infant acquires from the mother during breast-feeding. Generally, most drugs taken by the mother either inadvertently or for therapy achieve appreciable concentrations in breast milk. In most instances, however, they do not present a problem to the infant. If the drug is one that could have adverse effects on the baby, timing breast-feeding to coincide with trough concentrations in the mother may be useful. The American Academy of Pediatrics statement (*Pe-*

diatrics 1994;93:137) reviews drugs contraindicated in the breast-feeding mother.

American Academy of Pediatrics Committee on Drugs: The transfer of drugs and other chemicals into human milk. Pediatrics 1994;93:137.

American Academy of Pediatrics Committee on Substance Abuse: Drug-exposed infants. Pediatrics 1995;96:364.

American Academy of Pediatrics Committee on Substance Abuse: Fetal alcohol syndrome and fetal alcohol effects. Pediatrics 1993;91:1004.

Brooks-Gunn J et al: Effects of in utero drug exposure on children's development. Arch Pediatr Adolesc Med 1994;148:33.

Chasnoff IJ (editor): Chemical dependency and pregnancy. Clin Perinatol 1991;18:1.

Clarren SK, Smith DW: The fetal alcohol syndrome. N Engl J Med 1978;298:1063.

Olds DL et al: Intellectual impairment in children of women who smoke cigarettes during pregnancy. Pediatrics 1994;93:221.

Pearson MA et al: Toluene embryopathy: Delineation of the phenotype and comparison with fetal alcohol syndrome. Pediatrics 1994;93:211.

Ryan RM et al: Meconium analysis for improved identification of infants exposed to cocaine in utero. J Pediatr 1994;125:435.

Singer LT et al: Increased incidence of intraventricular hemorrhage and developmental delay in cocaine-exposed, very low birth weight infants. J Pediatr 1994;124:765.

Zuckerman B, Frank DA: Prenatal cocaine exposure: Nine years later. J Pediatr 1994;124:731.

RENAL DISORDERS

Renal function is dependent on postconceptual age. The glomerular filtration rate (GFR) is 20 mL/min/1.73 m^2 in term neonates and 10–13 mL/min/1.73 m^2 in infants 28–30 weeks of gestation. The velocity of maturation after birth is also dependent on postconceptual age. Creatinine can be used as a clinical marker of GFR. Values over the first month of life are shown in Table 2–27. Creatinine at birth reflects the maternal level and should decrease slowly over the first 3–4 weeks. An increasing serum creatinine is never normal. The ability to concentrate urine and retain sodium is also dependent on gestational age. Infants less than 28–30 weeks of gestation are compromised in this respect and, if not observed carefully, can become dehydrated and hyponatremic. Preterm infants also have an increased bicarbonate excretion and have a low tubular maximum for glucose (approximately 120 mg/dL).

RENAL FAILURE

Renal failure is most commonly seen in the setting of birth asphyxia, hypovolemia, or shock from any cause. The normal rate of urine flow is 1–3 mL/kg/h. After a hypoxic or ischemic insult, acute tubular necrosis may ensue. Typically, there are 2–3 days of anuria or oliguria associated with hematuria, proteinuria, and a rise in serum creatinine. The period of anuria or oliguria is followed by a period of polyuria and then gradual recovery. During the polyuric phase, excessive urine sodium and bicarbonate losses may be seen. The initial step in management is restoration of the infant's volume status with colloid as needed. Then, restriction of fluids to insensible water loss (40–60 mL/kg/d) without added electrolytes, plus milliliter-for-milliliter urine replacement, should be instituted. Serum and urine electrolytes and body weights should be followed frequently. These measures should be continued through the polyuric phase. After urine output has been reestablished, urine replacement should be decreased to a ratio of between three-fourths and one-half milliliter for each milliliter of urine output to see if the infant has regained normal function. If so, the infant can be returned to maintenance fluids. Finally, many of these infants do experience fluid overload and should be allowed to diurese back to birth weight. Hyperkalemia, which may become life-threatening, may occur in this situation despite the lack of added intravenous potassium. If the serum potassium reaches 7–7.5, specific therapy (ie, sodium bicarbonate, 1–2 meq/kg infusion; glucose and insulin infusion, with 1 U of insulin for every 3 g of glucose adminstered; and binding resins) should be started. Calcium gluconate (100-mg/kg bolus) can also be helpful in the face of an arrhythmia resulting from hyperkalemia. Peritoneal dialysis is occasionally needed for the management of neonatal acute renal failure.

URINARY TRACT ANOMALIES

Abdominal masses in the newborn are most frequently caused by renal enlargement. Most common is a multicystic/dysplastic kidney; congenital hydronephrosis is second in frequency. Chromosomal abnormalities and syndromes with multiple anom-

Table 2–27. Normal values of serum creatinine (mg/dL).

Gestational Age at Birth (weeks)	Postnatal Age (d)	
	0–2	28
<28	1.2	0.7
29–32	1.1	0.6
33–36	1.1	0.45
33–42	0.8	0.3

alies frequently include renal abnormalities. An ultrasound examination is the first step in diagnosis. In pregnancies with oligohydramnios, renal agenesis or obstruction secondary to posterior urethral valves should be considered. Only bilateral disease or disease in a solitary kidney is associated with oligohydramnios, significant morbidity, and death. Such infants will generally also have pulmonary hypoplasia and die from pulmonary rather than renal insufficiency. The frequent use of prenatal ultrasonography identifies infants with renal anomalies (most often hydronephrosis) prior to birth. Postnatal evaluation of these infants should include a renal ultrasound scan and a voiding cystourethrogram. Until genitourinary reflux is ruled out, these infants should receive antibiotic prophylaxis.

RENAL VEIN THROMBOSIS

Renal vein thrombosis is seen most frequently in infants of diabetic mothers and in the context of dehydration and polycythemia. Of particular concern is the IDM infant, prone to hypercoagulability, who is also polycythemic. If fetal distress is superimposed on these problems, prompt reduction in blood viscosity is indicated. Thrombosis usually begins in intrarenal venules and can extend into larger veins. Clinically, there may be an enlarged kidney, with blood and protein in the urine. With bilateral renal vein thrombosis, anuria ensues. Diagnosis can be confirmed with an ultrasound examination of the kidneys. Treatment involves correcting the predisposing condition and systemic heparinization for the thrombosis. Prognosis is usually good with return of normal renal function. However, some infants will develop systemic hypertension.

Bueva A, Guignard J-P: Renal function in preterm neonates. Pediatr Res 1994;36:572.

Downing GJ et al: Kidney function in very low birth weight infants with furosemide-related renal calcifications at ages 1 to 2 years. J Pediatr 1992;120:599.

Fine RN: Diagnosis and treatment of fetal urinary tract abnormalities. J Pediatr 1992;121:333.

Gloor JM: Management of prenatally detected fetal hydronephrosis. Mayo Clin Proc 1995;70:145.

Karlowicz MG, Adelman RD: Acute renal failure in the neonate. Clin Perinatol 1992;19:139.

Schmidt B et al: Neonatal thrombotic disease: Prevention, diagnosis, and treatment. J Pediatr 1988;113:407.

Shackelford GD et al: Imaging the urinary tract. Clin Perinatol 1992;19:85.

BRAIN AND NEUROLOGIC DISORDERS

HYPOXIC-ISCHEMIC ENCEPHALOPATHY

The clinical correlate of perinatal oxygen deprivation is hypoxic-ischemic encephalopathy.

Diagnosis

Prenatal history, including abnormalities in antepartum testing, fetal distress with or without passage of meconium during labor, and low scalp pH (<7.15) are important in identifying infants at risk for hypoxic-ischemic encephalopathy. Apgar scores, the rapidity of the response of the infant to resuscitation, the amount of resuscitation needed, and cord acid-base status (pH <7.0) are other important features to note. Clinical features of hypoxic-ischemic encephalopathy progress over time:

(1) Birth to 12 hours: decreased level of consciousness, poor tone, decreased spontaneous movement, periodic breathing or apnea, and possible seizures.

(2) 12–24 hours: more seizures, apneic spells, jitteriness, and weakness.

(3) After 24 hours: decreased level of consciousness, further respiratory abnormalities (progressive apnea), onset of brain stem signs (oculomotor and pupillary disturbances), poor feeding, and hypotonia.

The severity of clinical signs and the length of time the signs persist correlate with the severity of the insult. Other evaluations helpful in assessing severity in the term infant include EEG, CT scan, and evoked responses. As experience in the use of magnetic resonance imaging is gained, this technique may also prove useful. Markedly abnormal EEGs with voltage suppression and slowing evolving into a burst-suppression pattern are seen with severe clinical symptomatology. A CT scan early in the course may demonstrate diffuse hypodensity, whereas later scans may demonstrate brain atrophy and focal ischemic lesions. Visual and somatosensory evoked potentials provide information about function. In most instances, it is not necessary to use all these tests, but some are obtained to confirm an ominous prognosis.

Treatment

The critical management issue in infants with hypoxic-ischemic encephalopathy is to maintain adequate delivery of oxygen to the already injured brain by supporting a normal PaO_2 and blood pressure. Glucose should be administered to maintain a normal serum glucose. Modest fluid restriction should be maintained to avoid exacerbating cerebral edema, and seizures should be controlled with phenobarbital and other anticonvulsants as needed. No other specific therapy (eg, steroids, osmotic agents) has been shown to be helpful in improving the outcome in hypoxic-ischemic encephalopathy. However, new therapies, including oxygen free radical inhibitors and scavengers, excitatory amino acid antagonists, and calcium channel blockers, are currently under investigation.

Prognosis

Fetal heart rate tracings, cord pH, and 1-minute and 5-minute Apgar scores are not very precise predictors of long-term outcome. Apgar scores of 0–3 at 5 minutes in term infants result in an 8% risk of death in the first year of life and a 1% risk of cerebral palsy among survivors. A 10-minute Apgar of 0–3 predicts death in the first year in 18% of cases and cerebral palsy among survivors in 5%; at 15 minutes, 48% and 9%, respectively; at 20 minutes, 59% and 57%, respectively. The single best predictor of outcome is the severity of clinical hypoxic-ischemic encephalopathy (severe symptomatology carries a 75% chance of death and 100% rate of neurologic sequelae among survivors). The major sequela of hypoxic-ischemic encephalopathy is cerebral palsy with or without associated mental retardation and epilepsy. Other prognostic features include prolonged seizures refractory to therapy, markedly abnormal EEGs, and CT scans with evidence of major ischemic injury.

INTRACRANIAL HEMORRHAGE

1. SUBDURAL HEMORRHAGE

Subdural hemorrhage is related to birth trauma; the bleeding is caused by tears in the veins that bridge the subdural space. Prospective studies relating incidence to specific obstetric complications are not available.

The most common site of subdural bleeding is rupture of superficial cerebral veins with blood over the cerebral convexities. These hemorrhages can be asymptomatic or cause seizures with onset on days 2–3 of life, vomiting, irritability, and lethargy. Associated findings include retinal hemorrhages and a full fontanelle. Diagnosis is confirmed by CT scan. Specific treatment entailing needle drainage of the subdural space is rarely necessary. Most infants survive, with 75% normal on follow-up.

2. PRIMARY SUBARACHNOID HEMORRHAGE

Primary subarachnoid hemorrhage is the most common type of neonatal intracranial hemorrhage. In the term infant, it can be related to trauma of delivery, whereas subarachnoid hemorrhage in the preterm infant is seen in association with germinal matrix hemorrhage. Clinically, these hemorrhages can be asymptomatic or present with seizures and irritability on day 2 or, rarely, a massive hemorrhage with rapid downhill course. The seizures associated with subarachnoid hemorrhage are very characteristic—usually brief, with a normal examination interictally. Diagnosis can be suspected on a spinal tap and confirmed with CT scan. Long-term follow-up is uniformly good.

3. PERIVENTRICULAR-INTRAVENTRICULAR HEMORRHAGE

Periventricular-intraventricular hemorrhage is a lesion seen almost exclusively in premature infants. The incidence is 20–30% in infants of less than 31 weeks of gestation and 1500 g. Bleeding is most commonly seen in the subependymal germinal matrix (a region of undifferentiated cells). Bleeding can extend into the ventricular cavity. The proposed pathogenesis of bleeding is presented in Figure 2–6. The critical event is likely ischemia/reperfusion injury to the capillaries in the germinal matrix that occurs in the immediate perinatal period. The actual amount of bleeding is also influenced by a variety of factors that affect the pressure gradient across the injured capillary wall. This pathogenetic scheme also applies to intraparenchymal bleeding (venous infarction in a region rendered ischemic) and periventricular leukomalacia (ischemic white matter injury in a watershed region of arterial supply).

Diagnosis

Up to 50% of hemorrhages occur at less than 24 hours of age, and virtually all occur by the fourth day. The clinical syndrome ranges from rapid deterioration (coma, hypoventilation, decerebrate posturing, fixed pupils, bulging fontanelle, hypotension, acidosis, acute drop in hematocrit) to a more gradual deterioration with more subtle neurologic changes to absence of any specific physiologic or neurologic signs.

Diagnosis can be confirmed by real-time ultrasound scan. This can be performed whenever bleeding is clinically suspected. If symptoms are absent, routine scanning should be done at 4–7 days in all infants of less than 31 weeks of gestation or in more mature infants in whom bleeding is suspected. Hemorrhages are graded as follows: (1) grade I—germinal matrix hemorrhage only, (2) grade II—intraventricular bleeding without ventricular enlargement, (3) grade III—intraventricular bleeding with ventricular enlargement, and (4) grade IV—any infant with intraparenchymal bleeding. The amount of bleeding is minor (grade I or II) in 75% of infants and major in 25% of infants who suffer from this complication.

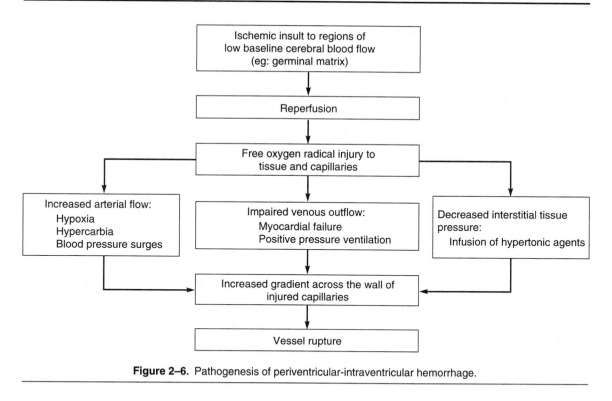

Figure 2–6. Pathogenesis of periventricular-intraventricular hemorrhage.

Follow-up ultrasound examinations are based on the results of the initial scan. Infants with no bleeding or germinal matrix hemorrhage require only a single late scan at 4–6 weeks of age to look for periventricular leukomalacia. Any infant with blood in the ventricular system is at risk for posthemorrhagic ventriculomegaly. Most commonly, this is the result of impaired absorption of cerebrospinal fluid, but can also occur secondary to obstructive phenomena. An initial follow-up scan should be done at 2 weeks of age. Those infants with intraventricular bleeding and ventricular enlargement should be followed up serially every 7–10 days until ventricular enlargement stabilizes or decreases. Infants without ventriculomegaly should have one additional scan at 4–6 weeks.

Treatment

During the acute hemorrhage, supportive treatment—restoration of volume and hematocrit, oxygenation, and ventilation—should be provided to avoid further cerebral ischemia. Progressive posthemorrhagic hydrocephalus (if it develops) can sometimes be controlled by decreasing the production of cerebrospinal fluid (furosemide 1 mg/kg/d, plus acetazolamide, increasing doses from 25–100 mg/kg/d) or by removal of cerebrospinal fluid (daily lumbar punctures). The process is usually self-limited and spontaneously resolves; the placement of a ventriculoperitoneal shunt is usually not needed.

Early treatment with medications or serial spinal taps does not appear to alter the incidence of ultimately needing a shunt, but may contribute to an improved long-term neurologic outcome.

The incidence of periventricular-intraventricular hemorrhage has progressively declined since the late 1970s. In addition, there has been a shift in severity toward less severe forms.

Improved obstetric and neonatal care resulting in less asphyxia, improved fluid management, and improved ventilator therapy have clearly had an important role in this trend. Postnatal administration of vitamin E or indomethacin has shown some effect in decreasing the incidence and, to a lesser extent, the severity of periventricular-intraventricular hemorrhage. However, since this entity is likely a perinatal event, antenatal therapies should be a more effective approach than agents given postnatally. Both corticosteroids and phenobarbital given prior to birth have demonstrated efficacy in decreasing the incidence and severity of periventricular-intraventricular hemorrhage.

Prognosis

There is no mortality as a result of grade I and II hemorrhages, whereas grade III and IV hemorrhages carry a mortality rate of 10–20%. Ventriculomegaly is rarely seen with grade I hemorrhages but is seen in 54–87% of grade II–IV hemorrhages. Very few of these infants will require a ventriculoperitoneal shunt. Long-term neurologic sequelae are seen no more frequently in infants with grade I and II hemorrhages than in preterm infants without bleeding. In infants with grade III and IV hemorrhages, severe sequelae occur in 20–25% of cases, mild sequelae in 35% of cases, and no sequelae in 40% of cases. The presence of severe periventricular leukomalacia, large parenchymal bleeds, and progressive ventriculomegaly greatly increases the risk of neurologic sequelae.

SEIZURES

Newborns rarely have well-organized tonic-clonic seizures because of their incomplete cortical organization and a preponderance of inhibitory synapses. The most common type of seizure is characterized by a constellation of findings, including horizontal deviation of the eyes with or without jerking; eyelid blinking or fluttering; sucking, smacking, drooling, and other oral-buccal movements; swimming, rowing, or paddling movements; and apneic spells. Strictly tonic or multifocal clonic episodes are also seen.

Table 2–28. Differential diagnosis of neonatal seizures.

Diagnosis	Comment
Hypoxic-ischemic encephalopathy	Most common cause (60%) onset in first 24 h
Intracranial hemorrhage	Up to 15% of cases, periventricular-intraventricular hemorrhage, subdural or subarachnoid bleeding
Infection	12% of cases
Hypoglycemia	Small for gestational age, infant of a diabetic mother (IDM)
Hypocalcemia, hypomagnesemia	Infant of low birth weight, IDM
Hyponatremia	Rare, seen with syndrome of inappropriate secretion of antidiuretic hormone (SIADH)
Disorders of amino and organic acid metabolism, hyperammonemia	Associated acidosis, altered level of consciousness
Pyridoxine dependency	Seizures refractory to routine therapy; cessation of seizures after administration of pyridoxine
Developmental defects	Other anomalies, chromosomal syndromes
Drug withdrawal	
No cause found	10% of cases

Diagnosis

Differential diagnosis of neonatal seizures is presented in Table 2–28. Information regarding antenatal drug use and the presence of birth asphyxia or trauma and family history (regarding inherited disorders) should be obtained. Physical examination focuses on neurologic features, other signs of drug withdrawal, concurrent signs of infection, dysmorphic features, and intrauterine growth. Screening workup should include blood glucose, ionized calcium, and electrolytes in all cases. Further workup is dependent on diagnoses suggested by the history and physical examination. If there is any suspicion of infection, a spinal tap should be done. Hemorrhages and structural disease of the central nervous system can be addressed with real-time ultrasound and CT scan. Metabolic workup should be pursued when appropriate. EEG should be done; the presence of spike discharges must be noted and the background wave pattern evaluated.

Treatment

Adequate ventilation and perfusion should be ensured. Hypoglycemia should be treated immediately with a 2 mL/kg infusion of $D_{10}W$, followed by 6 mg/kg/min of $D_{10}W$ (100 mL/kg/d). Other treatments, such as calcium or magnesium infusion and antibiotics, are indicated to treat hypocalcemia, hypomagnesemia, and suspected infection. Electrolyte abnormalities should be corrected. Phenobarbital, 20 mg/kg intravenously, should be administered to stop seizures. Supplemental doses of 5 mg/kg can be used if seizures persist, up to a total of 40 mg/kg. In most cases, phenobarbital controls seizures. If seizures continue, therapy with phenytoin, sodium valproate, or lorazepam may be indicated. For refractory seizures, a trial of pyridoxine is indicated.

Prognosis

Outcome is related to the underlying cause of the seizure. The outcomes for hypoxic-ischemic encephalopathy and intracranial hemorrhage have been discussed. In these settings, seizures that are difficult to control carry a poor prognosis for normal development. Seizures resulting from hypoglycemia, infection of the central nervous system, some inborn errors of metabolism, and developmental defects also have a high rate of poor outcome. Seizures caused by hypocalcemia or isolated subarachnoid hemorrhage generally resolve without sequelae.

Abdel-Rahman A, Rosenberg AA: Prevention of intraventricular hemorrhage in the premature infant. Clin Perinatol 1994;21:505.

Batton DG et al: Current gestational age–related incidence of major intraventricular hemorrhage. J Pediatr 1994;125:623.

Bernes SM, Kaplan AM: Evolution of neonatal seizures. Pediatr Clin North Am 1994;41:1069.

Fish WH et al: Effects of intramuscular vitamin E on mortality and intracranial hemorrhage in neonates of 1000 grams or less. Pediatrics 1990;85:578.

Freeman JM, Nelson KB: Intrapartum asphyxia and cerebral palsy. Pediatrics 1988;82:240.

Kaempf JW et al: Antenatal phenobarbital for the prevention of periventricular and intraventricular hemorrhage: A double-blind, randomized, placebo-controlled, multi-hospital trial. J Pediatr 1990;117:933.

Kuban KCK, Leviton A: Cerebral palsy. N Engl J Med 1994;330:188.

Leviton A et al: Antenatal corticosteroids appear to reduce the risk of postnatal germinal matrix hemorrhage in intubated low birth weight newborns. Pediatrics 1993; 91:1083.

Low JA et al: Newborn complications after intrapartum asphyxia with metabolic acidosis in the term fetus. Am J Obstet Gynecol 1994;170:1081.

Low JA et al: Newborn complications after intrapartum asphyxia with metabolic acidosis in the preterm fetus. Am J Obstet Gynecol 1995;172:805.

Ment LR et al: Low-dose indomethacin and prevention of intraventricular hemorrhage: A multicenter randomized trial. Pediatrics 1994;93:543.

Ment LR et al: Antenatal steroids, delivery mode, and intraventricular hemorrhage in preterm infants. Am J Obstet Gynecol 1995;172:795.

Nelson KB, Emery ES III: Birth asphyxia and the neonatal brain: What do we know and when do we know it? Clin Perinatol 1993;20:327.

Novotny EJ: Neonatal seizures. Semin Perinatol 1993; 17:351.

Palmer C, Vannucci RC: Potential new therapies for perinatal cerebral hypoxia-ischemia. Clin Perinatol 1993; 20:411.

Papile LA et al: Incidence and evaluation of subependymal and intraventricular hemorrhage: A study of infants with birth weights less than 1500 grams. J Pediatr 1978;92:529.

Philip AGS et al: Intraventricular hemorrhage in preterm infants: Declining incidence in the 1980's. Pediatrics 1989;84:797.

Robertson CMT, Finer NN: Long-term follow-up of term neonates with perinatal asphyxia. Clin Perinatol 1993;20:483.

Rogers B et al: Cystic periventricular leukomalacia and type of cerebral palsy in preterm infants. J Pediatr 1994;125:S1.

Scheller JM, Nelson KB: Does cesarean delivery prevent cerebral palsy or other neurologic problems of childhood? Obstet Gynecol 1994;83:624.

Vannucci RC et al: Carbon dioxide protects the perinatal brain from hypoxic-ischemic damage: An experimental study in the immature rat. Pediatrics 1995;95:868.

Volpe JJ: Neonatal seizures: Current concepts and revised classification. Pediatrics 1989;84:422.

CONGENITAL ANOMALIES

Major congenital malformations are seen in 1.5% of live births and account for 22% of perinatal deaths, 18% of stillbirths, and 27% of neonatal deaths. This topic is discussed in detail in Chapter 32.

The individual **inborn errors of metabolism** are rare, but collectively all such disorders create significant clinical problems. The diseases are considered in detail in Chapter 31, but the diagnoses should be entertained in infants that present with sepsis-like syndromes, recurrent hypoglycemia, neurologic syndromes (seizures, altered levels of consciousness), and unexplained acidosis.

Burton BK et al: Inborn errors of metabolism: The clinical diagnosis in early infancy. Pediatrics 1987;79:359.

Czeizel AE: Prevention of congenital abnormalities by periconceptional multivitamin supplementation. Br Med J 1993;306:1645.

Goodman SI, Greene CL: Inborn errors as causes of acute disease in infancy. Semin Perinatol 1991;15(Suppl 1):31.

Graham JM Jr (editor): Fetal clinical genetics. Clin Perinatol 1990;17:4.

Graham JM Jr (editor): Fetal dysmorphology. Clin Perinatol 1990;17:3.

Graham JM: Clinical approach to human structural defects. Semin Perinatol 1991;15(Suppl 1):2.

Jones KL (editor): *Smith's Recognizable Patterns of Human Malformation,* 4th ed. Saunders, 1988.

Lie RT et al: A population-based study of the risk of recurrence of birth defects. N Engl J Med 1994;331:1.

Maestri NE et al: Prospective treatment of urea cycle disorders. J Pediatr 1991;119:923.

REFERENCES

American Academy of Pediatrics: *Guidelines for Perinatal Care,* 3rd ed. American Academy of Pediatrics, 1992.

Avery GB, Fletcher MA, MacDonald MG (editors): *Neonatology: Pathophysiology and Management of the Newborn,* 4th ed. Lippincott, 1994.

Ballard RA (editor): *Pediatric Care of the ICN Graduate.* Saunders, 1988.

Boynton BR, Carlo WA, Jobe AH (editors): *New Therapies for Neonatal Respiratory Failure.* Cambridge Univ Press, 1994.

Briggs GG et al (editors): *Drugs in Pregnancy and Lactation,* 4th ed. Williams & Wilkins, 1994.

Gabbe SG, Niebyl JR, Simpson JL (editors): *Obstetrics: Normal and Problem Pregnancies,* 3rd ed. Churchill Livingstone, 1996.

Goldsmith JP, Karotkin EH (editors): *Assisted Ventilation of the Neonate,* 3rd ed. Saunders, 1996.

Jones KL (editor): *Smith's Recognizable Patterns of Human Malformation,* 4th ed. Saunders, 1988.

Jones MD Jr, Gleason CA, Lipstein SN (editors): *Hospital Care of the Recovering NICU Infant.* Williams & Wilkins, 1991.

Klaus MH, Fanaroff AA (editors): *Care of the High-Risk Neonate,* 4th ed. Saunders, 1993.

Long WA (editor): *Fetal and Neonatal Cardiology.* Saunders, 1990.

Remington JS, Klein JO (editors): *Infectious Diseases of the Fetus and Newborn Infant,* 4th ed. Saunders, 1995.

Tsang RC et al (editors): *Nutritional Needs of the Preterm Infant.* Williams & Wilkins, 1993.

Volpe JJ (editor): *Neurology of the Newborn,* 3rd ed. Saunders, 1995.

Young TE, Mangum OB (editors): *Neofax 95. A Manual of Drugs Used in Neonatal Care,* 8th ed. Ross Laboratories, 1995.

Behavioral Disorders & Developmental Variations

3

Edward Godson, MD

Behavioral disorders and concerns about variations in behavior encompass a wide range of issues concerning the growth and development of children. Most recently, disorders and variations in behavior and development have emerged as significant problems in pediatric practice. Most of the issues discussed below are not new to the practitioner. However, with increasing knowledge of neurologic and behavioral organization of children, newer concepts of these disorders are evolving, and different approaches to diagnosis and management are emerging.

The prevailing view of variations in behavior is that they reflect a blend of intrinsic biologic characteristics of the child and the environment with which the child interacts. This chapter first reviews behavior and temperament. It then focuses on those variations in development which frequently are of concern to parents. The discussion is organized in the following manner: colic, feeding disorders, nonepileptic paroxysmal events, sleep disturbances, and temper tantrums and associated behaviors.

Greydanus DE, Wolraich ML (editors): *Behavioral Pediatrics.* Springer, 1992.
Jenkins S et al: Continuities of common behaviour problems in preschool children. J Child Psychol Psychiatry 1984;25:75.

NORMALITY & TEMPERAMENT

In considering each of the behaviors listed above, one is immediately confronted by what is considered "normal." What is the relationship between the parent and the child? What are the parents' expectations, and what does the child bring, intrinsically, to this relationship? Critical to understanding these behaviors is an understanding of what is meant by *normal* and an understanding of childhood temperament. The physician confronted by a disturbance in physiologic function is usually able to define what is normal from a physiologic viewpoint and what is clearly abnormal. In contrast, such an all-or-none, yes/no approach is counterproductive in dealing with the prob-

lems we are concerned with in this chapter. By labeling many of these behaviors as "disorders," we imply *abnormality* and so may give rise to a behavior disorder where none previously existed. The approach of this chapter is to view the behaviors described here as encompassing a continuum of responses by the child to a variety of internal and external experiences.

The goal, for example, is not to "cure" crying or nightmares (once underlying disease has been excluded) but rather to help the parent and child understand what is wrong and to facilitate a functional approach to management in the specific context in which crying or nightmares occur. In other words, the approach should be to adjust to the child as the child adapts to his or her environment and to avoid pharmacologic management whenever possible.

An associated phenomenon to be considered when addressing variations in behavior is **temperament.** The concept of temperament has been of interest to philosophers and writers since ancient times. The Greeks proposed four temperament types: choleric, sanguine, melancholic, and phlegmatic. In more recent times, accepted folk wisdom defined *temperament* as being a genetically influenced behavioral disposition that is stable over time. Although there are a number of proposed models of temperament, the one usually used by pediatricians in clinical practice is the model developed by Thomas and Chess.

Thomas & Chess Model

Thomas and Chess describe temperament as being the "how" of behavior, as distinguished from motivation, the "why," and the abilities, the "what," of behavior. Temperament is an independent psychologic attribute that is expressed as a response to some external stimulus and must always be considered in terms of the social context in which it is expressed. Moreover, the influence of temperament is bidirectional—that is, the effect of a particular experience will be influenced by the child's temperament, and the child's temperament will affect the responses of those in the child's environment. Temperament is therefore the style with which the child interacts with the environment.

Since the Thomas and Chess model is an interactive one, the perceptions and expectations of parents must always be taken into consideration when a child is evaluated. A child that one parent might describe as being hyperactive would not be so for another parent. This can be expanded to include all the temperament dimensions. Thus, the concept of "goodness of fit" comes into play. For example, if the parents want and expect their child to be predictable and that is not the child's temperament (behavioral style), what emerges is a lack of "goodness of fit" and a potential source of tension. This may be expressed as the parents' perceiving the child as being "bad" or having a "behavioral disorder" rather than as a variation of development that must be addressed in terms of both the child and the child's environment. An appreciation of this phenomenon is important, because the physician may be able to enhance the parents' understanding of the child and beneficially influence their responses to the child's behavior. When there is a "goodness of fit," there will be less tension and stress, more harmony, and the potential for enhanced development not only of the child but also for the family. When there is not a "goodness of fit," the stage is set for tension and stress that can result in parental anger, disappointment, and frustration and conflict with the child.

The other models of temperament are more frequently used in child development research. These include the work of Rothbart, Buss and Plomin, and Goldsmith and Campos (Table 3–1). It is important to recognize that all seek to identify those characteristics in the child's behavior that are intrinsic to the child and lead him or her to respond to the world in a unique manner. One child may be highly emotional, another less so ("calmer") in response to a variety of stressful or pleasant experiences. One child may be perceived as being hyperactive by one parent but not by the other. One child may tolerate change easily, while another has great difficulty in adapting to change. One child may tolerate discomfort more easily than another. One child may be sociable, whereas another may be more retiring and reticent. What is important for the clinician is to recognize that each child brings some intrinsic, biologically based traits to his environment and that they are neither good nor bad, right nor wrong, normal nor abnormal. Instead, they are part of the child and must be recognized and respected as such. Thus, as one looks at variations in development, one should move away from the illness model and consider this construct as a means of understanding the nature of the child's behavior and its influence on the parent-child relationship.

Barr RG: Normality—A clinically useless concept: The case of infant crying and colic. J Dev Behav Pediatr 1993;14:264.

Goldsmith HH et al: Roundtable: What is temperament? Four approaches. Child Dev 1987;58:505.

Prior M: Childhood temperament. J Child Psychol Psychiatry 1992;33:249.

Thomas A, Chess S: *Temperament and Development.* Brunner/Mazel, 1977.

COMMON DEVELOPMENTAL CONCERNS

COLIC

The "syndrome" of colic is described as severe and paroxysmal crying that occurs mainly in the late afternoon. The infant's knees are abducted to the abdomen, with expulsion of flatus, the abdomen is distended, the facies "pained," the fists clenched, and there is minimal response to attempts at soothing. Among the difficulties for all concerned is the definition of this variation from normal behavior, its cause, and its treatment. Much of the problem lies in the name itself. The word *colic* is derived from Greek *kolikos* ("pertaining to the colon"). Thus, while colic has been attributed to a disturbance of the gastrointestinal tract, this has never been proved. Colic is a behavioral sign or symptom that begins in the first few weeks of life and usually peaks at 2 or 3 months. However, in about 30–40% of cases, colic continues into the fourth and fifth months.

Crying is considered a normal phenomenon of infancy and is present in all racial and ethnic groups around the world. Studies in the United States have reported that among most middle-class infants, crying increases in duration until 6 weeks of age and

Table 3–1. Theories of temperament.

Thomas and Chess	Temperament is an independent psychologic attribute, biologically determined, which is expressed as a response to an external stimulus. It is the child's behavioral style: an interactive model.
Rothbart	Temperament is a a function of biologically based individual differences in reactivity and self-regulation. It is subsumed under the concept of "personality" and goes beyond mere "behavioral style."
Buss and Plomin	Temperament is a set of genetically determined personality traits that appear early in life and are different from other inherited and acquired personality traits.
Goldsmith and Campos	Temperament is the individual's differences in the probability of experiencing emotions and arousal.

gradually declines at about 4 months to baseline. At about 2 weeks of age, crying lasts an average of about 2 hours per day, increases to about 3 hours per day by 6 weeks, and gradually decreases to about 1 hour per day by 3 months. It is noted that normal crying can be modulated somewhat by a sensitive caretaker's intervention.

Excessive crying—or colic—in the absence of any physical disorder has a similar pattern, but the duration and intensity of crying are more prolonged. The most common definition of colic is the one used by Wessel: a colicky infant is one who is healthy and well fed but cries for more than 3 hours a day, for more than 3 days a week, and for more than 3 weeks—commonly referred to as the "rule of threes." A "healthy child" is the operative concept. The infant with colic has no definable physiologic disorder. Thus, before the "diagnosis" of colic can be made, the pediatrician needs to rule out diseases that might be causing the symptom.

Among the myriad suggested causes of colic are intolerance to cow's milk proteins, intestinal gas, gastrointestinal motility, immaturity of the gastrointestinal and neurologic systems, or the caretaker's style of feeding. With the exception of the relatively few infants who respond to elimination of cow's milk from the infant's or the mother's diet, there has been little firm evidence of an association with gastrointestinal disorders. There have been pharmacologic attempts to eliminate gas with simethicone and to slow gut motility with the use of dicyclomine. Simethicone has not been shown to ameliorate the behavior. Dicyclomine has been associated with apnea in infants and is contraindicated.

This then leaves characteristics intrinsic to the child, such as temperament, and parental caretaking patterns as contributing to colic. Behavioral states have three features: (1) they are self-organizing— that is, they are maintained until it is necessary to shift to another one; (2) they are stable over several minutes; and (3) the same stimulus elicits a state-specific response that is different from other states. There is a crying state, a quiet alert state, an active alert state, a transitional state, and a state of deep sleep, among others. The states of importance with respect to colic are the crying state and transitional states. During transition from one state to another, infant behavior may be more easily influenced. Once an infant is in a stable state (ie, crying), it becomes more difficult to bring about a change (ie, soothe). How these transitions are accomplished is probably influenced by the infant's temperament as well as his neurologic maturity. Some infants move from one state to another easily and can be easily diverted; other infants sustain a particular state and may be resistant to change.

The other component that needs to be considered with the colicky infant is the feeding and handling behavior of the caretaker. Colic is a behavioral phenomenon that involves interaction between the infant and the caretaker. Different caretakers perceive, interpret, and respond to crying behavior differently. If the caretaker perceives the crying infant as being spoiled and demanding and is not sensitive or knowledgeable of the infant's cues and rhythms, or is hurried, or is somewhat "rough" with the baby, the infant's ability to organize himself, soothe himself, or respond to the caretaker's attempts at soothing may be compromised. On the other hand, if the temperament of an infant with colic is understood and the rhythms and cues can be deciphered, the crying can be anticipated and the caretaker should be able to intervene appropriately before the behavior becomes "organized" in the crying state and more difficult to extinguish.

Management

There are a number of approaches that can be taken toward management of the infant with colic.

(1) The parent needs to be educated about the normal developmental characteristics of crying behavior and made aware that crying increases normally into the second month and abates usually by the third to fourth months.

(2) The pediatrician needs to reassure the parent, after having taken a complete history and performed a physical examination, that the infant is not "sick." Although these behaviors are stressful, they are a normal variant of crying and are usually self-limited. This discussion can be facilitated by having the parent keep a diary of crying and weight gain. If there is a diurnal pattern and adequate weight gain, an underlying disease process is less likely to be present. Parental anxiety must be relieved, as it may be a factor contributing to the problem.

(3) For the parents to be able to soothe and comfort the infant, they need to learn and interpret the baby's cues. The pediatrician can be helpful in this process while observing and monitoring the infant's behavior and devising interventions aimed at calming both the infant and the parents. The clinician can suggest changes in the parents' behavior to include creation of a quiet environment without excessive handling. Rhythmic stimulation such as a gentle swing or gentle rocking, music, drives in the car, or walks in the stroller may be particularly helpful, especially if the parents are able to anticipate the onset of the crying before it becomes fixed. Another approach is to change the feeding technique so that the infant is not rushed, has ample opportunity to burp, and, if necessary, to be fed more frequently so as to decrease gastric distention if that seems to be contributing to the problem.

(4) In the past, medications such as phenobarbital elixir and dicyclomine have been used and found to be somewhat helpful. Presently, however, they have been discontinued.

(5) For colicky babies refractory to behavioral

management, a trial of changing the feedings by eliminating cow's milk from the formula or from the mother's diet if she is nursing may be indicated.

Barr RG: Colic and gas. In: *Pediatric Gastrointestinal Disease: Pathophysiology, Diagnosis, and Management.* Walker WA et al (editors). BC Decker, 1991.

Barr RG, Geertsma MA: Colic: The pain perplex. In: *Pain in Infants, Children and Adolescents.* Schechter NL, Berde CB, Yaster M (editors). Williams & Wilkins, 1993.

Carey WB: "Colic": Primary excessive crying as an infant-environmental interaction. Pediatr Clin North Am 1984;31:993.

Miller AR, Barr RG: Infantile colic: Is it a gut issue? Pediatr Clin North Am 1991;38:1407.

FEEDING DISORDERS

This cluster of behaviors occurs in two forms: overeating, leading to obesity; and undereating, leading to inadequate weight gain. Eating disorders are not uncommon in adolescents, in whom one may encounter marked obesity or anorexia nervosa and bulimia. Concerns about poor feeding and failure to gain weight in infants and young children are also among the more common complaints brought to the pediatrician. A healthy-appearing infant who is well nourished is a source of pride to most parents and in our society is the mark of good parenting. The focus of this section will be on the infant who does not eat. Eating disorders of adolescence are covered elsewhere.

The reasons that children have feeding problems are varied. The common denominator, however, is usually food refusal. Infants and young children may refuse to eat because they find eating aversive (eg, it hurts or is frightening); they may have had unpleasant experiences (emotional or physiologic) associated with eating; they may be depressed; or they may be engaged in a developmental conflict with their caretaker which is being played out in the arena of feeding. The child—more commonly the infant—may also refuse to eat if the rhythm of the feeding experience with the caretaker is not harmonious.

The child who has had an esophageal atresia repair and has a stricture—or even a mild narrowing of the esophagus—may find eating uncomfortable or even painful. The very young infant with severe oral candidiasis will refuse to eat because it hurts. The child who has had a choking experience associated with feeding may be terrified to eat (oral motor dysfunction or aspiration). The child who is forced to eat by a maltreating parent or an overzealous caretaker may come to refuse feeds, as may the child who is threatened. The child who may have tasted foods that he or she does not like or which were associated with some discomfort will refuse to eat those foods or foods in general.

Children who are depressed express this psychologic state in a variety of ways, one of which may be through food refusal. Food refusal may develop when the infant's cues around feeding are not correctly interpreted by the parent. The baby who needs to burp more frequently or the one who needs time between bites, but instead is rushed, will often passively refuse to eat. On the other hand, some will be more active refusers and will turn their heads away to avoid the feeder, may spit out food, or push food away.

Chatoor and coworkers have adopted a developmental and interactive view of the feeding experience. They consider the various stages through which the child normally progresses: establishment of homeostasis (0–2 months), attachment (2–6 months), and separation and individuation (6 months to 3 years). During the establishment of homeostasis, feeding can be most easily accomplished when the parent allows the infant to determine the timing, amount, pacing, and preference of food intake. During the attachment phase, allowing the infant to control the feeding permits the parent to effectively engage the infant in a positive manner. This provides the basis for the separation and individuation phase.

When there is a disturbance in the parent-child relationship at any of these developmental levels, there may ensue difficulty in feeding, with both the parent and the child contributing to the dysfunctional interaction. One of the most striking manifestations of food refusal occurs during the stage of separation and individuation. If the parent seeks to impose his or her will on the child through intrusive and controlling feeding behavior while at the same time the child is striving to achieve autonomy, conflict may arise. The scenario then observed is of the parent forcing food on the child while the child refuses to eat. This often leads to extreme parental frustration and anger at the child. At the same time, the child may be inadequately nourished and developmentally and emotionally thwarted.

When the pediatrician is attempting to sort out the factors contributing to the complaint of food refusal (feeding disorder), it is essential to obtain a complete history, including a social history. This should include information concerning the parents' perception of the child's behaviors and their expectations of the child. Second, a complete physical examination needs to be performed, with considerable emphasis on oral-motor behavior and the pursuit of other findings suggesting neurologic dysfunction or anatomic or physiologic abnormality that could make feeding difficult. As part of this evaluation, the child's emotional state and developmental level must be determined. This is particularly important if there is concern about depression or if there is a history of developmental delays. If there is evidence for these disturbances, a more complete behavioral evaluation needs to be obtained. If there is evidence for oral-motor difficulty, evaluation by an occupational thera-pist is warranted. Third, the feeding interaction needs to be observed. Finally, the physician needs to help the parent understand that in the face of a normal ex-amination, infants and children may indeed have dif-ferent styles of eating and food preferences and may refuse foods they do not like. This is not necessarily abnormal but rather reflects temperamental differ-ences and variations in the child's way of processing olfactory, gustatory, and tactile stimuli.

Management

The goal of intervention is to identify factors con-tributing to the disturbance and to work with the par-ent and child to alter the circumstances leading to the difficulty. This may mean that the parents must learn to view the child's behavior differently and not im-pose their expectations and desires on an unwilling child. On the other hand, the child's behavior may need to be modified in order for the parent to be able to appropriately nourish and nurture the baby.

When the chief complaint is failure to gain weight or failure to thrive, a somewhat different approach should be taken. A child who is failing to gain weight is one whose weight is falling across the percentile curves of weight by 2 SD or who has a persistent de-viation below the expected or established weight curve. The differential diagnosis should include food refusal as contributing to the problem but also must take into consideration medical disturbances and is-sues of maltreatment. The essential reason children do not gain weight is that they are not being ade-quately nourished for whatever reason. They may have excessive losses as a result of vomiting or diar-rhea; they may not be given adequate food, or the amount they receive may not meet their physiologic needs; or they may not be efficiently utilizing the nu-trients they are receiving. Failure to gain weight is usually the result of a combination of several of these factors. As with the case of the food-refusing child, a complete history and physical examination must be performed. A comprehensive psychosocial and de-velopmental history should be obtained along with observation of the feeding experience.

Basic laboratory studies include a complete blood count, erythrocyte sedimentation rate, urinalysis and urine culture, blood urea nitrogen, serum electrolytes and creatinine, and stool for ova and parasites and to look for evidence of malabsorption. Some practition-ers also include liver and thyroid profiles.

Recognizing that the cause of failure to gain weight is multifactorial, the approach toward diagno-sis and treatment needs to be broad-based and multi-disciplinary. Because of its complexity, no one disci-pline has sufficient skills to comprehensively evaluate the child and family. Thus, a team should be used that consists of a physician, a nurse, a social worker, and a dietitian as well as occupational and physical therapists, developmentalists, and psycholo-gists as required. In this way, a diagnosis can be ar-rived at and a comprehensive treatment and monitor-ing plan can be developed.

The overall goals for the management of the child with poor weight gain are to establish a normal pat-tern of weight gain and to facilitate improved family functioning. Guidelines to accomplishing these goals include the following:

(1) Establishing a comprehensive diagnosis that considers all the factors contributing to the poor weight gain.

(2) Monitoring the feeding interaction and assur-ing appropriate weight gain.

(3) Monitoring the developmental progress of the child and changes in the family dynamics that facili-tate optimal weight gain and psychosocial develop-ment.

(4) Provision of support to the family as they seek to help the child.

Frank D, Zeisel SH: Failure to thrive. Pediatr Clin North Am 1988;35:1187.
Goldbloom RR: Failure to thrive. Pediatr Clin North Am 1982;29:151.
Macht J: *Poor Eaters.* Plenum, 1990.
Stevenson RD: Failure to thrive. In: *Behavioral Pediatrics.* Greydanus DE, Wolraich ML (editors). Springer, 1992.

SLEEP DISORDERS

It is estimated that 20–30% of children experience sleep problems severe enough to cause concern to their families. These problems are usually divided into three groups: (1) night-time attacks (parasom-nias), (2) sleeplessness (insomnias or dyssomnias), and (3) excessive sleepiness during the day. We will discuss parasomnias and dyssomnias here. Research and clinical experience during the last 3 decades have added greatly to our understanding of sleep problems, many of which can be explained in terms of the physiology of sleep and individual circadian rhythms. Sleep is a complex physiologic process that is influenced by intrinsic biologic properties, individ-ual temperamental characteristics, cultural norms and expectations, and environmental conditions.

Normal sleep is made up of two cycling, distinctly different states that have been identified clinically and with the use of **polysomnography,** which con-sists of electroencephalography, electro-oculography, and electromyelography. The two states are rapid eye movement (REM) sleep and non–rapid eye move-ment (NREM) sleep. REM sleep is a very active state physiologically and mentally and is characterized by both deep and light sleep. Muscle tone is reduced, al-though the sleeper may twitch and grimace. The reg-ulation of temperature, blood pressure, heart rate, and respirations has increased variability, whereas higher cortical functions appear active. Dreaming is closely associated with REM sleep. REM cycles last about 90 minutes at intervals during the night but are most frequent during the latter half of the night.

NREM sleep is what we think of as sleep and is divided into four stages. In the process of falling asleep, the individual enters stage 1, light sleep, which is characterized by reduced bodily movements, eye rolling, and sometimes opening and closing of the eyelids. Stage 2 sleep is characterized by slowing of eye movements, slowing of respirations and heart rate, and weakening of the muscles but with repositioning of the body. Some dreaming may occur in this stage. Most mature sleepers spend about half of their sleeping time in this stage. Stages 3 and 4 (also called delta or slow-wave sleep) are similar. They are the deepest NREM sleep stages, during which the sleeper's body is relaxed, breathing is slow and shallow, and the heart rate is slow. Night-time sleep consists of repeated alternating episodes of NREM and REM sleep.

The onset of sleep occurs when the individual enters NREM stage 1 sleep. The individual then progresses to NREM stage 2 and on to NREM stages 3 and 4. The deepest NREM sleep occurs during the first 1–3 hours after going to sleep, with transitions to NREM stage 2 sleep and brief awakenings. REM and NREM stage 2 sleep cycles occur during the latter part of the night and are also interspersed with brief awakenings. The importance of understanding these patterns is that during NREM deep sleep, parasomnias occur; and during REM sleep, dreaming and nightmares occur.

1. PARASOMNIAS

Parasomnias are undesirable physical night-time attacks that are disorders of arousal from deep NREM sleep. Of all the sleep disorders, they are probably the most frightening for parents. The parasomnias include night terrors (pavor nocturnus), sleepwalking (somnambulism), nocturnal seizures, and nightmares.

Night terrors commonly occur within 2 hours after falling asleep, during the deepest stage of NREM sleep, and are often associated with sleepwalking. They are reported in about 3% of children. During a night terror, the child may sit up in bed screaming and thrashing about, with rapid breathing, tachycardia, and sweating. The child often has a glazed look in his eyes and is essentially incoherent. During the episode, the child seems not to be helped by, and may even resist, parental attempts at comforting. The attack may last for several minutes to half an hour, after which the child goes back to sleep and has no memory of the event the next day. It is critical for parents to be reassured that the child is not in pain and that they should let the episode run its course. However, there is an association between fatigue and emotional and psychosocial stress. Therefore, maintaining adequate sleep and decreasing daytime stresses become critical. In this context, behavioral approaches have been found to be most helpful. Although the condition is benign, treatment is important, first to allay parents' fears and second to prevent sleepwalking, which can result in injury. The parents should determine when the episode usually occurs and awaken the child to full arousal about 15 minutes before that time. After 4–5 minutes, the child is allowed to return to sleep. The waking is discontinued once the terrors stop, which, in most circumstances, is within a week. It should be remembered that sleepwalking can occur independently of night terrors and is another disorder of arousal. Under all of these conditions, the parents need to create an environment such that the child will not endanger himself or others. In the most severe cases, pharmacologic interventions have been used, but only on a temporary basis. Dahl suggests 25–50 mg of imipramine at bedtime as a window for more longlasting behavioral approaches which are used to increase the total amount of sleep, to identify the causes of sleep disruption, and to address the sources of anxiety and stress.

Nightmares, in contrast to night terrors, are frightening dreams that typically are followed by awakening and occur during REM sleep, usually in the latter part of the night. The peak occurrence is in the age group from 3 to 5 years, with an incidence between 25% and 50%. A child who awakens during these episodes is usually alert. He or she often can describe the frightening images, recall the dream, and talk about it during the day. The child seeks and will respond positively to parental reassurance. Moreover, the child will often have difficulty going back to sleep and will want to stay with the parents. By and large, nightmares are self-limited and need little treatment. However, if the child has recurrent nightmares, the pediatrician may have to make a more extensive investigation. Nightmares are often associated with stressful or frightening daytime events or anxieties that may include frightening television programs, traumatic life events, and chronic stresses in the family such as discord between the mother and father. These may need to be addressed if the child is to be helped. In more severe cases, a psychologist or psychiatrist may need to be consulted.

2. DYSSOMNIAS

The second group of disturbances includes the insomnias or dyssomnias, namely, problems of going to sleep and night-time awakenings. While the parasomnias are frightening to most parents, the dyssomnias tend to be annoying and frustrating. Among other things, they can result in daytime fatigue of both the parents and the child, parental discord about management, and family disruption. There are a number of factors that contribute to disturbances of sleep. First, there is the influence of infant feeding. The quantity and timing of feeds in the first years of life will influence night-time awakening. Most infants beyond 6 months of age can go through the night without being fed. Thus, it must be considered that, under normal circumstances, night waking for feeds is a learned behavior and is a function of the child's arousal and the parents' response to that arousal. Second, co-sleeping can play a role in night waking. In many cultures, co-sleeping is an accepted behavior. However, when it intrudes on the parents' rest and their sexual relationship, it can be a problem. Third, child-rearing approaches and the practices by which bedtime is initiated can influence settling in for the night as well as awakening and staying awake at night. If the child learns that going to sleep is always associated with a pleasant parental behavior such as rocking, singing, or nursing, if and when he or she arouses at night and the parent is not available, going back to sleep can be difficult. Fourth, the child's temperament is another factor contributing to sleep. It has been reported that children with low sensory thresholds and less rhythmicity are more prone to night waking. Fifth, children who have had perinatal difficulties have a greater incidence of night waking and difficulties returning to sleep. Finally, psychosocial stressors can play a role in night waking.

Management

There are a variety of approaches to the management of children with dyssomnias, but there is general agreement that it is not acceptable to allow the child to "cry it out." Basic to all the strategies is obtaining a detailed sleep history and diary to which both parents contribute. Problems often arise when parents try to get the child to sleep at a time when the child is not biologically ready for sleep. For example, a child put down too early will lie awake and cry (late sleep phase), or the parents may wait too long, resulting in crankiness and early awakening and disrupted nap times (early sleep phase). Second, a complete medical and psychosocial history should be obtained and a physical examination performed. If these data do not provide adequate information, some clinicians use polysomnography for diagnostic purposes.

A helpful developmental approach to management of these sleep difficulties is suggested by Largo (see references for other approaches). He advocates that the child's individual sleep behavior characteristics have to be taken into account and parental expectations and fears need to be identified and addressed. Counseling is then provided on the following premises:

(1) Sleep is a highly active and organized process that matures during the first years of life. One-week-old infants sleep about 16½ hours a day, with 10 of those hours being at night, whereas a 2-year-old sleeps a total of 13 hours a day, with only 1 of those hours being during the day.

(2) Individual circadian rhythms do not change immediately and require consistency and regularity over a period of time before change will occur.

(3) The duration of sleep for a given individual does not vary significantly, but there are large variations among different children.

(4) The duration of night-time sleep is negatively correlated with daytime sleep, and bedtimes and awakening times are positively correlated with each other.

(5) Night waking occurs in 40–60% of infants and young children. If the child does not cry or wake up the parents, such behavior should not be considered a sleep disturbance.

In working with parents, it is important to point out unrealistic expectations with regard to sleep behavior and identify and seek to correct inconsistencies in parental behavior around sleep. The inadvertent behaviors that parents use to reinforce the undesired sleep and waking behavior need to be identified and the parents educated. Parents need to set distinct limits for the child while acknowledging the child's individual biologic rhythms. At the same time, they need to be sure not to get caught up in the child's attempts to prolong bedtime or his attempts to engage them during night-time awakenings. Putting a child to bed after prolonged rocking, feeding, or when the child has already fallen asleep frequently results in disturbances of settling down at night or going back to sleep after a night-time awakening. The establishment of clear bedtime rituals, placing the child in bed before he is asleep, and creating a quiet, secure bedtime environment are essential if sleep problems are to be avoided and can also be used in treating them if they arise.

For the child who has a delayed sleep phase—difficulty in both falling asleep and waking at desired times but no difficulty at later times—a regular schedule and consistent, nonstimulating bedtime rituals must be provided. Approaches used to alter the child's behavior include having the parents withdraw the attention elicited by the wakeful child and by positive reinforcement of the desired behavior. Another strategy to alter this sleep pattern is to gradually move the bedtime hour up and awaken the child earlier in the morning. However, it must be remembered that there is nothing intrinsically normal or abnormal in this pattern. It only becomes a problem when it differs from what the parents want.

Some children are afraid to go to sleep. The parent needs to help the child identify what is frightening about going to sleep and may need to stay near the child as he goes to sleep, reassuring him that he is safe and that mommy and daddy will not let anything happen to him. Over a period of time, the child can be reassured and the parent may not need to be so involved. This also applies to night-time awakenings.

The key to management of children who have difficulty going to sleep or who awaken during the night and disturb others is to recognize that both the child and the parent play significant roles in initiating and sustaining what may be an undesirable behavior. Thus, it becomes important for the physician and parents to understand normal sleep patterns, the parents' responses that inadvertently reinforce undesirable sleep behavior, and the child's individual temperament traits.

Adair RH, Bauchner H: Sleep problems in childhood. Curr Probl Pediatr 1993;23:147.

Dahl RE: The pharmacologic treatment of sleep disorders. Psychiatr Clin North Am 1992;15:161.

Ferber R: Sleeplessness, night awakening, and night crying in the infant and toddler. Pediatr Rev 1987;9:69.

Lozoff B, Zuckerman B: Sleep problems in children. Pediatr Rev 1988;10:17.

Mahowald MW, Rosen GM: Parasomnias in children. Pediatrician 1990;17:21.

Richman N: Recent progress in understanding and treatment of sleep disorders. Adv Dev Behav Pediatr 1986;7:45.

Sladkin K, Brown LW: Sleep disorders in children and adolescents. In: *Behavioral Pediatrics.* Greydanus DE, Wolraich ML (editors). Springer, 1992.

TEMPER TANTRUMS & BREATH-HOLDING SPELLS

1. TEMPER TANTRUMS

Temper tantrums as an expression of anger and frustration are common between 12 months and 4 years of age, occurring about once a week in 50–80% of children in this age group. The behavior is characterized by the child lying or throwing himself down, kicking and screaming, on occasion throwing things or hitting, and occasionally holding his breath. These behaviors can usually be considered normal as the young child seeks to achieve mastery over his environment and autonomy in his actions. They are often a reflection of immaturity as the child strives to accomplish age-appropriate developmental tasks and meets with difficulty because of a lack of fine and gross motor skills, language development, impulsiveness, or restrictions placed by the parents. In the home, these behaviors can be annoying for parents, but they can be managed. In public, they serve as an embarrassment.

It is not clear why some children have tantrums whereas others do not. Under normal circumstances, this is probably related to the child's temperament. Some children tolerate frustration well, are able to persevere at tasks, and cope with difficulties relatively easily; others have a much greater problem dealing with experiences they may not understand and are still too immature to cope with. Tantrums can

be minimized with an understanding of the child's temperament and what the child is trying to communicate as well as a commitment to supporting the child's drive to master his feelings. Appropriate intervention can also provide an opportunity for enhancing the child's growth. It should be remembered that the tantrum is a loss of control on the child's part and a blow to the self-image, which is frightening for the child. Therefore, the parent and the physician need to view these behaviors within the child's developmental context rather than from a negative, adversarial, angry viewpoint.

Management

Several suggestions can be offered for parents and physicians in managing these normal responses to frustrations and anger:

(1) Minimize the need to say "no" by "child-proofing" the environment such that fewer restrictions need to be placed on the child and thus there is less chance for conflict to arise.

(2) Use distraction when frustration increases, direct the child to other, less frustrating activities, and reward the child's positive response.

(3) Present choices and options within the limits of what is acceptable so that the child does have a chance to practice mastery and autonomy.

(4) Fight only those battles that clearly need to be won and avoid those that set up an unnecessary conflict that may serve no significant purpose and may create more problems.

(5) Do not abandon the preschool child when a tantrum occurs, and stay in close proximity during the episode without intruding. At times, the child may need to be contained in order to gain control, and the parent should be willing and able to help. For the older child, suggest that the child go to his or her room until he or she settles down. No threats or arguments should be used, since they serve no purpose.

(6) Do not use negative terms when the tantrum is occurring. Instead, point out that the child is out of control and give praise when he or she regains control.

(7) Never let a child hurt himself or others.

(8) Do not "hold a grudge" after the tantrum is over. However, the child's demands leading to the tantrum should not be granted.

(9) Seek to maintain an environment that provides positive reinforcement for desired behavior. Do not overreact to undesired behavior, but set reasonable limits and provide responsible direction for the child.

Approximately 5–20% of young children have severe temper tantrums that go beyond what is considered normal. Tantrums become a problem that must be dealt with when they are very frequent and disrupt the family or when the child uses them as more than an expression of frustration. Such tantrums are often the result of a disturbance in the parent-child interaction. They may have their origin in poor parenting skills, with a lack of limit-setting and permissiveness, or may be part of a larger behavioral or developmental disorder. They may also emerge under adverse socioeconomic conditions, in circumstances of maternal depression and family dysfunction, or when the child is in poor health. The pediatrician can serve an important role by helping the parents identify the underlying conditions leading to the behavioral outburst and by acknowledging the parents' feelings of anger, shame, and frustration. The parents can then help develop strategies to extinguish the behavior. If there are significant disturbances in the family, referral to a psychologist or psychiatrist is appropriate while the pediatrician continues to support and work with the family.

2. BREATH-HOLDING SPELLS

While temper tantrums can be frustrating and annoying to parents, breath-holding spells can be terrifying. DiMario maintains that the name for this behavior is a misnomer in that it connotes volitional behavior resulting in prolonged inspiration. Instead, it occurs during expiration and is reflexive in nature. This is a paroxysmal event occurring in 0.1–5% of healthy children aged 6 months to 6 years. The spells usually start during the first year of life, often in response to anger or a mild injury. The child is provoked, starts to cry—briefly or for a considerable time—and then becomes noiseless. This is followed by a color change. Spells have been described as either pallid (acyanotic) or cyanotic, with the latter usually associated with anger and the former usually with an injury such as a fall. Following the period of noiselessness, the spell may resolve or the child may lose consciousness or, in severe cases, may become limp and progress to opisthotonos and body jerks and urinary incontinence. Only rarely does a spell proceed to asystole or a seizure.

For the child with frequent spells, disorders such as seizures, orthostatic hypotension, obstructive sleep apnea, abnormalities of the central nervous system, tumors, familial dysautonomia, and Rett's syndrome need to be considered. There is also an association between breath-holding spells, pica, and iron deficiency anemia. These conditions can be ruled out on the basis of the history, the physical examination, and appropriate laboratory studies. Once it has been determined that the child is essentially healthy, the primary form of treatment is for the pediatrician to reassure the parents that the problem will spontaneously resolve with time. There are no prophylactic medications. However, atropine, 0.01 mg/kg per dose, has been used to prevent spells accompanied by bradycardia or asystole.

Thus, the focus of treatment is behavioral. Parents should be taught to handle the spells in a matter-of-fact manner and monitor the child for any untoward events. The reality is that parents cannot completely protect their child from upsetting and frustrating events and probably should not try to do so. Instead, as in the case of temper tantrums, parents need to help the child control responses to frustrating and difficult events, using some of the techniques previously described. Moreover, they need to be careful not to be too permissive and submit to the child's every whim for fear the child might have a "spell." Such behavior can hamper the child's emotional and cognitive development and may be harmful to the parent-child relationship. If a syncopal event should occur, the child should be placed in a lateral, supine position to protect his head from injury and to avoid aspiration. Cardiopulmonary resuscitation should be avoided, although maintaining a patent oral airway is essential.

DiMario FJ Jr: Breath-holding spells in childhood. Am J Dis Child 1992;146:125.

Needlman R, Howard B, Zuckerman B: Temper tantrums: When to worry. Contemp Pediatr 1989;6:12.

Needlman R, Stevenson J, Zuckerman B: Psychosocial correlates of severe temper tantrums. J Dev Behav Pediatr 1991;12:77.

SUMMARY

This chapter has focused on several of the more common complaints about behavior encountered by those who care for children. It is important to understand that these behavioral "disorders" are, by and large, normal variations in behavior. They are a reflection of each child's individual biologic and temperament traits and the parental response to these characteristics as they are behaviorally expressed. The health provider should recognize there are no "cures" but that there are strategies that can enhance the parental understanding of the child and his or her relationship to the environment. Thus, diagnosis and management of these conditions require a comprehensive and often transdisciplinary approach. The health provider can play a major role in diagnosis and, when possible, in coordinating the child's evaluation, interpreting the results to the family, and providing reassurance and ongoing support.

4

Developmental Disorders

Bonnie W. Camp, MD, PhD, & Elizabeth B. Kozleski, EdD

This chapter considers problems in development of cognitive and social competence. Competence is usually defined by comparing performance levels of an individual child with some norm derived from evaluating many children of the same age. Other standards of competence include comparison of the child's performance level with that of the adult norm and comparison of the child's present skills with skills needed to accomplish a given task or engage in a specific activity. Functional problems of children with mental retardation are discussed in this chapter; however, the main emphasis is on the larger group of children with learning and behavior problems that may or may not be associated with mental retardation.

Measurement of developmental competence is patterned on concepts of measuring intelligence. Although there is continued controversy over the extent to which heredity and environment determine intelligence, assessment of competence can be more usefully discussed independently of this issue. Assessment of competence hinges on the recognition that (1) children are able to perform increasingly more complex and difficult tasks as they get older; and (2) when tested at ages fairly close together, individual children tend to have a similar standing in relation to other children from one age to the next. By evaluating a child's performance on a variety of tasks requiring skills such as reasoning, abstract thinking, judgment, and planning and by determining how the child compares with other children of the same age, it is usually possible to predict school performance. Such assessments provide the basis for deriving an intelligence quotient and also may have implications for social behavior.

Measures of intelligence may be thought of as measures of general competence that attempt to determine what a child has learned in the process of exposure to an environment that provides unsystematic opportunities for learning that are grossly similar within a given culture. Anything that limits the breadth, variety, and depth of exposure or the ability of a child to profit from such exposure may place limits on the learning a given child will achieve in a given period. Anything that increases systematic exposure or increases breadth, variety, and depth of exposure potentially enhances learning.

Both biologic and psychosocial factors can increase or interfere with the growth-promoting effect of a child's performance. Assessment of a child's general developmental or intellectual standing relative to other children sheds no light on the cause of the child's performance; consequently, it is important to determine whether an intelligence test gives a representative estimate of the child's usual functioning and whether other information might provide an explanation for low scores. Differences in experiential background often account for low scores of children from nondominant cultures given standard intelligence tests. Such explanations, however, do not necessarily alter the predictive value of scores from intelligence tests.

A variety of delays or deficiencies in the development of specific cognitive competence have also been identified and may or may not be associated with deficiencies in general competence. The most significant of these are associated with failure to acquire basic academic skills such as reading, writing, and arithmetic. Specific measures of competence are usually measures of achievement in areas where systematic instruction has been given (eg, music lessons, arithmetic lessons). Here again, both biologic and psychosocial factors (eg, "musical talent," "math aptitude") may facilitate or interfere with development of competence in these specific areas. Measures of relative standing in specific areas of achievement correlate well with measures of intelligence. This correlation provides the basis for determining a child's expected level of achievement, whereas the discrepancy between expected and actual levels of achievement is a key factor for differential diagnosis in children with developmental problems.

Traditionally, social and emotional aspects of development have not been conceptualized as a dimension of competence. However, it is increasingly recognized that social competence is an important concept for assessing some aspects of social and emotional development. This is particularly true for aspects of behavior and social interaction such as empathy, distractibility, activity level, and aggression, which show strong, regular progression with age and which are associated with what has traditionally been termed cognitive development.

The Role of Special Education

Federal law mandates that all children with disabilities, ages 3–21, are entitled to a free and appropriate public school education. Federal funding assists local educational agencies in meeting the specifics of the law. Although educational opportunities for persons with some types of disabilities have been available in this country for over 100 years, it was not until the passage of PL 94-142 in 1975 that all children with disabilities were guaranteed access to a free and appropriate public school education. In 1990, this bill was reauthorized and renamed as the Individuals With Disabilities Education Act (IDEA). Under this law, special education students are to receive an education based on a curriculum that can be modified and adapted to meet their unique needs. These needs are presumed to vary based on student age, preferences, ethnicity, family values, learning characteristics, physical capabilities, student motivation, and the demands of subsequent environments in which the student will be expected to perform. IDEA incorporates seven key elements: (1) access to free and appropriate public education, (2) individualization of the educational experience, (3) the right to be educated in the least restrictive environment, (4) the provision of related services, (5) guidelines for the determination of a disability, (6) protection of student and parent rights, and (7) the principles of state and local responsibilities (Overton, 1992). Under IDEA, students may receive one of the following labels: specific learning disability, seriously emotionally disturbed, deaf, deaf-blind, hard of hearing, mentally retarded, multi-handicapped, orthopedically impaired, other health impaired, speech impaired, or visually handicapped.

The due process component of the law allows parents to participate in and to challenge educational decisions made regarding their children. Multidisciplinary teams of professionals along with parents are required to determine placement in programs and to determine the types and amounts of educational services. Within the identification and assessment component, local school districts have developed policies and procedures that result in services such as Child Find, prereferral building level teams, multidisciplinary assessments, and staffings. In general, children tend to be overreferred for assessment and staffing into special education at the elementary level and underreferred at the secondary level.

Child Find, mandated by PL 94-142, requires that each district locate and assess all children and other young people from birth through age 21 who may have a disability. Child Find is typically implemented as an outreach program both within the school and in the community. Advertisements in local media encourage parents of children with perceived problems to come to local screening clinics. As a result of the screening, some children are referred for full assessments. If, as a result of a complete assessment, a multidisciplinary team concludes that the child has a disability according to federal and state guidelines and the child is age 3–21, services deemed necessary by the team must be provided by the local school system even if the child is enrolled in a private school.

Passage of PL 99-457

PL 99-457, passed in 1986, extends all rights and protections of PL 94-142 to children with disabilities through age 5 (Widerstrom, Mowder, and Sandall, 1991). This law has embraced the notion of families as a focus of intervention rather than children alone (eg, the development of an individualized educational plan [IEP] that includes a family component). Rather than focus on the child, an IFSP (individualized family service plan) has been mandated that places an emphasis on working with the family's needs rather than developing a treatment plan for the child only. Since this bill was passed, much attention has been paid to family involvement and the development of integrated preschool programs. Furthermore, this law has encouraged school systems to focus on early intervention.

Overton T: *Assessment in Special Education: An Applied Approach.* Macmillan, 1992.
Widerstrom AH, Mowder BA, Sandall S: *At Risk and Handicapped Newborns and Infants: Developmental Assessment and Intervention.* Prentice-Hall, 1991.

GENERAL PRINCIPLES IN EVALUATING COGNITIVE & SOCIAL COMPETENCE

Developmental evaluation should include (1) data that demonstrate a child's level of cognitive and social competence in both general and specific areas, (2) data that will assist in making an etiologic diagnosis, and (3) data relevant to management planning. An interdisciplinary team is often employed to develop the database and a plan for management; this is the most thorough and effective approach. In addition to the pediatrician, the team usually includes a psychologist, social worker, educational specialist, and speech and language specialist. Assistance is also often needed from health care specialists in nursing, physical therapy, occupational therapy, ophthalmology, audiology, nutrition, and dentistry. Where an organized, functioning team is not available, the primary care physician can achieve similar results by requesting consultations from various professionals and obtaining information from other sources such as school personnel. It is also possible for the primary care physician to develop the minimal database needed for initial assessment with only limited reliance on outside sources. The following discussion presents suggestions to assist the primary care physician in developing this database through use of questionnaires and screening tests when assistance from other professionals is limited or unavailable.

History

A. Medical History: The medical history should focus on aspects of pregnancy, labor, and delivery that are likely to produce damage to the child's central nervous system (eg, use of drugs or x-rays during pregnancy; neonatal infections, asphyxia, elevated bilirubin levels). Later evidence of central nervous system insults or injury, failure to thrive, chronic illnesses, hospitalizations, or abuse may also contribute significantly to a child's performance at school age. Neonatal records are often an important source of information, since they may reveal information forgotten by or unknown to parents. Recent studies have focused on ways of combining psychosocial information about families from birth certificates to assess the risk for later problems in development.

B. Developmental History: The developmental history should include information about the age at which various milestones were passed, especially those pertaining to speech and language. Inability to use meaningful words other than "dada," "mama," "bye-bye," and "hello" by 18 months and inability to speak in short phrases by 24 months have been reported in association with specific learning disability as well as general slow learning and mental retardation. Development of motor skills is also important, particularly in assessing mental retardation, but deviance or delay in motor development may also be present in other conditions such as cerebral palsy and neuromuscular disorders. Information about sleep patterns, problems of temperament such as excessive crying or hyperactivity, and general problems may also be helpful.

C. Family History: Specific information regarding central nervous system disorders, mental retardation, epilepsy, or evidence of school problems or specific learning disabilities in other family members should be included. Details of the mother's pregnancy history, including stillbirths, deaths, and other problems, may also be helpful.

D. Educational & Learning History: In preschool children, considerable information can be obtained from a description of something the child has learned in an informal setting. If the child has been placed in a formal preschool setting, information should be obtained regarding the type of preschool and the child's relationships with other children and with teachers. Teachers can often give an excellent description of the child's performance and behavior in the classroom environment, and such assessments, even in the preschool period, are often as good as tests in predicting later problems.

After a child has reached school age, the educational history should include details of grade placement, special education evaluations and placement, repetition of grades, and other details of academic performance and participation in special programs. Most school systems routinely test students at specific grade levels using standardized group-administered tests. These tests, which are typically administered to whole classes in the spring of the academic year, measure academic progress in reading, math, science, and social studies. Student performance is then compared with a representative sample of peers across the country who are enrolled at the same grade. Achievement scores are reported in terms of grade level attainment. For example, a 3.2 grade level means that a student is working at the third grade, second month level in a particular curriculum area. Achievement scores may also be reported as percentiles, where a student's performance is measured against other students of the same age or grade level. As a hypothetical example, suppose that Eric earned a percentile of 50. This means that 50% of the students of the same age or grade level as Eric who took the same test scored at or below Eric's score. Thus, percentile scores show only the student's performance relative to other students who took the same test. Usually, percentiles are based on the performance of a large number of students representing a national sample. When using percentiles, it is critical to make sure that the student in question is similar to those students in the standardization sample.

Although group-administered, standardized tests measure student skills in academic areas, they are rarely of great value in determining a student's specific areas of academic strength and weakness. When group-administered achievement scores differ more than 1 year from a student's grade placement—or where achievement scores show a scatter of more than 1 year between scores—it may be advisable to refer that child to the child study team at the student's school to determine whether further testing is necessary to investigate the possibility that a disability is interfering with the student's ability to perform effectively.

Although a child's achievement scores can help to identify that a problem in school is occurring, it does not necessarily imply that the child has a disability that is compromising the ability to perform. Issues such as how instruction is being provided, whether the instructional delivery is appropriate for the child's learning needs, and whether the content of instruction fits the context of the student's experience must be addressed in order to determine what course of action should be taken to support the child. Information about the child's academic achievement should provide information regarding learning patterns, ability to attend to tasks, motivation to attend to new material, interest areas, and preferences for learning activities. Furthermore, when test scores are available, it is critical to determine whether the test was group-administered or individually administered. Information regarding the student's emotional reactions to school situations should focus on whether the student's behavior is appropriate to the social as well as academic contexts of school. Responses to corrections and failures reveal a great deal about one's perception of oneself as a capable learner. In the absence of a psychologist or educational specialist to provide this information, direct contact with school personnel is imperative for the primary care physician. Telephone conversations with the school nurse, teacher, social worker, or other professionals are very helpful in obtaining a clear picture of the child's school performance and behavior. Written reports from teachers using questionnaires that systematically address the most common types of learning problems can be of great assistance.

E. Psychosocial History: Family problems and parental characteristics often interfere with development of both cognitive and social competence and foster deviant behavior in the child. Children of hostile, rejecting, highly authoritarian parents tend to be the most severely affected; these children often show advanced competence at 1 year of age but a progressive decline in competence beginning around 4 years of age. Children of nurturing parents with highly authoritarian parenting practices often do better; however, children of nurturing parents who are firm and verbal in providing guidance and setting standards without being rigidly authoritarian show advanced competence that increases with age. Parents who provide little nurturance or sense of belonging, who are too lax or too harsh in punishment, or who fail to supervise their children tend to have children who show early evidence of aggressive behavior problems that persist into adolescence and adulthood.

Because developmental and behavior problems in the child are often provoked by and associated with problems within the family or seem to be associated with a lack of family support for developing new skills, a good psychosocial history is an essential part of any developmental evaluation. Ideally, this should include assessment of the family's ability to promote cognitive and social development, which includes, as a minimum, information regarding the parents' linguistic and cultural background, quality of verbal interaction, disciplinary practices (use of positive reinforcement to shape behavior, reliance on physical punishment or limited use of reasoning or verbal explanations in discipline), ability to set standards, neglect, reliance on parenting practices that interfere

with or inhibit development, family instability, marital discord, a hostile attitude toward the child, limitations in cognitive and social competence, depression, signs of maladjustment (eg, alcoholism, chronic unemployment, criminal or psychiatric problems), and general stress in the parents and chaos in the family that may contribute to and intensify developmental problems in the child.

In examining only the child, it is often difficult to distinguish behavior disorders associated with family problems from developmental disorders due to immaturity or alteration in development of the neurologic system. This difficulty has resulted in diagnosis by exclusion; that is, psychosocial assessment is used to determine whether there are social or emotional factors in the child's environment that can account for the observed learning or behavior problems. This is a practical approach in middle-class families, since it is often possible to ascertain that the family is reasonably stable and able to provide adequate support and stimulation to the child. Diagnosis by exclusion is, however, a very unsatisfactory approach for dealing with children from lower socioeconomic families, that is, the majority of children with behavior problems. The need for better assessment of these children is particularly acute, since they often have delays in both social and cognitive development and combinations of developmental delay and behavior problems. Ninety percent of children who later show mental or emotional disorders are normal at birth and appear to be casualties of inadequate or pathologic environments.

At present, the most commonly used approach to family assessment is a global, clinical social history. Some of this information is usually included in the history obtained by the primary care physician. In most instances, however, a social worker will provide the most thorough and complete analysis. In preschool children, it is often helpful to supplement the usual clinical social history with the HOME (*home observation for measurement of the environment*) interview assessment of Bradley and Caldwell (see references, below). This is the most thoroughly studied approach to the systematic evaluation of the growth-promoting aspects of the child's environment. This interview, which requires a home visit, is used to identify economically disadvantaged families unlikely to support development in their children. It may be performed by any trained person but is usually done by a social worker or nurse. A shorter, questionnaire version of the HOME interview, the Home Screening Questionnaire (HSQ), provides most of the information obtained from the longer interview version and can be administered and scored by the pediatrician during a clinic or office visit. Although it has not yet been studied widely enough to determine its clinical usefulness, the HSQ appears to be a promising tool for use by the primary care physician. Neither scale is expected to be useful in evaluating children from middle or upper socioeconomic families.

Badger E, Burne D, Vietze P: Maternal risk factors as predictors of development outcome in early childhood. Infant Ment Health J 1981;2:33.

Bradley RH, Caldwell BM: Pediatric usefulness of home assessment. In: *Advances in Behavioral Pediatrics,* Vol 2. Camp BW (editor). JAI Press, 1981.

Coons CE et al: *The Home Screening Questionnaire Reference Manual.* LADOCA, 1981.

Physical & Neurologic Examination

It is essential that a thorough physical and neurologic examination be performed. A number of children will demonstrate neurologic "soft signs," such as clumsiness, right-left confusion, disordered temporal orientation, overflow phenomena, choreiform movements, and finger agnosia. Although "soft signs" are commonly associated with school learning and behavior problems, the significance of these signs is controversial because they are also found in children who have no other problems and because most appear to represent delay in maturation rather than dysfunction. PANESS (*physical and neurologic examination for soft signs*), a standardized neurologic examination, has been studied and shows promising results for systematic evaluation of "soft signs."

In addition, recent studies linking minor physical anomalies with behavior disorders in childhood have prompted physicians to examine for the presence of dysmorphic features such as abnormal palmar creases, syndactyly, unruly hair, malformed ears, skin tags, and facial abnormalities. Although these features are commonly seen in children with mental retardation, the implications of their presence in nonretarded children are not fully understood.

Holden EW, Tarnowski KJ, Prinz RJ: Reliability of neurobiological soft signs in children: Reevaluation of the PANESS. J Abnorm Child Psychol 1982;10:163.

Sensory Function

All children in whom developmental delay or mental retardation is suspected should be examined for visual and auditory problems. In infants and young children, sensory deficits may be mistaken for retardation. Retarded children often have sensory deficits in addition to their retardation, and this increases the complexity of their problem. In most nonretarded, school-age children, vision and hearing can be satisfactorily evaluated by the usual screening methods and referral made to a specialist for further evaluation of children with abnormal screening results.

A variety of vision problems have been proposed as causes of reading problems, most without substantial research support. Learning to read can be accomplished quite satisfactorily with limited visual acuity. Although it is important that visual defects be corrected to improve the child's overall functioning, it is generally agreed that learning problems are seldom linked to refractive errors. Difficulty with convergence at near point, however, may interfere significantly with the process of reading and should receive careful evaluation.

Hearing loss has a significant impact on language development and may be associated with severe learning and behavior problems. In the past, deaf children have often been mistakenly labeled retarded. Losses in the high-frequency range may be associated with problems in discriminating speech sounds necessary for school learning. Others may have problems differentiating speech sounds despite normal hearing.

Emotional & Social Behavior

Although some information can be obtained directly from the child through interviews, play, and projective testing, typically one must rely on interviews with parents and reports from school personnel to obtain a picture of the child's social competence. Much of this information is obtained by social workers, psychologists, or psychiatrists. In evaluating reports of problem behavior at home and at school, it is helpful to assess the degree of deviance by comparing an individual child's behavior with children in general. Large studies of normal children indicate that most children show a few signs of deviant behavior. The truly deviant child, however, usually demonstrates this in a variety of ways. It is especially important to seek information about positive attributes, because these appear to be more powerful indicators of later mental health than negative attributes are of later maladjustment. Three of the most important positive attributes are school attendance (regardless of performance), positive peer relations, and nondelinquency.

General adaptation and development of self-help are often included in developmental assessments of preschool children. Beginning around age 4 years (when abstract reasoning becomes the dominant factor in measures of cognitive development), it becomes increasingly important to include some assessment of general adaptation in the differential diagnosis of mental retardation. Children from minority cultures who perform poorly on IQ tests often appear less retarded when general adaptation is evaluated.

Rating scales of behavior, such as the ACTeRS scale (ADD-H: Comprehensive Teachers Rating Scale) (Table 4–1) for identifying children with attention-deficit disorder, are important tools for assessing school behavior. The ACTeRS scale has been designed to identify clusters of problems in the areas of attention, hyperactivity, social skills, and oppositional behavior. Norms to assess the degree of de-

Table 4–1.

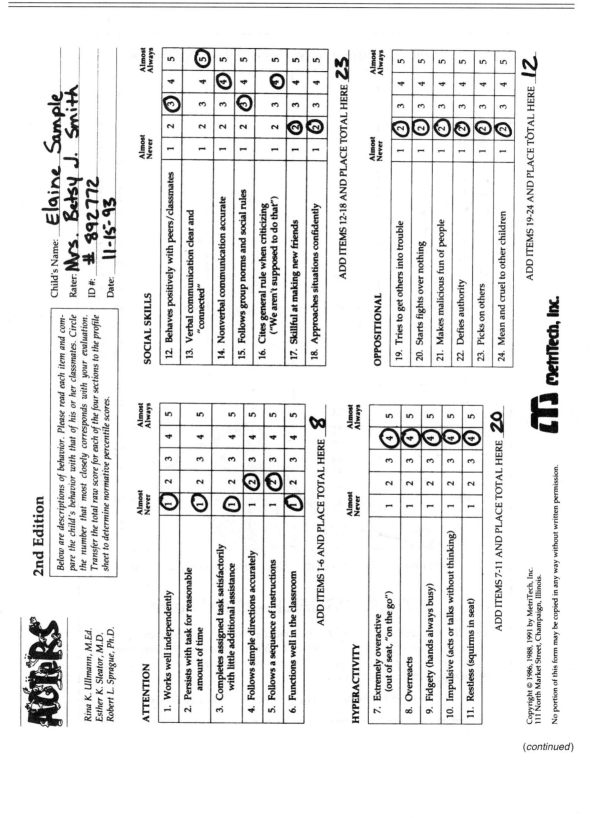

ACTeRS
2nd Edition

Rina K. Ullmann, M.Ed.
Esther K. Sleator, M.D.
Robert L. Sprague, Ph.D.

Below are descriptions of behavior. Please read each item and compare the child's behavior with that of his or her classmates. Circle the number that most closely corresponds with your evaluation. Transfer the total raw score for each of the four sections to the profile sheet to determine normative percentile scores.

Child's Name: Elaine Sample
Rater: Mrs. Betsy J. Smith
ID #: 892772
Date: 11-15-93

ATTENTION

	Almost Never 1	2	3	4	Almost Always 5
1. Works well independently	①	2	3	4	5
2. Persists with task for reasonable amount of time	①	2	3	4	5
3. Completes assigned task satisfactorily with little additional assistance	①	2	3	4	5
4. Follows simple directions accurately	1	②	3	4	5
5. Follows a sequence of instructions	1	②	3	4	5
6. Functions well in the classroom	①	2	3	4	5

ADD ITEMS 1-6 AND PLACE TOTAL HERE **8**

HYPERACTIVITY

	Almost Never 1	2	3	4	Almost Always 5
7. Extremely overactive (out of seat, "on the go")	1	2	3	④	5
8. Overreacts	1	2	3	④	5
9. Fidgety (hands always busy)	1	2	3	④	5
10. Impulsive (acts or talks without thinking)	1	2	3	④	5
11. Restless (squirms in seat)	1	2	3	④	5

ADD ITEMS 7-11 AND PLACE TOTAL HERE **20**

SOCIAL SKILLS

	Almost Never 1	2	3	4	Almost Always 5
12. Behaves positively with peers/classmates	1	2	③	4	5
13. Verbal communication clear and "connected"	1	2	3	4	⑤
14. Nonverbal communication accurate	1	2	3	④	5
15. Follows group norms and social rules	1	2	③	4	5
16. Cites general rule when criticizing ("We aren't supposed to do that")	1	2	3	④	5
17. Skillful at making new friends	1	②	3	4	5
18. Approaches situations confidently	1	②	3	4	5

ADD ITEMS 12-18 AND PLACE TOTAL HERE **23**

OPPOSITIONAL

	Almost Never 1	2	3	4	Almost Always 5
19. Tries to get others into trouble	1	②	3	4	5
20. Starts fights over nothing	1	②	3	4	5
21. Makes malicious fun of people	1	②	3	4	5
22. Defies authority	1	②	3	4	5
23. Picks on others	1	②	3	4	5
24. Mean and cruel to other children	1	②	3	4	5

ADD ITEMS 19-24 AND PLACE TOTAL HERE **12**

MetriTech, Inc.

(continued)

Table 4–1. (continued)

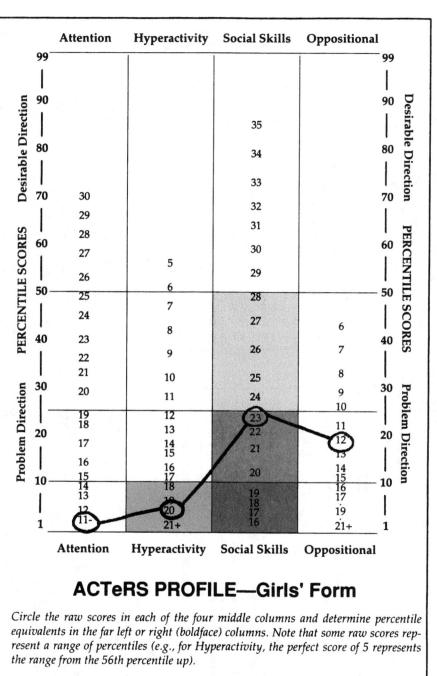

ACTeRS PROFILE—Girls' Form

Circle the raw scores in each of the four middle columns and determine percentile equivalents in the far left or right (boldface) columns. Note that some raw scores represent a range of percentiles (e.g., for Hyperactivity, the perfect score of 5 represents the range from the 56th percentile up).

viance are available. The ACTeRS scale is readily acceptable to teachers and can be used by primary care physicians to assess the need for and response to stimulant medication.

A scale for obtaining teacher and parent ratings of general behavior is also useful for identifying children with deviant behavior other than distractibility and hyperactivity and for assessing the degree and amount of prosocial behavior. Several such scales are available for assessing children as early as 2 years of age. The most commonly used scale with both parent and teacher forms is the Child Behavior Checklist (Achenbach).

Information about social and emotional behavior should include anecdotal details about ability to discriminate among a variety of roles and to perform socially within the boundaries imposed by those roles. For instance, the social skills necessary to interact effectively with peers may include, depending on the child's chronologic age, the ability to share, to take turns, to negotiate conflict, and to understand and use humor effectively. These social skills shift somewhat when the child is asked to interact with adults in positions of authority. The child needs to be able to understand the social rules for conduct in the classroom, for example, and to respond to direction, to time limits, and to feedback within the social context prescribed by adults. These skills are culturally influenced, and the child who has had little opportunity to acquire them may be labeled as a behavior problem. The behavioral expectations of classroom environments are complex and require repeated exposures to meet those expectations. Classroom procedures and rules vary dramatically from teacher to teacher, and the consistency with which they are followed is also teacher-dependent.

In addition to the social skills component of the social and emotional domain, two other factors must be accounted for in considering a child's social and emotional profile: attention to task and motivation. Attention to task is a major component of information processing and is frequently related to cognitive ability. However, inadequate or developmentally atypical capacity to attend to task may suggest emotional lability rather than cognitive disability. Attention to task may be viewed as a three- stage process. First, a child must be able to focus attention on a particular set of salient stimuli; second, the child must be able to sustain that attention over a span of time; and last, the child must be able to complete tasks. The inability of a child to perform any one of these components of attention to task may result from stress and anxiety imposed by a lack of predictability and routine in the classroom or home environment. Because children vary in their ability to handle disruption and multiple environments, information about the number of environments in which they are expected to participate daily or over the course of the week may suggest the need to restructure either the

quantity or the quality of the environment. Children's responses to success, correction, and failure often assist teachers in understanding how to motivate children to perform successively more difficult tasks. It is advisable to gather information about performance in more than the school environment in order to form a complete picture of social competence.

Family & Social Resources

The type, extent, and cost of educational and counseling services available to the child and family, the family's ability to support and carry through with treatment plans, and other community resources should be assessed early in the evaluation. These factors often limit or modify the treatment plan developed for a child. Sixty percent of families presenting children for evaluation of learning problems have clear-cut social and emotional problems that need to be assessed and addressed as an integral part of treatment planning for the child. Much of this information will be derived from the psychosocial history. In addition, however, the primary care physician should become familiar with resources in the community for family assessment and counseling.

Intelligence

Even though intelligence is perceived and understood in widely variable ways by education theorists, intelligence tests usually present increasingly difficult questions tapping general knowledge, reasoning, judgment, and organization of analytic skills that are expected to develop in the course of experiences encountered by most children in the process of growing up. Where children have grossly different experiences from those in the standard population, their scores may be expected to vary upward or downward. Originally, the IQ score obtained from such tests represented the percentage of expected growth a child had reached at a given age. This was derived by the following equation:

$$\textbf{(Mental age/chronologic age)} \times \textbf{100}$$

Scores on most modern tests can still be reported in terms of mental age/chronologic age, but the most widely used tests yield IQ scores that represent a child's relative distance from the average child in standard score units.

In the preschool period, the principal diagnostic tests in general use are the Bayley Scales of Infant Development (for children under 42 months of age), the Stanford-Binet Intelligence Scale, the McCarthy Scales of Children's Abilities (for children 3 years of age and older), and the Kaufman Assessment Battery for Children (K-ABC). These are all individually administered tests, given by trained personnel. The screening tests used most commonly in the preschool period are the Denver II (Frankenburg, 1992); the Revised Developmental Screening Inventory

(Knobloch, 1980); and, among older preschool children, the Early Screening Inventory (Meisels, 1983). Table 4–2 provides a summary of the screening tests discussed in this chapter.

Several assessment methods are also available to capitalize on the caretaker's knowledge of the infant or preschool child. Procedures such as the Kent Infant Development Scale (KIDS; Reuter, 1990) for children under 12 months of age and the Child Development Inventory (Ireton, 1995) for children over 15 months of age use the caretaker's report to assess the child's general development, including cognitive, gross motor, fine motor, expressive language, self-help, and personal/social development. These procedures have several advantages. They provide for the inclusion of a large number of items at each age, are based on behavior readily observable at home, do not require extensive training for administration, and can be used to plan and monitor appropriate intervention at home. Disadvantages include potential inaccuracy in the caretaker's reply and bias in reporting.

The Wechsler scales (Wechsler Adult Intelligence Scale [WAIS], Wechsler Intelligence Scale for Children III [WISC-III], and Wechsler Preschool and Primary Scale of Intelligence–Revised [WPPSI-R]), the Stanford-Binet Intelligence Scale, and the Kaufman Assessment Battery for Children (K-ABC) are the most widely used individual intelligence tests for school-age and older children. The Stanford-Binet test is a highly verbal test with nonverbal items intermingled. The Wechsler scales are subdivided into six verbal and six nonverbal tests so that a verbal IQ and performance IQ can both be obtained as well as an IQ based on the full test (full-scale IQ). The Kaufman Battery is designed to assess differences in simultaneous and sequential processing of information as well as differences between aptitude and achievement. It is commonly thought that intelligence tests can reveal the potential for higher functioning, especially when scatter (the pattern of high and low scores) is examined carefully, and both the K-ABC and Wechsler scales lend themselves particularly well to this task.

The standardized, individually administered tests

Table 4–2. Recommendations for use of assessment procedures.

Name	Type of Test	Age Range	Administered by
Bayley Scales of Infant Development	Development	1–42 mo	Professional
Beery Test of Visual-Motor Integration	Visual-motor	2–15 y	Professional
Denver II	Development	3 mo–6 y	Trained screener
Developmental Profile II (DPII)	Development	0–9 y	Trained screener
Early Screening Inventory	Development	4–6 y	Trained screener
Kaufmann Assessment Battery for Children (K-ABC)	Intelligence and achievement	2.5–12.5 y	Professional
Kaufmann Brief Intelligence Test (K-BIT)	Intelligence	4 y–adult	Trained screener
Kent Infant Development Scale (KIDS)	Development	0–1 y	Caretaker response
McCarthy Scales of Children's Abilities	Intelligence	2.5–8.5 y	Professional
Minnesota Child Development Inventory (MCDI)	Development	1–6 y	Caretaker response
Scales of Independent Behavior	Adaptive behavior	All ages	Professional
Slosson Intelligence Test	Intelligence	4.5 y–adult	Trained screener
Stanford-Binet Intelligence Scale	Intelligence	2 y–adult	Professional
Vineland Adaptive Behavior Scales	Adaptive behavior	All ages	Professional
Wechsler Preschool & Primary Scale of Intelligence–Revised (WPPSI-R)	Intelligence	3 y–7 y, 3 mo	Professional
Wechsler Intelligence Scale for Children–III (WISC-III)	Intelligence	6–16 y	Professional
Wide Range Achievement Test 3	Achievement: reading, spelling, math, visual-perceptual	5 y–adult	Trained screener
Woodcock-Johnson Psych-Educational Battery	Aptitude and achievement	3 y–adult	Professional

of intelligence discussed above require extensive training for proper administration and are usually administered by trained psychologists. The Kaufman Brief Intelligence Test (K-BIT), the Slosson Intelligence Test, and the Peabody Picture Vocabulary Test are screening tests designed for use by nonprofessionals, including office assistants and primary care physicians.

Achievement

Achievement usually refers to performance in specific school-related areas in which a child has received instruction. In the preschool period, achievement is seldom distinguished from general development. By the time the child enters kindergarten, however, a variety of procedures are available for assessing readiness. In a child with a mental age of 6 years, two of the best predictors for readiness to enter the first grade are the ability to engage in sustained task-oriented behavior and the knowledge of letter names and sounds. A number of procedures are available to assess school readiness, and in recent years, testing programs have been specifically designed for early identification of children with learning disabilities. Although results of these programs appear to be about as accurate as teacher assessments of kindergarten performance, many feel that the programs represent an important advance. Most of the early identification testing programs are designed for use in schools or by psychologists. Several procedures are also available for use by primary care physicians in screening for school readiness at the time of well-child visits in the 4½- to 5½-year age range. These include the developmental screening tests described previously and the preschool portions of the Wide Range Achievement Test 3 (WRAT-3; see later in this section).

For school-age children, scores on a variety of achievement tests are often available through routine classroom testing done at school, and results of such testing should be included in the educational history. Where low scores are obtained, individual testing should be performed before accepting the results as representative of the child's ability. Many school systems with special education services can administer individual tests of achievement and, with permission from the parents, give the test scores to the primary care physician. However, test scores in and of themselves do not constitute evidence of the presence of developmental disorders unless the test scores have been interpreted carefully by a trained educational specialist or school psychologist. Individually administered achievement tests such as the Woodcock-Johnson Psychoeducational Battery–Revised (Woodcock, 1990) are used to analyze more closely a learner's performance. The use of complex and lengthy tools such as the Woodcock-Johnson test and the validity of the results of such an assessment rest heavily on the skills and abilities of the examiner to

interpret test performance and scores on as many as 27 subtests. Analysis of discrepancies between subtests on this assessment tool assist the educational diagnostician in determining whether, for instance, discrepancies between orally identifying sight words and comprehending text are indicative of a disability or reflective of the developmental nature of these different skills.

Research on the interaction between cognitive processes, such as measured by intelligence tests, and achievement has led to the understanding that three components of cognition are particularly important for school learning and achievement: attention, memory, and the coordination of these processes. The ability to focus and sustain attention over time on events or tasks that are prescribed in school is a fundamental academic skill. Although some children may fail to focus or sustain attention because of interfering emotional factors, another group appears to be unable to manage this cognitive function for other reasons. For this group of children, failure to attend successfully appears to be related to an inability to determine the salient features of a task, that is, what, when, and how a task needs to be accomplished and what procedures must be brought to bear to complete it. In other words, these children lack the ability to think about their thinking and to contrive or activate problem-solving procedures that will guide their performance of a given task. In the problem-solving sequence, these children have a tendency to break down in any one of several areas: (1) problem identification ("What is it I need to do here?"); (2) organization of strategies; (3) generalization from other, similar situations; (4) attainment of logical solutions; and (5) critical analysis and evaluation. Furthermore, in the problem-solving task, an inability to attend simultaneously to the task as well as monitor their performance and differentially allot attention to various elements of the task plagues many of these learners.

Another group of learners may have trouble because of limited ability to store or retrieve information. Cognitive psychologists discuss this problem in terms of storage capacity, or how much information an individual can maintain in either short-term or long-term memory banks. Where capacity is not at issue, retrieval proposes a second stumbling block. Children may lack a complex semantic retrieval system that enables them to access stored information from multiple avenues. Teachers often report anecdotally about these learners in terms somewhat as follows: "I know he knows it. He could do it all last week, but this week it's as if he never learned it." Additional problems may arise if attention, processing, and retrieval are not well coordinated. Patterns of performance on tests that assess these cognitive abilities may indicate that the child has a specific learning disability in one or more cognitive functions.

Individually administered achievement tests, in

conjunction with measures of intelligence, are used to look at whether discrepancies between academic achievement and individual potential exist and whether these discrepancies may be attributable to some form of learning disability.

Academic achievement is additionally dependent on environmental factors that are not necessarily measured through achievement tests. These factors include cultural background and experience, motivation to achieve, expectancy for success, and instruction that accounts for these variables. A thorough diagnostic evaluation should address these concerns. Unfortunately, many children who are referred to a pediatrician for evaluation have no current achievement test scores in their school records. This is particularly true for children referred because of behavior problems. When an educational specialist or psychologist is unavailable to provide this information, the primary care physician may wish to test patients through the use of a screening test such as the Wide Range Achievement Test 3 (Wilkinson, 1993). Because of the limited number of test items on this screening device, the validity of the results is somewhat questionable. However, by using this screening device, physicians can determine whether further testing is desirable for assessing whether a child is having difficulties in school because of cognitive or behavioral disorders.

Adaptive Behavior

Assessment of adaptive behavior is seldom addressed directly in children unless a child is suspected of being mentally retarded. Because poor performance on a cognitive test may result from many factors, it is essential that the accuracy of low scores be confirmed by assessment of functional level in everyday living. Scales such as the Vineland Adaptive Behavior Scales and the Scales of Independent Behavior are questionnaires and structured interview methods for assessing the child's developmental level in areas such as social interaction, communication, personal living, and community living.

Perceptual-Motor Function

In the early school years, a number of children with delays in copying and drawing skills also demonstrate problems in learning to read. These problems have been variously termed visual-perceptual and visual-motor problems, and their presence in children beyond 7–9 years of age has often been thought to indicate the existence of central nervous system dysfunction, although this inference is controversial. There is a relationship between visual-perceptual problems and reading problems in the early school years; as children get older, however, reading achievement becomes more and more related to intelligence, even when the perceptual problems persist. Furthermore, perceptual problems are common among children from families in lower socioeconomic groups and even among children whose only

history is confinement to bed for more than 2 months during the preschool years.

Because performance on tests of copying skills is highly correlated with intelligence, such tests are most useful when there is a discrepancy between the developmental level demonstrated on visual-perceptual tests and general intelligence. Methods for assessing the degree of this discrepancy are not as well developed as for assessing the discrepancy between IQ and achievement. At a practical level, however, these problems may be severe enough to interfere with learning the skills of printing and writing. In the latter case, it is usually more helpful to analyze the child's writing, but several visual-perceptual tests, such as the Beery Test of Visual-Motor Integration, are commonly used to examine copying skills per se.

Speech & Language

Speech and language delays are common in mentally retarded children but may also occur in children with average or above-average intelligence. A number of children who appear to have specific learning problems, on closer evaluation, show evidence of delay in language development or an articulation problem (or both). These problems can limit academic achievement in areas that depend on verbal skills (eg, reading). Speech and language delays in preschool children and methods for evaluating them have been discussed previously (see Chapter 1). Most children should reach the adult proficiency level in language by 7–8 years of age, at which time evaluation of language skills typically becomes merged with evaluation of verbal intelligence. Scores on tests such as the Wechsler scale or the Stanford-Binet test reflect language skills as well as intelligence. Specialized tests for assessing components of receptive and expressive language and language processing skills are also available.

Motivation

Clinical assessment of motivation has received little attention despite mounting evidence that motivation is a key factor in determining how a child will use whatever time and help are provided for learning new skills. Studies of achievement motivation have suggested that two main motivational types can be identified: those who are challenged by moderately difficult tasks and respond to success and those who are primarily motivated to avoid failure and will attempt only very easy tasks, in which failure is unlikely, or very difficult ones, in which failure carries no stigma. One of the major shifts that occurs in the age range of 5–7 years is from motivational dependence on social and external rewards to internal motivation for mastery of skills. Some children make this shift poorly or not at all and fail to learn in the usual academic climate, which emphasizes mastery and competition. Often these are the children who seem primarily motivated to avoid failure and who need liberal support from external sources (praise, concrete incentives) just for trying. Although motivational immaturity is seldom the principal problem, it is often a major determinant of how well a child will respond or progress in an educational program.

Achenbach TM: *The Child Behavior Checklist.* University of Vermont Press, 1991.

Beery KE: *Revised Administration, Scoring, and Teaching Manual for the Developmental Test of Visual-Motor Integration.* Modern Curriculum Press, 1982.

Bruininks RH et al: *Scales of Independent Behavior.* DLM Teaching Resources, 1984.

Frankenburg WK: *The Denver II*: A major revision and restandardization of the Denver Developmental Screening Test. Pediatrics 1992;89:91.

Ireton H: *Child Development Inventory.* Behavior Science Systems, 1995.

Knobloch H, Steven F, Malone AF: *Manual of Developmental Diagnosis.* Harper, 1980.

Meisels SJ, Wiske MS: *Early Screening Inventory.* Teachers College, 1983.

Reuter J, Bickett L: *The Kent Infant Development Scale.* Kent Developmental Metrics, 1990.

Sparrow SS et al: *Vineland Adaptive Behavior Scales: Interview Edition, Survey Form Manual.* American Guidance Service, 1984.

Wilkinson GS: *Wide Range Achievement Test 3.* Jastak, 1993.

Woodcock R: *Woodcock-Johnson Psychoeducational Battery–Revised.* Teaching Resources, 1990.

EVALUATING THE DISCREPANCY BETWEEN INTELLIGENCE & ACHIEVEMENT

The differential diagnosis of competence problems necessitates an evaluation of the significance of the discrepancy between expected achievement based on measures of general competence (intelligence) and actual achievement in specific areas of academic performance.

The US Office of Education defines the discrepancy between achievement and IQ as significant when achievement is below 50% of expected grade level. The lowest level of achievement commensurate with age and intelligence is calculated by the following formula:

$$\text{Age}[(\text{IQ}/300) + 0.17] - 2.5 = \text{lowest grade}$$

For an 8-year-old child with an IQ of 100, this formula indicates that a grade level of 1.5 is the lowest score that would be commensurate with age and intelligence. If this child's achievement test scores are below grade level 1.5, there is a significant discrepancy. If he or she is at grade level 1.5 or higher, the discrepancy is not significant. Some difference between expected and actual achievement represents normal variation, whereas a significant discrepancy

is defined in terms of an unusual degree of difference. Individual school districts are free to adopt their own criteria for determining how large this discrepancy must be for a child to qualify for special services.

TEMPERAMENTAL TRAITS & REACTIONS TO DEVELOPMENTAL CRISES

During the ages of 5–7 years and 10–13 years, major developmental changes occur in most children. In the 5- to 7-year period, children enter school, begin to develop operational thought, and shift from associative thinking to use of verbal mediation activity in learning and thinking. The 10- to 13-year period heralds the onset of puberty, entrance into junior high school, and development of formal operational thought. Inflections in the growth curve for intelligence occur during both periods, and there is a dramatic increase in a cluster of behavior problems that appear to be phase-specific reactions to the developmental changes occurring during these periods. These problems include restless sleep, disturbing dreams, physical timidity, irritability, overdependence, and jealousy. Emotional turbulence during one of these periods may or may not be associated with turbulence during the other period, and its occurrence in either does not seem to be indicative of serious long-term problems.

Often there is overlap between these phase-specific reactions and temperamental traits, which include characteristics such as shyness, oversensitiveness, somberness, and reserve. Both phase-specific reactions and temperamental traits may be a source of conflict between parents and children, but they do not in themselves indicate the presence of serious emotional disturbance. They usually resolve with support, and the child does not need treatment.

Kohlberg L, LaCrosse J, Ricks D: The predictability of adult mental health from childhood behavior. In: *Manual of Child Psychopathology.* Wolman BB (editor). McGraw-Hill, 1972.

DISORDERS IN DEVELOPMENT OF COGNITIVE COMPETENCE (See Table 4–3.)

SPECIFIC LEARNING DISORDERS

Essentials of Diagnosis

- Significant discrepancy between estimated intelli-

Table 4–3. Differential diagnosis of learning problems.

Type of Learning Problem	Characteristics	Treatment Issues
Disorders with IQ-achievement discrepancy Specific learning disorders: Reading/spelling (dyslexia)	Achievement is below IQ in an isolated area. The disorder is not caused by sensory impairment. Other areas are at level of expectancy. Achievement is below expectancy only in reading/spelling.	Individualized instruction (often tutoring) in area of weakness should be provided. Normalized educational experiences in other areas are indicated. Specific instruction in reading/spelling/language arts is indicated. The child often exhibits generalized deficits in language processing. The child may have problems in math because of reading.
Arithmetic (dyscalculia)	Achievement is below expectancy only in arithmetic.	Specific instruction in math is indicated. Dsycalculia may be difficult to separate from a reading or writing disorder.
Writing (dysgraphia)	Achievement is below expectancy in written work.	Status of visual functioning must be clarified. Specific treatment for handwriting skills is indicated. Dysgraphia is often difficult to separate from dyslexia.
Hyperflexia	The child begins reading at a very early age (eg, 2 y). The child may appear autistic or show unusual discrepancies in abilities.	Comprehensive assessment and treatment in several areas of weakness is necessary. The prognosis for the autistic child is relatively good.
Nonspecific learning disorders: Underachievement	Achievement is below IQ in several areas. Underachievement may be caused by environmental, behavioral (eg, ADHD), motivational, or situational problems, or to school absence.	The child often has emotional/behavior problems as well.
Generalized learning disability	Achievement is below IQ in several areas. The disability is not caused by sensory impairment. The disability is often accompanied by evidence of visual/perceptual/motor difficulties. Associated environmental, emotional/behavioral, or motivational problems are often present.	Unusual combinations of discrepant functioning may be a reflection of abnormal brain functioning.
Disorders without IQ-achievement discrepancy Slow learner	IQ and achievement are commensurate but at low-normal to below-normal levels.	Learning is slow but steady with appropriate programming.
Mental retardation	Both IQ and achievement are more than 2 SD below average.	
Educable	IQ is usually 50–70.	The child is capable of achieving rudiments of literacy.
Trainable	IQ is usually below 50.	The child is capable of acquiring preacademic and vocational skills.

gence (usually verbal) and achievement in one or more areas.

- Achievement commensurate with intelligence in one or more academic areas.
- No evidence of sensory deficits.

- Either presence or absence (often absence) of behavior problems.

General Considerations

Specific problems may be experienced in any area

of academic achievement, but the most common problems involve reading or spelling (dyslexia). Frequent but less common problems are specific to arithmetic (dyscalculia) or writing (dysgraphia). Intelligence is usually average or above average, but the key element in making the diagnosis is demonstrating a discrepancy between actual achievement and expected achievement in a specific area. (See previous section on discrepancy.)

Descriptive Classification

A. Reading & Spelling Disorders (Developmental Dyslexia): Dyslexia is the most common type of specific learning disorder. It occurs more frequently in boys than in girls (3:1), and in 34% of cases there is a strong family history, especially among the male relatives. Speech and language problems and problems in sequencing are the most common developmental problems associated with specific reading disorders. A variety of developmental problems such as clumsiness and incoordination, directional confusion, right-left confusion, disordered temporal orientation, and difficulties in naming colors and in recognizing the meaning of pictures have been reported in children with specific reading problems. These are of lesser importance than the speech and language problems and may be related more to intelligence than to reading disorder per se. A history of delays in speech and language development is present in at least one-third of cases. This involves delays such as failure to use meaningful words other than "mama," "dada," "hello," and "bye-bye" until after 18 months of age and failure to use two-word phrases by 24 months of age. Although evidence of associated neurologic deficit or differential use of the right versus the left hemisphere can be demonstrated in some children, such results of neurologic investigations have generally contributed little to treatment or prognosis.

Traditionally, the definition of specific reading disorder (dyslexia) included failure to learn to read despite adequate sensory apparatus, conventional instruction, average intelligence, and sociocultural opportunity. Such diagnosis by exclusion was an attempt to distinguish between "unexpected" reading failure and reading failure that could be explained by a more general or pervasive factor, such as mental subnormality, cultural or educational deprivation, sensory defects, or emotional disturbance. With this approach, most children with reading problems tend to be excluded from the diagnosis of specific reading disorder—that is, their reading problems are attributed to the fact that they are slightly below average in intelligence, come from economically disadvantaged homes, or have emotional and behavior problems. Yet many in this large group show reading achievement below expectancy for their mental age; and in neurologic status, cognitive functioning, and other areas of achievement they are indistinguishable

from the group defined in the traditional sense as having specific reading disorder. In addition, the presence of a significant discrepancy between actual and expected achievement is the only characteristic that is common to members of highly specific etiologic groups such as those with genetic dyslexia diagnosed on the basis of linkage studies.

Consequently, current thinking endorses the concept that subtypes of reading disability should first be described in terms of clear-cut characteristics irrespective of etiologic considerations. There have been two major approaches to this subtyping. One approach attempts to distinguish among different problems on the basis of analysis of reading and spelling errors; this has led to subtyping into two groups based on whether performance indicates heavier reliance on auditory-sequential-phonologic skills (auditory reader) or on-visual-spatial-imagery (visual reader). The other approach uses associated disabilities such as those in language, perceptual-motor skills, and memory to distinguish the following probable subtypes: (1) a language disorder group with defects in understanding and expression of oral language; (2) a dyscoordination group with defects in speech articulation, copying skills, and understanding of oral language; (3) a visual-spatial-perceptual disorder group with visual, perceptual, and visual-constructive problems but intact oral language; and (4) a group with dysphonemic sequencing disorder.

B. Mathematics Disorders (Developmental Dyscalculia): Mathematics disorders have been studied primarily in relation to the developmental Gerstmann syndrome (dyscalculia, right-left disorientation, and finger agnosia) and often have been considered to be part of a reading disorder. However, limited studies of school children who demonstrate a significant discrepancy between actual and expected achievement in arithmetic suggest that a specific syndrome of mathematical disability does exist and affects approximately 6% of the population. Developmental disorder is distinguished from acquired disorder by the absence of clearly defined brain damage and neurologic findings in the former.

Several forms have been described and are characterized by difficulty in verbalizing, writing, reading, manipulating, or understanding mathematical operations. In individuals whose difficulties are confined to performance on numerical tests, signs of neurologic abnormalities tend to be few. In those who are unable to read or write numbers, the disorder may be associated with general disorders in reading and writing as well as mathematics, so that a learning disorder specific to mathematics may be difficult to demonstrate.

C. Writing Disorders (Developmental Dysgraphia): Children with reading problems often have illegible handwriting as well as spelling problems. In younger children, problems due to immature perceptual-motor development (eg, mirror writing, reversal of letters, and poor construction of letters) are common. Some children will have problems confined to illegible handwriting, inaccurate copying, or inability to transmit sequences of verbal information to paper. In some of these instances, illegibility is associated with mild cerebral palsy or general problems in fine motor coordination. Whether encountered alone or in combination with reading or math disability, specific training is often required to correct the penmanship problems.

A common syndrome seen in students during late elementary and junior high school involves not only elements of poor handwriting (slow, illegible, poor spatial organization) but also deficits in memory, expressive language, organization of ideas, and fluency. This has been termed "developmental output failure"; it is usually manifested by overall reduced productivity, with refusals to complete work, failure to submit assignments, and "forgetting" to do homework.

Left-handed children deserve special attention because they have frequently had poor instruction. In most instances, their problems in penmanship will improve with appropriate instruction. Despite common belief to the contrary, there is little evidence associating left-handedness with any kind of deficiency.

Etiologic Classification

Both psychobiologic and sociopsychologic factors appear to play a major causative role in specific learning disabilities. The group of children who fail to learn despite conventional instruction, adequate familial-cultural opportunity, and adequate intelligence have generally been thought to represent an idiopathic or genetically based syndrome. This group has been distinguished from children with emotionally, educationally, or culturally based limitations on the one hand and those with disorders secondary to sensory defects, brain damage, or mental retardation on the other.

In the idiopathic group, the term *minimal brain dysfunction* (MBD) has often been applied when neurologic "soft signs," poor motor coordination, and distractibility are present along with learning problems in children of average or above-average intelligence. The term has also been applied indiscriminately to children who show any one of these features alone, but the clinical picture of children with the full picture described above provides the most convincing evidence for attributing the problem to some type of neurologic handicap. However, because extensive research has failed to provide substantial evidence of dysfunction and because many of the characteristics are common in preschool children and tend to be present only in younger learning-disabled children, many have abandoned the concept of minimal brain damage altogether in favor of the view that the neurologic problem is one of immaturity.

Clinical Findings

A family history often reveals affected family members, especially among the males. Findings on physical examination are usually normal, and those on neurologic examination are normal except for the presence of "soft signs." Behavior problems may or may not be present. Intelligence test results often indicate average or above-average intelligence on nonverbal tests and may or may not show some decrease in verbal IQ. In contrast, achievement in the affected area of learning is significantly below nonverbal intelligence and sometimes below verbal intelligence. Achievement in nonaffected areas tends to progress normally. Vision and hearing are usually normal, although deficits in processing auditory sequential information are often noted on extensive testing.

Although reading disorders are common among brain-injured children (18–40%), a reading disorder is not necessarily associated with other evidence of altered cortical functioning. Furthermore, educational, language, and other psychometric tests are often of no help in distinguishing poor readers who are brain-injured from poor readers who are not brain-injured. Electroencephalography, CT scanning, and a variety of other procedures have been used in the past with little or no success.

Differential Diagnosis

The term *specific learning disability* is primarily a descriptive one that distinguishes between specific learning disorder, general learning disorder (slow learner), or mental retardation. Etiologic diagnosis is more difficult. The most important distinction is whether there is a strong family history, inadequate educational background, sociocultural disadvantage, or evidence of brain damage.

Treatment

There have been many claims that instruction should be tailored to the subtype of reading disorder, but research has generally failed to support this claim. In part, this may result from the fact that discussions of reading instruction often deal only with questions of content. In this regard, there are basically three approaches to teaching children to read. First, many special educators use a bottom-up approach to developing reading skills. That is, children learn to identify letters, to match sounds and letters, to develop a basic sight word vocabulary, to apply sound/letter matches to novel words, and finally to read words in text. Variations of this model include the use of syllabary (or rebus) systems to begin to decode meaning and to learn to read from left to right. With children who seem to need additional cues to discriminate between letters and words, initial, modified alphabets may be used or words may be color-coded. This task analytic approach has been favored by special educators based on the presumption that breaking down reading into simpler discrimination tasks that lend themselves to routinized practice drills would increase the learner's success rate.

A second approach to teaching reading is based on the notion that learning to read is essentially a language development task and therefore follows the same developmental sequence that occurs when young children learn to speak. Thus, reading is taught from a holistic perspective in which teachers help children to link words that describe the world around them to print. Children are exposed to repeated readings of simple books and encouraged to read along with the teacher. Comprehension rather than word recall is stressed. This approach to reading also stresses the concurrent development of writing, since writing is the expressive aspect of the reading process. Rather than focus on the mechanics of spelling, children are urged to write using invented spelling to understand the notion of words as visual referents to the language we speak.

In a recent meta-analysis of research that analyzed the effectiveness of these two approaches to reading, Stahl and Miller (1989) found little evidence that favored either the bottom-up or the whole language approach to reading. These researchers concluded, as have many other reading and learning disabilities specialists, that careful assessment of individual learner needs should dictate the types of strategies used to help a child learn to read. There is evidence that a third approach based on an interactive model that combines attention to the graphophonemic elements of text (phonics) as well as to the semantic and experiential elements of comprehension may be the most efficient means of teaching a child to read.

It is evident from considering the various structures of the reading programs and strategies used in teaching that the number of possible approaches to reading instruction is quite large. With the variety of approaches available, selection of the best approach for a particular child may require a series of learning trials. Most children will begin to demonstrate learning after four to six lessons. General principles for promoting progress, however, include introduction of some phonics or word attack skills at some level of teaching; mastery of early, less difficult material before proceeding to more difficult material; and continuation of instruction over a long enough period for results to be long-lasting. Approximately 40 lessons are required before most children will register a substantial and enduring gain in reading skills. More rapid increases are sometimes reported, but these can often be attributed to spuriously depressed initial scores.

A minority of children will fail to learn to read or perform successfully in academic subjects despite individual instruction. For these children, a focus on goals that will ensure the maximum amount of independence as adults is vital even in the primary grades. Special education efficacy studies (eg, Kavale, 1982; Shepard, 1983) suggest that much of special education has not adequately addressed outcomes for the community (ie, employment and independent living), or for individuals (ie, heightened self-esteem, community membership status), or for schools (ie, efficient delivery of service). In seven statewide studies, less than 50% of the graduates of special education programs were employed full time. More than 50% of each sample earned less than minimum wage, and more than 60% of the graduates continued to live at home after graduation. Thus, outcome data from graduates of special programs suggest that the special education programs need to incorporate content and experiences to prepare young people to access employment and independent living opportunities in their own communities.

Several approaches to drug therapy for children with reading disability have been proposed, but none have yet received adequate study to warrant their recommendation. Furthermore, drug therapy prescribed for attention-deficit disorder, if successful, may be expected to alter impulsive and distractible behavior but typically does not "cure" the learning problems if these are present. At best, the climate for learning is improved, but educational progress will still depend primarily on the quality and amount of instruction provided to the child.

Prognosis

With or without individual instruction, only a minority of children remain nonreaders into adulthood. There are, however, many adolescents and adults who read poorly. Ultimate level of skill usually depends on the child's intelligence, the type and amount of individual instruction provided, the severity of retardation, the age at which remediation is begun, motivation, and several other factors including the child's general emotional state. In some adults, poor spelling may be the only stigma of a childhood reading problem, whereas other adults may continue to show evidence of problems in reading and general language skills as well. Even with individual instruction, progress is often slow, sometimes slower than progress being made by children described as slow learners. In children with specific learning disorder, however, progress in nonaffected areas of achievement tends to proceed at a normal pace.

Kavale KA, Glass GV: The efficacy of special education interventions and practices: A compendium of meta-analysis findings. Focus Except Child 1982;15:1.

Kosc L: Developmental dyscalculia. J Learn Disab 1974;7:164.

Myklebust HR (editor): *Progress in Learning Disabilities,* Vols 1–5. Grune & Stratton, 1983.

Rutter M (editor): *Developmental Neuropsychiatry.* Guilford, 1983.

Schain RJ: *Neurology of Childhood Learning Disorders.* Williams & Wilkins, 1972.

Shepard LA, Smith LA, Vojir CP: Characteristics of pupils identified as learning disabled. J Spec Educ 1983;16:73.

Stahl S, Miller P: Whole language and language experience: Approaches for beginning reading: A quantitative research synthesis. Rev Educ Res 1989;59:87.

SLOW LEARNER

Essentials of Diagnosis

- Achievement below average.
- No mental retardation but IQ often below average.
- No significant discrepancy between IQ and achievement.
- Performance usually poor in all subjects.
- School progress at a slower rate than average but nevertheless continuous.

General Considerations

The average IQ of children in this group tends to be in the 80s. Approximately 11% have definite evidence of neurologic dysfunction, 25% show questionable neurologic findings, and 60% have difficulty in copying forms. Clumsiness, motor impersistence, and right-left confusion are twice as common in this group as in children with specific learning disorders. Forty percent tend to have at least one sign of language delay (eg, first phrases after 24 months). The frequency of neurodevelopmental problems increases in children with lower IQs.

Clinical Findings

The most important characteristic of the slow learner is the lack of a significant discrepancy between intelligence and achievement. These children are often low-average to borderline in intelligence, and achievement is slow but commensurate with mental age. Usually the child is slow in all areas of achievement, but achievement in one area may be slower than in others. The lower the child's intelligence, the more one is likely to find evidence of neurodevelopmental problems and associated behavior problems. The history often reveals evidence of developmental delays, especially in the language area. A family history of school problems may or may not be present. In the absence of a positive family history, problems during the pregnancy, advanced maternal age, or difficulties in the newborn period are often cited as possible causes of early brain damage that might explain the appearance of such a child in a well-educated family. In many instances, however, the mother's educational and cognitive level will be consistent with that of the child whether signs of neurodevelopmental delay are present or not.

Treatment

Educational programming that uses community, school, work, and family as the conceptual organizers for planning curriculum often makes more sense for slow learners than the traditional academic curriculum. Families are frequently asked to participate in curriculum planning by reporting what they would like their child to be able to do 3 years from now in terms of accessing and participating in community activities, developing effective job habits, and participating in family recreational activities. By including the family in educational planning, recognition and acceptance of the child's capacities is made easier. Counseling or short-term psychotherapy can assist the family in dealing with feelings of denial or guilt. Often the school has developed an appropriate educational plan for the child, and treatment needs to be directed toward helping the family accept the school's plan.

Prognosis

Given an appropriate educational opportunity to progress at their own rate, slow learners tend to make steady progress commensurate with their mental age. In many instances, long-term follow-up may show that these children actually make better progress in their areas of deficiency than do children with specific learning disorders.

NONSPECIFIC & EMOTIONALLY BASED LEARNING DISORDERS

Essentials of Diagnosis

- Usually, average or above-average intelligence.
- Significant discrepancy between intelligence and achievement, often in more than one academic area.
- Frequent association with emotional or behavior problems.
- Frequent incidence among children from culturally disadvantaged homes and large families.

General Considerations

Included in this group are the large numbers of children with learning disorders in association with psychiatric disorders and familial-cultural problems of motivation. A significant discrepancy between intelligence and achievement may exist in one or more areas, or the child may be generally slow. Family problems are usually apparent, and children frequently come from culturally disadvantaged homes and large families. These children have many of the same educational needs as children with more specific problems—and often more—but they have, unfortunately, been excluded from federal funding for education of the learning disabled.

This group also includes children with wide discrepancies in functioning that result from or appear to result from altered brain function, with or without attendant emotional or behavior problems. Reduced functioning in several areas without significant IQ impairment is frequently observed in children with documented neurologic disorders (eg, epilepsy, structural lesions, head injury).

Differential Diagnosis

Differentiation from specific learning disabilities is made primarily on the basis of motivational and emotional problems and a lack of specificity of learning problems in children with average or above-average intelligence. Slow learners or mentally retarded children with emotional problems may be indistinguishable. The most difficult differential diagnosis is between specific reading disabilities in an emotionally disturbed child and an emotionally based learning disability concentrated in the language area.

Children with documented head injury or brain damage may not present a diagnostic problem. Often, however, the pattern of performance on psychologic tests, particularly those that are sensitive to disturbance in cortical functioning, may be the only available evidence pointing to brain dysfunction. Neurologic tests such as EEGs or CT scans are seldom beneficial in making a diagnosis.

Treatment

School systems are required by federal law to provide services to students who, through school-based diagnostic procedures, are labeled as emotionally disturbed. Services range from the development and implementation of behavior modification programs to full-day classes that serve students with these disorders. Curriculum components generally include manipulations of the instructional environment such as shortened or simplified academic tasks, cooperative learning groups, and contingency management strategies. A second curriculum component focus is on the management of aggressive or out-of-control behaviors through cognitive behavior modification and behavior control training. In addition, curriculum that addresses the development of social and affective skills should be a component of programming. A final ingredient in programs for students with emotional problems is counseling. The effectiveness of these programs is generally related to the skills of the multidisciplinary team assigned to the program. Services should reflect the needs of the student rather than a generic approach that treats all children with emotional disturbance in a similar fashion.

MENTAL RETARDATION

Essentials of Diagnosis

- Significantly limited intelligence (≥ 2 SD below average [IQ of <70]).
- Adaptation significantly below age level.
- Possible presence of sensory defects not responsible for delay.
- Onset in the developmental period.

General Considerations

Mental retardation is a descriptive term defined as significantly subaverage intellectual functioning existing concurrently with deficits of adaptive behavior and manifested during the developmental period. Significantly subaverage intelligence is defined as 2 SD or more below average (IQ below 70 on the Wechsler scales or below 69 on the Stanford-Binet test) and by definition affects approximately 2–3% of the general population. An additional 6% are considered borderline in intelligence (IQ of 70–79). Adaptive deficiency is less easily evaluated.

About 10% of the retarded population are identified during infancy and early childhood. Most fall in the moderate to profound retardation group (IQ below 50), and most of them have clear-cut evidence of brain damage, genetic disorder, or other pathologic conditions. Moderate to profound retardation is distributed equally among different socioeconomic groups but is more common in males than in females.

The remaining 90% of the retarded population tend to be mildly retarded (IQ of 50–69), and most are not identified before entering school, partly because limited efforts are made at earlier identification. The great majority of those with mild handicaps are diagnosed as cultural-familial retardates. They entral nervous system injury, and they come from families characterized by low intelligence and low socioeconomic status. Many who are mildly handicapped and identified primarily during the school years eventually blend into society and become at least marginally adequate citizens. There is a preponderance of males at all levels of retardation, except for those with organic disorders that are diagnosed after age 5 years.

Mildly retarded children (IQ 50–69) usually are considered educable and in many instances are able to blend into society with minimal or no protective custody. Moderately retarded children (IQ 30–49) are considered trainable but require protective care (sheltered workshop, guardian, group home). More recently, the public schools have been required to provide services to members of this group. Severely to profoundly retarded children (IQ <30) usually require continuous care, and this group often includes the most severely deformed, nonambulatory, and minimally communicative individuals. Educational programs at all levels of disability stress providing an appropriate education in the least restricted, most normalized environment.

Etiologic Considerations

Mental retardation is a descriptive diagnosis with a wide variety of causes. Many of the causative factors that can be identified are essentially untreatable. The basic database will be helpful in deciding how far to pursue an etiologic diagnosis.

A. Genetic:

Inborn errors of metabolism—Aminoacidopathies, cerebral lipidoses, mucopolysaccharidoses, disorders of carbohydrate metabolism.

2. Chromosome disorders—Autosomal disorders, sex chromosome disorders such as fragile X syndrome.

B. Intrauterine: Congenital infections, placental-fetal malfunction, complications of pregnancy (maternal malnutrition, pre-eclampsia–eclampsia, use of drugs or radiation, intrauterine growth retardation).

C. Perinatal: Prematurity, postmaturity, metabolic disorders (hypoglycemia, hyperbilirubinemia).

D. Postnatal: Endocrinopathies, metabolic disorders, trauma, infections, poisoning, abuse.

E. Cultural-Familial: Low family intelligence, low socioeconomic status, environmental deprivation.

Clinical Findings

A. History: In infants and preschool children with developmental delays, there may be evidence of a genetic syndrome or factors in the prenatal or perinatal period that can account for delay. Often, however, there will also be evidence of maternal deprivation or neglect, particularly among children who are only mildly or moderately delayed. The older the child at the time of diagnosis, the more likely that retardation will be explained by deficiencies in early experience or by familial-cultural factors. Even when there are other family members with similar problems, a genetic basis for the retardation cannot be established unequivocally. Children who are not diagnosed until after entering school often have a history of normal development in the first 2 years, and siblings may show a similar decline in relative competency as they get older. Children who come from nondominant cultural backgrounds often show adequate functioning on measures of adaptation despite poor performance on standard intelligence tests. If behavior problems, especially disruptive and antisocial behavior, are absent, children who show relatively better adaptability than intelligence tend to blend into society after leaving school.

B. Symptoms & Signs: In mental retardation, the developmental or intellectual performance is at least 2 SD below the mean, and there is accompanying evidence of significant limitations in adaptability. In preschool children, developmental delay on screening tests may be the principal presenting finding. Sensory defects are also common, as are speech and language problems, motor handicaps, neurodevelopmental delays, seizure disorders, and behavior problems. Serious family problems are also common, and frequently the mentally retarded child merely appears to be enough slower than other members of the family to be identified as retarded rather than borderline or dull normal. If the child is examined adequately, signs of significant developmental delay including deficiencies in adaptation will often be evident by age 2 years.

Once the child reaches school age, general adaptation and achievement in all areas tend to be low but commensurate with mental age. Children with low IQs who are not retarded on measures of adaptation should not be diagnosed as mentally retarded. Occasionally, a mildly retarded or borderline child will show a significant discrepancy between actual and expected achievement in one academic area more than in others. This may technically represent a specific learning disability; however, if the child's overall intelligence is low enough (IQ below 70), special education will be indicated anyway. Idiot savants have been described as showing extraordinary ability in a circumscribed area while functioning on a mentally retarded level in all other ways. Neglect, abuse, and other family experiences damaging to growth may result in bizarre forms of behavior and emotional disturbance that are difficult to distinguish from autistic or psychotic behavior. Mentally retarded children are often transparent mirrors of disturbances going on within the family. The appearance of unusual behavior, sexual acting out, or bizarre activity in an otherwise stable retarded child is often an indication of a disturbance in the family.

C. Special Studies: General rules for ordering tests include (1) laboratory testing for treatable conditions when an etiologic diagnosis is unknown, for example, use of an amino acid or organic acid screen; and (2) ordering other tests such as electroencephalography, skull films, and chromosome studies only if clinical findings suggest specific syndromes or problems.

Differential Diagnosis

After a descriptive diagnosis is made, the basic database should provide enough information so that a decision can be made on how far to pursue an etiologic diagnosis. It is particularly important to distinguish the deaf, blind, and orthopedically handicapped from the mentally retarded. This is often difficult, since many retarded children also have sensory and orthopedic handicaps. It is also often difficult to differentiate between autism and retardation in very young children, particularly when family and social background indicates deprivation or neglect. Usually, however, the young retarded child shows delay in all areas of development, whereas the autistic child may be normal in motor development but show bizarre behavior and serious delays in language development.

Management

Mental retardation usually is diagnosed only after a significant period of developmental delay has been observed. The older the child at the time of diagnosis, the less the likelihood of reversing the signs of retardation even when a treatable cause can be identified. Prevention is therefore the only significant approach to treatment at present. A screening program for early detection of inborn errors of metabolism and institution of treatment before significant damage to the nervous system can occur represents the model approach to the problem of mental retardation. This same model has been used in developing preventive programs for children at risk for familial-cultural retardation. Controlled studies of stimulation programs for infants in sociocultural groups with high rates of mental retardation have shown significant long-range results after termination of the program when (1) parents have been involved in the program, (2) the infant participated in the program frequently (once every 2 weeks or more), and (3) the program continued for at least 2 years. Head Start has also been shown to decrease the number of children in special education classes and to increase the number of children from high-risk populations who remain in school.

In most instances, however, management of the retarded child does not involve treatment of the retardation per se but must be directed toward (1) assessing the impact on the family and providing support and psychotherapy, (2) providing protection for the child, (3) providing education and rehabilitation to maximize the child's potential, and (4) providing treatment of associated medical, emotional, and behavior problems.

A. Impact on the Family: The diagnosis of mental retardation is an event for which few families are prepared. Often parents can assess the mental age of their child within a few months but still refuse to accept the implications of this information. The tact and sensitivity with which the initial discussion of developmental delay is broached can determine how early the family will allow appropriate treatment, education, and rehabilitation to be started; thus, the primary care physician should be alert to parents' initial questions about developmental delay. A second opinion or repeated evaluation is almost mandatory when the impression of significant developmental delay arises unexpectedly from screening tests or school observations. After the diagnosis is confirmed, the family will need continued assistance and support in adjusting to the diagnosis and in making contact with community resources.

Retarded children and adults can successfully remain within the family in most instances, but they usually require a host of family and community support services. These often include social services, infant education programs, and occupational and physical therapy programs and services for handicapped infants that begin as early as the newborn period. In school-age children, most services are organized through the public school systems, but the primary care physician may be called on to assist in difficult situations.

Once a severely handicapped child is "accepted" by the family, family resources may be totally consumed by care of the child, often to the detriment of normal siblings. Professionals involved with these families should provide help in developing priorities and alleviating parental guilt at being unable to do everything everyone suggests for the child. Less severely handicapped children are often less acceptable to the family, with resulting conflict and emotional disturbance as parents attempt to deny or seek more ego-syntonic diagnoses and explanations for the child's delays. Parental difficulty in accepting evidence of mild retardation often leads them to seek more than one evaluation as they pass through a mourning process and eventually develop more realistic expectations for the child. Parent support groups have been particularly helpful to families with retarded children.

B. Protection, Education, & Rehabilitation: The schools have responsibility for providing educational services to students with mental retardation ages 3–21 in the least restrictive, most normalized environment in which the student can be reasonably expected to receive educational benefit. Regardless of the extent of the individual's disability, the judicial system has interpreted the provisions of PL 94-142 to mean that *all* children—even those with the most profound mental retardation—must be served through the local public school system. Students with disabilities who are enrolled in private or parochial schools are also entitled to receive services through the local public school system. As a result, most metropolitan, suburban, and small school districts provide services for these students in their local public schools. In communities where regional or state residential services for individuals with mental retardation are provided, children living in these institutions are generally transported to classrooms located in public school buildings. Multidisciplinary teams trained to work with these individuals have responsibility for such health care procedures as catheterization, tube feeding, and so on. Motor and language therapists work in concert with special education teachers to provide functional educational programs that focus on increasing levels of personal care, daily living skills, social interaction, and communication. Many schools provide opportunities for interaction with nondisabled peers to increase the quality of life and natural supports for individuals with profound disabilities as well as increase the capacity of children without disabilities to understand and appreciate the full spectrum of human diversity. Where children with mental retardation have additional cognitive capacities, the opportunities for interaction with typical peers are increased. However, the curriculum continues to focus on functional, independent living skills.

As children with mental retardation become adolescents, educational personnel are mandated by law to focus on the transition from school to adult life. Thus, multidisciplinary teams must write specific goals that address support or independent work and residential needs into individualized educational plans. Adult human service agencies must be involved in these transition plans by the time the student reaches the age of 16. Passed in 1990, the Americans With Disabilities Act (ADA) ensures that employers must make accommodations for workers with disabilities, including individuals with mental retardation. Furthermore, ADA specifies that transportation systems and businesses that serve the public must provide access and services to individuals with all types of disabilities. Human service agencies funded to provide resources and services to adults with developmental disabilities, including mental retardation, continue to serve more and more profoundly disabled individuals in nonsheltered environments. Although many adults with developmental disabilities will continue to require individual support and training throughout their lives, these supports will most likely be provided in typical rather than sheltered environments.

C. Treatment of Associated Medical, Emotional, & Behavior Problems: Sensory, motor, and orthopedic handicaps and other medical problems should be treated appropriately. The most controversial area of management concerns the use of psychotropic medication for treatment of emotional and behavior problems, especially in institutionalized retarded children. Although most of these medications are approved primarily for use in treatment of psychotic conditions, the phenothiazines in particular have been used extensively in behavioral management of retarded persons.

Psychotropic medication practices have often resulted in too much being given for too long a time to too many institutionalized children. Frequently, several psychotropic drugs are given at the same time. Some children may be so heavily drugged that they are unable to respond maximally to educational and rehabilitative programs. These practices are often based on claims that the response to neuroleptic and psychotropic medications is altered in retarded children, but other evidence supports the interpretation that psychotropic medication often represents a "chemical straitjacket," which is used as a substitute for adequate personnel to provide more appropriate care. It is uncertain whether attention-deficit disorder in mentally retarded children should be treated with stimulant medication. Some children appear to become worse with treatment (as do many psychotic children), whereas stimulant medication appears to be the treatment of choice for others. As children are withdrawn from heavy medication with phenothiazines and other major psychotropic drugs, symptoms such as dyskinesia may emerge, that is, withdrawal emergent symptoms, which require diagnosis and treatment in themselves. The most serious of these is tardive dyskinesia, which may also appear during treatment.

To avoid misuse of psychotropic medication in the mentally retarded, (1) a diagnosis of the emotional or behavior problem should be made and an appropriate drug and dosage selected on the basis of the diagno-

sis; and (2) the patient's response to the medication should be carefully monitored by the physician through direct evaluation and observation as well as review of reports provided by caretakers.

MOTOR HANDICAPS

A variety of nonspecific problems in development of motor coordination has been observed in children with learning disorders and also as isolated problems. Mental retardation, cerebral palsy, or a neuromuscular disorder is also present in many cases. A larger group, estimated at about 6–7% of the population, shows clumsiness, awkwardness, choreiform movements, or generally poor coordination but no signs of systemic disease except for an increased incidence of other "soft signs" on neurologic examination. Many of the children in this group also show evidence of learning problems, and the motor problems have been cited as evidence of a neurologic basis for the learning problems. However, as with "soft signs" in general, this interpretation is controversial.

Clumsiness and awkwardness have also been reported in association with attention-deficit disorder. In this instance, treatment with stimulant medications has frequently been accompanied by improvement in motor coordination. Occupational and physical therapy are often recommended for these children, although there are no adequately controlled studies with data to support the efficacy of these approaches for improving educational achievement. There is clear evidence that instruction in reading is better than perceptual-motor training in improving reading ability irrespective of the child's motor status. The whole area of mild motor disability has received so little formal scrutiny, however, that much is yet to be learned about ways of identifying and ameliorating developmental impairments in motor skills.

Connolly K: Motor development and motor disability. In: *Developmental Psychiatry.* Rutter M (editor). Heinemann, 1980.

Henderson A: Research in occupational therapy and physical therapy with children. In: *Advances in Behavioral Pediatrics,* Vol 2. Camp BW (editor). JAI Press, 1981.

DEVELOPMENTAL-ADAPTATIONAL PROBLEMS

Developmental-adaptational problems are behavior problems that in normal children decline steadily with age either from infancy or from their appearance in the preschool years. Manifestations include fears, distractibility, hyperactivity, destructiveness, lying, negativism, temper tantrums, enuresis, and thumbsucking. Children with these manifestations often show no maladjustment later in life; absence of these manifestations does not rule out later maladjustment. The gradual decline in these behavior problems is associated with maturation of cognitive competence, including not only intelligence but moral maturity and ego development as well. When deficiencies in social character and cognitive adaptability persist in children beyond the early school years, they are more likely to have a poor prognosis.

ATTENTION-DEFICIT HYPERACTIVITY DISORDER

Essentials of Diagnosis

- Distractibility, short attention span, hyperactivity, impulsivity.
- Duration of longer than 6 months.
- No association with psychosis.
- Association with aggressive behavior, sometimes but not always present.
- Onset before age 7 years.
- Present in more than one setting.

General Considerations

Attention-deficit hyperactivity disorder is characterized by heightened distractibility, short attention span, and impulsiveness. The rate of incidence is about 5%, and the disorder is more common in boys than in girls. Most of the children previously labeled hyperactive or said to have minimal brain dysfunction are children with attention-deficit hyperactivity disorder. In normal children, attention span and ability to concentrate on cognitive tasks increase throughout childhood. Ability of preschool children to engage in sustained task-oriented behavior is one of the most reliable predictors of later school performance. Some evidence suggests that even in infants, attention span may be an early indication of later cognitive performance. In older children, attentiveness is one of the major characteristics of competent children with good peer relations.

The child who persists in immature forms of attentional behavior after age mates have matured is noticeably out of phase in cognitively stressful situations such as school. In these circumstances, children may appear driven to aimless, purposeless activity. Some children also show hyperactive behavior at home, on the playground, and in the physician's office, as well as in the classroom; others may show problems only under cognitive stress. Some children with attention-deficit hyperactivity disorder have also been described as hypoactive rather than hyperactive.

In evaluating behavior problems, it is important to determine whether aggressive behavior problems or conduct disorders are also present. This mixture of behavior problems is common. It is not clear whether the presence of aggressive behavior alters the short-term response to treatment. However, long-term prognosis is poorer in those who have a mixed disorder than in those whose behavior problems are confined to distractibility, impulsiveness, and short attention span.

The causes of attention-deficit hyperactivity disorder are not well understood, although there is evidence of a genetic or constitutional basis for the problem in many children. The diagnosis is largely descriptive, but it carries the implication that specific causes of distractibility and short attention span (eg, neurologic insult or injury, emotional trauma, psychosis, depression) have been eliminated. Immaturity in development of the central nervous system is one of the most likely underlying causes of the problem. However, children who show the functional disorder may or may not have evidence of "soft signs" on neurologic examination or abnormal findings on electroencephalography. The presence of neurodevelopmental signs has not been consistently related to treatment outcome.

Clinical Findings

A. History: The most important diagnostic information comes from a description of behavior in the classroom and teacher ratings on a scale such as the ACTeRS (see Table 4–1). Ratings on this scale that fall below the 10th percentile on attention, hyperactivity, or both, regardless of ratings on the other scales, are usually indicative of attention-deficit hyperactivity disorder. If problems with attention or hyperactivity are not evident at school, it is very unlikely that the child has attention-deficit hyperactivity disorder. Physicians worried about teacher bias in completing the rating will often find that ratings obtained from several teachers will show similar results. However, ratings completed by parents may or may not show deviance. It is useful to review information about oppositional behavior and social skills and obtain information about intelligence and academic performance, because many children also show other behavior or learning problems. The most common other behavior problem encountered among children with attention-deficit disorder is aggressive behavior or oppositional defiant disorder. The family history is often positive for similar problems in childhood, particularly among male relatives. Children with attention-deficit disorder are frequently described as active, colicky infants, and typically parents can recall many incidents indicating distractibility and hyperactivity in the preschool period. Attention-deficit hyperactivity disorder is usually first recognized as a problem after a child enters school. The diagnosis can sometimes be made with great confidence in preschool children, but many of these children are primarily in need of improved parental management.

B. Symptoms & Signs: The neurologic examination may or may not show signs of neurologic immaturity. There are usually no sensory impairments. A significant number of children also have learning problems that may be general or specific, usually depending on the child's level of intelligence. Attention-deficit hyperactivity disorder occurs at all intellectual levels, but among children of average intelligence with behavior problems confined to the attention-deficit hyperactivity disorder syndrome, achievement is often adequate despite teacher complaints that the child is "not learning." When a learning problem accompanies a behavior problem, the problems should be addressed separately.

Family problems may contribute to attention-deficit hyperactivity disorder and increase the difficulty of treatment, especially in children who show aggressive behavior. Attention-deficit disorder is excluded when a diagnosis of childhood psychotic disorder has been made, but the diagnosis may be made in mentally retarded children.

C. Special Studies: Tests measuring continuous performance or vigilance have been widely used in research on attention-deficit hyperactivity disorder. These tests usually require that the child look for occurrences of one specified design among many, either on a page or sequentially flashing on a screen. Two such systems with norms are commercially available for electronic administration of a vigilance test; nevertheless, the clinical application of these procedures is incompletely worked out. No other special tests aid in diagnosis. If there is a question of seizure disorder or clear-cut evidence of neurologic disorder, investigation of these conditions is indicated.

Treatment

Two major effective forms of treatment are behavior modification programs in the classroom and stimulant drugs (methylphenidate [Ritalin], dextroamphetamine [Dexedrine; many others], pemoline [Cylert]). Drug treatment, if effective, tends to have more dramatic results than behavior modification.

Approximately 50–80% of children with attention-deficit hyperactivity disorder are responsive to stimulant drug therapy. Dose-response studies on methylphenidate suggest that a dose of 0.3 mg/kg produces optimal cognitive improvement (concentration) as well as significant improvement in social behavior. Greater improvement in social behavior can be achieved with higher doses, but this occurs at the expense of some loss in concentration. Peak action usually occurs 2 hours after ingestion, and most effects have dissipated after 6 hours. The usual regimen is to start with an early morning dose, followed by a dose at noon if needed. Morning activities often require the most concentration, and the noon dose may be unnecessary. If problems at home are also severe, a third dose may be given in the late afternoon.

Medication on weekends and during school holidays should be tailored to the needs of the child and family. Dextroamphetamine and methylphenidate are similar in onset and duration of action, and most children who respond to one will respond to the other. Pemoline appears to be somewhat different in onset of action, and doses often require adjustment over a longer period of time.

Drug "holidays" are an important part of chronic drug therapy with psychotropic drugs. Medication should be withdrawn for at least 2 weeks of each year to determine whether therapy needs to be continued. Two convenient times for this are summer vacations and spring holidays. In the latter case, a week at home without medication can precede a week at school without medication.

The most common adverse reactions are decreased appetite, headache, stomachache, increased emotional lability, and insomnia. When these side effects appear early in the course of treatment, they are often transient or respond to dosage reduction. It is sometimes difficult to determine whether or not they are indeed medication-related; however, when in doubt, the best approach is to stop or change the medication. All of the stimulants have the potential for exacerbating motor and phonic tics and Tourette's syndrome. Dextroamphetamine is contraindicated in the presence of moderate to severe hypertension, and methylphenidate should be used cautiously in the presence of hypertension. Pemoline is contraindicated in patients with impaired hepatic function. Methylphenidate has been implicated as lowering the threshold for seizures, though a prospective study of a small number of seizure patients did not show this effect. Pemoline has also been associated with development of seizures and elevation of liver enzymes. Decrements in predicted growth have been reported with long-term administration of stimulants, and though a causal relationship has not been established, growth should be carefully monitored.

"Rebound" effects—the appearance of symptoms in exaggerated form when "the medicine wears off"—is a common experience. This is often especially marked in children who have a dramatic response to medication. These effects can frequently be modified by use of a sustained-release form of medication or addition of a small dose of medication after school. In most cases, the family may or may not choose to give medication on the weekend; however, it is usually most beneficial to give medication on weekends in patients who have significant rebound effects.

Monitoring for side effects should be continuous. Weekly teacher reports (ACTeRS scale) during the first month are helpful for monitoring and evaluating treatment. The child should be reevaluated at 1 month to determine whether the response is sufficient to justify continuing with medication.

Behavior modification programs are often tailored

to an individual child's situation. Planning an individualized program usually involves the services of a psychologist or educational specialist. Think Aloud, a general cognitive behavior modification program for improving self-control in children 6–8 years of age, can be used in an office setting. Typically, it has been carried out by special teachers, psychologists, social workers, or other mental health workers but can be used by an intelligent parent or interested physician.

Prognosis

With or without treatment, the long-term outcome is better in the more intelligent children with stable families and uncomplicated attention-deficit hyperactivity disorder. These children often require only short-term treatment (usually 2 years or less). In recent years, increasing emphasis has been placed on recognizing and treating adolescents and adults who continue to be symptomatic.

Camp BW, Bash MAS: *Think Aloud: Increasing Social and Cognitive Skills—A Problem Solving Program for Children.* Research Press, 1981.

Ingersoll B: *Your Hyperactive Child: A Parent's Guide to Coping With Attention Deficit Disorders.* Doubleday, 1988.

Wender PH: *The Hyperactive Child, Adolescent, and Adult.* Oxford Univ Press, 1987.

AGGRESSIVE ANTISOCIAL BEHAVIOR PROBLEMS

Essentials of Diagnosis

- Fighting and physically attacking other children or adults.
- Behavior often boisterous, disruptive, and argumentative, with a "chip on the shoulder" attitude.
- Probable evidence of family disturbance or disharmony.
- Frequent coexistence of poor achievement in children over 10 years of age.
- Higher incidence among less intelligent children.

General Considerations

Destructive, aggressive behavior is common in preschool children but declines significantly with the developmental shift at 5–7 years of age. Nevertheless, it is one of the most malignant behavior problems of childhood. It is more common in boys than in girls. By age 6–8, most normal children have shown a marked decrease in aggressive behavior. A significant number of those who continue to show aggressive behavior after 8 years of age will be aggressive in adolescence. Aggressive behavior is less likely to persist in children who identify with the values of one or both parents. Family disharmony and distur-

bance are the most important contemporaneous instigators of aggressive behavior problems at school.

Clinical Findings

A. History: Active destructive behavior is often seen at an early age and is frequently accompanied by risk-taking and other forms of behavior that make the child difficult to manage. The parents are often characterized as too strict or too lax, providing the child with little supervision or sense of belonging, and often openly rejecting the child. Aggressive behavior by the parents often complicates the diagnosis, since the child may be merely imitating the parents' behavior. Aggressive children of aggressive parents, however, often reject the parents' values even as they imitate the parents' behavior.

B. Symptoms & Signs: The most important information is from teacher, parent, and other reports of aggressive, antisocial, or disruptive behavior. Because some aggressive behavior is present in most children, only teacher and parent rating scales for general behavior that show increases of at least 1.5 SD above normal in amount of aggressive behavior should be considered significant. Neurologic examination usually shows normal results. Intelligence may be average or above average, but aggressive problems occur more frequently in children with lower IQs. Achievement may be average in the first few years of school but shows a steady decline after third grade, frequently accompanied by truancy. Learning delays in all areas are common in the aggressive delinquent adolescent, but 26% show evidence of specific learning disorders. (Most children with specific learning disability are not aggressive, however.) In early school years, the cognitive pattern of aggressive boys tends to show more impulsiveness and less verbal mediation activity than that of normal boys. By adolescence, the typical antisocial, aggressive boy shows a characteristic pattern of decreased verbal intelligence relative to nonverbal, impulsive stereotyped thinking and immaturity in ego development.

Treatment

Large-scale delinquency prevention programs for young aggressive boys have been unsuccessful even when they provided remedial reading instruction as well as counseling and family support. Small-scale behavior modification programs have had some success in normalizing cognitive and social behavior or slowing the increase in delinquent behavior. Psychotherapy and other methods of treatment have met with more modest success.

Behavior modification or other treatment programs are typically designed and monitored by psychologists or child psychiatrists. For younger children (6–8 years of age), the Think Aloud program has been used successfully by teachers, psychologists, social workers, and other mental health workers to help normalize both cognitive and social behavior at school.

When attention-deficit disorder accompanies aggressive behavior problems, stimulant medication is sometimes helpful in decreasing general disruptive behavior as well as impulsiveness and distractibility, but the response may be quite variable.

Camp BW, Ray RS: Aggression. In: *Cognitive Behavior Therapy for Children.* Meyers A, Craighead LW (editors). Plenum, 1984.

Lefkowitz MM et al: *Growing Up to Be Violent.* Pergamon, 1977.

REFERENCES

Levine MD et al: *Developmental and Behavioral Pediatrics.* Saunders, 1983.

Mussen PH (editor): *Carmichael's Manual of Child Psychology,* Vols 1–4. Wiley, 1983.

Parker S, Zuckerman B (editors): *Behavioral and Developmental Pediatrics: A Handbook for Primary Care.* Little, Brown, 1995.

Reynolds CR, Mann L (editors): *Encyclopedia of Special Education,* Vols 1–3. Wiley, 1987.

Adolescence

5

David W. Kaplan, MD, MPH, & Kathleen A. Mammel, MD

Adolescence is a unique period of rapid physical, emotional, cognitive, and social growth and development bridging childhood and adulthood. Generally, adolescence begins at age 11–12 years and ends between ages 18 and 21. Most teenagers complete puberty by ages 16–18 years; in Western society, however, for educational and cultural reasons, the adolescent period is prolonged to allow for further psychosocial development before the young person assumes adult responsibilities.

The developmental passage from childhood to adulthood encompasses the following steps: (1) completing puberty and somatic growth; (2) developing socially, emotionally, and cognitively—moving from concrete to abstract thinking; (3) establishing an independent identity and separating from the family; and (4) preparing for a career or vocation.

DEMOGRAPHY

In the United States in 1995, there were 18 million adolescents between the ages of 15 and 19 years and 17.9 million between 20 and 24 years of age. Adolescents and young adults (15–24 years of age) constitute 13.7% of the US population.

MORTALITY DATA

There has been a remarkable decrease in the mortality rate among 15- to 24-year-olds during this century. Deaths resulting from infectious diseases such as tuberculosis, influenza, and pneumonia, which were common at the beginning of the century, are rare events today. During the last 20 years, there have been changes not only in the major causes of death in the adolescent and young adult population but also in disease-specific mortality rates. Deaths due to motor vehicle crashes, suicide, and homicide have increased 300–400%. For the adolescent population, cultural and environmental rather than organic factors pose the greatest threats of death. For every 15- to 19-year-old who dies of cancer, 8.6 die as a re-sult of an unintentional injury.* For every teenager who dies of heart disease, 8 die as a result of homicide; and for every teenager who dies of kidney disease, 84 commit suicide.

The three leading causes of death (Figure 5–1) in the adolescent population (ages 15–19 years) in 1992 were unintentional injuries (43.3–78% of all unintentional injuries were caused by motor vehicle crashes), suicides (12.8%), and homicides (22.9%). These three causes of violent death accounted for 79% of all adolescent deaths among 15- to 19-year-olds. Homocide is the leading cause of death for black adolescents aged 15–19 years, accounting for 53.2% of all deaths. Deaths resulting from homocide among black 15- to 19-year-old adolescents increased 300% between 1983 and 1992. In 1992, 41.2% of all mortality among adolescent males aged 15–19 years was due to homocide and suicide. Although deaths from automobile crashes have decreased over the last few years, alcohol use remains the underlying cause of most teenage motor vehicle deaths. Almost two-thirds of motor vehicle deaths involving young drinking drivers occur on Friday, Saturday, or Sunday, and 70% occur between 8:00 PM and 4:00 AM.

Deaths due to unintentional injury, homicide, and suicide among adolescents and young adults are distressing not only because of their violent nature but also because they are largely preventable.

MORBIDITY DATA

During the mid 1970s and 1980s, demographic and economic changes in the American family have had a profound effect on many children and adoles-

---

*The term *injury* is preferable to *accidents,* which implies "an act of God" or "bad luck." Injuries during this period most commonly are related to motor vehicle accidents, drownings, falls, and fires. Injuries comprise three elements: the host (who is affected), the agent (the direct cause), and the environment (where, when, and under what conditions).

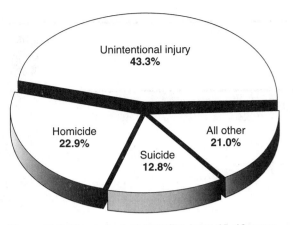

Figure 5–1. Percentage of mortality, ages 15–19 years, 1992.

cents. Between 1955 and 1980, the divorce rate rose from about 400,000 to nearly 1.2 million a year. Between 1960 and 1984, the number of children involved in divorce each year increased from 460,000 to 1.1 million. In 1990, 25% of children were living in single-parent homes, compared with 12% in 1970. In 1991, 45.6% of black, 39.8% of Hispanic, and 16.1% of white children under 18 years of age lived in families with incomes below the poverty level.

The major causes of morbidity during adolescence are primarily psychosocial: unintended pregnancy, sexually transmitted disease, substance abuse, smoking, dropping out of school, depression, running away from home, physical violence, and juvenile delinquency. High-risk behavior in one area is often associated with or may lead to problems in another area (Figure 5–2). For example, teenagers who live in a dysfunctional family (eg, having problems related to parental alcoholism or physical or sexual abuse) are much more likely than other teenagers to be depressed. A depressed teenager is at greater risk for abusing drugs or alcohol, having academic difficulties, running away from home, getting involved sexually as a means of seeking the attention and affection they are not receiving at home, acquiring a sexually transmitted disease, having an unintended pregnancy, or committing suicide.

Early identification of the teenager at risk for these problems is important to prevent the immediate complications and future associated problems. The early indicators of an adolescent at high risk for problems related to depression include the following:

(1) Decline in school performance.
(2) Excessive school absences or cutting class.

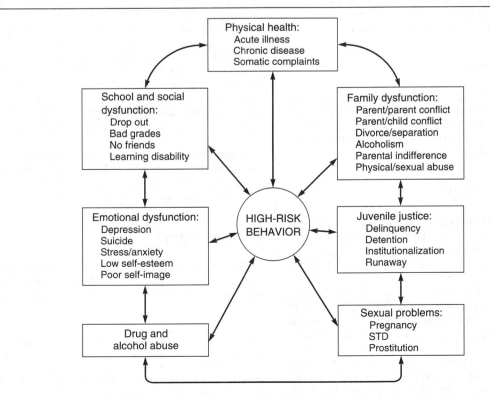

Figure 5–2. Interrelation of high-risk adolescent behavior.

(3) Frequent or persistent psychosomatic complaints.

(4) Changes in sleeping or eating habits.

(5) Difficulty in concentrating or persistent boredom.

(6) Signs or symptoms of depression, extreme stress, or anxiety.

(7) Withdrawal from friends or family, or change to a new group of friends.

(8) Unusually severe violent or rebellious behavior, or radical personality change.

(9) Conflict with parents.

(10) Sexual acting out.

(11) Conflicts with the law.

(12) Suicidal thoughts or preoccupation with themes of death.

(13) Drug and alcohol abuse.

(14) Running away from home.

American Academy of Pediatrics Committee on Adolescence: Firearms and adolescents. Pediatrics 1992; 89:784.

Dryfoos JG: *Adolescents at Risk: Prevalence and Prevention.* Oxford Univ Press, 1990.

Hechinger FM: *Fateful Choices: Healthy Youth for the 21st Century.* Carnegie Corporation of New York, 1992.

Millstein SG, Petersen AC, Nightingale EO: *Promoting the Health of Adolescents: New Directions for the Twenty-First Century.* Oxford Univ Press, 1993.

Rogers DE (editor): Cornell Health Policy Conference: Adolescents at risk. J Adolesc Health 1991;12:585.

Wood DL et al: Access to medical care for children and adolescents in the United States. Pediatrics 1990;86:666.

DELIVERY OF HEALTH SERVICES

How, where, why, and when adolescents seek health care depend on a number of factors: ability to pay for care, distance to health care facilities, availability of transportation, accessibility of services, time out of school, and privacy. Many common teenage health problems—such as unintended pregnancy, sexually transmitted disease, the need for contraception, substance abuse, and depression and other emotional problems—have moral or ethical implications. Teenagers are often reluctant to confide in their parents for fear of punishment or disapproval. Recognizing this reality, health care providers have set up many specialized programs, such as teenage family planning clinics, drop-in centers, sexually transmitted disease clinics, hot lines, and adolescent clinics. For the physician, establishing a trusting and confidential relationship is basic to meeting an adolescent patient's health care needs. A patient who senses the physician will inform the parents about a confidential problem may lie or fail to disclose information essential for proper diagnosis and treatment.

GUIDELINES FOR ADOLESCENT PREVENTIVE SERVICES

In 1992, the American Medical Association released a comprehensive set of guidelines for adolescent care to promote healthful lifestyles and physical and emotional well-being. These guidelines for adolescent preventive services (GAPS) cover screening, health guidance, immunizations, and delivery of health care services. The guidelines have four goals: (1) to deter adolescents from participating in behaviors that jeopardize health; (2) to detect physical, emotional, and behavioral problems early and to intervene immediately; (3) to reinforce and encourage behaviors that promote healthful living; and (4) to provide immunizations against infectious diseases. The guidelines recommend that all adolescents between the ages of 11 and 21 should have annual routine health visits. The health services provided should be developmentally appropriate and culturally sensitive, and confidentiality between patient and physician should be ensured. A complete schedule of the recommended guidelines is shown in Figure 5–3A.

RELATING TO THE ADOLESCENT PATIENT

Adolescence is one of the physically healthiest periods in an individual's life. The challenge of caring for adolescents does not lie in managing complex organic disease but in accommodating to the changing and developing cognitive, emotional, and psychosocial growth that influences health behavior.

How the physician initially approaches the adolescent may determine the success or failure of the visit. The physician should behave simply and honestly, without an authoritarian or excessively "professional" manner. Because the self-esteem of many young adolescents is fragile, the physician must be careful not to overpower and intimidate the patient. To establish a comfortable and trusting relationship, the physician should strive to present the image of an ordinary person who has special training and skills.

Because onset and termination of puberty may vary considerably from individual to individual, chronologic age may be a poor indicator of expected physical, physiologic, and emotional development. In communicating with an adolescent, the physician must be especially sensitive to the patient's develop-

Preventive Health Services by Age and Procedure

Adolescents and young adults have a unique set of health care needs. The recommendations for Guidelines for Adolescent Services (GAPS) emphasize annual clinical preventive services visits that address both the developmental and psychosocial aspects of health, in addition to traditional biomedical conditions. These recommendations were developed by the American Medical Association with contributions from a Scientific Advisory Panel, comprised of national experts, as well as representatives of primary care medical organizations and the health insurance industry. The body of scientific evidence indicates that the periodicity and content of preventive services can be important in promoting the health and well-being of adolescents.

Procedure	Early				Middle			Late			
Age of Adolescent	11	12	13	14	15	16	17	18	19	20	21
Health Guidance											
Parenting*			——●——			●					
Development	●	●	●	●	●	●	●	●	●	●	●
Diet and Physical Activity	●	●	●	●	●	●	●	●	●	●	●
Healthy Lifestyle**	●	●	●	●	●	●	●	●	●	●	●
Injury Prevention	●	●	●	●	●	●	●	●	●	●	●
Screening											
History											
Eating Disorders	●	●	●	●	●	●	●	●	●	●	●
Sexual Activity***	●	●	●	●	●	●	●	●	●	●	●
Alcohol and Other Drug Use	●	●	●	●	●	●	●	●	●	●	●
Tobacco Use	●	●	●	●	●	●	●	●	●	●	●
Abuse	●	●	●	●	●	●	●	●	●	●	●
School Performance	●	●	●	●	●	●	●	●	●	●	●
Depression	●	●	●	●	●	●	●	●	●	●	●
Risk for Suicide	●	●	●	●	●	●	●	●	●	●	●
Physical Assessment											
Blood Pressure	●	●	●	●	●	●	●	●	●	●	●
BMI	●	●	●	●	●	●	●	●	●	●	●
Comprehensive Exam			——●——			●				●	
Tests											
Cholesterol			———1———			—1—				—1—	
TB			———2———			—2—				—2—	
GC, Chlamydia, Syphilis, & HPV			———3———			—3—				—3—	
HIV			———4———			—4—				—4—	
Pap Smear			———5———			—5—				—5—	
Immunizations											
MMR		—●—									
Td		—●—				——○——					
Hep B		—●—				——6——				——6——	
Hep A			———7———			——7——				——7——	
Varicella			———8———			——8——				——8——	

1. Screening test performed once if family history is positive for early cardiovascular disease or hyperlipidemia.
2. Screen if positive for exposure to active TB or lives/works in high-risk situation, eg homeless shelter, jail, health care facility.
3. Screen at least annually if sexually active.
4. Screen if high risk for infection.
5. Screen annually if sexually active or if 18 years or older.
6. Vaccinate any adolescent not previously vaccinated.
7. Vaccinate if at risk for hepatitis A infection.
8. Offer vaccine if no reliable history of chicken pox or previous immunization.
* A parent health guidance visit is recommended during early and middle adolescence.
** Includes counseling regarding sexual behavior and avoidance of tobacco, alcohol, and other drug use.
*** Includes history of unintended pregnancy and STD.
○ Do not give if administered in last five years.

A

Figure 5–3. *A:* Guidelines for preventive health services. (Reproduced, with permission, from *AMA Guidelines for Adolescent Preventive Services: Recommendations and Rationale.* American Medical Association, 1995.)

TEEN HEALTH HISTORY

This information is *strictly confidential.* Its purpose is to help your caregiver give you better care. We request that you fil out the form completely, but you may skip any question that you do not wish to answer.

NAME _____ DATE _____

FIRST   MIDDLE INITIAL   LAST

BIRTHDATE _____ AGE _____ GRADE _____ Name that you like to be called _____

1. Why did you come to the clinic today? _____

_____

_____

Medical History   **STRICTLY CONFIDENTIAL**

2. Are you allergic to any medicines? . . . .   YES NO
   Name of medicines _____
3. Are you taking any medicines now? . . . .   YES NO
   Name of medicines _____
4. Do you have any long-term health conditions? . . . .   YES NO
   Conditions _____
5. Date or age at your last tetanus (or dT) shot _____

School Information

6. What grade do you usually make in English? _____
   (Example: A, B, C, D, E, F)
7. What grade do you usually make in Math? _____
8. How many days were you absent from school last semester? _____
9. How many days were you absent last semester because of illness? _____
10. How do you get along at school? _____

1	2	3	4	5	6	7
TERRIBLE						GREAT

11. Have you ever been suspended? . . . .   YES NO
12. Have you ever dropped out of school? . . . .   YES NO
13. Do you plan to graduate from high school? . . . .   YES NO

Job/Career Information

14. Are you working? . . . .   YES NO
    If YES, what is your job? _____
    How many hours do you work per week? _____
15. What are your future plans or career goals? _____

Family Information

16. Who do you live with? (Check all that apply.)
    _____ Both natural parents   _____ Stepmother   _____ Brother(s)-ages: _____
    _____ Mother   _____ Stepfather   _____ Sister(s)-ages: _____
    _____ Father   _____ Guardian   _____ Other: Explain _____
    _____ Adoptive parents   _____ Alone
17. Have there been any changes in your family? Check all that apply.
    _____ a. Marriage   _____ d. Serious illness   _____ g. Births
    _____ b. Separation   _____ e. Loss of job   _____ h. Deaths
    _____ c. Divorce   _____ f. Move to new home   _____ i. Other
18. Father's/stepfather's occupation or job: _____
    Mother's/stepmother's occupation or job: _____

B

(continued)

Figure 5–3. *B:* Adolescent medical history questionnaire.

19. How do you get along at home?

| 1 TERRIBLE | 2 | 3 | 4 | 5 | 6 | 7 GREAT |

20. Have you ever run away from home? .... YES NO
21. Have you ever lived in foster care or an institution? .... YES NO

Self Information

22. On the whole, how do you like yourself?

| 1 NOT VERY MUCH | 2 | 3 | 4 | 5 | 6 | 7 A LOT |

23. What do you do best?_____
24. If you could, what would you like to change about yourself? _____
_____

25. List any habits you would like to break. _____

26. Do you feel people expect too much from you? .... YES NO
27. How do you get along with your friends/peers?

| 1 TERRIBLE | 2 | 3 | 4 | 5 | 6 | 7 GREAT |

28. Do you feel you have friends you can count on? .... YES NO
29. Have you ever felt really sad or depressed for more than 3 days in a row? .. YES NO
30. Have you ever thought of suicide as a solution to your problems? .... YES NO
31. Have you gotten into any trouble because of your anger/temper? .... YES NO

Health Concern

32. On a scale of 1–7, how would you rate your general health?

| 1 TERRIBLE | 2 | 3 | 4 | 5 | 6 | 7 GREAT |

33. Do you have any questions or concerns about any of the following? (Check those that apply.)

____ Height/weight
____ Blood pressure
____ Head/headaches
____ Dizziness/passing out
____ Eyes/vision
____ Ears/hearing/earaches
____ Nose/frequent colds
____ Mouth/teeth
____ Neck/back
____ Chest/breathing/coughing
____ Breasts
____ Heart
____ Stomach/pain/vomiting
____ Diarrhea/constipation

____ Skin rash
____ Arms, legs/muscle or joint pain
____ Frequent or painful urination
____ Wetting the bed
____ Sexual organs/genitals
____ Trouble sleeping
____ Tiredness
____ Diet food/appetite
____ Eating disorder
____ Smoking/drugs/alcohol
____ Future plans/jobs
____ Worried about parents

____ Family violence/physical abuse
____ Feeling down or depressed
____ Dating
____ Sex
____ Worried about VD/STD
____ Masturbation
____ Sexual abuse/rape
____ Having children/parenting/adoption
____ Cancer/or dying
____ Other (explain) _____
_____

Health Behavior Information

34. Have you lost or gained any weight in the last year? .... YES NO
    Gained ( ) How much? _____
    Lost ( ) How much? _____
35. In the past year, have you tried to lose weight or control your weight by vomiting, taking diet pills or laxatives, or starving yourself? .... YES NO
36. Do you ever drive after drinking or when high? .... YES NO
37. Do you ever smoke cigarettes or use snuff or chewing tobacco? .... YES NO
38. Do you ever smoke marijuana? .... YES NO
39. Do you ever drink alcoholic beverages? .... YES NO
40. Do you ever use street drugs (speed, cocaine, acid, crack, etc.)? .... YES NO
41. Does anyone in your household smoke? .... YES NO
42. Does anyone in your family have a problem with drugs or alcohol? .... YES NO

Figure 5–3. *B:* (continued)

43. Have you ever been in trouble with the police or the law? . . . .   YES NO
44. Have you begun dating? . . . .   YES NO
45. Do you currently have a boyfriend or girlfriend? . . . .   YES NO
    If YES, how old is he/she? _____
46. Do you think you might be gay/lesbian/homosexual? . . . .   YES NO
47. Have you ever had sex (sexual intercourse)? . . . .   YES NO
48. Are you interested in receiving information on preventing pregnancy? . . . . . .   YES NO
49. If you have had sex, are you (or your partner) using any kind of birth control?   YES NO
50. If you have had sex, have you ever been treated for gonorrhea or chlamydia
    or any other sexually transmitted disease? . . . .   YES NO

For males only
51. Have you been taught how to use a condom correctly? . . . .   YES NO
52. If you have had sex, do you use a condom every time or almost every time?   YES NO
53. Have you ever fathered a child? . . . .   YES NO

For females only
54. How old were you when your periods began? . . . .   _____
55. What date did your last period start? . . . .   _____
56. Are your periods regular (once a month)? . . . .   YES NO
57. Do you have painful or excessively heavy periods? . . . .   YES NO
58. Have you ever had a vaginal infection or been treated for a female disorder?   YES NO
59. Do you think you might be pregnant? . . . .   YES NO
60. Have you ever been pregnant? . . . .   YES NO

Everyone
61. Do you have any other problems you would like to discuss with the caregiver?   YES NO

Past Medical History
62. Were you born prematurely or did you have any serious problems as an infant?   YES NO
63. Are you allergic to any medicines? . . . .   YES NO
    If YES, what? _____

64. List any medications that you are taking and the problems for which the
    medication was given:

MEDICATION	REASON	HOW LONG
_____	_____	_____
_____	_____	_____
_____	_____	_____

65. Have you ever been hospitalized? . . . .   YES NO
    If YES, describe your problem and your age at the time.

AGE	PROBLEM
_____	_____
_____	_____
_____	_____

66. Have you had any injuries? . . . .   YES NO
    If YES, describe the injury and your age when it occurred.

AGE	KIND OF INJURY
_____	_____
_____	_____

67. Have you had any serious illnesses? . . . .   YES NO
    If YES, state the kind of illness and your age when it started.

AGE	ILLNESS
_____	_____
_____	_____

(continued)

Figure 5–3. *B:* (continued)

Family History

Have any members of your family, alive or dead (parents, grandparents, uncles, aunts, brothers or sisters), had any of the following problems? If YES, please state the age of the person when the condition occurred and the person's relationship to you.

	PROBLEM	YES	NO	DON'T KNOW	AGE	RELATIONSHIP
A.	Seizure disorder Epilepsy					
B.	Mental retardation Birth defects					
C.	Migraine headaches					
D.	High blood pressure High cholesterol					
E.	Heart attack or stroke at less than age 60					
F.	Lung disease Tuberculosis					
G.	Liver or intestinal disease					
H.	Kidney disease					
I.	Allergies Asthma Eczema					
J.	Arthritis					
K.	Diabetes					
L.	Endocrine problems Other glandular problems					
M.	Obesity Eating disorder					
N.	Cancer					
O.	Blood disorders Sickle cell anemia					
P.	Emotional problems Suicide					
Q.	Alcoholism Drug problems					

Figure 5–3. *B:* (continued)

mental level, recognizing that physical appearance and chronologic age may not give an accurate assessment of cognitive development. Talking to a teenager as a child or, at the other extreme, as an adult, may interfere with communication and cause the patient to lose confidence in the provider.

Working with teenagers can be draining emotionally. Adolescents have a unique ability to identify hidden emotional vulnerabilities. The physician who has a personal need to control patients or foster dependency may be disappointed in caring for teenagers. Because teenagers are consumed with their own emotional needs, they rarely provide the physician with the ego rewards that younger or older patients do.

The physician should be sensitive to the issue of countertransference, the emotional reaction elicited in the physician by the adolescent. How the physician relates to the adolescent patient often depends on personal characteristics of the physician. This is especially true of physicians treating families with parent-adolescent conflicts. It is common for young physicians to overidentify with the teenage patient and for older physicians to see the conflict from the parents' perspective. Overidentification with the parents is readily sensed by the teenager, who is likely to view the physician as just another authority figure who cannot understand the problems of being a teenager. Assuming a parental-authoritarian role as a physician and lecturing the adolescent not only is counterproductive but also may seriously jeopardize establishing a working relationship with the patient. In the case of the young physician, overidentification with the teenager may cause the parents to become extremely defensive about their parenting role and discount the experience and ability of the physician.

THE SETTING

Adolescents respond positively to a setting and services that communicate a sensitivity to their age. For instance, a pediatrician's waiting room scattered with toddler's toys and examination tables too short for a young adult make adolescent patients feel that they have outgrown the practice. Similarly, a waiting room filled with geriatric or pregnant patients can make a teenager feel out of place. An examination room designed with adolescents in mind and special appointment times may be useful in engaging this age group.

It is not uncommon to see a new teenage patient who has absolutely no interest in being there, especially when the teenager is brought in for evaluation of drug and alcohol use, parent-adolescent conflict, school failure, depression, or a suspected eating disorder. Even in cases of acute physical illness, the adolescent may feel anxiety about having a physical examination, especially if the teenager is overly

modest, is worried about having blood drawn, or simply fears the unknown. If future visits are to be successful, the physician must spend time on the first visit to give the teenager a sense of trust and an opportunity to feel comfortable.

CONFIDENTIALITY

It is helpful at the beginning of the visit to talk with the adolescent and the parents about what to expect. The physician should address the issue of confidentiality, telling the parents that two meetings—one with the teenager alone and one only with the parents—will take place. Adequate time must be spent with both the patient and the parents, or important information may be missed. At the beginning of the interview with the patient, it is useful to say, "I am likely to ask you some personal questions. This is not because I am trying to snoop into your private life, but because these questions may be important to your health. I want to assure you that what we talk about is confidential, just between the two of us. If there is something I feel we should discuss with your parents, I will ask your permission first, unless I feel it is life-threatening."

THE STRUCTURE OF THE VISIT

Caring for adolescents is a time-intensive process. In many adolescent practices, a 40–50% no-show rate is not unusual, making scheduling complex. In addition, it is not uncommon for an adolescent to come in without an appointment because of a seemingly minor complaint. Because of issues related to confidentiality, teenagers may initially conceal their real concern. For example, a healthy-appearing 15-year-old girl may walk in with the chief complaint of a sore throat but actually be worried about being pregnant. What initially appeared to be a 10-minute visit for a throat culture may turn into a 1-hour visit spent counseling an anxious pregnant teenager.

By the age of 11 or 12, patients should be seen alone, without a parent. This gives them an opportunity to ask questions they may be embarrassed to ask in front of a parent. Because of the physical changes that take place in early puberty, some adolescents are too self-conscious to undress in front of a parent (and sometimes the physician). If an adolescent comes in willingly, either for an acute illness or a routine physical examination, it may be helpful to meet with the adolescent and parent together to obtain the history. In the case of angry adolescents who are brought in against their will, it is useful to meet with the parents and adolescent just long enough to have the parents describe the conflict and state their concerns. This meeting should last no longer than 3–5 minutes, and then the adolescent should be seen alone. This approach conveys that the physician is primarily interested in the adolescent patient, yet gives the physician an opportunity to acknowledge the parents' anger and the fact that the patient probably didn't want to come in the first place.

The Interview

The first few minutes of the interview may dictate the success of the visit—whether or not a trusting relationship can be established. Taking a few minutes getting to know the patient is time well spent. For example, immediately asking a teenager who is brought in for suspected marijuana use "Do you smoke marijuana?" confirms the adolescent's negative preconceptions about the physician and the purpose of the visit.

It is preferable to spend a few minutes asking nonthreatening questions. Examples are: "Tell me a little bit about yourself so I can get to know you." "What do you like to do most?" "Least?" "What are your friends like?" Neutral questions help defuse some of the patient's anger and anxiety. Examples are: "How has your health been?" "What kinds of serious accidents or injuries have you had?" Toward the end of the interview, the physician can ask more directed questions about psychosocial concerns.

Medical history questionnaires for the patient and the parents are very useful in collecting the necessary historical data and making the visit as efficient as possible (Figure 5–3B). Although the history questionnaire is helpful, the physician must spend sufficient time to get to know the patient and establish a meaningful relationship.

The history should include an assessment of progress with psychodevelopmental tasks and of behaviors that are potentially detrimental to health. The review of systems should include questions about the following:

(1) Nutrition: number and balance of meals; calcium, iron, cholesterol intake.

(2) Sleep: number of hours, problems with insomnia or frequent waking.

(3) Seat belt or helmet: regularity of use.

(4) Self-care: knowledge of testicular or breast self-examination, dental hygiene, and exercise.

(5) Family relationships: parents, siblings, relatives.

(6) Peers: best friend, involvement in group activities, boyfriends, girlfriends.

(7) School: attendance, grades, activities.

(8) Educational and vocational interests: college, career, short-term and long-term vocational plans.

(9) Tobacco: use of cigarettes, snuff, chewing tobacco.

(10) Substance abuse: frequency, extent, and history of alcohol and drug use.

(11) Sexuality: sexual activity, contraceptive use, pregnancies, history of sexually transmitted disease, number of sexual partners, risk for HIV infection.

(12) Emotional health: signs of depression and excessive stress.

The physician's personal attention and interest is likely to be a new experience for the teenager, who has probably received medical care only through a parent. The teenager should leave the visit with a sense of having a personal physician.

Physical Examination

During early adolescence, many teenagers may be shy and modest, especially if examined by a physician of the opposite sex. The examiner should address this concern directly, because it can be allayed by acknowledging the uneasiness verbally and explaining the purpose of the examination—for example, "Many boys that I see who are your age are embarrassed to have their penis and testes (balls) examined. This is an important part of the examination for a couple of reasons. First, I want to make sure that there aren't any physical problems, and second, it helps me determine if your development is proceeding normally." This also introduces the subject of sexual development for discussion.

A pictorial chart of sexual development (Figures 5–4 and 5–5) is extremely useful in showing the patient how development is proceeding and what changes to expect in the future. The chart shows the relationship between height, breast development, menstruation, and pubic hair growth in the female and between height, penis and testes development, and pubic hair growth in the male. Although many teenagers do not openly admit that they are interested in this subject, they are usually attentive during the discussion. This discussion is particularly useful in counseling teenagers who lag behind their peers in physical development.

Because teenagers are especially sensitive about their changing bodies, it is useful to comment on the findings during the physical examination—for example, "Your heart sounds fine. I am examining your breasts and feel a small lump under your right breast. This is very common during puberty in boys. It is called gynecomastia and should disappear in 6 months to a year. Don't worry, you are not turning into a girl."

The question of the appropriate age for the first pelvic examination often arises. The following are indications for a pelvic examination in a teenage girl:

(1) Sexual intercourse. (The pelvic examination should be done for purposes of contraceptive counseling and to rule out sexually transmitted disease.)

(2) Abnormal vaginal discharge.

(3) Menstrual irregularities, such as amenorrhea, hypermenorrhea, dysmenorrhea.

(4) Suspicion of anatomic abnormalities, such as diethylstilbestrol exposure, imperforate hymen.

(5) Pelvic pain.

(6) Patient request of an examination.

If a teenage girl has not been sexually active and

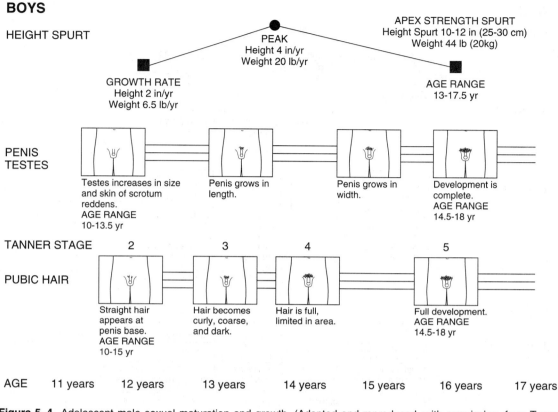

Figure 5–4. Adolescent male sexual maturation and growth. (Adapted and reproduced, with permission, from Tanner JM: *Growth at Adolescence.* Blackwell, 1962.)

has no gynecologic complaints or abnormalities, a pelvic examination is usually not necessary until about age 18.

Elster AB, Kuznets NJ: *AMA Guidelines for Adolescent Preventive Services.* Williams & Wilkins, 1994.

English A: Treating adolescents: Legal and ethical considerations. Med Clin North Am 1990;74:1097.

Green M (editor): *Bright Futures: Guidelines for Health Supervision of Infants, Children, and Adolescents.* National Center for Education in Maternal and Child Health, 1994.

Society for Adolescent Medicine: Access to health care for adolescents. J Adolesc Health 1991;13:162.

GROWTH & DEVELOPMENT

PUBERTY

Pubertal growth and physical development are a result of activation of the hypothalamic-pituitary go-nadal axis in late childhood. Before the onset of puberty, pituitary and gonadal hormones remain at very low levels. With the onset of puberty, the inhibition of gonadotropin-releasing hormone (GnRH) in the hypothalamus is removed, allowing pulsatile production and release of the gonadotropins, luteinizing hormone (LH) and follicle-stimulating hormone (FSH). In early to middle adolescence, there is an increase in pulse frequency and amplitude of LH and FSH secretion, which stimulates the gonads to produce sex steroids (estrogen or testosterone). In the female, FSH stimulates ovarian maturation, granulosa cell function, and estradiol secretion. LH is important in ovulation and is also involved in corpus luteum formation and progesterone secretion. Initially, estradiol has an inhibitory effect on the release of LH and FSH. Eventually, estradiol becomes stimulatory, and the secretions of LH and FSH become cyclic. There is a progressive increase in estradiol, resulting in maturation of the female genital tract and breast development.

In the male, LH stimulates the interstitial cells of the testes, which produce testosterone. FSH stimulates the production of spermatocytes in the presence of testosterone. The testes also produce inhibin, a

GIRLS

HEIGHT SPURT

PEAK
Height 3 in/yr
Weight 17.5 lb/yr

GROWTH RATE
Height 2 in/yr
Weight 6 lb/yr

AGE RANGE
11.5-16.5 yr

MENARCHE

Age Range 10-16.5 yr
Average Height 62.5 in (158.5 cm)
Average Weight 106 lb (48 kg)

BREAST

Breast buds begin. AGE RANGE 8-13 yr

Breast and areola grow.

Nipple and areola form separate mound, protruding from breast.

Areola rejoins breast contour and development is complete. AGE RANGE 12.5-18.5 yr

TANNER STAGE: 2 3 4 5

PUBIC HAIR

Initial hair is straight and fine. AGE RANGE 8-14 yr

Pubic hair coarsens, darkens and spreads.

Hair looks like adults but limited in area.

Inverted triangular pattern is established AGE RANGE 12.5-16.5 yr

AGE: 11 years 12 years 13 years 14 years 15 years

Figure 5–5. Adolescent female sexual maturation and growth. (Adapted and reproduced, with permission, from Tanner JM: *Growth at Adolescence.* Blackwell, 1962.)

Sertoli cell protein that also inhibits the secretion of FSH. During puberty, circulating testosterone increases more than 20-fold. Levels of testosterone correlate with the physical stages of puberty and the degree of skeletal maturation.

PHYSICAL GROWTH

During adolescence, a teenager's weight doubles, and height increases by 15–20%. During puberty, major organs double in size, with the exception of lymphoid tissue, which decreases in mass. Before puberty, there is little difference in muscular strength between boys and girls. The body's musculature increases both in size and strength during puberty, with maximal strength lagging behind the increase in size by many months. Boys attain greater strength and mass, and strength continues to increase into late puberty. Although motor coordination lags behind growth in stature and musculature, it continues to improve as strength develops.

The pubertal growth spurt begins nearly 2 years earlier in girls than in boys. Girls reach their peak height velocity (PHV) between 11½ and 12 years of age; boys, between 13½ and 14 years of age. Linear growth at peak velocity is 9.5 cm/y + 1.5 cm for boys and 8.3 cm/y + 1.2 cm for girls. Pubertal growth usually takes 2–4 years and continues longer in boys than in girls. By age 11 years in girls and age 12 in boys, 83–89% of ultimate height has been attained. An additional 18–23 cm (7–9 in.) in females and 25–30 cm (10–12 in.) in males will be achieved during further pubertal growth. Following menarche, growth is rarely more than 5–7.5 cm (2–3 in.).

Boys increase the quantity of body fat before beginning the height spurt. They then lose fat until the growth spurt has finished and gradually again increase in fat. Muscle mass doubles between ages 10 and 17 years. Girls, by contrast, gradually store fat from about age 6 and do not decrease the quantity of fat, although its location changes, with an increase of subcutaneous fat in the region of the pelvis, breasts, and upper back.

SEXUAL MATURATION

Tanner's scale of sexual maturation is useful clinically to categorize genital development. Tanner staging includes age ranges of normal development and specific descriptions for each stage of pubic hair growth, penis and testis development in boys, and breast maturation in girls. Figures 5–4 and 5–5 graphically represent this chronologic development with reference to each Tanner stage. Tanner stage I is prepuberty; stage V, adult maturity. In stage II there is sparse, fine, nonpigmented, downy pubic hair; in stage III, the hair becomes pigmented and curly and increases in amount; and in stage IV, the hair is adult in texture but limited in area. The appearance of pubic hair precedes that of axillary hair by more than 1 year. Male genital development begins with stage II, in which the testes become larger and the scrotal skin reddens and coarsens. In stage III, the penis lengthens; and in stage IV, the penis enlarges in general size and the scrotal skin becomes pigmented.

Female breast development follows a predictable sequence. Small, raised breast buds appear in stage II. In stage III, there is general enlargement and raising of breast and areolar tissue. The areola and papilla (nipple) form a separate mound from the breast in stage IV, and in stage V the areola assumes the same contour as the breast.

Great variability exists in the timing and onset of puberty and growth, and psychosocial development does not necessarily parallel physical changes. Because of this variability, chronologic age is a poor indication of physiologic and psychosocial development during adolescence. Skeletal maturation correlates well with biologic maturity and pubertal development.

Teenagers have been entering puberty at increasingly earlier ages during the last century because of better nutrition and improved socioeconomic conditions. The age at menarche has decreased by about 4 months per decade during the last century. In the United States, the average age at menarche is 12¾ years. Frisch has shown that among girls reaching menarche, the average weight is 48 kg (106 lb), and the average height is 158.5 cm (62.5 in.). However, menarche may be delayed until age 16 or begin as early as age 10. Although the first measurable sign of puberty in girls is the beginning of the height spurt, the first conspicuous sign usually is development of breast buds between the ages of 8 and 11 years. Although breast development usually antedates the growth of pubic hair, in some normal girls the reverse may occur. A common concern for girls at this time is whether the breasts will be of the right size and shape, especially since it is not unusual for one breast to grow faster than the other. Among girls, the growth spurt starts at about age 9 years and reaches a peak at age 11½, usually at stage III-IV breast development and stage III pubic hair development. However, the height spurt may start as early as age 8 years in early maturers or as late as age 11½ in late maturers. The spurt usually ends by age 14. Girls who mature early will reach their PHV sooner and attain their final height earlier. Girls who mature late will attain a greater ultimate height because of the longer period of growth before the growth spurt. Final height is related to skeletal age at onset of puberty as well as genetic factors. The height spurt correlates more closely with breast developmental stages than with pubic hair stages.

The first sign of puberty in the male, usually between the ages of 10 and 12, is scrotal and testicular growth. The appearance of pubic hair is usually an early event in puberty but can occur any time between ages 10 and 15 years. The penis begins to grow significantly a year or so after the onset of testicular and pubic hair development, usually between the ages of 10 and 13½. The first ejaculation is a notable event and usually occurs about 1 year after initiation of testicular growth, but its timing is highly variable. About 90% of boys have this experience between the ages of 11 and 15 years. Gynecomastia, a hard nodule under the nipple, occurs in a majority of boys, with a peak incidence between ages 14 and 15 years. Gynecomastia usually disappears within 2 years. The height spurt begins at age 11 but increases rapidly between the ages of 12 and 13, with the PHV reached at age 13½ years. However, the height spurt may start at age 10 in early maturers or as late as age 13–14 in late maturers. The period of pubertal development lasts much longer in boys and may not be completed until age 18 years. The height velocity is higher in males (8–11 cm/y) than females (6½–9½ cm/y). The development of axillary hair, deepening of the voice, and the development of chest hair in boys usually occurs in mid puberty, about 2 years after onset of growth of pubic hair. Facial and body hair begin to increase at ages 16–17 years.

Litt IF: Pubertal and psychosocial development: Implications for pediatricians. Pediatr Rev 1995;16:243.

Tanner JM: *Growth at Adolescence.* Blackwell, 1962.

Tanner JM, Davies PW: Clinical longitudinal standards for height and height velocity for North American children. J Pediatr 1985;107:317.

PSYCHOSOCIAL DEVELOPMENT

Adolescents are struggling to find out who they are, what they want to do in the future, and, in relation to that goal, what their personal strengths and weaknesses are. These questions arise primarily because teenagers are in the process of establishing their own identity. Adolescence is a period of progressive individuation and separation from the family. Because of the rapid physical, emotional, cognitive, and social growth occurring during adolescence, it is useful to divide the period into three sequential phases of development. Early adolescence occurs roughly between ages 10 and 13; middle adolescence, between ages 14 and 16; and late adolescence, at age 17 and later.

Early Adolescence

Early adolescence (ages 10–13) is characterized by rapid growth and development of secondary sex characteristics. Young adolescents are often preoccupied with the physical changes taking place in their bodies. Because of these rapid physical changes, body image, self-concept, and self-esteem fluctuate dramatically. Concerns about how their growth and development deviate from that of their friends may be a great worry, especially short stature in boys and delayed breast development or delayed menarche in girls. Although there is a certain curiosity about sexuality, young adolescents tend to feel much more comfortable with members of the same sex. As the young teenager begins to become more independent and family ties loosen, allegiance shifts from parents to peers, who become much more important. Young teenagers still think concretely and cannot easily conceptualize about the future. They may have vague and unrealistic professional goals, such as becoming a lead singer in a rock group or a famous movie star. Only through the experiences encountered in later adolescence do they become more realistic.

Middle Adolescence

During middle adolescence (14–16 years), as the rapid pubertal growth of early adolescence decreases, teenagers begin to adjust and become more comfortable with their "new" bodies. Intense emotions and wide swings in mood are typical. Although some teenagers go through this experience relatively peacefully, others struggle desperately. Cognitively, teenagers move from concrete thinking to formal operations and develop the ability to think abstractly. With this new mental power comes a sense of omnipotence and a belief that the world can be changed by merely thinking about it. Sexually active teenagers may believe they do not need to worry about using contraception because they "can't get pregnant—it won't happen to me." Sixteen-year-old drivers believe that they are the best drivers in the world and think the insurance industry is conspiring against them by charging such high rates for automobile insurance. With the onset of the ability to think abstractly, teenagers begin to see themselves as others see them and may become extremely self-centered. Because they are establishing their own identities, relationships with other people, including peers, are primarily narcissistic, and experimenting with different images is quite common. Peers determine the standards for identification, behavior, activities, and fashion and provide emotional support, intimacy, empathy, and the sharing of guilt and anxiety during

the struggle for autonomy. The struggle for independence and autonomy is often a difficult and stressful period for both the teenager and the parents.

As sexuality increases in importance, midadolescents may begin dating and experimenting with sex. Relationships usually tend to be one-sided and narcissistic. By age 18, nearly half of American females and two-thirds of males have had intercourse.

Late Adolescence

Late adolescents (17 years and older) are much less self-centered and begin caring much more about others. Social relationships shift from the peer group to the individual. Dating becomes much more intimate. The older adolescent becomes more independent from the family. The ability to think abstractly allows older adolescents to think more realistically in terms of future plans, actions, and careers. Older adolescents have very rigid concepts of what is right and what is wrong. This is a period of idealism.

Homosexuality in Adolescence

Homosexual characteristics appear to be established before adolescence. Sexual orientation develops during early childhood. One's gender identity is established by age 2, and a sense of masculinity or femininity usually solidifies by age 5 or 6. Homosexual adults describe homosexual feelings during late childhood and early adolescence, years before engaging in overt homosexual acts.

Although only 5–10% of American young people acknowledge having had homosexual experiences and only 5% feel that they are or could be gay, homosexual experimentation is common, especially during early and middle adolescence. Experimentation may include mutual masturbation and fondling the genitals and does not by itself cause or lead to adult homosexuality. Theories about the etiology of homosexuality include genetic, hormonal, environmental, and psychologic models; however, there is no definitive explanation for the development of homosexual behavior.

The development of homosexual identity in adolescence commonly progresses through three stages. The adolescent feels "different," develops a crush on a person of the same sex without clear self-awareness of a gay identity, and then goes through a "coming-out" phase in which the homosexual identity is defined for the individual and revealed to others. The coming-out phase may be a very difficult period for the young person and the family. The young adolescent is afraid of society's bias and seeks to reject homosexual feelings. This struggle with identity may include episodes of both homosexual and heterosexual promiscuity, sexually transmitted disease, depression, substance abuse, attempted suicide, school avoidance and failure, running away from home, and other crises.

In a clinical setting, the issue of homosexual identity most often surfaces as a result of a teenager being seen for a sexually transmitted disease, family conflict, school problem, attempted suicide, or substance abuse rather than as a result of a consultation about sexual orientation. Pediatricians should be aware of the psychosocial and medical implications of homosexual identity and be sensitive to the possibility of these problems in gay adolescents. The successful management of these problems depends on the physician's ability to gain the trust of the gay adolescent and on a knowledge of the wide range of medical and psychologic problems for which gay adolescents may be at risk. Pediatricians must be nonjudgmental in posing sexual questions if they are to be effective in encouraging the teenager to share concerns. Physicians who for religious or other personal reasons cannot be objective must refer the patient to another professional for treatment and counseling.

Adams GR et al (editors): *Biology of Adolescent Behavior and Development.* Sage, 1989.

American Academy of Pediatrics Committee on Adolescence: Homosexuality and adolescence. Pediatrics 1993; 92:631.

Levine M et al (editors): *Developmental Behavioral Pediatrics,* 2nd ed. Saunders, 1992.

Milstein SG et al: Health-risk behaviors and health concerns among young adolescents. Pediatrics 1992;3:422.

Remafedi G et al: Demography of sexual orientation in adolescents. Pediatrics 1992 89:714.

Remafedi G: Fundamental issues in the care of homosexual youth. Med Clin North Am 1990;74:1169.

Vaughan VC, Litt IF: *Child and Adolescent Development: Clinical Implications.* Saunders, 1990.

BEHAVIOR & PSYCHOLOGIC HEALTH

It is not unusual for adolescents to seek medical attention for seemingly minor complaints. During early adolescence, teenagers may worry about normal developmental changes such as gynecomastia. Teenagers may present with vague symptoms—the hidden agenda may be concerns about pregnancy or a sexually transmitted disease. Adolescents with emotional disorders often present with somatic symptoms—for example, abdominal pain, headaches, dizziness or syncope, fatigue, sleep problems, chest pain—that appear to have no biologic cause. The emotional basis of such a complaint may be varied: somatoform disorder, depression, or stress and anxiety.

PSYCHOPHYSIOLOGIC SYMPTOMS & CONVERSION REACTIONS

The most common somatoform disorders during adolescence are conversion disorders or conversion reactions. (A conversion reaction is a psychophysiologic process in which unpleasant feelings, especially anxiety, depression, and guilt, are communicated through a physical symptom.) Psychophysiologic symptoms result when anxiety activates the autonomic nervous system, resulting in tachycardia, hyperventilation, and vasoconstriction. The emotional feeling may be threatening or unacceptable to the individual, who expresses it as a physical symptom rather than verbally. This process is unconscious, and the anxiety or unpleasant feeling is dissipated by the somatic symptom. The degree to which the conversion symptom lessens anxiety, depression, or the unpleasant feeling is referred to as "primary gain." Conversion symptoms not only diminish unpleasant feelings but also remove the adolescent from conflict or an uncomfortable situation. This removal is referred to as "secondary gain." Secondary gain may intensify the symptoms, especially with increased attention from concerned parents and friends. Adolescents with conversion symptoms tend to have overprotective parents and become increasingly dependent on their parents as the symptom becomes the major focus of both the parents' and the adolescent's life.

Clinical Findings

The symptom may appear at times of stress, such as parental conflict, serious illness in a parent or grandparent, or change in school. Nervous, gastrointestinal, and cardiovascular systems are frequently involved, such as paresthesias, anesthesia, paralysis, dizziness, syncope, hyperventilation, abdominal pain, nausea, and vomiting. Specific symptoms may reflect existing or previous illness (eg, pseudoseizures in adolescents with epilepsy) or modeling of a close relative's symptom (eg, chest pain in a boy whose grandfather died of a heart attack).

Conversion symptoms tend to be more common in girls than boys. They occur in children and adolescents from all socioeconomic levels; however, the complexity of the symptom may vary with the sophistication and cognitive level of the patient.

Differential Diagnosis

In cases of suspected conversion reaction, history and physical findings are usually inconsistent with anatomic and physiologic concepts. Conversion symptoms are exhibited most frequently at times of stress and in the presence of individuals meaningful to the patient. The patient often exhibits a characteristic personality pattern, including egocentricity, labile emotional states, and dramatic and attention-seeking behaviors.

Conversion reactions are differentiated from hypochondriasis, which is a preoccupation with the fear of developing—or the belief that one has—a serious illness. In hypochondriacal patients, despite medical reassurance that there is no evidence of disease, the patient's (or parents') fear persists. Although adolescents generally regard their symptoms (even minor complaints) with great concern, adolescents with hypochondriasis cannot be reassured that they are healthy. Over time, the fear of one disease may be replaced with concern about another. In contrast to patients with conversion symptoms, who seem relieved if an organic cause is considered, patients with hypochondriasis become more anxious when such a cause is considered.

Malingering is uncommon during adolescence. The malingering patient consciously and intentionally produces false or exaggerated physical or psychologic symptoms. Such patients are motivated by external incentives, such as avoiding work, evading criminal prosecution, obtaining drugs, or obtaining financial compensation. These patients may be hostile and aloof. Parents of patients with conversion disorders and malingering have a similar reaction to illness. They have an unconscious psychologic need to have sick children and reinforce their child's behavior.

Somatic delusions are physical symptoms that accompany other signs of mental illness. Examples are visual or auditory hallucinations, delusions, incoherence or loosening of associations, rapid shifts of affect, and confusion. The symptoms are often peculiar or unusual.

Treatment

Because the symptom is perceived as being physical, pediatricians are often the most appropriate professionals to care for a patient with a conversion symptom. The physician must plan what further tests need to be done to complete the physical evaluation. It is critical from the onset for the physician to emphasize to the patient and the family that both physical and emotional causes of the symptom need to be considered. The relationship between physical causes of emotional pain and emotional causes of physical pain needs to be described to the family, using examples such as stress causing an ulcer or making a severe headache worse. The patient should be encouraged to understand that the symptom may persist and that at least a short-term goal is to continue normal daily activities in school and with friends. Medication is rarely helpful in relieving or resolving the symptom. If the family is accepting of psychologic referral as part of the evaluation, this is often the initial step for psychotherapy. If the family resists psychiatric or psychologic referral, the pediatrician may need to begin to deal with some of the emotional factors responsible for the persistent symptom while building rapport with the patient and family so that they may accept psychologic referral in the future. Regular weekly appointments should be set up with the patient and parents. During the sessions, the teenager should be seen first and encouraged to talk about school, friends, the relationship with the parents, and the stresses and pressures of life. Discussion of the symptom itself should be minimized; however, the physician should be supportive and never suggest that the pain is not real. As the parents gain further insight into the cause of the symptom, they will become less indulgent of the complaints, facilitating the resumption of normal activities. If management is successful, the adolescent will acquire increased coping skills and become more independent, with decreasing secondary gain.

If the symptom continues to interfere with daily activities, school attendance, participation in extracurricular activities, and involvement with peers and if the patient and parents feel that no progress is being made, psychologic referral is definitely indicated. A psychotherapist experienced in treating adolescents with conversion reactions is in the best position to establish a strong therapeutic relationship with the patient and family. After referral is made, the pediatrician should continue to follow the patient to ensure compliance with psychotherapy.

American Psychiatric Association: *Diagnostic and Statistical Manual of Mental Disorders,* 4th ed. American Psychiatric Press, 1994.

Prazer G: Conversion reactions in adolescents. Pediatr Rev 1987;8:279.

DEPRESSION
(See also Chapter 7.)

Symptoms of clinical depression—such as lethargy, loss of interest, sleep disturbances, decreased energy, feelings of worthlessness, and difficulty concentrating—can be common during the normal emotional mood swings of adolescence. The intensity of feelings—often in response to seemingly trivial events such as a poor grade on an examination or not being invited to a party—makes it difficult to differentiate a serious depression from normal sadness or dejection. In a less serious depression, sadness or unhappiness associated with problems of everyday life is generally short-lived. The symptoms usually result in only minor impairment in school, social activities, and relationships with others. With reassurance the teenager should return to a normal affect within a few days.

Clinical Findings

Serious depression in adolescents may present in several ways. The presentation may be similar to that in adults, with vegetative signs such as depressed mood nearly every day, crying spells or inability to cry, discouragement, irritability, a sense of emptiness and meaninglessness, negative expectations of oneself and the environment, low self-esteem, isolation, a feeling of helplessness, markedly diminished interest or pleasure in most activities, significant weight loss or weight gain, insomnia or hypersomnia, fatigue or loss of energy, feelings of worthlessness, and diminished ability to think or concentrate. However, it is not unusual for a serious depression to be masked because the teenager cannot tolerate the severe feelings of sadness. Such a teenager may present with recurrent or persistent psychosomatic complaints, such as abdominal pain, chest pain, headache, lethargy, weight loss, dizziness and syncope, or other nonspecific symptoms. Other behavioral manifestations of masked depression include truancy, running away from home, defiance of authorities, self-destructive behavior, vandalism, drug and alcohol abuse, sexual acting out, and delinquency.

Differential Diagnosis

The pediatrician must first recognize that the teenager may be suffering from an affective disorder. A complete history and physical examination, including a careful review of the patient's past medical and psychosocial history, should be performed. The family history should be explored for psychiatric problems.

The teenager should be questioned directly about any specific symptoms of depression, such as extreme lethargy, decreased energy, feelings of worthlessness, problems sleeping, changes in eating habits, difficulty concentrating, periods of uncontrollable crying, prolonged sadness and unhappiness, suicidal thoughts, or preoccupation with death. The history should include an assessment of the student's school performance. The physician looks for signs of academic deterioration, excessive absences or cutting class, changes in work or other outside activities, and changes in the family (eg, separation, divorce, serious illness, loss of employment by a parent, a recent move to a new school, increasing quarrels or fights with parents, the death of a close relative). The teenager may have withdrawn from friends or family or switched allegiance to a new group of friends. The physician should seek to develop a history of drug and alcohol abuse, conflicts with the law, sexual acting out, running away from home, unusually violent or rebellious behavior, or radical personality change. Patients with vague somatic complaints (eg, headaches, abdominal pain, dizzy spells, chest pain, joint pains, concerns about having a fatal illness, a "positive review of systems") often have an underlying affective disorder.

Because a number of physical disorders can mimic, cause, or exacerbate major depression, adolescents presenting with significant symptoms of depression deserve a thorough medical evaluation to rule out any contributing or underlying medical illness. Among the medical conditions associated with affective disorders are eating disorders (anorexia nervosa and bulimia), organic disorders of the central nervous system (tumors, vascular lesions, closed head trauma, and subdural hematomas), metabolic and endocrinologic disorders (systemic lupus erythematosus, hypothyroidism, hyperthyroidism, Wilson's disease, hyperparathyroidism, Cushing's syndrome, Addison's disease, premenstrual syndrome), infections (infectious mononucleosis, syphilis), and mitral valve prolapse. In addition, over 200 drugs have been reported to cause depressive symptoms. Marijuana use, phencyclidine abuse, amphetamine withdrawal, and excessive caffeine intake can cause symptoms of depression. Common prescription medications used by this age group (eg, birth control pills) and anticonvulsants may be responsible for depressive symptoms.

Most physical disorders presenting with symptoms of depression are usually evident by the presenting history, the past medical history, and the physical examination. However, some routine laboratory studies are indicated, including a complete blood count and determination of sedimentation rate, urinalysis, serum electrolytes, blood urea nitrogen (BUN), serum calcium; thyroxine and thyroid-stimulating hormone, VDRL or rapid plasma reagin (RPR), and liver enzymes. Although metabolic markers such as abnormal secretion of cortisol, growth hormone, and thyrotropin-releasing hormone have been useful in confirming major depression in adults, these neurobiologic markers are less reliable in adolescents.

The risk of depression appears to be greatest in families with a history of depression of early onset and a chronicity of depressive symptoms. Depression of early onset and bipolar illness are more likely to occur in families with a strong multigenerational history of depression. The lifetime risk of depressive illness in first-degree relatives of adult depressed patients has been estimated to be between 18% and 30%.

Treatment

The primary care physician may be able to counsel adolescents and parents if an underlying depression is mild or seems to be the result of an acute identifiable personal loss or frustration and if the patient is not contemplating suicide or at risk for other life-threatening behaviors. If there is evidence of a longstanding depressive disorder, suicidal thoughts, or psychotic thinking, or if the physician does not feel competent or has no interest in counseling the patient, a psychologic referral should be made. In uncomplicated depressions that are a reaction to life stresses or interpersonal conflicts, helping the adolescent put things in proper perspective may be enormously beneficial. Encouraging the adolescent to verbalize thoughts, understand emotional responses, and examine unrealistic attitudes and beliefs can help the patient find an appropriate solution to the problem that led to the depression.

Counseling involves establishing and maintaining a positive supportive relationship; following the patient at least weekly; remaining accessible to the patient at all times; encouraging the patient to express emotions openly, defining the problem and clarifying negative feelings, thoughts, and expectations; setting realistic goals; helping to negotiate interpersonal crises; teaching assertiveness and social skills; reassessing the depression as it is expressed; and staying alert to the possibility of suicide.

Patients with a clinical course consistent with bipolar disease or who have a significant depression that is unresponsive to supportive counseling, should be referred to a psychiatrist for evaluation of antidepressant medication.

Brent DA: Depression and suicide in children and adolescents. Pediatr Rev 1993;14:380.

Hodgman CH, McAnarney ER: Adolescent depression and suicide: Rising problems. Hosp Pract (Off Ed) 1992; 27;73.

Jensen PS, Ryan ND, Prien R: Psychopharmacology of child and adolescent major depression: Present status and future directions. J Child Adolesc Psychopharmacol 1992;2:31.

ADOLESCENT SUICIDE
(See also Chapter 7.)

In 1992, there were 4693 suicides among people 15–24 years of age: 1847 suicides among those 15–19 and 2846 among those 20–24. In the younger group, males had a rate 7.8 times higher than females, and white males had the highest rate, 18.4 per 100,000. The incidence of unsuccessful suicide attempts is three times higher in females than in males. The estimated ratio of attempted suicides to actual suicides is estimated to be 100:1–50:1. Among actual suicides, firearms are the leading cause of death for both males and females, used in over 67% of suicides.

With the normal mood swings of adolescence, short periods of depression are common. At some time, a teenager may have thoughts of suicide. Normal depressive mood swings during this period rarely interfere with sleeping, eating, or participating in normal activities. Acute depressive reactions (transient grief responses) to the loss (death or separation) of a close family member or friend may result in depression lasting for weeks or even months. An adolescent who is unable to work through this grief can become increasingly depressed. A teenager who is unable to keep up with schoolwork, does not participate in normal social activities, withdraws socially, has sleep and appetite disturbances, and has feelings of hopelessness and helplessness should be considered to be at increased risk for suicide.

Another group of suicidal adolescents is composed of angry teenagers attempting to influence others by their actions, usually the parents. They may be only mildly depressed and may not have a longstanding wish to die. Teenagers in this group, usually females, may "attempt suicide" or make a "suicidal gesture" as a way to get back at someone or gain attention by scaring another person.

The last group of adolescents at risk for suicide is made up of teenagers with a serious psychiatric problem such as acute schizophrenia or a true psychotic depressive disorder.

Risk Assessment

The physician must determine the extent of the teenager's depression and risk of inflicting self-harm. The evaluation should include interviews with both the teenager and the family. The history should include the medical, social, emotional, and academic background. (See Table 7–16, Clinical Interview to Assess Suicide Risk.) The physician should inquire about (1) common signs of depression; (2) recent events that could be at the root of an underlying depression; (3) evidence of longstanding problems in the home, at school, or with peers; (4) drug or substance use and abuse; (5) signs of psychotic thinking, such as delusions or hallucinations; and (6) evidence of masked depression, such as rebellious behavior, running away from home, reckless driving, or other acting out behavior. When seeing depressed patients, the physician should always inquire about thoughts of suicide: "Are things ever so bad that life doesn't seem worth living?" If the response is positive, a more specific question should be asked: "Have you thought of taking your life?" If the patient has thoughts of suicide, the immediacy of risk can be assessed by determining if there is a concrete, feasible plan. Although patients who are at greatest risk have a concrete plan that can be carried out in the near future—especially if they have rehearsed the plan—the physician should not dismiss the potential risk of suicide in the adolescent who does not describe a specific plan. The physician should pay attention to "gut feelings." There may be subtle nonverbal signs that the patient is at greater risk than is apparent on the surface.

Treatment

The primary care physician is often in a unique position to identify an adolescent at risk for suicide, because many teenagers who attempt suicide seek medical attention in the weeks preceding the attempt. These visits are often for vague somatic complaints or subtle signs of depression. If there is evidence of depression, the physician must assess the severity of the depression and suicidal risk. The pediatrician should always seek emergency psychologic consultation for any teenager who is severely depressed, psychotic, or acutely suicidal. It is the psychologist's or psychiatrist's responsibility to assess the seriousness of suicidal ideation and decide whether hospitalization or outpatient treatment is most appropriate. Adolescents with mild depression and at low risk for suicide should be followed closely, and the extent of the depression should be assessed on an ongoing basis. If at any point it appears that the patient is worsening or the teenager is not responding to supportive counseling, referral should be made.

American Academy of Pediatrics Committee on School Health: The potentially suicidal student in the school setting. Pediatrics 1990;86:481.
Blumenthal SJ. Youth suicide: The physician's role in suicide prevention. JAMA 1990;264:3194.
Crumley FE: Substance abuse and adolescent suicidal behavior. JAMA 1990;263:3051.
Kellerman AL et al: Suicide in the home in relation to gun ownership. N Engl J Med 1992;327:467.
Shaffer D et al: Preventing teenage suicide: A critical review. J Am Acad Child Adolesc Psychiatry 1988;27:675.

SUBSTANCE ABUSE

Substance abuse is a complex problem for adolescents and the broader society. See Chapter 6 for an in-depth look at this issue.

EATING DISORDERS
(See also Chapter 7.)

The prevalence of anorexia nervosa among adolescents has steadily risen over the past 4 decades. At a rate of 0.48% for 15- to 19-year-olds, anorexia nervosa is now the third leading chronic condition of female adolescents, after obesity and asthma. During the 1980s, 1–5% of adolescent girls met strict DSM-III-R criteria for bulimia nervosa. There are many more teens with disordered eating who do not meet full DSM-IV (Table 5–1) criteria for anorexia nervosa or bulimia nervosa (because weight is not a full 15% below expected weight, or menses have elapsed for less than 3 months, or they purge but do not binge), but who have as much emotional distress as those who meet strict diagnostic criteria. The preponderance of eating disorders among higher socioeconomic groups is changing, and eating disorders are found in all social classes. The causes of eating disorders remain unclear. There are contributing psychosocial and cultural factors, for example, the current emphasis on thinness and the "superwoman" image in today's society. The genetic component and the neuroendocrine/hypothalamic role is being investigated.

A teenager with anorexia is unlikely to present to the physician of her own accord, because denial of illness is one of the components of the syndrome.

Table 5–1. Diagnostic criteria for eating disorders.

Anorexia nervosa
Weight loss or failure to gain weight during growth such that weight is 15% below norm for age and height
Fear of weight gain or obesity despite being underweight
Disturbed body image: feels all or part of body is fat even when severely underweight, or self-evaluation overly influenced by body image
Interruption of menstrual cycles for at least 3 months
Bulimia nervosa
Repeated binge eating (excessive number of calories in short period of time accompanied by the perception that one lacks control over eating)
Recurrent compensatory behaviors to prevent weight gain (self-induced emesis; use of laxatives, diuretics, or emetics; excessive exercise, or severely restricted intake)
Binge eating and compensatory behaviors both occurring at least twice a week for 3 months or more
Self-evaluation overly influenced by body image
Not occurring exclusively as part of anorexia nervosa

Modified and reproduced from American Psychiatric Association: *Diagnostic and Statistical Manual of Mental Disorders,* 4th ed. APA Press, 1994.

She may present because of fatigue, abdominal pain, nausea, fainting spells, hair loss, amenorrhea, or at the urgings of an astute school nurse or coach. Bulimics, however, may present on their own and may feel relieved to share their burden with someone.

Clinical Findings
A. Symptoms & Signs: The diagnosis of anorexia nervosa or bulimia nervosa is largely based on history; specific diagnostic criteria are given in Table 5–1; however, the clinician is cautioned to have a low threshold of suspicion so that the opportunity for early intervention in subclinical cases will not be missed. The history needs to include the presenting symptoms; weight history, including desired weight; dietary intake, unusual eating behaviors, or avoided foods; history of any compensatory behaviors, such as vomiting, excessive exercise, or use of diet pills, diuretics, emetics, or laxatives; and menstrual history for irregular cycles, secondary amenorrhea, or delay in anticipated menarche. The social history may provide clues to a perfectionistic drive in anorexics, impulsiveness in bulimics (eg, substance abuse, sexual promiscuity), or family dysfunction. Review of systems should focus on symptoms of possible complications of the above behaviors and on symptoms of other diseases in the differential diagnosis. The use of the Eating Attitudes Test (EAT) and the Eating Disorder Inventory (EDI) may aid in diagnosis.

The physical examination is most often normal, but this does not rule out the diagnosis of an eating disorder. The anorexic may hide under layers of bulky clothing, but the loss of subcutaneous tissue becomes apparent when the patient disrobes. The anorexic's weight is the indicator of actual loss. Hypothermia, bradycardia, or hypotension may be evident when the anorexic's vital signs are assessed. Other findings in anorexia include dry skin, presence of fine, downy hair on the body or an increase in pigmentation of body hair, limpness and loss of sheen in the scalp hair, excoriation over the sacral spine from excessive sit-ups, prominent ribs, atrophied breasts, scaphoid abdomen, palpable hard stool in the rectal vault, cold extremities, squaring off of the convergence of the thighs, or edema of the extremities. Bulimics are usually of normal weight or within 10 lb of normal (under or over). In patients with self-induced emesis, there may be loss of tooth enamel, particularly on the posterior aspect of the front teeth, or calluses on the dorsum of the fingers.

B. Laboratory Findings: The goal of laboratory tests is to exclude other diagnoses and assess the patient's status. Most laboratory studies do not change until late in the disease. It is useful to obtain a complete blood count to assess nutritional status, a sedimentation rate to help exclude inflammatory bowel disease or collagen-vascular disease, and electrolyte studies to detect the presence of hypochloremic alkalosis and hypokalemia due to vomiting or of metabolic acidosis due to laxative abuse. A urinalysis may show concentrated urine or, late in anorexia nervosa, loss of urine concentrating ability. Serum total protein and albumin are usually normal until late. Prealbumin, transferrin, or C3 complement levels can help assess the degree of malnutrition. Bone densitometry should be done at baseline for severely malnourished teens, especially those with a prolonged history or delayed growth. Serum calcium, phosphorus, and magnesium should be closely followed during refeeding, since they may quickly become depleted resulting in a medical emergency. Other laboratory studies, such as thyroid function tests, chest x-ray, ECG, upper gastrointestinal series, or CT scan of the head need only be done as indicated by the presentation.

Differential Diagnosis

The causes of weight loss are legion. Causes such as cancer, collagen-vascular disease, diabetes mellitus, hyperthyroidism, malabsorptive syndromes, inflammatory bowel disease, or chronic renal, pulmonary, or cardiac disease warrant consideration in the suspected anorexic; however, in patients with these disorders there may be weight loss but no associated disturbance of body image or fear of obesity. Several psychiatric disturbances, including depression, may be associated with loss of appetite and weight loss. Some unusual central nervous system disorders may present like bulimia, but again there is no distorted body image or overconcern with body shape or weight.

Complications

Eating disorders can result in severe consequences

to nearly every system of the body (Table 5–2). The most common complications, however, are fluid and electrolyte abnormalities or constipation. Recently, reduced bone mineral density and cortical atrophy of the brain have been appreciated as significant and early consequences of anorexia nervosa in adolescents; long-term implications are still under investigation. Growth retardation can also occur. In addition, there may be long-term difficulties with eating and weight management.

Treatment

First, the diagnosis must be discussed with the patient and her parents. The patient needs to know that the clinician appreciates her struggle, aims to restore her to health, will not let her become fat, and will help her to regain control. The parents need to understand that eating disorders are symptoms of underlying issues, often a family problem, and that the family is very important to the solution. They need to see that although the presenting symptoms are physical, eating disorders are psychiatric disorders and require the intervention of mental health practitioners. With this age group, it is important to have a mental health

Table 5–2. Complications of eating disorders.

Cardiovascular	↑Liver function tests (fatty
Bradycardia	infiltration of the liver)
Postural hypotension	**Hematologic**
Arrhythmia, sudden death	Leukopenia
Congestive heart failure	Anemia
(during refeeding)	Thrombocytopenia
Pericardial effusion	↓ESR
Mitral valve prolapse	Impaired cell-mediated
ECG abnormalities	immunity
(prolonged QT, low	**Metabolic**
voltage, T-wave abnormal-	Dehydration
ities, conduction defects)	Acidosis
Endocrine	Hypokalemia
↓LH, FSH	Hyponatremia
↓T_3,↑rT_3; normal T_4, TSH	Hypochloremia
Irregular menses	Hypochloremic alkalosis
Amenorrhea	Hypocalcemia
Hypercortisolism	Hypophosphatemia
Growth retardation	Hypomagnesemia
Sort stature	Hypercarotenemia
Delayed puberty	**Neurologic**
Gastrointestinal	Cortical atrophy
Dental erosion	Peripheral neuropathy
Parotid swelling	Seizures
Esophagitis, esophageal	Thermoregulatory abnormal-
tears	ities
Delayed gastric emptying	↓REM and slow-wave sleep
Gastric dilatation (rarely rup-	**Renal**
ture)	Hematuria
Pancreatitis	Proteinuria
Constipation	↓Renal concentrating ability
Diarrhea (laxative abuse)	**Skeletal**
Superior mesenteric artery	Osteopenia
syndrome	Fractures
Hypercholesterolemia	

ESR = erythrocyte sedimentation rate; REM = rapid eye movement.

practitioner who is skilled in family therapy and has experience with adolescents (see Chapter 7).

Restoration of the nutritional and physiologic state is an early goal of treatment, because the patient may need to gain weight before she can deal effectively with her fear of fatness or other issues. A dietitian is helpful in establishing a refeeding program. The patient may not be in any metabolic danger at the time of presentation, and provided the weight can be stabilized, she may not require hospitalization but rather regular outpatient visits with medical and mental health professionals. An individualized contract can be drawn up and signed by the patient. This contract addresses such issues as long-term weight goals, rate of weight gain, amount of exercise, frequency of visits and of laboratory tests, minimal weight signaling the need for hospitalization, and consequences of failed weight goals. At each medical visit, the patient should be weighed in only a gown after she voids. Body mass index (BMI) can be followed over time (Figure 5–6). The long-term goal is to achieve a weight at which menstruation can take place; in general, 90% of ideal body weight is required, but not alone sufficient, to restore menstruation. Vital signs and chest and abdominal examinations should also be conducted at each visit, and the height and the triceps skinfold should be monitored over time.

Most often, the patient can eat sufficient amounts to replace nutrient deficits and to gain weight. High-calorie fluid supplements may be added if weekly weight goals are missed. It is best not to tell the patient that she must take in a certain number of calories, because she is already fixated on calories. Rather, plans can be developed with the assistance of the dietitian; the planned diets contain sufficient calories to gain 0.5–2 lb/wk (2–3 lb/wk for inpatients). In extremely malnourished and noncompliant hospitalized patients, nasogastric tube feedings or hyperalimentation may be necessary initially. With severe anorexics, one must be on the watch for congestive heart failure caused by refeeding too rapidly. In addition, serum phosphate levels should be followed, because there may be a shift from serum to cells during conversion to anabolic metabolism.

Drug therapy—including appetite stimulants or suppressants, antidepressants, anxiolytics, and anticonvulsants—has been investigated in a number of studies, but the results to date are equivocal. Antidepressants may be helpful in select patients but need to be carefully monitored in cachectic patients. Selective serotonin reuptake inhibitors are often helpful in medically stable anorexics and have been shown to reduce the frequency of binging and purging, as well as obsessive food thoughts, in bulimics.

Hospitalization may become necessary for medical or psychiatric reasons (Table 5–3). In addition, the patient may require hospitalization not because she is medically unstable or in emotional crisis but because she is out of control or making no progress as an outpatient and thus requires more intensive treatment.

Prognosis

Outcome is difficult to predict because there have been few long-term studies and there is little standardization of criteria and variables. It appears that 40–60% of significantly ill anorexics will make a good physical and psychosocial recovery and that 75% will gain weight. The mortality rate ranges from 0–19% and is at least 5% in those receiving therapy. For bulimia, the literature is even younger, and the outcome appears less favorable. As few as 40–50% of treated bulimics are felt to be cured, and there is a greater likelihood of serious medical complications, death, and risk of suicide than for anorexics who do not manifest bulimic behavior. Recently, however, more attention has focused on eating disorders, and the lay public is becoming more aware of them. For this reason, the disease is being recognized earlier than before.

American Psychiatric Association: *Diagnostic and Statistical Manual of Mental Disorders,* 4th ed. American Psychiatric Press, 1994.

Commerci GD: Eating disorders in adolescents. Pediatr Rev 1988;10:37.

FBNC Study Group: Fluoxetine in the treatment of bulimia nervosa: A multicenter, placebo-controlled, double-blind trial. Arch Gen Psychiatry 1992;49:139.

Fisher M et al: Eating disorders in adolescents: A background paper. J Adolesc Health 1995;16:420.

Kaye WH: An open trial of fluoxetine in patients with anorexia nervosa. J Clin Psychiatry 1991;52:464.

Kreipe RE, Uphoff M: Treatment and outcome of adolescents with anorexia nervosa. Adolescent Medicine: State of the Art Reviews 1992;3:519.

Kreipe RE et al: Eating disorders in adolescents: A position paper of the Society for Adolescent Medicine. J Adolesc Health 1995;16:476.

Palla B, Litt IF: Medical complications of eating disorders in adolescents. Pediatrics 1988;81:613.

Williams RL: Use of the Eating Attitudes Test and Eating Disorder Inventory in adolescents. J Adolesc Health Care 1987;8:266.

EXOGENOUS OBESITY

Obesity is the presence of excessive body fat, or weight 20% above desirable weight if the excess weight is due to fat. Body weight is most commonly used to quantitate obesity; however, this is a function of age, sex, height, frame, and Tanner stage. In children under 6–7 years of age, body weight tends to underestimate fatness, and in adolescents it overestimates fatness. Although underwater weights may be the most accurate measure of lean body mass, this weighing procedure is not frequently available. Triceps skinfold thickness is the most practical way to measure obesity in children and teenagers, but repro-

A

AGE	MALES							FEMALES					
(yr)	5th	10th	25th	50th	75th	90th	95th	5th	10th	25th	50th	75th	90th	95th
6	13.0	13.6	14.4	15.3	16.0	17.7	18.7	12.8	13.5	14.0	15.0	16.0	16.9	17.3
7	13.3	13.9	14.7	15.7	16.7	18.5	19.9	13.1	13.8	14.5	15.6	16.8	18.4	19.2
8	13.6	14.2	15.1	16.1	17.4	19.4	21.1	13.5	14.2	15.1	16.2	17.7	19.9	21.1
9	14.0	14.5	15.5	16.6	18.1	20.4	22.3	13.9	14.6	15.6	16.9	18.7	21.3	23.0
10	14.5	14.9	15.9	17.1	18.9	21.3	23.4	14.4	15.1	16.2	17.5	19.6	22.7	24.8
11	15.0	15.3	16.4	17.6	19.7	22.2	24.5	14.9	15.5	16.7	18.2	20.4	23.8	26.3
12	15.5	15.8	16.9	18.2	20.4	23.1	25.5	15.3	16.0	17.3	18.8	21.2	24.8	27.7
13	16.0	16.3	17.4	18.8	21.1	24.0	26.5	15.8	16.4	17.8	19.3	21.9	25.6	28.8
14	16.5	16.9	18.0	19.4	21.9	24.8	27.3	16.2	16.8	18.2	19.9	22.5	26.1	29.6
15	17.0	17.5	18.7	20.1	22.5	25.6	28.0	16.6	17.2	18.6	20.3	23.0	26.5	30.2
16	17.4	18.0	19.2	20.8	23.2	26.3	28.6	16.9	17.5	18.9	20.7	23.5	26.7	30.6
17	17.8	18.5	19.8	21.4	23.8	26.9	29.2	17.1	17.8	19.2	21.0	23.8	26.9	30.9
18-20	18.6	19.7	21.0	23.0	25.3	28.4	30.5	17.6	18.4	19.7	21.6	24.3	27.2	31.2
21-23	19.0	20.0	21.4	23.6	26.0	29.0	31.2	17.7	18.5	19.8	21.8	24.4	27.7	31.5

B

Figure 5–6. A: Nomogram for determining body mass index (BMI) from height and weight. A straight-edge connecting weight and height allows one to read BMI (weight in kg [height in m]²). The three dots on the left side of the BMI line represent 50th percentile values for females aged 20 years (*top*), 15 years (*middle*), and 10 years (*bottom*). The dots on the right side are for similar-aged males. **B:** Percentile values for BMI (kg/m²). (**A** and **B** reproduced, with permission, from Forbes GR: Nutrition and growth. In: *Textbook of Adolescent Medicine.* McAnarney ER et al [editors]. Saunders, 1992.)

Table 5–3. Indications for hospitalization of an adolescent with an eating disorder.

Medical
Weight < 75% of ideal body weight
Severe metabolic disturbance
    Heart rate < 40 beats/min
    Temperature < 36°C
    Systolic blood pressure < 70 mm Hg
    Serum K$^+$ < 2.5 meq/L despite oral K$^+$ replacement
    Severe dehydration
Cardiac arrhythmia
Arrested growth and development
Acute food refusal
Severe binging and purging
Failure to respond to outpatient treatment
Psychiatric
Severe depression or risk of suicide
Psychosis
Family crisis
Failure to comply with a therapeutic contract, or inadequate response to outpatient treatment

ducibility is in question. A triceps skinfold measurement of more than 1 SD above the mean (85th percentile) defines obesity, and one at the 95th percentile indicates superobesity (Figure 5–7). The BMI (weight [kg] divided by height squared [m^2]), used to assess obesity in adults correlates less well with the percentage of body fat in children and adolescents than skinfold thickness (Figure 5–7).

Background

Obesity is the most common nutritional disorder of children in the United States, and the prevalence of obesity increases significantly between the elementary and high school years. If a child enters adolescence obese, the odds are 4:1 against later achievement of normal weight; but if a child leaves adolescence obese, the odds are 28:1 against later normal weight. The National Children and Youth Fitness Study, parts I and II, completed in 1987, demonstrated a decline in fitness of fifth through twelfth graders and first through fourth graders, respectively. When these results were compared with those of a 1960s National Center for Health Statistics study, an increase in skinfold measurements was found. The reduction in fitness has paralleled a rise in hours of television watched by children. Factors known to increase the risk of a child's being obese include having obese parents and being an only child. The associated medical risks of obesity include pediatric and adult hypertension, elevated triglyceride levels, cerebrovascular accidents, diabetes mellitus, gallbladder disease, slipped capital-femoral epiphyses, degenerative arthritis, and pregnancy complications. The psychosocial hazards of obesity tend to be the greatest consequence for adolescents, who may experience alienation, distorted peer relations, poor self-esteem, guilt, depression, or altered body image.

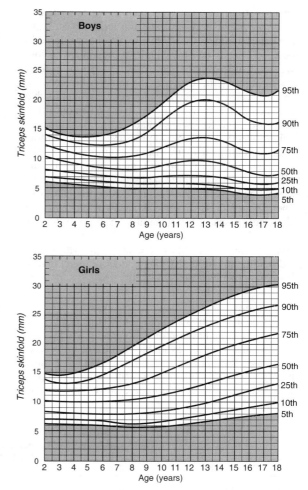

Figure 5–7. Triceps skinfold thickness in boys and girls 2–18 years. (Reproduced, with permission, from Ross Laboratories. Adapted from Johnson CL et al: Basic data on anthropometric measurements and angular measurements of the hip and knee joints for selected age groups, 1–74 years of age, United States, 1971–1975. *Vital and Health Statistics,* Series 11, No. 219. [PHS] 81-1669, 1981. © 1983 Ross Laboratories, Columbus, OH 43216. May be copied for individual patient use.)

Diagnosis

A triceps skinfold measurement of more than 1 SD above the mean or weight 20% over ideal body weight indicates obesity. An adolescent with a BMI above the 85th percentile is considered to be at risk of overweight; weight above the 95th percentile is considered overweight. Patients can be identified as at risk for obesity based on current weight relative to height, growth and weight trend, and weight of family members. The history should include onset of obesity, eating and exercise habits, amount of time spent in sedentary activities such as watching television, previous successful and unsuccessful attempts at weight loss, and family history of obesity. In addition, one needs to assess patients' readiness to lose weight, that is, whether patients are aware of or deny a weight problem; recognize the relationship between food, activity, and weight; and recognize factors that they could change in their own lives. When obesity is diagnosed, the following database can be collected: height; weight; BMI; blood pressure; triceps skinfold measurement; fat distribution; examination of the skin, thyroid, heart, and abdomen; hematocrit; and urinalysis. This database helps the physician assess the patient's status and exclude endocrine causes of obesity. Endocrine causes, such as hypothyroidism or Cushing's disease, can generally be excluded on the basis of history and physical examination. If an adolescent is healthy and has no delay of growth or sexual maturation, an underlying endocrinologic, neurologic, or genetic cause is unlikely.

Treatment

For poorly motivated patients, it is probably best to provide some basic information about weight control and make oneself available for future visits, so as not to set the patient up for failure. For the more highly motivated patient, treatment should be appropriate to age and developmental level and should produce a significant reduction in body weight. The adolescent should be taught appropriate eating and exercise habits to maintain a weight reduction yet meet nutrition needs for growth and development.

Anorectic drugs, fasting, and bypass surgery do not have a role in the management of obese adolescents. An age-appropriate behavior modification program incorporating good dietary counseling and exercise is optimal (Table 5–4). Diet or exercise alone is not nearly as effective. Guidelines that group foods in categories according to their caloric density may be appreciated by adolescents who hate to count calories. Lifestyle activity, such as walking and taking the stairs, may be more effective in the long run than regimented exercise programs. Behavior modification components—such as recording one's eating and activity in a notebook, receiving systematic reinforcement for behavior changes, and restructuring how one sees oneself or plans for success—are especially helpful. Behavioral treatment involving parents has been shown to improve long-term maintenance of weight loss in children. One must recognize, however, that no program has the high success rate desired and that the problem of adolescent obesity must be examined further.

Arden MA: Obesity. In: *Textbook of Adolescent Medicine.* McAnarney ER et al (editors). Saunders, 1992.

Table 5–4. Program components for weight control interventions.

Component	Specific Aspects

Physical activity
  1. Cardiovascular fitness
  2. High-calorie equivalent
	Frequency: 3 or 4 times a week.
	Intensity: 50–60% maximal ability (55–65% maximum heart rate).
	Duration: 15 minutes at start of program, building to 30–40 minutes.
	Mode: Use large muscle activity, eg, walking, jogging, swimming, cycling.
	Interests: Encourage a wide variety of recreational activities.
	Enjoyment: Focus on the fun of movement and the enjoyment of being physically active.

Nutritional education	Teach critical aspects of quality nutrition, ie, food groups, serving requirements, and variety. Develop an understanding of caloric balance; calories in versus calories out. Alert children to resist the pressures of media advertising. Instruct on role of snacks and ideas for "good" snacking. Assist children with balancing fast-food eating and caloric intake. Teach children to reduce intake of high-calorie, low-nutrition foods.

Behavior modification
  1. Change eating habits
  2. Increase habitual physical activity
	Identify those cues that affect eating, eg, location of meals, size of plates, food in easy-to-see places.
	Identify behavior that negatively affects weight control: speed of eating, chronic second portions, high-calorie food choices, "pickiness."
	Contract for increased levels of activity, using record cards or activity contracts.
	Develop strategies to encourage more functional activity, eg, walking to school, taking stairs, sitting rather than lying.
	Develop interests in a variety of recreational areas: tennis, dancing, skating.
	Identify cues that lead to inactivity: frequent TV watching, lying down after school or meals, friends who do not like active play.

Modified and reproduced, with permission, from Ward DS Bar-Or O: Role of the physician and physical education teacher in the treatment of obesity at school. Pediatrician 1986:13:44.

Bandini LG: Obesity in the adolescent. Adolesc Med: State Art Rev 1992;3:459.

Epstein LH et al: Ten-year follow-up of behavioral, family-based treatment for obese children. JAMA 1990;264: 2519.

Raithel KS: Are American children really unfit? Physician Sports Med 1988;16:146.

Rees JM: Management of obesity in adolescence. Med Clin North Am 1990;74:1275.

SCHOOL AVOIDANCE

Any teenager who has missed more than 1 week of school for a physical illness or symptom—and whose clinical picture is inconsistent with a serious illness—should be suspected of harboring primary or secondary emotional factors that contribute to the absence. Investigation of absences may show a pattern, such as missing morning classes or missing the same days at the beginning or end of the week. Emotional factors for school absenteeism are usually attributed to physical symptoms in this age group.

School avoidance should be suspected in children who are consistently absent in spite of parents' and professionals' attempts to encourage school attendance. Adolescents with school avoidance problems often have a history of excessive absences or separation difficulties as a younger child. There may also be a record of recurrent somatic complaints. Parents of a school avoider often feel at a loss about how to compel their adolescent to attend school, may lack the sophistication to distinguish malingering from illness, or may have an underlying need to keep the teenager at home.

A complete history and physical should be performed, reviewing the past medical, educational, and psychiatric history. Signs of emotional problems should be explored. After obtaining permission from the patient and parents, the physician may find it helpful to speak directly with school officials and some key teachers. There may be problems with particular teachers or subjects; environmental factors at the school (eg, fears of physical violence, problems with intimidation). Some students get so far behind academically that they see no way of catching up and feel overwhelmed. The adolescent may have a long history of separation anxiety, dating back to a traumatic separation from the mother. Separation anxiety may persist and be manifested in subconscious worries that something may happen to the mother while the teenager is at school.

The school nurse may give useful information, including the number of visits to the nurse during the last school year. An important part of the history is how the parents respond to the absences and somatic complaint. There may be a subconscious attempt to keep the adolescent at home, which may be coupled with secondary gains (increased parental attention) for remaining at home.

Treatment

The importance of going back to school after a period of school avoidance in the next 2 or 3 days needs to be emphasized. The pediatrician should facilitate this process by offering to speak with school officials to excuse missed examinations, homework, and papers. The pediatrician should speak directly with teachers who are punitive. The objective is to make the transition back to school as easy as possible. The longer adolescents stay out of school, the more anxious they may become about returning, and the more difficult the return becomes. If an illness or symptoms become so severe that an adolescent cannot go to school, both the patient and the parents must be informed that a visit to the doctor's office is necessary. The physician focuses visits on the parents as much as on the adolescent to alleviate any parental guilt about sending the child to school. If the adolescent cannot stay in school, hospitalization should be recommended for an in-depth medical and psychiatric evaluation. Parents should be cautioned about the possibility of relapse after school holidays, summer vacation, or an acute illness.

Klerman LV: School absence: A health perspective. Pediatr Clin North Am 1988;35:1253.

SCHOOL FAILURE

When children graduate from grade school to middle school or junior high school, the amount and complexity of course work increase significantly. This occurs at about the same time as the rapid physical, social, and emotional changes of puberty. To perform well academically, young adolescents must have the needed cognitive ability, study habits, concentration, motivation, interest, and emotional focus. Academic failure presenting at adolescence has a broad differential: (1) limited intellectual abilities, (2) specific learning disabilities, (3) depression or emotional problems, (4) physical causes such as visual or hearing problems, (5) excessive school absenteeism secondary to chronic disease such as asthma or neurologic dysfunction, (6) lack of ability to concentrate, (7) attention-deficit disorder, (8) lack of motivation, and (9) drug and alcohol problems. Each of these possible causes must be explored in depth (Table 5–5).

A thorough history, physical examination, appropriate laboratory studies, and educational and psychologic testing should be performed. A detailed medical history is taken to look for the presence of chronic disease or sensory deficits. School avoidance (see previous discussion) should be ruled out. A history of an attention-deficit disorder or use of stimu-

Table 5–5. A classification of common developmental dysfunctions in adolescence.

Dysfunction	Subtypes	Frequent Manifestations[1]
1. Attention deficits	a. Primary b. Secondary (to anxiety or poor information processing) c. Situational (only evident in certain settings)	Weak attention to detail; distractibility; impulsivity, restlessness; task impersistence; performance inconsistency; organizational problems; reduced working capacity
2. Memory impairments	a. Generalized retrieval problems b. Modality-specific retrieval problems c. Attention-retention deficiencies	Deficient, undependable, or slow recall of data from long- or short-term memory Problems with revisualization or auditory, motor, or sequential recall Poor recall associated with superficial initial registration
3. Language disorders	a. Receptive b. Expressive	Poor verbal and reading comprehension; poor listening; trouble following directions and explanations Problems with word finding, sentence formulation Difficulty with written expression
4. Higher order cognitive disabilities	a. Inferential weakness b. Poor verbal reasoning c. Poor nonverbal reasoning d. Difficulty with abstraction, symbolization e. Weak generalization and rule application	Problems understanding and assimilating new concepts; tendency to think "concretely" delays in mathematics, reading comprehension, science, social studies
5. Fine motor incoordination	a. Eye:hand coordination problems b. Impaired propriokinesthetic feedback c. Dyspraxia d. Motor memory impairment	Slow, labored, sometimes illegible writing; awkward pencil grip; dyssynchrony between cognitive tempo and writing speed; output failure—reduced productivity
6. Organizational deficiencies	a. Temporal-sequential disorientation b. Material disarray c. Integrative dysfunction d. Resynthesis problems e. Attentional disorganization	Problems with time allocation, schedules, planning, arranging ideas in writing Tendency to lose, misplace, forget books, papers; trouble organizing notebook Varying inability to integrate data from multiple sources or sensory modalities Trouble extracting most salient details, retelling and adapting data to current demands Impulsivity, erratic tempo, poor self-monitoring, careless errors
7. Socialization disabilities	a. Wide range of subtypes, including conduct disorder, social impulsivity, impaired social cognition or feedback, egocentricity	Antisocial behaviors; delinquency; withdrawal; excessive dependency on peer support

Modified and reproduced, with permission, from Levine MD, Zallen BG: Learning disorders of adolescence. Pediatr Clin North Am 1984;31:2.

[1]Manifestations are likely to vary somewhat depending on compensatory strengths, quality of educational experience, and motivation.

lant medication in the past may be an indication of ongoing problems with concentration. Educational records, including previous educational and intelligence testing, are important background information. The emotional history may reveal past episodes of counseling for depression or other significant psychiatric problems. The presence of conflict in the family, such as divorce or alcoholism, may play an important role, distracting the adolescent from academic responsibilities. There may be a history of school problems in other siblings or family members.

Treatment

Treatment depends on the cause. Management must be individualized to address specific needs, foster strengths, and implement a feasible program. For children with specific learning disabilities, an individual prescription for regular and special educa-

tional courses, teachers, and extracurricular activities is important. Counseling helps these adolescents gain coping skills, raise self-esteem, and develop socialization skills. If there is a history of hyperactivity or attention-deficit disorder along with poor ability to concentrate, a trial of stimulant medication (eg, methylphenidate hydrochloride, dextroamphetamine sulfate) may be useful. If the teenager appears to be depressed or if other serious emotional problems are uncovered, further psychologic evaluation should be recommended.

Lerner JW: Eductional interventions in learning disabilities. J Am Acad Child Adolesc Psychiatry 1989;28:326.

Levine M: *Keeping a Head in School: A Student's Book About Learning Abilities and Learning Disorders.* Educators Publishing Service, 1990.

Levine MD, Zallen BG: The learning disorders of adolescence: Organic and nonorganic failure to strive. Pediatr Clin North Am 1984;31:345.

Pelham WE et al: Relative efficacy of long acting stimulants on children with attention deficit–hyperactivity disorder. Pediatrics 1990;86:226.

BREAST DISORDERS

The breast examination should become part of the routine physical examination in females as soon as breast budding occurs. The preadolescent comes to see breast examination as a routine part of health care, and it provides an opportunity to reassure her about any concerns she may have. The breast examination begins with inspection of the breasts for symmetry and Tanner stage. Asymmetric breast development is common in adolescents, who need reassurance that the asymmetry usually becomes less apparent as development progresses. Unusual causes of breast asymmetry that may require further intervention include unilateral breast hypoplasia, amastia, or absence of the pectoralis major muscle. In addition, unilateral virginal hypertrophy (massive enlargement of the breast during puberty) may result in significant asymmetry.

Palpation of the breasts can be performed with the patient in the supine position and the patient's ipsilateral arm placed behind her head. The examiner palpates the breast tissue with the flat of the fingers in concentric circles from the sternum, clavicle, and axilla in to the areola. The areola should be gently compressed to check for discharge.

Instructions for breast self-examination and its purpose can be given to older adolescents during this portion of the physical examination, and the patient should be encouraged to begin monthly self-examination after each menstrual flow.

BREAST MASSES

Most breast masses in adolescents are benign (Table 5–6); however, approximately 150 cases of adenocarcinoma are reported each year in the United States in women under 25 years of age. Fibroadenomas account for 90% of breast lumps in teenagers seen in referral clinics; the remainder are cysts. In practice, cysts may account for as many as 60% of breast masses in adolescents, but they are readily diagnosed, and many resolve spontaneously.

Fibroadenoma

Fibroadenoma presents as a rubbery, well-demarcated, slowly growing, nontender mass that may oc-

TABLE 5–6. Breast masses in adolescent females.

Most common	Rare
Benign fibroadenoma	Lymphangioma
Breast cyst	Hemangioma
Less common	Neurofibromatosis
Giant (juvenile) fibroadenoma	Dermatofibromatosis
Virginal (juvenile) hypertrophy	Papillomatosis
Breast abscess	Papilloma sarcoidosis
Lipoma	Nipple adenoma
Hematoma	Nipple keratoma
Malignant potential	Mammary duct estasia
Adenocarcinoma	Intraductal granuloma
Invasive ductal carcinoma	Galactocele
Intraductal papilloma	Metastatic disease
Cystosarcoma phyllodes	Other

Reproduced, with permission, from Beach RK: Breast disorders. In: McAnarney ER et al: *Textbook of Adolescent Medicine.* WB Saunders, 1992.

cur in any quadrant but is most commonly found in the upper outer quadrant of the breast. Most are less than 5 cm in diameter. In 25% of cases, there are multiple or recurrent lesions. Quiescence can be expected after the teenage years.

Cysts

Breast cysts are generally tender and spongy, with exacerbation of symptoms premenstrually and abatement just after. Often they are multiple. Spontaneous regression occurs over two or three menstrual cycles in about 50% of cases.

It is reasonable to follow breast masses that are consistent with fibroadenoma or cyst in adolescents for two or three menstrual cycles. About 25% of fibroadenomas become smaller, and about 50% of cysts resolve. If there is no change in a presumed fibroadenoma after this time, an ultrasound study will differentiate a solid tumor from a cyst. Patients with solid tumors over 2.5 cm in diameter should be referred for excisional biopsy. Those with tumors less than 2.5 cm in diameter may be followed every 3–6 months, since many will shrink or remain the same. Persistent cystic lesions may be drained by needle aspiration. Patients with suspicious lesions should be referred immediately to a breast surgeon (Table 5–7).

Fibrocystic Breasts

Fibrocystic breasts (or fibrocystic breast disease) is sometimes seen in older adolescents but is more common in women in their third and fourth decades. It is characterized by cyclic tenderness and nodularity bilaterally and is believed to be influenced by the estrogen-progesterone balance.

Reassuring the young woman about the benign nature of the process and emphasizing the importance of breast self-examination may be all that is needed. Oral contraceptives reduce the risk of fibrocystic breast disease and may be appropriate for the sexually active female with a personal history of breast cyst or family history of fibrocystic breasts. Studies

Table 5–7. Breast lesions.

Adenocarcinoma	Hard, nonmobile, well-circumscribed, painless mass; generally indolent clinical course; occurs also in males but less frequently.
Cystosarcoma phyllodes	Firm, rubbery mass that may suddenly enlarge; associated with skin necrosis; most often benign.
Giant juvenile fibroadenoma	Remarkable large fibroadenoma with overlying dilated superficial veins; accounts for 5–10% of fibroadenomas in adolescents; benign but requires excision to prevent breast atrophy and for cosmetic reasons.
Intraductal papilloma	A cylindrical tumor arising from the ductal epithelium; often subareolar but may be in the periphery of the breast in adolescents, with associated nipple discharge. Most are benign but require excision for cytologic diagnosis.
Fat necrosis	Localized inflammatory process in one breast; follows trauma in about half of cases. Subsequent scarring may be confused with cancer.
Virginal or juvenile hypertrophy	Massive enlargement of both breasts or less often, one breast; attributed to end-organ hypersensitivity to normal hormonal levels just before or within a few years after menarche.
Miscellaneous	Fibroma, galactocele, hemangioma, intraductal granuloma, interstitial fibrosis, keratoma, lipoma, granular cell myoblastoma, papilloma, sclerosing adenosis.

have shown no association between methylxanthines and fibrocystic breasts; however, some women report reduced symptoms when they discontinue caffeine intake. The efficacy of vitamin E remains unknown.

Breast Abscess

The female with a breast abscess usually complains of unilateral breast pain, and examination reveals overlying inflammatory changes. Often the examination is misleading in that the infection may extend much deeper than suspected. A palpable mass is found only late in the course. Although breast-feeding is the most common cause of mastitis, trauma and eczema involving the areola are frequent factors in teenagers. *Staphylococcus aureus* is the most common cause, but other aerobic and anaerobic organisms have also been implicated.

Cyclic mastodynia, fibrocystic disease, or chest wall pain may also be causes of breast pain, but there should be no associated inflammatory signs.

Fluctuant abscesses should be surgically incised and drained. Oral antibiotics with appropriate coverage (dicloxacillin or a cephalosporin) should be given for 2–4 weeks. In addition, ice packs for the first 24 hours and heat thereafter may relieve symptoms.

GALACTORRHEA

In teenagers, galactorrhea, or inappropriate nipple discharge, is most often benign; however, a careful history and workup are necessary. Prolactinomas are the most common pathologic cause of galactorrhea in adolescents of both sexes and generally present as failure of sexual maturation. Hypothyroidism is the second most common cause in the adolescent years but has only been reported in girls, usually prepubertally.

Galactorrhea may be present after spontaneous or induced abortions as well as postpartum. Numerous prescribed and illicit drugs are associated with galactorrhea (Table 5–8). In addition, stimulation of the

Table 5–8. Drugs associated with breast symptoms (glalactorrhea, gynecomastia, pain, mass).

Street drugs (illicit or abused)
  Amphetamines
  Marihuana
  Mebrobamate
  Opiates
    Codeine
    Heroin
    Morphine
Hormones or related drugs
  Bromocriptine withdrawal
  Estrogens
  Human chorionic gonadotropin
  Methyltestosterone
  Oral contraceptives
  Tamoxifen
Cancer drugs
  Busulfan
  Vincristine
Prescription medications
  Amitriptyline
  Chlordiazepoxide
  Chlorpromazine
  Cimetidine
  Diazepam
  Digoxin
  Fluphenazine
  Haloperidol
  Imipramine
  Isoniazid
  Mesoridazine
  Methylodopa
  Perphenazine
  Phenothiazines
  Reserpine
  Spironolactone
  Thiethylperazine
  Thioxanthines
  Tricyclic antidepressants
  Trifluoperazine
  Trimeprazine

Modified and reproduced, with permission, from Beach RK: Routine breast exams: A chance to reassure, guide, and protect. Contemp Pediatr 1987;4:70.

intercostal nerves (following surgery or due to herpes zoster), stimulation of the nipples, endocrine disorders (hypothyroidism, pituitary prolactinoma), central nervous system disorders (hypothalamic injury), or significant emotional distress may produce galactorrhea (Table 5–9).

Clinical Findings

If there is no history of pregnancy or drug use, thyroid-stimulating hormone (TSH) and prolactin levels should be determined. An elevated TSH confirms the diagnosis of hypothyroidism. An elevated prolactin and normal TSH, often accompanied by amenorrhea, suggest a hypothalamic or pituitary tumor, and CT scan or MRI is indicated. When the prolactin level is normal, uncommon causes such as adrenal, renal, or ovarian tumors should be considered. The female with a negative workup and persistent galactorrhea may be followed with menstrual history and prolactin level every 6–12 months. In many cases, symptoms resolve spontaneously, and no diagnosis is made. The female with an elevated prolactin but negative prolactinoma workup may be treated with bromocriptine if her symptoms are bothersome or may be observed with CT scan or MRI every 18 months for several years. Males with a negative workup and normal puberty need to be intensively followed. Males with elevated prolactin levels deserve a CT scan or MRI every 12–18 months even if the galactorrhea resolves, as there is a significant risk of harboring a pituitary adenoma.

Treatment

Treatment of galactorrhea depends on the underlying cause. Prolactinomas may be surgically removed or suppressed with bromocriptine. Bromocriptine may also be beneficial to some amenorrheic females with normal prolactin levels.

GYNECOMASTIA

Gynecomastia is a common concern of male adolescents, most of whom (60–70%) develop transient subareolar breast tissue during Tanner stages II and III. Proposed causes include testosterone-estrogen imbalance, increased prolactin level, or abnormal serum binding protein levels.

Clinical Findings

In type I idiopathic gynecomastia, the adolescent presents with a unilateral (20% bilateral), tender, firm mass beneath the areola. More generalized breast enlargement is classified as type II. Pseudogynecomastia refers to excessive fat tissue or prominent pectoralis muscles.

Differential Diagnosis

Gynecomastia may be drug-induced (see Table 5–8). Testicular, adrenal, or pituitary tumors, Klinefelter's syndrome, primary hypogonadism, thyroid or hepatic dysfunction, or malnutrition may also be associated with gynecomastia (Table 5–10).

Treatment

If gynecomastia is idiopathic, reassurance of the common and benign nature of the process is given. Resolution may take several months to 2 years. Medical reduction has been achieved with pharmacotherapeutic agents, such as dihydrotestosterone heptanoate, danazol, clomiphene citrate, and tamoxifen citrate, but these should be reserved for those with no

Table 5–9. Causes of galactorrhea.

Hypothalamic disorders
  Functional
    Postpartum
    Without pregnancy
  Pathologic
    Iinfiltrative
      Sarcoid
      Histiocytosis X
      Hypothalamic tumors
    Section of pituitary stalk
Drug therapy
  Tranquilizers
  Tricyclic antidepressants
  Methyldopa
  Rauwolfia alkaloids
  Oral contraceptives
  Estrogens
Neoplasms
  Pituitary tumors
    Prolactin secretion only
    Prolactin and ACTH secretion (Cushing's disease)
    Growth hormone secretion with or without prolactin
      secretion (acromegaly)
  Ectopic prolactin-secreting tumors
Hypothyroidism
Neorogenic stimulation
  Breast stimulation
  Chest wall lesions (herpes zoster, thoracotomy)

Modified and reproduced, with permission, from Fraser WM, Blackard WG: Medical conditions that affect the breast and lactation. Clin Obstet Gynecol 1975;18:51.

Table 5–10. Disorders associated with gynecomastia.

Klinefelter's syndrome
Traumatic paraplegia
Male pseudohermaphroditism
Testicular feminization syndrome
Reifenstein's syndrome
17-Ketosteroid reductase deficiency
Endocrine tumors (seminoma, Leydig cell tumor, teratoma, feminizing adrenal tumor, hepatoma, leukemia, hemophilia, bronchogenic carcinoma, leprosy, etc)
Hypothyroidism
Hyperthyroidism
Cirrhosis
Herpes zoster
Friedreich's ataxia

decrease in breast size after 2 years. Surgery is reserved for those with significant psychologic trauma or severe breast enlargement.

Beach RK: Routine breast exams: A chance to reassure, guide, and protect. Contemp Pediatr 1987 (Oct);4:70.

Mahoney CP: Adolescent gynecomastia: Differential diagnosis and management. Pediatr Clin North Am 1990;37:1389.

Neinstein LS, Atkinson J, Diament M: Prevalence and longitudinal study of breast masses in adolescents. J Adolesc Health 1993;13:277.

Rohn RD: Galactorrhea in the adolescent. J Adolesc Health Care 1984;5:37.

GYNECOLOGIC DISORDERS IN ADOLESCENCE

MENSTRUAL PHYSIOLOGY

The menstrual cycle is divided into three phases: follicular, ovulatory, and luteal. During the follicular phase, pulsatile gonadotropin-releasing hormone (GnRH) stimulates anterior pituitary secretion of follicle-stimulating hormone (FSH) and luteinizing hormone (LH). Under the influence of FSH and LH, a dominant follicle emerges by days 5–7 of the menstrual cycle, and the others become atretic. Rising estradiol levels cause proliferation of the endometrium. By midfollicular phase, FSH is beginning to decline secondary to estradiol-mediated negative feedback, while LH continues to rise as a result of estradiol-mediated positive feedback.

There has been a proliferation of LH receptors on the follicle, and it secretes more estradiol in the periovulatory phase, resulting in further proliferation of the endometrium. The rising LH initiates progesterone secretion and the luteinization of the granulosa cells of the follicle. Progesterone in turn stimulates LH and FSH further. This leads to the LH surge, which causes the follicle to rupture and expel the oocyte.

During the luteal phase, the pulsatile release of GnRH occurs less frequently, and LH and FSH gradually decline. The corpus luteum secretes progesterone and 17-hydroxyprogesterone. The endometrium enters the secretory phase in response to rising levels of estrogen and progesterone, with maturation 8–9 days after ovulation. If there is no pregnancy or placental human chorionic gonadotropin (hCG), luteolysis begins; estrogen and progesterone levels decline; and the endometrial lining is shed as menstrual flow (Figure 5–8).

Figure 5–8. Physiology of the normal ovulatory menstrual cycle; gonadotropin secretion, ovarian hormone production, follicular maturation, and endometrial changes during one cycle. FSH = follicle-stimulating hormone, LH = luteinizing hormone. (Reproduced, with permission, from Emans SJH, Goldstein DP: *Pediatric & Adolescent Gynecology,* 3rd ed. Little, Brown, 1990.)

PELVIC EXAMINATION

A pelvic examination may be indicated to evaluate abdominal pain or menstrual disorders or to detect a suspected sexually transmitted disease in the adolescent. In addition, by approximately 16–18 years of age, a pelvic examination should be performed to obtain the first Papanicolaou (Pap) smear and ensure normal reproductive anatomy if annual pelvic examination has not yet been initiated. The adolescent may be apprehensive about the first examination. It should not be rushed, and an explanation of the procedure and its purpose should precede it. The patient can be encouraged to relax by slow, deep breathing and by relaxation of her lower abdominal and inner thigh muscles. A young adolescent may wish to have her mother present during the examination, but the history should be taken privately. A female chaperone should be present for male examiners.

The pelvic examination begins by placing the patient in the dorsal lithotomy position after equipment and supplies are ready (Table 5–11). The examiner inspects the external genitalia, noting the pubic hair maturity rating, the size of the clitoris (2–5 mm is normal), Skene's glands just inside the urethral meatus, and Bartholin's glands at 4 o'clock and 8 o'clock outside the hymenal ring. In cases of alleged sexual abuse or assault, the horizontal measurement of the relaxed prepubertal hymenal opening should be taken, and the presence of any lacerations, bruises, scarring, or synechiae about the hymen, vulva, or anus should be noted.

A vaginal speculum of the appropriate size is then inserted at a 45-degree twist and angled 45 degrees downward. (A medium Pederson speculum is most often used in sexually experienced patients; a narrow Huffman is used for virginal patients. A pediatric speculum may be necessary in examining children.) The vaginal walls are inspected for estrinization, inflammation, or lesions. The cervix should be dull pink. Cervical ectropion is commonly seen in adolescents; the columnar epithelium extends outside the cervical os onto the face of the cervix until later adolescence, when it recedes.

Specimens are obtained, including a wet preparation for leukocytes, trichomonads, and "clue cells"; potassium hydroxide preparation for yeast; cervical swab for gonorrhea culture; endocervical and cervi-

cal (transition zone from columnar to squamous epithelium) samples for Papanicolaou smear; and, last, a cervical swab for *Chlamydia* antigen detection testing. A cervical brush provides a higher yield of cells for the endocervical Papanicolaou slide. Papanicolaou smears should be interpreted by a cytopathologist at a laboratory employing the Bethesda system of classification.

The speculum is then removed, and the bimanual examination is performed to assess uterine size and position, adnexal enlargement or tenderness, or cervical motion tenderness. Rectovaginal examination may be helpful in assessing uterine size or detecting beading from endometriosis.

MENSTRUAL DISORDERS

1. AMENORRHEA

Amenorrhea is the lack of menses when normally anticipated. **Primary amenorrhea** is delay in menarche such that there are no menstrual periods or secondary sex characteristics by 14 years of age or no menses in the presence of secondary sex characteristics by 16 years of age. Constitutional delay is normal pubertal progression at a delayed onset or rate. **Secondary amenorrhea** is defined as the absence of menses for at least three cycles after regular cycles have been present. In some instances, evaluation should begin immediately, without waiting for the specified age or duration of lapsed periods, such as in patients with suspected pregnancy, short stature with the stigmata of Turner's syndrome, or an anatomic defect.

Evaluation for Primary Amenorrhea

Primary amenorrhea may be the result of anatomic abnormalities, chromosomal deviations, or physiologic delay (Table 5–12).

The history should include whether puberty has commenced, level of exercise, presence of stressors, and the age at menarche for female relatives. A careful physical examination should be done, noting the percent of ideal body weight for height and age, Tanner stage, vaginal patency, presence of the uterus (assessed through rectoabdominal examination or ultrasonography if pelvic examination is not appropriate), signs of virilization (acne, clitoromegaly of >5 mm, hirsutism), or stigmata of Turner's syndrome (<60 in. tall, shield-like chest, widely spaced nipples, increased carrying angle of the arms, webbed neck). The examiner keeps in mind that adrenal androgens are largely responsible for axillary and pubic hair and that estrogen is responsible for breast development; maturation of the external genitalia, vagina, and uterus; and menstruation. If pelvic examination reveals normal female external genitalia and pelvic or-

---

Table 5–11. Items for pelvic exam tray.

Medium and virginal speculums (warm)
Gloves
Applicator sticks, sterile
Sigmoidoscopy swabs to remove excess discharge
Cervical spatulas, cervical brushes
Microscope slides and cover slips (frosted and labeled)
Centrifuge tube or test tube (if swab is to be placed in drop of saline and slide prepared later)
NaCl dropper bottle
KOH dropper bottle
Slide container to send to lab
Gonorrhea culture plate (room temperature)
Chlamydia culture tube or antigen detection kit
Lubricant
Kleenex
Hemoccult cards
pH paper

Table 5–12. Causes of amenorrhea.

Hypothalamic pituitary axis
  Hypothalamic repression
    Emotional stress
    Depression
    Chronic disease
    Weight loss
    Obesity
    Severe dieting
    Strenuous athletics
    Drugs (post birth control pills, phenothiazines)
  CNS lesion
    Pituitary lesion: adenoma, prolactinoma
    Craniopharyngioma and other brainstem, parasellar
      tumors
    Head injury with hypothalamic contusion
    Infiltrative process (sarcoidosis)
    Vascular disease (hypothalamic vasculitis)
  Congenital conditions[1]
    Kallmann' syndrome
Ovaries
  Gonadal dysgenesis[1]
    Turner's syndrome (XO)
    Mosaic (XX/XO)
  Injury to ovary
    Autoimmune disease (may include thyroid, adrenal,
      islet cells)
    Infection (mumps, oophoritis)
    Toxins (alkylating chemotherapeutic agents)
    Irradiation
    Trauma, torsion (rare)
  Polycystic ovary syndrome (Stein-Leventhal) (virilization
    may be present)
  Ovarian failure
    Premature menopause (may result from causes of
      ovarian injury)
    Resistant ovary
    Variant of gonadal dysgenesis (mosaic)
Uterovaginal outflow tract
  Müllerian dysgenesis[1]
    Congenital deformity or absence of uterus, uterine
      tubes, or vagina
  Imperforate hymen, transverse vaginal septum, vaginal
    agenesis, agenesis of the cervix[1]
  Testicular feminization (absent uterus)[1]
  Uterine lining defect
    Asherman's syndrome (intrauterine synechiae
      postcurettage or endometritis)
    TB, brucellosis
**Defect in hormone synthesis or action (virilization may
be present)**
  Adrenal hyperplasia[1]
  Cushing's disease
  Adrenal tumor
  Ovarian tumor (rare)
  Drugs (steroids, ACTH)

[1]Indicates condition that usually presents as primary amenorrhea.

gans, the physician may order a vaginal smear for estrogen influence or a challenge of medroxyprogesterone acetate (Provera), 10 mg orally twice daily for 5 days (Figure 5–9). If the vaginal smear shows estrogen influence or if withdrawal bleeding occurs within 5–7 days after administration of medroxyprogesterone, normal anatomy and adequate estrogen effect are implied. Determination of serum LH level helps to rule out polycystic ovary syndrome; if this test is normal, reassurance may be given and the developmental process followed every few months. If estrogen is insufficient (atrophic vaginal smear or no withdrawal bleeding), serum gonadotropin (FSH and LH) levels should be determined. Low levels of gonadotropins indicate a more severe hypothalamic suppression, perhaps due to anorexia nervosa, chronic disease, or a central nervous system tumor. Involvement of a gynecologist and endocrinologist is helpful at this point. If gonadotropin levels are high, ovarian failure or gonadal dysgenesis is implied, and karyotype should clarify the cause. Absence of any sign of puberty by 14 years of age indicates inadequate estrogen, and the physician should check FSH, LH, and karyotype first before testing for estrogen effect.

If signs of virilization are present (Figure 5–10), obtaining testosterone and dihydroepiandrostenedione sulfate (DHEAS) will help to separate polycystic ovaries (PCO) from adrenal causes of virilization and amenorrhea. Although elevation of testosterone and DHEAS occurs in virilized patients with PCO, it is not as dramatic as with androgen-producing adrenal or ovarian tumors, adrenal hyperplasia, or Cushing's syndrome or disease. Endocrinologic consultation will assist in differentiating the latter causes. **Polycystic ovaries** is a spectrum of disorders not necessarily accompanied by classic symptoms of obesity, hirsutism, oligomenorrhea, and infertility. Although a classic LH:FSH ratio of 3:1 is described in PCO, up to 20% of patients do not have elevated LH levels. Because of insufficient FSH, androstenedione cannot be converted to estradiol in the ovarian follicle, and anovulation and production of excess androgens result. These patients can be given progesterone, 10 mg daily, for the first 10 days of each month to allow withdrawal flow if there is no evidence of progressive hirsutism and the ovaries are normal in size. Oral contraceptive pills, containing a less androgenic progestin (Demulen, Orthocept), are an alternative treatment. Hirsute patients should have serum testosterone, DHEAS, and a lipid profile checked. If the patient wishes to become pregnant, she should be referred to a gynecologist for clomiphene citrate or menotropins.

If physical examination reveals an absent uterus (see Figure 5–10), karyotype should be performed to differentiate testicular feminization from mullerian duct defect, because these two entities are managed differently.

Evaluation & Treatment of Secondary Amenorrhea

Secondary amenorrhea results when there is unopposed estrogen, maintaining the endometrium in the proliferative phase. The most common causes are pregnancy, stress, or PCO syndrome. The history should focus on issues of stress, chronic illness, drugs, weight change, strenuous exercise, sexual ac-

Figure 5–9. Evaluation of primary amenorrhea in a normal female. FSH = follicle-stimulating hormone, IBW = ideal body weight, LH = luteinizing hormone. (Modified from Roberta K Beach, MD.)

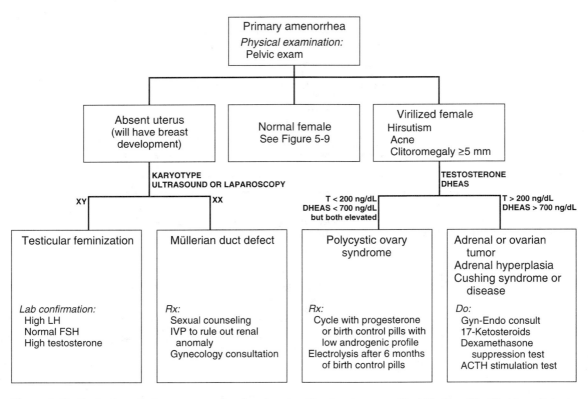

Figure 5–10. Evaluation of primary amenorrhea in a female without a uterus or with virilization. (Modified from Roberta K Beach, MD.)

tivity, and contraceptive use. A review of systems should include questions about headaches, visual changes, and galactorrhea. Physical examination should include a careful funduscopic examination, examination of visual fields, palpation of the thyroid, determination of blood pressure and heart rate, compression of the areola to check for galactorrhea, and a search for signs of androgen excess (eg, hirsutism, clitoromegaly, severe acne, ovarian enlargement).

The first laboratory study obtained is a pregnancy test, even if the patient denies sexual activity. If there is no pregnancy, a progesterone challenge (medroxyprogesterone acetate, 10 mg orally twice daily for 5 days) should be done to determine whether the patient has an estrogen-primed uterus that will respond with withdrawal bleeding 5–7 days later (Figure 5–11).

Most patients who have withdrawal flow after progesterone have mild hypothalamic suppression due to weight change, athletics, stress, or illness; however, disorders such as PCO, adrenal disorders, ovarian tumors, thyroid disease, and diabetes mellitus should be excluded by history and physical examination and appropriate laboratory studies. (See the section on primary amenorrhea and Figure 5–11.)

If there is no withdrawal flow after the progesterone challenge (see Figure 5–11), serum levels of estradiol, FSH, LH, and prolactin should be checked. An elevated FSH level accompanied by a low estrogen level implies ovarian failure, in which case blood for antiovarian antibodies should be obtained and laparoscopy considered. If gonadotropin levels are low or normal and the estradiol level is low, hypothalamic amenorrhea is likely; however, one must consider the possibilities of a central nervous system tumor (prolactinoma), pituitary infarction from postpartum hemorrhage or sickle cell anemia, uterine synechia, or chronic disease. Further evaluation may be necessary.

2. DYSMENORRHEA

Dysmenorrhea is the most common gynecologic complaint of adolescent girls, with an incidence of about 60%. Yet many teenage girls do not seek help from a physician, relying instead on female relatives, friends, and the media for advice. Therefore, the physician should ask about "menstrual cramps" when taking a review of systems. In this era of prostaglandin inhibitors, much can be done to alleviate suffering (Table 5–13).

Dysmenorrhea can be divided into primary and

Figure 5–11. Evaluation of secondary amenorrhea. ACTH = adrenocorticotropic hormone, ESR = erythrocyte sedimentation rate, FSH = follicle-stimulating hormone, LH = luteinizing hormone, TSH = thyroid-stimulating hormone, U/A = urinalysis. (Modified from Mammel KA: Secondary amenorrhea. In: *Pediatric Decision Making,* 3rd ed. Berman S [editor]. Decker, 1995.)

Table 5–13. Prostaglandin inhibitors used for dysmenorrhea.

Generic Name	Trade Name	Preparations Available (mg)[1]
Aspirin	Many	325, 500
Ibuprofen	Motrin	200, 300, 400, 600, 800
	Rufen	400, 600, 800
	Advil, Nuprin Medipren	200
Mefenamic acid	Ponstel	250
Naproxen	Naprosyn	250, 375, 500
	Aleve	200
Naproxen sodium	Anaprox	275, 550

[1]Take as directed at onset of menstrual cramps or flow, then every 6–8 hours thereafter.

secondary dysmenorrhea on the basis of whether or not there is underlying pelvic disease.

Primary dysmenorrhea, in which no pelvic disease is detectable, can be further subdivided into **primary spasmodic dysmenorrhea** and **psychogenic dysmenorrhea** (Table 5–14). Primary spasmodic dysmenorrhea accounts for 80% of cases of adolescent dysmenorrhea and most often affects women under 25 years of age.

Pelvic examination is normal in females with primary spasmodic or psychogenic dysmenorrhea. The pelvic examination has diagnostic benefits and provides an opportunity to educate and reassure the patient about her normal reproductive function. However, if the patient has never been sexually active and the history is consistent with primary spasmodic dysmenorrhea, a trial of a prostaglandin inhibitor is reasonable. If the patient is sexually active or if there is no response to a prostaglandin inhibitor, pelvic examination is indicated.

Secondary dysmenorrhea is menstrual pain due to an underlying pelvic lesion (see Table 5–14). Although uncommon in adolescents, when present it is most often due to infection or **endometriosis.** Endometriosis is not limited to adults, as once thought; in one study of adolescent females with chronic pelvic pain, more than 40% who had not received a definitive diagnosis by the third visit were found to have endometriosis.

The clinician evaluating a patient with secondary dysmenorrhea should take a sexual history and conduct a pelvic examination even if the patient is not sexually active. Culture for gonococci, *Chlamydia* antigen detection test, CBC, determination of the erythrocyte sedimentation rate, and pregnancy test should be done. Gynecologic consultation is indicated to look for endometriosis or congenital problems by ultrasonography, hysteroscopy, or laparoscopy. Treatment depends on the cause (see Table 5–14).

3. DYSFUNCTIONAL UTERINE BLEEDING

Dysfunctional uterine bleeding (DUB) may consist of hypermenorrhea or polymenorrhea. It results when an endometrium that has proliferated under unopposed estrogen stimulation finally begins to slough, but incompletely, causing irregular, painless bleeding. The unopposed estrogen stimulation occurs during anovulatory cycles, common in younger adolescents who have not been menstruating for long but occurring also in older adolescents during times of stress or illness.

Clinical Findings

Typically, the adolescent has had several years of regular cycles and then begins to have menses every 2 weeks, or complains of bleeding for 2–3 weeks after 2–3 months of amenorrhea. A past history of painless, irregular periods at intervals of less than 3 weeks may also be elicited. Bleeding for more than 10 days should be considered abnormal. Dysfunctional uterine bleeding must be considered a diagnosis of exclusion (Table 5–15).

Management

A pregnancy test and pelvic examination with appropriate cultures should be performed in sexually active patients. A CBC, including a platelet count, should also be obtained. The history and physical findings may suggest the need for additional coagulation or hormonal studies. Coagulation studies should be done if the patient presents with severe bleeding or within 1 year of menarche. Management depends on the severity of the problem (Table 5–16). It is important to treat for a minimum of 3–4 months to progressively reduce the endometrium to baseline height.

4. MITTELSCHMERZ

Mittelschmerz is the name given to the pain caused by irritation of the peritoneum due to spillage of fluid from the ruptured follicular cyst at the time of ovulation. The patient presents with a history of midcycle, unilateral dull or aching abdominal pain lasting a few minutes or as long as 8 hours. This pain rarely mimics the acute abdominal findings of appendicitis, torsion or rupture of an ovarian cyst, or ectopic pregnancy. The patient should be reassured and treated symptomatically. If the findings are severe enough to warrant consideration of the above diagnoses, laparoscopy may be done to rule them out.

5. PREMENSTRUAL SYNDROME

Premenstrual syndrome (PMS) has received much

Table 5–14. Dysmenorrhea in the adolescent.

Primary Dysmenorrhea—no pelvic pathology

	Etiology	Onset and Duration	Symptoms	Pelvic Exam	Treatment
Primary spasmodic	Excessive amount of prostaglandin F2α, which attaches to myometrium causing uterine contractions, hypoxia, and ischemia. Also, directly sensitizes pain receptors.	Begins with onset of flow or just prior and lasts 1–2 days. Does not start until 6–18 months after menarche, when cycles become ovulatory.	Lower abdominal cramps radiating to lower back and thighs. Associated nausea, vomiting diarrhea, and urinary frequency also due to excess prostaglandins.	Normal. May wait to examine if never sexually active and history is consistent with primary spasmodic dysmenorrhea.	Mild—heating pad, warm baths, nonprescription analgesics. Moderate—severe: prostaglandin inhibitors at onset of flow or pain. Oral contraceptives for sexually active patients.
Psychogenic	May have history of sexual abuse or may have difficulty adjusting to womanhood. May have secondary gain from school or work avoidance.	Starts at menarche. Pain begins with anticipation of menses and lasts throughout flow.	Abdominal cramps.	Normal.	Educate regarding normal menstrual function. Reassure that pain does not indicate pathology. Relaxation techniques and biofeedback. Counseling to understand underlying issues.

Secondary Dysmenorrhea—underlying pathology present. (Always perform pelvic exam if secondary dysmenorrhea suspected or patient is sexually active. Gonorrhea culture, test for chlamydia, CBC, and ESR should be obtained.)

	Etiology	Onset and Duration	Symptoms	Pelvic Exam	Treatment
Infection	Most often due to a sexually transmitted disease such as chlamydia or gonorrhea.	Recent onset of pelvic cramps.	Pelvic cramps, excessive bleeding, intermenstrual spotting or vaginal discharge.	Mucopurulent or purulent discharge from cervical os, cervical friability, cervical motion tenderness, adnexal tenderness, positive culture for STD.	Appropriate antibiotics.
Endometriosis	Aberrant implants of endometrial tissue in pelvis or abdomen; may result from reflux.	Generally starts more than 2 years after menarche.	Pelvic pain, may occur intermenstrually.	Two thirds are tender on exam especially during late luteal phase.	Hormonal suppression by oral contraceptives or danazol. Surgery may be necessary for extensive disease.
Complication of pregnancy	Spontaneous abortion, ectopic pregnancy.	Acute onset.	Pelvic cramps associated with a delay in menses.	Positive hCG, enlarged uterus or adnexal mass.	Immediate gynecologic consult.
Congenital anomalies	Transverse vaginal septum, septate uterus, or cervical stenosis.	Onset at menarche.	Pelvic cramps.	Underlying congenital anomaly may be apparent. May require exam under anesthesia.	Gynecologic consult for ultrasound, hysteroscopy, or laparoscopy.
IUD	Increased uterine contractions, or increase risk for pelvic infection.	Onset after placement of IUD or acutely if due to infection.	Pelvic cramps, heavy menstrual bleeding, may have vaginal discharge.	Normal, or see infection earlier.	Prostaglandin inhibitors of mefenamic acid may be drug of choice because it also reduces flow. Appropriate antibiotics and consider removal of IUD if infection is present.
Pelvic adhesions	Previous abdominal surgery or pelvic inflammatory disease.	Delayed onset after surgery or PID.	Abdominal pain, may or may not be associated with menstrual cycles; possible alteration in bowel pattern.	Variable.	Surgery.

Table 5–15. Differential diagnosis of dysfunctional uterine bleeding in adolescents.

Pelvic inflammatory disease or cervicitis
Complication of pregnancy: ectopic pregnancy, threatened abortion, incomplete abortion, missed abortion
Breakthrough bleeding on oral contraceptives
Blood dyscrasias: iron deficiency, thrombocytopenia, coagulaopathy, von Willebrand's disease, leukemia
Endocrine disorders: hypothyroidism, hyperthyroidism, diabetes mellitus, adrenal disease, hyperprolactinemia
Trauma
Foreign body
Uterine, vaginal, ovarian, abnormalities: carcinoma, fibroids, adenosis from DES, premature menopause

Reproduced, with permission, from Merenstein GB, Kaplan DW, Rosenberg AA (editors): *Handbook of Pediatrics,* 17th ed. Appleton & Lange, 1994.

attention in the lay press. The term is applied to a cluster of physical and psychologic symptoms that are temporally related to the week preceding menstruation and are alleviated by the onset of menses. PMS should be distinguished from common premenstrual molimina (fluid retention, breast tenderness),

depression, idiopathic cyclic edema, premenstrual dysphoric disorder, fibromyalgia, chronic fatigue syndrome, and psychosomatic disorders. This may be difficult because of the diversity of symptoms ascribed to PMS and the variability from month to month in the same patient. Premenstrual symptoms most commonly cited include emotional lability, anxiety, poor concentration, impaired judgment, gastrointestinal symptoms, hot flashes, and hypoglycemic symptoms. Previously thought to be a disorder limited to adult women, recent studies indicate that adolescents also experience premenstrual symptoms. Although a number of causes have been proposed (progesterone deficiency, hyperprolactinemia, estrogen excess or imbalance of the estrogen:progesterone ratio, vitamin B_{12} deficiency, fluid retention, low endorphins, prostaglandins, hypoglycemia, psychosomatic factors), none has been proved. There may be some hormonal role; women who have undergone hysterectomy but not oophorectomy may have cyclic symptoms resembling PMS, whereas postmenopausal women have no such symptoms. Several treatments have been advocated, but

Table 5–16. Management of dysfunctional bleeding (DUB).[1]

	Mild	Moderate	Severe
Characteristics	Hct>33% or Hb>11 g/dL Shortened intervals or heavy flow	Hct 27–33% or Hb 9–11 g/dL Moderately heavy and prolonged cycles, or persistently short intervals	Hct <27% or Hb<9 g/dL (or dropping orthostatic symptoms and signs Heavy vaginal bleeding
Acute treatment	Menstrual calendar Iron supplementation Nonsteroidal anti-inflammatory drug with menses may help reduce flow. Consider OCPs if patient is sexually active and desires contraception (standard once-daily dose).	OCPs (1/35) up to 4 pills per day and taper over 2–3 weeks; may need antiemetic. Bleeding should stop in a few days. Expect withdrawal flow a few days after last dose.	Fluids, blood transfusion prn. Hospitalize. *For hemostasis, consider:* conjugated estrogens (Premarin) 25 mg IV q 4–6 h x 24 h bleeding stops; antiemetic. *Then:* OCPs (1/35) cycle 4 pills/d x 4d 3 pills/d x 4 d 2 pills/d x 17 d withdrawal bleeding x 7 days[3]
Long-term management	*Monitor* menstrual calendar and Hb *Follow-up* in 2 months	*Cycle with either:* Medroxyprogesterone acetate 10 mg orally twice a day for 10 days starting day 14 of each cycle for 3–6 months *or* OCPs (1/35)[2] for 3–6 months beginning the Sunday after withdrawal bleeding starts. Iron supplementation. *Monitor:* HB *Follow-up* within 2–3 weeks and every 3 months	*Next:* OCPs (1/50)[4] cycle (using 28-d packs) for 3 months. Begin the Sunday after withdrawal bleeding begins. Length of use dependent on resolution of anemia. *Monitor:* Hb *Follow-up* within 2–3 weeks and every 3 months.

[1]Diagnosis: Prolonged painless menses (>8 days); heavy flow (>6 tampons/pads per day); short cycles (<21 days); no other cause found.
[2]Triphasic OCP is acceptable.
[3]This schedule will use three 21-day packages.
[4]Use pill with 50 µg of ethinyl estradiol for first 3 months, then 30–35 µg monophasic or triphasic pill.
OCPs = oral contraceptive pills.
Modified from Blythe M: Common menstrual problems. Part 3. Abnormal uterine bleeding. Adolescent Health Update 1992;4:1.

none has conferred consistent benefits. Education is the most useful measure at this time. The patient can keep a calendar of symptoms for several months, and proper eating, exercise, and sleep can be stressed. Salt restriction or mild diuretics can be prescribed for patients with fluid retention. Oral contraceptives or prostaglandin inhibitors may be beneficial for some women. Tricyclic antidepressants do not have a role in the treatment of this disorder.

6. OVARIAN CYSTS

Functional cysts account for 20–50% of ovarian tumors in adolescents and are a variation of the normal physiologic process. They may be asymptomatic or may cause menstrual irregularity, constipation, or urinary frequency. Functional cysts, unless large, rarely cause abdominal pain; however, torsion or hemorrhage of an ovarian cyst may present as an acute or subacute abdomen. **Follicular cysts** account for the majority of ovarian cysts. They are produced every cycle but occasionally are not resorbed. **Follicular cysts** are unilateral, usually not larger than 4 cm in diameter, and resolve spontaneously. If the patient is asymptomatic, she can be given oral contraceptives containing 50 μg of estrogen for suppression and examined monthly. The patient should be referred to a gynecologist for laparoscopy if she is premenarcheal; if the cyst has a solid component or is larger than 5 cm by ultrasonography; if there are symptoms or signs suggestive of hemorrhage or torsion; or if the cyst fails to regress after two or three menstrual cycles. **Lutein cysts** occur less commonly and may be 5–10 cm in diameter. The patient may have associated amenorrhea or, as the cyst becomes atretic, heavy vaginal bleeding. The patient may be monitored on suppression with oral contraceptives for 3 months but should have a laparoscopy if the cyst is larger than 5 cm or if there is pain or bleeding from the cyst.

7. ENDOMETRIOSIS

See Secondary Dysmenorrhea, earlier.

Beach RK: Relieving the pain of menstrual cramps. Contemp Pediatr 1986;3:115.

Blythe M: Common menstrual problems: Part 1: Management in the pediatric practice. Adolesc Health Update 1991;3:1.

Blythe M: Common menstrual problems: Part 2: Amenorrhea and oligomenorrhea. Adolesc Health Update 1991;4:1.

Blythe M: Common menstrual problems. Part 3: Abnormal uterine bleeding. Adolesc Health Update 1992;4:1.

Davis GD, Thillet E, Lindemann J: Clinical characteristics of adolescent endometriosis J Adolesc Health 1993; 14:362.

Emans SJH, Goldstein DP: *Pediatric and Adolescent Gynecology*. Little, Brown, 1990.

Ginsburg KA: A practical approach to diagnosing PMS. Intern Med 1995 (June):47.

Grumbach MM: The neuroendocrinology of puberty. Hosp Pract 1980 (March);15:51.

Mansfield MJ, Emans SJ: Anorexia nervosa, athletics, and amenorrhea. Pediatr Clin North Am 1989;36:533.

National Cancer Institute Workshop: The 1988 Bethesda system for reporting cervical/vaginal cytological diagnoses. JAMA 1989;262:931.

Neinstein LS: Menstrual problems in adolescents. Med Clin North Am 1990;74:1181.

Polaneczky MM, Slap GB: Menstrual disorders in the adolescent: Amenorrhea. Pediatr Rev 1992;13:43.

Speroff L, Glass RH, Kase NG (editors): *Clinical Gynecologic Endocrinology and Infertility,* 4th ed. Williams & Wilkins, 1989.

Strasburger VC (editor): Adolescent gynecology. Pediatr Clin North Am 1989;38:3.

CONTRACEPTION

Sexually active adolescent females wait an average of 1 year before seeking contraception; however, 50% of teen pregnancies in the United States occur in the first 6 months after sexual activity begins. Sexuality, contraception, and pregnancy prevention are areas with which the pediatrician has become familiar out of necessity.

Abstinence & Decision Making

Adolescents may have poorly formulated skills for making decisions of any kind and often benefit from a decision-making framework that can be applied to a variety of situations, particularly those involving peer pressure. For younger adolescents, this framework can be made more concrete by providing written materials on which the adolescent fills in alternatives and their consequences.

Many adolescents have given little thought to how they feel about their developing sexuality or how they would handle sexual situations. As a result, sexual intercourse may be initiated because the individuals are ill-prepared to handle a situation. By talking with teenagers about their alternatives to sexual intercourse and its implications (unintended pregnancy; sexually transmitted diseases; possible emotional trauma; effects on education, career, and income; and responsibilities if a pregnancy occurs), physicians can help them make informed decisions before they find themselves in a dilemma.

Teenagers need to be aware that 50% of all teenagers have not engaged in sexual intercourse. Abstinence is the most commonly used method of birth control. If an adolescent chooses to remain abstinent, the clinician should reinforce the decision. It is also prudent to encourage adolescents to use contraception at the time they do initiate sexual intercourse.

Condoms & Spermicides

Barrier methods of contraception have gained popularity—even among adolescents—as a result of the educational and marketing efforts driven by the AIDS epidemic. In 1988, 55% of sexually active 15- to 19-year-old males reported using a condom at first intercourse, and 57% at last intercourse—compared with about 20% of 17- to 19-year-old males in 1979. Regardless of whether another method is used, all sexually active adolescents should be counseled to use condoms. Condoms also offer protection against sexually transmitted diseases by preventing the transmission of gonococci, chlamydia, spirochetes, hepatitis virion particles, and possibly HIV. Spermicides containing nonoxynol-9 have virucidal and bactericidal effects. Aside from the diaphragm and cervical cap, barrier methods do not require a medical visit or prescription and are widely available (Table 5–17). The polyurethane vaginal pouch, or "female condom," is now available. Although it has pregnancy

and sexually transmitted disease prevention properties similar to those of the male condom, its higher cost and more difficult insertion make it unlikely to appeal to adolescents.

Oral Contraceptives

Oral contraceptives have a three-pronged mechanism of action: (1) suppression of ovulation; (2) thickening of the cervical mucus, thereby making sperm penetration more difficult; and (3) atrophy of the endometrium, which diminishes the chance of implantation. The latter two actions are progestin effects.

A. Combination Oral Contraceptives: Combination oral contraceptives are birth control pills containing both estrogen and progestin. Ethinyl estradiol and mestranol (which is converted to ethinyl estradiol by the liver before it is pharmacologically active) are the two estrogens currently used in oral contraceptives in the United States. An oral contraceptive containing 30–35 µg of ethinyl estradiol is most often prescribed to adolescents beginning to take birth control pills. A number of different pro-

Table 5–17. Lowest expected, typical, and lowest reported failure rates during the first year of use of a method of contraception, United States. Percentage of women experiencing an accidental pregnancy in the first year of use.

Method	Lowest Expected[1]	Typical[2]	Lowest Reported[3]
Chance	85	85	43.1
Spermicides[4]	3	21	0
Sponge			
Parous women	9	28	27.7
Nulliparous women		18	133.9
Cervical cap[5]	6	18	8
Diaphragm	6	18	2.1
Condom[6]	2	12	4.2
Pill			
Combined	0.1		0
Progestogen only	0.5		1.1
Depot medroxyprogesterone acetate	0.3	0.3	0
Levonorgestrel implants (Norplant System)	0.04	0.04	0

Modified and reproduced, with permission, from Hatcher RA et al: *Contraceptive Technology 1990–1992,* 15th rev ed. Irvington, 1990.
[1]Among couples who initiate use of a method (not necessarily for the first time) and who use it *perfectly* (both consistently and correctly); the authors' best guess of the percentage expected to experience an accidental pregnancy during the first year if they do not stop use for any other reason.
[2]Among *typical* couples who initiate use of a method (not necessarily for the first time), the percentage who experience an accidental pregnancy during the first year if they do not stop use for any other reason.
[3]In the literature on contraceptive failure, the *lowest* reported percentage who experienced an accidental pregnancy during the first year following initiation of use (not necessarily for the first time) if they did not stop use for any other reason.
[4]Foams and vaginal suppositories.
[5]With spermicidal cream or jelly.
[6]Without spermicides.

gestins are used in oral contraceptives and differ in their estrogenic, antiestrogenic, and androgenic effects. Triphasic oral contraceptives were introduced in the United States in 1984. Their main advantage is a 35–39% lower progestin dose over the course of the month, resulting in fewer progestin-related metabolic effects such as those on lipids, blood pressure, and carbohydrate metabolism. Disadvantages include confusion due to the multiple pill colors and a breakthrough bleeding rate that is comparable to or somewhat greater than that of low-dose monophasic counterparts. As estrogen doses decreased in oral contraceptives, the androgenic side effects of progestins became more apparent, leading to the development of three progestins (desogestrel, gestodene, and norgestimate). These "new" progestins in combination with ethinyl estradiol or mestranol are now being introduced in the United States (after about 10 years of use in Europe). To date, clinical evaluations show virtually identical efficacy rates in pregnancy prevention, very similar metabolic and side effects, and the same noncontraceptive benefits as previous combination pills. Their less androgenic profile may benefit patients with PCO or androgenic side effects.

B. Minipill: Minipills contain progestins found in combination oral contraceptives—but in smaller doses—and no estrogen. Their chief use is in women who experience unacceptable estrogen-related side effects with combination oral contraceptives. Their lack of estrogen, however, is also responsible for the main side effect, that of less predictable menstrual patterns. For this reason, and because minipills are not as effective as combination oral contraceptives, they are a poor choice for adolescents. Their mechanism of action relies on the progestin-mediated actions, and ovulation is suppressed in only 15–40% of cycles.

C. Indications & Contraindications: Combined oral contraceptives may be the method of choice for sexually active adolescents, who frequently have unplanned intercourse; however, the patient must be able to comply with a daily dosing regimen. Most states allow oral contraceptives to be prescribed to minors confidentially. Ideally, it is best to wait until six to 12 regular menstrual cycles have occurred before beginning oral contraceptives; however, if the teenager is already sexually active, the medical and social risks of pregnancy probably outweigh the risks of oral contraceptives.

Oral contraceptives may also be used to treat dysmenorrhea (see earlier).

Contraindications to combined oral contraceptives can be categorized as absolute and relative (Table 5–18). When use of estrogenic agents is contraindicated, progestin-only pills are an alternative.

D. Beginning Birth Control Pills & Follow-up: Before a patient begins taking oral contraceptives, a careful menstrual history, medical history, and family medical history should be taken. In addi-

Table 5–18. Contraindications to combined birth control pills.

Absolute contraindications
History of thrombophlebitis, thromboembolic disorder, cerebrovascular disease, ischemic heart disease
Known or suspected carcinoma of the breast or estrogen-dependent neoplasia
Known or suspected pregnancy
History of benign or malignant liver tumor
Undiagnosed abnormal vaginal bleeding

Strong relative contraindications
Severe vascular or migraine headaches
Hypertension
Diabetes
Active gallbladder disease
Mononucleosis, acute phase
Sickle cell disease or sickle C disease
Upcoming major surgery
Long-leg cast or major injury to lower leg
Known impaired liver function at present time
Completion of term pregnancy within past 10–14 days

Modified and reproduced, with permission, from Breedlove B, Judy B, Martin N (editors): *Contraceptive Technology 1988–1989*, 14th rev ed. Irvington Publishers, 1988.

tion, baseline weight and blood pressure should be established, breast and pelvic examination should be performed, and specimens for urinalysis, Papanicolaou smear, gonorrhea culture, and chlamydial culture or antigen detection test obtained.

If there are no contraindications (see Table 5–18), the patient may begin her first pack of pills with her next menstrual period (either the first Sunday after flow begins or the first day of flow, depending on the brand). A triphasic or a low-dose combined oral contraceptive is used for those without contraindications to use of estrogen. With adolescents, it is wise to use 28-day packs rather than 21-day packs to reduce the chance of missing pills. The patient should be instructed on the use of her pills and on the possible risks and side effects and their warning signs. To ensure protection, she should use a back-up method, such as condoms and foam, for the first 2 weeks. In addition, the patient should be advised to use condoms at every intercourse to prevent sexually transmitted diseases. A follow-up visit in 1 month and then every 2–3 months for the first year may improve compliance, since teenagers often discontinue birth control pills because of nonmedical reasons or minor side effects. Teenagers may need reassurance about the safety of birth control pills and their added benefits (Table 5–19).

E. Management of Side Effects: A different type of combined oral contraceptive should be tried if a patient has a persistent minor side effect for more than the first 2–3 months. Adjustments should be made on the basis of hormonal effects (Table 5–20). Changes are most often made for persistent breakthrough bleeding not related to missed pills.

Table 5–19. Noncontraceptive health benefits of oral contraceptive pills.

Protection against life-threatening conditions
Ovarian cancer
Endometrial cancer
Pelvic inflammatory disease
Ectopic pregnancy
Morbidity and mortality due to unintended pregnancies

Alleviate conditions affecting quality of life
Iron deficiency anemia
Benign breast disease
Dysmenorrhea
Irregular cycles
Functional ovarian cysts
Premenstrual syndrome

Mounting evidence
Improved bone density

Injectable Hormonal Contraceptives

The depot form of medroxyprogesterone acetate (DMPA) was approved by the FDA as a long-acting injectable progestational contraceptive in 1992. It is given as a 150-mg deep intramuscular injection into the gluteal or deltoid muscle every 12 weeks with a 2-week grace period. The first injection should be given within the first 5 days of the menstrual cycle to ensure immediate contraceptive protection. DMPA works chiefly by blocking the LH surge, thereby suppressing ovulation, but it also thickens cervical mucus and alters the endometrium to inhibit ovum implantation. With a failure rate of less than 0.3%, minimal compliance issues, long- acting nature, reversibility, lack of interference with intercourse, and lack of estrogen-related side effects, it may be an at-

Table 5–20. Pill side effects: hormone etiology.

Estrogen Excess	Progestin Excess	Androgen Excess	Estrogen Deficiency	Progestin Deficiency
1. Nausea, dizziness	1. Increased appetite and weight gain (noncyclic)	1. Increased appetite and weight gain (noncyclic)	1. Irritability, nervousness	1. Late breakthrough bleeding and spotting
2. Edema and abdominal or leg pain with cyclic weight gain, bloating	2. Tiredness, fatigue, and weakness	2. Hirsutism	2. Hot flushes, vasomotor symptoms	2. Heavy menstrual flow and clots
3. Leukorrhea	3. Depression	3. Acne	3. Uterine prolapse, pelvic relaxation symptoms	3. Delayed onset of menses
4. Increased leiomyoma size	4. Decreased libido	4. Oily skin, rash	4. Early and midcycle spotting	4. Dysmenorrhea
5. Chloasma	5. Oily scalp, acne	5. Increased libido	5. Decreased amount of menstrual flow	5. Weight loss
6. Uterine cramps	6. Loss of hair	6. Cholestatic jaundice	6. No withdrawal bleeding	
7. Irritability, depression	7. Cholestatic jaundice	7. Pruritus	7. Decreased libido	
8. Increased fat deposition	8. Decreased length of menstrual flow		8. Diminished breast size	
9. Cervical extrophia	9. Hypertension?		9. Dry vaginal mucosa, atrophic vaginitis, and dyspareunia	
10. Poor contact lens fit	10. Headaches between Pill packages		10. Headaches	
11. Telangiectasia	11. Candidal vaginitis/cervicitis		11. Depression	
12. Vascular-type headache	12. Increased breast size (alveolar tissue)			
13. Hypertension?	13. Breast tenderness			
14. Lactation suppression	14. Decreased carbohydrate tolerance			
15. Headaches while taking the Pill	15. Dilated leg veins			
16. Cystic breast changes	16. Pelvic congestion syndrome			
17. Breast tenderness				
18. Increased breast size (ductal and fatty tissue and fluid retention)				
19. Thrombophlebitis				
20. Cerebrovascular accidents				
21. Myocardial infarction				
22. Hepatic adenoma				
23. Cyclic weight gain				

Adapted and reproduced, with permission, from: Dickey RP: Medical approaches to reproductive regulation: The pill. ACOG Semin Fam Plan 1974; Table II:21; Dickey RP: *Managing Contraceptive Pill Patients,* 4th ed. Creative Infomatics, 1984; and Hatcher RA et al: *Contraceptive Technology, 1986–1987,* 13th rev ed. Irvington, 1987.

tractive contraceptive for many adolescents, particularly for those who consider its 50% rate of amenorrhea at 1 year of use a desirable side effect or for whom estrogens are contraindicated. Patients should be warned about unpredictable menstrual patterns, the possibility of weight gain or mood changes, and the potential for decreased bone density, which remains under investigation. DMPA may reduce intravascular sickling and increase hemoglobin and red cell survival in patients with sickle cell disease. Moreover, DMPA may be the preferred method for patients with seizure disorders, since it has been found to reduce the number of seizures in some. A recent World Health Organization case-control study concluded that there was no increased risk of liver cancer or invasive squamous cell cervical cancer among users of DMPA, and the risk of endometrial and ovarian cancers was reduced. No statistically significant increased risk of breast cancer has been determined by large studies.

The levonorgestrel-containing nonbiodegradable subdermal implant (Norplant), which is inserted under the skin of the upper arm using a trocar, became available for contraception in the United States in 1991. It is highly effective for 5 years, with pregnancy rates ranging from 0.04 per 100 woman-years in the first year of use to 1.1 per 100 woman-years in the fifth year. It acts through ovulation inhibition and thickening of the cervical mucus. Menstrual irregularities (including prolonged bleeding, intermenstrual spotting, and amenorrhea) are the most common side effects, although headache, acne, weight gain or loss, and depression may occur as well. Its ease of use, lack of compliance issues, high efficacy, and long-term protection make the subdermal implant an ideal contraceptive for adolescents who can tolerate the menstrual irregularities.

Contraceptive Methods *Not* Usually Recommended for Teenagers

Adolescents should understand the menstrual cycle and be taught either that there is no "safe" period or that ovulation occurs 2 weeks before the next menstrual period and may be difficult to predict. Because teenagers frequently have irregular cycles and because sexual intercourse is often spontaneous and unplanned, the rhythm or calendar method is not effective for them. Adolescents also need to be educated that withdrawal is not a reliable method of contraception. Because diaphragms and cervical caps require not only a professional fitting with prescription, but also patient comfort and skill with the insertion technique and concomitant use of spermicides, they have low popularity among teenagers. Intrauterine devices (IUDs) carry an increased risk (within 3 months of insertion) of sexually transmitted diseases and pelvic inflammatory disease and its serious sequelae (infertility, ectopic pregnancy).Therefore, nulligravidity and behaviors that put one at risk of sexu-

ally transmitted diseases are contraindications to the use of IUDs, eliminating many adolescents. Sterilization should be viewed as a permanent method of contraception and therefore is not suitable for teenagers.

American Academy of Pediatrics Committee on Adolescence: Contraception and adolescents. Pediatrics 1990; 86:134.

Beach RK: Contraception for adolescents: Part 1. Adolesc Health Update 1994;7(1):1.

Beach RK: Contraception for adolescents: Part 2. Adolesc Health Update 1995;7(2):1.

Dickey RP: *Managing Contraceptive Pill Patients.* Creative Infomatics, 1993.

Grimes D (editor): Subdermal implants: A new approach to contraception. Contraception Rep 1991;2:4, 10.

Grimes D (editor): Depot medroxyprogesterone acetate: An overview of DMPA and its FDA approval. Contraception Rep 1992;3:4.

Grimes D (editor): Contraception and adolescents. Contraception Rep 1995;6:4.

Hatcher RE et al: The pill: Combined oral contraceptives. In: *Contraceptive Technology,* 16th ed. Irvington, 1994.

Holder AR: Legal issues in adolescent sexual health. AM:STARS 1992;3:257.

Sikand A, Fisher M: The role of barrier contraceptives in prevention of pregnancy and disease in adolescents. AM:STARS 1992;3:223.

PREGNANCY

More than 1 million teenage girls become pregnant in the United States each year. The overall teen pregnancy rate remained steady at 11% of US females aged 15–19 throughout the 1980s, although the birth rate increased from a low of 50.2 per 1000 females 15–19 years old in 1986 to 59.9 per 1000 in 1990. About 45% of 15- to 19-year-old females are sexually active, and more than one-third of these become pregnant within 2 years after onset of sexual activity. More than 80% of these pregnancies are unintended, and about 68% of pregnancies in women under 20 years of age are out of wedlock.

Young maternal age and associated maternal risk factors have been linked to adverse neonatal outcome, including higher rates of low birth weight babies (<2500 g) and neonatal mortality. The psychosocial consequences for the teenage mother and her infant are listed in Table 5–21. Teenagers who are pregnant require additional support from their caregivers, and clinics for young mothers may be the best providers.

Presentation

Adolescents may present with delayed or missed menses or may even request a pregnancy test, but often they present with an unrelated concern or have a hidden agenda. Because of the high level of denial, they may come in with complaints of abdominal pain, urinary frequency, dizziness, or other nonspe-

Table 5–21. Psychosocial consequences of pregnancy for the adolescent mother and her infant.

Mother	Infant
Increased morbidity related to pregnancy	Greater health risks
Greater risk of toxemia, anemia, prolonged labor, premature labor	Increased chance of low birth weight or prematurity
Increased chance of miscarriages, stillbirths	Increased risk of infant death
Increased change of maternal mortality	Increased risk of injury and hospitalization by age 5
Decreased educational attainment	Decreased academic achievement
Less likely to get high school diploma, go to college, or graduate	Lower cognitive scores
	Decreased development
Lower occupational attainment and prestige	Greater chance of being behind grade or needing remedial help
Less chance of stable employment (some resolution over time)	Lower chance of advanced academics
Lower job satisfaction	Lower academic aptitude as a teenager and perhaps a higher probability of dropping out of school
Lower income/wages	
Greater dependence on public assistance	
Less stable marital relationships	Psychosocial consequences
Higher rates of single parenthood	Greater risk of behavior problems
Earlier marriage (though less common than in the past)	Poverty
	Higher probability of living in a nonintact home while in high school
Accelerated pace of marriage, separation, divorce, and remarriage	Greater risk of adolescent pregnancy
Faster pace of subsequent childbearing	
High rate of repeat unintended pregnancy	
More births out of marriage	
Closer spacing of births	
Larger families	

cific symptoms and have no concern about pregnancy. A history of symptoms such as weight gain, engorged breasts, an unusually light or mistimed period, and urinary frequency can be sought, but the adolescent may not have noted these signs of pregnancy. Denial also contributes to the delay in seeking prenatal care. Only about one-third of adolescents receive prenatal care in the first trimester. Clinicians need to have a low threshold for suspicion of pregnancy. If there is any suspicion, a urine pregnancy test should be obtained.

Diagnosis

History, as above, and physical examination may assist in making the diagnosis of pregnancy. Bluish coloring and softening of the cervix may be noted on speculum examination. The uterine fundus may be palpable on abdominal examination if sufficient time has elapsed. If uterine size on bimanual examination does not correspond to dates, one must consider ectopic pregnancy, incomplete or missed abortion, twin gestation, or inaccurate dates.

Laboratory tests for human chorionic gonadotropin (hCG) are simple to perform and are usually diagnostic. Enzyme-linked immunoassay test kits specific for the β-hCG subunit and sensitive to less than 50 mIU/mL of hCG can be performed on urine (preferably the first morning voided specimen, because it is more concentrated) in less than 5 minutes, and are accurate within 12 days after conception. Serum radioimmunoassay is also specific for the beta subunit, is accurate within 7 days after conception, and is helpful in ruling out ectopic pregnancy or threatened abortion. Serum radioreceptor assay may cross-react with LH, is accurate within 14 days after conception, and may be used to confirm a normal pregnancy. Slide agglutination tests are more difficult to read, less sensitive than the above tests, and cross-react with LH. Home pregnancy tests are relatively accurate, particularly when positive; however, they are expensive and have fairly complex instructions that many teenagers have difficulty following. Also, they may preclude obtaining counseling, early entry into prenatal care, or detection of ectopic pregnancy or threatened abortion.

The timing of pregnancy tests is important, since hCG levels initially rise after conception, peak at about 60–70 days, then drop to levels not detected by routine office slide tests after 16–20 weeks.

Special Issues in Management

When an adolescent presents for pregnancy testing, it is wise to find out what she hopes the results will be and what she thinks she will do before performing the test. If she wants to be pregnant and the test is negative, further counseling about the implications of teen pregnancy should be undertaken. For those who do not wish to be pregnant, this is a good time to begin contraception because teens who present for a pregnancy test that is negative have a high risk of pregnancy in the next 2 years.

If the adolescent is pregnant, the physician must discuss her support systems and her options with her (abortion, adoption, raising the baby). Many teenagers need help in telling and involving their parents. It is important to remain available for further assistance with decision making. If the patient knows what she wants to do, she should be referred to the appropriate resources. Since teenagers are often ambivalent about their plans and may have a high level of denial, it is prudent to follow up in 1 week to be certain that a decision has been made and to help the patient obtain prenatal care if she has chosen to continue the pregnancy.

Maternal age alone is not responsible for low birth weight and poor fetal outcome; rather, low maternal prepregnancy weight, poor weight gain, delay in prenatal care, low socioeconomic status, and black race also are contributing factors. The poor nutritional status of some teenagers and their erratic diets, smoking, drinking, or substance abuse, and high prevalence of sexually transmitted diseases play a role. Teenagers are also at greater risk of eclampsia–pre-eclampsia, iron deficiency anemia, cephalopelvic disproportion, prolonged labor, premature labor, and maternal death. Early prenatal care and good nutrition can make a difference with a number of these problems.

Because of the high risk of a second unintended pregnancy within the next 2 years, postpartum contraceptive counseling and follow-up are imperative. Pregnancy prevention is the most cost-effective means of reducing the consequences of teenage pregnancy. Sexual decision making, contraceptive counseling, and close follow-up of sexually active adolescents of both sexes can make a difference. Adolescents who receive sexuality and contraceptive education are not more likely to have intercourse but are less likely to become pregnant than their counterparts who do not receive such instruction.

Ammerman S, Shafer MA, Snyder D: Ectopic pregnancy in adolescents: A clinical review for pediatricians. J Pediatr 1990;117:677.

Klerman LV, Horwitz SM: Reducing the adverse consequences of adolesent pregnancy and parenting: The role of service programs. AM:STARS 1992;3:299.

McAnarney ER, Hendee WR: Adolescent pregnancy and its consequences. JAMA 1989;262:74.

Stevens-Simon C, Fullar SA, McAnarney ER: Teenage pregnancy: Caring for adolescent mothers with their infants in pediatric settings. Clin Pediatr 1989;28:282.

VULVOVAGINITIS

Vaginitis may be due to pathogens or to indigenous flora after a change in milieu of the vagina. *Candida* vulvovaginitis and bacterial vaginosis (formerly called *Gardnerella, Haemophilus,* or nonspecific vaginitis) may be found in patients who are not sexually active. These are examples of indigenous flora that may cause infection. Bacterial vaginosis, however, is more prevalent in those who are sexually active. In sexually active patients, *Trichomonas* infection or cervicitis due to sexually transmitted pathogens must be considered (see section on sexually transmitted diseases, later). For this reason, sexually active patients or suspected victims of sexual abuse should have appropriate specimens taken to detect sexually transmitted disease even if yeast forms are present or bacterial vaginosis is identified.

1. PHYSIOLOGIC LEUKORRHEA

Leukorrhea is the normal vaginal discharge that begins around the time of menarche. The discharge is typically clear or whitish, and its consistency may vary according to cyclic hormonal influences. There should be no odor. Girls in early adolescence may have concerns about such a discharge and need reassurance that it is normal. This may be a good time to tell girls that there is no need for douching. If a vaginal wet preparation is examined, a few squamous epithelial cells may be revealed, but there should be fewer than five polymorphonuclear cells per high-power field.

2. CANDIDAL VULVOVAGINITIS

Candidal vulvovaginitis is caused by yeast. It typically occurs after a course of antibiotics, after which the normal perineal flora are altered and yeast is allowed to proliferate. Diabetics, patients with compromised immune systems, and those who are pregnant or receiving oral contraceptives are more prone to develop candidal infections.

Clinical Findings

The patient usually complains of vulvar pruritus or dyspareunia and a cheesy vaginal discharge, frequently beginning the week prior to menses. Examination of the vulva reveals an erythematous mucosa, sometimes with excoriation, and a thick, white, cheesy discharge. The discharge may be adherent to the walls of the vagina, which will also be inflamed if the infection is internal. Leukocytes may be seen on a wet preparation, and potassium hydroxide preparation may reveal budding yeast or mycelia. No "clue cells" should be seen. Often the vaginal preparations are unhelpful, and the patient should be treated on the basis of the clinical examination. Vaginal culture for yeast is usually unnecessary.

Treatment

Butoconazole, clotrimazole, miconazole, terconazole, or tioconazole vaginal creams or suppositories designed for three or seven nightly doses are effective in most patients. Some patients require a longer course of treatment. Fluconazole (150 mg once orally) is also effective and may be beneficial on a monthly prophylactic basis for women with recurring infections. Patients with recurrent episodes should be given prophylactic treatment whenever they take antibiotics. It may be helpful to simultaneously treat the partners of sexually active patients with recurrent candidal infections.

3. BACTERIAL VAGINOSIS

Bacterial vaginosis may be caused by any of the indigenous vaginal flora, such as *Gardnerella, Bacteroides, Peptococcus,* or lactobacilli.

Clinical Findings

The patient generally complains of malodorous mild discharge. On examination, a thin, homogeneous, grayish-white discharge is found adherent to the vaginal wall with diffuse vaginal erythema. A whiff test, in which a drop of potassium hydroxide is added to a smear of the discharge on a slide, results in the release of amines, causing a fishy odor. Wet preparation reveals an abundance of "clue cells" (vaginal epithelial cells stippled with adherent bacteria) and small pleomorphic rods.

Treatment

Treatment for bacterial vaginosis is with metronidazole (500 mg orally twice a day for 7 days) or clindamycin (300 mg orally twice a day for 7 days). Topical metronidazole or clindamycin may also be effective. Ampicillin (500 mg orally four times a day for 7 days) is the alternative for pregnant patients.

4. OTHER CAUSES OF VULVOVAGINITIS

Sexually Transmitted Diseases

Sexually transmitted diseases are an important cause of vaginal discharge in adolescents. (See Chapter 39.) One should obtain appropriate cultures whenever an adolescent complains of vaginal discharge, even when the cervix appears normal.

Foreign Body Vaginitis

Foreign bodies—most commonly retained tampons—cause extremely malodorous vaginal discharges. Treatment consists of removal, for which ring forceps may be useful. Further treatment is generally not necessary.

Allergic or Contact Vaginitis

Bubble baths, feminine hygiene sprays, or vaginal contraceptive foams or suppositories may cause chemical irritation of the vaginal mucosa. Discontinuing use of the offending agent is indicated.

REFERENCES

Adams GR et al (editors): *Biology of Adolescent Behavior and Development.* Sage, 1989.

Adolescent Health Update, Vol 8. American Academy of Pediatrics, 1996.

Adolescent Medicine: State of the Art Reviews. Hanley & Belfus. [Series.]

Blum RW (editor): *Chronic Illness and Disabilities in Childhood and Adolescence.* Grune & Stratton, 1984.

Blumenthal SJ, Kupfer DJ: *Suicide Over the Life Cycle: Risk Factors, Assessment, and Treatment of Suicidal Patients.* American Psychiatric Press, 1990.

Christophersen ER, Levine MD (editors): Development and behavior: Older children and adolescents. Pediatr Clin North Am 1992;39:3.

Dickey RP: *Managing Contraceptive Pill Patients.* Creative Infomatics, 1993.

Dryfoos JG: *Adolescents at Risk: Prevalence and Prevention.* Oxford University Press, 1990.

Emans SJH, Goldstein DP: *Pediatric and Adolescent Gynecology.* Little, Brown, 1990.

Erickson EH: *Identity: Youth and Crisis.* Norton, 1968.

Farrow JA (editor): Adolescent medicine. Med Clin North Am 1990;74:5.

Friedman SB, Fisher M, Schonberg SK (editors): *Comprehensive Adolescent Health Care.* Quality Medical Publishing, 1992.

Furstenberg FF Jr, Brooks-Gunn J, Morgan SP: *Adolescent Mothers in Later Life.* Cambridge Univ Press, 1987.

Greydanus DE: *Caring for Your Adolescent, Ages 12 to 21.* Bantam, 1991.

Guidelines for Adolescent Preventive Services: American Medical Association, 1992.

Hatcher RA et al: *Contraceptive Technology,* 16th ed. Irvington, 1994.

Hechinger FM: *Fateful Choices: Healthy Youth for the 21st Century.* Carnegie Corporation of New York, 1992.

Hendee WR (editor): *The Health of Adolescents: Understanding and Facilitating Biological, Behavioral, and Social Development.* Jossey-Bass, 1991.

Hergenroeder AC, Garrick JG (editors): Sports medicine. Pediatr Clin North Am 1990;37:5.

Hoffman A: *Adolescent Medicine.* Appleton & Lange, 1989.

Holder AR: *Legal Issues in Pediatrics and Adolescent Medicine.* Yale Univ Press, 1985.

Holmes KK et al (editors): *Sexually Transmitted Diseases,* 2nd ed. McGraw-Hill, 1990.

Jessor R, Donovan JE, Costa FM: *Beyond Adolescence: Problem Behavior and Young Adult Development.* Cambridge Univ Press, 1991.

Jones RL: *Black Adolescents.* Cobb & Henry, 1989.

Journal of Adolescent Health. Official Publication of the Society for Adolescent Medicine. Litt IF (editor-in-chief). Elsevier. [Series.]

Kagan J, Coles R: *Twelve to Sixteen: Early Adolescence.* Norton, 1972.

Katchadourian H: *The Biology of Adolescence.* Freeman, 1977.

Lerner JW: Educational interventions in learning disabilities. J Am Acad Child Adolesc Psychiatry 1989;28:326.

Lerner RM et al (editors): *Encyclopedia of Adolescence.* Garland, 1991.

Levine M: *Keeping a Head in School: A Student's Book About Learning Abilities and Learning Disorders.* Educators Publishing Service, 1990.

Levine M et al (editors): *Developmental Behavioral Pediatrics,* 2nd ed. Saunders, 1992.

Litt IF: *Evaluation of the Adolescent Patient.* Hanley & Belfus, 1990.

McAnarney ER et al (editors): *Textbook of Adolescent Medicine.* Saunders, 1992.

Meeks JE: *The Fragile Alliances.* Krieger, 1980.

Miller D: *The Age Between: Adolescence and Therapy.* Aronson, 1983.

Millstein SG, Petersen AC, Nightingale EO: *Promoting the Health of Adolescents: New Directions for the Twenty-First Century.* Oxford Univ Press, 1993.

Muuss RE: *Theories of Adolescence,* 3rd ed. Random House, 1975.

Neinstein LS: *Adolescent Health Care: A Practical Guide,* 2nd ed. Urban & Schwarzenberg, 1991.

Speroff L, Glass RH, Kase NG: *Clinical Gynecologic Endocrinology and Infertility.* Williams & Wilkins, 1989.

Tanner JM: *Growth at Adolescence.* Blackwell, 1962.

Vaughan VC, Litt IF: *Child and Adolescent Development: Clinical Implications.* Saunders, 1990.

6 Adolescent Substance Abuse

Trina Menden Anglin, MD, PhD*

INTRODUCTION

Definitions

"Substance abuse" denotes a pathologic use of psychoactive drugs or alcohol. The American Psychiatric Association defines **substance abuse** as a maladaptive pattern of use leading to clinically significant impairment or distress that includes at least one of the following criteria: (1) recurrent substance use resulting in failure to fulfill major role obligations at work, school, or home; (2) recurrent substance use in physically hazardous circumstances; (3) recurrent legal problems associated with psychoactive substances; or (4) continued substance use despite persistent or recurrent social or interpersonal problems caused or exacerbated by the effects of the substance.

Substance dependence carries a more restrictive definition and includes cognitive, behavioral, and physiologic features. A formal diagnosis means that three of the following seven criteria have occurred within the preceding 12 months and have led to clinically significant impairment or distress: (1) tolerance; (2) withdrawal syndrome or need to escalate the use of a specific substance to relieve or avert withdrawal symptoms; (3) use of a larger amount or extending use over a longer time period than intended; (4) persistent desire or unsuccessful attempts to reduce or control use; (5) a great deal of time spent in activities necessary to obtain the substance, to use it, or to recover from its effects; (6) forgoing or reducing important social, occupational, or recreational activities because of substance use; (7) continuing use of a substance despite knowledge that it is causing or exacerbating a persistent or recurrent physical or psychological problem.

Table 6–1 demonstrates that all major classes of substances are associated with dependence and indicates which substances evoke syndromes of intoxication and withdrawal. In addition, many adolescents demonstrate polysubstance abuse. A significant proportion of persons who use tobacco, alcohol, marijuana, and cocaine report at least one indicator of dependence (75%, 14%, 23%, and 29%, respectively). These percentages are much higher for daily users (91%, 48%, 60%, 79%, respectively).

American Psychiatric Association: *Diagnostic and Statistical Manual of Mental Disorders,* 4th ed. American Psychiatric Association, 1994.

Centers for Disease Control and Prevention: Symptoms of substance dependence associated with use of cigarettes, alcohol, and illicit drugs—United States, 1991–1992. MMWR 1995;44:830.

Etiology

The cause of substance abuse and dependence is complicated and multifactorial. It is based on the interaction between biologic and environmental conditions. A biologic vulnerability to alcohol and drug addiction is caused by inheritance of certain genetic codes that affect neurotransmitters in ways that are not completely understood. Certain heritable personality dimensions—novelty seeking, failure to avoid harm, and low reward dependence—are thought to be associated with monoamine neurotransmitters. These neurotransmitters—dopamine, serotonin, and norepinephrine—are themselves associated with neuropharmacologic effects of intoxication with and withdrawal from several major classes of substances (eg, psychostimulants such as cocaine and amphetamines, hallucinogens, nicotine, and alcohol). Moreover, a synthesis theory of addiction considers dopaminergic fibers of the medial forebrain bundle and its nuclei and projection fields to serve as a final common pathway of psychomotor activation for the brain's reinforcement circuits for a variety of substances associated with compulsive self-administration.

Persons with the personality traits just outlined, which frequently manifest during childhood, are at higher risk for developing substance abuse and conduct disorders. Early aggressive behavior also ap-

---

*Portions of this chapter were adapted from a previous work by the author, Interviewing guidelines for the clinical evaluation of adolescent substance abuse. Pediatr Clin North Am 1987;34(2):381. Permission to adapt and to update this work for publication as a chapter in this book has been granted by WB Saunders.

Table 6–1. Major classes of substances associated with dependence, intoxication, and withdrawal.

	Dependence	Intoxication	Withdrawal
Alcohol	X	X	X
Amphetamines	X	X	X
Cannabis	X	X	
Cocaine	X	X	X
Hallucinogens	X	X	
Inhalants	X	X	
Nicotine	X		X
Opioids	X	X	X
Phencyclidine	X	X	
Sedatives, hypnotics, anxiolytics	X	X	X

Adapted with permission by the American Psychiatric Association, from *Diagnostic and Statistical Manual of Mental Disorders,* 4th ed. American Psychiatric Association, 1994:177.

pears to be linked to the development of conduct disorder and substance abuse.

Poor parenting skills and lack of supervision, low levels of familial nurturance and high levels of familial conflict, and familial modeling of substance use increase the likelihood that an adolescent will abuse substances. Adolescents tend to associate with peers who are already similar to them, but who may promote actual substance use behavior through modeling and supplying of drugs and alcohol.

Hawkins JD, Catalano RF, Miller JY: Risk and protective factors for alcohol and other drug problems in adolescence and early adulthood: Implications for substance abuse prevention. Psychol Bull 1992;112:64.

Meyer RE: Biology of psychoactive substance dependence disorders: Opiates, cocaine, and ethanol. In: *Textbook of Psychopharmacology.* Schatzberg AF, Nemeroff CB (editors). American Psychiatric Press, 1995.

Miller NS, Gold MS: A hypothesis for a common neurochemical basis for alcohol and drug disorders. Psychiatr Clin North Am 1993;16:105.

Newlin DB: Alcohol challenge in high-risk individuals. In: *The Development of Alcohol Problems: Exploring the Biopsychosocial Matrix of Risk.* Zucker R, Boyd G, Howard J (editors). NIAAA, US Department of Health and Human Services (NIH Publication No. 94-3495), 1994.

Patton LH: Adolescent substance abuse: Risk factors and protective factors. Pediatr Clin North Am 1995;42:283.

Problems Linked With Substance Abuse

Most adolescents who have used alcohol and drugs do not develop dependency. In fact, experimental use of alcohol and even marijuana may be considered normative experiences for teenagers living in the United States, because such large proportions of young people have tried these substances at least once. Youngsters who experiment with substances but do not use them on a regular basis have been found to demonstrate better psychological adjustment than adolescents who by the age of 18 have never experimented with any drugs. However,

teenagers who use substances frequently are not well adjusted and demonstrate emotional distress, a sense of alienation from others, and poor impulse control.

Many other serious adolescent problems are linked to the use of alcohol and drugs. These include nonintentional trauma such as motor vehicle accidents, drownings, and falls, and interpersonal violence such as fights between peers and among family members, and homicide. Teenagers who were victimized by physical or sexual abuse during childhood, or whose families are riddled by conflict, are at heightened risk for substance abuse. Certain common mental health problems, including depression, suicidal behavior, and anxiety disorders, are frequently associated with substance abuse.

A definite relationship exists between conduct disorder and delinquency, and substance use. However, it is probable that adolescents with attention-deficit hyperactivity disorder are *not* at higher risk for substance abuse unless they also demonstrate evidence for a conduct disorder. Even though covariance between sexual activity and substance abuse has not been consistently demonstrated, especially among urban African-American adolescents, there appear to be clear associations between sexual activity and use of tobacco, alcohol, and illicit substances among younger adolescents. Although pregnant and parenting adolescents may be at relatively high risk for alcohol and illicit substance use, they also tend to limit their use of alcohol, marijuana, and other illicit substances voluntarily and substantially during pregnancy.

Armentano ME: Assessment, diagnosis, and treatment of the dually diagnosed adolescent. Pediatr Clin North Am 1995;42:479.

Kokotailo PK et al: Cigarette, alcohol, and other drug use by school-age pregnant adolescents: Prevalence, detection, and associated risk factors. Pediatrics 1992;90:328.

Lohr MJ et al: Factors related to substance use by pregnant, school-age adolescents. J Adolesc Health 1992;13:475.

Miller NS, Fine J: Current epidemiology of comorbidity of psychiatric and addictive disorders. Psychiatr Clin North Am 1993;16:1.

Millstein SG et al: Health-risk behaviors and health concerns among young adolescents. Pediatrics 1992;89:422.

Shedler J, Block J: Adolescent drug use and psychological health: A longitudinal inquiry. In: *Annual Progress in Child Psychiatry and Child Development 1991*. Chess S, Hertzig ME (editors). Brunner/Mazel Publishers, 1992.

Stanton B et al: Early initiation of sex and its lack of association with risk behaviors among adolescent African-Americans. Pediatrics 1993;92:13.

Stowell RJA, Estroff TW: Psychiatric disorders in substance-abusing adolescent inpatients: A pilot study. J Am Acad Child Adolesc Psychiatr 1992;31:1036.

SCOPE OF ADOLESCENT SUBSTANCE USE

The most useful and widely cited information regarding adolescent substance use in the United States comes from a national self-reporting, annual survey of eighth, tenth, and twelfth graders conducted by the University of Michigan's Institute for Social Research. After about a 12-year decline in the use of illicit substances, a resurgence in use has occurred since about 1991–1992. It is thought that this discouraging reversal may reflect the declining public attention that drug abuse is receiving in this country as other societal issues have emerged. Table 6–2 summarizes current patterns of use. Lifetime prevalence indicates experimental use, 30-day prevalence points toward probable misuse, and daily use indicates actual substance abuse and probable dependence.

Physicians can use the national data to help estimate the prevalence of substance use and substance abuse by the teenagers they encounter. However, local communities may have patterns of substance use that differ from national averages, and different groups of teenagers may also display differing patterns of use.

CONTEXT OF EVALUATION

All teenagers should be screened for their risk of harmful substance use as part of health maintenance care or health supervision, upon entering into mental health counseling, as part of the evaluation process for poor or deteriorating scholastic performance, and as part of the intake process into the juvenile justice system. Opportunities for health maintenance visits for adolescents include examinations for school and camp, preparticipation sports evaluations, and preemployment examinations. A physician who has known a teenager since childhood should not slip into complacency regarding evaluation of the patient's psychosocial status. All teenagers deserve periodic reassessment of their psychosocial development and functioning. Screening for substance use and abuse should be routinely included as part of an adoles-

Table 6–2. Prevalence of substance use among adolescents during 1995.[1]

	Lifetime (%)	30-day (%)	Daily (%)
Alcohol			
8th grade	54	25	0.7
10th grade	70	39	1.7
12th grade	81	51	3.5
Binging pattern in past 2 weeks			
8th grade		14	
10th grade		24	
12th grade		30	
Been drunk			
8th grade	25	8.3	0.2
10th grade	47	21	0.6
12th grade	63	33	1.3
Any illicit drug			
8th grade	28	12	—
10th grade	41	20	—
12th grade	48	24	—
Any illicit drug other than marijuana			
8th grade	18	6.5	—
10th grade	24	8.9	—
12th grade	28	10	—
Marijuana			
8th grade	20	9.1	0.8
10th grade	34	17	2.8
12th grade	42	21	4.6
Inhalants			
8th grade	22	6.1	0.2
10th grade	19	3.5	0.1
12th grade	17	3.2	0.1
Total cocaine			
8th grade	4.2	1.2	0.1
10th grade	5.0	1.7	0.1
12th grade	6.0	1.8	0.2
Stimulants			
8th grade	13	4.2	0.2
10th grade	17	5.3	0.2
12th grade	15	4.0	0.3
Hallucinogens			
8th grade	5.23	1.7	0.1
10th grade	9.3	3.3	<0.1
12th grade	13	4.4	0.1
Tranquilizers			
8th grade	4.5	1.2	<0.1
10th grade	6.0	1.7	<0.1
12th grade	7.1	1.8	<0.1
Steroids			
8th grade	2.0	0.6	<0.1
10th grade	2.0	0.6	0.1
12th grade	2.3	0.7	0.2

[1]Information is summarized from a press release. The University of Michigan, News and Information Services, The Monitoring the Future Study. December 11, 1995.

Selected categories of substances are presented. This table omits barbiturates, heroin, and other opioids, and subclasses of cocaine, stimulants, inhalants, and hallucinogens. Percentages are rounded to the nearest whole number for prevalence figures of at least 10%. One decimal place is preserved for smaller percentage figures.

cent's general psychosocial assessment. In addition, adolescents with chronic diseases and disabilities are not immune from substance use and abuse.

Physicians need to consider substance abuse when adolescent patients report fatigue, recurrent abdominal pain, chest pain, palpitations, headache, chronic cough, persistent nasal congestion, and recurrent sore throats.

Concerned family members or school personnel may request that an adolescent be evaluated specifically for substance abuse or more generally for dysfunctional behavior or deteriorating school performance. Parents may request help spontaneously, or under duress, from school officials because of a child's behavior problems or evidence of substance use while at school.

Teenagers who are experiencing dysfunctional consequences from substance abuse are unlikely to directly request evaluation and intervention. Although youngsters are unlikely to appear for scheduled appointments intoxicated or high, it is nevertheless possible, and physicians should be alert for overt and subtle signs of alcohol and drug effects.

Physicians may also become aware of a possible substance abuse problem when they need to prescribe medication and review instructions for its use. Pharmaceuticals that interact with alcohol are good examples, such as oral metronidazole for treatment of trichomoniasis and bacterial vaginosis and antihistamines available over-the-counter for allergic rhinitis. Teenagers who drink alcohol frequently disclose this information to clinicians as part of this discussion.

Teenagers are frequently brought to the emergency department either because they are acutely intoxicated or because they are experiencing an adverse or withdrawal reaction from ingesting drugs or alcohol. Adolescents may also require repair of injuries sustained while intoxicated. In these circumstances, physicians will be able to document the substance use through interview, physical findings, and toxicologic testing of urine.

INTERVIEWING TECHNIQUES

General strategies for interviewing adolescents are addressed in Chapter 5. Suggested techniques for interviewing adolescents about substance use are summarized in Table 6–3. The remainder of this section focuses on strategies helpful for interviewing adolescents who are actually experiencing substance abuse.

Youngsters who abuse substances may resort to several defenses as they struggle to conceal their problem. These behaviors are not directed personally at the physician. They occur if an adolescent feels that continuation of substance use is being threatened. The interviewer will gain respect from the adolescent by recognizing and acknowledging these be-

Table 6–3. Suggested interviewing techniques.

- Interview the adolescent privately.
- Discuss the parameters of confidentiality.
- Avoid parental subterfuge.
- Ask open-ended questions.
- Do not barrage the adolescent with questions.
- Do not lecture or moralize.
- Be sensitive to the adolescent's responsiveness to your style and to specific questions. Determine what types of information the adolescent would like to learn or verify, and then provide it.
- If the adolescent has no questions, offer information that is developmentally appropriate, using the technique of generalization.

haviors as protective strategies and returning the interview to its appropriate course.

For example, a frightened or angry adolescent may show resistance by refusing to answer questions. The interviewer can frequently cut through this behavior by describing what is occurring in a warm, empathic way. "You seem quite upset (angry, unhappy) about coming here today. I can understand your not wanting to come"—allow the adolescent to respond briefly—"but even though you feel that way, we have a job to do." Angry adolescents may also use profanity or vulgar language to express themselves or to attempt to discomfit the interviewer. Calmly accepting the language by acknowledging its use is an appropriate response.

Adolescents who abuse substances may also attempt to divert attention from themselves. One tactic is to disclose another family member's problem behavior, such as physical abuse or parental drinking. This information is obviously valuable for the clinical evaluation. However, for the time being, it must remain tangential to the interviewer's focus. It is appropriate to acknowledge receiving the information by saying, "I can understand your being upset (concerned) about that. Let's talk about it a little later (at our next visit). Right now, however, I need to ask you . . ."

Adolescents who abuse substances may minimize their involvement or distort factual information. The parents frequently perceive them as liars. These behaviors are actually strategies that help the adolescent maintain the pattern of use. It is important to let the adolescent know that the attempted deception has not succeeded. During an initial assessment, however, direct confrontation is usually counterproductive. For example, if the adolescent presents obviously inconsistent information, the physician might say, "That doesn't make sense. Earlier you said that . . . (your mother said that . . .) Now you are telling me. . . . It just doesn't add up." Attempts to mislead the interviewer should be made part of the assessment record.

PSYCHOSOCIAL ASSESSMENT

A general psychosocial assessment of an adolescent provides the infrastructure for addressing actual substance use. It helps to determine what roles, if any, psychoactive substance use plays in the adolescent's life. Information should be gathered that will help determine whether an adolescent is at risk for abusing substances, is making satisfactory developmental progress, or has experienced any negative consequences from substance abuse. Table 6–4 outlines the key substantive areas of exploration.

Substance abuse interferes with an adolescent's development. It interferes with reality testing and learning how to make sound decisions. It can exaggerate the egocentric world view of adolescents and, based on the psychoactive properties of the substances used, make the teenager alternate between sensations of grandeur and loss of control. Adolescents who abuse substances lose opportunities for growth by failing to address their academic, environmental, and vocational responsibilities, and they are not able to define work and play roles. They may isolate themselves in a subgroup that is internally cohesive but negativistic and incongruent with wider societal, community, and familial goals. Although teenagers who abuse substances may feel liberated from societal constraints, they are actually more dependent on their families and society as they fail to make psychoemotional developmental progress.

Assessment of adolescent substance abuse can be difficult for the following reasons:

1. Compared with adults, adolescents have a relatively short history of substance use and have not always experienced many negative consequences from it.
2. There is normative acceptance of excessive levels of alcohol and drug use among groups of substance-abusing young people, so that an adolescent who consumes similar quantities will not consider the behavior abnormal or deviant.
3. The psychological, familial, and social dysfunction that frequently accompanies a substance abuse problem may have existed previously or may have been exacerbated by it.
4. Most adolescents' cognitive skills are not yet fully developed. Self-definition and effective problem-solving skills may be limited by the adolescent's cognitive immaturity.

Table 6–4. Substantive areas of psychosocial assessment.

- Home and family relationships (constellation, shared activities, respect for parents, organization of family's daily life, isolation, conflict, breaking of family rules, running away)
- Family history (use by parents, sibs, and relatives)
- School (performance and classroom placement, attendance, behavior, ability to concentrate and remember, involvement in sports and extracurricular activities)
- Peers (developmental appropriateness, shared activities, fighting, substance use, involvement in gang activities and gang membership, legal involvement, motor vehicle accidents and traffic citations)
- Sexual behavior (romantic involvement, use by boyfriend/girlfriend, risk for pregnancy/fatherhood and sexually transmitted infections, number of partners, prostitution, trading sex for drugs)
- Leisure activities (fun, relaxation, preferred music and video genres, community organizations and service)
- Employment (position, schedule, disposition of earnings)
- Role of religion (religiosity of parents and of adolescent, any unique beliefs associated with their religion's tenets, involvement with youth group activities)
- Physical health (general health and somatic concerns, symptoms of withdrawal, toxic reactions to specific drugs and to alcohol, overdoses, blackouts, history of trauma and injuries, bulimic binging and purging)
- History of victimization by abuse (physical, sexual)
- Motor vehicle history (driving record, accidents and near misses, traffic citations)
- Access to weapons (family, peers, firearm ownership)
- Police and court involvement (probation status, history of illegal activities, incarceration, pattern of charges and offenses)
- Mental health (depression and moods, alienation, anxiety, hallucinations, suicidal ideation and attempts, anger, impulsivity, history of intervention and hospitalization)
- Aspirations and goals for the future (hopes and plans for beyond high school)
- Self-perception (self-liking and satisfaction with current life)

SUBSTANCE USE HISTORY

Order of Interview Process

The interviewer should discuss more general lifestyle questions before inquiring about use of substances. There are two important reasons for this sequence. The first is that the teenager needs time to develop or renew a relationship with the physician before being asked to discuss a sensitive subject. The second reason is that the physician will be able to use general psychosocial information as a database to help determine how much at risk an adolescent may be for substance abuse. This information will help to determine how deeply the physician must probe in this section of the interview.

One strategy that can provide order to the interview process and improve the quality of information gathered is to start with the least socially frowned-on substances and then move on to more sensitive substances. Questions about use of tobacco are considered a mildly sensitive area, because use of such products, including cigarettes and smokeless tobacco, is so common among adolescents in the United States. In fact, tobacco sales to minors is illegal. (Individual states are starting to legislate more restrictive statutes aimed at limiting minors' use of tobacco, and the FDA has stated an intent to regulate the access and appeal of tobacco products to minors.)

Alcohol is next on the continuum. Again, drinking by teenagers can almost be considered normative, but the sensitivity is somewhat intensified because purchase of alcoholic beverages by minors carries clear legal sanctions.

Inquiry about marijuana is the next step. Use of this substance may be considered more sensitive than use of alcohol, because marijuana is an illicit substance for adults as well as for minors. Furthermore, teenagers' parents are far less likely to use marijuana than to drink alcoholic beverages. This gulf increases adult social (and consequently societal) disapproval. Even though 31% of 1994's senior high school class in the United States used marijuana during the preceding 12 months, this figure represents only 42% of the proportion of high school seniors who had used alcohol during the same period. This relatively lower percentage of use is consistent with decreased social acceptability and contributes to its greater sensitivity as a topic of discussion.

Finally, the interviewer should ask about the use of other illicit drugs, reviewing major techniques of use (eg, pills, smoking, sniffing or huffing, snorting, injecting), as well as classes of drugs.

In summation, this organization of the interview provides a natural order of progression, moving from the socially accepted to the socially tolerated to the socially disapproved to the overtly illegal.

Initial Exploration

People who abuse substances tend to minimize their involvement with them. On the other hand, substance abusers will provide a valid history if they trust and respect the interviewer. In particular, most teenagers whose lifestyles do not revolve around substance use provide sufficient information about their use of alcohol and drugs to allow the physician to complete an accurate evaluation. It is critical, however, for the physician to establish an appropriate atmosphere for the interview and to convey an impression of trustworthiness and sincerity.

The purpose of initial exploratory inquiries is to help establish the tone of this section of the interview. During this process, the medical clinician may be tested by the adolescent patient. If the interviewer appears to register disapproval, dismay, or condescension in reaction to initial disclosure statements, it is doubtful that the adolescent will provide accurate information about substance use. The physician will have failed the teenager's test and will not be deemed trustworthy or credible. In addition, the interviewer can measure the adolescent's willingness to offer information during this exploratory phase.

Exploratory issues are phenomenologic—they address the adolescent's perceptions of how widely drugs and alcohol are used by other teenagers. Specifically, the physician can inquire about whether many students at the teenager's school are "into drinking or doing drugs." If someone wanted to buy marijuana, crack, or uppers, how easy would it be? What happens at parties and social occasions that the

teenager has heard about? Or at parties the teenager has personally attended? This approach is less threatening because it does not ask for information about personal involvement.

Elements of a Formal Substance Use History

The goal of this set of questions is to determine the quality and depth of the relationship that the adolescent has with substances. Minimal time is needed to discuss these issues with a teenage patient who is functioning well and who admits to little or no use of alcohol and drugs. These questions are very useful, however, when the physician needs to explore an adolescent's use of substances more intensively. Table 6–5 summarizes the elements of a substance use history.

When asking an adolescent to discuss personal use of alcohol and drugs, it is less threatening to establish a historical perspective. Before addressing current use patterns, find out about the teenager's first experiences with alcohol and with marijuana. "Tell me about the first time you ever had anything to drink. What was it like?" "When was the first time that you ever got really high?" With these questions, the interviewer is trying both to help the teenager disclose accurate information and to determine whether the adolescent is preoccupied with the experience of getting high. Although one cannot ask specific questions that directly address the latter goal, one can frequently document this preoccupation through the adolescent's enthusiastic descriptions of what it feels like to be "high."

The interviewer should gradually move the questions forward to the present time. "About how much are you drinking now compared to last fall when school started?" In identifying patterns of use, the physician will need to learn how frequently the adolescent uses particular substances and how much is consumed at a time. "How many times did you get high in the last month?" Forced multiple choice an-

---

Table 6–5. Elements of a substance use history.

- First use: age, circumstances, feeling effects
- Past substance use patterns
- Current motivation to use (perceived benefits of use)
- Current feeling effects of use (include both pleasant and negative experiences)
- Current patterns of use (substances used, frequency, binging behavior, circumstances of use)
- Current frequency of intoxication or becoming "high"
- Tolerance (How much alcohol does it take to get high now? What about 6 months ago? A year ago?)
- Substance of choice
- Personal limits to categories of substances willing to try
- How substance obtained
- Financial resources
- Dealing activities
- Perceptions of significant others about use (family members, peers, boyfriend or girlfriend)

swers are a useful strategy for adolescents who find it difficult to answer spontaneously. For example, one could provide the choices: "About once every month, Saturday nights only, or three times a week?" When was the last time the teenager got high? Is the adolescent using drugs or alcohol on school nights or only on weekends?

It may be less threatening to determine approximate quantities of substances consumed by using the concept of tolerance rather than asking for this information directly. Increasing tolerance for specific agents is associated with increasing use. Tolerance can be addressed historically by determining how much it takes to get a little high and how much to get really high. Have the teenager compare these amounts with what was necessary to get high 6 months ago and 1 year ago.

The physician should learn about the circumstances of use. Does the teenager use substances only during parties or also when alone? Has the teenager ever used at school? What does the adolescent gain from the experience of becoming high? Examples of possible questions that can explore this experience follow. "What is it like to be high?" "Has anything really good ever happened while you've been high?" "What does getting high do for you?" The appetitive effects of substances serve as an important motivator to continue use once a person experiences pleasurable sensations.

Another important area concerns the benefits that substance use may offer the teenager. Does intoxication relieve negative pressures and enhance the ability to relax? Teenagers who have learned to use substances for anxiety relief are at special risk for developing more serious problems. In addition, they have not been able to learn healthy mechanisms for coping with stress or for addressing troublesome issues. A possible exploratory question is, "How do you make yourself feel better when you're really upset or nervous about something?"

The concept outlined above—that adolescents who use substances perceive benefits from their use—has been elaborated into a brief screening instrument. The five items that compose the empirically validated scale can be incorporated into the clinical interview by asking the teenager how much drugs and alcohol help make it easier to relax, be friendly, be with friends who drink or do drugs, forget problems, and feel good about oneself. When used in this manner, these questions are meant to enrich clinical information and to help youngsters gain insight into their relationships with substances.

Learning how a teenager obtains drugs and alcohol may not be possible unless a trusting relationship has developed. To obtain supplies, youngsters who have become substance-dependent frequently resort to deviant and illegal behaviors, such as stealing, dealing, and prostitution. An adolescent engaging in such activities obviously has a very serious problem. (How-

ever, some adolescent dealers may not use substances in order to retain a sharp business acumen.) There is an excellent chance that such an adolescent will exhibit dysfunctional behavior in other areas. Even though an adolescent may vociferously deny stealing from parents, it may be this very behavior that finally forces parents to seek help. Some exploratory questions include, "How much do you spend a week on drugs?" (Try to be as specific as possible, naming drugs that you know the adolescent favors.) "Have you ever needed to borrow money or take something that didn't belong to you so you could get a supply?" "Have you ever traded sex for drugs?" "Have you ever gotten into trouble with the law trying to get drugs?" "How much do you deal?"

It is frequently enlightening to learn who is concerned about an adolescent's use of alcohol and drugs. The concerns of family members, friends, and romantic partners who worry that an adolescent may be using alcohol or drugs excessively are usually accurate. The physician should be aware, however, that heightened media publicity about drug use may overly sensitize cautious parents about an adolescent's experimentation. A teenager who abuses substances may be able to admit that a parent is anxious about the use even while minimizing or belittling the concern. It is unusual, however, for a substance-abusing adolescent to admit spontaneously that the involvement is dysfunctional even when use has caused significant problems.

Dysfunctional Consequences

Even though adolescents who are abusing alcohol and drugs may not recognize dysfunctional consequences associated with the abuse, medical clinicians can play an important role by pointing out to both the family and the adolescent that use has caused problems. The impact of associating a negative consequence with use of substances is more powerful if it occurs close to the time that the consequence occurred. For example, during recovery from the ill effects of an overdose or acute intoxication, the adolescent and family may be more receptive to intervention. The need for an emergency room visit or hospitalization for substance associated trauma, behavioral aberration, or mental status impairment is a medical consequence that a physician should target. Such episodes can be helpful in convincing a family that a substance abuse problem exists; that is, when people are frightened, they feel vulnerable and perhaps more open to offers of help. For example, most adolescents admitted to inpatient substance abuse treatment programs are in crisis. However, the parents have usually been aware of the substance abuse for 1–2 years.

In summation, substance-abusing teenagers and their families may be more receptive to help during times of acute crisis than they are at other times. The unfortunate corollary is that they may not seek help until a crisis erupts.

The physician should seek other common consequences associated with the use of substances by focused interview questions. Table 6–6 outlines areas that should be explored.

SYNTHESIZING INTERVIEW INFORMATION

The accuracy of an adolescent's substance use history should be judged by indirect measures. The physician can compare the adolescent's individual history of use of substances with empirical information that supports the "stage theory." It has been demonstrated that most adolescents follow a specific sequence of substance use. They rarely begin with an illicit drug—the usual sequence is beer or wine, tobacco or hard liquor, and marijuana. Escalation of alcohol intake may occur following initiation of marijuana use. The use of these substances precedes involvement with other illicit drugs, such as cocaine. For example, if there is evidence that a youngster has used amphetamines but denies having used anything else, this information is not consistent with empirically described patterns. Even though a youngster may have a substance of choice, other drugs previously used on a regular basis are not usually abandoned. More likely is an addition, not a substitution. However, adolescents may avoid categories of substances that have caused unpleasant or frightening effects in prior experience.

Dimensions of adolescent substance use can also be categorized by a transitional framework. The first stage, *initiation,* represents experimental use, or the transition from a nonuser to a user. The second stage is *continuation* of a certain class of substances; this stage may represent substance abuse. *Maintenance and progression within a class of substances* is usu-

ally dependent on the practices of an adolescent's peer group. However, individual adolescents may start using more concentrated forms of a substance, such as drinking distilled liquor rather than beer, injecting cocaine rather than snorting. The fourth stage of the continuation is *progression across drug classes.* It represents polysubstance abuse and dependence. Adolescents may also have *regression, cessation, and relapse cycles.*

The physician can determine the severity of an adolescent's substance abuse by determining what stage the pattern of use represents, and by placing this information into the context of the adolescent's general psychosocial functioning.

Dusenbury L, Khuri E, Millman RB: Adolescent substance abuse: A sociodevelopmental perspective. In: *Substance Abuse: A Comprehensive Textbook,* 2nd ed. Lowinson JH et al (editors). Williams & Wilkins, 1992.

Kandel D, Yamaguchi K: From beer to crack: Developmental patterns of drug involvement. Am J Public Health 1993;83:851.

CONFIDENTIALITY

Confidentiality of patient care is a maxim of adolescent medicine. In general, medical clinicians honor the confidentiality of adolescent patients unless there is concern that the adolescent is engaging in life-jeopardizing or serious health-compromising behavior. Substance abuse is clearly a health-compromising behavior. Most physicians would agree that parents need to be included in the process if an adolescent is experiencing serious behavioral dysfunction from substance use or if referral to a treatment program is necessary. However, state laws vary regarding the need for parental consent for treatment. Statutes in 46 states permit minors to consent to treatment of drug and alcohol abuse, but 28 states have placed various limitations on minors' ability to consent, which include age restrictions and mandated physician notification of parents. In practice, the problem of reimbursement for treatment services usually necessitates parental involvement.

Substance misuse may represent a different circumstance. For example, a physician may be faced with the realization that an adolescent drives while intoxicated or accepts automobile rides from an intoxicated driver. The parents do not seem aware of these practices. Except for this risky behavior, the teenager appears to be functioning well. How can the physician intervene effectively? Should the parents be warned? In this situation, the clinician may well decide that directly informing the parents would be counterproductive. An alternative approach is to involve the parents and the adolescent in a discussion of prevention of unsafe driving practices and "passengership." Have the family unit decide how it

Table 6–6. Exploration for consequences of substance use.[1]

Medical and physical
  Somatic symptoms
  Blackouts
  Trauma and unintentional injury
  Visits to emergency facility for intoxication or overdose
Social
  Motor vehicle accidents and near misses
  Conflict with family
  Loss of friends
  Loss of romantic relationship
  Fighting
  Impulsive sexual behavior
  Destruction of property
  Theft
  School failure
  Disciplinary action (DUI, other legal involvement, school suspension, dropped from sports team)

[1]Note that these common examples are embedded in the psychosocial history.

would handle a request from an intoxicated adolescent for help getting home. The physician can help parents and teenagers prepare to deal with risky situations that are frequently part of the maturational process in this society.

English A: Legal aspects of care. In: *Textbook of Adolescent Medicine.* McAnarney ER et al (editors). WB Saunders, 1992.

Gans, JE (editor): *Confidential Health Services for Adolescents.* American Medical Association, 1993.

CLINICAL SCREENING INSTRUMENTS

Physicians who lack the time to conduct more comprehensive interviews of adolescents may use formal clinical screening instruments, which include both interview and written questionnaire formats and provide a highly structured and time-efficient approach to screening. More detailed instruments can also yield severity scores. In contrast, the detailed clinical interview, as outlined in earlier sections, is descriptive, open-ended, and interactive. If conducted skillfully, it can also offer a contextual richness that is missing from more structured approaches. In clinical settings, a written questionnaire cannot be administered in the absence of interaction between the patient and the clinician. In addition, it is helpful if the instrument also considers general psychosocial functioning. Both interview and questionnaire approaches to the process of assessment can help the physician achieve the following goals: to describe the teenager's presenting problems clearly; to identify the pattern of behavioral, psychologic and physiologic conditions associated with substance use; and to determine whether referral to an appropriate facility for further evaluation and intervention is indicated.

Kaminer Y, Bukstein O, Tarter RE: The teen-addiction severity index: Rationale and reliability. Int J Addict 1991;26:219.

Rahdert ER (editor): *The Adolescent Assessment/Referral System Manual.* US Department of Health and Human Services, Alcohol, Drug Abuse and Mental Health Administration, National Institute on Drug Abuse, DHHS Publication # (ADM) 91-1735, 1991.

Riggs SG, Alario AJ: Adolescent substance use. Instructor's Guide. In: *The Project ADEPT Curriculum for Primary Care Physician Training,* Dubé CE et al (editors). Project ADEPT, Brown University, 1989.

Tarter RE: Evaluation and treatment of adolescent substance abuse: A decision tree method. Am J Drug Alcohol Abuse 1990;16:1.

Werner MJ, Hoover A: Early identification, screening, and brief intervention for adolescent alcohol use. Arch Pediatr Adolesc Med 1995;149:1241.

Winters KC: Development of an adolescent alcohol and other drug abuse screening scale: Personal experience screening questionnaire. Addictive Behav 1992;17:479.

PHYSICAL & PHYSIOLOGICAL SCREENING OF ADOLESCENTS WHO HAVE USED SUBSTANCES

Medical Assessment

Unless an adolescent is experiencing the effects of an overdose and seeks help from a free clinic or hospital emergency department, it is unusual to be able to diagnose substance abuse by physical examination findings. Individuals experiencing acute effects, overdoses, and withdrawal from alcohol and specific classes of drugs will demonstrate recognized constellations of physical and mental status findings. (The acute medical presentations of specific substances of abuse are summarized in Chapter 12.) Table 6–7 lists chronic or recurrent physical symptoms and mental health problems that may cause an adolescent substance user to seek medical care or that may be disclosed during a review of systems. Certain chronic symptoms are clearly linked to specific classes of substances, but others are more general and may be caused by more than one type of substance.

Some symptoms represent the acute effects of use (eg, cocaine and amphetamines cause tachycardia), and some represent complications of use. For example, cocaine can cause cardiac arrhythmias, which

Table 6–7. Recurrent physical symptoms and mental health problems that may be related to substance use.

General	Neurologic
Fatigue	Headaches
Poor appetite	Blackouts (amnesia)
Weight loss	Lightheadedness and vertigo
Malnutrition	Syncope
Fever	Ataxia
Insomnia	Peripheral neuropathy
Increased sleeping	Seizures
Nightmares	Head injury
	Cognitive dysfunction
Respiratory	
Pharyngitis	**Hormonal and reproductive**
Cough	Abnormal menstrual cycles
Laryngitis	Male sexual dysfunction
Bronchitis	Male gynecomastia
Wheezing	
	Skin
Mucous membranes and nose	Skin infections
	Scars from injection sites and
Conjunctival irritation	trauma
Nasal congestion	
Nosebleeds	**Psychiatric**
Sinusitis	Depression and suicidality
	Mania
Cardiac	Irritability
Tachycardia	Violent outbursts
Palpitations	Anxiety
Chest pain	Panic attacks
Hypertension	Hallucinations
	Psychosis
Gastrointestinal	Depersonalization and
Abdominal pain	derealization
Vomiting	Eating disorders
Constipation	Personality disorders

can be experienced as palpitations, as well as constriction of blood vessels supplying the heart, which can cause chest pain. Chronic use of toluene can cause cerebellar ataxia and chronic inhalation of aliphatic hydrocarbons can result in a small fiber peripheral neuropathy. Other symptoms, such as weight loss, fatigue and disordered sleep, may either be specific for certain classes of psychoactive substances, or represent more general indicators of substance abuse.

A medical evaluation, including a thorough physical and neurologic examination, is recommended as part of the assessment process for adolescent substance abusers. It has several goals. First, many teenagers who have used substances do not receive regular health care and deserve age-appropriate screening and immunizations. Second, although organ system damage is unusual among adolescent substance abusers, it can occur. Substance abusers with specific symptoms should be evaluated carefully to ensure that complications of substance use are not causing them. For example, youngsters with upper abdominal pain may have alcohol-related gastritis or pancreatitis. Finally, young people who abuse substances are at risk for multiple problems, largely because of their lifestyles. For example, they are at risk for sexually transmitted infections, pregnancy, and sexual assault. They also experience disproportionately high rates of nonintentional injury. Chronic users of certain classes of drugs may be at risk for malnutrition.

General inspection may disclose the odor of tobacco or marijuana smoke, alcohol, or hydrocarbons; inspection of the skin may reveal scars from track marks, resolved skin infections, or multiple episodes of trauma (eg, cigarette burns, ecchymoses, lacerations) and tobacco-stained fingers.

No laboratory markers exist that can identify adolescents who chronically abuse specific classes of substances; however, users of anabolic androgenic steroids may have an increased red blood cell mass. In contrast, adult alcoholics may demonstrate elevation of certain hepatic enzymes (γ-glutamyl transpeptidase [GGTP], serum glutamic-oxaloacetic transaminase [SGOT]), an increased mean volume of red blood cells (MCV), and changes in high-density lipoproteins. However, none of these physiologic changes is sensitive or specific enough to serve as a marker for alcoholism. No similar laboratory parameters have been identified in persons of any age who have used other categories of substances.

For these reasons, routine laboratory testing to search for standing physiologic changes is not recommended. Adolescent substance abusers may be nutritionally deficient, however, and should be screened for anemia, along with appropriate laboratory and imaging assessment of symptoms and abnormal physical findings. Adolescents who inject drugs should be screened for hepatitis B and C and

for HIV infection. They are also at risk for multiple medical complications such as cellulitis, osteomyelitis, thrombophlebitis, pneumonia, brain abscess, and chronic liver disease. Debilitated and homeless adolescents should be screened for tuberculosis. Finally, substance-abusing adolescents should be screened for problems such as sexually transmitted infections and hepatitis A, because their behavior enhances their risk.

Alling FA: Detoxification and treatment of acute sequelae. In: *Substance Abuse: A Comprehensive Textbook,* 2nd ed. Lowinson JH et al (editors). Williams & Wilkins, 1992.

Dackis CA, Gold MS: Psychiatric hospitals for treatment of dual diagnosis. In: *Substance Abuse: A Comprehensive Textbook,* 2nd ed. Lowinson JH et al (editors). Williams & Wilkins, 1992.

Novick DM: The medically ill substance abuser. In: *Substance Abuse: A Comprehensive Textbook,* 2nd ed. Lowinson JH et al (editors). Williams & Wilkins, 1992.

Pharmacologic Testing

Pharmacologic or drug screening of body fluids for substances of abuse is a technologically sophisticated but controversial procedure. Public and institutional policies that mandate involuntary, obligatory, and random urine testing for substances of abuse continue to be debated. However, this section discusses the pharmacologic testing of individual teenagers for clinical or diagnostic purposes. Drug testing can only differentiate between persons who have used a drug, and those who have not. Drug tests cannot provide information about the abuse of or dependence on drugs or about any related physical or mental impairment. In contrast, blood alcohol levels are correlated with degrees of neurologic impairment. Furthermore, because most substances and their metabolic products have relatively short half-lives, the time window following exposure during which they can be detected is limited. Therefore, a negative test cannot guarantee that the adolescent does not use substances. Retention times, or ability to detect the substance after last use, vary by class of substance and range from 2–14 hours (alcohol) to 2–4 days (cocaine metabolites—acute use), to 2–8 days (occasional use of marijuana), to 14–42 days (chronic use of marijuana).

There are several clinical circumstances that necessitate drug screening in adolescents: psychiatric symptoms and acute-onset behavior states, coma and less severe mental status changes, seizures, arrhythmias and chest pain, and recurrent and unexplained nonintentional trauma (eg, motor vehicle accidents and falls). Patients with recurrent respiratory symptoms and unexplained somatic symptoms may also merit drug testing. Many physicians would obtain drug tests on adolescents in legal-social crises such as running away and engaging in delinquent behaviors. Teenagers with these problems are considered to be at high risk for substance abuse. Finally, based on historical circumstance, many adolescents who sustain trauma serious enough to warrant care by a hospital emergency department should undergo pharmacologic testing for alcohol and drugs as part of their visit. Even trauma patients whose blood alcohol concentrations are nil may be at risk for psychoactive substance abuse disorders.

Pharmacologic testing for drugs is not recommended as part of routine adolescent health care. Screening by interview has been found to be more sensitive than testing body fluids, because it also explores the possibility of use in the past. Even though some substance-using adolescents will not accurately describe their usage patterns at a first interview, obtaining drug tests on youngsters who show no acute behavioral problems or physical symptoms is usually counterproductive. Merely confronting substance abusers with objective evidence of their use (eg, positive drug tests) appears to have little impact on behavior and offers little chance in a medical setting to motivate them to stop using. Pharmacologic testing should be incorporated into a comprehensive plan of assessment rather than being conducted independently.

If an anxious parent or institutional authority requests a drug screen on an asymptomatic adolescent, the information outlined above should be conveyed. The physician should determine what consequences would occur if the results of the drug screen were positive and if they were negative. The intent is often to document use of illicit substances in order to take disciplinary action.

A 1989 statement from the American Academy of Pediatrics reminds us that physicians' roles in this area should be counseling and treatment, not police work. Therefore, physicians in clinical practice should not perform drug testing for the primary purpose of detecting illegal use. The physician must present and discuss the screening request with the adolescent and explain the reasons for the request. Assuming that the adolescent is mentally competent, informed consent should be obtained. Parental permission for testing is not sufficient for involuntary screening of a mentally competent teenager. It can be predicted that if the adolescent agrees to drug testing, the results will be negative. Refusing to submit to testing may well arouse suspicion of recent substance use. However, the physician will be more likely to retain the trust of the adolescent for future encounters with the health care system.

If the decision is made to proceed with drug testing, the physician must be cognizant of the four stages of screening. Errors at any stage can lead to inappropriate management and may have legal ramifications. The first stage, preparation of the "donor" (the adolescent), and the fourth stage, clinical application of the laboratory results, have been discussed previously. The remainder of this discussion focuses on the technical aspects of drug screening.

Urine screening provides the best way of identifying illicit substances in the body. Special attention must be paid to collection of the urine specimen, especially if the results may have punitive or disciplinary consequences or affect employability or eligibility for participation in sports programs. In general, the specimen should be obtained under direct observation and under circumstances that minimize opportunity for tampering (eg, no sink in the room, minimal clothing and personal belongings allowed in the room, noting urine color and temperature, using a colored disinfectant in the toilet bowl water, and labeling and holding the urine specimen in a secure refrigerator). Measurement of urine pH, specific gravity, and creatinine are also helpful in detecting adulteration.

The third stage of urine screening is the laboratory analysis. Drug testing must be conducted by an accredited laboratory, which will perform two types of tests: screening and confirmatory. Screening tests are highly sensitive and are usually efficient and relatively inexpensive. Confirmatory tests on specimens that screen positive are more specific, complex, labor-intensive, and expensive. Two independent test methods are often used to confirm positive screens. Several techniques are available for use by modern laboratories to analyze specimens for various compounds. To screen for all classes of substances of abuse, laboratories may need to use more than one method. Current techniques include enzyme immunoassay (EIA), such as the enzyme-multiplied immunoassay test (EMIT), radioimmunoassay (RIA), and fluorescent polarization immunoassay (FPIA), thin-layer chromatography (TLC) (sensitivity can be enhanced by use of high-power thin-layer chromatography [HPTLC]), and gas-liquid chromatography (equipped with a nitrogen-phosphorous detector).

Enzyme immunoassay is frequently used to screen for a panel of drugs; it is relatively inexpensive, does not require extraction of drugs from body fluids, is sufficiently sensitive, and is adaptable for high-volume automated screening. However, a variety of licit medications can produce false positive results through antibody cross-reactions. Some laboratories use thin-layer chromatography for routine drug screening because it is inexpensive. However, it may not be sufficiently sensitive to detect such common drugs as marijuana, PCP (phencyclidine hydrochloride), and LSD and may not detect low levels of cocaine, barbiturates, and opioids. Gas chromatography and mass spectrometry are used as a combined technique to confirm positive screening results. This technique is highly sensitive and specific and is the only test admissible as evidence of substance use in most courts of law. Routine testing methods cannot usually detect solvents and other abused inhalants. Radioimmunoassay is usually used as the preliminary screen for anabolic androgenic steroids, which are not included in routine laboratory panels. Chemical analyses of sweat patches and hair can detect drug use over a long time period and may prove useful for drug use surveillance in treatment programs and as part of court-ordered supervision. However, the risk of false-positive results is high.

Schwartz RH: Testing for drugs of abuse: Controversies and techniques. Adolesc Med: State Art Rev 1993; 4:353.

Verebey K: Diagnostic laboratory: Screening for drug abuse. In: *Substance Abuse: A Comprehensive Textbook.* Lowinson JL et al (editors). Williams & Wilkins, 1992.

Woolf AD, Shannon MW: Clinical toxicology for the pediatrician. Pediatr Clin North Am 1995;42:317.

COUNSELING STRATEGIES FOR REFERRAL OF ADOLESCENTS WITH SUBSTANCE ABUSE PROBLEMS

Most medical clinicians will not—and probably should not—assume the responsibility for actual treatment of substance-abusing adolescents and their families. However, they can employ counseling strategies to ensure effective communication and referral. Many substance-abusing adolescents and even their families have not previously considered substance use to be a source of concern, even though it is objectively associated with dysfunctional consequences. These teenagers and their families may be less able to accept the recommendation that treatment would be helpful. Using the "stages of change" model, these individuals may be placed into the "precontemplative" stage, which describes the substance use pattern prior to any active consideration of change. The physician may need to modify the counseling goal for these youngsters and their families and may need to accept success in calling their attention to the substance abuse as a problem behavior, which may allow them to proceed to the "contemplation" stage. Although individuals in this stage are clearly considering addressing the substance abuse problem, they also experience motivational conflict and ambivalence and may need bolstering of their self-perceived efficacy.

The physician's goal for teenagers and their families who are at this second stage is to move them forward to the "determination" or "preparation" substage of contemplation, and finally to an "action stage," in which they make active attempts to change. A successful counseling outcome for these adolescents and their families would be acceptance of the screening evaluation and follow-through with the recommendation for full assessment and therapeutic intervention.

Counseling strategies that the physician can use to help teenagers and their families make the transition to a substance abuse treatment agency are summa-

rized in Table 6–8 and elaborated in the text that follows.

First, the physician should permit the adolescent to describe perceptions of the substance use and the problems it may be causing. Regardless of the adolescent's perceptions, the physician should then summarize the information gathered during the assessment. This approach shows respect for the adolescent and allows the physician to make adjustments in communication style so as to respond most effectively to the adolescent's concerns. In addition to preparing the adolescent and family for future steps, summarization ensures that the physician understands the historical information and can communicate the problem accurately. A descriptive summary provides a clear statement of the problem behaviors to the adolescent and family. It is helpful to outline dysfunctional behavior in the context of substance use. The following example illustrates this process:

> I know that many teenagers occasionally smoke marijuana. However, since this school year started, you have been using marijuana more frequently than you did last year, and a lot of things have happened that have aroused my concern. First, you haven't been feeling well—you are tired all the time, and have been coughing. Second, school isn't going well for you. You've already been suspended twice for fighting, you dropped out of the debating club and quit soccer, and your grades are down. Third, you were really shaken up last week by that traffic accident. And fourth, you have been feeling very sad, and other people see you as being angry all the time. I am very worried about you.

Following communication of concern, the next step is to provide clear information without moralizing or lecturing.

Table 6–8. Counseling strategies.

- Allow the adolescent to verbalize his or her understanding of the substance use.
- Summarize information disclosed as part of the interview and from any collateral sources, using a nonconfrontational style.
- Clarify the problem behaviors regarding the substance use.
- Provide clear information about dysfunctional consequences, including medical and psychosocial problems that have resulted from substance use; do not moralize.
- Communicate concern for the adolescent's well-being.
- Allow the adolescent and family to express their responses to your summary and synthesis of the problems.
- Clarify your role in the evaluation and intervention process.
- Provide concrete assistance to the adolescent and family to enhance the likelihood that successful completion of a referral to a treatment agency will occur.
  1. If necessary assume responsibility for acting as an intermediary between the adolescent and the parents.
  2. Assume responsibility for initiating the referral to a treatment agency.

When a person becomes really involved with drinking or doing drugs, without realizing it, or even wanting it to happen, the alcohol and drugs can take over a person's life. This is what I believe is happening to you.

At this point, the teenager may again need a chance to respond. Do not expect your assessment to be automatically accepted by either the teenager or the family even if the adolescent is experiencing serious dysfunction.

Clarify your role as you facilitate the referral process. Try not to allow the teenager and family to perceive the referral as rejection by you. Two techniques you can use to avoid this issue are commitment to continued appropriate involvement with the adolescent and personalization of the referral process:

> I believe that it would really help you to feel better if you and your family learned more about substance dependence and enrolled in a treatment program for teenagers who have problems with drugs and alcohol. I would like you to meet a friend of mine who knows a lot about teenagers, families, and the problems that drugs and alcohol can cause. I don't have the background to give you really expert help for this problem. I will continue to be here for you as your doctor, but you also need counseling help.

It may be necessary to provide concrete assistance in facilitating referral to a treatment agency. The physician should be familiar with community resources and the philosophies of treatment of various programs, the actual services they provide, and their fee schedules. Establish personal contact with program staff members. Teenagers and families often feel overwhelmed and powerless when they are confronted with serious problems. Your status as their physician will help provide the stimulus they need to complete the referral successfully. You may want the patient or family to telephone the counseling professional or treatment agency from your office. Ask the family to call you after their first appointment. Let them know that you will have the agency or counselor contact you if the adolescent misses the first appointment.

Werner MJ: Principles of brief intervention for adolescent alcohol, tobacco, and other drug use. Pediatr Clin North Am 1995;42:335.

TREATMENT SERVICES

Teenagers require professional treatment for substance use if they develop physical, social, or emotional problems. Broad treatment goals include the elimination of substance abuse and any accompanying undesirable behaviors and restoration of the teenager to a healthy functional status.

There are several categories of treatment programs for adolescents who abuse substances, but all are based on the "disease" model of substance dependency and incorporate the 12-step approach of Alcoholics Anonymous and Narcotics Anonymous. Virtually all treatment programs in the United States share the belief that treatment begins with cessation of use and requires stable maintenance of sobriety or abstinence, and they have the goal of a substance-free lifestyle. Individual programs have historically offered the same treatment package to all clients, regardless of the characteristics and needs of the adolescent. Client-treatment matching is a newer approach that grades treatment options to individual teenagers' problems and needs.

Outpatient counseling programs are most appropriate for motivated teenagers without other significant mental health problems and who have no withdrawal risk. More intensive outpatient programs (eg, day treatment) are also available for adolescents who require more structure. Inpatient substance abuse treatment programs represent the most intensive format for patients who require a 24-hour structured setting. They provide medical and nursing care, and detoxification services, as well as counseling, education, and family activities.

Dual diagnosis inpatient units are able to integrate and address the needs of teenagers who have both psychiatric or behavioral problems and substance abuse problems. Treatment may include the prescription of such psychotropic agents as antidepressants, lithium, and neuroleptics.

Adolescents who require inpatient treatment for substance abuse problems are also expected to attend outpatient after-care programs. A residential program may be necessary if the risk of relapse is high.

Evaluation studies have shown that substance abuse treatment does help promote abstinence and improve social behavior. However, a significant proportion of patients quit treatment and levels of use frequently reescalate within 1–2 years. Adolescent patients with mood disorders and who receive prescribed psychotropic medication are most likely to complete substance abuse treatment and patients with conduct disorders are most likely to quit treatment.

Bergmann PE, Smith MB, Hoffman NG: Adolescent treatment: Implications for assessment, practice guidelines, and outcome management. Pediatr Clin North Am 1995;42:453.

Blood L, Cornwall A: Pretreatment variables that predict completion of an adolescent substance abuse treatment program. J Nervous Ment Dis 1994;182:14.

Catalano RF, Hawkins JD, Wells EA, Miller J: Evaluation of the effectiveness of adolescent drug abuse treatment, assessment of risks for relapse, and promising approaches for relapse prevention. Int J Addict 1990–91; 25:1085.

TOBACCO

Prevalence of Use

Although the proportion of adolescents who smoke cigarettes had been gradually decreasing between 1974 and 1992, a more recent upswing has occurred among eighth, tenth and twelfth graders. Although Table 6–9 outlines current adolescent smoking rates, cigarette use frequently starts during late childhood (10 years or age or younger). This table demonstrates the high probability of experimental use progressing to daily use, which is associated with addiction to nicotine.

Over the past decade, adolescent use of smokeless tobacco has also aroused concern. In 1995, more than 30% of US high school seniors had used smokeless tobacco at least once, 12% had used it within the preceding 30 days, and more than 3.5% had done so on a daily basis. Regular use by younger students, although lower, is also concerning. In 1995, about 7% of eighth graders and 10% of tenth graders had used smokeless tobacco within the preceding 30 days. White male adolescents, especially those living in rural and small communities, appear to be at highest risk for using smokeless tobacco.

Despite the high prevalence of tobacco use among adolescents, only 25% of teenagers and young adults overall and 50% of current daily smokers report receiving topical counseling by a health care provider about cigarette smoking. Parallel figures for health counseling about smokeless tobacco are 12% overall and 48% for current daily users.

Nicotine Dependence

Regular use of tobacco is now defined as nicotine dependence. Although nicotine has harmful health effects in its own right, including the promotion of atherosclerosis, coronary artery disease, and cerebrovascular and peripheral vascular disease (probably because it stimulates sympathetic ganglia, releases catecholamines, and activates chemoreceptors in the aortic and carotid bodies), multiple other physiologically active toxic substances found in cured tobacco products and tobacco smoke are chiefly responsible for the development of local cancers, chronic lung disease, susceptibility to respiratory tract infection, and exacerbation of reactive airway disease.

Adolescents may be particularly susceptible to initiating and maintaining smoking. The long latency period to the development of cardiovascular disease and malignancy makes these problems appear unreal or hypothetical to adolescents, who have not yet developed the skills of formal operational thinking (see Chapters 5 and 7). Second, smoking does not cause significant mental or motor impairment, as do most other categories of substance use; on the contrary, nicotine may actually enhance cognitive and motor performance. Finally, adolescents (and children) may be more easily entrapped than adults by tobacco companies' advertising campaigns and marketing strategies.

Although nicotine may initially cause a mild euphoria, tolerance for this pleasurable sensation develops rapidly. Nicotine has been found to release dopamine in the reinforcement areas of the brain. However, it is postulated that negative reinforcement is largely responsible for nicotine dependence; that is, smokers need to use nicotine for relief of withdrawal symptoms. Ritual behaviors associated with smoking (eg, smoking following a meal) are considered secondary positive reinforcers.

Nicotine is readily absorbed through the skin and all mucosal surfaces. Given the large pulmonary surface for absorption and the ability to bypass the venous circulation, inhalation of nicotine through cigarette smoking is the most efficient way to raise nicotine blood levels. Inhalation is also the most addictive form of nicotine use. Physiologically, nicotine causes release of catecholamines, with a secondary increased heart rate, peripheral vasoconstriction, and a fine tremor. Individuals unused to nicotine may develop nausea and vomiting, lightheadedness, and vertigo. Nicotine also exerts the following nervous system effects: facilitation of attention and memory, speed and accuracy of motor function, appetite suppression, and self-reported relaxation of mood.

Nicotine withdrawal causes a specific syndrome that includes mood changes and physiologic symptoms and signs. Withdrawal symptoms can start abruptly within 2 hours after the last nicotine use, which may help to explain heavy smokers' compulsive need to smoke. (The approximate half-life of nicotine is 2 hours.) Adverse changes in mood and in cognitive and motor performance peak within 1–3

Table 6–9. Prevalence of cigarette smoking among adolescents in 1995.[1]

	8th Grade (%)	10th Grade (%)	12th Grade (%)
Lifetime	46	58	64
30-day	19	28	34
Daily	9	16	22
≥ ½ pack/day	3	8	12

[1]Information summarized from a press release. The University of Michigan, New and Information Services, The Monitoring the Future Study. December 11, 1995.

days of withdrawal and gradually subside over several days to several weeks. Persons who withdraw from nicotine also experience a decrease in heart rate, blood pressure, and measured levels of epinephrine, norepinephrine and cortisol, and increased peripheral blood flow. Common mood changes include irritability and anxiety. Individuals also experience restlessness, difficulty concentrating, and hunger, which can result in weight gain. They "crave" nicotine and have a strong urge to smoke. These symptoms of withdrawal quickly resolve with the resumption of nicotine intake.

Counseling Strategies to Help Adolescents Quit Smoking

One should not assume that all teenagers who smoke want to continue. More than 50% of adolescents who smoke regularly have attempted to quit. Unfortunately, less than 25% of adolescents who try to quit smoking without help manage to abstain for at least 6 months. Based on data from adults, we know that most smokers who are able to quit do so on their own, frequently using a "cold turkey" approach.

Although no data are available for adolescents, firm advice from a physician has been found to influence adult smokers to quit. Success rates increase when physicians formalize brief protocols for themselves and their office staff for use with every patient who smokes. Table 6–10 outlines specific steps to help adolescent patients quit smoking. The clinician should remember that individuals must be motivated to quit smoking, but motivation by itself is not sufficient. Learning how to use coping skills to prevent relapse is perhaps the most important element of successful smoking cessation. Positive feedback regarding even small successes is also helpful. Finally, to help prevent relapse, it is important for individuals who are trying to quit smoking to have a smoke-free environment.

Pharmacologic Treatment of Nicotine Dependence

Two types of nicotine replacement systems are available by prescription and are recommended to control symptoms of withdrawal in adults who smoke at least 20 cigarettes a day or who smoke their first cigarette within 30 minutes of waking and who express a clear motivation to quit. Although these agents have not been tested for safety or efficacy in adolescents and are FDA-approved only for adults, selected adolescent patients may benefit from such a prescription in combination with counseling. Almost 30% of adolescents believe that medication to make quitting easier would be useful in helping teenagers to stop smoking.

Nicotine polacrilex gum was introduced about 20 years ago. If used correctly (slow chewing followed by lodging or "parking" the gum in the vestibule of the oral cavity for mucosal absorption), this technique is able to produce low and slowly rising levels of nicotine for weaning. A new piece should be used every 1–2 hours while awake. Two dosage strengths are available, and the weaning process may take 2–3 months. Although controlled trials with adults have demonstrated enhanced cessation rates for smoking compared with placebo, clinical use is problematic. Many patients do not use the gum correctly, and many do not receive counseling to help prevent relapse.

Transdermal nicotine patches offer several advantages for persons interested in smoking cessation. The constant slow transdermal absorption of nicotine produces a steady state concentration that effectively relieves most withdrawal symptoms; the patches are easy to use, which enhances patient compliance; and side effects are minimal (local erythema and contact dermatitis; sleeping difficulties, which are relieved by using an intermittent patch). However, the dosing is inflexible, and a relatively long interval of 4–6 hours is necessary to reach plasma levels high enough to alleviate symptoms of nicotine withdrawal. The total duration of patch therapy is usually 6–8 weeks. In adults, controlled clinical trials yielded 6-month abstinence rates of 22–42%. Counseling, including both cognitive and behavioral strategies, remains essential in helping persons to stop smoking.

A variety of pharmacologic agents have been used in adults to help reduce craving and relieve the anxiety and depression commonly associated with nicotine withdrawal. They include clonidine, anxiolytics such as buspirone, and antidepressants such as fluoxetine. However, there is either inconsistent information or little published data regarding the efficacy of these agents in promoting smoking cessation. Anticholinergic drugs such as transcutaneous scopolamine have been reported to reduce nicotine craving and withdrawal symptoms. Lobeline, which has been available for many years without prescription, is a weak nicotine receptor agonist. However, there is no evidence for lobeline's efficacy in helping individuals to quit smoking.

Centers for Disease Control and Prevention: Health care provider advice on tobacco use to persons aged 10–22 years—United States, 1993. MMWR 1995;44:826.

Epps RP, Manley MW, Glynn TJ: Tobacco use among adolescents. Pediatr Clin North Am 1995;42:389.

Evans N et al: Influence of tobacco marketing and exposure to smokers on adolescent susceptibility to smoking. J Natl Cancer Inst 1995;87:1538.

Fiore MC et al: Tobacco dependence and the nicotine patch. JAMA 1992;268:2687.

Institute of Medicine: *Growing Up Tobacco Free. Preventing Nicotine Addiction in Children and Youths.* National Academy Press, 1994.

Jarvik ME, Schneider NG: Nicotine. In: *Substance Abuse: A Comprehensive Textbook,* 2nd ed. Lowinson JH et al (editors). Williams & Wilkins, 1992.

Miller NS, Cocores JA: Nicotine dependence: Diagnosis,

Table 6–10. Clinical steps to help adolescent patients quit smoking.

Ask all preadolescents and adolescent patients whether they or their friends smoke or use smokeless tobacco.
• How old were they when they first tried smoking?
• How old were they when they first started to smoke regularly?
• What made them start smoking?
• Why do they continue to smoke? (eg, stress and anxiety, friends smoke, bored, something to do)
• Where do they smoke? (at home, at school, at work, with friends)
• Where do they obtain their cigarettes? (Note that it is illegal for minors to purchase tobacco products, and, conversely, for vendors to sell tobacco products to minors.)
• How soon after waking do they have their first cigarette?
• How much do they enjoy smoking?
• Have they ever tried to quit? What happened?
• Do their parents or siblings smoke?
• What do their parents think about their smoking?
• Safety: Have they ever fallen asleep while smoking? Ever smoked in bed? Ever been burned?
• How interested are they in stopping smoking?
• What do they know about the health effects of tobacco use? Where did they learn this information? Have they learned about tobacco in school? Does their school provide a program that enhances teenagers' ability to handle uncomfortable social situations?

Advise all teenagers who smoke to stop. (Note that physicians should also advise parents who smoke to stop, regardless of their children's ages.)
• State your advice clearly but nonjudgmentally.
• Personalize your messages to quit, based on the adolescent's activities and developmental status.
    1. General messages for adolescents can include cosmetic reasons (bad breath, stained teeth and fingers, smelly clothes, burned clothes and furniture), cost (what they could do with money saved), lack of independence (being controlled by cigarettes), hampered sports performance through compromised respiratory function, sore throats, cough, and more frequent respiratory infections.
    2. It is easier to stop now than it will be when they are older. Most adults who smoke wish they had never started, and would like to stop smoking.
    3. Teenagers with reactive airway disease: more difficult to control.
    4. For adolescents starting oral contraceptive pills: increased risks for thromboembolic phenomena. (The actual risk in adolescents is low, and counseling shouldn't place adolescents in the position of choosing continuation of smoking over effective pregnancy prevention.)
    5. Pregnant teenagers: risk of an unhealthy newborn with low birth weight; increased rate of fetal death; as parents, smoking provides a poor role model; exposure to smoke can harm their children's health through respiratory infections.

Assist the patient in stopping.
• Establish a quit date. Negotiate with the adolescent for a date within the next 2–4 weeks. Acknowledge that no time is ideal.
• Provide self-help materials, and review them with the adolescent. (Materials are available from the National Cancer Institute and from local chapters of the American Heart Association, the March of Dimes, and the American Respiratory Diseases Association.)
• Establish a "No Smoking" contract with the patient. It should be developed together, and personalized. Its format can be written or oral, sealed with a handshake.
• Help the adolescent to solve problems in advance.
    1. Rehearse through role play how to respond to social situations where other adolescents may be smoking.
    2. How to handle irritability
    3. How to handle "cravings"
    4. How to handle hunger
    5. How to help satisfy need for oral activity
    6. How to help satisfy need for hand activity
• Encourage participation in activities incompatible with smoking (eg, athletic activities)
• Suggest having a friend or family member with whom to quit. (This suggestion to promote successful smoking cessation was the one made most frequently by adolescents.)
• If the parent is aware of the adolescent's smoking and the adolescent want the parent's encouragement, involve the parent. If the adolescent and parent have a conflict-ridden relationship, the adolescent may be alienated by a parent's comments or advice.
• For adolescents who don't want to stop smoking or who deny that they might have a problem with nicotine dependence:
    1. Try not to alienate them with a "hard sell." You want them to return as your patients.
    2 Consider an independent substance abuse program.
    3. Consider having them complete a motivational questionnaire that measures nicotine dependence. (Note that these materials were developed primarily for adults.)
        a. National Cancer Institute pamphlet "Why do you smoke?" (available from 800-4-CANCER)
        b. Fagerström Test for Nicotine Dependence (a six-item questionnaire with scores ranging from 0 to 10 that is included as part of the item entry for nicotine polacrilex in the *Physicians' Desk Reference*)

Arrange follow-up visits.
• Schedule a brief follow-up visit within 1–2 weeks following the quit date.
    1. Provide positive reinforcement if the adolescent was successful, and encouragement if the adolescent was not successful in stopping, or has relapsed.
    2. Determine circumstances of any relapse.
    3. Review strategies to help prevent future relapse.
    4. Discuss any patient concerns.
• With the patient's permission, call (or have a member of the office staff call) or write the adolescent within 1 week after the visit, reminding the patient of the quit date and reinforcing the decision to stop smoking.
• Schedule a second brief follow-up visit within 1 month.

chemistry, and pharmacologic treatments. Pediatr Rev 1993;14:275.

National Institutes of Health, National Cancer Institute: *Tobacco and the Clinician. Interventions for Medical and Dental Practice.* US Department of Health and Human Services (NIH Publication No. 94-3693), January, 1994.

US Department of Health and Human Services: *Preventing Tobacco Use among Young People: A Report of the Surgeon General.* US Government Printing Office, 1994.

ANABOLIC ANDROGENIC STEROIDS

Although professional athletes have used anabolic androgenic steroids for at least 4 decades to enhance performance, physical appearance and fighting ability, concern about adolescent use is more recent. Table 6–2 shows that in 1994, 2.4% of high school seniors had used anabolic steroids at least once, and 0.9% reported use within the previous month. Male students are at higher risk than female students (about 5% compared with 1–2% lifetime use). About 50% of male students who use anabolic steroids first tried them by the tenth grade. Adolescent students who use anabolic steroids are also likely to use tobacco products, alcohol, marijuana, and cocaine and to engage in other problem and high-risk behaviors. Clinicians should suspect use of anabolic steroids in adolescents who lift weights, are body builders, or who play sports that reward muscle mass and strength.

Several forms of synthetic anabolic androgenic steroids exist. Although formulations approved by the FDA are legitimately used to replace endogenous testosterone, to enhance serum complement factors in the treatment of hereditary angioneurotic edema, to treat anemias caused by deficient red blood cell production, and to treat endometriosis, fibrocystic breast disease, and advanced breast cancer in postmenopausal women, it is illegal to prescribe anabolic androgenic steroids for athletic or cosmetic purposes. Testosterone and its derivatives are Schedule III controlled substances. Most persons who use these compounds illicitly obtain them from smuggled foreign sources and from veterinary suppliers. Both parenteral and oral formulations are available. The latter have a shorter half-life but impose a greater risk of hepatotoxicity. Users tend to take anabolic androgenic steroids in cycles of 4–18 weeks interspersed with "drug holidays." The daily dose can range from 2 to 200 times the pharmacologic doses recommended for treatment of medical problems. Some users "stack," or use multiple compounds simultaneously. Increasing the size of the dose over time is called "pyramiding."

Medical Consequences of Use

Several medical consequences are recognized for high-dose use of anabolic androgenic steroids. However, few well-designed studies are available, so that much of our information comes from clinical series and case reports. Athletes who use anabolic steroids believe that these agents promote muscle growth and enhance muscle capacity, increase strength and endurance, and quicken recovery from exercise, which together permit athletes to engage in more frequent workouts and to exercise at a higher intensity. Although these peripheral effects on muscle function are theoretically possible, it has been difficult to distinguish them from anabolic steroids' effects on the central nervous system, which may drive individuals' motivation for heightened performance, so that observed physical changes are secondary. Small measured changes in muscle function may confer a competitive advantage. It has been observed clinically, however, that individuals who use anabolic steroids do increase their lean body mass and improve their strength if they engage in high-intensity resistance training and maintain an adequate protein intake.

Other medical effects of high-dose anabolic androgenic steroids are less desirable. High doses induce hypogonadotropic hypogonadism, which for males results in a significant decrease in testicular volume and oligospermia. Although probably reversible, these effects can persist for long periods. High circulating levels of testosterone in younger adolescents who have not yet completed longitudinal growth can promote early epiphyseal closure with consequent foreshortened stature and premature virilization. Adolescent males may develop gynecomastia as a feminizing side effect, which results from the peripheral conversion of testosterone to estrogen. They can also have too frequent or persistent penile erections. Virilizing effects in females are largely irreversible and include hirsutism, male pattern baldness, coarsening of the voice, and clitoral enlargement. Females also develop menstrual irregularity. Both males and females can develop significant seborrhea and acne.

Users of anabolic androgenic steroids frequently develop hepatic dysfunction. Oral agents produce cholestasis, and users may develop cholestatic jaundice. Serum levels of liver enzymes can also rise, but this phenomenon is probably transient. Individuals using androgens for long-term legitimate medical treatment appear to be at risk for peliosis hepatis (blood-filled cysts in the liver) and for hepatocellular carcinoma.

Persons who use anabolic steroids may also be at risk for cardiovascular disease. The HDL:LDL cholesterol ratio is reversed, which may accelerate atherosclerosis. They may also be at risk for thromboembolic phenomena, partly because of increased red cell mass, potentiated platelet aggregation, and high estrogen levels. Sodium retention may cause edema and heightened blood pressure. It is also possible that use of anabolic steroids enhances the risk for cardiomyopathy, tendon rupture, and prostatic hypertrophy.

Anabolic steroids have important psychoactive effects. They can provide a sensation of euphoria and increased libido. Individuals who use anabolic steroids are also at risk for aggressive behaviors, including fighting and purposeful destruction of property. They are prone to impulsivity and impaired judgment, as well as feelings of irritation and hostility with urges to harm others. Although no single psychiatric syndrome has been linked with the use of anabolic androgenic steroids, some users have met criteria for bipolar disorder and others have exhibited paranoid thoughts and delusions, grandiose delusions, auditory hallucinations, and other psychotic features. Some users have experienced anxiety, panic attacks, depression, and suicidal ideation.

Users of anabolic steroids may meet psychiatric criteria for drug dependence. Over time, they take larger doses, complete more cycles of use, and are unable to stop use, even if they experience significant negative side effects or want to stop the practice. Those who stop use, either on a cyclical or a permanent basis, are highly likely to experience symptoms consistent with an abstinence syndrome, which include drug craving, dissatisfaction with body image, headaches, fatigue, depressed mood, restlessness and insomnia, anorexia, and decreased libido. It is during times of withdrawal that users of anabolic steroids appear most likely to use other illicit substances, perhaps in an attempt to ameliorate the symptoms of withdrawal.

Brower KJ: Anabolic steroids. Psychiatr Clin North Am 1993;16:97.

DuRant RH et al: Use of multiple drugs among adolescents who use anabolic steroids. N Engl J Med 1993;328:922.

Middleman AB et al: High-risk behaviors among high school students in Massachusetts who use anabolic steroids. Pediatrics 1995;96:268.

CLINICAL PREVENTION OF ADOLESCENT SUBSTANCE ABUSE

The major focus of this chapter has been the identification and counseling of substance-abusing adolescents. Because substance abuse has a complex, multifactorial etiology, primary prevention strategies must have multiple components and be provided at home and school, through the community, and in physicians' offices. The following discussion emphasizes what medical clinicians can accomplish as part of patient care activities. They may be able to provide effective health counseling regarding use of alcohol and drugs if they adapt the strategies of successful classroom-based primary prevention programs—social influence resistance training in conjunction with social competence skill development. This approach also reinforces information already taught at school. Teaching methods include discussion, behavior modeling and role play, practice sessions, and a public commitment not to use.

Medical clinicians should ask every adolescent about use of alcohol and drugs at every health supervision visit. Rather than just lecturing or distributing a written brochure, the physician should engage the adolescent in a relevant conversation; personalized interactions are more effective. For example, the physician can ask an adolescent going out for football, "What have you heard about steroids?" In this way, the adolescent's knowledge can be gauged and accurate cautionary information can be communicated as part of the conversation. The medical clinician can provide positive reinforcement for correct knowledge and a decision not to try steroids and, if necessary, can use the opportunity to attempt to modify an adolescent's favorable attitude toward steroid use.

Older adolescents with expectations of a positive outcome from substance use are more likely to use more heavily, but frequently decrease their substance use when their specific beliefs are challenged. Role play helps adolescents to practice decision-making and social skills and can easily be conducted by a physician. For example, the teenager can play the role of a peer encouraging acceptance of a cigarette, and the physician can demonstrate socially gracious and humorous refusal techniques.

Physicians have a second important role to play in the primary prevention of adolescent substance abuse. They can promote social attachment, which is a strong protective factor against substance abuse and other adolescent problem behaviors. For example, physicians can identify children who may be at risk for future substance abuse because of familial issues, and they direct the parents to programs that enhance parenting skills (consistent nurturance and discipline) and to substance abuse and mental health treatment. In addition, physicians can assist all families in setting standards of prosocial behavior and can help adolescents to develop meaning for and direction in their lives and to promote involvement in school and constructive community activities.

Anglin TM: Life skills training for adolescent health promotion. Adolesc Health Update, American Academy of Pediatrics 1993;5:1.

Bruvold WH: A meta-analysis of adolescent smoking prevention programs. Am J Public Health 1993;83:872.

Botvin GJ, Baker E, Dusenbury L, Botvin EM, Diaz T: Long-term follow-up results of a randomized drug abuse prevention trial in a white middle-class population. JAMA 1995;273:1106.

Hawkins JD, Catalano RF, Miller JY: Risk and protective factors for alcohol and other drug problems in adolescence and early adulthood: Implications for substance abuse prevention. Psychol Bull 1992;112:64.

Kumpfer KL, Hopkins R: Prevention. Current research and trends. Psychiatr Clin North Am 1993;16:11.

REFERENCES

Gullotta TP, Adams GR, Montemayor R (editors): *Substance Misuse in Adolescence.* Sage Publications, 1994.

Kaminer Y: *Adolescent Substance Abuse. A Comprehensive Guide to Theory and Practice.* Plenum Medical Book Company, 1994.

Lowinson JL et al (editors): *Substance Abuse: A Comprehensive Textbook,* 2nd ed. Williams & Wilkins, 1992.

Rogers PD, Werner MJ (editors): Substance Abuse. Pediatr Clin North Am 1995;42(2):241.

Psychosocial Aspects of Pediatrics & Psychiatric Disorders

7

R. Barkley Clark, MD

FAMILY LIFE

FAMILY FUNCTIONS

The structure of families has changed in recent years with the increase in the number of single-parent homes, reconstituted families, alternative lifestyles, and the decline in extended families. Despite these changes, the nuclear family continues to play a vital role in meeting the needs of society and of individual family members. The family serves the following functions: (1) the rearing of offspring to become autonomous adults, and eventually competent parents; and (2) meeting the needs of individual family members for nurturing, protection, feedback, recognition (mirroring), promoting adaptive behaviors, and emotional closeness and support. Evidence suggests that the lifestyle preferences of the parent figure(s) are less important to healthy development than is the ability of the parent(s) to perform parental functions consistently.

THE PARENTAL UNIT

The cornerstone of family functioning is the parental unit, which must serve as the source of leadership and power. The parental unit must meet the emotional and physical needs of other, more dependent family members while at the same time defining the norms of behavior that will lead to adaptive, independent functioning in the future. In short, the ways in which the parental unit exercises its leadership roles determine in large part the health or sickness of the family and its individual members.

Parenthood is emotionally and physically draining, and parents must have their own source of support to function as providers and setters of limits for the family. In the case of a two-parent unit, the partners provide the necessary emotional support, respite, and adult companionship for each other. The "women's movement" has helped men broaden their parental roles and personal identities to include more nurturing activities. Single parents often have no "in-house" source of adult support; in such cases, unfortunately, the child is at risk of becoming a pseudoadult companion to the single parent.

The lack of a solid partnership can be an important factor in virtually any child-centered problem. To function successfully as a parental unit, the couple must find the marriage mutually satisfying through mutual (1) nurturing and affirmation, (2) trust and respect, (3) conflict recognition and resolution, and (4) intimacy and sexual satisfaction.

When the parental unit is weakened by dissatisfaction or by persistent conflict, children are at risk of becoming the focus of parental conflict. In effect, the child becomes the focus of parental attention and concern, thus "detouring" the conflict within the marriage unit onto the child. The parental concern about the child distracts the parents from their own marital problems, and the child ends up functioning as a buffer between the parents. Questions designed to screen the quality of the marital and parental relationship are outlined in the section on screening for psychosocial problems and disorders.

Barker P: Healthy families and their development. In: *Basic Family Therapy.* Oxford Univ Press, 1992.

Martin A: *The Lesbian and Gay Parents' Handbook.* HarperCollins, 1993.

Miller DA: *Coping When a Parent Is Gay.* Rosen Publishing Group, 1993.

ISSUES IN PARENTHOOD

In rearing children, parents undertake a potentially rewarding but often tiring and frustrating task. The greatest pitfalls in parenting involve (1) physical and emotional exhaustion, and (2) unfulfilled expectations about having children. All of these can be provided in part by a partner who shares in the parenting responsibilities. Primary caregivers are also partly replenished emotionally by their child's responsiveness (in the form of smiles and excitement in the presence of the parent) and by memories of the care they received from their own parents. Children who are developmentally disabled or temperamentally difficult consume more parental energy and may not be as emotionally responsive and rewarding. The parent who had inadequate care as a child can call on fewer positive memories to help replenish energy stores.

Parental exhaustion decreases the parent's emotional and physical responsiveness toward the child and brings about a state of anger and frustration. A mild consequence may be a state of tension—a more extreme one, child abuse and neglect.

The second major pitfall in parenting comes from the disappointment of unfulfilled expectations. Parents want their children to be healthy, competent, and happy. They hope to meet the child's needs and, in doing so, feel a sense of accomplishment and fulfillment.

Parents may have unrealistic fantasies about their children that may serve to satisfy their own unmet needs for admiration and respect. Such fantasies may include basking in the glow of a child's exceptional achievements. Parents may fantasize that their children will thank them for all of their hard work in parenting and may even hope to be loved by their children in ways that will relieve the pain and loneliness of their own lives.

Parents who have children with illnesses, disabilities, or temperamental difficulties have to adjust their expectations so that they can realistically meet the child's special needs. That adjustment involves grieving over the loss of the child that was hoped for but did not materialize. For the individual whose hope was to compensate for personal unhappiness through parenthood, raising children can become an exercise in futility and a burden to the child unable to meet the parent's needs.

Each new phase of child development presents unique challenges. In infancy, irregular sleep-wake cycles and the necessity for constant care become physically exhausting, especially to a single parent. The physical demands are even greater if the child is not easily soothed.

During the toddler years, the child's striving for autonomy and independence can be misunderstood. To parents, the behavioral opposition and verbal "noes" of toddlers can seem like a rejection of parental caretaking. The resulting pain and anger may be expressed either in irritation with the child or in attempts to smooth the relationship by giving in to the child's demands. In the former case, the child's autonomous strivings are met with parental displeasure; in the latter, the child becomes a tyrant.

In the later preschool years, parents are faced with competitive challenges from their children. A sense of humor and perspective, combined with a solid marital relationship, allows parents to balance respect for the child's wishes to be "big" with the ability to set firm limits that maintain boundaries between the private lives of the parents (eg, the parents' bedroom) and their children.

During the elementary school years, parents must come to grips with allowing their children to experience the challenges that await them outside the home and family. Parental support of skill development must be balanced with realistic definitions of success. Persistent separation anxiety on the part of parents and unrealistic standards of performance can contribute to a child's anxiety during school years.

Adolescence presents new challenges to parents. The early adolescent has unpredictable changes of mood, intense attachment to peers, and a self-centered point of view, all of which deprive parents of the positive feedback they once enjoyed from the child who wanted to please the parents. Not since infancy and the toddler years have parents received so little gratitude for their efforts. And, as in toddler years, parents must remind themselves that what may seem to be a rebuff is in fact a further step along the child's road to independence. Like parents of toddlers, the parents of young adolescents need to support autonomy while preventing tyranny and disaster.

The sexual interests of the middle adolescent can elicit parental reactions related to parents' own concerns about sexuality, ranging from pride to fear to envy to sexual stimulation.

Finally, as the late adolescent prepares to leave home, parents face the sense of loss and grief associated with the launching of offspring into the world.

PSYCHOSOCIAL ASSESSMENT OF CHILDREN & FAMILIES

Five percent to 15% of children in the United States are affected by psychiatric disorders, and nearly 50% of pediatric office visits are related to psychosocial or developmental problems. These statistics underscore the importance of psychosocial problems in children and their families.

SCREENING FOR PSYCHOSOCIAL PROBLEMS & PSYCHIATRIC DISORDERS WITHIN THE CONTEXT OF HEALTH MAINTENANCE

The most efficient indicator in screening for psychosocial problems is the history provided by caregivers. Psychosocial information can be obtained from three sources: checklists, general questioning, and direct questioning.

The 35-item pediatric symptom checklist (Table 7–1) screens children 6–12 years of age for psychosocial dysfunction. The checklist is to be completed in the waiting room by a parent or other caregiver. Each item is rated by the parents as "often" (2 points), "sometimes" (1 point), or "never" present (0 points). The information can be used in two ways: first, as a psychosocial review of symptoms and point of departure for the discussion of problems that "often" or "sometimes" occur; and second, as a general screening device, with a total score of 28 or higher indicating a need for in-depth psychosocial evaluation of the child.

Five questions comprising the mnemonic device "PSYCH" can be addressed to parents as a means of uncovering areas of concern. These same questions can be slightly rephrased and then directed to children as well.

(1) *P*arent-child interaction: How are things going with you and your child?

(2) *S*chool: How are things going in school? (Academically and behaviorally.)

(3) *Y*outh: How are things with peer relationships?

(4) *C*asa: How are things going at home? (Including siblings, the marriage, and parents as individuals.)

(5) *H*appiness: Describe your child's mood? (Comfortable and happy, versus tense and unhappy.)

Directed questions regarding age-appropriate behavior norms can then be reviewed. Concerns about infant attachment, "the terrible twos," childhood fears, school problems, and adolescent behavioral problems can in this way be brought into the open for further discussion.

ASSESSMENT OF PSYCHOSOCIAL SIGNS & SYMPTOMS

When an emotional or behavioral sign or symptom is present, a thorough psychosocial evaluation is indicated. Data must be collected from caregivers, the child, and sometimes school personnel and others acquainted with the child's functioning. At least 30 minutes should be scheduled to cover the items listed in Table 7–2.

It is useful to see the parents and the patient first together, then the parents alone, and then the child alone. This sequence enables the physician to observe interactions among family members and give the parents and the child an opportunity to speak confidentially about their concerns. Parents and children often feel shame and guilt about some personal inadequacy they perceive to be causing the problem. The physician can ease that burden and facilitate the assessment by acknowledging that the family is trying to cope and that the ultimate task of assessment is to seek solutions and not to assign blame. An attitude of nonjudgmental inquiry can be captured in supportive statements such as "Let's see if we can figure out what might be happening."

History of the Presenting Problem

First, obtain a detailed description of the problem. When did it start? Were there unusual stresses at that time? How is the child's life and the family's functioning affected? What does the child say about the problem? What attempts have been made to alleviate the problem? Do the parties have any opinions about the cause of the problem? Questions to screen for other psychosocial problems, listed in Table 7–2, can be asked when additional information is sought.

Interviewing the Preschool Child

Preschool children are often distressed when separated from their parents, and they do not describe their problems in detail, so they are best interviewed with their parents. As the parents discuss their concerns, the physician can look for the following behaviors:

(1) Does the child use the parent as a source of security and support appropriately?

(2) Does the 2- to 5-year-old warm up to the strange environment and begin to explore the room and even interact with the physician from a distance?

(3) How does the child relate to toys that are offered?

(4) What is the child's activity level?

(5) Does the child display unusual mannerisms (eg, intense clinging, stereotypical motor behaviors)?

(6) Does the child disrupt or control the interview?

(7) Does the parent attempt to place appropriate limits on behavior? How does the child respond?

It is helpful to have toy figures available which the child can use to portray emotional states and interpersonal interactions. After hearing the history from the parents and after observing the child, the physician may question the 3- to 5-year-old about toy figures who appear to be feeling sad, worried, angry, or bossy. Children aged 3–5 are frequently able to confirm important interpersonal relationships and attitudes in their symbolic play activities.

Interviewing the School-Age Child

Most school-age children have mastered separation anxiety sufficiently to tolerate at least a brief interview with the physician. In addition, they have important information to share about their own worries.

The child should be told beforehand by the parents or physician (or both) that the doctor will wish to talk to the child about his or her feelings. School-age children understand and even appreciate parental concern about unhappiness, worries, and difficulty in getting along with people, and they are usually willing to discuss their perceptions of these problems.

At the outset, it is useful to restate that the interview is to explore the child's own opinions about certain issues raised by the parents. Rapport can be

Table 7–1. Pediatric symptom checklist.[1] Parents are asked to indicate which category—Never, Sometimes, or Often—best fits their child, with 0, 1, or 2 points assigned to each answer, respectively. For interpretation of scores, see text.

	Never	Sometimes	Often
1. Complains of aches or pains			
2. Spends more time alone			
3. Tires easily, little energy			
4. Fidgets, is unable to sit still			
5. Has trouble with a teacher			
6. Is less interested in school			
7. Acts as if driven by a motor			
8. Daydreams too much			
9. Is distracted easily			
10. Is afraid of new situations			
11. Feels sad, unhappy			
12. Is irritable, angry			
13. Feels hopeless			
14. Has trouble concentrating			
15. Has less interest in friends			
16. Fights with other children			
17. Is absent from school			
18. Experiences a drop in school grades			
19. Is down on himself or herself			
20. Visits doctor, with doctor finding nothing wrong			
21. Has trouble with sleeping			
22. Worries a lot			
23. Wants to be with you more than before			
24. Feels he or she is bad			
25. Takes unnecessary risks			
26. Gets hurt frequently			
27. Seems to be having less fun			
28. Acts younger than children the same age			
29. Does not listen to rules			
30. Does not show feelings			
31. Does not understand other people's feelings			
32. Teases others			
33. Blames others for his or her troubles			
34. Takes things that belong to others			
35. Refuses to share			

[1]Modified and reproduced, with permission, from Murphy JM, Jellinek M: Screening for psychosocial dysfunction in economically disadvantaged and minority children: Further validation of the pediatric symptom checklist. AM J Orthopsychiatry 1988;58:450. Copyright © 1988 by the American Orthopsychiatric Association.

Table 7–2. Screening for psychosocial problems.

Developmental history
1. Review the landmarks of psychosocial development
2. Summarize the child's temperamental traits
3. Review stressful life events and the child's reactions to them
   a. Separations
   b. Losses
   c. Marital conflict
   d. Illnesses, injuries, and hospitalizations
4. Obtain details of past mental health problems and their treatment

Family history
1. Marital history
   a. Overall satisfaction with the marriage
   b. Conflicts or disagreements within the relationship
   c. Quantity and quality of time together away from children
   d. Whether the child comes between or is a source of conflict between the parents
   e. Marital history prior to having children
2. Parenting history
   a. Feelings about parenthood
   b. Whether parents feel united in dealing with the child
   c. "Division of labor" in parenting
   d. Parental energy or stress level
   e. Sleeping arrangements
   f. Privacy
   g. Attitudes about discipline
   h. Interference with discipline from outside the family (eg, ex-spouses, grandparents)
3. Stresses on the family
   a. Problems with employment
   b. Financial problems
   c. Changes of residence
   d. Illness, injuries, and deaths
4. Family history of mental health problems
   a. Depression? Who?
   b. Suicide attempts? Who?
   c. Psychiatric hospitalizations? Who?
   d. "Nervous breakdowns"? Who?
   e. Substance abuse or problems? Who?
   f. Nervousness or anxiety? Who?

Observation of parents
1. Do they agree on the existence of the problem or concern?
2. Are they uncooperative or antagonistic about the evaluation?
3. Does the parent appear depressed or overwhelmed?
4. Can the parents present a coherent picture of the problem and their family life?
5. Do the parents accept some responsibility for the child's problems, or do they blame forces outside the family and beyond their control?
6. Do they appear burdened with guilt about the child's problem?

Observation of the child
1. Does the child acknowledge the existence of a problem or concern?
2. Does the child want help?
3. Is the child uncooperative or antagonistic about the assessment?
4. What is the child's predominant mood or attitude?
5. What does the child wish could be different (eg, "three wishes")?
6. Does the child display unusual behavior (activity level, mannerisms, fearfulness)?
7. What is the child's apparent cognitive level?

Observation of parent-child interaction
1. Do the parents show concern about the child's feelings?
2. Does the child control or disrupt the joint interview?
3. Does the child respond to parental limits and control?
4. Do the parents inappropriately answer questions addressed to the child?
5. Is there obvious tension between family members?

Data from other sources
1. Waiting room observations by office staff
2. School (teacher, nurse, social worker, counselor)
3. Department of social services

enhanced by asking if the child has ever talked with anyone before about how he or she feels. If the answer is "yes," the child may explain more about what he or she liked or did not like about that discussion. If the child has never before talked about personal feelings with a professional, the physician can acknowledge that it is often not easy to talk with "a stranger" about some kinds of problems.

The physician should then ascertain whether the child agrees a problem exists (eg, unhappiness, worry, "not getting along"). If that is so, the physician should ask what the child can say about the magnitude of the problem, how it affects the child and the family, and what seems to be the cause.

Asking directly about how mom and dad get along can yield significant information about parental conflicts. A kinetic family drawing—"Draw your family and have everyone doing and saying something"— can provide clues to how the child fits into the family and how members of the family interact. Questions

about school can yield information about life outside the home and with peers. Questions about worries, unhappy feelings, and what makes the child angry can develop unsuspected clues to the child's emotional life. Asking a child to make "three wishes" can help to uncover important concerns that may not have been apparent from the history ("Let's pretend you could have anything or change anything. What would you wish for and why?").

At the end of the child interview, it is important to share or reiterate the salient points derived from the interview and to state that the next step is to talk with the parents about ways to make things better for the child. At that time, it is good to discuss any concerns or misgivings that the child might have about sharing information with parents so that the child's right to privacy is not arbitrarily violated. Most children want to make things better and therefore will allow the physician to share appropriate concerns with the parents.

Interviewing the Adolescent

Because the developmental task of adolescence is to fashion an identity separate from that of the parents, the physician must show respect for the patient's point of view. That process begins with the patient's participating in the format for the evaluation—meeting first alone with the physician, together with the parents, or after the physician has talked further with the parents. The parents need to be told why this is necessary, and the patient is then informed of the parents' expressed concern and the physician's wish to help the family determine whether a problem does, in fact, exist.

The issue of confidentiality must be approached forthrightly at the first interview. A good policy is to say, "What we talk about today is between you and me unless we decide someone should know or unless it appears to me that you might be in some danger."

The interview might then start with a restatement of the parents' concern. The patient is then encouraged to describe the situation in his or her own words. The physician should then ask questions about:

(1) Predominant mood state.

(2) Nature of relationships with family members.

(3) Level of satisfaction with school and peer relationships.

(4) Plans for the future.

(5) Drug and alcohol use.

(6) Worries or concerns.

(7) Biggest "stumbling block" in the adolescent's life.

(8) What the adolescent would like to be different.

In closing the interview, it is important that the physician review the salient points and discuss a plan for either further investigation or ways of dealing with the problem.

Murphy JM et al: Screening for psychosocial dysfunction in pediatric practice. Clin Pediatr 1992;31:660.

DIAGNOSTIC FORMULATION & INTERPRETATION OF FINDINGS

Diagnosis starts with a description of the presenting problem, which is then scrutinized in the context of the child's age, developmental needs and tasks, temperament, the stresses and strains on the child and the family, and the functioning of the family system. The physician develops a diagnostic hypothesis, which is then considered in the following perspectives:

(1) The behavior as described is within the range of normal, given the child's developmental level.

(2) The behavior is a temperamental variation.

(3) The behavior is the result of nervous system dysfunction.

(4) The behavior is a normal reaction to stressful circumstances (eg, medical illness, change in family structure, loss of a loved one).

(5) The problem is primarily caused by family dysfunction.

(6) The problem is a manifestation of a psychiatric disorder.

(7) Some combination of the above.

The physician's interpretation of the findings is then presented to the family. The interpretive process includes the following components: (1) an explanation of how the presenting problem or symptom is a reflection of a hypothesized cause (eg, children frequently display a disturbance in conduct in the wake of stressful circumstances or become bossy or demanding when parent and child roles are not defined clearly enough); and (2) a suggested plan of interaction that is based on the hypothesized mechanism.

A joint plan—physician, parents, and child—is then formulated to address the developmental needs of the child in light of the family structure and stresses. If a plan cannot be developed with a reasonable amount of effort by the parties, the question of referral to a mental health practitioner should be raised.

DEVELOPMENTAL DISTURBANCES & CONCERNS

Developmental disturbances are variations in normal child development that cause distress or concern on the part of adult caregivers. As a result, parents frequently contact their physicians with questions about the "terrible twos," childhood fears and anxieties, and adolescent rebellion. In these circumstances, the health care provider is faced with making the correct diagnosis, educating the concerned parents about normal developmental variations, and then (when needed) finding strategies to help the distressed parents facilitate normal parent-child interaction.

THE PUSHY PRESCHOOLER

The push for independence and autonomy that begins in the second year of life can pose problems for parents who are uncertain or insecure about their own role as parents. Preschool children typically want to have their way even when it poses a danger or breaches generational boundaries. Many children try to decide when and what the family eats, what time they go to bed, and who sleeps in which bed. In short, preschool children can be quite demanding, pushy, and bossy—all as part of their rudimentary push to become independent.

The formidable task for parents is to respect the child's wish for self-determination while setting limits and providing guidance so that the child does not become tyrannical or out of control. Parents who are having difficulty placing limits on their child's behavior will present with one of the following types of complaints:

(1) "Discipline won't work with this child."

(2) "I can't get her to do what I ask without getting mad."

(3) "He says, 'I don't have to do it if I don't want to.'"

(4) "She won't sleep in her own bed."

(5) "Other children his age don't like him. He always wants his way."

(6) "Is this child hyperactive?"

Parents who have difficulty saying "no" calmly yet firmly may be emotionally drained and lack the energy to say "no" effectively, or they may believe that conflicts and disagreements in interpersonal relationships must be avoided. In the former case, parental depression or emotional exhaustion from working and single parenthood is common. In the latter case, the parent typically overidentifies with the frustrated child's distress and is then reminded of painful conflicts or unhappiness in his or her own life. Keeping the child "happy" (ie, avoiding conflict) keeps the parent from feeling distressed and unhappy.

In planning interventions, the physician must educate the parents about the sometimes pushy nature of children who are "feeling their oats." With that explanation comes the need for external limits, because a child's judgment and self-control are as yet underdeveloped. Parents need to know that a child's disappointment and frustration with limits do not mean poor parenting or an unhappy child.

Parents who are emotionally depleted or depressed need to be cared for themselves, either through rest, emotional support, and assistance with parenting or through professional care for their depression.

In the case of a parent who avoids conflict, the physician should suggest addressing one or two discipline problems. For example, if toys are not picked up after a reminder, they are put away out of the child's reach for some announced period of time. Likewise, if a meal is not eaten within a reasonable and specified time limit, the food is taken away and snacks are withheld until the next meal. As the parent begins to feel more comfortably in control, the child's behavior typically becomes less oppositional; at this point, the parent should use positive reinforcement, such as "I like the way you picked up your toys—let's read a story together."

Lieberman AF: The challenges of being (and raising) a toddler. In: *The Emotional Life of the Toddler.* Free Press, 1993.

CHILDHOOD FEARS & ANXIETIES

Childhood is a time of both excitement and worry—the latter manifested by fears and anxieties.

In a study of nearly 500 randomly selected families, mothers reported that about 43% of their children had displayed at least seven fears or worries between 6 and 12 years of age. The vast majority of childhood fears are not associated with psychologic disorders; in fact, the fearful stimuli tend to evolve and change with age in a developmental sequence (see Table 7–3) and, overall, tend to decrease in frequency with age (Spence, 1993).

Although the manifestations of many developmental anxieties, such as separation distress and fear of the dark, may wax and wane over months or years, most specific childhood fears are transient (days to weeks in duration) and not associated with significant interference with daily life. In most cases, all that is needed is to reassure the parents about the developmental nature of fears; the parents, in turn, can then reassure their children that they will be fine even though they feel frightened at times. Fears become a source of greater concern to health care providers when they appear outside the normal developmental sequence of fears, when they are persistent, when they cause severe distress, or when they interfere with adaptive functioning, such as poor attendance at school or avoidance of peer relationships. Approximately 2–3% of children have fears significant enough to require specific mental health interventions.

Spence SH, McCathie H: The stability of fears in children: A two-year prospective study: A research note. J Child Psychol Psychiatry 1993;34:579.

ADOLESCENT REBELLION & TURMOIL

Surveys of large adolescent populations confirm that adolescence is not the turbulent state depicted in individual clinical case studies. General theoretic impressions and sampling bias at one time tended to exaggerate the turmoil of normal adolescence.

A longitudinal study of normal suburban middle-

Table 7–3. Sequence of developmental anxieties.

Age at First Appearance	Source of Anxieties
Early infancy	Sudden loud noises, unpredictable stimuli, loss of postural support, heights
1 y	Stranger, unfamiliar situations and objects. Beginning of separation distress.
2–6 y	Animals, darkness, imaginary creatures (ghosts and monsters)
School age	Bodily injury, physical danger. Fear of loss of loved one.
Teens and adulthood	Fear of failure (eg, test anxiety), concerns about social acceptance, loss of a loved one, physical danger, natural disasters

class boys through their high school years identified only 21% as experiencing tumultuous unrest. On closer inspection, this population was distinguished from the remainder of the sample by lower socioeconomic status, more overt marital conflicts in the family, and a higher than normal incidence of mental illness in the family. Overall, approximately 20% of normal adolescents have a stormy course; another 20% progress continuously and smoothly through adolescence; and the remainder show normal overall adjustment but have had temporary difficulty during times of stress. Eighty percent of adolescents adjust successfully with no signs and symptoms of emotional disturbances unless confronted with clear socioenvironmental stressors.

When behavioral deviance or a clearly psychopathologic disorder is identified in adolescence, those problems tend not to remit with time. In short, adolescents with significant problems do not outgrow them. Continuity does, therefore, seem to exist between adolescent and adult psychopathology.

PSYCHIATRIC DISORDERS

Psychiatric disturbances are classified on the basis of descriptive and phenomenologic data (American Psychiatric Association, 1994) rather than presumed or hypothesized etiologic mechanisms.

A *psychiatric disorder* is defined as a cluster of symptoms (ie, emotions, behaviors, psychologic states) that occur with statistically significant frequency within the identified population; furthermore, the symptoms are associated with subjective distress or maladaptive behavior. This definition presumes that the individual's symptoms are of such intensity, persistence, and duration that the ability to adapt to life's challenges is compromised.

About 10% of children and adolescents are personally affected by psychiatric disorders. As a general rule, these children will benefit from treatment by professionals experienced in the treatment of psychiatric disturbances.

American Psychiatric Association: *Diagnostic and Statistical Manual of Mental Disorders,* 4th ed. American Psychiatric Press, 1994.

DISTURBANCES IN PARENT-INFANT INTERACTION

Primary Caregiver Dysfunction

Primary caregiver dysfunction can be defined as a failure to provide parenting functions (usually, but not necessarily, by the mother) because of parental vulnerability or disability, with the result that the parent is unable to meet the caretaking or developmental needs of the child. Although these parents have no single psychiatric diagnosis (in fact, they may not be formally diagnosable at all), they can manifest anxiety, distress, exhaustion, anger, or indifference in relation to the tasks of child care. Caregiver dysfunction can result in a number of symptoms that are presented to the health care provider, usually within the first 6 months of life (Table 7–4).

These individuals frequently have difficult psychosocial histories, find themselves currently without emotional or physical support, and have many unmet personal needs of their own (see Table 7–5). Characteristics of the child may also contribute to the parent's failure to "tune in and turn on" to the child's needs. Risk factors include prematurity, perinatal complications, birth defects, multiple births, and a difficult temperament. These characteristics frequently define the child as different, defective, or disappointing in the parent's eyes.

Clinical Findings

The diagnosis of caregiver dysfunction is made by interviewing the parents and in observing the interaction between parent and child. The child should be evaluated for organic disorders that could explain the presenting symptoms.

A history directed toward identification of specific parental risk factors should be obtained directly from the parent (Table 7–5), with particular reference to feelings of stress or being overwhelmed by the caretaking needs of the child or by the demands of daily life. Attention should be paid to the parent's description of the child and to parental symptoms of anxiety or depression manifest by tenseness, irritability, fatigability, tearfulness, sleep disturbance, and a wish to avoid or withdraw from daily activities.

In observing the parent-child interaction, the physician should look for reciprocity, mutual enthusiasm, and enjoyment in the relationship, as opposed to pathologic signs of tension, irritability, or apathy on either side of the relationship.

Differential Diagnosis

Physical disorders that may explain the presenting symptoms must be ruled out, but it should also be

Table 7–4. Signs and symptoms suggesting primary caregiver dysfunction.

Failure to thrive
Feeding problems
Delays in development
Signs of abuse
Frequent physician visits, especially for nonspecific concerns
Excessive parental worry about illness in the child
Inadequate physical care
Child perceived as "difficult to deal with"
Sleep problems

Table 7–5. Parental risk factors contributing to primary caregiver dysfunction.

History of inadequate relations with own mother
Isolation from an adult support system (eg, single parent)
Psychiatric disorders (particularly acute or chronic depression)
Chronic psychosocial or cognitive dysfunctions (eg, unstable relationships, school problems, legal problems, employment problems)
Unresolved grief over past losses
Marital discord
Poverty or financial problems
Personal or family illnesses
Unwanted or difficult pregnancy
Current life stresses (eg, loss of a relationship, recent illness, job loss)

noted that caregiver dysfunction and organic disease not infrequently coexist.

Complications

Unrecognized parental dysfunction can result in disorders of attachment, nonorganic failure to thrive, child abuse, later behavioral problems in the child, and another generation of children who will themselves probably display caregiver dysfunction as parents.

Treatment

Treatment is focused primarily on supporting and educating the parents. The physician should empathize, explaining that being a parent is difficult and tiring work and that it requires health, energy, and emotional support. The task is to help the parent feel well physically and emotionally and then to facilitate the development of appropriate child care skills. Any underlying medical or psychiatric disorder the parent may have should be treated, and a social support system for the parent should be found. Parenting skills are taught and positively reinforced over time.

Prognosis

The prognosis depends greatly on the ability of the parent to view professional support and education as helpful rather than critical or indifferent.

Lieberman AF, Zeanah CH: Disorders of attachment in infancy. Child Adolesc Psychiatr Clin North Am 1995; 4:571.

PERVASIVE DEVELOPMENTAL DISORDERS & SCHIZOPHRENIA

Pervasive developmental disorders (PDDs) and childhood schizophrenia are a group of early-onset, severe neuropsychiatric disorders that were once referred to as childhood psychoses. Today, PDDs (including autism) are categorized separately from childhood schizophrenia on the basis of clinical dif-

ferences and family histories. *Pervasive developmental disorder* is a term that actually denotes a group of disorders with the common finding of impairment in socialization.

1. AUTISTIC DISORDER

Essentials of Diagnosis

- Profound deficits in social responsiveness and interpersonal relatedness.
- Abnormal speech and language development.
- Behavioral peculiarities.
- Onset in infancy or early childhood.

General Considerations

Autism is uncommon, with an incidence of approximately 4:10,000 school-age children. More boys than girls are affected (3–4:1).

Although the cause of autism remains unknown, central nervous system dysfunction is suggested by the increased incidence of autism in populations affected by perinatal problems: rubella, phenylketonuria, tuberous sclerosis, infantile spasms, encephalitis, and fragile X syndrome. In addition, studies of twins reveal over 90% concordance for autism in monozygotic twins compared to 24% in dizygotic twins. No consistent psychopathologic pattern is seen in the parents of autistic children, although 25% of families with an autistic child have other family members with language-related disorders.

Clinical Findings

Profound deficits in reciprocal social interaction—for example, delayed or absent social smile, failure to anticipate interaction with caregivers, and a lack of attention to a primary caregiver's face—are often evident even in the first year of life. In toddlers, findings include deficiencies in imitative play and a relative lack of interest in interpersonal interactions. Language development is often quite delayed. In fact, children are often first referred for evaluation because they appear to lack responsiveness to spoken language and are presumed to be hearing-impaired. When speech does begin to develop, it frequently is not used for meaningful symbolic communication but is instead echolalic and nonsensical.

Autistic children often display peculiar interests, bizarre responses to sensory stimuli; repetitive, stereotypic motor behaviors (eg, twirling, hand flapping); odd posturing; self-injurious behavior; abnormal patterns of eating and sleeping; and unpredictable mood changes. About 70% have IQs of less than 70.

Differential Diagnosis

Although autism and mental retardation often coexist, the vast majority of mentally retarded children do not show the essential characteristics of autism. A hearing or visual impairment must be ruled out with appropriate screening. Children with developmental speech and language disorders typically show better interpersonal interactions than autistic children. Youngsters should be investigated for metabolic disorders and fragile X syndrome.

Complications

Approximately 25% of autistic individuals eventually develop a seizure disorder. Some autistic adolescents who have higher cognitive skills become depressed as they become partially aware of their deficits.

Treatment

Behaviorally oriented special education or day treatment programs are vital in helping the autistic child acquire more appropriate social, linguistic, self-care, and cognitive skills. The goal is to normalize the child's behavior and adaptive social skills.

Antipsychotic medications (particularly haloperidol in doses of 0.5–4 mg/d) can modify a variety of disruptive symptoms, including hyperactivity, aggressiveness, and negativism, making the child more accessible to education. Fenfluramine may help the few autistic children with elevated serotonin, but stimulants can sometimes make the symptoms of autism more severe. Naltrexone may help control self-injurious behavior. Parents and families need strong support as well as education in coping with the disorder.

Prognosis

Autism is a lifelong disorder with an overall poor prognosis. Approximately one-sixth of autistic children become gainfully employed as adults, and another one-sixth are able to function in sheltered workshops and halfway houses. Two-thirds need ongoing supervision and support. The best prognosis is seen in children who have normal, testable intelligence and who have developed significant symbolic language skills by the age of 5 years.

Klin A, Volkmar FR: Autism and the pervasive developmental disorders. Child Adolesc Psychiatr Clin North Am 1995;4:617.

Mauk JE: Autism and pervasive developmental disorders. Pediatr Clin North Am 1993;40:567.

2. NONAUTISTIC PERVASIVE DEVELOPMENTAL DISORDERS

Essentials of Diagnosis
- Some degree of persistent social impairment.
- Onset by early childhood.

General Considerations

Children with nonautistic pervasive developmental disorders display a wide range of deficits in social and language skills that is similar to that in children with autism. In the past, many of these children would have been classed in the group manifesting "atypical development." Children with nonautistic pervasive developmental disorders probably outnumber autistic children by as much as 2–3:1.

Clinical Findings

These autistic-like children include those with Asperger's syndrome, childhood disintegrative disorder, Rett syndrome, and pervasive developmental disorder, not otherwise specified (PDD, NOS) (see Table 7–6).

Differential Diagnosis

Specific developmental speech and language disorders should be distinguished. Hearing impairment should be ruled out with appropriate screening.

Treatment

The backbone of treatment for PDD, NOS is special education services designed to inculcate more appropriate social and language skills. Family education and support are important.

Some children may benefit from mental health treatment for depression as they become aware of their deficiencies. Psychoactive medications may be helpful for specific target symptoms.

Table 7–6. Characteristics of nonautistic pervasive developmental disorders.

Disorder	Age at Onset	Clinical Features
Asperger's syndrome	Early childhood	"Odd" males with normal intelligence, motor clumsiness, eccentric interests, and a limited ability to appreciate social nuances
Childhood disintegrative disorder	3–4 y	Profound deterioration to severe autism
Rett syndrome	5 mo	Females with reduced head circumference and loss of social relatedness who develop stereotyped hand movements and have impaired language and mental functioning
Pervasive developmental disorder, not otherwise specified	Preschool years	Two to three times more common than autism, with similar but less severe symptoms

Prognosis

The prognosis is variable, depending on the severity of social and language deficits.

Klin A, Volkmar FR: Autism and the pervasive developmental disorders. Child Adolesc Psychiatr Clin North Am 1995;4:617.

Towbin KE: PDD, NOS: A review and guidelines for clinical care. Child Adolesc Psychiatr Clin North Am 1994;3:149.

3. CHILDHOOD SCHIZOPHRENIA

Essentials of Diagnosis

- Rambling or illogical speech patterns.
- Bizarre thought content.
- Hallucinations, delusions, or both.

General Considerations

Childhood schizophrenia is probably the more severe form of the spectrum of schizophrenic disorders. It affects only 1–2 children in every 10,000 of the population under 15 years of age, and boys outnumber girls approximately 2:1. Childhood schizophrenia appears to be genetically related to the adult type of schizophrenia.

Clinical Findings

Affected children display many of the symptoms of adults with schizophrenia. Hallucinations or delusions, bizarre and morbid thought content, or rambling and illogical speech are typical. These children tend to withdraw into an internal world of fantasy and may then behave as though the fantasy were, in fact, external reality. They generally have difficulty with schoolwork and with peer relationships. The vast majority of childhood schizophrenics have had nonspecific psychiatric symptoms or symptoms of delayed development for months or years prior to the onset of their overtly psychotic symptoms (Fish, 1992).

Differential Diagnosis

Psychotic symptoms in children under 8 years of age must be differentiated from normal vivid fantasy life. Rambling speech and bizarre thought content can be helpful distinguishing factors. Learning disabilities should also be identified. In psychotic adolescents, mania is differentiated by observation of high levels of energy, excitement, and irritability. Any youngster presenting with new psychotic symptoms requires a medical evaluation that includes a physical and neurologic examination; drug screen; metabolic screen for endocrinopathies, Wilson's disease, and delirium; and an MRI and EEG.

Treatment

The treatment of childhood schizophrenia focuses on four main areas: (1) ameliorating active psychotic symptoms, (2) teaching appropriate social and cognitive skills, (3) reducing the risk of relapse of psychotic symptoms, and (4) providing support and education to parents and family members. Antipsychotic medications and a supportive, reality-oriented focus in relationships can help in reducing hallucinations, delusions, frightening thoughts, and social withdrawal. Teaching appropriate life skills is probably best accomplished in a special education program or a day treatment setting. Support for the family emphasizes the importance of clear, focused communication and an emotionally calm climate in preventing recurrences of overtly psychotic symptoms in schizophrenic individuals.

Prognosis

Childhood schizophrenia is generally considered a chronic disorder with exacerbations and remissions in active psychotic symptoms. It is generally believed that earlier onset (prior to age 13 years) and poor premorbid functioning (oddness or eccentricity) predict a poorer prognosis.

Caplan R: Childhood schizophrenia: Assessment and treatment. Child Adolesc Psychiatr Clin North Am 1994; 3:15.

Fish B et al: Infants at risk for schizophrenia: Sequelae of a genetic neurointegrative defect. Arch Gen Psychiatry 1992;49:221.

Werry JS, McClellan JM: Predicting outcome in child and adolescent (early onset) schizophrenia and bipolar disorder. J Am Acad Child Adolesc Psychiatry 1992;31:147.

MOOD DISORDERS

1. DEPRESSION IN CHILDREN & ADOLESCENTS

Essentials of Diagnosis

- Dysphoric mood or depressed appearance, persisting for days to weeks at a time.

General Considerations

The term *depression* can denote an emotional state, a symptom, or a clinical syndrome. All three are now well-recognized entities in children and adolescents.

Depression is as frequent in boys as in girls. The incidence of depression in children increases with age, from 1–3% before puberty to 3–6% of adolescents (McCracken, 1992). The incidence of depression in children is significantly higher when other family members have been affected by depressive disorders.

Clinical Findings

Clinical depression can be defined as a persistent state of unhappiness or misery that interferes with pleasure or productivity. The signs and symptoms of depression are surprisingly constant from early childhood to adolescence and adulthood (Table 7–7). The dysphoria of depression in children and adolescents is equally likely to be an irritable mood state as it is to be a down mood (Biederman, 1995).

Typically, a child or adolescent with depression begins to look unhappy and may make comments such as "I have no friends . . . life is boring . . . there is nothing I can do to make things better . . . I wish I were dead." There is usually a change in behavior patterns that includes social isolation, deterioration in schoolwork, loss of interest in usual activities, and flashes of intense anger and irritability. Sleep and appetite patterns frequently change, and the child may complain of tiredness and somatic pain.

Differential Diagnosis

Youngsters with clinical depression can be identified by actively questioning them about depressive symptoms. Children are often more accurate in assessing their own mood state than are their caretakers. When symptoms are numerous, persistent, and intense, a diagnosis of major depressive disorder is appropriate. When symptoms are fewer and of less intensity but have persisted for months or years, a diagnosis of dysthymic disorder is made. When depressive symptoms are milder and of relatively short duration and clearly follow some stressful life event, a diagnosis of adjustment disorder with depressed mood is proper.

Children with attention-deficit disorders, conduct disorders, and developmental disabilities can become quite "demoralized" or "reactively depressed" by their chronic difficulties in life. There are also substantial rates of comorbidity of depression with attention-deficit hyperactivity disorder, conduct disorder, anxiety disorders, eating disorders, and substance abuse disorders (McCauley, 1993). Medically ill patients also have an increased incidence of depression. Every child and adolescent with a depressed mood state should be questioned about victimization by child abuse. Depressed adolescents should be screened for hypothyroidism and substance abuse.

Complications

Because the emotional pain associated with severe depression can be intensely distressing, suicide may be considered. In addition, adolescents have a propensity to avoid the pain of depression through substance abuse or excitement-seeking behaviors (eg, "partying," negativism and defiance, reckless behavior).

Treatment

The treatment of depression focuses on two issues: (1) helping those in the environment to respond more effectively to the child's emotional needs, and (2) ameliorating the child's depressive symptoms. Efforts are made to resolve conflicts between family members and to increase the opportunity for enjoyable time together. Attitudes, expectations, and disciplinary methods are evaluated. The child is encouraged to become involved in activities and to pursue opportunities for maximizing skills and talents. Individual psychotherapy can increase the patient's awareness of care and concern on the part of adults. It also helps the young person to identify, label, and verbalize feelings and misperceptions.

When the symptoms of depression are severe, persistent, and disabling, antidepressant medication can be of help, especially when there is a family history of depressive disorder responding to these drugs. However, controlled studies have not shown tricyclic antidepressants to be superior to placebo in children and adolescents with major depression (Ambrosini, 1993).

Prognosis

A growing body of follow-up data strongly suggests that depression in children and adolescents is a chronic condition that requires monitoring over time (Rao, 1995). In addition, approximately one-third of preadolescents with major depression manifest bipolar disorder at 2-year follow-up (Geller, 1994).

Table 7–7. Clinical manifestations of depression in children and adolescents.

Depressive Symptom	Clinical Manifestations
Dysphoric mood	Tearfulness; sad, downturned expression; unhappiness; slumped posture; quick temper; irritability; anger
Anhedonia	Loss of interest and enthusiasm in play, socializing, school, and usual activities; boredom; loss of pleasure
Fatigability	Lethargy and tiredness; no play after school
Morbid ideation	Self-deprecating thoughts, statements; thoughts of disaster, abandonment, death, suicide, or hopelessness
Somatic symptoms	Changes in sleep or appetite patterns; difficulty in concentrating; bodily complaints, particularly headache and stomachache

Ambrosini PJ et al: Antidepressant treatments in children and adolescents: Affective disorders. J Am Acad Child Adolesc Psychiatry 1993;32:1.

Biederman J et al: Psychiatric comorbidity among referred juveniles with major depression: Fact or artifact? J Am Acad Child Adolesc Psychiatry 1995;34:579.

Geller B et al: Rate and predictors of prepubertal bipolarity during follow-up of 6 to 12 year old depressed children. J Am Acad Child Adolesc Psychiatry 1994;33:461.

Kovacs M et al: Childhood onset dysthymic disorder: Clinical features and prospective naturalistic outcome. Arch Gen Psychiatry 1994;51:365.

McCauley E et al: Depression in young people: Initial presentation and clinical course. J Am Acad Child Adolesc Psychiatry 1993;32:714.

McCracken JT: The epidemiology of child and adolescent mood disorders. Psychiatr Clin North Am 1992;1:53.

Mood disorders in children and adolescence. The Harvard Mental Health Lett 1993;10(4 and 5).

Rao U et al: Unipolar depression in adolescents: Clinical outcome in adulthood. J Am Acad Child Adolesc Psychiatry 1995;34:566.

2. BIPOLAR DISORDER

Essentials of Diagnosis

- Periods of abnormally and persistently elevated, expansive, or irritable mood and heightened levels of energy and activity. Not caused by prescribed or illicit drugs.

General Considerations

Bipolar disorder (previously referred to as manic-depressive disease) is an episodic mood disorder manifested by distinct periods of both manic and depressive episodes or, less commonly, manic episodes alone. Children and adolescents often present with a variable course of mood instability combined with problems with conduct and impulse control, with or without substance abuse. At least 20% of bipolar adults experience the onset of symptoms before the age of 20 years. The onset of bipolar disorder before puberty is thought to be infrequent, while the lifetime prevalence of bipolar disorder in mid to late adolescence appears to approach 1% (Lewinsohn, 1995).

Clinical Findings

In 70% of patients, the first symptoms are primarily those of depression; in the remainder, manic, hypomanic, or mixed states dominate the symptom presentation. Manic patients present a variable pattern of elevated, expansive, or irritable mood, along with more rapid speech, higher energy levels, some difficulty in sustaining concentration, and a decreased need for sleep. Patients often do not recognize that there is any problem with their mood or behavior. The clinical picture can be quite dramatic, with florid psychotic symptoms of delusions and hallucinations (a full-blown manic psychosis), more subtle changes in mood or behavior (cyclothymia), or milder symptoms of psychomotor activation seen with hypomania.

Differential Diagnosis

Diagnostic considerations must include an acute organic process, particularly substance abuse disorder. Hyperthyroidism should be ruled out. In prepubescent children, mania may be difficult to differentiate from attention-deficit hyperactivity disorder (ADHD) and other disruptive behavior disorders. Intense and prolonged rages or dysphoria and some periodicity of symptom activity suggest bipolar disorder (Wozniak, 1995). Table 7–8 further defines points of differentiation between bipolar disorder, ADHD, and conduct disorder.

Complications

The poor judgment associated with manic episodes predisposes to dangerous, impulsive, and sometimes criminal activities. Affective disorders are associated with a 30-fold greater incidence of successful suicide.

Treatment & Prognosis

Most patients with bipolar disease respond to treatment with mood-stabilizing medications (lithium and/or valproate), supportive psychotherapy, and education about the recurrent nature of the illness (Kafantaris, 1995).

Fristad MA et al: Bipolar disorder in children and adolescents. Child Adolesc Psychiatr Clin North Am 1992; 1:13.

Kafantaris V: Treatment of bipolar disorder in children and adolescence. J Am Acad Child Adolesc Psychiatry 1995;34:732.

Kovacs M, Pollock M: Bipolar disorder and comorbid conduct disorder in childhood and adolescence. J Am Child Adolesc Psychiatry 1995;34:715.

Lewinsohn PM et al: Bipolar disorder in a community sample of older adolescents: Prevalence, phenomenology, comorbidity, and course. J Am Acad Child Adolesc Psychiatry 1995;34:454.

Wozniak J et al: Mania-like symptoms suggestive of childhood onset bipolar disorder in clinically referred children. J Am Acad Child Adolesc Psychiatry 1995;34:867.

CONDUCT DISORDERS

Essentials of Diagnosis

A persistent pattern of behavior includes the following:

- Defiance of authority.
- Violating the rights of others or society's norms.
- Aggressive behavior toward others.

General Considerations

Disorders of conduct affect approximately 9% of males and 2% of females under the age of 18 years. This is a very heterogeneous population, with significant overlap among attention-deficit hyperactivity disorder, learning disabilities, and family dysfunction. Many of these individuals have "difficult temperaments" and come from broken homes where domestic violence, child abuse, drug abuse, shifting parental figures, and poverty are environmental risk factors. Harsh parental discipline with physical pun-

Table 7–8. Differentiating behavior disorders.

	ADHD[1]	Conduct Disorder	Bipolar Disorder
School problems	Yes	Yes	Yes
Behavior problems	Yes	Yes	Yes
Defiant attitude	Occasional	Constant	Episodic
Motor restlessness	Constant	May be present	May wax and wane
Impulsivity	Constant	May be present	May wax and wane
Distractibility	Constant	May be present	May wax and wane
Anger expression	Short-lived (minutes)	Plans revenge	Intense rages (minutes to hours)
Thought content	May be immature	Blames others	Morbid or grandiose ideas
Sleep disturbance	May be present	No	May wax and wane
Self-deprecation	Briefly, with criticism	No	Prolonged, with or without suicidal ideation
Obsessed with ideas	No	No	Yes
Hallucinations	No	No	Diagnostic, if present
Family history	May be a history of school problems	May be a history of antisocial behavior	May be a history of mood disorders

[1]ADHD = attention-deficit hyperactivity disorder.

ishment appears to lead to more aggressive behavior in children and adolescents (Weiss, 1992).

Clinical Findings

The typical child with conduct disorder is a boy with tempestuous social and academic difficulties. Defiance of authority, fighting, tantrums, running away, school failure, and destruction of property are common symptoms. With increasing age, fire setting and stealing may occur, followed in adolescence by truancy, vandalism, and substance abuse. Hyperactive, aggressive, and uncooperative behavior patterns in the preschool and early school years tend to predict conduct disorder in adolescence with a high degree of accuracy. The risk for conduct disorder increases with inconsistent and severe parental disciplinary techniques, parental alcoholism, and parental antisocial behavior.

Differential Diagnosis

Young people with conduct disorders—especially those with more violent histories—have an increased incidence of neurologic signs and symptoms, psychomotor seizures, psychotic symptoms, mood disorders, attention-deficit hyperactivity disorder, and learning disabilities. Efforts should be made to identify these associated disorders (Table 7–8).

Treatment

Treatment is difficult and not very effective. Efforts should be made to stabilize the environment and improve functioning within the home, particularly as it relates to disciplinary techniques. Any associated neurologic, psychiatric, or educational disorders should be treated specifically. In severe cases, residential treatment may be needed.

Prognosis

The prognosis is poor, especially for children who present with onset before age 10 years, who display a diversity of antisocial behaviors across multiple settings, and who are raised in an environment characterized by parental antisocial behavior, alcoholism, and conflict. Nearly half of such children become antisocial as adults. Antisocial behavior in childhood tends to predict a diagnosable psychiatric disorder in adulthood with a high degree of accuracy.

Kazdin AE: *Conduct Disorders in Childhood and Adolescence,* 2nd ed. Sage, 1995.
Weiss B et al: Some consequences of early harsh discipline: Child aggression and a maladaptive social information processing style. Child Dev 1992;63:1321.

ANXIETY DISORDERS

1. ANXIETY-BASED SCHOOL REFUSAL (School Avoidance)

Essentials of Diagnosis

- A persistent pattern of school avoidance related to symptoms of anxiety.

- Prominent somatic symptoms of anxiety on school mornings, with the symptoms resolving if the child is allowed to remain at home.
- No organic medical disorder that accounts for the child's symptoms.

General Considerations

Anxiety-based school refusal, or school phobia, is a clinical syndrome rather than a diagnostic entity. It refers to a pattern of school nonattendance resulting from symptoms of anxiety. The anxiety may be related to a dread of leaving home (ie, separation anxiety), a fear of some aspect of school (ie, "true" school phobia), or a fear of feeling exposed or embarrassed at school (ie, social phobia). In most cases, anxiety-based school refusal represents a prototype of persistent, developmentally inappropriate separation anxiety in which the child feels anxious being away from primary caregivers. It affects boys and girls with approximately equal frequency, and there appear to be peaks in the incidence at the ages of 6 and 7 years, again at 10–11 years of age, and finally in early adolescence.

Clinical Findings

In preadolescent children, school refusal often begins after some clear precipitating stress, such as an illness in the child or a parent or the birth of a sibling. The child's anxiety is then manifested either as somatic symptoms or in displacement of the child's anxiety onto some aspect of the school environment that the child perceives as frightening.

The symptoms often represent somatic manifestations of anxiety, such as dizziness, nausea, and stomach distress. Characteristically, the somatic symptoms become more prominent as the time to leave for school approaches and then remit if the child is allowed to remain at home for the day. In older children, the onset of school refusal is more insidious and is often associated with symptoms of social withdrawal and depression. There is an increased incidence of anxiety and mood disorders in these families.

Differential Diagnosis

The differential diagnosis of school nonattendance is set forth in Table 7–9. Medical disorders that may be causing the somatic symptoms must be ruled out. One should investigate the possibility of "good reasons" for staying home, for example, in the case of a child who is being intimidated by bullying students or an abusive teacher. Children with learning disabilities may wish to stay home to avoid the sense of failure they experience at school. Normal children may also have very transient episodes of wanting to stay at home while they struggle with some internal conflict. Finally, truants are to be differentiated on the basis of their chronic noncompliance with adult

Table 7–9. Differential diagnosis of school nonattendance.[1]

I. Emotional or anxiety-based school refusal[2]
  A. Separation anxiety disorder (50–80% of anxious refusers)
  B. Overanxious disorder
  C. Mood/depressive disorder (with or without comorbid anxiety)
  D. Social anxiety
  E. Simple phobia
  F. Panic disorder
  G. Psychosis ("voices" say not to attend)
II. Truancy[3] behavior disorders
  A. Oppositional defiant disorder, conduct disorder
  B. Substance abuse disorders
III. "Realistic" school refusal
  A. Learning disability, unaddressed or undetected
  B. Marauding students (including gangs)
  C. Psychologically abusive teacher
  D. Family-sanctioned nonattendance
    1. For companionship
    2. For child care
    3. To supplement family income
  E. Socioculturally sanctioned nonattendance (school is not valued)
  F. Homosexual attraction, gender concerns
IV. Undiagnosed medical condition (including pregnancy)

[1]Medically unexplained absence of more than 2 weeks.
[2]Subjectively distressed child who generally stays at home.
[3]Non subjectively distressed and not at home.

authority and their preference for being with peers rather than at home.

Complications

The longer a child remains out of school, the more difficult it is to return and the more strained the relationship between child and parent becomes. Many parents of nonattending children feel tyrannized by their defiant, clinging child. Children often feel accused of "making up" their symptoms, leading to further antagonism between the child, parents, and medical caregivers.

Treatment

The cornerstone of treatment is helping the child to confront anxiety and overcome it by returning to school. This requires a strong alliance between the parents and the health care provider that is built on trust. The parent must understand that no underlying medical disorder exists, that the child's symptoms are a manifestation of anxiety, and that the basic problem is anxiety that must be faced to be overcome. Parents must be reminded that being good parents in this case means helping a child to face a distressing experience. Children must be reassured that their symptoms are caused by "worry" and that they will be overcome upon return to school.

A plan for returning the child to school is then developed with parents and school personnel. The child is brought to school by someone not likely to waver in the face of the child's distress—for example, the father or an older sibling. If significant symptoms develop at school, the child should be checked by the school nurse and then returned to class after a brief rest. The parents must be reassured that school staff will handle the situation at school and that school personnel can reach the child's primary health care provider if any questions arise.

In cases in which parents are unable to enter into that kind of treatment contract, more in-depth mental health assistance must be provided as a way of supporting autonomy in family members. For children with more severe symptoms of separation or panic anxiety or major depression, tricyclic antidepressants or a brief course of a high-potency benzodiazepine may be an important adjunct to the behavioral treatment.

Prognosis

Although the vast majority of preadolescent children can be effectively returned to school, the long-term prognosis is more questionable. Recent studies suggest that a history of school refusal is significantly more frequent in adults with "neuroticism," panic anxiety, and agoraphobia than in the general population. Thus, there may be some correlation between symptoms of school refusal in childhood and the development of psychiatric disorders in adulthood.

Bell-Dolan D, Brazeal T: Separation anxiety disorder, overanxious disorder, and school refusal. Child Adolesc Psychiatr Clin North Am 1993;2:563.

Berg I: Absence from school and mental health. Br J Psychiatry 1992;161:154.

Kutcher S et al: Pharmacotherapy: Approaches and applications. In: *Anxiety Disorders in Children and Adolescents.* March JS (editor). Guilford, 1995.

2. THE OVERLY ANXIOUS CHILD

Transient developmental fears are common in early childhood. Therefore, the person evaluating the clinical significance of anxiety symptoms in children must consider the age of the child, the developmental fears that can normally be expected at that age, the form of the symptoms and their duration, and the degree to which the symptoms disrupt the child's life.

Anxiety can be manifested either directly or indirectly, as shown in Table 7–10. The characteristics of anxiety disorders in childhood are listed in Table 7–11. Community-based studies of school-age children and adolescents suggest that nearly 10% of children have some type of anxiety disorder. The differential diagnosis of symptoms of anxiety is presented in Table 7–12.

The treatment of the overanxious child frequently involves interventions at more than one level. Of greatest importance, the child's family and school environment should be evaluated for marital discord,

Table 7–10. Signs and symptoms of anxiety in children.

Direct manifestations of anxiety
　Psychologic manifestations:
　　Fears and worries
　　Uneasiness and apprehension
　　Frightening themes in play and fantasy
　Psychomotor manifestations:
　　Motoric restlessness and hyperactivity
　　Sleep disturbances
　　Decreased concentration
　Psychophysiologic manifestations:
　　Autonomic hyperarousal
　　　Dizziness and light-headedness
　　　Palpitations
　　　Shortness of breath
　　　Flushing, sweating, dry mouth
　　　Nausea and vomiting
　　　Panic
　　Headaches and stomachaches
Indirect manifestations of anxiety
　Increased dependence on home and parents
　Avoidance of anxiety-producing stimuli
　Decreased school performance
　Increased self-doubt and irritability
　Ritualistic behaviors (eg, washing, counting)

family violence, harsh or inappropriate disciplinary methods, or emotional overstimulation. The child's experience of anxiety and its relationship to life events are explored, and the child is taught specific cognitive and behavioral techniques needed to confront the anxiety. Finally, when severe separation or panic anxiety appears to play a prominent role in the child's anxiety disorder or when the child has persistent obsessive-compulsive disorder, psychopharma-

Table 7–11. Anxiety disorders in children and adolescents.

Disorder	Major Clinical Manifestations
Separation anxiety disorder	Developmentally inappropriate wish to maintain proximity with caretakers; morbid worry of threats to family integrity; intense homesickness
Generalized anxiety disorder	Intense worry, often about future events
Social phobia	Painful shyness or self-consciousness; fear of humiliation with public scrutiny
Simple phobia	Avoidance of specific feared stimuli
Panic disorder	Unprovoked, intense fear with sympathetic hyperarousal, and often palpitations and/or hyperventilation
Post-traumatic stress disorder	Fear of a recurrence of an intense, anxiety-provoking experience, causing sympathetic hyperarousal, avoidance or reminders, and the reexperiencing of aspects of the traumatic event

Table 7–12. Differential diagnosis of symptoms of anxiety.

I. **Normal developmental anxiety**
   A. Stranger anxiety (5 mo to 2½ y, with a peak at 6–12 mo)
   B. Separation anxiety (7 mo to 4 y, with a peak at 18–36 mo)
   C. The child is fearful or even phobic of the dark and monsters (3–6 y)
II. **"Appropriate" anxiety**
   A. Anticipating a painful or frightening experience
   B. Avoidance of a reminder of a painful or frightening experience
   C. Child abuse
III. **Anxiety disorder (see Table 7–11),** with or without other comorbid psychiatric disorders
IV. **Substance abuse**
V. **Medications and recreational drugs**
   A. Caffeinism (including colas and chocolate)
   B. Sympathomimetic agents
   C. Idiosyncratic drug reactions
VI. **Hypermetabolic or hyperarousal states**
   A. Hyperthyroidism
   B. Pheochromocytoma
   C. Anemia
   D. Hypoglycemia
   E. Hypoxemia
VII. **Cardiac abnormality**
   A. Dysrhythmia
   B. High-output state
   C. Mitral valve prolapse

cologic agents may be helpful (Popper, 1993). Selective serotonin reuptake inhibitors may be helpful across a broad spectrum of anxiety symptoms (Birmayer, 1994). The long-term prognosis for these disorders is largely unknown.

Birmayer B et al: Fluoxetine for childhood anxiety disorders. J Am Acad Child Adolesc Psychiatry 1994;33:993.

March JS (editor): *Anxiety Disorders in Children and Adolescents.* Guilford, 1995.

Popper CW: Psychopharmacologic treatment of anxiety disorders in adolescents and children. J Clin Psychiatry 1993;54(Suppl):52.

3. POST-TRAUMATIC STRESS DISORDER

Essentials of Diagnosis

- Signs and symptoms of autonomic hyperarousal.
- Avoidant behaviors.
- Flashbacks to a traumatic event.
- All of the above following the occurrence of traumatic events such as natural disasters, unexpected personal tragedies, and ongoing interpersonal violence.

General Considerations

Long-overdue attention is now being paid to the horrific effects of family and community violence on the psychologic development of children and adolescents. Some 40% of urban adolescents report having experienced or witnessed frightening violent events.

As many as 25% of youth exposed to violence develop symptoms of post-traumatic stress (Singer, 1995).

Clinical Findings

Children who have been psychically traumatized show persistent evidence of fear and anxiety. They are hypervigilant to the possibility of recurrence of a traumatic event. In addition, they regress developmentally and experience fears of strangers, of the dark, and of being alone. They avoid reminders of the traumatic event.

In addition, children frequently reexperience elements of the traumatic events in frightening dreams and intrusive daytime flashbacks. In their symbolic play, one can often notice a monotonous repetition of some aspect of the traumatic event.

Treatment

The cornerstone of treatment for post-traumatic stress disorder is the intense education of the child and family regarding the nature of post-traumatic stress disorder so that the child's emotional reactions and regressive behavior are not mistakenly viewed as "crazy" or "manipulative." Support, reassurance, repeated explanations, and understanding are all needed. Specific fears will wane with time, and behavioral desensitization may help. A supportive relationship with a caretaking adult is essential. For children with more severe symptoms, a variety of psychoactive medications, including mood stabilizers, clonidine, propranolol, and antidepressants—singly or in combination—can be helpful in ameliorating symptoms of autonomic hyperarousal.

Prognosis

Children who have experienced psychic trauma often harbor significant emotional scars. At 4- to 5-year follow-ups, many children continue to have vivid and frightening memories and dreams and a pessimistic view of the future. Evidence is growing to support a connection between victimization in childhood and unstable personality and mood disorders in later life.

Amaya-Jackson L, March JS: Posttraumatic stress disorder. In: *Anxiety Disorders in Children and Adolescents.* March JS (editor). Guilford, 1995.

Pynoos RS: Traumatic stress and developmental psychopathology in children and adolescents. Rev Psychiatry 1993;12:205.

Singer MI et al: Adolescent's exposure to violence and associated symptoms of psychological trauma. JAMA 1995;273:477.

SOMATOFORM DISORDERS

Essentials of Diagnosis

- A symptom suggesting physical dysfunction.
- No known physical disorder accounting for the symptom.

- Symptoms cause distressor dysfunction.
- Symptoms are not voluntarily maintained.

Clinical Findings

Somatoform disorders are a group of conditions that suggest the presence of physical illness or disability for which no organic cause can be ascertained, although neither the patient nor the caretaker is consciously fabricating the symptoms. The category includes conversion disorder, hypochondriasis, somatization disorder, somatoform pain disorder, and body dysmorphic disorder (see Table 7–13).

Conversion symptoms most frequently occur in school-age children and adolescents. Their exact incidence is unclear, but in pediatric practice they are probably more often seen as transient symptoms rather than as chronic disorders requiring help from mental health practitioners. The appearance of the conversion symptom is thought to be an expression of underlying psychologic conflict or stress. Although children can present with a variety of symptoms, many presentations initially suggest a disorder of neurologic or sensory origin. Symptoms include unusual sensory phenomena, paralysis, and movement or seizure-like disorders.

In the classic case of conversion disorder, the child's symptom complex and examination are not consistent with the clinical manifestations of any organic disease process. In addition, the symptoms frequently begin as an intercurrent illness within the context of a family experiencing significant stress, such as serious illness, a death, or family discord. On closer examination, the child's symptoms are often found to resemble symptoms present in other significant family members. Children with conversion symptoms often, but not always, have some secondary gain associated with their symptoms.

A number of reports have pointed to the increased association of conversion symptoms with sexual overstimulation or sexual abuse. Health care providers should always keep that possibility in mind.

Differential Diagnosis

It is sometimes not possible to be sure that the symptoms are not caused by an underlying disease process. In such cases, follow-up observation is required to see whether further symptoms evolve.

Somatic symptoms can be prominent in children with anxiety and depressive disorders (Table 7–13). The child's mood state and associated symptoms of avoidance are helpful indicators in determining whether such disorders are present. Occasionally, psychotic children present with somatic preoccupations and even somatic delusions.

Treatment

In most cases, conversion symptoms resolve quickly when the child and family are reassured that the symptom is a way of reacting to identifiable stresses in the child's life. The child is encouraged to continue with daily activities as normally as possible, knowing that the symptom will resolve when the stress is resolved.

If identifiable stresses are not clearly understood or if the symptom does not resolve with reassurance, further investigation by a mental health professional is indicated. When the more chronic somatoform disorders evolve in children and adolescents, treatment with appropriate psychopharmacologic agents may be helpful (Hollander, 1993).

Hollander E: Pharmacologic treatment of obsessive-compulsive spectrum disorders. Psychiatr Times 1993;10:36.
Nemzer ED: Somatoform disorders. In: *Child and Adolescent Psychiatry: A Comprehensive Textbook.* Lewis M (editor). Williams & Wilkins, 1991.

ADJUSTMENT DISORDERS

Children's lives are filled with stresses and changes, most of which are not of their choosing. The list is endless, but the most frequent and most disturbing stresses for children and adolescents include marital discord or dissolution, family illness, the loss of a loved one, or a change of residence.

When faced with stress, children can manifest many different symptoms, including changes in mood, changes in behavior, and physical complaints. Key findings include the following: (1) the precipitating event or circumstance is identifiable; (2) the symptoms have appeared since the occurrence of the stressful event; (3) the intensity of the child's reac-

Table 7–13. Somatoform disorders in children and adolescents.

Disorder	Major Clinical Manifestations
Conversion disorder	Symptom onset follows psychologically stressful event; symptoms express unconscious feelings and result in secondary gain
Hypochondriasis	Preoccupation with worry that physical symptoms manifest an unrecognized and threatening condition; medical assurance does not provide relief from worry
Somatization disorder	Long standing preoccupation with multiple somatic symptoms
Somatoform pain disorder	Preoccupation with pain that results in distress or impairment beyond what would be expected from physical findings
Body dysmorphic disorder	Preoccupation with an imagined defect in personal appearance

tion is not severe and disabling; and (4) the reaction does not persist beyond a few months. The range of symptoms of patients with adjustment disorders are listed in Table 7–14.

Differential Diagnosis

When symptoms are clearly a reaction to an identifiable stressor but are severe, persistent, or disabling, depressive, anxiety, and conduct disorders must be considered.

Treatment

The mainstay of treatment is the doctor's assurance that the emotional or behavioral change is a predictable consequence of the stressful events. Such a statement serves both to validate the child's reaction and to encourage the child to talk about feelings associated with the stressful occurrence and its aftermath. Parents are asked to understand the child's reaction and encourage the appropriate verbal expression of feelings, while also defining boundaries for behavior that prevent the child from feeling out of control.

Prognosis

The duration of symptoms in adjustment reactions depends on the severity of the stress, the child's personal sensitivity to stress, and the support system available to the child. The prognosis is generally good when these children feel understood by someone to whom they can express their feelings. Nonetheless, the loss of a parent or the breakup of a marriage can lead to years of intermittent distress in normal children. In addition, the precipitating stressful event may uncover a more chronic vulnerability to anxiety or depression.

Tomb DA: Adjustment disorder. In: *Child and Adolescent Psychiatry: A Comprehensive Textbook.* Lewis M (editor). Williams & Wilkins, 1991.

ELIMINATION DISORDERS

1. ENURESIS

Essentials of Diagnosis

- Involuntary urinary incontinence in a child 5 years of age or older.

- No physical abnormality causing the urinary incontinence.

General Considerations

Enuresis is the involuntary passage of urine into bedclothes or undergarments. At least 90% of enuretic children have primary nocturnal enuresis—that is, they wet only at night during sleep, and they have never had a sustained period of dryness. Diurnal enuresis (daytime wetting) is much less common, as is secondary enuresis, which develops after a child has had a sustained period of bladder control. The latter two varieties are much more frequently associated with emotional stress, anxiety, and psychiatric disorders. Primary nocturnal enuresis is generally viewed as a developmental disorder or maturational lag that is infrequently associated with a significant psychopathologic disorder.

Clinical Findings

Primary nocturnal enuresis is common (Table 7–15). The incidence is three times higher in boys than in girls. With each year that passes, a proportion of nighttime wetters stop wetting without any form of treatment. The family history in such cases frequently reveals other members—especially fathers—who have had prolonged nighttime bed-wetting problems.

Although the cause of primary nocturnal enuresis is not established, it appears to be related to maturational delay of sleep and arousal mechanisms or to delay in development of increased bladder capacity.

Daytime wetting most often occurs in timid and shy children or in children with attention-deficit disorder. It occurs with about equal frequency in boys and girls, and 60–80% of daytime wetters also wet at night.

Secondary enuresis typically follows a stressful event, such as the birth of a sibling, a significant loss, or discord within the family. The symptom can be seen as the result of regression in response to stress or as a more symbolic expression of the child's feelings.

Differential Diagnosis

The differential diagnosis includes neurologic ab-

Table 7–14. Signs and symptoms of adjustment reactions.

Irritable, angry mood
Anxious, worried mood
Unhappy, depressed mood
Angry resistance to authority
Fatigue
Aches and pains
Decreased school performance
Social withdrawal
Any combination of the above

Table 7–15. Incidence of enuresis in children.

Age (y)	Primary Nocturnal Enuresis (%)	Occasional Daytime Enuresis (%)
5	15	8
7–8	7	—
10	3–5	—
12	2–3	1
14	1	—

normalities, seizure disorders, diabetes mellitus, and abnormalities of the urinary tract. Obtaining a urinalysis and urine culture and observing the child's urinary stream can essentially rule out the vast majority of organic causes of enuresis. Some children with daytime wetting can have "difficult" temperamental variations or overt depression.

Complications

The most common complication of enuresis is low self-esteem in response to criticism from caregivers.

Treatment

The most important aspect of treatment for children with primary nocturnal enuresis is reassuring the family and child that the symptom is a developmental lag and not indicative of emotional problems or "bad" behavior. Treatment can then be pursued if this largely "cosmetic" problem is a source of concern for the child. If the child chooses to pursue treatment, positive motivation is an important precondition to successful intervention.

Treatment can begin with a program of bladder exercises such as holding urine as long as possible during the day and then starting and stopping the urine stream during micturition. In addition, the child is instructed to practice getting up from bed and going to the bathroom at bedtime. The child lies down, counts to 50, gets up, goes to the bathroom, and tries to urinate. The child repeats this procedure 10–20 times each night before retiring. The combination of these procedures is helpful in perhaps 30–40% of children with nighttime wetting. For the remainder, an alerting buzzer that sounds early in the bed-wetting process is helpful to about 70% of children. The child is instructed to get up and go to the bathroom and finish emptying the bladder if the alarm goes off.

For others, a trial of imipramine is worthwhile at dosages of 25–50 mg at bedtime for children under 12 years of age and 50–75 mg for older children. Imipramine generally provides satisfactory results in about 70% of children. Unfortunately, many patients relapse once the drug is stopped; thus, its primary use is for camp or overnight visits, when a temporary period of dryness is important. Desmopressin acetate, 20–40 µg intranasally at bedtime, can result in complete remission of nocturnal enuresis in 50% of children so long as they continue the treatment.

Mental health treatment is more often needed for children with daytime wetting or secondary enuresis. The focus is on the verbal expression of feelings that may be associated with perpetuation of the symptom.

Howe AC, Walker CE: Behavioral management of toilet training, enuresis, and encopresis. Pediatr Clin North Am 1992;39:413.

Reiner WG: Enuresis in child psychiatric practice. Child Adolesc Psychiatr Clin North Am 1995;4:453.

2. FUNCTIONAL ENCOPRESIS

Essentials of Diagnosis

- Fecal incontinence in a child 4 years of age or older. Not caused by physical abnormality.

General Considerations

Functional encopresis is defined as the repeated, usually involuntary passage of feces in inappropriate places in a child at least 4 years of age. It affects approximately 1–1.5% of school-age children—boys four times as commonly as girls. Functional fecal incontinence is rare in adolescence.

Clinical Findings

Functional encopresis can be divided into four types: retentive, continuous, discontinuous, and "toilet phobia."

In **retentive encopresis**—also called psychogenic megacolon—the child withholds bowel movements, leading to the development of constipation, fecal impaction, and the seepage of soft or liquid feces into the underclothing. Marked constipation and painful defecation often contribute to a vicious cycle of withholding—larger impaction—further seepage. These children often have a history of crossing their legs to resist the urge to defecate and of infrequent bowel movements large enough to stop up the toilet, and they are found on examination to have large fecal masses in their rectal vaults. Most of these children are distressed by the soiling that occurs.

Children with **continuous encopresis** have never gained primary control of bowel function. Usually, the bowel movement is randomly deposited in underclothing without regard to social norms. Typically, the family structure does not encourage organization and skill training, and for that reason the child has never had adequate consistent bowel training. These children and their parents are more apt to be socially or intellectually disadvantaged.

Children with **discontinuous encopresis** have a clear history of having attained an extended period of normal bowel control. Loss of control often occurs in response to a stressful event, such as the birth of a sibling, a separation, family illness, or marital disharmony. These children then begin to put feces in "irritating places" as an expression of anger or of a wish to be perceived as younger. Typically, these children display relative indifference to the symptom.

In the infrequent case of "toilet phobia," a relatively young child views the toilet as a frightening structure to be avoided. These children may view the bowel movement as an extension of themselves, which is then swept away in a frightening manner. They may have the thought that they, too, may be swept away "down the toilet."

Differential Diagnosis

The main differential diagnosis involves the medical causes of constipation and retentive encopresis. Hirschsprung's disease can be ruled out with reasonable certainty by the history of passing large-caliber bowel movements in the past. Neurologic disorders, hypothyroidism, hypercalcemia, and diseases of smooth muscle must be considered as well. The child should be examined for anal fissures, which tend to encourage the withholding of bowel movement.

In addition, fecal soiling can be a presenting symptom in childhood depression and is sometimes a concomitant finding in children with attention-deficit hyperactivity disorder.

Treatment

Identifying the type of encopresis is important in treatment planning. Another important variable is the child's own concern and level of distress about the symptom. Children who display denial or indifference about their symptoms are much harder to treat. Children with coexisting depression or attention-deficit hyperactivity disorder need to be treated for those conditions prior to focusing treatment on the symptom of soiling.

With the most common type of encopresis—the retentive type—efforts are made to soften stool so that constipation and painful defecation do not perpetuate the behavior. These children are then taught to overcome the problem by adopting a regular schedule of postprandial sessions on the toilet. A system of positive reinforcement can be added in which the child is rewarded for each day with no soiled underclothes. The responsibility for rinsing own soiled clothing and depositing it in the appropriate receptacle rests with the child. In the case of continuous fecal soiling, the family is taught to train the child. For toilet phobia, a progressive series of rewarded desensitization steps is necessary.

Children with discontinuous soiling that persists over a number of weeks often need psychotherapy to help them recognize and express their anger and wish to be dependent verbally rather than by fecal soiling.

Prognosis

While the ultimate prognosis is excellent, parental distress and parent-child conflict may be great prior to the cessation of symptoms. The natural history of soiling is that it resolves by adolescence in all but the most severely disturbed teenagers.

Howe AC, Walker CE: Behavioral management of toilet training, enuresis, and encopresis. Pediatr Clin North Am 1992;39:413.

Mikkelson EJ: Modern approaches to enuresis and encopresis. In: *Child and Adolescent Psychiatry: A Comprehensive Textbook.* Lewis M (editor). Williams & Wilkins, 1991.

SUICIDE IN CHILDREN & ADOLESCENTS

Suicide has become the third leading cause of death among people 15–24 years of age. The suicide rate among adolescents 15–19 years of age quadrupled—from approximately 2.7 to 11.3 per 100,000—over the last 40 years. For children 14 years of age and younger, the rate of completed suicide is low but has increased by 120%, from 0.8 to 1.7 per 100,000 from 1980 to 1992 (*JAMA,* 1995).

Adolescent girls make three to four times the number of suicide attempts as do boys of the same age. On the other hand, suicide attempts of adolescent males are more lethal—the number of completed suicides is three to four times greater in males than in females. Firearms are the most commonly used method in successful suicides, accounting for 40–60% of cases; hanging, carbon monoxide poisoning, and drug overdoses each account for approximately 10–15% of completed suicides. Among young people, there are perhaps 50–100 suicide attempts for every completed suicide. Each year, approximately 25% of high school students seriously consider suicide, 15% make a plan, 8% make some type of attempt, and 2% come to medical attention because of a suicide attempt.

Suicide is associated with psychopathologic disorder and should not be viewed as a philosophic choice about life or death. Over 50% of suicides occur in young people who are sad, despairing, or depressed; another 20% are described as angry, with the suicide attempt occurring rather impulsively. Substance abuse is implicated in at least 20% of suicides.

The vast majority of young people who commit suicide give some clue to their distress or their tentative plans to commit suicide. Most show signs of depression, such as social withdrawal, loss of interest in activities, and an irritable or depressed mood. Over 60% make comments such as "I wish I were dead" or "I just can't deal with this any longer" within the 24 hours prior to death. In one study, nearly 70% of subjects experienced a crisis event, such as a loss, a failure, or an arrest prior to completed suicide.

Assessment of Suicide Risk

The best assessment of suicide risk comes from a high index of suspicion and a direct interview with the patient and "significant others" such as family members, peers, and teachers. A format for the interview for the adolescent is provided in Table 7–16.

The highest risk of suicide is associated with older white adolescent boys who express an intention to die, especially when they are away from other family members. Previous suicide attempts, a written note,

Table 7–16. Clinical interview to assess suicide risk.

1. An observation or change has been noted.
2. How have you been feeling (inside/emotionally)?
3. Have you had periods of feeling down or discouraged?
   a. How often?
   b. How long?
   c. How severe?
4. Do they interfere with your life?
   a. Daily activities?
   b. School or work?
   c. Sleep or appetite (or both)?
   d. Family life?
5. Do you have feelings of
   a. Self-criticism or worthlessness?
   b. Helplessness?
   c. Hopelessness?
   d. Wanting to give up?
6. Are the feelings ever so strong that life does not seem worth living? Have you had thoughts of suicide?
   a. Are you having thoughts of suicide now?
   b. How persistent are they?
   c. How much effort does it take to resist?
   d. Can you tolerate the pain you are feeling?
7. Have you made any plans to carry out suicide?
   a. What are the plans?
   b. Have you taken any tentative action (eg, obtaining a gun or rope, stockpiling pills)?
   c. As you have thought about suicide, how have you viewed the idea of death?
8. What deters you from trying suicide?
9. If the suicidal feelings are subsiding, could you resist the feelings if they returned?
10. Is there someone you can turn to for help at those times? Who?
11. Has the idea of suicide come up in the past?
    a. How often?
    b. When and under what circumstances?
    c. What has happened at those times?
12. Can you tolerate the pain that you are feeling right now?

and a viable plan for suicide with the availability of lethal means are high-risk factors. Signs and symptoms of major depression, a family history of suicide, a recent death in the family, and a view of death as a relief from the pain in their lives are further risk factors. Persons who have little or no family support, are facing a crisis in their lives at work or school, or refuse to agree not to commit suicide are also at high risk.

Principles of Intervention

The health care provider (1) must consider any suicide attempt a serious matter; (2) must not allow the patient to be left alone; (3) must make an effort to understand the young person's pain and convey a desire to help; (4) must meet with the patient and the family, both alone and together, and listen carefully to their problems and perceptions; and (5) must let these patients know that their pain and feelings of hopelessness are understood. At the same time, the health care provider should express the firm conviction that with the assistance of mental health professionals, solutions can be found.

These patients should be hospitalized if there appears to be a high potential for suicide, if they are severely depressed or intoxicated, if the family does not appear properly concerned, or if there are practical limitations to providing supervision and support and ensuring safety. Doubts about the necessity for hospitalization should be resolved in favor of that decision.

Any decision to send the patient home without hospitalization should be made only after consultation with a mental health expert. The decision should rest on a decrease in the risk of suicide and the family's ability to provide 24-hour supervision. The patient's home must be "sterilized" of guns, pills, knives, and razor blades, and the patient should be restricted from driving for at least the first 24 hours. The focus is on providing support and easing the emotional strain. Phone contact must be available, and the family must be committed to a plan for mental health treatment.

Finally, the physician should be aware of his or her own emotional reactions to dealing with potentially suicidal adolescents and their families. Because the assessment takes considerable time and energy, the physician should be on guard against becoming tired, irritable, or angry. The parents should not be blamed. The physician need not be afraid of precipitating suicide by direct and frank discussions of suicidal risk.

Hendin H: Psychodynamics of suicide, with particular reference to the young. Am J Psychiatry 1991;148:1150.
Suicide among children, adolescents, and young adults—United States, 1980–1992. JAMA 1995;274:451. (Editorial.)

THE CHRONICALLY ILL CHILD

Reactions to Chronic Illness or Disability

Five percent to 10% of children experience a prolonged period of illness or disability during childhood, and the psychosocial effects of that illness are often profound for the child and the family. Although the specific impact of illness on children and their families depends on the characteristics of the illness, the age of the child, and premorbid functioning, it can be expected that both the child and the parents will go through predictable stages toward eventual acceptance of the disease state. Shock and disbelief at the time of diagnosis give way in time to anger and to mourning the loss of the normal, healthy child. It may take months for a family to come to accept the disease, to cope with the stresses, and to resume normal life to the extent possible. These stages resemble those that follow the loss of a loved one. If anxiety and guilt remain prominent within the family, a pattern of overprotection can evolve. Likewise, when the illness is not accepted as a reality to be dealt with, a pattern of denial may become prominent. The clinical manifestations of these patterns of behavior are set forth in Table 7–17.

Assistance From Health Care Providers

A. Educate the Patient and Family: Children and their families should be given information about the illness, including its course and treatment, at frequent intervals. Factual, open discussions minimize the anxieties that are created by family secrets about the illness. The explanation should be comprehensible to all, and time should be set aside for questions and answers. The setting can be created with the invitation "Let's take some time together to review the situation again."

B. Prepare the Child for Changes and Procedures: The physician should explain what can be expected with a new turn in the illness or with upcoming medical procedures. This explanation enables the child to anticipate and in turn to master the new development and promotes trust between the patient and the health care providers.

C. Encourage the Normalization of Activities: The child should attend school and play with peers as much as the illness allows. At the same time, parents should be encouraged to apply the same rules of discipline and behavior to the ill child as are applied to normal siblings.

D. Encourage Compensatory Activities, Interests, and Skill Development: For example, a child whose athletic development has been interrupted by the disability might pursue the acquisition of computer skills.

E. Promote Self-Reliance: The health care provider should guide and encourage parents in helping ill children assume responsibility for some aspects of their medical care.

F. Periodically Review Family Coping: From time to time, the physician should ask, "How is everyone doing with this?" The feelings of the patient, the parents, and other children in the family are explored as well as concerns about finances and the status of the marriage. Feelings of fear, guilt, anger, and grief should be watched for and accepted as normal reactions to difficult circumstances.

G. Recommend Support Groups: Lay support groups for the patient and family should be used to the fullest extent.

Long-Term Coping

The process of coping with a chronic illness is an ongoing one. Each change in the course of the illness and each new developmental stage for the child presents new challenges. With each step comes the need for new and painful acceptance of the disease and its limitations.

Lavigne JV, Faier-Routman J: Psychological adjustment to pediatric physical disorders: A meta-analytic review. J Pediatr Psychol 1992;17:133.
McGrath PJ, McAlpine L: Psychological perspectives on pediatric pain. J Pediatr 1993;122(Suppl):2.

THE TERMINALLY ILL CHILD

The diagnosis of fatal illness in a child is a severe blow, even to families who have reason to suspect that outcome. Most parents face the news of a fatal illness as the worst experience of their lives, and although parents want and need to know the truth, they are best told in piecemeal fashion beginning with temporizing phrases such as "The news is not good—it's a life-threatening illness." The parents' reactions and questions can then be scrutinized for clues to how much they want to be told at any one time. Parents' reactions then proceed in a sequence of grief, including initial shock and disbelief lasting days to weeks, followed by anger, despair, and guilt over weeks to months, ending in acceptance of the loss.

Although children probably do not fully understand the permanency of death until about 8 years of age, most ill children experience a sense of danger and doom that is associated with death before that age. Even so, the question of whether to tell a child about the fatal nature of a disease should, in most cases, be answered in the affirmative unless the parents object. Refusal of the adults to tell the child—especially when the adults themselves are very sad—

Table 7–17. Patterns of coping with chronic illness.

Overprotection
Persistent anxiety or guilt
Few friends and peer activities
Poor school attendance
Overconcern with somatic symptoms
Secondary gain from the illness
Effective coping
Realistic acceptance of limits imposed by illness
Normalization of daily activities with peers, play, and school
Denial
Lack of acceptance of the illness
Poor medical compliance
Risk-taking behaviors
Lack of parental follow-through with medical instructions
General pattern of acting-out behavior

leads to a "conspiracy of silence" that increases fear of the unknown in the child and leads to feelings of loneliness and isolation at the time of greatest need. In fact, children who are able to discuss their illness with family members are less depressed, have fewer behavior problems, have higher self-esteem, feel closer to their families, and adapt better to the rigors of their disease and its treatment.

Children are very observant and intuitive when it comes to understanding their illness and its general prognosis. At the same time, their primary concerns are the effects of the illness on everyday life, feeling sick, and limitations on normal activities. Children are also keenly aware of the family's reactions and are reluctant to bring up issues they know are upsetting to their parents. Whenever possible, parents should be encouraged to discuss the child's illness and to answer questions openly and honestly, including exploration of the child's fears and fantasies. Such interactions promote closeness and relieve the child's sense of isolation. Even with these active attempts to promote effective sharing between the child and the family, ill children frequently experience fear, anxiety, irritability, and anger over their illness and guilt over causing family distress. Sleep disturbances, tears, and clingy, dependent behavior are not infrequent or abnormal.

The siblings of dying children are also significantly affected by the stress imposed on the family. They feel neglected and deprived because of the time their parents must spend with the sick child. Anger and jealousy then give rise to feelings of guilt over having such "bad" feelings about their sick sibling.

After the child dies, the period of bereavement may last up to 3 years. Family members may need outside help in dealing with their grief through supportive counseling services.

Grollman EA: *Talking About Death: A Dialogue Between Parent and Child.* Beacon, 1990.
Leach P: Will I die? Parenting 1993 (April): 105.

EFFECTS OF MARITAL DISSOLUTION

Currently, about 40% of families are destined to divorce. Seventy-five percent of divorced parents remarry, and another 50% divorce a second time. Approximately 90% of single parents are mothers, and about 50% of their children have little or no contact with the father.

Clinical Effects of Divorce

The adverse emotional effects of divorce are far-reaching for both adults and children. Many women who have been through a divorce report that it takes 3 years for a sense of order and stability to return.

There are significant effects on the parent-child relationship. First, there is a decrease in parenting capacity, which is manifested in irregularity of daily schedules, flares of temper, decreased emotional sensitivity and support of the child, inconsistent discipline, and decreased pleasure in the parent-child relationship. A tendency exists for the divorced parent to look to the child as a source of emotional support. Younger children become inappropriately close to their parents by acting as "little helpers" and parental advisors. Adolescents, on the other hand, may rebel in order to distance themselves from the emotional needs of their distressed parents.

The effects of divorce on children are most dramatically seen in the 2 years following dissolution of the marriage. Few children experience the dissolution of even turbulent marriages as a relief, because the breakup of the nuclear family is perceived as a loss of the structure that provides for their safety and support. Children would rarely choose divorce as a solution for their parents' problems.

The effects of divorce on children vary with the child's age and developmental level. Most preschoolers display a behavioral regression, experiencing fears of separation at night and when they are with baby-sitters. In addition, sleep disturbances and irritability toward parents, peers, and siblings are common. In children aged 5–8, grief, sadness, and tears predominate. These children are heartbroken and wish for reconciliation of the parents. Approximately 50% experience a decrease in school performance. In children aged 9–12, anger is the predominant affect, with the child blaming and taking sides against one or another parent. At the same time, a child at this age is at greatest risk of becoming a surrogate companion. In adolescence, anger and depression go hand in hand. In addition, teenagers are at risk of developing a sense of pessimism about their own future involvement in intimate relationships because of what they have been through in their own families.

Outcome

The most favorable outcome is for the parents to put aside old conflicts and resume caretaking relationships with their children. Younger children actually fare best, particularly when they have a support network (eg, siblings, grandparents) during the time when parents are preoccupied with their own problems. When the parents have their own adult support network, the children are not so apt to be burdened with the responsibility of caring for the parents.

At 5-year follow-up, nearly 33% of children of divorced parents are moderately depressed. At 10-year follow-up, 40% of such children report worry, underachievement, self-deprecation, and lingering anger. Upon reaching adulthood, most survivors of divorce fear repeating their parents' unhappy marriages.

Wallerstein JS: The long-term effects of divorce on children: A review. J Am Acad Child Adolesc Psychiatry 1991;30:349.

OVERVIEW OF PEDIATRIC PSYCHOPHARMACOLOGY

As with any medication, the risks versus the benefits of administering psychoactive medications must be carefully considered with the child's guardian. Not only should a diagnosable psychiatric disorder be present, but that disorder must be significantly interfering with psychosocial development, interpersonal relationships, or the patient's sense of personal well-being before intervention with psychoactive drugs can be justified. Informed consent should be given by the guardian, and noted in the record. One must remember that psychopharmacologic agents are never the only treatment for any psychiatric disorder.

A few rules of thumb apply to the use of psychoactive medications in children and adolescents. First, identify target symptoms that can be followed to evaluate the efficacy of the treatment. When initiating treatment, start with low doses and increase slowly, monitoring the side effects along with effects of the medication on the target symptoms. Divided daily doses are the rule with children and adolescents. When psychoactive medications are to be discontinued, dosages should be tapered over 2–4 weeks in order to minimize withdrawal effects.

Table 7–18 presents an overview of the clinical conditions for which psychopharmacologic agents might be considered as part of a treatment plan. In the column of "probable" indications are listed those agents whose efficacy has been established in controlled drug trials or after substantial clinical experience. The column of "possible" indications consists of agents for which uncontrolled, preliminary clinical investigations have suggested some therapeutic efficacy.

In the text that follows, the major classes of psychopharmacologic agents with probable clinical indications in child and adolescent psychiatric practice are represented. The more commonly prescribed drugs from each class are reviewed with reference to

Table 7–18. Indications for psychopharmacologic interventions in children and adolescents.[1]

Condition	Probable	Possible
ADHD	Psychostimulants, tricyclics, clonidine, bupropion	Neuroleptics, guanfacine, venlafaxine
ADD without H		Psychostimulants
Anorexia nervosa		SSRIs
Autistic disorder	Haloperidol, clomipramine, clonidine	Other neuroleptics, naltrexone
Bipolar disorder	Lithium, neuroleptics	Carbamazepine, valproate
Bulimia nervosa	SSRI's tricyclics	
Major depressive disorder		SSRIs, tricyclics, buproprion, lithium, venlafaxine
Nonspecific sedation	Diphenhydramine	
Panic disorder	Tricyclics	High-potency benzodiazepines, SSRIs
Post-traumatic stress disorder		SSRIs, beta-blockers, clonidine, lithium, carbamazepine, high-potency benzodiazepines, tricyclics
Obsessive-compulsive disorder	Clomipramine, SSRIs	
Schizophrenia	Neuroleptics	Atypical neuroleptics
Self-injurious behavior	Naltrexone	Neuroleptics, SSRIs
Separation anxiety disorder	Tricyclics	High-potency benzodiazepines, SSRIs
Severely aggressive behavior	Neuroleptics, lithium, carbamazepine	Beta-blockers, clonidine
Tourette's disorder	Haloperidol	Clonidine, tricyclics, clomipramine, SSRIs, guanfacine

[1]ADHD = attention-deficit hyperactivity disorder, SSRIs = selective serotonin reuptake inhibitors.

indications, relative contraindications, initial medical screening procedures (in addition to a general pediatric examination), dosage, adverse effects, drug interactions, and medical follow-up recommendations.

PSYCHOSTIMULANTS

Methylphenidate

A. Indications: Psychostimulants are the drugs of first choice for treating attention-deficit hyperactivity disorder (ADHD) in children and adolescents. Approximately 75% of ADHD children exhibit improved attention span, decreased hyperactivity, and decreased impulsivity when given stimulant medications. Up to 75% of children with ADHD who do not respond favorably to one stimulant will respond to another. Attention-deficit disorder (ADD) without hyperactivity appears to be somewhat responsive to the stimulant medications also.

B. Relative Contraindications: Methylphenidate is contraindicated in individuals with a personal or family history of motor tics or Tourette's syndrome. It is also contraindicated if other members of the family have known and untreated substance abuse disorders.

C. Initial Medical Screening: One should search for a history of personal or family motor tics or Tourette's syndrome. The child should be observed for involuntary movements. Height, weight, pulse, and blood pressure should be recorded.

D. Dosage: The regimen calls for 0.2–0.5 mg/kg per dose (usually 5–20 mg), administered before school and at noon, with or without another dose at 4 PM. The dose is titrated upward weekly, checking for clinical effects. Administration on weekends and during vacations is determined by the need at those times. The duration of action is approximately 3–4 hours. The sustained-release preparation (Ritalin-SR) is not as effective in some children, and the duration of action may not be as long as the purported equivalent of 10 mg of methylphenidate in the morning and at noon.

E. Adverse Effects: Often dose-related and time-limited.

1. Common adverse effects—Anorexia, weight loss, abdominal distress, headache, insomnia, dysphoria and tearfulness, irritability, lethargy or "zombie-like" appearance, mild tachycardia, mild elevation in blood pressure.

2. Less common effects—Interdose rebound of ADHD symptoms, emergence of motor tics or Tourette's syndrome, behavioral stereotypy, seizures, significant tachycardia or hypertension, depression, mania, psychotic symptoms. Reduced growth velocity is seen only during active administration. Growth rebound occurs during periods of discontinuation. There is usually no significant compromise of ulti-

mate height. Psychostimulants do not appear to predispose to future substance abuse.

F. Drug Interactions: Additive stimulant effects are seen with sympathomimetic amines (ephedrine, pseudoephedrine).

G. Medical Follow-up: Pulse, blood pressure, height, and weight should be recorded every 3–4 months and at times of dosage increases. Assess for abnormal movements at each visit.

Dextroamphetamine Sulfate

Indications, contraindications, medical screening and follow-up procedures, adverse effects, and drug interactions are the same as for methylphenidate (see above). The dosage is 2.5–10 mg per dose, administered twice daily before school and at noon, with or without another dose at 4 PM. A sustained-release preparation (Dexedrine Spansules) may have clinical effects for up to 8 hours.

Pemoline

A. Indications: Indications are as for methylphenidate and dextroamphetamine. The onset of effect may occur more gradually over 2–4 weeks.

B. Relative Contraindications: As for methylphenidate, plus history of hepatic dysfunction or disease.

C. Initial Medical Screening: As for methylphenidate, plus liver function tests.

D. Dosage: The longer half-life of pemoline allows for the administration of a single dose each morning. The usual starting dose of 37.5 mg is increased weekly by 18.75 mg to the desired clinical effect or to a maximum daily dose of 112.5 mg.

E. Adverse Effects: Generally as for methylphenidate, but with fewer cardiovascular effects and less interdose rebound. Elevated liver enzymes occur in 1–3% of children receiving pemoline; hepatotoxic effects appear to be reversible with drug discontinuation.

F. Drug Interactions: As for methylphenidate.

G. Medical Follow-up: As for methylphenidate, plus liver function tests every 6 months.

TRICYCLIC ANTIDEPRESSANTS

Imipramine

A. Indications: Imipramine is the most frequently prescribed antidepressant in children and adolescents. It has clinical efficacy in the treatment of ADHD, panic disorder, anxiety-based school refusal, separation anxiety disorder, bulimia, primary nocturnal enuresis, night terrors, and sleepwalking. It may be helpful in major depression in children and adolescents.

B. Relative Contraindications: Known cardiac disease or arrhythmia, undiagnosed syncope, known seizure disorder, family history of sudden cardiac death or cardiomyopathy, known electrolyte abnormality (with binging and purging).

C. Initial Medical Screening: The family history should be searched for sudden cardiac death and the patient's history for cardiac disease, arrhythmias, syncope, seizure disorder, or congenital hearing loss (associated with prolonged QT interval). Other screening procedures include serum electrolytes and BUN (with patients who have eating disorders), cardiac examination, and a baseline ECG.

D. Dosage: Daily dosage requirements vary considerably with different clinical disorders. Enuresis and sleep disorders can generally be treated with 25–75 mg of imipramine at bedtime, depending on the size of the child. Treatment for ADHD often requires 1–3 mg/kg/d in two divided doses. The treatment of major depressive disorder and the anxiety disorders in children and adolescents frequently requires 3–5 mg/kg/d in two divided doses. The onset of clinical effect may take 4–6 weeks to occur.

The starting dose is 1 mg/kg/d. Dosage increases of 25% are made every 4 or 5 days as tolerated to 3 mg/kg/d. Regular cardiovascular and electrocardiographic monitoring is required with each dosage increase above 3 mg/kg/d. Therapeutic antidepressant effect is most clearly associated with steady-state plasma levels of imipramine plus desipramine (see below) ranging between 150 and 300 ng/mL.

E. Adverse Effects:

1. Cardiotoxic effects—The cardiotoxic effects of tricyclic antidepressants appear to be more frequent in children and adolescents than in adults. In addition to anticholinergic effects, tricyclic antidepressants have quinidine-like effects that result in slowing of cardiac conduction. Increased plasma levels appear to be weakly associated with an increased risk of cardiac conduction abnormalities. Steady-state plasma levels of desipramine or of desipramine plus imipramine should therefore not exceed 300 ng/mL. In addition, each dosage increase above 3 mg/kg/d must be carefully monitored with pulse, blood pressure, and repeat ECGs. Upper limits for cardiovascular parameters when administering tricyclic antidepressants to children and adolescents are listed in Table 7–19.

2. Anticholinergic effects—Tachycardia, dry mouth, stuffy nose, blurred vision, constipation, sweating, vasomotor instability, withdrawal syndrome (gastrointestinal distress and psychomotor activation).

3. Other effects—Orthostatic hypotension, lowered seizure threshold, increased appetite and weight gain, sedation, irritability and psychomotor agitation, rash (often associated with yellow dye No. 5), headache, abdominal complaints, sleep disturbance and nightmares, mania.

F. Drug Interactions: Tricyclic antidepressants may potentiate the effects of central nervous system depressants and stimulants; barbiturates and

Table 7–19. Upper limits of cardiovascular parameters with tricyclic antidepressants.

Heart rate	≤130/min
Systolic blood pressure	≤130 mm Hg
Diastolic blood pressure	≤85 mm Hg
PR interval	≤0.20 s
QRS interval	≤0.12 s, or no more than 30% over baseline
QT corrected	≤0.45 s

cigarette smoking may decrease plasma levels; phenothiazines, methylphenidate, and oral contraceptives may increase plasma levels; tachycardia may be more pronounced with marihuana.

G. Medical Follow-up: Pulse and blood pressure with each dosage increase up to 3 mg/kg/d; pulse, blood pressure, and ECG with each dosage increase above 3 mg/kg/d; height, weight, pulse, blood pressure, and ECG every 3–4 months at steady state.

Desipramine

A. Indications: As for imipramine, but often preferred over that drug because of fewer anticholinergic side effects. Suppression of tics in Tourette's syndrome has recently been reported.

B. Relative Contraindications: As for imipramine.

C. Initial Medical Screening: As for imipramine.

D. Dosage: As for imipramine. Steady-state plasma levels of desipramine should be between 150 and 300 ng/mL. Plasma levels above 300 ng/mL or total doses greater than 5 mg/kg/d should be avoided. As with imipramine, careful attention must be paid to pulse, blood pressure, and ECG with dosage increases above 3 mg/kg/d.

E. Adverse Effects: As for imipramine, except less prominent anticholinergic effects. There has also been concern about five unexplained instances of sudden death in children taking desipramine. The evidence to date does not support a causal link (Biederman, 1995).

F. Drug Interactions: As for imipramine.

G. Medical Follow-up: As for imipramine.

Nortriptyline

Indications, contraindications, initial medical screening procedures, and drug interactions are as listed above for imipramine.

A. Dosage: Daily dosage for major depressive disorder ranges from 0.5 to 2 mg/kg/d in two divided doses. Therapeutic antidepressant effects appear to be associated with plasma levels between 60 and 100 ng/mL in children.

B. Adverse Effects: As for imipramine, but with fewer anticholinergic effects. Daily doses should not exceed 2 mg/kg/d, and plasma levels should not exceed 150 ng/mL.

C. Medical Follow-up: Careful cardiac monitoring with dosage increases.

Clomipramine

A. Indications: Clomipramine has been shown to be effective in the treatment of obsessive-compulsive disorder in children and adolescents, resulting in moderate to marked symptomatic improvement in 75% of individuals by week 5 of treatment. The effects of clomipramine in the management of obsessive-compulsive disorder appear to be independent of the drug's antidepressant effect. Clomipramine also appears to be helpful in reducing the repetitive, ritualized behaviors of some autistic children (Gordon, 1993).

B. Relative Contraindications: As for imipramine.

C. Initial Medical Screening: As for imipramine, plus liver function tests.

D. Dosage: The initial daily dose of 1 mg/kg/d is advanced gradually to a target dose of approximately 3 mg/kg/d (with a maximum daily dose of 200 mg/d). Therapeutic blood levels are not yet established. In prepubertal children, daily doses are given in two divided doses.

E. Adverse Effects: As for imipramine. Some hepatotoxicity has been noted. Clomipramine appears to be as well tolerated as desipramine or imipramine.

F. Drug Interactions: As for imipramine.

G. Medical Follow-up: As for imipramine.

SELECTIVE SEROTONIN REUPTAKE INHIBITORS (SSRIs)

Fluoxetine

A. Indications: Fluoxetine is a nontricyclic SSRI that is receiving great clinical attention because of its favorable side effect profile, its relative lack of cardiotoxicity, and its wide margin of safety in overdose situations. It is probably indicated in the treatment of major depressive disorder in adolescents, particularly when there may be a greater risk of drug overdose. Fluoxetine also appears to be helpful in child and adolescent anxiety disorders (especially obsessive-compulsive disorder) and eating disorders.

B. Relative Contraindications: Known liver disease or bipolar disorder.

C. Initial Medical Screening: General medical examination only.

D. Dosage: The major metabolites of fluoxetine have half-lives of approximately 1 week. This allows for once-daily or even alternate-day dosing. The initial daily dose of 5–10 mg is increased by 5–10 mg every 1–2 weeks as tolerated to a maximum dose of 40 mg/d. Antidepressant response is generally achieved in adolescents on daily doses of 20–40 mg by the sixth week of treatment. Fluoxetine is usually administered as a single morning dose but may be divided into morning and noon doses if side effects so dictate.

E. Adverse Effects: Often dose-related and time-limited; gastrointestinal distress, nausea, headache, tremulousness, anorexia and weight loss, insomnia. Adverse behavioral activation can occur in approximately 20% of children taking SSRIs. This can include irritability, social disinhibition, restlessness, and emotional excitability (Tierney, 1995).

F. Drug Interactions: All SSRIs inhibit the efficiency of the hepatic P450 microsomal enzyme system. This can lead to higher than expected blood levels of other drugs, including antidepressants, antiarrhythmics, antipsychotics, beta-blockers, opiates, and the antihistamines terfenadine and astemizole ("The P450 Family," 1995). Tryptophan may result in a serotoninergic syndrome of psychomotor agitation and gastrointestinal distress.

G. Medical Follow-up: General medical examination with weight and blood pressure.

Sertraline & Paroxetine

A. Indications: As for fluoxetine.

B. Relative Contraindications: As for fluoxetine.

C. Initial Medical Screening: General medical examination.

D. Dosage: Both sertraline and paroxetine have shorter half-lives (approximately 1–2 days) than fluoxetine (approximately 1 week). This still generally allows for once-daily dosing, usually in the morning. Therapeutic doses of sertraline range from 50 to 150 mg/d, while therapeutic doses of paroxetine range from 10 to 40 mg/d.

E. Adverse Effects: As for fluoxetine.

F. Drug Interactions: As for fluoxetine, but sertraline may inhibit cytochrome P450 hepatic enzymes *less* than do fluoxetine and paroxetine.

G. Medical Follow-up: As for fluoxetine.

OTHER ANTIDEPRESSANTS

Bupropion

A. Indications: Bupropion is a nontricyclic antidepressant that is receiving favorable attention for its therapeutic effects with major depressive disorder in adolescents and with ADHD in children and adolescents (Barrickman, 1995). Like the SSRIs, bupropion has very few anticholinergic or cardiotoxic effects.

B. Relative Contraindications: History of seizure disorder. Teratogenic effects are uncertain.

C. Initial Medical Screening: General medical examination if there is a history of seizures.

D. Dosage: The dosage is not well established, but the range is thought to be from 150 to 375 mg/d in two or three divided doses. The maximum daily dosage in adolescents should be less than 450 mg.

E. Adverse Effects: Psychomotor activation (agitation or restlessness), headache, gastrointestinal distress, nausea, anorexia with weight loss, insomnia, tremulousness, precipitation of mania, and the induction of seizures with doses above 450 mg/d.

F. Drug Interactions: Uncertain.

G. Medical Follow-up: General medical examination.

Venlafaxine

A. Indications: Venlafaxine is a nontricyclic non-SSRI antidepressant that inhibits reuptake of serotonin and norepinephrine. It appears to be a useful antidepressant in children and adolescents, and perhaps also in ADHD.

B. Relative Contraindications: None known.

C. Initial Medical Screening: No specific issues.

D. Dosage: Not well established for children; 50–200 mg/d, divided into two doses, is probably appropriate.

E. Adverse Effects: Has had fewer anticholinergic, antihistaminic, and antiadrenergic side effects than the tricyclic antidepressants. The most common adverse effects were nausea, nervousness, and sweating. Like other antidepressants, venlafaxine can induce a manic switch in depressed bipolar patients.

F. Drug Interactions: Weak inhibitor of hepatic cytochrome P450 enzymes.

G. Medical Follow-up: No specific issues known.

NEUROLEPTICS

The neuroleptics—also known as antipsychotics—are most clearly indicated for the psychotic symptoms in schizophrenia. They are also used for acute mania and as an adjunct to antidepressants in the treatment of psychotic depression (with delusions or hallucinations). They can be used very cautiously in refractory ADHD and in individuals with markedly aggressive behavioral problems.

Haloperidol

A. Indications: Haloperidol can also suppress tics in Tourette's syndrome and specific target symptoms in autistic disorder.

B. Relative Contraindications: Haloperidol is contraindicated in patients with a history of poorly controlled seizures, cardiac arrhythmias, or agranulocytosis, previous neuroleptic malignant syndrome, or tardive dyskinesia.

C. Initial Medical Screening: One should observe and examine for abnormal movements and establish baseline CBC and liver function tests. An ECG should be taken if there is a history of cardiac disease or arrhythmia.

D. Dosage: Conservative treatment starts with 0.5–1 mg/d in two daily doses, increasing by 0.5 mg every 3–5 days to clinical effect, side effects, or a maximum daily dose of 4 mg. Daily doses above 4 mg should be reserved for the most disturbed and refractory patients. Antipsychotic effects may take 2–3 weeks to become fully apparent.

E. Adverse Effects: The two most troublesome adverse effects are cognitive slowing resulting from sedation and/or extrapyramidal syndromes. The high-potency neuroleptics (eg, haloperidol) cause less sedation but have a greater frequency of extrapyramidal effects. The low-potency neuroleptics (eg, thioridazine) can cause greater sedation but fewer extrapyramidal effects. In any case, sedation, cognitive slowing, and extrapyramidal effects all tend to be dose-related. Because of the risk of tardive dyskinesia, neuroleptic medications should be reserved for children and adolescents for whom less harmful treatments are not available.

1. Extrapyramidal syndromes—Acute dystonic reactions are tonic muscle spasms, often of the tongue, jaw, or neck, which may result in such dramatically distressing symptoms as oculogyric crisis, torticollis, and even opisthotonos. The onset usually occurs within days after a dosage change and may occur in up to 25% of children treated with neuroleptics. Thioridazine is much less frequently associated with dystonic reactions. Acute neuroleptic-induced dystonias are quickly relieved by anticholinergics such as diphenhydramine.

2. Pseudoparkinsonism—Pseudoparkinsonism is usually manifested 1–4 weeks after the start of treatment. It presents as muscle stiffness, cogwheel rigidity, masked facies, bradykinesia, drooling, and occasionally pill-rolling tremor. Anticholinergic medications or dosage reductions are helpful.

3. Akathisia—Akathisia is usually manifested after 1–6 weeks of treatment. It presents as a very unpleasant feeling of driven motor restlessness that ranges from vague muscular discomfort to a markedly dysphoric agitation with frantic pacing. Anticholinergic agents or beta-blockers are sometimes helpful.

4. Neuroleptic malignant syndrome—This is a medical emergency manifested by severe muscular rigidity, altered sensorium, hyperpyrexia, autonomic lability, and myoglobinemia. Mortality rates have been reported as high as 30%.

5. "Rabbit syndrome"—This is a rare parkinsonian-like tremor of the mouth that develops late, presenting as rapid chewing-like movements similar to what is observed in rabbits.

6. Withdrawal symptoms—Dyskinesias are reversible movement disorders that appear following the withdrawal of neuroleptic drugs. They occur in up to 25% of children exposed to neuroleptics for 1 year and in approximately 50% of those exposed to neuroleptics for 2½ years. After withdrawal of the drug, dyskinetic movements develop within 1–4 weeks and may then persist for months before resolving.

7. Tardive dyskinesias—Tardive dyskinesias are the dreaded late-developing, irreversible movement disorders that appear after long-term use of neuroleptic medications. They most often present as choreoathetoid movements of the tongue and mouth but may also involve the extremities and trunk. The risk of tardive dyskinesia is thought to be small in patients exposed to neuroleptics for less than 6 months. There is no effective treatment.

8. Other adverse effects of neuroleptics—Orthostatic hypotension, cardiac arrhythmias, anticholinergic effects, weight gain, irregular menses, gynecomastia (even galactorrhea), sexual dysfunction, photosensitivity, rashes, lowered seizure threshold, hepatic dysfunction, blood dyscrasias.

F. Drug Interactions: Potentiation of central nervous system depressant effects or the anticholinergic effects of other drugs may occur, as well as increased plasma levels of antidepressants.

G. Medical Follow-up: One should examine the patient at least every 3 months for signs of tardive dyskinesia.

Thioridazine

Thioridazine is effective in the treatment of psychotic disorders and severely aggressive disorders. It is not helpful for Tourette's syndrome.

The relative contraindications and initial medical screening are as for haloperidol. The dose ranges from 20 to 200 mg/d, divided into two doses. The adverse effects resemble those for haloperidol, although thioridazine is considered less likely to cause acute dystonic reactions and pseudoparkinsonian effects. In doses above 800 mg/d, thioridazine is associated with retinitis pigmentosa. Drug interactions and medical follow-up are as for haloperidol.

ATYPICAL NEUROLEPTICS

Risperidone

Risperidone blocks type 2 serotonin in addition to type 2 dopamine receptors. Adult schizophrenics given 2–8 mg/d of risperidone had better symptom relief and fewer side effects than those treated with conventional neuroleptics. Anecdotal reports suggest that similar results may be obtained in adolescents with schizophrenia (Quintana, 1995). The initial dose is 1–6 mg/d, divided into two doses. The relative contraindications, initial medical screening, adverse effects, drug interactions, and medical follow-up are as for haloperidol.

Clozapine

Clozapine blocks type 2 dopamine receptors weakly and is virtually free from extrapyramidal side effects, apparently including tardive dyskinesia. It was very effective in some 40% of chronic adult schizophrenics who did not respond to conventional neuroleptics. It has an important non–dose-related adverse effect, agranulocytosis, in 0.5–2% of subjects. Of 200 subjects who developed agranulocytosis, 7 died. There are case reports of benefit from clozapine in child and adolescent schizophrenics resistant to other treatment.

Any history of leukopenia, or concurrent treatment with carbamazepine, is a relative contraindication. Initial medical screening is with a CBC and liver function tests. The daily dose is 200–600 mg, divided between two doses. Because of the risk of neutropenia, patients taking clozapine must be registered with the clozapine registry and a WBC count must be obtained weekly, before a 1-week supply of the drug is dispensed. If the WBC count falls below 3000, clozapine is usually discontinued. Other side effects include sedation, weight gain, and increased salivation. The incidence of seizures increases with doses above 600 mg/d.

MOOD STABILIZERS

Lithium Carbonate

A. Indications: Lithium remains a front-line drug in the treatment of bipolar mood disorder. It may be helpful also in the treatment of patients with severely aggressive symptoms, emotionally unstable behavior disorders, and behaviorally disturbed children whose parents are known lithium responders. Lithium has sometimes been shown to have an augmenting effect when combined with SSRIs in individuals with treatment-resistant depression and obsessive-compulsive disorder.

B. Relative Contraindications: Lithium is contraindicated in patients with known renal, thyroid, or cardiac disease; those at high risk for dehydration and electrolyte imbalance (eg, vomiting and purging); and those at risk of pregnancy (teratogenic effects).

C. Initial Medical Screening: General medical screening with pulse, blood pressure, height, and weight; CBC; serum electrolytes, BUN, and creatinine; and thyroid function tests with TSH.

D. Dosage: Oral doses of lithium up to 1800 mg/d are frequently necessary to maintain therapeutic blood levels of 1–1.5 meq/L. Daily dosage is generally given in three divided doses—or two doses with sustained-release lithium preparations. Lithium blood level samples should be drawn 12 hours after the last dose.

E. Adverse Effects:

1. Lithium toxicity—Lithium has a low therapeutic index—that is, blood levels required for therapeutic effects are close to blood levels that produce toxic symptoms. Mild symptoms of toxicity include increased tremor, gastrointestinal distress, neuromuscular irritability, and altered consciousness that can be seen with blood levels above 1.5 meq/L. Moderate to severe symptoms of lithium toxicity are associated with blood levels above 2 meq/L.

2. Common lithium side effects—Intention tremor, gastrointestinal distress (including nausea and vomiting and sometimes diarrhea), polyuria and polydipsia, drowsiness, malaise, weight gain, acne, granulocytosis.

3. Uncommon lithium side effects—Lithium-induced hypothyroidism, chronic renal disease, unknown effects on developing bone.

F. Drug Interactions: Excessive salt intake and salt restriction should be avoided. Thiazide diuretics and nonsteroidal anti-inflammatory agents (except aspirin and acetaminophen) lead to increased lithium levels. Precautions against dehydration are required in hot weather and with vigorous exercise.

G. Medical Follow-up: Serum lithium levels should be measured 5–7 days following a change in dosage and then monthly at steady state; serum creatinine and TSH concentrations should be determined every 3–4 months.

Valproate

A. Indications: Valproate is a front-line medication for bipolar disorder in adults. Its efficacy in acute mania equals that of lithium, but it is generally better tolerated. Valproate is more effective than lithium in patients with rapid bipolar cycling (more than four cycles per year) and in patients with mixed states (coexisting symptoms of depression and mania). Valproate may be more effective than lithium in adolescents with bipolar disorder because they often have rapid cycling and mixed states.

B. Relative Contraindications: Liver dysfunction.

C. Initial Medical Screening: CBC and liver function tests.

D. Dosage: Usually starts at 15 mg/kg/d and is increased in increments of 5–10 mg/kg/d every 1–2 weeks to a range of 500–1500 mg/d, divided into two or three doses. Trough levels in the range of 80–120 µg/mL are thought to be therapeutic.

E. Adverse Effects: Ten percent to 20% of patients experience sedation and/or anorexia, particularly early in treatment or if the dose is increased too rapidly. Gastrointestinal upset occurs in 25% of patients and, when severe, can usually be treated with cimetidine. Increased appetite and weight gain can be problematic for adolescents. Blurred vision,

headache, hair loss, and tremor occur occasionally. Slight elevations in transaminases are frequent. Severe idiosyncratic hepatitis, pancreatitis, and agranulocytosis occur only rarely.

F. Medical Follow-up: Serum alanine transaminase should be checked every 3–4 weeks for 3–4 months. Subsequently, alanine transaminase, CBC, and trough valproate levels should be obtained every 3–4 months.

ALPHA-ADRENERGIC AGONISTS

Clonidine

A. Indications: Clonidine is a nonselective, alpha-adrenergic agonist that has been found to be clinically useful in decreasing states of hyperarousal. It seems to be particularly helpful as an adjunct to methylphenidate in children with ADHD when the history is of very early onset of marked hyperactivity, aggression, and oppositional behavior. Bedtime doses of clonidine can be helpful with the delayed onset of sleep that can be seen with ADHD or stimulant medication effects (Wilens, 1994). It is also frequently effective in the treatment of ADHD and tics in Tourette's syndrome and in states of hyperarousal associated with post-traumatic stress disorder. Clonidine also appears helpful with ADHD-like symptoms in some autistic children (Frankhauser, 1992).

B. Relative Contraindications: Clonidine is contraindicated in patients with known renal or cardiovascular disease and those with a family or personal history of depression.

C. Initial Medical Screening: The pulse and blood pressure should be recorded and a baseline ECG taken.

D. Dosage: Initial dosage of clonidine is 0.05 mg at bedtime; that dose is increased after 3–5 days by giving 0.05 mg also in the morning; and further dosage increases are made by adding 0.05 mg alternating in the morning, at noon, or in the evening every 3–5 days to a maximum total daily dose of 0.3 mg (3–5 µg/kg/d) in three or four divided doses per day. The half-life of clonidine is in the range of 3–4 hours. Although a clinical response generally becomes apparent by about 4 weeks, treatment effects may increase over 2–3 months. Therapeutic doses of methylphenidate can frequently be decreased by 30–50% when used in conjunction with clonidine.

Transdermal administration of clonidine using a skin patch can be quite effective but may result in significant skin irritation in 40% of cases. Patches are generally changed every 5 days.

E. Adverse Effects: Sedation can be prominent. Other side effects include fatigability, mild hypotension, increased appetite and weight gain, headache, sleep disturbance, gastrointestinal distress, skin irritation with transdermal administration, and rebound hypertension with abrupt withdrawal. Bradycardia can occasionally be pronounced.

F. Drug Interactions: Increased sedation with central nervous system depressants; possible cardiotoxicity with cocaine; increased anticholinergic toxicity.

G. Medical Follow-up: Pulse and blood pressure should be recorded every 2 weeks for 2 months, and then every 3 months. The discontinuation of clonidine should occur gradually, at a rate of 0.05 mg every 3 days, to avoid rebound hypertension. Blood pressure should be monitored during the withdrawal.

Guanfacine

Guanfacine is a selective agonist for alpha$_{2A}$-adrenergic receptors with advantages over the nonselective agonist clonidine. Guanfacine is less sedating, is less hypotensive, and has a longer half-life, allowing for twice-daily dosing. Case reports find guanfacine effective in ADHD (Hunt, 1995) and Tourette's disorder with comorbid ADHD (Chappel, 1995).

Relative contraindications are as for clonidine. An initial medical screening should record pulse and blood pressure. The dose is 2–4 mg/d, divided into two or three doses. Adverse effects include transient headaches and/or stomachaches in 25% of patients. Sedation and hypertension are mild. For medical follow-up, pulse and blood pressure should be checked every 1–2 weeks for 2 months, and then at 3-month intervals.

BETA-ADRENERGIC BLOCKERS

Propranolol

A. Indications: Propranolol is a nonselective beta-adrenoceptor blocking agent that reduces peripheral autonomic tone and in that way ameliorates the somatic symptoms of anxiety, including palpitations, tremulousness, sweating, and blushing. Propranolol appears to have clinical efficacy in the treatment of performance anxiety (stage fright), post-traumatic stress disorder, episodic outbursts of rage, lithium-induced tremor, and neuroleptic-induced akathisia.

B. Relative Contraindications: Propranolol should not be given to patients with a history of diabetes, cardiovascular disease, reactive airway disease, and depression.

C. Initial Medical Screening: Pulse and blood pressure should be recorded, as well as the fasting blood sugar in patients with a family history of diabetes.

D. Dosage: Daily doses for prepubertal children range from 10 to 120 mg/d and for adolescents from 20 to 300 mg/d. Blood pressure should be kept above 90/60 mm Hg in adolescents, and the pulse

should be kept above 60/min. The drug is usually given in three divided daily doses.

E. Adverse Effects: Sedation, fatigue, bradycardia, hypotension, bronchospasm, depression, sleep disturbance, hypoglycemia in diabetics, sexual dysfunction.

F. Drug Interactions: Propranolol may inhibit the action of sympathomimetics and xanthines.

G. Medical Follow-up: Pulse and blood pressure must be closely monitored.

OPIOID ANTAGONIST

Naltrexone

A. Indications: Naltrexone is helpful in some cases of autistic disorder and in the management of self-injurious behavior in autistic and mentally retarded individuals.

B. Dosage: A single oral daily dose of 0.5–1.5 mg/kg has been found to decrease self-injurious behavior, social withdrawal, hyperactivity, and stereotypy.

C. Adverse Effects: Sedation.

Alvir J et al: Clozapine induced agranulocytosis. N Engl J Med 1993;329:162.

Barrickman LL et al: Bupropion vs. methylphenidate in the treatment of ADHD. J Am Acad Child Adolesc Psychiatry 1995;34:649.

Biederman J et al: Estimation of the association between desipramine and the risk for sudden death in 5–14 yr old children. J Clin Psychiatry 1995;56:87.

Birmayer B et al: Fluoxetine for childhood anxiety disorders. J Am Acad Child Adolesc Psychiatry 1994;33:993.

Campbell M et al: Lithium in hospitalized aggressive children with conduct disorder: A double blind and placebo-controlled study. J Am Acad Child Adolesc Psychiatry 1995;34:445.

Chappel PB et al: Guanfacine treatment of comorbid ADHD and Tourette's syndrome: Preliminary clinical experience. J Am Acad Child Adolesc Psychiatry 1995;34:140.

Crewe HK et al: The effects of SSRI's on cytochrome P4502D6 (CYP2D6) activity in human liver microenzymes. Br J Clin Pharmacol 1992;34:262.

Frankhauser MP et al: A double-blind, placebo controlled study of the efficacy of transdermal clonidine in autism. J Clin Psychiatry 1992;53:77.

Gordon CT et al: A double-blind comparison of clomipramine, desipramine, and placebo in the treatment of autistic disorder. Arch Gen Psychiatry 1993;50:441.

Hunt RD et al: An open trial of guanfacine in the treatment of ADHD. J Am Acad Child Adolesc Psychiatry 1995;34:50.

Morton WA et al: Venlafaxine: A structurally unique and novel antidepressant. Ann Pharmacother 1995;29:387.

The P450 family. Biol Ther Psychiatry Newsl 1995;18:29.

Pickar D, Hsiao JK: Clozapine treatment of schizophrenia. JAMA 1995;274:981.

Quintana H, Keshavan M: Case study: Risperidone in children and adolescents with schizophrenia. J Am Acad Child Adolesc Psychiatry 1995;34:1292.

Remschmidt H et al: An open trial of clozapine in 36 adolescents with schizophrenia. J Child Adolesc Psychopharmacol 1994;4:31.

Risperidone. Biol Ther Psychiatry Newsl 1993;16:45.

Settle EC: Bupropion: Update 1993. Int Drug Ther Newsl 1993;28:29.

Tierney E et al: Sertraline for major depression in children and adolescents: Preliminary clinical experience. J Child Adolesc Psychopharmacol 1995;5:13.

Venlafaxine offers an alternative to stimulants. Clin Psychiatry News 1995 (July):p 5.

West SA et al: An open trial of valproate in the treatment of adolescent mania. J Child Adolesc Psychopharmacol 1994;4:263.

Wilens T et al: Nortriptyline in the treatment of ADHD: A chart review of 58 cases. J Am Acad Child Adolesc Psychiatry 1993;32:343.

Wilens T et al: Clonidine for sleep disturbances associated with ADHD. J Am Acad Child Adolesc Psychiatry 1994;33:424.

8

Child Abuse & Neglect

Richard D. Krugman, MD

The problem of child abuse and neglect, barely recognized as a significant problem in the earliest editions of this textbook, has grown to a problem of such serious proportions that the United States Advisory Board on Child Abuse and Neglect called the present state of the nation's ability to protect children a "national emergency." What Kempe and colleagues called "battered child syndrome" was thought to affect 749 children in the United States in 1960. The best data now suggest that 2–2.5% of American children are abused or neglected annually. In 1994, there were just over 3 million reports of abuse and neglect, with 1.2 million of these substantiated by child protective service agencies. This dramatic increase in cases has resulted from significantly increased recognition of the problem by professionals, in part from the influence of mandatory reporting statutes; a broadening of the definition of abuse and neglect from the original "battered child" concept; and changes in the demography and social structure of families and neighborhoods over the past several decades. Abuse and neglect of children are best considered in an ecologic perspective that recognizes the individual, family, social, and psychologic influences that come together to contribute to the problem. For most pediatric health care professionals, however, their involvement will be limited to individual cases. This chapter, therefore, focuses on the knowledge necessary for the recognition, intervention, and follow-up of the more common forms of child maltreatment and highlight the role of pediatric professionals in prevention.

FORMS OF CHILD MALTREATMENT

It should be noted that the forms of maltreatment briefly described in the text that follows may occur either within or outside the family. The proportion of intrafamilial to extrafamilial cases varies with the type of abuse as well as the gender and age of the child.

Physical Abuse

Physical abuse, or nonaccidental trauma, occurs when injury is inflicted on children, most often by a caretaker but occasionally by strangers. The most common manifestations of physical abuse include bruises, burns, fractures, and head and abdominal injuries. A small but significant number of unexpected deaths of infants and children are related to physical abuse.

Sexual Abuse

Sexual abuse is defined as the engaging of dependent, developmentally immature children in sexual activities that they do not fully comprehend and to which they cannot give informed consent or which violate the laws and taboos of a society. It includes pedophilia and all forms of incest, and rape. It also involves fondling, oral-genital contact, and all forms of intercourse, exhibitionism, voyeurism, and the involvement of children in the production of pornography.

Emotional Abuse

Emotional abuse—or, more broadly, "psychologic abuse"—has been defined as the rejection, ignoring, criticizing, isolation, or terrorizing of children, all of which have the effect of eroding their self-esteem. The most common form is verbal abuse or denigration.

Physical Neglect

Physical neglect is the failure to provide the necessities of food, clothing, shelter, and a safe environment in which children can grow and develop normally. Although associated with poverty, these cases involve a more serious problem than just absence of financial resources. There is often a component of emotional neglect and an inability to recognize and respond to the needs of the child.

Emotional Neglect

The most common feature of emotional neglect is the absence of normal parent-child attachment and a subsequent inability to recognize and respond to an infant's or child's needs. The most common manifestation of emotional neglect in infancy is nutritional (nonorganic) failure to thrive.

Medical Care Neglect

Medical care neglect is failure to provide needed treatment to infants or children who have generally life-threatening or other serious medical conditions.

Münchausen Syndrome by Proxy

This is a relatively unusual disorder in which a caretaker, usually the mother, either simulates or creates the symptoms or signs of illness in the child.

RECOGNITION OF ABUSE & NEGLECT

Recognition of abuse and neglect of children can occur only if the possibility is entertained in the differential diagnosis of the condition for which the child is brought for care. The approach to the family should be supportive, empathic, and nonaccusatory. The person who brings the child for care may not have any involvement in the abuse. Approximately one-third of the incidents of child abuse occur in extrafamilial settings. Nevertheless, the assumption that the caretaker is "nice," combined with failure to raise the possibility of abuse can be costly, even fatal. Nearly 95% of the American public is aware of the existence of child abuse and neglect. Raising the possibility that a child has been abused in a neutral, calm manner is *not* the same as accusing the caretaker of being the abuser. The health professional who is examining the child can explain to the family that there are several reasons that might explain the injuries or abuse-related symptoms the child has. If the family (or whoever brings the child for evaluation) is not involved, they will welcome a report and investigation.

History

The medical diagnosis of **physical abuse** is based on the presence of a "discrepant history." The history offered by the caretaker does not accord with the clinical findings. The "discrepancy" may exist because there is no history, a partial history, changing histories over time, or simply an illogical or improbable history. The presence of a discrepant history should lead to a request for consultation with a multidisciplinary child protection team or a report to the child protective services agency mandated by state law to receive and investigate reports of suspected child abuse and neglect. It may take a social services or law enforcement investigation and home visit to sort out the circumstances of the child's injuries. Other features that are present in many abuse cases are listed in Table 8–1.

Sexual abuse may present in three different ways. (1) The child may be brought in for routine care or for an acute problem, and sexual abuse may be suspected by the examining professional as a result of the history obtained or physical findings found. (2) The parent or other caretaker may bring the child

Table 8–1. Common historical features in abuse cases.

Discrepant history
Delay in seeking care
Stressed caretaker
Behavior by child that triggered assault
History of abuse in caretaker's childhood
Unrealistic expectations of caretaker for child
Social isolation of caretaker
Pattern of increased severity of injury if no intervention
Use of multiple hospitals or caretakers for injuries to child

to the pediatric health care provider because of a suspicion that the child may have been sexually abused, asking for an examination to "rule in or rule out" the possibility. (3) The child may be referred by child protective services or law enforcement personnel for an evidentiary examination following disclosure by the child or an allegation by a parent or third party. Table 8–2 lists the numerous ways sexual abuse may present in children. It should be emphasized that with the exception of certain sexually transmitted diseases and forensic laboratory findings, none of these presentations is specific. They should, however, raise the possibility of abuse and lead the practitioner to ask about the possibility of abuse—again, in a compassionate, nonaccusatory way. The American Academy of Pediatrics has recently published guidelines for the evaluation of child sexual abuse by primary care physicians.

Emotional abuse may cause nonspecific symptoms in children. Loss of self-esteem or self-confidence, sleep disturbances, somatic symptoms (eg, headaches, stomachaches), hypervigilance, or avoidant or phobic behaviors (eg, refusal to go to school or running away) may be presenting symptoms or complaints. Emotional abuse can occur in the

Table 8–2. Presentations of sexual abuse.

General or direct statements about sexual abuse
Sexualized play in developmentally immature children
Medical conditions
    Recurrent abdominal pain
    Genital, urethral, or anal trauma
    Sexually transmitted diseases
    Recurrent urinary tract infections
    Enuresis or encopresis
    Pregnancy
Behavioral changes
    Sleep disturbances (eg, nightmares, night terrors)
    Appetite disturbances (eg, anorexia, bulimia)
    Neurotic or conduct disorders
    Withdrawal, guilt, or depression
    Temper tantrums, aggressive behavior
    Suicidal or runaway threats or behaviors
    Hysterical or conversion reactions
    Excessive masturbation
School problems
Substance abuse
Promiscuity, prostitution
Sexual abuse of other children by the victim

home or in day care, school, sports team, or other settings.

Neglect of children is not easily documented on history. **Physical neglect**—which must be differentiated from the effects of poverty—will be present even after the provision of adequate social services to families in financial need. Neglectful parents appear to have an inability to recognize the physical or emotional states of their children. Emotionally neglectful parents respond differently to their children than do nurturing parents. A baby's cry may be perceived as an expression of anger at the parent, which can then be ignored. If hunger cries are misinterpreted in this way, the infant may not get adequate food, leading to failure to thrive.

The history offered in cases of **failure to thrive** is often discrepant with the findings as well. Infants who have dropped below the third percentile or who have experienced a significant deceleration in the growth curve are probably not receiving adequate amounts and appropriate types of food, in spite of a history that the infant takes adequate amounts of formula daily. In such cases, out-of-home placement is usually followed by a dramatic weight gain.

The hallmark of cases of **Münchausen syndrome by proxy** is that children have repeated visits to health care providers for unexplained illnesses. When the physician begins to think that the child he is seeing is a possible subject for a "case report," it may be time to think of this possibility.

Physical Findings

The physical findings of **physically abused** children include bruises, burns, lacerations, scars, bony deformities, alopecia, dental trauma, and, in the case of head or abdominal trauma, findings consistent with these injuries. The bruises of physically abused children are sometimes patterned (eg, belt marks, looped electric cord marks, oval grab marks) and are usually found over the soft tissue areas of the body. Toddlers or older children who sustain accidental bruising usually do so over bony prominences. *Any* bruise in an infant not yet developmentally able to be mobile should be viewed with concern. Lacerations of the frenulum and bruising of the lips are associated with forced feeding. Burns may also exhibit pathognomonic features. Scald burns in stocking or glove distribution, immersion burns of the buttocks, sometimes with a "doughnut hole" area of sparing, and cigarette burns are most common. The absence of splash marks or a pattern consistent with a spillage are helpful in differentiating accidental from nonaccidental burns.

The physical findings of **sexually abused children** have been reviewed recently in two atlases. It is important to realize that children who are victims of sexual abuse may have no physical findings attributable to the abuse. Similarly, there are abnormalities of the genital and rectal regions that are nonspecific and, in the absence of a history, mean little or nothing. Children who present to the practitioner with the symptoms and signs of sexually transmitted diseases should be strongly suspected of having been sexually abused. The presence of gonorrhea or syphilis in children after the perinatal period is diagnostic of sexual abuse. Chlamydial infection, HSV-2 infections, trichomoniasis, and venereal warts in children all are probably sexually transmitted, although the course and duration of these perinatally acquired infections may be protracted. This possibility must be considered as part of the evaluation.

Children with nonorganic **failure to thrive** have an absence of subcutaneous fat in the cheeks, buttocks, and extremities. If the condition has persisted for some time, they may also appear and act depressed. Older children who have been emotionally neglected for long periods may also have short stature ("deprivation dwarfism"). The head circumference in children with emotional neglect and failure to thrive is usually normal, giving these children the appearance of relative macrocephaly. If the head circumference has also decreased in its relative percentiles, the likelihood of more serious and possibly permanent developmental delay is greater.

Children with Münchausen syndrome by proxy present, if they are ill, with the physical findings of whatever illness is factitiously induced. Among reported presentations are children with dehydration resulting from induced diarrhea or vomiting, the signs of sepsis when contaminated material is injected into the child, or signs of poisoning.

Radiologic & Laboratory Findings

Certain radiologic findings are strong indicators of **physical abuse:** Metaphysial "corner" or "bucket handle" fractures of the long bones in infants, spiral fractures of the long bones in nonambulatory infants, and multiple fractures of the ribs or long bones at different stages of healing are examples. These findings should trigger a search for an explanation. Skeletal surveys are particularly useful in preverbal children who are suspected of being abused. CT or MRI findings of subdural hemorrhage in infants are highly correlated with abuse, especially after the advent of infant seat restraint laws, which have dramatically reduced the incidence of head trauma in infants. Ultrasound is useful in the delineation of abdominal injuries in children, but it is not useful in the diagnosis of subdural hematomas.

Coagulation studies are useful in children who have many bruises at different ages. Various types of coagulopathy may confuse the diagnostic picture, but abuse and coagulopathy are independent entities. There is as much abuse seen in hemophilia clinics as in the general population.

Several recent reviews have discussed the differentiation of physical abuse from **osteogenesis imperfecta.** The radiologic findings are different in most cases, but there may be variants that are difficult to diagnose. If the approach to these cases—as in all cases of suspected abuse—is compassionate, empathic, and nonaccusatory, the potential harm of "mislabeling" a parent as abusive will be avoided when, in fact, the child has another physical disorder that allows signs of trauma with normal childhood activity.

The **forensic evaluation** of sexually abused children requires a setting that permits the evaluation to be done in a way that will prevent further trauma to the child. If there is a history that the child has been involved in abuse that included the possibility of ejaculation within 72 hours, an examination looking for semen, acid phosphatase, or other forensic evidence should be performed according to published protocols. If there is no recent evidence of an acute sexual encounter, the laboratory findings would be limited to a search for sexually transmitted diseases. Chlamydial infection and gonorrhea are the most common examples. Syphilis, trichomoniasis, herpetic infection, and venereal warts are also noted as sequelae of sexual abuse. HIV infection has also been reported. The laboratory evaluation of sexually abused children should be modified depending on the history of the type of contact and the epidemiology of these infectious agents in the community.

Children with **failure to thrive** should not have an extensive workup. A CBC, urinalysis, and serum electrolyte panel are sufficient screening tests. A skeletal survey may be helpful in diagnosing the minority of these children who are also physically abused. The best "test" for the condition, however, is placement in a setting in which the child can be fed "ad lib" and the weight monitored. Hospital or foster care management may be appropriate. Weight gain may not occur for several days to a week in severe cases.

Any child with polymicrobial sepsis, recurrent apnea, chronic dehydration of unknown cause, or other highly unusual laboratory findings should be suspected of having Münchausen syndrome by proxy.

MANAGEMENT & REPORTING OF ABUSE & NEGLECT

Physical injuries should of course be treated. If the child has a **sexually transmitted disease,** this should be treated immediately. Children with **failure to thrive** on the basis of emotional neglect need to be placed in a setting where they can be fed. If weight gain does not occur within a reasonable time, further evaluation for the myriad of organic causes of failure to thrive can be instituted.

In every state in the United States, practitioners (and many other professionals who come in contact with children) are "mandated reporters." If abuse or neglect is suspected, a report must be made to the local or state agency designated to take and investigate these reports. In most cases, this will be a child protective services agency. Law enforcement personnel may also receive reports. The purpose of the report is to permit professionals to gather enough information to assess whether the environment in which the child is placed is safe. Many hospitals and communities have child protection teams available for consultation when there are questions about diagnosis or management. A list of pediatric consultants in child abuse is available from the American Academy of Pediatrics.

The reporting of **emotional abuse,** except in extreme cases, is not likely to be responded to by most child protection agencies. Practitioners can encourage parents to get involved with parent effectiveness training programs (eg, Parents as First Teachers, Parents Anonymous) or seek mental health consultation to help them in this area.

If **Münchausen syndrome by proxy** is suspected, judicial involvement is usually required, either to obtain permission for video surveillance of the parent-child interaction in the hospital or to place the child out of the home environment to see whether the "illness" resolves.

PREVENTION OF ABUSE & NEGLECT

Physical abuse is preventable in many cases. Extensive experience and evaluation of high-risk families has shown that the provision of "home visitor" services to families at risk can prevent physical abuse of children. These services can be provided by public health nurses or trained paraprofessionals. This makes it as easy for the family to pick up the telephone and ask for help *before* they abuse a child as it is for a neighbor or the physician to report an episode of abuse after it has occurred. Parent education and anticipatory guidance, particularly with respect to handling of situations that stress parents (eg, crying, toilet training), may also be helpful.

The prevention of **sexual abuse** is more difficult. Most efforts in this area involve training children to protect themselves and their "private parts" from harm. These programs are useful in individual cases but in general are not as efficacious as necessary. More rational approaches to prevention will place the responsibility for prevention on the adults who supervise children than on the children themselves.

Efforts to prevent **emotional abuse** of children have been undertaken through extensive media campaigns. No data are available to assess the effectiveness of this approach.

REFERENCES

American Academy of Pediatrics: Guidelines for the evaluation of sexual abuse of children. Pediatrics 1991; 87:254.

Heger A, Emans SJ: *Evaluation of the Sexually Abused Child.* Oxford Univ Press, 1992.

Ludwig S, Kornberg AE (editors): *Child Abuse: A Medical Reference,* 2nd ed. Churchill Livingstone, 1992.

Monteleone JA, Brodeur AE (editors): *Child Maltreatment: A Clinical Guide and Reference.* Mosby, 1994.

Olds D: Home visitation for pregnant women and parents of young children. Am J Dis Child 1992;146:704.

Ambulatory Pediatrics

9

Roxann M. Headley, MD, & James V. Lustig, MD

Pediatrics is concerned with disorders of physical and psychologic development, prevention of disease, and enabling a child to reach his or her full potential. Pediatric services are provided in an outpatient setting and emphasize preventive health care services. This chapter emphasizes some of the unique aspects of the pediatric patient and the orientation a caregiver must take to provide a child with comprehensive, longitudinal care. Guidelines are offered for the health supervision visit, chronic disease follow-up, and consultations. Special attention is paid to the problems of telephone triage, fever, and growth reduction.

PEDIATRIC HISTORY

The pediatric history is unique in that children do not usually provide their own history. Instead, the parents interpret the child's actions to the physician, who then reinterprets the parents' summary. The sometimes vague exposition of complaints offered by parents who bring children to the office can confuse the nature of the symptoms and the sequence in which they appeared. These vague complaints are often really statements of the parents' own concerns about the child's progress. Instead of hearing that Andy has had a "warm, red, tender, swollen knee for 2 days," the pediatrician is more likely to hear that Andy has not played well this week or that he no longer wants to play on the soccer team. Many visits are precipitated by problems at school, such as poor grades or poor peer relationships. To distinguish organic from nonorganic illness and to intervene appropriately without subjecting the child to unnecessary testing, the physician must understand the family and its hopes and concerns for the child. It is often necessary to ask specifically what problems the parent wishes to address in order to determine what really precipitated the office visit. It is essential to obtain as much of the history as possible directly from the patient. Direct histories not only provide firsthand information but also give the child a degree of control over a potentially threatening situation and may reveal familial dysfunction.

Obtaining a comprehensive pediatric history is time-consuming. Many offices provide questionnaires for parents to complete before the child's visit. Data for questionnaires should make an outpatient visit more productive, allowing the physician to address problems in detail, while reviewing and dismissing areas that are not a problem. Questionnaires presented to patients via computer may be more productive than a face-to-face interview in revealing sensitive parts of the history, according to some recent studies. However, failure to study and assimilate this information prior to the visit may lead to hostility on the part of the parent/patient who feels that his or her time has been wasted.

Those elements of the history which are important over a long period must be readily accessible. In some practices, such information is kept on a summary sheet, as illustrated in Figure 9–1. This contains demographic data, a problem list, chronic medications, allergies, previous hospitalizations, and a listing of consultants. It is usually not feasible to maintain immunization data on the front sheet because of the detail that must be kept for the National Vaccine Injury Act. A second page for immunization data is preferable.

The components of a comprehensive pediatric history are listed in Table 9–1. Ideally, these components should be obtained at the first office visit. The first four items are included on the summary page. Items 5 and 6 occur with each episodic care visit. The remainder are updated at each health supervision visit.

Name _____ Nickname _____ D.O.B. _____
Mother _____ Father _____ Sibs _____
S.S. # _____ Insurance _____

Chronic Problems			Chronic Medications		
Date of onset	Description	Date resolved	Start date		Stop date
				Allergies:	
Date	**Hospitalizations/Injuries/Procedures**		Date	**Consultants**	

Figure 9–1. Use of a summary sheet such as this at the front of the record facilitates reorienting the caregiver and his or her partners to the patient. Some practices keep track of health supervision visits on this sheet to tell the physician whether the child is likely to have received the appropriate preventive services. Previously, many practices recorded the administration of immunizations on this sheet. However, a second page that lists data required by the National Vaccine Injury Act may be more useful. When a true allergy is identified, remember to have the patient wear a medical alert bracelet and obtain an epinephrine kit, if appropriate.

PEDIATRIC PHYSICAL EXAMINATION

In approaching the child, adequate time must be taken to allow the child to become familiar with the examiner. Interactions and instructions must be age-appropriate and developmentally appropriate so that the child understands what is occurring and what is expected. A gentle approach, friendly manner, and quiet voice help establish a setting that yields a productive physical examination without unduly threatening the child. Those areas in which the child's cooperation is needed should be addressed first. Painful or unpleasant procedures should be postponed until

Table 9–1. Components of the pediatric historical database.[1]

Demographic data	Name, date of birth, social security number, sex, race, parents' names (first and last), siblings' names, patient's nickname, and payor mechanism
Problem list	Major or significant problems, including the dates of onset and resolution
Allergies	Offending agent, the nature of the reaction, the treatment needed, and the date
Chronic medications	Name, concentration, dose, and frequency of chronically used medications
Reasons for visit	The patient's or parents' concerns, stated in their own words, serve as the focus for the visit
Present illness	A crisp, chronologic summary of the problems necessitating a visit, including the duration progression, exacerbating factors, ameliorating interventions, and associations
Past history state of health	A statement regarding the child's functionality and general well-being, including a summary record of past significant illnesses, injuries, hospitalizations, and procedures
Screening procedures	Results of all screening procedures and actions taken should be maintained as a distinct part of the medical record, including newborn screening, vision and hearing screening, any health screen, or screening laboratory tests (developmental screening results are maintained in the development section)
Birth history	Maternal health during pregnancy, medications, street drugs used, complications of pregnancy; duration and ease of labor; form of delivery; analgesics/anesthetics used; need for monitoring; and labor complications. Infant's birth weight, gestational age, Apgar scores, and problems in the neonatal period
Diet	Eating patterns, likes and dislikes, use of vitamins, and relative amounts of carbohydrates, fat, and protein in the diet
Immunizations	Date of each immunization administered, vaccine manufacturer and lot number, and name of the person administering the vaccine; previous reaction and contraindication to immunization (eg, immunodeficiency or an evolving neurologic problem) should be documented
Family history	Information about the illnesses of relatives, preferably in the form of a family tree
Social history	Family constellation, relationship, parents' educational background, religious preference, and the role of the child in the family; socioeconomic profile of the family to identify resources available to the child, access to services that may be needed, and anticipated stressors
Development	(1) Attainment of developmental milestones (including developmental testing results); (2) social habits and milestones (toilet habits, play, major activities, sleep patterns, discipline, development of relationships); (3) school progress and documentation of specific achievements and grades
Sexual history	Familial sexual attitudes, sex education, sexual development, sexual activity, sexually transmitted diseases, and birth control measures
Review of systems (ROS)	This area tends to be overlooked because of the work required to obtain a complete ROS and integrate data into the patient's problems list and care plan. A focused ROS is essential if any problem is to be addressed adequately. For example, if a child is wheezing, it is important to know whether ventilatory support was required in the newborn period, whether there is an antecedent or concurrent illness or chronic diarrhea, or whether the patient demonstrated failure to thrive. In such a case, it is also important for the examiner to determine whether an atopic diathesis, cardiac disease, chronic or nighttime cough or symptoms exacerbated by exercise are present

[1]The components of this table should be included in a child's medical record, structured to allow easy review and updating.

the end of the examination. If the physician is unable to establish rapport with the child, the process should proceed efficiently, quickly, and systematically.

Because the history is often incomplete and because young children may perceive the examination as threatening and become fussy, inspection is very important. The examiner should make observations throughout the visit, paying special attention to how the child interacts with the environment. Observation also affords the examiner a chance to assess parent-child interactions.

Clothing should be removed slowly and gently to avoid chilling or threatening the child. Modesty, whenever a child exhibits it, should be respected, and drapes should be provided. Both boys and girls should be offered a chaperon whenever a stressful or painful procedure is performed.

Examination tables are convenient, but a parent's

lap is a safe haven for a young child. An adequate examination, for most purposes, can be conducted on a "table" formed by the parent's and examiner's legs as they sit facing each other.

The nature of the physical examination changes as the child develops; Table 9–2 illustrates some of the goals of the physical exam as a physician approaches a preventive services visit for a 2-month-old child compared to a 14-year-old adolescent.

Bates B et al: *A Guide to Physical Diagnosis,* 6th ed. Lippincott, 1995.

Zitelli BJ, David HW (editors): *Atlas of Pediatric Physical Diagnosis,* 2nd ed. Mosby, 1992.

PREVENTIVE HEALTH CARE SERVICES

One of several timetables for preventive care services (from the American Academy of Pediatrics' [AAP's] Committee on Practice and Ambulatory Medicine) is illustrated in Figure 9–2. In areas where efficacy data are lacking, expert opinion has been used as the basis for these plans. For example, while immunizations have been shown to be effective, there is disagreement about which metabolic diseases should be screened on a routine basis. Anticipatory guidance is being actively studied, and programs to decrease poisonings, increase the use of car seats, and decrease smoking appear to be effective. While the guidelines serve as an important framework for basic services, the practitioner should individualize actual services according to the child's needs.

The preventive services visit should be structured to review both acute and chronic problems and to anticipate future developments. New issues such as developmental progress, family structure, or an organic problem such as a limp are elicited through an interim history. Vision and hearing should be objectively assessed at intervals. Development is similarly subjectively assessed at each visit and objectively assessed at intervals or if there is any question of appropriate progress. Laboratory evaluation may also be part of the visit. The physical examination in the first year of life focuses on possible physical anomalies. In subsequent years, the exam focuses on physical development, the progress of any existing disease, and alterations in growth. At each visit, growth is carefully documented and the growth chart is brought up to date (see Chapter 1). The final major portion of the health maintenance visit is anticipatory guidance. This section of the visit enables the health care provider to address issues which will arise, such as the need to childproof the house as a child becomes mobile, and issues like drug and tobacco use.

American Academy of Pediatrics, Committee on Psychosocial Aspects of Child and Family Health: *Guidelines for Health Supervision III,* 3rd ed. American Academy of Pediatrics, 1996.

Green M: *Bright Futures: Guidelines for Health Supervision of Infants, Children, and Adolescents.* National Center for Education in Maternal and Child Health, 1994.

Report of the US Preventive Services Task Force: *Guide to Clinical Preventive Services,* 2nd ed. International Medical Publishing, 1996.

Table 9–2. The focused physical examination, comparing the emphasis within each organ system for exams of a 2-month-old and a 14-year-old.

System	2-Month-Old	14-Year-Old
Growth	Length, weight, head circumference	Height, weight
Head, eye, ear, nose, & throat	Fontanelles, sutures, intact palate, red reflex, tear ducts, ear pits/deformities	Fundi, dentition
Skin	Birthmarks	Acne, distribution of hair, sequelae of sun exposure
Neck	Sinus tract, residua of torticollis	Thyroid
Chest		Breast development[1]
Cardiovascular	Murmurs, pulses	Blood pressure
Extremities	Physical deformities, proportion	Muscular development
Genitalia	Normal anatomy, descent of testes	Tanner staging[1]
Neurologic	Body position, tone, reflexes	Coordination, abstract reasoning

[1]Some physicians teach breast and testicular self-examination during the physical exam.

Committee on Practice and Ambulatory Medicine

Each child and family is unique; therefore, these **Recommendations for Preventive Pediatric Health Care** are designed for the care of children who are receiving competent parenting, have no manifestations of any important health problems, and are growing and developing in satisfactory fashion. **Additional visits may become necessary** if circumstances suggest variations from normal.

These guidlines represent a consensus by the Committee on Practice and Ambulatory Medicine in consultation with national committees and sections of the American Academy of Pediatrics. The Committee emphasizes the great importance of **continuity of care** in comprehensive health supervision and the need to avoid **fragmentation of care**.

A **prenatal visit** is recommended for parents who are at high risk, for first-time parents, and for those who request a conference. The prenatal visit should include anticipatory guidance and pertinent medical history. Every infant should have a newborn evaluation after birth.

Age[4]	INFANCY[3]								EARLY CHILDHOOD[3]					MIDDLE CHILDHOOD[3]				ADOLESCENCE[3]											
	New-born[1]	2-4 d[2]	By 1mo	2 mo	4 mo	6 mo	9 mo	12 mo	15 mo	18 mo	24 mo	3y	4y	5y	6y	8y	10y	11y	12y	13y	14y	15y	16y	17y	18y	19y	20y	21y
History																												
Initial/Interval	•	•	•	•	•	•	•	•	•	•	•	•	•	•	•	•	•	•	•	•	•	•	•	•	•	•	•	•
Measurements																												
Height / Weight	•	•	•	•	•	•	•	•	•	•	•	•	•	•	•	•	•	•	•	•	•	•	•	•	•	•	•	•
Head Circumference	•	•	•	•	•	•	•	•																				
Blood Pressure												•	•	•	•	•	•	•	•	•	•	•	•	•	•	•	•	•
Sensory Screening																												
Vision	S	S	S	S	S	S	S	S	S	S	S	O[5]	O	O	S	S	O	S	O	S	S	O	S	S	O	S	S	S
Hearing[6]	S/O	S	S	S	S	S	S	S	S	S	S	O	O	O	S	S	O	S	O	S	S	O	S	S	O	S	S	S
Developmntl./ Behavioral Assessment[7]	•	•	•	•	•	•	•	•	•	•	•	•	•	•	•	•	•	•	•	•	•	•	•	•	•	•	•	•
Physical Examination[8]	•	•	•	•	•	•	•	•	•	•	•	•	•	•	•	•	•	•	•	•	•	•	•	•	•	•	•	•
Procedures- General [9]																												
Hereditary/ Metabolic Screening[10]	←	→	•																									
Immunization[11]	←	→		•	•	•		←	→		←	→		←				•			←	→						
Lead Screen.[12]							←	→		•																		
Hematocrit or Hemoglobin			←			→								←						13								→
Urinalysis										•				←						14								→
Procedures- Patients at Risk																												
Tuberculin Test[15]								★	★	★	★	★	★	★	★	★	★	★	★	★	★	★	★	★	★	★	★	★
Cholesterol Screening[16]												★	★	★	★	★	★	★	★	★	★	★	★	★	★	★	★	★
STD Screening[17]																		★	★	★	★	★	★	★	★	★	★	★
Pelvic Exam[18]																		★	★	★	★	★	★	←★	★ 18	★	→	★
Anticipatory Guidance[19]	•	•	•	•	•	•	•	•	•	•	•	•	•	•	•	•	•	•	•	•	•	•	•	•	•	•	•	•
Injury Prevention[20]	•	•	•	•	•	•	•	•	•	•	•	•	•	•	•	•	•	•	•	•	•	•	•	•	•	•	•	•
Initial Dental Referral[21]									←		→																	

Key: • = to be performed   S = subjective, by history   ◄——► = the range during which a service may be provided,
  ★ = to be performed for   O = objective, by a standard   with the dot indicating the preferred age.
    patients at risk   testing method

NB: Special chemical, immunologic, and endocrine testing is usually carried out upon specific indications. Testing other than newborn (eg. inborn errors of metabolism, sickle disease, etc.) is discretionary with the physician.

The recommendations in this publication do not indicate an exclusive course of treatment or serve as a standard of medical care. Variations, taking into account individual circumstances, may be appropriate. *(continued)*

Figure 9–2. Recommendations for preventive pediatric health care.

1. Breastfeeding encouraged and instruction and support offered.
2. For newborns discharged in less than 48 hours after delivery.
3. Developmental, psychosocial, and chronic disease issues for children and adolescents may require frequent counseling and treatment visits separate from preventive care visits.
4. If a child comes under care for the first time at any point on the schedule, or if any items are not accomplished at the suggested age, the schedule should be brought up to date at the earliest possible time.
5. If the patient is uncooperative, rescreen within six months.
6. Some experts recommend objective appraisal of hearing in the newborn period. The Joint Committee on Infant Hearing has identified patients at significant risk for hearing loss. All children meeting these criteria should be objectively screened. See the Joint Committee on Infant Hearing 1994 Position Statement.
7. By history and appropriate physical examination: if suspicious, by specific objective developmental testing.
8. At each visit, a complete physical examination is essential, with infant totally unclothed, older child undressed and suitably draped.
9. These may be modified, depending upon entry point into schedule and individual need.
10. Metabolic screening (eg. thyroid, hemoglobinopathies, PKU, galactosemia) should be done according to state law.
11. Schedule(s) per the Committee on Infectious Diseases, published periodically in *Pediatrics*. Every visit should be an opportunity to update and complete a child's immunizations.
12. Blood lead screen per AAP statement "Lead Poisoning: From Screening to Primary Prevention" (1993).
13. All menstruating adolescents should be screened.
14. Conduct dipstick urinalysis for leukocytes for male and female adolescents.
15. TB testing per AAP statement "Screening for Tuberculosis in Infants and Children" (1994). Testing should be done upon recognition of high risk factors. If results are negative but high risk situation continues, testing should be repeated on an annual basis.
16. Cholesterol screening for high risk patients per AAP "Statement on Cholesterol" (1992). If family history cannot be ascertained and other risk factors are present, screening should be at the discretion of the physician.
17. All sexually active patients should be screened for sexually transmitted diseases (STDs).
18. All sexually active females should have a pelvic examination. A pelvic examination and routine pap smear should be offered as part of preventive health maintenance between the ages of 18 and 21 years.
19. Appropriate discussion and counseling should be an integral part of each visit for care.
20. From birth to age 12, refer to AAP's injury prevention program (TIPP[3]) as described in "A Guide to Safety Counseling in Office Practice" (1994).
21. Earlier initial dental evaluations may be appropriate for some children. Subsequent examinations as prescribed by dentist.

Figure 9–2. (continued)

HEALTH SUPERVISION VISIT

GROWTH PARAMETERS

Height, weight, and head circumference are carefully measured and plotted at each visit during the first 3 years. (Growth charts may be found in Chapter 1.) To ensure accurate weight measurements for longitudinal comparisons, infants should be undressed completely and young children should be dressed only in underpants. A recumbent length is plotted on the birth to 36-month chart, and when the child is old enough to be measured upright, parameters are plotted on the 2- to 18-year growth chart. If circumferential head growth has been steady for the first 2 years, routine measurement may be suspended. However, should a central nervous system problem exist or develop, or should the child manifest failure to thrive, this measurement continues to have utility. Tracking the growth velocity for each of these parameters allows the early recognition of deviations from the normal pattern.

BLOOD PRESSURE

Blood pressure screening is recommended beginning at 3 years of age. To obtain an accurate measurement, the cuff must cover two-thirds of the upper arm. The reading should be compared against age-related normals (Table 9–3). Blood pressure varies with height and weight, and there is some difference between the sexes, especially in the newborn and the older teenager. If the child has any renal or cardiac abnormality, a blood pressure reading must be obtained at each visit, regardless of the age.

Report of the Second Task Force on Blood Pressure Control in Children. National Heart, Lung, and Blood Institute, 1987.

Table 9–3. 90th percentile values of blood pressure.[1]

	Newborn	Age (years)							
		1	**3**	**6**	**9**	**12**	**15**	**18**
Systolic (mm Hg)	76–87	105	106	111	115	121	127–129	127–136
Diastolic (mm Hg)	68	68	68	70	74	77	79–82	80–84

[1]Ranges reflect differences in the sexes, with average values for males being at the high end of the range. (Adapted from *Report of the Second Task Force on Blood Pressure Control in Children.* National Heart, Lung, and Blood Institute, 1987.)

HEARING AND VISION

Infants should be observed to focus on an object, usually the face. An ophthalmoscopic examination of the anterior chamber checks for bleeding that may have occurred during birth. The presence of bilateral red reflexes rules out opacification from congenital cataracts or retinoblastoma. Beginning at 3 years of age, office screening of vision using Allen cards or the Snellen Illiterate E chart should be attempted. Each eye is tested separately. Credit is given for a line on which the child gets more than 50% correct. If the child is unable to follow the instructions, re-screen in 6 months. Because visual acuity improves with age, results of the test are interpreted using the cutoff values in Table 9–4. The corneal light reflex test may be performed at any age to screen for alignment of the eyes; a cover test allows for a functional look for strabismus. Both of these exams are described in Chapter 15.

In the newborn period, any infant who is at high risk for hearing loss by history should be tested. Pure tone audiometry in the office setting can be tested beginning at 3 years of age. (See Chapter 17 for more details.)

US Public Health Service: Vision screening in children. Am Fam Physician 1994;50:587.

DEVELOPMENTAL/BEHAVIORAL ASSESSMENT

At each visit, development of the child is assessed by using a parent-answered questionnaire or an interview or by testing the child. During the first 5 years

Table 9–4. Age-appropriate visual acuity.[1]

Age (years)	Minimal Acceptable Acuity
3	20/40
4	20/30
5	20/20

[1]Refer to an ophthalmologist if minimal acuity is not met at a given age or if there is a difference in scores of two or more lines between the eyes.

of life, a formal screening test, such as the Denver II, should be administered periodically in order to objectively define development. Other screening tests should be used as needed. For example, a 3-year-old boy who has difficulty saying certain sounds could be assessed against norms for age by using the Denver Articulation Screening Examination. The school-age child's cognitive function is assessed indirectly through academic achievement and his or her emotional well-being is screened by interview and observation. Behaviors appropriate for age are reviewed at each visit and sometimes observed. These behaviors include feeding, sleep, elimination, self-stimulating behaviors (thumb sucking, rocking, head banging, masturbation), and recurrent pain syndromes (headache, chest pain, abdominal pain, limb pain). Recognition of the child's temperament and knowledge of discipline techniques used by the family will allow the primary care provider to sensitively counsel around behavioral issues.

LABORATORY SCREENING

Newborn Screening

All 50 states in the United States mandate newborn screening for phenylketonuria (PKU) and congenital hypothyroidism (CH). PKU occurs once in every 15,000 live births, while CH is present in 1 of 4500 live births. Both diseases result in severe mental retardation, but early treatment maintains cognitive function in the normal range. Other diseases tested vary from state to state but may include galactosemia, homocystinuria, biotinidase deficiency, neuroblastoma, congenital adrenal hyperplasia, cystic fibrosis, and sickle cell anemia. Although some diseases are rare, the burden of suffering caused by these diseases is high, and effectiveness of early intervention is, for the most part, quite good. It must be remembered that screening does not equal diagnosis. Cases may be missed (false-negatives), and if symptoms of disease are present despite a negative test, an infant should be tested further. Because cutoff values of the tests are selected to reduce the number of patients missed who truly have the disease (false-negatives) and because of administrative or laboratory errors, false-positives are expected. If the screening test is reported as positive, results must be confirmed and parental anxiety addressed. The comprehensive database in the patient's chart should include the screening status, even if the child transferred into the practice beyond the newborn period.

Lead Toxicity

The developing infant and child are at special risk for the adverse effects of lead exposure. While acute or chronic high blood lead levels (>55 µg/dL) can produce multiorgan system effects (colic, nausea, nephritis, muscle aches, encephalopathy, seizures, headache, anemia), numerous studies have demonstrated that even children with low levels (10–25 µg/dL) can have more behavior problems, more learning disabilities, and lower IQs than cohorts with levels below 10 µg/dL. Furthermore, the effect persists into adulthood. The primary source of lead exposure in this country remains lead-based paint, even though its use has been banned since 1977. Probably because of environmental control such as the elimination of leaded gasolines and paints, as well as educational interventions, lead levels nationally have declined from a mean of 16 µg/dL in 1976 to about 5 µg/dL today. However, considerable variation exists in different parts of the United States.

Children may be screened by questionnaire for possible environmental risk factors at the time of health supervision visits between the ages of 6 months and 6 years. (See the sample questionnaire from the Centers for Disease Control and Prevention shown in Table 9–5.) Although the questionnaire is of limited use in identifying high-risk children, it can make families aware of risk factors. If any of these risks are present, a blood lead level should be obtained. In addition, routine screening of blood lead levels should be performed on all children at 9–12 months and at 2 years of age, regardless of the presence or absence of historical risk factors. A venous sample is preferred over a capillary specimen. Blood lead levels below 10 µg/dL are acceptable. Children with confirmed blood levels over 15 µg/dL should be evaluated for environmental exposure and development. If they are iron-deficient, supplemental iron is given. Chelation of lead should be considered for levels above 25 µg/dL and is urgently required for levels of 70 µg/dL or more. As more data are collected, low-risk communities may be identified where routine blood lead screening is unnecessary.

Anemia

Iron deficiency is the most common cause of anemia in young children, although the incidence has declined in recent years due, in large part, to the use of iron-fortified formulas until 1 year of age. Infants born prematurely, in a multiple pregnancy, or to iron-deficient mothers have an increased risk for iron deficiency. Asymptomatic iron deficiency anemia in the young child has been associated with impaired behavior and development, with deficits persisting into school age despite correction of the anemia. Therefore, screening of infants at 9 months of age seems reasonable. The Canadian Task Force recommends screening in the first week and at 9 months of age only those infants born prematurely. A screening hematocrit is also recommended for pregnant teenagers, because low maternal hemoglobin levels have been associated with low birth weight, prematurity, and high perinatal mortality.

Hypercholesterolemia/Hyperlipidemia

Blood screening of cholesterol and lipoproteins in children should be based on risk factors. If a parent has a cholesterol level above 240 mg/dL, the child should be screened by 2–3 years of age. If there is a history of cardiovascular disease in a parent or grandparent before 55 years of age, a complete lipoprotein analysis (fasting cholesterol, high-density lipoproteins [HDLs], low-density lipoproteins [LDLs], triglycerides) should be measured in the child. For all children, a prudent diet is advised (see p 225).

Bacteriuria

Controversy surrounds screening asymptomatic children for bacteriuria. For infant males, the prevalence of asymptomatic bacteriuria is 2–4%, and for early grade school girls it is 5–6%. It is assumed that detection and treatment of asymptomatic bacteriuria may prevent pyelonephritis and the possible subsequent development of renal scarring. This has not been proven. The dipstick urinalysis, including the nitrite test for bacteriuria and the leukocyte esterase test for pyuria, is an inexpensive screening test, but the 20% false-positive rate indicates that children must be rescreened or the urine must be cultured, thereby increasing the cost substantially. Nevertheless, the AAP and others recommend a screening urinalysis for all children around 5 years of age.

Table 9–5. Lead exposure screening questionnaire.[1]

Does your child—

1. Live in or regularly visit a house with peeling or chipping paint built before 1960? This could include a day care center, preschool, the home of a babysitter or relative, etc.
2. Live in or regularly visit a house built before 1960 with recent, ongoing, or planned renovation or remodeling?
3. Have a brother or sister, housemate, or playmate being followed up or treated for lead poisoning (ie, blood level ≥15 µg/dL)?
4. Live with an adult whose job or hobby involves exposure to lead?
5. Live near an active lead smelter, battery recycling plant, or other industry likely to release lead?

---

[1]From the Centers for Disease Control and Prevention.

Tuberculosis

In 1993, there were 2301 new cases of tuberculosis reported in children in the United States. Identification of groups most at risk to contract tuberculosis reduces the number of children who need to be screened. High-risk infants, children, and adolescents include those with infectious or high-risk contacts; those who are immunosuppressed, including human immunodeficiency virus (HIV)–positive persons; those who are from areas of high prevalence (Asia, Pacific Islands); those with a chest radiograph suggesting disease; and those with clinical symptoms. The Mantoux test (purified protein derivative [PPD]) is the recommended screening test beginning as early as 12 months of age and repeating yearly if the risk persists. The tine test should not be used.

Teenaged females who are sexually active or 18 years of age or older should have an annual Papanicolaou smear. All sexually active patients should be historically screened for sexually transmitted diseases (STDs), and males with symptoms should be cultured. Because females are often not symptomatic, gonococcal and chlamydial cultures are appropriate at the time of each Pap smear.

American Academy of Pediatrics, Committee on Environmental Health: Lead poisoning: From screening to primary prevention. Pediatrics 1993;92:176.

American Academy of Pediatrics, Committee on Genetics: Issues in newborn screening. Pediatrics 1992;89:345.

Kemper K et al: The case against screening urinalyses for asymptomatic bacteriuria in child. Am J Dis Child 1992;146:343.

National Cholesterol Expert Panel on Blood Cholesterol Levels in Children and Adolescents: Highlights of the report of the Expert Panel on Blood Cholesterol Levels in Children and Adolescents. Pediatrics 1992;89:495.

Oski FA: Iron deficiency in infancy and childhood. N Engl J Med 1993;329:190.

Peter G (editor): *1994 Red Book: Report of the Committee on Infectious Diseases,* 23rd ed. American Academy of Pediatrics, 1994.

Report of the US Preventive Services Task Force: *Guide to Clinical Preventive Services,* 2nd ed. International Medical Publishing, 1996.

ANTICIPATORY GUIDANCE

A major portion of the health supervision visit is anticipatory guidance. This section of the visit enables the health care provider to turn the parents' attention (and the older child's attention) to issues that will arise, such as the need to childproof the home as a child becomes mobile. Guidance must be appropriate to age. Topics may be discussed by the physician, they may be delegated to the office nurse, printed materials may be sent home, or a combination of presentations may be used. Areas of guidance include diet, injury prevention, development, behavior, and health promotion. Injury prevention is discussed here; other topics may be referenced in other sections of the book.

Injury Prevention

Injuries are the leading cause of death for children and adolescents after the first year of life. For young people aged 15–24 years, injuries are responsible for more than 75% of deaths (Figure 9–3C). Each year, 16 million visits to emergency departments occur as a result of pediatric injuries and more than 500,000 children are hospitalized.

Health care providers have a responsibility to injury prevention through patient/family education, support of community safety efforts, and identification of the child/family at risk. Education in the form of office-based counseling for injury prevention should be part of each health supervision visit and can be reinforced at episodic visits. Counseling should focus on problems that are frequent and age-appropriate, such as poison prevention for the toddler and firearm safety for the adolescent. Advice should be specific, for example, advise families to keep medications out of a child's reach as opposed to telling them to poison-proof the home. Passive strategies of prevention should be emphasized, as these are more effective than active strategies; for example, encouraging the use of childproof cupboard latches to prevent poisoning will be more effective than instructing parents to watch their children closely.

A parent-answered questionnaire assessing the safety of the home, such as The Injury Prevention Program (TIPP) from the AAP (Publications Department, 141 Northwest Point Blvd, PO Box 927, Elk Grove Village, IL 60007; phone 1-800-433-9016), can be completed while families are waiting for the physician. Advice can then be tailored to the specific needs of each family, with reinforcement from age-specific TIPP handouts.

Advocacy on behalf of children and adolescents for safety legislation and community safety programs means extending passive strategies to the entire community. For example, bicycle safety helmets can prevent 85% of head injuries. A community program in Seattle to promote the use of bicycle helmets has resulted in an increase in helmet use, from 2% to nearly 40%. The health care provider also has the responsibility to anticipate problems and work to prevent them. For example, the primary care provider is in an ideal position to screen for emotional problems, such as adolescent depression, and intervene before an injury, such as a motor vehicle accident or an attempted suicide related to drinking and driving, occurs. In the case of physical injury to a young child, the physician must be ever-vigilant, recognizing that some injuries may be intentional or may be the result of neglect.

A. Motor Vehicle Injuries: The foremost killer and crippler of children in the United States is the motor vehicle. Car safety seats are required in this

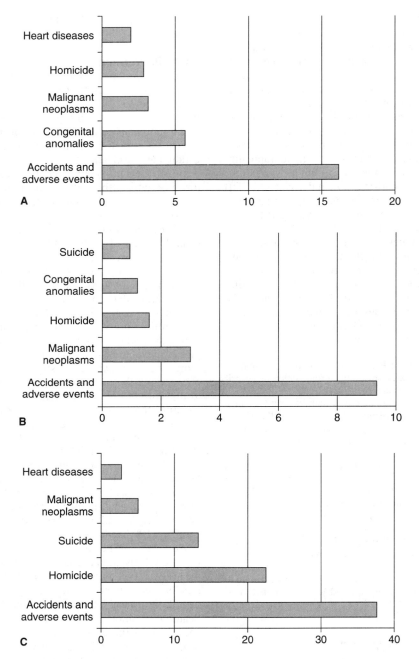

Figure 9–3. Leading causes of death in children **(A)** 1–4 years, **(B)** 5–14 years, and **(C)** 15–24 years of age (the 1992 rate per 100,000 population). (From the National Center for Health Statistics.)

country, and their use could reduce fatalities and hospitalizations by at least 50%. The type of safety seat to be used depends on the child's weight:

- Less than 20 lb: Rear-facing infant seat, avoiding seats with airbags
- 20–40 lb: Forward-facing toddler seat

- 40–60 lb: Shield booster seat with lap belt
- Over 60 lb: Regular lap belt
- Over 48 in.: Shoulder strap with lap belt

The leading cause of injury death among children aged 5–9 years is the motor vehicle–pedestrian collision. When the child is a motor vehicle occupant in a crash, the case-fatality rate is 1.0%; when the child is the pedestrian in a motor vehicle collision, the case-fatality rate increases threefold.

B. Bicycle Injuries: Head trauma accounts for three-quarters of all bicycle-related fatalities. More than 85% of brain injuries can be prevented through the use of bicycle helmets.

C. Firearm Injuries: On average, 14 children and adolescents each day are killed by firearms in the United States. Injuries from firearms are more frequent for young people aged 15–24 years than for any other pediatric or adult age group, and black males are especially vulnerable. Many firearm deaths may be unintentional, but the majority are the result of homicide or suicide. The risk of suicide is five times greater if there is a gun in the home. Although handguns are often kept in homes for protection, a gun is more likely to kill a family member or a friend than an intruder. The most effective way to prevent firearm injuries is to remove guns from the home. However, if families keep firearms at home, they should be advised to store them in a locked container and to store ammunition separately.

D. Drowning/Near-Drowning: Children between the ages of 1 and 3 years have the highest rate of drowning. In some warm-weather states (especially Arizona, California, Florida), drowning deaths exceed the number of deaths caused by motor vehicle or pedestrian accidents. For every death by drowning, six children are hospitalized and up to 10% of survivors suffer severe brain damage. Children under 1 year of age are most likely to drown in the bathtub, for children 1–4 years it is most often in the home swimming pool, and for school-age children and teens drowning occurs most often in outside bodies of water. Home pools must be securely fenced, and parents should know cardiopulmonary resuscitation (CPR). School-age children should be taught to swim, but should always be supervised.

E. Burn Injuries: Burns are the leading cause of childhood injury-related death within the home. Burn injuries include the categories of smoke inhalation and contact, scald, electrical, chemical, and ultraviolet burns, with scald burns being the most common type of pediatric burn. While the majority of scald burns involve foods and beverages, nearly one-quarter come from tap water, thus the recommendation to set hot water heaters to less than 54 °C. The greatest number of deaths result from smoke inhalation. Smoke detectors can prevent 85% of the injuries and deaths caused by fires in the home.

Monthly Vital Statistics Report. Centers for Disease Control and Prevention, 1995; page 43.

Committee on Injury and Poison Prevention: Office-based counseling for injury prevention. Pediatrics 1994; 94:566.

Hazinski MF et al: Pediatric injury prevention. Ann Emerg Med 1993;22:456.

PRUDENT DIET

Iron-fortified formula or breast milk (with attention to dietary iron intake) should be used for the first year of life, after which a transition to whole cow's milk can be made. Because of continued rapid growth and high energy needs, children should continue to drink whole milk until 2 years of age. Baby foods are generally introduced around 6 months of age.

By 2 years of age, a prudent diet employs diverse food sources, encourages high-fiber foods, limits sodium intake, and limits fat intake. Specific nutrient guidelines include:

- Carbohydrates: approximately 55% of total calories
- Protein: approximately 15–20% of total calories
- Total fat: less than 30% of total calories
- Saturated fat: less than 10% of total calories
- Cholesterol: less than 300 mg/d

IMMUNIZATIONS

A child's immunization status can easily be monitored in the medical record database. Additionally, parents should keep a record book. The immunization schedule and details are presented in Chapter 10.

To improve immunization rates, health care providers must be willing to give immunizations at every type of visit, including acute care visits. Education regarding the safety of immunizations during minor illnesses needs to reach both parents and health care providers. Flexible appointment scheduling, short waiting times, and repeated emphasis on the importance and timing of immunizations can remove some of the barriers to ensuring that children are protected as early in life as possible.

GROUP HEALTH SUPERVISION VISIT

An alternative model for providing health supervision is the group setting. Four or more parents and their children together receive 45 minutes of health education, followed by 15 minutes of individual time for examination and immunizations. The group model allows for more discussion of health care topics. Parents bring their children to more well-child visits, and between these visits they seek less advice than those whose care is provided in the traditional manner.

OTHER TYPES OF OFFICE VISITS

In addition to the health supervision visit, already reviewed, the office physician provides care under other formats.

ACUTE CARE VISITS

The acute care visit must be an efficient, structured routine. Office personnel should determine the reason for the visit, obtain a brief synopsis of the child's symptoms, and list known drug allergies. The physician should document the events related to the present problem together with a physical examination. The record should include a diagnosis and supporting laboratory data. Treatments and follow-up instructions must be recorded, including when to return to the office if the problem is not ameliorated.

PRENATAL VISITS

Ideally, a family's first trip to the pediatrician's office should occur before the birth of the baby. A prenatal visit goes a long way toward establishing trust and enables the physician to learn about a family's desires, concerns, and fears regarding the anticipated birth of a child. If the infant develops a problem during the newborn period, the physician who has not already met the family may have difficulty establishing rapport. Prenatal visits should be conducted in a relaxed atmosphere, with both parents present whenever possible.

Since the family is probably new to the practice, the prenatal visit provides an easy way to acquaint them with the manner in which the practice is conducted, its hours of operation, after-hours coverage, appointment scheduling, and billing. Parents want to know to whom they will speak when they call the office, when they may bring in children for acute care visits, and how their concerns will be met.

PRESCHOOL VISITS

Development, elimination patterns, social behavior, and diet should be assessed at preschool visits. Development and social behavior will affect the child's adjustment to school. Control of bladder and bowel functions is important to successful school entry; vision and hearing should be screened at this time. Subsequent visits should include assessment of the school performance, anticipated problems, and a critical review of both growth and development. One

of the sequelae for single-parent families or families in which both parents work is that the preschool visit is often too late to address the issues of separation and independence, as children may already have been in preschool programs or day care settings. Families should be advised of the goals of a "preschool" visit and should be encouraged to come in prior to having their child out of the home, whether the reason be the start of kindergarten or day care.

SPORT PHYSICALS

A physical examination is often needed before participation in organized sports programs. Time should be allotted not only to perform the physical exam but also to ask questions about the safety of the activities. What kind of protective equipment is provided? Are the supervisors and coaches trained to instruct children? What health care facilities are available? Will the patient require medication during competition (eg, beta-agonists for the patient with exercise-induced asthma)? Will the patient be exposed to unnecessary hazards, such as taking a turn at bat without a safety helmet or performing on the balance beam without a spotter? Does the program emphasize teamwork and skills, or is competition more important? Answering these questions can protect the child during an important part of childhood and at the same time ensure the child a joyful learning experience.

CHRONIC DISEASE FOLLOW-UP

A chronic illness is defined as one that has been present for more than 3 months. When both parental report and physical examination are used to find cases of chronic disease, rates are 25% for children and 35% for youths. Only about 10% of those children with chronic conditions will have a functional impairment. The most common chronic disease by parental report is asthma.

Children with chronic problems need special services and need to be followed up in a systematic manner to ensure that their needs are met. For example, records should be kept of all medications as well as immunizations for children with even moderate asthma. The family's comprehension of what to do in the event of wheezing must be brought up to date. Records of peak expiratory flow rates and pulmonary function should be kept. The child's environment should be reviewed at each visit, as families tend to relax their vigilance about environmental control when things are going well. Activity levels and the appearance of exercise-induced bronchospasm should be noted. A flow sheet used for children with asthma is illustrated in Figure 9–4, and similar flow sheets could be generated for other conditions.

Chronic problems often mean chronic medications and the need to monitor their use. Some offices enter a note in the patient's chart whenever a prescription is refilled. A useful alternative is a medication summary page, which allows easy visualization of the dosing and usage history plus space for notes such as when the anticonvulsant level was last checked and what it was (Figure 9–5).

Desquin BW et al: Comprehensive care of the child with a chronic condition. Curr Probl Pediatr 1994;24:230.

Jessop DF, Stein REK: Consistent but not the same—Effect of method on chronic condition rates. Arch Pediatr Adolesc Med 1995;149:1105.

COUNSELING

Topics amenable to office counseling include family stress such as separation, divorce, or remarriage; school problems; death; or parenting. Generally, 45 minutes allows adequate time for the therapeutic process to evolve, and this time should be protected from interruption. The young child is usually interviewed together with the parent. School-age children and adolescents benefit from time alone with the physician. After assessing the situation in one or two sessions, the primary care physician must decide whether the child's/family's needs are within his or her area of expertise or whether a referral to another professional, such as a psychologist or a learning specialist, would be appropriate.

Asthma Flow Sheet

Date	Jan	Feb	Mar	Apr	May	June	July	Aug
Medications								
Cromolyn	qid	> > >	> > >	tid	> > >	> > >	qid	> > >
Beta-agonist	Alb bid	> > >	> > >	Rescue	> > >	> > >	bid	> > >
Theophylline								
Steroids								
Inhaled							bid	
Pulse							5 days	
Chronic								
Atropine like								
Hospitalization								
E D visit							x 1	
School missed		1 day		3 days				
EIB						Soccer		
PEFR	85%			100%		83%	68%	
Spirometry					Normal			
Shots								
Education	PEFR	Exposures		Spacer	Sports			

Figure 9–4. Representative flow sheet for longitudinal follow-up of chronic disease. Alb = albuterol, ED = emergency department, EIB = exercise-induced bronchospasm, PEFR = peak expiratory flow rate, nml = normal.

MEDICATION

	Date					Notes
	Last filled					
	# Renewals					
	Approved by					
	Called by					
	Pharmacy					
	Phone #					

Figure 9–5. Medication summary sheet.

CONSULTATIONS*

Referring Source

Children may be referred to a general pediatrician for consultation by (1) a parent who desires a second opinion regarding a specific problem; (2) another physician, such as a subspecialist or a family physician; (3) other professionals, such as dentists, school officials, psychologists, or social workers; or (4) an insurance company that requests a second opinion. Consultations usually require one or two 45- to 60-minute appointments. When the patient is referred to a pediatric consultant, the number of visits and the degree of service should be specified. A screening questionnaire, completed in advance, should delineate the patient's physical, intellectual, and emotional problems and serve as an initial database.

A. Evaluation Only: The consultant can do a diagnostic evaluation on a patient and tell the parents nothing except that the findings will be discussed with their primary physician. However, parents generally do not like this approach. They are paying for the consultation, and they prefer to hear something directly from the expert.

B. Evaluation and Interpretation: After the evaluation is completed, the consultant usually discusses the diagnosis and the causes of the problems with the family. Recommendations for therapy can be reviewed in general terms and with the clear understanding that the referring physician will be coordinating the therapy. A specific return appointment date with the referring physician should be given. The consultant may be called on periodically to reassess the response to therapy and to offer revised recommendations.

C. Evaluation and Treatment of an Isolated Problem: Often, the referring physician wants the consultant to assume responsibility for management of the problem that is the subject of referral. This usually happens with treatable problems that will require only two to four visits (eg, recurrent headaches, encopresis, failure to thrive). The consultant should clearly define and support the referring physician's role as the continuing provider of health supervision and acute illness care during this interval. When the problem is resolved, the patient should be returned to the referring physician for resumption of care.

Communication With the Referring Source

Communication is the key to a satisfactory referral process. The pediatric consultant should send the referral source a brief note acknowledging the referral and requesting any additional information that may be available. The final consultation report should be sent promptly, with content appropriate for the referring source. School officials usually want to know only whether the patient is physically healthy or, if not, what their responsibility is. A referring physician expects a full report that will be helpful in treating the patient. Recommendations should therefore be specific (drugs, dosages, other forms of therapy, duration of therapy, specific laboratory tests, the frequency of these tests, etc). A copy of or reference to a recent review article on the subject will also be appreciated.

A medical evaluation should not contain personal comments so that it can serve as an official report for anyone who might request a copy of it in the future. A copy can also be sent to the family for their records. Some cases require a brief telephone report in addition to the written report. These cases include situations in which the patient needs to return to the referring physician before a consultation report can be sent, the patient needs to be referred to an additional specialist, or a question exists about proper disposition.

At the end of the consultation, the parents should be told when the patient should see the primary physician—usually in 1–2 weeks. Positive comments about the referring physician's competence and judg-

---

*Contributed by Barton D. Schmitt, MD.

ment should be made. The parents must feel confident that the primary physician can provide the necessary follow-up care. If the referring physician had tentatively made the correct diagnosis prior to referral, the consultant's corroboration should be made clear to the parents and recorded in the consultation report.

Bailie MD et al: Making consultation and referrals count. Contemp Pediatr 1988;5:96.

TELEPHONE TRIAGING & ADVICE*

The physician is the person best qualified to give medical advice, both in the office and over the phone. However, most questions require only routine answers and can be handled by a trained office nurse. Office policies about medical advice over the phone should be standardized. Routine instructions for handling minor infections, minor injuries, reactions to immunizations, infant feeding problems, newborn care, and prescriptions refills are easy to communicate to parents if they are written down in an office protocol book. The protocol book should also specify the point at which each problem requires an office visit. This decision depends on (1) the type of symptom, (2) the duration of the symptom, (3) the age of the patient, (4) whether or not the patient acts "very sick," (5) an assessment of the calling parent's anxiety, and (6) the presence of any underlying chronic disease. (For example, most patients under 1 year of age with diarrhea *and* vomiting need to be examined.) After telephone baseline data are gathered, the nurse must be able to decide whether the child needs to be seen immediately, should be seen later by appointment, or can be safely cared for at home. The nurse should err on the side of seeing the patient when in doubt. For all calls, pertinent telephone data should be entered on a form that will go into the patient's chart.

It is helpful if parents understand two general telephone rules: (1) The nurse will screen all calls during office hours except emergency calls, and (2) nighttime calls should be restricted to emergencies or urgent problems that cannot wait until morning. Many routine calls come from anxious, inexperienced parents who need reassurance and acceptance, not criticism. Their conversation with the nurse should help to build confidence. Parents can be asked what they had considered doing, and that plan of action should be endorsed if possible. If parents are helped to become more confident and independent in these matters, unnecessary visits will be less frequent. However, the conversation should convey the message that telephone calls are important and that the parent is free to call whenever he or she is concerned.

The physician directly accepts some calls: (1) emergency calls from parents, (2) calls from physicians and other professionals, (3) calls regarding hospitalized patients, (4) long-distance calls, (5) calls from a parent who demands to talk to the physician, and (6) calls whose import the nurse is unclear about. Telephone calls that come after the office is closed may be handled in the same way. A nurse, either one from the practice or one contracted through a commercial telephone service, can take the call initially. The physician must be available as backup to the nurse.

There are four other methods of dealing with telephone calls, none of which serves as an acceptable alternative to having an office nurse screen calls and give telephone advice: (1) The physician can accept calls at any time throughout the day. These interruptions are unacceptable to most physicians and to most families who are in the office. (2) The physician can have a telephone hour at the beginning, middle, and end of the day and accept only emergency calls at other times. The disadvantages of this approach are that some parents must then wait for answers to urgent questions, and the physician lengthens his or her day with many routine calls. (3) The physician may charge for telephone advice. This decreases the number of calls, but in the process it may discourage important calls and thus interfere with preventive pediatrics. (4) The physician can allow various nonmedical office personnel to accept telephone calls randomly themselves. This approach would result in inconsistent medical advice and could be dangerous. The physician is, of course, legally liable for any harm to a patient caused by improper advice given over the phone by employees.

Recorded telephone advice is also an option for practices. A dedicated phone line or menu allows the caller to access the latest message. Messages, which can be changed as often as desired, can keep families appraised of the latest illness going around in the community, how to handle it at home, and when to bring their child in, or they may give information about upcoming services, for example, when the influenza vaccine will be available and who should receive it. Recently, commercial services have become available that allow the caller to choose from a list of hundreds of prerecorded health topics. In this way, families may get the information they need, such as how to handle a sunburn, without needing to speak directly to a member of the office staff.

---

*Contributed by Barton D. Schmitt, MD.

Schmitt BD: *Pediatric Telephone Advice,* 2nd ed. Little, Brown, 1994.

FEVER*

Pediatricians are called on daily to evaluate children with fever. *Fever* is defined as a rectal temperature over 38 °C, an oral temperature over 37.5 °C, or an axillary temperature over 37 °C.

Body temperature normally fluctuates during the day and may be 0.5 °C below normal in the morning, progressing to 0.5 °C above normal in the evening. Mild elevation of 1–1.5 °C can be caused by exercise, excessive clothing, a hot bath, or hot weather. Anderson (1990) found that bottle or breast feedings tend to raise the infant's temperature for about 30 minutes or more. Warm food or drink can elevate an oral temperature; therefore, if one of these causes is suspected, the temperature should be taken again in 30 minutes, after eliminating the possible cause.

Fever is a symptom, not a disease. It occurs when there is a rise in the hypothalamic set-point (caused by infection, malignancy, collagen-vascular disease, some drugs, etc), when the body's heat production or environmental heat exceeds heat loss mechanisms (as in malignant hyperthermia, excessive environmental heat), or when heat loss mechanisms are defective (as in ectodermal dysplasia). The vast majority of fevers are caused by viral illness and last 2–3 days. There is a direct relationship between fever magnitude and serious bacterial infection. Teething does not cause fever over 38.4 °C.

Fever causes no harm, such as brain damage, when it is less than 41.7 °C. Fortunately, the brain's thermostat keeps untreated fevers resulting from infection below 41.1 °C. While all children have fever on occasion, only 4% develop a febrile convulsion. This type of seizure is generally harmless.

Guidelines for Evaluating Children With Fever

A. See Immediately If:
- The child is under 2 months old.
- The fever is over 40.1 °C.
- The child is crying inconsolably or whimpering.
- The child cries when moved or otherwise touched by the parent.
- The child is difficult to awaken.
- The neck is stiff.
- Any purple spots are present on the skin.
- Breathing is difficult, and no better after the nose is cleared.
- The child is drooling saliva and is unable to swallow anything.

- A convulsion has occurred.
- The child acts or looks very sick.

B. See Within 24 Hours If:
- The child is 2–4 months old (unless fever occurs within 48 hours of a diphtheria-pertussis-tetanus [DPT] vaccine and the infant has no other serious symptoms).
- The fever exceeds 40 °C (especially if the child is under 3 years old).
- Burning or pain occurs with urination.
- The fever has been present more than 24 hours without an obvious cause or location of infection.
- The fever went away for more than 24 hours and then returned.
- The fever has been present for more than 72 hours.

Treatment of Fever

A. "Fever Phobia" and the Overtreatment of Fever:
Fever phobia is a term that describes the parents' anxious response to the fevers that all children experience. Schmitt's study (1980) found that 80% of parents thought fevers between 40 and 41.1 °C cause brain damage. About 20% of parents thought that if they did not treat the fever, it would keep going higher. Neither of these statements is true. Because of these misconceptions, many parents treat low-grade fevers unnecessarily. Teaching parents about fever can reduce the number of telephone calls and visits to the doctor.

B. Acetaminophen:
Acetaminophen is indicated for children older than 2 months of age if the fever is over 39 °C and/or the child is uncomfortable. It can be given every 4–6 hours and will reduce the fever by 1–2 °C within 2 hours of the dose. Antipyretics do not bring the temperature down to normal unless the fever was low-grade to begin with.

C. Liquid Ibuprofen:
Ibuprofen and acetaminophen are similar in safety and in their ability to lower fever. Ibuprofen lasts 6–8 hours, compared with 4–6 hours for acetaminophen. Parents should be cautioned that the milligram-per-kilogram dosing and the concentration of these drugs are different.

D. Cautions About Aspirin:
Aspirin should not be used for fever, because several studies have linked its use during viral illnesses (especially chickenpox and influenza) to Reye's syndrome.

E. Sponging for Fever:
Indications for immediate sponging with lukewarm water (never alcohol) are febrile delirium, febrile seizure, or any fever over 41.1 °C. For other children, sponging is rarely necessary. Acetaminophen should always be given 30 minutes prior to sponging. Until acetaminophen has taken effect, sponging will only cause shivering, which may ultimately raise the temperature. Heat stroke requires immediate cold-water sponging (antipyretics are not beneficial).

F. Other Measures:
Extra fluids should be encouraged. Body fluids are lost during fever because

---

*Contributed by Barton D. Schmitt, MD.

of sweating, and the increased respiratory rate associated with fever means increased insensible losses through respiratory vapors.

Types of Thermometers

Glass (with mercury) thermometers are inexpensive, but they record the temperature slowly and are often hard to read. Oral temperatures are accurate, provided that no hot or cold drinks or food has been consumed in the preceding 10 minutes. Axillary temperatures are the least accurate, but better than no measurement. Although rectal temperatures are the most accurate, they are uncomfortable and embarrassing for older children, and may perforate the rectum if improperly inserted. They are usually reserved for children under age 5. The thermometer must be left in place for 2 minutes for rectal, 3 minutes for oral, and 5–6 minutes for axillary temperatures.

Digital thermometers measure quickly and, in some studies, are more accurate than glass thermometers.

Tympanic thermometers read the temperature of the eardrum and are at least as accurate as the rectal temperature. Temperatures are measured in less than 2 seconds without discomfort, and the cooperation of the child is not essential.

Liquid crystal strips applied to the forehead and temperature-sensitive pacifiers are inaccurate and miss fevers in many children. Touching the forehead also tends to miss mild fevers.

Anderson ES et al: Factors influencing the body temperature of 3- to 4-month-old infants at home during the day. Arch Dis Child 1990;65:1308.

Beach P, McCormick D: Fever and tympanic thermometry. Clin Pediatr 1991;30(Suppl):1.

Schmitt BD: Fever phobia: Misconceptions of parents about fever. Am J Dis Child 1980;134:176.

EVALUATION OF THE FEBRILE CHILD AND "OUTPATIENT" BACTEREMIA

Every day, febrile children are evaluated by health care providers. Those at increased risk for serious bacterial illness must be identified and treated appropriately.

ESSENTIALS OF DIAGNOSIS

- Child less than 3 years of age with fever
- No focal infection found on physical examination

GENERAL CONSIDERATIONS

Children under the age of 3 years who present with a fever but no obvious source of infection present a special challenge to physicians. Both minor illnesses and serious bacterial infections (SBIs; sepsis, meningitis, urinary tract infections, pneumonia, septic arthritis/osteomyelitis, enteritis) are common at this age.

Bacterial pathogens most commonly seen in the infant less than 2 months of age are group B streptococcus and *Escherichia coli*. *Streptococcus pneumoniae* and *Haemophilus influenzae* type b are more commonly encountered in older children, although the incidence of *H influenzae* type b disease has fallen dramatically since the institution of this vaccine for infants. Other pathogens responsible for invasive disease include *Staphylococcus aureus, Salmonella* spp, and other gram-negative organisms.

In general, as the height of the fever increases, the risk of SBI increases. In infants younger than 30 days (Bonadio et al, 1990), the rate of SBI was found to be 4.4% for temperatures 38.1–39 °C, 7.6% for 39.1–39.9 °C, and 18% for temperatures of 40 °C or more. Various studies report the risk of occult bacteremia in children 3–36 months of age with fever without source to be from 3% to 11%.

MANAGEMENT

For infants and children less than 3 years of age with fever without source, Baraff et al (1993) proposed the following:

(1) Hospitalize any child who appears toxic.

(2) Hospitalize the newborn who is under 4 weeks of age. Infants under 1 month of age should have a sepsis workup and be hospitalized, even though the risk of SBI, if they meet the low-risk criteria below, is quite small. Generally, the hospitalized infant is placed on parenteral antibiotics pending culture results; however, they could also be observed in the hospital without antibiotics.

(3) Identify the "low-risk" febrile infant (1–3 months of age):

- Nontoxic
- Previously healthy
- No bacterial focus on examination (except otitis media)
- Good social situation
- WBC count 5000–15,000/mm^3; fewer than 1500 bands/mm^3 (In general, the higher the WBC count or the higher the absolute neutrophil count, the greater the likelihood of bacteremia. When the WBC count exceeds 15,000/mm^3, the probability of bacteremia increases fivefold.)
- Urinalysis with fewer than 5 WBCs per high-power field (hpf)

- If diarrhea is present, fewer than 5 WBCs per hpf in stool

Manage the low-risk infant (1–3 months of age), whose probability of an SBI is 0.2%, as an outpatient with one of two options: (a) Culture urine; reevaluate in 24 hours. (b) Culture blood, urine, and cerebrospinal fluid; administer ceftriaxone, 50 mg/kg; reevaluate in 24 hours. Parenteral antibiotics are more effective than oral antibiotics.

(4) Hospitalize the non–low-risk febrile infant.

(5) Determine the temperature of the previously healthy child who is 3 months to 3 years of age. If the fever is below 39.0 °C, use antipyretics and follow up. If the temperature is 39.0 °C or above, obtain a WBC count. If the count is at least 15,000/mm^3, obtain a blood culture and treat with ceftriaxone, 50 mg/kg. Males under 6 months of age and females under 2 years of age should also have a urine specimen, by either catheter or suprapubic tap, sent for culture. Chest x-ray and stool culture are useful only if indicated by history or examination.

FOLLOW-UP

Infants and children with positive blood or cerebrospinal fluid cultures should be admitted and treated with parenteral antibiotics. If the blood culture grows nonresistant *S pneumoniae* and the child is afebrile at the follow-up visit, outpatient therapy with oral amoxicillin or penicillin is adequate. Urinary tract infections may also be treated on an outpatient basis with oral antibiotics, based on sensitivities, if the child is afebrile.

Baraff LJ et al: Practice guidelines for the management of infants and children with 0 to 36 months of age with fever without source. Pediatrics 1993;92:1.

Bonadio WA, Romine K, Gyuro J: Relationship of fever magnitude to rate of serious bacterial infections in neonates. J Pediatr 1990;116:733.

GROWTH DEFICIENCY (FAILURE TO THRIVE)

Growth deficiency, formerly termed failure to thrive, occurs when there is a deceleration of growth velocity resulting in crossing two major percentile lines on the growth chart, or when a height-to-weight plot is lower than the fifth percentile. Because growth is so rapid in the first 6 months of life, care providers should be concerned if there is no weight gain over a 2-month period. Growth deficiency is present in about 8% of the pediatric population.

UNDERNUTRITION

Undernutrition is at the core of growth deficiency. In cases historically termed nonorganic failure to thrive, undernutrition is a result of environmental factors and aberrant caretaker-child interaction. For those cases previously termed organic failure to thrive, undernutrition occurs as a result of major organ system disease (eg, renal failure, congenital heart disease, hypothyroidism).

GROWTH CHART

Specific patterns of growth deficiency point to differing causes. In **type I growth deficiency,** the head circumference is preserved while the weight is depressed more than the height. This is the most common growth deficiency and results from inadequate caloric intake, excessive loss of calories, excessive utilization of calories, or inability to use calories peripherally. The majority of these cases result from inadequate delivery of calories. This may be the result of financial constraints, lack of caretaker understanding, poor caretaker-child interaction, abnormal feeding patterns, or a combination of these factors. **Type II growth deficiency,** which is associated with genetically determined short stature, endocrinopathies, constitutional growth delay, or various forms of dwarfism, is characterized by normal head circumference and proportional diminution of height and weight. In **type III growth deficiency,** all three parameters of growth are depressed. This pattern is associated with central nervous system abnormalities, chromosomal defects, and in utero or perinatal insults.

INITIAL EVALUATION

The history and the physical examination will identify the cause of growth reduction in the vast majority of cases. The history includes the following: (1) birth (rule out intrauterine growth retardation, anoxia, congenital infection), (2) feeding and nutrition (difficulty sucking, chewing, swallowing; feeding patterns; intake of formula, milk, juice, solids), (3) stooling and voiding (diarrhea, constipation, vomiting, poor urine stream), (4) growth pattern (several points on the growth chart are crucial), (5) recurrent infections, (6) hospitalizations, (7) HIV risk factors, (8) development, (9) social factors (family composition, financial status, supports, stresses), (10) family factors (inherited diseases, heights and weights of relatives), and (11) review of systems.

The physical examination should scrutinize for organic disease or evidence of abuse or neglect: dysmorphic features, skin lesions, neck mass, adventitial breath sounds, heart murmur, abdominal mass, and neuromuscular tone and strength. Throughout the evaluation, observation is made of the caretaker-child interaction and the level of family functioning. A formal developmental screening test, such as the Denver II, completes the initial office evaluation.

Table 9–6. Acceptable weight gain by age.

Age (months)	Weight Gain (g/d)
Birth to 3	20–30
3–6	15–20
6–9	10–15
9–12	6–11
12–18	5–8
18–24	3–7

FURTHER EVALUATION

A battery of screening laboratory tests cannot substitute for a thorough initial evaluation. Tests should be ordered based on the history and physical examination findings, for example, stool for fat examination if a history of diarrhea suggests malabsorption. A prospective 3-day diet record should be a standard part of the evaluation. This has utility in assessing undernutrition, even when there is organic disease. The diet history is evaluated by a pediatric dietitian for calories, protein, and micronutrients as well as for the pattern of eating.

TREATMENT

A successful treatment plan addresses the child's diet and eating patterns, the child's development, family/caretaker strengths and weaknesses, and any organic disease. High-calorie diets and frequent monitoring (initially, every 1–2 weeks) are essential. Acceptable weight gain varies by age (Table 9–6).

The child with a growth deficiency may also be developmentally delayed because of living in an environment that fails to promote development or as a consequence of nutrient deprivation effect on the brain. Restoring nutrition does not fully reverse the deficit, but does reduce the long-term consequences.

Education in nutrition and child development as well as psychosocial support of the primary caretaker is essential. If family dysfunction is mild, behavior modification and counseling will be useful. Day care may benefit the child by providing a structured environment for all activities, including eating. If family dysfunction is severe, refer to the local Department of Social Services, which can help provide structure and assistance to the family. Rarely, the child may need to be removed, at least temporarily, from the home.

Previously, the child with growth deficiency was separated from the mother, hospitalized, and then returned home, without modifying the environment that may have contributed to the problem. Today hospitalization is reserved for dehydration or starvation, evidence of abuse or willful neglect, an illness that compromises a child's ability to eat, or an impending foster care placement.

Colloton M: Investigating failure to thrive. J Am Acad Pediatr Adolesc 1989;2:359.

Frank DA, Zeisel SH: Failure to thrive. Pediatr Clin North Am 1988;35:1187.

Weston JA: Growth deficiency. In: *Pediatric Decision Making,* 3rd ed. Berman S (editor). 1996, in press.

10

Immunization

Eric A.F. Simoes, MD, DCH, & Jessie R. Groothuis, MD

The routine use of immunization has become an integral part of pediatric practice in the United States over the last 50 years. Despite problems arising out of complacency, increased cost, and threats of litigation, vaccinations continue to be a critical feature of well child care.

Immunization is intended to prevent either the primary manifestations of infection with a particular organism or secondary phenomena resulting from that infection. Any calculation of benefit must take into account the likelihood that the illness will occur in a defined population or individual as well as the likelihood that the vaccination will prevent that illness. This benefit must be weighed against the risk to the individual child. It is the obligation of the physician to present this information to the parents or legal guardian in lay terminology and to record their understanding of the information and their consent to immunization.The recommendations for use of immunizations outlined in this chapter are current. However, as technology and our understanding of the epidemiology of vaccine-preventable diseases change, the recommendations will also change. The most useful sources for current information are listed below:

(1) *Morbidity and Mortality Weekly Report.* Published weekly by the Centers For Disease Control and Prevention (CDC), Atlanta 30333. *MMWR* contains recommendations of the United States Public Health Service Advisory Committee on Immunization Practices (ACIP).

(2) *Report of the Committee on Infectious Diseases.* Published at 2- to 3-year intervals by the American Academy of Pediatrics, the *Red Book* is available from the American Academy of Pediatrics (AAP). Updates are published in the journal *Pediatrics.*

STANDARDS FOR PEDIATRIC IMMUNIZATION PRACTICES

Although 97–98% of children in the United States are vaccinated by or shortly after school entry, as many as 37–56% of the more than 8 million 2-year-olds in this country are not fully immunized. Low immunization coverage has been attributed to difficulties in reaching socioeconomic groups, including the urban poor and racial and ethnic minorities. However, the health care delivery system appears to bear much of the responsibility for low immunization coverage as well. Parents seeking immunization for their children face significant barriers; not all providers take advantage of opportunities to administer vaccines, and inadequate or absent third-party payment for immunizations further reduces coverage. Standards for Pediatric Immunization Practices (Table 10–1) and a guide to Contraindications and Precautions to Immunization (Table 10–2) reflect the current recommendations of the Advisory Committee on Immunization Practices and the Committee of Infectious Diseases of the American Academy of Pediatrics.

Standards for pediatric immunization practices. MMWR 1993;42(RR-5):1.

SAFETY OF IMMUNIZATION

VACCINE FACTORS

The safety standards for all vaccines licensed for use in the United States are established by the Food and Drug Administration (FDA) and involve regular examination of manufacturing techniques as well as

Table 10–1. Standards for pediatric immunization practices.

1. Immunization services are readily available.
2. There are no barriers or unnecessary prerequisites to the receipt of vaccines.
3. Immunization services are available free or for a minimal fee.
4. Providers use all clinical encounters to screen and, when indicated, vaccinate children.
5. Providers educate parents and guardians about immunization in general terms.
6. Providers question parents or guardians about contraindications and, before vaccinating a child, inform them in specific terms about the risks and benefits of the vaccinations their child is to receive.
7. Providers follow only true contraindications.
8. Providers administer simultaneously all vaccine doses for which a child is eligible at the time of each visit.
9. Providers use accurate and complete recording procedures.
10. Providers co-schedule immunization appointments in conjunction with appointments for other child health services.
11. Providers report adverse events following vaccination promptly, accurately, and completely.
12. Providers operate a tracking system.
13. Providers adhere to appropriate procedures for vaccine management.
14. Providers conduct semiannual audits to assess immunization coverage levels and to review immunization records in patient populations they serve.
15. Providers maintain up-to-date, easily retrievable medical protocols at all locations where vaccines are administered.
16. Providers practice patient-oriented and community-based approaches.
17. Vaccines are administered by properly trained persons.
18. Providers receive ongoing education and training regarding current immunization recommendations.

production lots of vaccine. There have been no incidents of bacterial or viral contamination of vaccines at the factory level in the United States for decades.

FACTORS RELATED TO VACCINE ADMINISTRATION

The use of disposable syringes and needles or some other form of single-dose delivery of vaccine is preferred to minimize the opportunity for contamination. If reusable glass syringes are used, they must be thoroughly cleaned and autoclaved after each use. If autoclaving is not possible, either dry heat of 170 °C for 2 hours or boiling for 30 minutes is an acceptable alternative. A 70% solution of alcohol is appropriate for disinfection of the stopper of the vaccine container and of the skin at the injection site.

The manufacturer's recommendations for route and site of administration of injectable vaccines are critical for safety and efficacy. All vaccines containing an adjuvant must be administered intramuscularly to avoid granuloma formation or necrosis. Such injections should be given in the anterolateral thigh (not intragluteally) in infants (<15 months of age) and may be given in the deltoid or triceps in older children. A 22-gauge needle 1–1¼ in. long is recommended for children, but a 25-gauge ⅝-in. needle may be sufficient for young infants. Aqueous vaccines may be administered intramuscularly, subcutaneously, or intradermally. For subcutaneous or intradermal injections, a 25-gauge ½- to ¾-in. needle is recommended. Good injection technique, including aspiration prior to injection, must always be practiced. A separate syringe and needle should be used for each vaccine.

It is safe to administer many combinations of vaccines simultaneously without increasing the risk of adverse effects (see individual preparations below for further discussion). Inactivated vaccines (with the exception of cholera and yellow fever) can be given simultaneously or at any time after a different vaccine. Whenever possible, live-virus vaccines, if not administered on the same day, should be given at least 30 days apart. If an immunoglobulin has been administered, live-virus vaccination should be delayed 6–10 months to avoid interference with the immune response.

HOST FACTORS

Healthy Children

Minor acute illnesses, with or without low-grade fever, are not contraindications to vaccination, since there is no evidence that vaccination under these conditions increases the rate of adverse effects or decreases efficacy. A moderate to severe febrile illness is reason to postpone vaccination. Routine physical examination and taking temperatures are not prerequisites for vaccinating apparently healthy infants and children.

Children With Chronic Illnesses

Most chronic diseases are not contraindications to vaccination; in fact, children with chronic diseases may be at greater risk of complications from vaccine-preventable diseases, such as influenza and pneumococcal infections. Premature infants are a good example. It is clear that they should be immunized according to their chronologic, not gestational, age. Vaccine doses should not be reduced for preterm or low birth weight infants. The one exception to this rule may be children with progressive central nervous system disorders. Vaccination may be deferred or avoided entirely for them, whereas children with static central nervous system diseases are candidates for vaccination.

Immunodeficient Children

Congenitally immunodeficient children should not be immunized with live-virus or live-bacteria vaccines. Depending on the nature of the immunodefi-

Table 10–2. Guide to contraindications and precautions to vaccinations.

GENERAL FOR ALL VACCINES (DTP/DTaP, OPV, IPV, MMR, Hib, HBV, VZV)

Contraindications	Not contraindications
Anaphylactic reaction to a vaccine contraindicates further doses of that vaccine Anaphylactic reaction to a vaccine constituent contraindicates the use of vaccines containing that substance Moderate or severe acute illnesses with or without a fever	Mild to moderate local reaction (soreness, redness, swelling) following a dose of an injectable antigen Mild acute illness with or without low-grade fever Current antimicrobial therapy Convalescent phase of illnesses Prematurity (same dosage and indications as for normal, full-term infants) History of penicillin or other nonspecific allergies or family history of such allergies

DTP/DTaP

Contraindication	Not contraindications
Encephalopathy within 7 days of administration of the previous dose of DTP **Precautions[1]** Fever of $\geq$40.5 °C (105 °F) or high-pitched cry within 48 h after vaccination with a prior dose of DTP Collapse or shock-like state (hypotonic-hyporesponsive episode) within 48 h after receiving a prior dose of DTP Seizures within 3 d of receiving a prior dose of DTP (see footnote 2 regarding management of children with a personal history of seizures at any time) Progressive seizure disorder or encephalopathy Persistent, inconsolable crying lasting $\geq$3 h within 48 h of receiving a prior dose of DTP	Temperature <40.5 °C (105 °F) following the previous dose of DTP Family history of convulsions[2] Family history of sudden infant death syndrome Family history of an adverse event following DTP administration

OPV[3]

Contraindications	Not contraindications
Infection with HIV or a household contact with HIV Known immunodeficiency (hematologic and solid tumors, congenital immunodeficiency, long-term immunosuppressive therapy) Immunodeficient household contact **Precaution[1]** Pregnancy	Breast-feeding Current antimicrobial therapy Diarrhea

(continued)

ciency, other vaccines are safe. However, these may fail to evoke an immune response. Children with cancer and children being treated with corticosteroids or other immunosuppressive agents should not be vaccinated with live-virus or live-bacteria vaccines. This contraindication does not apply if the malignancy is in remission and chemotherapy has not been administered for at least 90 days. In addition, previously healthy children who are being treated with low to moderate doses of corticosteroids for less than 14 days, children receiving low to moderate doses of alternate-day corticosteroids, children being maintained on physiologic corticosteroid therapy without other immunodeficiency, and children using only topical inhaled, or intra-articular corticosteroids may receive live vaccines safely. These guidelines apply to children with documented HIV infection, with the exception that live measles, mumps, and rubella vaccinations are recommended, whereas oral poliovirus vaccine is not. No distinction is made between children with asymptomatic or symptomatic HIV infection. Siblings and household contacts of a child who is immunodeficient should not receive oral poliovirus vaccine unless the immunodeficient child has been successfully immunized against poliomyelitis. If that is not the case, the siblings should receive inactivated poliovirus vaccine (IPV). Measles, mumps, and rubella (MMR) vaccines are not contraindicated under these circumstances.

Allergic or Hypersensitive Children

Hypersensitivity reactions are rare following vaccination. They are generally attributable to a trace component of the vaccine rather than to the antigen itself. MMR, IPV, and varicella-zoster vaccine (VZV) contain microgram quantities of neomycin, and IPV also contains trace amounts of streptomycin. Children with known anaphylactic responses to these antibiotics should not be given these vaccines. Trace quantities of egg antigens may be present in influenza measles, mumps, and yellow fever vaccines. Children who have had anaphylactic reactions to eggs should not be given these vaccines. Children with less serious reactions to eggs may generally be safely immunized with these products. If doubt exists about the nature of a child's egg sensitivity, a skin testing procedure is outlined in the *Red Book*.

Table 10–2. (continued)

IPV

Contraindication
Anaphylactic reaction to neomycin or streptomycin
Precaution[1]
Pregnancy

MMR[3]

Contraindications	**Not contraindications**
Anaphylactic reactions to egg ingestion and to neomycin[4]	Tuberculosis or positive skin test
Pregnancy	Simultaneous TB skin testing[5]
Known immunodeficiency except HIV (hematologic and solid	Breast-feeding
tumors, congenital immunodeficiency, long-term	Pregnancy of mother or recipient
immunosuppressive therapy)	Immunodeficient family member or household contact
Precaution[1]	Infection with HIV (including children)
Recent (within 3 mo) immune globulin administration	Nonanaphylactic reactions to eggs or neomycin

Hib

Contraindications
None identified

HBV

Contraindications	**Not a contraindication**
None identified	Pregnancy

VZV

Contraindications	**Not contraindications**
Same as for OPV	Steroids <2 mg/kg/d of prednisone
Neomycin allergy	Salicylates

[1]The events or conditions listed as precautions, although not contraindications, should be carefully reviewed. The benefits and risks of administering a specific vaccine to an individual under the circumstances should be considered. If the risks are believed to outweigh the benefits, the immunization should be withheld; if the benefits are believed to outweigh the risks (eg, during an outbreak or foreign travel), the immunization should be given. Whether and when to administer DTP to children with proved or suspected underlying neurologic disorders should be decided on an individual basis. It is prudent on theoretical grounds to avoid vaccinating pregnant women. However, if immediate protection against poliomyelitis is needed, OPV, not IPV, is recommended.
[2]Acetaminophen given prior to administering DTP and thereafter every 4 h for 24 h should be considered for children with a personal or family history of convulsions in siblings or parents.
[3]There is a theoretical risk that the administration of multiple live virus vaccines (OPV, MMR) within 30 d of one another if not given on the same day will result in a suboptimal immune response. There are no data to substantiate this.
[4]Persons with a history of anaphylactic reactions following egg ingestion should be vaccinated only with extreme caution. Protocols have been developed for vaccinating such persons and should be consulted. (J Pediatr 1983;102:196; J Pediatr 1988;113:504).
[5]Measles vaccinations may temporarily suppress tuberculin reactivity. If testing cannot be done the day of MMR vaccination, the test should be postponed for 4–6 wk.

Borkowsky W et al: Cell-mediated and humoral immune responses in children infected with human immunodeficiency virus during the first few years of life. J Pediatr 1992;120:371.

General recommendations on immunization: Recommendations of the Immunization Practices Advisory Committee (ACIP). MMWR 1994;43:RR-1.

Immunization of children infected with human immunodeficiency virus: Supplementary ACIP statement. MMWR 1988;37:181.

1996 Red Book: Report of the Committee on Infectious Diseases, 24th ed. American Academy of Pediatrics, 1996.

THE COMPOSITION OF IMMUNIZING AGENTS

ACTIVE IMMUNIZATION

Although each vaccine is unique, the practitioner should be familiar with the general constituents of a vaccine. The antigenic component, or immunogen, may be a single well-defined entity, such as tetanus toxoid, or it may be a mixture of defined entities, such as the capsular polysaccharides of pneumococcal vaccine. The immunogen may be a live attenuated organism such as measles vaccine, or it may be whole killed organisms such as the IPV. The antigenic component may be a complex of killed disrupted organisms and products, as in pertussis vaccine. All antigens are not equally capable of inducing an immunologic response in all hosts. The factors influencing host responses include genetic variability in immune responsiveness, age at first exposure to the antigen, residual maternal antibody, and any prior experience with the antigen. A small proportion of children receiving certain antigens simply do not mount a response that is capable of conferring protection. For this reason, every vaccine has a definable failure rate.

The immunogen is suspended or dissolved in a fluid, like sterile water or saline. The fluid may be more complex, such as tissue culture medium, and may contain constituents from the biologic system used to produce the immunogen. Most vaccines contain materials to preserve or stabilize the immunogen, particularly mercurials. In addition, trace amounts of antibiotics such as neomycin may be present to prevent bacterial overgrowth.

Some vaccines contain adjuvants such as alum, aluminum hydroxide, and aluminum phosphate, which are nonspecific immune stimulants. They also help to retain the immunogen in a "depot site" for a prolonged time, thus increasing the antigenic stimulation.

Finally, despite rigorous testing and high standards of mechanical and biologic purity and stability, vaccines may contain unwanted and undetectable antigens and other materials. Although unlikely, vaccine administration could have unforeseen adverse consequences. Thus, vaccines should be administered where there is ready access to emergency resuscitative equipment and drugs (epinephrine, antihistamines).

PASSIVE IMMUNIZATION

Immune globulin (IG) is derived from pooled donations of large numbers of individuals (more than 1000 per lot). IG is prepared by alcohol fractionation, is sterile, and will not transmit any infectious agents (including hepatitis B virus and HIV). IG is a 16.5% solution consisting primarily of immunoglobulin G with very small amounts of immunoglobulins A and M.

ROUTINE CHILDHOOD IMMUNIZATIONS

See Table 10–3 for a detailed schedule of routine immunizations for normal infants and children. Even if the interval elapsed between doses in a series of immunizations is longer than recommended, that series can be resumed as if no interruption had taken place; it is not necessary to begin the series again.

Children with an unknown vaccination status should be considered unprotected. Table 10–4 presents recommended schedules for children who did not start vaccination at the recommended time during the first year of life. Variations from these schedules may be necessitated by epidemiologic or individual clinical circumstances.

Safe Handling of Vaccines

The numerous vaccines and other immunologic substances, such as antibody preparations and immunoglobulins for routine use by the practitioner, vary in correct storage temperatures. Vaccines that require routine freezing are varicella and oral polio vaccine. Yellow fever vaccine may also be stored frozen. Consult individual product package inserts for detailed information on storage conditions and shelf life.

Casto DT, Brunell PA: Safe handling of vaccines. Pediatrics 1991;87:108.

DIPHTHERIA

Diphtheria toxoid is prepared by the formaldehyde inactivation of diphtheria toxin. The toxoid content of the several available preparations varies and is measured in limit of flocculation (Lf) units. The protective efficacy of diphtheria toxoid has never been measured on a mass scale but is estimated to be greater than 85%.

Preparations Available

(1) Diphtheria toxoid is used only when tetanus toxoid and pertussis vaccine are both contraindicated. It contains 10–12 Lf units per immunizing dose.

(2) Diphtheria-tetanus (DT) (pediatric) is used when pertussis vaccine is contraindicated. DT contains 6.7–12.5 Lf units of diphtheria toxoid per dose. Pediatric DT should not be used in adults because of potentially severe adverse reactions.

(3) Tetanus-diphtheria (Td) (adult) is for use in persons 7 years of age or older and contains 2 Lf units or less of diphtheria toxoid. It is less likely to produce local reactions while still eliciting a good immunogenic response in this population.

(4) Diphtheria-tetanus-pertussis (DTP) is the standard immunizing agent for healthy children and contains 6.7–12.5 Lf units of diphtheria toxoid per dose.

(5) Diphtheria-tetanus-acellular pertussis (DTaP) contains 6.7–12.5 Lf units of diphtheria toxins per dose. It is licensed for use only as the fourth or fifth dose of the DPT series in children at least 12 months of age, provided 6 months have elapsed since the third DPT.

Dosage & Schedule of Administration

The above preparations are administered intramus-

Table 10–3. Recommended Childhood Immunization Schedule United States, July–December 1996.
Vaccines are listed under the routinely recommended ages. Bars indicate range of acceptable ages for vaccination.
Shaded bars indicate *catch-up vaccination:* at 11–12 years of age, hepatitis B vaccine should be administered to children not previously vaccinated, and Varicella Zoster Virus vaccine should be administered to children not previously vaccinated who lack a relaible history of chickenpox.

Age Vaccine	Birth	1 mo	2 mos	4 mos	6 mos	12 mos	15 mos	18 mos	4–6 yrs	11–12 yrs	14–16 yrs
Hepatitis B[1,2]	HepB-1										
			Hep B-2		Hep B-3					Hep B[2]	
Diphtheria, Tetanus, Pertussis[3]			DTP	DTP	DTP	DTP[3] (DTaP at 15+ m)			DTP or DTaP	Td	
H. influenzae type b[4]			Hib	Hib	Hib[4]	Hib[4]					
Polio[5]			OPV[5]	OPV	OPV				OPV		
Measles, Mumps, Rubella[6]						MMR			MMR[6] or MMR[6]		
Varicella Zoster Virus Vaccine[7]						Var				Var[7]	

Approved by the Advisory Committee on Immunization Practices (ACIP), the American Academy of Pediatrics (AAP), and the American Academy of Family Pysicians (AAFP).

[1]*Infants born to HBsAg-negative mothers* should receive 2.5 μg of Merck vaccine (Recombivax HB) or 10 μg of SmithKline Beecham (SB) vaccine (Engerix-B). The 2nd dose should be administered ≥1 mo after the 1st dose.

Infants born to HBsAg-positive mothers should receive 0.5 mL hepatitis B immune globulin (HBIG) within 12 hrs of birth, and either 5 μg of Merck vaccine (Recombivax HB) or 10 μg of SB vaccine (Engerix-B) at a separate site. The 2nd dose is recommended at 1–2 mos of age and the 3rd dose at 6 mos of age.

Infants born to mothers whose HBsAg status is unknown should receive either 5 μg of Merck vaccine (Recombivax HB) or 10 μg of SB vaccine (Engerix-B) within 12 hrs of birth. The 2nd dose of vaccine is recommended at 1 mo of age and the 3rd dose at 6 mos of age.

[2]Adolescents who have not previously received 3 doses of hepatitis B vaccine should initiate or complete the series at the 11–12 year-old visit. The 2nd dose should be administered at least 1 mo after the 1st dose, and the 3rd dose should be administered at least 4 mos after the 1st dose and at least 2 mos after the 2nd dose.

[3]DTP4 may be administered at 12 mos of age, if at least 6 mos have elapsed since DTP3. DTaP (diphtheria and tetanus toxoids and acellular pertussis vaccine) is licensed for the 4th and/or 5th vaccine dose(s) for children aged ≥15 mos and may be preferred for these doses in this age group. Td (tetanus and diphtheria toxoids, absorbed, for adult use) is recomended at 11–12 years of age if at least 5 years have elapsed since the last dose of DTP, DTaP, or DT.

[4]Three *H. influenzae* type b (Hib) conjugate vaccines are licensed for infant use. If PRP-OMP (PedvaxHIB[Merck]) is administered at 2 and 4 mos of age, a dose at 6 mos is not required. After completing the primary series, any Hib conjugate vaccine may be used as a booster.

[5]Oral poliovirus vaccine (OPV) is recommended for routine infant vaccination. Inactivated poliovirus vaccine (IPV) is recommended for persons with a congenital or acquired immune deficiency disease or an altered immune status as a result of disease or immunosuppressive therapy, as well as their household contacts, and is an acceptable alternative for other persons. The primary 3-dose series for IPV should be given with a minimum interval of 4 wks between the 1st and 2nd doses and 6 mos between the 2nd and 3rd doses.

[6]The 2nd dose of MMR is routinely recommended at 4–6 yrs of age or at 11–12 yrs of age, but may be administered at any visit, provided at least 1 mo has elapsed since receipt of the 1st dose.

[7]Varicella zoster virus vaccine (Var) can be administered to susceptible children any time after 12 months of age. Unvaccinated children who lack a reliable history of chickenpox should be vaccinated at the 11–12 year-old visit.

cularly in a dose of 0.5 mL. Administration of these adsorbed preparations by jet injection may be associated with more local reactions. See Table 10–3 for the routine schedule and Table 10–4 for those children not appropriately immunized during the first year of life.

Adverse Effects

No significant adverse reactions have been associated with diphtheria toxoid alone.

Antibody Preparations

Equine diphtheria antitoxin is available for treatment

Table 10–4. Recommended immunization schedules for normal children not immunized in their first year of life.

Recommended Time/Age	Immunizations[1]	Comments
YOUNGER THAN 7 YEARS		
First visit	DTP, OPV, MMR HbCV[2] VZV[3]	MMR if child ≥15 mo old; VZV if child is ≥12 mo old; tuberculin testing may be done at same time. For children aged 15–59 mo, can be given simultaneously with DTP and other vaccines (at separate sites).[4]
Interval after first visit 2 mo	DTP, OPV, (HbCV)[5]	Second and third dose of HbCV is indicated only in children whose first dose was received when younger than 15 mo.
4 mo	DTP (HbCV)	Third dose of OPV is not indicated in the United States but is desirable in other geographic areas where polio is endemic.
10–16 mo	DTP, (DTaP),[6] OPV	OPV is not necessary if third dose was given earlier.
4–6 y (at or before school entry)	DTP, (DTaP),[6] OPV (MMR)[7]	DTP is not necessary if the fourth dose was given after the fourth birthday; OPV is not necessary if the third dose was given after the fourth birthday.
11–12 y	MMR	At entry to middle school or junior high.
10 y later	Td	Repeat every 10 y throughout life.
7 YEARS AND OLDER[7,8]		
First visit	Td, OPV, MMR[9]	
Interval after first visit 2 mo	Td, OPV	
8–14 mo	Td, OPV	
11–12 y	MMR	At entry to middle school or junior high
10 y later	Td	Repeat every 10 y throughout life.

[1]Abbreviations are explained in footnote 4 of Table 10–3.
[2]See *Haemophilus influenzae* vaccination section.
[3]VZV may be given after 12 mo of age to the 13th birthday in children without a reliable chickenpox or vaccination history.
[4]The initial three doses of DTP can be given at 1- to 2-mo intervals; hence, for the child in whom immunization is initiated at age 15 mo or older, one visit could be eliminated by giving DTP, OPV, and MMR and HBV at the first visit; DTP and HbCV at the second visit (1 mo later); and DTP, HBV, and OPV at the third visit (2 mo after the first visit). Subsequent doses of DTP and OPV 10–16 mo after the first visit are still indicated. HbCV, MMR, DTP, and HBV can be given simultaneously at separate sites if failure of the patient to return for future immunizations is a concern.
[5]Please see section on hepatitis B vaccine for discussion of recommendations by the AAP and ACIP.
[6]DTaP is recommended only if three prior doses of DTP have been administered.
[7]The ACIP recommends MMR at this time.
[8]If person is ≥18 y old, routine poliovirus vaccination is not indicated in the United States.
[9]Minimal interval between doses of MMR is 1 mo.

of diphtheria. Dosage depends on the size and location of the diphtheritic membrane and an estimate of the patient's level of intoxication. Before proceeding with the use of this preparation, the presence or absence of equine serum sensitivity must be determined using conjunctival (1:10 dilution) or intradermal (1:100 dilution) tests. If present, desensitization must be undertaken. If absent, the following doses are suggested:

Site	Duration of Lesion	Toxic?	Dose (U)
Pharyngeal or laryngeal	≤48 h	—	20,000–40,000
Nasopharyngeal	—	—	40,000–60,000
Extensive or brawny swelling of the neck	≥72 h	Yes	80,000–100,000
Cutaneous	—	—	20,000–40,000

TETANUS

Tetanus toxoid is prepared by inactivating the toxin with formaldehyde. Its activity is measured in Lf units and is generally 4–10 Lf units per immunizing dose for adsorbed products and 4–5 Lf units per dose for the fluid product. The protective efficacy of tetanus toxoid has never been measured in any large study, but it is believed to be high.

Preparations Available

(1) Tetanus toxoid (fluid) is used rarely, only when rapid immunization is desirable.

(2) Tetanus toxoid adsorbed on aluminum phosphate is the standard single antigen "booster" toxoid.

(3) Tetanus-diphtheria (pediatric DT and adult Td) is discussed above.

(4) Diphtheria-tetanus-pertussis (DTP).

(5) Diphtheria-tetanus-acellular pertussis (DTaP).

(6) Diphtheria-tetanus-pertussis–*Haemophilus in-*

fluenzae b (DTP-Hib) is discussed later in the section on Hib.

Dosage & Schedule of Administration

The above preparations are administered intramuscularly in a dose of 0.5 mL. See Table 10–3 for the routine schedule and Table 10–4 for children not appropriately immunized during the first year of life. A booster dose of tetanus-diphtheria (Td) should be scheduled at 11–12 years of age or at 14–16 years of age and every 10 years thereafter to protect against tetanus and diphtheria.

Adverse Effects

Significant reactions to tetanus toxoid, historically an extremely safe preparation, are very unusual. Some older individuals who have had repeated doses may experience severe local reactions.

Antibody Preparations

Tetanus immune globulin (TIG) is indicated in the management of tetanus-prone wounds in individuals who have had an uncertain number or fewer than three tetanus immunizations. Persons immunized within 10 years need not receive TIG, regardless of the nature of their wound. The dose is 250–500 U (one or two vials) intramuscularly.

PERTUSSIS

Pertussis vaccines currently used in the United States for initial immunization are killed whole-cell preparations. Recently, two acellular formulations of DTP (DTaP) have been licensed for use by the FDA for the fourth and fifth doses. Currently available DTP preparations have a protective efficacy of about 60–80% after three doses depending on the source. Further epidemiologic evidence of the efficacy of pertussis vaccine is provided by the observation of a large increase in reported pertussis cases in Great Britain and Japan after those two countries reduced or abandoned use of the vaccine.

Preparations Available

(1) Pertussis vaccine (adsorbed) is manufactured by the Division of Biologic Products, Michigan Department of Public Health, for use within that state. It may be obtained for other use by consultation with the department.

(2) Diphtheria-tetanus-pertussis (DTP).

(3) Diphtheria-tetanus-acellular pertussis (DTaP)

(4) Diphtheria-tetanus-pertussis–*Haemophilus influenzae* b (DTP-Hib).

Dosage & Schedule of Administration

Each of the available preparations is administered in a dose of 0.5 mL intramuscularly. See Table 10–3 for the routine schedule and Table 10–4 for those children not appropriately immunized during the first year of life.

Adverse Effects

A large number of adverse reactions have been attributed to pertussis vaccine. These can be divided into three categories: local reactions, mild to moderate systemic reactions, and severe systemic reactions. The estimated rates of these reactions within the first 48 hours after vaccination are shown in Table 10–5. The only absolute contraindications to the further use of pertussis vaccine are an anaphylactic reaction to the vaccine or a severe acute neurologic illness within 7 days after vaccination (see Table 10–2). Precaution is urged for the following associations: a convulsion within 3 days; persistent, severe, inconsolable screaming or crying for over 3 hours or a high-pitched cry within 48 hours; a hypotonic-hyporesponsive episode within 48 hours; an unexplained temperature rise to 40.5 °C within 48 hours.

Controversy continues regarding the causation of serious neurologic illness by pertussis vaccine. A reassessment of the only large-scale case-control study with enough statistical power to examine this issue— the British National Childhood Encephalopathy Study (NCES)—has led to a reappraisal of the relationship. This controversy has engendered two epidemics: In the United Kingdom and Japan, alleged DTP-associated deaths or encephalopathy caused DTP vaccination rates to fall dramatically, resulting in epidemics of pertussis; whereas in the United States, an epidemic of DTP-associated litigation

Table 10–5. Frequency of common adverse events within 48 h after DTP.[1]

Adverse Event	Frequency:Dose
Local	
Pain	1:2
Swelling >2.4 cm	2:5
Redness >2.4 cm	1:3
Mild to moderate systemic	
Fever ≥38 °C	1:2
Fretfulness	1:2
Drowsiness	1:3
Anorexia	1:5
Vomiting	1:15
Severe	
Persistent crying (3 h)	1:100
High-pitched unusual crying	1:900
Fever ≥40.5 °C	1:330
Hypotonic, hyporesponsive episodes	1:1750
Seizures	1:1750

[1]These data are derived from 15,752 DTP immunizations. (Modified from Cody CL et al: Nature and rates of adverse reactions associated with DTP and ET immunizations in infants and children. Pediatrics 1981;68:650.)

threatens to overwhelm the National Vaccine Injury Compensation Program.

A causal relationship is almost impossible to establish for three reasons: (1) no specific clinical sign, neuropathologic change, or laboratory test has been consistently described in neurologic illnesses temporally associated with DTP vaccination; (2) any assessment of prior neurologic normality is hampered by the young age of the infants; and (3) there is no biologic plausibility—that is, there is no animal model and no convincing evidence that *Bordetella pertussis* or any of its components or products is neurotoxic. Thus, the British NCES conducted between 1976 and 1979 sought to assess the temporal relationship between DTP vaccination and permanent brain damage. It was calculated that while the attributable risk for serious acute neurologic injury ranges from less than 1 per 1 million to 1:140,000, the risk for permanent brain damage is even lower if indeed there is any risk at all. This reassessment, along with new studies, has led the American Academy of Pediatrics, the Canadian National Advisory Committee, and the British Pediatric Association to conclude that pertussis vaccine has not been proved to be the cause of brain damage and to reaffirm the safety and effectiveness of routine whole-cell pertussis vaccine in immunization programs for infants and children.

On July 3, 1991, the National Academy of Sciences Institute of Medicine released a report entitled *Adverse Effects of Pertussis and Rubella Vaccines* in response to a congressional request to review evidence about serious adverse events and immunization with pertussis and rubella vaccines. The committee concluded that the vaccine was causally related to only four adverse events: acute encephalopathy, the range of excess risk being nil to 10.5 per 1 million immunizations; shock (and unusual shock-like state), 3.5–291 cases per 100,000 immunizations; anaphylaxis, 2 cases per 100,000 injections of DTP; and protracted, inconsolable crying, 0.1–6% of recipients. Thus, although epidemiologic evidence may be consistent with a causal relationship, there is no plausible, biological evidence for a role of pertussis toxin in severe DTP reactions.

DIPHTHERIA-TETANUS-PERTUSSIS (DTP)

Diphtheria and tetanus toxoids and pertussis vaccine (DTP) constitute the recommended vehicle for the vaccination of healthy infants against the three diseases. It has been in wide use in the United States for more than 40 years. It has the combined clinical efficacy of the three single-dose preparations, and the efficacy of pertussis vaccine may even be enhanced by the adjuvant effect of the diphtheria and tetanus toxoids. It can be safely and effectively administered simultaneously with OPV or IPV, MMR, HBV and the *Haemophilus influenzae* type b vaccines.

Preparations Available

Each dose of combined diphtheria and tetanus toxoids and whole-cell pertussis vaccine contains 6.7–12.5 Lf units of diphtheria toxoid, 5 Lf units of tetanus toxoid, and not more than 16 opacity units of pertussis vaccine adsorbed with one of several adjuvants (alum, aluminum phosphate, or aluminum hydroxide, depending on the manufacturer).

Dosage & Schedule of Administration

DTP is administered in a dose of 0.5 mL intramuscularly. See Table 10–3 for the routine schedule and Table 10–4 for children not appropriately immunized during the first year of life.

Adverse Effects; Antibody Preparations

See above with the individual component vaccines.

American Academy of Pediatrics Committee on Infectious Diseases: The relationship between pertussis vaccine and brain damage: Reassessment. Pediatrics 1991;88: 397.

Blumberg DA et al: Severe reactions associated with diphtheria-tetanus-pertussis vaccine: Detailed study of children with seizures, hypotonic-hyporesponsive episodes, high fevers, and persistent crying. Pediatrics 1993;91: 1158.

Child Neurology Society: Report of the Therapeutics and Technology Assessment Subcommittee of the American Academy of Neurology. Assessment: DTP vaccination. Neurology 1992;42:471.

Diphtheria, tetanus, and pertussis: Recommendations for vaccine use and other preventive measures. Recommendations of the Immunization Practices Advisory Committee (ACIP). MMWR 1991;40(RR-10):1.

Howson CP, Fineberg HV: The ricochet of magic bullets: Summary of the institute of medicine report, *Adverse Effects of Pertussis and Rubella Vaccines.* Pediatrics 1992;89:318.

Onorato IM et al: Efficacy of whole-cell pertussis vaccine in preschool children in the United States. JAMA 1992;267:2745.

DIPHTHERIA-TETANUS & ACELLULAR PERTUSSIS VACCINE

Two basic types of acellular (DTaP) vaccines have been studied: The T-type vaccines are produced by extraction and purification of *B pertussis* cultures. In contrast, the B-type vaccines contain combinations of pertussis toxin (PT), filamentous hemagglutinin (FHA), pertactin (Prn), and fimbriae (Fim). It has been hypothesized that immunity against PT alone may be sufficient to protect against pertussis, but this view has been challenged, and it has been claimed that FHA, Prn, and Fim antibodies may be required for optimal protection.

Efficacy trials of various acellular pertussis vaccines in Japan and Sweden have established a twofold to 10-fold lesser frequency of "minor" adverse events compared with the whole-cell vaccine, good immunogenicity, and a protective efficacy ranging from 54% to 95%. On the basis of those trials and smaller ones in the United States, the FDA has licensed use of two DTaP vaccines for use as a fourth and fifth dose in children 12 months to 7 years of age, only after they receive three primary doses of DTP, and if 6 months have elapsed since the third DPT. DTaP (connaught) has been licensed for use in the routine schedule for use in infants at 2, 4 and 6 months.

Preparations Available

(1) Diphtheria-tetanus-acellular pertussis (Lederle/Takeda) contains 7.5 Lf units of diphtheria toxoid, 5 Lf units of tetanus toxoid, and 300 hemagglutinating units of Takeda acellular pertussis component, adsorbed to aluminum hydroxide and aluminum phosphate.

(2) Diphtheria-tetanus-acellular pertussis (Connaught/Biken) contains 6.7 Lf units of diphtheria toxoid, 5 Lf units of tetanus toxoid, 23.4 µg of inactivated PT, and 23.4 µg of FHA, absorbed to aluminum potassium sulfate.

Dosage & Schedule of Administration

DTaP is administered in a dose of 0.5 mL intramuscularly. See Table 10–3 for the routine schedule and Table 10–4 for the procedure in children not immunized during the first year.

DTaP is licensed for use only as the fourth and fifth doses for children who have received three prior doses of DTP and are between 12 months and 7 years of age if 6 months has elapsed since DPT3.

Adverse Effects

Local reactions, fever, and other mild systemic events occur with one-fourth to two-thirds the frequency noted following whole- cell DTP vaccination. Moderate to severe systemic events, including fever of 40.5 °C, persistent inconsolable crying lasting 3 hours or more, and hypotonic-hyporesponsive episodes, are less frequent than with whole-cell DTP. These are without sequelae. Severe neurologic events have not been temporally associated with DTaP vaccinations in limited use in the United States.

Blennow M et al: Adverse reactions and serologic response to a booster dose of acellular pertussis vaccine in children immunized with acellular or whole-cell vaccine as infants. Pediatrics 1989;84:62.

Edwards KM: Acellular pertussis vaccines: A solution to the pertussis problem? J Infect Dis 1993;168:15.

Feldman S et al: Comparison of acellular (B type) and whole-cell pertussis-component diphtheria-tetanus-pertussis vaccines as the first booster immunization in 15 to 24 month-old children. J Pediatr 1992:857.

Pertussis vaccination: Acellular pertussis vaccines for reinforcing and booster use: Supplementary ACIP statement. Recommendations of the Immunization Practices Advisory Committee (ACIP). MMWR 1992;41(RR-1):1.

Pichichero ME et al: Safety and immunogenicity of an acellular pertussis vaccine booster in 15 to 20 month-old children previously immunized with acellular or whole-cell pertussis vaccine as infants. Pediatrics 1993;91:756.

Committee on Infectious Diseases. The relations between pertussis vaccine and central nervous system sequelae; continuing assessment. Pediatrics 1996;97:279–281.

POLIOMYELITIS

Vaccines directed against poliovirus infections have largely eliminated the naturally occurring disease in developed countries. In the United States, the number of reported cases of paralytic poliomyelitis has fallen from more than 18,000 in 1954 to 0–10 per year currently. Despite—or perhaps because of—this extraordinary success, controversy continues over the appropriate poliovirus vaccine for mass usage. Live attenuated oral poliovirus vaccine (OPV) (Sabin) is prepared via passage in monkey kidney cells or human diploid cells, depending on the manufacturer. Inactivated injectable poliovirus vaccine (IPV) (Salk) is grown in human diploid cells and inactivated by formaldehyde. A newer preparation, injectable poliovirus vaccine of enhanced potency (IPV-E) (van Wezel), has a higher content of antigens than the old IPV, and field trials have demonstrated that fewer doses of IPV-E are required to attain immunity comparable to that achieved by OPV or IPV.

IPV is incapable of causing poliomyelitis by virtue of being inactivated, whereas OPV can cause such cases rarely. The rate of this in the United States is 3–5 cases of paralytic disease per 10 million doses of OPV distributed. Ninety-three percent of recipient cases and 76% of all vaccine-associated paralytic poliomyelitis (VAPP) occur after administration of the first or second dose of OPV. The risk of paralysis in the immunodeficient recipient may be as much as 2000 times that in normals. IPV cannot multiply in the gut as OPV does—in theory, not protecting against intestinal infection with wild virus, as OPV does—and thus cannot produce "secondary vaccination" of close contacts of vaccinees. IPV, however, produces a much higher serologic response than OPV, a higher booster response at lower prevaccination levels, and an equivalent mucosal response. IPV has the practical advantage of not requiring freezing for storage, as OPV does. However, the mass administration of OPV requires no needles and syringes.

Weighing all the advantages and disadvantages of each vaccine, the Institute of Medicine, the National Academy of Sciences, and the Committee on Infectious Diseases of the American Academy of Pediatrics all continue to recommend the use of OPV under most circumstances in the United States. Exceptions include immunodeficient recipients (including HIV-positive persons), recipients with immunodeficient persons or unimmunized adults in their households, and unvaccinated adults, all of whom should receive IPV. In addition, anyone who is informed of the risks and benefits of OPV should be permitted to elect to receive IPV if prepared to commit to a full schedule of vaccination with that preparation. This recommendation is regularly reexamined and could be changed if the epidemiology of poliomyelitis in the United States changes. The AAP/ACIP is considering a sequential IPV-OPV schedule in order to reduce the incidence of VAPP. Recommendations are imminent.

Preparations Available

(1) Inactivated injectable poliovirus vaccine of enhanced potency (IPV-E) contains 40, 8, and 32 D-antigen units, respectively, of types 1, 2, and 3 poliovirus.

(2) Trivalent live attenuated oral poliovirus vaccine (OPV) contains at least $10^{5.4}$, $10^{4.5}$, and $10^{5.2}$ $TCID_{50}$ of attenuated Sabin strains of poliovirus types 1, 2, and 3, respectively.

Dosage & Schedule of Administration

A. IPV-E: This is the only vaccine preparation available and is administered in a dose of 0.5 mL subcutaneously. Combination vaccines DPT–IPV-E are not yet licensed in the United States.

B. OPV: A single thawed ampule is given orally for each dose. See Table 10–3 for the routine schedule and Table 10–4 for children not appropriately immunized during the first year of life.

Adverse Effects

IPV has essentially no adverse effects associated with it other than possible rare hypersensitivity reactions to trace quantities of antibiotics. OPV carries a risk of vaccine-associated paralytic disease for immunodeficient recipients, immunodeficient contacts of recipients, and unvaccinated healthy adult contacts of recipients.

American Academy of Pediatrics Committee on Infectious Diseases: Administration of the third dose of oral poliomyelitis vaccine at 6 to 18 months of age. Pediatrics 1994;94:774.

Faden H et al: Long-term immunity to poliovirus in children immunized with live attenuated and enhanced-potency inactivated trivalent poliovirus vaccines. J Infect Dis 1993;168:453.

Onorato IM et al: Mucosal immunity induced by enhanced-potency inactivated and oral polio vaccines. J Infect Dis 1991;163:1.

Patriarca PA et al: Factors affecting the immunogenicity of oral poliovirus vaccine in developing countries: Rev Rev Infect Dis 1991;13:926.

Simoes EA, Abzug MJ: Enteroviruses: Issues in poliomyelitis immunization and perinatal enterovirus infections. Curr Opin Infect Dis 1993;6:547.

MEASLES

Routine measles vaccination was introduced in the United States in 1963. Since 1976, the Moraten strain vaccine has been used. In 1979, an improved stabilizer was added that made the vaccine more heat-stable.

After the introduction of measles vaccine, the annual number of reported cases in the United States decreased from about 500,000 in 1963 to 1497 in 1983. During 1989, there was a resurgence of measles, with 18,000 cases and 41 deaths reported; that trend intensified in 1990, with more than 27,000 cases and over 60 deaths. The major reasons for the increase in cases and resulting deaths are failure to provide vaccine to preschool children 15 months of age or older, the presence in the community of susceptible children under 15 months of age, and the accumulation of appropriately vaccinated but nonimmune individuals (primary vaccine failures: 2–10%) in schools and colleges. These reasons have led to recommendations for the routine revaccination of all children.

Given the efficacy rate of the current vaccine (>95%), the elimination of indigenous measles from the United States is an attainable public health goal. Currently, 5–7% of all cases reported each year are either acquired outside the United States or result from exposure to such a case. About one-third of reported indigenous cases are judged to be potentially preventable. An additional 28% occur in persons who would not have been immunized by virtue of age or exemption, and the remainder of cases occur in persons with a history of adequate vaccination. An aggressive two-dose campaign directed at ensuring that all eligible children are immunized at the appropriate ages would reduce the number of cases and might eliminate indigenous transmission completely.

Preparations Available

The Moraten strain is derived from the Edmonston B strain after multiple passages in chick embryo tissue culture and contains 1000–5000 $TCID_{50}$ of the United States Reference Measles Virus. The Moraten strain is equally effective in combination: with mumps vaccine (MM), with rubella vaccine (MR), and with mumps and rubella vaccines (MMR).

Dosage & Schedule
of Administration

A. Routine Vaccination: Under ordinary circumstances, the first dose of measles vaccine should be given as MMR to 12-month-old or 15-month-old children. A dose of 0.5 mL, whether alone or in combination, should be given subcutaneously. The recommended age for the second vaccination with MMR varies: 4–6 years (ACIP) or 11–12 years (AAP). The advantages of the former recommendation are that implementation is easy, there is no extra cost for physician visits, and elementary schools have an extensive tracking system to ensure compliance. The advantage of the later age of vaccination is that it has a rapid impact, since it is closer to the age when outbreaks occur. The individual practitioner can adopt either recommendation but may be preempted in this decision by laws mandating revaccination at school entry. Timing of MMR when immune globulin has been administered depends on the child's age as well as the type and route of administration. Consult the AAP *Red Book* for specific recommendations. The interval ranges between 3 and 11 months.

B. Vaccination in High-Risk Areas: A *high-risk area* has been defined by the ACIP as (1) a county with over five cases among preschool children during each of the last 5 years; (2) a county with a recent outbreak among preschool children; or (3) a city with a large unvaccinated population. In high-risk areas, age at primary vaccination may be lowered to 12 months, and the second dose should be administered at 4–6 or 11–12 years of age.

C. Revaccination Under Other Circumstances: Persons entering colleges and other institutions for education beyond high school, medical personnel beginning employment, and persons traveling abroad should have documentation of immunity to measles, defined as receipt of two doses of measles vaccine after their first birthday, birth before 1957, or a documented measles history or immunity. Children traveling to endemic areas should be immunized as if they were in an outbreak area (see next section).

D. Outbreak Control: An *outbreak* is defined in a community whenever a single case of measles is documented. Control depends on immediate protection of all susceptible persons (defined as persons who have no documented immunity to measles). In the case of unvaccinated individuals, the following recommendations hold: (1) 6–11 months of age: monovalent measles vaccine (or MMR) if cases are occurring in children less than 1 year old, followed by MMR at 15 months and again at 4–6 or 11–12 years; and (2) 12 months of age or older: MMR followed by revaccination at the recommended times.

A child with an unclear or unknown vaccination history should be reimmunized with MMR. Anyone with a known exposure who is not certain of receiving two doses of MMR should receive an additional dose. Measles vaccination is contraindicated in pregnant women, women intending to become pregnant within the next 90 days, immunocompromised persons (except those with HIV infection), and persons with anaphylactic egg or neomycin allergy. Children with minor acute illnesses (including febrile illnesses), nonanaphylactic egg allergy, or a history of tuberculosis should be immunized. Monovalent measles or MMR may be safely administered simultaneously with DTP and OPV.

Adverse Effects

Between 5% and 15% of vaccinees become febrile to 39.5 °C or higher about 1 week after vaccination, and 5% may develop a transient morbilliform rash. Encephalitis and other central nervous system conditions are reported to occur at a frequency of 1 case per 3 million doses in the United States. This rate is lower than the rate of these conditions in the general unvaccinated population, implying that the relationship between them and measles vaccination may not be causal. Recent reports have suggested that there may be a slightly increased risk for febrile convulsions in children with a family or personal history of seizures. A case of fatal measles vaccine strain pneumonia has been reported in an HIV-infected man who received MMR. The ACIP is reevaluating the recommendation for HIV-infected individuals.

Antibody Preparations

If a child is seen within 72 hours of exposure, vaccination is the preferred method of protection. IG, given at a dose of 0.25 mL/kg (0.5 mL/kg in the immunocompromised) intramuscularly, is effective in preventing or modifying measles if it is given within 6 days after exposure.

American Academy of Pediatrics Committee on Infectious Diseases: Recommended timing of routine measles immunization for children who have recently received immune globulin preparations. Pediatrics 1994;95:682.

Halsey NA: Increased mortality after high titer measles vaccines: Too much of a good thing. Pediatr Infect Dis J 1993;12:462.

Markowitz LE et al: Patterns of transmission in measles outbreaks in the United States, 1985–1986. N Engl J Med 1989;320:75.

1996 Red Book: Report of the Committee on Infectious Diseases, 24th ed. American Academy of Pediatrics, 1996.

CDC Measles pneumonitis following measles-mumps-rubella vaccination of a patient with HIV infection, 1993 MMWR 1996;45:603–606.

MUMPS

The mumps vaccine has dramatically reduced the incidence of this infection and its complications in the United States. Since its routine use from 1977, mumps decreased from 152,000 cases in 1968 to a low of 2982 cases in 1985. The incidence has subsequently increased, with outbreaks occurring in highly vaccinated populations scattered throughout the country.

Preparations Available

The Jeryl Lynn Strain is the only preparation available as monovalent vaccine. It is prepared from virus isolated from a child and passaged in embryonated hens' eggs and in chick embryo tissue culture. It contains the equivalent of over 20,000 $TCID_{50}$ of the United States Reference Mumps Virus. The Jeryl Lynn vaccine is also available in combination with measles vaccine (MM), with rubella vaccine, and with measles and rubella vaccines (MMR).

Dosage & Schedule of Administration

Mumps vaccine is given to children in the combination vaccine MMR at the age of 15 months and again at 4–6 or 11–12 years of age. Despite the over 95% efficacy of the mumps vaccine, outbreaks have been reported in highly vaccinated populations. Most cases were attributed to primary vaccine failure. It is hoped that the two-dose schedule will prevent these outbreaks. As monovalent vaccine, it is safe and effective if given after the first birthday. The dose of either monovalent or MMR vaccines is 0.5 mL, given subcutaneously. Use of the monovalent vaccine is limited to susceptibles with proved immunity to the other constituents of MMR. Revaccination with mumps vaccine or any of the vaccines in MMR is not harmful. Anyone with an unclear vaccination history should therefore be immunized. The same recommendations and contraindications apply to mumps vaccine as to measles vaccine (see above).

Adverse Effects

Illnesses after mumps vaccination are rare and include parotitis, low-grade fever, and orchitis. In 1989, a nationwide surveillance of neurologic complications after mumps vaccine was conducted in Japan. There were at least 311 cases of mild aseptic meningitis (96 had vaccine-type mumps virus in the cerebrospinal fluid) among 630,157 recipients. There were no sequelae. It may be more common than was previously suspected (1–4 cases per 10,000 vaccinations).

Fujinaga T et al: A prefecture-wide survey of mumps meningitis associated with measles, mumps and rubella vaccine. Pediatr Infect Dis J 1991;10:204.

Hersh BS et al: Mumps outbreak in a highly vaccinated population. J Pediatr 1991;119:187.

King JC et al: Measles, mumps and rubella antibodies in vaccinated Baltimore children. Am J Dis Child 1993; 147:558.

Mumps prevention. Recommendations of the Immunization Practices Advisory Committee (ACIP). MMWR 1989; 38:388, 397.

RUBELLA

The use of rubella vaccine represents an important deviation from the public health philosophy underlying the other vaccines discussed in this chapter. It is not intended to protect individuals from the consequences of rubella infection, but rather to prevent congenital rubella syndrome. In the United States, the approach has been to vaccinate young children. The intent is to reduce transmission to susceptible women of childbearing age via a herd immunity effect. Immunity lasts for at least 15 years. Other countries, notably the United Kingdom, vaccinate pubertal girls (aged 11–14). The relative efficacy of these two strategies in the prevention of congenital rubella syndrome is not clear.

With the use of rubella vaccines since 1970, rubella incidence rates have declined more than 95% to an all-time low of 225 cases reported to the CDC in 1988. However, approximately 10% of young adults are now susceptible to rubella. Outbreaks have occurred in settings where adult susceptibles congregated (eg, prisons, colleges). In most cases, failure to vaccinate susceptible persons, not vaccine failure, was implicated.

Preparations Available

(1) The RA 27/3 strain is the only vaccine available in the United States. It is grown in human diploid cells. Each dose contains more than 1000 $TCID_{50}$ of the United States Reference Rubella Virus. The RA 27/3 strain is available in combined preparations with measles vaccine (MR), mumps vaccine, and measles and mumps vaccines (MMR).

Dosage & Schedule of Administration

Either the monovalent or combined forms should be administered subcutaneously in a dose of 0.5 mL. Current practice is to use MMR vaccine at 15 months of age and at 4–6 or 11–12 years of age. A person can be considered immune only with documentation of either serologic immunity to rubella or vaccination with at least one dose of rubella vaccine after 1 year of age. A clinical diagnosis of rubella is unacceptable. Susceptible pubertal girls and postpubertal women identified by premarital or prenatal screening should also be immunized. All susceptible adults in institutional settings (including colleges), day care center personnel, military personnel, and hospital and health care personnel should be immunized. Whenever rubella vaccination is offered to a woman of childbearing age, pregnancy should be ruled out and the woman advised to prevent conception during the 90 days following vaccination.

It has been estimated that the risk of serious malformations attributable to giving the RA 27/3 vaccine to pregnant women is from nil to 1.6%. This is much less than the over 20% risk of congenital rubella syndrome after maternal infection in the first trimester of pregnancy.

Adverse Effects

In children, adverse effects from rubella vaccination are very unusual. Five percent to 15% of children develop rash, fever, or lymphadenopathy 5–12 days after vaccination. Rash also occurs alone or as a mild rubella illness in 2–4% of adults. Arthralgia and arthritis occur in 10–25% of adult vaccinees. Chronic arthritis may be causally related to RA 27/3 vaccinations. Rare complications include peripheral neuritis and neuropathy, transverse myelitis, and diffuse myelitis.

Best JM: Rubella vaccines: Past, present and future. Epidemiol Infect 1991;107:17.

Herrmann KL: Rubella in the United States: Toward a strategy for disease control and elimination. Epidemiol Infect 1991;107:55.

Howson CP, Fineberg HV: Adverse events following pertussis and rubella vaccines. JAMA 1992;267:392.

Recommended childhood immunization schedule—United States 1995. MMWR 1995;44:1.

HAEMOPHILUS INFLUENZAE TYPE b INFECTION

The first vaccine licensed against *Haemophilus influenzae* type b in the United States was composed of the capsular polysaccharide of *H influenzae* type b polyribosylribitol phosphate (PRP). This vaccine, which became available in 1985 for children between 2 and 5 years of age, was moderately effective in preventing *H influenzae* type b disease. Conjugation of the PRP with protein carriers confers T cell–dependent characteristics on the vaccine and enhances the immunologic response to PRP in infancy. Since 1994, four conjugate vaccines and a combination vaccine (DTP-Hib, Tetramune) have been licensed for children (Table 10–6).

Studies in infants aged 2–6 months demonstrated the immunogenicity of each of these vaccines except PRP-D, which is harmful to children over 12 months of age. A geometric mean titer (GMT) of 1 μg/mL of antipolysaccharide antibody 3 weeks postvaccination has correlated with long-term protection from invasive disease. After three doses at ages 2, 4, and 6 months, each of the three vaccines—HbOC, PRP-OMP, and PRP-T—produces protective levels of antibody. Regardless of the vaccine used in the primary series, booster vaccination of children over age 12 months with any licensed vaccine elicits an adequate response. Furthermore, each vaccine is immunogenic, as a single dose given after 15 months of age. Limited information on interchangeability of different Hib vaccines suggests that any combination of the three doses of Hib conjugate vaccines will provide adequate protection.

Clinical trials for all three conjugate vaccines among infants 2–6 months of age have been published. These studies form the basis for the FDA approval of vaccine use and new recommendations by the American Academy of Pediatrics and the Immunization Practices Advisory Committee on the use of *Haemophilus* type b conjugate vaccines. Because of the differences in the immunogenic response and the different regimens used in these trials, the recommendations for use of HbOC, PRP-T and PRP-OMP differ and are summarized in Table 10–7.

The FDA has recently licensed HbOC-DTP (Tetramune) for use in infants as young as 2 months of age. Antibody responses are comparable to HbOC and DTP administered separately. If the exact conjugate vaccine previously administered is unknown, it is recommended that at least three doses of conjugate vaccine be administered to children between 2 and 6 months of age. Unvaccinated or partially vaccinated children younger than 24 months of age who experience invasive *H influenzae* type b disease should receive a complete series of vaccinations. Children over the age of 24 months mount an adequate immune response to invasive *H influenzae* type b disease and do not require further vaccinations. Unimmunized children 5 years of age or older with a chronic illness that is known to be associated with in-

Table 10–6. *Haemophilus influenzae* type b conjugate vaccines for children.

Vaccine	Trade Name and Manufacturer	Polysaccharide	Linkage	Protein Carrier
PRP-D[1]	ProHIBiT (Connaught)	Medium	6-carbon	Diphtheria toxoid
HbOC	HibTITER (Lederle-Praxis)	Small	None	CMR[197] mutant *Corynebacterium diphtheriae* toxin protein
PRP-OMP	PedvaxHIB (Merck & Co)	Medium	Thioether	*Neisseria meningitidis* outer membrane protein complex
PRP-T	ActHIB OmniHIB (Pasteur Merieux Vaccines)	Large	6-carbon	Tetanus toxoid
HbOC-DTP	Tetramune (Lederle-Praxis)	Small	None	See above for HbOC

[1]Limited to children over 12 mo of age.

Table 10–7. Schedule for Hib conjugate vaccine administration.

Vaccine	Age at First Vaccination (mo)	Primary Series	Booster
HbOC or PRP-T[1]	2–6	3 doses 2 mo apart	12–15 mo
	7–11	2 doses 2 mo apart	12–18 mo
	12–14	1 dose	2 mo later
	15–59	1 dose	—
PRP-OMP	2–6	2 doses 2 mo apart	12–15 mo
	7–11	2 doses 2 mo apart	12–18 mo
	12–14	1 dose	2 mo later
	15–59	1 dose	—

[1]TETRAMUNE may be administered by the same schedule for primary immunization as HbOC or PRP-T (when the series begins at 2–6 mo of age). A booster dose of DTP or DTaP should be administered at 4–6 y of age, before kindergarten or elementary school. This booster is not necessary if the fourth vaccinating dose was administered after the fourth birthday.

vasive *H influenzae* type b disease, such as sickle cell anemia and asplenia, should be given a single dose of any of the licensed conjugate vaccines. Regardless of the regimen implemented, it is crucial to complete the series, since cases of invasive *H influenzae* type b disease have been described in partially vaccinated children.

Preparations Available
See Table 10–6.

Dosage & Schedule of Administration
Regardless of which preparation is used, 0.5 mL should be given intramuscularly.

Adverse Effects
These are the first vaccines for which the FDA requires active surveillance for adverse reactions after licensure. Fewer than 5% of those immunized develop systemic reactions (including fever) to the vaccine. About 25% of recipients develop local reactions. Adverse events following the second dose of PRP-OMP are more frequent than following the first dose and more frequent following the third dose of HbOC than following the first two doses. There have been no reports of more severe reactions.

American Academy of Pediatrics Committee on Infectious Diseases: *Haemophilus influenzae* type b conjugate vaccines: Recommendations for immunization with recently and previously licensed vaccines. Pediatrics 1993; 92:480.

Bulkow LR et al: Comparative immunogenicity of four *Haemophilus influenzae* type b conjugate vaccines in Alaska native infants. Pediatr Infect Dis J 1993;12:484.

Decker MD et al: Responses of children to booster immunization with their primary conjugate *Haemophilus influenzae* type B vaccine or with polyribosylribitol phosphate conjugated with diphtheria toxoid. J Pediatr 1993;122:410.

Recommendations for use of haemophilus b conjugate vaccines and a combined diphtheria, tetanus, pertussis, and *Haemophilus* b vaccine: Recommendations of the advisory committee on immunization practices (ACIP). MMWR 1993;42:1.

Vadheim CM et al: Effectiveness and safety of an *Haemophilus influenzae* type b conjugate vaccine (PRP-T) in young infants. Pediatrics 1993;92:272.

HEPATITIS B

The first hepatitis B vaccine was licensed in the United States in 1981 as a means of preventing infection via percutaneous and sexual exposure routes. Subsequent studies have shown it to be more than 85% effective in preventing perinatally acquired infection and 80–95% effective in preventing most postnatally acquired infections.

In 1988, the American College of Obstetrics and Gynecology recommended that all pregnant women be routinely screened for hepatitis B surface antigen (HBsAg). Women with positive reactions are highly likely to transmit the infection to their offspring. The use of hepatitis B vaccine with hepatitis B immune globulin (HBIG) as postexposure prophylaxis is established as an effective means of interrupting mother-to-infant transmission, except for the 2–3% of infants who acquire hepatitis B in utero.

Several risk categories have been identified as target populations for pre-exposure vaccination. Those that are relevant to physicians caring for children include clients and staff in institutions for the developmentally delayed, clients and staff of hemodialysis units, recipients of clotting factor concentrates, homosexually active males, users of illicit injectable drugs, household contacts of chronic hepatitis B carriers, and all health care personnel. With the exception of high-risk neonates, all persons identified as high risk should be screened for markers of past infection and immunized if they are proved susceptible. Since vaccines consist of a purified inactive subunit of the virus and are not infectious, they are not contraindicated in immunosuppressed individuals or in pregnant women.

Each year about 300,000 persons in the United

States are infected with hepatitis B virus; 50% of these develop clinical hepatitis, 10,000 are hospitalized, and an estimated 20,000–30,000 become chronic carriers. The risk of carriage varies inversely with age; thus, although only 1–3% of the infections occur in children under 5 years of age, they account for 20–30% of new carriers each year. Chronic carriers are at 12–300 times greater risk than noncarriers of developing primary liver cancer, and 25% develop chronic active hepatitis that progresses to cirrhosis over 5–20 years.

Hepatitis B vaccine is highly immunogenic in children and young adults; seroconversion rates are 95% or more, and higher titers are obtained when vaccination is begun later in infancy or childhood and with longer intervals between the second and third doses. The protective efficacy of hepatitis B vaccine correlates well with antibody levels, and virtually all persons with 10 mIU/mL or more are protected in clinical trials.

Universal child vaccination with hepatitis B vaccine has recently been recommended both by the ACIP and the AAP. When resources are limited, the AAP recommends giving the highest priority to immunization of high-risk infants and children, followed by all infants, adolescents in high-risk areas, and, finally, all adolescents. The AAP has recently published recommendations for the prevention of hepatitis B infections in school settings.

Optimally, two intramuscular doses of hepatitis B vaccine are needed. Increasing the interval between the first and second doses has little effect on immunogenicity, but longer intervals between the last two doses (4–12 months) results in higher titers of anti-HBs. Thus, adequate responses and seroconversion rates are achieved with doses administered at birth, 1 month, and 6 months; or birth, 2 months, and 6 months; or 2 months, 4 months, and 6 months. Simultaneous administration with other vaccines at different sites is safe and efficacious.

Preparations Available

Recombinant vaccine, licensed in 1986, is the only vaccine type available. It is immunologically indistinguishable from the HBsAg found in chronic carriers. Two vaccines, adsorbed with aluminum hydroxide and thimerosal, are licensed: Recombivax HB (Merck Sharpe & Dohme), containing 10 μg/mL; and Engerix-B (SmithKline Beecham), containing 20 μg/mL.

Dosage & Schedule of Administration

Note: Hepatitis B vaccine should be given only in the deltoid muscle for adolescents and children and in the anterolateral thigh muscle for infants and neonates. Administration intradermally or in the buttocks has resulted in poor immune response in some individuals, and these sites are not recommended.

A. Neonatal: Infants of HBsAg-positive mothers should be cleansed of the bloody products of conception in the delivery room. Both hepatitis B vaccine (see Table 10–8) and hepatitis B immune globulin (HBIG, 0.5 mL intramuscularly) should be administered simultaneously at different sites as soon as the baby is physiologically stable, preferably in the delivery room or within 12 hours after birth. The vaccine should be repeated at 1 month and 6 months. At 12–15 months of age, immunized infants should be tested for antibody to HBsAg (anti-HBs). If the anti-HBs is positive, vaccination has been effective. If negative, HBsAg should be tested for, and if positive, immunization has failed and the infant is a chronic carrier. If both HBsAg and anti-HBs are negative, a fourth dose of vaccine should be adminis-

Table 10–8. Hepatitis B vaccine schedule and dosage.

	Vaccine Dose		
	Recombivax HB	Engerix-B	Schedule: Doses at Ages
Infants of HBsAg-negative mothers[1]	0.25 mL	0.5 mL	0–2 d, 1–2 mo, and 6–18 mo
Older children <11 y (not vaccinated at birth)	0.25 mL	0.5 mL	1–2, 4, and 6–18 mo[2]
Infants of HBsAg-positive mothers (HBIG 0.5 mL should also be given)	0.5 mL	0.5 mL	Day 0, 1 mo, and 6 mo
Children and adolescents aged 11–19 y	0.5 mL	1.0 mL	Day 0, 1 mo, and 6 mo; or day 0, 2 mo, and 4 mo
Immunosuppressed persons and dialysis patients	1.0 mL[3]	2.0 mL[4]	

[1]Infants of mothers with unknown HBsAg status should be tested at delivery. The infant should receive hepatitis B vaccine within 12 h after birth in a dose appropriate for infants born to HBsAg-positive mothers. Preterm infants should receive vaccine at a weight of 2000 g or more.
[2]May be given along with routine vaccinations.
[3]Special formulation containing 40 μg/mL at day 0, 1 mo, and 6 mo.
[4]Two doses of 1 mL at one site in a four-dose schedule at day 0 and at 1, 2, and 6 mo.

tered, followed by the same testing sequence in another 30 days.

For infants born to HBsAg-negative mothers, the first dose should be administered in the newborn period—or, if this is not possible, at least before 2 months of age. The doses and schedule for routine vaccination of these infants are shown in Table 10–8. For preterm infants born to HBsAg-negative mothers with birth weights of less than 2000 g, initiation of hepatitis B vaccination should be delayed until the infant weighs 2000 g or more.

Infants born to mothers with unknown HBsAg status should receive hepatitis B vaccine within 12 hours of birth in the dose for infants born to HBsAg-positive mothers. If the mother's HBsAg is positive, the infant should receive HBIG as soon as possible and within 7 days after birth. (HBIG has been shown to be effective if given within 12 hours after birth.) The infant should then receive the remainder of the vaccinations as for an infant of an HBsAg-positive mother. If the mother is found to be HBsAg-negative, the infant should receive routine hepatitis B vaccinations.

If maternal screening is not possible, the infant should receive the first dose within 12 hours after birth, the second at 1–2 months of age, and the third at 6 months.

B. Older Children and Adolescents: Both the AAP and ACIP recommend vaccination of adolescents. Resources permitting, the universal immunization of all adolescents is recommended. (See Table 10–8 for dosages and schedules.)

C. Immunosuppressed Persons and Dialysis Patients: Hemodialysis patients and other immunocompromised persons should be vaccinated with larger doses or increased numbers of doses (or both) (see Table 10–8).

D. Lapsed Hepatitis B Immunization: The three-dose series can be completed regardless of the interval from the last vaccine dose. No need exists to start the series over or to test routinely for anti-HBs unless the child's mother is HBsAg-positive.

Vaccination in the perinatal period could prevent 22,000 cases of acute HBV infection and a maximum of 6000 chronic HBV infections annually. However, it is estimated that 300,000 persons become infected with HBV and 20,000–30,000 become chronic carriers annually. The dose of vaccine in children is half that of adolescents. Compliance with vaccination is better in infancy than in adolescence.

E. Postexposure Prophylaxis: Postexposure prophylaxis is indicated in individuals with inadvertent percutaneous or permucosal exposure to HBsAg-positive blood, sexual exposure to an HBsAg-positive individual, or household exposure of an infant under 12 months of age to a caregiver with acute hepatitis B. Unvaccinated individuals should receive HBIG (0.06 mL/kg—maximum 5 mL—within 24 hours [its value after 7 days is unknown]) and the

first dose of hepatitis B vaccine at a separate site or within 7 days of exposure. Previously vaccinated persons should be retested for anti-HBs. If levels are adequate ($\geq$10 mIU/mL), no treatment is necessary. If levels are inadequate, a booster dose is required. In individuals who cannot be tested, a dose of HBIG should be given. A known nonresponder should receive either two doses of HBIG (1 month apart) or one dose of HBIG and one of vaccine. If the patient becomes a chronic carrier, all household contacts should also receive vaccination.

Adverse Effects

The overall rate of adverse effects is low and minor, and effects include fever (1–6%) and pain at the injection site (3–29%). Despite vaccination of approximately 2.5 million persons with recombinant vaccine, no excess risk of Guillain-Barré syndrome has been observed.

Antibody Preparations

HBIG is prepared from HIV-negative donors with high titers of HBs antibody and has an anti-HBs titer of greater than 1:100,000 by radioimmunoassay. The Cohn fractionation process used to prepare this product inactivates HIV, and there is no evidence for HIV transmission by HBIG. The use of HBIG is described above.

American Academy of Pediatrics Committee on Infectious Diseases: Universal hepatitis B immunizations. Pediatrics 1992;89:745.

American Academy of Pediatrics Committee on Infectious Diseases: Prevention of hepatitis B virus infection in school setting. Pediatrics 1993;91:848.

Greenberg DP et al: Pediatric experience with recombinant hepatitis B vaccines and relevant safety and immunogenicity studies. Pediatr Infect Dis J 1993;12:438.

Halsey NA et al: Discussion of Immunization Practices Advisory Committee/American Academy Of Pediatrics recommendations for universal infant hepatitis B vaccination. Pediatr Infect Dis J 1993;12:446.

Margolis HS et al: Prevention of acute and chronic liver disease through immunization: Hepatitis B and beyond. J Infect Dis 1993;168:9.

Update on timing of hepatitis B vaccination for premature infants and for children with lapsed immunization. Pediatrics 1994;94:403.

VARICELLA

About 4 million cases of varicella occur annually in the United States, mostly in children less than 10 years of age. A live attenuated varicella-zoster vaccine (VZV) was developed in Japan in the 1970s and licensed in the United States by the FDA in 1995 for children over 12 months of age.

Preparation Available

A cell-free preparation of OKA strain VZV is produced and marketed in the United States (Merck & Company). Each dose of VZV contains not less than 1350 plaque-forming units of VZV and trace amounts of neomycin in a lyophilized form. Storage in a freezer with a temperature of −15 °C (5 °F) or colder provides a shelf life of 15 months. VZV must be administered within 30 minutes of thawing and reconstitution.

Dosage and Schedule of Administration

In healthy children, a single dose of VZV results in a seroconversion rate of more than 95%. These antibodies persist for up to 20 years following immunization. One dose (0.5 mL) of VZV is recommended for immunization for all healthy children 12 months to 13 years who lack a history of varicella. Children over 13 years require two doses of VZV 1 month apart. VZV may be given simultaneously with MMR at separate sites. If not given simultaneously, the interval between administration of VZV and MMR must be greater than 1 month. Simultaneous VZV administration probably does not affect the immune response to other childhood vaccines, although further immunogenicity studies are needed.

Adverse Events

About 5% of children and 10% of adults develop a mild VZV-related maculopapular or varicella-form rash. Local reactions occur in 25% of patients and consist of transient pain, tenderness, or redness. Herpes zoster occurs no more frequently in patients who receive VZV than in those who had natural varicella. VZV should not be administered within at least 5 months after receipt of immune globulin or other blood products.

Contraindications

See Table 10–2 for contraindications to VZV administration. Contraindications include hypersensitivity or allergy to any VZV component, including neomycin. VZV is also contraindicated in children with cancers involving the bone marrow or in children who are immunodeficient (eg, those with congenital, heredity conditions; those on immunosuppressive therapy). It is recommended that VZV be avoided during pregnancy and in those with active untreated tuberculosis. Because VZV is attenuated and produces mild disease, it has been suggested that VZV might actually be preferable in some, immunocompromised groups.

Antibody Preparations

Varicella-zoster immune globulin (VZIG) is prepared from plasma from persons known to have high titers of antivaricella antibody. It is indicated for high-risk susceptible persons who are exposed to varicella, such as immunocompromised individuals, healthy adults 25 years of age or older, pregnant women, newborns whose mothers develop varicella 5 days prior to delivery and within 48 hours after delivery, and hospitalized premature infants of less than 28 weeks' gestational age. *Exposure* is defined as a household contact or playmate contact (over 1 h/d), hospital contact (in the same contiguous room or ward), or a newborn contact. *Susceptibility* is defined as the absence of anti-VZV antibody by a sensitive test. VZIG must be administered within 96 hours after exposure. Newborns should be given one vial (125 U) intramuscularly. The dose for all others is 125 U/10 kg body weight intramuscularly (maximum dose, 625 U). VZIG should be readministered following reexposure of susceptible persons if more than 2 weeks has elapsed since a prior dose of VZIG.

American Academy of Pediatrics Committee on Infectious Diseases: Recommendations for the use of live attentuated varicella vaccine. Pediatrics 1995;95:79.

Arbeter AM et al: Immunization of children with acute lymphoblastic leukemia with live attenuated varicella vaccine without complete suspension of chemotherapy. Pediatrics 1990;85:338.

Diaz PS et al: Lack of transmission of the live attenuated varicella vaccine virus to immunocompromised children after immunization of their sibling. Pediatrics 1991;87:166.

Krause PR, Kleinman DM. Efficiacy immunogenicity, safety and use of live attenuate chickenpox vaccine. J. Pediatric 1995;127:518–25

White CJ et al: Varicella vaccine (VARIVAX) in healthy children and adolescents: Results from clinical trials 1987 to 1989. Pediatrics 1991;87:604.

VACCINATIONS FOR SPECIAL SITUATIONS

INFLUENZA

Influenza occurs each winter and early spring, often associated with significant morbidity and mortality rates in certain high-risk persons. These include children with hemoglobinopathies and with chronic cardiac, pulmonary (including asthma), metabolic, renal, and immunosuppressive diseases. Children and teenagers receiving long-term aspirin therapy should also receive the vaccine, as well as household members (including children) of persons in high-risk groups. The vaccine may be administered to children over 6 months of age. Physicians should identify high-risk children in their practices and encourage parents to seek influenza vaccination for these children each fall. In pandemic years, it may be important to advocate vaccination in all children regardless of their usual state of health. Influenza vaccination has a 65–80% efficacy in protecting against disease.

Each year recommendations are formulated in the spring and summer regarding the constituents of influenza vaccine for the coming season. These recommendations are based on the results of surveillance in Asia and the southern hemisphere during the spring and summer. The vaccine each year is a trivalent inactivated vaccine containing antigens from two strains of influenza A and one strain of influenza B. Influenza vaccine virus is grown in hens' eggs and formalin-inactivated. These whole-virus preparations may be further treated with detergents to produce split (subvirion) or purified–surface antigen vaccines.

Influenza causes serious illness in very young children, especially because of the ear and sinopulmonary bacterial superinfections, which often follow influenza. Unfortunately, the trivalent inactivated vaccine may have limited efficacy in this age group. Protection is short-lived and often incomplete. Live attenuated influenza A and B vaccines are being produced by genetic reassortment. A live cold-adapted type A vaccine administered intranasally has been shown to be safe and immunogenic in children as young as 6 months of age. Studies are under way to determine whether combinations of live and inactivated vaccines are immunogenic in young children.

Preparations Available

Several manufacturers produce similar vaccines each year. Whole-virus vaccines produce unacceptably high rates of adverse reactions in children and are therefore contraindicated. Only split-virus (subvirion) or purified–surface antigen preparations should be used. These are also effective in adults and adolescents.

Dosage & Schedule of Administration

Children under 6 months of age should not routinely be immunized. Two doses are recommended for children under 9 years of age who are receiving influenza vaccine for the first time. The dosage for children 6–35 months of age is 0.25 mL (two doses 4–6 weeks apart) and for older children is 0.5 mL, given once intramuscularly. Split-virus vaccine should be used for children under 12 years of age and either split or whole virus after 12 years. The recommended site of vaccination is the anterolateral aspect of the thigh for younger children and the deltoid for older children. Since this vaccine is inactivated, pregnancy is not an absolute contraindication to its use.

Adverse Effects

A small proportion of children will experience some systemic toxicity, consisting of fever, malaise, and myalgias. These symptoms generally begin 6–12 hours after vaccination and may last 24–48 hours. Cases of Guillain-Barré syndrome followed the swine influenza vaccination program in 1976–1977, but careful study showed no association with that vaccine in children and young adults, nor in any age with subsequent vaccines. In patients with anaphylactic egg allergies in whom influenza vaccination is indicated, a protocol for influenza vaccination has been referenced below.

Groothuis JR et al: Immunization of high-risk infants younger than 18 months of age with split-product influenza vaccine. Pediatrics 1991;87:823.

Gruber WC et al: Comparison of monovalent and trivalent live attenuated influenza vaccines in young children. J Infect Dis 1993;168:53.

Murphy KR, Strunk RC: Safe administration of influenza vaccine in asthmatic children sensitive to egg proteins. J Pediatr 1985;106:9313.

Prevention and control of influenza: Recommendations of the Advisory Committee on Immunization Practices (ACIP). MMWR 1995;44(RR-3):1.

PNEUMOCOCCAL INFECTIONS

Infections with *Streptococcus pneumoniae* cause significant morbidity and mortality in certain high-risk groups of children. These include children with anatomic and functional asplenia (including sickle cell disease), nephrotic syndrome, chronic renal failure, cerebrospinal fluid leaks, and immunosuppression (including those with HIV infection complement deficiencies and organ transplants). The vaccine is of limited efficacy in children under 2 years of age. It is not indicated for children having only recurrent upper respiratory tract infections such as otitis media or sinusitis. The protective efficacy of the vaccine in high-risk children has not been well studied but is presumed to be about 60%, based on extrapolation from investigations in adults. In persons over 5 years of age, the overall efficacy has been estimated to be 57% (95% CI = 45–66%). The currently used 23-valent vaccine was licensed in 1983. Conjugate pneumococcal vaccines that may work in young children are undergoing clinical trials.

Preparations Available

The standard dose of currently available vaccines contains 25 μg each of the purified capsular polysaccharide antigen of 23 serotypes of *S pneumoniae*. These 23 types cause 88% of the bacteremic and meningitic pneumococcal disease in adults and nearly 100% in children in the United States—and nearly 85% of acute pneumococcal otitis media in children. Cross-reactive antibody responses may protect against an additional 8% of bacteremic serotypes in adults.

Dosage & Schedule of Administration

The dose is 0.5 mL, given intramuscularly or subcutaneously. If splenectomy or immunosuppression can be anticipated, the vaccine should be given at least 2 weeks previously. Routine revaccination is not indicated because of an increased risk of adverse reactions. Children who received their initial vaccination during chemotherapy for Hodgkin's disease should be revaccinated 3–4 months after cessation of chemotherapy. Revaccination may be considered after 3–5 years in children at high risk of fatal pneumococcal infection such as those with sickle cell anemia, nephrotic syndrome, renal failure, organ transplants, or asplenia. Pregnant women should generally not be vaccinated. Vaccination is not a substitute for antibiotic prophylaxis in certain high-risk children.

Adverse Effects

Fifty percent of all vaccine recipients develop pain and redness at the injection site. Fewer than 1% develop systemic side effects such as fever and myalgia. Anaphylaxis is rare.

Antibody Preparations

Most authorities recommend the routine use of IGIV in agammaglobulinemic patients and in some patients with HIV infection, in part to prevent pneumococcal disease.

Butler JC et al: Pneumococcal polysaccharide vaccine efficacy: An evaluation of current recommendations. JAMA 1993;270:1826.

Jorgensen JH et al: Serotypes of respiratory isolates of *Streptococcus pneumoniae* compared with the capsular types included in the current pneumococcal vaccine. J Infect Dis 1991;163:644.

Opravil M et al: Poor antibody response after tetanus and pneumococcal vaccination in immunocompromised, HIV-infected patients. Clin Exp Immunol 1991;84:185.

Pneumococcal polysaccharide vaccine. MMWR 1989;38:64, 73.

RABIES

Human rabies has been rare in the United States over the last several decades, but animal rabies persists in many feral animal species throughout the country, and domestic animals may be secondarily infected. Travelers to developing countries, where dogs are a major vector, account for about 70% of cases of human rabies in the United States. The risk of rabies transmission is highly dependent on the nature of the animal-to-human contact (the risk of rabies after a bite is 50 times the risk after a scratch from a rabid animal), the species of animal involved (in the United States, 3–20% of bats are positive for rabies and 12–70% of raccoons, skunks, or foxes, but only 0.01% of rodents are positive), and the locale of the incident. Local public health officials are well versed in the epidemiology of animal rabies in their jurisdictions and should be consulted before any postexposure rabies prophylaxis is undertaken. First, they can avert unnecessary vaccination. Second, they

can assist in the proper handling of the animal if confinement or testing is appropriate. Third, they can supply needed biologicals that may not be routinely stocked in hospitals, offices, or pharmacies. In some jurisdictions, these biologicals are supplied at no expense to the recipient if the use is authorized by the appropriate public health official. In order to facilitate discussion, the physician should have the following information at hand: the species of animal, whether it is available for testing or confinement, the nature of the attack (provoked or unprovoked), and the nature of the exposure (bite, scratch, lick, aerosol of saliva, etc). Confinement and observation of the biting animal are appropriate *only* when that animal is either a dog or a cat and appears well.

Pre-exposure prophylaxis is indicated for veterinarians, animal handlers, and any persons, including children, whose work or home environment potentially places them in close contact with animal species in which rabies is endemic—bats, skunks, raccoons, and foxes. Travelers visiting foreign areas of enzootic rabies for over 30 days should also receive a primary course of vaccination.

Preparations Available

(1) Human diploid cell rabies vaccine (HDCV) is prepared from the Pitman-Moore strain of rabies virus grown in human diploid cell culture, concentrated by ultracentrifugation and inactivated with β-propionolactone. It is supplied in two forms: a single-dose vial of 1 mL, when reconstituted for intramuscular use; and a single-dose vial of 0.1 mL for intradermal use.

(2) Rabies vaccine, adsorbed (RVA), was licensed in March 1988 and is distributed by the Biologics Products Program, Michigan Department of Public Health. It is produced from the Kissling strain of rabies virus, grown on fetal rhesus lung diploid cell culture, inactivated with β-propionolactone and adsorbed to aluminum phosphate.

Dosage & Schedule of Administration

Both types are equally safe and efficacious for both pre- exposure and postexposure prophylaxis when given intramuscularly. Only the HDCV has been evaluated for the intradermal route.

A. Primary Pre-exposure Vaccination:

1. Intramuscular route—This consists of three intramuscular injections in the deltoid area of 1 mL of HDCV or RVA on days 0, 7, and 21 or 28. The intragluteal route of administration is not recommended because of a poor immunologic response.

2. Intradermal route—The intradermal route has been recommended as an alternative mode of vaccination and consists of three intradermal doses of 0.1 mL of HDCV (RVA cannot be used) in the area over the deltoid on days 0, 7, and 21 or 28. *Note:* Concomitant chloroquine phosphate use (for malaria chemoprophylaxis) interferes with the antibody response to intradermal vaccination with HDCV, but not with the intramuscular mode of vaccination. Thus, when simultaneous rabies and malaria prophylaxis is indicated, the intramuscular mode of vaccination is preferred.

B. Postexposure Prophylaxis:

1. In unvaccinated individuals—The wound should be immediately and thoroughly cleansed with soap and water. As soon as possible after the exposure (and up to 7 days after the first dose of vaccine), administer 20 IU/kg of rabies immune globulin (RIG) intramuscularly (if possible, half the dose should be infiltrated around the wound and the other half given intramuscularly in the gluteal area). At a different site—also as soon as possible after exposure—administer the first dose of HDCV. Four subsequent doses of HDCV should be given on days 3, 7, 14, and 28. The World Health Organization (WHO) recommends an additional dose on day 90, but the ACIP does not recommend this practice.

2. In previously vaccinated individuals—The wound should be cleaned with soap and water. RIG is not necessary, and only two doses of HDCV or RVA, 1 mL intramuscularly on days 0 and 3 are needed.

C. Booster Vaccination:

1. Pre-exposure booster doses of vaccine—Travelers living or visiting (for more than 30 days) in areas where rabies is enzootic in dogs should have a serum sample tested for rabies antibody every 2 years. If the titer is less than 1:5 for complete neutralization by the rapid fluorescent focus inhibition test, a booster dose should be administered.

Adverse Effects

HDCV is relatively free of side effects. Approximately 30–74% of adults experience pain, swelling, or erythema at the injection site, 7% have headache, 5% have nausea, and 4% have fever. Children complain of side effects less frequently. Allergic reactions occur chiefly after booster doses. The rate of anaphylaxis is estimated to be 1 per 10,000 doses. An immune complex–like reaction occurs in about 6% of persons 2–21 days after receiving booster doses of HDCV.

Travelers to countries where rabies is enzootic in dogs may need rabies vaccine immediately and may have to use indigenously available vaccines and antisera. In many developing countries, the only vaccines readily available may be nerve tissue vaccines (NTV) derived from the brains of adult animals or suckling mice, and the antirabies sera may be of equine origin. While the antisera have complication rates of only 1–6%, the NTV may induce neuroparalytic reactions in 1:2000 to 1:200 vaccinees; this is a significant risk and may motivate pre-exposure vaccination with the HDCV prior to travel.

Antibody Preparations

Rabies immune globulin is prepared from the plasma of human volunteers hyperimmunized with rabies vaccine. The rabies- neutralizing antibody content is 150 IU/mL, supplied in 2mL or 10mL vials. It is very safe. Usage is described above.

Berlin BS: Rabies vaccine adsorbed: Neutralizing antibody titers after three-dose pre-exposure vaccination. Am J Public Health 1990;80:476.

Chutivongse S et al: Postexposure prophylaxis for rabies with antiserum and intradermal vaccination. Lancet 1990;335:896.

Fishbein DB et al: Rabies. N Engl J Med 1992;329:1632.

Rabies prevention: United States, 1991. MMWR 1990; 40(RR-3):1.

Reid-Sanden FL et al: Administration of rabies vaccine in the gluteal area: A continuing problem. Arch Intern Med 1991;151:821.

World Health Organization expert committee on rabies. WHO Tech Rep Ser 1992;824:1.

TYPHOID FEVER

Typhoid vaccines have shown variable efficacy in field trials. Protection is inversely related to inoculum size in laboratory-based volunteer studies, which may be why some field trials have been disappointing. Three vaccines are available in the United States: a heat- and phenol-inactivated whole bacterial vaccine for parenteral use; an acetone-inactivated vaccine, available only to the armed forces; and a live attenuated vaccine for oral use (Ty21a). The inactivated vaccines have been in use for many decades, and their protective efficacy ranges from 51–76% (heat- and phenol-inactivated) to 66–94% (acetone-inactivated). However, they frequently cause marked systemic and local adverse reactions. The Ty21a vaccine has demonstrated equivalent efficacy in trials in Egypt and Chile (59–94%), and the reaction rates have been low. Moderate protection against invasive *Salmonella typhi* has been demonstrated for 2–5 years following vaccination.

Routine typhoid vaccination is not recommended in the United States. It is indicated for use in children who reside in a household with a proved typhoid carrier or in children who are going to reside in an endemic area. The oral vaccine is most commonly used. However, noncompliance with dosing instructions occurs frequently, and correct usage should be stressed. Although the vaccine is not approved for use in children under 6 years of age, a liquid formulation was found to be safe and immunogenic (70% seroconversion) in children aged 2–6 years. Travelers should be advised, however, that since neither vaccine offers total protection, careful selection of food and drink is imperative.

Preparations Available

(1) Parenteral killed vaccine is a saline suspension

of heat- and phenol-inactivated *S typhi* organisms at a concentration of not less than 10^9 bacteria per milliliter. It is supplied in multidose vials of 5, 10, or 20 mL.

(2) Oral live attenuated vaccine is supplied as enteric-coated capsules and contains the attenuated strain *S typhi* Ty21a.

Dosage & Schedule of Administration

The parenteral vaccine is given subcutaneously in a series of two injections of 0.5 mL each (for children ≥10 years of age) or 0.25 mL (children <10 years of age), 4 weeks or more apart, with booster doses every 3 years if residence in an endemic area continues. The booster dose is 0.5 mL (age ≥10 years) or 0.25 mL (age <10 years) subcutaneously or 0.1 mL intradermally.

The dose of the oral preparation is one capsule a day on alternate days to a total of four capsules, taken before meals. The capsules should be kept refrigerated. A full course of four capsules is recommended every 2–5 years if exposure continues. This vaccine is not approved for children under 6 years of age, and capsules should not be dispensed from a package that has been opened beforehand.

Adverse Reactions

The parenteral vaccine produces 1–2 days of severe discomfort at the injection site in 6–40% of vaccinees, causing missed school or work in 13–24% of vaccinated individuals. Fever and other systemic reactions occur in 15–30% of vaccinees. The only contraindication is a previous severe reaction to parenteral typhoid vaccination. It can be used in immunocompromised individuals.

The oral preparation rarely produces side effects; the most common ones are abdominal discomfort, nausea, and vomiting. This vaccine should not be used in immunocompromised individuals.

Black RE et al: Efficacy of one or two doses of Ty21a *Salmonella typhi* vaccine in enteric-coated capsules in a controlled field trial. Chilean Typhoid Committee. Vaccine 1990;8:81.

Cryz SJ et al: Safety and immunogenicity of *Salmonella typhi* Ty21a vaccine in young Thai children. Infect Immun 1993;61:1149.

Rahman S et al: Use of oral typhoid vaccine strain Ty21a in a New York state travel immunization facility. Am J Trop Med Hyg 1993;48:823.

Typhoid immunization: Recommendations of the Immunization Practices Advisory Committee (ACIP). MMWR 1990;39(RR-10):1.

MENINGOCOCCAL DISEASE

A quadrivalent vaccine containing 50 μg each of purified bacterial polysaccharide antigen from capsular groups A, C, Y, and W135 is available in the United States. Since meningococcal infection is not endemic in the United States, routine use of this vaccine is unnecessary. However, functionally or anatomically asplenic children should be vaccinated, and vaccination should be considered also for children deficient in the terminal components of complement. It will protect travelers to countries with hyperepidemic or endemic disease. The group A component is immunogenic in children over 3 months of age and the group C component in those over 24 months of age. The dose is 0.5 mL given once subcutaneously. In epidemic situations, children under 18 months of age have been vaccinated with two doses 3 months apart. In general, the vaccine should not be administered to such children before their second birthday. Adverse reactions are unusual, consisting of local pain and erythema at the injection site. The antibody levels decline after 5 years and are unaffected by booster doses. Sustained protection may require the development of vaccines that induce T-cell memory.

Andreoni J et al: Vaccination and the role of capsular polysaccharide antibody in prevention of recurrent meningococcal disease in late complement component-deficient individuals. J Infect Dis 1993;168:227.

Ceesay SJ et al: Decline in meningococcal antibody levels in African children 5 years after vaccination and the lack of an effect of booster immunization. J Infect Dis 1993;167:1212.

Laboratory-based surveillance for meningococcal disease in selected areas, United States, 1989–1991. MMWR 1993;42:21.

Meningococcal vaccines. MMWR 1985;34:255.

1994 Red Book: Report of the Committee on Infectious Diseases, 23rd ed. American Academy of Pediatrics, 1994: p 327.

CHOLERA

The currently available cholera vaccine is a phenol-killed whole bacterial cell preparation. Its use is limited because it has a maximum protective efficacy of only 50% with a duration of protection of only 3–6 months. It is no longer required by any country. Vaccination frequently results in redness and pain at the injection site, and fever, malaise, and myalgia occur approximately 1% of the time. The vaccine may be administered subcutaneously or intramuscularly. A primary series consists of two doses at least 1 week apart. Boosters may need to be given as frequently as every 6 months. For the quantity to be administered, see below. Vaccine should not be given to children under 6 months of age.

	Age at Immunization		
	6 mo to 4 y	5–10 y	>10 y
Dose	0.2 mL	0.3 mL	0.5 mL

Since *Vibrio cholerae* is not invasive and secretory IgA (sIgA) is crucial, the newer vaccines are administered orally. Two oral nonliving vaccines (one consisting solely of killed whole vibrios and the other in combination with the B subunit of cholera toxin) are safe and immunogenic. In field trials in Bangladesh, the protective efficacy was only 55–60% over 2 years of follow-up. Additional live oral vaccines are being developed against cholera by either deleting genes coding for virulence factors or expressing the genes coding for O antigens of *V cholerae* O1 in an *S typhi* carrier vaccine strain Ty21a. These approaches show promise, and an improved oral vaccine may be available in the next few years.

Imported cholera associated with a newly described toxigenic *Vibrio cholerae* 0139 strain—California, 1993. MMWR 1993;42:501.

Quiding M et al: Intestinal immune responses in humans: Oral cholera vaccination induces strong intestinal antibody responses and interferon-gamma production and evokes local immunological memory. J Clin Invest 1991;88:143.

1994 Red Book: Report of the Committee on Infectious Disease, 23rd ed. American Academy of Pediatrics, 1994: p 69.

Sack DA et al: Antibody responses after immunization with killed oral cholera vaccines during the 1985 vaccine field trial in Bangladesh. J Infect Dis 1991;164:407.

Tacket CO et al: Safety, immunogenicity, and efficacy against cholera challenge in humans of a typhoid-cholera hybrid vaccine derived from *Salmonella typhi* Ty21a. Infect Immun 1990;58:1620.

PLAGUE

Plague vaccine is composed of inactivated whole bacteria (*Yersinia pestis*). It should be used in children who reside in or are traveling to endemic areas. It should be administered intramuscularly according to the following dosage schedule:

	Age (y)			
	<1	1–4	5–10	>10
Day 0	0.1 mL	0.2 mL	0.3 mL	0.5 mL
Day 30	0.1 mL	0.2 mL	0.3 mL	0.5 mL
Days 60–120	0.04 mL	0.08 mL	0.12 mL	0.2 mL

Booster doses in the amount of the last dose listed above should be given at 6-month intervals until five doses have been given, and boosters should then be given at intervals of 1–2 years as long as the child resides in the endemic area.

Plague vaccine. Recommendations of the Immunization Practices Advisory Committee (ACIP). MMWR 1982; 31:301.

TUBERCULOSIS

BCG vaccine consists of live attenuated *Mycobacterium bovis*. BCG is not currently indicated for mass use in the United States, chiefly because of doubts about its efficacy. BCG may be useful in tuberculin-negative infants or older children residing in households where untreated or poorly treated individuals with active infection with isoniazid- and rifampin-resistant *M tuberculosis* also reside. BCG may be indicated in infants or children living under constant exposure (where >1% of the population develops new-onset tuberculosis annually) without access to prophylaxis and treatment. BCG reduces the risk of TB meningitis and disseminated TB in pediatric populations. It is given intradermally in a dose of 0.05 mL for newborns and 0.1 mL for all other children. Mantoux testing is advised 2–3 months later, and revaccination is advised if the test is negative. Adverse effects occur in 1–10% of healthy individuals and include ulceration, regional lymph node enlargement, and lupus vulgaris. The vaccine may cause disseminated or fatal infection in immunocompromised individuals, including those with HIV infection, and is therefore contraindicated in such persons. To ensure that those infected with TB are evaluated, a 5-mm or greater cutoff for a positive Mantoux test is taken. In immune-competent persons, the cutoff is 10 mm or above. BCG almost invariably causes its recipients to be tuberculin-positive. However, in a child with a history of BCG vaccination who is being investigated for tuberculosis as a case contact, a positive Mantoux test should be interpreted as indicating infection with *M tuberculosis,* essentially ignoring the history of BCG vaccination.

BCG is the most widely used vaccine in the world and has been administered to over 2.5 billion people with a low incidence of serious complications. It is cheap, can be given any time after birth, sensitizes the vaccinated individual for 5–50 years, and stimulates both B-cell and T-cell immune responses.

Clarke A, Rudd P: Neonatal BCG immunisation. Arch Dis Child 1992;67:473.

Essential components of a tuberculosis prevention and control program. MMWR 1995:44(RR-11):1.

Management of persons exposed to multidrug-resistant tuberculosis. MMWR 1992;41(RR-11):61.

Tuberculosis and human immunodeficiency virus infection: Recommendation of the Advisory Committee for the Elimination of Tuberculosis (ACET). MMWR 1989; 38:236, 243.

The role of BCG vaccine in the prevention and control of tuberculosis in the US: A joint statement by the Advisory Committee for Elimination of Tuberculosis, MMWR 1996;45:(RR-4).

YELLOW FEVER

Immunization against yellow fever is indicated for children as young as 6 months of age traveling to endemic areas or to countries that require it for entry, but generally it should be delayed until age 9 months or older. Public health authorities maintain updated information on these requirements and must be consulted. Yellow fever vaccine is a live vaccine made from the 17D yellow fever attenuated virus strain grown in chick embryos. It is contraindicated in infants less than 4 months of age, in pregnant women, in persons with anaphylactic egg allergy, and in immunocompromised individuals. It can only be administered at licensed yellow fever vaccination sites (usually public health departments). The dose is standardized to 1000 mouse LD_{50} units by the WHO. The package insert must therefore be consulted to determine the appropriate volume to be administered (generally 0.5 mL). It is injected subcutaneously. The International Health Regulations require revaccination at 10-year intervals, but immunity may last 30–35 years and is probably lifelong. Adverse reactions are generally mild—consisting of fever, headache, and myalgia 5–10 days after vaccination—and are uncommon, occurring in 2–5% of vaccinees. Rarely, encephalitis occurs within 30 days following vaccination (two cases reported after more than 24 million doses have been given in the United States). This is more likely to occur in infants less than 6 months of age. Yellow fever and cholera vaccines, when given simultaneously or less than 3 weeks apart, each interfere with the immune response of the other. These two vaccines should be administered at least 3 weeks apart. There is no contraindication to giving other live-virus vaccines simultaneously with yellow fever vaccine.

Yellow fever vaccine: Recommendations of the Immunization Practices Advisory Committee (ACIP). MMWR 1990;39(RR-6):1.

PASSIVE IMMUNIZATION

Immune globulin (IG) is indicated as replacement therapy in antibody deficiency disorders at a dose of 0.6 mL/kg/mo. It may prevent or modify infection with hepatitis A virus if administered in a dose of 0.02 mL/kg within 14 days after exposure. Measles infection may be prevented or modified in a susceptible person if IG is given in a dose of 0.25 mL/kg within 6 days of exposure. Special forms of IG include tetanus immune globulin (TIG), hepatitis B immune globulin (HBIG), rabies immune globulin (RIG), and varicella-zoster immune globulin (VZIG). These are obtained from donors known to have high titers of antibody against the organism in question. Their use has been described in appropriate sections

above. IG is administered via the intramuscular route only (IGIM). The dose varies depending on the clinical indication.

Adverse reactions include pain at the injection site, headache, chills, dyspnea, nausea, and anaphylaxis, although all but the first are rare.

There is also an immune globulin (IGIV), for intravenous use. Its primary indications are for replacement therapy in antibody-deficient individuals, for the treatment of Kawasaki disease, and for the treatment of some patients with idiopathic thrombocytopenic purpura and other autoimmune diseases. IGIV may also be beneficial in some children with HIV infection. It must only be administered intravenously. Adverse reactions include headache, flushing, diaphoresis, hypotension, fever, nausea, vomiting, and anaphylaxis. Specific antibody-enriched IGIV have also been developed for the prevention and treatment of virus infections: cytomegalovirus immune globulin (CMVIG) for prevention and treatment of CMV disease and respiratory syncytial virus immune globulin (RSVIG) for prevention of RSV illness in high-risk children.

Finally, there are some immune globulins of animal origin available for use in certain specific situations. These include botulism antitoxins, diphtheria antitoxin, and snake and spider antivenins. A variety of adverse reactions, including acute febrile responses, anaphylaxis, and serum sickness, may develop as a result of the use of these products. Their use should therefore be restricted to appropriate clinical circumstances. A schedule for hypersensitivity testing and desensitization for antisera of equine origin can be found in the *Red Book.*

LEGAL ISSUES IN IMMUNIZATION

The National Childhood Vaccine Injury Act of 1986 became effective as of October 1, 1988. The Act set up two programs, the National Vaccine Program (NVP) and the National Vaccine Injury Compensation Program (NVICP). The purpose was to provide "no-fault" compensation for persons found to have been injured by certain vaccines. It provides that liability claims against those who administer or manufacture vaccines must go before a federal compensation board before a civil suit may be filed. Compensation may be sought for certain events following certain immunizations within specified time intervals. Legal representatives (parents, guardians) must reject the judgment rendered by this compensation board before a civil suit may be filed in either state or federal court. The compensation system is now funded by a continuing surcharge levied against the manufacturers for each dose of the specified vaccines.

To receive compensation for injury from vaccines, the injured person or his or her representative must (1) go through the NVICP; (2) present evidence of death or residual effects lasting longer than 6 months and expenses greater than $1000; (3) must file a claim within 3 years after onset of the first symptoms or within 2 years after death; and (4) supply medical records or sworn affidavits in support of the claim.

Following a claim, the secretary of the Department of Health and Human Services, the defendant, evaluates the petition. Compensation is recommended if there is no alternative cause and the injury is a listed reportable event (see MMWR reference, below)—or, if the injury was not a reportable event, a vaccine was the proximate cause. Once a decision is made, the petitioner can accept or reject it within 90 days. If petitioner accepts the decision, no claim can thereafter be filed against the manufacturer or the vaccine provider. If the claim is not accepted, civil relief is available through the tort system, but the manufacturer cannot be sued for failure to warn the vaccinee of the risks associated with the product.

The Act imposes specific record-keeping and adverse reaction reporting duties on physicians who administer vaccines. For each dose administered, the medical record of the vaccinee or some other permanent record maintained in the administrator's office must set forth (1) the date of administration; (2) the name of the manufacturer and lot number of the vaccine; and (3) the name, work address, and title of the person administering the vaccine. Physicians administering the specified vaccines are also obliged by the Act to report any of the specified reactions to the Vaccine Adverse Events Reporting System (VAERS)—call 1-800-822-7967 for forms. Compensation forms from the NVICP may be obtained by calling 1-800-338-2382. The Act provides no penalty for failure to report.

Vaccine information materials are available from the CDC to meet the requirements of the Act. There are separate short (1500–2000-word) forms for DTP, MMR, and poliovirus vaccines. Patients or parents are legally required to sign these forms if the vaccine is purchased on a federal contract. Informed consent is also needed for physicians who wish to be fully covered by the vaccine compensation program.

National Childhood Vaccine Injury Act: Requirements for permanent vaccination records and for reporting of selected events after vaccination. MMWR 1988;37:197.

Normal Childhood Nutrition & Its Disorders

11

K. Michael Hambridge, MB, B. Chir, ScD, & Nancy F. Krebs, MD, MS

NUTRITIONAL REQUIREMENTS

NUTRITION & GROWTH

The nutrient requirements of the child are influenced substantially by the rate of growth, body composition, and composition of new growth. These factors vary with the age of the subject and are especially important during early postnatal life. Growth rates are higher in early infancy than at any other stage of the life cycle, including the peak of the adolescent growth spurt (Table 11–1). These rates decline rapidly starting in the second month of postnatal life (proportionately later in the premature infant). Because of a more rapid rate of growth in early infancy, nutrient requirements for males are slightly higher than those for females.

Nutrient requirements also depend on body composition. In the adult, the brain, which accounts for only 2% of body weight, contributes 19% to the total basal energy expenditure. In contrast, in a term neonate, the brain accounts for 10% of body weight and for 44% of total energy needs under basal conditions. Thus, in the young infant, total basal energy expenditure and the energy requirement of the brain are relatively high.

Composition of new weight gain is a third factor that influences nutrient requirements and changes the nutrient requirements with age. For example, fat accounts for about 40% of weight gain between birth and 4 months but for only 3% between 24 and 36 months. The corresponding figures for protein are 11% and 21%; for water, 45% and 68%. The high physiologic rate of fat deposition in early infancy has implications not only for energy requirements but also for the optimal composition of infant feeds.

Because of the high nutrient requirements for growth and the body composition, the young infant is especially vulnerable to undernutrition. Slowed physical growth rate is an early and prominent sign of undernutrition in the young infant. The limited fat

stores of the very young infant mean that energy reserves are unusually restricted. The relatively large size and continued growth of the brain render the central nervous system especially vulnerable to the effects of malnutrition in early postnatal life.

ENERGY

The major determinants of energy expenditure are basal metabolism, metabolic response to food, physical activity, and growth. In addition, the efficiency of energy utilization may be a significant factor, and thermoregulation may contribute in extremes of ambient temperature if the body is inadequately clothed. Because adequate data on requirements for physical activity in infants and children are not available and because individual growth requirements are variable, recommendations have been based on calculations of actual intakes by healthy subjects. The distinct recent trend toward lower figures for infants reflects a move away from hypercaloric and possibly inappropriate feeding practices that were in vogue between 1930 and 1970, when the growth data giving rise to the National Center for Health Statistics (NCHS) standards were collected. Suggested guidelines for energy intake of infants and young children are given in Table 11–2. Also included in this table are carefully calculated energy intakes of fully breast-fed infants, which have been verified recently in a number of centers. Though the growth pattern of breast-fed infants tends to differ from that of formula-fed infants, growth velocity during the first 3 months typically equals or exceeds the 50th percentile for the NCHS grids. Calculations of energy requirements based on recent direct measurement of energy expenditure in normal infants accord well with the intakes of breast-fed infants. The recommended energy intakes of the Food and Nutrition Board, National Academy of Sciences, National Research Council (10th edition) are not synonymous with requirements. Moreover, the RDAs do not take into account the rapid changes in requirements that occur over the course of infancy, especially in the first 6 months. For these reasons,

Table 11–1. Changes in growth rate, energy required for growth, and body composition in infants and young child.

Age (mo)	Growth Rage (g/d)			Energy Requirements for Growth (kcal/kg/d)	Body Composition[1]		
	Male	Both	Female		Water	Protein	Fat
0–0.25		0 (See note 2.)			75	11.5	11
0.25–1	40		35	50			
1–2	35		30	25			
2–3	28		25	16			
3–6		20		10	60	11.5	26
6–9		15					
9–12		12					
12–18		8					
18–36		6		2	61	16	21

[1]Data from Fomon SJ (editor): *Infant Nutrition,* 2nd ed. Saunders, 1974.
[2]Birth weight is regained by 10 d. Weight loss of more than 10% of birth weight indicates dehydration or malnutrition; this applies to both formula-fed and breast-fed infants.

this source cannot be recommended for calculating nutrient requirements of infants.

After the first 4 years, energy requirements expressed on a body weight basis fall progressively to 40 kcal/kg/d by the end of adolescence. Approximate daily energy requirements can be calculated by adding 100 kcal/y to a base of 1000 kcal at 1 year of age. Appetite and growth are reliable indices of caloric needs of most healthy children, but intake also depends, to some extent, on the energy density of the formula. Individual energy requirements of normal infants and children vary considerably, and malnutrition and disease add enormously to this variation. Basal energy requirements for the premature infant are approximately 120 kcal/kg/d.

One method of calculating requirements for malnourished patients is to base these on the ideal body weight (IBW; ie, 50th percentile weight for patients length/height–age or 50th percentile weight-for-height) rather than actual weight. Alternatively, the extra requirement kcal/d for "catch-up" growth can be calculated as:

$$\frac{5 \times \text{weight (g) deficit below IBW}}{\text{interval (days) for correction of deficit}}$$

where 5 kcal is the energy cost of each gram of new tissue deposited.

These calculations should be adjusted on an ongoing basis according to the growth response.

Heining MJ et al: Energy and protein intakes of breast-fed and formula-fed infants during the first year of life and

Table 11–2. Recommendations for energy and protein intake.[1]

	Energy (kcal/kg/d)			Protein (g/kg/d)	
	Based on Measurements of Energy Expenditure	Intake From Human Milk	Guidelines for Average Replacement	Intake From Human Milk	Guidelines for Average Requirements
10 d to 1 mo	—	105	120	2.05	2.5
1–2 mo	110	110	115	1.75	2.25
2–3 mo	95	105	105	1.36	2.25
3–4 mo	95	75–85	95	1.20	2.0
4–6 mo	95	75–85	95	1.05	1.7
6–12 mo	85	70	90	—	1.5
1–2 y	85	—	90	—	1.2
2–3 y	85	—	90	—	1.1
3–5 y	—	—	90	—	1.1

[1]Compiled from Krebs NF et al: Growth and intakes of energy and zinc in infants fed human milk. J Pediatr 1994;124:32–9; Garza C, Butte NF: Energy intakes of human milk-fed infants during the first year. J Pediatr 1990;117:(S)124.

their association with growth velocity: The Darling Study. Am J Clin Nutr 1993;58:152.

World Health Organization: Report of a Joint FAO/WHO/UNO Expert Consultation: Energy and Protein Requirements. WHO Tech Rep Ser No. 724, 1985;724.

PROTEIN

Only amino acids and ammonium compounds are usable as sources of nitrogen in human nutrition. Amino acids are provided by dietary protein. Dietary protein is hydrolyzed by pepsin in the stomach and by pancreatic trypsin digestion in the lumen of the small intestine. This is followed by peptidase digestion by pancreatic and intestinal peptidases. Nitrogen is absorbed from the gut lumen as amino acids and via short-peptide carrier systems. Absorption of nitrogen is more efficient from synthetic diets that contain peptides in addition to amino acids. Some intact proteins can be absorbed in early postnatal life and may result in allergies to these proteins. The liver plays a central role in amino acid metabolism, including regulation of the absorbed amino acids. Excess amino acids, including essential amino acids, are degraded in the liver—except for the branched-chain amino acids, which pass into the systemic circulation and are taken up primarily by muscle. Insulin stimulates this uptake and suppresses muscle protein catabolism. Protein turnover rates far exceed intake, indicating a marked reutilization of amino acids. However, some of these amino acids released from protein turnover are degraded. After removal of the amino group, the keto acids are either utilized directly for energy or converted to carbohydrate and fat. Nitrogen is excreted primarily via the kidney as urea.

All the body's protein plays a role in body structure or function. Because there are no true stores of body protein, a regular dietary supply is necessary, and any loss of protein decreases functional capacity. In infants and children, optimal growth depends on an adequate dietary protein supply. Relatively subtle effects of protein deficiency are now recognized—especially those affecting tissues with rapid protein turnover rates, such as the immune system and the gastrointestinal mucosa.

In relation to body weight, protein synthesis rates, protein turnover rates, and increments in body protein are exceptionally high in the infant, especially the premature infant. Eighty percent of the dietary protein requirement of the premature infant is utilized for growth, compared with only 20% in the 1-year-old child. Protein requirements expressed on a body weight basis decline rapidly across infancy as growth velocity decreases. The figures given in Table 11–2, which are derived chiefly from the report of the Joint FAO/WHO/UNO Expert Committee and are similar to those published in *Recommended Dietary Allowances* (10th edition), deliver a comfortable margin above the quantity provided in breast milk. The recommendations for premature infants weighing less than 1500 g is 3 g/kg/d or more.

Protein requirements increase in the presence of unusual cutaneous or enteral losses, burns, trauma, and severe sepsis. Requirements also increase during times of catch-up growth accompanying recovery from malnutrition (approximately 0.2 g of protein per gram of new tissue deposited). In a young infant during rapid recovery, this could amount to as much as 1–2 g/kg/d of extra requirement. By 1 year of age, this is unlikely to be more than 0.5 g of protein/kg/d. Circumstances in which the intake of protein may be deficient include low-protein supplements (eg, fruit juices) in the breast-fed infant, protein malabsorption (cystic fibrosis), or the use of a low-protein weaning food (eg, cassava) as the dietary staple.

The quality of protein depends on its amino acid composition. Infants require 43% of protein as essential amino acids, and children require 36%. Eight essential amino acids cannot be synthesized by adults: isoleucine, leucine, lysine, methionine, phenylalanine, threonine, tryptophan, and valine. Histidine may be added to this list. Cysteine and tyrosine are considered partially essential because their rates of synthesis are limited and may be inadequate in certain circumstances. During early development, rates of synthesis of cysteine, tyrosine, and perhaps taurine do not provide sufficient amounts of these substances. Taurine is a substrate in the conjugation of bile acids, and taurine supplements have been reported to improve fat absorption in preterm infants and in infants with cystic fibrosis. Taurine supplements have been reported to improve auditory brain stem–evoked potentials in preterm infants. Lack of an essential amino acid leads to weight loss within 1–2 weeks. Wheat and rice are deficient in lysine, and legumes are deficient in methionine. Appropriate mixtures of vegetable protein are therefore necessary to achieve high protein quality.

Glutamine is another important example of a nonessential amino acid whose synthesis is inadequate under certain abnormal circumstances. The integrity of the enterocyte, for example, may be dependent on addition of glutamine to parenteral nutrition in infants who cannot tolerate any enteral intake.

Because the mechanisms for removal of excess nitrogen are efficient, moderate excesses of protein are not harmful and may help to ensure an adequate supply of certain micronutrients. Adverse effects of excessive protein intakes may include increased calcium losses in urine and, over a life span, increased loss of renal mass. A gross excess of protein may cause elevated blood urea nitrogen, acidosis, hyperammonemia, and, in the premature infant, failure to thrive, lethargy, and fever.

Heining MJ et al: Energy and protein intakes of breast-fed and formula-fed infants during the first year of life and their association with growth velocity: The Darling study. Am J Clin Nutr 1993;58:152.

Souba WW: Intestinal glutamine metabolism and nutrition. J Nutr Biochem 1993;4:2.

LIPIDS

Fats are the main dietary energy source for infants and account for up to 50% of energy in human milk. Over 98% of these fats are in the form of triglycerides, which have an energy density of 9 calories per gram. Fats can be efficiently stored in adipose tissue with a minimal energy cost of storage. This is especially important in the young infant. Fats are required for the absorption of fat-soluble vitamins and for myelination of the central nervous system. Fat also provides essential fatty acids (EFA) necessary for brain development, for phospholipids in cell membranes, and for the synthesis of prostaglandins and leukotrienes. The EFA are polyunsaturated fatty acids derived from linoleic acid ($18:2\omega6$, ie, 18 carbons and two double bonds with the first located 6C from the methyl [omega] end) and linolenic acid ($18:3\omega3$) by elongation and further desaturation. Among these are arachidonic acid ($20:4\omega6$), which can be obtained from dietary linoleic acid and is present primarily in membrane phospholipids. Oxygenation of arachidonic acid through the lipoxygenase pathway yields leukotrienes, and oxygenation through the cyclooxygenase pathway yields prostaglandins. Important derivatives of linolenic acid are eicosapentaenoic acid ($20:6\omega3$) and docosahexaenoic acid ($22:6\omega3$), which is found in human milk and brain lipids. Visual acuity of formula-fed premature infants is improved with the addition of $20:6\omega3$, which is not derived readily from $18:3\omega3$.

Clinical features of EFA $\omega6$ deficiency include growth failure, abnormal scaliness, erythematous skin lesions, decreased capillary resistance, increased fragility of erythrocytes, thrombocytopenia, poor wound healing, and increased susceptibility to infection. The clinical features of deficiency of $\omega3$ fatty acids are less well defined, but dermatitis and neurologic abnormalities—including blurred vision, peripheral neuropathy, and weakness—have been reported. Marine oil–supplemented formula improves visual acuity of preterm infants through 4 months of age by improving docosahexaenoic acid status. Fatty fish are the best dietary source of $\omega3$ fatty acids. A high intake of fatty fish is associated with a decrease in platelet adhesiveness and decreased inflammatory response.

Up to 5–10% of fatty acids in human milk are polyunsaturated. Most of these are $\omega6$ series, but long-chain $\omega3$ fatty acids are also present. Breast milk also contains about 40% of fatty acids as monounsaturates, primarily oleic acid ($18:1$) and up to 10% of total fatty acids as medium-chain triglycerides (MCT). In general, the percentage of calories derived from fat is a little lower in infant formulas than in human milk. Typically, these formulas contain a relatively high percentage of linoleic acid but very little long-chain $\omega3$. The American Academy of Pediatrics recommends that infants receive a minimum of 30% of calories from fat, including a minimum of 1.7% of total calories from $\omega6$ fatty acids and 0.5% of calories from $\omega3$. Providing up to 40–50% of energy requirements as fats is desirable at this age. In contrast, children older than 2 years should derive a *maximum* of 30% of total calories from fat and no more than 10% of calories either from saturated fats or polyunsaturated fats.

Triglycerides are hydrolyzed to monoglycerides, free fatty acids, and glycerol in the lumen of the gut. Substantial hydrolysis of triglycerides in milk formulas occurs in the stomach by the action of lingual and gastric lipases. Pancreatic lipases and bile salt levels are relatively low in early postnatal life, but breast milk contains a bile salt–stimulated lipase that is effective in the lumen of the duodenum. Bile salts promote the formation of the colipase-lipase complex, which adheres to the triglycerides prior to hydrolysis. Bile salts also have a major role in the emulsification of fatty acids, allowing their passage through the unstirred water layer to the surface of the mucosal cell. After passage into the enterocyte, long-chain ($\geq C_{12}$) fatty acids and monoglycerides are reesterified to triglycerides and are packaged with phospholipids, cholesterol, and protein into chylomicrons, which are transported in the lymphatics to the systemic circulation. At the capillary endothelial surfaces in adipose and muscle tissue, lipoprotein lipase (LPL) hydrolyzes triglycerides from chylomicrons, releasing free fatty acids and glycerol, which are taken up by the adjacent cells. LPL also hydrolyzes triglycerides synthesized in the liver and transported to peripheral tissues as very low density lipoproteins.

β-Oxidation of fatty acids takes place in the mitochondria of muscle and liver. Carnitine is necessary for oxidation of the fatty acids, which must cross the mitochondrial membranes as acylcarnitine. Carnitine is synthesized in the human liver and kidney from lysine and methionine. Carnitine needs of infants are met by breast milk or formulas, and carnitine has recently been added to soy-based formulas but is not present in intravenous infusates. In the liver, substantial quantities of fatty acids are converted to ketone bodies, which are then released into the circulation and provide an important source of fuel for the brain in the young infant.

Medium-chain triglycerides (MCT C_8 and C_{10}, ie, energy density 7.6 kcal/g) are sufficiently soluble that micelle formation is not required for them to diffuse through the unstirred water layer. They are much more readily absorbed than long-chain triglycerides and are then transported directly to the liver via the portal circulation. MCTs are rapidly metabolized in the liver, undergoing β-oxidation or ketogenesis. They do not require carnitine to enter the mitochondria. Ketones are formed from MCT even when provided orally. MCTs are useful for patients with luminal phase defects (eg, cirrhosis), absorptive defects (eg, short bowel syndrome), and chronic inflammatory bowel disease. The potential side effects of MCT administration include diarrhea when they are given in large quantities, high octanoic acid levels in patients with cirrhosis, and, if they are the only source of lipids, deficiency of EFA.

Carlson SE: Visual acuity development in healthy preterm infants: Effects of marine oil supplementation. Am J Clin Nutr 1993;58:35.

CARBOHYDRATES

The energy density of carbohydrate is 4 kcal/g. Approximately 40% of caloric intake in human milk is in the form of lactose, or "milk sugar." The percentage of energy from lactose in cow's milk is only 20%, but infant formulas generally provide a somewhat higher percentage of energy from carbohydrates than does human milk.

After the first 2 years of life, 60% or more of energy requirements should be derived from carbohydrates, including no more than 10% from simple sugars. These dietary guidelines are, unfortunately, not reflected in the diets of North American children, who typically derive 25% of energy from sucrose and less than 20% from complex carbohydrates. Diets high in complex carbohydrates are, however, typical for most of the world's population of children.

The rate at which lactase hydrolyzes lactose to glucose and galactose in the brush border determines how quickly milk carbohydrates are absorbed. Lactase levels are highest in young infants, declining by more than 50% later in the first year. Lactase levels decline further with age, especially in children who are not of northern European descent. Many black and Hispanic children cannot consume large amounts of dairy products without some evidence of lactose intolerance, such as flatulence and loose stools. Lactase is located predominantly at the tip of the intestinal villi, where it is especially vulnerable to the effects of gastroenteritis or malnutrition. Thus, it may be helpful to avoid giving lactose-containing foods to children recovering from gastroenteritis or malnutrition, though this is not universally necessary. Galactose is preferentially converted to glycogen in the liver prior to conversion to glucose for subsequent oxidation. Infants with galactosemia, an inborn metabolic disease caused by deficient galactose-1-phos-

phate uridyltransferase, require a lactose-free diet starting in the neonatal period.

Starch is broken down in the lumen of the gut into disaccharides and oligosaccharides, which are hydrolyzed into glucose by maltase, isomaltase, and glucoamylase in the brush border. Glucoamylase, which hydrolyzes oligosaccharides of 4–9 glucose units, is located predominantly at the base of the villi, where it may be protected from partial villus atrophy. Glucose polymers of this length are used extensively in special infant formulas and for caloric supplementation. Advantages include a relatively low osmolar effect in the lumen of the intestine as well as relatively easy hydrolysis by the compromised mucosa. Glucose and galactose are absorbed actively with sodium. This provides the theoretic basis for the composition of oral rehydration solutions in the management of diarrhea. The glucose enhances the absorption of sodium (and thus of water) and also supplies some energy.

During and immediately following a meal, plasma glucose levels are maintained by glucose absorption. If less than 10% of dietary energy is provided by carbohydrate, ketosis results. Within 2–4 hours after a meal, maintenance of plasma glucose depends increasingly on utilization of hepatic glycogen stores. These provide only 100–150 g glucose in the adult and only 6 g in the neonate. Subsequently, until the next meal, there is progressive dependence on gluconeogenesis. Glucose is the principal fuel for the brain and is a necessary energy source for certain other tissues, including red and white blood cells.

Children and adolescents in North America consume large quantities of sucrose (table sugar) in such items as soft drinks, candy, syrups, and sweetened breakfast cereals. Average consumption by adolescents is 210 lb/y. A high intake of sucrose predisposes to obesity and is a major risk factor for dental caries. Sucrase hydrolyzes sucrose to glucose and fructose in the brush border of the small intestine. Fructose is absorbed more slowly than and independently of glucose by a facilitated diffusion process. This characteristic provides a distinct advantage. Neither fructose nor galactose stimulates insulin secretion. Fructose, however, is easily converted to hepatic triglycerides, which may be especially undesirable in malnourished subjects.

Dietary fiber can be classified into two major types: nondigested carbohydrate (β1–4 linkages) and noncarbohydrate (lignin). Insoluble fibers (cellulose, hemicellulose, and lignin) increase stool bulk and water content and decrease gut transit time. They may to some extent impair mineral absorption. Soluble fibers (pectins, mucilages, oat bran) bind bile acids and reduce lipid and cholesterol absorption. Pectins also slow gastric emptying and the rate of nutrient absorption. Fiber intakes are quite low in North America. Few data regarding the fiber needs of children are available.

MAJOR MINERALS
(See Table 11–3 for recommended intakes.)

Calcium

The major dietary sources of calcium are milk and other dairy products. Although some calcium is available from other sources, including fortified cereals, it is difficult to achieve an adequate intake of calcium if dairy products are excluded from the diet. In such cases, a calcium supplement may be desirable. Average calcium absorption, which depends on calcium status and intake, is 20–30%, but calcium absorption from human milk is 60%. Absorption is enhanced by lactose, glucose, and protein and is impaired by phytate, fiber, oxalate, and unabsorbed fat. Control of calcium absorption is exerted primarily by changes in levels of 1,25-dihydroxycholecalciferol, which are increased in response to an increase in circulating parathyroid hormone (PTH). PTH, which is secreted in response to a fall in plasma ionized calcium, also increases the release of calcium from bone. Calcium is excreted primarily via the kidney. It is the most abundant mineral in the body, and more than 99% is in the skeleton. Many vital cellular processes depend on calcium, especially changes in cytosolic free calcium levels. Changes in these levels also occur in various pathologic states and can grossly disturb intracellular metabolism. A defi- ciency in dietary calcium can occur in premature infants and lactating adolescents as a result of a restricted milk intake and also in patients with steatorrhea. The effect is a decrease in bone density, possibly progressing to rickets. Bone density increases with increasing calcium intake up to daily intakes of more than 1000 mg in adolescents. Maximizing bone density at this stage of the life cycle has important implications for minimizing postmenopausal osteoporosis.

Johnston CC et al: Calcium supplementation and increases in bone mineral density in children. N Engl J Med 1992;327:82.
Kreipe RE: Bone mineral density in adolescents. Pediatr Ann 1995;24:308.
Rubin K et al: Predictors of axial and peripheral bone mineral density in healthy children and adolescents, with special attention to the role of puberty. J Pediatr 1993;123:863.

Phosphorus

Phosphorus is abundant in meats, eggs, dairy products, grains, legumes, and nuts. Phosphorus levels are high in processed foods and very high in colas and other soft drinks. Approximately 80% of dietary phosphorus is absorbed; the kidney is responsible for homeostatic control. PTH decreases tubular reabsorption of phosphorus. More than 85% of body

Table 11–3. Suggested dietary intakes of minerals and trace elements.[1]

Nutrient	Premature Infant[2]	Term Infant	Children >1 y
Sodium		50 mg/kg/d (2 mmol/kg/d)	250–500 (10–20 mmol/d)
Potassium		80 mg/kg/d (2 mmol/kg/d)	800 (20 mmol/d)
Chloride		70 mg/kg/d (2 mmol/kg/d)	700 (20 mmol/d)
Calcium	180	400 (200) (See note 3.)	800
Phosphorus	150	300 (100) (See note 3.)	600
Magnesium	15	40	100
Iron	2 (after first 1–2 mo)	1 mg/kg/d ($\leq$0.1) (See note 3.) (after 2 mo)	10 (18 in adolescence)
Zinc	1.5	$4 \rightarrow 2$ ($2 \rightarrow 0.75$)	2–10
Copper	0.12	0.2–0.4	0.5–2
Selenium	0.003	0.01–0.03	0.03–0.1
Iodine	0.001	0.05	0.07–0.15

[1]Amounts expressed in mg/d unless otherwise indicated.
[2]The figures in this column indicate mg/kg/d.
[3]Amounts in parentheses are for the fully breast-fed infant aged less than 4–6 mo.

phosphorus is in bone. Phosphorus is also a component of many organic compounds that have a vital role in metabolism, including ATP and 2,3-diphosphoglycerate. Many of the clinical effects of phosphorus depletion are attributable to cellular energy depletion from lack of ATP or to cellular anoxia secondary to impaired release of oxygen from hemoglobin. Other key compounds containing phosphorus include cell membrane phospholipids and nucleotides.

Nutritional phosphorus deficiency is rare but has been documented in very premature infants fed human milk—in whom it can cause osteoporosis and rickets—and in patients undergoing rehabilitation from protein-energy malnutrition. Nonnutritional causes of phosphorus depletion include the ingestion of phosphorus- binding antacids. Severe hypophosphatemia results from a deficiency together with an acute extracellular to intracellular shift in phosphorus. This shift can be triggered by a glucose load, by insulin, or during nutritional rehabilitation of the malnourished patient. Phosphorus deficiency affects most organ systems, including muscle (weakness progressing to rhabdomyolysis), cellular components of blood (both physiologic and functional changes), the gastrointestinal system, the central nervous system, and bone (bone pain, osteomalacia, rickets). Respiratory insufficiency may result from weakness of the diaphragm. Phosphate depletion in the premature infant can cause hypercalcemia. Phosphorus depletion can be treated with phosphorus salts, cola drinks, or skim milk. Phosphorus excess may cause neonatal tetany due to decreased calcium. Phosphorus retention in chronic renal disease leads to metabolic bone disease.

Fouser L: Disorders of calcium, phosphorus and magnesium. Pediatr Ann 1995;24:38.

Magnesium

Two-thirds of dietary magnesium is derived from vegetables, cereals, and nuts. The kidney exerts very effective control of magnesium homeostasis. When intake is low, excretion is minimal, and intracellular levels are maintained very effectively. Magnesium is the second most abundant intracellular cation; 50% is in bone. Levels in the cell cytosol are 10 times those of the extracellular fluids and are especially high in mitochondria. Magnesium activates many enzymes, especially phosphorus-hydrolyzing and transferring enzymes involved in energy metabolism. Magnesium also plays major roles in nucleic acid metabolism.

Dietary magnesium deficiency is not recognized except as a component of protein-energy malnutrition, but magnesium depletion may occur secondary to renal disease or intestinal malabsorption. Clinical effects include increased neuromuscular excitability, muscle fasciculation and tremors, personality changes, neurologic abnormalities, and electrocardiographic changes (depression of ST segment and T waves). Disturbances of PTH metabolism can cause secondary hypocalcemia. Acute states of magnesium depletion can be treated with a 50% solution of $MgSO_4$ providing 0.3–0.5 meq of magnesium per kilogram (3–6 meq maximum) given intravenously over 3 hours and repeated over the remainder of a 24-hour period. Magnesium excess can cause respiratory depression, lethargy, and coma.

Sodium

In the United States and western Europe, only 10% of sodium intake is derived directly from food. Fifteen percent is derived from cooking and 75% from processed foods. The 10% derived from unprocessed foods is more than adequate to meet the normal requirement. Current dietary recommendations include a reduction from the typical intakes of North Americans, in which the ratio of sodium to potassium is 2:1; this ratio is 0.25:1 in other societies and in other mammalian species. High sodium:potassium ratios have been implicated in the pathogenesis of hypertension, especially if the intake of dietary calcium is low. Fifteen percent of the population may be susceptible to adverse effects from high sodium:potassium ratios. The sodium intake of breast-fed infants, while adequate (4–6 mmol/d), is low in comparison to that of most formula-fed infants.

Excessive sweating or cystic fibrosis may increase sodium requirements. Sodium deficiency, which occurs most commonly as a result of diarrhea and vomiting, causes dehydration. Anorexia, vomiting, and mental apathy may result from chronic depletion of sodium chloride. Hyponatremic and hypernatremic dehydration are discussed in Chapter 40.

Severe malnutrition and severe stress or hypermetabolism can disturb the ionic gradient across cell membranes and lead to an excess in intracellular sodium, which can adversely affect cellular metabolism. Sodium should be administered only with great caution in these circumstances.

Avner ED: Clinical disorders of water metabolism: Hyponatremia and hypernatremia. Pediatr Ann 1995;24:23.

Chloride

The intake and homeostasis of dietary chloride are closely linked with those of sodium. However, chloride is itself important in the physiologic mechanisms of the kidney and of the gut. Active chloride transport in the ascending loop of Henle is necessary for the passive reabsorption of sodium. Thus, a deficiency of chloride leads to a decrease in the absorption of sodium in the ascending loop of Henle and an increase in the amount of sodium presented to the lumen of the distal tube. This sodium is exchanged for H^+ and K^+, which can result in hypokalemic alkalosis.

Infants fed formulas low in chloride have experienced a nutritional deficiency of chloride. Other causes of chloride deficiency include cystic fibrosis, pyloric stenosis and other causes of vomiting, familial chloride diarrhea, chronic diuretic (furosemide) therapy, and Bartter's syndrome. Chloride deficiency has been associated with failure to thrive and may especially affect head growth. Other clinical features may include anorexia, lethargy, muscle weakness, vomiting, dehydration, and hypovolemia. Laboratory features include hypochloremia, hypokalemia, metabolic alkalosis, and hyperreninemia. Urine chloride levels depend on the cause of the depletion.

Malloy MH et al: Hypochloremic metabolic alkalosis from ingestion of a chloride deficient infant formula: Outcome 9 and 10 years later. Pediatrics 1991;87:811.

Potassium

Potassium is readily available in unprocessed foods, including nuts, whole grains, meats and fish, beans, bananas, and orange juice. Relatively high potassium intakes are encouraged except in the presence of renal failure. The kidneys control potassium homeostasis via the aldosterone-renin-angiotensin endocrine system. Potassium is the principal intracellular cation. The amount of total body potassium, therefore, depends on lean body mass. Potassium deficiency occurs in protein-energy malnutrition and, if not aggressively treated during the acute management stage, can be a cause of sudden death from cardiac failure. Because of loss of lean body mass, excessive potassium is excreted in the urine in any catabolic state. Again, this requires aggressive replenishment during recovery. In acidosis, intracellular potassium is exchanged for H^+. Potassium, thus shifted into the extracellular fluid, is subsequently lost in the urine, and total body potassium is depleted (eg, in diabetic ketoacidosis) despite normal or elevated levels of plasma potassium. Other prominent causes of potassium deficiency include diarrhea and the use of diuretics. The effects of potassium deficiency are muscle weakness, mental confusion, and sudden death from arrhythmias. Electrocardiographic findings include depression of the ST segment and low T waves. Hyperkalemia may result from renal insufficiency.

TRACE ELEMENTS

Trace elements that have a recognized role in human nutrition are iron, iodine, zinc, copper, selenium, manganese, molybdenum, chromium, cobalt (as a component of vitamin B_{12}), and fluoride. Dietary requirements of trace elements are summarized in Table 11–3. Iron deficiency is discussed in Chapter 21. In general, good dietary sources of trace elements include human milk, meats, shellfish, legumes, nuts, and whole-grain cereals. Fish are a good source

of selenium. Absorption of iron, zinc, copper, and probably other trace elements from human milk is especially favorable; the breast-fed infant does not normally require other sources of trace elements, including iron, for the first 4–6 months. Factors affecting the absorption of trace elements include the quantity of that trace element in the diet; dietary factors that form insoluble complexes (phytate, fiber, phosphate, oxalate); factors affecting oxidation state (ascorbic acid increases iron absorption and decreases copper absorption); chemical form (heme versus nonheme iron); competitive inhibition at mucosal cell (interactions of iron, zinc, and copper); and host factors (including nutritional status, diarrhea, impaired mucosal function). The gastrointestinal tract is the major site of homeostatic control for iron and zinc, the liver for copper, the intestinal tract and liver for manganese, and the kidneys for selenium, chromium, and iodine.

Deficiencies of iron, zinc, and possibly copper occur in the free-living population; in certain geochemical areas, the same is true of iodine and selenium. Infants fed cow's milk are at risk for deficiencies in iron and copper. Excessive losses, factors impairing absorption, or iatrogenic factors can cause deficiencies of iron, zinc, or copper. Deficiencies in these elements, as well as selenium, chromium, manganese, and molybdenum, have been associated with the use of synthetic diets, especially intravenous feeding. Protein-energy malnutrition may be complicated by deficiencies in iron, zinc, copper, selenium, or chromium. Finally, deficiencies in zinc, copper, iron, and molybdenum occur as a result of specific inborn metabolic diseases affecting the metabolism of these elements.

Hambidge KM: Trace element deficiencies in childhood. In: *Textbook of Pediatric Nutrition,* 2nd ed. Suskind RM, Suskind LL (editors). Raven, 1993.

Zinc

Zinc is a component of many enzymes, plays multiple roles in nucleic acid metabolism and protein synthesis, and is important for membrane structure and function. Causes of zinc deficiency include diets low in available zinc during periods of rapid growth in infancy and childhood, synthetic oral or intravenous diets lacking adequate zinc supplements, diseases associated with impaired absorption (eg, regional enteritis) or excessive losses (eg, chronic diarrhea) of zinc, and one or more inborn diseases of zinc metabolism. Zinc deficiency may be a factor of secondary importance in some cases of anorexia nervosa. Clinical effects of a mild deficiency include impaired growth and poor appetite. More severe cases are characterized by changes in mood, irritability, and lethargy. Impairment of the immune system, especially T-cell function, has been linked to increased susceptibility to infection. The most severe cases are characterized by an acro-orificial skin rash, usually accompanied by diarrhea and alopecia. These features occur in patients with acrodermatitis enteropathica, an inborn error of zinc metabolism; in those undergoing intravenous feeding without adequate zinc supplements; and in some premature breast-fed infants whose mothers have a defect in the secretion of zinc by the mammary gland. Plasma zinc collected before breakfast is below 6 µmol/L (40 µg/dL) in cases of severe zinc deficiency and 6–9 µmol/L (40–60 µg/dL) in cases of moderate zinc deficiency. In cases of mild zinc deficiency, plasma zinc concentrations may be within the normal range (9–15 µmol/L). Moderate hypozincemia occurs in response to release of interleukin-1 and in pregnancy even when zinc intake is adequate. Suspected dietary zinc deficiency can be treated with 1 mg/kg/d of zinc for 3 months (eg, 4.5 mg of $ZnSO_4 \cdot 7H_2O$ per kilogram per day), preferably administered separately from meals and from iron supplements. Sustained clinical remissions in acrodermatitis enteropathica are usually achieved with 30–50 mg Zn^{2+} per day, but larger quantities may be required.

Goldenberg RL et al: Zinc supplementation in pregnancy increases birthweight and head circumference in infants. JAMA 1995;274:463.

Copper

Copper is a vital component of several oxidative enzymes, including cytochrome c oxidase, the terminal oxidase in the electron transport chain; cytosolic and mitochondrial superoxide dismutases, which have key roles in the body defense against free radicals; lysyl oxidase, which is necessary for the cross-linking of elastin and collagen; and ferroxidases (including ceruloplasmin) necessary for the oxidation of ferrous storage iron to ferric iron prior to attachment to transferrin for transport to the red cell precursors in the bone marrow. Cu^{2+} is highly reactive and must be transported in the circulation tightly bound to ceruloplasmin so that its oxidative potential (when it is free or loosely bound) can be contained.

Copper deficiency may occur in the following circumstances: in premature infants fed milk preparations low in copper; in association with prolonged feeding with unmodified cow's milk; in association with more generalized malnutritional states; in patients maintained on prolonged total parenteral nutrition without copper supplementation; and secondary to intestinal malabsorption states or prolonged diarrhea.

Osteoporosis is an early finding. Later skeletal changes include enlargement of costochondral cartilages, cupping and flaring of long-bone metaphyses, and spontaneous fractures of the ribs. The radiologic findings must be distinguished from battering (not symmetric), rickets, and scurvy. Neutropenia and hypochromic anemia are other early manifestations. The anemia is unresponsive to iron therapy. Very se-

vere central nervous system disease is present in Menkes' steely (kinky) hair syndrome, in which a profound copper deficiency state results from a specific X-linked inherited defect in cellular metabolism of copper.

A low plasma copper or ceruloplasmin level helps confirm the diagnosis of copper deficiency. However, these levels are normally very low in the young infant, especially the premature infant, and are higher than adult values in later infancy and early childhood. Hence, carefully age-matched normal data are necessary for comparison. Interleukin-1 grossly elevates ceruloplasmin and copper levels; these levels are also very high in pregnancy.

Copper deficiency can be treated with a 1% solution of copper sulfate (2 mg of the salt or 500 µg of elemental copper per day for infants).

Harris ED: Menkes' disease: Perspective and update in a fatal copper disorder. Nutr Rev 1993;51:235.

Selenium

Selenium is an essential component of glutathione peroxidase, which catalyzes the reduction of hydrogen peroxide to water in the cell cytosol by the addition of reducing equivalents derived from glutathione. Hence, selenium plays an important role in the body's defenses against free radicals.

Selenium deficiency is now recognized as the major etiologic factor in Keshan disease, an often fatal cardiomyopathy affecting primarily infants, children, and young women in a large area of China where there is a severe geochemical deficiency of selenium. Similar cases have been identified in the United States in patients maintained on long-term total parenteral nutrition without adequate selenium supplements. Other patients receiving parenteral nutritional support have manifested selenium deficiency with incapacitating skeletal muscle pain and tenderness. Macrocytosis and loss of hair pigment occur in milder states of selenium deficiency. Blood levels are especially low in premature infants with bronchopulmonary dysplasia. It appears that the selenium intake of infants, especially premature infants, is suboptimal and is likely to be increased in the near future.

A plasma selenium level less than 0.5 µmol/L (<40 µg/L) is compatible with mild selenium deficiency; a level less than 0.12 µmol/L (<10 µg/L) indicates a possible severe selenium deficiency.

Litov RE, Combs GF Jr: Selenium in pediatric nutrition. Pediatrics 1991;87:339.

Iodine

Endemic goiter resulting from iodine deficiency has been eradicated in North America by effective prophylactic measures but continues to be a major health problem in many developing countries. Goiter occurs when iodine intake or excretion in urine is less than 20 μg/d. Most goitrous persons are clinically euthyroid. Maternal iodine deficiency causes endemic cretinism in about 5–15% of neonates who develop endemic goiters.

"Neurologic" endemic cretinism, seen clinically in most regions, is characterized by severe mental retardation, deaf-mutism, spastic diplegia, and strabismus. Clinical evidence of hypothyroidism is usually absent, and it is thought that the neurologic damage may be due to a direct effect of fetal iodine deficiency or to an imbalance between T_4 (low) and T_3 (normal or elevated). "Myxedematous" endemic cretinism predominates in some central African countries. Signs of congenital hypothyroidism are seen in this type. Milder neurologic damage occurs in many other cases of endemic neonatal goiter.

In North American countries, the use of iodized salt has been highly effective in preventing goiter. In areas where endemic goiter occurs, intramuscular depot injections of iodized oil have also been used extensively for prevention.

Fluoride Supplementation

When fluoride is incorporated into the hydroxyapatite matrix of dentin, it affords an inexpensive and effective means of helping to prevent dental caries. Fluoride is most effectively administered in the drinking water, but in infancy and childhood, fluoride in vitamin preparations or tablets serves the same purpose. Ready-made formulas provide less than 0.3 ppm. The well-recognized benefits of topical fluoride supplementation must be viewed in light of an increasing incidence of fluorosis in US children. Fluorosis is characterized by an increased porosity (undermineralization) of the enamel and is evident clinically as discoloration of the teeth. Recommendations for fluoride supplementation in infants have recently been revised (Table 11–4). The American Academy of Pediatrics Committee on Nutrition favors supplementation initiated shortly after birth in breast-fed infants (0.25 mg/d), but recognizes the view that initiation of supplements at 6 months may provide adequate protection.

American Academy of Pediatrics Committee on Nutrition: *Pediatric Nutrition Handbook,* 3rd ed. American Academy of Pediatrics, 1993.
Fomon SJ: In: *Nutrition of Normal Infants.* Mosby, 1993.

Table 11–4. Supplemental fluoride recommendations (mg/d).[1]

Age	Concentration of Fluoride in Drinking Water		
	<0.3 ppm	0.3–0.6 ppm	>0.6 ppm
6 mo to 3y	0.25	0	0
3–6 y	0.5	0.25	0
6–16 y	1	0.5	0

[1]From Council on Dental Therapeutics, 1994.

VITAMINS

1. FAT-SOLUBLE VITAMINS

Because they are insoluble in water, the fat-soluble vitamins require digestion and absorption of dietary fat and a carrier system for transport in the blood. Deficiencies in these vitamins develop more slowly than deficiencies in water-soluble vitamins because the body accumulates stores of fat-soluble vitamins. Excessive intakes carry a considerable potential for toxicity (Table 11–5).

Udall JN, Greene HL: Vitamin update. Pediatr Rev 1992;13:185.

Vitamin A

Dietary sources of vitamin A include dairy products, fortified margarine, eggs, liver, meats, fish oils, and corn. The vitamin A precursor β-carotene occurs in abundance in yellow and green vegetables. Dietary retinyl palmitate requires hydrolysis by pancreatic

Table 11–5. Effects of vitamin toxicity.

Thiamin
(Very rare.) Anaphylaxis; respiratory depression
Riboflavin
None
Pyridoxine
Sensory neuropathy at doses >500 mg/d
Niacin
Histamine release → cutaneous vasodilation; cardiac arrhythmias; cholestatic jaundice; gastrointestinal disturbance; hyperuricemia; glucose intolerance
Pantothenic acid
Diarrhea
Biotin
None
Folate
May mask B_{12} deficiency, hypersensitivity
Cobalamin
None
Vitamin C
Interference with copper absorption; decreased tolerance to hypoxia, increased oxalic acid excretion
Carnitine
None recognized
Vitamin A
(>20,000 IU/d): Vomiting, increased intracranial pressure (psuedotumor cerebri); irritability; headaches; insomnia; emotional lability; dry, desquamating skin; myalgia and arthralgia; abdominal pain; hepatosplenomegaly; cortical thickening of bones of hands and feet.
Vitamin D
(>40,000 IU/d: Hypercalcemia; vomiting; constipation; nephrocalcinosis
Vitamin E
? 25–100 mg/kg/d IV: Necrotizing enterocolitis and liver toxicity (but probably due to polysorbate 80 used as a solubilizer)
Vitamin K
Lipid-soluble vitamin K: Very low order of toxicity. *Water-soluble, synthetic vitamin K:* Vomiting, porphyrinuria; albuminuria; hemolytic anemia; hemoglobinuria; hyperbilirubinemia (do not give to neonates)

and intestinal hydrolases. β-Carotene is cleaved in the intestinal mucosal cells by dioxygenase to yield two molecules of retinal (retinaldehyde), which is then reduced to retinol (vitamin A alcohol). Carotene appears to have an important physiologic role in its own right as a powerful antioxidant.

Retinol is reesterified in the mucosal cells and transported in chylomicrons to the liver, where it is stored. From the liver, vitamin A is transported to the rest of the body attached to retinol-binding protein complexed to prealbumin. Retinol-binding protein may be decreased in liver disease or in protein-energy malnutrition. Circulating retinol-binding protein may be increased in chronic renal failure.

Vitamin A has a critical role in the photochemical basis of vision. The photosensitive pigment rhodopsin is formed from retinal and a protein called opsin. Vitamin A also modifies differentiation and proliferation of epithelial cells, especially in the respiratory tract. Vitamin A is necessary for glycoprotein synthesis and for the integrity of the immune system and may affect gene expression. Retinol can be irreversibly oxidized to retinoic acid, which is effective in glycoprotein synthesis but is ineffective for vision.

Vitamin A deficiency occurs in premature infants, in association with intravenous nutrition with inadequate vitamin A supplements, and in association with protein-energy malnutrition, when the manifestations are frequently made more severe by measles. Other causes of vitamin A deficiency are cultural factors (failure to grow vegetables even when practical, eg, in Central America and the Philippines), fat malabsorption syndromes (including biliary atresia), giardiasis, and cystic fibrosis.

The classic features of vitamin A deficiency are primarily related to the eye and vision. Night blindness progresses to xerosis (dryness of cornea and conjunctiva), xerophthalmia (extreme dryness of the conjunctiva), Bitot's spots, keratomalacia (clouding and softening of the cornea), ulceration and perforation of the cornea, prolapse of the lens and iris, and eventually blindness. Vitamin A deficiency is the leading cause of irreversible blindness in children worldwide. Other features of vitamin A deficiency can include follicular hyperkeratosis (dry, thickened, rough skin), pruritus, growth retardation, increased susceptibility to infection, anemia, and hepatosplenomegaly. Vitamin A treatment of children with measles in developing countries has been associated with reductions in morbidity and mortality.

Serum levels of retinol below 20 μg/dL are considered low; a level below 10 μg/dL indicates deficiency. A ratio of retinol:retinol-binding protein below 0.7 is also indicative of vitamin A deficiency.

Suggested intakes of vitamin A are summarized in Table 11–6. Therapy of xerophthalmia requires 50,000–100,000 IU orally or intramuscularly. The standard maintenance dose in fat malabsorption syn-

Table 11–6. Suggested intakes of vitamins.

	Premature Infants[1] (per kg/d)	Term Infants[1] (per day)	Adults[2] (per day)
Thiamin (mg)	0.35	12	1.5
Riboflavin (mg)	0.2	0.5	1.7
Pyridoxine (mg)	0.2	0.6	2.0
Niacin (mg NE)[3]	7	17 (NE)	19 (NE)
Pantothenic acid (mg)	2	5	4–7
Biotin (μg)	6	20	30–100
Folic acid (μg)	50	140	400
Cobalamin (μg)	0.3	1	2.0
Vitamin A (μg RE)[4]	500	700	1000
Vitamin C (mg)	25	80	60
Vitamin D (μg) (cholecalciferol)	4 (160 IU)	10 (400 IU)	5
Vitamin E (mg) (α-tocopherol)	3 (See note 5.)	7	10
Vitamin K (μg)	80	20	80

[1]Based on recent recommendations for intravenous vitamins. (Green HL Hambige KM, Schanler R, Tsang RC: Guidelines for the use of vitamins, trace elements, calcium, magnesium, and phosphorus in infants and children receiving total parenteral nutrition: Report of the Subcommittee on Pediatric Parenteral Nutrient Requirements from the Committee on Clinical Practice Issues of The American Society for Clinical Nutrition. Am J Clin Nutr 1988;48:1324 © AM J Clin Nutr. American Society for Clinical Nutrition.)
[2]Based on *Recommended Dietary Allowances*, 10th ed. National Research Council, National Academy Press, 1989, (except for folate).
[3]NE = Niacin equivalents.
[4]RE = Retinol equivalents (1 μg of retinol or 6 mg of ß-carotene = 1 RE; 1 IU = 0.3 μg of retinol).
[5]Oral doses up to 25 mg/d are now frequently used with the expectation that this may help to combat oxidant stress.

dromes is 2500–5000 IU (800–1600 μg). Doses as high as 25,000–50,000 IU/d may be needed, but monitoring to avoid toxicity is essential. Vitamin A can be provided in these circumstances as a water-soluble preparation, Aquasol A (1 mL = 50,000 IU). The effects of vitamin A toxicity are summarized in Table 11–5.

American Academy of Pediatrics Committee on Infectious Diseases: Vitamin A treatment of measles. Pediatrics 1993;91:1014.
Fawzi WW et al: Vitamin A supplementation and child mortality: A meta-analysis. JAMA 1993;269:898.

Vitamin D

Vitamin D requirements are normally met primarily from ultraviolet radiation of dehydrocholesterol in the skin with the formation of cholecalciferol (vitamin D_3). Similarly, vitamin D_2, or ergocalciferol, is derived from radiation of ergosterol. Vitamin D is transported from the skin to the liver attached to a specific carrier protein. The primary dietary source is vitamin D–fortified milk and formulas. Egg yolk and fatty fish contain some vitamin D. Vitamin D absorption depends on normal fat absorption. Absorbed vitamin D is transported to the liver in chylomicrons. Vitamins D_2 and D_3 undergo 25-hydroxylation in the liver and then 1α-hydroxylation in kidney proximal tubules to yield 25-hydroxycholecalciferol and 1,25-dihydroxycholecalciferol, respectively. Parathyroid hormone activates the 1α-hydroxylase enzyme in the kidney. Calcifediol (25-hydroxycholecalciferol) is the major circulating form of vitamin D. Calcitriol (1,25-dihydroxycholecalciferol) is the biologically active form of vitamin D. Calcitriol stimulates the intestinal absorption of calcium and phosphate, the renal reabsorption of filtered calcium, and the mobilization of calcium and phosphorus from bone.

Vitamin D deficiency results from lack of adequate sunlight coupled with a low dietary intake. An infant requires only 30 minutes per week of total body sun exposure or 2 hours per week of head exposure to maintain adequate vitamin D status. The breast-fed infant can acquire sufficient vitamin D from human milk if the mother's vitamin D status is optimal. Otherwise, a vitamin D supplement is required to avoid risk of rickets. In the United States, cow's milk and infant formulas are routinely supplemented with vitamin D. Nutritional rickets may occur in older infants and children who are not exposed to the sun or whose skin is deeply pigmented and who do not drink vitamin D–fortified milk.

Vitamin D deficiency also occurs in fat malabsorption syndromes, including small intestinal disease, cholestasis, and lymphatic obstruction. Use of P-450–stimulating drugs may decrease hydroxylated vitamin D, which can also be decreased by hepatic and renal disease and by inborn errors of metabolism. End-organ unresponsiveness to calcitriol may also occur.

The clinical effects of vitamin D deficiency are osteomalacia (adults) or rickets (children), in which there is an accumulation in bone of osteoid (matrix) with reduced calcification. Cartilage fails to mature and calcify. The effects include craniotabes, rachitic rosary, pigeon breast, bowed legs, delayed eruption of teeth and enamel defects, Harrison's groove, scoliosis, kyphosis, dwarfism, painful bones, fractures, anorexia, and weakness. X-ray findings include cupping, fraying, and flaring of metaphyses; the loss of sharp definition of bone trabeculae accounts for the general decrease in skeletal radiodensity. The diagnosis is supported by characteristic radiologic abnormalities of the skeleton, low serum phosphorus levels, high serum alkaline phosphatase levels, and high parathyroid hormone levels. The diagnosis can be confirmed by a low level of serum 25-hydroxycholecalciferol.

Rickets is treated with 1600–5000 IU/d of vitamin D_3 (1 IU = 0.25 μg). If this is poorly absorbed, 25-hydroxycholecalciferol, 2 μg/kg/d, or 1,25-dihydroxycholecalciferol, 0.05–0.2 μg/kg/d, is given. Renal osteodystrophy is treated with 1,25-dihydroxycholecalciferol (calcitriol).

Suggested dietary intakes for vitamin D are summarized in Table 11–6 and toxic effects in Table 11–5.

Hillman LS: Mineral and vitamin D adequacy in infants fed human milk or formula between 6 and 12 months of age. J Pediatr 1990;117:134.
Fraser DR: Vitamin D. Lancet 1995;345:104.

Vitamin E

Vegetable oils provide the main dietary source of vitamin E. Coconut and olive oils, however, are low in vitamin E. Some vitamin E is present in cereals, dairy products, and eggs. Activity may decrease with processing, storage, or heating. Vitamin E is a family of compounds, the tocopherols. There are four major forms: alpha, gamma, beta, and delta; α-tocopherol has the highest biologic activity. Vitamin E can donate an electron to a free radical molecule to stop oxidant reactions. Oxidized vitamin E is then reduced by ascorbic acid or glutathione. The reduced tocopherol is able to "scavenge" another free radical. The nutrients that participate in antioxidant defenses include β-carotene, vitamin C, selenium, copper, manganese, and zinc. Vitamin E is located at specific sites in the cell to protect polyunsaturated fatty acids in the membrane lipids from lipid peroxidation and to protect thiol groups and nucleic acids. Vitamin E also functions as a cell membrane stabilizer, may function in the electron transport chain, and may modulate chromosomal expression.

Vitamin E deficiency may occur in the following circumstances: in the premature infant; in cholestatic liver disease, pancreatic insufficiency (including cystic fibrosis), abetalipoproteinemia, and short bowel syndrome; as an isolated inborn error of vitamin E metabolism; and perhaps as a result of increased utilization due to oxidant stress.

Vitamin E deficiency shortens red cell half-life and may cause hemolytic anemia. Chronic vitamin E deficiency secondary to malabsorption results in a progressive neurologic disorder with loss of deep tendon reflexes, loss of coordination, loss of perception of vibration and position sensation, abnormalities in eye movements, weakness, scoliosis, and degeneration of the retina. In premature infants, vitamin E deficiency may contribute to oxidant injury of the lung, retina, and brain (brain hemorrhage). These putative adverse effects in the premature infant require confirmation.

Vitamin E nutritional status can be partially assessed with serum vitamin E (normal range for children is 3–15 µg/mL). The ratio of serum vitamin E to total serum lipid is normally more than 0.8 mg/g. Hydrogen peroxide–induced hemolysis is also used as a test of vitamin E status.

Suggested intakes are summarized in Table 11–6. Requirements increase if dietary polyunsaturated fatty acids (PUFA) increase (there is a need for 0.4–0.5 mg of vitamin E per gram of PUFA in the diet). One international unit = 1 mg of dl-α-tocopheryl acetate.

Large oral doses (up to 100 IU/kg/d) of vitamin E correct the deficiency resulting from most malabsorption syndromes. Intramuscular injections (5–7 mg/kg/wk) may be necessary in some cases of cholestatic liver disease. For abetalipoproteinemia, 100–200 IU/kg/d of vitamin E are needed. Vitamin E therapy in ischemia-reperfusion injury and in the prevention of intracranial hemorrhage in the preterm infant remains experimental. Toxic effects of vitamin E are summarized in Table 11–5.

Meydani M: Vitamin E. Lancet 1995;345:170.

Vitamin K

Vitamin K_1 (phylloquinone) is obtained from leafy vegetables, soybean oil, fruits, seeds, and cow's milk. Vitamin K_2 (menaquinone), which has 60% of the activity of K_1, is synthesized by intestinal bacteria. K_2 may be a major source of vitamin K in infants and young children, but less is produced in the intestine of the breast-fed infant.

Vitamin K is necessary for the post-translational carboxylation of glutamic acid residues of the vitamin K–dependent coagulation proteins. Carboxylation allows these proteins to bind calcium, leading to activation of the clotting factors. Thus, vitamin K is necessary for the maintenance of normal plasma levels of coagulation factors II (prothrombin), VII, IX, and X and is also necessary for maintenance of normal levels of the anticoagulation protein C. Vitamin K deficiency occurs in newborns, especially those who are breast-fed and who do not receive vitamin K prophylaxis at delivery. This deficiency results in hemorrhagic disease of the newborn. Later, vitamin K deficiency may result from fat malabsorption syndromes and the use of nonabsorbed antibiotics and anticoagulant drugs (eg, warfarin). Clinical features are hemorrhage into the skin (purpura), gastrointestinal tract, genital urinary tract, gingiva, lungs, joints, and central nervous system, which may be fatal. Vitamin K status can be assessed with plasma levels of protein-induced vitamin K absence or by prothrombin time.

Vitamin K requirements are summarized in Table 11–6. Newborns require prophylactic intramuscular vitamin K (0.5–1 mg). For older children with acute bleeding, 3–10 mg of vitamin K is given intramuscularly or intravenously. For chronic malabsorption syndromes, 2.5 mg twice weekly to 5 mg/d is given orally. To reverse warfarin effect, 50–100 mg of intravenous vitamin K is given. Toxic effects are summarized in Table 11–5.

Shearer MJ: Vitamin K. Lancet 1995;345:229.

2. WATER-SOLUBLE VITAMINS

Deficiencies of water-soluble vitamins are much less common in the United States because infant formulas and many foods are fortified, particularly with B vitamins. Most bread and wheat products are now routinely fortified with B vitamins. There is now conclusive evidence that folic acid supplements (400 µg/d) during the periconceptional period provide a strong protective effect for neural lobe defects. A good dietary intake of folate, which is likely to result from conformity with current dietary guidelines, also results in significant protection. A good dietary intake of folate as well as a multivitamin supplement in the periconceptional period may also afford protection against neuroectodermal brain tumors in young children.

The danger of toxicity from water-soluble vitamins is not as great because excesses can be excreted in the urine. However, deficiencies in these vitamins can also develop more quickly than deficiencies in fat-soluble vitamins because of the limited stores.

Additional salient details are summarized in Tables 11–6 to 11–11. Although dietary intake of the water-soluble vitamins on a daily basis is not necessary, these vitamins, with the exception of vitamin B_{12}, are not stored in the body.

Carnitine is synthesized in the liver and kidneys from lysine and methionine. In certain circumstances (Table 11–10), however, synthesis is inadequate, and carnitine can then be considered a vitamin. A dietary supply of other organic compounds, such as inositol, may also be required in certain circumstances.

Bunin GR et al: Relation between maternal diet and subsequent primitive neuroectodermal brain tumors in young children. N Engl J Med 1993;329:526.

Recommendations for use of folic acid to reduce number of spina bifida cases and other neural tube defects. MMWR 1992;41:1.

INFANT FEEDING

BREAST-FEEDING

Breast-feeding, one of the most important influences on children's health worldwide, provides optimal nutrition for the normal infant during the early

Table 11–7. Summary of biologic roles
of water-soluble vitamins.

**B vitamins involved in production of energy
of metabolism**
Thiamin (B_1)
  Thiamin pyrophosphate is coenzyme in oxidative decar-
  boxylation (pyruvate dehydrogenase, α-ketoglu-
  tarate dehydrogenase, and transketolase)
Riboflavin (B_2)
  Coenzyme of several flavoproteins (eg, flavin
  mononucleotide [FMN} and flavin adenine dinucleotide
  [FAD]) involved in oxidative/electron transfer enzyme
  systems
Niacin
  Hydrogen-carrying coenzymes: nicotinamide-adenine
  dinucleotide (NAD), nicotinamide-adenine dinucleo-
  tide phosphate (NADP); decisive role in intermediary
  metabolism
Pantothenic acid
  Major component of coenzyme A
Biotin
  Component of several carboxylase enzymes involved
  in fat and carbohydrate metabolism
Hematopoietic B vitamins
Folic acid
  Tetrahydrofolate has essential role in one-carbon trans-
  fers. Essential role in purine and pyramidine synthesis;
  deficiency → arrest of cell division (especially bone
  marrow and intestine)
Cobalamin (B_{12})
  Methyl cobalamin (cytoplasm): synthesis of methionine
  with simultaneous synthesis of tetrahydrofolate
  (reason for megaloblastic anemia in B_{12} deficiency).
  Adenosyl cobalamin (mitochondria) is coenzyme for
  mutases and dehydratases.
Other B vitamins
Pyridoxine (B_6)
  Prosthetic group of transaminases, etc, involved in
  amino acid interconversions; prostaglandin and heme
  synthesis; central nervous system function; carbohydrate metabolism; immune development
Other water-soluble vitamins
L-Ascorbic acid (C)
  Strong reducing agent—probably involved in all hydrox-
  ylations. roles include collagen synthesis; phenylalanine → tyrosine; trypophan → 5-OH tryptophan;
  dopamine → norepinephrine; Fe^{3+}; folic acid →
  folinic acid; cholesterol → bile acids; leukocyte function; interferon production; carnitine synthesis. Copper
  metabolism; reduces oxidized vitamin E.
Carnitine
  Transfer of long-chain fatty acids from cytosol to mitochondria (necessary for ß-oxidation)

Table 11–8. Major dietary sources of water-soluble vitamins.

Thiamin
  Whole grains, cereals (including fortification), lean pork,
  legumes
Riboflavin
  Dairy products, meat, poultry, wheat germ, leafy
  vegetables
Pyridoxine
  All foods
Niacin
  Meats, poultry, fish, legumes, wheat, all foods except fats,
  synthesized in body from tryptophan
Pantothenic acid
  Ubiquitous
Biotin
  Yeast, liver, kidneys, legumes, nuts, egg yolks (synthe-
  sized by intestinal bacteria)
Folic Acid
  Leafy vegetables (lost in cooking), fruits, whole grains,
  wheat germ, orange juice, beans, nuts
Cobalamin
  Eggs, dairy products, liver, meats; none in plants
Vitamin C
  Fresh fruits and vegetables
Carnitine
  Meats, dairy products, none in plants

mune composition of human milk. Additional differences of physiologic importance continue to be identified; recently identified examples include the substantial quantities of taurine and docosahexaenoic
acid found in human milk. Furthermore, the relationship developed through breast-feeding can be an important part of early maternal interactions with the
infant and provides a source of security and comfort
to the infant.

In the last decade, breast-feeding has been reestablished as the predominant mode of feeding the young
infant in the United States. Unfortunately, breast-
feeding rates remain low among several subpopula-
tions of women, including low-income, minority, and

Table 11–9. Circumstances in which the possibility of vitamin
deficiencies merit particular consideration.

Circumstance	Possible Deficiency
Prematurity	All vitamins
Protein-energy malnutrition	B_1, B_2, folate, A
Synthetic diets (including total parenternal nutrition	All vitamins
Inherited disorders	Folate, B_{12} D, carnitine
Vitamin-drug interactions	B_6, biotin, folate, B_{12}, carni- tine, fat-soluble vitamins
Fat malabsorbtion syndrome	Fat-soluble vitamins
Breast-feeding	B_1,[1] folate,[2] B_{12},[3] D,[4] K[5]
Periconceptional	Folate

[1]Alcoholic or malnourished mother.
[2]Folate-deficient mother.
[3]Vegan mother.
[4]Infant not exposed to sunlight and mother's vitamin D status
suboptimal.
[5]Maternal status poor; neonatal prophylaxis omitted.

months of life. Numerous immunoactive immunologic factors in breast milk (including secretory
IgA, lysozyme, lactoferrin, bifidus factor, and macrophages) help to provide protection against gastrointestinal and upper respiratory infections. In developing countries, lack of refrigeration and contaminated
water supplies frequently make formula feeding especially hazardous. Allergic diseases are less common among infants who have been breast-fed. Although formulas have improved progressively and
are made to resemble breast milk as closely as possible, it is impossible to mimic the nutritional or im-

Table 11–10. Causes of deficiencies in water-soluble vitamins.

Thiamin
Infantile beriberi; seen in infants breast-fed by mothers with history of alcoholism or poor diet; has been described as complication of total parenteral nutrition (TPN); protein-energy malnutrition; prematurity
Riboflavin
General undernutrition; prematurity; inactivation in TPN solutions exposed to light
Pyridoxine
Prematurity (these infants may not convert pyridoxine → pyridoxal-5-P); B_6 dependency syndromes; drugs (isoniazid); heat-treated formulas (historical)
Niacin
Maize or millet diets (high leucine and low tryptophan intakes); prematurity
Pantothenic acid
None
Biotin
Suppressed intestinal flora and impaired intestinal absorption
Folic acid
Prematurity; seen in term breast-fed infants whose mothers are folate-deficient and in term infants fed unsupplemented processed cow's milk or goat's milk; kwashiorkor; chronic overcooking; malabsorption of folate because of a congenital defect; sprue; celiac disease; drugs (phenytoin)
Increased requirements: chronic hemolytic anemias, diarrhea, malignancies, hypermetabolic states, infections, extensive skin disease, cirrhosis, pregnancy
Cobalamin
Rare; seen in breast-fed infants of mothers with latent pernicious anemia or who are on an unsupplemented strict vegetarian diet; absence of luminal proteases; congenital malabsorption of B_{12}
Vitamin C
Prematurity; maternal megadoses during pregnancy → deficiency in infants; lack of fresh fruits or vegetables; seen in infants fed formula and pasteurized cow's milk (historical)
Carnitine
Seen in premature infants fed unsupplemented soy formula or fed intravenously; dialysis; inherited deficits in carnitine synthesis; organic acidemias; valproic acid

Table 11–11. Clinical features of deficiencies in water-soluble vitamins.

Thiamin
Infantile beriberi (cardiac; aphonic; pseudomeningitic)
Riboflavin
Cheilosis; angular stomatitis; glossitis; soreness and burning of lips and mouth; dermatitis of nasolabial fold and genitals; ± ocular signs (photophobia → indistinct vision)
Pyridoxine
Listlessness; irritability; seizures; gastrointestinal disturbance; anemia; cheilosis; glossitis
Niacin
Pellagra (weakness; lassitude; dermatitis of exposed areas; diarrhea; dementia)
Pantothenic acid
Weakness; gastrointestinal disturbance; burning feet.
Biotin
Scaly dermatitis; alopecia; irritability; lethargy
Folate
Megaloblastic anemia; neutropenia; thrombocytopenia; growth retardation; delayed maturation of central nervous system in infants; diarrhea (mucosal ulcerations); glossitis; jaundice; mild splenomegaly; neural tube defects
Cobalamin
Megaloblastic anemia; neurologic degeneration
Vitamin C
Anorexia, irritability, apathy, pallor; fever; tachycardia; diarrhea; failure to thrive; increased susceptibility to infections; hemorrhages under skin, mucous membranes, into joints and under periosteum; long-bone tenderness; costochondral beading
Carnitine
Increased serum triglycerides and free fatty acids; decreasd ketones; fatty liver; hypoglycemia; genetic: progressive muscle weakness or cardiomyopathy or hypoglycemia

young mothers; many mothers face obstacles in maintaining lactation once they return to work. Skilled use of a breast pump, particularly an electric one, may help to maintain lactation in these circumstances.

Absolute contraindications to breast-feeding are rare. They include tuberculosis (in the mother) and galactosemia (in the infant). Although breast milk may serve as a vehicle for transmission of HIV, preliminary evidence suggests this is not a major route of transmission. Current recommendations are that HIV-infected mothers in developed countries refrain from breast-feeding because of the widely available, safe alternatives. In developing countries, the risk of HIV infection via breast milk is generally considered less than the known benefits of breast-feeding, particularly when alternative feeding methods may be hazardous.

The premature infant under 1500 g may benefit

from the addition of a milk fortifier, particularly to increase the density of protein, energy, calcium, and phosphorus. Breast-fed infants with cystic fibrosis may need an energy and protein supplement unless exogenous pancreatic enzymes are provided.

Management of Breast-feeding

Because most of today's grandmothers bottle-fed their children, the "art" of breast-feeding is no longer automatically passed from mother to daughter. Hence, the role of the health professional in supporting and promoting breast-feeding is of greater importance. Organizations such as the La Leche League have been effective in promoting breast-feeding as well as in providing education and support for mothers and health professionals alike.

Perinatal hospital routines and follow-up pediatric care have a great impact on the successful initiation of breast-feeding. Breast-feeding is promoted by prenatal and postpartum education, frequent mother-baby contact after delivery, one-on-one advice about breast-feeding technique, demand feeding, rooming-in, avoidance of bottle supplements, early follow-up after delivery, maternal confidence, family support, adequate maternity leave, and good advice about common problems such as sore nipples. Breast-feeding is undermined by mother and baby separations, feeding babies in the nursery at night, routinely offering supplemental bottles, conflicting advice from staff, incorrect infant positioning and latch-on, scheduled feedings, lack of maternal confidence or support, delayed follow-up, early return to employment, and inaccurate advice for common breast-feeding difficulties.

It is important for the mother to know that very few women are unable to nurse their babies. The newborn is generally fed ad libitum every 2–3 hours, with longer intervals (4–5 hours) at night. Thus, a newborn infant nurses at least eight to 10 times a day, so that a generous milk supply is stimulated. This frequency is not an indication of inadequate lactation. Mothers also frequently need to be reassured about stooling pattern. In early stages, a loose stool is often passed with each feeding; later (at 3–4 months of age), there may be an interval of several days between stools. Failure to pass several stools a day in the early weeks of breast-feeding suggests inadequate milk intake and supply.

Expressing milk may be indicated if the mother returns to her job or if the infant is premature, cannot suck adequately, or is hospitalized. Modern electric breast pumps are very effective and can be borrowed or rented.

Technique of Breast-feeding

Breast-feeding can be started after delivery as soon as both mother and baby are stable. Correct positioning and breast-feeding technique are necessary to ensure effective nipple stimulation and optimal breast emptying with minimal nipple discomfort.

If the mother wishes to nurse while sitting, the infant should be elevated to the height of the breast and turned completely to face the mother, so that their abdomens touch. The mother's arms supporting the infant should be held tightly at her side, bringing the baby's head in line with her breast. The breast should be supported by the lower fingers of her free hand, with the nipple compressed between the thumb and index fingers to make it more protractile. The infant's initial licking and mouthing of the nipple helps make it more erect. When the infant opens its mouth, the mother should rapidly insert as much nipple and areola as possible.

Some breast-fed infants fail to thrive. The most common cause of early failure to thrive is poorly managed mammary engorgement, which rapidly decreases milk supply. Unrelieved engorgement can result from inappropriately long intervals between feeding, improper infant suckling, a nondemanding infant, sore nipples, maternal or infant illness, nursing from only one breast, and latching difficulties. The mother's ignorance of technique, inappropriate feeding routines, and inadequate amounts of fluid and rest for the mother all can be factors. Some infants are too sleepy to do well on an ad libitum regimen and, in particular, may need waking to feed at night. Primary lactation failure is rare but does occur. Some decline in weight for age percentiles after 3 months should not necessarily be interpreted as an indication of inadequate nutrition, because the commonly used percentile charts have been constructed primarily from data on infants who have been formula-fed.

Rigid time restrictions should not be imposed. Sensible guidelines are 5 minutes per breast at each feeding the first day, 10 minutes on each side at each feeding the second day, and approximately 15 minutes per side thereafter. A vigorous infant can obtain most of the available milk in 5–7 minutes, but additional sucking time ensures breast emptying and ongoing milk production and satisfies the infant's sucking urge. The side on which feeding is commenced should be alternated. The mother may break suction gently after nursing by inserting her finger between the baby's gums.

Follow-up

Individualized assessment before discharge should identify the mothers and infants needing additional support. All cases require early follow-up after discharge. The onset of copious milk secretion between the second and fourth postpartum day is a critical time in the establishment of lactation. Failure to empty the breasts during this time can cause engorgement secondary to unrelieved pressure in the mammary gland, which quickly leads to diminished milk production.

Common Problems

Mild nipple tenderness requires attention to proper positioning of the infant and correct latch-on. Ancillary measures include nursing for shorter periods, beginning feedings on the less sore side, air drying the nipples well after nursing, and the application of lanolin cream. Severe nipple pain and cracking usually indicate improper infant attachment. Temporary pumping, which is well tolerated, may be needed.

Breast-feeding jaundice is exaggerated physiologic jaundice associated with inadequate intake of breast milk, infrequent stooling, and unsatisfactory weight gain. If possible, the jaundice should be managed by increasing the frequency of nursing and, if necessary, augmenting the infant's sucking with regular breast pumping. Supplemental feedings may be necessary, but care should be taken not to decrease breast milk production further.

In a small percentage of breast-fed infants, breast milk jaundice is caused by an unidentified property of the milk that inhibits conjugation of bilirubin. In severe cases, interruption of breast-feeding for 24–36 hours may be necessary. The mother's breast should be emptied with an electric breast pump during this period.

Maternal mastitis should be suspected when a nursing mother complains of a flu-like illness with local breast tenderness. Antibiotic therapy providing coverage against β-lactamase– producing organisms should be given for 10 days. Analgesics may be necessary, but breast-feeding should be continued. Breast pumping may be a helpful adjunctive therapy.

Maternal Drug Use

Many factors play a role in determining the effects of maternal drug therapy on the nursing infant, including the route of administration, dosage, molecular weight, pH, and protein binding. In general, any drug prescribed therapeutically to newborns can be consumed via breast milk without ill effect. Very few therapeutic drugs are absolutely contraindicated; these include radioactive compounds, antimetabolites, lithium, diazepam, chloramphenicol, antithyroid drugs, and tetracycline. For up-to-date information, a regional drug center should be consulted.

Maternal use of illicit or recreational drugs is a contraindication to breast-feeding. If a woman is unable to discontinue drug use, she should not breast-feed. Expression of milk for a feeding or two after use of a drug is not an acceptable compromise. The breast-fed infants of mothers taking methadone (but no alcohol or other drugs) as part of a treatment program have generally not experienced ill effects when the daily maternal methadone dose is under 40 mg.

Nutrient Composition

The nutrient composition of human milk is summarized and compared with that of cow's milk and formulas in Table 11–12. Outstanding characteristics include (1) the relatively low protein content, which is, however, quite adequate for the normal infant; (2) a generous but not excessive quantity of essential fatty acids; (3) the presence of long-chain unsaturated fatty acids of the ω3 series, of which docosahexaenoic acid is thought to be especially important; (4) a relatively low sodium and solute load; and (5) the lower concentration of calcium, iron, and

Table 11–12. The composition of milk (per 100 kcal).

Nutrient (Unit)	Minimal Level Recommended[1]	Mature Human Milk	Typical Commercial Formula	Cow's Milk (Mean)
Protein (g)	1.8 (See note 2.)	1.3–1.6	2.3	5.1
Fat (g)	3.3 (See note 3.)	5	5.3	5.7
Carbohydrate (g)	—	10.3	10.8	7.3
Linoleic acid (mg)	300	560	2300	125
Vitamin A (IU)	250	250	300	216
Vitamin D (IU)	40	3	63	3
Vitamin E (IU)	0.3 FT 0.7 LBW 1 g of linoleic	0.3	2	0.1
Vitamin K (μg)	4	2	9	5
Vitamin C (mg)	8	7.8	8.1	2.3
Thiamine (μg)	40	25	80	59
Riboflavin (μg)	60	60	100	252
Niacin (μg)	250	250	1200	131
Vitamin B_6 (μg)	15 μg of protein	15	63	66
Folic acid (μg)	4	4	10	8
Pantothenic acid (μg)	300	300	450	489
Vitamin B_{12} (μg)	0.15	0.15	0.25	0.56
Biotin (μg)	1.5	1	2.5	3.1
Inositol (mg)	4	20	5.5	20
Choline (mg)	7	13	10	23
Calcium (mg)	5	50	75	186
Phosphorus (mg)	25	25	65	145
Magnesium (mg)	6	6	8	20
Iron (mg)	1	0.1	1.5 in fortified	0.08
Iodine (μg)	5	4–9	10	7
Copper (μg)	60	25–60	80	20
Zinc (mg)	0.5	0.1–0.5	0.65	0.6
Manganese (μg)	5	1.5	5–160	3
Sodium (meq)	0.9	1	1.7	3.3
Potassium (meq)	2.1	2.1	2.7	6
Chloride (meq)	1.6	1.6	2.3	4.6
Osmolarity (mosm)	—	11.3	16–18.4	40

[1]Committee on Nutrition, American Academy of Pediatrics.
[2]Protein of nutritional quality equal to casein.
[3]Includes 300 mg of essential fatty acids.

zinc, which with the very favorable absorption provides adequate quantities of these nutrients to the normal breast-fed infant for 4–6 months despite the relatively low intakes.

Weaning

Weaning can take place according to the needs and desires of both infant and mother. Gradual weaning, starting typically after 4–6 months, is preferred. Bottle feedings (or cup feedings) are increased progressively over a period of several weeks as breast feedings are omitted.

American Academy of Pediatrics Committee on Drugs: Transfer of drugs and other chemical to human milk. Pediatrics 1994;93:137.

Cunningham AS, Jelliffe DB, Jelliffe EFP: Breast-feeding and health in the 1980s: A global epidemiologic review. 1991;118:659.

Freed GL, Landers SC, Schanler RJ: A practical guide to successful breast-feeding management. Am J Dis Child 1991;145:917.

Krebs NF et al: Growth and intakes of energy and zinc in infants fed human milk. J Pediatr 1994;124:32.

Losch M et al: Impact of attitudes on maternal decisions regarding infant feeding. J Pediatr 1995;126:507.

Oxtoby MJ: Human immunodeficiency virus and other viruses in human milk: Placing the issues in broader perspective. Pediatr Infect Dis J 1988;7:825.

SPECIAL DIETARY PRODUCTS FOR INFANTS

Feeding During the Second 6 Months

The standard (iron-fortified) infant formulas are suitable for use in the second 6 months. These formulas are preferred to unmodified cow's milk, which may be introduced cautiously after 9 months of age.

Soy Protein Formulas

The major indication for the use of soy protein formulas is lactose intolerance. For example, it is reasonable to recommend a soy protein formula during recovery from acute gastroenteritis for a period of 2–4 weeks. A lactose-free cow's milk–based formula is also available (Lactofree, Mead Johnson). Soy protein formulas are also used frequently in cases of suspected intolerance to cow's milk protein. However, infants who have true cow's milk protein intolerance may also be intolerant of soy protein. Many infants in the United States are currently fed soy protein formulas without good reason.

Semielemental Formulas

These formulas include Pregestimil (Mead Johnson), Nutramigen (Mead Johnson), and Alimentum (Ross). The major nitrogen source of each of these products is casein hydrolysate, supplemented with selected amino acids. Each contains an abundance of EFA from vegetable oil; Pregestimil and Alimentum also provide substantial amounts of medium-chain triglycerides (MCT). Pregestimil contains corn syrup solids; Nutramigen contains sucrose, which also provides part of the carbohydrate content in Alimentum.

These formulas are invaluable in a wide variety of malabsorption syndromes, including short bowel syndromes and some cases of chronic diarrhea and cystic fibrosis. They are also effective in feeding infants who cannot tolerate cow's milk and soy protein.

Formula Supplements

The most useful formula supplements are MCT oil and Polycose™ (Ross), both of which may be used to increase the energy density of a formula. Often it is more appropriate, however, to increase the concentration of the formula and thus increase the density of all nutrients.

Special Formulas

Special formulas include those in which one component, often an amino acid, is reduced in concentration or removed for the dietary management of specific inborn metabolic diseases. Also included under this heading is Amin-Aid (American McGaw).

Complete information regarding the composition of these special formulas, the standard infant formulas, and special formulas for premature infants can be found in standard reference texts such as the Harriet Lane handbook (*A Manual for Pediatric House Officers,*)* and in the manufacturer's literature.

PRUDENT DIET

A prudent diet should be encouraged for all children 2 years of age and older: children with high cholesterol levels tend to become adults with high cholesterol levels and are likely, therefore, to have an increased risk of coronary heart disease. Nutritional habits are formed early in life; dietary intervention may, therefore, be exceptionally effective when started in early childhood.

Salient features of a prudent diet include the following:

(1) Total fat should constitute less than 30% of caloric intake, with saturated fats and polyunsaturated fats providing less than 10% each. Thus, monounsaturated fats should provide 10% or more of caloric intake from fat.

(2) Cholesterol intake should be less than 100 mg/1000 kcal/d, to a maximum of 300 mg/d.

(3) Carbohydrates should provide 60% or more of

---

*References: (1) Fomon SJ et al: Formulas for older infants. J Pediatr 1990;11:690. (2) Greene MG: *The Harriet Lane Handbook,* 12th ed. Mosby–Year Book, 1991.

daily caloric intake, with 50% or more in the form of complex carbohydrates (ie, no more than 10% in the form of simple sugars). A high-fiber diet is also recommended.

(4) The diet should be nutritionally complete, include a variety of foods, and be adequate for optimal growth and activity.

(5) A low salt intake is advised.

The consumption of lean cuts of meats and poultry should be encouraged. Fish should be broiled or baked. Skim milk, soft margarine, and vegetable oils (especially olive oil) should be used. Consumption of egg yolks should be limited to two or three occasions per week. Whole-grain bread and cereals and plentiful amounts of fruits and vegetables are recommended. The consumption of processed foods, soft drinks, desserts, and candy should be limited.

A prudent diet should be only one component of counseling on lifestyles for children. Other aspects are the maintenance of ideal body weight, a regular exercise program, avoidance of smoking, and screening for hypertension. Universal screening for total cholesterol is controversial. Current recommendations are to routinely screen those children who have a positive family history of premature cardiovascular disease, although this approach will identify only about 50% of those with significantly elevated cholesterol levels. If the result is high ($\geq$200 mg/dL), a lipoprotein analysis should be obtained.

American Academy of Pediatrics Committee on Nutrition: Statement on cholesterol. Pediatrics 1992;90:469.

Lund EK et al: Dietary fat intake and plasma lipid levels in adolescents. Eur J Clin Nutr 1992;46:857.

National Cholesterol Education Program Coordinating Committee: *Highlights of the Report of the Expert Panel on Blood Cholesterol Levels in Children and Adolescents.* National Heart, Lung, and Blood Institute Information Center, 1991.

INTRAVENOUS NUTRITION

INDICATIONS

Supplemental Peripheral Nutrition

Supplemental peripheral nutrition is indicated when complete enteral feeding is not possible or desirable (eg, in the premature infant of very low birth weight during the first few days of postnatal life or in the malnourished surgical patient during the early postoperative period). Short-term partial intravenous feeding via a peripheral vein is a preferred alternative to dextrose and electrolyte solutions alone. Because of the osmolality of the solutions required, it is usu-

ally impossible to achieve total parenteral nutrition via a peripheral vein.

Total Parenteral Nutrition

Total parenteral nutrition (TPN) should be provided only when clearly indicated. Apart from the expense, numerous risks are associated with this method of feeding (see below). In addition, the powerful homeostatic control mechanisms provided by the intestine and the liver are bypassed. Even when TPN is indicated, every effort should be made to provide at least a minimum of nutrients enterally to help preserve the integrity of the gastrointestinal mucosa and of gastrointestinal function.

The primary indication for TPN is the loss of function of the gastrointestinal tract that prohibits the provision of more than a small proportion of required nutrients by the enteral route. Important examples include short bowel syndrome, some congenital defects of the gastrointestinal tract, and prematurity.

CATHETER SELECTION & POSITION

The Broviac is the catheter of choice for long-term intravenous nutrition. For periods of up to 3–4 weeks, a percutaneous central venous catheter threaded into the superior vena cava from a peripheral vein can be used. For the infusion of dextrose concentrations higher than 12.5%, the tip of the catheter should be located in the superior vena cava or right atrium. After placement, a chest x-ray must be obtained to check this position. If the catheter is to be used for nutrition and medications, a double-line catheter should be inserted.

COMPLICATIONS

Mechanical Complications

A. Related to Catheter Insertion or to Erosion of Catheter Through a Major Blood Vessel: There is an extensive list of complications involving trauma to adjacent tissues and organs, including damage to the brachial plexus, hydrothorax, pneumothorax, hemothorax, and cerebrospinal fluid penetration. The catheter may slip, especially if care is not taken at the time of dressing or tubing change. The patient may manipulate the line.

B. Clotting of the Catheter: Addition of heparin (1 U/mL) to the solution is an effective means of preventing this complication. If a catheter does become occluded urokinase can be administered for clot lysis.

C. Related to Composition of Infusate: Calcium phosphate precipitation is a major problem if excess amounts of calcium or phosphorus are administered. The quantities of calcium and phosphate that can be added to the infusate vary widely, depending on the particular commercial amino acid source. Factors that increase the risk of calcium phosphate precipitation include increasing pH and decreasing concentrations of amino acids. Precipitation of medications incompatible with TPN or lipids can also cause clotting.

Septic Complications

Septic complications are the most common cause of nonelective catheter removal, but strict use of aseptic technique and once-daily entry into the catheter at tubing change can result in greatly reduced rates of line sepsis. *For this reason, strict adherence to the standardized nursing protocol (for nurses and physicians) is mandatory.*

Metabolic Complications

A wide variety of metabolic complications associated with TPN has been documented. Many of these have been related to deficiencies or excesses of specific nutrients. The incidence of these complications has decreased as a result of improvements in amino acid solutions and lipid emulsions and a better understanding of how to achieve appropriate intakes of most nutrients. However, specific deficiencies still occur, especially in the premature infant. Avoidance of deficiencies and excesses and of metabolic disorders requires careful attention to the nutrient balance, electrolyte composition, and delivery rate of the infusate and careful monitoring, especially when the composition or delivery rate is changed.

Currently, the most challenging metabolic complication is cholestasis, particularly common in premature infants of very low birth weight. Amino acids competing for and blocking bile acid receptors at the hepatocyte appear to be one critical factor in the pathogenesis of this disorder. Complete lack of oral feeding, sepsis, free radical damage, or toxic factors present in TPN solutions may contribute to this problem. Amino acid solutions with added cysteine decrease cholestasis. Maneuvers that *may* minimize cholestasis include administering some enteral feedings (even if very small) as soon as feasible, protecting the TPN solutions from light, and alternating relatively larger doses with lower doses of amino acids every other day (eg, 1 g/kg/d alternating with 3 g/kg/d rather than administering 2 g/kg/d).

NUTRIENT REQUIREMENTS & DELIVERY

Energy

When patients are fed intravenously, no fat and carbohydrate intakes are unabsorbed, and no energy is used in nutrient absorption. These factors account for at least 7% of energy in the diet of the enterally fed subject. The intravenously fed patient also expends less energy in physical activity because of the impediment to mobility. Average energy requirements are therefore at least 7% lower in children fed intravenously, and the decrease in activity probably increases this figure to a total reduction of 10–15%. Caloric guidelines for the intravenous feeding of infants and young children are as follows:

Age (mo)	Requirments (kcal/kg/d)
2–4	100–110
4–36	90–100
4–36	75–80

These guidelines are averages; individuals vary considerably. Some older infants require 70 kcal/kg/d or less and on higher intravenous intakes will become obese. A multitude of factors can significantly increase the energy requirement, including exposure to a cold environment, fever, sepsis, burns, trauma, cardiac or pulmonary disease, and "catch-up" growth after malnutrition.

With few exceptions, such as some cases of respiratory insufficiency, at least 60% of energy requirements is provided as glucose. Up to 40% of calories may be provided by intravenous fat emulsions.

Dextrose

The energy density of intravenous dextrose (monohydrate) is 3.4 kcal/g. Thus, a 10% solution of dextrose in water ($D_{10}W$) provides 0.34 kcal/mL. Dextrose is the main exogenous energy source provided by total intravenous feeding. Intravenous dextrose suppresses gluconeogenesis and provides a substrate that can be oxidized directly, especially by the brain, red and white blood cells, and wounds. Because of the high osmolality of dextrose solutions ($D_{10}W$ yields 505 mosm/kg H_2O), concentrations greater than 10–12.5% cannot be delivered via a peripheral vein or improperly positioned central line.

The amount of glucose supplied is determined by the rate of administration as well as the dextrose concentration. Consequently, it is important to calculate the desired glucose load in planning dextrose infusions.

The standard initial quantity of dextrose administered is 10 g/kg/d, which provides 34 kcal/kg/d. This is typically, but not necessarily, provided as 100 mL/kg/d of $D_{10}W$. Tolerance to intravenous dextrose normally increases rapidly, primarily because hepatic production of endogenous glucose is suppressed. Dextrose can be increased by 2.5 g/kg/d. Standard final infusates for infants usually contain $D_{20}W$, but if necessary (especially at low flow rates), concentrations up to $D_{30}W$ or greater may be used. Such high concentrations should be delivered only into the superior vena cava or right atrium. Tolerance to intravenous dextrose loads is markedly diminished in the premature neonate and in patients in hypermetabolic states.

Problems associated with intravenous dextrose administration include hyperglycemia, hyperosmolality, and glucosuria (with osmotic diuresis and dehydration). Possible causes of unexpected hyperglycemia include the following: (1) inadvertent infusion of higher glucose concentrations than ordered; (2) uneven flow rate; (3) sepsis; (4) a stress situation; and (5) pancreatitis. Intravenous insulin reduces hyperglycemia but does not increase glucose oxidation rates; it may also decrease the oxidation of fatty acids, resulting in less energy for metabolism. Hence, insulin should be used very cautiously. A standard intravenous dose is 1 U/4 g of carbohydrate, but much smaller quantities may be adequate.

Hypoglycemia may occur after an abrupt decrease in or cessation of intravenous glucose. When cyclic intravenous nutrition is provided, the intravenous glucose load should be decreased steadily for 1–2 hours prior to discontinuing the infusate. If the central line must be removed, the intravenous dextrose should be gradually tapered over several hours.

The maximum oxidation rate of infused dextrose in infants is 18 g/kg/d (less if given with ≥3 g of lipid/kg/d). The corresponding rates at 6 years, at 10 years, and in adult life are 13, 8, and 4.3 g/kg/d, respectively. The very low birth weight neonate seldom tolerates more than 8–12 g/kg/d. Quantities of exogenous dextrose in excess of maximal glucose oxidation rates are used initially to replace depleted glycogen stores; hepatic lipogenesis occurs thereafter. Excess hepatic lipogenesis may lead to a fatty liver. Lipogenesis results in release of carbon dioxide, which when added to the amount of carbon dioxide produced by glucose oxidation (which is 40% greater than that produced by lipid oxidation) may elevate the $PaCO_2$ and aggravate respiratory insufficiency or impede weaning from a respirator.

Lipids

Several commercial fat emulsions are now available for intravenous use. All consist of more than 50% linoleic acid and 4–9% linolenic acid. It is recognized that this high level of linoleic is far from ideal except when small quantities of lipid are being given to prevent a deficiency in EFA. Ultimately, improved emulsions are anticipated. The level of lipoprotein lipase (LPL) activity is the rate-limiting factor in the metabolism and clearance of fat emulsions from the circulation. LPL activity is inhibited or decreased by malnutrition, leukotrienes, immaturity, growth hormone, hypercholesterolemia, hyperphospholipidemia, and theophylline. LPL activity is enhanced by glucose, insulin, lipid, catecholamines, and exercise. Heparin releases LPL from the endothelium into the circulation and enhances the rate of hydrolysis and clearance of triglycerides. In small premature infants, low-dose heparin infusions may increase tolerance to intravenous lipid emulsion. Because 10% and 20% lipid emulsions contain the same concentrations of phospholipids, a 10% solution delivers more phospholipid per gram of lipid than a 20% solution. Twenty percent lipid emulsions are preferred for all patients.

The advantages of using fat emulsions to provide up to 40% of caloric intake include the following:

(1) The energy density, which is 2 kcal/mL for 20% emulsions, allows more energy to be provided when fluid volume is restricted.

(2) The low osmolality is (280 mosm/kg H_2O) is of special value when using a peripheral line.

(3) Deficiencies in EFA can be prevented.

(4) The production of CO_2 is 40% lower per unit of energy, an important consideration in cases of pulmonary insufficiency.

(5) The energy cost of fat storage is negligible (energy does not have to be synthesized from dextrose).

(6) The risk of fatty liver is decreased because of decreased hepatic lipogenesis from dextrose.

Potential disadvantages of fat emulsions include the following:

(1) Impairment of function of lymphocytes, neutrophils, macrophages, and the reticuloendothelial system.

(2) Coagulation defects, including thrombocytopenia, elevated prothrombin time (PT), and partial thromboplastin time (PTT).

(3) Decrease in pulmonary oxygen diffusion.

(4) Competition with bilirubin and drugs for albumin binding sites.

(5) Increase in LDL cholesterol.

In general, these adverse effects can be avoided by starting with modest quantities and advancing cautiously in light of results of triglyceride monitoring and clinical circumstances. In cases of severe sepsis, special caution is required to ensure that the lipid is effectively metabolized. Continuous monitoring with long-term use is also essential.

Start with 1 g/kg/d. Advance every 1–2 days by 0.5–1 g/kg/d up to 2.5 g/kg/d in an infant and 3.5 g/kg/d in a child. Check serum triglycerides before starting and before and after increasing dose. Request results the same day. As a general rule, do not increase dose if serum triglyceride is greater than 250 mg/dL during infusion (150 mg/dL in neonates and septic patients). Clearance 4 hours postinfusion should also be monitored (<150 mg/dL).

Note: Linoleic acid must constitute 2–3% of caloric intake (300 mg linoleic acid per 100 kcal) so that a deficiency in EFA can be avoided. Linolenic acid (1%) is also needed and is adequately supplied when linoleic acid needs are met.

Nitrogen

One gram of nitrogen is yielded by 6.25 g of protein (1 g of protein contains 16% nitrogen). Caloric density of protein is equal to 4 kcal/g.

A. Protein Requirements: Protein requirements for intravenous feeding are the same as those for normal oral feeding (see Table 11–2).

B. Protein-Energy Interactions: There are important interactions between protein and energy requirements. A positive nitrogen balance cannot be achieved on a hypocaloric diet, because protein will be catabolized for energy. When energy intakes are low, the administration of some amino acid does, however, improve the severity of the negative nitrogen balance. Conversely, when nitrogen intake is low, the provision of calories improves nitrogen balance to some extent. In infants, the energy necessary to minimize nitrogen loss associated with an amino acid–free diet is approximately 70 kcal/kg/d. At this level of energy intake, a positive nitrogen balance can be achieved to a degree that depends on the level of nitrogen intake and is independent of further increase in energy intake.

In infants receiving about 50 kcal/kg/d, increasing protein intake up to 3 g/kg/d improves the nitrogen balance. In these circumstances, therefore, a ratio of grams of nitrogen per kilocalorie as low as 1:100 can be advantageous. However, at higher levels of energy intake, ratios of 1:250 to 1:150 or more are optimal. Although these ratios provide a useful crude check, they are not usually the best means of determining protein requirements.

C. Intravenous Amino Acid Solutions: Nitrogen requirements are provided by one of the commercially available amino acid solutions. All of the standard preparations are equally good sources of amino acids. There is some preliminary evidence, however, that the use of Trophamine is associated with superior nitrogen retention and less hepatotoxicity. The putative benefits of Trophamine are likely attributable in part to the cysteine that can be added to the solution immediately before use. Forty milligrams of cysteine is added for each gram of Trophamine. Thus, 1 L of 2% solution requires an addition of 800 mg of cysteine. Cysteine provides a good source of taurine.

Normally, the final infusate contains 2–3% amino acids, depending on the rate of infusion. In the very low birth weight or severely malnourished infant, the initial amount should be 1 g/kg/d.

Because of the high osmolality of amino acid solutions, the concentration should not be advanced beyond 2% in peripheral vein infusates.

D. Monitoring: Monitoring for tolerance of the intravenous amino acid solutions should include routine blood urea nitrogen (BUN). Serum alkaline phosphatase, γ-glutamyltransferase, and bilirubin should be monitored to detect the onset of cholestatic liver disease.

E. Special Amino Acid Preparations: Some solutions are designed to provide high concentrations of branched-chain amino acids. These solutions are expensive and should not be ordered without a specific reason, which does not include their routine use in liver disease. They may be indicated in hepatic failure, especially in the presence of encephalopathy, and are also undergoing experimental use in multisystem organ failure. In this circumstance, the branched-chain amino acids are given as a source of metabolizable energy, providing up to 25% of energy intake. Solutions containing only essential amino acids have some application in the management of patients with renal failure.

F. Albumin: Albumin (0.5–1 g/kg per dose) can be added to the infusate when clinically indicated to restore blood volume or oncotic pressure. If the origin of hypoalbuminemia is considered to be primarily nutritional, however, the hypoalbuminemia should be managed by careful nutritional rehabilitation rather than by intravenous administration of albumin. Albumin is deficient in isoleucine and tryptophan and has too long a half-life (15–20 days) to be considered a useful nutritional source of amino acids.

Minerals & Electrolytes

A. Calcium, Phosphorus, & Magnesium: The results of two recent studies have indicated that the intravenously fed premature and term infant should be given relatively high amounts of calcium and phosphorus. Current recommendations are as follows: calcium, 500–600 mg/L; phosphorus, 400–450 mg/L; and magnesium, 50–70 mg/L. After the age of 1 year, the recommendations are as follows: calcium, 200–400 mg/L; phosphorus, 150–300 mg/L; and magnesium, 20–40 mg/L. The calcium:phosphorus ratio should be 1.3:1 by weight or 1:1 by molar ratio. These recommendations are deliberately presented on a per liter infusate basis to avoid inadvertent administration of concentrations of calcium and phosphorus that are high enough to precipitate in the tubing. During periods of fluid restriction, care must be taken not to inadvertently increase the concentration of calcium and phosphorus in the infusate. These recommendations assume an average fluid intake of 120–150 mL/kg/d and an infusate of 25 g of amino acid per liter. With lower amino acid concentrations, the concentrations of calcium and phosphorus should be decreased.

B. Electrolytes: Standard recommendations are given in Figure 11–1. After chloride requirements are met, the remainder of the anion required to balance the cation should be given as acetate to avoid the possibility of acidosis resulting from excessive chloride. The required concentrations of electrolytes depend to some extent on the flow rate of the infusate and must be modified if flow rates are unusually low or high and if there are specific indications in individual patients. Intravenous sodium should be administered very sparingly in the severely malnourished patient because of impaired membrane function and high intracellular sodium levels. Conversely, generous quantities of potassium are indicated. Re-

PEDIATRIC PARENTERAL NUTRITION (PN) ORDER FORM Imprint Patient Plate

Weight of patient _____kg Central line_____ Peripheral line _____ _____

Rate _____

	Standard Order	Modifications To Standard Order	*Adjustments for Neonates and Premature Infants (Circle these when required and cross out corresponding items* under "standard order")
Protein (as amino acid)* _____	g%		*Use trophamine and cysteine for patients in level II and III nurseries who have a central line or are on a day 6 of peripheral therapy.
Dextrose _____	g%		
Na _____	30 meq/L		
K _____	25 meq/L		
Cl _____	20 meq/L		
Acetate _____	45 meq/L		
Ca (as gluconate) (10 mM Ca/L) _____	20 meq/L		
Mg (as sulfate) _____	3 meq/L		
P_____	10 meq/L		
MVI Pediatric _____	*5.0 mL/d		*2 mL/kg/d for patients < 2.5 kg
Zinc _____	*1.0 mg/L		*Zn: 400 µg/kg/d < 2 kg body weight 250 µg/kg/d others < 3 mo old
Copper _____	200 µg /L		
Manganese _____	5.0 µg/L		
Chromium _____	2.0 µg/L		
Selenium _____	20.0 µg/L		
Iodide _____	10 µg/L		
Heparin _____	1000 Units/L		
Cysteine (40 mg/g trophamine)*_____	mg/L		*Use only with trophamine

Pharmacy will automatically account for electrolytes provided in amino acid preparation.

Changes in Na or K to be made as: Cl only___, or Acetate only___, Cl: Acetate 1:1__, or other

Cl: Acetate ratio (specify_____).

Date:_____ Signature:_____M.D.

Figure 11–1. Example of pediatric parenteral nutrition order. Standard recommendations for minerals and trace elements are indicated.

placement electrolytes and fluids should be delivered via a separate infusate.

C. Trace Elements: Recommended intravenous intakes of trace elements are given in Figure 11–1.

When intravenous nutrition is supplemental or limited to less than 2 weeks, only zinc need routinely be added.

Intravenous copper requirements are relatively low in the young infant because of the presence of hepatic copper stores. These are significant even in the 28-week fetus. Circulating levels of copper and manganese should be monitored in the presence of cholestatic liver disease. If monitoring is not feasible, temporary withdrawal of added copper and manganese is advisable. Copper and manganese are excreted primarily in the bile, but selenium, chromium, and molybdenum are excreted primarily in the urine. These trace elements, therefore, should be administered with caution in the presence of renal failure.

For patients on long-term parenteral nutrition, a dose of 1 µg/kg/d of iodine avoids any risk of iodine deficiency and does not increase the risk of toxicity from accidental absorption of topical iodine-containing preparations.

Although low doses of iron are routinely added in some centers to the intravenous infusate for infants and children, no official recommendation has been made because of the lack of adequate published data regarding compatibility. Iron added to the infusate should be in a diluted form of iron dextran in a concentration of 1 mg/L. After 2 months of age, maintenance intravenous iron requirements for the term infant are approximately 100 µg/kg/d intravenously. After the first month, the premature infant requires up to 200 µg/kg/d intravenously. Although overload is unlikely to occur during short-term parenteral nutrition, a surreptitious accumulation of extra iron could occur if parenteral nutrition is prolonged. This risk is enhanced if the patient has received blood transfusions. A second concern is that the potential for free iron is increased in malnourished infants with low transferrin levels. Excess iron is thought to enhance the risk of gram-negative septicemia. Iron has powerful oxidant properties and can enhance the demand for antioxidants, especially vitamin E. None of these concerns appear to preclude the routine use of iron supplements during intravenous nutrition, but they do emphasize the need for a conservative attitude in determining dosage schedules.

Currently, intravenous infusates are contaminated with aluminum. In infants, aluminum accumulation in bone after 3 weeks of intravenous feeding can be marked. Aluminum intakes should be measured when possible, especially in the premature infant and in the infant or child with impaired renal function.

Vitamins

Recommendations for intravenous vitamin intakes are given in Table 11–6. MVI Pediatric (Armour) meets the guidelines for term infants. The recommended dose of MVI Pediatric for premature infants is 2 mL (40%) of a single-dose vial per kilogram per day. This formulation is not optimal (too little vitamin A, excessive amounts of water-soluble vitamins), but it is currently the best available.

Intravenous lipid preparations contain enough tocopherol to effect total blood tocopherol levels. The majority of tocopherol in soybean oil emulsion is γ-tocopherol, which has substantially less biologic activity than α-tocopherol, which is present in safflower oil emulsions. Premature infants may possibly be susceptible to liver damage from excessive intakes of vitamin E. The intravenous administration of 25–100 mg/d of α-tocopherol acetate for as little as 1 week has been associated with coagulopathy and progressive liver failure in several infants of very low birth weight. The toxicity was due to the solubilizer, polysorbate 80, rather than to the α-tocopherol.

Recent data indicate that a dose of 40 IU/kg/d of vitamin D (maximum 400 IU/d) is adequate for both term and preterm infants.

Fluid Requirements

The initial fluid volume and subsequent increments in flow rate are determined by basic fluid requirements, the clinical status of the patient, and the extent to which additional fluid administration can be tolerated and may be required to achieve adequate nutrient intake. Calculation of initial fluid volumes to be administered should be based on standard pediatric practice. Tolerance of higher flow rates must be determined on an individual basis. If replacement fluids are required for ongoing abnormal losses, these should be administered via a separate line.

Ordering

An example of a parenteral nutrition order form for pediatrics is given in Figure 11–1. Orders should be reviewed daily when changes are made and when the patient is acutely ill.

Monitoring

Vital signs should be checked at each shift.

With central catheter in situ and fever more than 38 °C, peripheral and central line blood cultures, urine cultures, complete physical examination, and examination of intravenous entry point are required. Instability of vital signs, elevated white blood cell count with left shift, and glycosuria suggest sepsis. Removal of the central venous catheter should be considered if patient is toxic or unresponsive to antibiotics (the patient must be weaned of high-dose dextrose prior to removal of the catheter).

A. Physical Examination: Monitor especially for hepatomegaly (differential diagnoses include fluid overload, congestive heart failure, steatosis, and hepatitis) and edema (differential diagnoses: fluid overload, congestive heart failure, hypoalbuminemia, thrombosis of superior vena cava).

B. Intake/Output Record: Calories and volume delivered should be calculated from previous day's intake and output sheets (that which was delivered rather than that which was ordered). The following should be recorded on flow sheets: intravenous, enteral, and total fluid (mL/kg/d); dextrose (g/kg/d); protein (g/kg/d); lipids (g/kg/d); energy (kcal/kg/d).

C. Growth, Urine, & Blood: Routine monitoring guidelines given in Table 11–13 are only a guide. These are minimum requirements, except in the very long-term stable patients. Individual variables should be monitored more frequently as indicated, as should additional variables or clinical indications. For example, a blood ammonia should be ordered in an infant

Table 11–13. Routine monitoring summary.

Variables	Acute Stage	Long-Term
Growth		
Weight	Daily	Weekly
Length	Weekly	
Head circumference	Weekly	
Urine		
Glucose (dipstick)	With each void	With changes in intake or status
Specific gravity	Void	
Volume	Daily	
Blood		
Glucose	4 h after changes,[1] then daily × 2	Weekly
Na^+, K^+, Cl^-, CO_2, BUN	Daily for 2 d after changes,[1] then twice weekly	Weekly
Ca^{2+}, Mg^{2+}, P	Initially, then twice weekly	Weekly
Total protein, albumin, bilirubin, AST, and alkaline phosphatase	Initially , then weekly	Every other week
Zinc and copper	Initially	Monthly
Triglycerides	Initially, 1 d after changes,[1] then weekly	Weekly
CBC	Initially, then twice weekly; according to clinical indications (see text)	Twice weekly

[1]Changes include alterations in concentration or flow rate.

with lethargy, pallor, poor growth, acidosis, azotemia, and elevated liver enzymes.

Greene HL et al: Guidelines for the use of vitamins, trace elements, calcium, magnesium, and phosphorus in infants and children receiving total parenteral nutrition: Report of the Subcommittee on Pediatric Parenteral Nutrient Requirements from the Committee on Clinical Practice Issues of the American Society for Clinical Nutrition. Am J Clin Nutr 1988;48:1324.

Heird WC: Parenteral support of the hospitalized child. In: *Textbook of Pediatric Nutrition.* Suskind R , Suskind LL (editors). Raven, 1993.

INTENSIVE CARE NUTRITION

Severe stress of any kind (eg, large surface area and deep burns, major trauma, major surgery, sepsis) results in common metabolic changes that require special understanding and nutritional management. First, several hormones are increased, including thyroid hormone, catecholamines, cortisol, and glucagon. These hormones, acting directly on peripheral tissues or indirectly through an increase in peripheral insulin resistance (as a result, insulin concentration may actually increase), produce hypermetabolism, increased protein catabolism, and hyperglycemia. These effects develop rapidly, from seconds for the catecholamines, to minutes for insulin and glucagon, to hours for thyroid and cortisol. Rapid measurements of these hormones and their metabolic effects are not available for routine clinical management, so the clinician must know that their concentration changes and metabolic effects are going to be present, highly variable, and significant, requiring special management early in the course of stressful events to counter their adverse effects on fuel metabolism. Early and aggressive intravenous and enteral nutrition are essential, with an emphasis on providing an increased supply of amino acids, particularly the branched-chain amino acids. Trials of insulin infusion, including coinfusion of growth hormone and insulin-like growth factor–I, are under way. The goal of such aggressive, early treatment is to provide an excess of nonprotein calories (favoring lipids over glucose) and amino acids to preserve essential protein structures.

Allison SP: Overview: Substrate and acute catabolism. In: *Organ Metabolism and Nutrition.* Kinney JM, Tucker HN (editors). Raven, 1994 107.

Provision of Nutrients in Hypermetabolic States

The most important principle is to continue enteral feeding whenever possible, so that the integrity of the enterocytes can be maintained. The increase in energy requirements varies according to the severity of hypermetabolism and its cause. Requirements are highest in burn patients, but major trauma and severe sepsis increase energy expenditure by 20–50%.

The uncontrolled muscle proteolysis and negative nitrogen balance that are characteristic of the hypermetabolic state cannot be counteracted totally by aggressive nutrition support, but the adverse effects can be attenuated. Negative nitrogen balance can be improved by providing 1½ to two times the basal protein requirement for that age. Larger quantities are unlikely to improve nitrogen balance, and they require substantial energy expenditure for oxidation and will increase CO_2 production. Additional amounts (up to 25% of caloric needs) of branched-chain amino acids (enteral or parenteral) are currently being used as an energy source for skeletal muscle.

Another major metabolic aberration in stress-induced, hypermetabolic states is persistent, uncontrolled hepatic gluconeogenesis, often producing markedly elevated blood glucose concentrations. Gluconeogenesis is not switched off—as would normally be expected—by the administration of intravenous dextrose; in fact, dextrose administration tends to aggravate hyperglycemia and increase hepatic lipogenesis. In some patients (especially those who develop multisystem organ failure), only very modest quantities (<45% of energy requirements) will be tolerated. If severe hyperglycemia and glycosuria occur, temporary insulin therapy is necessary. However, the putative effects of insulin in hypermetabolic states are complex and not well clarified. Hypermetabolism is characterized by insulin resistance. Furthermore, insulin requires the simultaneous administration of greater-than-normal amounts (up to 25% of energy needs) of amino acids to limit or partially reverse the uncontrolled muscle catabolism and gluconeogenesis. Theoretically, insulin administration could decrease lipolysis and thus deprive the hypermetabolic patient of some of the major sources of utilizable endogenous fuel.

Although lipolysis is increased in hypermetabolic states, β-oxidation of fatty acids also is increased, at least initially. Intravenous lipids usually can be metabolized well in early stages, and up to 50% of energy may be provided as lipid. Metabolically, lipid is the preferred fuel in patients with severe sepsis. Lipid tolerance deteriorates in advanced multisystem organ failure.

The metabolic and nutritional advantages of lipid as a fuel must be balanced against potential adverse effects in the septic child. These may include some impairment of the function of lymphocytes, neutrophils, and macrophages and possible coagulation defects. It is important to monitor these factors closely (including triglyceride, PT, PTT, and platelets) and not to administer fat emulsion in excess of quantities that can be cleared effectively from the circulation.

McClave SA, Snider HL: Understanding the metabolic response to critical illness: Factors that cause patients to deviate from the expected pattern of hypermetabolism. New Horizons 1994;2:139.

Much interest recently has focused on the potential benefits of glutamine during acute stress. Glutamine is a nonessential amino acid which is an important source of nitrogen for nucleic acid synthesis. It becomes conditionally essential and serves as a preferred energy source for certain tissues, including enterocytes. Supplementation with glutamine, orally or parenterally, has been associated with lessened bacterial translocation from the gut, improved nitrogen balance, and improved tolerance to enteral feeds in critically ill patients. Although most studies have been undertaken in adults, trials in pediatric bone marrow transplant patients and in children with short bowel syndrome are under way.

Tremel H et al: Glutamine dipeptide–supplemented parenteral nutrition maintains intestinal function in the critically ill. Gastroenterology 1994;107:1595.

Emergencies, Injuries, & Poisoning — 12

F. Keith Battan, MD, Richard C. Dart, MD, PhD, & Barry H. Rumack, MD

EMERGENCIES & INJURIES

F. Keith Battan, MD

Pediatric emergency medicine as a subspecialty has developed over the past 12–14 years to provide resuscitation and urgent care of infants, children, and adolescents. The body of research literature in this field is growing rapidly. The *EMS-C (Emergency Medical Services for Children) movement,* exists to enhance the care of the severely ill or injured child: community injury prevention, prehospital care by emergency medical technicians and paramedics, hospital-based stabilization and critical care, and rehabilitation. Trauma is the leading cause of death among children over 1 year of age.

Isaacman DJ, Davis HW: Pediatric emergency medicine: State of the art. Pediatrics 1993;91:587.

Lohr KN, Durch JS (editors): Emergency Medical Services for Children, Report to the Nation from the Institute of Medicine, Committee on Pediatric Emergency Medical Services. National Academy Press, 1993. (This reference describes the goals and activities of the EMS-C nationwide effort.)

Nelson DS et al: Spectrum and frequency of pediatric illness presenting to a general community hospital emergency department. Pediatrics 1992;90:5.

ESTIMATION FORMULAS		
Estimated body weight (kg)	=	(Age in years $\times$ 2) + 8
Median blood pressure (systolic)	=	(Age in years $\times$ 2) + 90
5th percentile systolic blood pressure (hypotension)	=	(Age in years $\times$ 2) + 70
Endotracheal tube size	=	$\dfrac{\text{(Age in years + 16)}}{4}$

ADVANCED LIFE SUPPORT FOR INFANTS & CHILDREN

Children may present in cardiopulmonary failure from a wide variety of causes, mainly respiratory disorders. Regardless of the primary origin, a systematic approach allows rapid determination of the patient's physiologic status followed by initiation of resuscitative measures. The goal of rapid assessment and intervention is not necessarily to make a specific etiologic diagnosis but to determine the degree of physiologic derangement—Is there respiratory failure? Is there shock?—and then to intervene promptly to ensure adequate oxygenation, ventilation, and circulation.

Children who become apneic and pulseless virtually never survive without neurologic devastation. When progressive deterioration leads to bradycardia and ultimately to asystole, sufficient hypoxic and ischemic insult to the brain and other vital organs has occurred to make neurologic recovery extremely unlikely. Children who respond to ventilation and oxygenation alone or to less than 5 minutes of advanced life support are much more likely to survive neurologically intact. Therefore, it is essential to recognize the child who is at risk for progressing to cardiopulmonary arrest and to provide aggressive intervention.

THE ABCs OF RESUSCITATION

Severely ill children should be rapidly evaluated in a sequence of *a*irway patency, *b*reathing adequacy, and *c*irculation integrity. Derangement in each must be corrected *before* proceeding to the next function. Thus, if a child's airway is obstructed, one must open the airway (eg, by head positioning and the chin lift maneuver) before assessing breathing and then circulation.

Airway

Look, listen, and feel for airway patency: (1) *Look* for signs of obstruction such as inspiratory work or suprasternal retractions. Rapidly assess the level of consciousness. A patient with significant airway obstruction will have an altered level of consciousness, such as agitation or unresponsiveness. (2) *Listen* for adventitious breath sounds such as stridor, snoring, or gurgling. (3) *Feel* for air movement with your face near the child's mouth and nose.

The airway is managed initially by noninvasive means such as chin lift, suctioning, or bag-valve-mask ventilation, then by invasive maneuvers such as endotracheal intubation or cricothyroidotomy. If neck injury is suspected, the cervical spine must be immobilized. (See Approach to the Pediatric Trauma Patient below.) The following discussion assumes that basic life support techniques are known.

Knowledge of pediatric anatomic differences will help assess and manage the airway. Infants are obligate nasal breathers; therefore, secretions or blood can cause significant distress. Children's tongues are large relative to their oral cavities, and the larynx is high and anteriorly located. In unconscious children, prolapse of the tongue into the posterior pharynx is the most common cause of airway obstruction.

A. Place the head in the "sniffing position" (Figure 12–1). The neck should be slightly flexed and the head gently extended so as to bring the face forward. This position aligns the oral, pharyngeal, and tracheal planes (Figure 12–2). The head should be repositioned if airway obstruction persists after head tilt and jaw thrust. In an infant, the relatively large occiput puts the head in a sniffing position when supine; in an older child, more head extension is necessary. Avoid hyperextension of the neck, especially in infants.

B. Perform the chin lift or jaw thrust maneuver (Figure 12–3). Lift the chin upward while avoiding pressure on the submental triangle, or lift the jaw by traction upward on the angle of the jaw. Jaw thrust without head tilt should be done if cervical spine injury is possible.

C. Suction the mouth of secretions, blood, and foreign material.

D. Remove visible foreign bodies, using the fingers or a Magill forceps—visualizing by means of a laryngoscope if necessary. Blind finger sweeps should *not* be done.

E. Insert an oropharyngeal or, in the conscious patient, a nasopharyngeal airway to relieve upper airway obstruction due to prolapse of the tongue and mandibular block of tissue into the posterior pharynx

Figure 12–1. Opening the airway with the head tilt-chin lift maneuver. One hand is used to tilt the head, extending the neck. The index finger of the rescuer's other hand lifts the mandible outward by lifting on the chin. Head tilt should not be performed if cervical spine injury is suspected. (Reproduced, with permission, from *Textbook of Pediatric Life Support.* © 1994, American Heart Association.)

Figure 12–2. Correct positioning of the child more than 2 years of age for ventilation and tracheal intubation. **A:** With the patient on a flat surface (eg, bed or table), the oral (O), pharyngeal (P), and tracheal (T) axes pass through three divergent planes. **B:** A folded sheet or towel placed under the occiput of the head aligns the pharyngeal and tracheal axes. **C:** Extension of the atlanto-occipital joint results in alignment of the oral, pharyngeal, and tracheal axes. (Reproduced, with permission from Cote and Todres in *Textbook of Pediatric Life Support.* © 1994, American Heart Association.)

(Figures 12–4 and 12–5). The correct size for an oropharyngeal airway is obtained by measuring from the upper central gumline to the angle of the jaw. Nasopharyngeal airways should fit snugly but not tightly within the nares and are sized from the nares to the tragus.

Breathing

Assessment of respiratory status is largely accomplished by *inspection*. (1) *Look* for adequate and symmetric chest rise and fall, respiratory rate, increased work of breathing including retractions, flaring, and grunting, skin color, and tracheal deviation. (2) *Listen* for adventitious breath sounds such as wheezing. Auscultate for air entry, symmetry of breath sounds, and rales. (3) *Feel* for subcutaneous crepitus.

If there is no or inadequate spontaneous breathing, initiate positive-pressure ventilation with bag-valve-mask ventilation and 100% oxygen. *Universal precautions should be maintained during resuscitations.* If some respiratory effort is present, coordinate bagging with the patient's efforts. Adequacy of ventilation is reflected in adequate rise and fall of the chest and auscultation of good air entry bilaterally. The presence of asymmetric breath sounds in a child in cardiac arrest or in severe distress suggests pneumothorax and is an indication for needle thoracostomy. In infants, the transmission of breath sounds throughout the chest may impair the ability to auscultate the presence of a pneumothorax. If the chest does not rise and fall easily with bagging, one should reposition the airway and repeat the maneuvers in the "airway" section. Perform airway foreign body maneuvers if the airway remains obstructed, including visualizing the airway with a laryngoscope and using Magill forceps. *Note:* Effective oxygenation and ventilation are the keys to successful resuscitation.

Intubate the trachea, with cricoid pressure (Sellick maneuver) in patients unresponsive to bag-mask ventilation, those in coma, those who require airway protection, or those who will require prolonged ventilation. Advanced airway management techniques are described in the references accompanying this section. Cricothyroidotomy is rarely necessary. (See Approach to the Pediatric Trauma Patient.)

Circulation

Clinical assessment of hemodynamic status can be done rapidly. The diagnosis of shock can and should be made by clinical examination before the blood pressure is measured.

A. Pulses: Check heart rate and adequacy of peripheral pulses. Pulses can be bounding in the early phases of septic shock, or weak and thready in hypoperfusion states. Tachycardia is a nonspecific sign of distress, whereas bradycardia for age is a prearrest sign and necessitates aggressive resuscitation.

B. Extremities: If distal extremities are cool, locate the proximal point at which they become warm to assess the severity of shock. For example, a child whose extremities are cool distal to the elbows and knees is severely hypoperfused.

C. Capillary Refill Time: This is an important indicator of perfusion. A refill time longer than 2.0 seconds is abnormal unless the child is cold.

Figure 12–3. Opening the airway with the jaw-thrust maneuver. The airway is opened by lifting the angle of the mandible. The rescuer uses two or three fingers of each hand to lift the jaw while the remaining fingers guide the jaw upward and outward. (Reproduced, with permission, from *Textbook of Pediatric Life Support.* © 1994, American Heart Association.)

D. Mental Status: Hypoxia, hypercarbia, or ischemia will result in altered mentation.

E. Skin Color: Cyanosis is a late finding in children owing to their relative anemia. Compromised cardiopulmonary status can be reflected in pallor or in gray, mottled, or ashen skin colors.

F. Blood Pressure: Determination of blood pressure is not necessary to make the diagnosis of shock. It is important to remember that shock or inadequate perfusion of vital organs may be present before the blood pressure falls below the normal limits for age. As intravascular volume falls, peripheral vascular resistance increases so that blood pressure is maintained until there is 25–30% depletion of blood volume—followed by a precipitous and often irreversible deterioration into shock (Figure 12–6). Shock that occurs with signs of decreased perfusion (eg, tachycardia and delayed capillary refill time) but normal blood pressure is **compensated shock.** When blood pressure also falls, **decompensated shock** is present. The appropriate-sized cuff must be used to obtain an accurate blood pressure.

MANAGEMENT OF SHOCK

Intravenous access is essential but can be difficult to establish in the volume-contracted patient. First attempts should be for peripheral access, especially the antecubital veins, with attempts limited to 90 seconds. Central cannulation—depending on individual preference and expertise—follows quickly. Alternatives are percutaneous cannulation of femoral, subclavian, or internal or external jugular veins; cut-

down at antecubital, femoral, or saphenous sites; or intraosseous lines (Figure 12–7). Consider intraosseous needle placement in any severely ill child when venous access cannot be rapidly established. Use short, wide-bore catheters to allow maximal flow rates. Children in shock and other severely ill children should have two intravenous sites started. In newborns, the umbilical veins may be cannulated.

Consider arterial access if beat-to-beat monitoring, frequent arterial blood gas determinations, or laboratory tests will be needed.

Differentiation of Shock States & Initial Therapy

Therapy for inadequate circulation is based on the cause of circulatory failure.

A. Hypovolemic Shock: The most common type of shock in the pediatric population is hypovolemic. Common causes include dehydration from vomiting and diarrhea, diabetes, or heat illness; hemorrhage; and loss of plasma from burns or trauma. Initial therapy is with isotonic crystalloid solution, that is, lactated Ringer's solution or normal saline solution. Give 20 mL/kg body weight, repeated as necessary, with frequent reassessments, until perfusion normalizes. Children tolerate large volumes of fluid replacement—up to and over the full circulating blood volume of 80 mL/kg can be given safely with appropriate monitoring. Blood product replacement may be necessary in trauma patients not responding to two boluses of crystalloid solution. Pressors are generally not required in simple hypovolemic states.

B. Distributive Shock: Distributive shock represents relative hypovolemia from increased vascular

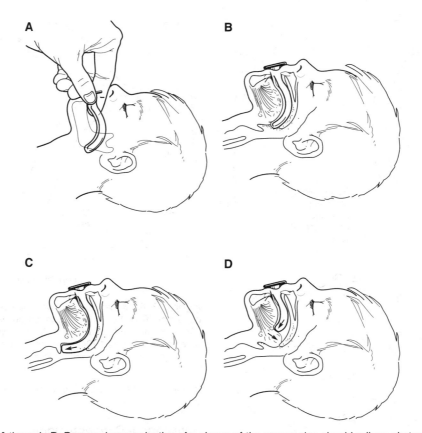

Figure 12–4. **A** through **D**: Proper airway selection. An airway of the proper size should relieve obstruction caused by the tongue without damaging laryngeal structures. The appropriate size can be estimated by holding the airway next to the child's face **(A)**: The tip of the airway should end just cephalad to the angle of the mandible **(broken line)**, resulting in proper alignment with the glottic opening **(B)**: If the oral airway inserted is too large, the tip will align posterior to the angle of the mandible **(C)** and obstruct the glottic opening by pushing the epiglottis down *(arrow)*. If the oral airway inserted is too small, the tip will align well above the angle of the mandible **(D)** and exacerbate airway obstruction by pushing the tongue into the oropharynx *(D, arrows)*. (Adapted, with permission, from Cote and Todres in *Textbook of Pediatric Life Support*. © 1994, American Heart Association.)

capacitance of circulating volume. Examples are sepsis, anaphylaxis, and central nervous system injury. Initial therapy is again by isotonic volume replacement, but pressors may be necessary if perfusion does not normalize after delivery of two 20 mL/kg boluses of fluid.

C. Cardiogenic Shock: Cardiogenic shock can occur as a complication of congenital heart disease, myocarditis, arrhythmias, ingestions (eg, clonidine, tricyclic antidepressants), from serious infections, or as a sequela of shock due to any cause. The diagnosis is suggested by any of the following signs: abnormal cardiac rhythm, distended neck veins, rales, abnormal heart sounds such as an S_3 or S_4, friction rub, narrow pulse pressure, or hepatomegaly. Chest radiographs will show cardiomegaly and pulmonary edema—not seen in shock due to other causes. An initial bolus of crystalloid may be given, but dopamine or other pressors, and possibly agents to re-

duce afterload, are necessary to improve perfusion. Full cardiopulmonary monitoring is essential.

Children in cardiogenic or distributive shock must be admitted to a pediatric intensive care unit.

Observation & Further Management

Reassess perfusion immediately after each bolus of fluid to determine additional fluid needs. Serial central venous pressure determinations or a chest radiograph may aid clinical assessments to help determine volume status. Place a Foley catheter to monitor urine output.

Caution must be exercised with volume replacement if intracranial pressure is potentially elevated, such as in severe head injury or meningitis. Even in such situations, however, *intravascular volume must be restored, as reflected by adequate peripheral per-*

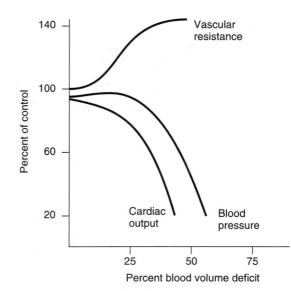

Figure 12–6. Model for cardiovascular response to hypovolemia from hemorrhage (based on normative data). (Reproduced, with permission, from *Textbook of Pediatric Life Support*. © 1994, American Heart Association.)

Figure 12–5. *A:* Nasopharyngeaal airway. A shortened endotracheal tube may be substituted (to reduce resistance). *B:* Placement of a nasopharyngeal airway. Note that the standard 15-mm adapter must be firmly reinserted into the endotracheal tube. *C:* Cut-off endotracheal tube used as a nasopharyngeal airway. (Reproduced, with permission, from *Textbook of Pediatric Life Support*. © 1994, American Heart Association.)

fusion, to achieve adequate cerebral perfusion pressure.

Summary of Cardiopulmonary Resuscitation

Assess the ABCs in sequential fashion, and begin interventions as soon as a derangement is detected—before assessing the next system. After each intervention, it is essential that each system be *reassessed* to ensure improvement and to avoid deterioration.

Bell LM: Shock. In: Fleisher GR, Ludwig S (editors). *Textbook of Pediatric Emergency Medicine,* Williams & Wilkins, 1993.

Carcillo JA, Davis AL, Zaritsky A: Role of early fluid resuscitation in pediatric septic shock. JAMA 1991; 266:1242.

Chameides L, Hazinski MF (editors): *Textbook of Pediatric Advanced Life Support.* American Heart Association/American Academy of Pediatrics, 1994.

Silverman BK (editor): *Textbook of Advanced Pediatric Life Support.* APLS Joint Task Force: American College of Emergency Physicians/American Academy of Pediatrics, 1993.

EMERGENCY PEDIATRIC DRUGS

Careful attention to airway and breathing remains the mainstay of pediatric resuscitation. Drugs should

Tibial tuberosity

Anterior border

90° to
medial surface

Figure 12–7. Intraosseous cannulation technique. (Reproduced, with permission, from *Textbook of Pediatric Life Support.* © 1994, American Heart Association.)

be considered only after optimal oxygenation and ventilation have been accomplished and, in general, only if hemodynamic compromise exists. Rapid delivery to the central circulation is essential. Infuse medications close to the catheter's hub and flush in with saline to achieve the most rapid systemic effects. If no intravenous or IO access is achievable, some drugs may be given by endotracheal tube (Table 12–1). The use of preprinted resuscitation drug charts or length/dose resuscitation tapes (Broselow tapes) speeds drug dose and equipment determinations and helps eliminate dosing errors.

Selected emergency drugs used in pediatrics are summarized in Table 12–2.

American Heart Association, Subcommittee on Pediatric Resuscitation: Pediatric Basic and Advanced Life Support. JAMA 1992;268(16):2251.

DeBehnke DJ et al: Use of cardiopulmonary bypass, high-dose epinephrine, and standard-dose epinephrine in resuscitation from post-countershock electromechanical dissociation. Ann Emerg Med 1992;21:1051.

Dieckmann RA, Vardis R: High-dose epinephrine in pediatric out-of-hospital cardiopulmonary arrest. Pediatrics 1995;95:901.

Goetting MG, Paradis NA: High-dose epinephrine improves outcome from pediatric cardiac arrest. Ann Emerg Med 1991;20:22.

APPROACH TO THE SEVERELY ILL CHILD

Often a child presents in cardiorespiratory failure of unknown cause. Occasionally, an unstable patient presents with a known diagnosis, such as a child known to have asthma in status asthmaticus and respiratory failure, or a child with known congenital heart disease. The initial approach is identical, however, and designed to rapidly identify and reverse life-threatening conditions.

Preparation for Emergency Management

Resuscitation of a severely ill child requires action simultaneously at two levels: a rapid cardiopulmonary assessment, with indicated stabilizing measures while initiating monitoring and venous access (sometimes called "lifelines"). A method of accomplishing these concurrent goals is outlined below.

A. If advance notice of the patient's arrival has been received from prehospital providers or via telephone, prepare a resuscitation room and summon appropriate personnel as needed, such as a neurosurgeon for an unresponsive child after severe head

Table 12–1. Emergency drugs that can be given by endotracheal tube.

Lidocaine
Naloxone
Epinephrine
Atropine

Table 12–2. Emergency pediatric drugs.

Drug	Indications	Dosage and Route	Comment
Atropine	1. Bradycardia, especially cardiac in origin 2. Vagally mediated bradycardia, eg, during laryngoscopy and intubation 3. Anticholinesterase poisoning 4. Asystole, after epinephrine use	0.01–0.02 mg/kg (minimum, 0.1 mg; maximum, 1–2 mg) IV, IO, ET. May repeat every 5 minutes.	Atropine may be useful in hemodynamically significant primary cardiac-based bradycardias. Because of paradoxical bradycardia sometimes seen in infants, a minimum dose of 0.1 mg is recommended by the American Heart Association. Epinephrine is the first-line drug in pediatrics for bradycardia caused by hypoxia or ischemia.
Bicarbonate	1. Documented metabolic acidosis 2. Hyperkalemia	1 meq/kg IV or IO; by arterial blood gas: $1.3 \times$ kg $\times$ base deficit. May repeat every 5 minutes.	Infuse slowly. Sodium bicarbonate will be effective only if the patient is adequately oxygenated, ventilated, and perfused. Has some adverse side effects.
Calcium chloride 10%	1. Documented hypocalcemia 2. Calcium channel blocker overdose 3. Hyperkalemia, hypermagnesemia	10–30 mg/kg slowly IV, preferably centrally, IO	Calcium is no longer indicated for asystole. Potent tissue necrosis results if infiltration occurs. Use with caution.
Epinephrine	1. Bradycardia, especially hypoxic-ischemic 2. Hypotension (by infusion) 3. Asystole 4. Fine ventricular fibrillation refractory to initial defibrillation 5. Pulseless electrical activity 6. Anaphylaxis	Bradycardia and first dose in arrests: 0.01 mg/kg IV or IO of 1:10,000 solution. Second and subsequent doses in arrests: 0.1–0.2 mg/kg IV or IO of 1:1000 solution. Repeat every 3 minutes. ET: 0.1 mg/kg of 1:1000 solution. SC: .01 mg/kg 1:1000 solution (= 0.01 mL/kg) (anaphylactic shock). Maximum dose: 0.3–0.5 mL. Infusion: 0.1–1 µg/kg	Epinephrine is the single most important drug in pediatric resuscitation. Evidence from animal studies and small series of human subjects indicates that the present recommended dose may be insufficient and that doses of 0.1–0.3 mg/kg may be optimal. A randomized controlled trial has not been done.
Glucose	1. Hypoglycemia 2. Altered mental status (empiric) 3. With insulin, for hyperkalemia	0.5–1 g/kg IV, IO. May repeat as necessary	Neonates: 2 mL/kg D_{10}W. Older child: 2–4 mL/kg D_{25}W, 6–10 mL/kg D_{10}W
Naloxone	1. Opiate overdose 2. Altered mental status (empiric)	< 10 kg: 0.1 mg/kg IV, IO, ET > 10 kg: 0.01 mg/kg IV, IO, ET. May repeat as necessary.	Side effects are few. A dose of 2 mg may be given in young children, 4 mg in adolescents. Repeat as necessary, or as constant infusion in narcotic overdoses.

ET = endotracheally, IO = intraosseously, IV = intravenously, SC = subcutaneously.

injury or a radiology technician for assessment of line and tube placement.

B. Assign team responsibilities, including a team leader plus others designated to manage the airway, perform chest compressions, achieve access, draw blood for laboratory studies, place monitors, gather additional historical data, and provide family support.

C. Age-appropriate equipment should be made ready, including a cardiorespiratory monitor, pulse oximeter, and appropriate blood pressure cuff. Age- and weight-based laryngoscope blades, endotracheal tubes, nasogastric tubes, and indwelling urinary catheter should be assembled for rapid access. See Table 12–3 for sizes.

Reception & Assessment

When the patient arrives, the team leader begins a rapid assessment as team members perform their preassigned tasks. If the patient is received from prehospital care providers, careful attention must be paid to their report, since they have information that they alone have observed. Interventions and medications should be ordered only by the team leader to avoid confusion, and the leader should refrain from personally performing distracting procedures. A complete record should be kept of events, including medications, timing of interventions, and response to intervention.

A. All Cases: In addition to cardiac compressions and ventilation, ensure that the following are instituted.

Table 12–3. Equipment sizes and estimated weight by age.

Age (years)	Weight (kg)	Endotracheal Tube Size (mm)[1]	Laryngoscope Blade	Chest Tube (F)	Foley (F)
Premature	1–2.5	2.5 uncuffed	0	8	5
Term newborn	3	3.0	0–1	10	8
1	10	3.5–4.0	1	18	8
2	12	4.5	1	18	10
3	14	4.5	1	20	10
4	16	5.0	2	22	10
5	18	5.0–5.5	2	24	10
6	20	5.5	2	26	12
7	22	5.5–6.0	2	26	12
8	24	6.0 cuffed	2	28	14
10	32	6.0–6.5 cuffed	2–3	30	14
Adolescent	50	7.0 cuffed	3	36	14
Adult	70	8.0 cuffed	3	40	14

[1]Internal diameter.

1. 100% oxygen
2. Cardiorespiratory monitoring
3. Pulse oximetry and end-tidal CO_2 monitor, if available
4. Intravenous (peripheral, intraosseous, or central) access within 90 seconds
5. Blood drawn and sent
6. Full vital signs obtained
7. Clothes removed
8. Foley catheter and nasogastric tube inserted
9. Complete history
10. Notify needed consultants
11. Family support

B. As Appropriate:

1. Immobilize neck.
2. Have chest x-ray taken for line and tube placement.
3. Insert arterial line.

APPROACH TO THE PEDIATRIC TRAUMA PATIENT

Injuries, including motor vehicle crashes, falls, burns, and immersions, account for the greatest num-ber of deaths among children over 1 year of age. Pediatricians must be cognizant of this sobering statistic, become involved, and work with injury prevention specialists, prehospital providers, and emergency and critical care physicians and nurses to reduce this terrible loss. An organized team approach to the seriously injured child, using preassigned roles as above, will optimize outcomes. Accurate, timed records are invaluable. A calm atmosphere in the receiving unit will contribute to thoughtful care. Compiling a problem list helps determine priorities in timing of definitive care. Assignment of a pediatric trauma score assists in triage decisions and prognosis. Conscious children are terribly frightened by serious injury; constant reassurance can help alleviate anxiety. Analgesia and sedation can and should be given to appropriately stable patients. Parents often feel angry and guilty and require ongoing support from the services of social workers or Child Life workers (therapists knowledgeable about child development) whenever possible.

The past decade has seen the emergence of designated pediatric trauma centers, where dedicated teams of *pediatric* specialists in trauma surgery, orthopedics, neurosurgery, critical care, and emergency pediatrics combine to provide optimal multidisciplinary care. Because most children with severe injuries are not seen in these centers, however, pediatricians and others must be able to provide initial assessment and stabilization of the child with life-threatening injuries before transport to a referral center.

Mechanism of Injury

The mechanism of injury is important in evaluation. Document the time of occurrence, the type of energy transfer to the child (eg, hit by a car, rapid deceleration), secondary injury at impact if the child was thrown by the initial impact, appearance of the child at the scene according to bystanders, interventions performed, and clinical condition during transport. The report of EMS personnel is invaluable. All information of this type must be forwarded with the patient to the referral facility.

Initial Assessment & Management

Children die from injuries during three distinct time periods: at the scene, usually from irreparable central nervous system injury, disruption of major vessels, or airway compromise; within minutes to hours after the injury, usually from intracranial hemorrhage, hemopneumothorax, liver or spleen injury, or bleeding from multiple sites; and much later, usually in intensive care units, from multiorgan failure. It is this middle group that can benefit most from expeditious management—hence the term "golden hour" of trauma. Most (98%) children who reach a hospital survive until discharge, and most deaths from trauma in children are due to head injuries. Therefore, cerebral resuscitation must be the foremost consideration when treating seriously injured children. The ultimate measure of outcome is the child's eventual level of functioning.

There is a method for evaluating injured patients in a systematic way that provides a rapid assessment and stabilization phase, followed by a head-to-toe examination and definitive care phase. These are called the primary and secondary surveys, respectively.

PRIMARY SURVEY

The primary survey is designed to rapidly identify and *immediately treat* physiologic derangements. It is the *resuscitation* phase. Priorities are still *a*irway, *b*reathing, and *c*irculation, but with important further considerations in the trauma setting:

Airway, with cervical spine control
Breathing
Circulation, with hemorrhage control
Disability (neurologic deficit)
Exposure (undress the patient completely and examine)

Evaluation and treatment of the ABCs are as discussed previously. Modifications in the trauma setting will be added here. Trauma in children is predominantly blunt, although penetrating trauma does occur. Head and abdominal injuries are particularly important in the pediatric age group.

Airway

Failure to manage the airway appropriately is the most common cause of preventable death. Administer 100% high-flow oxygen to all patients. During assessment and management of the airway, one should provide cervical spine protection, initially by manual in-line immobilization (not traction). A hard cervical spine collar is then applied, and the head is taped to a backboard, surrounded by some means of cushioning (eg, rolled blankets) to further immobilize the head and allow log-rolling of the child in case of vomiting. The body must also be secured to the backboard.

Assess the airway for patency as before. Head positioning must avoid flexion or extension of the neck—eg, use jaw thrust rather than chin lift. Suction the mouth and pharynx free of blood, foreign material, or secretions, and remove loose teeth. Insert a nasopharyngeal or oropharyngeal airway if upper airway noises are heard or obstruction from posterior prolapse of the tongue occurs. A child with a depressed level of consciousness or a need for prolonged ventilation, hyperventilation, or operative intervention requires endotracheal intubation after bag-mask preoxygenation. Orotracheal intubation is the route of choice and is possible without cervical spine manipulation. Nasotracheal intubation may be possible in the children 12 years or older with spontaneous respirations—if not contraindicated by midfacial injury with the possibility of cribriform plate disruption. Rarely, if tracheal intubation cannot be accomplished—particularly in the setting of massive midfacial trauma—cricothyroidotomy may be necessary. Needle cricothyroidotomy using a large-bore catheter through the cricothyroid membrane is the procedure of choice in the younger patient (less than 12 years). Operative revision will be needed for formal controlled tracheostomy.

Breathing

Most ventilatory problems are adequately resolved by the airway maneuvers previously described and by positive-pressure ventilation. Breathing assessment is as described previously: One should assess for an adequate rate and for symmetric chest rise, increased work of breathing, color, tracheal deviation, deformity, or penetrating wounds. Sources of traumatic pulmonary compromise include pneumothorax, hemothorax, pulmonary contusion, flail segments, and central nervous system depression. Asymmetric breath sounds, particularly if tracheal deviation or bradycardia is present, suggests pneumothorax, probably under tension. To evacuate the pneumothorax, insert a large-bore catheter-over-needle attached to a syringe over the fourth rib in the anterior axillary line into the pleural cavity and withdraw air. If a pneumothorax or hemothorax was present, place a chest tube. Insertion should be over the rib to avoid the neurovascular bundle. Open pneumothoraces can be treated temporarily by taping petrolatum-impregnated gauze on three sides over the wound, creating a flap valve.

After airway and breathing have been stabilized, hemodynamic status may be addressed.

Circulation

Ongoing hemorrhage, external or internal, gives pediatric trauma some of its unique anxiety-provoking character. During the assessment of circulation, intravenous access should be achieved, preferably at two sites. If peripheral access is not readily available, a central line, cutdown, or intraosseous line should be established. A cardiorespiratory monitor should be applied early in the resuscitation. Blood pressure measurements should be recorded at frequent intervals. Determine hematocrit, blood type and crossmatch, liver function tests, and serum amylase.

External hemorrhage can be controlled by direct pressure. To avoid damage to adjoining nerves and vessels, avoid placing hemostats on vessels, except in the scalp.

Determination of the site of internal hemorrhage can be challenging. Sites include the chest, abdomen, retroperitoneum, pelvis, and thighs. Bleeding into the intracranial vault rarely causes shock in children except in infants. The aid of an experienced pediatric trauma surgeon and radiologic studies—principally double-contrast computed tomography (CT)—help to locate the site of internal bleeding.

Suspect cardiac tamponade after penetrating or crush injury to the chest if shock, narrowed pulse pressure, distended neck veins, hepatomegaly, or muffled heart sounds are present. Treat with rapid volume infusion and pericardiocentesis.

Treat signs of poor perfusion vigorously: A tachycardic child with a capillary refill time of 3 seconds is *in shock and sustaining vital organ insults.* Remember that hypotension is a late finding. Volume replacement is initially accomplished by rapid infusion of isotonic crystalloid at 20 mL/kg of body weight, followed by 10 mL/kg of packed red blood cells if perfusion does not normalize after two crystalloid bolus infusions.

Reassessment should be done rapidly following the initial bolus. If clinical signs of perfusion have not normalized, repeat the bolus. Lack of response or later signs of hypovolemia suggest the need for blood transfusion and possible surgical exploration. Blood loss at the scene and ongoing losses should be replaced on a 3:1 basis with crystalloid solution.

A common problem is the brain-injured child who is at risk for cerebral edema and intracranial hypertension and who is also hypovolemic. In such cases, circulating volume must be restored to ensure adequate cerebral perfusion; therefore, fluid replacement is required until perfusion normalizes and fluid restriction may be instituted thereafter.

Disability

A brief neurologic examination is performed to assess pupillary size and reaction to light and the level of consciousness. The level of consciousness can be reproducibly characterized by the AVPU system (Table 12–4). Pediatric Glasgow Coma Scale assessments should be done as part of the secondary survey (Table 12–5; see below). Changes in intracranial pressure or cerebral perfusion are eventually reflected in changes in these scales.

Exposure

Significant injuries can be missed unless the child is completely undressed and examined fully, front and back. Movement can be minimized by cutting away clothing as necessary. Because of their high ratio of surface area to body mass, infants and children cool rapidly. Because hypothermia compromises outcome, it is necessary to monitor the body temperature and use warming techniques as necessary.

Monitoring

Cardiopulmonary monitors with pulse oximetry should be applied immediately. At the completion of the primary phase, additional "tubes" should be placed.

A. Nasogastric or Orogastric Tube: Children's stomachs should be assumed to be full at all times, and gastric distention from positive-pressure ventilation increases the chance of vomiting and aspiration.

B. Urinary Catheter: An indwelling urinary bladder catheter should be placed to monitor urine output. Contraindications are based on the risk of urethral transection; signs include blood at the meatus or in the scrotum or a displaced prostate detected on rectal examination. Urine should be tested for blood. Urine output should exceed 1 mL/kg/h.

SECONDARY SURVEY

After the resuscitation phase, a head-to-toe examination should be performed to reveal all injuries and determine priorities for definitive care.

Skin

Search for lacerations, hematomas, swelling, and abrasions. Remove foreign material, and cleanse as necessary. Cutaneous signs may indicate underlying pathology (eg, a flank hematoma overlying a renal

Table 12–4. AVPU system for evaluation of level of consciousness.

A	Alert
V	Responsive to *Voice*
P	Responsive to *Pain*
U	*Unresponsive*

Table 12–5. Glasgow Coma Scale.

Eye opening response	
Spontaneous	4
To speech	3
To pain	2
None	1
Verbal response	
Oriented	5
Confused conversation	4
Inappropriate words	3
Incomprehensible sounds	2
None	1
Best upper limb motor response	
Obeys	6
Localizes	5
Withdraws	4
Flexion in response to pain	3
Extension in response to pain	2
None	1

contusion), although surface signs may be absent with significant internal injury. Skin changes may evolve. Make certain that the child's tetanus immunization status is current.

Head

Check for hemotympanum and for clear or bloody discharge from the nares from cerebrospinal fluid leak. Battle's sign and raccoon eyes are late signs of basilar skull fracture. Explore wounds, excluding foreign bodies and defects in galea or skull. Closed head injury is most commonly encountered. CT scan of the head has become an integral part of evaluation for altered level of consciousness, seizure after trauma, or focal neurologic findings (see below).

Spine

Cervical spine injury must be ruled out in all but verbal, alert children who have no history of transient neurologic impairments, who can deny neck pain and tenderness to palpation, and who have a normal neurologic examination. Symmetric voluntary movement of the extremities must be observed. A cross-table neck radiograph is obtained initially, followed by anterior-posterior and odontoid views. "Normal" studies do not exclude significant injury, which can be bony or ligamentous, or of the spinal cord itself. Therefore, leave obtunded children in cervical spine precautions until the child has awakened and an appropriate neurologic examination can be performed. The entire thoracolumbar spine must also be palpated and areas of pain or tenderness examined by radiography.

Chest

Pneumothoraces are detected and decompressed during the primary survey. Hemothoraces can occur with rib fractures and intercostal vessel injury, large pulmonary vessel injury, or pulmonary laceration. Tracheobronchial disruption is suggested by large continued air leak despite chest tube decompression. With large energy transfer, pulmonary contusion can occur, requiring ventilatory support. Myocardial contusions are unusual in children.

Abdomen

Blunt abdominal injury is very common in multisystem injuries. Significant injury can exist without cutaneous signs or instability of vital signs. Tenderness, guarding, distention, lack of bowel sounds, or hemodynamic instability mandates immediate evaluation by a pediatric trauma surgeon. Injury to solid viscera frequently can be managed nonoperatively in hemodynamically stable patients; however, intestinal perforation or hypotension requires operative treatment. Serial examinations and CT scan—or, in unstable patients, diagnostic peritoneal lavage—provide diagnostic help. Elevated liver function tests have good specificity but only fair sensitivity for hepatic injury.

Pelvis

Pelvic fractures are classically manifested by pain, crepitus, and abnormal motion. Pelvic fracture is a relative contraindication to urethral catheter insertion. Perform a rectal examination, noting prostate position in boys, tone, and tenderness. Stool should be tested for blood. Orthopedic consultation is indicated if pelvic fracture is suspected.

Genitourinary

If urethral transection is suspected (see above), perform a urethrogram before catheter placement. Diagnostic imaging of the child with hematuria is evolving, with CT scan becoming the modality of choice. Intravenous pyelograms are performed at some centers. Management of kidney injury is largely nonoperative except for renal pedicle injuries.

Extremities

Long bone fractures are common but rarely lifethreatening. Test for pulses, perfusion, and sensation. Neurovascular compromise requires immediate orthopedic consultation. Careful palpation and serial examination will reveal orthopedic injuries requiring diagnostic imaging and treatment. Delayed diagnosis of fracture is not uncommon when children are comatose; re-examination is key to avoid missing previously occult fractures.

Neurologic

Most children who die of multisystem trauma die of head injuries, therefore principles of neurointensive care are of primary importance in continued trauma care. Significant injuries include cerebral edema, subdural and epidural hematomas, parenchymal hemorrhages, and spinal cord injury. A full sensorimotor examination should be performed, noting pupillary size and extraocular movements. Deficits require immediate neurosurgical consultation. Extensor or flexor posturing represents intracranial hypertension (not seizure activity) until proved otherwise and should be treated with hyperventilation, adequate but not excessive volume resuscitation, and consideration of diuretics, usually mannitol. Normal peripheral perfusion must be assured before fluid restriction is started to optimize cerebral perfusion. Level of consciousness by the AVPU system or Glasgow Coma Scale (see Tables 12–4 and 12–5) should be serially assessed. Seizure activity warrants exclusion of significant intracranial injury. Acute spinal cord injury may benefit from high-dose methylprednisolone therapy. Corticosteroids are not indicated in traumatic head injuries.

HEAD INJURY

Closed head injuries range from minor asymptomatic head injuries without sequelae to intracranial hemorrhage and subsequent death. Head injury, including the shaken-baby syndrome, is common in child abuse. Most deaths following multiple trauma are from head injury. Even following minor closed head injury, many parents are appropriately concerned about neurologic sequelae, including subtle neuropsychiatric differences. Children may be classified clinically at the time of initial evaluation as having mild, moderate, or severe head injury (Table 12–6).

Assessment

The considerations discussed above in the care of the trauma patient apply here. The history should include the time and mechanism of injury. How far did the child fall and onto what surface? Was there loss of consciousness? Does the child remember events preceding, during, and following the injury? What have been the levels of consciousness and activity since the injury? Has there been vomiting, headache, ataxia, or visual symptoms?

The physical examination should be complete, keeping in mind the mechanism of injury, and should include a detailed neurologic examination. Look for associated injuries such as mandibular fracture, scalp or skull injury, or cervical spine injury. Cerebrospinal fluid leak from the ears or nose, or the two later-appearing signs of periorbital hematomas (raccoon eyes) and Battle's sign imply a basilar skull fracture. Obtain vital signs and assess the level of consciousness by the AVPU system (see Table 12–4) or by the Glasgow Coma scale (see Table 12–5) in children over 3 years of age, noting irritability or lethargy; pupillary equality, size, and reaction to light; funduscopic examination; reflexes; body posture; and rectal tone. Always consider child abuse; the injuries observed should be consistent with the history.

Radiographic studies may be indicated. Plain films are useful chiefly for assessing depressed skull fractures or penetrating head trauma. Major morbidity does not stem from skull fracture per se but rather from the associated intracranial injury. The presence of a skull fracture on plain films increases the likelihood of finding a serious intracranial injury demonstrated by CT scanning. CT scan should be performed in the child with a history of significant impact, with persistent vomiting, or with an abnormal or lateralizing neurologic examination, including an abnormal mental status that does not quickly return to normal.

CONCUSSION

A concussion injury is defined as a brief loss or alteration of consciousness followed by a return to the normal state. There is no anatomic damage to brain tissue. There are no focal findings on detailed neurologic examination. There may be pallor, amnesia, or several episodes of vomiting. Disposition is based on the clinical course and suitability of follow-up. If the level of consciousness is normal or improving, the patient may be discharged when neurologically normal after a period of observation. Parents should assess the child at home every 3–4 hours for the first 24–36 hours, and return if the child exhibits altered level of consciousness, persistent vomiting, gait disturbances, unequal pupils, seizures, or increasing headache, or if the parents have any concerns.

CONTUSION

A bruise of the brain matter is a contusion. There is a decrease in level of consciousness, and focal

Table 12–6. Clinical classification of head-injured patients.

Mild	No loss of consciousness or amnesia, alert and oriented. Asymptomatic or with only slight headache and dizziness
Moderate	Possible findings: history of loss of consciousness, amnesia; post-traumatic seizures, vomiting, more than slight headache, listlessness, lethargy
Severe	Possible findings: disoriented, unable to follow commands, decreasing level of consciousness, focal neurologic signs, penetrating skull injury or depressed skull fracture

Reproduced, with permission, from: Rosenthal BW, Bergman I: Intracranial injury after moderate head trauma in children. J Pediatr 1989;115:346.

findings are present that correspond to the area of the brain that is injured. These patients require CT scan, a period of observation, and consideration of neurosurgical consultation.

ACUTE INTRACRANIAL HYPERTENSION

Close observation by medical and nursing personnel will detect early signs and symptoms of intracranial pressure (ICP) elevation. Early recognition is essential to avoid disastrous outcomes. Serious intracranial pathology after closed head injury includes subdural or epidural hematomas, parenchymal hemorrhage, diffuse axonal injury, and cerebral edema. In addition to traumatic causes, ICP elevation with or without herniation syndromes may be seen in spontaneous intracranial hemorrhage, central nervous system infection, hydrocephalus, ruptured arteriovenous malformation, metabolic derangement (eg, diabetic ketoacidosis), or tumor. Symptoms include headache, diplopia, vomiting, agitation, gait difficulties, and a progressively decreasing level of consciousness. Other signs may include stiff neck, cranial nerve palsies, and progressive hemiparesis. Cushing's triad (bradycardia, hypertension, and irregular respirations) is a late and pre-arrest finding. Papilledema is also a *late* finding. Lumbar puncture should not be performed before CT scan if there is concern about ICP elevation because of the risk of precipitating herniation.

Therapy for ICP elevation must be swift and aggressive. Strict attention to the ABCs is paramount. Controlled rapid sequence intubation with appropriate sedation, muscle relaxation, and agents to reduce the ICP elevation that accompanies intubation is followed by hyperventilation and avoidance of hypoxemia. Mannitol (0.5 g/kg intravenously), an osmotic diuretic, will reduce brain water, as will furosemide (0.1–0.2 mg/kg intravenously). These measures effectively reduce cerebral blood flow and acutely lower intracranial pressure. Normal arterial blood pressure and peripheral perfusion should be maintained by fluid infusion and pressors, if necessary. Adjunctive measures include elevating the head of the bed 30 degrees, treating hyperpyrexia and pain, and maintaining the head in a midline position. Obtain immediate neurosurgical evaluation. Further details about management of intracranial hypertension (cerebral edema) are presented in Chapter 13.

DISPOSITION FOR CHILDREN WITH CLOSED HEAD INJURY

Patients with mild head injury as defined in Table 12–6 may be discharged with detailed written instructions—after a period of brief observation—if the examination remains normal and parental supervision and follow-up are appropriate. Some children with moderate head injury will require admission or prolonged observation. If the patient responds to voice commands and mental status is gradually improving over a period of several hours, in-hospital observation may be done without further radiographic studies. If the mental status deteriorates, however, CT scan and neurosurgical consultation are indicated. If the CT scan is normal and if the physical findings normalize, these children may also be discharged after a period of observation.

Patients with severe head injury require cerebral resuscitation, evaluation by a neurosurgeon, and admission to hospital.

Aldrich EF et al: Diffuse brain swelling in severely head-injured children. J Neurosurg 1992;76:450.

Bracken MB et al: A randomized, controlled trial of methylprednisolone or naloxone in the treatment of acute spinal cord injury. N Engl J Med 1990;322:1405.

Gnauck K et al: Emergency intubation of the pediatric medical patient: Use of anesthetic agents in the emergency department. Ann Emerg Med 1994;23:1242.

Jaffe D, Wesson D: Emergency management of blunt trauma in children. N Engl J Med 1991;324:1447.

Kharasch SJ et al: The routine use of radiography and arterial blood gases in the evaluation of blunt trauma in children. Ann Emerg Med 1994;23:212.

McGrory BJ et al: Acute fractures and dislocations of the cervical spine in children and adolescents. J Bone Joint Surg 1993;75[Am]:988.

Moulton SL et al: Operative intervention for pediatric liver injuries: Avoiding delays in treatment. J Pediatr Surg 1992;27:958.

Orenstein JB et al: Delayed diagnosis of pediatric cervical spine injury. Pediatrics 1992;89:1185.

Pigula FA et al: The effect of hypotension and hypoxia on children with severe head injuries. J Pediatr Surg 1993;28:310.

Pons P: Head trauma. In: Rosen P et al (editors). *Emergency Medicine: Concepts and Clinical Practice,* 3rd ed. CV Mosby, 1992.

Rosenthal BW, Bergman I: Intracranial injury after moderate head trauma in children. J Pediatr 1989;115:346.

Trunkey DD (editor): *Textbook of Advanced Trauma Life Support Course.* American College of Surgeons Committee on Trauma, 1993.

BURNS

Thermal injury is a major cause of accidental death and disfigurement in children. Pain, morbidity, the association with child abuse, and the preventable nature of burns constitute an area of major concern in pediatrics. Common causes include hot water or food, appliances, flames, grills, and curling irons.

Burns occur commonly in toddlers—in boys more frequently than in girls.

Electrical Burns

Even brief contact with a high-voltage source will result in a contact burn. If an arc is created with passage of current through the body, the pattern of the thermal injury will depend on the path of the current; therefore, a thorough search should be made for an exit wound and intervening injuries. Extensive damage to deep tissues may occur. Current traversing the heart may cause nonperfusing arrhythmias. Neurologic effects of electrical burns can be immediate, such as confusion, disorientation, and peripheral nerve injury; secondary; or late, such as impaired concentration or memory.

Electric cords are a common source of these injuries. Typically, an infant or toddler bites an electric cord, sustaining burns to the oral commissure that appear gray and necrotic, with surrounding erythema. Delayed coagulation around the mouth may occur, and as the burn heals, sloughing of eschar may lead to brisk bleeding.

EVALUATION OF THE BURNED PATIENT

Classification

Burns are classified clinically according to the nature of the burn and the extent and thickness of the burn; associated injuries are ascertained in the initial evaluation.

Superficial burns are easily recognized and treated. They are painful, dry, red, and hypersensitive. Sunburn is a common example. Healing occurs with minimal damage to epidermis. At the other end of the spectrum are **full-thickness burns** affecting all epidermal and dermal elements, leaving avascular skin. The wound is dry, depressed, leathery in appearance, and without sensation. Unless skin grafting is provided, the scar will be hard, uneven, and fibrotic. **Partial-thickness burns** are further classified as superficial or deep, depending on appearance and healing time, with each subgroup treated differently. Superficial partial-thickness burns are red and may blister. Deep partial-thickness burns are white and dry, blanch with pressure, and have decreased sensitivity to pain.

Management

Burn management depends on the depth and extent of thermal injury. Burn extent can be classified as major or minor. Minor burns are less than 10% of the body surface area for superficial and partial-thickness burns, or less than 2% if full-thickness burns. Burns of the hands, feet, face, eyes, ears, and perineum are considered major.

A. Superficial and Partial-Thickness Burns:
These injuries can generally be treated in the outpatient setting. Superficial burns are treated with cool compresses and analgesia. Treatment of partial-thickness burns with blisters consists of aseptic debridement, antiseptic cleansing, and topical antimicrobial coverage. Blisters appear early in deeper partial-thickness burns and if open should be debrided. After debridement, the wound should be cleansed with dilute (1–5%) povidone-iodine solution, thoroughly washed with normal saline, and covered with topical antibiotic, commonly silver sulfadiazine. The wound should be protected with a bulky dressing and reexamined within 24 hours and serially thereafter, depending on the course. Wounds with a potential for causing loss of function or scarring—especially wounds of the hand or digits—should be promptly referred to a burn surgeon.

B. Full-Thickness and Deep or Extensive Partial-Thickness Burns: Major burns place particular importance on the ABCs of trauma management. Early establishment of an artificial airway is critical with oral or nasal burns because of their association with inhalation injuries and critical airway narrowing.

BURN RESUSCITATION PROTOCOL
- Secure the airway
- Administer 100% oxygen
- Assist ventilation if necessary
- Remove all clothing
- Stop the burning process
- Irrigate chemical burns
- Establish IV access
- Restore intravascular volume
- Perform complete examination

The trauma resuscitation protocol outlined previously in Primary Survey should be followed. There may be inhalation injury from carbon monoxide, cyanide, or other toxic products if flames were present. A nasogastric tube and bladder catheter should be placed. The secondary survey should ascertain whether any other injuries are present, including those suggestive of abuse.

Fluid administration is based on several principles. Capillary permeability is markedly increased. Fluid needs are based on percentage of body surface area burned, depth, and age. Maintaining normal intravascular pressure and replacing fluid losses are essential. Figure 12–8 shows percentages of body surface area by body part in infants and children. The Parkland formula for fluid therapy is 4 mL/kg per percent body surface area burned for the first 24 hours, with half in the first 8 hours, in addition to maintenance rates. Acutely, however, fluid resuscitation should be based on clinical assessment of volume depletion as described above.

Indications for admission include major burns as defined above; uncertainty of follow-up; suspicion of abuse; presence of upper airway injury; explosion, inhalation, electrical, or chemical burns; burns associated with fractures; or the need for parenteral pain control. Children with chronic metabolic or connec-

Infant Less Than One Year of Age

Name_____ Age_____ Ward_____

1st-degree erythema
not to be included.

2nd-degree   3rd-degree

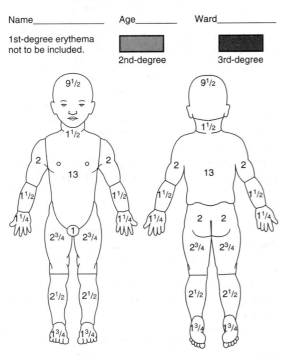

Variations From Adults Distribution in
Infants and Children (in Percent).

	New-born	1 Year	5 Years	10 Years
Head	19	17	13	11
Both thighs	11	13	16	17
Both lower legs	10	10	11	12
Neck	2			
Anterior trunk	13			
Posterior trunk	13			
Both upper arms	8	These percentages		
Both lower arms	6	remain constant at		
Both hands	5	all ages		
Both buttocks	6			
Both feet	7			
Genitalia	1			
	100			

Figure 12–8. Lund and Browder modification of Berkow's scale for estimating extent of burns. (The table under the illustration is after Berkow.)

tive tissue diseases and infants deserve hospitalization.

Deitch EA: The management of burns. N Engl J Med 1990;323:1249.

Joffe MD: Burns. In: *Textbook of Pediatric Emergency Medicine,* 3rd ed. Fleisher G, Ludwig S (editors). Williams & Wilkins, 1993.

Powell EC, Tanz RR: Comparison of childhood burns associated with use of microwave ovens and conventional stoves. Pediatrics 1993;91:344.

HEAT PROSTRATION

Heat injury and illness cover a spectrum from mild cramps to life-threatening heat stroke. **Heat cramps** are characterized by brief, severe cramping (not rigidity) of skeletal or abdominal muscles following exertion. Core temperature is normal or only slightly elevated. Heat cramps may be associated with a relative sodium deficiency. Mild cases can be treated with oral salt-containing solutions; more severe cases require intravenous infusion of normal saline solution. **Heat exhaustion** is manifested by constitutional symptoms after exposure to heat and humidity. Patients continue to sweat, and core temperature is again normal or only slightly increased. Patients with heat exhaustion have varying proportions of salt and water depletion. Presenting symptoms and signs include weakness, fatigue, headache, disorientation, thirst, nausea and vomiting, and occasionally muscle cramps. Shock may be present. There should be no major central nervous system dysfunction. Treat with intravenous fluids, modified by measured electrolyte levels. Both heat cramps and heat exhaustion can be avoided with acclimatization and liberal water and salt intake during exercise.

Heat stroke represents failure of thermoregulation and is a life-threatening emergency. The diagnosis is based on a rectal temperature of over 40 °C with associated neurologic signs in a patient with an exposure history. Lack of sweating is *not* a necessary criterion. Symptoms are similar to those of heat exhaustion, but central nervous system dysfunction is more prominent. Patients with heat stroke are often incoherent and combative. In more severe cases, coma, seizures, nuchal rigidity, and posturing may be present. Patients can have high, low, or normal cardiac output. Cellular hypoxia, enzyme denaturation and inactivation, and disrupted cell membranes lead to global end-organ derangements: rhabdomyolysis, myocardial necrosis, acute tubular necrosis, hepatic degeneration, adult respiratory distress syndrome, and disseminated intravascular coagulation. Other complications include vomiting, shivering, sodium and potassium derangements, renal failure, and shock. Consider infectious causes, malignant hyperthermia, and neuroleptic malignant syndrome in the differential diagnosis.

Heat Stroke Management

A. Immediately cool body with cool water mist, ice, fans, or other cooling device.

B. Maintain the airway if comatose, giving 100% oxygen.

C. Administer intravenous fluids: Isotonic fluid for hypotension, 5% dextrose/50% normal saline for maintenance. Consider central venous pressure determination.

D. Cardiac monitor, continuous rectal temperatures, Foley catheter, nasogastric tube.

E. Obtain laboratory tests: Complete blood count, electrolytes, glucose, creatinine, prothrombin time and partial thromboplastin time, creatine kinase, liver function tests, arterial blood gases, urinalysis, and serum calcium, magnesium, and phosphate.

F. Admit to pediatric intensive care unit.

Thompson AE: Environmental emergencies. In: Fleisher GR, Ludwig S (editors). *Textbook of Pediatric Emergency Medicine,* 3rd ed. Williams & Wilkins, 1993.

Yarbrough B: Heat illness. In: Rosen P et al (editors). *Emergency Medicine: Concepts and Clinical Practice,* 3rd ed. CV Mosby, 1992.

HYPOTHERMIA

Hypothermia in children, defined as core temperature less than 35 °C, is frequently associated with cold water submersion accidents. Many other disorders cause incidental hypothermia, including sepsis, metabolic derangements, ingestions, central nervous system disorders, and endocrinopathies. Neonates, trauma victims, intoxicated patients, and the chronically disabled are particularly at risk. Diagnosis requires maintaining a high index of suspicion, particularly in temperate climates. Mortality rates are high and are related to the underlying disorder.

As core temperature falls, a variety of mechanisms begin to conserve and produce heat. Peripheral vasoconstriction allows optimal maintenance of core temperature. Heat production can be increased by a hypothalamic-mediated increase in muscle tone and metabolism. When shivering begins, heat production increases to two to four times basal levels.

Clinical Findings

Clinical manifestations of hypothermia depend on the severity of body temperature depression. Severe cases (< 28 °C) mimic death: Patients are pale or cyanotic, pupils may be fixed and dilated, muscles are rigid, and there may be no palpable pulses. Heart rates as low as 4–6/minute may provide adequate perfusion, however, because of the lowered metabolic needs in severe hypothermia. If these findings are *primarily* a result of hypothermia and not postmortem changes, the fact of death cannot be ascertained until the patient has been rewarmed and remains unresponsive to resuscitative efforts. Children with a core temperature as low as 19 °C have survived neurologically intact.

Treatment

A. General Supportive Measures: Management of patients with hypothermia is complex but largely supportive. Hypothermia must be documented by continuously monitoring with a low-reading rectal thermometer. Patients must be handled gently, since the hypothermic myocardium is exquisitely sensitive and prone to arrhythmias. Ventricular fibrillation may occur spontaneously or as a result of minor handling or invasive procedures. If asystole or ventricular fibrillation is present on the cardiac monitor, perform chest compressions and use standard pediatric advanced life support techniques and medications. Spontaneous reversion to sinus rhythm at 28–30 °C may occur as rewarming proceeds.

B. Rewarming:

1. *Passive* rewarming, such as covering with blankets, is appropriate only for mild cases (> 33 °C).

2. *Active* rewarming is achieved by external or core rewarming techniques. **External rewarming** methods include warming lights, thermal mattresses or electric warming blankets, immersion in warm baths, and hot water bottles or warmed bags of intravenous solutions. One must be aware of the potential for core temperature "afterdrop" as warmed peripheral acidemic blood is distributed to the core circulation. **Core rewarming** techniques are optimal and include the delivery of warmed, humidified oxygen and the use of warmed (to 40 °C) fluids for intravenous replacement, peritoneal dialysis, bladder irrigation, and mediastinal lavage. Hemodialysis and extracorporeal blood rewarming achieve controlled core rewarming, can stabilize volume and electrolyte disturbances, and are maximally effective (Table 12–7).

Table 12–7. Management of hypothermia.

General measures
- Administer warmed and humidified 100% oxygen.
- Monitor core temperature, heart and respiratory rates, and blood pressure continuously.
- Consider central venous pressure determination.

Laboratory studies
- Complete blood count.
- Serum electrolytes, glucose, creatinine, amylase.
- Prothrombin time, partial thromboplastin time.
- Arterial blood gases.
- Consider toxicology screen.

Treatment
- Correct hypoxemia, hypercapnia, pH < 7.2, clotting abnormalities, and glucose and electrolyte disturbances.
- Start rewarming techniques: passive, active (core and external), depending on degree of hypothermia.
- Replace intravascular volume with intravenous normal saline or lactated Ringer's injection at 43 °C.
- Treat asystole and ventricular fibrillation per ALS protocols. Cardiac massage should be continued at least until core temperature reaches 30 °C, when defibrillation is more likely to be effective.

Gentilello LM, et al: Continuous arteriovenous rewarming: Rapid reversal of hypothermia in critically ill patients. J Trauma 1992;32:316.

Thompson AE: Environmental emergencies. In: Fleisher GR, Ludwig S:(editors). *Textbook of Pediatric Emergency Medicine,* 3rd ed. Williams & Wilkins,1993.

Weinberg AD: Hypothermia. Ann Emerg Med 1993; 22:370.

DROWNING

Drowning is the second most common cause of death by unintentional injury among children. Water hazards are ubiquitous and include lakes and streams, swimming pools, bathtubs, and even toilets, buckets, and washing machines. Risk factors include epilepsy, alcohol, intentional trauma, and lack of supervision. Males predominate in submersion deaths, as in most other accidental deaths. All pediatric care providers must make efforts to prevent these needless tragedies.

Submersion incidents are classified according to outcome: drownings are those with death occurring within 24 hours; survival for over 24 hours constitutes near-drowning. Major morbidity stems from pulmonary and central nervous system insult. Fresh water aspiration results in pulmonary surfactant disruption and membrane leak, with subsequent pulmonary edema. Salt-water aspiration creates an osmotic gradient for the influx of water into the lungs. However, the type of water aspirated generally has little clinical significance. Laryngospasm or breath-holding may lead to loss of consciousness and cardiovascular collapse before aspiration can occur.

Anoxia from laryngospasm or aspiration leads to irreversible central nervous system damage after only 4–6 minutes. If a child falls through ice or directly into icy water, cerebral metabolism may be sufficiently slowed by hypothermia to provide some protection from anoxic damage.

Cardiovascular changes include myocardial depression and arrhythmias. Electrolyte alterations are generally slight. Unless hemolysis occurs, hemoglobin concentrations also change only slightly.

Assessment & Management

Depending on the duration of submersion and any protective hypothermia effects, children may appear clinically dead or completely normal. Observation over time assists with prognosis. The normothermic apneic and pulseless child in the emergency department will probably not survive to discharge or will be left with severe neurologic deficits. Until a determination of brain death can be made, however, aggressive resuscitation is appropriate.

One should keep in mind possible associated injuries, such as the possibility of the adolescent who dives into shallow water and sustains neck injury. Core temperature should be monitored continuously with a low-reading rectal thermometer.

For children who appear well initially, observation for 12–24 hours will detect late decompensation in gas exchange. An abnormal chest radiograph, abnormal arterial blood gases, or hypoxemia by pulse oximetry indicates the need for treatment with supplemental oxygen, cardiopulmonary monitoring, and frequent reassessment. Serially assess the degree of respiratory distress and mental status. Signs of pulmonary infection may appear many hours after the submersion event.

Patients who are in coma and who require mechanical ventilation have a high risk of anoxic encephalopathy. The value of therapy with hyperventilation, corticosteroids, intentional hypothermia, and barbiturates continues to be debated.

Bratton SL et al: Serial neurologic examinations after near drowning and outcome. Arch Pediatr Adolesc Med 1994;148:167.

Quan L: Drowning issues in resuscitation. Ann Emerg Med 1993;22(pt 2):366.

Quan L et al: Pediatric submersions: Prehospital predictors of outcome. Pediatrics 1992;90:909.

Yamamoto LG et al: A one-year series of pediatric ED water-related injuries: The Hawaii EMS-C project. Pediatr Emerg Care 1992:8:129.

BITES: ANIMAL & HUMAN

Bites account for a large number of visits to the emergency department. Most fatalities are due to dog bites. However, the majority of infected bite wounds are from human and cat bites.

Dog Bites

Boys are bitten more frequently than girls, and the dog is known by the victim in most cases. Younger children have a higher incidence of head and neck wounds, whereas school-age children are bitten most often on the upper extremities.

Dog bites are cared for in a similar fashion to other wounds: high-pressure, high-volume irrigation with normal saline, debridement of any devitalized tissue and removal of foreign matter, and tetanus prophylaxis. The risk of rabies is low in developed countries, but rabies prophylaxis should be considered when appropriate. Wounds should be sutured only if necessary for cosmetic reasons. Prophylactic antibiotics have not been shown to decrease rates of infection in low-risk dog bite wounds not involving the hands or feet. If a bite involves a joint, periosteum, or neurovascular bundle, prompt orthopedic surgery consultation should be obtained.

Pathogens that infect dog bites include *Pasteurella*

multocida, streptococci, staphylococci, and anaerobes. Infected dog bites can be treated with penicillin for *P multocida,* and broad-spectrum coverage can be provided by amoxicillin and clavulanic acid. Complications of dog bites include central nervous system infections, septic arthritis, osteomyelitis, endocarditis, and sepsis.

Cat Bites

Cat-inflicted wounds occur more frequently in girls, and their principal complication is infection. Wound management is similar to that for dog bites. Cat wounds should not be sutured except when absolutely necessary for cosmetic reasons. Cat bites create a puncture-wound inoculum, and prophylactic antibiotics (penicillin or amoxicillin and clavulanic acid [Augmentin]) are recommended. *P multocida* is the most common pathogen.

Human Bites

Most human bites occur during assaults. *P multocida* is not a known pathogen in human bites. Cultures most commonly grow streptococci, anaerobes, staphylococci, and *Eikenella corrodens.* Hand wounds and deep wounds should be treated with coverage against *E corrodens* and gram-positive pathogens by a penicillinase-resistant penicillin. Wound management is the same as for dog bites. Only severe lacerations involving the face should be sutured. Other wounds can be managed by delayed primary closure or healing by second intention.

A major complication of human bite wounds is infection of the metacarpophalangeal joints. Clenched-fist injuries from human bites should be evaluated by a hand surgeon. Operative debridement is followed in many cases by intravenous antibiotics.

Avner JR et al: Dog bites in urban children. Pediatrics 1991;88:55.

Dire DJ: Cat bite wounds: Risk factors for infection. Ann Emerg Med 1991;20:973.

Leung AKC et al: Human bites in children. Pediatr Emerg Care 992;8:255.

Zubowicz VN et al: Management of early human bites of the hand: A prospective randomized study. Plast Reconstruct Surg 1991;88:111.

POISONING

Richard C. Dart, MD, PhD, &
Barry H. Rumack, MD

Poisonings, the fourth most common cause of death in children, result from the complex interaction of the agent, the child, and the family environment. The peak incidence is at age 2 years. Most ingestions occur in children under 5 years of age as a result of insecure storage of drugs, household chemicals, etc. Twenty-five percent of children will have a second episode of ingestion within 1 year following the first one. Repeated poisonings may require intervention on the child's behalf. Accidental poisonings are unusual after age 5 years. "Poisonings" in older children and adolescents usually represent manipulative behavior, chemical or drug abuse, or genuine suicide attempts.

Litovitz TL et al: 1994 annual report of the American Association of Poison Control Center's Toxic Exposure Surveillance System. Am J Emerg Med 1995;13:551.

PREVENTING CHILDHOOD POISONINGS

Each year, children are accidentally poisoned by medicines, polishes, insecticides, drain cleaners, bleaches, household chemicals, and garage products. It is the responsibility of adults to make sure that children are not exposed to potentially toxic substances.

Here are some suggestions for parents:

1. Insist on packages with safety closures and learn how to use them properly.

2. Keep household cleaning supplies, medicines, garage products, and insecticides out of the reach and sight of your child. Lock them up whenever possible.

3. Never store food and cleaning products together. Store medicine and chemicals in original containers and never in food or beverage containers.

4. Avoid taking medicine in your child's presence. Children love to imitate. Always call medicine by its proper name. Never suggest that medicine is "candy"—especially aspirin and children's vitamins.

5. Read the label on all products and heed warnings and cautions. Never use medicine from an unlabeled or unreadable container. Never pour medicine in a darkened area where the label cannot be clearly seen.

6. If you are interrupted while using a product, take it with you—it takes only a few seconds for your child to get into it.

7. Know what your child can do physically. For example, if you have a crawling infant, keep household products stored above floor level, not beneath the kitchen sink.

8. Keep the phone number of your doctor, poison center, hospital, police department, and fire department or paramedic emergency rescue squad near the phone.

PHARMACOLOGIC PRINCIPLES OF TOXICOLOGY

In the evaluation of the poisoned patient, it is important to compare the anticipated pharmacologic or toxic effects with the clinical presentation of the patient. If the history is that the patient ingested phenobarbital 30 minutes ago but the clinical examination reveals dilated pupils, tachycardia, dry mouth, absent bowel sounds, and active hallucinations—clearly anticholinergic toxicity—diagnosis and therapy should proceed accordingly. Knowledge of the pharmacokinetics of the toxic agent helps the physician to plan a rational approach to definitive care after necessary life-supporting measures have been instituted.

LD50, MLD

Estimates of the LD50 or MLD (minimum lethal dose) of a substance derived from animal studies are of little clinical value, since it is usually impossible to accurately determine *the amount* swallowed *or absorbed,* the metabolic status of the patient, or where the patient's response to the agent will *be atypical.* Furthermore, these values are often not valid in humans even if the history is accurate.

Half-Life ($t_{1/2}$)

The $t_{1/2}$ of an agent must be interpreted carefully. Most published $t_{1/2}$ values are for therapeutic dosages. The $t_{1/2}$ may increase as the quantity of the ingested substance increases for many common intoxicants such as barbiturates, salicylates, and phenytoin. One cannot rely on the published it$_{1/2}$ for salicylate (2 hours) to assume rapid elimination of the drug. In an acute salicylate overdose (150 mg/kg), the apparent $t_{1/2}$ is prolonged to 24–30 hours.

Volume of Distribution (V_d)

The volume of distribution (V_d) of a drug is obtained by dividing the amount of drug absorbed by the blood level. With theophylline, for example, this is 0.46 L/kg body weight, or 32 L in an adult. Ethchlorvynol, a lipophilic drug, on the other hand, distributes well beyond total body water. Because the calculation produces a volume above body weight (300 L in an adult, five times the body weight in children), this figure is frequently referred to as an **apparent volume of distribution,** a designation shared by many drugs (Table 12–8).

The V_d can be useful in predicting which drugs will be removed by dialysis or exchange transfusion. When a drug is differentially concentrated in body lipids or is heavily tissue- or protein-bound and has a high volume of distribution, only a small proportion of the drug will be in the free form and thus accessible to diuresis, dialysis, or exchange transfusion. On the other hand, a drug that is water-soluble and has a low volume of distribution may cross the dialysis membrane well and also respond to diuresis. In general, methods of extracorporeal elimination are not effective for toxic agents with a V_d greater than 1 L/kg.

Metabolism & Excretion

The route of excretion or detoxification is important for planning treatment. Methanol, for example, is metabolized to the toxic product, formic acid. This metabolic step may be blocked by ethanol. Long-acting barbiturates are metabolized chiefly in the liver but are also partially excreted in the urine, which means that forced diuresis will increase excretion. Secobarbital, a short-acting barbiturate, is poorly excreted in the urine and has a larger V_d, making forced diuresis ineffective.

Blood Levels

Care of the poisoned patient should never be guided solely by laboratory measurements. Treatment should be directed first by the clinical signs and symptoms, followed by more specific therapy based on laboratory determinations. Clinical information may speed the identification of a poison by the laboratory pathologist.

Table 12–8. Some examples of pK_a and V_d.[1]

Drug	pK_a	Diuresis	Dialysis	Apparent V_d
Amobarbital	7.9	No	No	200–300% body weight
Amphetamine	9.8	No	Yes	60% body weight
Aspirin	3.5	Alkaline	Yes	15–40% body weight
Chlorpromazine	9.3	No	No	40–50 L/kg (2800–3500% body weight)
Codeine	8.2	No	No	5–10 L/kg (350–700% body weight)
Desipramine	10.2	No	No	30–40 L/kg (2100–2800% body weight)
Ethchlorvynol	8.7	No	No	5–10 L/kg (350–700% body weight)
Glutethimide	4.5	No	No	10–20 L/kg (700–1400% body weight)
Isoniazid	3.5	Alkaline	Yes	61% body weight
Methadone	8.3	No	No	5–10 L/kg (350–700% body weight)
Methicillin	2.8	No	Yes	60% body weight
Phenobarbital	7.4	Alkaline	Yes	75% body weight
Phenytoin	8.3	No	No	60–80% body weight
Tetracycline	7.7	No	No	200–300% body weight

[1]See Table 41–2 for additional V_d values.

Handling of Specimens

A. Vomitus and Gastric Lavage Fluid: Collect, place in separate containers, and send to the laboratory initial material recovered. Send also an aliquot of the remainder, and make a "best guess" estimate of its volume. Include material appearing to be pill fragments.

B. Blood: Determine specifically what type of container and anticoagulant are required before drawing the sample.

C. Urine: Collect an initial sample of 100 mL for analysis. Subsequently, timed 6- to 12-hour collections may be useful in determining the excretion rate of the agent.

GENERAL TREATMENT
OF POISONING

The telephone is often the first contact in pediatric poisoning. Proper telephone management can reduce morbidity and prevent unwarranted or excessive treatment. The decision to refer the patient is based on the identity and dose of the ingested agent, the age of the child, the time of day, the reliability of the parent, and whether child neglect or endangerment is suspected.

Initial Telephone Contact

Basic information that should be *written down* at the first telephone contact includes the patient's name, age, weight, address and telephone number, the agent and amount of agent ingested, the patient's present condition, and the time elapsed since ingestion or other exposure.

Use the history to evaluate the urgency of the situation and decide whether immediate emergency transportation to a health facility is indicated. If immediate danger does not exist, the physician should obtain more details about the suspected toxic agent. It may be difficult to obtain an accurate history. Obtain names of drugs or ingredients, manufacturers, prescription numbers, names and phone numbers of prescribing physician and pharmacy, and so on. Find out whether the substance was shared among several children, whether it had been recently purchased, who had last used it, how full it was, and how much was spilled. If one is unsure of the significance of an exposure, consultation with a certified Poison Control Center is recommended.

FIRST AID FOR POISONING
(Advice for Parents)

Always keep syrup of ipecac in your home. Determine whether activated charcoal for home use is available in your area, and store it with the ipecac if obtainable. The ipecac is used to induce vomiting;

the activated charcoal is used to adsorb poisons. Use them only as instructed by your Poison Control Center or doctor.

Inhaled Poisons

If smoke, gas, or fumes have been inhaled, immediately drag or carry the patient to fresh air. Then call the poison center or your doctor. Do not enter an area where there are poisonous fumes. Too often the rescuer becomes a victim as well.

Poisons on the Skin

If the poison has been spilled on the skin or clothing, remove the clothing and flood the involved parts with water. Wash with soapy water and rinse thoroughly. Then call the Poison Control Center or your doctor.

Swallowed Poisons

If the substance swallowed is a medicine, give nothing. Milk or water should be immediately administered to any patient who has ingested a strongly acid or alkaline agent. Do not give more than 15 mL/kg (250 mL maximum in a child weighing 16 kg or more). Do not induce vomiting in patients who are comatose, convulsing, or who have lost the gag reflex. If emesis is induced on the way to the hospital, syrup of ipecac should be administered as described in the section on prevention of absorption (see p 307). *Caution:* Antidote labels on products may be incorrect. Do not give salt, vinegar, or lemon juice. Call before doing anything else.

Poisons in the Eye

Rinse out the eye with plain water before the patient arrives at the emergency room. Use plain tap water—do not try to neutralize acids or alkalies. Pour water into the eye from a drinking glass or pitcher for 15–20 minutes. Then transport the patient to the hospital.

Bring the Poison to the Hospital

Everything in the vicinity of the patient that may be a cause of poisoning should be brought along.

Poison Information

Up-to-date data on ingredients of commercial products and medications can usually be obtained from a certified regional poison center and through *POISINDEX Information System.* It is important to have the actual container at hand if the manufacturer is called. In some cases, the experience of the company physician may be of value in management. *Caution:* Antidote information on labels of commercial products may be incorrect or inappropriate.

Follow-up

In over 95% of cases of ingestion of potentially toxic substances by children, a trip to the hospital is not required. In these cases, it is important to call the parent at 1 and 4 hours after an ingestion. If the child has actually ingested an additional unknown agent and develops symptoms, a change in management may be needed, including transportation to the hospital. An additional call should be made 24 hours after the ingestion to begin the process of poison prevention.

Poison Prevention Over the Telephone

Start with a few simple questions about storage of hazardous substances in the home. The following is a partial list of potentially poisonous substances that must be stored safely if there are small children in the home: drain-cleaning crystals or liquid, dishwasher soap and cleaning supplies, paints and paint thinners, garden spray and other insecticide materials, automobile products, and all medications.

If there are problems that may lead to further episodes of poisoning, the parents should be seen or a public health nurse sent to the home.

PREVENTION OF POISONING

A major goal of pediatricians is to reduce the number of accidental ingestions in the high-risk age group under 5 years of age. A systematic poison education effort should be part of the routine care of every patient. Parents of very young children should be encouraged to search the house and identify all hazardous substances that should be removed from the home or locked up.

The section entitled "Preventing Childhood Poisonings," reproduced on p 303, may be copied from this book and given to parents along with a bottle of syrup of ipecac at the 6-month checkup.* Reinforcement should occur at the 1-year checkup to make certain that adequate poison-proofing measures have been instituted and maintained.

INITIAL EMERGENCY DEPARTMENT CONTACT

Make Certain the Patient Is Breathing

As in all emergencies, the principles of treatment are attention to airway, breathing, and circulation. These are sometimes overlooked under the stressful conditions of a severe pediatric poisoning.

Treat Shock

Initial therapy of the hypotensive patient should consist of laying the patient flat and administering

isotonic solutions. Vasopressors should be reserved for poisoned patients in shock who do not respond to these standard measures.

Treat Burns

Burns may occur following exposure to strong acid or strong alkaline agents or petroleum distillates. Burned areas should be decontaminated by flooding with sterile saline solution or water. A burn unit should be consulted if more than minimal burn damage has been sustained. Skin decontamination should be performed in a patient with cutaneous exposure. Emergency department personnel in contact with a patient who has been contaminated (with an organophosphate insecticide, for example) should themselves be decontaminated if their skin or clothing becomes contaminated.

Take a Pertinent History

The history should be taken from the parents and all individuals present at the scene. It may be crucial to determine all of the kinds of poisons in the home. These may include drugs used by family members, chemicals associated with the hobbies or occupations of family members, or the purity of the water supply. Unusual dietary or medication habits or other clues to the possible cause of poisoning should also be investigated.

Assess Coma, Hyperactivity, & Withdrawal

It is useful to determine the level of coma, the degree of hyperactivity, or the severity of withdrawal symptoms as a means of assessing the efficacy of treatment.

A. Determine the Level of Coma: Coma is graded on a scale of 0–4:

0 Asleep but can be aroused and can answer questions.

1 Comatose: withdraws from painful stimuli; reflexes intact.

2 Comatose: does not withdraw from painful stimuli; most reflexes intact; no respiratory or circulatory depression.

3 Comatose: most or all reflexes absent; no depression of respiration or circulation.

4 Comatose: reflexes absent; respiratory depression with cyanosis, circulatory failure, or shock.

B. Determine the Degree of Hyperactivity:

1+ Restlessness, irritability, insomnia, tremor, hyperflexia, sweating, mydriasis, flushing.

2+ Confusion, hyperactivity, hypertension, tachypnea, tachycardia, extrasystoles, sweating, mydriasis, flushing, mild hyperpyrexia.

---

*No request for permission to reproduce the text is necessary, provided it is done without modification.

3+ Delirium, mania, self-injury, marked hypertension, tachycardia, cardiac arrhythmias, hyperpyrexia.

4+ The above symptoms and signs plus convulsions, coma, circulatory collapse.

C. Determine the Severity of Narcotic Withdrawal Symptoms: Score the following findings on a scale of 0–2:

Diarrhea	Hyperactive bowel
Insomnia	Restlessness
Dilated pupils	Sounds
Lacrimation	Tachycardia
Gooseflesh	Hypertension
Muscle cramps	Yawning

A score of 1–5 represents mild, 6–10 moderate, and 11–15 severe withdrawal symptoms.

Seizures, which are unusual in narcotic withdrawal, indicate severe withdrawal problems.

DEFINITIVE THERAPY OF POISONING

Prevention of Absorption

A. Emesis: Induced vomiting is *contraindicated* in patients who are comatose, convulsing, have lost the gag reflex, or have ingested strong acids, strong bases, some hydrocarbons, *or sharp objects.* In the case of hydrocarbons, vomiting should be induced if more than 1 mL/kg has been ingested or if the substance contains heavy metals.

1. Ipecac method–Adult dose, 30 mL; pediatric dose, 15 mL. Give orally and repeat once in 20 minutes if necessary. The procedure is as follows:

a. Give ipecac orally.

b. Follow with up to 6 oz of water or whatever fluid the child will drink.

c. Keep the patient ambulatory.

d. After 20 minutes, repeat the dose if vomiting has not occurred.

2. Other emetics–The only approved oral emetic agent is syrup of ipecac. Use of sodium chloride may lead to lethal hypernatremia. Apomorphine should not be used because its depressant effect outlasts the duration of reversal by naloxone. Other emetic agents, such as mustard and soap, are not as effective as syrup of ipecac and should be avoided.

B. Lavage: If the patient is or is becoming unconscious, is convulsing, or has lost the gag reflex, gastric lavage following endotracheal or nasotracheal intubation should be performed rather than induction of vomiting. Lavage is less effective than emesis if a small (8–16F) tube is utilized but not if the recommended 28–36F Ewald tube is used. The tube should be inserted orally, and lavage should be with warm saline solution in a small child to avoid hyponatremia or hypothermia. Save the initial aspirate for laboratory determination and lavage until the returns have been clear for 1 liter. Monitor the amount of fluid given. The amount instilled should approximate the amount removed.

Emesis and lavage recover an average of about 30% of the stomach contents. Although these procedures may be helpful in reducing the amount of material available for absorption, approximately 70% of an ingested dose will remain. Additional measures such as charcoal and cathartics should be instituted to prevent further absorption.

C. Charcoal: Thirty grams of charcoal should be made into a slurry with a minimum of 240 mL of diluent. Give 1–2 g/kg (maximum, 100 g) per dose. The charcoal may be in an aqueous slurry or mixed with a saline cathartic or sorbitol.

Repeating the dose of activated charcoal may be useful for those agents that undergo enterohepatic circulation or those that slow passage through the gastrointestinal tract. When multiple doses of activated charcoal are given, repeated doses of sorbitol or saline cathartics should *not* be given. Repeated doses of cathartics may cause electrolyte imbalances and fluid loss. Charcoal dosing is repeated every 2–6 hours until charcoal is passed per rectum.

The patient may regurgitate some of the charcoal, but 70% is usually retained. Charcoal has been shown to reduce the half-life of an agent even when it is given after the intravenous administration of phenobarbital or theophylline.

D. Catharsis: *Caution:* Despite their widespread use, cathartics have not been shown to improve outcome. The use of cathartics should therefore be limited to patients in whom they can be safely used. In particular, do not give cathartics containing magnesium or phosphate to patients in renal failure. Pneumonitis may occur following aspiration of oil-based cathartics.

Acceptable cathartics include magnesium sulfate or sodium sulfate (250 mg/kg/dose orally [maximum, 30 g]); magnesium citrate (4 mL/kg/dose [maximum, 300 mL]); and sorbitol (1–1.5 g/kg/dose, of a 35% solution, for children over 1 year of age [maximum, 50 g/dose]). Sorbitol should be administered in a health care facility so that fluid and electrolyte status can be monitored, especially in children.

E. Whole Gut Lavage: Whole bowel lavage utilizes an orally administered, nonabsorbable hypertonic solution such as Colyte or Golytely. The use of this procedure in poisoned patients remains controversial. Preliminary recommendations for use of whole bowel irrigation include sustained-release preparations, mechanical movement of items through the bowel (eg, cocaine packets), and substances poorly absorbed by charcoal (lithium, iron). Underlying bowel pathology and functional obstruction are relative contraindications to its use.

Kulig K et al: Management of acutely poisoned patients without gastric emptying. Ann Emerg Med 1985;14:562.

Phillips S, Gomez H, Brent J: Pediatric gastrointestinal decontamination in acute toxin ingestion. J Clin Pharmacol 1993;33:497.

Tenenbein M, Cohen S, Sitar DS: Efficacy of ipecac-induced emesis, orogastric lavage and activated charcoal for acute drug overdose. Ann Emerg Med 1987;16:838.

Enhancement of Urinary Excretion

Urinary excretion of certain substances can be hastened by urinary alkalinization or dialysis. In the past, forced diuresis or forced alkaline diuresis was used. While these have been abandoned because of their high complication rates, it is important to make certain that the patient is not volume-depleted. Volume-depleted patients should receive a normal saline bolus of 10–20 mL/kg, followed by sufficient intravenous fluid administration to maintain urine output at 2–3 mL/kg/h.

A. Urinary alkalinization:

1. Alkaline diuresis–Urinary alkalinization should be chosen on the basis of the substance's pK_a, so that ionized drug will be trapped in the tubular lumen and not reabsorbed (see Table 12–8). Thus, if the pK_a is less than 7.5, urinary alkalinization is appropriate; if it is over 8.0, this technique is not usually beneficial. The pK_a is sometimes included along with general drug information. Urinary alkalinization can usually be achieved with sodium bicarbonate. It is well to observe for potassium depletion, caused by the shift of potassium intracellularly. Follow serum K^+ and observe for electrocardiographic (ECG) evidence of hypokalemia.

B. Dialysis: Hemodialysis (or peritoneal dialysis if hemodialysis is unavailable) is useful in the poisonings listed below. Dialysis should be considered part of supportive care if the patient satisfies any of the following criteria:

1. Clinical criteria–

a. Stage 3 or 4 coma or hyperactivity that is caused by a dialyzable drug and cannot be treated by conservative means.

b. Hypotension threatening renal or hepatic function that cannot be corrected by adjusting circulating volume.

c. Marked hyperosmolality or severe acid-base or electrolyte disturbances not responding to therapy.

d. Marked hypothermia or hyperthermia not responding to therapy.

2. Immediate dialysis–Immediate dialysis may be considered in ethylene glycol and methanol poisoning only if acidosis is refractory and blood levels of ethanol of 100 mg/dL are consistently maintained during dialysis.

3. Dialysis indicated on basis of condition of patient–(In general, dialyze if patient is in coma deeper than level 3.)

Alcohols	Bromides	Paraldehyde
Ammonia	Calcium	Potassium
Amphetamines	Chloral	Quinidine
Anilines	hydrate	Quinine
Antibiotics	Fluorides	Salicylates
Barbiturates	Iodides	Strychnine
(long-acting)	Isoniazid	Thiocyanates
Boric Acid	Meprobamate	

(Other drugs may be dialyzable, but the information should be verified prior to institution of dialysis therapy.)

4. Dialysis not indicated except for support–Therapy consists of intensive care.

Antidepressants	Heroin and other opioids
(cyclics and	Methaqualone
MAO inhibitors)	Methyprylon
Antihistamines	Oxazepam
Barbiturates	Phenothiazines
(short-acting)	Phenytoin
Chlordiazepoxide	Synthetic anticholiner-
Diazepam	gics and belladonna
Digitalis and	compounds
related drugs	
Diphenoxylate	
with atropine	

Salicylates generally respond very well to intensive alkaline diuretic therapy, but if complications such as renal failure or pulmonary edema develop, hemodialysis alone or with hemoperfusion may be helpful.

Peritoneal dialysis and **exchange transfusion** may be more useful in small children than hemodialysis, as much for fluid and electrolyte homeostasis as for poison removal.

Hemoperfusion

Perfusion of blood through charcoal- or resin-filled devices has theoretical advantages for some poisons, but is often difficult to arrange on an emergent basis. Contact your nephrology service to determine availability and expertise in this modality.

MANAGEMENT OF SPECIFIC COMMON POISONS

Unless otherwise contraindicated, syrup of ipecac should be given to all conscious patients poisoned by the substances listed in the following section, particularly if it can be administered at home within 1 hour after ingestion. Whenever possible, patients should be evaluated regarding the need for emesis, which depends on the severity of the exposure. Gastric lavage after an endotracheal tube is inserted is usually indicated for comatose patients.

ACETAMINOPHEN
(Paracetamol)

Overdosage of acetaminophen can cause severe hepatotoxicity. The incidence of hepatotoxicity in adults and adolescents has been reported to be 10 times higher than in young children; in the latter group, only three of 4187 patients under the age of 5 years developed hepatotoxicity.

Acetaminophen is normally metabolized in the liver. A small percentage of the drug goes through a pathway leading to a toxic metabolite. Normally, this nucleophilic reactant is removed harmlessly by conjugation with glutathione. In overdosage, the supply of glutathione becomes exhausted, and the metabolite may bind covalently to components of liver cells to produce necrosis.

Treatment

Treatment is to supply a surrogate glutathione by giving acetylcysteine. In the United States, it may only be given orally. Consultation on difficult cases may be obtained from the Rocky Mountain Poison Center (1-800-525-6115). Blood levels should be obtained as soon as possible after 4 hours and plotted on Figure 12–9. Acetylcysteine is administered to patients whose acetaminophen levels plot in the toxic range on the nomogram (see Figure 12–9). Preliminary evidence suggests that acetylcysteine may also be of use even after 24 hours post ingestion.

The dose is 140 mg/kg orally, diluted to a 5% solution in sweet fruit juice or carbonated soft drink. The primary problems associated with administration are nausea and vomiting. After this loading dose, 70 mg/kg should be administered orally every 4 hours for 72 hours. AST (aspartate transaminase), ALT (alanine transaminase), serum bilirubin, and plasma prothrombin time should be followed daily.

Parker D et al: Safety of late acetylcysteine treatment in paracetamol poisoning. Hum Exp Toxicol 1990;9:25.

Peterson RG, Rumack BH: Pharmacokinetics of acetaminophen in children. Pediatrics 1978;62:877.

Rumack BH et al: Acetaminophen overdose. Arch Intern Med 1981;141:380.

Smilkstein M et al: Efficacy of oral *N*-acetylcysteine in the treatment of acetaminophen overdose. N Engl J Med 1988;319:1557.

ALCOHOL, ETHYL
(Ethanol)

Alcoholic beverages, tinctures, cosmetics, and rubbing alcohol are common sources of poisoning in children. Concomitant exposure to other depressant drugs increases the seriousness of the intoxication. (Blood levels cited are for adults; comparable figures for children are not available. In most states, alcohol levels of 50–80 mg/dL are considered compatible

Figure 12–9. Semilogarithmic plot of plasma acetaminophen levels versus time. (Modified and reproduced, with permission, from Rumack BH, Matthew H: Acetaminophen poisoning and toxicity. Pediatrics 1975; 55:871.)

with impaired faculties, and levels of 80–150 mg/dL are considered evidence of intoxication.)

50–150 mg/dL: Incoordination, slow reaction time, and blurred vision.
150–300 mg/dL: Visual impairment, staggering, and slurred speech. Marked hypoglycemia may be present.
300–500 mg/dL: Marked incoordination, stupor, hypoglycemia, and convulsions.
>500 mg/dL: Coma and death, except in individuals who have developed tolerance.

Complete absorption of alcohol requires 30 minutes to 6 hours, depending upon the volume, the presence of food, the time spent in consuming the alcohol, etc. The rate of metabolic degradation is constant (about 20 mg/h in an adult). Less than 10% is excreted in the urine. Absolute ethanol, 1 mL/kg, results in a peak blood level of about 100 mg/dL in 1 hour after ingestion. Acute intoxication and chronic alcoholism increase the risk of subarachnoid hemorrhage.

Treatment

Management of hypoglycemia and acidosis is usually the only measure required. Start an intravenous drip of D_5W or $D_{10}W$ if blood glucose is under 60 mg/dL. Fructose has been suggested as an accelerator of metabolism, but it may cause vomiting, intensify lactic acidosis, and decrease blood volume via osmotic diuresis. Glucagon does not correct the hypoglycemia, because hepatic glycogen stores are reduced. Oxygen saturation should be measured and oxygen given in serious overdose because death is usually caused by respiratory failure. In severe cases, cerebral edema should be treated with dexamethasone, 0.1 mg/kg intravenously every 4–6 hours. Dialysis is indicated in life-threatening intoxication.

Hammond K, Rumack B, Rodgerson D: Blood ethanol. JAMA 1973;226:63.
Leung AKC: Ethyl alcohol ingestions in children. Clin Pediatr (Phila) 1986;25:617.
Scherger DL et al: Ethyl alcohol (ethanol)-containing cologne, perfume, and aftershave ingestions in children. Am J Dis Child 1988;142:630.

AMPHETAMINES & RELATED DRUGS (Methamphetamine)

Clinical Presentation

A. Acute Poisoning: Amphetamine poisoning is common because of the widespread availability of "diet pills" and the use of "speed," "crank," "crystal," and "ice" by adolescents. (Care must be taken in the interpretation of slang terms because they have multiple meanings.) Symptoms include central nervous system stimulation, anxiety, hyperactivity, hyperpyrexia, hypertension, abdominal cramps, nausea and vomiting, and inability to void urine. Severe cases may include rhabdomyolysis. A toxic psychosis indistinguishable from paranoid schizophrenia may occur.

B. Chronic Poisoning: Chronic amphetamine users develop tolerance; more than 1500 mg of intravenous methamphetamine can be used daily. Hyperactivity, disorganization, and euphoria are followed by exhaustion, depression, and coma lasting 2–3 days. Heavy users, taking more than 100 mg/d, have restlessness, incoordination of thought, insomnia, nervousness, irritability, and visual hallucinations. Psychosis may be precipitated by the chronic administration of high doses. Depression, weakness, tremors, gastrointestinal complaints, and suicidal thoughts occur frequently.

Treatment

Standard decontamination procedures should be used: gastric emptying followed by charcoal in recent ingestions; activated charcoal alone if ingestion occurred hours earlier. The treatment of choice is diazepam. If this fails to reduce hyperactivity, chlorpromazine (0.5–1 mg/kg intravenously) may be given and repeated in 30 minutes. A maximum daily dose of 2.5–6 mg/kg may be used. Chlorpromazine may produce hypotension. In case of extreme agitation or hallucinations, droperidol (0.1 mg/kg/dose) or haloperidol (up to 0.1 mg/kg) parenterally has been used. When combinations of amphetamines and barbiturates (diet pills) are used, the action of the amphetamines begins first, followed by a depression caused by the barbiturates. In these cases, treatment with additional barbiturates is contraindicated because of the risk of respiratory failure.

Chronic users may be withdrawn rapidly from amphetamines. On the other hand, if amphetamine-barbiturate combination tablets have been used, the barbiturates must be withdrawn gradually to prevent withdrawal seizures. Psychiatric treatment should be provided.

Broscoe JG et al: Pemoline-induced choreoathetosis and rhabdomyolysis. Med Toxicol 1988;3:72.
Gary NE, Saidi P: Methamphetamine intoxication. Am J Med 1978;64:537.
Hong R, Matsuyama E, Nur K: Cardiomyopathy associated with the smoking of crystal methamphetamine. JAMA 1991;265:1152.
Jackson JG: The hazards of smokable methamphetamine. N Engl J Med 1989;321:907.
Stek AM et al: Maternal and fetal cardiovascular responses to methamphetamine in the pregnant sheep. Am J Obstet Gynecol 1993;169:888.

ANESTHETICS, LOCAL

Intoxication from local anesthetics may be associated with central nervous system stimulation, acidosis, delirium, ataxia, shock, convulsions, and death. Methemoglobinuria has been reported following local dental analgesia.

Local anesthetics used in obstetrics cross the placental barrier and are not efficiently metabolized by the fetal liver. Mepivacaine, lidocaine, and bupivacaine can cause fetal bradycardia, neonatal depression, and death. Prilocaine causes methemoglobinemia, which should be treated if levels in the blood exceed 40% or if the patient is symptomatic.

Accidental injection of mepivacaine into the head of the fetus during paracervical anesthesia has caused neonatal asphyxia, cyanosis, acidosis, bradycardia, convulsions, and death.

Treatment

If the anesthetic has been ingested, induced vomiting should be followed by activated charcoal. Mucous membranes should be carefully cleansed. Oxygen administration, with assisted ventilation if necessary, is indicated. Methemoglobinemia is treated with methylene blue, 1%, 0.2 mL/kg (1–2 mg/kg/dose) intravenously over 5–10 minutes; this should promptly relieve the cyanosis. Acidosis may be treated with sodium bicarbonate, seizures with diazepam, bradycardia with atropine. Therapeutic levels of mepivacaine, lidocaine, and procaine are less than 5 μg/mL.

Amitai Y, Whitesell L, Lovejoy FH: Death following accidental lidocaine overdose in a child. N Engl J Med 1986; 314:181.

Bozynski MEA, Rubarth LB, Patel JA: Lidocaine toxicity after maternal pudendal anesthesia in a term infant with fetal distress. Am J Perinatol 1987;4:164.

ANTIHISTAMINES

Although antihistamines typically cause central nervous system depression, children often react paradoxically with excitement, hallucinations, delirium, ataxia, tremors, and convulsions followed by central nervous system depression, respiratory failure, or cardiovascular collapse. Anticholinergic effects such as dry mouth, fixed dilated pupils, flushed face, fever, and hallucinations may be prominent.

Antihistamines are widely available in allergy, sleep, cold, and antiemetic preparations, and many are supplied in sustained-release forms, which increases the likelihood of dangerous overdoses. They are absorbed rapidly and metabolized by the liver, lungs, and kidneys. A potentially toxic dose is 10–50 mg/kg of the most commonly used antihistamines, but toxic reactions have occurred at much lower doses.

Treatment

Activated charcoal should be used to reduce drug absorption. Emetics may be ineffective if the antihistamine is structurally related to phenothiazines. A cathartic is indicated for sustained-release preparations. Physostigmine, 0.5–2 mg slowly intravenously, dramatically reverses the central and peripheral anticholinergic effects of antihistamines, but it should be used only for diagnostic purposes. Diazepam, 0.1–0.2 mg/kg intravenously, can be used to control seizures. Forced diuresis is not helpful. Exchange transfusion was reported effective in one case.

Cetaruk EW, Aaron CK: Hazards of nonprescription medications. Emerg Med Clin North Am 1994;12:483.

Richmond M, Seger D: Central anticholinergic syndrome in a child: A case report. J Emerg Med 1985;3:453.

Rumack BH et al: Ornade and anticholinergic toxicity, hypertension, hallucinations and arrhythmia. Clin Toxicol 1974;7:573.

Tobin JR et al: Astemizole-induced cardiac conduction disturbances in a child. JAMA 1991;266:2737.

ARSENIC

Clinical Presentation

A. Acute Poisoning: Abdominal pain, vomiting, watery and bloody diarrhea, cardiovascular collapse, paresthesias, neck pain, and garlic odor on breath occur. Convulsions, coma, anuria, and exfoliative dermatitis are later signs. Inhalation may cause pulmonary edema. Death is the result of cardiovascular collapse.

B. Chronic Poisoning: Anorexia, generalized weakness, giddiness, colic, abdominal pain, polyneuritis, dermatitis, nail changes, alopecia, and anemia often develop.

Arsenic is commonly used in insecticides (fruit tree or tobacco sprays), rodenticides, weed killers, and wallpaper. It is well absorbed primarily through the gastrointestinal and respiratory tracts, but skin absorption may occur. Arsenic can be found in the urine, hair, and nails by laboratory testing.

Highly toxic soluble derivatives of this compound, such as sodium arsenite, are frequently found in liquid preparations and can cause death in as many as 65% of victims. The alkyl methanearsonates found in "persistent" or "preemergence" type weed killers are relatively less soluble and less toxic. Poisonings with a liquid arsenical preparation that does not contain alkyl methanearsonate compounds should be considered potentially lethal. Patients with clinical signs other than gastroenteritis should be treated until laboratory tests indicate that treatment is no longer necessary.

Treatment

In acute poisoning, induce vomiting and administer activated charcoal. Then immediately give dimercaprol (BAL), 2.5 mg/kg intramuscularly, and follow with 2 mg/kg intramuscularly every 4 hours. The dimercaprol-arsenic complex is dialyzable. A second choice is succimer. The initial dose is 10 mg/kg every 8 hours for 5 days. A third choice is penicillamine, 100 mg/kg orally to a maximum of 1 g/d in four divided doses.

Chronic arsenic intoxication should be treated with succimer or penicillamine. Collect a 24-hour baseline urine specimen and then begin chelation. If the 24-hour urine arsenic level is greater than 50 µg, continue chelation for 5 days. After 10 days, repeat the 5-day cycle once or twice depending on how soon the urine arsenic level falls below 50 µg/24 h.

Donofrio PD et al: Acute arsenic intoxication presenting as Guillain-Barré-like syndrome. Muscle Nerve 1987;10: 114.

Fournier L et al: 2,3-Dimercaptosuccinic acid treatment of heavy metal poisoning in humans. Med Toxicol 1988; 3:499.

Peterson RG, Rumack BH: Arsenic poisoning treated with D-penicillamine. J Pediatr 1977;91:661.

BARBITURATES

The toxic effects of barbiturates include confusion, poor coordination, coma, miotic or fixed dilated pupils, and increased or (more commonly) decreased respiratory effort. Respiratory acidosis is commonly associated with pulmonary atelectasis, and hypotension occurs frequently in severely poisoned patients. Ingestion of more than 6 mg/kg of long-acting or 3 mg/kg of short-acting barbiturates is usually toxic; however, chronic users of barbiturates can tolerate blood levels up to 25 mg/dL.

Treatment

If the patient is awake, vomiting should be induced and activated charcoal should be given. Careful, conservative management with emphasis on maintaining a clear airway, adequate ventilation, and control of hypotension is critical. Urinary alkalinization and the use of multiple-dose charcoal may decrease the elimination half-life of phenobarbital but have not been shown to alter the clinical course. Hemodialysis is not useful in the treatment of poisoning with short-acting barbiturates. Analeptics are contraindicated.

Amitai Y, Degani Y: Treatment of phenobarbital poisoning with multiple dose activated charcoal in an infant. J Emerg Med 1990;8:449.

Groschel D, Gerstein A, Rosenbaum J: Skin lesions as a diagnostic aid in barbiturate poisoning. N Engl J Med 1970;283:409.

Zawada ET et al: Advances in the hemodialysis management of phenobarbital overdose. South Med J 1983;76:6.

BELLADONNA ALKALOIDS
(Atropine, Jimsonweed, Potato Leaves, Scopolamine, Stramonium)

The effects of anticholinergic compounds include dry mouth; thirst; decreased sweating with hot, dry, red skin; high fever; and tachycardia that may be preceded by bradycardia. The pupils are dilated, and vision is blurred. Speech and swallowing may be impaired. Hallucinations, delirium, and coma are common. Leukocytosis may occur, confusing the diagnosis.

Atropinism has been caused by normal doses of atropine or homatropine eye drops, especially in children with Down's syndrome. Many common plants and over-the-counter sleeping medications contain belladonna alkaloids.

Treatment

Emesis or lavage should be followed by activated charcoal and cathartics. Gastric emptying is slowed by anticholinergics, so that gastric decontamination may be useful even if delayed. Physostigmine, 0.5–2 mg slowly intravenously (can be repeated every 30 minutes as needed), dramatically reverses the central and peripheral signs of atropinism but should be used only as a diagnostic agent. Neostigmine is ineffective because it does not enter the central nervous system. High fever must be controlled. Catheterization may be needed if the patient cannot void.

Beech M, Hell C, Nightingale P: Central anticholinergic syndrome. Lancet 1987;1:1089.

Fitzgerald DA et al: Seizures associated with 1% cyclopentolate eyedrops. J Paediatr Child Health 1990;26:106.

CARBON MONOXIDE

The degree of toxicity correlates well with the carboxyhemoglobin level taken soon after acute exposure but not after oxygen has been given or when there has been some time since exposure. Onset of symptoms may be more rapid and more severe if the patient lives at a high altitude, has a high respiratory rate (ie, infants), is pregnant, or has myocardial insufficiency or lung disease. Normal blood may contain up to 5% carboxyhemoglobin.

The most prominent early symptom is headache. Proteinuria, glycosuria, elevated serum aminotransferase levels, or ECG changes may be present in the acute phase. Permanent cardiac, liver, renal, or central nervous system damage occasionally occurs. The outcome of severe poisoning may be complete recovery, vegetative state, or any degree of mental injury between these extremes. The primary mental deficits are neuropsychiatric.

Treatment

The biologic half-life of carbon monoxide on room air is approximately 200–300 minutes; on 100% oxygen, it is 60–90 minutes. Hyperbaric oxygen therapy at 2–2.5 atm of oxygen shortens the half-life to 30 minutes. After the level has been reduced to near zero, therapy is aimed at the nonspecific sequelae of anoxia. Dexamethasone, 0.1 mg/kg intravenously or intramuscularly every 4–6 hours, should be added if cerebral edema develops.

Crocker PJ, Walker JS: Pediatric carbon monoxide toxicity. J Emerg Med 1985;3:443.

Farrow JR et al: Fetal death due to nonlethal maternal carbon monoxide poisoning. J Forensic Sci 1990;35:1448.

Raphael JC et al: Trial of normobaric and hyperbaric oxygen for acute carbon monoxide intoxication. Lancet 1989;2:414.

Thom SR et al: Delayed neuropsychologic sequelae after carbon monoxide poisoning: Prevention by treatment with hyperbaric oxygen. Ann Emerg Med 1995;25:474.

CAUSTICS

1. ACIDS
(Hydrochloric, Hydrofluoric, Nitric, & Sulfuric Acids; Sodium Bisulfate)

Strong acids are commonly found in metal and toilet bowl cleaners, batteries, and other products. Hydrofluoric acid is the most toxic and hydrochloric acid the least toxic of these household substances. However, even a few drops can be fatal if aspirated into the trachea.

Painful swallowing, mucous membrane burns, bloody emesis, abdominal pain, respiratory distress due to edema of the epiglottis, thirst, shock, and renal failure can occur. Coma and convulsions sometimes are seen terminally. Residual lesions include esophageal, gastric, and pyloric strictures as well as scars of the cornea, skin, and oropharynx.

Hydrofluoric acid is a particularly dangerous poison. Dermal exposure creates a penetrating burn that can progress for hours or days. Large dermal exposure or ingestion may produce life-threatening hypocalcemia as well as burn reactions.

Treatment

Emetics and lavage are contraindicated. Water or milk (<15 mL/kg) are used to dilute the acid, because a heat-producing chemical reaction does not occur. Take care not to induce emesis by excessive fluid administration. Alkalies should not be used. Burned areas of the skin, mucous membranes, or eyes should be washed with copious amounts of warm water. Opioids for pain may be needed. An endotracheal

tube may be required to alleviate laryngeal edema. Esophagoscopy should be performed if the patient has significant burns or difficulty in swallowing. Acids are likely to produce gastric burns or esophageal burns. Evidence is not conclusive, but corticosteroids have not proved to be of use.

Hydrofluoric acid burns on skin are treated with 10% calcium gluconate gel or calcium gluconate infusion. Severe exposure may require large doses of intravenous calcium. Therapy should be guided by calcium levels, the ECG, and clinical signs.

2. BASES
(Clinitest Tablets, Clorox, Drano, Liquid-Plumr, Purex, Sani-Clor)

Alkalies produce more severe injuries than acids. Some substances, such as Clinitest Tablets or Drano, are quite toxic, whereas the chlorinated bleaches (3–6% solutions of sodium hypochlorite) are usually not toxic. When sodium hypochlorite comes in contact with acid in the stomach, hypochlorous acid, which is very irritating to the mucous membrane and skin, is formed. Rapid inactivation of this substance prevents systemic toxicity. Chlorinated beaches, when mixed with a strong acid (toilet bowl cleaners) or ammonia, may produce irritating chlorine or chloramine gas.

Alkalies can burn the skin, mucous membranes, and eyes. Respiratory distress may be due to edema of the epiglottis, pulmonary edema resulting from inhalation of fumes, or pneumonia. Mediastinitis or other intercurrent infections or shock can occur. Perforation of the esophagus or stomach is rare.

Treatment

The skin and mucous membranes should be cleansed with copious amounts of water. A local anesthetic can be instilled in the eye if necessary to alleviate blepharospasm. The eye should be irrigated for at least 20–30 minutes. Ophthalmologic consultation should be obtained for all alkaline eye burns.

Ingestions should be treated with water as a diluent. Routine esophagoscopy is no longer indicated to rule out burns of the esophagus due to chlorinated bleaches unless an unusually large amount has been ingested or the patient is symptomatic. The absence of oral lesions does not rule out the possibility of laryngeal or esophageal burns following granular alkali ingestion. The use of corticosteroids is controversial but has not been shown to improve long-term outcome. Antibiotics may be needed if mediastinitis is likely, but they should not be used prophylactically.

Gaudreault P et al: Predictability of esophageal injury from signs and symptoms: A study of caustic ingestion in 378 children. Pediatrics 1983;71:767.

Lovejoy FH Jr: Corrosive injury of the esophagus in children: Failure of corticosteroid treatment reemphasizes prevention. (Editorial.) N Engl J Med 1990;323:668.

Nuutinen M et al: Consequences of caustic ingestion in children. Acta Pediatr 1994;83:1200.

COCAINE

Most street cocaine is adulterated. Cocaine is absorbed intranasally or via inhalation or ingestion. Effects are noted almost immediately when the drug is taken intravenously or smoked. Peak effects are delayed for about an hour when the drug is taken orally or nasally. Cocaine prevents the reuptake of endogenous catecholamines, thereby causing an initial sympathetic discharge, followed by catechol depletion after chronic abuse.

Clinical Findings

A local anesthetic and vasoconstrictor, cocaine is also a potent stimulant to both the central nervous system and the cardiovascular system. The initial tachycardia, hyperpnea, hypertension, and stimulation of the central nervous system are often followed by coma, seizures, hypotension, and respiratory depression. In severe cases, various dysrhythmias may be seen, including sinus tachycardia, atrial arrhythmias, premature ventricular contractions, bigeminy, and ventricular fibrillation. If large doses are taken intravenously, cardiac failure, dysrhythmias, or hyperthermia may result in death.

Treatment

Testing for cocaine in blood or plasma is generally not clinically useful, but a qualitative analysis of the urine may aid in confirming the diagnosis. For severe cases, an ECG is indicated. When a teenager is suspected of being a "body packer," x-rays of the gastrointestinal tract are warranted. Cocaine is usually smoked or taken intranasally or intravenously; for this reason, decontamination is seldom possible. When cocaine is taken orally, lavage may be indicated, depending on the potential for seizures or loss of gag reflex. Activated charcoal may also be indicated. For body packers, whole bowel lavage may be useful in passing the packets quickly. Seizures may be treated with intravenous diazepam titrated to response or intravenous phenytoin (loading dose 10–15 mg/kg, maintenance 4–7 mg/kg/24 h). Hypotension may be treated with standard agents. However, because cocaine abuse may deplete norepinephrine, an indirect agent such as dopamine may be less effective than a direct agent such as norepinephrine. Agitation is best treated with diazepam.

Azuma SD, Chasnoff IJ: Outcome of children prenatally exposed to cocaine and other drugs: A path analysis of three-year data. Pediatr 1993;92:396.

Durand DJ, Espinoza AM, Nickerson BT: Association be-

tween prenatal cocaine exposure and sudden infant death syndrome. J Pediatr 1990;117:909.

Fitzmaurice LS et al: TAC use and absorption of cocaine in a pediatric emergency department. Ann Emerg Med 1990;19:515.

King TA et al: Neurologic manifestations of in utero cocaine exposure in near-term and term infants. Pediatrics 1995;96:259.

Mott SH, Packer RJ, Soldin SJ. Neurologic manifestations of cocaine exposure in childhood. Pediatr 1994;93:557.

CONTRACEPTIVE PILLS

The only known toxic effects following acute ingestion of oral contraceptive agents are nausea, vomiting, and vaginal bleeding in girls.

COSMETICS & RELATED PRODUCTS

The relative toxicities of commonly ingested products in this group are listed in Table 12–9.

Permanent wave neutralizers may contain bromates, peroxides, or perborates. Bromates have been removed from most products because they can cause nausea, vomiting, abdominal pain, shock, hemolysis, renal failure, and convulsions. Perborate can cause boric acid poisoning. Four grams of bromate salts is potentially lethal.

Poisoning is treated by induced emesis or gastric lavage with 1% sodium thiosulfate followed by demulcents to relieve gastric irritation. Sodium bicarbonate, 2%, in the lavage fluid may reduce hydrobromic acid formation. Sodium thiosulfate, 1%, 100–500 mL, can be given intravenously, but methylene blue should not be used to treat methemoglobinemia in this situation, because it increases the toxicity of bromates. Dialysis is indicated in renal failure but does not enhance excretion of bromate.

Fingernail polish removers used to contain toluene, but now usually have an acetone base, which

Table 12–9. Relative toxicities of cosmetics and similar products.

High toxicity	Low toxicity
Permanent wave neutralizers	Perfume
	Hair removers
	Deodorants
Modern toxicity	Bath salts
Fingernail polish	
Fingernail polish remover	**No toxicity**
Metallic hair dyes	Liquid makeup
Home permanent wave lotion	Vegetable hair dye
	Cleansing cream
Bath oil	Hair dressing
Shaving lotion	(nonalcoholic)
Hair tonic (alcoholic)	Hand lotion or cream
Cologne, toilet water	Lipstick

does not require specific treatment other than monitoring central nervous system status.

Cobalt, copper, cadmium, iron, lead, nickel, silver, bismuth, and tin are sometimes found in metallic hair dyes. In large amounts, they can cause skin sensitization, urticaria, dermatitis, eye damage, vertigo, hypertension, asthma, methemoglobinemia, tremors, convulsions, and coma. Treatment for ingestions is to administer demulcents and, only with large amounts, the appropriate antidote for the heavy metal involved.

Home permanent wave lotions, hair straighteners, and hair removers usually contain thioglycolic acid salts, which cause alkaline irritation and perhaps central nervous system depression.

Shaving lotion, hair tonic, hair straighteners, cologne, and toilet water contain denatured alcohol, which can cause central nervous system depression and hypoglycemia.

Deodorants usually consist of an antibacterial agent in a cream base. Antiperspirants are aluminum salts, which frequently cause skin sensitization. Zirconium oxide can cause granulomas in the axilla with chronic use.

Fischer H, Caurdy-Bess L: Scalp burns from a permanent wave product. Clin Pediatr (Phila) 1990;29:53.

Lehman AJ: Health aspects of common chemicals used in hair-waving preparations. JAMA 1949;41:842.

CYCLIC ANTIDEPRESSANTS

Cyclic antidepressants (eg, amitriptyline, imipramine) have a very low toxic:therapeutic ratio, and even a moderate overdose can have serious effects. Cyclic antidepressant overdosage causes dysrhythmias, coma, convulsions, hypertension (and, later, hypotension), and hallucinations. These may be life-threatening and require rapid intervention. One agent, amoxapine, differs in that it causes fewer cardiovascular complications, but it has a higher incidence of seizures.

Treatment

An ECG should be taken in all patients. If dysrhythmias are demonstrated, the patient should be admitted and monitored until free of irregularity for 24 hours. Another indication for monitoring is persistent tachycardia of more than 110 beats/min plus additional findings of anticholinergic toxicity. The onset of dysrhythmias is rare beyond 24 hours after ingestion.

Alkalinization with sodium bicarbonate, 0.5 meq/kg intravenously, or hyperventilation may dramatically reverse ventricular dysrhythmias and narrow the QRS interval. Phenytoin or lidocaine may be added for treatment of arrhythmias. Sodium bicarbonate should be administered to all patients with significant dysrhythmias to achieve a pH of 7.5–7.6. Forced diuresis is contraindicated. A QRS interval greater than 100 ms specifically identifies patients at risk to develop dysrhythmias. Diazepam should be given for convulsions.

Hypotension is a major problem. Cyclic antidepressants block the reuptake of catecholamines, thereby producing initial hypertension followed by hypotension. Treatment with physostigmine is not effective. Vasopressors are generally effective. Dopamine is the agent of choice because it is readily available. If dopamine is ineffective, norepinephrine (0.1–1 µg/kg/min, titrated to response) should be added. Diuresis and hemodialysis are not effective. Decontamination should include gastric lavage and administration of activated charcoal.

Ellison DW, Pentel PR: Clinical features and consequences of seizures due to cyclic antidepressant overdose. Am J Emerg Med 1989;7:5.

Lavoie RW, Gansert CG, Weiss RE: Value of initial ECG findings and plasma drug levels in cyclic antidepressant overdose. Ann Emerg Med 1990;19:696.

Liebelt EL, Francis PD, Woolf AD: ECG lead aVR versus QRS interval in predicting seizures and arrhythmias in acute tricyclic antidepressant toxicity. Ann Emerg Med 1995;26:195.

DIGITALIS & OTHER CARDIAC GLYCOSIDES

Features include nausea, vomiting, diarrhea, headache, delirium, confusion, and, occasionally, coma. Cardiac irregularities such as atrial fibrillation, paroxysmal atrial tachycardia, and atrial flutter often occur. Death usually is the result of ventricular fibrillation. Transplacental intoxication by digitalis has been reported.

Treatment

If vomiting has not occurred, induce emesis or provide lavage followed by charcoal and cathartics. Potassium should not be given in acute overdosage unless there is laboratory evidence of hypokalemia. In acute overdosage, hyperkalemia is more common.

The patient must be monitored carefully for ECG changes. Every type of dysrhythmia has been reported in digitalis intoxication. The correction of acidosis better demonstrates the degree of potassium deficiency present. Bradycardias have been treated with atropine. Phenytoin, lidocaine, magnesium salts (not in renal failure), amiodarone, and bretylium have been used to correct arrhythmias.

Definitive treatment is with digoxin antibody fragments (digoxin immune Fab). Indications for Fab use include ventricular dysrhythmias and progressive bradydysrhythmia. Techniques of determining dosage are described in product literature.

Antman EM et al: Treatment of 150 cases of life-threatening digitalis intoxication with digoxin-specific Fab antibody fragments. Circulation 1990;81:1744.

Kaufman J et al: Use of digoxin Fab immune fragments in a seven-day-old infant. Pediatr Emerg Care 1990;6:118.

DIPHENOXYLATE HYDROCHLORIDE (Lomotil)

Lomotil contains diphenoxylate hydrochloride, a synthetic narcotic, and atropine sulfate. Early signs of Lomotil intoxication are due to its anticholinergic effect and consist of fever, facial flush, tachypnea, and lethargy. However, the miotic effect of the narcotic predominates. Later, hypothermia, increasing central nervous system depression, and loss of the facial flush occur. Seizures are probably secondary to hypoxia. Small amounts are potentially lethal in children; it is contraindicated in children under age 2 years.

Treatment

Prolonged monitoring (24 hours) with pulse oximetry is sufficient in most cases. If respiratory depression occurs, an airway should be established with an endotracheal tube. Gastric lavage and administration of activated charcoal may be useful because of the prolonged delay in gastric emptying time.

Naloxone hydrochloride (0.4–2 mg intravenously in children and adults) should be given. A transient improvement in respiration may be followed by respiratory depression. Repeated doses may be required because the duration of action of diphenoxylate is considerably longer than that of naloxone. The anticholinergic effects do not usually require treatment.

Al Ragheb et al: A case of fatal Lomotil overdosage. Med Sci Law 1982;22:210.

Rumack BH, Temple AR: Lomotil poisoning. Pediatrics 1974;53:495.

DISINFECTANTS & DEODORIZERS

1. NAPHTHALENE

Naphthalene is commonly found in mothballs, disinfectants, and deodorizers. Naphthalene's toxicity is often not fully appreciated. It is absorbed not only when ingested but also through the skin and lungs. It is potentially hazardous to store baby clothes in naphthalene, because baby oil is an excellent solvent that may increase dermal absorption.

Metabolic products of naphthalene may cause severe hemolytic anemia, similar to that due to primaquine toxicity, 2–7 days after ingestion. Other physical findings include vomiting, diarrhea, jaundice, oliguria, anuria, coma, and convulsions. The urine may contain hemoglobin, protein, and casts.

Treatment

Induced vomiting should be followed by activated charcoal and a cathartic. Urinary alkalinization may prevent blocking of the renal tubules by acid hematin crystals. Anuria may persist for 1–2 weeks and still be completely reversible.

Ostlere L, Amos R, Wass JAH: Haemolytic anaemia associated with ingestion of naphthalene-containing anointing oil. Postgrad Med J 1988;64:444.

Picchioni AL: Mothball poisoning in children. Am J Hosp Pharm 1960;17:303.

2. p-DICHLOROBENZENE, PHENOLIC ACIDS, & OTHERS

Disinfectants and deodorizers containing p-dichlorobenzene or sodium sulfate are much less toxic than those containing naphthalene. Disinfectants containing phenolic acids are highly toxic, especially if they contain a borate ion. Phenol precipitates tissue proteins and causes respiratory alkalosis followed by metabolic acidosis. Some phenols cause methemoglobinemia.

Local gangrene occurs after prolonged contact with tissue. Phenol is readily absorbed from the gastrointestinal tract, causing diffuse capillary damage and, in some cases, methemoglobinemia. Pentachlorophenol, which has been used in terminal rinsing of diapers, has caused infant fatalities.

The toxicity of alkalies, quaternary ammonium compounds, pine oil, and halogenated disinfectants varies with the concentration of active ingredients. Wick deodorizers are usually of moderate toxicity. Iodophor disinfectants are the safest. Spray deodorizers are not usually toxic, because a child is not likely to swallow a very large dose.

Manifestations of acute quaternary ammonium compound ingestion include diaphoresis, strong irritation, thirst, vomiting, diarrhea, cyanosis, hyperactivity, coma, convulsions, hypotension, abdominal pain, and pulmonary edema. Acute liver or renal failure may develop later.

Treatment

Activated charcoal may be used prior to gastric lavage. Castor oil dissolves phenol and may retard its absorption. This property of castor oil, however, has not been proved clinically. Mineral oil and alcohol are contraindicated because they increase the gastric absorption of phenol. A cathartic may be useful. The metabolic acidosis must be carefully managed. Anticonvulsants or measures to treat shock may be needed.

Because phenols are absorbed through the skin, exposed areas should be irrigated copiously with water. Undiluted polyethylene glycol may be a useful solvent as well.

Mucklow ES: Accidental feeding of dilute antiseptic solution (chlorhexidine 0.05% with cetrimide 1%) to five babies. Hum Toxicol 1988;7:567.

Pegg SP, Campbell DC: Children's burns due to cresol. Burns 1985;11:294.

Van Berkel M, de Wolff FA: Survival after acute benzalkonium chloride poisoning. Hum Toxicol 1988;7:191.

DISK BATTERY

Small, flat, smooth disk-shaped batteries measure between 10 and 25 mm in diameter. About 69% of them pass through the gastrointestinal tract in 48 hours and 85% in 72 hours. Some may become entrapped. These batteries contain caustic materials and heavy metals.

Batteries impacted in the esophagus may cause symptoms of refusal to take food, increased salivation, vomiting with or without blood, and pain or discomfort. Aspiration into the trachea may also occur. Fatalities have been reported in association with esophageal perforation.

When a history of disk battery ingestion is obtained, x-rays of the entire respiratory tract and gastrointestinal tract should be taken so that the battery can be located and the proper therapy determined.

Treatment

If the disk battery is located in the esophagus, it must be removed immediately. If the battery has been in the esophagus for more than 24 hours, the risk of caustic burn is greater.

Location of the disk battery below the esophagus has been associated with tissue damage, but the course has been benign in most cases. Perforated Meckel's diverticulum has been the major complication. It may take as long as 7 days for spontaneous passage to occur, and lack of movement in the gastrointestinal tract may not require removal in an asymptomatic patient. Some have suggested repeated x-rays and surgical intervention if passage of the battery pauses, but this approach may be excessive. Batteries that have opened in the gastrointestinal tract have been associated with some toxicity due to mercury, but the patients have recovered.

Emesis is ineffective in removal of the battery from the stomach. Asymptomatic patients may simply be observed and stools examined for passage of the battery. If the battery has not passed within 7 days or if the patient becomes symptomatic, x-rays should be repeated. If the battery has come apart or appears not to be moving, a purgative, enema, or nonabsorbable intestinal lavage solution should be administered. If these methods are not successful, surgical intervention may be required. Levels of heavy metals (mainly of mercury) should be measured in patients in whom the battery has opened or symptoms have developed.

Litovitz TL Schmitz BF: Ingestion of cylindrical and button batteries: an analysis of 2382 cases. Pediatrics 1992; 89:747.

Mank TGK et al: Mercury poisoning after disc-battery ingestion. Hum Toxicol 1987;6:179.

Rumack BH, Rumack CM: Disk battery ingestion. JAMA 1983;249:2509.

HYDROCARBONS
(Benzene, Charcoal Lighter Fluid, Gasoline, Kerosene, Petroleum Distillates, Turpentine)

Ingestion may cause irritation of mucous membranes, vomiting, blood-tinged diarrhea, respiratory distress, cyanosis, tachycardia, and fever. Although a small amount of certain hydrocarbons (10 mL) is potentially fatal, patients have survived ingestion of several ounces of other petroleum distillates. The more aromatic a hydrocarbon and the lower its viscosity rating, the more potentially toxic it is. Benzene, gasoline, kerosene, and red seal oil furniture polish are the most dangerous. A dose exceeding 1 mL/kg is likely to cause central nervous system depression. A history of coughing or choking, as well as vomiting, suggests aspiration with resulting hydrocarbon pneumonia. This is an acute hemorrhagic necrotizing disease that usually develops within 24 hours of the ingestion and resolves without sequelae in 3–5 days. However, several weeks may be required for full resolution of a hydrocarbon pneumonia. Pneumonia may be caused by the aspiration of a few drops of petroleum distillate into the lung or by absorption from the circulatory system. Pulmonary edema and hemorrhage, cardiac dilatation and dysrhythmias, hepatosplenomegaly, proteinuria, and hematuria can occur following large overdoses. Hypoglycemia is occasionally present. A chest film may reveal pneumonia within hours after the ingestion. An abnormal urinalysis in a child with a previously normal urinary tract suggests a large overdose.

Treatment

Both emetics and lavage should be avoided when only a small amount has been ingested. It is impossible to do a "cautious gastric lavage" unless a cuffed endotracheal tube is inserted. Under these circumstances, gastric lavage may be done using saline. Following lavage, magnesium or sodium sulfate should be left in the stomach. (Mineral oil should not be given, because it is capable of causing a low-grade lipoid pneumonia.)

Emetics are probably preferable to gastric lavage if massive ingestion has occurred. Epinephrine should not be used with halogenated hydrocarbons because it may affect an already sensitized myocardium. Analeptic drugs are contraindicated. The usefulness of corticosteroids is debated, and antibiotics should be reserved for patients with infections. Oxygen and mist are helpful. Extracorporeal membrane oxygenation has been successful in at least two cases of failure with standard therapy.

Anas N, Namasonthi V, Ginsburg C: Criteria for hospitalizing children who have ingested products containing hydrocarbons. JAMA 1981;246:840.

Bysani GK, Rucoba RJ, Noah ZL. Treatment of hydrocarbon pneumonitis. High frequency jet ventilation as an alternative to extracorporeal membrane oxygenation. Chest 1994;106:300.

Weber TR et al: Prolonged extracorporeal support for nonneonatal respiratory failure. J Pediatr Surg 1992;27:1100.

IBUPROFEN

Most exposures in children do not produce symptoms. In one study, for example, children ingesting up to 2.4 g remained asymptomatic. When symptoms occur, the most common are abdominal pain, vomiting, drowsiness, and lethargy. In rare cases, apnea (especially in young children), seizures, metabolic acidosis, and central nervous system depression leading to coma have occurred.

Treatment

If a child has ingested less than 100 mg/kg, dilution with water or milk may be all that is necessary to minimize the gastrointestinal upset. In children, the volume of liquid used for dilution should be less than 4 oz. When the ingested amount is more than 400 mg/kg, there is a potential for seizures or central nervous system depression; therefore, gastric lavage may be preferred to emesis. If the ingested amount is between 100 and 400 mg/kg, emesis may be of equal value. Activated charcoal and a cathartic may also be of some value. There is no specific antidote. Neither alkalinization of the urine nor hemodialysis has been proved helpful.

Hall AH, Rumack BH: Treatment of patients with ibuprofen overdose. Ann Emerg Med 1988;17:185.

Hall AH et al: Ibuprofen overdose: A prospective study. West J Med 1988;148:653.

Jenkinson ML et al: The relationship between plasma ibuprofen concentrations and toxicity in acute ibuprofen overdose. Hum Toxicol 1988;7:319.

INSECT STINGS
(Bee, Wasp, & Hornet)

Insect stings are painful but not usually dangerous; however, death from anaphylaxis may occur.

Bee venom, has hemolytic, neurotoxic, and histamine-like activities that can on rare occasions cause hemoglobinuria and severe anaphylactoid reactions.

Treatment

The physician should remove the stinger, taking care not to squeeze the attached venom sac. For allergic reactions, epinephrine 1:1000 solution, 0.01 mL/kg, should be administered intravenously or subcutaneously above the site of the sting. Three to four whiffs from an isoproterenol aerosol inhaler may be given at 3- to 4-minute intervals as needed. Corticosteroids (hydrocortisone), 100 mg intravenously, and diphenhydramine, 1.5 mg/kg intravenously, are useful ancillary drugs but have no immediate effect. Ephedrine or antihistamines may be used for 2 or 3 days to prevent recurrence of symptoms.

A patient who has had a potentially life-threatening insect sting should be desensitized against the Hymenoptera group, because the honey bee, wasp, hornet, and yellow jacket have common antigens in their venom.

For the more usual stings, cold compresses, aspirin, and diphenhydramine 1 mg/kg orally, are sufficient.

Barsky HE: Stinging insect allergy: Avoidance, identification, and treatment. Postgrad Med J 1987;82:157.

Reisman RE, Livingstone A: Late-onset allergic reactions, including serum sickness after insect stings. J Allergy Clin Immunol 1989;84:331.

INSECTICIDES

The petroleum distillates or other organic solvents used in these products are often as toxic as the pesticide. Unless otherwise indicated, induced vomiting or gastric lavage after insertion of an endotracheal tube is warranted.

DePalma AE, Kwalich DS, Zukerberg N: Pesticide poisoning in children. JAMA 1970;211:1979.

Rumack BH, Spoerke DG, Smolinske SC (editors): POISINDEX Information System. Micromedex, Inc, Denver, Colorado. [Published quarterly.]

1. CHLORINATED HYDROCARBONS (Aldrin, Carbinol, Chlordane, DDT, Dieldrin, Endrin, Heptachlor, Lindane, Toxaphene, etc)

Signs of intoxication include salivation, gastrointestinal irritability, abdominal pain, vomiting, diarrhea, central nervous system depression, and convulsions. Inhalation exposure causes irritation of the eyes, nose, and throat; blurred vision; cough; and pulmonary edema.

Chlorinated hydrocarbons are absorbed through

the skin, respiratory tract, and gastrointestinal tract. Decontamination of skin with soap and evacuation of the stomach contents are critical. All contaminated clothing should be removed. Castor oil, milk, and other substances containing fats or oils should not be left in the stomach because they increase absorption of the chlorinated hydrocarbons. Convulsions should be treated with diazepam, 0.1–0.3 mg/kg intravenously. Epinephrine should not be used because it may cause cardiac arrhythmias.

2. ORGANOPHOSPHATE (CHOLINESTERASE-INHIBITING) INSECTICIDES (Chlorthion, Co-Ral, DFP, Diazinon, Malathion, Paraoxon, Parathion, Phosdrin, TEPP, Thio-TEPP, etc)

Dizziness, headache, blurred vision, miosis, tearing, salivation, nausea, vomiting, diarrhea, hyperglycemia, cyanosis, sense of constriction of the chest, dyspnea, sweating, weakness, muscular twitching, convulsions, loss of reflexes and sphincter control, and coma can occur.

The clinical findings are the result of cholinesterase inhibition, which causes an accumulation of acetylcholine. The onset of symptoms occurs within 12 hours of the exposure. Red cell cholinesterase levels should be measured as soon as possible. (Some normal individuals have a low serum cholinesterase level.) Normal values vary in different laboratories. In general, a decrease of red cell cholinesterase to below 25% of normal indicates significant exposure.

Repeated low-grade exposure may result in sudden, acute toxic reactions. This syndrome usually occurs after repeated household spraying rather than agricultural exposure.

Although all organophosphates act by inhibiting cholinesterase activity, they vary greatly in their toxicity. Parathion, for example, is 100 times more toxic than malathion. The toxicity is influenced by the specific compound, the type of formulation (liquid or solid), the vehicle, and the route of absorption (lungs, skin, or gastrointestinal tract).

Treatment

Atropine plus a cholinesterase reactivator, pralidoxime, is an antidote for organophosphate insecticide poisoning. After assessment and management of the ABCs, large doses of atropine should be given and repeated every few minutes until signs of atropinism are present. An appropriate starting dose of atropine is 2–4 mg intravenously in an adult and 0.05 mg/kg in a child. The patient should receive enough atropine to stop secretions (approximately 10 times the normal dose). Severe poisoning may require gram quantities of atropine per 24 hours.

Because atropine antagonizes the muscarinic parasympathetic effects of the organophosphates but does not affect the nicotinic receptor, it does not improve muscular weakness. Pralidoxime should also be given immediately in more severe cases and repeated every 6–12 hours as needed (25–50 mg/kg diluted to 5% and infused over 5–30 minutes at a rate of no more than 500 mg/min). Pralidoxime should be used in addition to—not in place of—atropine if red cell cholinesterase is less than 25% of normal. Pralidoxime is most useful within 48 hours after the exposure but has shown some effects 2–6 days later. Morphine, theophylline, aminophylline, succinylcholine, and tranquilizers of the reserpine and phenothiazine types are contraindicated. Hyperglycemia is common in severe poisonings.

Decontamination of skin, nails, hair, and clothing with soapy water is extremely important. Decontamination must be done carefully to avoid abrasions, which increase organophosphate absorption.

Bardin PG, Van Eeden SF: Organophosphate poisoning: Grading the severity and comparing treatment between atropine and glycopyrrolate. Crit Care Med 1990;8:956.

Borowitz SM: Prolonged organophosphate toxicity in a 26-month-old child. J Pediatr 1988;112:302.

Chaturvedi AK et al: Toxicological evaluation of a poisoning attributed to ingestion of malathion inspect spray and correlation with in vitro inhibition of cholinesterases. Hum Toxicol 1989;8:11.

3. CARBAMATES (Carbaryl, Sevin, Zectran, etc)

Carbamate insecticides are reversible inhibitors of cholinesterase. The signs and symptoms of intoxication are similar to those associated with organophosphate poisoning but are generally less severe. Atropine titrated to effect is sufficient treatment. Pralidoxime should not be used with carbaryl poisoning but is of value with other carbamates. In combined exposures to organophosphates, give atropine but reserve pralidoxime for cases in which the red cell cholinesterase is depressed below 25% of normal or marked effects of nicotinic receptor stimulation are present.

Harris LW et al: The relationship between oxime induced reactivation of carbamylated acetylcholinesterase and antidotal efficacy against carbamate intoxication. Toxicol Appl Pharmacol 1989;98:128.

4. BOTANICAL INSECTICIDES (Black Flag Bug Killer, Black Leaf CPR Insect Killer, Flit Aerosol House & Garden Insect Killer, French's Flea Powder, Raid, etc)

Allergic reactions, asthma-like symptoms, coma, and convulsions have been seen. Pyrethrins, allethrin, ryania, and rotenone do not commonly cause signs of toxicity. Antihistamines, short-acting barbiturates, and atropine are helpful as symptomatic treatment.

IRON

Five stages of intoxication occur following iron intoxication: (1) Hemorrhagic gastroenteritis, which occurs 30–60 minutes after ingestion and may be associated with shock, acidosis, coagulation defects, and coma. This phase usually lasts 4–6 hours. (2) Phase of improvement, lasting 2–12 hours, during which patient looks better. (3) Delayed shock, which may occur 12–48 hours after ingestion and is usually associated with a serum iron level greater than 500 μg/dL. Metabolic acidosis, fever, leukocytosis, and coma may also be present. (4) Liver damage with hepatic failure. (5) Residual pyloric stenosis, which may develop about 4 weeks after the ingestion.

Once iron is absorbed from the gastrointestinal tract, it is not normally eliminated in feces but may be partially excreted in the urine, giving it a red color prior to chelation. A reddish discoloration of the urine suggests a serum iron level greater than 350 μg/dL.

Treatment

Gastrointestinal decontamination is based on clinical assessment. Syrup of ipecac may be administered at home, with appropriate follow-up, provided the history does not warrant an emergency department visit. The patient should be referred to a health care facility if symptomatic or if the history indicates toxic amounts. Gastric lavage and whole bowel irrigation should be considered in these patients.

Shock must be treated in the usual manner. Sodium bicarbonate or Fleet's Phospho-Soda left in the stomach to form the insoluble phosphate or carbonate have not shown clinical benefit and have caused lethal hypernatremia or hyperphosphatemia. Deferoxamine, a specific chelating agent for iron, is a useful adjunct in the treatment of severe iron poisoning. It forms a soluble complex that is excreted in the urine. It is contraindicated in patients with renal failure unless dialysis can be used. Institute intravenous deferoxamine chelation therapy if the patient is symptomatic and a serum iron determination cannot be readily obtained, or if the peak serum iron exceeds 400 μg/dL (62.6 μmol/L) at 4–5 hours after ingestion.

Deferoxamine should not be delayed until serum iron levels are available in serious cases of poisoning. Intravenous administration is indicated if the patient is in shock, in which case it should be given at a dosage of 15 mg/kg/h. Infusion rates up to 35 mg/kg/h have been used in life-threatening poisonings. Rapid intravenous administration can cause hypotension, facial flushing, urticaria, tachycardia, and shock. Deferoxamine, 90 mg/kg intramuscularly every 8 hours (maximum, 1 g), may be given if intravenous access cannot be established, but the procedure is painful. The drug should not be given orally. The indications for discontinuation of deferoxamine have not been clearly delineated. Generally, it can be stopped after 12–24 hours if the acidosis has resolved and the patient is improving.

Hemodialysis, peritoneal dialysis, or exchange transfusion can be used to increase the excretion of the dialyzable complex. Urine output should be monitored and urine sediment examined for evidence of renal tubular damage. Initial laboratory studies should include blood typing and cross-matching; total protein; serum iron, sodium, potassium, and chloride; CO_2; pH; and liver function tests. Serum iron levels fall rapidly even if deferoxamine is not given.

After the acute episode, liver function studies and an upper gastrointestinal series are indicated to rule out residual damage.

Chyka DA, Butler AY: Assessment of acute iron poisoning by laboratory and clinical observations. Am J Emerg Med 1993;11:99.

Mann KV et al: Management of acute iron overdose. Clin Pharm 1989;8:428.

Schauben JL et al: Iron poisoning: Report of three cases and a review of therapeutic intervention. J Emerg Med 1990;8:309.

LEAD

Lead poisoning causes vague symptoms, including weakness, irritability, weight loss, vomiting, personality changes, ataxia, constipation, headache, and colicky abdominal pain. Late manifestations consist of retarded development, convulsions, and coma associated with increased intracranial pressure. The latter is a medical emergency.

Plumbism usually occurs insidiously in children under 5 years of age. The most likely sources of lead include flaking leaded paint, artist's paints, fruit tree sprays, solder, brass alloys, home-glazed pottery, and fumes from burning batteries. Only paint containing less than 1% lead is safe for interior use (furniture, toys, etc). Repetitive ingestions of small amounts of lead are far more serious than a single massive exposure. Toxic effects are likely to occur if more than 0.5 mg of lead per day is absorbed.

Blood lead levels are used to assess the severity of exposure. A complete blood count and serum ferritin concentration should be obtained; iron deficiency increases absorption of lead. Glycosuria, proteinuria, hematuria, and aminoaciduria occur frequently. Blood lead levels usually exceed 80 µg/dL in symptomatic patients. Abnormal blood lead levels should be repeated in asymptomatic patients to rule out laboratory error. Specimens must be meticulously obtained in acid-washed containers. A normocytic, slightly hypochromic anemia with basophilic stippling of the red cells and reticulocytosis may be present in plumbism. Stippling of red blood cells is absent in cases involving only recent ingestion.

The cerebrospinal fluid protein is elevated, and the white cell count is usually less than 100 cells/mL. Cerebrospinal fluid pressure may be elevated in patients with encephalopathy; lumbar punctures must be performed cautiously to prevent herniation.

Treatment

Standard gastrointestinal decontamination is indicated if an acute ingestion has occurred or lead is noted on the abdominal x-ray. Succimer is 2,3-dimercaptosuccinic acid, an orally administered chelator approved for use in children only and reported to be as efficacious as calcium edetate. Treatment for children with blood lead levels of 20–45 µg/dL has not been determined. Succimer should be initiated at blood lead levels over 45 µg/dL. The initial dose is 10 mg/kg (350 mg/m^2) every 8 hours for 5 days. The same dose is then given every 12 hours for 14 days. At least 2 weeks should elapse between courses. Blood lead levels increase somewhat ("rebound") after discontinuation of therapy. Courses of dimercaprol (4 mg/kg/dose) and calcium edetate may still be used but are no longer the preferred method, except in cases of lead encephalopathy.

Anticonvulsants may be needed. Mannitol or corticosteroids and volume restriction are indicated in patients with encephalopathy. A high-calcium, high-phosphorus diet and large doses of vitamin D may remove lead from the blood by depositing it in the bones. A public health team should evaluate the source of the lead. Necessary corrections should be completed before the child is returned home.

Chisholm J et al: Recognition and management of children with increased lead absorption. Arch Dis Child 1979; 54:249.

Graziano JG et al: Controlled study of meso-2,3-dimercaptosuccinicacid for the management of childhood lead intoxication. J Pediatr 1992;120:133.

Lin-Fu J: Lead exposure among children: A reassessment. N Engl J Med 1979;300:731.

Needleman HL et al: The long term effects of exposure to low doses of lead in childhood: An 11-year follow-up report. N Engl J Med 1990;322:83.

MUSHROOMS

Toxic mushrooms are often difficult to distinguish from edible varieties. Symptoms vary with the species ingested, time of year, stage of maturity, quantity eaten, method of preparation, and interval since ingestion. A mushroom that is toxic to one individual may not be toxic for another. Drinking alcohol and eating certain mushrooms may cause a reaction similar to that seen with disulfiram and alcohol. Cooking destroys some toxins but not the deadly one produced by *Amanita phalloides,* which is responsible for 90% of deaths due to mushroom poisoning. Mushrooms toxins are absorbed relatively slowly. Onset of symptoms within 2 hours of ingestion suggests muscarinic toxin, whereas a delay of symptoms for 6–48 hours after ingestion strongly suggests *Amanita* (amatoxin) poisoning. Patients who have ingested *A phalloides* may relapse and die of hepatic or renal failure following initial improvement.

Mushroom poisoning may be manifested by muscarinic symptoms (salivation, vomiting, diarrhea, cramping abdominal pain, tenesmus, miosis, and dyspnea), coma, convulsions, hallucinations, hemolysis, and delayed hepatic and renal failure.

Treatment

Induce vomiting and follow with activated charcoal and a saline cathartic. If the patient has muscarinic signs, give atropine, 0.05 mg/kg intramuscularly (0.02 mg/kg in toddlers), and repeat as needed (usually every 30 minutes) to keep the patient atropinized. Atropine, however, is only used when there are cholinergic effects and not for all mushrooms. Hypoglycemia is most likely to occur in patients with delayed onset of symptoms. Try to identify the mushroom if the patient is symptomatic. Local botanical gardens, university departments of botany, and societies of mycologists may be able to help. Supportive care is usually all that is needed except in the case of A phalloides, where penicillin, silibinin, or hemodialysis may be indicated.

Lampe KF, McCann MA: Differential diagnosis of poisoning by North American mushrooms, with particular emphasis on *Amanita phalloides*-like intoxication. Ann Emerg Med 1987;16:956.

Spoerke DG, Rumack BH (editors): *Mushroom Poisoning, Diagnosis and Treatment,* 2nd ed. CRC Press, 1994.

NITRITES, NITRATES, ANILINE, PENTACHLOROPHENOL, & DINITROPHENOL

Nausea, vertigo, vomiting, cyanosis (methemoglobinemia), cramping abdominal pain, tachycardia, cardiovascular collapse, tachypnea, coma, shock, convulsions, and death are possible manifestations of nitrite or nitrate poisoning.

Nitrite and nitrate compounds found in the home include amyl nitrite, butyl nitrates, isobutyl nitrates, nitroglycerin, pentaerythritol tetranitrate, sodium nitrite, nitrobenzene, and phenazopyridine. Pentachlorophenol and dinitrophenol, which are found in wood preservatives, produce methemoglobinemia and high fever because of uncoupling of oxidative phosphorylation. Headache, dizziness, and bradycardia have been reported. High concentrations of nitrites in water or spinach have been the most common cause of nitrite-induced methemoglobinemia. Symptoms do not usually occur until 15–50% of the hemoglobin has been converted to methemoglobin. A rapid test is to compare a drop of normal blood with the patient's blood on a dry filter paper. Brown discoloration of the patient's blood indicates a methemoglobin level of more than 15%.

Treatment

Induce vomiting, administer activated charcoal, and follow with a cathartic. Decontaminate affected skin with soap and water. Oxygen and artificial respiration may be needed. If the blood methemoglobin level exceeds 30%, or if levels cannot be obtained and the patient is symptomatic, give a 1% solution of methylene blue, 0.2 mL/kg intravenously over 5–10 minutes. Avoid perivascular infiltration, because it causes necrosis of the skin and subcutaneous tissues. A dramatic change in the degree of cyanosis should occur. Transfusion is occasionally necessary. Epinephrine and other vasoconstrictors are contraindicated. If reflex bradycardia occurs, atropine should be used.

Bardoczky GI, Wathieu M, D'Hollander A: Prilocaine-induced methemoglobinemia evidenced by pulse oximetry. Acta Anaesthesiol Scand 1990;34:162.

Caudill L, Walbridge J, Kuhn G: Methemoglobinemia as a cause of coma. Ann Emerg Med 1990;19:677.

Kaplan A et al: Methaemoglobinaemia due to accidental sodium nitrite poisoning: Report of 10 cases. S Afr Med J 1990;77:300.

OPIOIDS*
(Codeine, Heroin, Methadone, Morphine, Propoxyphene)

Opioid-related medical problems may include drug addiction, withdrawal in a newborn infant, and accidental overdoses. Unlike other narcotics, methadone is readily absorbed from the gastrointestinal tract. Most opioids, including heroin, methadone, meperidine, morphine, and codeine, are excreted in the urine within 24 hours and can be readily detected.

Adolescent narcotic addicts often have other medical problems, including cellulitis, abscesses, thrombophlebitis, tetanus, infective endocarditis, HIV infection, tuberculosis, hepatitis, malaria, foreign body emboli, thrombosis of pulmonary arterioles, diabetes mellitus, obstetric complications, nephropathy, and peptic ulcer.

Treatment of Overdosage

Opioids can cause respiratory depression, stridor, coma, increased oropharyngeal secretions, sinus bradycardia, and urinary retention. Pulmonary edema rarely occurs in children; deaths usually result from aspiration of gastric contents, respiratory arrest, and cerebral edema, singly or in combination. Convulsions may occur with propoxyphene overdosage.

Although suggested doses for naloxone hydrochloride range from 0.01 to 0.1 mg/kg, it is generally unnecessary to calculate the dosage on this basis. This extremely safe antidote should be given in sufficient quantity to reverse opioid binding sites. For children under 1 year of age, 1 ampule (0.4 mg) should be given initially; if there is no response, give five more ampules (2 mg) rapidly. Older children should be given 0.4–0.8 mg, followed by 2.0–4.0 mg if there is no response. An improvement in respiratory status may be followed by respiratory depression, because the depressant action of narcotics may last 24–48 hours but the antagonist's duration of action is less than 1 hour. Neonates poisoned in utero may require 10–30 µg/kg to reverse the effect.

Withdrawal in the Addict

The severity of withdrawal signs should be evaluated as explained on p 000. Seizures and hallucinations are almost always associated with concomitant withdrawal from sedative-hypnotics.

Diazepam, 10 mg every 6 hours orally, has been recommended for the treatment of mild narcotic withdrawal in ambulatory adolescents. Management of withdrawal in the confirmed addict may be accomplished with the administration of clonidine, by substitution with methadone, or with reintroduction of the original addicting agent, if available through a

---

*Diphenoxylate poisoning is discussed on p 000.

supervised drug withdrawal program. A tapered course over 3 weeks will accomplish this goal. Death rarely, if ever, occurs. The abrupt discontinuation of narcotics (cold turkey method) is not recommended and may cause severe physical withdrawal signs.

Withdrawal in the Newborn

A newborn infant in narcotic withdrawal is usually small for gestational age and demonstrates yawning, sneezing, decreased Moro reflex, hunger but uncoordinated sucking action, jitteriness, tremor, constant movement, a shrill protracted cry, increased tendon reflexes, convulsions, vomiting, fever, watery diarrhea, cyanosis, dehydration, vasomotor instability, seizure, and collapse. The onset of symptoms commonly begins in the first 48 hours but may be delayed as long as 8 days depending upon the timing of the mother's last fix and her predelivery medication. The diagnosis can be easily confirmed by identifying the narcotic in the urine of the mother and baby.

Several methods of treatment have been suggested for narcotic withdrawal in the newborn. Phenobarbital, 8 mg/kg/d intramuscularly or orally in four doses for 4 days and then reduced by one third every 2 days as signs decrease, may be continued for as long as 3 weeks. Methadone may be necessary in those infants with congenital methadone addiction who are not controlled in their withdrawal by large doses of phenobarbital. Dosage should be 0.5 mg/kg/d in two divided doses but can be gradually increased as needed. Slow tapering off may be necessary over 4 weeks for methadone addiction.

It is not clear whether prophylactic treatment with these drugs decreases the complication rate. The mortality rate of untreated narcotic withdrawal in the newborn may be as high as 45%.

AAP Committee on Drugs: Emergency drug doses for infants and children and naloxone use in newborns: Clarification. Pediatrics 1989;83:803.

Bradberry JC, Raebel MA: Continuous infusion of naloxone in the treatment of narcotic overdose. Drug Intell Clin Pharm 1981;15:945.

Reddy AM, Harper RG, Stern G: Observations on heroin and methadone withdrawal in newborn. Pediatrics 1971; 48:353.

PHENOTHIAZINES
(Chlorpromazine, Prochlorperazine, Trifluoperazine)

Clinical Presentations

A. Extrapyramidal Crisis: Episodes characterized by torticollis, stiffening of the body, spasticity, poor speech, catatonia, and inability to communicate although conscious are typical manifestations. These episodes usually last a few seconds to a few minutes but have rarely caused death. Extrapyramidal crises may represent idiosyncratic reactions and are aggravated by dehydration. The signs and symptoms occur most often in children who have received prochlorperazine. They are commonly mistaken for psychotic episodes.

B. Overdose: Lethargy and deep prolonged coma commonly occur. Promazine, chlorpromazine, and prochlorperazine are the drugs most likely to cause respiratory depression and precipitous drops in blood pressure. Occasionally, paradoxic hyperactivity and extrapyramidal signs as well as hyperglycemia and acetonemia are present. Seizures are uncommon.

Treatment

Extrapyramidal signs are alleviated within minutes by the slow intravenous administration of diphenhydramine, 1–2 mg/kg (maximum, 50 mg), or benztropine mesylate, 1–2 mg intravenously (1 mg/min). No other treatment is usually indicated.

Patients with overdoses should be treated conservatively. Vomiting should be induced with ipecac followed by administration of activated charcoal. Emetics are often unsuccessful because phenothiazines are potent antiemetics; gastric lavage may be the only practical way to remove gastric contents. Hypotension may be treated with standard agents, starting with isotonic saline administration. Agitation is best treated with diazepam. Neuroleptic malignant syndrome may be treated with dantrolene, 1 mg/kg (maximum, 50 mg) every 12 hours.

Baker PB et al: Hyperthermia, hypertension, hypertonia, and coma in massive thioridazine overdose. Am J Emerg Med 1988;6:346.

Sanders KM, Minnema AM, Murray GB: Low incidence of extrapyramidal symptoms in treatment of delirium with intravenous haloperidol and lorazepam in the intensive care unit. J Intens Care Med 1989;4:201.

PLANTS

Many common ornamental, garden, and wild plants are potentially toxic. Only in a few cases will small amounts of a plant cause severe illness or death. Table 12–10 lists the most toxic plants, symptoms and signs of poisoning, and treatment.

Frohne D, Pfander HJ: *A Colour Atlas of Poisonous Plants.* Wolfe, 1984.

Lampe KF, McCann MA: *AMA Handbook of Poisonous and Injurious Plants.* American Medical Association, 1985.

Table 12–10. Poisoning due to plants.[1]

	Symptoms and Signs	Treatment
Arum family: *Caladium, Dieffenbachia,* calla lily, dumb cane (oxalic acid)	Burning of mucous membranes and airway obstruction secondary to edema caused by calcium oxalate crystals.	Accessible areas should be thoroughly washed. Corticosteroids relieve airway obstruction. Apply cold packs to affected mucous membranes.
Castor bean plant (ricin—a toxalbumin) Jequinty bean (abrin—a toxalbumin)	Mucous membrane irritation, nausea, vomiting, bloody diarrhea, blurred vision, circulatory collapse, acute hemolytic anemia, convulsions, uremia.	Fluid and electrolyte monitoring. Saline cathartic. Forced alkaline diuresis will prevent complications due to hemagglutination and hemolysis.
Foxglove, lily of the valley, and oleander[2]	Nausea, diarrhea, visual disturbances, and cardiac irregularities (eg, heart block).	See treatment for digitalis drugs in text (p 307)
Jimsonweed: See Belladonna Alkaloids, p 304	Mydnasis, dry mouth, tachycardia, and hallucinations.	Atropine.
Larkspur (ajacine, *Delphinium,* delphinine)	Nausea and vomiting, irritability, muscular paralysis, and CNS depression.	Symptomatic. Atropine may be helpful.
Monkshood (aconite)	Numbness of mucous membranes, visual disturbances, tingling, dizziness, tinnitus, hypotension, bradycardia, and convulsions.	Activated charcoal, oxygen. Atropine is probably helpful.
Poison hemlock (coniine)	Mydnasis, trembling, dizziness, bradycardia. CNS depression, muscular paralysis, and convulsions. Death is due to respiratory paralysis.	Symptomatic. Oxygen and cardiac monitoring equipment are desirable. Assisted respiration is often necessary. Give anticonvulsants if needed.
Rhododendron (grayanotoxin)	Abdominal cramps, vomiting, severe diarrhea, muscular paralysis, CNS and circulatory depression. Hypertension with very large doses.	Atropine can prevent bradycardia. Epinephrine is contraindicated. Antihypertensives may be needed.
Yellow jessamine (active ingredient, geisemine, is related to strychnine)	Restlessness, convulsions, muscular paralysis, and respiratory depression.	Symptomatic. Because of the relation to strychnine, activated charcoal and diazepam for seizures is worth trying.

[1]Many other plants cause minor irritation but are not likely to cause serious problems unless large amounts are ingested. See Lampe KF, McCann MA: *AMA Handbook of Poisonous and Injurious Plants.* American Medical Association, 1985. See also Rumack BH, Spoerke DG (editors): *POISINDEX® Information System.* Micromedex, IAC, Denver, Colorado. [Published quarterly.]
[2]Done AK: Ornamental and deadly. Emerg Med (April) 1973;5:255.

PSYCHOTROPIC DRUGS

Psychotropic drugs consist of four general classes: stimulants (amphetamines, cocaine), depressants (eg, narcotics, barbiturates), antidepressants and tranquilizers, and hallucinogens (eg, LSD, PCP).

The following clinical findings are commonly seen in patients abusing drugs:

Stimulants. Agitation, euphoria, grandiose feelings, tachycardia, fever, abdominal cramps, visual and auditory hallucinations, mydriasis, coma, convulsions, and respiratory depression.

Depressants. Emotional lability, ataxia, diplopia, nystagmus, vertigo, poor accommodation, respiratory depression, coma, apnea, and convulsions. Dilatation of conjunctival blood vessels suggests marijuana ingestion. Narcotics cause miotic pupils and, occasionally, pulmonary edema.

Antidepressants and tranquilizers. Hypotension, lethargy, respiratory depression, coma, and extrapyramidal reactions.

Hallucinogens and psychoactive drugs. Belladonna alkaloids cause mydriasis, dry mouth, nausea, vomiting, urinary retention, confusion, disorientation, paranoid delusions, hallucinations, fever, hypotension, aggressive behavior, convulsions, and coma. **Psychoactive drugs** such as LSD cause mydriasis, unexplained bizarre behavior, hallucinations, and generalized undifferentiated psychotic behavior.

See also other entries discussed in alphabetic sequence in this chapter.

Management of the Patient Who Abuses Drugs

Only a small percentage of the persons using drugs come to the attention of physicians; those who do are usually suffering from adverse reactions such as panic states, drug psychoses, homicidal or suicidal thoughts, or respiratory depression.

Even with cooperative patients, an accurate history is difficult to obtain. The user often does not really know what drug has been taken or how much. "Street drugs" are almost always adulterated with one or more other compounds. Multiple drugs are often taken together, making it impossible to clinically define the type of drug. Friends may be a useful source of information. A drug history is most easily obtained in a quiet spot by a gentle, nonthreatening, honest examiner.

The general appearance, skin, lymphatics, cardiorespiratory status, gastrointestinal tract, and central nervous system should be stressed during the physical examination, because they often provide clues suggesting drug abuse. A drug history should not be taken from an adolescent in the parents' presence.

Hallucinogens are not life-threatening unless the patient is frankly homicidal or suicidal. A specific diagnosis is usually not necessary for management; instead, the presenting signs and symptoms are treated. Does the patient appear intoxicated? In withdrawal? "Flashing back?" Is some illness or injury (eg, head trauma) being masked by a drug effect? (Remember that a known drug user may still have hallucinations from meningoencephalitis.)

The signs and symptoms in a given patient are a function of not only the drug and the dose but also the level of acquired tolerance, the "setting," the patient's physical condition and personality traits, the potentiating effects of other drugs, and many other factors.

A common drug problem is the "bad trip," which is usually a panic reaction. This is best managed by "talking the patient down" and minimizing auditory and visual stimuli. Sitting with a friend while the drug effect dissipates may be the best treatment that can be offered. This may take several hours. The physician's job is not to terminate the drug effect but to help the patient over the bad experience.

Drug therapy is often unnecessary and may complicate the clinical course of a patient with a panic reaction. Although phenothiazines have been commonly used to treat "bad trips," they should be avoided if the specific drug is not known, because they may enhance toxicity or produce unwanted side effects. Diazepam is the drug of choice if a sedative effect is required. Physical restraints are rarely indicated and usually increase the patient's panic reaction.

For treatment of life-threatening drug abuse, consult the section on the specific drug elsewhere in this chapter and the section on general management at the beginning of the chapter.

After the acute episode, the physician must decide whether psychiatric referral is indicated; in general, patients who have made suicidal gestures or attempts and adolescents who are not communicating with their families should be referred.

Cohen S: The "angel dust" states: Phencyclidine. Pediatr Rev 1979;1:17.
Smith D et al: PCP problems and prevention. J Psychedelic Drugs 1980;12:181.

SALICYLATES

The use of childproof containers and publicity regarding accidental poisoning have reduced the incidence of acute salicylate poisoning. Nevertheless, serious intoxication still occurs and must be regarded as an emergency.

Salicylates uncouple oxidative phosphorylation, leading to increased heat production, excessive sweating, and dehydration. They also interfere with glucose metabolism and may cause hypoglycemia or hyperglycemia. Respiratory center stimulation occurs early.

Patients usually have signs of hyperventilation, sweating, dehydration, and fever. Vomiting and diarrhea sometimes occur. In severe cases, disorientation, convulsions, and coma may develop.

The severity of acute intoxication can in some measure be judged by serum salicylate levels (Figure 12–10). High levels are always dangerous irrespective of clinical signs, and low levels may be misleading in chronic cases. Other laboratory values usually indicate metabolic acidosis despite hyperventilation; low serum K^+ values; and often abnormal serum glucose levels.

Salicylate poisoning is classified as mild when plasma pH is greater than 7.4 and urine pH is greater than 6.0; as moderate when plasma pH is greater than 7.4 and urine pH is less than 6.0; and as severe when plasma pH is less than 7.4 and urine pH is less than 6.0.

In mild and moderate poisoning, stimulation of the respiratory center produces respiratory alkalosis. In severe intoxication (seen in severe acute ingestion with high salicylate levels and in chronic toxicity with lower levels), respiratory response is unable to overcome the metabolic overdose.

Once the urine becomes acidic, progressively smaller amounts of salicylate are excreted. Until this process is reversed, the half-life will remain prolonged, because metabolism contributes little to the removal of salicylate.

Chronic severe poisoning may be seen as early as 3 days after a regimen of salicylate is begun. Find-

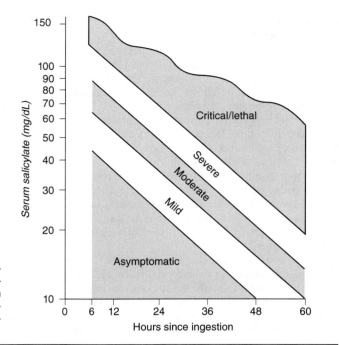

Figure 12–10. Nomogram relating serum salicylate concentration and expected severity of intoxication at varying intervals following ingestion of a single dose of salicylate. (Redrawn and reproduced, with permission, from Done AK: Salicylate intoxication. Pediatrics 1960;26:800.)

ings usually include vomiting, diarrhea, and dehydration.

Treatment

Charcoal binds salicylates well and, after emesis or lavage, should be given for acute ingestions. Mild poisoning may require only the administration of oral fluids and confirmation that the salicylate level is falling. Moderate poisoning is reflected by moderate dehydration and depletion of potassium. Fluids must be administered to correct dehydration and produce urine with a pH of greater than 7.0 at a rate of 2–3 mL/kg/h. Initial intravenous solutions should be isotonic, with sodium bicarbonate constituting half the electrolyte content. Once the patient is rehydrated, the solution can contain more free water and approximately 40 meq of potassium per liter.

Severe ingestion is marked by major dehydration in cases of chronic poisoning. Symptoms may be confused with those of Reye's syndrome, encephalopathy, and metabolic acidosis. Salicylate levels may even be in the "therapeutic range." Major fluid correction of dehydration is required. Once this has been accomplished, hypokalemia must be corrected and sodium bicarbonate given. Usual requirements are sodium bicarbonate, 1–2 meq/kg/h over the first 6–8 hours, and K+, 20–40 meq/L. A urine flow of 2–3 mL/kg/h should be established.

Vitamin K should be administered, although bleeding is rare except in severely poisoned patients.

Renal failure or pulmonary edema is an indication for dialysis. Hemodialysis is most effective and peritoneal dialysis relatively ineffective. Acetazolamide should not be used.

Keller RE, Schwab RA, Krenzelok EP: Contribution of sorbitol combined with activated charcoal in prevention of salicylate absorption. Ann Emerg Med 1990;19:654.
Snodgrass W et al: Salicylate toxicity following therapeutic doses in young children. Clin Toxicol 1981;18:247.

SCORPION STINGS

Scorpion stings are common in arid areas of the southwestern USA. Scorpion venom is more toxic than most snake venoms, but only minute amounts are injected. Although neurologic manifestations may last a week, most clinical signs subside within 24–48 hours.

The most common scorpions in the USA are members of the *Vejovis, Hadrurus, Androctonus,* and *Centruroides* species. Stings by the first three produce edema and pain. Stings by *Centruroides* cause tingling or burning paresthesias that begin at the site of the sting; other findings include hypersalivation, restlessness, muscular fasciculation, abdominal cramps, opisthotonos, convulsions, urinary incontinence, and respiratory failure.

Treatment

Sedation is the primary therapy. In severe cases, the airway may become compromised by secretions and weakness of respiratory muscles. Endotracheal intubation may be required. Patients may require treatment for seizures, hypertension, or tachycardia.

The prognosis is good as long as the airway is managed appropriately.

Bond GR: Antivenom administration for *Centruroides* scorpion sting: Risks, benefits. (Abstract.) Vet Hum Toxicol 1990;32:367.

Rachesky IJ et al: Treatments for *Centruroides exilicauda* envenomation. Am J Dis Child 1984;138:1136.

SNAKEBITE

Despite the lethal potential of venomous snakes, human morbidity and mortality rates are surprisingly low. The outcome depends on the size of the child, the site of the bite, the degree of envenomation, the type of snake, and the effectiveness of treatment.

Ninety-eight percent of poisonous snakebites in the USA are caused by pit vipers (rattlesnakes, water moccasins, and copperheads). A few are caused by elapids (coral snakes), and occasional bites occur from cobras and other nonindigenous exotic snakes kept as pets. Snake venom is a complex mixture of enzymes, peptides, and proteins that may have predominantly cytotoxic, neurotoxic, hemotoxic, or cardiotoxic effects but other effects as well. Up to 25% of bites by pit vipers do not result in venom injection.

Pit viper venom is predominantly caused by a severe local reaction with pain, discoloration, and edema, as well as hemorrhage.

Swelling and pain occur soon after rattlesnake bite and are a certain indication that envenomation has occurred. During the first few hours, swelling and ecchymosis extend proximally from the bite. The bite is often obvious as a double puncture mark surrounded by ecchymosis. Hematemesis, melena, hemoptysis, and other manifestations of coagulopathy develop in severe cases. Respiratory difficulty and shock are the ultimate causes of death. Even in fatal rattlesnake bite, there is usually a period of 6–8 hours between the bite and death; there is, therefore, usually enough time to start effective treatment.

Coral snake envenomation causes little local pain, swelling, or necrosis, and systemic reactions are often delayed. The signs of coral snake envenomation include bulbar paralysis, dysphagia, and dysphoria; these may appear in 5–10 hours and may be followed by total peripheral paralysis and death in 24 hours.

Treatment

Children in snake-infested areas should wear boots and long trousers, should not walk barefoot, and should be cautioned not to explore under ledges or in holes.

The treatment of snakebite envenomation is controversial, but the following approach seems most useful.

A. Emergency (First Aid) Treatment: The most important first aid measure is transportation to a medical facility. Splint the affected extremity and minimize the patient's motion. Tourniquets and ice packs are contraindicated. Incision and suction are not useful for either crotalid or elapid snake bite. High vacuum suction (Extractor) has been shown to remove venom in a rabbit model. Its value in humans is unknown.

B. Definitive Medical Management: Blood should be drawn for hematocrit, clotting time and platelet function, and serum electrolyte determinations. Establish two secure intravenous sites for the administration of antivenin and other medications.

Specific antivenin is indicated when signs of progressive envenomation are present. Polyvalent pit viper antivenin and eastern coral snake antivenin (Wyeth Laboratories) are available from hospital pharmacies. There is no antivenin for the western coral snake. If horse serum sensitivity tests are negative, antivenin should be given intravenously over 1 hour. For pit vipers, give 5–8 vials for minimal, 8–15 vials for moderate, and 15 or more vials for severe envenomation. Dilute each vial to 50–200 mL. (Antivenin should not be given intramuscularly or subcutaneously.) Epinephrine, 0.3 mL of 1:1000 solution, should be drawn up in a syringe before antivenin is administered. Hemorrhage, pain, and shock are rapidly diminished by adequate amounts of antivenin. For coral snakes, give three to five vials of antivenin in 250–500 mL of isotonic saline solution. An additional three to five vials may be required.

Codeine, 1–1.5 mg/kg per dose orally, or meperidine, 0.6–1.5 mg/kg per dose orally or intramuscularly, is necessary to control pain. Cryotherapy is contraindicated because it commonly causes additional tissue damage. Early physiotherapy minimizes contractures. In rare cases, fasciotomy to relieve pressure within muscular compartments is required. The evaluation of function as well as of pulses will better predict the need for fasciotomy. Corticosteroids (hydrocortisone, 1–2 g intravenously every 4–6 hours) are useful in the treatment of serum sickness or anaphylactic shock. Antibiotics are not needed unless clinical signs of infection occur. Tetanus status should be evaluated and treated, if needed.

Kitchens CS, Van Mierop LHS: Envenomation by the eastern coral snake *(Micrurus fulvius)*: A study of 39 victims. JAMA 1987;258:1615.

Russell FE: *Snake Venom Poisoning.* Scholium International, 1983.

SOAPS & DETERGENTS

1. SOAPS

Soap is made from salts of fatty acids. Some toilet soap bars contain both soap and detergent. Ingestion of soap bars may cause vomiting and diarrhea, but they have a low toxicity. Induced emesis is unnecessary.

2. DETERGENTS

Detergents are nonsoap synthetic products used for cleaning purposes because of their surfactant properties. Commercial products include granules, powders, and liquids. Dishwasher detergents are very alkaline and can cause caustic burns. Low concentrations of bleaching and antibacterial agents as well as enzymes are found in many preparations. The pure compounds are moderately toxic, but the concentration used is too small to alter the product's toxicity significantly, although occasional primary or allergic irritative phenomena have been noted in housewives and in employees manufacturing these products.

Cationic Detergents (Ceepryn, Diaperene, Phemerol, Zephiran)

Cationic detergents in dilute solutions (0.5%) cause mucosal irritation, but higher concentrations (10–15%) may cause caustic burns to mucosa. Clinical effects include nausea, vomiting, collapse, coma, and convulsions. As little as 2.25 g of some cationic agents have caused death in an adult. In four cases, 100–400 mg/kg of benzalkonium chloride caused death. Cationic detergents are rapidly inactivated by tissues and ordinary soap.

Because of the caustic potential and rapid onset of seizures, emesis is not recommended. Activated charcoal and a cathartic should be administered. Anticonvulsants may be needed.

Anionic Detergents

Most common household detergents are anionic. Laundry compounds have water softener (sodium phosphate) added, which is a strong irritant and may reduce ionized calcium. Anionic detergents irritate the skin by removing natural oils. Although ingestion causes diarrhea, intestinal distention, and vomiting, no fatalities have been reported.

The only treatment usually required is to discontinue use if skin irritation occurs and replace fluids and electrolytes. Induced vomiting is not indicated following ingestion of electric dishwasher detergent, because of its alkalinity. Dilute with water or milk.

Nonionic Detergents (Brij Products; Tritons X-45, X-100, X-102, & X-144)

These compounds include lauryl, stearyl, and oleyl alcohols and octyl phenol. They have a minimal irritating effect on the skin and are almost nontoxic when swallowed.

Deichmann WB, Gerarde HW: Hazards of alkaline laundry detergents. JAMA 1972;220:1014.

Enzyme detergents. (Editorial.) Br Med J 1970;1:518.

Jeven JE: Severe dermatitis and "biological" detergents. Br Med J 1970;1:299.

SPIDER BITES

Most medically important bites in the USA are caused by the black widow spider (*Latrodectus mactans*) and the North American brown recluse (violin) spider (*Loxosceles reclusa*). It is helpful if positive identification of the spider can be made, since many spider bites may mimic those of the brown recluse spider.

Black Widow Spider

The black widow spider is endemic to nearly all areas of the United States. The initial bite causes sharp fleeting pain. Local and systemic muscular cramping, abdominal pain, nausea and vomiting, and shock can occur. Convulsions are more commonly seen in small children. Systemic signs of black widow spider bite may be confused with other causes of acute abdomen. Although paresthesias, nervousness, and transient muscle spasms may persist for weeks in survivors, recovery from the acute phase is generally complete within 3 days. In contrast to popular opinion, death is extremely rare.

Most authors recommend calcium gluconate as initial therapy (50 mg/kg intravenously per dose, up to 250 mg/kg/24 h), although it is often not effective and the effects are of short duration. Methocarbamol (15 mg/kg orally) or diazepam titrated to effect is useful. Morphine or barbiturates may occasionally be needed for control of pain or restlessness, but they increase the possibility of respiratory depression. Antivenin is available but should be reserved for severe cases in which the above therapies have failed. Local treatment of the bite is not helpful.

Brown Recluse Spider (Violin Spider)

The North American brown recluse spider is most commonly seen in the central and midwestern areas of the United States. Its bite characteristically produces a localized reaction with progressively severe pain within 24 hours. The initial bleb on an erythematous ischemic base is replaced by a black eschar within 1 week. This eschar separates in 2–5 weeks, leaving an ulcer that heals slowly. Systemic signs include cyanosis, morbilliform rash, fever, chills, malaise, weakness, nausea and vomiting, joint pains, hemolytic reactions with hemoglobinuria, jaundice, and delirium. Fatalities are rare. Fatal disseminated intravascular coagulation has been reported.

Although of unproved efficacy, the following therapies have been used: dexamethasone, 4 mg intravenously four times a day, during the acute phase; polymorphonuclear leukocyte inhibitors, such as dapsone or colchicine, and oxygen applied to the bite site; and total excision of the lesion to the fascial level.

Alario A et al: Cutaneous necrosis following a spider bite: A case report and review. Pediatrics 1987;79:618.

Vorse H: Disseminated intravascular coagulopathy following fatal brown spider bite. J Pediatr 1971;80:1035.

Wasserman GS, Anderson PC: Loxoscelism and necrotic arachnidism. J Tox Clin Toxicol 1984;21:451.

Yarbrough BE: Current treatment of brown recluse spider bites. Curr Concepts Wound Care 1987;Winter:4.

THYROID PREPARATIONS
(Thyroid Desiccated, Sodium Levothyroxine)

Ingestion of the equivalent of 50–150 g of desiccated thyroid can cause signs of hyperthyroidism, including irritability, mydriasis, hyperpyrexia, tachycardia, and diarrhea. Maximal clinical effect occurs about 9 days after ingestion—several days after the protein-bound iodine level has fallen dramatically.

Induce vomiting. If the patient develops clinical signs of toxicity, propranolol, 0.01–0.1 mg/kg (maximum, 1 mg), is useful because of its antiadrenergic activity.

Golightly LK et al: Clinical effects of accidental levothyroxine ingestion in children. Am J Dis Child 1987;141:1025.

Gorman RL et al: High anxiety-low toxicity: A massive T_4 ingestion. Pediatrics 1988;82:666.

VITAMINS

Accidental ingestion of excessive amounts of vitamins rarely causes significant problems. Occasional cases of hypervitaminosis A and D do occur, however, particularly in patients with poor hepatic or renal function. The fluoride contained in many multivitamin preparations is not a realistic hazard, because a 2- or 3-year-old child could eat 100 tablets, containing 1 mg of sodium fluoride per tablet, without producing serious symptoms. Iron poisoning has been reported with multiple vitamin tablets containing iron. Pyridoxine abuse has caused neuropathies; nicotinic acid, myopathy.

Dalton K, Dalton MJT: Characteristics of pyridoxine overdose neuropathy syndrome. Acta Neurol Scand 1987;76:8.

Dean BS, Krenzelok EP: Multiple vitamins and vitamins with iron: Accidental poisoning in children. Vet Hum Toxicol 1988;30:23.

DiPalma JR, Ritchie DM: Vitamin toxicity. Ann Rev Pharm Tox 1977;17:133.

Litin SC, Anderson CF: Nicotinic acid-associated myopathy: A report of three cases. Am J Med 1989;86:481.

WARFARIN

Warfarin is used as a rodenticide. It causes hypoprothrombinemia and capillary injury. It is readily absorbed from the gastrointestinal tract but is absorbed poorly through the skin. A dose of 0.5 mg/kg of warfarin may be toxic in a child. A prothrombin time is helpful in establishing the severity of the poisoning.

Treatment consists of induced vomiting followed by a saline cathartic. If bleeding occurs or the prothrombin time is prolonged, give 1–5 mg of vitamin K_1 (phytonadione) intramuscularly or subcutaneously. For large ingestions with established toxicity, 0.6 mg/kg may be given.

A new group of long-acting anticoagulant rodenticides (brodifacoum, difenacoum, bromadiolone, diphacinone, pinone, valone, and coumatetralyl) have been a more serious toxicologic problem than warfarin. They also cause hypoprothrombinemia and a bleeding diathesis that responds to phytonadione, though the anticoagulant activity may persist for periods ranging from 6 weeks to several months. Treatment with vitamin K_1 may be needed for weeks.

Smolinske SC et al: Superwarfarin poisoning in children: A prospective study. Pediatrics 1989;84:490.

REFERENCES

Arena JM, Drew RH: *Poisoning: Toxicology, Symptoms, Treatments,* 5th ed. CC Thomas, 1986.

Baselt RC, Cravey RH: *Disposition of Toxic Drugs and Chemicals in Man,* 3rd ed. Year Book, 1989.

Bayer MJ, Rumack BH, Wanke L: *Toxicologic Emergencies: A Manual of Diagnosis and Management.* Brady-Prentice Hall, 1983.

Bresinsky A, Besl H: *A Colour Atlas of Poisonous Fungi: A Handbook for Pharmacists, Doctors, and Biologists.* Wolfe, 1990.

Clayton GD, Clayton FE: *Patty's Industrial Hygiene and Toxicology,* vol 2, 4th ed, Wiley-Interscience, 1993.

Doull J, Klaassen C, Amdur M (editors): *Cassarett and Doull's Toxicology: The Basic Science of Poisons,* 4th ed. Macmillan, 1991.

Ellenhorn MJ, Barceloux DG: *Medical Toxicology: Diagnosis and Treatment of Human Poisoning.* Elsevier, 1988.

Finkel AJ (editor): *Hamilton & Hardy's Industrial Toxicology,* 4th ed. Publishing Sciences Group, 1983.

Goldfrank LR et al: *Goldfrank's Toxicologic Emergencies,* 4th ed. Appleton-Century-Crofts, 1990.

Grant WM: *Toxicology of the Eye,* 3rd ed. CC Thomas, 1986.

Haddad LM, Winchester JF: *Poisoning and Drug Overdose,* 2nd ed. WB Saunders, 1990.

Koren G: *Maternal-Fetal Toxicology: A Clinician's Guide.* Marcel Dekker, 1990.

Lampe KF, McCann MA: *AMA Handbook of Poisonous and Injurious Plants.* American Medical Association, 1985.

Olson KR (editor): *Poisoning and Drug Overdose.* Appleton & Lange, 1990.

Rumack BH, Spoerke DG, Smolinske SC (editors): *POISINDEX Information System.* Micromedex, Inc, Denver, Colorado. [Published quarterly.]

Critical Care

13

Emily L. Dobyns, MD, Anthony G. Durmowicz, MD, Desmond B. Henry, MD,
Stanley Loftness, MD, & Kurt R. Stenmark, MD

INTRODUCTION

Pediatric critical care has evolved into a subspecialty devoted to the understanding of the pathophysiology of life-threatening diseases and to the development of technical facilities for monitoring and treating these patients. The patients often require the attention of multiple specialized services such as an emergency transport service, stabilization in the emergency department, operative treatment, and nutritional support. It is the high level of interdisciplinary collaboration and communication that has improved patient survival in the ICU.

Children are resilient and have tremendous recovery potential, in many cases recovering from injuries that adults would not survive. They may, however, be nonverbal, uncooperative, and unable to understand their illness or the hospital environment, and thus may require the services provided by social workers, psychiatrists, physical therapists, and speech therapists to help their families and themselves cope with their illness. The dynamic features of continuing growth and development must always be factored into the patient and family needs.

The pediatric intensive care unit provides the specialized environment, equipment, and specialists needed to evaluate, diagnose, and treat critically ill patients on a 24-hour basis. This unit permits close observation by experienced team members, thereby permitting rapid responses to changes in the patients' acuity. In many cases, these changes can be anticipated and management plans altered accordingly.

American Academy of Pediatrics Committee on Hospital Care: Guidelines and levels of care for pediatric intensive care units. Crit Care Med 1993;21:1077.

Hazinski MF: Physician-nurse interaction in the paediatric intensive care unit. In: *Textbook of Pediatric Critical Care.* Holbrook PR (editor). Saunders, 1993.

Pollack MM: Outcome analysis. In: *Textbook of Pediatric Critical Care.* Holbrook PR (editor). Saunders, 1993.

ACRONYMS USED IN THIS CHAPTER

ARDS	Adult respiratory distress syndrome
CPAP	Continuous positive airway pressure
CPP	Cerebral perfusion pressure
CT	Computed tomography
ECG	Electrocardiogram
ECMO	Extracorporeal membrane oxygenation
EMLA	Eutectic mixture of lidocaine 2.5% and prilocaine 2.5%
FEV_1	Forced expiratory volume in 1 second
FRC	Functional residual capacity
ICP	Intracranial pressure
ICU	Intensive care unit
IL	Interleukin
IMV	Intermittent mandatory ventilation
MAP	Mean arterial pressure
MRI	Magnetic resonance imaging
NO	Nitric oxide
NSAID	Nonsteroidal anti-inflammatory drug
PCA	Patient-controlled analgesia
PEEP	Positive end-expiratory pressure
PERF	Peak expiratory flow rate
PICU	Pediatric intensive care unit
PVR	Pulmonary vascular resistance
REM	Rapid eye movement
SIMV	Synchronized intermittent mandatory ventilation

ACUTE RESPIRATORY FAILURE

Respiratory failure is defined as inability of the respiratory system to deliver adequate oxygen or to remove CO_2 from the circulation, leading to arterial hypoxia, hypercapnia, or both. It accounts for approximately 50% of deaths of children under 1 year of age. Infants are at higher risk for respiratory failure because their thoracic cage is soft and provides an unstable base for the ribs. Intercostal muscles are poorly developed, so children cannot achieve the "bucket handle" motion that characterizes adult breathing. Furthermore, the diaphragm is less effective in infants because it is relatively flat and short and has fewer type I muscle fibers. During REM sleep, the ventilatory movements of the rib cage become uncoordinated and out of phase with those of the diaphragm. The infant's trachea is only one-third the diameter of the adult trachea, so a 1-mm thickening of the respiratory mucosa causes a 75% reduction in cross-sectional area in the infant airway, compared to only a 20% reduction in the adult airway. Finally, children's alveoli are smaller and have a greater tendency to collapse and cause atelectasis.

Respiratory failure can be classified into two types, which usually coexist in variable proportion. The PaO_2 is low in both, while the $PaCO_2$ is high only in Type II patients (Table 13–1). Type I is the failure of the lung to oxygenate the blood and occurs in three situations: (1) The most common is a **ventilation/perfusion defect** (V/Q mismatch), which occurs when blood flows to parts of the lung that are poorly ventilated or underventilated. (2) **Diffusion defects** are caused by thickened alveolar membrane or a buildup of interstitial fluid at the alveolar-capillary junction. (3) **Intrapulmonary shunt** occurs when blood flows through areas of the lung that are never ventilated.

Type II respiratory failure generally results from alveolar hypoventilation and is usually secondary (Table 13–1). Hypoxemia is not always related to respiratory failure. Right-to-left cardiac shunts, high altitude with its low ambient oxygen concentration, and the production of methemoglobin all may produce severe hypoxemia with normal respiratory function.

Clinical Findings

A. Symptoms & Signs: The clinical findings in respiratory failure are caused by the low PaO_2, high $PaCO_2$, and pH changes affecting the lungs, heart, kidneys, and brain. Clinical features of progressive respiratory failure are summarized in Table 13–2. Hypercapnia depresses the central nervous system, and the resulting acidemia depresses myocardial function. Patients in respiratory failure can exhibit significant changes in central nervous system and cardiac function (Table 13–2). Features of respiratory failure are not always clinically evident, and some signs or symptoms may have nonrespiratory causes. Furthermore, a strictly clinical assessment of arterial hypoxemia or hypercapnia is not reliable. Thus, precise assessment of oxygenation and ventilatory adequacy must be based on both clinical and laboratory data.

B. Laboratory Findings: Laboratory findings are often helpful in gauging the severity and acuity of respiratory failure. Arterial oxygen saturation can be measured continuously and noninvasively by pulse oximetry. Readings may be affected by poor perfusion, hyperbilirubinemia, severe anemia, methemoglobinemia, and hypercapnia. Nevertheless, oximetry should be used in the assessment and management of all patients with suspected respiratory failure. Capnography provides a continuous noninvasive measure of $PaCO_2$. End-tidal CO_2 ($ETCO_2$) approximates alveolar CO_2. $ETCO_2$ may be falsely lowered in severe respiratory disease as a result of increased dead space. Despite this limitation, $ETCO_2$ provides a trend for assessing the disease process over time. Because of this discrepancy and the ongoing need to assess the acid-base status of the patient, **arterial blood gas measurement** remains the best means for assessment of acute respiratory failure. Arterial blood gases give information on the acid-base status (with a measured pH and calculated bicarbonate level) as well as the PaO_2 and $PaCO_2$) in the patient. The

Table 13–1. Types of respiratory failure.

Findings	Causes	Examples
Type I Hypoxia Decreased PaO_2 Normal $PaCO_2$	Ventilation/perfusion defect	Positional (supine in bed), adult respiratory distress syndrome (ARDS), atelectasis, pneumonia, pulmonary embolus, bronchopulmonary dysplasia
	Diffusion impairment	Pulmonary edema, ARDS, interstitial pneumonia
	Shunt	Pulmonary arteriovenous malformation, congenital adenomatoid malformation
Type II Hypoxia Hypercapnia Decreased PaO_2 Increased $PaCO_2$	Hypoventilation	Neuromuscular disease (polio, Guillain-Barré syndrome), head trauma, sedation, chest wall dysfunction (burns), kyphosis, severe reactive airways

Table 13–2. Clinical criteria for respiratory failure.

Respiratory
  Wheezing
  Expiratory grunting
  Decreased or absent breath sounds
  Flaring of alae nasi
  Retractions of chest wall
  Tachypnea, bradypnea, or apnea
  Cyanosis
Cerebral
  Restlessness
  Irritability
  Headache
  Confusion
  Convulsions
  Coma
Cardiac
  Bradycardia or excessive tachycardia
  Hypotension or hypertension
General
  Fatigue
  Sweating

$PaCO_2$ is a sensitive measure of ventilation and is inversely related to the minute ventilation (Figure 13–1). Knowing the arterial blood gas values and the inspired oxygen concentration enables one to calculate several parameters that may be helpful in determining the efficiency of gas exchange. The difference between alveolar oxygen concentration and the arterial oxygen value is the **alveolar-arterial oxygen difference** ($AaDO_2$). The $AaDO_2$ is less than 15 mm Hg under normal conditions, and it increases with increasing inspired oxygen concentrations to about 100 mm Hg in normal patients breathing 100% oxygen. Diffusion impairment, shunts, and V/Q mismatches all cause increased $AaDO_2$ (Table 13–3).

In addition to the calculation of the $AaDO_2$, assessment of the intrapulmonary shunting (that percentage of pulmonary blood flow which passes through nonventilated areas of the lung) may be helpful. Normal individuals have less than a 5% physiologic shunt from bronchial, thebesian, and coronary circulations. Shunt fractions greater than 15% usually indicate the need for aggressive respiratory support. When intrapulmonary shunt reaches 50% of pulmonary blood flow, PaO_2 does not increase regardless of the amount of supplemental oxygen used.

Dead space ventilation is that part of the breath in the conducting air passages plus the alveolar volume which is ventilated but not perfused by the pulmonary circulation. Dead space ventilation is increased in bronchopulmonary dysplasia, V/Q mismatches, pulmonary interstitial emphysema, pulmonary embolism, and many other entities. Decreasing dead space ventilation depends on its cause, but such methods as tracheostomy in patients with chronic respiratory failure or streptokinase therapy in persons with pulmonary emboli are examples.

Treatment

A. Oxygen Supplementation: Patients with hypoxemia induced by respiratory failure may respond to supplemental oxygen administration alone (Table 13–4). Those with hypoventilation and diffusion defects respond better than patients with shunts or V/Q mismatches. Severe V/Q mismatches often do not respond to anything but aggressive airway management and mechanical ventilation. Patients with a decreased functional residual capacity (FRC)—the amount of air left in the lungs at the end of passive expiration—often respond to the delivery of continuous positive airway pressure (CPAP), 5–10 cm H_2O by either mask or endotracheal tube. This improves oxygenation by increasing FRC to above closing capacity (closing capacity is the combination of the expiratory reserve volume and closing volume and represents the volume that the FRC must exceed during tidal breathing to prevent closure of airways). Patients with severe hypoxemia, hypoventilation, or apnea require assistance with bag and mask ventilation until the airway is intubated. Ventilation may be maintained for some time with a mask of the proper size, but gastric distention, emesis, and inadequate tidal volumes are possible complications. An artificial airway may be lifesaving for patients who fail to respond to simple oxygen supplements.

B. Intubation: Intubation of the trachea in infants and children requires experienced personnel and the right equipment. A patient in respiratory failure whose airway must be stabilized should first be properly positioned to facilitate air exchange while supplemental oxygen is given. The sniffing position is used in infants. Head extension with jaw thrust is used in older children without neck injuries. If obstructed by secretions or vomitus, the airway must be cleared by suction. When not obstructed by a foreign body or epiglottitis, airways should open with proper positioning and placement of an oral or nasopharyngeal airway of the correct size. Conscious patients tolerate nasal airways better than oral airways. As each step is taken, it is imperative to monitor changes in chest movement, airway and breath sounds, skin color, and mental status. Patients with a normal airway may be intubated under intravenous anesthesia by experienced physicians (Table 13–5). Patients with obstructed upper airways (eg, patients with croup, epiglottitis, foreign bodies, or subglottic stenosis) should be awake when intubated unless trained airway specialists decide otherwise.

The size of the endotracheal tube is of critical importance in pediatrics (see Table 11–3 for sizes). Too large a tube can cause pressure necrosis of the tissues in the subglottic region. (This is the narrowest portion of the upper airway in children—in contrast to

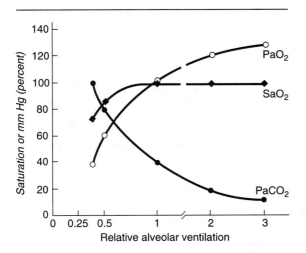

Figure 13–1. Relationship between alveolar ventilation, arterial oxygen saturation (SaO_2), and partial pressures of oxygen and CO_2 in the arterial blood (PaO_2 and $PaCO_2$, respectively). (Reproduced, with permission, from Pagtakhan RD, Chernicic V: Respiratory failure in the pediatric patient. Pediatr Rev 1982;3:244.)

Table 13–3. Pulmonary status equations.

Pio_2 = (barometric pressure − 47) × % inspired oxygen concentration
$Aado_2$ = $Pio_2 - (Paco_2/R) - Pao_2$ (normal = 5–15 mm Hg)
Co_2 = $(1.34 \times$ hemoglobin $\times Sao_2) + (0.003 \times Pao_2)$
Do_2 = $Cao_2 \times CI \times 10$ (normal 620 ± 50 mL/min/m²)
Oxygen consumption $(\dot{V}o_2) = (Cao_2 - Cvo_2) \times CI \times 10$ (normal 120–200 mL/min/m²)

$$\frac{Qs}{Qt} = \frac{Cco_2 - Cao_2}{Cco_2 - Cvo_2} \qquad \text{(normal <5\%)}$$

$$Vd = \frac{(Paco_2 - Peco_2)}{(Pcco_2)} \qquad \text{(normal approximately 2 mL/kg)}$$

$$Compliance = \frac{Volume\ (tidal\ volume)}{Pressure\ (PIP - PEEP)} \qquad \text{(normals vary with age)}$$

$Aado_2$ = Alveolar-arterial oxygen difference (mm Hg)
Cao_2 = Oxygen content of arterial blood (mL/dL)
Cco_2 = Oxygen content of pulmonary capillary blood (mL/dL)
CI = Cardiac index (L/min)
Co_2 = Oxygen content of the blood (mL/dL)
Cvo_2 = Oxygen content of mixed venous blood (mL/dL)
Do_2 = Oxygen delivery (mL/min)
$Paco_2$ = Partial pressure of carbon dioxide in arterial blood (mm Hg)
Pao_2 = Partial pressure of oxygen in arterial blood (mm Hg)
$Pcco_2$ = Partial pressure of carbon dioxide in capillary blood (mm Hg)
$Peco_2$ = Partial pressure of carbon dioxide in expired air (mm Hg)
Pio_2 = Partial pressure of oxygen in inspired air (mm Hg)
PIP = Peak inspiratory pressure
Qs/Qt = Intrapulmonary shunt (in patients without cardiac shunt) (%)
R = Respiratory quotient (usually 0.8)
Sao_2 = Arterial oxygen saturation (fractional)
Vd = Physiologic dead space (anatomic dead space + alveolar dead space) (mL)
Ve = Expiratory minute volume (L/min)
$\dot{V}o_2$ = Oxygen consumption per minute

Table 13–4. Supplemental oxygen therapy.

Source	Maximum % O_2	Range of Flow Rates	Advantages	Disadvantages
Nasal cannula	35–40%	0.125–4 L/min	Easily applied, relatively comfortable	Uncomfortable at higher flow rates, requires open nasal airways, easily dislodged, lower % O_2, nosebleeds
Simple mask	50–60%	5–10 L/min	Higher % O_2, good for mouth breathers	Uncomfortable, dangerous for patients with poor airway control and at risk for emesis, hard to give airway care, unsure of % O_2
Face tent	40–60%	8–10 L/min	Higher % O_2, good for mouth breathers, less restrictive	Uncomfortable, dangerous for patients with poor airway control and at risk for emesis, hard to give airway care, unsure of % O_2
Rebreathing mask	80–90%	5–10 L/min	Higher % O_2, good for mouth breathers, highest O_2 concentration	Uncomfortable, dangerous for patients with poor airway control and at risk for emesis, hard to give airway care, unsure of % O_2
Oxyhood	90–100%	5–10 L/min (mixed at wall)	Stable and accurate O_2 concentration	Temperature regulation, hard to give airway care

Table 13–5. Drugs commonly used for controlled intubation.

Drug	Dose (mg/kg)	Advantages	Disadvantages
Atropine	0.02; minimum of 0.1	Blocks bradycardia, dries secretions	Tachycardia, fever, histamine release, seizures, coma
Thiopental	3–5	Fast onset, short duration of action	Vascular irritant, negative inotropic, no analgesic properties, histamine release (avoid in asthma), induces porphyria
Ketamine	1–2 IV 4–8 IM	Fast onset, positive inotropic	Increased bronchorrhea, increased pulmonary and systemic vascular resistance, increased intracranial pressure, emergence problems
Succinylcholine (depolarizing muscle relaxant)	1–2	Fast onset, short duration of action	Bradycardia (premedicate with atropine); fasciculations; contraindicated in burns, hyperkalemia, massive trauma, and various neurologic disorders
Pancuronium (nondepolarizing muscle relaxant)	0.1	Lasts 40–60 min, can be given by continuous infusion, reversible	Slow onset (2–3 min), tachycardia
Vecuronium (nondepolarizing muscle relaxant)	0.1	Lasts 20–30 min, can be given by continuous infusion, reversible	Slow onset (2–3 min)

the glottis in adults.) The scarring that follows necrosis can cause permanent stenosis of the subglottic region, requiring tracheostomy or cricoid split for repair. Too small an endotracheal tube can result in inadequate pulmonary toilet and excessive air leak around the endotracheal tube, making optimal ventilation and oxygenation difficult. There are many ways to calculate the size of the endotracheal tube that is appropriate for a child. Two useful methods are (1) measuring the height with a Broselow tape and then reading the endotracheal tube size off the tape or (2) in children over 2 years of age, tube size = (16 + age [in years])/4. Patients under 8 years of age should have uncuffed endotracheal tubes.

After placement of the endotracheal tube, breath sounds should be evaluated for bilateral equality. One should then check for a leak between the endotracheal tube and the larynx. To do this, connect a pressure-monitored anesthesia bag to the circuit and allow it to inflate, creating positive pressure. Check for the leak by auscultating over the throat, noting the pressure at which air escapes around the endotracheal tube. Leaks of 15–20 cm H_2O are acceptable. Larger leaks (>20 cm H_2O) are acceptable only in patients having severe lung disease and poor compliance and requiring high pressures to achieve ventilation. In this situation, one must be aware of the possible postextubation complications of subglottic stenosis in the patient. A chest x-ray is necessary for final assessment of endotracheal tube placement.

Demling RH, Knox JB: Basic concepts of lung function and dysfunction: Oxygenation, ventilation, and mechanics. New Horizons 1993;1:362.

Heffner JE: Tracheal intubation in mechanically ventilated patients. Clin Chest Med 1988;9:23.
Katz R, Pollack M, Spady D: Cardiopulmonary abnormalities in severe acute respiratory failure. J Pediatr 1984; 104:357.
Pagtakhan RD, Pasterkamp H: Intensive care for respiratory disorders. In: *Disorders of the Respiratory Tract in Children,* 5th ed. Chernick V (editor). Saunders, 1990.
Prevoznik SJ: Intubation of the trachea. In: *Introduction to Anesthesia,* 7th ed. Dripps RD, Eckenhoff JE, Vandam LD (editors). Saunders, 1988.
Raphaely RC: Acute respiratory failure in infants and children. Pediatr Ann 1986;15:315.

MECHANICAL VENTILATION

The increased compliance of an infant's chest wall, the increasing number of alveoli until approximately the age of 8, the small size of the airways, and the lack of collateral ventilation make pediatric ventilation challenging. Mechanical ventilators are designed to facilitate movement of air into and out of the lungs and to deliver oxygen. They use either positive pressure to "pump" the lungs full of gas or negative pressure to "suck" air into the lungs, much like the diaphragm does. This section deals with the more commonly used positive-pressure mechanical ventilators that are most appropriate for acute situations.

Pressure Ventilators

Pressure-limited, time-cycled ventilation is increasingly used to ventilate older children and adults to minimize barotrauma. In pressure-limited ventilators, air flow is generated at the start of the inspiratory cycle and continues until a preset pressure is reached. Pressure is maintained until, at the end of the inspiratory time, the exhalation valve opens. Pressure ventilators provide intermittent mandatory ventilation (IMV) so that, when set to 15 breaths per minute, the machine delivers a breath every 4 seconds. Newer ventilators can provide synchronized pressure-limited ventilation. The advantages of pressure-limited ventilators lie in their ability to support spontaneous respirations with continuous gas flow, their avoidance of barotrauma by limiting the pressure of breaths, and their relatively simple operation. The main disadvantages are the possibility of inadequate tidal volumes, especially during periods of rapidly changing lung compliance.

Volume Ventilators

Reduced working volumes and low-compliance ventilator tubing now allow volume ventilators to be used in patients of any age. With these ventilators, a standard tidal volume is set (10–15 mL/kg), and the inspiratory time is set either to an absolute value (0.3–1.5 seconds) or to a percentage of the respiratory cycle. In contrast to pressure-limited ventilators, volume-limited ventilators deliver a preset tidal volume. The pressure generated in response to a preset tidal volume will therefore change as lung compliance changes. There is usually a pressure limit dial where a preset pressure can be set above which the ventilator breath will be halted. This is a safety mechanism to avoid dangerously high lung inflation pressures. These ventilators may function in either an intermittent (IMV) or synchronized (SIMV) fashion. SIMV allows a window of time during which a patient's inspiratory effort will initiate the delivery of a tidal volume and is often helpful in patients breathing spontaneously. Volume ventilators are volume-limited and either volume-cycled or time-cycled. They may provide either continuous flow through the system, allowing uninterrupted access of fresh gas to the patient (which decreases the work of breathing, especially in young infants) or flow that is held in check until an inspiratory effort opens a demand valve.

Volume ventilators may have as added variables an inspiratory hold or pressure support. The advantages of volume ventilators include ensured delivery of a preset volume, compliance measurements, and availability of SIMV. Disadvantages of some volume ventilators include possible increased barotrauma from excessive delivery pressure and lack of a continuous flow system.

Positive End-Expiratory Pressure

All mechanical ventilators open their expiratory limbs at the end of inspiration until a preset pressure is achieved; this is the positive end-expiratory pressure (PEEP) value. During ventilation of normal lungs, "physiologic" PEEP is felt to be 2–4 cm H_2O pressure. In disease states, a higher PEEP may in-

crease the FRC, open previously collapsed alveoli, increase mean airway pressure (MAP), and improve oxygenation. A higher PEEP, though often valuable, may cause CO_2 retention, barotrauma with extrapleural air leaks, decreased central venous return, decreased cardiac output, and increased intracranial pressure. CPAP is the lowest expiratory pressure a spontaneously breathing patient achieves and for practical purposes is synonymous with PEEP. PEEP and CPAP have an optimal setting for each individual patient, maximally improving FRC and V/Q mismatches while not causing the problems associated with excessive intrathoracic pressure (see earlier). Multiple parameters have been proposed with varying success to define *optimal PEEP*. Variables that should be considered in determining appropriate PEEP include PaO_2, central venous pressure, and cardiac output. PEEP should be decreased for pulmonary leak and cerebral edema and may need to be increased for pneumonia, pulmonary edema, and adult respiratory distress syndrome.

Ventilator Management

Mechanical ventilators affect both ventilation and oxygenation. Ventilation is related to alveolar minute volume. On a pressure ventilator, the minute volume is directly related to rate and peak inspiratory pressure; on a volume ventilator, it is related to rate and tidal volume. Thus, increased rate, tidal volume, or peak inspiratory pressure will increase ventilation and should decrease the $PaCO_2$. Changes in oxygenation other than those resulting from the concentration of delivered oxygen depend in part on the variables that determine MAP or the average of all the pressures experienced by the lung in one respiratory cycle. These include PEEP, inspiratory time, and the peak inspiratory pressure delivered. By increasing any of these settings, one achieves an elevation in MAP and, up to a point, an increase in oxygenation. One must remember that increasing these settings can worsen V/Q mismatches, decrease cardiac output, and decrease oxygen delivery to the tissue. Therefore, the changes resulting in elevated MAP do not always improve arterial oxygenation or oxygen delivery.

The intubated patient deserves attention directed toward improving comfort and decreasing anxiety. Chloral hydrate, benzodiazepines, and narcotics have been used. Continuous infusions of the short-acting benzodiazepines and opioids create a steady state of sedation. Occasionally, patients are so agitated that ventilation and oxygenation suffer. In these cases, muscle paralysis may facilitate oxygenation and ventilation. The nondepolarizing neuromuscular blocking agents pancuronium bromide and vecuronium bromide are most commonly used for this purpose. They may be given as necessary or as continuous infusions. When giving muscle relaxants, one must be prepared to provide, by mechanical means, ventilation and oxygenation to the patient who previously breathed spontaneously; in most cases, ventilatory support must be increased.

Monitoring the Ventilated Patient

Ventilated patients must be monitored for respiratory rate and activity, chest wall movement, and quality of breath sounds. Oxygenation should be measured either by arterial blood gases or by transmission oximetry with lightweight digital or earlobe probes. O_2 (PtO_2) or CO_2 ($PtcO_2$) can be measured transcutaneously with sufficient accuracy in younger patients with good skin perfusion. $PaCO_2$ may also be assessed by monitoring end-tidal CO_2 ($PetCO_2$). This is done by placing a gas-sampling port on the endotracheal tube and analyzing expired gas for $PetCO_2$. This technique appears to be more valuable in patients with large tidal volumes, and its accuracy improves with more proximal sampling, that is, closer to the airways. $PetCO_2$ values may differ from measured $PaCO_2$ and are most useful for following relative fluctuations in $PaCO_2$.

The ventilator itself has many variables. The most common are tidal volume, minute ventilation, peak inspiratory pressure, and inspiratory and expiratory time. MAP should be monitored in mechanically ventilated patients and maintained as low as possible to achieve adequate oxygenation and ventilation. Work of breathing and oxygen consumption may also be measured; these measurements may be helpful in making ventilator changes in chronically ventilated patients. While technologic advances in monitoring provide more data, they do not substitute for the physical examination and good clinical judgment.

Alternative Methods of Ventilation

High-frequency jet ventilation with passive expiration (300–3000/min) and high-frequency oscillation with active expiration (300–1800/min) have been used to manage select groups of neonates and older pediatric patients, including those suffering from major pulmonary barotrauma (air leaks, pulmonary interstitial emphysema), respiratory distress syndrome, and congenital diaphragmatic hernia. These techniques have also been used to manage patients who have undergone operative procedures on airway structures, so that MAP can be maintained with lower peak inspiratory pressure, thus helping prevent postoperative air leaks at the surgical site.

Pressure-controlled inverse ratio ventilation and permissive hypercapnia have also been used successfully to manage severe respiratory failure such as that seen in adult respiratory distress syndrome. These techniques allow maintenance of high MAP while reducing peak inspiratory pressure and the incidence of barotrauma to as low a level as possible.

The use of fluorocarbon-based liquids to both oxygenate and remove CO_2 in children with severe lung injury is presently undergoing clinical trials. Potential benefits of liquid ventilation include reduction of barotrauma, better lung expansion and compliance, and better pulmonary toilet.

Arnold JH et al: High frequency oscillatory ventilation in pediatric respiratory failure. Crit Care Med 1993;21:272.

Betit P, Thompson JE, Benjamin PK: Mechanical ventilation. In: *Neonatal and Pediatric Respiratory Care,* 2nd ed. Koff PB, Eitzman D, Neu J (editors). Mosby–Year Book, 1993.

Demling RH, Knox JB: Basic concepts of lung function and dysfunction: Oxygenation, ventilation, and mechanics. New Horizons 1993;1:362.

Hickling KG, Henderson SJ, Jackson R: Low mortality associated with low volume pressure limited ventilation with permissive hypercapnia in severe ARDS. Intensive Care Med 1990;16:372.

Marini JJ, Ravenscraft SA: Mean airway pressure: Physiologic determinants and clinical importance. (Two parts.) Crit Care Med 1992;20:1461, 1604.

Martin LD et al: Principles of respiratory support and mechanical ventilation. In: *Textbook of Pediatric Intensive Care,* 2nd ed. Rogers MC (editor). Williams & Wilkins, 1992.

Shaffer TH, Wolfson MR, Clark LC Jr: Liquid ventilation. Pediatr Pulmonol 1992;14:102.

ADULT RESPIRATORY DISTRESS SYNDROME (ARDS)

ARDS is a syndrome of acute respiratory failure characterized by increased pulmonary capillary permeability and pulmonary edema that results in refractory hypoxemia, decreased lung compliance, and bilateral diffuse alveolar infiltrates on chest radiography. ARDS accounts for approximately 1% of PICU admissions.

ARDS may be precipitated by a variety of insults (Table 13–6), of which infection is the most common. Despite the diversity of causes, the clinical presentation is remarkably similar in most cases.

An expanded definition of *ARDS* or *acute lung injury* has been developed to define the clinical features better. First, the severity of acute lung injury is scored through assessments of arterial oxygenation

Table 13–6. Adult respiratory distress syndrome risk factors.

Direct Lung Injury	Indirect Lung Injury
Aspiration of gastric contents	Sepsis syndrome
Inhalation of toxic fumes	Multiple trauma
Near-drowning	Multiple transfusions
Oxygen toxicity	Fat embolism
Pulmonary contusion	Shock
Pneumonia: bacterial, viral, other	Pancreatitis
	Drug overdoses (especially aspirin, opioids, tricyclic antidepressants, barbiturates)
	Burns

(PaO_2/FiO_2), chest radiographs, static lung compliance, and the level of PEEP required. Second, because the clinical disorder or disorders that led to the development of acute lung injury clearly influence the patient's prognosis for recovery, precise definition of the underlying problem becomes important. For instance, although the average mortality rate in this population is 45–60%, the rate is quite variable and appears dependent on the associated clinical disorder, with mortality rates of 90% in ARDS associated with sepsis and only 10% in ARDS associated with fat embolism. The third part of the definition specifies the failure of organs other than the lung. The importance of nonpulmonary organ failure is of major importance in the outcome of the ARDS patient. For instance, concomitant hepatic failure and ARDS are associated with an almost 100% mortality rate. In fact, any combination of three organs that have failed for more than 7 days carries a 98% mortality rate.

Thus, a more quantitative definition of *pulmonary* and *nonpulmonary organ failure,* including the associated clinical disorders, is critical for establishing the actual incidence of ARDS and for determining the prognosis for recovery.

Clinical Presentation & Pathophysiology

ARDS can be roughly divided into four clinical phases (Table 13–7). In the earliest phase, the patient may exhibit dyspnea and tachypnea with a relatively normal PO_2 and a hyperventilation-induced respiratory alkalosis. No significant abnormalities are noted on physical or radiologic examination of the chest. Experimental studies suggest that neutrophils accumulate in the lungs at this stage and that their products damage lung endothelium. Over the next few hours, hypoxemia increases and respiratory distress becomes clinically apparent, with cyanosis, tachycardia, irritability, and dyspnea. Radiographic evidence of early parenchymal change is noted by "fluffy" alveolar infiltrates initially appearing in dependent lung fields, indicative of pulmonary edema. The edema fluid typically has a high concentration of protein (75–95% of plasma protein concentration) which is characteristic of an increased-permeability

Table 13–7. Pathophysiologic changes of modern adult respiratory distress syndrome (low-pressure pulmonary edema).[1]

Radiographic Change	Clinical Findings	Physiologic Change	Pathologic Change
Phase 1 (early changes) Normal radiograph	Dyspnea, tachypnea, normal chest examination	Mild pulmonary hypertension, normoxemic or mild hypoxemia, hypercapnia	Neutrophil sequestration, no clear tissue damage
Phase 2 (onset of parenchymal changes)[2] Patchy alveolar infiltrates beginning in dependent lung No perivascular cuffs (unless a component of high-pressure edema is present) Normal heart size	Dyspnea, tachypnea, cyanosis, tachycardia, course rales	Pulmonary hypertension, normal wedge pressure, increased lung permeability, increased lung water, increasing shunt, progressive decrease in compliance, moderate to severe hypoxemia	Neutrophil infiltration, vascular congestion, fibrin strands, platelet clumps, alveolar septal edema, intra-alveolar protein, white cells, type I epithelial drainage
Phase 3 (acute respiratory failure with progression, 2–10 d) Diffuse alveolar infiltrates Air bronchograms Decreased lung volume No bronchovascular cuffs Normal heart	Tachypnea, tachycardia, hyperdynamic state, sepsis syndrome, signs of consolidation, diffuse rhonchi	Phase 2 changes persist. Progression of symptoms, increasing shunt fraction, further decrease in compliance, increased minute ventilation, impaired oxygen extraction of hemoglobin.	Increased interstitial and alveolar inflammatory exudate with neutrophil and mononuclear cells, type II cell proliferation, beginning fibroblast proliferation, thromboembolic occlusion
Phase 4 (pulmonary fibrosis, pneumonia with progression, >10 d)[3] Persistent diffuse infiltrates Superimposed new pneumonic infiltrates Recurrent pneumothorax Normal heart size Enlargement with pulmonale	Symptoms as above, recurrent sepsis, evidence of multiple organ system failure	Phase 3 changes persist. Recurrent pneumonia, progressive lung restriction, impaired tissue oxygenation. Multiple organ system failure.	Type II cell hyperplasia, interstitial thickening; infiltration of lymphocytes, macrophages, fibroblasts; loculated pneumonia or interstitial fibrosis; medial thickening and remodeling of arterioles

[1]Modified slightly and reproduced, with permission, from Demling RH: Adult respiratory distress syndrome: Current concepts. New Horizons 1993;1:388.
[2]The process is readily reversible at this stage if the initiating factor is controlled.
[3]Multiple organ system failure is common. The mortality rate is greater than 80% at this stage, since resolution is more difficult.

edema and differentiates it from cardiogenic or hydrostatic pulmonary edema. Epithelial injury in ARDS lowers the threshold for alveolar edema and impairs gas exchange. If patients can reabsorb the alveolar edema within 12 hours of formation, alveolar epithelial function remains reasonably intact and there is an excellent chance for recovery. In contrast, patients who have no change in edema fluid content or protein concentration in the first 12 hours after onset of mechanical ventilation have a much higher mortality rate. Pulmonary hypertension, decreases in lung compliance, and increases in airway resistance are also noted. Clinical studies suggest that airway resistance may be increased in 50% of patients with ARDS.

Type II cell and fibroblast proliferation occur in the interstitium of the lung during the subacute phase of ARDS (5–10 days after lung injury). Decreased lung volumes and signs of consolidation are noted clinically and radiographically. Worsening of the hypoxemia with an increasing shunt fraction as well as a further decrease in lung compliance are noted. Some patients develop an accelerated fibrosing alveolitis in which there is a marked increase in fibroblasts and collagen formation in the interstitium. The mechanisms responsible for these changes are not clear. Current investigation centers on the role of growth and differentiation factors such as transforming growth factor β and platelet-derived growth factor released by resident and nonresident lung cells such as alveolar macrophages, mast cells, neutrophils, alveolar type II cells, and fibroblasts.

During the chronic phase of ARDS (10–14 days after lung injury), there is fibrosis, emphysema, and pulmonary vascular obliteration. Patients usually do not have as severe an oxygenation defect as they did in the acute phase, and the requirements for PEEP may decline. Patients have large amounts of dead space and may require a high minute ventilation. Their compliance remains low, perhaps because of pulmonary fibrosis and insufficient surface-active material.

Secondary infections are common in the subacute and chronic phases of ARDS and significantly influence the outcome. The mechanisms responsible for increased host susceptibility to infection during this phase are not well understood.

The mortality rates in the late phase of ARDS exceed 80%. Death is usually caused by multiple organ failure and systemic hemodynamic instability rather than by hypoxia.

Treatment

A. Ventilatory Support: An FiO_2 greater than 50% over 24 hours can cause lung injury to ARDS patients, so positive-pressure ventilation and PEEP are used to improve oxygenation. Ventilation is best on a volume ventilator because of rapidly changing compliance of the lungs. Poor compliance may result in high peak inspiratory pressure. PEEP is used to open collapsed alveoli, reduce shunting, and increase FRC above the closing volume. All these measures decrease dead space ventilation and may improve oxygenation. The PEEP that provides the best combination of oxygenation, lung compliance, cardiac output, and lowered intrapulmonary shunt is found by increasing the PEEP by increments (2–3 cm H_2O every 30 minutes) until pulmonary and hemodynamic measurements fit the patient's requirements. PEEPs of 15–25 cm H_2O have been used successfully in some patients. Before increasing PEEP, one should optimize conditions by making sure that the intravascular volume is appropriate, the endotracheal tube does not leak, and the patient is well sedated or paralyzed. A Qs/Qt of less than 15%, oxygen saturations greater than 90% on an FiO_2 of less than 60%, and a good cardiac output may signal the end point of PEEP adjustments.

Blood gases (PaO_2 and $PaCO_2$) should not be normalized at the cost of injuring the lung with high pressures and high concentrations of oxygen. Permissive hypercapnia in the face of normal blood pH is acceptable. Newer ventilator strategies (discussed above) are also being tried in an attempt to decrease lung injury. These include primarily a switch from volume-controlled to pressure-controlled ventilation.

B. Hemodynamic Support: Hemodynamic support is directed toward increasing perfusion and oxygen delivery. Volume expansion is achieved by giving packed red blood cells to maintain the hematocrit between 40% and 50% and by giving either colloid or crystalloid solutions to nonanemic volume-depleted patients. There is no one recommendation on the type of fluid to give the nonanemic patient. Certainly, colloids should be used in patients with low intravascular oncotic pressures as estimated by reduced total protein or albumin concentrations. In all other ARDS patients, however, the optimal fluid resuscitation has not been well established. Use of inotropic drugs is often necessary. The most effective inotropic dosages should be determined by monitoring blood pressure, urinary output, cardiac output, pulmonary and systemic vascular resistances, and the patient's gas exchange.

C. Control of Infection: Prevention or early treatment of infection is an extremely important aspect of the management of ARDS.

D. Pharmacotherapy: Drug therapies have not proved particularly successful in ARDS. Clinical studies have not shown that steroids, ibuprofen, or indomethacin benefit ARDS patients. Vasodilators such as nitroglycerin, sodium nitroprusside, prostaglandin E_1 and I_2, and calcium channel blockers have all been used to combat pulmonary vasoconstriction, but their use is frequently limited by the development of systemic hypotension. As yet, there is no clear evidence suggesting that these drugs have beneficial effects. Some enthusiasm exists for the treatment of patients with antibodies specific to circulating mediators of sepsis and lung injury. Anti–tumor necrosis factor antibodies and interleukin receptor antagonists are examples.

E. Monitoring: Multiorgan system monitoring is needed in patients with ARDS. Ventilation can be assessed by monitoring arterial blood gases, oxygen saturation, and end-tidal CO_2. Lung compliance should be known as increases in PEEP or tidal volume are made. Obtaining chest films daily is important for patients receiving vigorous support because severe ARDS is associated with a 40–60% incidence of air leaks. Hemodynamic monitoring should include, at a minimum, central venous monitoring to determine volume status; if PEEPs greater than 12 cm H_2O are used, a pulmonary artery catheter is recommended. Surveillance for infection or sepsis is important because secondary infections are common and increase the mortality rate strikingly. Renal, liver, and gastrointestinal function need close attention because of the great likelihood of multiple organ dysfunction.

F. Alternative Management: New techniques have evolved in the respiratory treatment of ARDS. **High-frequency ventilation** has proved helpful only in patients with large air leaks, although more and better trials evaluating the efficacy of high-frequency oscillatory or jet ventilation are needed. Surfactant replacement therapy has been tried with some success in patients with ARDS. Surfactant replacement, in some instances, improves lung compliance and allows patients' lungs to be ventilated at a smaller FiO_2, with weaning from mechanical ventilation earlier than in nontreated patients. Prospective randomized trials are needed. Pediatric patients with severe ARDS who received **extracorporeal membrane oxygenation** (**ECMO**) have better survival rates than historical controls. There is currently a prospective study evaluating venovenous ECMO as treatment for ARDS. The results of that study are not complete, but to date the data show no difference between the control and the ECMO-treated groups. Criteria for selecting which patients should receive these new therapies have not been established. Very recent reports have demonstrated that inhaled **nitric oxide** (**NO**) may be beneficial in ARDS. This effect is based on the ability of NO to reduce pulmonary artery pressure and to improve the matching of ventilation with perfusion without producing systemic vasodilation. Patient selection and efficacy of these new therapies have yet to be established, but many of them are being documented in prospective randomized clinical trials.

G. Follow-up: The follow-up of pediatric ARDS patients is limited. One report of 10 children followed 1–4 years after severe ARDS showed 3 still symptomatic and 7 with hypoxemia at rest. Until further information is available, all patients with a history of ARDS need close follow-up of pulmonary function.

Abman SH et al: Acute effects of iNO in children with severe hypoxemic respiratory failure. J Pediatr 1994; 124:881.

Bersten A, Sibald WJ: Acute lung injury in septic shock. Crit Care Clin 1989;5:49.

Demling RH: Adult respiratory distress syndrome: Current concepts. New Horizons 1993;1:388.

Downey GP, Fiolkow L, Fukushima T: Initial interaction of leukocytes within the microvasculature: Deformability, adhesion, and transmigration. New Horizons 1995; 3:219.

Edelson JD: Epithelial dysfunction in acute lung injury. New Horizons 1995;3:229.

Enhorning G: Surfactant replacement in adult respiratory distress syndrome. Am Rev Respir Dis 1989;140:281.

Holcroft JW, Vassar MJ, Weber CJ: Prostaglandin E and survival in patients with the adult respiratory syndrome. Ann Surg 1986;203:371.

Knaus WA, Wagner DP: Multiple systems organ failure: Epidemiology and prognosis. Crit Care Clin 1989;5:221.

Luce JM et al: Ineffectiveness of high-dose methylprednisolone in preventing parenchymal lung injury and improving mortality in patients with septic shock. Am Rev Respir Dis 1988;136:62.

MacNaughton PD, Evans TW: Management of adult respiratory distress syndrome. Lancet 1992;339:469.

Marini JJ: Ventilation of the acute respiratory distress syndrome: Looking for Mr. Goodmode. Anesthesiology 1994;40:972.

Murray JF et al: An expanded definition of the adult respiratory distress syndrome. Am Rev Respir Dis 1988; 138:720.

Nichols DG, Rogers MC: Adult respiratory distress syndrome. In: *Textbook of Pediatric Intensive Care.* Rogers MC (editor). Williams & Wilkins, 1987.

Pinsky MR: The effects of mechanical ventilation on the cardiovascular system. Crit Care Med 1990;6:660.

Repine JE: Scientific perspectives on adult respiratory distress syndrome. Lancet 1992;339:466.

Rossaint R et al: Inhaled nitric oxide for the adult respiratory distress syndrome. N Engl J Med 1993;328:399.

Royal JA, Levin DL: Adult respiratory distress syndrome in pediatric patients. 1. Clinical aspects, pathophysiology, and mechanisms of lung injury. J Pediatr 1988; 112:169.

Royal JA, Levin DL: Adult respiratory distress syndrome in pediatric patients. 2. Management. J Pediatr 1988; 112:335.

Snyder LS et al: Failure of lung repair following acute lung injury: Regulation of the fibroproliferative response. (Two parts.) Chest 1990;98:733, 989.

Weg JG et al: Safety and potential efficacy of an aerosolized surfactant in human sepsis-induced adult respiratory distress syndrome. Chest 1994;105:195.

Weiner-Kronish JP, Gropper MA, Matthay MA: The adult respiratory distress syndrome: Definition and prognosis, pathogenesis and treatment. Br J Anaesth 1990;65:107.

ASTHMA (LIFE-THREATENING)

Status asthmaticus may be defined as reversible small airway obstruction that is refractory to sympathomimetic and anti-inflammatory agents and which may progress to respiratory failure without prompt and aggressive intervention. Life-threatening asthma is caused by severe bronchospasm, excessive mucous secretion, inflammation, and edema of the airways. Reversal of these mechanisms is the key to successful treatment. Status asthmaticus remains a common diagnosis among children admitted to the ICU, and asthma continues to be associated with a surprisingly high mortality rate.

The physical examination helps determine the severity of illness. Accessory muscle (sternocleidomastoid) use correlates well with an FEV_1 and peak expiratory flow rates (PEFRs) less than 50% of normal predicted values. A paradoxic pulse of over 22 mm Hg has been correlated with elevated $PaCO_2$ levels. The absence of wheezing may be misleading because, in order to produce a wheezing sound, the patient must take in a certain amount of air. The arterial blood gas remains the single most important laboratory determination in the evaluation of a child in severe status asthmaticus. Patients with severe respiratory distress, signs of exhaustion, alterations in consciousness, elevated $PaCO_2$, or acidosis should be admitted to the PICU.

Treatment

Because of inadequate minute ventilation and V/Q mismatching, severe asthmatics are almost always hypoxemic and should receive supplemental humidified oxygen immediately.

A. Pharmacotherapy:

1. Nebulized β_2-agonist therapy such as with albuterol or terbutaline remains first-line therapy to reverse acute bronchoconstriction. If the patient is in severe distress and has poor inspiratory flow rates, thus preventing adequate delivery of nebulized medication, subcutaneous injection of epinephrine or terbutaline may be required. The frequency of β_2-agonist administration varies according to the severity of the patient's symptoms and the occurrence of adverse side effects. Albuterol may be given continuously by nebulization, usually without serious side effects. However, the heart rate and blood pressure of these patients should be closely monitored, as excessive tachycardia and ventricular ectopy may occur.

2. Theophylline confers additional benefit when given with steroids and β_2-agonists. Besides bronchodilation, it decreases mucociliary inflammatory mediators and reduces microvascular permeability. When the decision to add theophylline to high-dose β_2-agonist therapy for severe status asthmaticus is being weighed, the increased risk of serious side effects such as tachycardia and cardiac arrhythmias must be considered.

3. Systemic corticosteroids speed the resolution of severe asthma exacerbations refractory to bronchodilator therapy and should be given to all patients admitted to the hospital with severe asthma. The optimal dose is not known, although a frequently used dosage is 1 mg/kg of intravenous methylprednisolone every 6 hours. The acute complications of corticosteroid usage include gastrointestinal bleeding and perforations.

4. Nebulized **anticholinergic agents** are also recommended, at least as a trial, in severe asthmatics. In some patients, cholinergic-related bronchoconstriction is more marked than in others, so not all patients respond. Nebulized ipratropium bromide is the drug of choice. Atropine has more potential side effects than ipratropium bromide, for example, tachycardia, urinary retention, and pupillary dilation, but can be given up to every 6 hours.

5. Intravenous beta-agonists such as isoproterenol and terbutaline are used in children with severe airway obstruction and impending respiratory failure. Isoproterenol is a nonspecific beta-agonist whose use may lead to excessive tachycardia, myocardial ischemia, and arrhythmia. Terbutaline is more β_2-receptor–specific and usually causes fewer cardiac side effects. Patients placed on intravenous beta-agonist therapy should have indwelling arterial lines for continuous pressure and blood gas monitoring and have cardiac enzymes monitored for signs of myocardial damage.

B. Specific Drugs and Dosages:

1. Give humidified oxygen—Try to keep O_2 saturations at 90% or higher.

2. Beta-sympathomimetic therapy—Albuterol or terbutaline by nebulization (albuterol, 0.1 mg/kg per nebulization, up to 2.5 mg; or terbutaline, 0.1–0.2 mg/kg per nebulization, up to 4 mg). Albuterol may be given continuously at a dose of 0.5 mg/kg/h to a maximum of 15 mg/h.

3. Corticosteroids—Methylprednisolone, 2 mg/kg intravenously as a loading dose, then 1 mg/kg intravenously every 6 hours.

4. Intravenous aminophylline—Each 1 mg/kg of aminophylline given as a loading dose will increase the level by approximately 2 μg/dL. In a patient who has not previously received aminophylline or oral theophylline preparations, load with 7–8 mg/kg of aminophylline in an attempt to achieve a level of 15 μg/dL; then start a continuous infusion of aminophylline at a dosage of 0.8–1 mg/kg/h. Watch closely for toxicity (gastric upset, tachycardia, seizures) and follow levels closely, trying to maintain steady-state levels of 13–16 μg/dL.

5. Anticholinergic therapy—Atropine, 0.025–0.05 mg/kg per dose up to 2 mg every 6–8 hours by nebulization, or ipratropine bromide, 60–80 mg by metered-dose inhaler or 250 mg by nebulization every 6 hours, is useful in a select group of patients.

6. Intravenous beta-sympathomimetic therapy—This should be used only in patients who have not responded to the preceding steps and have worsening respiratory failure.

a. Terbutaline—Give 10 μg/kg over 10 minutes as a loading dose, then start an infusion at 0.1

µg/kg/min, increasing by increments of 0.1 µg/kg/min every 30 minutes until a response is achieved or side effects (tachycardia, tremor, nausea) become apparent.

b. Isoproterenol—Give 0.1 µg/kg/min, increasing by increments of 0.1 µg/kg/min to a maximum of 1 µg/kg/min, again titrating therapy to the patient's response or until side effects (tachycardia, arrhythmia) become a problem.

7. Intravenous administration of magnesium sulfate—This has been reported as an effective bronchodilator in adults with severe status asthmaticus. Its smooth muscle relaxation properties are probably caused by interference with calcium flux in the bronchial smooth muscle cell.

C. Mechanical Ventilation: If the above aggressive management regimen fails to result in significant improvement, mechanical ventilation may be necessary. In general, if there is steady deterioration (increased acidosis, rising $PaCO_2$), despite intensive therapy for asthma, the patient should be intubated and mechanically ventilated. Mechanical ventilation in asthmatics is difficult and by no means simplifies treatment. The goal of mechanical ventilation in an intubated asthmatic is to maintain adequate oxygenation and ventilation with the least amount of barotrauma until other therapies have had a chance to become effective. Airway obstruction from persistent bronchoconstriction remains a major problem because the constricted bronchus is lined with smooth muscle, and paralyzing drugs affect only skeletal muscle. The patient, once intubated, should remain paralyzed and sedated. A volume ventilator is necessary to deliver a reasonable tidal volume in patients with poor lung compliance. Expiratory time should be prolonged to avoid air trapping. The IMV rate may need to be lowered to allow proper expiration time. PEEP should be kept low. There are isolated reports of patients who require greater PEEP, but these are the exception. Aerosolized beta-agonists may be given through the ventilator circuit and should be administered as close to the endotracheal tube as possible.

Weaning the very ill asthmatic from ICU therapy should begin with ventilatory support and then with the aggressive drug therapy. Changes should be made slowly, because patients can rebound and worsen quickly.

D. Metabolic Changes in the Severe Asthmatic: Metabolic disorders may occur in the severe asthmatic. Hypercapnia, hypoxia, and a poor perfusion may lead to acidosis. Slow intravenous sodium bicarbonate therapy (1 meq/kg for pH <7.20) in the ventilated patient is a reasonable treatment of metabolic acidosis, although it may raise the $PaCO_2$. Hypokalemia is also a complication of beta-agonist therapy, and serum potassium needs to be monitored, especially in patients receiving nebulized beta-agonist drugs continuously.

E. Monitoring: Severe asthmatics should be monitored for heart rate, blood pressure, O_2 saturation, and arterial pH and $PaCO_2$. Ventilator monitoring must be meticulous, because increases in peak inspiratory pressure or decreases in pulmonary compliance may signal worsening bronchoconstriction or an extrapleural air leak. In addition, if the patient is mechanically ventilated and paralyzed, the degree of nerve block should be monitored using an electrical stimulator, as nondepolarizing agents given with corticosteroids can cause prolonged paralysis and muscle weakness. Chest films of ventilated asthmatics should be obtained daily.

Benatar SR: Fatal asthma. N Engl J Med 1986;314:423.

Helfaer MA et al: Lower airway disease: Bronchiolitis and asthma. In: *Textbook of Pediatric Intensive Care,* 2nd ed. Rogers MC (editor). Williams & Wilkins, 1992.

Jeene JW, Murphy S: Drug therapy for asthma: Research and clinical practice. In: *Lung Biology in Health and Disease,* Vol 5. Dekker, 1987, vol 5.

Koff PB, Durmowicz AG: Pharmacology. In: *Neonatal and Pediatric Respiratory Care,* 2nd ed. Koff PB, Eitzman D, Neu J (editors). Mosby–Year Book, 1993.

McFadden ER Jr: Dosages of corticosteroids in asthma. Am Rev Respir Dis 1993;147:1306.

Milgram H, Bender B: Current issues in the use of theophylline. Am Rev Respir Dis 1993;147:533.

National Asthma Education Program, Expert Panel Report: *Guidelines for the Diagnosis and Management of Asthma 1991.* National Heart, Lung, and Blood Institute, 1991.

Noppen M: Bronchodilating effect of intravenous magnesium sulfate in acute severe bronchial asthma. Chest 1990;97:373.

POSTOPERATIVE CARDIAC MANAGEMENT

The outcome for pediatric patients undergoing cardiac surgery has been improved by advances in surgical technique, myocardial preservation, and postoperative care. A clear understanding of the preoperative anatomy and dysfunction (ie, the existence of pulmonary hypertension in lesions associated with high pulmonary blood flow), the operative repair, the intraoperative events, and the postoperative hemodynamic and metabolic conditions is necessary for postoperative care.

Cardiopulmonary bypass and deep hypothermic arrest affect the function of multiple organs. Some of the effects most pertinent to postoperative care include increased total body water, transient myocardial dysfunction, gas exchange abnormalities, coagulation abnormalities, and hormonal and stress responses. In addition, general anesthesia is associated with atelectasis and decreased functional reserve capacity. Postoperative management seeks to minimize these adverse effects. Close monitoring of the patient allows early recognition and response to changing hemodynamic, respiratory, and metabolic status. Physical assessment of heart and breath sounds is helpful in detecting cardiac tamponade, pneumothorax, and signs of congestive heart failure.

Ventricular function is determined by measuring systemic arterial pressure and waveform, heart rate, skin color, extremity perfusion, peripheral pulses, urinary output, core temperature, and acid-base status. In some cases, cardiac output is measured by thermodilution with a pulmonary artery catheter. The factors that influence cardiac output (preload or end-diastolic volume, afterload or systolic wall tension, contractility, heart rate, rhythm) are assessed and manipulated as needed. If cardiac output is inadequate, the first approach should be to increase the blood volume so as to increase cardiac filling. A second approach is to reduce the cardiac afterload with a vasodilator such as nitroprusside. Inotropic agents (dopamine, amrinone, dobutamine) are added if these initial adjustments fail.

Conduction abnormalities are common in the postoperative period. They can be related to electrolyte abnormalities, rewarming following hypothermia, or injury to the conduction pathways. Since heart rate and rhythm can affect cardiac output, cardiac rhythm is continuously monitored by electrocardiography to detect arrhythmias rapidly. Tachycardia can be particularly detrimental, because it shortens diastolic filling (decreasing preload and reducing coronary artery perfusion) and increases myocardial oxygen demand. Treatment is directed first to the cause (eg, normalizing temperature and electrolytes, pain control) and may require specific antiarrhythmics or pacing.

Following surgery, the right ventricle can be small and stiff. Its function can be improved by reducing pulmonary vascular resistance (PVR). Pulmonary vascular tone can be reduced by giving oxygen and by manipulating gas exchange, pH, and lung volumes with mechanical ventilation. PVR can also be lowered by inducing a respiratory alkalosis by alterations in both ventilatory rate and volume. Maintaining appropriate lung volumes, especially FRC, is critical to reducing PVR. Compression of the pulmonary microvasculature by atelectasis and compression of the capillaries in the alveolar septum by hyperinflation are both associated with elevation of the PVR. Both of these extremes should be avoided by appropriate manipulation of tidal volume, PEEP, and inspiratory pressure. Postoperative pain management is easier in patients whose ventilation is mechanically maintained. This is needed to reduce stress and labile hemodynamic responses to pain. The patient's primary lesion and postoperative complications dictate how aggressively the patient can be weaned from the ventilator. Extubation is considered when the patient is hemodynamically stable, arrhythmias are controlled, reoperation is not planned, and the patient can maintain an airway with satisfactory gas exchange.

Anand KJS, Hansen DD, Hickey PR: Hormonal-metabolic stress response in neonates undergoing cardiac surgery. Anesthesiology 1990;73:661.

Castaneda AR, Mayer JE, Jonas RA: The neonate with critical congenital heart disease. Repair—A surgical challenge. J Thorac Cardiovasc Surg 1989;98:869.

Wieman DS et al: Perioperative respiratory management in cardiac surgery. Clin Chest Med 1993;14:283.

SHOCK

Shock may be defined as failure of the cardiovascular system to deliver critical substrates and to remove toxic metabolites. This failure leads to anaerobic metabolism in cells and ultimately to irreversible cellular damage. Shock has been categorized into a series of recognizable stages: compensated, uncompensated, and irreversible. Patients in compensated shock have relatively normal cardiac output and normal blood pressures but alterations in the microcirculation, which increase flow to some organs and reduce flow to others. In infants, compensatory increases in cardiac output are achieved primarily by tachycardia rather than by increases in stroke volume. Heart rates of 190–210/min are common in infants with compensated shock, but heart rates over 220/min raise the possibility of supraventricular tachycardia. In older patients, cardiac contractility (stroke volume) and heart rate increase to improve cardiac output. Blood pressure remains normal initially because of peripheral vasoconstriction and increased systemic vascular resistance. Thus, hypotension occurs late and is more characteristic of the uncompensated stage of shock. In the uncompensated stage, there is further deterioration of the oxygen and nutrient supply to the cells with subsequent cellular breakdown and release of toxic substances, causing further redistribution of flow. At this point, the patient is hypotensive, with poor cardiac output. Irreversible shock involving organ damage of the brain and heart is terminal.

The causes of shock are hypovolemic, cardiogenic, and distributive. Often, two or three of these occur together. **Hypovolemic shock** is caused by decreased circulating blood volume. This may result from loss of whole blood or plasma or from fluid loss from the kidney or gut. These patients usually have intact compensatory mechanisms which maintain normal blood pressure by increasing cardiac output and shunting blood away from certain organs. All these responses serve to protect blood flow to the heart and brain. Untreated, hypovolemic shock can progress to an irreversible stage.

Cardiogenic shock is an ominous state of decreased substrate delivery secondary to "pump failure." The causes include congenital heart disease, cardiac surgery (following cardioplegia and ventriculotomy), cardiomyopathy secondary to infection or toxins, and ischemic-reperfusion injuries. The patient's compensatory efforts (eg, release of catecholamines with increases in blood pressure, heart rate, and systemic vascular resistance) often have deleterious effects on an already stressed and injured myocardium.

"**Distributive shock**" is a catchall phrase for those cases that involve arterial and capillary shunting past tissue beds with an increase in venous capacitance. Examples include anaphylaxis and septic shock. Gram-negative septic shock appears to be mediated by endotoxins (lipopolysaccharides) and subsequent formation of cytokines (tumor necrosis factor, interleukin-1 [IL-1], IL-10)), eicosanoid products, bradykinin, and endorphins. These agents can directly mediate many of the manifestations of septic shock, and they also amplify the injury by attracting granulocytes and macrophages—cells that cause further epithelial injury, activate additional cells, and release mediators. Vasodilators (prostaglandin I_2, endorphins) predominate early, causing a drop in systemic vascular resistance. Cardiac output generally is increased to compensate for the decreased systemic vascular resistance. This phase has been described as "warm shock," since the skin remains well perfused and warm. As septic shock progresses, the heart is no longer able to maintain such a high output, and vasoconstrictors (thromboxane, leukotrienes, endothelin) predominate, with resultant decreased peripheral perfusion. Extremities become cool, urine output decreases, and oxygen delivery falls. The speed with which distributive shock progresses varies according to the cause; it can be quite fast in anaphylaxis and insidious in cases associated with gram-positive cocci.

Other Organ Involvement

Organ dysfunction during and after an episode of shock is common. Systems most often affected include the kidney, the blood coagulation system, the lungs, the central nervous system, the liver, and the gastrointestinal tract. The kidney responds to hypotension by increasing plasma renin and angiotensin concentrations, causing a decrease in glomerular filtration rate and urine output. This can progress to damage of the energy-consuming renal parenchyma, causing acute tubular necrosis. Coagulopathies may exist in any type of shock but are especially common in septic shock. They result from the release of mediators that activate the clotting cascade, leading ultimately to a consumptive coagulopathy. The central nervous system dysfunction is related to decreased cerebral perfusion pressure and thus to decreased substrate delivery to the brain. Liver dysfunction commonly occurs after shock and may be manifested by increases in liver enzymes or a bleeding diathesis. Gastrointestinal problems include ileus, bleeding (eg, gastritis, ulcers), and necrosis with sloughing of intestinal mucosa. These organ system complications

should be aggressively searched for after an episode of shock. Multiple organ system failure secondary to shock greatly increases the mortality rates.

Monitoring

Both noninvasive and invasive monitoring of the patient in shock provides information on the severity, progression, and response to treatment. Extremely valuable information can be derived from examination of the cardiovascular, central nervous, renal, musculoskeletal, and mucocutaneous systems.

A. Clinical Findings:

1. Cardiovascular system—Tachycardia is not always present even in profound hypotension. Hypotension occurs late in pediatric shock (mean systolic blood pressure for a child over 2 years of age can be estimated by adding 90 mm Hg to twice the age in years). An important part of the cardiovascular examination is simultaneous palpation of distal and proximal pulses. An increase in the amplitude difference of pulses between proximal arteries (carotid, brachial, femoral) and distal arteries (radial, posterior tibial, dorsalis pedis) can be palpated in early shock and reflects increased systemic vascular resistance. Distal pulses may be thready or absent even in the presence of normal blood pressure because of poor stroke volume compensated by tachycardia and increased systemic vascular resistance. In uncompensated shock, hypotension is present and proximal pulses are also diminished. Early shock causes peripheral cutaneous vasoconstriction, which preserves flow to vital organs.

2. Skin—Because of peripheral vasoconstriction, the skin is gray or ashen in newborns and pale and cold in older patients. Capillary refilling after blanching is slow (>3 seconds). Mottling of the skin may also be observed.

3. Musculoskeletal system—Decreased oxygen delivery to the musculoskeletal system produces hypotonia. Decreased spontaneous motor activity, flaccidity, and prostration are observed.

4. Urinary output—Urine output is directly proportionate to renal blood flow and the glomerular filtration rate. Catheterization of the bladder is necessary to give accurate and continuous information. (Normal urine output is ≥1 mL/kg/h; outputs <0.5 mL/kg/h are considered significantly decreased.)

5. Central nervous system—The patient's level of consciousness reflects the adequacy of cortical perfusion. When this is severely impaired, the infant or child fails to respond first to verbal stimuli, then to light touch, and finally to pain. Lack of motor response and failure to cry in response to venipuncture or lumbar puncture should alert the clinician to the severity of the situation. In uncompensated shock in the presence of hypotension, brain stem perfusion may be decreased. Poor thalamic perfusion can result in loss of sympathetic tone. Finally, poor medullary flow produces irregular respirations followed by gasping, apnea, and respiratory arrest.

B. Invasive Monitoring: Patients with poor cardiac output who are hypovolemic often need invasive monitoring for diagnostic and therapeutic reasons. Arterial catheters give constant blood pressure readings, and, to an experienced interpreter, the shape of the waveform is helpful in evaluating cardiac output. Central venous pressure monitoring gives useful information about relative changes in volume status as therapy is given. Central venous pressure monitoring does not provide information about absolute volume status because intravascular volume, which is considered preload, is most accurately inferred from left ventricular end-diastolic pressures. Therefore, intravascular volume is more accurately assessed by monitoring pulmonary capillary wedge pressure or left atrial pressure. Measurements of pulmonary capillary wedge pressure can be obtained with a pulmonary artery catheter. The pulmonary artery catheter provides additional valuable information on volume and cardiac status (Table 13–8) but is associated with a higher complication rate than central venous pressure lines. Measurements of arterial and mixed venous oxygen saturations, along with cardiac output data, are useful in calculating oxygen delivery, consumption, and extraction. Oxygen consumption is frequently reduced long before hypotension is present. With the use of a pulmonary artery catheter, the effects of manipulating hemoglobin, oxygen saturation, and cardiac output (the determinants of oxygen consumption and delivery) can be followed in attempts to achieve independence of oxygen delivery and consumption. Patients receiving significant inotropic or ventilatory support may also benefit from the placement of a pulmonary artery catheter.

Treatment
(See also p 000.)

A. Fluid Resuscitation: A timely infusion of fluids may reverse the shock in patients with hypovolemic and distributive shock. Patients with cardiogenic shock, however, may worsen when given intravenous fluids unnecessarily because of the diminished ability of the left ventricle to handle volume.

Initially, most patients tolerate crystalloid (salt solution), which is readily available and inexpensive. However, 4 hours after a crystalloid infusion, only 20% of the solution remains in the intravascular space. Patients with serious capillary leaks and ongoing plasma losses (eg, burn cases) should initially receive crystalloid, because in these cases colloid (protein and salt solution) leaks into the interstitium. The protein draws intravascular fluid into the interstitium, thus increasing ongoing losses. Patients with hypoalbuminemia or those with intact capillaries who need to retain volume in the intravascular space (eg, patients at risk for cerebral edema) probably benefit from colloid infusions. Experience with dextran (a starch compound dissolved in salt solution) is limited. The amount of fluids given should be governed by physical examination, cardiovascular status, and laboratory results. Patients with normal heart function tolerate increased volume better than those with poor function.

B. Pharmacotherapy: Inotropic support may be needed in patients unable to meet the increased demand for cardiac output. Dopamine can increase renal, coronary, and cerebral blood flow by its action on beta-receptors and dopaminergic receptors. At higher doses (15 µg/kg/min), alpha-vasoconstrictor actions predominate. Dobutamine is often added to dopamine. Indeed, dobutamine may be the drug of choice in low cardiac output states because—unlike dopamine—it increases stroke volume and therefore cardiac output while decreasing left ventricular wall tension and myocardial oxygen consumption. Norepinephrine can be used to increase peripheral vasoconstriction, especially in septic shock. Epinephrine should be used with caution because it increases heart rate and afterload, neither of which may be well

Table 13–8. Hemodynamic parameters.[1]

Parameter	Formula[2]	Normal Values	Units
Cardiac output	$CO = HR \times SV$	Wide age-dependent range	L/min
Cardiac index	$CI = CO/BSA$	3.5–5.5	$L/min/m^2$
Stroke index	$SI = SV/BSA$	30–60	mL/m^2
Systemic vascular resistance	$SVR = 79.9 \dfrac{(MAP - CVP)}{CI}$	800–1600	dyne s/cm^{-5}/m^2
Pulmonary vascular resistance	$PVR = 79.9 \dfrac{(MPAP - PCWP)}{CI}$	80–240	dyne s/cm^{-5}/m^2

[1]Formulas and normals from Katz RW, Pollack M, Weibley R: Pulmonary artery catheterization in pediatric intensive care. Adv Pediatr 1984;30:169.
[2]HR = heart rate, SV = stroke volume, BSA = body surface area, MAP = mean arterial pressure, CVP = central venous pressure, MPAP = mean pulmonary artery pressure, PCWP = pulmonary capillary wedge pressure.

tolerated in the failing heart. Amrinone is a phosphodiesterase inhibitor increasingly used in shock. It has actions similar to those of dobutamine, increasing cardiac output and decreasing systemic vascular resistance, right atrial pressure, pulmonary capillary wedge pressure, and pulmonary artery pressure. Patients with increased systemic vascular resistance receiving cardiotonic drugs may benefit from a direct vasodilator to reduce the systemic vascular resistance or afterload and increase cardiac contractility (Table 13–9).

Although infusions of endotoxin into experimental animals have demonstrated a major role for endotoxin in the pathophysiology of septic shock, recent human trials of antiendotoxins showed no improvement in survival. The agents tested were able to bind endotoxin, but not neutralize it. It is now thought that the inability to neutralize endotoxin may be related to the lack of efficacy seen in these early trials. Antagonists to endotoxin and IL-1 (an inflammatory mediator activated in sepsis) are currently being investigated. Early results in human trials have been disappointing, but may suggest some improvement in survival in adults with multiorgan dysfunction and sepsis. Antagonists to tumor necrosis factor and bradykinin are in early clinical trials. Ibuprofen, with

Table 13–9. Pharmacologic support of the shock patient.

Drug	Dose	Alpha-Adrenergic Effect[1]	Beta-Adrenergic Effect[1]	Vasodilator Effect	Actions and Advantages	Disadvantages
Dopamine	1–20 μg/kg/min	+ to +++ (dose-related)	+ to +++ (dose-related)	At low doses, renal vasodilation occurs (dopaminergic receptors)	Moderate inotrope, wide and safe dosage range, short half-life	May cause worsening of pulmonary vasoconstriction
Dobutamine	1–10 μg/kg/min	0	+++		Moderate inotrope, less chronotropic, fewer dysrhythmias than with isoproterenol or epinephrine	Marked variation among patients
Amrinone	Bolus, 0.75 mg/kg over 3 min; infusion, 5–10 μg/kg/min	0	0	Direct smooth muscle relaxant	Non–β-adrenergic inotrope, afterload reduction	Arrhythmias, thrombocytopenia, gastrointestinal complaints
Epinephrine	0.05–1 μg/kg/min	++ to +++ (dose-related)	+++		Significant increases in inotropy, chronotropy, and systemic vascular resistance	Tachycardia, dysrhythmias, renal ischemia, systemic and pulmonary vascular resistance
Isoproterenol	0.05–1 μg/kg/min	0	+++	Peripheral vasodilation	Significant increase in inotropy and chronotropy. Systemic vascular resistance can drop, and pulmonary vascular resistance should not increase and may decrease.	Significant myocardial oxygen consumption increases, tachycardia, dysrhythmia
Norepinephrine	0.05–1 μg/kg/min	+++	+++		Powerful vasoconstrictor (systemic and pulmonary); rarely used except possibly in patients with very low systemic vascular resistance or in conjunction with vasodilator	Reduced cardiac output if afterload is too high, renal ischemia
Nitroprusside	0.05–8 μg/kg/min	0	0	Arterial and venous dilation (smooth muscle relaxation)	Decreases systemic and pulmonary vascular resistance, very short-acting. Blood pressure returns to previous levels within 1–10 minutes after infusion is stopped.	Toxicities (thiocyanates and cyanide), increased intracranial pressure and ventilation/perfusion mismatch, methemoglobinemia, increased intracranial pressure

[1]0 = no effect, + = small effect, ++ = moderate effect, +++ = potent effect.

its ability to block cyclo-oxygenase (cyclo-oxygenase metabolites are known inflammatory mediators), has shown a trend toward stabilizing patients with septic shock, and clinical trials are planned. Recently, excess production of NO has been demonstrated to contribute to the hypotension and poor perfusion seen in shock. Analogues of L-arginine (L-NMA) have been used to block the production of NO in animal models of septic shock with some improvement in survival. Anecdotal use in adults with severe septic shock has demonstrated some success.

Corticosteroids, by virtue of their action on many mediators, are thought to play a role in shock and—based on positive results in animal models of septic shock—have been advocated for treatment of shock. Clinical trials of steroids in sepsis showed no difference in mortality rates between steroid-treated and placebo-treated groups. Two exceptions appear to be children with meningococcal meningitis and AIDS patients with *Pneumocystis* pneumonia. Both groups have shown improvement in oxygenation and a trend toward improved survival when treated with corticosteroids.

Bernard GR: Sepsis trials. Am J Respir Crit Care 1995; 152:4.

Bone RC, Balk RA, Cerra FB, and the ACCP/SCCM Consensus Conference Committee: Definitions for sepsis and organ failure and guidelines for the use of innovative therapies in sepsis. Chest 1992;101:1644.

ECMO has been considered in the treatment of shock in patients with recoverable cardiac and pulmonary function who require both pulmonary and cardiac support. Eight of 10 neonates with fulminant septic shock not responsive to conventional treatment survived after treatment. Further data are needed to determine the role of this modality in the treatment of shock.

Astiz ME, Rackow EC, Weil MH: Pathophysiology and treatment of circulatory shock. Crit Care Clin 1993; 9:183.

Boyd JL, Stanford GC, Chernow B: The pharmacotherapy of septic shock. Crit Care Clin 1989;5:133.

Burns KM: Vasoactive drug therapy in shock. Crit Care Nurs Clin North Am 1990;2:167.

Fields AI: Invasive hemodynamic monitoring in children. Clin Chest Med 1987;8:611.

Fink MP: Gastrointestinal mucosal injury in experimental models of shock, trauma, and sepsis. Crit Care Med 1991;19:627.

Katz RW, Pollack MM, Weibley RE: Pulmonary artery catheterization in pediatric intensive care. Adv Pediatr 1984;30:169.

Kilbourn RG et al: Reversal of endotoxin mediated shock by NG-methyl-L-arginine, an inhibitor of nitric oxide synthesis. Biochem Biophys Res Commun 1990;172: 1132.

Putterman C: Modern approaches to the therapy of septic shock. Am J Emerg Med 1990;8:152.

Shoemaker WC: Relationship of oxygen transport patients to the pathophysiology and therapy of shock states. Intensive Care Med 1987;13:230.

St John RC, Dorinsky PM: Immunologic therapy of ARDS, septic shock, and multiple organ failure. Chest 1993; 103:932.

Summers G: The clinical and hemodynamic presentation of the shock patient. Crit Care Nurs Clin North Am 1990;2:161.

Whitfield JM, Dobyns EL, Webb SA: Neonatal sepsis. In: *Textbook of Critical Care.* Holbrook PR (editor). Saunders, 1993.

Worthley L, Tyler P, Moran JL: A comparison of dopamine, dobutamine and isoproterenol in the treatment of shock. Intensive Care Med 1985;11:13.

INDICATIONS FOR CENTRAL VENOUS AND ARTERIAL CANNULATION

Placement of catheters into the central venous or arterial circulation may be justified for continuous assessment of intravascular volume, cardiac function, blood drawing for lab work or administration of volume, drugs, or hyperalimentation.

General Rules for Equipment Selection and Technique

(1) Vascular access equipment should be selected based on evaluation of the following: material; tendency to burr, buckle, or crimp; patient comfort; thrombogenicity; resistance to bacterial colonization; and price.

(2) Greater consistency and success can be achieved by restricting the variety, number of kits, and equipment.

(3) Open the kit and examine all components. This includes feeding the wire through the needle and filling all lines with normal saline to prevent air from entering the circulation.

(4) In the awake or sedated patient, greater success can be achieved if two people perform the procedure (in addition to those occupied with restraining or positioning the patient).

(5) Apply EMLA cream (eutectic mixture of lidocaine 2.5% and prilocaine 2.5%) to the area of puncture (45 minutes before the procedure) or infiltrate with an appropriate local anesthetic before prepping and draping the skin.

(6) Sterilize and drape the area around the point of entry.

(7) When searching for the vessel, make straight passes while maintaining slight negative pressure. Advance and withdraw the needle at the same speed. Frequently, the blood return will occur during withdrawal.

(8) Once there is free flow of venous blood into the syringe, remove the syringe without moving the needle and, if using the Seldinger technique, pass the

J wire through the needle. When appropriate, watch the ECG for arrhythmias, since they are frequently seen when the J wire touches the right side of the heart.

(9) Withdraw the needle over the J wire and clean the wire of blood.

(10) Make a nick with a No. 11 blade at the point where the J wire enters the skin. Pass the introducer and/or the intravascular catheter over the J wire.

(11) With the catheters in place, remove the wire along with the introducer.

(12) Check to make sure that blood can be drawn easily through the new line.

(13) Verify the position of the line on x-ray.

Points of Entry for Venous Line Placement

(1) **External jugular vein:** Place a soft cloth roll beneath the patient's shoulder and turn the head to the contralateral side (Figure 13–2). Valsalva's maneuver, Trendelenburg position, or occlusion of the vessel at the clavicular level are ways of temporarily increasing jugular distention and visibility. To overcome the problems of this vessel's mobility and thick wall, apply cephalic retraction of the skin over the

Figure 13–2. External jugular vein technique. (Reproduced, with permission, from Chameides L: *Textbook of Pediatric Advanced Life Support.* American Heart Association, 1988.)

vessel superior to the point of needle entry. Maintain gentle negative pressure in the syringe attached to the needle as it is advanced toward the vessel. Needle entry into the vessel lumen is usually signaled by a change in resistance followed by appearance of venous blood in the hub of the needle. Lay the needle along the side of the vessel and advance it a few more millimeters to ensure that the bevel of the needle is completely in the vessel lumen. Remove the syringe without moving the needle and pass a soft J wire into the vessel lumen. With manipulation, the J wire should pass into the central circulation. Remove the needle and pass the central line over the J wire.

(2) **Internal jugular vein:** Once the patient has been prepped, draped, and positioned as shown in Figure 13–3, feel for the trachea halfway between the angle of the jaw and the suprasternal notch and then feel lateral to the trachea for the carotid pulse. Just lateral to the carotid pulse, at a 30-degree angle from horizontal, insert a finder needle (25-gauge), aiming between the ipsilateral nipple and shoulder. Once venous return is established, remove the finder needle and repeat the procedure with the appropriate-size larger needle.

(3) **Subclavian entry:** After the patient has been prepped, draped, and positioned (Figure 13–4), move the needle flat along the chest, entering along the inferior edge of the clavicle just lateral to the midclavicular line and aiming for the suprasternal notch. Once venous return is established, use the Seldinger technique.

(4) **Femoral approach:** With the patient's leg slightly abducted (Figure 13–5), find the femoral artery 3–4 cm below the inguinal ligament. The femoral vein is just medial and parallel to the femoral artery. Insert the needle at a 30- to 45-degree angle. Once venous return is established, use the Seldinger technique.

(5) **Antecubital approach:** "PIC" (peripherally inserted catheter) lines (No. 2.8–4 French) are long, soft Silastic styleted catheters most commonly threaded from an antecubital vessel to the right atrium. These lines are not difficult to insert and are easy to dress and keep clean. They are suited for long-term use because they are less thrombogenic, tolerable for the patient, and good for infusion of hyperalimentation and drugs. In general, they are not suitable for obtaining blood for laboratory analysis.

General Rules for Cannulation of the Arterial System

(1) Rules 1–6 for the central venous system apply for the arterial system as well.

(2) The Seldinger technique can be applied for arterial tree cannulation.

(3) Most arteries can be cannulated percutaneously.

(4) Puncture the skin at the insertion site to elimi-

Figure 13–3. A: The internal jugular vein and its relationship to the surrounding anatomy. **B:** Technique of anterior internal jugular cannulation. (Reproduced, with permission, from Chameides L: *Textbook of Pediatric Advanced Life Support.* American Heart Association, 1988.)

Figure 13–4. Subclavian artery. **A:** Anatomy. **B:** Technique. (Reproduced, with permission, from Chameides L: *Textbook of Pediatric Advanced Life Support.* American Heart Association, 1988.)

nate any drag or resistance on the catheter advancement.

(5) Insert the cannula at a 30-degree angle to the skin surface, advancing at a slow rate toward the arterial pulse. Watch the hub of the cannula for a flash of arterial blood.

(6) When arterial flash is seen, lower the catheter to a 10-degree angle with the surface of the skin and advance the catheter into the lumen of the artery. If successful, pulsatile arterial flow will continue into the catheter. Advance an additional centimeter to make certain that the catheter is in the arterial lumen.

(7) Hold the catheter while removing the needle stylet. Arterial blood will pulse out of the catheter if the tip is in the arterial lumen.

(8) Advance the catheter into the lumen; attach a syringe containing normal saline with 1 U/mL of heparin; aspirate to make certain that there are no bubbles; and then gently flush the catheter.

(9) If arterial flow into the needle stylet stops during catheter advancement, advance this unit an additional centimeter. Remove the needle stylet and place it on a sterile surface. Pull the catheter out slowly. When the tip of the catheter flips into the arterial lu-

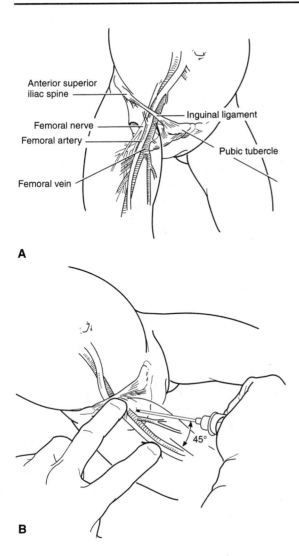

A

B

Figure 13–5. Femoral vein. **A:** Anatomy. **B:** Technique. (Reproduced, with permission, from Chameides L: *Textbook of Pediatric Advanced Life Support.* American Heart Association, 1988.)

men, the pulsatile arterial blood flow is seen. Rotate the catheter to ensure that the catheter is free within the vessel lumen, then advance the remainder of the catheter length into the vessel.

(10) Suture the catheter in place while ensuring that the arterial trace is not damped.

(11) Dress the insertion site with sterile gauze, and tape it to the skin.

Point of Entry for Arterial Line Placement

Always consider whether there is collateral arterial blood flow to the structures distal to the insertion

point. Allen's test must be done prior to radial or ulnar artery cannulation.

Arterial sites, listed in order of preference, include:

(1) Radial artery (nondominant arm first).

(2) Femoral artery (morbidity is the same as for the radial artery beyond the newborn period).

(3) Posterior tibial artery.

(4) Dorsalis pedis artery.

(5) Ulnar artery (if distal radial filling is present in that hand).

(6) Axillary artery.

(7) Brachial artery (poor collateral flow, used only during cardiac surgery in newborn-sized patients with arterial access limitations).

Final Considerations

(1) Patient benefit should outweigh any risks from central venous or arterial cannulation.

(2) Coagulation status of the patient at the time of placement and throughout the time of use must be considered, since deep venous and arterial thrombus formation is partially related to the patient's coagulation status.

(3) The incidence of catheter colonization and infection increases if central venous and arterial lines are left in for more than 6 days.

Agee KR, Balk RA: Central venous catheterization in the critically ill patient. Crit Care Clin 1992;8:677.
Allen EV: Thromboangiitis obliterans: Methods of diagnosis of chronic occlusive arterial lesions distal to the wrist with illustrative cases. Am J Med Sci 1929;178:237.
Clark VL, Kruse JA: Arterial catheterization. Crit Care Clin 1992;8:687.
Seldinger SI: Catheter placement of needle in percutaneous arteriography; a new technique. Acta Radiol 1953;39: 368.

CEREBRAL EDEMA

Cerebral edema is a major cause of morbidity and mortality in the PICU. Cerebal edema is generally broken down into three types. **Cytotoxic edema** is caused by direct cellular injury, usually as a consequence of hypoxia or anoxia. Cellular energy stores are depleted, and ionic pumps of the cell cease activity, causing fluid to accumulate in the cell. **Vasogenic edema** is the result of direct injury to the blood-brain barrier. When the tight junctions of the endothelium are injured, water and protein can extravasate into the interstitium of the brain. In traumatic head injury, this may be a major cause of edema. **Interstitial edema** is caused by an imbalance of cerebrospinal fluid production and reabsorption and is treatable with ventricular shunting.

Much of the damage to the brain from traumatic head injury is a result of direct damage to neurons and therefore is not influenced by intensive therapy.

The goal of ICU management is to decrease secondary injury to the brain resulting from hypoxia, hypoperfusion, and acidosis.

Clinical Findings

A. Symptoms & Signs: Patients with elevations in intracranial pressure (ICP) may develop headaches, vomiting, diplopia, seizures, and/or a decrease in Glasgow Coma Score. Physical findings include alterations in mental status, alterations in muscle tone and deep tendon reflexes, bradycardia, hypertension, and a bulging fontanelle or increase in head circumference (<12 months of age). Papilledema may take 8–12 hours to develop. The young patient may not demonstrate the Cushing reflex of hypertension, bradycardia, and decreased respirations.

B. ICP Monitoring (Table 13–10): The benefit of ICP monitoring is dependent on the cause of cerebral edema. ICP monitoring has shown potential benefit in acute head trauma and Reye's syndrome. Its use in cerebral hemorrhage, meningitis, and encephalitis is more controversial. No benefit has been shown in hypoxic-ischemic injuries, such as near-drowning or sudden infant death syndrome (SIDS).

Treatment

Treatment for ICP should be started when clinical evidence of its presence exists. Therapies can be broken down into basic and advanced therapies.

A. Basic Therapies: These therapies do not require the presence of an ICP monitor.

(1) Elevation of the head of the bed to 30 degrees, with the head maintained in the midline.

(2) Ventilation of the patient to maintain a P_{O_2} greater than 80 mm Hg and a P_{CO_2} of 25–30 mm Hg.

(3) Maintenance of the blood pressure in the normal range for age.

(4) Avoidance of hyperthermia, which increases cerebral metabolic rate.

(5) Avoidance of seizures, which increase cerebral oxygen consumption. Prophylactic anticonvulsants may be indicated, especially in head trauma.

(6) Paralysis and sedation should be used only if necessary to control ventilation and patient movement.

(7) Hypovolemia should be treated aggressively to maintain blood pressure. Raising the osmolality of the blood to between 300 and 310 mosm/kg will help slow the formation of edema and reduce the ICP. This can be accomplished through the use of mannitol, furosemide, and/or moderate fluid restriction.

(8) Lidocaine (1 mg/kg IV) given 1 minute before endotracheal tube suctioning blunts the ICP response to stimulation.

B. Advanced Therapies: These therapies are more controversial and require the continuous monitoring of ICP.

(1) Maintenance of the cerebral perfusion pressure (CPP = MAP – ICP) at 50 mm Hg or higher. The optimal pressure has not been established. Positive inotropic agents may be required to maintain the pressure.

(2) Barbiturate coma has been shown to be effective in controlling ICP, but not necessarily in improving outcome. The barbiturates are all negative inotropes and vasodilators and may decrease CPP.

(3) Moderate hypothermia and decompressive craniotomy have been shown to lower ICP, but not to improve outcome.

Outcome

Pupillary response is an important prognostic indicator, with a mortality rate of 50% associated with an absent unilateral response and 90% with an absent response bilaterally.

Chesnut RM: Secondary brain insults after head injury: Clinical perspectives. New Horizons 1995;3:366.

Ghayar J, Harini RJ: Management of pediatric head injury. Pediatr Clin North Am 1992;39:1093.

Lang EW, Chesnut RM: Intracranial pressure and cerebral

Table 13–10. Comparison of intracranial pressure monitoring techniques.

Type of Monitor	Placement	Advantages	Disadvantages
External (pressure-sensitive)	Over the skin of open anterior fontanelle	Noninvasive. Useful as trending device.	Very indirect measurement. Useful in limited age group.
Epidural (fiberoptic, hydraulic, and pneumatic)	Between skull and dura	Easy placement. Low risk of infection. Difficult to occlude.	Unable to draw off CSF fluid. May create epidural bleeding.
Subarachnoid (hydraulic or fiberoptic)	Between dura and brain substance	Easy placement. Low risk of infection.	May be occluded by debris. Unable to draw off CSF fluid. May give falsely low readings.
Intraventricular (hydraulic, fiberoptic)	Inside the lateral ventricle	Most direct measurement. Therapeutic if able to draw off CSF.[1]	Requires adequately sized lateral ventricles. Increased risk of bleeding and infection.

[1]CSF = cerebrospinal fluid.

perfusion pressure in severe head injury. New Horizons 1995;3:400.

Marshall LF, Marshall SB: Pharmacologic therapy: Promising clinical investigations. New Horizons 1995;3:573.

McGillicuday JE: Cerebral protection: Pathophysiology and treatment of increased intracranial pressure. Chest 1985;87:85.

Olshaker JS, Whye DW Jr: Head trauma. Emerg Med Clin North Am 1993;11:165.

Robertson CS, Cormio M: Cerebral metabolic management. New Horizons 1995;3:410.

Rosner MJ, Daughton S: Cerebral perfusion pressure management in head trauma. J Trauma 1990;30:933.

BRAIN RESUSCITATION

The subspecialty of neurologic intensive care has grown rapidly over the past 20 years, mainly as a result of longer survival of sicker patients and the more rapid transport of critically ill patients with head injuries. Interest in preventing and limiting hypoxic-ischemic damage following primary brain injury has increased dramatically. However, attempts to reverse this damage have met with little success. The role of hypoxia and ischemia in causing damage is related to the metabolic breakdown caused both by intracellular hypoxia and by the cascade of events that follows cell reperfusion.

Initial enthusiasm for the use of barbiturate coma to decrease cerebral metabolism has somewhat subsided. Barbiturates do not appear to selectively lower cerebral metabolism without lowering cerebral blood flow. They are now recommended for limited use to treat increased intracranial pressure, with close observation for potential hemodynamic instability induced by barbiturates.

Reperfusion injury in the ischemic region is believed to be related to free radical interaction with lipid membranes, DNA, and intracellular calcium, resulting in cellular damage. Animal research using free radical scavengers and calcium channel blockers show promising results, and human trials are being undertaken.

Recently, specific amino acids have been identified as excitatory neurotransmitters and are postulated to play a role in neurologic injury and seizures. Use of antagonists may be effective treatment and is being investigated.

One must keep in mind that respiratory arrest in the research setting causes more brain damage than does the global ischemia caused by circulatory arrest. This finding is worrisome, because the typical arrest in pediatrics is respiratory.

Kochanek PM: Novel pharmacologic approaches to brain resuscitation after cardiorespiratory arrest in the pediatric patient. Crit Care Clin 1988;4:661.

Krause GS: Brain cell death following ischemia and reperfusion: A proposed biochemical sequence. Crit Care Med 1988;16:714.

Rogers MC, Kirsch JR: Current concepts in brain resuscitation. JAMA 1989;261:3143.

Safar P: Resuscitation from clinical death: Pathophysiologic limits and therapeutic potentials. Crit Care Med 1988;16:923.

Sutton-Tyrrell K et al: Brain Resuscitation Clinical Trial Study Group: Risk monitoring of randomized trials in emergency medicine: Experience of the brain resuscitation clinical trial II. Am J Emerg Med 1991;9:112.

ETHICAL CONSIDERATIONS IN INTENSIVE CARE

Patient Autonomy

Although the pediatric patient is generally a minor, respect for the patient's rights and wishes should still play a part in the decision-making process. Whenever appropriate, the child should be included in discussions concerning the clinical problem and its management.

Brain Death

The limited pool of organ donation candidates and the increasing number of potential recipients has made the diagnosis of death prior to the cessation of physiologic function an imperative professional obligation. Currently, the diagnosis of brain death is fairly straightforward and accepted in all jurisdictions. It requires the following conditions:

(1) The absence of a primary remediable condition that might mimic brain death (eg, acute subdural hemorrhage). This generally requires a clear history or a CT scan.

(2) The absence of hypotension with consequent cerebral hypoperfusion that would alter cerebral activity.

(3) The absence of hypothermia, which would alter cerebral activity. Generally, this requires a temperature of greater than 35 °C.

(4) The absence of exposure to drugs or toxins that would mimic brain death. This generally requires a toxicology screen. Therapeutic levels of anticonvulsants and sedatives will not mimic brain death.

Once these conditions have been met, the brain death examination can be performed. This examination is designed to guarantee the absence of any cortical or brain stem activity. The following procedures must be performed:

(1) Assessment of cranial nerve function. Test the following reflexes: optic light, oculocalorics, oculocephalics, cough, gag, and corneal. Test for pain sensation on the face.

(2) Assessment of pain response. The body should be examined for the presence of purposeful withdrawal to pain. Caution must be exercised in the interpretation of spinal reflexes.

(3) Assessment of respiratory drive. A 3-minute apnea test should be performed starting with a PCO_2 of 55 mm Hg, and with the patient on 100% oxygen during the test.

Discontinuance of Life Support

In spite of advances in medicine, ICU patients are frequently at the limits of the physician's ability to sustain life. In the interests of the quality of life for the patient and the family, it is often necessary to consider the limitation or discontinuance of life-sustaining treatments. While the topic is too complex and patient variability is too great to allow for a comprehensive discussion of this topic, certain principles underlie the majority of such decisions:

(1) The patient should be considered terminal. Generally, this implies that continuation of life in the best of possible circumstances will be less than 1 year. In addition, some patients with no ability to meaningfully interact with their environment may also be considered.

(2) There must be single organ system failure that is not amenable to transplant (eg, the cerebral cortex) or multiple organ system failure.

(3) There must be a medical consensus among involved health care personnel as to these diagnoses. This requires the concurrence of at least two physicians as well as of nursing and social services personnel.

(4) The burden of continued existence—pain and suffering—should outweigh any potential gain of continued therapy.

(5) The patient, if appropriate and capable, and the patient's parents and guardians must be fully informed and in agreement with the course of action.

Hospital ethics committees may be of assistance in situations in which there is disagreement among health care providers.

Once the decision to limit or discontinue medical therapy has been agreed on, a course of action that is both humane and in compliance with good medical practice must be determined. All medical therapy may be considered to be extraordinary in certain circumstances.

These decisions cannot be considered irrevocable. If at any time the family or health care providers wish to reconsider the decision, full medical therapy should be reinstituted until the situation is clarified.

Nelson LJ, Nelson RM: Ethics and the provision of futile, harmful, or burdensome treatment to children. Crit Care Med 1992;20:427.

Task Force on Ethics of the Society of Critical Care Medicine: Consensus report on the ethics of foregoing life-sustaining treatments in the critically ill. Crit Care Med 1990;18:1435.

Truog RD, Fackler JC: Rethinking brain death. Crit Care Med 1992;20:1705.

NUTRITIONAL SUPPORT AFTER INJURY

Trauma, sepsis, and significant injury are associated with a variety of profound metabolic and physiologic responses. Nutritional status has an impact on in-hospital morbidity rates and mortality outcomes. Inadequate nutrition can impair wound healing and immune function and prevent early weaning from mechanical ventilation. Stress in critically ill children induces more than simple starvation. The hypermetabolic response seen during severe stress results in increased energy usage and endogenous nutrient requirement, especially protein. The metabolic needs of critically ill children are largely managed by intravenous hyperalimentation, tailored to meet stress and hypercatabolic states (qv).

Demling RH, DeBiasse MA: Micronutrients in critical illness. Crit Care Clin 1995;11:651.

Kinney JM: Metabolic responses of the critically ill patient. Crit Care Clin 1995;11:569.

Manning EMC, Shenkin A: Nutritional assessment in the critically ill. Crit Care Clin 1995;11:603.

McNurlan MA, Garlick PJ: Protein and amino acids in nutritional support. Crit Care Clin 1995;11:635.

Wojnar MM, Hawkins WG, Lang CH: Nutritional support of the septic patient. Crit Care Clin 1995;11:717.

PAIN & ANXIETY CONTROL
(See Table 13–11.)

Anxiety control and pain relief are two of the most important responsibilities of the critical care physician. Earlier perceptions that children do not require pain relief have drastically changed in response to documented proof of improved outcomes in children receiving appropriate pain relief. The anxiety of patients in the PICU is well known. These responses may interact to heighten fear and the perception of pain and may reach levels sufficient to cause deterioration in the patient's clinical condition. It is important to distinguish between anxiety and pain, since pharmacologic therapy may be directed at either one or both of these symptoms.

Sedation

Sedative (anxiolytic) drugs are used to induce calmness without producing sleep—although at high doses all anxiolytics will cause drowsiness and sleep. The five indications for the use of sedative drugs are (1) to allay fear and anxiety; (2) to manage acute confusional states; (3) to facilitate treatment or diagnostic procedures; (4) to facilitate mechanical ventilation; and (5) to obtund physiologic responses to stress, that is, reduce tachycardia, hypertension, or increases in intracranial pressure. In the ICU setting, a parenteral (intravenous bolus or infusion) preparation is essential to allow titration of clinical effects in

Table 13–11. Pain and anxiety control.

Drug	Dose and Method of Administration[1]	Advantages	Disadvantages	Usual Duration of Effect
Morphine	IV, 0.1 mg/kg; continuous infusion; 0.01–0.05 mg/kg/h	Excellent pain relief, reversible	Respiratory depression, hypotension, nausea, suppression of intestinal motility, histamine release	2–4 h
Meperidine	IV, 1 mg/kg	Good pain relief, reversible	Respiratory depression, histamine release, nausea, suppression of intestinal motility	2–4 h
Fentanyl	IV, 1–2 μg/kg; continuous infusion; 0.5–2 μg/kg/h	Excellent pain relief, reversible, short half-life	Respiratory depression, chest wall rigidity, severe nausea and vomiting	30 min
Diazepam	IV, 0.1 mg/kg	Sedation and seizure control	Respiratory depression, jaundice, phlebitis	1–3 h
Lorazepam	IV, 0.1 mg/kg	Longer half-life, sedation and seizure control	Nausea and vomiting, respiratory depression, phlebitis	2–4 h
Midazolam	IV, 0.1 mg/kg	Short half-life, only benzodiazepine given as continuous infusion	Respiratory depression	30–60 min

[1]IV administration is most common in the ICU. The effects of morphine, meperidine, and fentanyl are reversible by administration of naloxone (opioid antagonist).

the face of possible impaired organ dysfunction (cardiac, respiratory, hepatic, renal, etc). Sedatives fall into several classes, with the opioid and benzodiazepine classes serving as the mainstay of anxiety treatment in the ICU.

A. Benzodiazepines: Benzodiazepines possess anxiolytic, hypnotic, anticonvulsant, and skeletal muscle relaxant properties. Although their exact mode of action is not known, it appears to be located within the limbic system of the central nervous system and to involve the neuroinhibitory transmitter γ-aminobutyric acid. Most benzodiazepines are metabolized in the liver, with their metabolites subsequently excreted in the urine; thus, patients in liver failure are likely to have long elimination times.

Benzodiazepine overdosage can cause respiratory depression if given rapidly in high doses, and they potentiate the analgesic and respiratory depressive effects of opioids and barbiturates.

Three benzodiazepines with differing half-lives are presently used in the ICU setting.

1. Midazolam—Midazolam has the shortest half-life (1½–3½ hours) of the benzodiazepines and is the only benzodiazepine that should be administered as a continuous intravenous infusion. It produces excellent retrograde amnesia lasting for 20–40 minutes after a single intravenous dose. Therefore, it can be used either for short-term sedation or for "awake" procedures such as endoscopy or as a continuous infusion in the anxious, restless patient. The single intravenous dose is 0.1 mg/kg, while a continuous infusion should be started at a rate of 0.1

mg/kg/h after an initial loading dose of 0.1 mg/kg. The midazolam infusion dosage must be titrated upward to achieve the desired effect. Midazolam is not an analgesic, and if very high doses are being used without the proper effect and it is felt that analgesia is also needed, the dose of midazolam can usually be lowered by the concurrent use of small doses of an appropriate analgesic such as morphine or fentanyl. When administering midazolam or any other benzodiazepine, it is important to monitor cardiorespiratory status and have resuscitation facilities available.

2. Diazepam—Diazepam has a longer half-life than midazolam and can be given orally as well as by the intravenous route. Its disadvantage in the ICU is its intermediary metabolite, nordiazepam, which has a very long elimination half-life and may accumulate, causing prolonged sedation. It produces excellent anxiolysis and amnesia. Additionally, it is used to treat acute status epilepticus. The intravenous dose is 0.1 mg/kg and can be repeated every 15 minutes to achieve the desired effect or until undesirable side effects such as somnolence and respiratory depression occur.

3. Lorazepam—Lorazepam possesses the longest half-life of the three benzodiazepines discussed here and can be used to achieve sedation for as long as 6–8 hours. It has less effect on the cardiovascular and respiratory systems than other benzodiazepines and can be given orally, intravenously, or intramuscularly, with the intravenous route the most effective in the ICU setting. The intravenous dosage is 0.1 mg/kg. Lorazepam can also be used to treat acute status epilepticus.

B. Other Drugs:

1. Chloral hydrate—Chloral hydrate is an enteral sedative and hypnotic agent frequently used in children. After either oral or rectal administration, it is rapidly metabolized by the liver to its active form trichloroethanol, which has an 8-hour half-life. A sedative dose is 6–20 mg/kg per dose, usually given every 6–8 hours, while the hypnotic dose is up to 50 mg/kg with a maximum dose of 1 g. The hypnotic dose is frequently used to sedate young children for outpatient radiologic procedures such as CT scanning and MRI. There is little effect on respiration or blood pressure with therapeutic doses of chloral hydrate. The drug is irritating to mucus membranes, however, and may cause gastric upset if administered on an empty stomach.

2. Ketamine—Ketamine is a phencyclidine derivative that produces a trance-like state of immobility and amnesia known as "dissociative anesthesia." After intramuscular or intravenous administration, it causes central sympathetic nervous system stimulation with resultant increases in heart rate, blood pressure, and cardiac output. Respiration is not depressed at therapeutic doses. However, salivary and tracheobronchial mucous gland secretions are increased, so atropine should be administered 20 minutes prior to the ketamine. A distinct disadvantage of its use is the occurrence of unpleasant dreams or hallucinations, although the incidence is decreased in children compared to adults and can be reduced even further by the concurrent administration of a benzodiazepine. Because of its inotropic properties, it is useful for the sedation of certain critically ill patients whose condition is unstable. It is given as an intravenous injection of 1–2 mg/kg over 60 seconds, with supplementary doses of 0.5 mg/kg being required every 10–30 minutes to maintain an adequate level of anesthesia. Alternatively, it can be administered as an intramuscular injection of 5–10 mg/kg, which usually produces the desired level of anesthesia within 3–4 minutes. If prolonged anesthesia is required, ketamine can be administered by intravenous infusion at doses of 3–20 mg/kg/h.

3. Antihistamines—The antihistamines **diphenhydramine** and **hydroxyzine** can be used as sedatives but are not as effective as the benzodiazepines. Diphenhydramine produces sedation in only 50% of those treated. It can be given intravenously, intramuscularly, or orally at a dose of 1 mg/kg. Hydroxyzine can be given either intramuscularly or orally. It is frequently used concurrently with morphine or meperidine, adding anxiolysis and potentiating the effects of the opioid. The sedative effects of both drugs can last from 4 to 6 hours following a single dose.

4. Propofol—Propofol is an anesthetic induction agent whose main advantage is a rapid recovery time and no cumulative effects resulting from its rapid hepatic metabolism. It has no analgesic properties, frequently causes pain on injection, and causes a dose-related fall in blood pressure because of decreases in systemic vascular resistance. There are only a few clinical reports of its use as a sedative agent in pediatric patients, and the drug is very expensive. The sedative dose is 1 mg/kg as an intravenous bolus followed by an infusion of 1 mg/kg/h.

5. Barbiturates—Barbiturates (phenobarbital, thiopental) can cause direct myocardial and respiratory depression and are, in general, poor choices for sedation of seriously ill patients. Phenobarbital has a very long half-life (up to 4 days), and recovery from thiopental, though it is a "short-acting" barbiturate, can be prolonged because remobilization of tissue stores occurs.

Analgesia

A. Opioid Analgesics:

Opioid analgesics (morphine, fentanyl, codeine, meperidine) are the mainstays of therapy for most forms of acute severe pain as well as chronic cancer pain management. They possess both analgesic and dose-related sedative effects, although there is a range of plasma concentrations that produce analgesia without clouding of the sensorium. In addition, opioids can cause respiratory depression, nausea, pruritus, slowed intestinal motility, miosis, urinary retention, cough suppression, biliary spasm, and vasodilation. There is great individual variation in the dose of opioid required to produce adequate analgesia. Therefore, in the intensive care setting, a continuous infusion of morphine or fentanyl allows dosages to be easily titrated to achieve the desired effect.

In general, infants under 3 months of age are more susceptible to the respiratory depressant effects of opioids, and starting dosages for these patients should be about one-third to one-half the usual pediatric dose. Most opioids (except meperidine) have minimal cardiac depressive effects, and critically ill patients generally tolerate them well. Fentanyl does not cause the histamine release that morphine does and thus produces less vasodilation and drop in systemic blood pressure. Opioids are metabolized in the liver, with metabolites excreted in the urine. Thus, patients with hepatic or renal impairment may have a prolonged response to their administration. Patients who receive regular doses of opioids for 2 weeks or more frequently develop a physiologic dependence with the development of withdrawal symptoms (agitation, tachypnea, tachycardia, sweating, diarrhea) upon acute termination of the drug. In these patients, gradual tapering of the opioid dosage over a 5- to 10-day period will prevent withdrawal symptoms. As with any potent sedative or analgesic used in the ICU setting, appropriate patient monitoring (pulse oximetry, cardiorespiratory monitoring, blood pressure monitoring) should be used during the period of opioid administration, and equipment should be available to support prompt intervention if undesired side effects occur.

The ICU regimen for sedation and analgesia must be carefully modified when the patient is transferred to the ward or a lower vigilance area. Patients with baseline respiratory, hepatic, or renal insufficiencies are most predisposed to respiratory insufficiency from sedatives or opioid analgesics.

Patient-controlled analgesia (PCA) is a computer-controlled infusion pump for constant infusion or patient-controlled bolus infusion of opioid analgesics. The basal infusion mode is intended to provide a constant serum level of analgesic. The bolus mode allows the patient to self-administer, by pushing a button, additional doses for breakthrough pain. The patient is usually permitted six boluses an hour, with 10-minute blockouts. If the patient is using allotted hourly boluses, this usually means that the basal infusion rate is too low.

The patient must understand the concept of PCA in order to be a candidate for its use. There are circumstances in pediatrics in which it is appropriate for the nurse or parent to administer the bolus dose.

Naloxone reverses the analgesia, sedative, and respiratory depressive effects of opioid agonists. Its administration should again be titrated to achieve the desired effect (eg, reversal of respiratory depression, since full reversal using 0.01–0.02 mL/kg may cause acute anxiety, dysphoria, nausea, and vomiting). Furthermore, since the duration of effect of naloxone is shorter (30 minutes) than that of most opioids, the patient must be carefully observed for reappearance of the undesired effect.

B. Nonopioid Analgesics: Nonopioid analgesics used in the treatment of mild to moderate pain include acetaminophen, aspirin, and other nonsteroidal anti-inflammatory drugs (NSAIDs), such as ibuprofen and naproxen.

1. Acetaminophen—Acetaminophen is the most commonly used analgesic in pediatrics in the United States and is the drug of choice for mild to moderate pain because of its low toxicity and lack of effect on bleeding time. It is metabolized by the liver. Suggested doses are 10–15 mg/kg orally to approximately 10–20 mg/kg rectally every 4 hours.

2. Aspirin—Aspirin is also an effective analgesic for mild to moderate pain at doses of 10–15 mg/kg orally every 4 hours. However, its prolongation of bleeding time, association with Reye's syndrome, and propensity to cause gastric irritation limit its usefulness in pediatric practice. Aspirin and other NSAIDs are still useful, especially for pain of inflammatory origin, bone pain, and pain associated with rheumatic conditions.

3. Other NSAIDs—Ibuprofen and naproxen are both NSAIDs whose use has been limited in pediatrics to date. **Naproxen** is FDA-approved for children 2–12 years of age (5–7 mg/kg orally every 8–12 hours), while **ibuprofen** requires more frequent dosing intervals (4–10 mg/kg orally every 6–8 hours).

All of the NSAIDs have a therapeutic "ceiling"—that is, unlike opioids, which have a dose-related increase in potency, there is no increase in analgesic potency above the recommended dose. They all can cause gastritis and should be given with antacids or with meals. In addition, the analgesic effects of acetaminophen, aspirin, and other NSAIDs are additive to those of opioids. Thus, if additional analgesia is required, their use should be continued and an appropriate oral opioid (codeine, morphine) or parenteral opioid (morphine, fentanyl) begun.

American Academy of Pediatrics Committee on Drugs: Guidelines for monitoring and management of pediatric patients during and after sedation for diagnostic and therapeutic procedures. Pediatrics 1992;89:1110.

American Academy of Pediatrics Committee on Drugs and Committee on Environmental Health: Use of chloral hydrate for sedation in children. Pediatrics 1993;92:471.

Bailey PL et al: Frequent hypoxemia and apnea after sedation with midazolam and fentanyl. Anesthesiology 1990; 73:826.

Traynor LA: Midazolam-fentanyl sedation. (Letter.) Pediatrics 1991;88:1286.

Skin

14

Joseph G. Morelli, MD, & William L. Weston, MD

GENERAL PRINCIPLES OF DIAGNOSIS

Examination of the Skin

Examination of the skin requires that the entire surface of the body be palpated and inspected in good light. The onset and duration of each symptom should be recorded, together with a description of the primary lesion and any secondary changes, using the following terminology:

A. Primary Lesions (the First to Appear):

1. Macule—Any circumscribed color change in the skin that is flat. *Examples:* White (vitiligo), brown (café au lait spot), purple (petechia).

2. Papule—A solid, elevated area less than 1 cm in diameter whose top may be pointed, rounded, or flat. *Examples:* Acne, warts, small lesions of psoriasis.

3. Plaque—A solid, circumscribed area more than 1 cm in diameter, usually flat-topped. *Example:* Psoriasis.

4. Vesicle—A circumscribed, elevated lesion less than 1 cm in diameter and containing clear serous fluid. *Example:* Blisters of herpes simplex.

5. Bulla—A circumscribed, elevated lesion more than 1 cm in diameter and containing clear serous fluid. *Example:* Bullous erythema multiforme.

6. Pustule—A vesicle containing a purulent exudate. *Examples:* Acne, folliculitis.

7. Nodule—A deep-seated mass with indistinct borders that elevates the overlying epidermis. *Examples:* Tumors, granuloma annulare. If it moves with the skin on palpation, it is intradermal; if the skin moves over the nodule, it is subcutaneous.

8. Wheal—A circumscribed, flat-topped, firm elevation of skin resulting from tense edema of the papillary dermis. *Example:* Urticaria.

B. Secondary Changes:

1. Scales—Dry, thin plates of keratinized epidermal cells (stratum corneum). *Examples:* Psoriasis, ichthyosis.

2. Lichenification—Induration of skin with exaggerated skin lines and a shiny surface resulting from chronic rubbing of the skin. *Example:* Atopic dermatitis.

3. Erosion and oozing—A moist, circumscribed, slightly depressed area representing a blister base with the roof of the blister removed. *Examples:* Burns, bullous erythema multiforme. Most oral blisters present as erosions.

4. Crust—Dried exudate of plasma on the surface of the skin following acute dermatitis. *Examples:* Impetigo, contact dermatitis.

5. Fissure—A linear split in the skin extending through the epidermis into the dermis. *Example:* Angular cheilitis.

6. Scar—A flat, raised, or depressed area of fibrotic replacement of dermis or subcutaneous tissue. *Examples:* Acne scar, burn scar.

7. Atrophy—Depression of the skin surface caused by thinning of one or more layers of skin. *Example:* Lichen sclerosis et atrophicus.

C. Color: The lesion should be described as red, yellow, brown, tan, or blue. Particular attention should be given to the blanching of red or brown lesions. Failure to blanch suggests bleeding into the dermis (petechiae).

D. Configuration of Lesions: Clues to diagnosis may be obtained from the characteristic morphologic arrangement of primary or secondary lesions.

1. Annular (circular)—Annular nodules represent granuloma annulare; annular papules are more apt to be caused by dermatophyte infections.

2. Linear (straight line)—Linear papules represent lichen striatus; linear vesicles, incontinentia pigmenti; linear papules with burrows, scabies.

3. Grouped—Grouped vesicles occur in herpes simplex or zoster.

4. Discrete—Discrete lesions are independent of each other.

E. Distribution: It is useful to note whether the eruption is generalized, acral (hands, feet, buttocks, face), or localized to a specific skin region.

F. Description of Skin Lesions: Skin lesions are described in reverse order from that of their identification. One begins with distribution, configuration, color, secondary changes, and then primary lesion; for example, guttate psoriasis could be described as generalized discrete, red, scaly papules.

GENERAL PRINCIPLES
OF TREATMENT OF SKIN DISORDERS

TOPICAL THERAPY

Treatment should be simple and aimed at preserving or restoring the physiologic state of the skin. It is essential to keep in mind that one is treating the child and not the anxious parent or grandparent. Topical therapy is often preferred, because medication can be delivered in optimal concentrations at the exact site where it is needed.

Water is an important therapeutic agent, and optimally hydrated skin is soft and smooth. This occurs at approximately 60% environmental humidity. Because water evaporates readily from the cutaneous surface, skin hydration (stratum corneum of the epidermis) is dependent on the water concentration in the air, and sweating contributes little. However, if sweat is prevented from evaporating (eg, in the axilla, groin), local humidity and hydration of the skin are increased. As humidity falls below 15–20%, the stratum corneum shrinks and cracks; the epidermal barrier is lost and allows irritants to enter the skin and induce an inflammatory response. Replacement of water will correct this condition if evaporation is prevented. Therefore, dry and scaly skin is treated by soaking the skin in water for 5 minutes and then adding a barrier to evaporation (Table 14–1). Oils and ointments prevent evaporation for 8–12 hours, so they must be applied once or twice a day. In areas already occluded (axilla, diaper area), ointments or oils will merely increase retention of water and should not be used.

Overhydration (maceration) can also occur. As environmental humidity increases to 90–100%, the number of water molecules absorbed by the stratum corneum increases and the tight lipid junctions between the cells of the stratum corneum are gradually replaced by weak hydrogen bonds; the cells eventually become widely separated, and the epidermal barrier falls apart. This occurs in immersion foot, diaper areas, axillae, etc. It is desirable to enhance evaporation of water in these areas by air drying.

WET DRESSINGS

By placing the skin in an environment where the humidity is 100% and allowing the moisture to evap-

Table 14–1. Bases used for topical preparations.

Base	Combined With	Uses
Liquids		Wet dressings: relieve pruritus, vasoconstrict
	Powder	Shake lotions, drying pastes: relieve pruritus, vasoconstrict
	Grease and emulsifier; oil in water	Cream: penetrates quickly (10–15 min) and thus allows evaporation
	Excess grease and emulsifier; water in oil	Emollient cream: penetrates more slowly and thus retains moisture on skin
Grease		Ointments: occlusive (hold material on skin for prolonged time) and prevent evaporation of water
Gel		Transparent, colorless, semisolid emulsion: nongreasy, more drying and irritating than cream
Powder		Enhances evaporation

Characteristics of bases for topical preparations:
1. Most greases are triglycerides (eg, Aquaphor, petrolatum, Eucerin).
2. Oils are fluid fats (eg, Alpha Keri, olive oil, mineral oil).
3. True fats (eg, lard, animal fats) contain free fatty acids that increase in amount upon standing and cause irritation.
4. Ointments (eg, Aquaphor, petrolatum) should not be used in intertriginous areas such as the axillae, between the toes, and in the perineum, because they increase maceration. Lotions or creams are preferred in these areas.
5. Oils and ointments hold medication on the skin for long periods and are therefore ideal for barriers or prophylaxis and for dried areas of skin. Medication gets into the skin more slowly from ointments.
6. Creams carry medication into skin and are preferable for intertriginous dermatitis.
7. Solutions, gels, or lotions should be used for scalp treatments.

orate to 60%, pruritus is relieved. Evaporation of water stimulates cold-dependent nerve fibers in the skin and this may prevent the transmission of the itching sensation via pain fibers to the central nervous system. It also is vasoconstrictive, thereby helping to reduce the erythema and also decreasing the inflammatory cellular response.

Gauze of 20/12 mesh is commonly used for wet dressings. Parke-Davis 4-in. gauze comes in 100-yard rolls, and 5 yards is usually sufficient for application to the extremities. Curity 18-in. gauze can be used for application to the trunk. An alternative is to use the "two–long johns" technique, in which a pair of wet cotton long-sleeved and long-legged underwear is covered by a dry pair.

Warm but not hot water is used, and the gauze or long johns are soaked in the water and then wrung out until no more drops come out. The dressings are then wrapped around the extremities and fastened with a safety pin. The wet dressings are then covered with dry flannel or dry long johns, thereby slowing down the evaporation process but not completely retarding it, so that the wet dressings need to be changed only every 4–6 hours.

TOPICAL GLUCOCORTICOIDS

Twice-daily application of topical steroids is the mainstay of treatment for all forms of dermatitis (Table 14–2). Topical steroids can also be used under wet dressings. Wet dressings are removed every 4–6 hours and a topical steroid is applied; then the skin is covered again with wet dressings. If treatment is applied throughout the 24-hour period, maximum benefit is obtained after 72 hours; if treatment is applied only at night, maximum benefit is obtained after 7 days. When the condition has improved, the wet dressings are discontinued and a steroid ointment is applied twice daily. Daily application of steroids is not to be continued for more than 1 month. Only low-potency steroids (Table 14–2) are applied to the face or intertriginous areas.

Hepburn D, Yohn JJ, Weston WL: Topical glucocorticoid treatment in infants, children, and adolescents. Adv Dermatol 1994;9:225.

Table 14–2. Topical glucocorticoids.

	Concentrations (Percent)
Low potency[1] = 1–9 Hydrocortisone	0.5 and 1.0
Desonide	0.05
Moderate potency = 10–99 Mometasone furoate	0.1
Hydrocortisone valerate	0.2
Fluocinolone acetonide	0.025
Triamcinolone acetonide	0.01
Amcinonide	0.1
High potency = 100–499 Desoximetasone	0.25
Fluocinonide	0.05
Halcinonide	0.1
Super potency = 500–7500 Betamethasone dipropionate	0.05
Clobetasol propionate	0.05

[1]1% hydrocortisone is defined as having a potency of 1.

DISORDERS OF THE SKIN IN NEWBORNS

TRANSIENT DISEASES IN THE NEWBORN

Milia

Multiple white papules 1 mm in diameter scattered over the forehead, nose, and cheeks are present in up to 40% of newborn infants. Histologically, they represent superficial epidermal cysts filled with keratinous material associated with the developing pilosebaceous follicle. Their intraoral counterparts are called Epstein's pearls and are even more common than facial milia. All of these cystic structures spontaneously rupture and exfoliate their contents.

Sebaceous Gland Hyperplasia

Prominent yellow macules at the opening of each pilosebaceous follicle, predominantly over the nose, represent overgrowth of sebaceous glands in response to the same androgenic stimulation that occurs in adolescence.

Acne Neonatorum

Open and closed comedones, erythematous papules, and pustules identical in appearance to adolescent acne may occur in infants over the forehead, cheeks, and chin. The lesions may be present at birth but usually do not appear until 4–6 weeks of age. Spontaneous resolution occurs over a period of 6 months to 1 year. Rarely, neonatal acne may be a manifestation of a virilizing syndrome.

Harlequin Color Change

A cutaneous vascular phenomenon unique to neonates in the first week of life occurs when the infant (particularly one of low birth weight) is placed on one side. The dependent half develops an erythematous flush with a sharp demarcation at the midline, and the upper half of the body becomes pale. The color changes usually subside within a few seconds after the infant is placed supine but may persist for as long as 20 minutes.

Mottling

A lace-like pattern of dilated cutaneous vessels appears over the extremities and often the trunk of neonates exposed to lowered room temperature. This feature is transient and usually disappears completely upon rewarming.

Erythema Toxicum

Up to 50% of term infants develop erythema toxicum. Usually at 24–48 hours of age, blotchy erythematous macules 2–3 cm in diameter appear, most prominently on the chest but also on the back, face, and extremities. These are occasionally present at birth. Onset after 4–5 days of life is rare. The lesions vary in number from two or three up to as many as 100. Incidence is much higher in term infants than in premature ones. The macular erythema may fade within 24–48 hours or may progress to develop urticarial wheals in the center of the macules or, in 10% of cases, pustules. Examination of a Wright's-stained smear of the lesion will reveal numerous eosinophils. This may be accompanied by peripheral blood eosinophilia of up to 20%. All of the lesions fade and disappear by 5–7 days. A similar eruption in black newborns, benign pustular melanosis, has a neutrophilic predominance and leaves hyperpigmentation.

Sucking Blisters

Bullae, either intact or in the form of an erosion representing a blister base without inflammatory borders, may occur over the forearms, wrists, thumbs, or upper lip. These presumably result from vigorous sucking in utero. They resolve without complications.

Miliaria

Obstruction of the eccrine sweat ducts occurs often in neonates and produces one of two clinical pictures depending on the level of obstruction. **Miliaria crystallina** is characterized by tiny (1- to 2-mm), superficial grouped vesicles without erythema over intertriginous areas and adjacent skin (eg, neck, upper chest). Obstruction occurs in the stratum corneum portion of the eccrine duct. More commonly, obstruction of the eccrine duct deeper in the epidermis results in erythematous grouped papules in the same areas and is called **miliaria rubra.** Rarely, these may progress to pustules. Heat and high humidity predispose the patient to eccrine duct pore closure. Removal to a cooler environment is the treatment of choice.

Subcutaneous Fat Necrosis

Reddish or purple, sharply circumscribed, firm nodules occurring over the cheeks, buttocks, arms, and thighs and occurring between day 1 and day 7 in infants represent subcutaneous fat necrosis. Cold injury is thought to play an important role. These lesions resolve spontaneously over a period of weeks, although—as in all instances of fat necrosis—they may calcify.

Weston WL, Lane AT, Morelli JG: *Color Textbook of Pediatric Dermatology,* 2nd ed. Mosby–Year Book, 1996.

1. PIGMENT CELL BIRTHMARKS, NEVI, & MELANOMA

Birthmarks may involve an overgrowth of one or more of any of the normal components of skin: pigment cells, blood vessels, lymph vessels, etc. A nevus is a hamartoma of highly differentiated cells that retain their normal function.

Mongolian Spot

A blue-black macule found over the lumbosacral area in 90% of Native American, black, and Asian infants is called a mongolian spot. These spots are occasionally noted over the shoulders and back and may extend over the buttocks. Histologically, they consist of spindle-shaped pigment cells located deep in the dermis. The lesions fade somewhat with time, but some traces may persist into adult life.

Café au Lait Macule

A café au lait macule is a light brown, oval macule (dark brown on black skin) that may be found anywhere on the body. Ten percent of white and 22% of black children have café au lait spots greater than 1.5 cm in their longest diameter. These lesions persist throughout life and may increase in number with age. The presence of six or more such lesions over 1.5 cm in their longest diameter may represent a clue to neurofibromatosis 1 (NF-1). Patients with Albright's syndrome (Chapter 29) also have increased numbers of café au lait macules. Most newborns with NF-1 will acquire the macules later.

Spindle & Epithelioid Cell Nevus

A reddish-brown solitary nodule appearing on the face or upper arm of a child represents a spindle and epithelioid cell nevus. Histologically, it consists of pigment-producing cells of bizarre shape with numerous mitoses.

Melanoma

Pigmented lesions with variegated colors (red, white, blue), notched borders, and nonuniform, irregular surfaces should arouse a suspicion of melanoma. Ulceration and bleeding are advanced signs of melanoma. If melanoma is suspected, excisional biopsy for pathologic examination should be done as the treatment of choice.

Junctional Nevus & Compound Nevus

Dark brown or black macules, usually few in number at birth but becoming more numerous with age, represent junctional nevi. Histologically, these lesions are large clones of melanocytes at the junction of the epidermis and dermis. With aging, they may become raised (papules) and contain intradermal melanocytes, creating a compound nevus. Often the surface becomes irregular and roughened.

Brown to blue solitary papules with smooth surfaces represent intradermal nevi. When pigmentation is present deeper in the dermis, the lesions appear blue or blue-black and are called blue nevi.

Giant Pigmented Nevus (Bathing Trunk Nevus)

An irregular dark brown to black plaque over 10 cm in diameter represents a giant pigmented nevus. Often the lesions are of such size as to cover the entire trunk (bathing trunk nevi). Histologically, they are compound nevi. Transformation to malignant melanoma has been reported in as many as 10% of cases in some series, although the true incidence is probably much lower. Malignant change may occur at birth or at any time thereafter.

Tissue expanders may be useful in excision of large lesions. The risk of melanoma and the potential for cosmetic improvement should be carefully evaluated for each patient.

Angelucci D et al: Rapid perinatal growth mimicking malignant transformation in a giant congenital melanocytic nevus. Hum Pathol 1991;22:297.

From L: Congenital nevi: Let's be practical. Pediatr Dermatol 1992;9:345.

Mackie RM: Nevi as risk factors for melanoma. Pediatr Dermatol 1992;9:340.

Ruiz-Maldanado R et al: Giant pigmented nevi: Clinical, histologic, and therapeutic considerations. J Pediatr 1992;120:906.

2. VASCULAR BIRTHMARKS

Capillary Malformations

Flat vascular birthmarks can be divided into two types: those that are orange or light red (salmon patch) and those that are dark red or bluish-red (port wine stain).

A. Salmon Patch: The salmon patch is a light red macule found over the nape of the neck, upper eyelids, and glabella. Fifty percent of infants have such lesions over their necks. Eyelid lesions fade completely within 3–6 months; those on the nape of the neck fade somewhat but usually persist into adult life.

B. Port Wine Stain: Port wine stains are dark red or purple macules appearing anywhere on the body. A bilateral port wine stain or one covering the entire half of the face may be a clue to **Sturge-Weber syndrome,** which is characterized by seizures, mental retardation, glaucoma, and hemiplegia (Chapter 23). Most infants with smaller, unilateral port wine stains do not have Sturge-Weber syndrome.

Similarly, a port wine stain over an extremity may be associated with hypertrophy of the soft tissue and bone of that extremity (**Klippel-Trenaunay syndrome**).

The pulsed dye laser is the treatment of choice for infants and children with port wine stains.

Morelli JG et al: Initial lesion size is a critical factor in determining the response of port wine stains in children treated with the pulsed (450 microsecond) dye (585 nanometer) laser. Arch Pediatr Adolesc Med 1995; 149:1142.

Talman B et al: Portwine stains and the likelihood of ophthalmologic or CNS complications. Pediatrics 1991; 87:323.

Hemangioma

A red, rubbery nodule with a roughened surface is a hemangioma. The lesion is often not present at birth but is represented by a permanent blanched area on the skin that is supplanted at 2–4 weeks of age by red nodules. Histologically, these are benign tumors of capillary endothelial cells. Hemangiomas may be superficial, deep, or mixed. The terms *strawberry* and *cavernous* are misleading and should not be used. The biologic behavior of a hemangioma is the same despite its location. Fifty percent resolve spontaneously by age 5, 70% by age 7, 90% by age 9, and the rest by adolescence.

Hemangiomas resolve, leaving redundant skin, hypopigmentation, and telangiectasia. Local complications include superficial ulceration and secondary pyoderma.

Complications that require immediate treatment are (1) thrombocytopenia resulting from platelet trapping within the lesion (**Kasabach-Merritt syndrome**); (2) airway obstruction (hemangiomas of the head and neck are often associated with subglottic hemangiomas); (3) visual obstruction (with resulting amblyopia); and (4) cardiac decompensation (high-output failure). In these instances, the treatment of choice is with prednisone, 1–2 mg/kg orally daily or every other day for 4–6 weeks. Interferon alfa-2a has been used to treat serious hemangiomas unresponsive to prednisone. If the lesion is ulcerated or bleeding, pulsed dye laser treatment may be helpful.

Eskowitz RAB, Mulliken JB, Folkman J: Interferon alfa-2a therapy for life-threatening hemangiomas of infancy. N Engl J Med 1992;326:1456.

Esterly NB: Hemangiomas in infants and children: Clinical observation. Pediatr Dermatol 1992;9:353.

Garden JM, Bakus AD, Paller AS: Treatment of cutaneous hemangiomas by the flashlamp-pumped pulsed dye laser: Prospective analysis. J Pediatr 1992;120:555.

Morelli JG et al: Management of ulcerated hemangiomas in infancy. Arch Pediatr Adolesc Med 1994;148:1104.

Lymphangioma

Lymphangiomas are rubbery, skin-colored nodules occurring in the parotid area (cystic hygromas) or on the tongue. They often result in grotesque enlargement of soft tissues. Surgical excision is the only treatment available, although the results are not satisfactory.

3. EPIDERMAL BIRTHMARKS

Epidermal Nevus

Linear or groups of linear, warty, papular, unilateral lesions represent overgrowth of epidermis since birth. These areas may range from dirty yellow to brown or may be darkly pigmented. The histologic features of the lesions include thickening of the epidermis and elongation of the rete ridges and hyperkeratosis. Clinically, widespread lesions may be associated with focal motor seizures, mental subnormality, and skeletal anomalies.

Treatment once or twice daily with topical tretinoin 0.05% (retinoic acid [Retin-A]) will keep the lesions flat.

Rogers M: Epidermal nevi and the epidermal nevus syndrome: A review of 233 cases. Pediatr Dermatol 1992;9:342.

Nevus Comedonicus

The lesion known as nevus comedonicus consists of linear groups of widely dilated follicular openings plugged with keratin, giving the appearance of localized noninflammatory acne. The treatment of choice is surgical removal. If this is not feasible, topical retinoic acid is helpful.

Nevus Sebaceous

The nevus sebaceous of Jadassohn is a hamartoma of sebaceous glands and underlying apocrine glands that is diagnosed by the appearance at birth of a yellowish, hairless, smooth plaque in the scalp or on the face. The lesion may be contiguous with an epidermal nevus on the face and constitute part of the linear epidermal nevus syndrome.

Histologically, nevus sebaceous represents an overabundance of sebaceous glands without hair follicles. At puberty, with androgenic stimulation, the sebaceous cells in the nevus divide, expand their cellular volume, and synthesize sebum, resulting in a warty mass. Because 15% of these lesions become basal cell carcinomas after puberty, excision is recommended before puberty.

4. CONNECTIVE TISSUE BIRTHMARKS (Juvenile Elastoma, Collagenoma)

Connective tissue nevi are smooth, skin-colored papules 1–10 mm in diameter that are grouped on the trunk. A solitary, larger (5- to 10-cm) nodule is called a **shagreen patch** and is histologically indistinguishable from other connective tissue nevi that show thickened, abundant collagen bundles with or without associated increases of elastic tissue. Although the shagreen patch is a cutaneous clue to **tuberous sclerosis** (Chapter 23), the other connective tissue nevi occur as isolated events. These nevi remain throughout life, and no treatment is necessary.

HEREDITARY SKIN DISORDERS

The Ichthyoses

Ichthyosis is a term applied to several heritable diseases characterized by the presence of excessive scales on the skin. Major categories are listed in Table 14–3. Treatment consists of controlling scaling with Lac-Hydrin 12% applied once daily. Restoring water to the skin is also very helpful.

Paller AS: Laboratory tests for ichthyosis. Dermatol Clin 1994;12:99.

Table 14–3. Four major types of ichthyosis.

Name	Age at Onset	Clinical Features	Genetic Defect	Inheritance
Ichthyosis with normal epidermal turnover				
Ichthyosis vulgaris	Childhood	Fine scales, deep palmar and plantar markings	Filaggrin/profilaggrin	Autosomal dominant
X-linked ichthyosis	Birth	Palms and soles spared; thick scales that darken with age; corneal opacities in patients and carrier mothers	Cholesterol sulfatase	X-linked
Ichthyosis with increased epidermal turnover				
Epidermolytic hyperkeratosis	Birth	Verrucous, yellow scales in flexural areas and palms and soles	Keratins 1 and 10	Autosomal dominant
Lamellar ichthyosis	Birth; collodion baby	Erythroderma, ectropion, large coarse scales; thickened palms and soles	Transglutaminase 1	Autosomal recessive

Epidermolysis Bullosa

The diagnostic feature of this group of diseases is the formation of blisters in response to slight trauma. They can be divided into scarring and nonscarring types (Table 14–4).

Treatment usually consists of systemic antibiotics for infection, protective dressings of petrolatum or zinc oxide, and cooling the skin. If hands and feet are involved, reducing skin friction with 5% glutaraldehyde every 3 days is helpful.

Uitto J, Christiano AM: Inherited epidermolysis bullosa. Dermatol Clin 1993;11:549.

COMMON SKIN DISEASES IN INFANTS, CHILDREN, & ADOLESCENTS

ACNE

Essentials of Diagnosis

- Seen in newborns and adolescents.
- Inflammatory papules, open and closed comedones on surface.
- Face, upper chest and back involvement common.

Clinical Findings

The common forms of acne in pediatric patients occur at two ages: in the newborn period and in adolescence. Neonatal acne is a response to maternal an-drogen, first appearing at 4–6 weeks of age and lasting until 4–6 months of age. The lesions are primarily on the face, upper chest, and back, in a distribution similar to that seen in adolescent acne. It has been hypothesized, but not proved, that infants who have severe neonatal acne will develop severe adolescent acne.

The onset of adolescent acne is between ages 8 and 10 in 40% of children. The early lesions are usually limited to the face and are primarily closed comedones (whiteheads; see below). Eventually, 85% of adolescents will develop some form of acne.

Acne occurs in sebaceous follicles, which, unlike hair follicles, have large, abundant sebaceous glands and usually lack hair. They are located primarily on the face, upper chest, back, and penis. Obstruction of the sebaceous follicle opening produces the clinical lesion of acne. If the obstruction occurs at the follicular mouth, the clinical lesion is characterized by a wide, patulous opening filled with a plug of stratum corneum cells. This is the open comedone, or blackhead. Open comedones are the predominant clinical lesion in early adolescent acne. The black color is caused not by dirt but by oxidized melanin within the stratum corneum cellular plug. Open comedones do not often progress to inflammatory lesions. Closed comedones, or whiteheads, are caused by obstruction just beneath the follicular opening in the neck of the sebaceous follicle, which produces a cystic swelling of the follicular duct directly beneath the epidermis. The stratum corneum produced accumulates continuously within the cystic cavity. The resultant lesion is an enlarging sphere just beneath the skin surface. Most authorities believe that closed comedones are precursors of inflammatory acne. If open or closed

Table 14–4. Types of epidermolysis bullosa.

Name	Age at Onset	Clinical Features	Genetic Defect	Inheritance
Nonscarring types				
Epidermolysis bullosa simplex	Birth	Hemorrhagic blisters over the lower legs; cooling prevents blisters	Keratins 5 and 14	Autosomal dominant
Recurrent bullous eruption of the hands and feet (Weber-Cockayne syndrome)	First few years of life	Blisters brought out by walking		Autosomal dominant
Junctional bullous dermolysis (Herlitz's disease)	Birth	Erosions on legs, oral mucosa; severe peri-oral involvement	Laminin V	Autosomal recessive
Scarring types				
Epidermolysis bullosa dystrophica, dominant	Infancy	Numerous blisters on hands and feet; milia formation	Type VII collagen	Autosomal dominant
Epidermolysis bullosa dystrophica, recessive	Birth	Repeated episodes of blistering, secondary infection and scarring—"mitten hands and feet"	Type VII collagen	Autosomal recessive

comedones are the predominant lesions on the skin in adolescent acne, the condition is called **comedonal acne.**

In typical adolescent acne, several different types of lesions are present simultaneously, for example, open and closed comedones and inflammatory lesions such as papules, pustules, and cysts. Inflammatory lesions may also rarely occur as interconnecting, draining sinus tracts. Adolescents with cystic acne require prompt medical attention, since ruptured cysts and sinus tracts result in severe scar formation. New acne scars are highly vascular and have a reddish or purplish hue. Such scars return to normal skin color after several years. Acne scars may be depressed beneath the skin level, raised, or flat to the skin. In adolescents with a tendency toward keloid formation, keloidal scars can occur following acne lesions, particularly over the sternal area.

Differential Diagnosis

Consider rosacea, nevus comedonicus, flat warts, the angiofibromas of tuberous sclerosis, miliaria, and molluscum contagiosum.

Pathogenesis

The primary event in acne formation is obstruction of the sebaceous follicle. Ordinarily, the lining of such follicles contains one or two layers of stratum corneum cells, but in acne the stratum corneum is overproduced. This phenomenon is androgen-dependent in adolescent acne. The sebaceous follicles contain an enzyme, testosterone 5α-reductase, which converts plasma testosterone to dihydrotestosterone. This androgen is a potent stimulus for nuclear division of the follicular germinative cells and subsequently of excessive cell production. Thus, obstruction requires the presence of both circulating androgens and the converting enzyme. After the production or administration of androgens, there is a delay until cellular proliferation occurs and follicular obstruction subsequently appears.

The pathogenesis of inflammatory acne is not well understood. Undoubtedly, physical manipulation of a closed comedone could lead to rupture of the cavity contents into the dermis with a subsequent inflammatory response. Spontaneous inflammation also occurs in obstructed follicles, but the reason for this is unclear. An attractive hypothesis is that overgrowth of gram-positive bacteria in the obstructed follicle (either *Propionibacterium acnes* or *Staphylococcus epidermidis*) might stimulate factors that initiate inflammation. Overproduction of sebum and free fatty acid formation seem unlikely as causes of inflammation in acne as presently understood.

Adolescent acne may result from several external causes. Frictional acne caused by headbands, football helmets, or tight-fitting brassieres or other garments occurs predominantly underneath the area where the garment is worn. Oil-based cosmetics may be responsible for predominantly comedonal acne, and hair sprays may produce acne along the hair margin.

Drug-induced acne should be suspected in teenagers if all lesions are in the same stage at the same time and if involvement extends to the lower abdomen, lower back, arms, and legs. Drugs responsible for acne include corticotropin (ACTH), glucocorticoids, androgens, hydantoins, and isoniazid. They have the common property of elevating plasma testosterone.

Treatment

A. Topical Keratolytic Agents: The mainstay of acne therapy is the use of potent topical keratolytic agents applied to the skin to relieve follicular obstruction. Two classes of potent keratolytic agents are available: tretinoin (retinoic acid) and benzoyl peroxide gel. These have been found to be the most efficacious agents in the treatment of acne. Either agent may be used once daily, or the combination of retinoic acid cream applied to acne-bearing areas of the skin once daily in the evening and a benzoyl peroxide gel applied once daily in the morning may be used. This regimen will control 80–85% of adolescent acne.

B. Topical Antibiotics: Topical antibiotics are used to avoid the side effects caused by systemic antibiotics. Topical antibiotics are less effective than systemic antibiotics and at best are equivalent in potency to 250 mg of tetracycline orally once a day. One percent clindamycin phosphate solution is the most efficacious of all topical antibiotics. Some percutaneous absorption may occur rarely with this drug, resulting in diarrhea and colitis; 1.5% and 2% topical erythromycin solutions are effective; 1% topical tetracycline solution is minimally effective.

C. Systemic Antibiotics: Antibiotics that are concentrated in sebum, such as tetracycline and erythromycin, are very effective in inflammatory acne. The usual dose is 0.5–1 g taken once or twice daily on an empty stomach (nothing to eat 1 hour before or after the medication). Tetracycline or erythromycin should be continued for 2–3 months until the acne lesions are suppressed.

D. Oral Retinoids: An oral retinoid, 13-*cis*-retinoic acid (isotretinoin [Accutane]), offers the most efficacious treatment of severe cystic acne. The precise mechanism of its action is unknown, but decreased sebum production, decreased follicular obstruction, decreased skin bacteria, and general anti-inflammatory activities have been described. The initial dosage is 40 mg once or twice daily. This drug is not effective in comedonal acne or other mild forms of acne. Side effects include dryness and scaliness of the skin, dry lips, and, occasionally, dry eyes and dry nose. Up to 10% of patients experience mild, reversible hair loss. Elevated liver enzymes and blood lipids have rarely been described. Isotretinoin is teratogenic. Use in young women of childbearing age is not recommended unless strict adherence to manufacturer's guidelines is ensured.

E. Other Acne Treatments: There is no convincing evidence that dietary management, mild drying agents, abrasive scrubs, oral vitamin A, ultraviolet light, cryotherapy, or incision and drainage have any beneficial effects in the management of acne.

F. Avoidance of Cosmetics & Hair Spray: Acne can be aggravated by a variety of external factors that result in further obstruction of partially occluded sebaceous follicles. Discontinuing the use of oil-based cosmetics, face creams, and hair sprays may alleviate the comedonal component of acne within 4–6 weeks.

Patient Education & Follow-up Visits

It is important to explain the mechanism of acne and the treatment plan to adolescent patients. Time should be set aside at the first visit to answer the patient's questions. Explain that there will not be much improvement for 4–8 weeks. Establish guidelines for ideal control, and explain that the best the patient might achieve is one or two new pimples a month. No drug is available that will prevent an adolescent from ever having another acne lesion. A written education sheet is most useful.

Follow-up visits should be made every 6–8 weeks. The criterion for ideal control is a few lesions every 2 weeks. Explain again what medications are being used and what the treatment is intended to achieve, and question the patient to determine whether the medications are being used properly.

Clark C: Acne—General practice management. Practitioner 1993;237:162.

BACTERIAL INFECTIONS OF THE SKIN

Impetigo

Erosions covered by honey-colored crusts are diagnostic of impetigo. Staphylococci and group A streptococci are important pathogens in this disease, which histologically consists of superficial invasion of bacteria into the upper epidermis, forming a subcorneal pustule.

Patients should be treated with an antimicrobial agent effective against *Staphylococcus aureus* (β-lactamase–resistant penicillins or cephalosporins, clindamycin, amoxicillin-clavulanate) for 7–10 days. Topical mupirocin (tid) is also effective.

Dagan R: Impetigo in childhood: Changing epidemiology and new treatments. Pediatr Ann 1993;22:235.

Bullous Impetigo

All impetigo is bullous, with the blister forming just beneath the stratum corneum, but in "bullous impetigo" there is, in addition to the usual erosion covered by a honey-colored crust, a border filled with clear fluid. Staphylococci may be isolated from these lesions, and systemic signs of circulating exfoliatin are absent. "Bullous varicella" is a disorder that represents bullous impetigo as a superinfection in varicella lesions. Treatment with oral antistaphylococcal drugs for 7–10 days is effective. Application of cool compresses to debride crusts is a helpful symptomatic measure.

Ecthyma

Ecthyma is a firm, dry crust, surrounded by erythema, that exudes purulent material. It represents deep invasion by the streptococcus through the epidermis to the superficial dermis. Treatment is with systemic penicillin.

Cellulitis

Cellulitis is characterized by erythematous, hot, tender, ill- defined, edematous plaques accompanied by regional lymphadenopathy. Histologically, this disorder represents invasion of microorganisms into the lower dermis and sometimes beyond, with obstruction of local lymphatics. Group A β-hemolytic streptococci and coagulase-positive staphylococci are the most common causes; pneumococci and *Haemophilus influenzae* are rare causes. Staphylococcal infections are usually more localized and more likely to have a purulent center; streptococcal infections spread more rapidly, but these characteristics cannot be used to specify the infecting agent. An entry site of prior trauma or infection (eg, varicella) is often present. Septicemia is common, and treatment with the appropriate systemic antibiotic is indicated.

Sachs MK: Cutaneous cellulitis. Arch Dermatol 1991; 127:493.

Folliculitis

A pustule at a follicular opening represents folliculitis. If the pustule occurs at eccrine sweat orifices, it is correctly called **poritis**. Staphylococci and streptococci are the most frequent pathogens. Treatment consists of measures to remove follicular obstruction—either cool, wet compresses for 24 hours or keratolytics such as those used for acne.

Abscess

An abscess occurs deep in the skin, at the bottom of a follicle or an apocrine gland, and is diagnosed as an erythematous, firm, acutely tender nodule with ill-defined borders. Staphylococci are the most common organisms. Treatment consists of incision and drainage and systemic antibiotics.

Scalded Skin Syndrome

This entity consists of the sudden onset of bright red, acutely painful skin, most obvious periorally, periorbitally, and in the flexural areas of the neck, the axillae, the popliteal and antecubital areas, and the groin. The slightest pressure on the skin results in severe pain and separation of the epidermis, leaving a glistening layer (the stratum granulosum of the epidermis) beneath. The disease is caused by a circulating toxin (exfoliatin) elaborated by phage group II staphylococci. The site of action of the exfoliatin is the intracellular area of the granular layer, resulting in a separation of cells.

Scalded skin syndrome includes **Ritter's disease** of the newborn, toxic shock syndrome, and the mildest form, staphylococcal scarlet fever. (See also Bullous Impetigo, earlier.) In all of the forms of this entity, the causative staphylococci may be isolated not from the skin, but rather from the nasopharynx, an abscess, sinus blood culture, etc. Treatment consists of systemic administration of antistaphylococcal drugs.

Ben-Amitai D, Ashkenazi S: Bacterial skin infections in childhood. Pediatr Ann 1993;22:225.

FUNGAL INFECTIONS OF THE SKIN

1. DERMATOPHYTE INFECTIONS

Essentials of Diagnosis
- Red, scaly, round lesions.
- Hair loss with or without scaling in tinea capitis.

General Considerations

Dermatophytes become attached to the superficial layer of the epidermis, nails, and hair, where they proliferate. They grow mainly within the stratum corneum and do not invade the lower epidermis or dermis. Release of toxins from dermatophytes, especially those whose natural host is animals or soil, for example, *Microsporum canis* and *Trichophyton verrucosum,* results in dermatitis. Fungal infection should be suspected with any red and scaly lesion.

Classification & Diagnosis

A. Tinea Capitis: Thickened, broken-off hairs with erythema and scaling of underlying scalp are the distinguishing features (Table 14–5). In epidemic ringworm, hairs are broken off at the surface of the scalp, leaving a black dot appearance. Pustule formation and a boggy, fluctuant mass on the scalp occur in *M canis* and *Trichophyton tonsurans* infections. This mass, called a **kerion,** represents an exaggerated host response to the organism. Fungal culture should be performed in all cases of suspected tinea capitis.

B. Tinea Corporis: Tinea corporis presents either as annular marginated papules with a thin scale

Table 14–5. Clinical features of tinea capitis.

Most Common Organisms	Clinical Appearance	Microscopic Appearance in KOH
Trichophyton tonsurans (90%)	Hairs broken off 2–3 mm from follicle; "black dot"; no fluorescence	Hyphae and spores within hair
Microsporum canis (10%)	Thickened broken-off hairs that fluoresce yellow-green with Wood's lamp[1]	Small spores outside of hair; hyphae within hair

[1]Select fluorescent hairs for examination in KOH and culture.

and clear center or as an annular confluent dermatitis. The most common organisms are *Trichophyton mentagrophytes* and *M canis*. The diagnosis is made by scraping thin scales from the border of the lesion, dissolving them in 20% KOH, and examining for hyphae.

C. Tinea Cruris: Symmetric, sharply marginated lesions in inguinal areas are seen with tinea cruris. The most common organisms are *Trichophyton rubrum, T mentagrophytes,* and *Epidermophyton floccosum.*

D. Tinea Pedis: The diagnosis of tinea pedis in a prepubertal child must always be regarded with skepticism; atopic feet or contact dermatitis is a more likely diagnosis in this age group. Tinea pedis is seen most commonly in postpubertal males with blisters on the instep of the foot. Fissuring between the toes is occasionally seen.

E. Tinea Unguium (Onychomycosis): Loosening of the nail plate from the nail bed (onycholysis), giving a yellow discoloration, is the first sign of fungal invasion of the nails. Thickening of the distal nail plate then occurs, followed by scaling and a crumbly appearance of the entire nail plate surface. *T rubrum* and *T mentagrophytes* are the most common causes. The diagnosis is confirmed by KOH examination and fungal culture. Usually one or two nails are involved. If every nail is involved, psoriasis or lichen planus is a more likely diagnosis than fungal infection.

Treatment

The treatment of dermatophytosis is quite simple: *If hair or nails are involved, griseofulvin is the treatment of choice.* Topical antifungal agents do not enter hair or nails in sufficient concentration to clear the infection. The absorption of griseofulvin from the gastrointestinal tract is enhanced by a fatty meal; thus, whole milk or ice cream taken with the medication increases absorption. The dosage of griseofulvin is 20 mg/kg/d. With hair infections, cultures should be done every 4 weeks and treatment should be continued for 6–8 weeks following a negative culture. In nail infections, treat for a minimum of 3 months. The side effects are few, and the drug has been used successfully in the newborn period.

Tinea corporis, tinea pedis, and tinea cruris can be treated effectively with topical medication after careful inspection to make certain that the hair and nails are not involved. Treatment with clotrimazole (Lotrimin), miconazole (Micatin), econazole (Spectazole), or haloprogin (Halotex) applied twice daily for 3–4 weeks is recommended.

Degreef H: The treatment of superficial skin infections caused by dermatophytes. Curr Top Med Mycol 1992; 4:189.
Goldgeier MH: Fungal infections of the skin, hair and nails. Pediatr Ann 1993;22:253.

2. TINEA VERSICOLOR

Tinea versicolor is a superficial infection caused by *Pityrosporum orbiculare* (also called *Malassezia furfur,*) a yeast-like fungus. It characteristically causes polycyclic connected hypopigmented macules and very fine scales in areas of sun-induced pigmentation. In winter, the polycyclic macules appear reddish-brown.

Treatment consists of application of selenium sulfide (Selsun), 2.5% suspension, or topical antifungals. Selenium sulfide should be applied to the whole body and left on overnight. Treatment can be repeated again in 1 week and then monthly thereafter. It tends to be somewhat irritating, and the patient should be warned about this difficulty.

Borelli D, Jacobs PH, Nall L: Tinea versicolor: Epidemiological, clinical and therapeutic aspects. J Am Acad Dermatol 1991;25:300.

3. *CANDIDA ALBICANS* INFECTIONS (See Chapter 38.)

In addition to being a frequent invader in diaper dermatitis, *Candida albicans* also infects the oral mucosa, where it appears as thick white patches with an erythematous base (**thrush**); the angles of the mouth, where it causes fissures and white exudate (**perlèche**); and the cuticular region of the fingers, where thickening of the cuticle, dull red erythema, and distortion of growth of the nail plate suggest the diagnosis of candidal paronychia. Candida dermatitis is characterized by sharply defined erythematous patches, sometimes with eroded areas. Pustules, vesicles, or papules may be present as satellite lesions. Similar infections may be found in other moist areas, such as the axilla and in neck folds. This infection is

more common in children who have recently received antibiotics.

Nystatin (Mycostatin) is the drug of first choice for *C albicans* infections. It is supplied as an ointment, cream, or oral suspension. In diaper dermatitis, the cream form can be applied every 3–4 hours. In oral thrush, the suspension should be applied directly to the mucosa with the parent's finger or a cotton-tipped applicator, since it is not absorbed and acts topically. In candidal paronychia, nystatin is applied over the area, covered with occlusive plastic wrapping, and left on overnight after the application is made airtight. Haloprogin, miconazole, econazole nitrate, or clotrimazole are effective alternatives. Refractory candidiasis will respond to a brief course of oral fluconazole.

Thomas I: Superficial and deep candidiasis. Int J Dermatol 1993;32:778.

VIRAL INFECTIONS OF THE SKIN

Herpes Simplex

Grouped vesicles or grouped erosions suggest herpes simplex. The microscopic finding of epidermal giant cells after scraping the vesicle base with a No. 15 blade, smearing on a slide, and staining with Wright's stain (Tzanck smear) suggests herpes simplex or varicella-zoster. A rapid immunofluorescent test for HSV is available. In infants, lesions resulting from herpes simplex type 1 are seen on the gingiva and lips, periorbitally, or on the thumb in thumb suckers. Recurrent erosions in the mouth are usually aphthous stomatitis in children rather than recurrent herpes simplex. Herpes simplex type 2 is seen on the genitalia and in the mouth in adolescents. Cutaneous dissemination of herpes simplex occurs in patients with atopic dermatitis (**eczema herpeticum, Kaposi's varicelliform eruption**). The treatment of this and other herpesvirus infections is discussed in the infectious diseases section. In severe disseminated infection, oral acyclovir may be helpful.

Spruance SL: The natural history of recurrent oral-facial herpes simplex virus infection. Semin Dermatol 1992;11:200.

Varicella-Zoster

Grouped vesicles in a dermatome on the trunk or face suggest herpes zoster. Zoster in children may not be painful and usually has a mild course. In patients with compromised host resistance, the appearance of an erythematous border around the vesicles is a good prognostic sign. Conversely, large bullae without a tendency to crusting imply a poor host response to the virus. Varicella-zoster and herpes simplex lesions undergo the same series of changes: papule, vesicle, pustule, crust, slightly depressed scar. Varicella appears in crops, and many different stages of lesions are present at the same time.

Itching is usually the only symptom, and cool baths as frequently as necessary or drying lotions such as calamine lotion are sufficient to relieve symptoms. In immunosuppressed children, intravenous or oral acyclovir should be used.

Weller TH: Varicella and herpes zoster: A perspective and overview. J Infect Dis 1992:166(Suppl 1):1.
Whitley RJ: Therapeutic approaches to varicella-zoster virus infections. J Infect Dis 1992;166(Suppl 1):551.

HIV Infection

The average time of onset of skin lesions after perinatally acquired HIV infection is 4 months, and 11 months after transfusion-acquired HIV infection. Persistent oral candidiasis and recalcitrant candidal diaper rash are the most frequent cutaneous manifestations of infantile HIV infection. Severe or recurrent herpetic gingivostomatitis, herpes zoster, and molluscum contagiosum are seen. Recurrent staphylococcal pyodermas, tinea of the face, and onychomycosis are also observed. A generalized dermatitis with features of seborrhea is extremely common. In general, persistent, recurrent, or extensive skin infections should make one suspicious of HIV infection.

Prose NS: Cutaneous manifestations of pediatric HIV infections. Pediatr Dermatol 1992;9:326.
Smith KJ et al: Cutaneous findings in HIV-1 positive patients: A 42 month prospective study. J Am Acad Dermatol 1994;31:746.

Virus-Induced Tumors

A. Molluscum Contagiosum: Molluscum contagiosum consists of umbilicated, white or whitish-yellow papules in groups on the genitalia or trunk. They are common in sexually active adolescents as well as in infants and preschool children. Crushing a lesion between glass slides followed by microscopic examination after staining with Wright's stain will demonstrate epidermal cells with inclusions. Molluscum contagiosum is a poxvirus that induces the epidermis to proliferate, forming a pale papule.

Removal of the lesion with a sharp curette or knife is curative. This therapy may leave a small scar, and one must weigh the advantage of removal of lesions that will disappear in 2–3 years.

B. Warts: Warts are skin-colored papules with irregular (verrucous) surfaces. They are intraepidermal tumors caused by infection with human papillomavirus. This DNA virus induces the epidermal cells to proliferate, thus resulting in the warty growth.

No therapy for warts is ideal, and some types of therapy should be avoided because the recurrence rate of warts is high. Flat warts generally require no treatment. They may be considered a mild wart virus infection, and since they usually disappear within 6–9 months they are best left alone. This holds true

especially for all flat warts on the face. A good response to 0.05% tretinoin (Retin-A) cream, applied once daily for 3–4 weeks, has been reported.

The best treatment for the solitary **common ("vulgaris") wart** is to freeze it with liquid nitrogen. The liquid nitrogen should be allowed to drip from the cotton-tipped applicator onto the wart without pressure. Pressure exaggerates cold injury by causing vasoconstriction and may produce a deep ulcer and scar. Liquid nitrogen is applied by drip until the wart turns completely white and stays white for 20–25 seconds. Large and painful plantar warts are treated most effectively by applying 40% salicylic acid plaster cut with a scissors to fit the lesion. The sticky brown side of the plaster is placed against the lesion, taped on securely with adhesive tape, and left on for 5 days. The plaster is then removed, and the white necrotic warty tissue can be gently rubbed off with the finger and a new salicylic acid plaster applied. This procedure is repeated every 5 days, and the patient is seen every 2 weeks. Most plantar warts resolve in 2–4 weeks when treated in this way.

Sharp scalpel excision, electrosurgery, and laser surgery should be avoided, since the resulting scar often becomes a more difficult problem than the wart itself and there may be recurrence of the wart in the area of the scar.

Venereal warts (**condyloma acuminatum**) are best treated with 25% podophyllum resin (podophyllin) in alcohol or Podofilox, a lower concentration of purified podophyllin. These should be painted on the lesions and then washed off after 4 hours. Re-treatment in 7–10 days may be necessary. A wart not on the vulvar mucous membrane but on the adjacent skin should be treated as a common wart and frozen.

For isolated warts and periungual warts, cantharidin (Cantharone, Verr-Canth) is effective and painless in children. It causes a blister and sometimes is difficult to control. An undesirable complication is the appearance of warts along the margins of the cantharidin blister. Cantharidin is applied to the skin, allowed to dry, and covered with occlusive tape such as Blenderm for 24 hours.

No wart therapy is immediate and definitive, and recurrences are reported in more than 30% of cases even with the best care.

Bender ME: The protean manifestations of human papillomavirus infection. Arch Dermatol 1994;130:1429.
Williams H, Pottier A, Strachan D: The descriptive epidemiology of warts in British schoolchildren. Br J Dermatol 1993;128:504.

INSECT INFESTATIONS

These disorders are characterized generally by discrete red papules, nodules, and S-shaped burrows on the skin. Hand and foot involvement is common.

Scabies

Scabies is suggested by the appearance of linear burrows about the wrists, ankles, finger webs, areolas, anterior axillary folds, genitalia, or face (in infants). Often, there are excoriations, honey-colored crusts, and pustules from secondary infection. Identification of the female mite or her eggs and feces is necessary to confirm the diagnosis. Scrape an unscratched papule or burrow with a No. 15 blade and examine microscopically in immersion oil to confirm the diagnosis. In a child who is often scratching, scrape under the fingernails. Examine the parents for unscratched burrows.

Lindane (gamma benzene hexachloride; Kwell) and permethrin are excellent scabicides. However, since lindane is concentrated in the central nervous system, where toxicity from systemic absorption in infants has been reported, the following restricted use of this agent is recommended: (1) For adults and older children, one treatment of lindane lotion or cream applied to the entire body and left on for 4 hours, followed by shower, is sufficient. (2) Infants tend to have more organisms and many more lesions and may have to be re-treated in 7–10 days. All family members should be treated simultaneously. Permethrin 5% cream (Elimite) may be substituted for lindane in infants.

Paller AS: Scabies in infants and small children. Semin Dermatol 1993;12:3.

Pediculoses
(Louse Infestations)

Excoriated papules and pustules with a history of severe itching at night suggest infestation with the human body louse. This louse may be discovered in the seams of underwear but not on the body. In the scalp hair, the gelatinous nits of the head louse adhere tightly to the hair shaft. The pubic louse may be found crawling among pubic hairs, or blue-black macules may be found dispersed through the pubic region (maculae ceruleae). The pubic louse is often seen in the eyelashes of newborns.

Lindane (gamma benzene hexachloride; Kwell) has been the treatment of choice. The following use is recommended: For head lice, a shampoo preparation is left on the scalp for 5 minutes and rinsed out thoroughly. The hair is then combed with a fine-tooth comb to remove nits. This may be repeated in 7 days. Lindane cream or lotion applied to the body for 4 hours may be necessary for body lice, but washing the clothing in boiling water followed by ironing the seams with a hot iron usually eliminates the organisms. Permethrin 1% creme rinse is also efficacious for the elimination of lice.

Lindane cream or lotion applied to the pubic area for 24 hours is sufficient to treat pediculosis pubis. It may be repeated in 4–5 days.

Clare ER, Longyear LA: A comparative study of seven pediculicides and their packaged nit removal combs. J Pediatr Health Care 1993;7:55.

Janniger CK, Kuflik AS: Pediculosis capitis. Cutis 1993;51:407.

Papular Urticaria

Papular urticaria is characterized by grouped erythematous papules surrounded by an urticarial flare and distributed over the shoulders, upper arms, and buttocks in infants. These lesions represent delayed hypersensitivity reactions to stinging or biting insects and can be reproduced by patch testing with the offending insect. Fleas from dogs and cats are the usual offenders. Less commonly, mosquitoes, lice, scabies, and bird and grass mites are involved. The sensitivity is transient, lasting 4–6 months. The logical therapy is to remove the offending insect. Topical corticosteroids and oral antihistamines will control symptoms.

DERMATITIS*
(Eczema)

Essentials of Diagnosis

- Red skin with disruption of skin surface.
- Vesicles, crusting, or lichenification may be present.

General Considerations

The terms *dermatitis* and *eczema* are currently used interchangeably in dermatology, although the etymologic implication of eczema is "a boiling over" and the term originally denoted an acute weeping dermatosis. All forms of dermatitis, regardless of cause, may present with acute edema, erythema, and oozing with crusting, mild erythema alone, or lichenification. Lichenification is diagnosed by thickening of the skin with a shiny surface and exaggerated, deepened skin markings. It is the response of the skin to chronic rubbing or scratching.

Although the lesions of the various dermatoses are histologically indistinguishable, clinicians have nonetheless divided the disease group called dermatitis into several categories based on known causes in some cases and differing natural histories in others.

Atopic Dermatitis

Atopic dermatitis is not a clearly defined clinical entity but a general term for chronic superficial inflammation of the skin that can be applied to a heterogenous group of patients. Many (not all) patients go through three clinical phases. In the first, infantile

---

*From the perspective of a dermatologist. See also the discussion of atopic dermatitis in Chapter 33.

eczema, the dermatitis begins on the cheeks and scalp and frequently expresses itself as oval patches on the trunk, later involving the extensor surfaces of the extremities. The usual age at onset is 2–3 months, and this phase ends at age 18 months to 2 years. Only one-third of all infants with atopic eczema progress to phase 2—childhood or flexural eczema—in which the predominant involvement is in the antecubital and popliteal fossae, the neck, the wrists, and sometimes the hands or feet. This phase lasts from age 2 years to adolescence. Some children will have involvement of the soles of their feet only, with cracking, redness, and pain—the so-called **atopic feet.** Only a third of children with typical flexural eczema will progress to adolescent eczema, which is usually manifested by hand dermatitis only. Atopic dermatitis is quite unusual after age 30.

Atopic dermatitis has no known cause, and despite the high incidence of asthma and hay fever in these patients (30%) and their families (70%), evidence for allergy beyond this hereditary association is limited to testimonials. The case for food and inhalant allergens as specific causes of atopic dermatitis is not strong.

A few patients with atopic dermatitis have immunodeficiency with recurrent pyodermas, unusual susceptibility to herpes simplex and vaccinia virus, hyperimmunoglobulinemia E, defective neutrophil and monocyte chemotaxis, and impaired T-lymphocyte function. (See Chapter 28.)

A faulty epidermal barrier may predispose the patient with atopic dermatitis to itchy skin. Inability to hold water within the stratum corneum results in rapid evaporation of water, shrinking of the stratum corneum, and "cracks" in the epidermal barrier. Such skin forms an ineffective barrier to the entry of various irritants—and, indeed, it may be clinically useful to regard atopic dermatitis as a primary irritant contact dermatitis and simply tell the patient, "You have sensitive skin." Chronic atopic dermatitis is frequently secondarily infected with *S aureus* or *Streptococcus pyogenes.*

A. Treatment of Acute Stages: Application of wet dressings and topical corticosteroids is the treatment of choice for acute, weeping atopic eczema. A topical steroid preparation is applied four times daily and covered with wet dressings as outlined at the beginning of this chapter. Systemic antibiotics chosen on the basis of appropriate skin cultures may be necessary, since lesions in the acute stages are often secondarily infected.

B. Treatment of Chronic Stages: Treatment is aimed at avoiding irritants and restoring water to the skin. No soaps or harsh shampoos should be used, and the patient should avoid woolen or any rough clothing. Restoring water to the skin is important in atopic dermatitis. This can be accomplished by two baths daily, less than 5 minutes each, after which lubricating oils or ointments are applied.

Moisturel is a useful lubricant. Plain petrolatum and lards are often too greasy and may cause considerable sweat retention. Liberal use of Cetaphil lotion as a soap substitute four or five times a day is also satisfactory as a means of lubrication. A bedroom humidifier is often helpful. Topical corticosteroids should be limited to the less potent ones (see Table 14–2). Hydrocortisone ointment, 1% twice daily, is often sufficient. There is *never* any reason to use super- or high-potency corticosteroids in atopic dermatitis. In superinfected atopic dermatitis, systemic antibiotics for 10–14 days are necessary.

Treatment failures in chronic atopic dermatitis are most often the result of patient noncompliance. This is a frustrating disease for parent and child.

DeProst YD: Management of severe atopic dermatitis. Acta Derm-Venereol 1992;176:117.

Kay J et al: The prevalence of childhood atopic dermatitis in a general population. J Am Acad Dermatol 1994; 30:35.

Williams HC et al: The UK Working Party's diagnostic criteria for atopic dermatitis. I. Derivation of a minimum set of discriminators for atopic dermatitis. Br J Dermatol 1994;131:383.

Nummular Eczema

Nummular eczema is characterized by numerous symmetrically distributed coin-shaped patches of dermatitis, principally on the extremities. These may be acute, oozing, and crusted or dry and scaling. The disease lasts 9 months to 2 years. The differential diagnosis should include tinea corporis and atopic dermatitis.

The same topical measures should be used as for atopic dermatitis, although treatment is often more difficult.

Primary Irritant Contact Dermatitis (Diaper Dermatitis)

Contact dermatitis is of two types: primary irritant and allergic eczematous. Primary irritant dermatitis develops within a few hours, reaches peak severity at 24 hours, and then disappears. Allergic eczematous contact dermatitis (see below) has a delayed onset of 18 hours, peaks at 48–72 hours, and often lasts as long as 2–3 weeks, even if exposure to the offending antigen is discontinued.

Diaper dermatitis, the most common form of primary irritant contact dermatitis seen in pediatric practice, is caused by prolonged contact of the skin with urine and feces, which contain irritating chemicals such as urea and intestinal enzymes. The diagnosis of diaper dermatitis is based on the picture of erythema and thickening of the skin in the perineal area and the history of skin contact with urine or feces. In 80% of cases of diaper dermatitis lasting more than 3 days, the affected area is colonized with *Candida al-*

bicans even before the classic signs of a beefy red, sharply marginated dermatitis with satellite lesions appear.

Treatment consists of changing diapers frequently. Because rubber or plastic pants serve as occlusive dressings and prevent the evaporation of the contactant and enhance its penetration into the skin, they should be avoided as much as possible. Air drying is useful. Streptococcal perianal cellulitis should be included in the differential diagnosis. Treatment of longstanding diaper dermatitis should include application of nystatin (Mycostatin) or an imidazole cream with each diaper change.

Allergic Eczematous Contact Dermatitis (Poison Ivy Dermatitis)

Children often present with acute dermatitis with blister formation, oozing, and crusting. Blisters are often linear and of acute onset. Plants such as poison ivy, poison sumac, and poison oak cause most cases of allergic contact dermatitis in children.

Allergic contact dermatitis has all the features of delayed-type (T lymphocyte–mediated) hypersensitivity. Although many substances may cause such a reaction, nickel sulfate (metals), potassium dichromate, and neomycin are the most common causes. The true incidence of allergic contact dermatitis in children is not known.

Treatment of contact dermatitis in localized areas is with topical corticosteroids. In severe generalized involvement, prednisone, 1–2 mg/kg/d orally for 14–21 days, can be used.

Grerelink SA, Murrel DF, Olsen EA: Effectiveness of various barrier preparations in preventing and/or ameliorating experimentally produced *Toxicodendron* dermatitis. J Am Acad Dermatol 1992;27:182.

Seborrheic Dermatitis

Seborrheic dermatitis consists of an erythematous scaly dermatitis accompanied by overproduction of sebum occurring in areas rich in sebaceous glands, that is, the face, scalp, and perineum. This common condition occurs predominantly in the newborn and at puberty, the ages at which hormonal stimulation of sebum production is maximal. Although it is tempting to speculate that the overproduction of sebum causes the dermatitis, the exact relationship is unclear.

Seborrheic dermatitis on the scalp in infancy is often confused with atopic dermatitis, and only after other areas are involved or flexural involvement occurs is it clear that the diagnosis is atopic dermatitis. Psoriasis also occurs in seborrheic areas in older children and should always be considered in the differential diagnosis.

Seborrheic dermatitis responds well to topical corticosteroids; 1% hydrocortisone cream three times daily is often sufficient to control this disorder.

Dandruff

Physiologic scaling or mild seborrhea, in the form of greasy scalp scales, may be treated by medicated dandruff shampoos.

Dry Skin Dermatitis (Asteatotic Eczema, Xerosis)

Newborns and older children who live in arid climates are susceptible to dry skin, characterized by large cracked scales with erythematous borders. The stratum corneum is dependent on environmental humidity for its water, and below 30% environmental humidity the stratum corneum loses water, shrinks, and cracks. These cracks in the epidermal barrier allow irritating substances to enter the skin, predisposing the patient to dermatitis.

Treatment consists of increasing the water content of the skin's immediate external environment. House humidifiers are very useful. Two 5-minute baths a day with immediate application of oils or ointments (petrolatum) after the bath will allow the skin to retain water. Frequent soaping of the skin impairs its water-holding capacity and serves as an irritating alkali, and all soaps should therefore be avoided. Frequent use of emollients (eg, Cetaphil, Eucerin, Lubriderm, Moisturel) should be a major part of therapy.

Keratosis Pilaris

Follicular papules containing a white inspissated scale characterize keratosis pilaris. Individual lesions are discrete and may be red. They are prominent on the extensor surfaces of the upper arms and thighs and on the buttocks and cheeks. In severe cases, the lesions may be generalized. Such lesions are seen frequently in children with dry skin and have also been associated with atopic dermatitis and ichthyosis vulgaris.

Treatment is with keratolytics such as topical retinoic acid, lactic acid, or urea creams followed by skin hydration.

Pityriasis Alba

White, scaly macular areas with indistinct borders are seen over extensor surfaces of extremities and on the cheeks in children. Suntanning exaggerates these lesions. Histologic examination reveals a mild dermatitis. These lesions may be confused with tinea versicolor. There is no satisfactory treatment.

COMMON SKIN TUMORS

If the skin moves with the nodule on lateral palpation, the tumor is located within the dermis; if the skin moves over the nodule, it is subcutaneous. Table 14–6 lists the tumors according to these categories.

Table 14–6. Common skin tumors.

Intradermal
Epidermal inclusion cyst
Pilomatricoma
Dermatofibroma
Melanocytic nevus
Pyogenic granuloma
Neurofibroma
Granuloma annulare
Subcutaneous
Lipoma
Rheumatoid nodule

Table 14–7. Papulosquamous eruptions in children.

Psoriasis
Pityriasis rosea
Secondary syphilis
Lichen planus
Chronic parapsoriasis
Pityriasis rubra pilaris
Tinea corporis
Dermatomyositis
Lupus erythematosus

Epidermal Inclusion Cysts

Epidermal inclusion cysts are smooth, dome-shaped nodules in the skin that may grow to 2 cm in diameter. In infants, they may be found about the eyes and in older children and adolescents on the chest, back, or scalp. They are the most common superficial lumps in children. Treatment, if desired, is surgical excision.

Granuloma Annulare

Circles or semicircles of nontender intradermal nodules found over the lower legs and ankles, the dorsum of the hands and wrists, and the trunk, in that order, suggest granuloma annulare. Histologically, the disease appears as a central area of tissue death (necrobiosis) surrounded by macrophages and lymphocytes. No treatment is necessary. Lesions resolve spontaneously within 1–2 years in most children.

Pyogenic Granuloma

Rapid growth of a dark red papule with an ulcerated and crusted surface over 1–2 weeks following skin trauma suggests pyogenic granuloma. Histologically, this represents excessive new vessel formation with or without inflammation (granulation tissue). It is neither pyogenic nor granulomatous but should be regarded as an abnormal healing response. Pulsed dye laser or excision are the treatments of choice.

Keloids

Keloids are scars raised above the skin surface with many radial projections of scar tissue. They continue to enlarge over several years. They are often found on the face, earlobes, neck, chest, and back. Keloids show no racial predilection. Treatment includes intralesional injection with triamcinolone acetonide, 20 mg/mL, or excision and injection with corticosteroids.

PAPULOSQUAMOUS ERUPTIONS
(See Table 14–7.)

Papulosquamous eruptions are eruptions that consist of papules or plaques with varying degrees of scale.

Pityriasis Rosea

Erythematous papules that coalesce to form oval plaques preceded by a large oval plaque with central clearing and a scaly border (the herald patch) establish the diagnosis of pityriasis rosea. The herald patch has the appearance of ringworm and is often treated as such. It appears 1–30 days before the onset of the generalized papular eruption. The oval plaques are parallel in their long axis and follow Langer's lines of skin cleavage. In whites, the lesions are primarily on the trunk, accentuated in the axillary and inguinal areas. In blacks, lesions are primarily on the extremities. This disease is common in school-age children and adolescents and is presumed to be viral in origin. It lasts 6 weeks and may be pruritic the first 7–10 days. The major differential diagnosis is secondary syphilis, and a VDRL test should be done if syphilis is suspected. A chronic variant of this disease may last 2–3 years and is called **chronic parapsoriasis** or **pityriasis lichenoides chronicus.**

Exposing the skin to sunlight until a mild sunburn occurs (slight redness) will hasten the disappearance of lesions. Ordinarily, no treatment is necessary.

Ginsburg CM: Pityriasis rosea. Pediatr Infect Dis J 1991; 10:858.

Psoriasis

Psoriasis is characterized by erythematous papules covered by thick white scales. Guttate (drop-like) psoriasis is a common form in children that often follows an episode of streptococcal pharyngitis by 2–3 weeks. The sudden onset of small (3- to 8-mm) papules, which are seen predominantly over the trunk and quickly become covered with thick white scales, is characteristic of guttate psoriasis. Chronic psoriasis is marked by thick, large (5- to 10-cm) scaly plaques over the elbows, knees, scalp, and other sites of trauma. Pinpoint pits in the nail plate are seen as well as yellow discoloration of the nail plate resulting from onycholysis. Thickening of all 20 nails is an uncommon feature. The sacral and seborrheic areas are commonly involved. Psoriasis has no known cause and demonstrates active proliferation of epidermal cells, with a turnover time of 3–4 days versus 28 days for normal skin. These rapidly proliferating epidermal cells are producing excessive stratum corneum, giving rise to thick, opaque scales. Papulosquamous eruptions that present problems of differential diagnosis are listed in Table 14–7.

All therapy is aimed at diminishing epidermal turnover time. Sunlight or artificial ultraviolet light (UVL) alone will produce some improvement. Coal tar enhances the effect of UVL and hastens the disappearance of psoriatic lesions. Bathing with a bath product containing tar (eg, Balnetar) at night, followed by UVL the next day, may be sufficient in mild cases. In more severe psoriasis, 10% liquor carbonis detergens in petrolatum should be applied after the bath. The newer tar gels (Estar Gel, psoriGel) cause less staining and are most efficacious. They are applied twice daily for 6–8 weeks.

Crude coal tar therapy is messy and stains bedclothes, and patients may prefer to use topical corticosteroids. Penetration of topical corticosteroids through the enlarged epidermal barrier in psoriasis requires that more potent preparations be used, for example, fluocinonide 0.05% (Lidex) or triamcinolone 0.5% (Aristocort, Kenalog) two or three times daily.

Anthralin therapy is also useful. Anthralin is applied to the skin for a short contact time (eg, 20 minutes once daily) and then washed off with a neutral soap (eg, Dove). A 6-week course of treatment is recommended.

Scalp care using a tar shampoo requires leaving the shampoo on for 5 minutes, washing it off, and then shampooing with commercial shampoo to remove scales. It may be necessary to shampoo daily until scaling is reduced.

More severe cases of psoriasis are best treated by a dermatologist.

Krueger GG, Duvic M: Epidemiology of psoriasis: Clinical issues. J Invest Dermatol 1994;102:145.

HAIR LOSS
(Alopecia)

Hair loss in children (Table 14–8) imposes great emotional stress on the patient and the parent. A 60% hair loss in a single area is necessary before hair loss can be detected clinically. Examination should begin with the scalp to determine whether there are color changes or infiltrative changes. Hairs should be examined microscopically for breaking and structural defects and to see whether growing or resting hairs are being shed. Placing removed hairs in mounting fluid (Permount) on a glass microscope slide makes them easy to examine. Three diseases account for most cases of hair loss in children: alopecia areata, tinea capitis, and trichotillomania.

Alopecia Areata

Loss of every hair in a localized area is called alopecia areata. This is the most common cause of

Table 14–8. Other causes of hair loss in children.

Hair loss with scalp changes
Nodules and tumors:
  Nevus sebaceus
  Epidermal nevus
Thickening:
  Burn
Atrophy:
  Lupus erythematosus
  Lichen planus
Hair loss with hair shaft defects (hair fails to grow out enough to require haircuts)
Monilethrix—alternating bands of thin and thick areas
Trichorrhexis nodosa—nodules with fragmented hair
Trichorrhexis invaginata (bamboo hair)—intussusception of one hair into another
Pili torti—hair twisted 180 degrees, brittle
Pili annulati—alternating bands of light and dark pigmentation

hair loss in children. An immunologic pathogenic mechanism is suspected because dense infiltration of lymphocytes precedes hair loss. Ninety-five percent of children with alopecia areata completely regrow their hair within 12 months, although as many as 40% may have a relapse in 5–6 years. A rare and unusual form of alopecia areata begins at the occiput and proceeds along the hair margins to the frontal scalp. This variety, called **ophiasis,** often results in total scalp hair loss (**alopecia totalis**). The prognosis for regrowth in ophiasis is poor.

No treatment is indicated for alopecia areata. Systemic corticosteroids given to suppress the inflammatory response will result in hair growth, but the hair will fall out again when the drug is discontinued. In children with alopecia totalis, a wig is most helpful.

Tobin DJ et al: Antibodies to hair follicles in alopecia areata. J Invest Dermatol 1994;102:721.

Trichotillomania

Traumatic hair pulling causes the hair shafts to be broken off at different lengths, an ill-defined area of hair loss, petechiae around follicular openings, and a wrinkled hair shaft on microscopic examination. This may be merely habit or the result of severe anxiety in the child. Eyelashes and eyebrows rather than scalp hair may be pulled out. If the behavior has a long history, psychiatric evaluation may be helpful. Oiling the hair to make it slippery is an aid to behavior modification.

Grabe J, Arndt WM: Trichotillomania. Compr Psychiatry 1993;34:340.

REACTIVE ERYTHEMAS

Erythema Multiforme

Erythema multiforme begins with papules that later develop a dark center and then evolve into lesions with central blisters and the characteristic target lesions (iris lesions) with three concentric circles of color change. Primary injury is to endothelial cells, with later destruction of epidermal basal cells and blister formation. Erythema multiforme has sometimes been diagnosed in patients with severe mucous membrane involvement, but **Stevens-Johnson syndrome** is the usual term when severe involvement of conjunctiva, oral cavity, and genital mucosa also occur.

Many causes are suspected, particularly herpes simplex virus, sulfonamide drugs, and *Mycoplasma* infections. Recurrent erythema multiforme is usually associated with reactivation of herpes simplex virus. In the mild form, spontaneous healing occurs in 10–14 days, but Stevens-Johnson syndrome may last 6–8 weeks.

Treatment is symptomatic in uncomplicated erythema multiforme. Removal of offending drugs is an obvious measure. Oral antihistamines such as hydroxyzine, 2 mg/kg/d orally, are useful. Cool compresses and wet dressings will relieve pruritus. Steroids have not been demonstrated to be effective.

Weston WL: What is erythema multiforme? Pediatr Ann 1996;25:106.

Weston JA, Weston WL: The overdiagnosis of erythema multiforme. Pediatrics 1992;89:802.

Weston WL et al: Herpes simplex virus in childhood erythema multiforme. Pediatrics 1992;89:32.

Drug Eruptions

Drugs may produce urticarial, morbilliform, scarlatiniform, or bullous skin eruptions. Urticaria may appear within minutes after drug administration, but most reactions begin 7–14 days after the drug is first administered. These eruptions may occur in patients who have received these drugs for long periods, and eruptions continue for days after the drug has been discontinued. Drugs commonly implicated in skin reactions are listed in Table 14–9.

Breathnach SM, Hintner H: *Adverse Reactions in the Skin.* Blackwell, 1992.

MISCELLANEOUS SKIN DISORDERS ENCOUNTERED IN PEDIATRIC PRACTICE

Aphthous Stomatitis

Recurrent erosions on the gums, lips, tongue, palate, and buccal mucosa are often confused with herpes simplex. A smear of the base of such a lesion

Table 14–9. Common drug reactions.

Erythema multiforme/toxic epidermal necrolysis
  Sulfonamides
  Nonsteroidal anti-inflammatory drugs
  Anticonvulsants
Urticaria
  Penicillins
  Sulfonamides
  Barbiturates
  Opioids
Morbilliform eruption
  Penicillins
  Cephalosporins
  Sulfonamides
  Anticonvulsants
Photodermatitis
  Psoralens
  Tetracyclines
  Thiazides
  Sulfonamides

stained with Wright's stain will aid in ruling out herpes simplex by the absence of epithelial multinucleate giant cells. A culture for herpes simplex is also useful in this difficult differential diagnostic problem. It has been shown that recurrence of aphthous stomatitis correlates positively with lymphocyte-mediated cytotoxicity.

There is no specific therapy for this condition. Rinsing the mouth with liquid antacids will provide relief in most patients. Topical corticosteroids in a gel base (eg, fluocinonide gel) may provide some relief. In severe cases that interfere with eating, prednisone, 1 mg/kg/d orally for 3–5 days, will suffice to abort an episode.

Jasmin JR et al: Local treatment of minor aphthous ulceration in children. Am J Dis Child 1993;60:26.

Vitiligo

Vitiligo is characterized clinically by the development of areas of depigmentation. These are often symmetrical and occur mainly on extensor surfaces. The depigmentation results from a destruction of melanocytes. The basis for this destruction is unknown, but immunologically mediated damage is likely and vitiligo sometimes occurs in individuals with selective IgA deficiency, graft-versus-host disease or autoimmune endocrinopathies. Treatment is not very effective. Topical psoralens with UV irradiation are reserved for children over 12 years of age.

Jaisankar TJ, Baruah MC, Gorg BR: Vitiligo in children. Int J Dermatol 1992;31:621.

REFERENCES

Schachner L, Hansen R: *Pediatric Dermatology,* 2nd ed. Churchill Livingstone, 1996.

Weston WL, Lane AT, Morelli JG: *Color Textbook of Pediatric Dermatology,* 2nd ed. Mosby–Year Book, 1996.

Eye

15

Allan M. Eisenbaum, MD

For visual development to proceed normally, a child must experience a normal visual environment with well-aligned eyes that are free of visually threatening disease and significant refractive errors. The consequences of not meeting these requirements during the sensitive period of visual development in the first decade of life are strabismus and decreased vision.

COMMON NONSPECIFIC SIGNS & SYMPTOMS

There are several nonspecific signs and symptoms that are common as a chief complaint or item in the history of children with eye disease. These are often grouped together by the patient or parent.

Redness

Redness or injection of the bulbar conjunctiva or deeper vessels is very common. Causes include superficial or penetrating foreign bodies, infection, allergy, and conjunctivitis associated with systemic entities such as Stevens-Johnson syndrome or Kawasaki disease. Irritating, noxious agents also result in injection. Subconjunctival hemorrhage may be traumatic, associated with hematopoietic disease, vascular anomalies, or inflammatory processes (Table 15–1).

Tearing

In infants, tearing is usually due to nasolacrimal obstruction, but tearing may also be associated with glaucoma, in which case photophobia and blepharospasm may also be present. Inflammation, allergic and viral diseases, and corneal irritation can also cause tearing.

Discharge

Purulent discharge is usually associated with a bacterial conjunctivitis. Watery discharge occurs with viral infection, iritis, foreign bodies, and nasolacrimal obstruction. Mucoid discharge can be found with allergic conjunctivitis and nasolacrimal obstruction.

Pain

Pain in or about the eye may be due to foreign bodies, corneal abrasions, lacerations, acute infections of the globe, or adnexa, iritis, and glaucoma. Large refractive errors, poor accommodative ability, and sinus disease may manifest as headaches.

Photophobia

Acute aversion to light may occur with corneal abrasions, foreign bodies, and iritis. Photophobia is present in infants with glaucoma, albinism, and aniridia. Light-complected individuals may be light-sensitive. Photophobia is common after ocular surgery and pharmacologic dilatation of the pupil.

Leukocoria

Although not a common sign or complaint, leukocoria (a white pupil) is associated with serious conditions and requires prompt ophthalmologic consultation. Causes of leukocoria include retinoblastoma, retinopathy of prematurity, pupillary membrane, cataract, vitreous opacities, retinal detachment, and dysplasia (Figure 15–1).

REFRACTIVE ERRORS

Refractive error refers to the optical state of the eye. It is a physical characteristic such as height or weight and can be quantitated. Not all refractive errors require correction. There are three types of refractive errors: myopia, hyperopia, and astigmatism. Inequality of the refractive state between the two eyes can cause amblyopia (reduced vision without an appropriate organic lesion (see Amblyopia).

Myopia (Nearsightedness)

For the person with myopia, objects nearby are in focus; those at a distance are blurred. Typically, the onset of myopia is around 8 years of age. A myopic person may squint to produce a pinhole effect, which improves distance vision. Headaches are common. Divergent lenses provide clear distant vision.

Table 15–1. Differential diagnosis of redness of the eye in pediatric patients.

	Acute Conjunctivitis	Acute Iritis	Acute Glaucoma[1]	Corneal Abrasion
Incidence	Very common.	Uncommon.	Rare.	Fairly common.
Etiology	Usually bacterial; may be viral, fungal, or allergic.	Usually unknown; may be associated with juvenile rheumatoid arthritis.	Developmental defects or obstruction of aqueous drainage channels.	Foreign body; abrasion.
Redness	Diffuse injection of conjunctiva; greater toward fornices.	Purple-red; circum-corneal injection.	Often diffuse injection of bulbar conjunctiva.	Diffuse injection of conjunctiva.
Discharge	Moderate to heavy; mucoid or mucopurulent.	None.	None; tearing.	Watery.
Visual acuity	Normal.	Decreased.	Decreased.	Decreased.
Corneal transparency	Clear.	Clear or some haze.	Hazy; cornea enlarged in congenital form.	Variable haze. Positive fluorescein stain.
Anterior chamber depth	Normal.	Normal; cloudy.	Shallow; deep in congenital form.	Normal.
Pupil size	Normal.	Constricted.	Dilated.	Normal.
Intraocular pressure	Normal.	Usually normal; may be low or elevated.	Elevated.	Normal.
Conjunctival smear results	Causative organisms identified; numerous polymorphonuclear neutrophils found in bacterial infection; numerous mononuclear cells found in viral infection.	Normal.	Normal.	Normal.

[1]Primary narrow-angle glaucoma is very rare in children. Congenital glaucoma may not produce redness of the eye.

Hyperopia (Farsightedness)

Saying the hyperopic child is sighted for far (not near) is somewhat misleading, since the child can focus on near targets if the hyperopia is not excessive. Large amounts of uncorrected hyperopia can cause esotropia and amblyopia (see Amblyopia & Strabismus). Most children have a hyperopic refraction, which begins to diminish at about 8 years of age and does not require correction.

Astigmatism

Astigmatism is a refractive state in which there are two planes of focus within one eye. Large amounts of astigmatism not corrected at an early age can cause decreased vision from amblyopia, but proper refractive correction can prevent this.

EXAMINATION

Ophthalmic examination of the pediatric patient begins with a calm demeanor and reassuring voice. Having a parent present is invaluable. The examination includes a history, an assessment of visual acuity, an external examination, ocular alignment and motility, and an ophthalmoscopic examination. Less frequently measured is intraocular pressure. Testing of binocular status and near point is desirable.

Circumstances will dictate the use of ancillary procedures such as instilling fluorescein dye and radiologic tests (magnetic resonance imaging [MRI] and computed tomography [CT]). The electroretinogram and electro-oculography test retinal function. The vi-

Figure 15–1. Leukocoria of left eye with mild microphthalmia caused by retrolental membrane (persistent hyperplastic primary vitreous).

sually evoked response tests the function of the visual pathways. Visual field testing demonstrates the presence or absence of scotomata and visual field cuts.

History

Evaluation begins by obtaining the chief complaint and history of present illness. Past ocular history is obtained, as well as perinatal and developmental history and history of allergy. The family history should be explored for ocular disorders that may be familial or inherited.

Visual Acuity

Visual acuity testing is the single most important test of visual function and should be part of every general physical examination. The level of visual acuity should be documented after ocular trauma and before and after any treatment. Acuity should be tested in each eye individually. If latent nystagmus is present, vision of both eyes should be tested simultaneously, as well as each eye individually. Vision is recorded both without spectacles (uncorrected vision), and with spectacles in place (corrected vision). In older children who can cooperate, the use of a pinhole will improve vision in children not wearing the appropriate spectacle prescription.

The type of test used to determine acuity is dictated by the age of the child. In the sleeping newborn, the presence of a blepharospastic response to bright light is an adequate response. At 6 weeks of age, eye-to-eye contact with slow following movements can be detected. By 3 months, the infant should be fixing and following ocular movements at a distance of 2–3 feet. At 6 months of age, interest in movement across the room is the norm. Vision can be recorded for the presence or absence of fixing and following behavior and for whether vision is steady (unsteady when nystagmus is present) and maintained. Vision should be tested and recorded for each eye. Visual acuity can be quantified in infants using other techniques.

In the verbal child, the use of familiar icons will allow for a quantitative test. Four-year-olds are often ready to play the tumbling E game. Literate youngsters are tested with letters. Typical acuity levels in developmentally appropriate children are approximately 20/60 in 2½-year-olds, 20/40–20/30 in 3-year-olds, 20/30–20/25 in 4-year-olds, and 20/20 in literate 5-year-olds. Perhaps more important than the level of absolute visual acuity is the presence of a difference of acuity between the two eyes, which might indicate amblyopia, uncorrected refractive error, or a pathologic condition.

The practitioner should be aware of two situations complicated by nystagmus. Children who require a face turn or torticollis to quiet the nystagmus will record poor visual acuity results when tested in the absence of the compensatory head posture.

When latent nystagmus is present, acuity testing is particularly challenging (see Nystagmus). Nystagmus appears or worsens when an eye is occluded, degrading central vision. To minimize the nystagmus, the occluder should be held about 12 inches in front of the eye not being tested. Testing both eyes simultaneously without occlusion may record better acuity than either eye individually.

External Examination

Inspection of the anterior segment of the globe and its adnexa requires adequate illumination and often magnification. Immobilization of the child may be necessary. A drop of topical anesthetic may facilitate the examination. Assessment of the entire anterior segment except the trabecular meshwork is possible. In cases of suspected perforation of the globe, it may be best to keep the child at rest, patch and shield the eye, and keep the examination to a minimum to prevent expulsion of intraocular contents. In this setting, the child should be given nothing by mouth in case an eye examination under anesthesia may be required.

In cases of suspected foreign body, pulling down on the lower lid provides excellent visualization of the inferior cul-de-sac (palpebral conjunctiva). Visualizing the upper cul-de-sac and superior bulbar conjunctiva is possible by having the patient look inferiorly while the upper lid is pulled away from the globe. Illumination with a penlight is necessary. The upper lid should be everted to evaluate the superior tarsal conjunctiva by pulling the lid down at the lid margin while everting the lid back up on itself over a thin stick, such as a cotton applicator placed at the upper tarsal border of the lid (Figure 15–2).

When indicated to better evaluate the cornea, a small amount of fluorescein solution should be in-

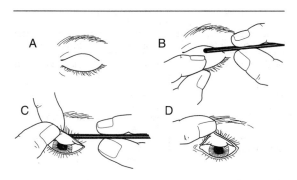

Figure 15–2. Eversion of the upper lid. **A:** The patient looks downward. **B:** The fingers pull the lid down, and a rod is placed on the upper tarsal border. **C:** The lid is pulled up over the rod. **D:** The lid is everted. (Redrawn and reproduced, with permission, from Liebman SD, Gellis SS [editors]: *The Pediatrician's Ophthalmology*. CV Mosby, 1966.)

stilled into the lower cul-de-sac. Blue light will cause the fluorescein to fluoresce yellow. Disease-specific staining patterns may be observed. For example, herpes simplex lesions of the corneal epithelium produce a dendrite. A foreign body lodged beneath the upper lid shows one or more vertical lines of stain on the cornea. Contact lens overwear produces a central staining pattern. A fine, scattered punctate pattern may indicate a viral keratitis or medication toxicity. Punctate erosions of the inferior third of the cornea can be seen with a staphylococcal blepharitis or exposure keratitis secondary to incomplete lid closure.

Alignment & Motility Evaluation

Alignment and motility should be tested, since amblyopia is associated with strabismus. Besides alignment, ocular rotations should be evaluated in the six cardinal positions of gaze (Table 15–2; Figure 15–3). A small toy is an interesting target to test ocular rotations in infants, whereas a penlight works well in older children.

Alignment can be assessed in several ways. In order of increasing accuracy, these methods are observation, the corneal light reflex test, and cover testing. **Observation** requires that an educated guess be made as to whether the eyes are properly aligned or not. **Corneal light reflex** evaluation (Hirschberg test) is performed by shining the beam of a light at the patient's eyes, observing the reflections off each cornea, and estimating whether these "reflexes" appear to be properly positioned. If the reflection of light is noted temporally on the cornea, esotropia is suspected (Figure 15–4). Nasal reflection of the light suggests exotropia. Neither of these tests is sensitive in differentiating pseudostrabismus from true strabismus.

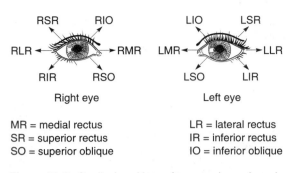

MR = medial rectus   LR = lateral rectus
SR = superior rectus   IR = inferior rectus
SO = superior oblique   IO = inferior oblique

Figure 15–3. Cardinal positions of gaze and muscles primarily tested in those fields of gaze. Arrow indicates position in which each muscle is tested.

Another way of evaluating alignment is with the **cover test,** in which the patient looks at a target while one eye is covered. If the uncovered eye is deviated inward (esotropia) or outward (exotropia), a corrective movement is made by the uncovered eye to refixate the target. The other eye is similarly tested. When the occluder is removed from the eye just uncovered, a refixation movement of that eye indicates a phoria or latent deviation. If the eye remains in a deviated position after removing the occluder, then a tropia is noted to be present (Figure 15–5).

Ophthalmoscopic Examination

A hand-held direct ophthalmoscope allows visualization of the ocular fundus. As the patient's pupil becomes more constricted, viewing the fundus becomes more difficult. Although it is taught that pupillary dilatation can precipitate an attack of angle closure glaucoma in the predisposed adult, children are not predisposed to angle closure. Exceptions include those with a dislocated lens or an eye previously compromised by a retrolental membrane, such as in retinopathy of prematurity. Therefore, if an adequate view of the fundus is precluded by a miotic pupil, the use of a dilating agent (eg, 2.5% phenylephrine, or 0.5% or 1% tropicamide) should provide adequate

Table 15–2. Function and innervation of each of the extraocular muscles.

Extraocular Muscle	Function	Innervation
Medial rectus	Adductor	Oculomotor (third)
Lateral rectus	Abduction	Abducens (sixth)
Inferior rectus	Depressor Adductor Extorter	Oculomotor
Superior rectus	Elevator Adductor Intorter	Oculomotor
Inferior oblique	Elevator Abductor Extorter	Oculomotor
Superior oblique	Depressor Abductor Intorter	Trochlear (fourth)

Figure 15–4. Lateral displacement of light reflection showing esotropia (internal deviation) of the right eye. Nasal displacement of the reflection would show exotropia (outward deviation).

Eyes straight (maintained in position by fusion).

Position of eye under cover in orthophoria (fusion-free position). The right eye under cover has not moved.

Position of eye under cover in esophoria (fusion-free position). Under cover, the right eye has deviated inward. Upon removal of cover, the right eye will immediately resume its straight-ahead position.

Position of eye under cover in exophoria (fusion-free position). Under cover, the right eye has deviated outward. Upon removal of the cover, the right eye will immediately resume its straight-ahead position.

Figure 15–5. Cover testing. The patient is directed to look at a target at eye level 6 m (20 feet) away. Note that in the presence of strabismus, the deviation will remain when the cover is removed. (From Vaughan DG, Asbury T, Riordan-Eva P: *General Ophthalmology,* 14th ed. Appleton & Lange, 1995:231.)

mydriasis (dilatation). In infants, a combination of 1% phenylephrine with 0.2% cyclopentolate is safer.

Ophthalmoscopy should include assessment of the clarity of the ocular media, that is, the quality of the red reflex. If an opacity is noted, the patient should be referred to an ophthalmologist. Structures to be observed include the optic disc, vessels, macular reflex, and retinal changes as well as the clarity of the vitreous media. By increasing the amount of plus lens dialed into the instrument, focus moves anteriorly from vitreous, lens, and finally to the cornea.

OCULAR TRAUMA

Foreign Bodies & Abrasions

Foreign bodies on the globe and palpebral conjunctiva of the lids usually cause discomfort and red eye. Magnification may be needed to discover the foreign body. Those that lodge on the palpebral conjunctiva of the upper lids are best viewed by everting the lid on itself and removing with a cotton applicator. The lower lid presents no problem with visual-

ization. After removal of a foreign body, no treatment is needed if there is no corneal abrasion.

When foreign bodies are noted on the bulbar conjunctiva or cornea, removal is facilitated by using a topical anesthetic. If the foreign body is not too adherent, it can be dislodged by using a stream of irrigation solution (dacriose or salt solution) or a cotton applicator. An antibiotic ointment is applied. For corneal involvement, a gentle pressure patch is applied. Ferrous corneal bodies often have an associated rust ring, which is removed under slit-lamp visualization.

Corneal abrasions are evaluated with fluorescein dye and treated with topical antibiotic and a pressure patch. A drop of a topical cycloplegic agent such as 2% homatropine or 0.25% scopolamine is useful to relieve the discomfort of ciliary spasm and iritis. Daily follow-up is required until healing is complete.

Suspected intraocular foreign bodies, and corneal and scleral lacerations, require emergency referral to an ophthalmologist. The diagnosis may be difficult to establish if the signs of obvious corneal perforation—shallow anterior chamber with hyphema and

Figure 15–6. Corneal laceration with irregular pupil and vitreous loss.

irregular pupil—are not present (Figure 15–6). In addition, nonradiopaque masses such as glass will not show up on x-ray.

INJURIES TO THE EYELIDS

Ecchymosis

Orbital and soft tissue trauma may produce the "black eye," which is ecchymosis (blue or purplish hemorrhagic areas) of the eyelids. The extent of the injury to the eye and orbit may not directly correlate with its appearance. Blowout fracture, which occurs from blunt trauma fracturing the walls of the orbit, must be suspected. Ocular motility must be assessed and the globe examined for injury, vascular embarrassment, and increased intraocular pressure. Cold compresses are used in the first 24 hours after trauma to reduce hemorrhage and swelling. Nonaccidental trauma needs to be considered when orbital trauma is poorly explained.

Lacerations

The lids and lacrimal apparatus are susceptible to laceration. Except for superficial lacerations away from the globe, repair is best performed in the operating room under general anesthesia. Special consideration must be given to lacerations involving the lid margin, to through-and-through lacerations, and to lacerations in which the levator muscle in the upper lid may be involved.

Burns

Eyelid burns can occur in toddlers who are struck by a lit cigarette. The cornea is often involved as well. These burns usually heal with topical antibiotic ointment. Severe burns, thermal or chemical, can cause scars resulting in cicatricial ectropion or entropion and scarring of the conjunctiva and cul-de-sacs.

Burns of the conjunctiva and cornea may be thermal, radiant, or chemical. Heat burns that are superficial will cause the eye to be painful, to tear, and to be injected. Care for these is with topical antibiotics and patching. Add a cycloplegic agent if corneal involvement is present, since ciliary spasm and iritis may accompany the injury.

Radiant energy causes an ultraviolet keratitis. Typical of this is the welder's burn or the burn occurring in a skier who did not wear goggles. The fluorescein dye pattern will show a uniformly stippled appearance of the corneal epithelium. Antibiotic ointment, pressure patches, and a cycloplegic agent, such as 5% homatropine, are usually curative within 24 hours.

Chemical burns with strong acid and alkaline agents can be blinding. Examples are exploding batteries, spilled drain cleaner, and bleach. Alkali burns may not cause significant injection since the conjunctival vessels become damaged. Alkali tends to penetrate deeper into ocular tissue than acids. Immediate treatment consists of copious irrigation as soon as possible after the injury. The patient should be referred to an ophthalmologist.

Cullom RD Jr, Chang B (editors): *The Wills Eye Manual. Office and Emergency Room Diagnosis and Treatment of Eye Disease,* 2nd ed. MA Friedberg, Christopher J Rapuano, founding editors. JB Lippincott, 1994:19.

Hyphema

Blunt trauma to the globe may cause bleeding within the anterior chamber from a ruptured vessel located near the root of the iris or in the angle. Bleeding may be microscopic or may fill the entire anterior chamber. Blunt trauma severe enough to cause a hyphema may be associated with other ocular injury, including iritis, retinal edema or detachment, and glaucoma. In sickle cell patients, even moderate elevations of intraocular pressure may quickly lead to optic atrophy. Therefore, these patients require extra vigilance in diagnosing and treating hyphema.

Management of hyphema in an otherwise uninjured patient should include evaluation of vision and integrity of the globe and orbit. A patch and shield should be placed over the eye, the head elevated, and arrangements made for ophthalmologic referral.

Nontraumatic causes of hyphema include juvenile xanthogranuloma, retinoblastoma, and blood dyscrasias.

Fong LP: Secondary hemorrhage in traumatic hyphema: Predictive factors for selective prophylaxis. Ophthalmology 1994;101:1583.
Teboul BK et al: Clinical evaluation of aminocaproic acid for managing traumatic hyphema in children. Ophthalmology 1995;102:1646.

Nonaccidental Trauma & Shaken Baby Syndrome

From an ocular standpoint, in both nonaccidental

trauma and shaken baby syndrome, the hallmark is retinal hemorrhage. The hemorrhages can be unilateral or bilateral and located in the posterior pole or periphery. Whereas retinal hemorrhages tend to resolve fairly quickly, those in the vitreous do not. If located over the macula, deprivational amblyopia may occur. Other ocular findings associated with nonaccidental trauma include lid ecchymosis, subconjunctival hemorrhage, and hyphema.

Buys YM et al: Retinal findings after head trauma in infants and young children. Ophthalmology 1992;99:1718.

Prevention of Ocular Injuries

Certain steps can be taken to avoid ocular injury. Fireworks and BB guns should be avoided. Safety goggles should be used in laboratories and industrial arts classes and when using snow blowers, power lawn mowers, power tools, and hammers and nails. Sports goggles and visors will prevent injuries in games using fast projectiles or where opponents may swing elbows or poke at the eye.

The one-eyed individual should be specifically advised about eye protection and counseled to avoid high-risk activities.

DISORDERS OF THE OCULAR STRUCTURES

Diseases of the Eyelids

Blepharitis is an inflammation of the lid margin characterized by crusty debris at the base of the lashes, varying degrees of erythema at the lid margins, and, in severe cases, secondary corneal changes such as punctate erosions, vascularization, and ulcers. When injected conjunctiva accompanies blepharitis, the condition is known as blepharoconjunctivitis. *Staphylococcus* is the most common bacterial cause. Treatment includes lid scrubs with a nonburning baby shampoo several times per week and application of a topical antibiotic ointment such as erythromycin or bacitracin at bedtime.

Pediculosis of the lids with *Phthirus pubis* reveals nits and adult lice when viewed microscopically. Mechanical removal and treating the lid margins with phospholine iodide can be effective. Other bodily areas of involvement must also be treated.

Localized staphylococcal infections of the glands of Zeis within the lid cause a sty or **hordeolum.** When the infection coalesces and points internally or externally, it may discharge itself or require incision. The lesion is tender and red. Warm compresses help to hasten the acute process. Some practitioners prescribe a topical antibiotic. Any coexisting blepharitis should be cleared up.

Chalazion is an inflammation of the meibomian glands, which may produce a tender, localized nodule over the tarsus of the upper or lower lid. In addi-

tion to a localized erythema of the corresponding palpebral conjunctiva, there may be a yellow lipogranuloma (Figure 15–7). Treatment includes warm compresses for 5–10 minutes at a time, four times per day, for up to 6 weeks. If incision and curetting are needed, the child will require a general anesthetic.

Viral Lid Disease

Herpes simplex blepharitis may affect the lids at the time of primary herpes simplex infection. Vesicular lesions with an erythematous base are seen. Treatment is with topical 1% trifluridine or 3% vidarabine. **Herpes zoster** causes vesicular disease in association with a skin eruption in the dermatome of the ophthalmic branch of the trigeminal nerve. In older children, treatment of ophthalmic herpes zoster with oral acyclovir or valacyclovir within 5 days of onset may reduce the morbidity. When vesicles are present on the tip of the nose with herpes zoster (Hutchinson's sign), ocular involvement including iritis may develop. Herpes simplex or herpes zoster can be diagnosed by rapid viral culture (24–48 hours). Impetigo is in the differential diagnosis of vesicular lid disease.

Molluscum contagiosum lesions are typically umbilicated papules. If near the lid margin, the lesions may shed and cause conjunctivitis. Cautery or excision of lesions at the lid margin is useful.

Baum J: Infections of the eye. Clin Infect Dis 1995;21:479.

Ptosis

Ptosis (droopy upper lid) may be congenital or acquired, but is usually congenital in children, owing to a defective levator muscle. Other causes of ptosis are Horner's syndrome, myasthenia gravis, lid injuries, and third nerve palsy. Moderate and severe ptosis requires surgical correction, mild cases less often. Ptosis may be associated with astigmatism and amblyopia.

Figure 15–7. Right upper lid chalazion.

DISORDERS OF THE NASOLACRIMAL SYSTEM

Nasolacrimal Duct Obstruction

Nasolacrimal obstruction occurs in up to 6% of infants. Most cases clear spontaneously. Signs and symptoms include a wet eye with mucoid discharge, irritated skin, and conjunctivitis. There may be obstruction in any part of the drainage system due to incomplete canalization of the duct or membranous obstructions.

Differential diagnosis of tearing includes congenital glaucoma, foreign bodies, and nasal pathology.

Massage over the duct may be beneficial by causing egress of debris from the nasolacrimal sac. Cleansing the lids and medial canthal area decreases the likelihood of infection and irritation. Antibiotics can decrease the discharge, but superinfection may occur. Probing is the mainstay of surgical treatment for nasolacrimal obstruction. Probing is successful 80% or more of the time, but the success rate decreases after the infant reaches 1 year. Other surgical procedures may be necessary when probings fail.

Kassoff J, Meyer D: Early office-based vs. late hospital-based nasolacrimal duct probing: A clinical decision analysis. Arch Ophthalmol 1995;113:1168.

Paul TO, Shepherd R: Congenital nasolacrimal duct obstruction: Natural history and the timing of optimal intervention. J Pediatr Ophthalmol Strabismus 1994; 31:362.

Congenital Dacryocystocele

Congenital dacryocystocele is another type of nasolacrimal obstruction seen in the newborn. The pathophysiology is thought to be due to obstructions proximal and distal to the nasolacrimal sac.

At birth, the nasolacrimal sac is distended and has a bluish hue, which often causes an erroneous diagnosis of hemangioma. The swollen sac is tense and displaces the medial canthus superiorly. Massage and warm compresses are sometimes effective, but often a probing (or repeated probings) of the involved nasolacrimal system is necessary to open the drainage apparatus.

Dacryocystitis

Acute and chronic dacryocystitis are typically bacterial and due to gram-positive organisms such as *Staphylococcus aureus, Streptococcus pneumoniae, Streptococcus pyogenes, Streptococcus viridans,* as well as *Moraxella catarrhalis,* and *Haemophilus* spp. Acute dacryocystitis presents with inflammation, swelling, tenderness, and pain over the involved lacrimal sac (located inferior to the medial canthal tendon). There may also be fever. When the infection is organized, it may point externally (Figure 15–8). A purulent discharge and tearing can be expected, since

Figure 15–8. Acute dacryocystitis in an 11-week-old infant.

the cause of infection is almost always nasolacrimal obstruction.

Signs of chronic dacryocystitis are mucopurulent debris on the lids and lashes, tearing and injected lid conjunctiva, and reflux of pus at the puncta when pressure is applied over the sac. Chronic dacryocystitis and recurrent episodes of low-grade dacryocystitis are due to nasolacrimal obstruction.

Treatment of acute dacryocystitis requires systemic antibiotics for severe cases. Oral antibiotics can be tried in milder cases. Topical antibiotic administration is adjunctive and also used with recurrent, chronic infections. Warm compresses are beneficial. Attempts at identifying the offending organism by culture and staining should be made when possible. If a pointing lesion is present, it can be incised and drained, although a fistula can result. After the acute episode subsides, and in chronic cases, the nasolacrimal obstruction must be relieved surgically.

DISEASES OF THE CONJUNCTIVA

Conjunctivitis may be infectious, allergic, or associated with systemic disease (Table 15–3).

Ophthalmia Neonatorum

Ophthalmia neonatorum (conjunctivitis in the newborn) occurs during the first month of life and is visually threatening if due to *Neisseria gonorrhoeae.* It is characterized by red, swollen lids and conjunctiva and by discharge (Figure 15–9). Ophthalmia neonatorum is caused by inflammation from silver nitrate prophylaxis given shortly after birth, bacterial (gonococcal, staphylococcal, pneumococcal), chlamydial, or viral. In developed countries, chlamydia is the most common cause. Herpes simplex is a rare but serious cause of neonatal conjunctivitis. Gram's stain, Giemsa stain for elementary bodies, enzyme

Table 15–3. Clinical and laboratory features of conjunctivitis.

	Viral	Bacterial	Chlamydial	Allergic
Itching	Minimal	Minimal	Minimal	Severe
Hyperemia	Generalized	Generalized	Generalized	Generalized
Tearing	Profuse	Moderate	Moderate	Moderate
Exudation	Minimal, mucoid	Profuse, purulent	Profuse, mucoid or mucopurulent	Minimal, slight mucus
Preauricular adenopathy	Common	Uncommon	Common only in inclusion conjunctivitis	None
Stained conjunctival smears and scrapings	Lymphocytes, plasma cells, multinucleated giant cells, eosinophilic intranuclear inclusions	Neutrophils, bacteria	Neutrophils, plasma cells, basophilic intracytoplasmic inclusions	Eosinophils
Associated sore throat and fever	Occasionally	Occasionally	Never	Never

Modified from Vaughan D, Asbury T, Riordan-Eva P: General Ophthalmology, 14th ed. Appleton & Lange, 1995.

immunoassay for chlamydia, and cultures aid in making an etiologic diagnosis.

Treatment of each of these infections requires specific systemic antibiotics since they can cause widespread serious infections in other organs. Parents of the infected infant should be examined and treated when a sexually associated pathogen is present.

Isenberg SJ et al: Povidone-iodine for ophthalmic neonatorum prophylaxis. Am J Ophthalmol 1994;118:701.

Bacterial Conjunctivitis

In general, bacterial conjunctivitis is accompanied by a purulent discharge and viral infection by a watery discharge. Common bacterial causes of conjunctivitis in older children include nontypable *Haemophilus* spp, *S pneumoniae, M catarrhalis,* and *S aureus.* If not associated with systemic illness, topical antibiotics such as erythromycin, polymyxin-bacitracin, or sulfacetamide are usually adequate. Systemic therapy is recommended for conjunctivitis associated with *N gonorrhoeae, Chlamydia trachomatis,* and *N meningitidis.*

Viral Conjunctivitis

Adenovirus is often associated with pharyngitis, a follicular reaction of the palpebral (lid) conjunctiva and preauricular nodes. Treatment is supportive. Herpes simplex virus may cause a conjunctivitis or blepharoconjunctivitis. Treatment with a topical antiherpes drug is indicated.

Allergic Conjunctivitis

Conjunctivitis may have an allergic cause. In hay fever conjunctivitis, the eyes are red and itchy with mucoid discharge. Symptomatic treatment with a combination topical vasoconstrictor-antihistamine (naphazoline-antazoline or ketoralac tromethamine) or 0.125% prednisolone may be useful. Corticosteroids should be used with caution because extended use in some patients causes glaucoma. Prolonged use of corticosteroids also causes cataracts.

Vernal conjunctivitis is a seasonal form of allergic conjunctivitis associated with tearing, itching, and a stringy discharge. It is more common in males. In the palpebral form, dramatic changes of the superior palpebral conjunctiva occur with cobblestone papillae (Figure 15–10). Corneal ulcers can occur. Topical treatments include 4% sodium cromolyn, 0.1% lodoxamide tromethamine, and a topical steroid. A form of vernal conjunctivitis occurs with nodules at the limbus. Contact lens wear may induce a conjunc-

Figure 15–9. Ophthalmia neonatorum in a 2-week-old infant caused by *Chlamydia trachomatis.*

Figure 15–10. Vernal conjunctivitis. "Cobblestone" papillae in superior tarsal conjunctive. (Courtesy of P Thygeson.) In: Vaughan D, Asbury T, Riordan-Eva P: *General Ophthalmology,* 14th ed. Appleton & Lange, 1995.)

Figure 15–11. Iris coloboma located inferiorly.

tivitis that appears similar to the palpebral form of vernal conjunctivitis.

Mucocutaneous Diseases

Conjunctivitis and conjunctival changes are seen in a number of systemic syndromes. Examples are erythema multiforme/Stevens-Johnson syndrome, Reiter's syndrome, and Kawasaki disease—the latter also associated with iritis. With Stevens-Johnson syndrome, conjunctival changes include erythema, vesicular lesions that frequently rupture, and symblepharon (adhesions) between the raw edges of the bulbar and palpebral conjunctiva. Management may include lubricants to provide comfort and to prevent adhesions of dry eye in the more severe cases of erythema multiforme. Cycloplegic agents and topical steroids are prescribed for iritis in Kawasaki disease.

Baum J: Infections of the eye. Clin Infect Dis 1995;21:479.
Power WJ et al: Analysis of the acute ophthalmic manifestations of the erythema multiforme/Stevens-Johnson syndrome/toxic epidermal necrolysis disease spectrum. Ophthalmology 1995;102:1669.

DISORDERS OF THE IRIS

Iris Coloboma

Iris coloboma is a developmental defect due to incomplete closure of the anterior embryonal fissure. The pupil will have an elongated shape reminiscent of a keyhole or cat's eye (Figure 15–11). The affected area is located inferonasally, but may extend posteriorly involving the retina and choroid. The effect on visual acuity is variable. Iris coloboma may be an isolated defect or may be associated with a number of chromosomal abnormalities and syndromes.

Aniridia

Aniridia is a bilateral disorder that includes absence of almost all of the iris and macular hypoplasia (Figure 15–12). Cataract, corneal changes, and glaucoma frequently are seen. Photophobia and nystagmus occur.

Aniridia may occur in an autosomal dominant or in a sporadic form that is associated with Wilms' tumor. Therefore, repeated examination and abdominal ultrasonography are indicated. The aniridia gene has been isolated to the 11p13 chromosome region. Aniridia, genitourinary abnormalities, and mental retardation have been linked to an 11p deletion.

Albinism

Albinism can have a profound effect on vision and can require low vision aids to enhance visual function. Albinism may be ocular or oculocutaneous and inherited by different modes, depending on the type. Bleeding problems occur in individuals with the Hermansky-Pudlak syndrome in which oculocutaneous albinism is associated with a platelet abnormality.

Figure 15–12. Bilateral aniridia. Iris remnants present temporally in each eye.

Iris color in albinism varies according to type and severity of albinism as well as the individual's race. Iris transillumination may be obvious or may require slit-lamp examination to detect focal areas of transillumination.

Other iris findings include heterochromia of the irides, which can be seen in congenital Horner's syndrome, after iritis, or with tumors and nevi of the iris. Acquired iris nodules, known as Lisch nodules, are seen in type I neurofibromatosis. When seen on slit-lamp examination, they are 1–2 mm in size and often beige in color, although their appearance can be variable. Iris xanthogranuloma occurring with juvenile xanthogranuloma can cause hyphema. Patients with juvenile xanthogranuloma should be evaluated by an ophthalmologist for ocular involvement.

Summers CG, King RA: Ophthalmic features of minimal pigment oculocutaneous albinism. Ophthalmology 1994;101:906.

GLAUCOMA

Glaucoma signifies increased intraocular pressure causing damage to ocular structures and loss of vision. Signs of glaucoma presenting within the first year of life include tearing, photophobia, corneal enlargement and clouding due to edema, and optic nerve cupping. Pediatric glaucomas can be congenital or acquired, unilateral or bilateral. Glaucoma may be inherited.

Glaucoma also occurs with ocular and systemic syndromes. Aniridia and anterior segment dysgenesis are examples. Systemic syndromes with glaucoma include Sturge-Weber syndrome, the oculocerebral renal syndrome of Lowe, and the Pierre-Robin sequence. Glaucoma can also occur with hyphema, iritis, lens dislocation, intraocular tumor, and retinopathy of prematurity. Treatment depends on the cause, but surgery is often the choice.

Ritch R, Shields MB, Krupin T (editors): *The Glaucomas,* 3 vols, 2nd ed. CV Mosby 1996.

UVEITIS

Inflammation of the uveal tract is called uveitis. It can be subdivided according to the uveal tissue primarily involved or by location, that is, anterior, intermediate, or posterior uveitis. Perhaps the most commonly diagnosed uveitis in childhood is traumatic iridocyclitis (iritis).

Anterior Uveitis

Iritis (anterior uveitis) is usually accompanied by injection, photophobia, pain, and blurred vision. An exception to this is iritis associated with juvenile rheumatoid arthritis. The eye is quiet and asymptomatic, but slit-lamp examination will reveal iritis.

Although iridocyclitis associated with juvenile rheumatoid arthritis occurs most often in girls with pauciarticular arthritis and a positive antinuclear antibody, all children with juvenile rheumatoid arthritis need to be screened. Treatment with topical corticosteroid and a cycloplegic agent is aimed at quieting the inflammation and preventing or delaying the onset of cataract and glaucoma.

Other causes of anterior uveitis in children include syphilis, tuberculosis, sarcoidosis, and Lyme disease, with all but the latter entity also causing posterior uveitis. There is also a substantial percentage of cases of unknown origin.

American Academy of Pediatrics Section on Rheumatology and Ophthalmology: Guidelines for ophthalmologic examinations in children with juvenile rheumatoid arthritis. Pediatrics 1993;92:295.

Posterior Uveitis

Choroiditis, retinitis, and chorioretinitis are the primary tissues that can be involved in posterior uveitis. Characteristic features occur with retinitis due to certain organisms. The scar of toxoplasmosis produces a white punched-out lesion with a hyperpigmented border. Contiguous white satellite lesions suggest reactivation of disease. A granular "salt-pepper" retinopathy is characteristic of rubella. In infants, toxoplasmosis, rubella, cytomegalovirus, herpes simplex (TORCH agents), and syphilis must be suspected in congenital infections which can cause chorioretinitis. Cytomegalovirus must be considered as a cause of retinitis in immunocompromised and HIV-infected children.

In toddlers and older youngsters, *Toxocara* infections occurring from ingesting contaminated soil cause a unilateral uveitis with vitreal inflammation and retinal detachment in some cases.

Intermediate Uveitis

Pars planitis is an intermediate uveitis, often of uncertain cause, which may present with vitreous floaters. Macular edema and decreased vision can result.

Retinoblastoma and other neoplasms can imitate uveitis causing a so-called "masquerade" syndrome.

Salvadore F et al: Cytomegalovirus retinitis in pediatric acquired immunodeficiency syndrome: Report of two cases. J Pediatr Ophthalmol Strabismus 1993;30:159.

DISORDERS OF THE CORNEA

Corneal trauma is dealt with under Ocular Trauma earlier in this chapter.

Conditions Causing Corneal Clouding

The differential diagnosis in a newborn presenting with a cloudy cornea includes forceps trauma, congenital glaucoma, infection, congenital malformation, and tumor. In older children, corneal clouding may be seen with mucopolysaccharidoses, Wilson's disease, and cystinosis. Infiltrates occur with virus infections, staphylococcal lid disease, corneal dystrophies, and interstitial keratitis due to congenital syphilis.

Microcornea & Megalocornea

Microcornea, a corneal diameter less than 10 mm, may be associated with other anterior segment malformations or a microphthalmic globe. Megalocornea, a corneal diameter of 12.5 mm or greater, should be considered to be caused by congenital glaucoma until proved otherwise.

Keratitis

Both herpes simplex and herpes zoster can infect the cornea causing a keratitis. When the epithelium breaks down, a dendritic or ameboid pattern can be seen with fluorescein staining. Corneal involvement with herpes simplex can be recurrent and lead to blindness. Topical antivirals, such as trifluridine or vidarabine, are indicated when herpes simplex infection is limited to the corneal epithelium. Topical corticosteroids may be a useful addition when there is stromal disease. The use of corticosteroids with herpetic disease should be undertaken by an ophthalmologist. Oral acyclovir started in the early phase (first 5 days) may be helpful in herpes zoster eye disease.

Adenovirus, which causes a conjunctivitis, may also cause a keratitis occurring 1–2 weeks after the onset of the conjunctivitis. Slit-lamp examination reveals white infiltrates beneath the corneal epithelium. Vision may be decreased. No treatment is necessary, since the keratitis is most often self-limiting.

Contact lens wearers are at risk for developing a severe vision-threatening keratitis due to the organism *Acanthamoeba*. Contaminated contact lens solution can be the carrier for this organism. Treatment is difficult and may require corneal transplantation.

Corneal Ulcers

Bacterial corneal ulcers in healthy youngsters who are not contact lens wearers are usually secondary to corneal trauma, that is, from corneal abrasion or a penetrating foreign body. Decreased vision, pain, injection, a white corneal infiltrate (ulcer), and hypopyon (pus in the anterior chamber) may all be present. Prompt referral to an ophthalmologist is necessary.

Dana MR et al: The indications for and outcome in pediatric keratoplasty: A multicenter study. Ophthalmology 1995;102:1129.

DISORDERS OF THE LENS

Lens disorders involve abnormality of clarity or position. Opacification—a cataract—can affect vision depending on the density, size, and location of the opacity within the lens. Visual potential is also influenced by age of onset and success with amblyopia treatment.

Cataracts

Cataracts in children may be unilateral or bilateral, may exist as isolated defects, or may be accompanied by other ocular pathology or systemic disease (Figure 15–13). Leukocoria, poor fixation, strabismus, or nystagmus or both may be the presenting complaint. In the newborn, absence of a red reflex should suggest the possibility of cataract, especially if the neonate is examined with a dilated pupil.

Sometimes the appearance of the cataract may suggest its cause. For example, anterior capsular cataracts are developmental, not related to infection or metabolic problems. Laboratory studies should include urinalysis for reducing substances (galactosemia), and cultures or serologic tests for toxoplasmosis, rubella, cytomegalovirus, herpes simplex, and syphilis. Calcium and phosphorus levels and urinalysis for amino acids are obtained to discover other inborn errors causing lens opacity.

Diagnosis and treatment of cataracts as soon as possible are necessary to prevent deprivational amblyopia from occurring. Cataracts that are visually significant require removal. Rehabilitation may be with an intraocular lens, contact lens, or spectacles.

Dislocated Lenses

Dislocated lenses usually are bilateral except when due to trauma. Subluxated lens cause refractive errors of large magnitude, which are difficult to correct. Other ophthalmologic concerns are pupillary block glaucoma and retinal detachment.

Dislocated lenses are associated with other ocular conditions and systemic syndromes, including Mar-

Figure 15–13. Cataract causing leukocoria.

fan syndrome, homocystinuria, Weill-Marchesani syndrome, sulfite oxidase deficiency, hyperlysinemia, syphilis, and Ehlers-Danlos syndrome. Workup and treatment are multidisciplinary (Figure 15–14).

Brady KM et al: Cataract surgery and intraocular lens implantation in children. Am J Ophthalmol 1995;120:1.

Salehpour D et al: The surgical management of nontraumatic ectopic lenses. J Pediatr Ophthalmol Strabismus 1996;33:8.

Scott MH et al: Autosomal dominant cataract: Interocular phenotypic variability. Ophthalmology 1994;101:866.

Wright KW, Matsumoto E, Edelman PM: Binocular fusion and stereopsis associated with early surgery for monocular congenital cataracts. Arch Ophthalmol 1992;110:1670.

DISORDERS OF THE RETINA

Retinopathy of Prematurity

The practitioner may confront diseases of the retina in the newborn period or shortly thereafter. Retinopathy of prematurity (ROP) continues to be a cause of blindness, especially for infants less than 28 weeks' gestation and weighing less than 1250 g. Premature infants with incomplete retinal vascularization are at risk for developing abnormal peripheral retinal vascularization, which may lead to retinal detachment in severe cases. However, most cases of ROP do not progress to retinal detachment and require no treatment.

The risk of developing visually threatening ROP is inversely proportional to birthweight and gestational age. Infants less than 1500 g at birth may develop visually threatening ROP. The role of supplemental oxygen as a causative agent in the development of ROP is still not fully understood. Duration of supplemental oxygen, but not level of oxygen, does correlate with the development of ROP. Other correlates are hyaline membrane disease, bronchopulmonary dysplasia, patent ductus arteriosus, apnea and bradycardia, intraventricular hemorrhage, and multiple births.

Screening guidelines and a uniform classification system have been adopted, which recommends the first retinal examination at 4–6 weeks of age (Table 15–4). Follow-up examinations are predicated by the findings and the risk of developing the disease. Treatment of stage III ROP (at threshold stage III+ disease) with cryotherapy has reduced by 50% the occurrence of visual loss. Laser therapy also arrests progression of ROP. In spite of treatment, there are still some cases that go on to develop blinding retinal detachment. Other findings associated with ROP include strabismus, amblyopia, myopia, and glaucoma.

Cryotherapy for Retinopathy of Prematurity Cooperative Group. The natural ocular outcome of premature birth and retinopathy: Status at 1 year. Arch Ophthalmol 1994;112:903.

Dobson V et al: Grating visual acuity in eyes with retinal residue of retinopathy of prematurity. Arch Ophthalmol 1995;113:1172.

Multicenter trial for cryotherapy for retinopathy of prematurity. 3½-year outcome—structure and function: Cryotherapy for Retinopathy of Prematurity Cooperative Group. Arch Ophthalmol 1993;111:339.

Schalij-Delfos NE et al: Screening for retinopathy of prematurity: Do former guidelines still apply? J Pediatr Ophthalmol Strabismus 1996;33:35.

Retinoblastoma

Retinoblastoma is the most common primary intraocular malignancy of childhood with an incidence of 1 in 15,000–20,000 live births. Most patients present before 3 years of age, with bilateral cases presenting earlier than unilateral.

Both sporadic and inherited forms of retinoblastoma occur. Inheritance is autosomal dominant with high penetrance. The disease may present as a solitary mass or as multiple tumors in one or both eyes. Inherited cases and some unilateral cases are due to a germinal mutation, whereas the unilateral cases with a solitary tumor are due to a somatic retinal mutation. In both cases, the mutation occurs in the region of the q14 band on chromosome 13. Individuals with a germinal mutation are at risk for the development of tu-

Figure 15–14. Subluxated lens. Lens dislocated superiorly. (From *Pediatric Ophthalmology and Strabismus.* Section 6. Basic Clinical Science Course 1994. American Academy of Ophthalmology, San Francisco, 1995:84.)

Table 15–4. Stages of retinopathy of prematurity.

Stage I	Demarcation line or border dividing the vascular from the avascular retina.
Stage II	Ridge. Line of previous stage acquires volume and rises above the surface retina to become a ridge.
Stage III	Ridge with extraretinal fibrovascular proliferation.
Stage IV	Subtotal retinal detachment.
Stage V	Total retinal detachment.

mors other than retinoblastoma (pineal tumors, osteosarcoma, and other soft tissue sarcomas).

The most common presenting sign in a child with previously undiagnosed retinoblastoma is leukocoria (see Figure 15–1). Others present with strabismus, red eye, glaucoma, or pseudohypopyon (pus in the anterior chamber).

Treatment of unilateral cases is usually enucleation, since at the time of presentation the eye is filled with tumor. In bilateral cases, it may be possible to salvage vision or an eye when the tumors are small enough to be amenable to treatment with photocoagulation, cryotherapy, or radiation. Eradication of tumor before infiltration into the optic nerve or choroid carries a good prognosis for survival. Treatment is multidisciplinary involving ophthalmology, oncology, radiology, pediatrics, and genetics.

Buckley EG, Heath H: Visual acuity after successful treatment of large macular retinoblastoma. J Pediatr Ophthalmol Strabismus 1992;29:103.

Molney BG, Robertson DM: Ancillary testing for metastasis in patients with newly diagnosed retinoblastoma. Am J Ophthalmol 1994;118:707.

Shields CL et al: Plaque radiotherapy in the management of retinoblastoma: Use as a primary and secondary treatment. Ophthalmology 1993;100:216.

Weiss AH et al: Visual outcomes of macular retinoblastoma after external beam radiation therapy. Ophthalmology 1994;101:1244.

Retinal Detachment

Retinal detachment occurs infrequently in children. Common causes are trauma and high myopia. Other causes in childhood are ROP, Marfan syndrome, and Stickler's syndrome.

Symptoms of detachment are floaters, flashing lights, and loss of visual field. However, children often cannot appreciate or verbalize their symptoms. A detachment may not be discovered until the child is referred after failing a vision screening examination, strabismus supervenes, or leukocoria is noted.

Treatment of retinal detachment is surgical.

DISEASES OF THE OPTIC NERVE

Optic nerve function is evaluated as part of the visual pathway by checking vision and pupillary response. Poor optic nerve function results in decreased central or peripheral vision, strabismus, and nystagmus.

The "swinging flashlight test" uses a consists of a light shined alternately in front of each pupil to check for an afferent pupillary defect. An abnormal response in the affected eye is noted by the pupil dilating when the light is directed into that eye. This results from poorer conduction along the optic nerve of the affected eye, which in turn results in less pupillary constriction than occurs if conduction were normal. Hippus, rhythmic dilating and constricting movements of the pupil, can be confused with an afferent pupillary defect, also known as a Marcus-Gunn pupillary defect.

The optic nerve is evaluated on the basis of size, shape, color, and vascularity. Occasionally, myelinization past the entrance of the optic nerve head appears white with a feathered edge (Figure 15–15). Myelinization onto the retina can be associated with myopia and amblyopia. Anatomic defects of the optic nerve such as **optic nerve hypoplasia** may be associated with absence of the septum pellucidum and hypothalamic-pituitary dysfunction (de Morsier's syndrome).

Since the optic nerve is an outgrowth of the brain, pathology of this structure often reflects central nervous system pathology.

Papilledema

Papilledema is associated with increased intracranial pressure. This appears as an elevated disc with indistinct margins, increased vessel diameter, and increased capillarity giving the disc a hyperemic appearance with surrounding hemorrhages.

Papillitis

Papillitis, seen as an inflamed optic nerve head on examination, is an optic neuritis and has the same appearance as the nerve head with papilledema. However, papillitis may be unilateral, whereas papilledema is almost always bilateral. Papillitis can be differentiated from papilledema by an afferent pupillary defect (Marcus-Gunn pupil) and its more pro-

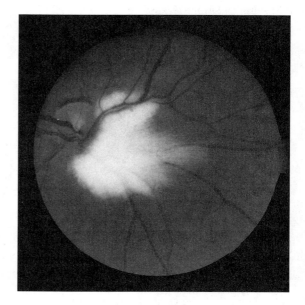

Figure 15–15. Myelinization extending from optic nerve superiorly onto the retina.

found effect on decreasing visual acuity and color vision and producing a central scotoma. Papilledema that is not yet chronic will not have as dramatic an effect on vision and will demonstrate an enlarged blind spot on visual field testing. Pseudopapilledema, a normal variant of the optic disc, shows the disc to appear elevated with indistinct margins and a normal vascular pattern.

Optic Atrophy

Optic atrophy, noted as pallor of the nerve head with loss of capillarity is most frequently seen in children after neurologic compromise during the perinatal period; for example, the ex-premature infant with an intraventricular bleed. Hydrocephalus, glioma of the nerve and optic foramen, craniostenosis, and neurologic disease and toxins such as methyl alcohol can cause optic atrophy as well as certain inborn errors of metabolism.

DISEASES OF THE ORBIT

Periorbital & Orbital Cellulitis

The fascia of the eyelids join with the fibrous orbital septum to isolate the orbit from the lids. Infections arising external to the orbital septum are termed **preseptal.** Preseptal **periorbital cellulitis,** which indicates infection of the structures around the eye, is characterized by lid edema, swelling, pain, and mild fever. It usually arises from a local exogenous source, such as an abrasion of the eyelid, other infections (hordeolum, dacryocystitis, chalazion), or from infected varicella or insect bite lesions. *S aureus* and *S pyogenes* are the most common pathogens from these sources. Preseptal infections in children less than 3 years of age also occur from bacteremia, although this is much less common since immunization became available to prevent *H influenzae* infections. *S pneumoniae* is still an occasional cause of this infection. Children with periorbital cellulitis from presumed bacteremia must be examined for additional foci of infection.

Infection of the orbit almost always arises from contiguous sinus infection, since the walls of three sinuses make up portions of the orbital walls and infection can breach these walls or extend by way of bridging veins. The orbital contents can develop a phlegmon **(orbital cellulitis),** or frank pus can develop in the orbit **(orbital abscess).** When the orbit is infected, the signs of periorbital infection are joined by proptosis, restricted eye movement, and pain with eye movement. Fever is usually high and hectic. CT or MRI imaging is required to establish the extent of the infection within the orbit. Sinus imaging should be obtained at the same time. The etiologic agents are those of acute or chronic sinusitis—respiratory flora and anaerobes. *S aureus* is also frequently implicated.

Therapy of preseptal infection is with systemic antibiotics. Treatment of orbital infections often requires surgical drainage in conjunction with intravenous antibiotics. Drainage of infected sinuses is often part of the therapy.

Tole DM, Anderton LS, Hayward JM: Orbital cellulitis demands early recognition, urgent admission and aggressive management. J Accid Emerg Med 1995;12(2):151.

Craniofacial Anomalies

Craniofacial anomalies can affect the orbit and visual system. Examples of changes associated with craniofacial disease involving the orbits are proptosis, corneal exposure, hypertelorism, strabismus, amblyopia, and lid coloboma.

Orbital Tumors

Both benign and malignant lesions occur in the orbit of children. The most common tumor is a **capillary hemangioma** (Figure 15–16). This type of tumor may be located superficially in the lid or deep in the orbit and can cause ptosis, refractive errors, and amblyopia. Deeper lesions may cause proptosis. Capillary hemangiomas occurring in infants initially increase in size before involuting at about 5 years of age. Therapy with corticosteroids is indicated if the lesion is large enough to cause amblyopia.

Orbital dermoid cysts vary in size and are usually found temporally at the brow and orbital rim or superonasally. These lesions are firm, well encapsulated, and mobile. Rupture of the cyst causes a severe inflammatory reaction. Treatment is by excision. **Lymphangioma** occurring in the orbit is typically poorly encapsulated, increases in size with upper respiratory infection, and is susceptible to hemorrhage. Other benign tumors of the orbit are orbital pseudotumor, neurofibroma, teratoma, and tumors arising from bone, connective tissue, and neural tissue.

Of grave concern is orbital **rhabdomyosarcoma,** the most common childhood primary orbital malig-

Figure 15–16. Right upper lid hemangioma causing ptosis. Note hemangioma of conjunctive.

nancy. This tumor grows rapidly and displaces the globe. The average age of onset is 7 years. Often the tumor is initially mistaken for orbital swelling due to insignificant trauma. Biopsy, with debulking of the tumor, radiation, and chemotherapy are required. With expeditious diagnosis and efficacious treatment, the survival rate of patients with orbital rhabdomyosarcoma approaches 90%.

Tumors metastatic to the orbit also occur—**neuroblastoma** being the most common. Presentation may be with proptosis, orbital ecchymosis ("raccoon eyes"), Horner's syndrome, or opsoclonus ("dancing eyes"). Ewing's sarcoma, leukemia, Burkitt's lymphoma, and the histiocytosis X group of diseases may involve the orbit.

Abramson DH, Notis CM: Visual acuity after radiation for orbital rhabdomyosarcoma. Am J Ophthalmol 1994; 118:808.

NYSTAGMUS

Nystagmus is rhythmic oscillations of the eyes. It may be unilateral or bilateral, more pronounced in one eye, or gaze-dependent. Nystagmus may be associated with esotropia or may occur with ocular lesions that cause deprivational amblyopia (ie, media opacities) or conditions in which the visual pathways are hypoplastic. Macular hypoplasia that occurs with aniridia or ocular albinism, and optic nerve hypoplasia both are associated with nystagmus. Nystagmus can also occur with normal ocular structures and seemingly normal central nervous system development. In the latter instance, the nystagmus may be blocked in certain positions of gaze, in which case a face turn or torticollis may develop. In latent nystagmus, the nystagmus is seen when one eye is occluded. This type of nystagmus is seen in patients with congenital esotropia. There may also be an associated amblyopia.

Most nystagmus presenting in childhood is of ocular origin, but central nervous system disease and, less frequently, inner ear disease are other causes. A central nervous system cause is likely when the nystagmus is vertical. Fundus examination should seek optic nerve abnormalities and the presence of a macular reflex, since optic nerve hypoplasia and macular hypoplasia both can cause nystagmus.

Evaluation of nystagmus begins with the pediatric ophthalmologist, since associated ocular pathology is common. Some types of nystagmus can be treated, usually with surgery; less frequently prisms are useful. Spasmus nutans, in which there is a rapid shimmering nystagmus with head bobbing and torticollis, is said to improve with time. Glioma of the hypothalamus mimics spasmus nutans.

Arnoldi KA, Tychsen L: Prevalence of intracranial lesions in children initially diagnosed with disconjugate nystagmus (spasmus nutans). J Pediatr Ophthalmol Strabismus 1995;32:296.

Mitchell PR: Diagnosis and management of abnormal head posture in congenital nystagmus. Am Orthop J 1995; 45:7.

AMBLYOPIA & STRABISMUS

Amblyopia

Amblyopia is a unilateral or bilateral reduction in central visual acuity due to the sensory deprivation of a well-formed retinal image that occurs with or without a visible organic lesion commensurate with the degree of visual loss. Amblyopia can occur only during the critical period of visual development that occurs during the first decade of life when the visual nervous system is plastic. Amblyopia is categorized into three types. **Strabismic amblyopia** may occur in the nondominant eye of a strabismic patient. **Refractive amblyopia** can occur in both eyes if significant refractive errors have been left untreated (ametropic or refractive amblyopia). Another type of refractive amblyopia may occur in the eye with the worse refractive error when there is an imbalance between the eyes (anisometropic amblyopia). **Deprivational amblyopia** occurs when lesions such as cataracts, media opacities, or complete ptosis preclude a formed retinal image. Of the three types of amblyopia, this form of amblyopia results in the worst vision.

The earlier that treatment of amblyopia is begun, the better is the chance of improving vision. Generally, treatment is discontinued after age 9 years. Amblyogenic factors such as refractive errors are addressed. Because of the extreme sensitivity of the visual nervous system in infants, congenital cataracts and media opacities must be diagnosed and treated within the first few weeks of life. Visual rehabilitation and amblyopia treatment must then be begun in order to foster visual development.

After eradicating amblyogenic factors, the mainstay of treatment is patching the sound eye.

Keech RV, Kutschke PJ: Upper age limit for the development of amblyopia. J Pediatr Ophthalmol Strabismus 1995;32:89.

Levartovsky S et al: Factors affecting long term results of successfully treated amblyopia: Age at beginning of treatment and age at cessation of monitoring. J Pediatr Ophthalmol Strabismus 1992;29:219.

Strabismus

Strabismus connotes a misalignment of the visual axes of the two eyes. Its prevalence in childhood is about 2–3%. Strabismus is categorized by the direction of the deviation and its frequency. Early diagnosis of strabismus and amblyopia provides the affected child with the best chance of reaching full visual potential. Strabismus may cause or be due to an amblyopia.

A misdiagnosis of strabismus, pseudostrabismus, can occur when relying on the corneal light reflex test. If the child has prominent epicanthal folds, pseudoesotropia may be erroneously diagnosed. An infant destined to be well aligned may appear intermittently esotropic, but this should occur less frequently over the first few months of life. By 5 or 6 months, the baby should be constantly well aligned. Children do not outgrow strabismus if it is truly present.

Beside its effect on visual development, strabismus may be a marker of other ocular or systemic disease. Twenty percent of patients with retinoblastoma present with strabismus. Patients with central nervous system causes such as hydrocephalus, space-occupying lesions, and an amaurotic (blind) eye can also present with strabismus. Note that in children younger than 3 or 4 years of age, blind eyes tend to assume an esodeviation, but after about age 4 an amaurotic eye tends to show an exotropic shift.

A. Esotropia: In esotropia, the visual axes of the eyes are excessively convergent. In terms of cause and treatment, esotropia can be categorized as to age of onset. **Congenital esotropia** (infantile esotropia) has its onset in the first year of life in healthy infants. The magnitude of the deviation is large. Strabismus surgery is the mainstay of treatment. To foster the development of binocularity, good alignment should be achieved by age 2 years.

Esotropia beginning in the first year is seen in the ex-premature infant or the child with a complicated perinatal history associated with central nervous system problems such as intracranial bleeds and periventricular leukomalacia. There are also syndromes with which esotropia is associated. In Möbius syndrome, there is a sixth nerve palsy causing esotropia associated with palsies of the seventh and twelfth cranial nerves and limb deformities. Duane's syndrome, which can affect both horizontal muscles, may be an isolated defect or may be associated with a multitude of systemic defects (eg, Goldenhar's syndrome). Children with unilateral paretic or restrictive causes of esotropia may develop face turns toward the affected eye.

The largest group of patients diagnosed with acquired esotropia are of the accommodative type. Onset of the deviation is usually between 2 and 5 years of age. The deviation is variable in magnitude and frequency and accompanied by amblyopia. With one type of **accommodative esotropia,** a high hyperopic refraction is associated. In another type of accommodative esotropia, the deviation is worse with near vision than with distant vision.

Treatment consists of glasses, amblyopia treatment, and sometimes surgery.

After age 5 years, any recent-onset esotropia should be noted with suspicion and central nervous system disease ruled out. Infratentorial masses, hydrocephalus, and demyelinating disease are causes of abducens palsy, which presents as an esotropia, lateral rectus paralysis or paresis, and face turn. The face turn is used to maintain binocularity away from the field of action of the paretic muscle. Papilledema is present with increased intracranial pressure. Besides the abducens' vulnerability to increased intracranial pressure, it is susceptible to infection and inflammation. Otitis media and Gradenigo's syndrome (inflammatory disease of the petrous bone) can cause a sixth nerve palsy. Less commonly, migraine and diabetes are considerations in children with sixth nerve palsy. Workup includes imaging studies and neurologic examination.

B. Exotropia: Exotropia in general does not present as many diagnostic pitfalls for the practitioner as esotropia. The visual axes of the two eyes are deviated in a divergent position. Usually the deviation begins intermittently and is seen after age 2 years. Congenital (infantile) exotropia is extremely rare in an otherwise healthy infant. Early-onset exotropia may be seen in infants and children with severe neurologic problems. Treatment considerations include surgery, patching, and occasionally glasses.

Kodsi SR, Youngle BR: Acquired oculomotor, trochlear and abducent cranial nerve palsies in pediatric patients. Am J Ophthalmol 1992;114:568.

Pickering JD et al: Alignment success following medical rectus recessions in normal and delayed children. J Pediatr Ophthalmol Strabismus 1995;32:225.

Shauly Y, Prager TC, Mazow ML: Clinical characteristics and long term results in infantile esotropia. Am J Ophthalmol 1994;117:183.

UNEXPLAINED DECREASED VISION IN INFANTS & CHILDREN

Some infants who are delayed in visual development during the first few months of life, but are otherwise normal neurologically, will reach an appropriate level of visual maturation.

Occult causes of poor vision in children include Leber's congenital amaurosis, which is a childhood form of retinitis pigmentosa; achromatopsia, the absence of cones from the retina; and optic nerve abnormalities including optic nerve hypoplasia and atrophy.

Cortical visual impairment in a child manifests as decreased visual attentiveness of varying degree. Cortical visual impairment can be congenital or acquired. Insults to the optic pathways and higher cortical visual centers are responsible. Asphyxia, trauma, and intracranial hemorrhage are some of the causes of cortical visual impairment.

Besides an ophthalmologic workup, an electroretinogram testing retinal function and a visually evoked response evaluating the visual pathways may be performed. Imaging studies of the brain and a pediatric neurologic evaluation may be useful. A low vision assessment may be indicated. Low-vision aids to enhance remaining vision include magnifiers for distance and near, closed-circuit television, and large-print material.

Chen TC et al: Development of object vision in infants with permanent cortical visual impairment. Am J Ophthalmol 1992;114:575.
Colenbrander A, Fletcher DC (guest editors): Low vision and vision rehabilitation. Ophthalmol Clin North Am 1994;27:27.
King KM, Cronin CM: Ocular findings in premature infants with grade IV intraventricular hemorrhage. J Pediatr Ophthalmol Strabismus 1993;30:84.

THE BLIND CHILD

Vision is the predominant sensory input. A child's development therefore will be profoundly affected by blindness or very poor vision. Although acquired blindness may give an individual the time to grow as a sighted person and make preparations as a nonsighted person if the loss of vision is slow and predicted, psychological consequences must be addressed. The child blind from birth or from very early childhood has had little or no opportunity to form impressions of the physical world with the benefit of sight.

Blind infants reach developmental landmarks on a different schedule from that of sighted children. In addition, some blind children are multiply handicapped. For example, the ex-premature child who is blind from ROP may also have cerebral palsy. Children with Usher's syndrome are both deaf and blind.

Blind children and their families should receive the benefit of knowledgeable therapists and support groups.

LEARNING DISABILITIES

Visits to the physician because of educational difficulties are common. Part of the evaluation of the youngster with learning disabilities and dyslexia are an ophthalmologic examination to rule out and treat any ocular disorders that could cause or contribute to academic difficulties. Most children with learning difficulties do not have a demonstrable problem on ophthalmic examination.

A multidisciplinary approach as suggested by the American Academy of Pediatrics, American Associations of Pediatric Ophthalmology and Strabismus, and the American Academy of Ophthalmology is recommended in evaluating children with learning disabilities. Although many therapies directed at "training the eyes" exist, scientific support for such approaches is weak.

Menacker SJ et al: Do tinted lenses improve the reading performance of dyslexic children? A cohort study. Arch Ophthalmol 1993;111:213.
Sadun AA: Dyslexia at the New York Times: (mis) Understanding of parallel visual processing. (Editorial.) Arch Ophthalmol 1992;110;933.

REFERENCES

Albert DM, Jakobiec FA (editors): *Principles and Practice of Ophthalmology,* 6 vols. WB Saunders, 1996.
Albert DM, Jakobiec FA (editors): *ATLAS of Clinical Ophthalmology.* WB Saunders, 1996.
American Academy of Ophthalmology: Pediatric Ophthalmology and Strabismus. Basic and Clinical Science Course. Section 6, 1994–1995. San Francisco, CA.
Cullom RD Jr, Chang B (editors): *The Wills Eye Manual Office and Emergency Room Diagnosis and Treatment of Eye Disease,* 2nd ed. MA Friedberg, CJ Rapuano founding editors. JB Lippincott, 1994.
Fraunfelder FT, Roy FH (editors): *Current Ocular Therapy 4.* WB Saunders, 1995.
Hart WM Jr (editor): *Adler's Physiology of the Eye,* 19th ed. Mosby-Year Book, 1992.
Isenberg SJ (editor): *The Eye in Infancy,* 2nd ed. CV Mosby, 1994.
Nussenblatt RB, Whitcup SM, Palestine AG (editors): *Uveitis Fundamentals and Clinical Practice,* 2nd ed. CV Mosby, 1996.

Ritch R, Shields MB, Krupin T (editors): *The Glaucomas,* 3 vols, 2nd ed. CV Mosby, 1996.
Stewart WM (editor): *Surgery of the Eyelid, Orbit and Lacrimal System,* 3 vols. American Academy of Ophthalmology, 1993, 1994, 1995.
Tasman W, Jaeger EA (editors): *Duane's Clinical Ophthalmology,* 6 vols. JB Lippincott, 1994. (1995 edition on CD-ROM.)
Vaughan DG, Asbury T, Riordan-Eva P: *General Ophthalmology,* 14th ed. Appleton & Lange, 1995.
von Noorden GK: *Binocular Vision and Ocular Motility: Theory and Management of Strabismus,* 4th ed. CV Mosby, 1990.
Walsh TJ: *Neuro-Ophthalmology: Clinical Signs and Symptoms,* 3rd ed. Lea & Febiger, 1992.
Wright KW (editor): *Pediatric Ophthalmology and Strabismus.* CV Mosby, l995.

Oral Medicine & Dentistry 16

R.B. Abrams, DDS, & W.A. Mueller, DMD

Disease in the oral cavity can have a profound effect on systemic health, and the converse is also true in that systemic disease can be reflected in the oral cavity. This chapter will discuss the interface between medicine and dentistry for the pediatric patient.

THE MOUTH OF THE NEWBORN & OF THE INFANT

The mouth of the newborn should be lined with an intact, smooth, moist and shiny mucosa. The alveolar ridges (Figure 16–1) should be continuous and relatively smooth. Within the alveolar bone are numerous tooth buds which at birth are mostly primary (baby) teeth with a few permanent teeth just starting.

Teeth

The primary teeth begin to form at approximately 6 weeks of gestation, and their calcification starts at some time in the second trimester. The permanent teeth are just beginning to develop at birth. There is enough development of permanent teeth to permit their damage by perinatal or antenatal trauma.

The primary teeth usually do not begin to erupt until approximately 6–7 months of age. However, on rare occasions (1:2000), teeth are present at birth (natal teeth) or erupt within the first month (neonatal teeth). These are most common in the anterior mandible and can be "real" primary teeth or supernumerary (extra) teeth. These can be differentiated radiographically. On occasion, these teeth will need to be removed to facilitate nursing, heal persistent ulceration of the ventral tongue, or eliminate the risk of aspiration. Consultation with a pediatric dentist is advisable.

Frena

There should be noticeable but small maxillary and mandibular labial frena (Figure 16–2). Sometimes these are slightly thick, but they are usually of no consequence. There may also be several small accessory frena farther posteriorly. The extreme is multiple thick tightly bound frena, as in oral–facial–digital syndrome.

Decisions about if and when a labial frenum should be surgically reduced are best left until adolescence. Many thick frena need not be corrected.

The tongue is connected to the floor of the mouth by the lingual frenum (Figures 16–1 and 16–3). This connection should not impede the free movement of the tongue. If the attachment is tight and high up on the alveolar ridge (Figure 16–4), it may restrict movement. This condition is called ankyloglossia (tongue–tie). If it needs to be surgically corrected, earlier (3–4 years) is better than later, but there is usually no urgency for surgery in the neonatal period.

The Palate

The palate of the newborn should be intact and continuous from the alveolar ridge anteriorly to the uvula (Figure 16–1). Cleft lip and palate are common defects (1:700). The cleft of the palate can be unilateral or bilateral (Figure 16–5). The cleft can involve just the alveolar ridge, as in Figure 16–5, or the ridge and entire palate. Clefts can be isolated soft palate defects also. This is common in the Robin anomalad. A final classification of cleft palate is submucous cleft, which is harder to detect. This is a muscular problem in the soft palate with no bony component. Sometimes affected children have a notched or bifid uvula.

Cleft lip and palate rehabilitation is an extensive program involving many specialties and can be lifelong. Owing to the complexity of the problem, children with cleft palate are best treated by a cleft palate team so that treatment can be coordinated among all the specialties.

Cleft lip and palate treatment begins immediately after birth with the fabrication of a palatal obturator to help the baby feed. This same appliance can be used to "mold" the alveolus closed once the initial lip repair has been accomplished. In the case of bilateral cleft lip and palate, the dentist will apply extraoral orthopedic traction to guide the protruding premaxilla back into the oral cavity to facilitate lip closure by the surgeon.

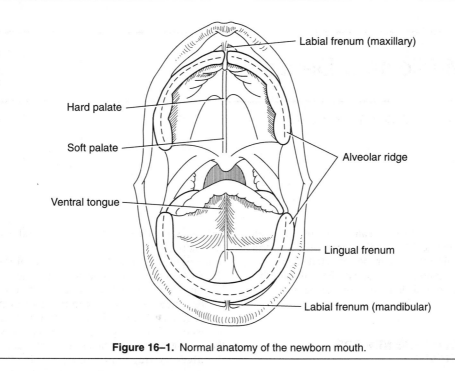

Figure 16–1. Normal anatomy of the newborn mouth.

Dental involvement in children with cleft palate is extensive and may extend over a lifetime. A cleft palate team is a good place to find expertise to deal with this problem.

Other Soft Tissue Variations

Other minor soft tissue variations can exist in the newborn mouth. Small (1–2 mm) round, smooth, whitish bumps can appear on the alveolar ridges or the palate. These are keratin cysts and are called Epstein's pearls or dental lamina cysts. They are benign and require no treatment since they usually disappear.

Some newborns may have small intraoral lymph-

Figure 16–2. The frena.

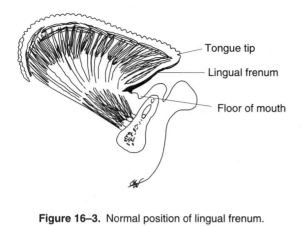

Figure 16–3. Normal position of lingual frenum.

angiomas on the alveolar ridge or the floor of the mouth. These and any other soft tissue variations that are more noticeable or larger than those just described should be evaluated by a dentist familiar with management of neonates.

Teething

A. Normal Eruption: As the child grows and begins to develop teeth, problems of teething may occur. Primary teeth generally begin to erupt at around 6 months of age. They are usually mandibular incisors but can be maxillary first and appear as early as 3–4 months or as late as 12–16 months. Concerns about sequence or timing of eruption should be discussed with a dentist comfortable with young children. There are many reported side effects from teething—diarrhea, drooling, fever, rash, and so on—but any real correlation is doubtful.

Common treatment for teething pain has been the application of a topical anesthetic or "teething gel." Most of these anesthetic agents contain benzocaine or, less commonly, lidocaine. They can cause pro-

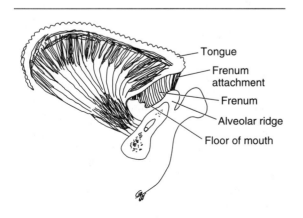

Figure 16–4. Ankyloglossia (tongue–tie).

found numbness of the entire oral cavity and pharynx. Suppression of the gag reflex can be a serious sequela. Systemic analgesia (acetaminophen or ibuprofen) is safer and more effective. Solid rubber or chilled fluid-filled teething toys are beneficial if only for distraction purposes. Massaging the gums can be very soothing.

Occasionally, a noticeable swelling of the gingiva is seen during teething. This condition can present as red to purple, round, raised, smooth lesions, which may be symptomatic but usually are not. They can appear in the anterior or posterior alveolar ridge and are always on the crest. These eruption cysts or eruption hematomas are fluid-filled areas immediately overlying an erupting tooth and generally disappear spontaneously. Any decision about surgical intervention is best left to a dental specialist.

B. Delayed Eruption: Premature loss of a primary tooth can cause either accelerated or delayed eruption of the underlying secondary tooth. Early eruption occurs if the permanent tooth is beginning its active eruption and the overlying primary tooth is removed. This generally occurs when the primary tooth is within 1 year of its normal time of exfoliation. If, however, loss of the primary tooth occurs more than 1 year before expected exfoliation, the permanent tooth will probably be delayed in eruption owing to healing that results in filling in of bone and gingiva over the permanent tooth. The loss of a primary tooth may cause adjacent teeth to tip into the space and lead to impaction of the underlying permanent tooth. A space maintainer should be placed by a dentist to keep this from happening.

Other local factors delaying or preventing eruption include supernumerary teeth, cysts, tumors, overretained primary teeth, ankylosed primary teeth, and impaction. A generalized delay in eruption may be due to endocrinopathies (hypothyroidism, hypopituitarism) or other systemic conditions (cleidocranial dysplasia, rickets, trisomy 21).

C. Ectopic Eruption: Ectopic eruption occurs if the position of an erupting tooth is abnormal. In severe instances, the order in which teeth erupt is affected. If the dental arch provides insufficient room for permanent teeth, they may erupt abnormally. In the mandible, lower incisors may be lingually placed to such an extent that the primary incisors do not exfoliate. The parents' concern about a "double row of teeth" may be the reason for the child's first dental visit. If the primary teeth are not loose, they should be removed by the dentist. If they are loose, they should be allowed to exfoliate naturally. In the maxilla, inadequate room for eruption of the permanent first molar may cause abnormal resorption of the distal root structures of the second primary molar. If the problem is severe, the permanent molar may even become caught under the unresorbed enamel crown of the deciduous molar and thus require extraction of the primary tooth and orthodontic repositioning of

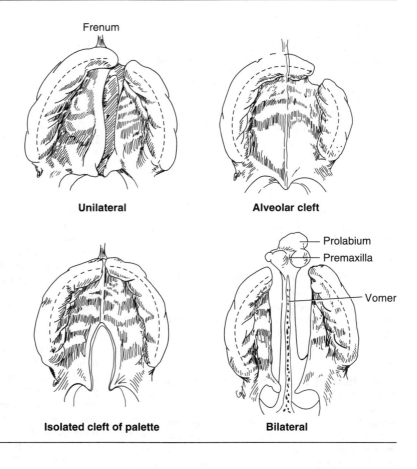

Figure 16–5. Types of clefts.

Labels in figure: Frenum, Unilateral, Alveolar cleft, Isolated cleft of palette, Bilateral, Prolabium, Premaxilla, Vomer

the permanent first molar after it has erupted. If it is not repositioned, the second premolar is likely to become impacted. If problems are detected early, the dentist may be able to redirect the permanent molar's eruption pathway so that the permanent first molar erupts correctly and the second primary molar is not lost.

D. Impaction: Impaction occurs when a tooth is prevented from erupting for any reason. The teeth most often affected are the third molars and the maxillary canines. Because patients with impacted third molars are at risk for developing ameloblastomas or dentigerous cysts, if these teeth are not surgically removed, the impacted third molar (along with its opposing third molar) should be removed after it has been determined that eruption will not be possible, however this may sometimes not be able to be assessed until the late teens. Maxillary canines should not be extracted because of their aesthetic importance and key role in dental occlusion. They can often be brought into correct alignment through surgical exposure and orthodontic treatment.

E. Other Variations: Failure of teeth to develop—a condition sometimes called congenitally missing teeth—is rare in the primary dentition. However, it occurs in about 5% of permanent dentitions,

with one or more of the third molars missing in about 25% of all individuals. The incidence of congenitally missing teeth varies among different genetic groups, but the most frequently missing are maxillary lateral incisors and mandibular second premolars.

Occasionally, there are extra teeth—most typically an extra (fourth) molar or extra (third) bicuspid. Mesiodentes, which are peg-shaped supernumerary teeth situated at the maxillary midline, are seen in about 5% of individuals and may interfere with eruption of permanent incisors. Mesiodentes should be considered for removal even if they do not erupt.

Dental Caries & Periodontal Disease

After teeth begin to erupt, they are at risk for dental caries (decay). Parents must be educated about dental diseases and their causes and consequences. Almost all dental disease can be prevented, so the earlier the parents are indoctrinated, the better chance the child has to be disease-free. The best time to introduce the idea of oral hygiene is during prenatal care, followed by strong reinforcement after delivery. The current recommendation of the American Academy of Pediatric Dentistry is for children to have their first dental visit between 12 and 18 months of age.

Dental caries and periodontal disease are among the most common of all infectious diseases. They are also among the most easily preventable. Oral hygiene for the infant can start at birth. The gums can be gently cleaned with a moist soft cloth. Once the teeth begin to erupt, oral hygiene must be practiced in earnest. Again, a soft moist cloth can be used after feeding to gently rub the teeth. A very small, very soft toothbrush can be used as well. Toothpaste at the start is not necessary.

Figure 16–6 demonstrates the conditions that must be met for dental caries to start. Once teeth are present, they can be attacked by acidogenic bacteria, especially *Streptococcus mutans*. Dental plaque accumulates on the surface of the teeth as an adherent film. As plaque grows, bacteria accumulate within it in close proximity to the tooth. The third necessary ingredient is a substrate for the bacteria. In the case of dental caries, carbohydrate—especially refined carbohydrates such as sucrose—is the most active in that the bacteria metabolize sucrose and produce considerable acid as a by–product. This acid promptly reduces the oral pH. The acidic environment causes the enamel of the teeth to dissolve, which is the beginning of caries. After the decay process has worked its way through the enamel, there is very little resistance to keep it from affecting the vital tissues (nerve) of the tooth. The tooth subsequently becomes necrotic, and an abscess occurs. Figure 16–7 demonstrates the progression of caries from the enamel through to the pulp and the subsequent formation of a dental abscess. This process is not always sympto-matic, but it can lead to severe pain, fever, and swelling.

In the early stages of decay, the tooth may be sensitive to temperature changes or especially sweets. At this point, the tooth can be repaired by removing the caries and "filling" the defect. As the decay progresses, more pain may be involved, and generally one needs the equivalent of root canal therapy to save the tooth. Once there is an abscess, with or without swelling, a choice must be made between root canal therapy and removal of the tooth. In the presence of cellulitis or facial space abscess, extraction is usually the treatment of choice.

Many people question the importance of the primary dentition. Baby teeth allow the child to eat properly, speak properly, have a good self-image, and preserve the space for the permanent dentition. Premature loss of primary teeth can cause major orthodontic and growth and development problems.

Preventing Dental Disease

To prevent dental caries, it is necessary to remove the bacteria on a regular basis. Brushing with a fluoride-containing toothpaste and flossing the teeth regularly (at least twice daily) will keep the oral flora to a minimum. A second step is to decrease the amount of substrate available to the bacteria. Limiting or eliminating refined carbohydrate is very effective (low sugar diets), as is limiting exposures to refined carbohydrates. The ideal schedule would be for a small "sugar" exposure at the end of each meal. The form of the substrate is important also. Caramels, licorice, raisins, gummy bears, and so on, are concentrated sugar and because of their sticky texture will remain on the teeth for much longer than the same sugar in liquid form. The child's primary care physician can play an invaluable role in disseminating this information and reinforcing these ideas.

Fluoride

The final step in fighting the spread of dental caries is to strengthen the tooth. The addition of fluoride helps to create a more resistant tooth. Systemic fluoride, whether from water fluoridation or dietary supplementation, is incorporated into the crystalline structure of the enamel and creates a stronger, more acid-resistant covering. Topically applied fluoride is important in interfering with oral flora metabolism and in remineralizing early carious lesions. Table 16–1 demonstrates the current systemic fluoride dose recommended by the American Academy of Pediatrics and the American Academy of Pediatric Dentistry. It is important not to exceed these recommendations. To do so may lead to fluorosis, which is an unsightly staining of the permanent teeth.

Topical fluoride therapy is used in addition to all other oral hygiene measures in certain high-risk children. Children allowed to take their bottle to bed and those who nurse at will and fall asleep nursing are at

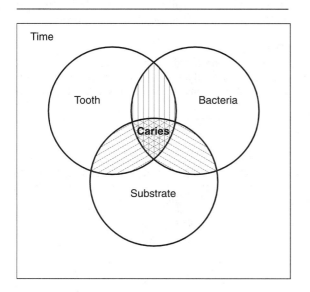

Figure 16–6. Conditions necessary for caries.

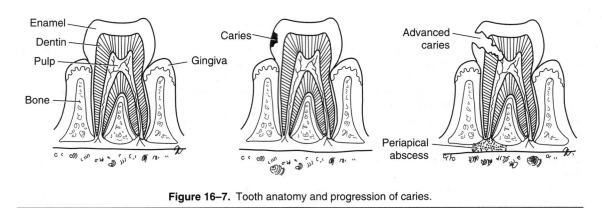

Figure 16–7. Tooth anatomy and progression of caries.

risk for nursing bottle caries. This particular type of decay involves mostly the maxillary incisors. When a child is lying in bed sucking on a bottle, the contents of the bottle are "trapped" between the backs of the front teeth and the tongue. This allows for more concentrated damage to the teeth as the acid produced by bacteria fails to dissipate. In addition, as the child falls asleep, salivary function decreases dramatically. This further endangers the teeth by eliminating the buffering capacity of saliva and its remineralizing potential. Topical fluoride may slow the decay process. In combination with eliminating high–risk nursing practices and instituting good oral hygiene, these infants may avoid serious dental problems.

Patients with chronically low oral pH may benefit from topical fluoride. This includes those with gastroesophageal reflux, bulimia, or salivary dysfunction from radiation, graft–versus–host disease, or autoimmune disease. Saliva is the most effective oral cavity buffer there is. It also helps remineralize minor enamel dissolution. Xerostomia can lead to rampant caries. These children must have dental care more routinely than healthy children. Multiply handicapped children who cannot accomplish or receive proper oral hygiene can also benefit from additional topical fluoride.

Table 16–1. Fluoride dosages based on tap water fluoride supply.

| Age (years) | Dose of Fluoride Administered (mg/d) | |
	If <0.03 ppm F in Drinking Water	If 0.3–0.7 ppm F in Drinking Water[1]
Birth to age 2	0.25	Nil
2–3 years	0.5	0.25
3–13 years	1	0.5

[1]If there is >0.7 ppm of fluoride in drinking water, no supplement is needed.

Note: There is a reported risk of fluorosis associated with the above regimen; however, no consensus has been reached about revising it. Until that is done, practitioners can consider halving the fluoride dosage until age 6 for children who are considered at low risk for caries.

Any child with a serious medical problem or handicapping condition should be referred to a pediatric dentist as early as possible.

Periodontal Disease

Periodontal disease is a problem with the supporting structures: bone, gums, and ligaments. It begins as an inflammation of the gum tissue adjacent to the tooth. Bacterial accumulation in the space between the tooth and gum (gingival sulcus) causes irritation that leads to inflamed tissue. This beginning phase is called gingivitis. As the inflammation spreads through the sulcus, there is more soft tissue involvement. Eventually, there is soft tissue destruction and loss of bone as disease spreads toward the apex of the tooth. This level of involvement is periodontitis and requires professional cleaning and often medication or surgery for correction. Figure 16–8 shows the different stages and progression of periodontal disease.

The prevention and initial management of periodontal disease in children involves the removal of bacteria from the teeth with proper oral hygiene.

Trauma

Managing orofacial trauma is a regular part of pediatric dentistry. Trauma often consists only of abrasions or lacerations of lips, gingiva, tongue, or mu-

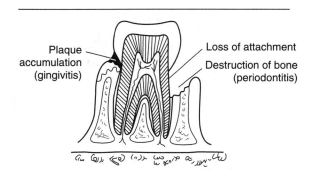

Figure 16–8. Periodontal disease.

cosa, including frena, with no hard tissue damage. The lacerations should be cleansed and inspected for foreign bodies and sutured where appropriate. Occasionally, radiographs of the tongue, lips, or cheeks are used to look for tooth fragments or other foreign bodies.

Tooth-related trauma can consist of displacement (luxation), fracture, or loss of teeth (avulsion). Figure 16–9 demonstrates the different luxation injuries, and Figure 16–10 shows the different degrees of tooth fracture.

The most innocent luxation injury is mobility without displacement (subluxation). Unless mobility is extensive, this condition can be followed without active intervention. An intrusive luxation in the primary dentition is usually observed for a period of time to discern whether the tooth or teeth in question will reerupt (see Figure 16–9). If after several months this has not occurred or if the area becomes infected, the teeth are usually removed. There is a 30% chance of damage to the permanent teeth with any intrusive injury of primary teeth. Permanent teeth intrusions are corrected with surgical or orthodontic repositioning of teeth and placement of a splint to stabilize the teeth. Stabilization is for 10–14 days. Root canal treatment may be necessary in the future. Lateral and extrusive luxations are generally repositioned and splinted also in permanent teeth. Severe luxations in any direction in primary teeth are treated with extraction.

Avulsed primary dentition is not replanted. The

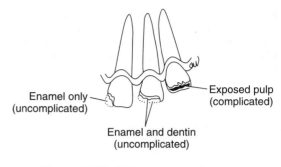

Figure 16–10. Patterns of crown fractures.

area is investigated for fractured roots or foreign bodies. Avulsed permanent teeth are gently cleansed and replanted with splinting. If replaced into the alveolar bone within 1 hour, these teeth have a good prognosis. The prognosis worsens rapidly with increased time outside of the mouth. Recent studies show that milk is the best storage and transport medium for avulsed teeth that will be replanted. Water, saline, and saliva can be used if milk is not accessible.

All luxated and replanted teeth need to be followed carefully and regularly by a dentist. These teeth can become abscessed or fused to the bone (ankylosed) at any time during the healing process.

Fractured teeth should be seen promptly by a dentist. Many need to be protected quickly to avoid sensitivity, pain, or infection from exposed pulp. If the fractured tooth is severe enough, it may require immediate root canal surgery.

All facial trauma needs to be evaluated for jaw fracture. Blows to the chin are among the most common childhood oral–facial traumas. They are also a leading cause of condylar fracture in the pediatric population. One should be suspicious of pain or deviation when the jaw is opened.

Dental Emergencies

Dental emergencies other than trauma usually present as pain or swelling due to advanced caries. Odontogenic pain usually responds to acetaminophen, ibuprofen, codeine, or, in severe cases, hydrocodone. As with teething, topical application of medicaments is of limited value.

Swelling confined to the gum tissue above or below the tooth is usually not an urgent situation. This "gumboil" or parulis represents infection that has spread outward from the root of the tooth through the bone and periosteum into the gum. Usually it will begin to drain and leave a fistulous tract. If the infection invades the facial spaces, cellulitis can occur. Swelling of the mid face, especially the bridge of the nose and the lower eyelid, is an urgent situation. All facial swelling needs to be evaluated by a dentist.

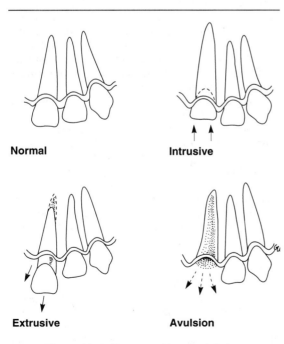

Figure 16–9. Patterns of luxation injuries.

Extraction of teeth or root canal therapy combined with antibiotics is the usual treatment. With extensive facial cellulitis, many young children will be admitted to hospital and managed with intravenous antibiotics.

Antibiotics in Pediatric Dentistry

Antibiotics of choice for odontogenic infection include penicillin G or V, or clindamycin for penicillin–allergic or refractory patients. When calculating the dose of oral antibiotics, one should keep in mind that penicillin and amoxicillin are only about 50% absorbed, so the dose should be chosen from the high end of the range. Intramuscular benzathine penicillin G is favored by many pediatric dentists because of the rapid rise in blood level that occurs with this preparation and the longer-acting feature.

Several patient groups require prophylactic antibiotic coverage prior to any invasive dental manipulation, including tooth cleaning. Cardiovascular patients at risk for subacute infective endocarditis are at the top of this list. The American Heart Association has made specific recommendations for premedication of cardiac patients. Immunosuppressed patients (oncology, HIV, post-transplant) also require coverage, as do children with indwelling central venous catheters. Patients with Broviac, Quinton, Hickman, etc, lines are routinely medicated prior to invasive dental treatment even though there are no reported dental-related catheter infections.

Children with a ventriculoperitoneal shunt may receive prophylaxis, though many practitioners refuse on the grounds that there is no circulatory connection to such a shunt and therefore no danger from bacteremia.

All of these children are premedicated using current American Heart Association guidelines. The most popular drug regimen is oral amoxicillin, 50 mg/kg 1 hour prior to appointment, followed by 25 mg/kg 6 hours later. Clindamycin is recommended for penicillin-allergic patients.

Selected orthopedic patients with prosthetic replacements will be "covered" with cephalosporins such as cephalexin, 1 g 1 hour before and 0.5 g 6 hours later. The dose is doubled at 60 lb.

The Pediatric Oncology Patient

The child with cancer needs to be evaluated by a dentist knowledgeable about pediatric oncology. The evaluation should be accomplished as soon after diagnosis and before chemotherapy as possible.

The aim of the consultation is to eliminate all existing and potential sources of infection before the child becomes neutropenic. Once chemotherapy begins, there is a brief interval before "counts" reach their nadir (7–10 days). Areas of concern to the dentist include abscessed teeth, teeth with extensive caries, soon to exfoliate teeth, ragged or broken teeth or fillings, and orthodontic appliances. Once the child becomes neutropenic, abscessed or infected or severely carious teeth can no longer be considered innocent, even if asymptomatic. Loose teeth that will soon exfoliate can also become a nidus for infection as well as a cause of bleeding if the patient becomes profoundly thrombocytopenic. Sharp, ragged teeth can be a source of irritation that can lead to infection. Chemotherapeutic drugs are cytotoxic to the oral mucosa. The oral mucosa becomes atrophic and ulcerates with ease (mucositis). This is painful and often leads to inadequate oral intake and nutrition. Once the mucosal barrier is breached by ulceration, the patient can become septic, especially with alpha–hemolytic streptococci and other mouth flora. Friction and damage to mucosa is the main concern with braces. Therefore, all orthodontic hardware is removed prior to chemotherapy.

The pediatric oncology patient should be monitored steadily during cancer therapy to screen for infection, manage oral bleeding, and control oral pain. These children can experience spontaneous oral hemorrhaging, especially when platelet counts are below 20,000/μL. Poor oral hygiene or areas of irritation can increase the chances of bleeding.

The child receiving radiation therapy to the head and neck is prone to develop extensive salivary dysfunction (xerostomia) if salivary tissue is in the path of the primary beam of radiation. This should be managed aggressively to avoid rapid extensive destruction of dentition. Customized fluoride applicators are used in this situation combined with close follow-up.

The child undergoing bone marrow transplantation must be similarly screened. These children may develop oral morbidity from an acute graft–versus–host reaction while they are in isolation before their marrow has become reconstituted. Long-term follow-up includes monitoring of growth, managing salivary dysfunction from total body radiation, and treatment of oral graft–versus–host disease.

The pediatric oncology patient also needs to be followed carefully after completion of therapy to manage oral and maxillofacial growth disturbances. Late effects of therapy are morphologic changes in tooth development (microdontia or extensive hypocalcification) and disturbances in eruption (no eruption, no root or delayed eruption). These side effects are seen in chemotherapy and radiation therapy patients, and must be managed by a dentist who is familiar with young children and their growth and development.

The Child With Hematologic Problems

The child with hemophilia needs the appropriate "factor" levels managed before and after any invasive dental procedures (including the administration of local anesthesia, even for simple fillings). The rule of thumb is 50% of factor activity for factor VIII deficiency and 25% for factor IX. Some patients with very mild factor VIII or von Willebrand's disease may respond to desmopressin acetate. Antifibrinolytic medications such as aminocaproic acid or tranexamic acid are used successfully after dental treatment. Postoperative bleeding can also be treated with a wide variety of topical medicaments such as Gelfoam and thrombin.

Anticoagulant Therapy

The pediatric patient receiving anticoagulant therapy must undergo dosage adjustment before invasive dental treatment. This is a relatively simple matter when dealing with heparin, with its short half-life of 4–6 hours. It is a much more difficult problem with warfarin and its half-life of 40–70 hours.

Diabetic Patients

Children who are insulin-dependent are prone to problems with dental treatment. The diabetic child has a reduced capacity to heal, a higher incidence of periodontal disease, and a higher caries rate. These children need to be followed carefully managed on a routine basis. Care must be taken not to disturb the regular cycle of eating and insulin dosage. Anxiety associated with dental appointments can cause a major upset in the diabetic child's routine. Postoperative pain or pain from dental abscess can cause patients not to eat. Warning not to eat until the numbness wears off or until the filling gets hard can also create imbalances in the patient's normal schedule of food intake and insulin dosage. Insulin levels must be adjusted to conform to treatment needs and vice versa. Children with diabetes need to be monitored for hypoglycemic episodes as well as diabetic ketoacidosis.

HIV Infection

The child with HIV infection is especially prone to opportunistic infections, especially oral candidiasis. There may be recurrent bouts of major oral ulceration and extensive gingivitis, which could lead to problems with nutrition and infection.

Arthritis

The child with juvenile rheumatoid arthritis can have major disturbances in oral and maxillofacial growth. This is especially true if the temporomandibular joint is involved. These children may experience extensive growth retardation in the mandible and develop a decreased oral opening. Dental care can be very difficult to accomplish. The arthritic child's medication regimen must also be considered prior to invasive dental treatment. Methotrexate, because of its immune suppression, and aspirin and nonsteroidal anti-inflammatory agents, because they disturb platelet function, are of concern to the dental practitioner.

Renal Disease

The pediatric patient with chronic renal disease usually has a greatly decreased incidence of dental caries. This is presumably due to increased salivary urea concentration. There is, however, an increased incidence of enamel hypoplasia and xerostomia. Uremic stomatitis was once a prevalent finding in renal patients, but not now. Oral ecchymosis and petechiae are common. The renal transplant child must be managed in light of its immunosuppressed status and should be monitored for any signs of neoplasm secondary to his immunosuppression.

Reactive Airway Disease

The child with severe reactive airway disease can be a management problem for the dental practitioner. Managing behavior and medications are the two major concerns. The stress of an invasive dental procedure can trigger a reactive airway episode. The patient receiving multiple medications, including corticosteroids, must be carefully managed through the stressful experience.

DENTAL REFERRAL

Referral to a dentist is appropriate whenever there is a question about a child's oral and maxillofacial health and development. Most pediatric dentists will want to see a child for a first visit between 12 and 18 months of age. The average child should be seen every 6 months for dental follow-up. This recommendation changes for any of the medically involved children whose problems are discussed in the text that precedes. They should be seen earlier and more frequently.

Close cooperation between physician and dentist can lead to improved outcomes for both the well child and the medically compromised child. Early intervention in the dental disease process will result in reduced morbidity and healthier children.

REFERENCES

Andreasen Jo, Andreasen FM: *Essentials of Traumatic Injuries to the Teeth.* Munksgaard, 1990.

Bardach J, Morris, HL:*Multidisciplinary Management of Cleft Lip and Palate.* Saunders, 1990.

Brodsky L, Holt L, Ritter-Schmidt D: *Craniofacial Anomalies: An Interdisciplinary Approach.* Mosby Year Book, 1992.

Little JW, Falace D: *Dental Management of the Medically Compromised Patient,* 4th ed. Mosby Year Book, 1993.

Nelson JD: *Pocket Book of Pediatric Antimicrobial Therapy,* 9th ed. Williams & Wilkins, 1991.

Pizzo PA, Poplack DG: *Principles and Practice of Pediatric Oncology,* 2nd ed. Lippincott, 1993.

Proffit WR: *Contemporary Orthodontics,* 2nd ed. Mosby Year Book, 1993.

Redding SW, Montgomery M: *Dentistry in Systemic Disease.* JBK Publishing, 1990.

Rose LF, Kaye D: *Internal Medicine for Dentistry,* 2nd ed. Mosby, 1990.

Schluger S et al: *Periodontal Diseases.* Lea & Febiger, 1990.

Wei SHY: *Pediatric Dentistry.* Lea & Febiger, 1988.

Ear, Nose, & Throat

17

Stephen Berman, MD, & Ken Chan, MD

THE EAR: DISEASES & DISORDERS

Infections of the ear represent a spectrum of diseases involving the structures of the outer ear (otitis externa), middle ear (otitis media), mastoid (mastoiditis), and inner ear (labyrinthitis).

OTITIS EXTERNA

General Considerations

Otitis externa is an inflammation of the skin lining the ear canal and surrounding soft tissue. The most common cause is the loss of the protective function of cerumen leading to maceration of the underlying skin. Other causes of otitis externa are trauma to the ear canal from using cotton-tipped applicators for cleaning or from poorly fitted ear plugs for swimming; contact dermatitis due to hair sprays, perfumes, or self-administered ear drops; and chronic drainage from a perforated tympanic membrane. The infections are often due to *Staphylococcus aureus* or *Pseudomonas aeruginosa.*

Clinical Findings

Pain and itching in the ear occur in otitis externa, especially with chewing or pressure on the tragus. Movement of the pinna or tragus causes considerable pain. Drainage may be minimal. The ear canal may be grossly swollen, and the patient may resist any attempt to insert an ear speculum. Debris is noticeable in the canal. It is often impossible to visualize the tympanic membrane. Hearing is normal unless complete occlusion has occurred.

Treatment

Topical treatment usually suffices. The crucial initial step is removal of the desquamated epithelium and moist cerumen. This debris can be irrigated out or suctioned out using warm Burow's solution (one packet of Domeboro Powder to 250 mL tap water) or normal saline. Once the ear canal is open, instill antibiotic-corticosteroid ear drops three or four times daily. The corticosteroid is needed to reduce the inflammatory response. In some cases, the canal may be too edematous to allow the ear drop to get in, and the use of an ear wick for the first few days may be extremely helpful. Oral antibiotics are indicated if any signs of invasiveness are present, such as fever, cellulitis of the auricles, or tender postauricular lymph nodes. Prescribe an antistaphylococcal antibiotic while awaiting the results of culture of the ear canal discharge. Systemic antibiotics alone without topical treatment may not clear up otitis externa. Analgesics—sometimes codeine—may be required temporarily.

During the acute phase, the patient should avoid swimming. A cotton ear plug is not helpful and may prolong the infection. Schedule a follow-up visit in 1 week to document an intact tympanic membrane. Children who have intact tympanic membranes and are predisposed to this problem should instill 2 or 3 drops of a 1:1 solution of white vinegar and 70% ethyl alcohol into their ears before and after swimming.

OTITIS MEDIA

Classification & Clinical Findings

Otitis media, an inflammation of the middle ear, is associated with a middle ear effusion (a collection of fluid in the middle ear space) or otorrhea (a discharge from the ear through a perforation in the tympanic membrane or ventilating tube). Otitis media can be further classified by its associated clinical symptoms otoscopic findings, duration, frequency, and complications into acute otitis media, otitis media with effusion (residual or persistent effusion), unresponsive otitis media, recurrent otitis media, otitis media with complications, and chronic suppurative otitis media.

Acute otitis media is commonly defined as inflammation of the middle ear presenting with rapid onset of symptoms such as otalgia, fever, irritability, anorexia, or vomiting. Otoscopic findings of middle ear inflammation include decreased tympanic membrane mobility, a bulging contour with impaired visibility of the ossicular landmarks, a yellow or red color, exudate on the membrane, and bullae. In acute otitis media, symptoms are nonspecific and often result from an associated viral upper respiratory infection. Therefore, the case definition of acute otitis media may be based on otoscopic findings of inflammation, regardless of other symptoms. Approximately one third of cases with otoscopic signs of inflammation and decreased mobility do not present with fever, pain, or irritability.

Otitis media with effusion is defined as an asymptomatic middle ear effusion, which may be associated with a "plugged ear" feeling. Findings that suggest otitis media with effusion include visualization of air-fluid levels, serous middle ear fluid, and diminished membrane mobility when the membrane is translucent. The presence of an effusion is associated with either a mild or moderate conductive hearing impairment of 15 dB or higher. Otitis media with effusion can also be associated with negative middle ear pressure, which is suggested by prominence of the lateral process, a more horizontal orientation of the malleus, and better mobility with negative compared to positive pressure.

Otitis media with residual effusion is characterized by the presence of an asymptomatic middle ear effusion without otoscopic signs of inflammation 3–16 weeks following the diagnosis of acute otitis. After 16 weeks this condition can be considered **otitis media with persistent effusion.**

Both acute otitis media and otitis media with effusion can be associated with decreased tympanic membrane mobility, a flat type B tympanogram and a conductive hearing loss. The distinguishing characteristics are the presence of symptoms and inflammation of the membrane. In an asymptomatic patient, it is difficult to distinguish acute otitis media from otitis media with effusion when the membrane appears opaque, thickened, and scarred. However, bacterial pathogens can be isolated frequently from effusions in these cases with opaque membranes regardless whether the fluid is purulent, serous, or mucoid.

Unresponsive acute otitis media is characterized by clinical signs and symptoms associated with otoscopic findings of inflammation that continue beyond 48 hours of therapy.

Recurrent acute otitis media can be defined as three new acute otitis media episodes within 6 months or four episodes during 1 year.

Otitis media with complications involves damage to the middle ear structures such as tympanosclerosis, retraction pockets, adhesions, ossicular erosion, cholesteatoma, and perforations as well as other intratemporal and intracranial complications. Tympanosclerosis is caused by chronic inflammation or trauma that produces granulation tissue, hyalinization, and calcification. The appearance of a small defect in the posterosuperior area of the pars tensa or in the pars flaccida suggests a retraction pocket. Retraction pockets occur when chronic inflammation and negative pressure in the middle ear space produce atrophy and atelectasis of the tympanic membrane.

Continued inflammation can cause adhesions between the retraction pocket and the ossicles. This condition, referred to as *adhesive otitis,* predisposes to formation of a cholesteatoma or fixation and erosion of the ossicles. Erosion of the ossicles results from osteitis and compromise of the blood supply. Ossicular discontinuity produces a hearing loss with a 25- to 50-dB threshold. A tympanogram with very high compliance indicates ossicular discontinuity. The presence of a greasy-looking mass or debris seen in a retraction pocket or perforation suggests cholesteatoma regardless of the presence of discharge. When a perforation is present, the condition is usually painless. If no infection is present, the middle ear cavity generally contains normal mucosa. If infection is superimposed, serous or purulent drainage will be seen, and the middle ear cavity may contain granulation tissue or even polyps. A conductive hearing loss is usually present, depending on the size and location of the perforation. The site of perforation is important. Central perforations are usually relatively safe from cholesteatoma formation. Peripheral perforations, especially in the pars flaccida, impose a risk for development of cholesteatoma because the ear canal epithelium adjacent to the perforation may invade it.

Chronic suppurative otitis media is defined as persistent otorrhea present longer than 6 weeks. Most often it occurs in children with tympanostomy tubes or tympanic membrane perforations. Occasionally, it is an accompanying sign for a cholesteatoma. Visualization of the tympanic membrane, meticulous culture of the drainage, and appropriate antimicrobial therapy are keys to management of cases not related to a cholesteatoma.

Pathogenesis

The pathogenesis of otitis media is a contest between the pathogen and the host, with factors influencing the outcome. The relative odds of the pathogen winning are increased when the infecting inoculum in the middle ear space is larger and the type of the pathogen has virulence factors that promote attachment to the respiratory epithelium. The odds of the host winning are enhanced when immune defenses and nonimmune defenses are fully functional.

A. Colonization: The pathogen gains a major advantage when the nasopharynx becomes heavily colonized with the otitis pathogens such as *Streptococcus pneumoniae, Haemophilus influenzae,* or

Moraxella catarrhalis. Colonization with these organisms increases the risk of subsequent otitis as well as recurrent episodes. Colonization with normal flora such as *Streptococcus viridans* may prevent recurrent otitis episodes by reducing the growth of *H influenzae* and *S pneumoniae.* Viral upper respiratory infections increase the colonization of the nasopharynx with *H influenzae* and other otitis pathogens, perhaps because of increased adherence to mucosa. Therefore, factors that increase the frequency of viral respiratory infections, such as child care attendance, later birth order, and absence of breastfeeding, promote colonization with otitis pathogens and predispose to otitis.

B. Aspiration into the Middle Ear Space: Aspiration of nasopharyngeal secretions containing an otitis pathogen into the middle ear space is promoted by factors that increase the positive pressure in the nasopharyngeal space (eg, nasal obstruction) or negative pressure in the middle ear space (eg, eustachian tube dysfunction). Concurrent viral respiratory infection or the irritation associated with passive smoking also promote attachment of the pathogen to respiratory epithelium in the middle ear space.

C. Host Immune Defenses: The host's immune response is the most effective defense against otitis. However, this response is a double-edged sword that damages normal tissue in the process of eradicating the pathogen. Children who experience recurrent or persistent otitis may have selective immune defense impairments to specific otitis pathogens.

D. Breastfeeding and Exposure to Passive Smoking: Two environmental factors that influence otitis are breastfeeding and exposure to passive smoke. Breastfeeding reduces the incidence of acute respiratory infections, prevents colonization with otitis pathogens with selective IgA antibody, and decreases the amount of contaminated secretions aspirated into the middle ear space because of sucking mechanisms. Alternatively, passive smoking increases the risk of persistent middle ear effusion by enhancing attachment by the pathogen, prolonging the inflammatory response and impeding drainage through the eustachian tube. For infants 12–18 months of age, each additional pack of cigarettes smoked at home is associated with an 11% increase in the amount time with a middle ear effusion.

Microbiology

The most common bacterial pathogens in acute otitis media are *S pneumoniae* and nontypable *H influenzae*—the same bacterial pathogens most frequently associated with sinusitis and pneumonia. Other bacterial pathogens include *M catarrhalis, Streptococcus pyogenes, S aureus,* gram-negative enteric organisms, and anaerobic organisms. The microbiologic causes of acute otitis media in early infancy differ from those in later life. The risk of gram-negative enteric infection is especially high in infants who are under 6 weeks of age and have been or are hospitalized in a neonatal intensive care nursery. In normal infants seen during the first 3 months of life, acute otitis media is caused by *S aureus* and *Chlamydia trachomatis* as well as *S pneumoniae, H influenzae* and *M catarrhalis.*

Middle ear aspirates of residual and persistent middle ear effusions often grow pathogenic organisms. The most common pathogens isolated from these effusions are *H influenzae, S pneumoniae, M catarrhalis* and *S pyogenes.* Most strains of *H influenzae* and *M catarrhalis* are β-lactamase-positive. The role of *S epidermidis* and diphtheroids is unclear.

Chronic suppurative otitis media is often caused by resistant organisms especially *Pseudomonas, S aureus,* anaerobes, and gram-negative enteric organisms.

Recently, resistant *S pneumoniae* is emerging as a more common pathogen in acute and unresponsive otitis as well as in persistent effusions and chronic suppurative otitis, especially in cases with ventilating tubes. In Washington, DC, Rodriguez and associates reported that 54% of children had a penicillin-resistant *S pneumoniae* or an ampicillin-resistant β-lactamase organism isolated from middle ear aspirates in acute otitis media. Among 62 resistant strains of *S pneumoniae* isolated from middle ear aspirates reported in Texas by Nelson and colleagues, intermediate penicillin resistance occurred in 56% and high resistance in 44%. Among the intermediate resistant strains, 42% were susceptible to trimethoprim-sulfamethoxazole, 68% to clarithromycin, 63% to erythromycin, and 8–90% for oral cephalosporins. Among highly resistant strains, none was susceptible to trimethoprim-sulfamethoxazole, 42% to clarithromycin, 23% to erythromycin, and 0–42% for oral cephalosporins. Ninety-five to 100% of intermediate and highly resistant strains were susceptible to clindamycin and rifampin. Children with resistant strains are often younger than 18 months and have more unresponsive infections.

Prior recent antibiotic treatment appears to increase the risk of the pathogen being a resistant *S pneumoniae.* The relation between viral and bacterial infection remains controversial. Since viruses have been isolated as the single agent in only 6% of middle ear aspirates with acute otitis media, it appears that viruses promote bacterial superinfection by impairing eustachian tube function and altering nasopharyngeal bacterial growth, as well as impairing host immune and nonimmune defenses.

Diagnosis

A. Pneumatic Otoscopy: Acute otitis media is commonly overdiagnosed. Errors in the diagnosis are related to physician and parental bias to treat a sick child with antibiotics, the temptation to diagnose acute otitis media without removing enough cerumen to adequately visualize the membrane, and the mistaken belief that a red membrane with normal mobility establishes the diagnosis of acute otitis media. In fact, a red membrane can be caused by the viral upper respiratory infection, the child's crying, or efforts to remove cerumen. Assuming that the clinician is using a pneumatic otoscope head and has an adequate view of the membrane (Figure 17–1), reasons why clinicians have difficulty in assessing membrane mobility include failure to achieve an adequate seal with the speculum, poor visualization due to low light intensity, and mistaking the ear canal wall for the membrane.

To assess mobility of the tympanic membrane, a pneumatic otoscope with a rubber suction bulb and tube is used. The speculum inserted into the patient's ear canal must be large enough to provide an airtight seal. Placing a piece of rubber tubing ⅛- to ¼-cm wide near the end of the ear speculum helps to create an adequate pneumatic seal. The diameter of the tubing should be appropriate to fit snugly on the speculum at the distance about ½ cm from its end (Figure 17–2). When the rubber bulb is squeezed, the tympanic membrane will flap briskly if no fluid is present (normal finding); if fluid is present in the middle ear space, the mobility of the tympanic membrane will be diminished. It is important to recognize that excessive pressures produced by the rubber bulb may create mobility of the tympanic membrane that is otherwise immobile. The ability to assess mobility is compromised by low light intensity. The problem of low light output is more likely to be restored by

Figure 17–2. **A**: Pneumatic otoscope with an operating lens attached. **B**: Ear curette. **C**: Overlapping lateral (left) and overhead view of a pneumatic otoscope head with an additional operating lens attached.

replacement of the otoscope bulb than by battery replacement.

B. Cerumen Removal: Cerumen removal is an essential skill for anyone who cares for children. Cerumen often prevents adequate visualization of the tympanic membrane. Impacted cerumen can also cause itching, pain, hearing loss, or otitis externa. Parents should be advised that earwax protects the ear (cerumen contains lysozymes and immunoglobulins that curtail infection) and will come out by itself; therefore, parents should never put anything into the ear canal to remove the ear wax.

All procedures to remove cerumen with a curet require immobilization to prevent injury of the ear canal. The physician should remove cerumen under direct vision through the operating head of an otoscope. When an operating microscope is not available, an alternative method is to use a size 00 ear curet through a size 3-mm speculum (for a 12-month-old) with a Welch Allyn fiberoptic pneumatic otoscope head that has been modified with an additional attached operating lens (catalog No. 20206) as shown in Figure 17–1. Frequently, cerumen that obstructs the view of the tympanic membrane can be pushed aside, the pneumatic seal reestablished, and mobility assessed without removing the speculum.

Irrigation can also be used to remove cerumen. Very hard cerumen may adhere to the wall of the ear canal and cause pain or bleeding if one attempts to remove it with a curet. This type of wax can be softened with Cerumenex or a few drops of detergent before irrigation is attempted. After 20 minutes, irrigation with a soft bulb syringe can be started with water warmed to 35–38 °C to prevent vertigo. A commercial jet tooth cleanser (eg, Water Pik) is also an excellent device for removing cerumen, but it is important to set it at low power (2 or less) to prevent damage to the intact tympanic membrane. A perforated tympanic membrane is a contraindication to

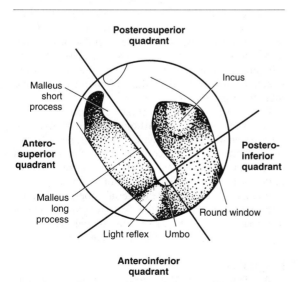

Figure 17–1. Schematic diagram of the left tympanic membrane. (Courtesy of the Department of Otolaryngology, University of Pittsburgh School of Medicine, and Eli Lilly and Co.)

any form of irrigation. In difficult cases, it may be necessary to use the expertise of an otolaryngologist.

C. Tympanometry: Tympanometry can be used to identify an effusion. It should not replace pneumatic otoscopy because it does not identify inflammation. Because of the compliance of the cartilaginous canal of the infants, tympanometry should be reserved for children over the age of 6 months. Tympanometry uses an electroacoustic impedance bridge to measure tympanic membrane compliance and display it in graphic form. Compliance is determined at specific air pressures (from +200 to –400 mm H_2O air pressure) that are created in the hermetically sealed external ear canal. The existing middle ear pressure can be measured by determining the ear canal pressure at which the tympanic membrane is most compliant. Because total visualization of the tympanic membrane is not necessary, tympanometry does not require removal of cerumen unless the canal is completely blocked.

Tympanograms can be classified into three major patterns, as shown in Figure 17–3. The type A pattern, characterized by maximum compliance at normal atmospheric pressure (0 mm H_2O air pressure), indicates a normal tympanic membrane, good auditory tube function, and absence of effusion. The type B pattern identifies a nonmobile tympanic membrane, which may be associated with middle ear effusion, perforation, patent ventilation tubes, or excessive and hard-packed cerumen. The type C pattern indicates an intact mobile tympanic membrane with poor auditory tube function and excessive negative pressure (> –150 mm H_2O air pressure) in the middle ear. Middle ear effusion is present in about 20% of patients with a type C pattern.

Treatment

An algorithm for the management of acute otitis media with effusion is presented in Figure 17–4.

A. Antibiotic Therapy: Few issues in clinical medicine are as controversial as antibiotic treatment of otitis media because of concern for the increasing prevalence of resistant organisms and questions about efficacy. Klein reviewed 11 studies that correlated the clinical response to antibiotic treatment with eradication of the pathogens. Only 38% of patients with acute otitis require antibiotic therapy for the resolution of clinical signs and symptoms. Sixty-two percent of the children treated with antibiotics that fail to eradicate the bacterial organism still appear to be clinically cured. Unfortunately, there are no clinical criteria that distinguish patients who will require antibiotic therapy to improve from patients that do not require therapy. Rosenfeld and associates published a meta-analysis of the results of 33 randomized placebo-controlled clinical trials of the effectiveness of antibiotics for the treatment of acute otitis media. Eighty-one percent (95% CI 69–94%) of patients who received a placebo became asymptomatic. Treatment with antibiotics increased the resolution rate by 13.7% (95% CI 8.2–19.2%). The type of antibiotic administered had no effect on outcome regardless of whether the antibiotic had better coverage of β-lactamase organisms.

Although most clinicians routinely treat acute otitis with antibiotics, it is also reasonable to individualize this decision and involve the family in the decision-making process. This assessment includes a trade-off among the risks of antibiotic treatment associated with an allergic reaction, significant side effect, and colonization and subsequent infection with

Figure 17–3. Type A tympanograms are characterized by maximum compliance at normal atmospheric pressure (0 mm H_2O air pressure). Type B tympanograms show little or no change in compliance of the tympanic membrane as air pressure in the external ear canal is varied. Type C tympanograms show near-normal compliance with significant negative middle ear pressures (typically more severe than –150 mm H_2O). (Reproduced, with permission, from Northern JL: Advanced techniques for measuring middle ear function. Pediatrics 1978;61:761.)

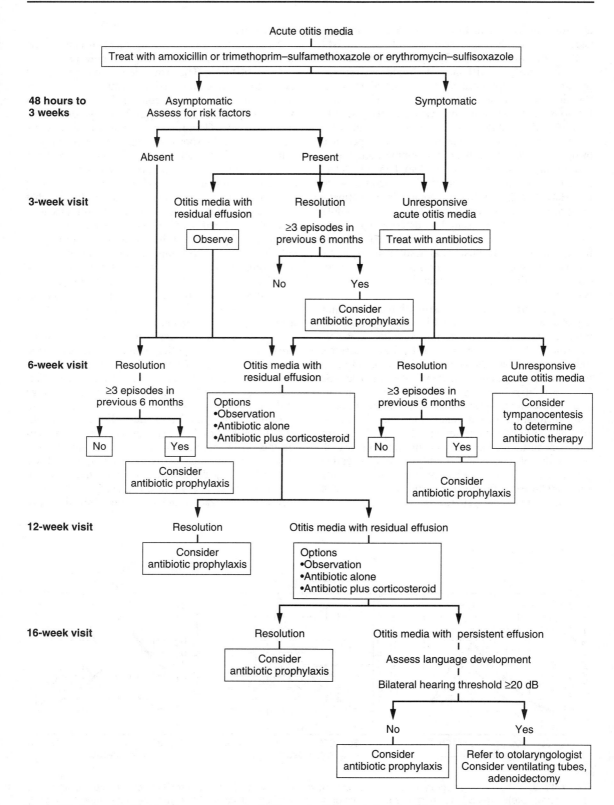

Figure 17–4. An algorithm for the management of otitis media. For prophylaxis in children with recurrent acute otitis media, see text. (From Berman S: Otitis media in children. N Engl J Med 1995;332:1561.)

an antibiotic-resistant pathogen versus the benefit of a more rapid clinical response in about 14% of patients. However, it is advisable to treat children younger than 1 year of age with antibiotics because of their higher risk of developing complications. Patients who fail to improve within 48–72 hours should be seen for a reassessment and also treated with antibiotics. It is best to avoid the antibiotic treatment dilemma as much as possible by not overdiagnosing acute otitis media.

First-line antibiotics for acute otitis media are amoxicillin, trimethoprim plus sulfamethoxazole, and erythromycin plus sulfisoxazole (Table 17–1). In most cases, third-generation cephalosporins, amoxicillin plus clavulanate, and clarithromycin, should not be used as first-line antibiotics for otitis in a normal child who is not allergic to amoxicillin or sulfa-containing antibiotics. These drugs should be reserved as second-line agents.

The optimal duration of therapy is unclear; 5–7 days appears to be as effective as 10–14 days. If the physician is concerned about an associated bacteremia or about compliance, the patient can be treated with an intramuscular injection of ceftriaxone or penicillin G. Procaine penicillin is similar to amoxicillin in its coverage of *H influenzae.* Antihistamines with or without decongestants are ineffective in the prevention or treatment of otitis media.

B. Pain Management: Children with pain related to acute otitis media may get relief from acetaminophen, ibuprofen, or topical therapy with Auralgan. In a randomized controlled trial, Auralgan ear drops were superior to olive oil in reducing pain.

Table 17–1. Drugs commonly used for acute otitis media, recurrent otitis media, and otitis media with effusion in children.

Therapy	Dosage
For acute otitis media	
Amoxicillin	40 mg/kg/d in three divided doses for 7–10 days
Erythromycin–sulfisoxazole	40 mg of erythromycin and 150 mg of sulfisoxazole/kg/d in four divided doses for 7–10 days
Trimethoprim–sulfamethoxazole	8 mg of trimethoprim and 40 mg of sulfamethoxazole/kg/d in two divided doses for 7–10 days
For recurrent otitis media	
Amoxicillin	20 mg/kg/d in one or two doses for 3–6 months
Sulfisoxazole	75 mg/kg/d in one or two doses for 3–6 months
For otitis media with effusion	
Antibiotic agent	Give as for acute otitis media, but for 14–21 days
Prednisone or prednisolone	1 mg/kg/d in two divided doses for 7 days

From Berman S: Otitis media in children. N Engl J Med 1995;332:1560.

When pain persists after antimicrobial treatment, tympanocentesis should be considered for pain relief and the identification of potential resistant organism.

C. Follow-up Visits: The optimal timing for follow-up visits depends on the child's response to therapy. Reassess children when symptoms of acute otitis media continue beyond 48 hours or reoccur prior to the next scheduled visit. The timing of a scheduled follow-up visit for children who become asymptomatic should be between 3 and 6 weeks. Follow-up visits for children with risk factors for treatment failure should be scheduled 3 weeks after initiating therapy. Risk factors include age under 15 months, a prior history of recurrent otitis media, or a history of antibiotic treatment of otitis media within the prior month. Follow-up visits for asymptomatic children without risk factors may be scheduled 6 weeks after initiating treatment.

D. Antibiotic Therapy for Unresponsive Acute Otitis Media: Unresponsive acute otitis media after 48 hours of initial antibiotic therapy occurs in about 10% of children. Unresponsive acute otitis media occurs more frequently when antibiotic therapy fails to eradicate pathogens than when pathogens are eradicated. However, organisms sensitive to initial therapy can be identified in about 20% of post-therapy aspirates. Persistent symptoms and otoscopic findings of inflammation are associated with higher viral isolation rates from middle ear aspirates.

Treat unresponsive acute otitis media in a child who has been treated initially with amoxicillin with trimethoprim plus sulfamethoxazole or erythromycin plus sulfisoxazole, and vice versa. The sequential administration of these antibiotics provides excellent coverage for most middle ear pathogens. Trimethoprim plus sulfamethoxazole and erythromycin plus sulfamethoxazole cover most β-lactamase-producing organisms resistant to amoxicillin such as *H influenzae, M catarrhalis,* and many strains of *S aureus,* while amoxicillin covers organisms resistant to trimethoprim plus sulfamethoxazole such as *S pyogenes,* group B streptococci, and enterococci. Third-generation cephalosporins and amoxicillin plus clavulanate offer minimal advantage in covering highly resistant pneumococcal organisms. These more expensive antibiotics are mainly useful as second-line therapy for children who are allergic to antibiotics containing penicillin or sulfa. If the child is allergic to amoxicillin but not cephalosporins, use a third-generation cephalosporin or clarithromycin to treat resistant otitis media. If the child is allergic to an antibiotic containing sulfa; use amoxicillin plus clavulanate, a third-generation cephalosporin, or clarithromycin when the otitis has not responded.

E. Tympanocentesis or Myringotomy: Tympanocentesis is performed by placing a needle through the tympanic membrane and aspirating the middle ear fluid. Myringotomy involves making an incision of the drum with a myringotomy knife to drain the fluid. Indications for a tympanocentesis or myringotomy are (1) acute otitis media in a hospitalized newborn, because the pathogens may be gram-negative; (2) acute otitis media in a patient with compromised host resistance, because the organism may be unusual; (3) painful bullae of the tympanic membrane; (4) a complete workup for presumed sepsis or meningitis; (5) unresponsive otitis media despite courses of two different antibiotics; and (6) acute mastoiditis.

Technique–

- **Premedication.** In the conditions mentioned, the pain associated with tympanocentesis is only slightly greater than the pain that already exists from acute inflammation of the tympanic membrane. Therefore, no premedication is generally indicated. The patient who is extremely difficult to hold may be premedicated with meperidine, 1 mg/kg intramuscularly.
- **Restraint.** The patient must be completely immobile while the incision is being made. A papoose board or a sheet can be used to immobilize the body. An extra attendant is required to hold the patient's head steady.
- **Site.** With an open-headed operating otoscope, the operator carefully selects a target. This is generally in the posteroinferior quadrant. This site prevents disruption of the ossicles during the procedure.
- **Aspiration.** An 8.8-cm spinal needle (No. 18 or No. 20) with a short bevel is attached to a 1-mL syringe. The plunger is removed from the syringe, and a suction tube is placed over the syringe opening. The spinal needle is bent at a slight angle so that its end is out of the operator's line of vision. The operator moves the needle toward the posteroinferior quadrant, inserting it through the tympanic membrane, and aspirates the middle ear effusion into the syringe. Aspirate should be directly placed onto culture plates for maximum recovery.

F. Management of Recurrent Otitis: The decision to administer antibiotic prophylaxis to children who have experienced three documented episodes of acute otitis media in a 6-month period should be individualized and the risks and benefits reviewed with the parents. Antibiotic prophylaxis is as effective as ventilating tubes at preventing new otitis episodes (see Table 17–1). However, neither intervention appears to make a major clinical difference with respect to a placebo. Antibiotic prophylaxis is marginally effective in reducing the frequency of otitis episodes. A meta-analysis of nine randomized controlled trials with 958 subjects compared the difference in the rate of occurrence of acute otitis media per patient month while receiving antibiotic prophylaxis with that of placebo controls.

Although antibiotic prophylaxis reduced the otitis rate by 44%, patients receiving antibiotics had a mean of only about one and one third fewer episodes per patient per year compared with those of controls. The increased risk of acquiring resistant *S pneumoniae* while on continuous prophylaxis is not clear. Administration of antibiotic therapy at the onset of upper respiratory infection symptoms rather than daily continuous therapy also decreases otitis episodes and may have less of an effect on colonization with resistant *S pneumoniae.*

Another approach to preventing recurrent otitis episodes is active immunization. Clinical trials of the newly developed conjugate pneumococcal vaccine to prevent acute otitis media episodes are currently underway. Consider immunizing children with recurrent otitis with influenza vaccine and in children older than 2 years with the 23-valent pneumococcal vaccine (Pneumovax).

Surgical options for the treatment of recurrent otitis media include tympanostomy with tube placement and adenoidectomy. Insertion of a tympanostomy tube is indicated when a child has failed antimicrobial prophylaxis at least twice during a respiratory season or has experienced six or more infections during a 6-year period. Tube insertion is also indicated in children with recurrent otitis superimposed on chronic otitis media with effusion that is unresponsive to medical therapy. Data are sufficient to support the role of adenoidectomy in the management of otitis media in selected children over the age of 3 years. The indication of adenoidectomy should be considered in conjunction with tube placement.

G. Management of Otitis Media With Residual and Persistent Effusions: The main reason to treat otitis media with effusion is concern about the negative effects of prolonged conductive hearing impairments on language development and academic functioning. Although the available data document a causal relationship between severe congenital or acquired hearing loss (usually sensorineural) and language development, the data fail to establish a causal relationship between conductive hearing loss associated with otitis media and subsequent hearing-related development. Data from multiple studies on the impact of conductive hearing impairment related to otitis report conflicting results.

The management options for otitis media with residual effusion present 6 weeks to 4 months include observation, antibiotics alone, and combination antibiotic and corticosteroid therapy. If combination therapy is selected, corticosteroid (prednisone) can be administered for 7 days combined with an antibiotic (trimethoprim-sulfamethoxazole or an alternative) for 14–21 days. Crushed prednisone tablets added to jelly are well tolerated. Children without a history of varicella who have been exposed in the prior month should not receive prednisone because of the potential risk of disseminated disease if on corticosteroid therapy. Prednisone side effects are similar to those noted in treating asthmatic episodes with short corticosteroid courses: increased appetite, fluid retention, occasional vomiting, and, in rare cases, marked behavior changes. If the patient clears the persistent middle ear effusion unilaterally or bilaterally, follow up the patient monthly and consider administering low-dose intermittent antibiotic prophylaxis with amoxicillin, 20 mg/kg/day, either one or two times daily or sulfisoxazole, 75 mg/kg/day, either one or two times daily for colds during the subsequent 3 months to prevent a recurrence of otitis media.

The guideline developed by the Agency for Health Care Policy and Research for the management of otitis media with effusion recommends that ventilating tubes be considered only after the effusion has persisted for at least 4 months and is accompanied by a documented bilateral hearing impairment of 20 dB or greater. When to place ventilating tubes should depend on the child's developmental and behavioral status as well as on parental preference.

Studies have established that children with otitis media with persistent effusion have a higher incidence of abnormalities such as cholesteatoma, adhesive otitis, retraction pockets, membrane atrophy, and persistent membrane perforation compared with children with no history of persistent effusion. However, the clinical usefulness of this association is limited, since there is no way to identify the small proportion of children with a history of persistent otitis who will sustain damage to the middle ear, and, more important, for whom the insertion of ventilating tubes does not prevent the damage from occurring. Daly reviewed data on the incidence of sequelae of otitis media with effusion treated with ventilating tube placement. The weighted average incidence of a retraction pocket was 4%, atelectasis 7%, tympanosclerosis 10%, membrane atrophy 8%, perforation 1%, and cholesteatoma 0.5%.

Current criteria for tube insertion in children with chronic otitis media with effusion unresponsive to medical therapy are bilateral effusion for at least 4 months and unilateral effusion for 6 months. Adenoidectomy cannot be recommended for children under 4 years of age for the treatment of persistent effusion alone because no data are currently available concerning its efficacy at this age.

Adenoidectomy for otitis media without signs of upper airway obstruction is usually considered as a second-line surgical intervention when a child requires multiple tube reinsertions. However, some surgeons advocate adenoidectomy as the primary surgical therapy. Children with a submucous cleft should not have an adenoidectomy because of the risk of velopharyngeal insufficiency and speech impairments. Tonsillectomy in combination with adenoidectomy is no more effective than adenoidectomy alone in treating persistent effusions and is therefore not recommended.

H. Management of Otitis Media With Perfo-

ration: Most perforations seen with acute otitis media heal within 2 weeks. When perforations fail to heal after 3–6 months, a surgical repair may be needed. Repair of the defect in the tympanic membrane is generally delayed until the child is older and the eustachian tube function has improved. A variety of procedures is available, such as paper patch, fat myringoplasty, and tympanoplasty. Tympanoplasty is generally deferred until age 7–9 years. The perforated eardrum can be repaired earlier if the nonperforated one remains free of infection and effusion for 1 year. Water activities should be limited to surface swimming, preferably with the use of an ear mold. Diving, jumping into the water, and underwater swimming should be avoided.

I. Management of Chronic Suppurative Otitis Media Without Cholesteatoma: The successful treatment of chronic suppurative otitis usually requires parenteral therapy using an antibiotic that covers *Pseudomonas* or anaerobes or both. The role of oral quinoline antibiotics effective against *Pseudomonas* infection for outpatient management is unclear because of possible side effects on growing cartilage in children.

Kenna and associates reported the long-term follow-up of 51 patients enrolled in a clinical trial of medical management of chronic suppurative otitis media with intravenous antibiotics effective against *Pseudomonas* infection. Among these patients, 78% had resolution of their otorrhea, and 22% required surgery either initially or because of recurrence of otorrhea. When a cholesteatoma is present, medical therapy is not effective. If the discharge does not respond to 2 weeks of aggressive therapy, the mastoiditis or cholesteatoma should be suspected. Serious central nervous system complications such as extradural abscess, subdural abscess, brain abscess, meningitis, labyrinthitis, or lateral sinus thrombophlebitis can occur with extension of this process. Therefore, patients with facial palsy, vertigo, or other central nervous system signs should be immediately referred to an otolaryngologist.

Berman S: Current concepts: Otitis media in children. N Engl J Med 1995;332:1560.

Berman S et al: Effectiveness of continuous versus intermittent amoxicillin to prevent episodes of otitis media. Pediatr Infect Dis J 1992;11:63.

Casselbrandt ML et al: Efficacy of antimicrobial prophylaxis and tympanostomy tube insertion for prevention of recurrent acute otitis media: Results of a randomized clinical trial. Pediatr Infect Dis J 1992;11:278.

Daly K: Risk factors for otitis media sequelae and chronicity. Ann Otol Rhinol Laryngol 1994;103:39.

Duncan B et al: Exclusive breast-feeding for at least 4 months protects against otitis media. Pediatrics 1993; 91:867.

Ey JL et al: Group Health Medical Associates: Passive smoke exposure and otitis media in the first year of life. Pediatrics 1995;95:670.

Gates GA: Adenoidectomy for otitis media with effusion. Ann Otol Rhinol Laryngol 1994;103:54.

Hathaway TJ, Katz HP, Dershewitz RA, Marx TJ: Acute otitis media: Who needs posttreatment follow-up? Pediatrics 1994;94(2):143.

Kenna MA, Rosane BA, Bluestone CD: Medical management of chronic suppurative otitis media without cholesteatoma in children: Update 1992. Am J Otol 1993; 14:469.

Klein JO: Microbiologic efficacy of antibacterial drugs for acute otitis media. Pediatr Infect Dis J 1993;12:973.

Nelson CT, Mason EO Jr, Kaplan SL: Activity of oral antibiotics in middle ear and sinus infections caused by penicillin-resistant *Streptococcus pneumoniae:* Implications for treatment. Pediatr Infect Dis J 1994:13:585.

Rosenfeld RM et al: Clinical efficacy of antimicrobial drugs for acute otitis media: Metaanalysis of 5400 children from 33 randomized trials. J Pediatr 1994;124:355.

Stool SE et al: Otitis media with effusion in young children: Clinical practice.

Williams RL et al: Use of antibiotics in preventing recurrent acute otitis media and in treating otitis media with effusion. JAMA 1993;270:1344.

MASTOIDITIS

General Considerations

Infection of the mastoid antrum and air cells can be associated with an episode of acute otitis media. Mastoiditis is unusual before age 2 years, when air cells begin to develop. The most common etiologic agents are *S pyogenes, S pneumoniae,* and *S aureus. H influenzae* causes mastoiditis much less frequently than might be expected. Other agents that can cause this disease include *Pseudomonas, Mycobacterium,* enteropathic gram-negative rods, and *M catarrhalis.* Anaerobic organisms appear to play a role in chronic mastoiditis; however, no data are available on how frequently they cause acute mastoiditis.

Clinical Findings

The principal complaints of patients with mastoiditis are usually postauricular pain and fever. On examination, the mastoid area often appears swollen and reddened. In the late stage, it may be fluctuant. The earliest finding is severe tenderness upon mastoid percussion.

Acute otitis media is almost always present. Late findings are a pinna that is pushed forward by postauricular swelling and an ear canal that is narrowed in the posterosuperior wall because of pressure from the mastoid abscess. In infants less than 1 year of age, the swelling occurs superior to the ear and pushes the pinna downward rather than outward. In the acute phase, there is diffuse inflammatory clouding of the mastoid cells as in every case of acute otitis media. Later there is evidence of bony destruction and resorption of the mastoid air cells. The best method to determine the extent of disease is by computed tomography (CT) scan.

Complications

Meningitis is a complication in up to 9% of cases of acute mastoiditis. This infection should be suspected when a child has high fever, stiff neck, severe headache, or other meningeal signs. A lumbar puncture should be performed to diagnose this condition. Brain abscess occurs in 2% of cases and may be associated with persistent headaches, recurring fever, or changes in sensorium.

Treatment

The patient with mastoiditis must be hospitalized because this disorder represents osteitis. Before therapy is initiated, tympanocentesis or myringotomy should be performed to obtain material for culture and also to relieve the pressure in the middle ear-mastoid space.

The initial management of uncomplicated acute mastoiditis includes intravenous antibiotic therapy. Results of gram-stained smears taken during tympanocentesis may help in the choice of antibiotics. Reasonable initial therapy is ceftriaxone with nafcillin or clindamycin. Indications for immediate surgery include clear evidence of a major complication such as meningitis, brain abscess, cavernous sinus thrombosis, acute suppurative labyrinthitis, or facial palsy. Some otolaryngologists consider the destruction of septation of the mastoid (coalescence) an indication for surgery as well. Duration of antibiotic therapy following mastoidectomy is dependent on the type of complication encountered. The prognosis is good if treatment is started early and continued until the process is inactive.

Myer CM: The diagnosis and management of mastoiditis. Pediatr Ann 1991;20:622.

ACUTE TRAUMA TO THE MIDDLE EAR

Head injuries, a blow to the ear canal, sudden impact with water, blast injuries, or the insertion of pointed instruments into the ear canal can lead to perforation of the tympanic membrane or hematoma of the middle ear. One study reported that 50% of serious penetrating wounds of the tympanic membrane were due to parental use of a cotton-tipped swab.

Treatment of middle ear hematomas consists mainly of watchful waiting. Prophylactic antibiotics are not necessary unless signs of superimposed infection appear. The prognosis for unimpaired hearing depends on whether or not the ossicles are dislocated or fractured in the process. The patient needs to be followed with audiometrics until hearing has returned to normal.

Traumatic perforations of the tympanic membrane often do not heal spontaneously, and the patient should be referred to an otolaryngologist. Perforations caused by a foreign body must be attended to immediately, especially if accompanied by vertigo.

EAR CANAL FOREIGN BODY

Numerous objects can be inserted into the ear canal by a child. If the object is large, wedged into place, or difficult to remove with available instruments, the patient should be referred to an otolaryngologist early rather than risk traumatizing the ear canal and causing edema that will require removing the foreign body under anesthesia.

HEMATOMA OF THE PINNA

Trauma to the earlobe can result in formation of a hematoma between the perichondrium and cartilage. The hematoma appears as a boggy purple swelling of the upper half of the earlobe. If this is unattended, it can cause pressure necrosis of the underlying cartilage and result in a boxer's "cauliflower ear." To prevent this cosmetic deformity, physicians should refer patients to an otolaryngologist for aspiration and the application of a carefully molded pressure dressing. Recurrent or persistent hematoma of the ear may require surgical drainage and insertion of a drain.

CONGENITAL EAR MALFORMATIONS

Agenesis of the external ear canal results in conductive hearing loss that requires evaluation in the first month of life by hearing specialists and an otolaryngologist.

"Lop ears" (Dumbo ears) lead to much teasing and ridicule. To prevent secondary emotional problems, they can be surgically corrected at age 5 or 6 years. The ear is of approximately adult size by then, and there is little risk of affecting growth of the tissues.

An ear is low-set if the upper pole is below eye level. This condition is often associated with renal malformations (eg, Potter's syndrome), and renal ultrasound examination is helpful.

Preauricular tags, ectopic cartilages, fistulas, sinuses, and cysts require surgical correction, mainly for cosmetic reasons. Children with any of the above findings should have their hearing tested. Most preauricular pits are asymptomatic. If one should become infected, the patient should receive antibiotic therapy and be referred to an otolaryngologist for eventual excision.

DETECTION & MANAGEMENT OF HEARING DEFICITS

Hearing deficits are classified as conductive, sensorineural, or mixed. **Conductive hearing loss** re-

sults from a blockage of the transmission of sound waves from the external auditory canal to the inner ear and is characterized by normal bone conduction and reduced air conduction hearing. In children, conductive losses are most often caused by middle ear effusion. **Sensorineural hearing loss** occurs when the auditory nerve or cochlear hair cells are damaged. **Mixed hearing loss** is characterized by components of both conductive and sensorineural loss. The criteria for normal hearing levels in children are lower than those in adults, since children are in the process of learning language. In children, a hearing loss of 15–30 dB is considered mild, 31–50 dB moderate, 51–80 dB severe, and 81–100 dB profound.

Conductive Hearing Loss

By far the greatest number of conductive hearing losses during childhood are caused by otitis media and its sequelae. Other causes include atresia, stenosis, or collapse of the ear canal; furuncle, cerumen, or foreign body in the ear; aural discharge; bony growths; otitis externa; perichondritis; and middle ear anomalies (eg, stapes fixation, ossicular malformation).

The average hearing loss due to middle ear effusion (whether serous, purulent, or mucoid) is 27–31 dB, the equivalent of a mild hearing loss. This loss may be intermittent in nature and may occur in one or both ears.

The American Academy of Pediatrics recommends that hearing be assessed and language development skills be monitored in children who have frequently recurring acute otitis media or middle ear effusion persisting longer than 3 months. The effects of hearing loss may be insidious and may not be discernible until the explosive phase of expressive language development occurs between 16 and 24 months of age; therefore, the optimal times for screening very young children are between 18 and 24 months. An acceptable tool for language screening at these ages is the Early Language Milestone (ELM) scale. Children 3, 4, and 5 years of age should also be screened for language delays.

To diminish the likelihood of a communication disorder developing, the physician should inform parents of a child with middle ear disease that the child's hearing may not be normal and should instruct the parents to (1) turn off sources of background noise (eg, televisions, radios, dishwashers) when speaking to the child; (2) focus on the child's face and gain his or her direct attention before speaking; (3) speak slightly louder than usual; and (4) have the teacher place the child in the front of the classroom.

Sensorineural Hearing Loss

Sensorineural hearing loss (SNHL) arises from a lesion in the cochlear structures of the inner ear or in the neural fibers of the auditory nerve (cranial nerve

VIII). Most sensorineural losses in children are congenital, with an estimated incidence of 1 in 750–1000 live births. Causes of SNHL can be classified as either congenital or postnatal and genetic versus nongenetic within each classification. Common congenital genetic causes include inner ear dysplasias and SNHL with and without associated abnormalities (eg, Usher's syndrome). Common postnatal genetic causes include SNHL with and without associated abnormalities (eg, Alport's and Klippel-Feil syndromes). Common congenital nongenetic causes are prenatal infections, teratogenic drugs, and perinatal injuries. Common postnatal nongenetic causes are infections, trauma, ototoxic drugs, metabolic disorders, neoplastic, and autoimmune diseases. Prior to the introduction of Hib vaccine, meningitis was the most common cause of acquired hearing loss, with deafness occurring in about 10% of children with bacterial meningitis. A "shot-gun" approach to the laboratory evaluation of SNHL is not warranted because of the low yield in such an approach.

The clinician needs to balance the cost-effectiveness of an evaluation and the medical-legal implications of a missed or delayed diagnosis.

In the past, the effect of unilateral deafness on school performance was thought to be insignificant. However, studies now show that more than one third of affected children fail one or more grades in school. Therefore, merely recommending preferential classroom seating for these children is no longer sufficient; they should be referred for full evaluation of their hearing needs.

Acquisition of language skills is more severely affected by bilateral than unilateral sensorineural hearing loss. The earlier the deafness occurs, the graver the consequences for language development; the earlier a sensorineural loss is detected and treated (by sound amplification and language habilitation), the better the chances of a good outcome.

Screening for Hearing Deficits

Screening procedures are established for early detection and diagnosis of hearing deficits. The need for identifying hearing impairment in infants was instituted in the 1970s with the formation of the high-risk registry. The latest stage of evolution is the Joint Committee's 1994 Position Statement (see Screening of Newborns below). It called for the use of auditory brain stem response screening, preferably before discharge from the hospital for neonates identified as being high risk. However, a Consensus Development Conference sponsored by the National Institutes of Health in 1993 recommended universal hearing screening of all neonates using evoked oto-acoustic emission testing. Although this position is not yet fully accepted by the pediatric and otolaryngologic communities, the trend for the future is for early universal screening. The procedures listed in the following text are meant to be a guide, and the confirmation of SNHL is dependent on audiologic testing.

A. Screening of Newborns: Preferably during the hospital stay, records of the infant's neonatal course and family history should be reviewed to determine whether the infant is at risk for SNHL. According to the 1990 Position Statement of the Joint Committee on Infant Screening, the following factors place infants at high risk: (1) family history of SNHL; (2) known or suspected maternal infections (eg, cytomegalovirus, rubella, herpes simplex, toxoplasmosis, syphilis); (3) craniofacial anomalies; (4) birth weight less than 1500 g; (5) hyperbilirubinemia at levels exceeding indications for exchange transfusion; (6) bacterial meningitis; (7) signs of severe asphyxia at birth (eg, Apgar scores of 0–3, failure to show spontaneous respiration by 10 minutes after birth, hypotonia persisting to 2 hours of age; (8) prolonged mechanical ventilation; and (9) stigmata of known syndrome. If any of these risk factors is present, the neonate should be screened preferably before discharge using auditory brain stem response audiometry. If results of the screening test are positive for hearing deficit, the audiologist should do further diagnostic testing.

B. Screening of Infants: The Joint Committee recommends a similar screening protocol for infants (29 days to 2 years) if one of the following risk criteria is identified. The risk criteria for this age group are (1) concerns regarding hearing, speech, language, or developmental delay; (2) bacterial meningitis; (3) neonatal risk factors listed above; (4) head trauma; (5) ototoxic drug use; (6) neurodegenerative disorders; and (7) childhood infectious diseases (eg, mumps, measles).

In the past, the parents' report of their infant's behavior was considered an adequate assessment of the infant's hearing. However, a deaf infant's behavior can appear normal and mislead the parents as well as the professional, especially if the infant has autosomal recessive deafness and is the firstborn child of carrier parents. The following office screening techniques should identify gross hearing losses, but they may or may not detect less severe hearing losses due to otitis media.

1. From birth to 4 months–In response to a sudden loud sound (70 dB or more) produced by a horn, clacker, or special electronic device, the infant should show a startle reflex or blink the eyes.

2. From 4 months to 2 years–While the infant is distracted with a toy or bright object, a noisemaker is sounded softly outside the field of vision at the child's waist level. Normal responses are as follows: at 4 months, there is widening of the eyes, interruption of other activity, and perhaps a slight turning of the head in the direction of the sound; at 6 months, the head turns toward the sound; at 9 months or older, the child is usually able to locate a sound originating from below as well as turn to the appropriate side; after 1 year, the child is able to locate sound whether it comes from below or above.

After responses to these soft sounds are noted, a loud horn or clacker should be used to produce an eye blink or startle reflex. This last maneuver is necessary because deaf children are very often visually alert and able to scan the environment so actively that their scanning can be mistaken for an appropriate response to the softer noise test. A deaf child will not blink in response to the loud sound. Consonant sounds such as "mama," "dada," "baba" should be present in speech by age 11 months. Children who fail to respond appropriately should be referred for audiologic assessment.

C. Screening of Older Children: When children reach 3 years of age, their hearing can be tested by earphones and pure tone audiometry. The test frequencies for screening are 1000 Hz, 2000 Hz, and 4000 Hz, with the same tone presented at each frequency. Normally, the screening level is 20 dB. If a sound- proof room is not available, the screening may be done at 25 dB. If the child does not respond at any one of the test frequencies in either ear, the test should be repeated within 1 week. Failures on rescreening should be referred for audiologic evaluation.

High-risk categories in older children include osteogenesis imperfecta and syndromes associated with deafness, such as Waardenburg's syndrome, Hurler's syndrome, Alport's syndrome, Treacher Collins' syndrome, Klippel-Feil syndrome, and fetal alcohol syndrome. Children with these disorders should receive audiologic evaluation as part of the complete workup. In addition, before any child is labeled as having mental retardation, autism, or severe behavior problems, the adequacy of his or her hearing must be determined. If a developmental speech delay is diagnosed, hearing should be tested as the first step in evaluating the language problem.

Referral

In addition to the referrals for audiologic testing mentioned in the preceding text, a child with confirmed hearing loss should be referred to an otolaryngologist for evaluation and further management. Any child failing the language screen should be referred to a speech pathologist for language evaluation. Home language enrichment programs for children with mild language delays can be directed by the physician or by a speech pathologist. Programs for the deaf child vary from aural to total communication; the latter includes elements of aural programs plus signing. Each program should be thoroughly scrutinized for its relevance to the deaf child's age and hearing level.

Prevention

Appropriate pediatric care may help prevent many causes of hearing deficits. Erythroblastosis fetalis can usually be prevented by the use of $Rh_o(D)$ immune globulin, and hyperbilirubinemia can be controlled by phototherapy and exchange transfusions. Congenital rubella infections can be prevented by the use of rubella vaccine, and immunizations for other childhood diseases (eg, mumps) effectively prevent hearing losses from those conditions.

Aminoglycosides and diuretics, especially in combination, are potentially ototoxic and should be used judiciously and monitored carefully, especially in premature infants and in patients with renal insufficiency.

Reduction of exposure to loud noise in the child's environment will prevent high-frequency hearing losses. Repeated exposure to loud music, firecrackers, or shots from guns or cap pistols can impair hearing.

Chan KH: Sensorineural hearing loss in children: Classification and evaluation. Otolaryngol Clin North Am 1994; 27:473.

THE NOSE & PARANASAL SINUSES

ACUTE VIRAL RHINITIS
(Common Cold)

The common cold is the most common pediatric infectious disease, and the incidence is higher in early childhood than in any other period of life. Children under age 5 have 6–12 colds per year. Upper respiratory infections may be caused by over 200 different viruses, including rhinovirus, coronavirus, adenovirus, influenza virus, parainfluenza virus, respiratory syncytial virus, and coxsackievirus.

Clinical Findings

The patient usually experiences a sudden onset of clear or mucoid rhinorrhea, nasal congestion, and fever. Mild sore throat and cough may also develop. Although the fever is usually low-grade in older children, in the first 5 or 6 years of life it can be as high as 40.6 °C without superinfection. The nose, throat, and tympanic membrane can appear red and inflamed.

The primary physician can use the following guidelines when screening children with a cold for elective surgery: Surgery is usually postponed if fever or cough is present. Surgery can proceed if the child has only a runny nose, sore throat, or ear infection. If anesthesia does not require intubation, surgery may be permitted even if the child has a cough, provided that findings on chest radiograph are normal.

Treatment

Treatment for the common cold is largely symptomatic. Acetaminophen or ibuprofen is helpful for fever, sore throat, or muscle aches. A stuffy, congested nose can be treated with normal saline nose drops (mix ¼ tsp table salt with 6 oz of water), 3 drops in each nostril. After several minutes, a suction bulb can be used to remove the secretions of the infant unable to blow the nose. If this procedure fails after several attempts and the stuffy nose still interferes with feeding or sleep, consider long-acting xylometazoline (Otrivin) or oxymetazoline (Afrin) 0.05% nose drops. Drops should be used only when the nose is congested and discontinued within 5 days to prevent rebound chemical rhinitis.

Antihistamines are not effective in relieving cold symptoms. In rhinoviral colds, increased levels of histamine are not observed. Antibiotics do not prevent superinfection and should not be used. Codeine and dextromethorphan should be discouraged because they do not alleviate the symptoms of acute cough. Parents should be instructed that fast breathing or difficult breathing with retraction are signs of a lower respiratory infection such as bronchiolitis or pneumonia.

Hutton N et al: Effectiveness of an antihistamine-decongestant combination for young children with the common cold: A randomized, controlled clinical trial. J Pediatr 1991;118:125.

Taylor JA et al: Efficacy of cough suppressants in children. J Pediatr 1993;122:799.

SINUSITIS

1. ACUTE SINUSITIS

General Considerations

Acute bacterial infection of the paranasal sinuses is called sinusitis. The maxillary and ethmoidal sinuses are most commonly involved when mucociliary clearance and drainage are impaired by an upper respiratory infection or allergic rhinitis. The ethmoid sinus is the only one that is significantly developed at birth. The maxillary sinus is rudimentary at birth and visible on x-ray film by 6 months. The frontal sinus is not visible until the child is 3–9 years of age. Clinical ethmoiditis does not usually occur until 6 months of age. About 50% of cases occur between 1 and 5 years of age, during which time the most common presenting sign is periorbital cellulitis. Maxillary sinusitis is seen clinically after 1 year of age. Frontal sinusitis is unusual before 10 years of age.

The pathogens that cause acute sinusitis are usually *S pneumoniae, H influenzae* (nontypable), *M catarrhalis,* and β-hemolytic streptococci. Rarely, anaerobic bacterial infections can cause fulminant frontal sinusitis. Viruses can be isolated in 10% of sinus aspirates, but their pathogenic role is unclear.

Clinical Findings

The clinical presentation of acute sinusitis in children may be either gradual or sudden. With the gradual presentation, nasal discharge or postnasal drip and daytime cough persist longer than 10 days. In addition, a low-grade fever is often present in association with malodorous breath or intermittent, painless morning periorbital swelling. Older patients may complain of a headache, a sense of facial fullness, or facial pain overlying the involved sinus. With the more sudden toxic presentation, the patient presents with a high fever and more severe pain or periorbital inflammation. Ethmoiditis causes retro-orbital pain; maxillary sinusitis causes upper molar or zygomatic pain; and frontal sinusitis causes pain above the eyebrow.

Physical examination reveals inflamed nasal mucosa, usually associated with nasal or postnasal mucopurulent discharge. Occasionally, there is percussion tenderness overlying the sinusitis. In ethmoiditis, the tenderness is elicited by pressing medially on the inner canthus of the eye. Tenderness of the eyeball may also be present. Maxillary sinusitis reveals percussion tenderness on the maxillary bone. Frontal sinusitis reveals percussion tenderness when the physician presses upward on the floor of the supraorbital ridge. Periorbital swelling or mild discoloration may be present. The examination should identify exudative tonsillitis, a nasal foreign body, or dental caries and poor dental hygiene. Transillumination of the sinuses is difficult to perform and not very helpful unless it is grossly asymmetric.

Consider a sinus aspiration for diagnostic purposes in patients with complications and in those with an immunosuppressive disease. Gram's stain or culture of nasal discharge does not correlate with cultures of sinus aspirates. If the patient is hospitalized because of complications, a blood culture should be obtained.

Imaging studies of the paranasal sinuses during an acute illness are not indicated except for the evaluation of complications. In the past, plain radiography was used to diagnose sinusitis when an air-fluid level or mucosal thickening greater than 4 mm is seen. Because of the cost of CT scanning, CT should be ordered in children with complications or lack of resolution following adequate antibiotic therapy. Findings consistent with sinusitis may be found in asymptomatic patients with colds or nasal allergies. Because of sensitivity and specificity issues relating to plain radiography, CT scans are generally used in younger children and plain radiographs are reserved for older children and adolescents.

Complications

The most common paranasal sinus to develop complications is the ethmoid sinus. Complications of ethmoiditis represent a continuum beginning with preseptal cellulitis. More serious complications include postseptal cellulitis, subperiosteal abscess, orbital abscess, and cavernous sinus thrombosis. These complications are associated with decreased extraocular movement, proptosis, chemosis, and altered visual acuity. The most common complication of frontal sinusitis is osteitis of the frontal bone, (Pott's puffy tumor). Intracranial extension leads to meningitis, epidural, subdural, and brain abscesses. The most common maxillary complication is cellulitis of the cheek. Rarely, osteomyelitis of the maxilla can develop.

Treatment

Patients with evidence of invasive infection or any central nervous system complications should be immediately hospitalized. Intravenous therapy with nafcillin or clindamycin, plus a third-generation cephalosporin such as cefotaxime should be initiated until culture results become available. Treat less severe cases of acute sinusitis with oral antibiotics for 10 days. Continue antibiotic treatment for another week if the patient has improved but is not totally asymptomatic. The usual antibiotic is amoxicillin, 15 mg/kg, three times per day. In areas where β-lactamase-positive pathogens are common or when the patient is allergic to penicillin, use trimethoprim-sulfamethoxazole, 5 mg/kg/dose twice daily, or erythromycin plus sulfamethoxazole, 10 mg/kg/dose three to four times daily. Additional possibilities include third-generation cephalosporins, amoxicillin-clavulanate, or clarithromycin. Failure to improve after 48 hours suggests a resistant organism or potential complication and is an indication to admit for parenteral therapy.

Topical decongestants and oral combinations are frequently used in acute sinusitis to promote drainage. Their effectiveness has not been proved, and concern has been raised about potential adverse effects related to impaired ciliary function, decreased blood flow to the mucosa, and reduced diffusion of antibiotic into the sinuses. Patients with underlying allergic rhinitis may benefit from intranasal cromolyn or corticosteroid nasal spray. Vasoconstrictor nose drops and spray are associated with rebound edema if used for more than 5–7 days.

Pain Management: A patient may require acetaminophen, ibuprofen, or occasionally even codeine temporarily to permit sleep until drainage of the obstructed sinus is achieved. The application of ice over the sinus may help to relieve pain.

2. RECURRENT OR CHRONIC SINUSITIS

Chronic or frequent episodes of sinusitis occur in a small group of patients. Recurrent and chronic sinusitis in infant and young children may be related to daycare attendance. Important factors to consider include allergies, anatomy, and host immunity. Mucosal inflammation leading to obstruction is most commonly caused by allergic rhinitis and occasionally is the result of nonallergic rhinitis. Rarely, chronic sinusitis is caused by anatomic variations such as septal deviation, polyp, or foreign body. In cases of chronic or recurrent pyogenic pansinusitis, poor host resistance (eg, an immune defect, Kartagener's syndrome, or cystic fibrosis), though rare, must be ruled out by immunoglobulin studies, cilia studies, and a sweat chloride test. Anaerobic and staphylococcal organisms are often responsible for chronic sinusitis. Evaluation by an allergist and an otolaryngologist may be useful in determining the underlying causes.

Surgical Treatment

A. Antra Lavage: This is generally regarded as a diagnostic procedure but may have some therapeutic value. An aspirate or an irrigation of the fluid from the maxillary sinus is retrieved either with a spinal needle or a curved-tip instrument under anesthesia. In the very young child, this may be the only procedure that can be performed.

B. Endoscopic Sinus Surgery: This method of surgical intervention was popularized in the 1980s. No data are available comparing the outcome of this surgical intervention with traditional surgical procedures. There are large variations in use of this procedure by otolaryngologists, especially in younger patients.

C. External Drainage: External ethmoidectomy and fronto-ethmoidectomy are used to manage complications arising from ethmoiditis and frontal sinusitis.

Dunham ME: New light on sinusitis. Contemp Pediatr 1994;11:102.

Gwaltney JM et al: Computed tomographic study of the common cold N Engl J Med 1994;330:25.

Poole MD: Pediatric sinusitis is not a surgical disease. Ear Nose Throat J 1992;71:622.

Wald ER: Sinusitis in children. N Engl J Med 1992; 326:319.

Wald ER: Purulent nasal discharge. Pediatr Infect Dis J 1991;10:329.

3. CHOANAL ATRESIA

Choanal atresia occurs bilaterally in 25% of affected children and unilaterally in 75%. Bilateral cases causes severe respiratory distress at birth. Unilateral atresia generally presents with unilateral chronic nasal discharge. A No. 8 soft rubber catheter should be passed through the nose and visualized in the oropharynx. If this procedure cannot be accomplished, a diagnosis of choanal atresia should be confirmed by radiographic study. The clinician should consider CHARGE syndrome association when choanal atresia is encountered.

An oral airway should be used when a newborn has been diagnosed with bilateral choanal atresia. An otolaryngologist should be consulted for possible surgery to repair the atresia or bypass the upper airway obstruction. Unilateral atresia is generally not corrected until later in life.

4. RECURRENT RHINITIS

Recurrent rhinitis is frequently in the office practice of pediatrics. A child is brought in frequently with the chief complaint that he or she has "one cold after another," has "constant colds," or "is always sick." Approximately two thirds of these children have recurrent colds, and the remaining third has either allergic rhinitis or recurrent sinusitis.

Allergic Rhinitis

The onset of "hay fever" is usually after a child is 2 years of age and has had adequate exposure to allergens. There is no fever or contagion among close contacts. The attacks include frequent sneezing, rubbing of the nose, and a profuse clear discharge. The nasal turbinates are swollen. The nasal smear demonstrates over 20% of the cells to be eosinophils. Nasal secretions should be collected only when the patient is symptomatic. Between attacks or after receiving antihistamines, the eosinophil smear may be falsely negative. A full discussion of vasoconstrictor nose drops beyond 5–7 days results in a rebound reaction and secondary nasal congestion (rhinitis medicamentosa). The offending nose drops should be discontinued.

Vasomotor Rhinitis

Some children react to sudden changes in environmental temperature with prolonged congestion and rhinorrhea. Air pollution (especially tobacco smoke) may be a factor. Oral decongestants can be used periodically to give symptomatic relief.

EPISTAXIS

The nose is a very vascular structure. In most cases, epistaxis (nosebleed) is due to mild trauma to the anterior portion of the nasal septum (Kiesselbach's area) usually due to vigorous nose rubbing, nose blowing, or nose picking. Less than 5% of children with recurrent epistaxis have a bleeding disorder. Examination of Kiesselbach's area usually reveals a red, raw surface with fresh clots or old crusts. Look for telangiectasia, hemangiomas, or varicosities.

Most patients do not need a hematologic workup, but bleeding tests are indicated if any of the following is present: a family history of a bleeding disorder, a past medical history of easy bleeding, spontaneous bleeding at other sites, bleeding that lasts for over 30 minutes or will not clot with direct pressure by the physician, onset before age 2 years, or a drop in hematocrit due to epistaxis. High blood pressure may also predispose to prolonged nosebleeds.

A nasopharyngeal angiofibroma may present as recurrent epistaxis. Adolescent males are almost exclusively affected. CT scan of the nasal cavity and nasopharynx is diagnostic.

Treatment

The following approach can be carried out in the office or given as phone advice: The patient should sit up and lean forward so as not to swallow the blood. The nasal cavity should be cleared of clots by blowing. The soft part of the nose is pinched firm enough to elicit pain, with pressure over the bleeding site being maintained for 5 minutes by the clock. If bleeding continues, the bleeding site needs to be visualized. A small piece of gelatin sponge (Gelfoam) or collagen sponge (Surgicel) can be inserted over the bleeding site.

The friability of the nasal vessels can be decreased with daily application of either petroleum-based or water-based ointment by cotton-tipped applicator. The lubricant is applied daily until 5 days have passed without a nosebleed, then weekly for 1 month, environment, humidification of the patient's room may be helpful. Aspirin should be avoided, as should vigorous blowing of the nose.

NASAL FURUNCLE

A nasal furuncle is an infection of a hair follicle in the anterior nares. Hair plucking or nose picking can provide a route of entry. The most common organism is *S aureus*. The diagnosis is made by finding an exquisitely tender, firm, red lump in the anterior naris. Treatment includes dicloxacillin or cephalexin orally for 5 days to prevent spread. The lesion should be gently incised and drained as soon as it points, usually with a needle. Topical bacitracin ointment may be of additional value. Since this lesion is in the drainage area of the cavernous sinus, the patient should be followed up closely until healing is complete. Parents should be advised never to pick or squeeze a furuncle in this location, nor should the physician. Associated cellulitis or spread requires hospitalization for administration of intravenous antibiotics.

NASAL SEPTUM SUBLUXATION

Newborn infants rarely have subluxation of the quadrangular cartilage of the septum. The top of the nose deviates to one side, and the inferior septal border deviates to the other. There is also leaning of the columella and instability of the nasal tip. This disorder must be distinguished from the more common transient flattening of the nose caused by the birth process. In the past, physicians were encouraged to reduce all subluxations in the nursery. Otolaryngologists are more likely to perform the reduction under anesthesia for the more difficult cases.

NASAL FRACTURE

Most blows to the nose result in swallowing and hematoma without fracture. A persistent nosebleed after trauma, crepitus or instability of the bones in the nasal bridge, and marked deviation of the nose to one side indicate a fracture. However, septal injury can be ruled out only by careful intranasal examination. Patients with suspected nasal fractures should referred to an otolaryngologist for definitive therapy. Resetting of the nasal fracture can be postponed up to 1 week without causing difficulty.

NASAL SEPTUM HEMATOMA

After nasal trauma, it is essential to examine the inside of the nose with a nasal speculum. Hematoma of the nasal septum imposes a considerable risk of pressure necrosis and resorption of the cartilage, leading to septal perforation or a saddle-back nose in adulthood. This diagnosis is confirmed by the abrupt onset of nasal obstruction following trauma and the presence of a boggy, widened nasal septum. The normal nasal septum is 2–4 mm thick.

Treatment consists of prompt referral to an otolaryngologist for evacuation of the hematoma and packing of the nose.

NASAL SEPTUM ABSCESS

A nasal septal abscess usually follows nasal trauma or a nasal furuncle. Examination reveals a fluctuant gray septal swelling, usually bilateral. The possible complications are the same as for nasal septal hematoma as well as spread of the infection to the central nervous system. Treatment consists of immediate hospitalization and incision and drainage by an otolaryngologist.

FOREIGN BODIES IN THE NOSE

There are many ways to remove nasal foreign bodies. The obvious first maneuver is vigorous nose blowing if the child is old enough. The key to nasal foreign body removal is topical anesthesia, nasal decongestion, good lighting, correct instrumentation, and physical restraint. Topical pontacaine or lidocaine can be used in young children without aerodigestive tract compromise. Nasal decongestion can be achieved by topical pseudoephedrine or oxymetazoline. When the child is properly restrained, most nasal foreign bodies can be removed using a pair of alligator forceps through an operating head otoscope. If the object seems inaccessible, is wedged in, or is quite large, the patient should be referred to an otolaryngologist without worsening its position through futile attempts.

THE THROAT

ACUTE STOMATITIS

Recurrent Aphthous Stomatitis ("Canker Sore")

The main finding is single (two or three at most) small (3–10 mm) ulcers on the inside of the lips and throughout the remainder of the mouth. There is usually no associated fever or cervical adenopathy. The ulcers are very painful and last 1–2 weeks. They may recur numerous times throughout a patient's lifespan. The cause is not known, although an allergic or autoimmune basis is suspected.

Treatment consists of coating the lesions with topical antacid or sucralfate four times daily. Topical corticosteroids, either in a dental paste, such as triamcinolone acetonide 0.1% (Kenalog in Orabase), or in a mouthwash administered four times daily also have efficacy. Pain can be symptomatically improved by a bland diet, avoiding salty or acid foods, switching from a bottle to a cup in infants, giving 2% viscous lidocaine prior to meals, and giving acetaminophen or even codeine at bedtime. If the child is not old enough to expectorate the lidocaine, it must not be used.

Herpes Simplex Gingivostomatitis

Approximately 1% of children who have their first encounter with the herpes simplex virus develop multiple (10 or more) small (1–3 mm) ulcers of the buccal mucosa, anterior pillars, inner lips, tongue, and especially the gingiva. The lesions are often associated with fever, tender cervical nodes, and generalized inflammation of the mouth. Affected children are commonly under 3 years of age. Herpes Simplex gingivostomatitis lasts 7–10 days. Severe dysphagia interferes with eating and drinking. Treatment is symptomatic as described for recurrent aphthous stomatitis (see earlier), with the exception that corticosteroids are contraindicated because they may result in spread of the infection. Early in the course, consider prescribing acyclovir suspension (200 mg/5 mL), 10 mg/kg/dose three times daily for 7 days. The patient must be followed up closely. Dehydration occasionally ensues despite liberal offerings of cold fluids, in which case the patient must be hospitalized so that the intravenous fluids can be administered. Herpetic laryngotracheitis is a rare complication.

Thrush

Oral candidiasis mainly affects infants and occasionally older children in a debilitated state. *Candida albicans* is a saprophyte that normally is not invasive unless the mouth is abraded. The use of broad-spectrum antibiotics may be a contributing factor. The symptoms include soreness of the mouth and refusal of feedings. Lesions consist of white curd-like plaques predominantly on the buccal mucosa. These plaques cannot be washed away after a water feeding.

Specific treatment consists of use of nystatin (Mycostatin) oral suspension, 1 mL four times daily for 1 week. This should be preceded by attempts to remove any large plaques with a moistened cotton-tipped applicator or piece of gauze.

Traumatic Oral Ulcers

Ulcers are a nonspecific response of the oral mucosa to trauma. Mechanical trauma most commonly occurs on the buccal mucosa secondary to accidentally biting it with the molars. Thermal trauma, as from very hot foods, can also cause ulcerative lesions. Chemical ulcers can be produced by mucosal contact with aspirin, caustics, and the like. Oral ulcers can also occur with leukemia or on a recurrent basis with cyclic neutropenia. These lesions usually need no treatment. The pain subsides in 2 or 3 days.

ACUTE VIRAL PHARYNGITIS & TONSILLITIS

More than 90% of cases of sore throat and fever in children are due to viral infections. Most children develop associated rhinorrhea and mild cough. The findings seldom give any clue to the particular viral agent, but six types of viral pharyngitis are sufficiently distinctive to support an educated guess about the specific cause.

Clinical Findings

A. Infectious Mononucleosis: The findings are an exudative tonsillitis, generalized cervical adenitis, and fever, usually in a teenage patient. A palpable spleen or axillary adenopathy adds weight to the diagnosis. The presence of more than 20% atypical lymphocytes on a peripheral blood smear or a positive mononucleosis spot test (Monospot) confirms the diagnosis, although the Monospot is fre-

quently negative in children under 5 years old. This diagnosis is often not considered until a patient with a presumptive diagnosis of streptococcal pharyngitis has failed to respond to 48 hours of treatment with penicillin.

B. Herpangina: Herpangina ulcers, 2–3 mm in size, are found on the anterior pillars and sometimes on the soft palate and uvula. There are no ulcers in the anterior mouth, as there are in herpes simplex. Herpangina is caused by several members of the coxsackie A group of viruses, and a patient can have up to five bouts of herpangina in a lifetime.

C. Lymphonodular Pharyngitis: The classic finding is small, yellow-white nodules in the same distribution as the small ulcers in herpangina. In this condition, which is caused by coxsackievirus A10, the nodules do not ulcerate.

D. Hand, Foot, and Mouth Disease: This entity is caused by coxsackieviruses A5, A10, and A16. Ulcers occur on the tongue and oral mucosa. Vesicles, which usually do not ulcerate, are found on the palms, soles, and interdigital areas.

E. Pharyngoconjunctival Fever: This disorder is caused by an adenovirus. Exudative tonsillitis, conjunctivitis, and fever are the main findings.

F. Rubeola: The prodrome of measles looks like any nonspecific viral respiratory infection until one closely examines the buccal mucosa and the inner aspects of the lower lip. Small white specks the size of salt granules on an erythematous base (Koplik's spots) found at these sites are pathognomonic of early measles.

Treatment

The treatment of acute viral pharyngitis is strictly symptomatic. Older children can gargle with warm saline solution or antacid solution (eg, Mylanta). Younger children can suck on hard candy (especially butterscotch). Analgesics and antipyretics are sometimes helpful. Antibiotics are not helpful.

McMillan JA et al: Pharyngitis associated with herpes simplex virus in college students. Pediatr Infect Dis J 1993; 12:280.
Nakayama M et al: Pharyngoconjunctival fever caused by adenovirus type 11. Pediatr Infect Dis J 1992;11:6.

ACUTE STREPTOCOCCAL PHARYNGITIS & TONSILLITIS

Approximately 10% of children with sore throat and fever have a streptococcal infection. Untreated streptococcal pharyngitis can result in acute rheumatic fever, glomerulonephritis, and suppurative complications (eg, cervical adenitis, peritonsillar abscess, otitis media, cellulitis, and septicemia). Vesicles and ulcers are suggestive of viral infection, whereas cervical adenitis, petechiae, a beefy-red

uvula, and a tonsillar exudate are suggestive of streptococcal infection; the only way to make a definitive
diagnosis is by obtaining a throat culture or a rapid
identification test. Rapid identification tests are very
specific but lack sensitivity. Therefore, a positive test
indicates infection, but a negative result requires confirmation with culture.

Treat cases of suspected or proved *S pyogenes* infection with a 10-day course of oral penicillin V potassium or cephalosporin such as cephalexin, or an
intramuscular injection of penicillin G benzathine.
Use erythromycin for patients with penicillin allergy.
Treatment failure after 10 days of penicillin V administered three times daily varies from 6% to 23%.
The small difference between the cure rates of penicillin and cephalosporins reported in the literature
may result from eradication of the carrier state rather
than treatment failures. Causes of treatment failure
include unrecognized carriers, poor compliance,
reacquisition of a different strain, inactivation of
penicillin by β-lactamase, or the development of tolerance by *S pyogenes*. Approximately 5% of *S pyogenes* are resistant to erythromycin. Remember that
trimethoprim-sulfamethoxazole is not an effective
antibiotic for *S pyogenes*. Children should receive 24
hours of therapy prior to returning to school.

If the child has a history of recurrent streptococcal
infection, one must document the presence of *S pyogenes* in an asymptomatic patient following a course
of therapy. If compliance or the antibiotic dosage
was questionable, treat with intramuscular penicillin;
otherwise treat with an antibiotic effective against
β-lactamase-producing organisms (amoxicillin plus
clavulanate, a cephalosporin, or erythromycin). If
this therapy fails to eradicate the organism, consider
a course of clindamycin for 10 days.

In general, the carrier state is harmless, not contagious, and self-limited (2–6 months). An attempt to
eradicate the carrier state is warranted only if the patient or another family member has frequent streptococcal infections or when a family member or patient
has a history of rheumatic fever or glomerulonephritis.

Also consider treatment for carriers who live in
closed or semiclosed community settings. If the patient had three or more documented infections within
6 months, consider instituting daily penicillin prophylaxis during the winter season. Refer patients for
tonsillectomy only when they continue to have frequent episodes or when persistently enlarged tonsils
cause chronic upper airway obstruction.

Other rare causes of acute nonviral pharyngitis are
Corynebacterium diphtheriae, Neisseria gonorrhoea,
group C streptococci, meningococci, *Chlamydia,
Francisella tularensis,* and *Mycoplasma pneumoniae.*

Denny FW: Tonsillopharyngitis 1994. Pediatr Rev 1994;
15:185.

Deutsch ES, Esaacson GC: Tonsils and adenoids: An update. Pediatr Rev 1995;16:17.
Pichiechero ME: Cephalosporins are superior to penicillin
for the treatment of streptococcal tonsillopharyngitis: Is
the difference worth it? Pediatr Infect Dis J 1993;
12:268.
Pichiechero ME et al: Comparative reliability of clinical,
culture, and antigen detection methods for the diagnosis
of group A beta-hemolytic streptococcal tonsillopharyngitis. Pediatr Ann 1992;21:798.

RECURRENT PHARYNGITIS

School-age children are occasionally brought to a
physician with a complaint of recurrent or persistent
sore throat. Fever and other systemic manifestations
are usually absent. There are three common causes of
this problem: mouth breathing, postnasal drip, and
school phobia.

Mouth breathing leads to dryness and irritation
of the throat, especially in areas of low humidity. Occasionally, children complain even upon awakening
that their lips are stuck to their teeth. The causes of
mouth breathing should be investigated. Symptomatic treatment consists of good hydration and environmental humidification.

Postnasal drip due to chronic sinusitis can lead to
continuous irritation of the throat. Examination reveals mucopurulent secretions descending from the
nasopharynx after the patient sniffs. The irritation is
largely due to repeated clearing of the throat.

Children with **school attendance problems** are
brought in repeatedly for sore throats, but physical
examination reveals a normal oropharynx and tonsillar area. The diagnosis is made by asking the parent
if the problem has been interfering with the child's
school attendance. The answer will be affirmative
and completely out of keeping with the degree of
symptoms. Management is described in Chapter 6.

Tanz RR et al: Clindamycin treatment of chronic pharyngeal carriage of group A streptococci. J Pediatr 1991;
119:123.

PERITONSILLAR CELLULITIS
OR ABSCESS
(Quinsy)

Tonsillar infection occasionally penetrates the tonsillar capsule, spreads to the surrounding tissues, and
causes peritonsillar cellulitis. If untreated, necrosis
occurs and a tonsillar abscess forms. This can occur
at any age. The most common cause is β-hemolytic
streptococci. Other pathogens are group D streptococci, α-hemolytic streptococci, *S pneumoniae,* and
anaerobes.

The patient complains of a severe sore throat even
before the physical findings become marked. A high

fever is usually present. The process is almost always unilateral. The tonsil bulges medially, and the anterior pillar is prominent. The soft palate and uvula on the involved side are edematous and displaced medially toward the uninvolved side. In severe cases, trismus, dysphagia, and, finally, drooling occur. The quality of the serious complication of inadequately treated peritonsillar abscess is a lateral pharyngeal abscess. This leads to fullness and tenderness of the lateral neck, as well as torticollis. Without intervention, the abscess eventually threatens life by airway obstruction or carotid artery erosion.

Frequently, it is clinically difficult to differentiate peritonsillar cellulitis from abscess. In adolescents, it is possible to aspirate the peritonsillar space to arrive at the diagnosis. However, it is reasonable to admit a child for 12–24 hours of intravenous antimicrobial therapy, since aggressive treatment in early cases of peritonsillar cellulitis usually aborts the process and prevents suppuration. The choice of parenteral therapy includes procaine penicillin and clindamycin. Failure to respond to therapy during the first 12–24 hours indicates the high probability of an abscess formation. An otolaryngologist should be consulted for incision and drainage under general anesthesia.

Recurrent peritonsillar abscesses are so uncommon (7%) that routine tonsillectomy for a single bout is not indicated. Hospitalized patients can be discharged on oral antibiotics when fever is resolved for 24 hours and they can swallow easily.

RETROPHARYNGEAL ABSCESS

Retropharyngeal nodes drain the adenoids, nasopharynx, and paranasal sinuses and can become infected. The most common causes are β-hemolytic streptococci and *S aureus*. If this pyogenic adenitis goes untreated, a retropharyngeal abscess forms. The process occurs most commonly during the first 2 years of life. Beyond this age, retropharyngeal abscess usually results from superinfection of a penetrating injury of the posterior wall of the oropharynx.

The diagnosis of retropharyngeal abscess should be strongly suspected in an infant with fever, respiratory symptoms, and neck hyperextension. Dysphagia, drooling, dyspnea, and gurgling respirations are also found and are due to impingement by the abscess. Prominent swelling on one side of the posterior pharyngeal wall confirms the diagnosis. Swelling usually stops at the midline because a medial raphe divides the prevertebral space. Lateral neck soft tissue films show the retropharyngeal space to be wider than the C4 vertebral body.

Although retropharyngeal abscess is a surgical emergency, frequently it cannot be distinguished from retropharyngeal adenitis. Immediate hospitalization and intravenous antimicrobial with a semisynthetic penicillin or clindamycin is the first step for

most cases. Immediate surgical drainage is required when a definite abscess is seen radiographically or when the airway is markedly compromised. In most instances, a period of 12–24 hours of antimicrobial therapy will help to differentiate the two entities. In the child with adenitis, fever will decrease and oral intake will increase. A child with retropharyngeal abscess will continue to deteriorate. A surgeon should incise and drain the abscess under general anesthesia to prevent its extension. The head should be kept down during incision to prevent aspiration of purulent material.

LUDWIG'S ANGINA

Ludwig's angina is a rapidly progressive cellulitis of the submandibular space. The submandibular space extends from the mucous membrane of the tongue to the muscular and fascial attachments of the hyoid bone. It is infrequently encountered in infants and children. The initiating factor in over 50% of cases is dental disease, including abscesses and extraction. Some patients have a history of lacerations and injuries to the floor of the mouth. Group A streptococci are the most common organisms identified, but other pathogens have been recovered.

The presenting symptoms are fever and tender swelling of the floor of the mouth. The tongue can become enlarged as well as tender and erythematous. Upward displacement of the tongue may cause dysphagia and drooling. Laboratory evaluation includes blood cultures and hypopharyngeal aspiration to attempt to identify the specific pathogen.

Treatment consists of giving high doses of intravenous clindamycin or ampicillin plus nafcillin until the results of cultures and sensitivity tests are available. Because the most common cause of death in Ludwig's angina is sudden airway obstruction, the patient must be monitored closely in the intensive care unit and intubation provided for progressive respiratory distress. Consult an otolaryngologist to identify and perform a drainage procedure.

ACUTE CERVICAL ADENITIS

General Considerations

Local infections of the ear, nose, and throat can spread to a regional node and cause a secondary inflammation there. The most commonly involved node is the jugulodigastric node, which drains the tonsillar area. The problem is most prevalent among preschool children.

A classic case involves a large, unilateral, solitary, tender node. About 70% of these cases are due to β-hemolytic streptococci, 20% are due to staphylococci, and the remainder may be due to viruses. *H influenzae* type B or anaerobes have rarely been reported as a cause. Surgeons report a higher incidence of staphylococcal infection except in newborns, but they see a greater proportion of atypical cases that have failed to respond to penicillin therapy and thus require incision and drainage.

The most common cause of invasion is from pharyngitis or tonsillitis. Other entry sites for pyogenic adenitis include periapical dental abscess (usually producing a submandibular adenitis), facial impetigo (infected cuts or bug bites), infected acne, and otitis externa (usually producing a preauricular adenitis).

Early treatment with antibiotics prevents many cases of pyogenic adenitis from progressing to suppuration. However, once fluctuation occurs, antibiotic therapy alone is not sufficient. When fluctuation or pointing is present and the purified protein derivative (PPD) skin test is negative, needle aspiration may promote resolution and surgery may not be needed. If not, the surgeon should incise and drain the abscess. Hospitalization is required only if the patient is toxic, dehydrated, dysphagic, dyspneic, or younger than 6 months of age.

Differential Diagnosis

A. Cat-Scratch Fever: Cat-scratch fever is frequently implicated in cases of chronic cervical adenopathy. The diagnosis is aided by the finding of a primary papule in approximately 61% of cases. in over 90% of cases, cat scratches are present or there is a history of contact with cats. The node is usually mildly tender. The cat-scratch skin test is helpful and relatively safe. Cat-scratch disease, caused by a pleomorphic gram-negative bacillus called *Afipia felis,* can be treated orally with rifampin (87% efficacy), ciprofloxacin (84% efficacy), or trimethoprim-sulfamethoxazole (58% efficacy). Intramuscular gentamicin is an acceptable alternative, which is about 73% effective.

B. Atypical Mycobacterial Infection: Cervical lymphadenitis can be caused by nontuberculous or atypical mycobacterium. The adenitis is often unilateral and indolent, developing over a prolonged period of time without systemic signs or much local pain. Atypical mycobacterial infections are often associated with PPD skin reactions less then 10 mm. A positive PPD can cause confusion regarding the possibility of tuberculosis. Fluctuant cervical nodes should be aspirated for Gram's stain and culture. Although treatment usually involves surgical excision, therapy with clarithromycin or rifampin may be tried.

C. Malignancy and Cervical Nodes: Malignant tumors usually are not suspected until the adenopathy persist despite treatment. Classically, the nodes are painless, nontender, and firm to hard in consistency. They may be fixed to underlying tissues. These nodes may occur as a single node, as unilateral multiple nodes in a chain, as bilateral cervical nodes, or as generalized adenopathy. Common malignancies

that may present in the neck include Hodgkin's disease, non-Hodgkin's lymphoma, rhabdomyosarcoma, and thyroid carcinoma.

D. Imitators of Adenitis: Several structures in the neck can become infected and resemble a node. The first three masses are of congenital origin and are listed in order of frequency.

1. Thyroglossal duct cyst–When superinfected, this congenital malformation can become acutely swollen. Helpful findings are the fact that it is in the midline, located between the hyoid bone and suprasternal notch, and moves upward when the tongue is stuck out or during swallowing. Occasionally, the cyst develops a sinus tract and opening just lateral to the midline.

2. Branchial cleft cyst–When superinfected, this can become a tender mass 3–5 cm in diameter. Aids to diagnosis are the fact that the mass is located along the anterior border of the sternocleidomastoid muscle and is smooth and fluctuant, as a cyst should be. Occasionally, it is attached to the overlying skin by a small dimple or a draining sinus tract.

3. Cystic hygroma–Most of these lymphatic cysts are located in the posterior triangle just above the clavicle. The mass is soft and compressible and can be transilluminated. Over 60% of hygromas are noted at birth, and the remainder are usually seen by the time the child is 2 years of age. If cysts become large enough, they can compromise swallowing and breathing.

4. Parotitis–The most common pitfall in differential diagnosis of cervical adenopathy is mistaking parotitis for adenitis. However, a swollen parotid crosses the angle of the jaw, is associated with preauricular percussion tenderness, is bilateral in 70% of cases, and there may frequently be a history of exposure to mumps and no mumps immunization. Submandibular parotitis can present a diagnostic dilemma.

5. Ranula–A ranula is a cyst in the floor of the mouth caused by obstruction of the ducts of the sublingual gland. A plunging ranula extends below the mylohyoid muscle and can present as a neck mass.

6. Sternocleidomastoid muscle hematoma–This cervical mass is noted at 2–4 weeks of age. On close examination, it is found to be part of the muscle body and not movable. An associated torticollis is usually confirmatory.

Gorenstein A, Somekh E: Suppurative cervical lymphadenitis: Treatment by needle aspirations. Pediatr Infect Dis J 1994;7:669.

Huebner RE et al: Usefulness of skin testing with mycobacterial antigens in children with cervical lymphadenopathy. Pediatr Infect Dis J 1992;11:450.

Margileth AM: Antibiotic therapy for cat-scratch disease: Clinical study of therapeutic outcome of 268 patients and a review of the literature. Pediatr Infect Dis J 1992;11:474.

SNORING, MOUTH BREATHING, & UPPER AIRWAY OBSTRUCTION

A child is sometimes brought in with the complaint that "he always breathes through his mouth," "he snores," "he can't sleep at night." When the severity of the snoring is in doubt, an audiotape or videotape during sleep may help. However, it cannot be used to accurately document the frequency and severity of upper airway obstruction.

Differential Diagnosis

A. Large Adenoids: Large adenoids can be suspected if the typical "adenoid facies" is encountered. The adenoids can be assessed by mirror examination, endoscopy or by radiographic studies.

B. Allergic Rhinitis: Severe cases of allergic rhinitis present like any other causes of nasal obstruction. History and physical examination will assist in the diagnosis.

C. Nasal Polyps: Polyps appear as glistening, gray to pink, jelly-like masses that are prominent just inside the anterior nares and occur singly or in clusters. They occur in cystic fibrosis and severe allergic rhinitis. Do not mistake the turbinates for polyps.

D. Other Causes: Persistent mouth breathing may be due to obstruction by nasopharyngeal tumor or by meningocele or encephalocele herniated into the nasal cavity. If unilateral nasal obstruction and epistaxis are frequent, juvenile angiofibroma should be suspected.

Diagnosis

A lateral neck radiograph or fiberoptic nasopharyngoscopy will help assess the relative size of the adenoids. When episodes of hypopnea or obstructive apnea, failure to thrive, or clinical signs of cardiac disease are present, a chest radiograph and electrocardiogram should be obtained. Children with severe snoring may also develop obstructive sleep apnea or hypopnea, which can be identified by a sleep study polysomnogram. **Obstructive apnea** is defined as periods when air flow stops for 6–10 seconds associated with respiratory effort or bradycardia or oxygen desaturation or termination with gasping and agitated arousal. Hypopnea is defined as loud snoring during sleep with periods of reduced airflow for 10 seconds or longer associated with oxygen desaturation or arousal. These are definitions for adults, since criteria for children are not established. A sleep study polysomnogram measures heart rate, oxygen saturation, oronasal airflow, chest wall movement, carbon dioxide, electrocardiogram, and electroencephalogram waves. Absent oronasal airflow with the presence of chest wall movement, oxygen desaturation, and bradycardia indicates obstruction sleep apnea.

Demain JG, Goetz DW: Pediatr adenoidal hypertrophy and nasal airway obstruction. Otolaryngol Head Neck Surg 1991;105:427.

Everett AD, Koch WC, Saulsbury FT: Failure to thrive due to obstructive sleep apnea. Clin Pediatr 1987;26:90.

TONSILLECTOMY & ADENOIDECTOMY (T&A)

Indications

The following conditions are indications for tonsillectomy with or without adenoidectomy: pulmonary conditions such as chronic hypoxia related to upper airway obstruction or hypopnea/obstructive sleep apnea, oral facial conditions such as mandibular growth abnormalities, dental malocclusion and swallowing disorders, speech abnormalities, and persistent or recurrent infections.

Chronic hypoxia related to upper airway obstruction can result in signs of right heart failure (cor pulmonale) or pulmonary hypertension. Obstructive sleep apnea presents with loud snoring during sleep with periods of respiratory pauses terminated with gasping and agitated arousal. In young children, sleep apnea should not be confused with restless sleep patterns, trained night feeders, and trained night crying. There is no consensus on the infectious criteria for tonsillectomy. Reasonable indications are four or more documented *S pyogenes* infections per year, documented *S pyogenes* carrier resistant to medical therapy, or six or more tonsillitis episodes per year or five or more per year for 2 years.

Adenoidectomy

The adenoids, composed of lymphoid tissue in the nasopharynx, are a component of Waldeyer's ring of lymphoid tissue with the palatine tonsils and lingual tonsils. Enlargement of the adenoids with or without infection can obstruct the upper airway, alter normal orofacial growth, and interfere with speech, swallowing, or the eustachian tube. Most children with prolonged mouth breathing eventually develop dental malocclusion and what has been termed an adenoidal facies. The face is pinched and the maxilla narrowed because the molding pressures of the orbicularis oris and buccinator muscles are unopposed by the tongue. The role of hypertrophy and chronic infection in the pathogenesis of sinusitis is unclear.

Indications

Indications for adenoidectomy with or without tonsillectomy include pulmonary conditions such as chronic hypoxia related to upper airway obstruction or hypopnea/obstructive sleep apnea; orofacial conditions such as mandibular growth abnormalities, dental malocclusion, and swallowing disorders; speech abnormalities, and persistent middle ear effusion.

Children with suspected velopharyngeal insufficiency such as those with cleft palate should not have an adenoidectomy except when there is a life-threatening obstruction.

Complications of T&A

The mortality rate associated with T&A varies from 0.004% to 0.006%; the rate of hemorrhage has been reported to vary from 0.49% to 4%. Some children with previously normal speech develop hypernasal speech. The emotional hazards of hospitalization and surgery in a child under 5 years of age have been well documented.

Contraindications to T&A

A. Short Palate: Adenoids should not be removed in a child with a cleft palate or submucous cleft palate, because of the risk of aggravating the velopharyngeal incompetence and causing hypernasal speech and nasal regurgitation. Occasionally, a "modified" adenoidectomy is performed in a child with marked obstructive sleep apnea who has a submucous cleft palate.

B. Bleeding Disorder: If a chronic bleeding disorder is present, it must be diagnosed and compensated for before T&A.

C. Acute Tonsillitis: A routine T&A should be postponed until an acute tonsillitis is resolved. This guideline may prevent superinfection of the wound.

Deutsch ES, Isaacson GC: Tonsils and adenoids: An update. Pediatr Rev 1995;16:17.

Paradise JL et al: Efficacy of tonsillectomy for recurrent throat infection in severely affected children. N Engl J Med 1984;310:674.

DISORDERS OF THE LIPS

Labial Sucking Tubercle

A small baby may present with a small callus in the mid upper lip. It usually is asymptomatic and disappears after cup feeding is initiated.

Cheilitis

Dry, cracked, scaling lips are usually due to sun or wind exposure. Contact dermatitis from mouthpieces or various woodwind or brass instruments has also been reported. Licking the lips accentuates the process, and the patient should be warned of this. Liberal use of lip balms gives excellent results.

Inclusion Cyst

Inclusion cysts, or retention cysts, are due to the obstruction of mucous glands or other mucous membrane structures. In the newborn, they occur on the hard palate or gums and are called Epstein's pearls. These small cysts resolve spontaneously in 1–2 months. In older children, inclusion cysts usually oc-

cur on the palate, uvula, or tonsillar pillars. They appear as taut, yellow sacs varying in size from 2 mm to 10 mm. Inclusion cysts that do not spontaneously resolve should undergo incision and drainage. Occasionally, a mucous cyst on the lower lip (mucocele) requires drainage for cosmetic reasons. Minor salivary glands are present at this site, and biting the lip may sever their ducts and initiate the problem.

DISORDERS OF THE TONGUE

Geographic Tongue (Benign Migratory Glossitis)

This condition of unknown cause is marked by circular or elliptical smooth areas on the tongue devoid of papillae and surrounded by a narrow ring of hyperkeratosis. The pattern can change from day to day. The lesions are painless and may last months to years. This puzzling disorder is benign, uncommon after age 6, and requires no treatment.

Fissured Tongue (Scrotal Tongue)

This condition is marked by numerous irregular fissures on the dorsum of the tongue. It occurs in approximately 1% of the population and is usually a dominant trait. It is also frequently seen in children with trisomy 21 and other retarded patients who have the habit of chewing on a protruded tongue.

Coated Tongue (Furry Tongue)

The tongue normally becomes coated if mastication is impaired and the patient is on a liquid or soft diet. Mouth breathing, fever, or dehydration can accentuate the process.

Macroglossia

Tongue hypertrophy and protrusion may be a clue to Beckwith-Wiedemann syndrome, glycogen storage disease, cretinism, Hurler's syndrome, lymphangioma, or hemangioma. Tongue reduction procedures should be considered in otherwise healthy subjects when macroglossia affects airway patency, eating, dental development, and normal mandibular growth. In trisomy 21, the normal-sized tongue protrudes because the oral cavity is small.

HALITOSIS

"Bad breath" is a puzzling and distressing complaint. In most cases, it is due to acute stomatitis, pharyngitis, or sinusitis. In children, there are two common causes of chronic halitosis: continual mouth breathing and thumb sucking or blanket sucking. In older children and adolescents, halitosis can be part of the presenting symptoms of chronic sinusitis. Unusual diverticulum, gastric bezoar, bronchiectasis, and lung abscess. In older children, the presence of orthodontic devices or dentures can cause halitosis if good dental hygiene is not maintained. Halitosis can also be caused by decaying food particles that are embedded in cryptic tonsils. In adolescents, tobacco use is a common cause. Also, offensive skin odors (eg, dirty feet) of long duration can become absorbed and excreted through the lungs. Mouthwashes and chewable breath fresheners give limited improvement. The cause must be uncovered to help the patient with chronic halitosis.

SALIVARY GLAND DISORDERS

Suppurative Parotitis

Suppurative parotitis is an unusual clinical disorder found chiefly in newborns and debilitated older patients. The parotid gland is swollen, tender, and often reddened. The diagnosis is made by expression of purulent material from Stensen's duct. The material should be smeared and cultured. Fever and leukocytosis may be present.

Treatment includes hospitalization and intravenous nafcillin because the most common causative organism is *S aureus*.

Recurrent Idiopathic Parotitis

Some children experience repeated episodes of parotid swelling that lasts 1–2 weeks and then resolves spontaneously. There is usually mild pain and often no fever. The process is most often unilateral, a fact that argues against an autoimmune process as the underlying cause and suggests instead some sort of obstructive process. Serum amylase is normal, which speaks against a diagnosis of viral parotitis, as can occur with mumps, parainfluenza, and other viral infections. As many as 10 episodes may occur from age 2 years on. Antibiotic prophylaxis may reduce the number of episodes. The problem usually resolves spontaneously at puberty.

Treatment includes analgesics if pain is present. A 4-day course of corticosteroids can be recommended if it can be initiated early in an attack. A second attack of parotid swelling without fever should result in referral to an otolaryngologist for a sialogram to rule out calculus of Stensen's duct. The usual finding is sialectasia. The sialogram seems to improve as the recurrence rate diminishes.

Tumors of the Parotid

Mixed tumors, hemangiomas, and leukemia can present in the parotid gland as a hard or persistent mass. The patient should be referred to an oncologist and a surgeon.

Ranula

A ranula is a retention cyst of a sublingual salivary gland. It is found on the floor of the mouth to one side of the lingual frenulum. Ranula has been described as resembling a frog's belly because it is thin-walled and contains a clear bluish fluid. Referral to an otolaryngologist for excision of the cyst and associated sublingual gland is the treatment of choice.

ORAL CONGENITAL MALFORMATIONS

Tongue-Tie

The tightness of the lingual frenulum varies greatly among normal people. A short frenulum prevents both protrusion and elevation of the tongue. A puckering of the midline of the tongue occurs with tongue movement. The condition in no way interferes with the ability to speak, because even children with ankyloglossia have normal speech.

Treatment consists of reassurance. Although there is no evidence to support it, clipping of the frenulum is sometimes recommended if the tongue does not protrude beyond the teeth or gums. If this degree of tongue-tie is associated with impairment of rapid articulation, the patient should be referred to an otolaryngologist for correction. Casual frenulum clipping can result in significant bleeding.

Cleft Lip & Cleft Palate

Cleft lip, cleft palate, or both conditions are found in 1 in 800 live births. They are readily diagnosed in the newborn nursery. Treatment requires a multidisciplinary team approach—plastic surgeons, otolaryngologist, audiologists, speech therapists, orthodontists, and prosthodontists. Cleft lip repair is usually performed before 3 months of age. Cleft palate repair is usually performed at about 12 months of age—this is essential to permit normal speech development, which should begin at this time. Approximately 90% of children with cleft palate have recurrent or persistent otitis media and must be carefully followed up for this problem. Some otolaryngologists recommend prophylactic tympanoplasty tubes. See discussion in Chapter 32 for details of management of cleft lip and palate.

Bifid Uvula & Submucous Cleft Palate

A bifid uvula is present in 3% of healthy children. However, there is a close association (as high as 75%) between this and submucous cleft palate. A submucous cleft can be diagnosed by noting a translucent zone in the middle of the soft palate. Palpation of the hard palate reveals absence of the posterior bony portion. Affected children have a 40% risk of developing persistent middle ear effusion. They also are at risk of incomplete closure of the palate, resulting in hypernasal speech. During feeding, some of these infants experience nasal regurgitation of food. Children with a submucous cleft palate that causes abnormal speech or nasal regurgitation of food need referral to a surgeon for repair.

High-Arched Palate

A high-arched palate is usually a genetic trait of no consequence. It is seen also in children who are chronic mouth breathers and in premature infants who undergo prolonged oral intubation. Some rare causes of high-arched palate are congenital disorders such as Marfan's syndrome, Treacher Collins' syndrome, and Ehlers-Danlos syndrome.

Robin (Pierre Robin) Sequence

This congenital malformation is characterized by the triad of micrognathia, cleft palate, and glossoptosis. Affected children present as emergencies in the newborn period because of infringement on the airway by the tongue. The main objective of treatment is to prevent asphyxia until the mandible becomes large enough to accommodate the tongue. In some cases, this objective can be achieved by leaving the child in a prone position while unattended. In severe cases, a tracheotomy is often required. The child requires close observation and careful feeding until the problem is outgrown.

18 Respiratory Tract & Mediastinum

Gary L. Larsen, MD, Steven H. Abman, MD, Leland L. Fan, MD, Jeffrey S. Wagener, MD, Carl W. White, MD, & Frank J. Accurso, MD

Pediatric pulmonary diseases are common, accounting for slightly less than 50% of deaths in children under 1 year of age and about 20% of all hospitalizations of children under 15 years of age. Approximately 7% of children suffer some sort of chronic disorder of the lower respiratory system.

Understanding the pathophysiology of pediatric pulmonary diseases requires an appreciation of the normal growth and development of the lung. These matters are dealt with here, followed by discussions of congenital and acquired diseases of the respiratory tract and mediastinum.

US Department of Health and Human Services, National Institutes of Health: Pediatric Respiratory Disorders. Department of Health and Human Services Publication No. (NIH) 86-2107, 1986.

GROWTH & DEVELOPMENT OF THE LUNG

The lung derives from the foregut during the fourth week of gestation. Subsequent branching leads to the development of the conducting airways (bronchial tree) by about 16 weeks of gestation. The terminal respiratory units—the gas-exchanging portion of the lung—develop from the latter third of gestation through the first few months after birth, when alveoli with adult morphology are formed. It is clear that alveoli increase in number throughout childhood, but the age at which this increase normally stops is controversial, with estimates ranging from 2 years to adolescence. The development of the pulmonary arterial system in general occurs with the development of the airways, whereas capillary proliferation in the terminal respiratory units occurs with the development of the alveoli.

At birth, the lung assumes the gas-exchanging function served by the placenta in utero, placing immediate stress on all components of the respiratory system. Abnormalities in the lung, respiratory muscles, chest wall, airway, respiratory controller, or pulmonary circulation may therefore present at birth. Postnatal survival depends, for example, on the development of the surfactant system to maintain airway stability and allow gas exchange. Immaturity of the surfactant system, often seen in infants of less than 35 weeks' gestational age, can result in severe respiratory morbidity in the immediate neonatal period as well as subsequent chronic lung disease. Persistent pulmonary hypertension of the newborn—the failure of the normal transition to a low-resistance pulmonary circulation at birth—can complicate a number of neonatal respiratory diseases.

Several mechanical properties of the respiratory system in infants increase the risk of respiratory compromise. The upper airway in infants is smaller and less firm than the upper airway in adults; therefore, obstruction in response to infection, inflammation, or foreign body is more likely. The greater compliance of the infant's chest wall allows for collapse or labored breathing when respiration is obstructed. In addition, the infant has fewer fatigue-resistant diaphragmatic muscle fibers, so respiratory muscle fatigue may occur earlier in response to an increased load.

Infants' airways are now thought capable of responding to bronchoactive agents. The mechanisms responsible for this are not completely understood but probably include contractile elements in the airway that respond to neural stimuli. Recent studies also suggest that genetic and environmental factors play a role in the development of airway reactivity. Pulmonary defense mechanisms, including cough, mucociliary clearance, and local and circulating components of the immune system, are present at birth.

Fagan DG, Emery JL: A review and restatement of some problems in histological interpretation of the infant lung. Semin Diagn Pathol 1992;9:13.

Langston C et al: Human lung growth in late gestation and in the neonate. Am Rev Respir Dis 1984;129:607.

Laros CD, Westermann CJJ: Dilatation, compensatory

growth, or both following pneumonectomy during childhood and adolescence. J Thorac Cardiovasc Surg 1987; 93:570.

Murray JF: The Normal Lung: *The Basis for Diagnosis and Treatment of Pulmonary Disease.* Saunders, 1986.

DIAGNOSTIC AIDS

PHYSICAL EXAMINATION OF THE RESPIRATORY TRACT

Assessing the rate, depth, ease, symmetry, and rhythm of respiration is critical to the detection of pulmonary disease. Attention should be given to tracheal position and thoracic configuration. Auscultation should be done to assess the quality of breath sounds and to detect the presence of abnormal sounds. Although there is confusion in the literature, the American Thoracic Society recommends classifying abnormal breath sounds as interrupted (fine or coarse crackles) or continuous (wheezing or rhonchi) sounds.

Extrapulmonary manifestations of pulmonary disease include growth failure, altered mental status (with hypoxemia or hypercapnia), cyanosis, clubbing, and osteoarthropathy. In a recent study of children with respiratory illness, abnormalities of attentiveness, consolability, respiratory effort, color, and movement had a good diagnostic accuracy in detecting hypoxemia. Evidence of cor pulmonale (loud pulmonic component of the second heart sound, hepatomegaly, elevated neck veins, and, rarely, peripheral edema) signifies advanced lung disease.

Respiratory disorders can be secondary to disease in other systems. It is therefore important to look for other conditions such as congenital heart disease (murmur, gallop), neuromuscular disease (muscle wasting, scoliosis), immunodeficiency (rash, diarrhea), and autoimmune disease or occult malignancy (arthritis, hepatosplenomegaly).

Accurso FJ, Eigen H, Loughlin GM: History and physical examination. In: *Respiratory Disease in Children—Diagnosis and Management.* Loughlin GM, Eigen H (editors). Williams & Wilkins, 1994.

Margolis PA et al: Accuracy of the clinical examination in detecting hypoxemia in infants with respiratory illness. J Pediatr 1994;124:552.

PULMONARY FUNCTION TESTS

Lung function tests can measure disease severity, define precipitants of symptoms, and evaluate therapy. They can help define the risks of anesthesia and surgery and assist in the planning of respiratory care in the postoperative period. For example, the range of normal values for a test may be wide, and the predicted normal values change dramatically with growth. For this reason, serial determinations of lung function are often more informative than a single determination. Patient cooperation is essential for almost all physiologic assessments. Most children are not able to perform the necessary maneuvers before 5–7 years of age. Despite these problems, tests of lung function may still contribute to the care of children.

Spirometers on which forced vital capacity can be recorded either as a volume-time tracing (spirogram) or a flow-volume curve are widely available. The patient inhales maximally, holds in inhalation for a short period, and then exhales as fast as possible for at least 3 seconds. The tracing produced by the exhalation shows forced vital capacity (FVC), which is the total amount of air that is exhaled from maximum inspiration, and the forced expiratory volume in the first second of the exhalation (FEV_1). The maximum midexpiratory flow rate (MMEF, or $FEF_{25-75\%}$), is the mean flow rate during the middle portion of the FVC maneuver. The FEV_1/FVC ratio is calculated from these absolute values; A ratio greater than 0.8 in children and young adults shows unlimited, normal airflow.

These basic tests of lung function differentiate obstructive from a restrictive process. Examples of obstructive processes include asthma, chronic bronchitis, and cystic fibrosis, whereas restrictive problems include chest wall deformities that limit lung expansion and interstitial processes due to collagen-vascular diseases, hypersensitivity pneumonitis, and interstitial fibrosis. Classically, diseases that obstruct airflow decrease the FEV_1 more than the FVC, so that the FEV_1/FVC ratio is low. In restrictive problems, however, the decreases in the FEV_1 and FVC are proportionate; thus, the ratio of FEV_1 to FVC is either normal or high. Clinical suspicion of a restrictive disease is usually an indication for referral to a tertiary care center.

The peak expiratory flow rate (PEFR, the maximal flow recorded during an FVC maneuver) can be assessed by hand-held devices. Patients can measure the PEFR at home at regular intervals and record the results in a diary, a practice that may be helpful in following the course of various pulmonary disorders, especially those that are difficult to control and require multiple medications (eg, steroid-dependent asthma). These devices can also be used to give patients with poor perception of their disease an awareness of a decrease in lung function, thus facilitating earlier treatment.

Cross D, Nelson HS: The role of the peak flow meter in the diagnosis and management of asthma. J Allergy Clin Immunol 1991;87:120.

Wenzel SE, Larsen GL: Assessment of lung function: Pulmonary function tests. In: *Allergy, Asthma, and Immunology from Infancy to Childhood,* 3rd ed. Bierman CW, Pearlman DS, Dhapiro GG, Busse, WW (editors). Saunders, 1995.

ARTERIAL BLOOD GASES & NONINVASIVE ASSESSMENT OF OXYGEN TENSION & SATURATION

Arterial blood gas determinations are the best indicators of gas exchange by the respiratory system. Assessment of blood gases is essential in critically ill children and may be used also for determining the severity of lung involvement in chronic conditions. Abnormalities in the respiratory controller, the conducting airways, the gas-exchanging portions of the lung, the pulmonary circulation, the respiratory muscles, and the chest wall affect blood gas measurements. In pediatrics, hypoxia (low PaO_2) most commonly results from mismatching of ventilation and perfusion. Hypercapnia (elevated $PaCO_2$) often results from increased work of breathing secondary to increased pulmonary resistance, decreased compliance, or an abnormal chest wall. Hypercapnia may also occur with normal lungs and a normal chest wall if there is a depressed respiratory controller or if respiratory muscles are weakened. Table 18–1 gives normal values for arterial pH, PaO_2, and $PaCO_2$ at sea level and at an altitude of 5000 feet.

The noninvasive, transcutaneous techniques of measuring oxygen saturation and PO_2 allow on-line monitoring in many different settings. Monitoring oxygen saturation in the intensive care unit is vital to anticipating respiratory failure in critically ill patients. As another example, desaturation during sleep is an important finding in patients with upper airway obstruction. The importance of evaluating the gas-exchanging portions of the lung make arterial blood gas measurements or noninvasive measurements of oxygen saturation an important part of the evaluation of any pediatric patient with suspected lung disease.

Hay WW Jr, Thilo E, Curlander JB: Pulse oximetry in neonatal medicine. Clin Perinatol 1991;18:441.

Levison H et al: Arterial blood gases, alveolar-arterial oxygen difference, and physiologic dead space in children and young adults. Am Rev Respir Dis 1970;101:972.

Table 18–1. Normal arterial blood gas values on room air.

	pH	Pao$_2$ (mm Hg)	Paco$_2$ (mm Hg)
Sea level	7.38–7.42	85–95	36–42
5000 feet	7.36–7.40	65–75	35–40

CULTURE OF MATERIAL FROM THE RESPIRATORY TRACT

Expectorated sputum is rarely available from patients under 5–6 years of age, but in older children a sputum Gram's stain showing significant numbers of organisms within neutrophils may indicate the pathogen present. Stains and cultures for bacteria from nasopharyngeal secretions are frequently misleading.

Cultures from the lower respiratory tract can be obtained by (1) tracheal aspiration through an endotracheal tube or through a rigid or fiberoptic bronchoscope, (2) transtracheal percutaneous aspiration, (3) lung puncture, or (4) the double-brush technique through the fiberoptic bronchoscope. The latter technique can be used to obtain endobronchial secretions in older critically ill or debilitated children large enough to accommodate the large (4.9 mm) bronchoscope required for the procedure.

Complications are most likely to occur with transtracheal percutaneous aspiration or lung puncture. These complications are related to a lack of experience by most physicians in using these techniques in children. The other methods, however, are more likely to produce samples contaminated with oropharyngeal flora and may not be the best guide to therapy. Lung puncture, directed to a consolidated area using physical examination, radiographic studies, or ultrasonography, is the favored approach in the child who deteriorates after initial antibiotic treatment or in the critically ill or immunocompromised child. Pneumothoraces (1–10% of cases) that follow lung puncture are usually small. Open lung biopsy, though a major intervention, should be considered in the worsening or critically ill child when other approaches have not been successful. In skilled hands, thoracoscopic lung biopsy may obviate the open procedure and some of its potential complications. Thoracentesis should be performed when pleural fluid is present, and complete cultures should be obtained. Blood glucose and lactate dehydrogenase should be drawn simultaneously for comparison with pleural fluid chemistries. Blood cultures provide specific diagnoses and must be obtained in children with acute pneumonia.

Specimen obtained by invasive means should be studies for the following: (1) viruses, (2) *Mycoplasma pneumoniae,* (3) *Chlamydia,* (4) *Legionella pneumophila,* (5) *Bordetella pertussis,* (6) fungi, (7) acid-fast bacteria, (8) anaerobes or other bacteria, and (9) *Pneumocystis carinii.* In addition, these specimens should be studied for potential pathogens using rapid diagnostic techniques such as immunofluorescent antibody and enzyme-linked immunosorbent assay (ELISA). Counterimmunoelectrophoresis performed on pleural fluid, serum, or concentrated urine may help identify disease due to *Streptococcus pneumoniae* or *Haemophilus influenzae.* Because these tests can be performed quickly, they may obviate further, more invasive studies.

Alpert BE, O'Sullivan BP, Panitch HB: Nonbronchoscopic approach to bronchoalveolar lavage in children with artificial airways. Pediatr Pulmonol 1992;13:38.

Koumbourlis AC, Kurland G: Nonbronchoscopic bronchoalveolar lavage in mechanically ventilated infants: Technique, efficacy, and applications. Pediatr Pulmon 1993;15:257.

Peter G: The child with pneumonia: Diagnostic and therapeutic considerations. Pediatr Infect Dis J 1988;7:453.

IMAGING OF THE RESPIRATORY TRACT

The plain chest radiograph remains one of the most important techniques for investigating suspected lung disease. Both frontal and lateral views should be obtained in most instances. Hyperaeration, best demonstrated in the lateral projection as flattening of the diaphragm, is a common finding because of the propensity of young children to develop small airways obstruction and the prevalence of asthma. Parenchymal changes may cause increased interstitial markings, consolidation, air bronchograms, or loss of diaphragm or heart contours. When pleural fluid is suspected, lateral decubitus films may be helpful in determining the extent and mobility of the fluid. When a foreign body is suspected, forced expiratory films may demonstrate focal air trapping and shift of the mediastinum to the contralateral side. Lateral neck films can be useful in assessing the size of adenoids and tonsils and also in differentiating croup from epiglottitis, the latter being associated with the "thumbprint" sign.

Barium swallow is indicated for patients with suspected aspiration so that the physician can look for swallowing dysfunction, tracheoesophageal fistula, gastroesophageal reflux, and achalasia. This technique is also very important in detecting vascular rings and slings, because most (not all) are also associated with esophageal compression. Airway fluoroscopy is another important tool for assessing both fixed airway obstruction (ie, subglottic stenosis) and dynamic airway obstruction (ie, tracheomalacia). Fluoroscopy of the diaphragm can detect paralysis by demonstrating paradoxic movement of the involved hemidiaphragm.

High-resolution computed tomography (CT scanning) is useful to evaluate diffuse infiltrative lung disease, metastatic disease, mediastinal masses, and chest wall disease. Magnetic resonance imaging (MRI) is useful for defining subtle or complex abnormalities and vascular rings. Ventilation/perfusion scans can provide information about regional ventilation and perfusion and can help detect vascular malformations and pulmonary emboli (rare in children). Pulmonary angiography is occasionally necessary to define the pulmonary vascular bed more precisely. Bronchography is rarely done in the United States, but can be useful in the specific circumstance when lobectomy is contemplated for suspected localized bronchiectasis.

Newman B: The pediatric chest. Radiol Clin North Am 1993;31:453.

BRONCHOSCOPY

The indications for laryngoscopy include undiagnosed hoarseness, stridor, and symptoms of obstructive sleep apnea; indications for bronchoscopy include wheezing, suspected foreign body, pneumonia, atelectasis, chronic cough, hemoptysis, and placement of an endotracheal tube and assessment of patency. In general, the more specific the indication, the higher the diagnostic yield.

Pediatric bronchoscopy instruments are either flexible fiberoptic or rigid open-tube. The advantages of using a flexible bronchoscope include the following: (1) the procedure can be done at the bedside with sedation and topical anesthetics and requires no general anesthesia; (2) evaluation of the upper airway can be done with little risk in patients who are awake; (3) the distal airways of intubated patients can be examined without removing the endotracheal tube; (4) the instrument can be used as an obturator to intubate a patient with a difficult upper airway; (5) endotracheal tube placement and patency can be checked; (6) assessment of airway dynamics is generally better; and (7) it is possible to examine more distal airways. The advantages of using a rigid instrument are (1) easier removal of foreign bodies (for this reason, rigid bronchoscopy remains the procedure of choice for suspected foreign body aspiration); (2) better airway control, which allows the patient to be ventilated through the bronchoscope; and (3) superior optics. The choice of procedures depends largely on the expertise available.

Bronchoalveolar lavage through a flexible bronchoscope is being used routinely in children to detect infection in both the immunocompetent and the immunocompromised host. Aspiration and hemorrhage are also suspected in the presence of lipid-and hemosiderin-laden macrophages, respectively. Transbronchial biopsy is being done often to look for infection and rejection in transplant patients and to diagnose other conditions such as sarcoidosis.

Perez CR, Wood RE: Update on pediatric flexible bronchoscopy. Pediatr Clin North Am 1994:441:385.

Schnellhase DE, Fan LL: Flexible endoscopy in the diagnosis and management of neonatal and pediatric airway and pulmonary disorders. Respir Care 1995;40:48.

GENERAL THERAPY OF PEDIATRIC LUNG DISEASES

OXYGEN THERAPY

Supplemental oxygen to increase arterial oxygen tension can be administered through an endotracheal tube during mechanical ventilation or through an inflatable anesthesia bag with a mask. In spontaneously breathing patients, delivery can be achieved by nasal cannula, head hood, or mask (including simple, rebreathing, nonrebreathing, or Venturi masks). The general goal of oxygen therapy is to achieve an arterial oxygen tension of 65–90 mm Hg or an oxygen saturation above 92%. The actual oxygen concentration achieved by nasal cannula or mask depends on the flow rate, the type of mask used, and the patient's age. Small changes in flow rate during oxygen administration by nasal cannula can lead to substantial changes in inspired oxygen concentration in young infants. The amount of oxygen required to correct hypoxemia may vary according to the child's activity. It is not unusual, for example, for an infant with chronic lung disease to require 0.75 L/min while awake but 1 L/min while asleep or feeding.

Although the head hood is an efficient device to deliver oxygen in young infants, the nasal cannula is used more often because it allows the infant greater activity. The cannula generally has nasal prongs that are inserted in the nares, but it can be modified by removing the prongs. This nasal catheter can then be taped under the nose or inserted in the nasopharynx. The flow through the nasal cannula should generally not exceed 3 L/min to avoid excessive drying of the nasal mucosa. Even at high flow rates, oxygen by nasal cannula rarely delivers inspired oxygen concentrations greater than 40–45%. In contrast, partial rebreathing and nonrebreathing masks or head hoods achieve inspired oxygen concentrations as high as 90–100%.

Because the physical findings of hypoxemia are subtle, the adequacy of oxygenation should be measured as the arterial oxygen tension or by transcutaneous PO_2 monitoring. In addition, oxygen saturation can be determined by oximetry. The advantages of the noninvasive methods (transcutaneous PO_2 and oximetry) include the ability to obtain continuous measurements during various normal activities and to avoid artifacts caused by crying or breath holding during attempts at arterial puncture. For children with chronic cardiopulmonary disorders that may require supplemental oxygen therapy (such as bronchopulmonary dysplasia or cystic fibrosis), frequent noninvasive assessments are essential to ensure the safety and adequacy of treatment.

Abman SH et al: Pulmonary vascular response to oxygen in infants with BPD. Pediatrics 1985;75:80.

National Conference on Oxygen Therapy. Chest 1984; 86:236.

INHALATION OF BRONCHODILATORS

Airway obstruction reversed by a bronchodilator, occurs cystic fibrosis, bronchiolitis, and bronchopulmonary dysplasia as well as in acute and chronic asthma.

The β-adrenergic agonists may be delivered by a metered-dose inhaler (MDI), a dry powder inhaler, or a nebulizer. MDIs are convenient to use and are best combined with spacing devices for children who lack the ability to coordinate actuation of the MDI with inhalation. On the other hand, the nebulizer is a more effective method of delivering medication to infants and young children. Several inhaled β_2-adrenergic agents that are more selective for the respiratory tract and have longer durations of action are now available (see Chapter 33 and discussion of asthma). In the treatment of acute episodes of airway obstruction, the inhaled adrenergic agents have been shown to be as effective as the injectable agents. In addition, delivery of the drug by the aerosol route fewer side effects. These drugs can be safely administered at home as long as both physician and family realize that a poor response to the agents may signify the need for corticosteroids to help restore β-adrenergic responsiveness.

Anticholinergic agents may also acutely decrease airway obstruction. Furthermore, they may yield a longer duration of bronchodilation than do many adrenergic agents. Selected patients may benefit from receiving both β-adrenergic and anticholinergic agents. In general, this class of drugs is most effective in the treatment of chronic bronchitis.

Goren A et al: Assessment of the ability of young children to use a powder inhaler device (Turbuhaler). Pediatr Pulmonol 1994;18:77.

Kerrebijn KF, van Essen-Zandvliet EEM, Neijens HJ: Effect of long-term treatment with inhaled corticosteroids and beta-agonists on the bronchial responsiveness in children with asthma. J Allergy Clin Immunol 1987; 79:653.

König P: Inhaled corticosteroids: Their present and future role in the management of asthma. J Allergy Clin Immunol 1988;82:297.

Levison H, Reilly PA, Worsley GH: Spacing devices and metered-dose inhalers in childhood asthma. J Pediatr 1985;107:662.

Nelson HS: Drug therapy: Beta-adrenergic bronchodilators. N Engl J Med 1995;333:.

PULMONARY PHYSIOTHERAPY

Chest physical therapy, with postural drainage, percussion, and forced expiratory maneuvers, has been widely used to improve the clearance of secretions, even though there are few studies of the efficacy of techniques used. Studies have suggested that chest physical therapy is not helpful in adults with uncomplicated pneumonias. Nevertheless, children with cystic fibrosis show less decline in pulmonary function if treated with traditional postural drainage and percussion than with directed coughing alone.

Postural drainage requires positioning of the patient to favor emptying each of the segmental bronchi. Percussion or vibration is used to loosen secretions and facilitate drainage. Physicians should carefully review the positions and the technique of percussion to perform this mode of therapy properly. In general, the patient spends 1–2 minutes in each of nine body positions (ie, 10–20 min for the duration of a treatment). Treatments may be given 1–4 times a day at home and sometimes more frequently in the hospital setting. Patients are encouraged to cough regularly during the procedure. Children who cannot be encouraged to cough may require pharyngeal suctioning by trained personnel.

"Blow bottles" that provide the patient feedback about respiratory efforts may also encourage deep breathing. This technique is particularly useful in patients recovering from surgery.

Reisman JJ et al: Role of conventional physiotherapy in cystic fibrosis. J Pediatr 1988;113:632.

AVOIDANCE OF ENVIRONMENTAL HAZARDS

Parents of normal children as well as those of children with respiratory disorders should be counseled about environmental hazards to the lung. The list of potential hazards includes small objects that may be aspirated, allergens that can precipitate respiratory symptoms in atopic children, and cigarette smoke.

The harmful effects of smoking in the home deserve special emphasis. Children from families where the parents and others smoke have decreased lung growth as well as decreased pulmonary function in comparison with children raised in homes where there are no smokers. Exposure of children to tobacco smoke also leads to an increased frequency of lower respiratory tract infections and an increased incidence of respiratory symptoms, including recurrent wheezing. Health care providers must increase their efforts to educate patients and their families about the hazards of smoking. Resources within the community that will help smokers give up the habit should be used as part of the routine health maintenance for all children.

American Academy of Pediatrics Committee on Environmental Hazards: Involuntary smoking: A hazard to children. Pediatrics 1986;77:755.

Weitzman M et al: Maternal smoking and childhood asthma. Pediatrics 1990;85:505.

DISORDERS OF THE CONDUCTING AIRWAYS

The conducting airways consist of the nose, mouth, pharynx, larynx, trachea, bronchi, and bronchioles. These airways direct inspired air to the gas exchange units of the lung; they do not participate in gas exchange themselves. Airflow obstruction in the conducting airways occurs by: (1) external compression (eg, vascular ring, tumor), (2) abnormalities of the airway structure itself (eg, congenital defects, thickening of an airway wall due to inflammation), or (3) material in the airway lumen (eg, foreign body, mucus).

Airway obstruction can be fixed (airflow limited in both the inspiratory and expiratory phases of respiration) or variable (airflow limited more in one phase of respiration than the other). Variable obstruction is common in children because their airways are more compliant and susceptible to dynamic compression. With variable extrathoracic airway obstruction (eg, croup), airflow limitation is greater during inspiration, leading to inspiratory stridor. With variable intrathoracic obstruction, limitation is greater during expiration, producing expiratory wheezing. Thus, determining the phase of respiration in which obstruction is greatest may be helpful in localizing the site of obstruction.

EXTRATHORACIC AIRWAY OBSTRUCTION

Patients with abnormalities of the extrathoracic airway may present with snoring and other symptoms of obstructive apnea, hoarseness, brassy cough, or stridor. The course of the illness may be acute (eg, infectious croup), recurrent (eg, spasmodic croup), chronic (eg, subglottic stenosis), or progressive (eg, laryngeal papillomatosis). Significant risk factors are difficult delivery, ductal ligation, and intubation. Examination should determine if obstructive symptoms are present at rest or with agitation, if they are positional, or if they are related to sleep. The presence of agitation, air hunger, severe retractions, cyanosis, lethargy, or coma should alert the physician to a potentially life-threatening condition that may require immediate airway intervention. Helpful diagnostic studies in the evaluation of upper airway obstruction include chest and lateral neck films, airway fluoroscopy, and barium swallow. An ECG can provide evidence of pulmonary hypertension in patients with chronic obstruction. Patients with symptoms of obstructive sleep apnea may benefit from polysomnography (measurements during sleep of the motion of the chest wall, airflow at the nose and mouth, heart rate, oxygen saturation, and selected electroencephalographic leads to stage sleep), which can help define the severity of the illness. In older children, pulmonary function tests can differentiate fixed from variable airflow obstruction and determine the site of variable obstruction. Direct laryngoscopy and bronchoscopy remain the procedures of choice to establish the precise diagnosis. Treatment should be directed at relieving airway obstruction and correcting the underlying condition if possible.

Tan HKK, Holinger LD: How to evaluate and manage stridor in children. J Respir Dis 1994;15:245.

INTRATHORACIC AIRWAY OBSTRUCTION

Patients with abnormalities of the intrathoracic airways usually present with wheezing that is most prominent during expiration. The history should include the following: (1) age at onset; (2) precipitating factors (eg, exercise, upper respiratory illnesses, allergens, choking while eating, etc); (3) course, that is, acute (bronchiolitis, foreign body), chronic (tracheomalacia, vascular ring), recurrent (reactive airways disease), or progressive (cystic fibrosis, bronchiolitis obliterans); (4) presence and nature of cough; (5) production of sputum; (6) previous response to bronchodilators; (7) symptoms with positional changes (vascular rings); and (8) involvement of other organ systems (malabsorption in cystic fibrosis).

Physical examination should include growth measurements and vital signs. The examiner should look for cyanosis or pallor, barrel-shaped chest, retractions and use of accessory muscles, and clubbing. Auscultation should define the pattern and timing of respiration, detect the presence of crackles and wheezing, and determine whether findings are localized or generalized.

Routine tests include plain chest films, a sweat test, and pulmonary function tests in older children. Other diagnostic studies are dictated by the history and physical findings. Treatment should be directed toward the primary cause of the obstruction but generally includes a trial of bronchodilators.

CONGENITAL DISORDERS OF THE EXTRATHORACIC AIRWAY

LARYNGOMALACIA

Laryngomalacia is a benign congenital disorder in which the cartilaginous support for the supraglottic structures is underdeveloped. It is the most common cause of persistent stridor in infants and usually is seen in the first 6 weeks of life. Stridor has been reported to be worse in the supine position, with increased activity, with upper respiratory infections, and during feeding; however, the clinical presentation can be variable. The condition usually improves with age and resolves by 2 years of age, but symptoms may persist for years. The diagnosis is established by direct laryngoscopy, in which inspiratory collapse of an "omega-shaped" epiglottis (with or without long, redundant arytenoids) is visualized. In mildly affected patients with a typical presentation (those without stridor at rest or retractions), this procedure may not be necessary. No treatment is needed except in the extremely rare circumstance of severe obstruction that requires airway intervention. These patients may have slight desaturation during sleep, the clinical importance of which is unknown.

Belmont JR, Grundfast K: Congenital laryngeal stridor (laryngomalacia): Etiologic factors and associated disorders. Ann Otol Rhinol Laryngol 1984;93:430.
Macfarlane PI, Olinsky A, Phelan PD: Proximal airway function 8 to 16 years after laryngomalacia: Follow-up flow-volume loop studies. J Pediatr 1985;107:216.
McCray PB et al: Hypoxia and hypercapnia in infants with mild laryngomalacia. Am J Dis Child 1988;142:896.

OTHER CONGENITAL PROBLEMS

Other congenital lesions of the larynx (laryngeal atresia, laryngeal web, laryngocele and cyst of the larynx, subglottic hemangioma, and laryngeal cleft) are rare. These disorders are best diagnosed by direct laryngoscopy. Laryngeal atresia obviously presents immediately after birth with severe respiratory distress and is usually fatal. Laryngeal web, representing fusion of the anterior portion of the true vocal cords, is associated with hoarseness, aphonia, and stridor. Surgical correction may be necessary, depending on the degree of airway obstruction.

Congenital cysts and laryngoceles are believed to have similar origin. Cysts are more superficial, whereas laryngoceles communicate with the interior of the larynx. Cysts are generally fluid-filled, whereas laryngoceles may be air- or fluid-filled. Airway obstruction is usually prominent and requires surgery or laser therapy.

Subglottic hemangiomas are seen in infancy with signs of upper airway obstruction and are often associated with similar lesions of the skin. Although these lesions tend to regress spontaneously, airway obstruction may require surgical treatment with laser or even tracheostomy.

Laryngeal cleft is a very rare condition resulting from failure of posterior cricoid fusion. Patients with this condition may have stridor but always aspirate severely, resulting in recurrent or chronic pneumonia and failure to thrive. Barium swallow is always positive for severe aspiration, but diagnosis can be very difficult even with direct laryngoscopy. Patients often require tracheostomy and gastrostomy, because surgical correction is not always successful.

Platzker ACG: Congenital and acquired disorders of the airway. Curr Opin Pediatr 1992;4:437.
Sie KCY, McGillT, Healy GB: Subglottic hemangioma; Ten years' experience with the carbon dioxide laser. Ann Otol Rhinol Laryngol 1994;103:167.

ACQUIRED DISORDERS OF THE EXTRATHORACIC AIRWAY

CROUP SYNDROME

Croup describes a series of acute inflammatory diseases of the larynx including viral croup (laryngotracheobronchitis), epiglottitis (supraglottitis), and bacterial tracheitis. These entities are the main differential diagnosis for patients with acute stridor, although spasmodic croup, angioneurotic edema, laryngeal or esophageal foreign body, and retropharyngeal abscess should be considered.

1. VIRAL CROUP

Viral croup generally affects younger children in the fall and early winter and is most often caused by parainfluenza virus type 1. Other organisms causing croup include parainfluenza virus types 2 and 3, respiratory syncytial virus, influenza virus, rubeola virus, adenovirus, and *Mycoplasma pneumoniae*. Although inflammation of the entire airway is usually present, edema formation in the subglottic space accounts for the predominant signs of upper airway obstruction.

Clinical Findings
A. Symptoms and Signs: There is usually a prodrome of upper respiratory tract symptoms followed by the development of a barking cough and stridor. Fever is usually absent or low grade, but may on occasion be as high as in patients with epiglottitis. Patients with mild disease may exhibit only stridor when agitated, but as obstruction worsens, symptoms may progress to stridor at rest, accompanied by retractions, air hunger, and cyanosis in severe cases. On examination, the presence of cough and the absence of drooling tend to favor the diagnosis of viral croup over epiglottitis.

B. Imaging: Lateral neck films can be diagnostically helpful by showing subglottic narrowing and a normal epiglottis. It is important to confirm that the epiglottis is normal by direct laryngoscopy, because the presentation of epiglottitis may be similar to that of croup. Although controversy exists regarding the safety of such a procedure, a recent study suggests that it is reasonably safe in patients with suspected viral croup. Direct inspection is necessary because some patients with suspected croup actually prove to have epiglottitis.

Treatment
Treatment of viral croup is supportive. Patients without stridor at rest may be managed as outpatients with mist therapy, oral hydration, and minimal handling. Although mist is believed to be helpful in relieving symptoms, the only clinical study done to date failed to demonstrate its effectiveness. Patients with stridor at rest require hospitalization. Appropriate hospital management includes the same therapy given to outpatients. In addition, oxygen should be administered with careful observation to patients demonstrating desaturation by pulse oximetry. Nebulized racemic epinephrine (0.5 mL of a 2.25% solution diluted with 1.5–3.5 mL of sterile water) has been shown to relieve airway obstruction for up to 2 hours, presumably by reducing edema. Nebulized L-Epinephrine (5 mL of 1:1000 solution) is also effective. Other, more pure alpha-agonists are also effective but are shorter-acting. The use of corticosteroids remains controversial; all controlled studies to date have had methodologic shortcomings. Nonetheless, the efficacy demonstrated in some studies, together with the lack of identified side effects, seems to justify a short course in severe cases (those patients not responding to racemic epinephrine). Dexamethasone (0.5–1 mg/kg [up to 10 mg] given orally or parenterally as a single dose or repeated in 12 h) is appropriate. Nebulized steroid may also be effective but is currently unavailable in the United States.

Patients with impending respiratory failure require an artificial airway. Although there is controversy regarding the choice between intubation and tracheostomy, recent studies suggest that intubation with an endotracheal tube of slightly smaller diameter than would ordinarily be used is reasonably safe.

Extubation should be accomplished within 2–3 days to minimize the risk of laryngeal injury. If the patient fails extubation, tracheostomy should be performed.

Prognosis

Most children with viral croup have an uneventful course and improve within a few days. Recent studies suggest that patients with a history of croup may have airway hyperreactivity. However, it has not been determined if this was present prior to the croup episode or if the croup episode itself altered airway function. Recurrence of croup occurs in some instances, implying airway hyperreactivity.

Husby S et al: Treatment of croup with nebulized steroid (budesonide): A double blind, placebo controlled study. Arch Dis Child 1993;68:352.

Kairys SW, Olmstead EM, O'Connor GT: Steroid treatment of laryngotracheitis: A meta-analysis of the evidence from randomized trials. Pediatrics 1989;83:683.

Ledwith CA, Shea LM, Maureo RD: Safety and efficacy of nebulized racemic epinephrine in conjunction with oral dexamethasone and mist in the outpatient treatment of croup. Ann Emerg Med 1995;25(3):331.

McEniery J et al: Review of intubation in severe laryngotracheobronchitis. Pediatrics 1991;87:847.

Waisman Y et al: Prospective randomized double-blind study comparing L-Epinephrine and racemic epinephrine aerosols in the treatment of laryngotracheitis (croup). Pediatrics 1992;89:302.

2. EPIGLOTTITIS

Epiglottitis is a true medical emergency. It is almost always caused by *Haemophilus influenzae* type B, although other organisms such as *Streptococcus pneumoniae* and groups A and C *Streptococcus pyogenes* have been implicated. Resulting inflammation and swelling of the supraglottic structures (epiglottis and arytenoids) can develop rapidly and lead to life-threatening upper airway obstruction. The incidence has decreased dramatically since the *Haemophilus influenzae* vaccine was introduced.

Clinical Findings

A. Symptoms and Signs: Typically, patients present with a rather sudden onset of fever, dysphagia, drooling, muffled voice, inspiratory retractions, cyanosis, and soft stridor. They often sit in a "sniffing dog" position, which gives them the best airway possible under the circumstances. Progression to total airway obstruction may occur and result in respiratory arrest.

B. Imaging: Diagnostically, lateral neck films may be helpful in demonstrating a classic "thumbprint" sign. Obtaining films, however, may delay important airway intervention. The definitive diagnosis is made by direct inspection of the epiglottis, a procedure that should be done by an experienced airway specialist under controlled conditions (usually the operating room). The typical findings are a cherry-red and swollen epiglottis and arytenoids.

Treatment

Once the diagnosis of epiglottitis is made, endotracheal intubation should be performed immediately. Most anesthesiologists favor the use of general anesthesia (but not muscle relaxants) to facilitate intubation. After an airway is established, cultures of the blood and epiglottis should be obtained and the patient started on appropriate intravenous antibiotics to cover *H influenzae* (ceftriaxone sodium, 150 mg/kg/d in two divided doses or equivalent cephalosporin).

Careful attention should be given to respiratory care of the intubated patient to prevent accidental extubation and tube obstruction. This includes adequate restraint, humidification, and frequent suctioning. Extubation can usually be accomplished in 24–48 hours, when direct inspection shows significant reduction in the size of the epiglottis. Some centers use the resolution of fever as a criterion for extubation. Intravenous antibiotics should be continued for 2–3 days, followed by oral antibiotics to complete a 10-day course.

If a physician who has little experience in treating airway disorders and is located far from a tertiary pediatric facility encounters a patient with epiglottitis, the following is recommended. Start the patient on oxygen, and assemble all the airway equipment available. Manipulate the patient as little as possible, and allow the child to remain sitting up. Enlist the help of the most experienced airway person available, or call a transport team. Carefully start an intravenous line, and give antibiotics. If the patient obstructs completely and suffers a respiratory arrest, attempt to establish an airway by any means possible: intubation, bag and mask ventilation, transtracheal ventilation with a large-bore angiocatheter attached to a 3-mm endotracheal tube adapter and resuscitation bag, or tracheostomy.

Complications

Complications related to H influenzae infection in other sites include pneumonia, cervical adenitis, and septic arthritis. Meningitis is extremely rare.

Prognosis

Prompt recognition and appropriate treatment usually results in rapid resolution of swelling and inflammation. Recurrence is unusual.

Cressman WR, Myer CM: Diagnosis and management of croup and epiglottitis. Pediatr Clin North Am 1994; 41:265.

Gorelick MH, Baker MD: Epiglottitis in children, 1979 through 992: Effects of *Haemophilus influenzae* type b immunization. Arch Pediatr Adolesc Med 1994;148:447.

3. BACTERIAL TRACHEITIS

Bacterial tracheitis (pseudomembranous croup) is a severe form of laryngotracheobronchitis. The organism most often isolated is *Staphylococcus aureus,* but organisms such as *H influenzae,* group A *Streptococcus pyogenes, Neisseria* species, and others have been reported. The disease probably represents localized mucosal invasion of bacteria in patients with primary viral croup, resulting in inflammatory edema, purulent secretions, and pseudomembranes. Although cultures of the tracheal secretions are frequently positive, blood cultures are almost always negative.

Clinical Findings

A. Symptoms and Signs: The early clinical picture is similar to that of viral croup. However, instead of gradual improvement, patients develop high fever, toxicity, and progressive upper airway obstruction that is unresponsive to standard croup therapy. The incidence of sudden respiratory arrest or progressive respiratory failure is very high; in such instances, airway intervention is required.

B. Laboratory Findings: The white cell count is usually elevated, with left shift. Cultures of tracheal secretions usually demonstrate one of the causative organisms.

C. Imaging: Lateral neck films show a normal epiglottis but often severe subglottic and tracheal narrowing. Frequently, irregularity of the contour of the proximal tracheal mucosa and pseudomembrane formation in the airway are present.

Treatment

Patients with suspected bacterial tracheitis should be managed in a similar fashion to those with epiglottitis. Because of the high incidence of respiratory arrest or progressive respiratory failure, intubation is almost always necessary. Once intubated, patients often have thick, purulent, obstructive tracheal secretions. Therefore, extreme care (adequate humidification, frequent suctioning, intensive care monitoring) is required to prevent endotracheal tube obstruction. Appropriate intravenous antibiotics to cover *S aureus, H influenzae,* and the other organisms are indicated. Because thick secretions persist for several days, the period of intubation required is longer for bacterial tracheitis than for epiglottitis.

Prognosis

Despite the severity of this illness, the reported mortality rate is very low.

Britto J et al: Systemic complications associated with bacterial tracheitis. Arch Dis Child 1996;74:249.

Hen J: Current management of upper airway obstruction. Pediatr Ann (April) 1986;15:274.

Liston SL et al: Bacterial tracheitis. Am J Dis Child 1983; 137:764.

Nelson WE: Bacterial croup: A historical perspective. J Pediatr 1984;105:52.

VOCAL CORD PARALYSIS

Unilateral or bilateral vocal cord paralysis may be congenital or, more commonly, result from injury to the recurrent laryngeal nerves. Risk factors for acquired paralysis include difficult delivery (especially face presentation), neck and thoracic surgery (eg, ductal ligation, repair of tracheoesophageal fistula), trauma, mediastinal masses, pulmonary hypertension, and central nervous system disease (eg, Arnold-Chiari malformation). Patients usually present with varying degrees of hoarseness, aspiration, or high-pitched stridor. Unilateral cord paralysis is more likely to occur on the left because of the longer course of the left recurrent laryngeal nerve and its proximity to major thoracic structures. Patients with unilateral paralysis are usually hoarse but rarely have stridor. With bilateral cord paralysis, the closer to midline the cords are positioned, the greater the airway obstruction; the more lateral the cords are positioned, the greater the tendency to aspirate and experience hoarseness or aphonia. With partial function (paresis), the adductor muscles tend to operate better than the abductors, with a resultant high-pitched inspiratory stridor and normal voice. Airway intervention (intubation, tracheostomy) is rarely indicated in unilateral paralysis but is often necessary for bilateral paralysis. Recovery is related to the severity of nerve injury and the potential for healing.

Cohen SR et al: Laryngeal paralysis in children: A long-term retrospective study. Ann Otol Rhinol Laryngol 1982;91:417.

Emery PJ, Fearon B: Vocal cord palsy in pediatric practice: A review of 71 cases. Int J Pediatr Otorhinolaryngol 1984;8:147.

Fan LL et al: Paralyzed left vocal cord associated with patent ductus arteriosus ligation. J Thorac Cardiovasc Surg 1989;98:611.

SUBGLOTTIC STENOSIS

Subglottic stenosis can be congenital or, more commonly, result from endotracheal intubation. Neonates and infants are particularly vulnerable to subglottic injury from intubation: the subglottis is the narrowest part of an infant's airway, and the cricoid cartilage, which supports the subglottis, is the only cartilage that completely encircles the airway. The clinical presentation may vary from patients who are totally asymptomatic to those who have typical evidence of severe upper airway obstruction. Patients with signs of stridor who fail extubation repeatedly are likely to have subglottic stenosis. As with other conditions, diagnosis is ultimately established by direct laryngoscopy and bronchoscopy. Tracheostomy is often required when airway compromise is severe. Although a number of surgical approaches to correct this problem have been tried, the failure rate is high. The most promising procedures are the "cricoid split," in which the cricoid cartilage is surgically opened (better for acquired than congenital lesions), and the laryngotracheoplasty, in which a cartilage graft from another source (eg, rib) is used to expand the framework.

Berkowitz RG: Experience with anterior cricoid split for infantile subglottic stenosis. Paediatr Child Health, 1994;(4):345.

Couser RJ et al: Effectiveness of dexamethasone in preventing extubation failure in preterm infants at increased risk for airway edema. J Pediatr 1992;121:591.

Pashley NRT, Fan LL: Laryngeal injury from endotracheal intubation in the neonate. In: *Bronchopulmonary Dysplasia.* Bancalari E, Stocker JT (editors). Hemisphere Publishing, 1988.

LARYNGEAL TRAUMA

Injury to the larynx may result from external trauma, such as automobile accidents, snowmobile accidents (clothesline injury), and hanging, or internal trauma, such as noxious inhalation (burns and caustic substances) and intubation. External trauma can cause laryngeal fracture, which requires an emergency tracheostomy to prevent death. After appropriate airway intervention, attention should be directed to debridement and closure of lacerations. Reduction of laryngeal fractures should be performed as soon as the patient is stabilized.

Myers EN: Assessing and repairing laryngeal injuries. J Respir Dis 1982;3:43.

LARYNGEAL PAPILLOMATOSIS

Papillomas of the larynx are benign, warty growths that are difficult to treat. The presumed cause is human papillomavirus infection. A substantial percentage of mothers of patients with laryngeal papillomas have a history of genital condyloma at the time of delivery, a fact suggesting that the virus is acquired at birth during passage through an infected birth canal.

The age at onset is usually 2–4 years, but the disease may present at any age. Patients usually develop hoarseness, croupy cough, or stridor that can lead to life-threatening airway obstruction. Diagnosis is established by direct laryngoscopy.

Treatment is directed at relieving airway obstruction, usually by surgical removal of the lesions. Oc-

casionally, tracheostomy is necessary when life-threatening obstruction or respiratory arrest occurs. Although a number of surgical procedures (laser, cup forceps, cryosurgery) have been used to remove papillomas, none is satisfactory: Recurrences are the rule, and repeated operations at frequent intervals to prevent airway compromise are required. Occasionally, the lesions spread down the trachea and bronchi, making surgical removal more difficult. The use of interferon therapy remains controversial. Fortunately, spontaneous remissions do occur, usually by puberty, so that the goal of therapy is to maintain an adequate airway until remission occurs.

McDonald GA, Strong MS: Respiratory papillomatosis: Keeping it under control. J Respir Dis 1984;5:36.

CONGENITAL DISORDERS OF THE INTRATHORACIC AIRWAYS

TRACHEOMALACIA

Tracheomalacia exists when the cartilaginous framework of the trachea is inadequate to maintain airway patency. Because cartilage of the infant airway is normally "soft," all infants may have some degree of dynamic collapse of the trachea during expiration, when pressure outside the trachea exceeds intraluminal pressure. In tracheomalacia, whether congenital or acquired, dynamic collapse leads to airway obstruction. The congenital variety may be isolated or associated with another developmental defect, such as tracheoesophageal fistula or vascular ring. It may be localized to part of the trachea or, more commonly, may involve the entire trachea as well as the remainder of the conducting airways. In severe cases, cartilage in the involved area may be missing or underdeveloped. The acquired variety has been associated with long-term ventilation of premature newborns that results in chronic tracheal injury.

Patients present with coarse wheezing, a prolonged expiratory phase, and a croupy cough, all of which increase with agitation and upper respiratory tract infections. Diagnosis can be made by cinefluoroscopy or bronchoscopy. Barium swallow may be indicated to rule out coexisting conditions. Usually, no treatment is indicated for the isolated condition, which generally improves over time. Coexisting lesions such as tracheoesophageal fistulas and vascular rings need primary repair. In severe cases of tracheomalacia, airway intervention by intubation or tracheostomy may be necessary; but this procedure alone is seldom satisfactory, because airway collapse continues to exist below the tip of the artificial airway. The application of continuous positive airway pressure through an artificial airway has occasionally been successful in stabilizing the collapsing airway.

Cogbill TH et al: Primary tracheomalacia. Ann Thorac Surg 1983;35:538.

Kanter et al: Treatment of severe tracheobronchomalacia with continuous positive airway pressure (CPAP). Anesthesiology 1982;57:54.

Sotomayor JL et al: Large-airway collapse due to acquired tracheobronchomalacia in infancy. Am J Dis Child 1986; 140:367.

VASCULAR RINGS & SLINGS

Vascular anomalies of the aorta and its branches and the pulmonary arteries may compress the trachea or esophagus. The most common varieties include double aortic arch, right aortic arch with left ligamentum arteriosum or patent ductus arteriosus, pulmonary sling, anomalous innominate or left carotid artery, and aberrant right subclavian artery.

All but the aberrant right subclavian artery are associated with tracheal compression and, therefore, present in infancy with symptoms of chronic airway obstruction including stridor, course wheezing, and croupy cough. Symptoms are often worse in the supine position. Respiratory compromise is most severe with double aortic arch and may lead to apnea, respiratory arrest, or even death. Esophageal compression, present in all but anomalous innominate or carotid artery, may result in feeding difficulties, including dysphagia and vomiting. Therefore, barium swallow demonstrating this esophageal compression forms the mainstay of establishing the diagnosis. In the case of anomalous innominate or carotid artery, diagnosis is best established by cinefluoroscopy, MRI, or bronchoscopy.

Patients with significant symptoms require surgical correction, especially those with double aortic arch. Some controversy exists regarding whether angiography is necessary to define the anatomy prior to surgery. Patients usually improve following correction but may have persistent but milder symptoms of airway obstruction due to associated tracheomalacia.

Ashraf H, Subramanian S: Identifying the hallmarks of vascular rings in children. J Respir Dis 1985;6:31.

BRONCHOGENIC CYSTS

Bronchogenic cysts generally occur in the middle mediastinum (see Mediastinal Masses) near the carina and adjacent to the major bronchi but can be found elsewhere in the lung as well. Sizes are variable, ranging between 2 and 10 cm. Cyst walls are thick and may contain pus, mucus, or blood. These develop from abnormal lung budding of the primitive foregut. They do not contain distal lung parenchyma and generally do not communicate with the airway.

Clinically, respiratory distress can appear acutely in early childhood or present as chronic wheezing, chronic cough, tachypnea, recurrent pneumonia, or stridor, depending on location, size, and the degree of airway compression. On physical examination, the trachea may deviate from the midline, and the percussion note over involved lobes may be hyperresonant. Breath sounds over such areas will also be decreased. Air trapping and hyperinflation of the affected lobes is found on chest x-ray film. Smaller lesions or those detected early may not be appreciated on chest x-ray film or may appear spherical. Initial assessment of a suspected bronchogenic cyst usually includes a barium swallow to demonstrate the presence of a mass. This study also helps determine whether the lesion communicates with the gastrointestinal tract. CT scans or ultrasonography can differentiate solid versus cystic mediastinal masses and define the cyst's relationship to the rest of the lung.

Treatment involves surgical resection of the bronchogenic cyst. Vigorous pulmonary physiotherapy is indicated in the postoperative period to prevent complications of the surgery (atelectasis, infection of lung distal to the site of resection of the cyst).

Nuchtern JG, Harberg FJ: Congenital lung cysts. Semin Pediatr Surg 1994;3(4):233.

Ribet ME, Copin MC, Gosselin B: Bronchogenic cysts of the mediastinum. J Thorac Cardiovasc Surg 1995; 109(5):1003.

ACQUIRED DISORDERS OF THE INTRATHORACIC AIRWAYS

FOREIGN BODY ASPIRATION

1. FOREIGN BODIES IN THE UPPER RESPIRATORY TRACT

Essentials of Diagnosis

- Acute onset of cyanosis and choking.
- Inability to vocalize or cough (complete obstruction) or with drooling and stridor (partial obstruction).

General Considerations

Foreign body aspiration contributes significantly to morbidity and mortality of early childhood, with many deaths resulting from upper airway obstruction each year. Children between 6 months and 4 years of age are at particularly high risk for foreign body aspiration.

Clinical Findings

Foreign bodies lodged within the esophagus may compress the airway and cause respiratory distress. More typically, the foreign body lodges in the supraglottic airway, triggering protective reflexes that attempt to dislodge the object and causing laryngospasm. Onset is generally abrupt, with a history of the child running with food or other object in the mouth or playing with seeds, small coins, toys or other objects. Poor "child proofing" in the home and cases in which an older sibling feeds age-inappropriate foods (eg, peanuts, hard candy, carrot slices) to the younger child are typical. If the obstruction is only partial, coughing, stridor, and the ability to vocalize may persist. If complete, an inability to cough or vocalize (aphonia) and cyanosis with marked distress are observed. If untreated, progressive cyanosis, loss of consciousness, seizures, bradycardia, and cardiopulmonary arrest follow.

Treatment

The emergency treatment of upper airway obstruction due to foreign body aspiration is somewhat controversial. In general, it is recommended that if partial obstruction is present, children should be allowed to use their own cough reflex to extrude the foreign body. If after a brief observation period, the obstruction increases or the airway becomes completely obstructed, acute intervention is required. The AAP and AHA distinguish between children under or over 1 year of age. A choking infant under age 1 should be placed face-down over the rescuer's arm, with the head positioned below the trunk. Five measured back blows are delivered rapidly between the infant's scapulas with the heel of the rescuer's hand. If obstruction persists, the infant should be rolled over and five rapid chest compressions performed (similar to CPR). This sequence is repeated until the obstruction is relieved. In children over age 1 year, abdominal thrusts (Heimlich maneuver) may be performed, with special care in younger children because of concern about possible intra-abdominal organ injury.

In both groups, blind probing of the airway to dislodge a foreign body is discouraged because of the risk of impaction. The airway may be opened by jaw thrust, and if the foreign body can be directly visualized, careful removal with the fingers or instruments (Magill forceps) can be attempted. Patients with persistent apnea and inability to achieve adequate ventilation may require emergency intubation, tracheostomy, or needle cricothyrotomy, depending on the setting and the rescuer's skills.

Abman SH et al: Emergency treatment of foreign body obstruction of the upper airway in children. J Emerg Med 1984;2:7.

Chameides L, Hazinski MF: (editors): *Textbook of Pediatric Advanced Life Support.* American Heart Association and American Academy of Pediatrics, 1990.

2. FOREIGN BODIES IN THE LOWER RESPIRATORY TRACT

Essentials of Diagnosis

- Sudden onset of coughing, wheezing, or respiratory distress.
- Asymmetric physical findings of decreased breath sounds or localized wheezing.
- Asymmetric radiographic findings, especially with forced expiratory view.

General Considerations

The problem with diagnosing foreign body aspiration of the lower respiratory tract is the lack of parental observations documenting an acute aspiration. The abrupt onset of cough, choking, or wheezing, especially in children between 6 months and 4 years who have access to high-risk objects such as peanuts, hard candy, small toys, and other objects, should heighten suspicion.

Clinical Findings

A. Symptoms and Signs: Clinically, the range of respiratory symptoms and signs varies, depending on the site of obstruction and the duration following the acute episode. For example, a large or central airway obstruction may cause marked distress and prompt early intervention. In contrast, if the foreign object remains in the lower respiratory tract, the acute cough or wheezing may diminish over time, only to recur later and present as chronic cough or persistent wheezing. Thus, foreign body aspiration should be suspected in children with chronic cough, persistent wheezing, or recurrent pneumonia. Longstanding foreign bodies may lead to bronchiectasis or lung abscess. On physical examination, asymmetric breath sounds or localized wheezing also suggest the presence of a foreign body.

B. Imaging: Inspiratory and forced expiratory chest x-rays should be obtained if foreign body aspiration is suspected. The latter study can be obtained in young children by manually compressing the abdomen during expiration. The initial inspiratory view may show localized hyperinflation due to the ball-valve effect of the foreign body, causing distal air trapping. A positive forced expiratory study shows a mediastinal shift away from the affected side. If airway obstruction is complete, atelectasis and related volume loss will be the major radiologic findings. Chest fluoroscopy is an alternative approach for detecting air trapping and mediastinal shift.

Treatment

If the imaging is positive, or despite negative imaging, clinical suspicion persists, further evaluation with bronchoscopy is indicated. Rigid bronchoscopy under general anesthesia is recommended. Flexible bronchoscopy may be helpful for follow-up evaluations (after the foreign object has been removed).

Children with suspected acute foreign body aspiration should be admitted to the hospital for evaluation and treatment. Chest postural drainage is no longer recommended because the foreign body may become dislodged and obstruct a major central airway. Bronchoscopy should not be delayed in children with respiratory distress but should be performed as soon as possible once the diagnosis is made, even in children with more chronic symptoms. Following the removal of the foreign body, β-adrenergic nebulization treatments followed by chest physiotherapy are recommended to help clear related mucus or bronchospasm. The relative dangers of missing a foreign body in the lower respiratory tract are much greater; these include the development of bronchiectasis and lung abscess over time. This risk justifies an aggressive approach to suspected foreign bodies in undocumented but suspicious cases.

Kosloske AM: Tracheobronchial foreign bodies in children: Back to the bronchoscope and a balloon. Pediatrics 1980;66:321.

Wood RE, Gauderer MWL: Flexible fiberoptic bronchoscopy in the management of tracheobronchial foreign bodies in children: The value of a combined approach with open tube bronchoscopy. J Pediatr Surg 1984; 19:693.

BRONCHITIS

Essentials of Diagnosis

- Cough that usually progresses from dry to productive.
- Rhonchi appearing predominantly during expiration.

General Considerations

Bronchitis refers to inflammation of the major conducting airways within the lung, which may be acute, chronic, or recurrent. As an isolated entity, this problem is probably unusual in children. However, inflammation within this section of the airways commonly occurs in association with disease processes involving other areas of the respiratory tract. In adults, the diagnosis of chronic bronchitis is based on a history of at least 3 months of productive cough occurring for 2 or more years, but no generally acceptable criteria for this diagnosis exist in children. A differential diagnosis for 3–4 weeks of cough and sputum production in a child is given in the text that follows.

Clinical Findings

A. Symptoms and Signs: An acute bronchitis usually begins as a dry, nonproductive cough that may be associated with other features of an upper respiratory illness of viral origin. The longer the cough persists, the more likely it is to become productive. In general, children with uncomplicated acute bronchitis appear nontoxic, and fever, if present, is low-grade. There are diffuse rhonchi predominantly during expiration. In uncomplicated acute bronchitis, mucus production decreases, and the cough disappears over a period of 7–10 days.

B. Laboratory Findings: The white blood count is usually normal and, if elevated, may suggest a viral infection. Pulmonary function tests may reveal variable degrees of airway obstruction.

C. Imaging: An x-ray examination of the chest may be normal or show a mild increase in bronchovascular markings.

Differential Diagnosis

Most attacks of acute bronchitis are caused by viral infections. Certain viral pathogens, such as the adenovirus, can produce a more severe clinical picture that resembles a pertussis-like illness. Bacteria that may produce disease in which bronchitis is a prominent symptom include *Bordetella pertussis, Mycobacterium tuberculosis, Corynebacterium diphtheriae,* and *M pneumoniae.*

Noninfectious diseases need to be considered in the evaluation of an acute bronchitis that differs from the clinical picture described above and in cases of chronic bronchitis or recurrent bronchitic episodes. Asthma may present as a persistent cough with little or no wheezing. Sinus infections may provide a source of persistent irritation to the respiratory tract and lead to a chronic cough. Cystic fibrosis, an immunodeficiency, or primary ciliary dyskinesia must also be considered if the bronchitis persists or recurs and if bronchiectasis is present or suspected. In the younger child, respiratory tract anomalies, foreign bodies, and recurrent aspiration must also be considered. Tobacco or marihuana smoking may contribute to this process in older children. In patients of all ages, the potential role of irritants within their environment must also be evaluated.

Complications

In otherwise healthy children, complications of an acute bronchitis secondary to a viral infection are few but include otitis media, sinusitis, and pneumonia.

Treatment

When bronchitis is secondary to an uncomplicated acute viral infection, supportive therapy (stressing adequate hydration, rest, and patience) is all that is necessary. Expectorants and cough suppressants, though commonly used, are seldom indicated. Avoidance of irritants during the viral infection may also decrease symptoms and morbidity. When the bronchitic syndrome is due to other underlying problems, the treatment must address the primary process.

Florman AL, Cushing AH, Umland ET: Rapid noninvasive techniques for determining etiology of bronchitis and pneumonia in infants and children. Clin Chest Med 1987;8:669.

Loughlin GM: Bronchitis. In: *Disorders of the Respiratory Tract in Children,* 5th ed. Chernick V, Kendig EL Jr (editors). Saunders, 1990.

Rossman CM, Newhouse MT: Primary ciliary dyskinesia: Evaluation and management. Pediatr Pulmonol 1988; 5:36.

BRONCHIOLITIS

Essentials of Diagnosis

- Young infant with acute onset of tachypnea, cough, rhinorrhea, and expiratory wheeze.

General Considerations

Bronchiolitis is a common cause for acute hospital admissions in under 2 years, especially during the winter months. Although respiratory syncytial virus is by far the most common pathogen, other viruses include parainfluenza, influenza, and adenovirus. *Mycoplasma, Chlamydia, Ureaplasma,* and *Pneumocystis* are other potential causes of wheezing-associated respiratory illness during early infancy. Major concerns include not only the acute effects of bronchiolitis but also the possible development of chronic airways hyperreactivity (asthma). In addition, bronchiolitis due to respiratory syncytial virus (RSV) infection contributes substantially to morbidity and mortality in children with underlying cardiopulmonary disorders, including bronchopulmonary dysplasia, cystic fibrosis, and congenital heart disease, especially when pulmonary hypertension is present.

Clinical Findings

A. Symptoms and Signs: The usual course of RSV bronchiolitis is 1–2 days of fever, rhinorrhea, and cough, followed by wheezing, tachypnea, and respiratory distress. Typically, the breathing pattern is shallow, with rapid respirations. Nasal flaring, cyanosis, retractions, and rales may be present, along with prolongation of the expiratory phase and wheezing, depending on the severity of illness. Some young infants present with apnea and little auscultatory findings but may subsequently develop rales, rhonchi, and expiratory wheezing.

B. Laboratory Findings: The peripheral white blood cell count may be normal or show a mild lymphocytosis.

C. Imaging: Chest x-ray findings typically include hyperinflation with mild interstitial infiltrates, but segmental atelectasis is not uncommon.

Treatment

Susceptibility to RSV in high-risk children can be reduced by antibody. Prevention by new vaccines is also being explored. Although most children infected with RSV bronchiolitis are readily managed as outpatients with supportive therapy, hospitalization is required in children younger than 2 months of age and in patients with hypoxemia in room air, a history of apnea, moderate tachypnea with feeding difficulties, marked respiratory distress with retractions, or underlying chronic cardiopulmonary disorders. Initial management includes an assessment of oxygenation and ventilation and, if hypoxemia is present, the administration of supplemental oxygen. Noninvasive measurements of oxygenation by oximeter should be used to assess the response to therapy and provide early warning of impending respiratory failure in infants. In one series, 7% of normal children admitted for viral bronchiolitis subsequently required mechanical ventilation; infants with bronchopulmonary dysplasia and cystic fibrosis hospitalized with RSV bronchiolitis develop respiratory failure at higher rates. Progressive respiratory distress (including progressive hypoxemia and hypercapnia) and apnea are common indications for admission to the intensive care unit and mechanical ventilation.

Intravenous fluids should be given to correct losses and poor intake, while carefully monitoring intake, output, and urinary specific gravity to avoid overhydration and the risk of fluid overload and pulmonary edema. Although β-adrenergic therapy and corticosteroids may attenuate airway obstruction, their use remains controversial and empiric, and patients should be assessed individually to determine the degree of responsiveness to drug therapy.

The availability of rapid diagnostic testing for RSV infection may allow for early intervention with antiviral therapy (ribavirin), especially in children with marked respiratory distress or chronic cardiopulmonary disease. Although ribavirin's efficacy remains unclear, its use is currently recommended for hospitalized infants with severe disease or with coexistent congenital heart disease, bronchopulmonary dysplasia, cystic fibrosis, immunodeficiencies, other chronic lung disorders, recent transplant recipients and patients undergoing chemotherapy. In addition, children younger than 6 weeks and those with underlying metabolic, neurologic, or congenital abnormalities should be considered for ribavirin therapy.

Preliminary data suggest that therapy with immune globulin with a high titer of antibodies against RSV may be effective in decreasing the risk for RSV lung infection. Clinical trials are underway to evaluate its potential usefulness.

Prognosis

Although the outcome in bronchiolitis is good for healthy children, the mortality rate in patients with cardiopulmonary disease can be high. In addition, recurrent episodes of wheezing may follow acute infection in almost half of the hospitalized infants.

Abman SH et al: Role of RSV in early hospitalizations for respiratory distress of young infants with cystic fibrosis. J Pediatr 1988;113:826.

Groothuis JR et al: Prophylactic administration of respiratory syncytial virus immune globulin to high-risk infants and young children. N Engl J Med 1993;329:1524.

MacDonald NE et al: RSV in infants with congenital heart disease. N Engl J Med 1982;307:397.

Makela J, Ruuskanen O: RSV in children. Curr Opin Pediatr 1994;6:17.

Wohl MEB: Bronchiolitis. In: *Disorders of the Respiratory Tract in Children,* 5th ed. Chernick V, Kendig EL Jr (editors). Saunders, 1990.

Zucker AR, Meadows WL: Pediatric critical care physicians' attitudes about guidelines for the use of ribavirin in critically ill children with RSV pneumonia. Crit Care Med 1995;23:767.

BRONCHIECTASIS

Essentials of Diagnosis

- Chronic cough with sputum production.
- Persistent abnormalities on physical examination of the chest.
- Persistent abnormalities on chest x-ray.

General Considerations

The term "bronchiectasis" means dilatation of bronchi. The dilatation may be regular, with the airway continuing to have a smooth outline (cylindric bronchiectasis); irregular, with areas of dilatation and constriction (varicose bronchiectasis); or marked, with destruction of structural components of the airway wall (saccular bronchiectasis). Although the incidence of the disease in the general population is low (< 0.5%), the morbidity associated with the more severe forms of bronchiectasis is significant. Medical treatment can halt the progression of a potentially reversible form (cylindric bronchiectasis) to an irreversible destructive airway disease (saccular bronchiectasis).

Bronchiectasis results from obstruction of the airway and poor drainage (from such causes as cystic fibrosis, foreign bodies), and infection. Either infection or obstruction occurring alone is unlikely to lead to the more severe forms of bronchiectasis. The combination of the two for a period of time, however, can cause bronchiectasis.

Clinical Findings

A. Symptoms and Signs: These range from chronic cough with early morning sputum production in an overtly healthy child, to recurrent pneumonia with or without hemoptysis in a chronically ill child. There may be a history of recurrent respiratory infections, dyspnea on exertion, and a productive cough precipitated by exercise. Some children present with recurrent fevers. Chronic cough, persistent atelectasis, and failure of a chest x-ray to clear after a respiratory infection are typical. On physical examination, digital clubbing may be seen, and there may be evidence of sinusitis. Persistent moist rales, rhonchi, and decreased air entry are often noted over the bronchiectatic area when saccular changes are present.

B. Laboratory Findings and Imaging: Cultures from the respiratory tract usually reveal mixed flora; *H influenzae* is a common isolate.

Chest films may be mildly abnormal with slightly increased bronchovascular markings or areas of atelectasis, or they may demonstrate cystic changes in one or more areas of the lung. The extent of bronchiectasis is best defined by high-resolution CT scan of the lung, which often reveals far wider involvement of lung than expected from the plain chest film. Bronchography is no longer widely used.

Pulmonary function testing often reveals an obstructive pattern even in the absence of asthma, cystic fibrosis, or other disease processes leading to airway obstruction. This obstruction may result from difficulty in clearing secretions. Evaluation of lung function after use of a bronchodilator is helpful in assessing the benefit a patient may have from bronchodilators. In addition, serial assessments of lung function help define the progression or resolution of the disease.

Differential Diagnosis

Bronchiectasis can develop in patients with cystic fibrosis, immunodeficiencies involving humoral immunity, and abnormal mucociliary clearance (primary ciliary dyskinesia). Recently, bronchiectasis has also been described in children with HIV infection. Recurrent aspiration of a foreign body must also be considered, especially when bronchiectatic changes are confined to one area of the lung.

Although congenital causes of bronchiectasis are relatively uncommon compared with the predisposing factors previously listed, they must still be considered in the differential diagnosis. Bronchiectasis may result from defective development of bronchial cartilage (Williams-Campbell syndrome) and developmental failure of elastic and muscular tissues of the trachea and bronchi (tracheobronchomegaly or Mounier-Kuhn syndrome. Bronchial stenosis, either congenital or acquired, also predisposes to bronchiectasis.

Complications

Major concerns are severe pneumonia, hemoptysis, and cor pulmonale. Less usual complications include abscesses of the lung or central nervous system as well as empyema and bronchopleural fistula.

Treatment

Initial management is medical and consists of antibiotics for bacterial pathogens present in the bronchiectatic areas of lung. In addition to use of antibiotics is optimal pulmonary physiotherapy, which consists of inhalation of bronchodilators followed by postural drainage and chest percussion to affected areas of lung. If present, sinusitis must also be vigorously treated.

Surgical removal of an area of lung that has severe saccular bronchiectasis is considered when the response to several months of optimal medical therapy has been poor. Other indications include extensive or repeated hemoptysis and recurrent pneumonia in one area of lung. In general, surgery is best performed when the bronchiectatic area is well localized and the rest of the lung appears normal. This is most likely in a child who has saccular bronchiectasis due to foreign body aspiration or a congenital defect. In general, children with more serious underlying disorders (cystic fibrosis, hypogammaglobulinemia) are likely to have bronchiectatic changes in several areas of the lung and are not good candidates for surgery.

Prognosis

This depends on the underlying cause and the severity of the bronchiectasis, the extent of lung involvement, and the response to medical management. As noted, good pulmonary hygiene and avoidance of infectious complications in the involved areas of lung may reverse cylindric bronchiectasis.

Amorosa JK et al: Bronchiectasis in children with lymphocytic interstitial pneumonia and acquired immune deficiency syndrome: Plain film and CT observations. Pediatr Radiol 1992;22:603.

Brown MA, Lemen RJ: Bronchiectasis. In: *Disorders of the Respiratory Tract in Children,* 5th ed. Chernick V, Kendig EL Jr (editors). Saunders, 1990.

BRONCHIOLITIS OBLITERANS

Bronchiolitis obliterans is characterized by obstruction of bronchi and bronchioles by fibrous tissue. The disorder follows damage to the lower respiratory tract, such as inhalation of toxic gases, infections (adenovirus, influenza virus, rubeola virus, *Bordetella, Mycoplasma*), connective tissue diseases, transplantation, and aspiration. Many episodes of bronchiolitis obliterans are idiopathic. Adenovirus-induced bronchiolitis obliterans occurs more frequently in the Native American population in Canada and in Polynesian children in New Zealand, suggesting that racial or socioeconomic factors predispose to this process.

Clinical Findings

A. Symptoms and Signs: Bronchiolitis obliterans should be considered when there is persistent cough, wheezing, or sputum production after an acute pneumonia. Prolonged rales or wheezing or persistent exercise intolerance following a pulmonary insult should also suggest this disease.

B. Laboratory Findings and Imaging: Chest x-ray abnormalities include evidence of localized or generalized air trapping as well as possibly nodular densities and alveolar opacification. Scattered areas of matched decreases in ventilation and perfusion are seen when the lung is scanned. Pulmonary angiograms reveal decreased vasculature in the area of lung involvement, whereas bronchograms demonstrate marked pruning of the bronchial tree. An assessment of lung function demonstrates an obstructive process that may be combined with evidence of restriction. Inhaled bronchodilators of corticosteroids provide little improvement in lung function.

Differential Diagnosis

Poorly treated asthma, cystic fibrosis, and bronchopulmonary dysplasia must be considered in children with persistent airway obstruction. A trial of medications (including bronchodilators and corticosteroids) may help to define the reversibility of the process when the primary differential is between asthma and bronchiolitis obliterans. Although the results of imaging and pulmonary function testing are very suggestive, the best way to establish a definitive diagnosis is by lung biopsy.

Complications

Sequelae of bronchiolitis obliterans include persistent airway obstruction, recurrent wheezing, bronchiectasis, chronic atelectasis, recurrent pneumonia, and unilateral hyperlucent lung syndrome.

Treatment

Supplemental oxygen should be given to patients with oxygen desaturation during normal activities or sleep. In addition, early treatment should be directed at preventing ongoing airway damage due to problems such as aspiration, which may be either the primary insult or an acquired problem secondary to marked hyperinflation. Other forms of treatment may be more difficult to evaluate in terms of effectiveness. Oral and inhaled bronchodilators may be helpful in reversing airway obstruction if there is a reactive component to the disease. Many children also receive at least one course of corticosteroid treatment in an attempt to reverse the obstruction or prevent ongoing damage. Antibiotics should be used as clinically indicated for pneumonia.

Prognosis

Prognosis may depend in part on the underlying cause as well as the age at which the insult occurred. The course varies from mild asthma-like symptoms to rapidly fatal deterioration despite therapy.

Hardy KA: Obliterative bronchiolitis. In: Pediatric Respiratory Disease. Hillman B (editor). Saunders, 1993.

BRONCHOPULMONARY DYSPLASIA

Essentials of Diagnosis
- Acute respiratory distress in first week of life.
- Required oxygen therapy or mechanical ventilation.
- Persistent respiratory abnormalities, including physical signs, radiographic findings, and increased oxygen requirement, after 1 month of age.

General Considerations
Bronchopulmonary dysplasia remains one of the most significant sequelae following the management of acute respiratory distress in the neonatal intensive care unit, with an incidence between 10% and 40% (depending on the criteria used for definition and the gestational age of the population base). This disease was first characterized in 1967 when Northway and coworkers reported the clinical, radiologic, and pathologic findings in a group of premature newborns who required prolonged mechanical ventilation and oxygen therapy to treat hyaline membrane disease. The progression from acute hyaline membrane disease to chronic lung disease was divided into four stages: acute respiratory distress shortly after birth, usually hyaline membrane disease (stage I); clinical and radiographic worsening of the acute lung disease, often due to increased pulmonary blood flow secondary to a patent ductus arteriosus (stage II); and progressive signs of chronic lung disease (stages III and IV).

The precise definition of bronchopulmonary dysplasia remains controversial. Clinically it is a chronic respiratory disorder of infancy that follows treatment during the first week of life for acute respiratory distress and is subsequently associated with persistent signs of respiratory distress, a requirement for supplemental oxygen, and radiographic abnormalities beyond 30 days of age. This broad definition does not accommodate some key issues, including the following: (1) although most of these children were premature and had hyaline membrane disease, full-term newborns with such disorders as meconium aspiration or persistent pulmonary hypertension can also develop bronchopulmonary dysplasia; (2) some severely preterm newborns require minimal ventilator support yet subsequently develop a prolonged oxygen requirement despite the absence of severe acute manifestations of respiratory failure; (3) newborns dying within the first weeks of life can already have the aggressive, fibroproliferative pathologic lesions that resemble bronchopulmonary dysplasia; and (4) physiologic abnormalities (increased airway resistance) and biochemical markers of lung injury (altered protease and antiprotease ratios, increased inflammatory cells and mediators), which are predictive of bronchopulmonary dysplasia, are already present in the first week of life.

Although the exact mechanisms leading to chronic lung disease are not completely understood, bronchopulmonary dysplasia represents the consequences of lung injury caused by oxygen toxicity, barotrauma, and inflammation superimposed on a susceptible, generally immature lung. The premature lung often makes too little of functional surfactant; furthermore, the antioxidant defense mechanisms are not sufficiently mature to protect the lung from the toxic oxygen metabolites generated from hyperoxia. Thus, abnormal lung mechanics due to structural immaturity, surfactant deficiency, atelectasis, and pulmonary edema–plus lung injury secondary to hyperoxia and mechanical ventilation–lead to further abnormalities of lung function, causing increases in ventilator and oxygen requirements and leading to a vicious circle that compounds the progression of lung injury. Excessive fluid administration, patent ductus arteriosus, pulmonary interstitial emphysema, pneumothorax, infection, and inflammatory stimuli secondary to lung injury or infection also play important roles in the pathogenesis of the disease.

Differential Diagnosis
The radiologic differential diagnosis includes meconium aspiration syndrome, congenital infection (such as cytomegalovirus or *Ureaplasma*), cystic adenomatoid malformation, recurrent aspiration, pulmonary lymphangiectasia, total anomalous pulmonary venous return, overhydration, or idiopathic pulmonary fibrosis.

Clinical Course & Treatment
The clinical course of infants with bronchopulmonary dysplasia ranges from a mild increased oxygen requirement that gradually resolves over a few months to more severe disease requiring chronic tracheostomy and mechanical ventilation for the first 2 years of life. In general, patients show slow, steady improvements in oxygen or ventilator requirements but can have frequent respiratory exacerbations leading to frequent or prolonged hospitalizations. Clinical management generally includes careful attention to growth, nutrition, metabolic status, development, neurologic status, and related problems, along with the various cardiopulmonary abnormalities described below.

Because increased airways resistance and bronchial hyperreactivity are common in infants with the disorder, various combinations of β-adrenergic agonists, aminophylline, corticosteroids, and cromolyn are commonly part of the treatment plan. Part of the rationale for the use of corticosteroids is to decrease lung inflammation and enhance responsiveness to β-adrenergic drugs, as in the treatment of severe asthma. Because thick secretions are common and may contribute to airway obstruction or recurrent atelectasis, chest physiotherapy following the administration of β-adrenergic agonists is commonly part of the regimen.

Although bronchial hyperreactivity in affected infants is well recognized, structural lesions (such as subglottic stenosis, vocal cord paralysis, tracheal stenosis, tracheomalacia, bronchial stenosis, granulomatous bronchial polyps, and others) often contribute to airflow limitation. This possibility suggests the need for careful bronchoscopic evaluations in children with significant involvement.

Infants often have recurrent pulmonary edema, which may be due to increased permeability of the injured pulmonary circulation or to increases in hydrostatic pressure if left ventricular dysfunction is present. In addition, salt and water retention secondary to chronic hypoxemia, hypercapnia, or other stimuli may be present. Chronic or intermittent diuretic therapy with furosemide, hydrochlorothiazide, and spironolactone is commonly used if there are rales or signs of persistent pulmonary edema, with acute improvement in lung function demonstrated by clinical studies. Unfortunately, diuretics often cause major side effects, including severe volume contraction, hypokalemia, alkalosis, and hyponatremia. Potassium and arginine chloride supplements are commonly required.

Infants often have pulmonary hypertension, and in many children, even mild hypoxia can cause significant elevations of pulmonary artery pressure. To minimize the harmful effects of hypoxia, the PaO_2 should be kept above 55–60 mm Hg. Because even intermittent hypoxia contributes to the development or progression of pulmonary hypertension and cor pulmonale, noninvasive assessments of oxygenation must be made during all activities, including the infant's waking, sleeping, and feeding periods. Serial electrocardiographic and echocardiographic studies monitor the development of right ventricular hypertrophy. If hypertrophy persists or develops where it previously was not present, intermittent hypoxia should be considered and further assessments of oxygenation pursued, especially while the infant sleeps. In addition, barium swallow, esophageal pH probe studies, bronchoscopy, and cardiac catheterization may reveal previously unsuspected cardiac or pulmonary lesions—aspiration, tracheomalacia, obstructive sleep apnea, anatomic cardiac lesions, etc—that contribute to the underlying pathophysiology. In addition, long-term care should include monitoring systemic hypertension and the development of left ventricular hypertrophy.

Nutritional problems in infants may be due to increased oxygen consumption, feeding difficulties, gastroesophageal reflux, and chronic hypoxia. Hypercaloric formulas and gastrostomies are often required to ensure adequate intake while avoiding overhydration. In addition, influenza vaccine is recommended. With the onset of acute wheezing secondary to suspected viral infection, rapid diagnostic testing for RSV infection may facilitate early treatment, which may diminish the late morbidity of bronchiolitis.

For children who remain ventilator-dependent, the authors believe that arterial CO_2 should be maintained below 60 mm Hg—even when pH is normal—because of the potential adverse effects of hypercapnia on salt and water retention, cardiac function, and perhaps pulmonary vascular tone. Changes in ventilator settings in children with severe lung disease should be slow, because the effects of many of the changes may not be manifested for days. These signs may include poor feeding, irritability, weight loss, vomiting, increased retractions, wheezing, and CO_2 retention. Medical staff should frequently meet with the parents to review progress and changes in treatment plans and thereby decrease some of the family stresses involved in caring for children with chronic severe disease. Patience, continued family support, attention to developmental issues, and speech and physical therapy help to improve the long-term outlook.

Prognosis

Although the mortality rate is high in infants with severe (stage IV) bronchopulmonary dysplasia, the long-term outlook is generally favorable. More time and further study is needed, however, to assess the impact in adolescence and early adulthood of such sequelae as persistent airway hyperreactivity, exercise intolerance, and perhaps abnormal lung growth. New therapeutic approaches such as surfactant replacement and high-frequency ventilation have not yet been shown to reduce the severity or incidence of bronchopulmonary dysplasia. The possible role of antioxidant therapy or specific anti-inflammatory agents must be pursued.

Abman SH, Groothuis JR: Pathophysiology and treatment of bronchopulmonary dysplasia: Current issues. Pediatr Clin North Am 1994;41:277.

Gerhardt T et al: Serial determination of pulmonary function in infants with chronic lung disease. J Pediatr 1987; 110:448.

Groneck P, Speer CP: Inflammatory mediators and bronchopulmonary dysplasia. Arch Dis Child 1995;73:F1.

Holtzman RB, Frank L (editors): *Bronchopulmonary Dysplasia.* Clinical Perinatology, Vol 19. Saunders, 1992.

Northway WH, Rosan RC, Porter DY: Pulmonary disease following respiratory therapy of hyaline membrane disease: Bronchopulmonary dysplasia. N Engl J Med 1967;276:357.

Northway WH et al: Late pulmonary sequelae of bronchopulmonary dysplasia. N Engl J Med 1990;323:1793.

O'Brodovich HM, Mellins RM: Bronchopulmonary dysplasia. Unresolved neonatal acute lung injury. Am Rev Respir Dis 1985;132:694.

CYSTIC FIBROSIS

Essentials of Diagnosis

- Sweat chloride greater than 60 mmol/L.
- Pulmonary, gastrointestinal, or hepatic dysfunction.

General Considerations

Cystic fibrosis is the most common lethal genetic disease in the United States, with an incidence of 1:2000–3000 white births. It is a major cause of pulmonary and gastrointestinal morbidity in children and a leading cause of death in early adulthood. Although cystic fibrosis causes abnormalities in the hepatic, gastrointestinal, and male reproductive systems, the lung disease is the major cause of morbidity and mortality. Almost all patients develop obstructive lung disease associated with chronic infection that leads to progressive loss of pulmonary function. The prognosis has improved steadily over the past 20 years, so that the median survival is now 28 years—perhaps as a result of use of antibiotics, better treatment of malabsorption, and the development of a network of special cystic fibrosis care centers. The centers usually use a multidisciplinary approach to patient care, which involves contributions from physicians, nurses, social workers, nutritionists, and physical or respiratory therapists.

The cystic fibrosis gene is on the long arm of human chromosome 7 and codes for the cystic fibrosis transmembrane conductance regulator (CFTR). The CFTR is involved in chloride channel activity. Approximately 75% of the mutations in cystic fibrosis patients correspond to a specific deletion of three base pairs, which results in the loss of a phenylalanine residue at amino acid position 508 of the CFTR. The remainder of the cystic fibrosis mutant gene pool consists of many different mutations. Part of the variability in clinical course in cystic fibrosis can be explained by differences in genotype.

Clinical Findings & Treatment

A. Clinical Presentations and Diagnosis: Fifteen percent of infants with cystic fibrosis present at birth with an intestinal obstruction known as meconium ileus. Abdominal distention and the presence of a thick, sticky meconium throughout the large colon on meglumine diatrizoate (Gastrografin) enema examination suggest the diagnosis. In the past, surgical removal of the meconium was common and often led to resection of bowel. However, improved techniques of enema administration under radiologic observation have reduced the need for surgery.

Roughly 50% of patients with cystic fibrosis present classically in infancy with failure to thrive, respiratory compromise, or both. The age at presentation, however, can be variable; some patients are not diagnosed until adulthood. Neonatal screening based on elevations of immunoreactive trypsinogen in the blood is an alternative method of case identification.

Whether the clinical suspicion of cystic fibrosis is based on meconium ileus, failure to thrive, recurrent respiratory infections, or elevated immunoreactive trypsinogen in infancy, the diagnosis is made only after a positive sweat test or demonstration of a genotype consistent with cystic fibrosis. The sweat of individuals with cystic fibrosis contains elevated concentrations of chloride and sodium. Although elevated sweat electrolytes are associated with other conditions, a positive sweat test combined with the clinical picture usually confirms the diagnosis. Laboratories routinely performing sweat tests give more reliable results than those that perform them only occasionally. The Gibson-Cooke quantitative technique is the only acceptable method. Measurements of electrical conductivity alone can be unreliable.

B. Gastrointestinal and Nutritional Findings and Treatment: Untreated patients with cystic fibrosis have abdominal distention and discomfort; bulky, greasy stools; and increased flatulence secondary to exocrine pancreatic insufficiency and malabsorption. Some infants present with hypoalbuminemia, anemia, edema, and hepatomegaly. Infants with severe protein-calorie malnutrition have particularly difficult courses, with high morbidity and mortality rates. Children and adults with cystic fibrosis are subject to intestinal blockage from inspissated stool. This "meconium ileus equivalent" is now most often treated with cathartics and enemas and only rarely requires surgery. Patients with cystic fibrosis are more prone to intussusception (especially of the appendix) than are normal individuals.

The cornerstone of gastrointestinal treatment is pancreatic enzyme supplementation. Patients are required to take the enzyme capsules with each meal and with snacks. Newer enzyme preparations contain more lipase per capsule than older preparations; therefore, patients take fewer capsules, making administration easier. Occasionally, enzyme supplementation alone does not control the malabsorption, and antacids are added to the regimen.

Individuals with cystic fibrosis may have fat-soluble vitamin deficiency, hypoalbuminemia, and poor growth with decreased stores of body fat. In the past, fat-restricted diets were recommended. It is now recognized that patients with cystic fibrosis need all the calories they can take, and unrestricted diets are now the norm in most centers. Moreover, caloric supplements, such as high-calorie commercial supplements or formulas or food modules (including Polycose and medium-chain triglycerides) are often added to the patient's diet. In patients who do not respond to oral supplementation, night-time nasogastric feeding or feeding by means of gastrostomy or jejunostomy has been tried. Although there is general agreement that quality of life is enhanced by improved nutrition, it is not known whether aggressive nutritional treatment increases longevity.

C. Pulmonary Findings and Treatment: Infants with cystic fibrosis frequently have respiratory compromise. Cough, tachypnea, rales, and wheezing are common findings. RSV infection is associated with marked morbidity in early infancy. Some patients develop cough only later in childhood or adolescence, but by adulthood almost all patients with cystic fibrosis have productive coughs. In more advanced disease, hemoptysis due to bronchiectasis, exercise limitation, and cor pulmonale may be present. Rales may be heard on physical examination. Clubbing also develops as the lung disease progresses.

Pulmonary function abnormalities initially show obstructive patterns with diminished flow rates and increased lung volumes. As the disease progresses, vital capacity is also affected. The incidence of airway reactivity in cystic fibrosis has been estimated to be 25–50%, several times the incidence in the general population. Initially, the airway is colonized with *Staphylococcus aureus*, but in most patients, *Pseudomonas aeruginosa* becomes predominant at some point. The acquisition of the characteristic mucoid *Pseudomonas* is associated with a more rapid decline in pulmonary function. In addition, infection with *Pseudomonas cepacia* has been associated with rapid deterioration and death. Pathologically, the earliest lesions involve hyperplasia of the mucus glands of the bronchial epithelium and mucosal and submucosal cellular infiltrates. Bronchiolectasis and bronchiectasis usually follow throughout all lung fields.

Treatment of the pulmonary disease in cystic fibrosis includes chest physical therapy, antibiotics, bronchodilators, and (more recently) anti-inflammatory agents. Each of these treatments is controversial. A recent study of postural drainage and percussion has demonstrated benefit over a 3-year period in patients receiving the therapy. This study has put the use of postural drainage on firmer ground. Although controlled trials have yielded ambiguous results, there is general agreement that antibiotics play a major role in pulmonary treatment. Antibiotics are used liberally in outpatient treatment (eg, with a change in cough or respiratory symptoms) and are used extensively during inpatient admissions. Recent studies have suggested a benefit from inhaled antibiotics. The high incidence of airway reactivity suggests an important treatment role for bronchodilators, yet some studies have shown paradoxic responses to these medications. The paradoxic responses may be related in part to the fact that the increasing compliance of large airways leads to earlier airway closure.

Current speculation on the development of lung disease in cystic fibrosis includes not only the effects of the bacterial pathogens but also the host response to such pathogens. If activated neutrophils or immune complexes are important in the genesis of the airway injury, then anti-inflammatory agents may be helpful. Although corticosteroids may be beneficial in patients with increased airway reactivity, a multicenter trial has identified complications, including glucose intolerance, the development of diabetes, and decreased linear growth. associated with alternate-day prednisone use.

A subgroup of patients with cystic fibrosis have frequent pulmonary exacerbations characterized by difficult breathing, increased sputum production, decreased exercise tolerance, and diminished pulmonary function. These patients often benefit from hospital treatment, including intensive physical therapy, intravenous antibiotics, bronchodilators, and concentrated efforts at nutritional rehabilitation. Increasingly, outpatient intravenous therapy is being used to shorten or eliminate the hospital stay.

D. Hepatic Disease: Although most patients with cystic fibrosis demonstrate cirrhosis at autopsy, only a small percentage develop portal hypertension. In these individuals, however, the clinical manifestations of the liver disease may be severe, with esophageal varices leading to life-threatening gastrointestinal bleeding and hypersplenism requiring splenic embolization.

E. Reproductive Tract Involvement: More than 95% of males with cystic fibrosis are infertile, a condition secondary to failure of development of the vas deferens. Cystic fibrosis is occasionally diagnosed through infertility evaluations in men with relatively mild involvement of the respiratory and gastrointestinal tracts. In general, women with cystic fibrosis are fertile, but pregnancy may place considerable stress on patients with limited pulmonary function.

Prognosis

The rate of progression of lung involvement usually determines survival. Most patients now reach adulthood. Recent reports of successful lung transplantation have been encouraging. In addition, new treatments are being developed based on improved understanding of the disease at the cellular and molecular levels. Along these lines, inhaled recombinant human DNase therapy has been shown to improve pulmonary function in cystic fibrosis. Gene therapy trials are already under way.

Aitken ML et al: Recombinant human DNase inhalation in normal subjects and patients with cystic fibrosis: A phase 1 study. JAMA 1992;267:1947.

Kerem B-S et al: Identification of the cystic fibrosis gene: Genetic analysis. Science 1989;245:1073.

Kerem E et al: The relation between genotype and phenotype in cystic fibrosis: Analysis of the most common mutation (delta F_{508}). N Engl J Med 1990;323:1517.

MacLusky I: Cystic fibrosis for the primary care pediatrician. Pediatr Ann 1993;22:541.

Stern RC: The primary care physician and the patient with cystic fibrosis.

CONGENITAL DISEASES INVOLVING ALVEOLI

The clinical spectrum of congenital lung disorders can vary widely, ranging from severe, life-threatening respiratory distress in the neonate (which typically occurs with cystic adenomatoid malformation and most cases of congenital lobar emphysema) to chronic cough, wheezing, or stridor in the older child (with bronchogenic cyst, for example) to incidental radiologic findings in patients with very mild symptoms. The following is a limited discussion of selected congenital structural lesions that involve or compromise alveoli.

PULMONARY AGENESIS & HYPOPLASIA

Pulmonary agenesis or hypoplasia represents absent or incomplete lung development, which generally reflects an intrauterine interruption or alteration of the normal sequence of embryologic events and may be associated with other congenital abnormalities.

With unilateral **pulmonary agenesis** (the complete absence of one lung), the trachea continues into a main bronchus and often has complete tracheal rings. The left lung is affected more often than the right. With compensatory postnatal growth over time, the remaining lung often herniates into the contralateral chest. Chest x-ray study shows a mediastinal shift toward the affected side, and vertebral abnormalities may be present. The outcome is primarily related to the severity of associated congenital lesions. About 50% of patients survive; the mortality rate is higher with agenesis of the right lung than of the left lung. This difference is probably not related to the higher incidence of associated anomalies but rather to a greater shift in the mediastinum that leads to tracheal compression and distortion.

Pulmonary hypoplasia is incomplete development of one or both lungs, resulting in the reduction of the number of bronchial branchings or a decrease in expected lung weight, volume, or DNA content. It is part of a spectrum with a gradual transition. Pulmonary hypoplasia may be present in up to 10–15% of perinatal autopsies. The pathogenesis of hypoplasia is multifactorial and includes the presence of an intrathoracic mass, resulting in lack of space for the lungs to grow, decreased size of the thorax, decreased fetal breathing movements, decreased blood flow to the lungs, or possibly a primary mesodermal defect affecting multiple organ systems. Congenital diaphragmatic hernia is the most common cause of

pulmonary hypoplasia, with an incidence of 1:2200 births. Other causes include extralobar sequestration, diaphragmatic eventration or hypoplasia, thoracic neuroblastoma, fetal hydrops, and fetal hydrochylothorax. Chest cage abnormalities, diaphragmatic elevation, oligohydramnios, chromosomal abnormalities, severe musculoskeletal disorders, and cardiac lesions also may lead to hypoplastic lungs. In addition, postnatal factors may play important roles; for example, infants with advanced bronchopulmonary dysplasia can have pulmonary hypoplasia.

Clinical Findings

A. Symptoms and Signs: The clinical presentation is highly variable and is related to the severity of hypoplasia as well as associated abnormalities. Frequently, lung hypoplasia is associated with pneumothorax. Some newborns present with perinatal stress, severe acute respiratory distress, and persistent pulmonary hypertension of the newborn secondary to primary pulmonary hypoplasia (without associated anomalies). Children with milder degrees of hypoplasia may present with chronic cough, tachypnea, wheezing, and recurrent pneumonia.

B. Laboratory Findings and Imaging: Chest x-ray findings include variable degrees of volume loss in a small hemithorax with mediastinal shift. Ventilation/perfusion scans, angiography, and bronchoscopy are often helpful in the clinical evaluation. The degree of respiratory impairment is defined by analysis of arterial blood gases.

Treatment & Prognosis

Treatment is primarily supportive and directed at the symptoms. The overall outcome is determined by the severity of underlying medical problems and the extent of the hypoplasia.

Langston C, Thurlbeck WM: Conditions altering normal lung growth and development. In: *Neonatal Pulmonary Care.* Thibeault DW, Gregory GA (editors). Appleton-Century-Crofts, 1986.

Phelan PD, Landau, LI, Olinsky A: Congenital malformations of the bronchi, lungs, diaphragm and rib cage. In: *Respiratory Illness in Children.* 3rd ed. Phelan PD, Landou LI, Olinsky A (editors). Blackwell Scientific, 1990.

Stocker JT et al: Cystic and congenital lung disease in the newborn. In: *Perspectives in Pediatric Pathology.* Vol 4. Rosenberg H, Bolande T (editors). Year Book, 1978.

PULMONARY SEQUESTRATION

Pulmonary sequestration is a localized mass of disorganized growth that is classified as either extralobar or intralobar. **Extralobar sequestration** is a mass of pulmonary parenchyma anatomically separate from the normal lung, with a distinct pleural investment. Its blood supply derives from either the systemic circulation (more typical), pulmonary vessels, or both. Although it can rarely communicate with the esophagus or stomach, it does not communicate directly with the tracheobronchial tree. Pathologically, extralobar sequestration appears as a solitary thoracic lesion near the diaphragm. Abdominal sites are rare. Size varies between 0.5 cm and 12 cm.

Histologic findings include uniformly dilated bronchioles, alveolar ducts, and alveoli. Occasionally, the bronchial structure appears normal; often, however, the cartilage in the wall is deficient, or no cartilage-containing structures can be found. On occasion, lymphangiectasia is found within the lesion. Extralobar sequestration can be associated with other anomalies, including bronchogenic cysts, heart defects, and diaphragmatic hernia.

Intralobar sequestration is an isolated segment of lung within the normal pleural investment but without connection to the tracheobronchial tree. The arterial supply is often provided by one or more arteries arising from the aorta or its branches. Intralobar sequestration is usually found within the lower lobes (98%) and is rarely associated with other congenital anomalies (less than 2% versus 50% with extralobar sequestration). It is rarely seen in the newborn period (unlike extralobar sequestration). Some have hypothesized that intralobar sequestration is an acquired lesion secondary to chronic infection. Clinical presentation includes chronic cough, wheezing or patients with "recurrent pneumonias." Rarely, intralobar sequestration can present with hemoptysis. Diagnosis is often made by angiography, demonstrating large systemic arteries perfusing the lesion. Treatment is by surgical resection.

Alivizatos P et al: Pulmonary sequestration complicated by anomalies of pulmonary venous return. J Pediatr Surg 1985;20:76.

Savic B et al: Lung sequestrations: Report of 7 cases and review of 540 published cases. Thorax 1979;34:96.

CONGENITAL LOBAR EMPHYSEMA

Congenital lobar emphysema (also known as infantile lobar emphysema, congenital localized emphysema, unilobar obstructive emphysema, or congenital hypertrophic lobar emphysema) presents in most patients as severe neonatal respiratory distress or as progressive respiratory impairment during the first year of life. Rarely, the mild or intermittent nature of the symptoms in older children or young adults results in a delayed diagnosis. Most patients are white males. Although the cause of congenital lobar emphysema is not well understood, some lesions exhibit bronchial cartilaginous dysplasia due to abnormal orientation or distribution of the bronchial cartilage. This leads to expiratory collapse, producing obstruction and the symptoms outlined below.

Clinical Findings

A. Symptoms and Signs: Clinical features include tachypnea, cyanosis, wheezing, retractions, and cough. Physical examination reveals decreased breath sounds on the affected side, perhaps with hyperresonance to percussion, mediastinal displacement, and bulging of the chest wall on the affected side.

B. Imaging: Radiologic findings include overdistention of the affected lobe, with wide separation of bronchovascular markings, collapse of adjacent lung, shift of the mediastinum away from the affected side, and a depressed diaphragm on the affected side. Other diagnostic studies include chest x-ray with fluoroscopy, ventilation/perfusion study, and perhaps CT scan followed by bronchoscopy with or without bronchography, angiography, and exploratory thoracotomy.

Differential Diagnosis

The differential diagnosis of congenital lobar emphysema includes pneumothorax, pneumatocele, atelectasis with compensatory hyperinflation, diaphragmatic hernia, and congenital cystic adenomatoid malformation. The most common site of involvement is the left upper lobe (42%) or right middle lobe (35%). Evaluation must differentiate regional obstructive emphysema from lobar hyperinflation secondary to an uncomplicated ball-valve mechanism due to extrinsic compression from a mass (eg, bronchogenic cyst, tumor, lymphadenopathy, foreign body, "pseudotumor" or plasma cell granuloma, vascular compression) or intrinsic obstruction from a mucus plug due to infection and inflammation from various causes.

Treatment

Management generally involves surgery, especially when respiratory distress is marked, with either segmental or complete lobectomy. Conservative management in less symptomatic older children may lead to an outcome not different from those treated surgically with lobectomy.

Eigen H et al: Congenital lobar emphysema: Long-term evaluation of surgically and conservatively treated children. Am Rev Respir Dis 1976;113:823.

Luck SR et al: Congenital bronchopulmonary malformations. Curr Probl Surg (April) 1986;23:245.

Man DWK et al: Congenital lobar emphysema: Problems in diagnosis and management. Arch Dis Child 1983;58:709.

McBride JT et al: Lung growth and airway function after lobectomy in infancy for congenital lobar emphysema. J Clin Invest 1980;66:962.

CONGENITAL CYSTIC ADENOMATOID MALFORMATION

Congenital cystic adenomatoid malformations are unilateral hamartomatous lesions that generally present as marked respiratory distress within the first days of life. This disorder accounts for 95% of cases of congenital cystic lung disease.

Right and left lungs are involved with equal frequency. These lesions appear as gland-like space-occupying masses or have an "adenomatoid" increase in terminal respiratory structures, forming intercommunicating cysts of various sizes, lined by cuboidal or ciliated pseudostratified columnar epithelium. They may have polypoid formations of mucosa, with focally increased elastic tissue in the cyst wall beneath the bronchial type of epithelium. Air passages appear malformed and tend to lack cartilage.

There are three types. Type 1 is most common (75%) and consists of single or multiple large cysts (1–5 cm in diameter) with features of mature lung tissue. Type 1 is amenable to surgical resection. A mediastinal shift is evident on examination or chest x-ray film in 80% of patients and can mimic infantile lobar emphysema. Approximately 75% of type 1 lesions are right-sided. A survival rate of 90% is generally reported.

Type 2 lesions (20% of cases) consist of multiple small cysts (0.5–1.5 cm) resembling dilated simple bronchioles and are often associated with other anomalies (60%), especially renal agenesis or dysgenesis, cardiac malformations, and intestinal atresia. Approximately 60% of type 2 lesions are on the left side. Mediastinal shift is evident less often than in type 1 (10%), and the survival rate is worse (40%).

Type 3 lesions consist of small cysts (0.5 cm). They appear as a bulky, firm mass. The reported survival rate is 50%.

Clinical Findings

A. Symptoms and Signs: Clinically, respiratory distress is noted soon after birth. Expansion of the cysts occurs with the onset of breathing and produces compression of normal lung areas with mediastinal herniation. Breath sounds are decreased. With type 3 lesions, dullness to percussion may be present. The disorder can present in older patients as a spontaneous pneumothorax or "pneumonia."

B. Imaging: In type 1, chest x-ray shows an intrapulmonary mass of soft tissue density with scattered radiolucent areas of varying sizes and shapes, usually with a mediastinal shift and pulmonary herniation. Placement of a radiopaque feeding tube into the stomach helps in the differentiation from diaphragmatic hernia. Type 2 lesions appear similar except that the cysts are smaller. Type 3 may appear as a solid homogeneous mass filling the hemithorax and causing a marked mediastinal shift.

Treatment

Treatment of types 1 and 3 is surgical removal of the affected lobe. Because type 2 is often associated with other severe anomalies, management may be more complex. Segmental resection is not feasible because smaller cysts may expand after removal of the more obviously affected area.

Adzick NS, Harrison MR, Glick PC: Fetal cystic adenomatoid malformation: Prenatal diagnosis and natural history. J Pediatr Surg 1985;20:483.

ACQUIRED DISORDERS INVOLVING ALVEOLI

BACTERIAL PNEUMONIA

Essentials of Diagnosis

- Fever of acute onset.
- Respiratory signs: cough, dyspnea, tachypnea, grunting, or retractions.
- Abnormal chest examination (rales or decreased breath sounds) or abnormal chest radiograph.

General Considerations

Bacterial pneumonia is inflammation of the lung classified according to the infecting organism. It usually develops when one or more of the defense mechanisms normally protecting the lung is inadequate. Patients with the following problems are particularly predisposed to this disease: aspiration, immunodeficiency or immunosuppression, congenital anomalies (intrapulmonary sequestration, tracheoesophageal fistula, cleft palate), abnormalities in mucus clearance (cystic fibrosis, ciliary dysfunction, tracheomalacia, bronchiectasis), congestive heart failure, and perinatal contamination.

Clinical Findings

A. Symptoms and Signs: The bacterial pathogen, severity of the disease, and age of the patient may cause substantial variations in the presenting manifestations of acute bacterial pneumonia. Infants may manifest few or nonspecific findings on history and physical examination. Immunocompetent older patients may not be extremely ill. Some patients may present with fever only or only with signs of generalized toxicity. Others may have additional symptoms or signs of (1) lower respiratory tract disease (respiratory distress, cough, sputum production), (2) pneumonia (rales, decreased breath sounds, dullness to percussion, abnormal tactile or vocal fremitus), or (3) pleural involvement (splinting, pain, friction rub, dullness to percussion). Some patients may manifest additional extrapulmonary findings, such as meningismus or abdominal pain, due to pneumonia itself. Others may have evidence of infection at other sites due to the same organism causing their pneumonia: meningitis, otitis media, sinusitis, pericarditis, epiglottitis, or abscesses.

B. Laboratory Findings: Elevated white blood cell counts (> 15,000/μL) frequently accompany bacterial pneumonia. However, a low white blood count (< 5000/μL) can be an ominous finding in this disease.

C. Imaging: Chest radiographic findings (lateral and frontal views) define bacterial pneumonia. Patchy infiltrates, atelectasis, hilar adenopathy, or pleural effusion may be observed. Films should be taken in the lateral decubitus position to identify pleural fluid. Complete lobar consolidation is not a common finding in infants and children. Severity of disease may not correlate with radiographic findings. Clinical resolution precedes resolution by chest x-ray.

D. Special Examinations: Invasive diagnostic procedures (transtracheal aspiration, bronchial brushing or washing, lung puncture, or open biopsy) should be undertaken in critically ill patients when other means do not adequately define etiology (see Culture of Material From the Respiratory Tract).

Differential Diagnosis

The differential diagnosis of bacterial pneumonia also varies with the age and immunocompetence of the host. The full spectrum of potential pathogens must be considered in each host and includes aerobic and anaerobic bacteria; acid-fast bacteria, including *Mycobacterium tuberculosis; Chlamydia trachomatis* and *Chlamydia psittaci; Rickettsia quintana* (Q fever); *Pneumocystis carinii; Bordetella pertussis; Mycoplasma pneumoniae; Legionella pneumophila* and respiratory viruses.

Noninfectious pulmonary disease (including gastric aspiration, foreign body aspiration, atelectasis, congenital malformations, congestive heart failure, malignant growths, tumors such as plasma cell granuloma, chronic interstitial lung diseases, and pulmonary hemosiderosis) should be considered in the differential diagnosis of localized or diffuse infiltrates. When effusions are present, additional noninfectious disorders such as collagen diseases, neoplasm, and pulmonary infarction should also be considered.

Complications

Empyema may occur frequently with staphylococcal and group A β-hemolytic streptococcal disease. Pneumococcal effusions have a more benign course. Distal sites of infection—meningitis, otitis media, sinusitis (especially of the ethmoids) and septicemia—may be present, particularly with disease due to *S pneumoniae* or *H influenzae*. Certain immunocom-

promised patients, such as those who have undergone splenectomy or who have hemoglobin SS or SC disease or thalassemia, are especially prone to overwhelming sepsis with these organisms. Distal infection of the bones, joints, or other organs (eg, liver abscess) may occur in certain hosts with specific organisms.

Treatment

Appropriate antimicrobial therapy varies according to which organisms are the likely cause of the bacterial pneumonia. Treatment should be guided by (1) Gram's stain of sputum, tracheobronchial secretions, or pleural fluid if available; (2) radiographic findings; and (3) age and known or suspected immunocompetence of the host. For initial coverage in a patient with an unknown pathogen, the physician should consider (1) appropriate penicillins or cephalosporins (or both) to cover gram-positive organisms, including *S aureus;* (2) an aminoglycoside to cover gram-negative enteric organisms (especially in the newborn or immunocompromised host); (3) suitable coverage for *H influenzae* in patients at risk; and (4) erythromycin to cover *M pneumoniae, Legionella pneumophila, Chlamydia* species, and *Ureaplasma.* Therapy is also guided by results of studies for bacterial and viral pathogens (see Culture of Material From the Respiratory Tract, p 430) and is based on other diagnostic studies (see below).

Additional therapeutic considerations include (1) oxygen, (2) humidification of inspired gases, (3) hydration and electrolyte supplementation, (4) oral hygiene, and (5) nutrition. Removal of pleural fluid for diagnostic purposes is indicated initially to guide antimicrobial therapy. Many feel that early chest tube drainage of empyema fluid due to *S aureus* is indicated. Empyema due to group A β-hemolytic streptococci or *H influenzae* can also necessitate chest tube drainage, whereas pleural effusions due to *S pneumoniae* rarely do. Repeated pleural taps should be considered in the patient who has persistent high fever for more than 10 days in association with significant pleural effusions. The persistence of organisms in this fluid or the persistence of toxicity, malaise, anorexia, and wasting in the patient suggests the potential need for pleural decortication, a procedure that can be made less morbid by thoracoscopy in skilled hands.

Endotracheal intubation or mechanical ventilation may be indicated in patients with respiratory failure or those too debilitated or overwhelmed to handle their secretions.

Prognosis

For the immunocompetent host in whom bacterial pneumonia is adequately recognized and treated, the survival rate is high. For example, the mortality rate from uncomplicated pneumococcal pneumonia is less than 1%. If the patient survives the initial illness, persistently abnormal pulmonary function following empyema is surprisingly uncommon, even when treatment has been delayed or inappropriate.

Austrian R: Confronting drug-resistant pathogenic bacteria: A report on the Rockefeller University workshop. N Engl J Med 1994;330:1247.

Peter G: The child with pneumonia: Diagnostic and therapeutic considerations. Pediatr Infect Dis J 1988;7:453.

Scheld WM, Mandell GL: Nosocomial pneumonia: Pathogenesis and recent advances in diagnosis and therapy. Rev Infect Dis 1991;13(Suppl 9):S743.

Schutze GE, Jacobs RF: Management of community-acquired bacterial pneumonia in hospitalized children. Pediatr Infect Dis J 1992;11:160.

Tomasz A: Multiple antibiotic-resistant pathogenic bacteria: A report on the Rockefeller University workshop. N Engl J Med 1994;330:1247.

VIRAL PNEUMONIA

Essentials of Diagnosis

- Upper respiratory infection prodrome (fever, coryza, cough, hoarseness).
- Wheezing or rales.
- Myalgia, malaise, headache (older children).

General Considerations

Viral pneumonia constitutes the majority of pediatric pulmonary infections. Respiratory syncytial virus (RSV), parainfluenza (1, 2, and 3) viruses, and influenza (A and B) viruses are responsible for more than 75% of infections. Neither severity of the disease or height of fever, radiographic findings, nor characteristics of cough or lung sounds reliably differentiate viral from bacterial pneumonias. Substantial pleural effusions, pneumatoceles, abscesses, lobar consolidation with lobar volume expansion, and "round" pneumonias are generally inconsistent with viral disease.

Clinical Findings

A. Symptoms and Signs: An upper respiratory infection frequently precedes the onset of lower respiratory disease due to viruses. Although wheezing or stridor may be prominent in viral disease, cough, signs of respiratory difficulty (retractions, grunting, nasal flaring) and physical findings (rales, decreased breath sounds) may not be distinguishable from those in bacterial pneumonia.

B. Laboratory Findings: The peripheral white blood cell count can be normal or slightly elevated and is not useful in distinguishing viral from bacterial disease. A markedly elevated neutrophil count, however, indicates that viral disease is less likely.

Rapid viral diagnostic tests, such as fluorescent antibody tests or ELISA for RSV, are increasingly available and should be performed on nasopharyngeal secretions to confirm this diagnosis in high-risk patients and for epidemiology or infection control. Rapid diagnosis of RSV infection does not preclude the possibility of concomitant infection with other pathogens.

C. Imaging: Chest radiographs frequently show perihilar streaking, increased interstitial markings, peribronchial cuffing, or patchy bronchopneumonia. Lobar consolidation may occur, however, as in bacterial pneumonia. Patients with adenovirus disease may have severe necrotizing pneumonias, resulting in the development of pneumatoceles. Hyperinflation of the lungs may occur when involvement of the small airways is prominent.

Differential Diagnosis

Considerations for the differential diagnosis of viral pneumonia are the same as those for bacterial pneumonia. In patients in whom wheezing is a prominent feature, the physician should consider asthma, airway obstruction caused by foreign body aspiration, acute bacterial or viral tracheitis, and parasitic disease.

Complications

Bronchiolitis obliterans or severe chronic respiratory failure may follow adenovirus pneumonia. Bronchiolitis or viral pneumonia may contribute to persistent reactive airway disease in some patients. Bronchiectasis, persistent interstitial lung diseases (fibrosis and desquamative interstitial pneumonitis), and unilateral hyperlucent lung (Swyer-James syndrome) may follow measles, adenovirus, and influenzal pneumonias. Viral pneumonia or laryngotracheobronchitis may predispose the patient to subsequent bacterial tracheitis or pneumonia as immediate sequelae. Plasma cell granuloma may develop as a rare sequela of viral or bacterial pneumonia.

Treatment

General supportive care for viral pneumonia does not differ from that for bacterial pneumonia. Patients can be quite ill and should be hospitalized according to the level of their illness. Because bacterial disease often cannot be definitively excluded, concomitant antibiotics may be indicated.

Patients at risk for life-threatening RSV infections, such as those with bronchopulmonary dysplasia or other severe pulmonary conditions, congenital heart disease, or significant immunocompromise, should be hospitalized and treated with ribavirin. Rapid viral diagnostic tests may be a useful guide for such therapy. These high-risk patients should be immunized annually against influenza A and B viruses. Despite immunization, however, influenza can still occur. When available epidemiologic data indicate an active influenza A infection in the community, rimantadine or amantadine hydrochloride should be considered early for high-risk infants and children who appear to be infected.

Children with suspected viral pneumonia should be placed in respiratory isolation.

Prognosis

Although most children with viral pneumonia recover uneventfully, worsening reactive airway disease, abnormal pulmonary function or chest radiographs, persistent respiratory insufficiency, and even death may occur in high-risk patients such as newborns or those with underlying lung, cardiac, or immunodeficiency disease. Patients with adenovirus infection or those concomitantly infected with RSV and second pathogens such as influenza, adenovirus, cytomegalovirus or *P carinii* also have a poorer prognosis.

Hall CB: Hospital-acquired pneumonia in children: The role of respiratory viruses. Semin Respir Infect 1987; 2:48.

Heidemann SM: Clinical characteristics of parainfluenza virus infection in hospitalized children. Pediatr Pulmonol 1992;13:86.

Khamapirad T, Glezen WP: Clinical and radiographic assessment of acute lower respiratory tract disease in infants and children. Semin Respir Infect 1987;2:130.

Stretton M et al: Intensive care course and outcome of patients infected with respiratory syncytial virus. Pediatr Pulmonol 1992;13:143.

Tristram DA et al: Simultaneous infection with respiratory syncytial virus and other respiratory pathogens. Am J Dis Child 1988;142:834.

CHLAMYDIAL PNEUMONIA

Essentials of Diagnosis

- Cough, tachypnea, rales, few wheezes, and no fever (most patients).
- Appropriate age: 2–12 weeks.
- Inclusion conjunctivitis eosinophilia, or elevated immunoglobulins, or both, can be seen.

General Considerations

Pulmonary disease due to *C trachomatis* usually evolves gradually as the infection descends the respiratory tract. Infants may appear quite well despite the presence of significant pulmonary illness. Infant infections are now at epidemic proportions in urban environments worldwide. Other sexually transmitted organisms such as *U urealyticum* may also be widespread and contribute to lung disease in infants. Unlike bacteria, the chlamydiae are unable to synthesize their own ATP and are sometimes called "energy parasites."

Clinical Findings

A. Symptoms and Signs: About 50% of patients with chlamydial pneumonia have active inclusion conjunctivitis or a history of it. Rhinopharyngitis with nasal discharge or otitis media may have occurred or be currently present. Female patients may have vulvovaginitis.

Cough is usually present. It can have a staccato character and resemble that accompanying pertussis. The infant is usually tachypneic. Scattered inspiratory rales are commonly heard, but wheezes are rarely present. Significant fever suggests another or additional diagnosis.

B. Laboratory Findings: Although patients may frequently be hypoxemic, CO_2 retention is not common. Absolute peripheral blood eosinophilia (400 cells/μL) has been observed in about 75% of patients. Serum immunoglobulins are usually abnormal. IgM is virtually always elevated, IgG is high in many, and IgA is less frequently abnormal. *C trachomatis* can usually be identified in nasopharyngeal washings using a fluorescent antibody or culture techniques.

C. Imaging: Chest radiographs may reveal diffuse interstitial and patchy alveolar infiltrates, peribronchial thickening, or focal consolidation. A small pleural reaction can be present. Despite the usual absence of wheezes, hyperexpansion is commonly present.

Differential Diagnosis

Bacterial, viral, and parasitic (*P carinii*) pneumonias should be considered. Premature infants and those with bronchopulmonary dysplasia may also have chlamydial or associated pneumonias.

Treatment

Erythromycin or sulfisoxazole therapy should be administered for 14 days. Hospitalization may be required for infants with significant respiratory distress, coughing paroxysms, or posttussive apnea. Oxygen therapy may be required for prolonged periods in some patients.

Prognosis

An increased incidence of obstructive airway disease and abnormal pulmonary function tests may occur for at least 7–8 years following infection.

Brayden RM et al: Apnea in infants with *Chlamydia trachomatis* pneumonia. Pediatr Infect Dis J 1987;6:423.

Grayston JT et al: A new respiratory pathogen: *Chlamydia pneumoniae,* strain TWAR. J Infect Dis 1990; 161:618.

Hammerschlag MR et al: Persistent infection with *Chlamydia pneumoniae* following acute respiratory infection. Clin Infect Dis 1992;14:178.

Katzman DK et al: The incidence of Chlamydia pneumoniae lower respiratory tract infections among university students in northern California. West J Med 1991: 155:136.

MYCOPLASMAL PNEUMONIA

Essentials of Diagnosis

- Fever (usually 39 °C).
- Cough.
- Appropriate age: over 5 years old.

General Considerations

M pneumoniae is a common cause of symptomatic pneumonia in older children. Endemic and epidemic infection can occur. The incubation period is long (2–3 weeks), and the onset of symptoms is slow. Although the lung is the primary infection site, a variety of extrapulmonary complications can arise.

Clinical Findings

A. Symptoms and Signs: Fever, cough, headache, and malaise are common symptoms as the illness evolves. Although cough is usually dry at the onset, sputum production may develop as the illness progresses. Sore throat, otitis media, otitis externa, and bullous myringitis may occur. Rales are frequently present on chest examination; decreased breath sounds or dullness to percussion over the involved area may be present.

B. Laboratory Findings: The peripheral blood leukocyte count and differential white blood cell count are usually normal. The cold hemagglutinin titer should be determined, because it may be elevated during the acute presentation. A titer of 1:64 or higher supports the diagnosis. Acute and convalescent titers for *M pneumoniae* demonstrating a fourfold or greater rise in specific antibodies confirm the diagnosis.

C. Imaging: Chest radiographs usually demonstrate interstitial or bronchopneumonic infiltrates, frequently in the middle or lower lobes. Pleural effusions are extremely uncommon.

Complications

Extrapulmonary involvement of the blood, central nervous system, skin, heart, or joints can occur. Direct Coombs-positive autoimmune hemolytic anemia, occasionally a life-threatening disorder, is the most common hematologic abnormality that can accompany *M pneumoniae* infection. Coagulation defects and thrombocytopenia can also occur. Cerebral infarction, meningoencephalitis, Guillain-Barré syndrome, cranial nerve involvement, and psychosis all have been described. A wide variety of skin rashes, including erythema multiforme and Stevens-Johnson syndrome, can occur. Myocarditis, pericarditis, and a rheumatic fever-like illness can also occur.

Treatment

Antibiotic therapy with erythromycin for 7–10 days usually shortens the course of illness. Supportive measures, including hydration, antipyretics, and bed rest, are helpful.

Prognosis

In the absence of the less common extrapulmonary complications, the outlook for recovery is excellent. The extent to which *M pneumoniae* can initiate or exacerbate chronic lung disease is not well understood, however.

Broughton RA: Infections due to *Mycoplasma pneumoniae* in childhood. Pediatr Infect Dis J 1986;5:71.

Leigh MW, Clyde WA Jr: Chlamydial and mycoplasmal pneumonias. Semin Respir Infect 1987;2:152.

McCracken GH Jr: Current status of antibiotic treatment for *Mycoplasma pneumoniae* infections. Pediatr Infect Dis J 1986;5:167.

Orlicek SL, Walker MS, Kuhls TL: Severe mycoplasma pneumonia in young children with Down syndrome. Clin Pediatr 1992;31:409.

TUBERCULOSIS

Essentials of Diagnosis

- Positive tuberculin skin test or anergic host.
- Positive culture for *Mycobacterium tuberculosis.*

General Considerations

There is a resurgence of tuberculosis in all age groups, including children. The clinical spectrum of tuberculosis includes a positive tuberculin skin test without evident disease, asymptomatic primary infection, the Ghon complex, bronchial obstruction with secondary collapse or obstructed airways, segmental lesions, calcified nodules, pleural effusions, progressive primary cavitating lesions, contiguous spread into adjacent thoracic structures, acute miliary tuberculosis, adult respiratory distress syndrome (ARDS), overwhelming reactivation infection in the immunocompromised host, occult lymphohematogenous spread, and metastatic extrapulmonary involvement at almost any site. Symptoms of airway obstruction, sometimes with secondary bacterial pneumonia resulting from hilar adenopathy, are common presenting features in children.

Clinical Findings

A. Symptoms and Signs: The most important aspect of the history is that of contact with an individual with tuberculosis. Frequently, this contact may be made through an elderly relative, a caretaker, or a person previously residing in a region with endemic tuberculosis or by travel to, or residence in, such an area by the patients themselves. Homeless and medically indigent children are also at high risk, as are those in contact with high-risk adults (AIDS patients, residents or employees of correctional institutions or nursing homes, intravenous or other drug users, and health care workers). Once exposed, pediatric patients at risk for developing active disease include infants and those with malnutrition, AIDS, diabetes mellitus, or immunosuppression (antitumor chemotherapy, corticosteroids). In suspected cases, the patient, immediate family, and suspected carriers of the disease should be tuberculin-tested. Spread is mainly respiratory, so isolated pulmonary parenchymal tuberculosis constitutes more than 95% of presenting cases. The primary focus, which is usually single, and the nodal involvement may or may not be radiographically visible. Because healing—rather than progression—is the usual course in the uncompromised host, a positive tuberculin test may be the only manifestation of disease.

The tuberculous complications listed previously most often occur during the first year of infection. Thereafter, infection remains quiescent until adolescence, when reactivation of pulmonary tuberculosis is common. At any stage, chronic cough, anorexia, weight loss or failure to gain weight, or fever are useful clinical signs if present. Except in cases with complications or advanced disease, physical findings are few. Most children with pulmonary tuberculosis are asymptomatic.

B. Laboratory Findings: A positive tuberculin skin test is defined as 10 mm or more of induration 48–72 hours after intradermal injection of 5 tuberculin units of PPD (purified protein derivative). Tine tests should not be used. Appropriate control skin tests, such as those for hypersensitivity to diphtheria/tetanus, mumps, *Candida albicans,* or Dermatophytin/trichophyton, should be applied at the same time the PPD is applied. If the patient fails to respond to PPD and all of the controls, the possibility of tuberculosis is not excluded.

Chest radiographs, both anteroposterior and lateral views, should be obtained in all suspected cases. Culture for *M tuberculosis* is critical for proving the diagnosis and for defining drug susceptibility. Early morning gastric lavage following an overnight fast should be performed on three occasions in infants and children with suspected active pulmonary tuberculosis prior to the onset of drug therapy when the severity of illness allows. Although stains for acid-fast bacilli on this material are of little value, this is the ideal culture site. Despite the increasing importance of isolating organisms because of multiple drug resistance, only 40% of children will yield positive cultures.

Sputum cultures from older children and adolescents are similarly useful. Stains and cultures of bronchial secretions are useful if bronchoscopy is performed in the patient's evaluation. When pleural effusions are present, pleural biopsy for cultures and histopathologic examination for granulomas or organisms most consistently provide diagnostic information. Meningeal involvement is a real possibility in young children, and lumbar puncture should be considered in their initial evaluation.

Differential Diagnosis

Fungal diseases that primarily affect the lungs such as histoplasmosis, coccidioidomycosis, cryptococcosis, and North American blastomycosis may resemble tuberculosis and should be excluded by appropriate serologic studies if the diagnosis is uncertain. Atypical tuberculous organisms may involve the lungs, especially in the immunocompromised patient. Depending on the presentation, diagnoses such as lymphoreticular and other malignancies, collagen-vascular disorders, or other pulmonary infections may be considered.

Complications

In addition to those listed above, lymphadenitis, meningitis, osteomyelitis, arthritis, enteritis, peritonitis, and renal, ocular, middle ear, and cutaneous disease may occur. The infant born to tuberculous parents is at great risk for developing illness. The possibility of life-threatening airway compromise must always be considered in patients with large mediastinal or hilar lesions.

Treatment

Because the risk of hepatitis due to isoniazid is extremely low in children, this drug is indicated in children with a positive tuberculin skin test. This greatly reduces the risk of subsequent active disease and complications with minimal morbidity. Isoniazid plus rifampin treatment for 6 months, plus pyrazinamide during the first 2 months, is indicated when the chest radiograph is abnormal or when there is extrapulmonary disease. Without pyrazinamide, isoniazid plus rifampin must be given for 9 months. In general, the more severe tuberculous complications are treated with a larger number of drugs. Enforced, directly observed therapy (twice weekly or greater) is indicated when noncompliance is suspected. Recommendations for antituberculosis chemotherapy, based on disease stage, are continuously being updated. The most current edition of *The Red Book of the American Academy of Pediatrics* is a reliable source for these protocols.

Corticosteroids are used to control inflammation in selected patients with (1) potentially life-threatening airway compression by lymph nodes, (2) acute pericardial effusion, (3) massive pleural effusion with mediastinal shift, and, possibly, (4) miliary tuberculosis with respiratory failure.

Prognosis

In patients with an intact immune system, modern antituberculous therapy offers good potential for recovery. The outlook for patients with immunodeficiencies, organisms resistant to multiple drugs, poor drug compliance, or advanced complications is guarded. Organisms resistant to multiple drugs are increasingly common. Resistance emerges either because the physician prescribes an inadequate regimen or because the patient discontinues medications. When resistance to or intolerance of isoniazid and rifampin prevents their use, cure rates are 50% or less.

American Academy of Pediatrics Committee on Infectious Diseases: Screening for tuberculosis in infants and children. Pediatrics 1994;93:131.

Snider D: Pregnancy and tuberculosis. Chest 1984; 86(Suppl 3):10S.

Starke JR: Current chemotherapy for tuberculosis in children. Infect Dis Clin North Am 1992;6:215.

Stark JR: Universal screening for tuberculosis infection: School's out! JAMA 1995;274:652.

Starke JR, Jacobs RF, Jereb J: Resurgence of tuberculosis in children. J Pediatr 1992;120:839.

Steinhoff MC, Lionel J: Treatment of tuberculosis in newborn infants and their mothers. Indian J Pediatr 1988; 55:240.

ASPIRATION PNEUMONIA

Essentials of Diagnosis

- Patient at risk.
- Fever.
- Cough.

General Considerations

The risk of aspiration pneumonia occurs in patients when anatomic defense mechanisms are impaired. These include patients with (1) seizures; (2) depressed sensorium; (3) recurrent gastroesophageal reflux, emesis, or gastrointestinal obstruction; (4) neuromuscular disorders with suck/swallow dysfunction; (5) anatomic abnormalities (laryngeal cleft, tracheoesophageal fistula, vocal cord paralysis); (6) debilitating illnesses, (7) occult brain stem lesions; (8) near-drowning; (9) nasogastric, endotracheal, or tracheostomy tubes; and (10) severe periodontal disease. Acute disease is commonly caused by bacteria present in the mouth (especially gram-negative anaerobes), and multiple organisms may concomitantly cause infection in many patients. Chronic aspiration often causes recurrent bouts of acute febrile pneumonia. It may also lead to chronic focal infiltrates, atelectasis, or illness resembling asthma or interstitial lung disease.

Clinical Findings

A. Symptoms and Signs: Acute onset of fever, cough, respiratory distress, or hypoxemia in a patient at risk suggests aspiration pneumonia. Chest physical findings, such as rales, rhonchi, or decreased breath sounds, may initially be limited to the lung region into which aspiration occurred. Although any region may be affected, the right side, especially the right upper lobe in the supine patient, is commonly affected. In patients with chronic aspiration, diffuse wheezing may occur. Generalized rales may also be present. Such patients may not develop acute febrile pneumonias.

B. Laboratory Findings and Imaging: Chest radiographs may reveal lobar consolidation or atelectasis and focal or generalized alveolar or interstitial infiltrates. In some patients with chronic aspiration, perihilar infiltrates with or without bilateral air trapping may be seen.

In severely ill patients with acute febrile illnesses, a bacteriologic diagnosis should be made. In addition to blood cultures, cultures of tracheobronchial secretions and bronchoalveolar lavage or lung puncture specimens may be desirable (see Culture of Material From the Respiratory Tract, p 430).

In patients with chronic aspiration pneumonitis, solid documentation of aspiration as the cause of illness may be elusive. Barium contrast studies may provide evidence of suck-swallow dysfunction, laryngeal cleft, occult tracheoesophageal fistula, or gastroesophageal reflux. Overnight or 24-hour esophageal pH probe studies may also help establish the latter. Although radionuclide scans are commonly used, the yield from such studies is disappointingly low. Rigid bronchoscopy in infants or flexible bronchoscopy in older children can be useful in (1) more definitively excluding tracheoesophageal fistula and (2) obtaining bronchoalveolar lavage specimens to search for lipid-laden macrophages as evidence of chronic aspiration.

Differential Diagnosis

In the acutely ill patient, routine bacterial, viral, or mycoplasmal pneumonias should be considered. In the chronically ill patient, the differential diagnoses may include disorders causing (1) recurrent pneumonia (eg, immunodeficiencies, ciliary dysfunction, foreign body, etc); (2) chronic wheezing; or (3) interstitial lung disorders (see Interstitial Lung Disease), depending on the presentation.

Complications

Empyema or lung abscess may result from acute aspiration pneumonia. Chronic disease may result in bronchiectasis.

Treatment

Antimicrobial therapy for acute aspiration pneumonia includes appropriate coverage for gram-negative anaerobic organisms. This might include, for example, intravenous penicillin G, 12 million u/m^2/d, *plus* metronidazole, imipenem, or a combination of a β-lactam drug and β-lactamase inhibitor. In hospital-acquired infections, additional coverage for methicillin-resistant *S aureus* and multiply resistant *P aeruginosa,* streptococci, and other organisms should be provided.

Treatment of recurrent and chronic aspiration pneumonia may include the following: (1) surgical correction of anatomic abnormalities; (2) improved oral hygiene; (3) improved hydration; and (4) inhaled bronchodilators, chest physical therapy, and suctioning. In patients with compromise of the central nervous system, exclusive feeding by gastrostomy and (in some) tracheostomy may be required to control airway secretions. Gastroesophageal reflux, often requiring surgical correction, is commonly present in such patients.

Prognosis

The outlook for patients with aspiration pneumonia is directly related to the disorder causing their aspiration.

Colombo JL, Hallberg TK, Sammut PH: Time course of lipid-laden macrophages with acute and recurrent milk aspiration in rabbits. Pediatr Pulmonol 1992;12:95.

Colombo JL, Hallberg TK: Recurrent aspiration in children: Lipid-laden alveolar macrophage quantitation. Pediatr Pulmonol 1987;3:86.

Finegold SM: Aspiration pneumonia. Rev Infect Dis 1991; 13(Suppl 9):S737.

Moran JR et al: Lipid-laden alveolar macrophage and lactose assay as markers of aspiration in neonates with lung disease. J Pediatr 1988;112:643.

PNEUMONIA IN THE IMMUNOCOMPROMISED HOST

General Considerations

The immunocompromised host with pneumonia may be infected with any common bacteria (streptococcus, staphylococcus, *M pneumoniae*) or with less common pathogens. These include parasites (*P carinii, Toxoplasma gondii*); fungi (*Aspergillus* species, mucormycosis, *Candida* species, *Cryptococcus neoformans*); viruses (cytomegalovirus; varicella-zoster, herpes simplex, influenza, or RSV; adenovirus); and gram-negative enteric and anaerobic bacteria, *Nocardia,* and *L pneumophila* and mycobacteria. Multiple organisms are commonly present.

Clinical Findings

A. Symptoms and Signs: Patients often present with subtle signs such as mild cough, tachypnea, or low-grade fever which can rapidly progress to fever, respiratory distress, and hypoxemia. An obvious portal of infection, such as an intravascular catheter, may predispose a patient to bacterial or fungal infection.

B. Laboratory Findings and Imaging: Fungal, parasitic, or bacterial infection, especially with antibiotic-resistant bacteria, should be suspected in the neutropenic child. Cultures of peripheral blood, sputum, tracheobronchial secretions, urine, nasopharynx or sinuses, bone marrow, pleural fluid, biopsied lymph nodes, or skin lesions or cultures through intravascular catheters should be obtained as soon as infection is suspected.

Invasive methods are commonly required to make a diagnosis. Appropriate samples should be obtained soon after a patient with pneumonia starts to respond to first-time treatment. The results of these procedures usually lead to important changes in empiric preoperative therapy. Sputum is frequently unavailable. Bronchoalveolar lavage frequently provides the diagnosis of one or more organisms and should be done early in evaluation. The combined use of a wash, brushing, and lavage has a high yield. In patients with rapidly advancing disease, open lung biopsy becomes more urgent. The morbidity and mortality rates of this procedure can be reduced by a thoracoscopic approach, when performed by a skilled operator. Because of the multiplicity of organisms that may cause disease, a comprehensive set of studies should be done on lavage or biopsy material. These consist of (1) rapid diagnostic studies, including fluorescent antibody studies for *Legionella;* rapid culture and antigen detection for viruses; (2) Gram's, acid-fast, and fungal stains; (3) cytologic examination for viral inclusions; (4) cultures for viruses, anaerobic and aerobic bacteria, fungi, mycobacteria, and *Legionella;* and (5) rapid immunofluorescent studies for *P carinii.*

Chest radiographs may be useful. Dyspnea and hypoxemia may be marked, however, despite minimal radiographic abnormalities in *P carinii* pneumonia.

Differential Diagnosis

The organisms causing disease vary with the type of immunocompromise present. For example, the splenectomized patient may be overwhelmed by infection with *S pneumoniae* or *H influenzae*. The infant receiving ACTH therapy may be more likely to have *P carinii* infection. The febrile, neutropenic child who has been receiving adequate doses of intravenous broad-spectrum antibiotics may have fungal disease or *Pneumocystis* pneumonia. The key to diagnosis, however, is to consider all possibilities of infection.

Depending on the form of immunocompromise, perhaps only one-half to two-thirds of new pulmonary infiltrates in such patients represent infection. The remainder is caused by: (1) pulmonary toxicity of radiation, oxygen, chemotherapy, or other drugs; (2) pulmonary disorders, including hemorrhage, embolism, atelectasis, aspiration, or ARDS (adult respiratory distress syndrome); (3) recurrence or extension of primary malignant growths or immunologic disorders; (4) transfusion reactions, leukostasis, or tumor cell lysis; or (5) interstitial lung disease, such as lymphocytic interstitial pneumonitis with HIV infection.

Complications

Respiratory failure, shock, multiple organ damage, disseminated infection, and death commonly occur in the infected, immunocompromised host.

Treatment

Broad-spectrum intravenous antibiotics are indicated early in febrile, neutropenic, or immunocompromised children. Trimethoprim-sulfamethoxazole (for *Pneumocystis*) and erythromycin (for *Legionella*) are also indicated early in the treatment of immunocompromised children before an organism is identified. Further therapy should be based on studies of specimens obtained from bronchoalveolar lavage or lung biopsy.

Prognosis

Prognosis is based on the severity of the underlying immunocompromise, appropriate early diagnosis and treatment, and the infecting organisms.

Barbour SD: AIDS of childhood. Pediatr Clin North Am 1987;34:247.

Frankel LR et al: Bronchoalveolar lavage for diagnosis of pneumonia in the immunocompromised child. Pediatrics 1988;81:785.

Glaser JH et al: Cytomegalovirus and Pneumocystis carinii pneumonia in children with acquired immunodeficiency syndrome. J Pediatr 1992;120:929.

Hughes WT et al: Successful intermittent chemoprophylaxis for Pneumocystis carinii pneumonitis. N Engl J Med 1987;316:1627.

Hughes WT: Pneumonia in the immunocompromised child. Semin Respir Infect 1987;2:177.

Martin WJ II: Diagnostic bronchoalveolar lavage in immunosuppressed patients with new pulmonary infiltrates. Mayo Clin Proc 1992;67:296.

Shaw NJ, Elton R, Eden OB: Pneumonia and pneumonitis in childhood malignancy. Acta Paediatr 1992;81:222.

Valteau D et al: Nonbacterial nonfungal interstitial pneumonitis following autologous bone marrow transplantation in children treated with high-dose chemotherapy without total-body irradiation. Transplantation 1988;45:737.

HYPERSENSITIVITY PNEUMONIA

Essentials of Diagnosis

- History of exposure (eg, birds, organic dusts or molds).
- Interstitial infiltrates on chest radiograph or diffuse rales.
- Recurrent cough, fever, wheezing, or weight loss can occur.

General Considerations

Hypersensitivity pneumonitis is a disease involving peripheral airways, interstitium, and alveoli. Both acute and chronic forms may occur. In children, the most common forms are brought on by exposure to birds or bird droppings (eg, pigeons, parakeets, parrots, doves). Inhalation of almost any organic dust, however, (moldy hay, compost, logs or tree bark, sawdust, or aerosols from humidifiers) can cause disease. Although uncommon in children, many of the latter present as occupational lung diseases in adults.

Clinical Findings

A. Symptoms and Signs: Episodic cough and fever can occur with acute exposures. Chronic exposure results in weight loss, fatigue, dyspnea, cyanosis, and, ultimately, respiratory failure.

B. Laboratory Findings: Acute exposures may be followed by polymorphonuclear leukocytosis with eosinophilia and evidence of airway obstruction on pulmonary function testing. Chronic disease results in a restrictive picture on lung function tests. Arterial blood gases may reveal hypoxemia with a decreased $PaCO_2$ and normal pH.

The serologic key to diagnosis is the finding of precipitins (precipitating IgG antibodies) to the organic dusts that contain avian proteins or fungal or bacterial antigens. However, exposure without related disease may cause the presence of precipitins.

Differential Diagnosis

Patients with primarily acute symptoms must be differentiated from patients with atopic asthma. Those with chronic symptoms must be distinguished from those with collagen-vascular, immunologic, or primary interstitial pulmonary disorders.

Complications

Prolonged exposure to offending antigens may result in pulmonary hypertension due to chronic hypoxemia, cor pulmonale, irreversible restrictive lung disease due to pulmonary fibrosis, or respiratory failure.

Treatment

Complete elimination of exposure to the offending antigens is required. Corticosteroids may hasten recovery.

Prognosis

With appropriate diagnosis and avoidance of offending antigens, the prognosis is excellent. A good prognosis, however, is dependent on early diagnosis before pulmonary damage is irreversible.

Carlsen K-H et al: Allergic alveolitis in a 12-year-old boy: Treatment with budesonide nebulizing solution. Pediatr Pulmonol 1992;12:257.

Eisenberg JD, Montanero A, Lee RG: Hypersensitivity pneumonitis in an infant. Pediatr Pulmonol 1992;12:186.

Levy MG, Fink JN: Hypersensitivity pneumonitis. Ann Allergy 1985;54:167.

O'Connell EJ et al: Childhood hypersensitivity pneumonitis (farmer's lung): Four cases in siblings with long-term follow-up. J Pediatr 1989;114:995.

INTERSTITIAL LUNG DISEASE

Essentials of Diagnosis

- Tachypnea, dyspnea, retractions, or hypoxemia.
- Cough or rales.
- Bilateral pulmonary infiltrates.

General Considerations

Interstitial lung disorders in children may have a wide variety of presentations, and these are often subtle and gradual in onset. Such disorders in the child are commonly caused by infection, immunodeficiency, aspiration, cardiac disease, or pulmonary vascular disease. Also unlike adults, children less commonly have primary pulmonary interstitial lung disorders (eg, desquamative, usual, or lymphocytic interstitial pneumonitis, etc), hypersensitivity pneumonitis, or collagen-vascular diseases.

Clinical Findings

A. Symptoms and Signs: Children may present with a chronic dry cough or a history of dyspnea on exertion. The child with more advanced disease may have increased dyspnea, tachypnea, retractions, cyanosis, clubbing, failure to thrive, or weight loss. Physical examination may reveal these findings, and dry ("Velcro") rales may be present on chest auscultation, especially at the lung bases.

B. Laboratory Findings and Imaging: Chest radiographs may be normal in up to 10–15% of patients. More commonly, diffuse or perihilar bilateral reticular interstitial infiltrates are present. Nodular and reticulonodular diseases are uncommon in children except in cases of HIV infection. Bilateral disease is the rule except in cases of infection and aspiration-related disorders, which may be unilateral.

On pulmonary function testing, interstitial disorders often show a restrictive pattern of decreased lung volumes, compliance, and diffusing capacity for carbon monoxide, whereas the FEV_1/FVC ratio may be normal or increased. However, exercise-induced hypoxemia is often the earliest detectable abnormality of lung function. Blood gas abnormalities may include hypoxemia, a low $PaCO_2$, and normal pH.

Many chronically ill patients can be investigated in a sequence: (1) "serologic," (2) bronchoscopic, and (3) biopsy steps. Although bronchoalveolar lavage may be useful in identifying patients with pulmonary hemosiderosis (hemosiderin-laden macrophages), aspiration (lipid-laden macrophages), and infectious disorders, lung biopsy is the most reliable method for definitive diagnosis.

During the initial phase, x-rays, barium swallow, tests of pulmonary function, skin tests (see Tuberculosis), complete blood count, ESR, sweat test for cystic fibrosis, ECG or echocardiogram, serum immunoglobulins, IgE, and other immunologic evaluations, sputum studies (see Pneumonia in the Immunocompromised Host, p 458), and serologic studies for Epstein-Barr virus, cytomegalovirus, *M pneumoniae, Chlamydia, Pneumocystis,* and *U urealyticum* may appropriately be considered and performed.

During the second phase, rigid bronchoscopy should be performed to exclude anatomic abnormalities and obtain multiple bronchial biopsies to examine cilia. At the same procedure, bronchoalveolar lavage for microbiology and cytology, preferably through a flexible bronchoscope and an endotracheal tube if the patient is large enough, should be done. In patients with static or slowly progressing disease, one can await results of bronchoscopic studies before proceeding further. In patients with acute, rapidly progressive disease, this stage should be combined with open lung biopsy. Special stains and cultures, immunofluorescence for immune complexes, and electron microscopy, should be processed. Although transbronchial biopsy may be useful in diagnosing a few disorders (eg, sarcoid), its overall usefulness in pediatrics is limited.

Differential Diagnosis

Malignant disorders (histiocytosis X, disseminated carcinoma), congenital disorders (Gaucher's disease, neurofibromatosis, tuberous sclerosis, familial interstitial lung disease), pulmonary hemosiderosis, pulmonary telangiectasia or lymphangiectasia, bronchiolitis obliterans, sarcoidosis, and ciliary dyskinesia should be considered in addition to the groups of disorders mentioned above.

Complications

Respiratory failure or pulmonary hypertension with cor pulmonale may occur.

Treatment

Therapy for interstitial lung disease due to infection, aspiration, or cardiac disorders should be directed at the primary disorder. Most of the primary pulmonary interstitial disorders are treated initially with daily prednisone (2 mg/kg/d) therapy for a period of 6 weeks to 6 months, depending on the severity of disease and the response. Many patients require even more prolonged therapy with alternate-day prednisone. Chloroquine (5–10 mg/kg/d) may be useful in selected disorders such as desquamative interstitial pneumonitis. Use of additional cytotoxic drugs (azathioprine, cyclophosphamide) has not been shown in a controlled fashion to be more beneficial than prednisone alone.

Prognosis

The prognosis is guarded in children with interstitial lung disease due to collagen-vascular and primary pulmonary interstitial diseases, immunodeficiency diseases, and cancer.

Bokulic RE, Hilman BC: Interstitial lung disease in children. Pediatr Clin North Am 1994;41(3):543.

Diaz RP, Bowman CM: Childhood interstitial lung disease. Semin Respir Med 1990;11:253.

Falloon J et al: Human immunodeficiency virus infection in children. J Pediatr 1989;114:1.

Fan LL et al: Clinical spectrum of chronic interstitial lung disease in children. J Pediatr 1992;121:867.

Fan LL, Langston C: Chronic interstitial lung disease in children. Pediatr Pulmonol 1993;16:184.

EOSINOPHILIC PNEUMONIA

Essentials of Diagnosis

- Pulmonary infiltrates, often migratory, on chest radiograph.
- Persistent cough; wheezes or rales on chest auscultation.
- Excessive eosinophils in peripheral blood or in lung biopsy specimens.

General Considerations

A spectrum of diseases should be considered under this heading: (1) transient pulmonary infiltrates with eosinophilia (Loffler's syndrome), (2) tropical eosinophilia, (3) pulmonary eosinophilia with asthma (allergic bronchopulmonary aspergillosis and related disorders), (4) hypereosinophilic mucoid impaction, (5) bronchocentric granulomatosis, and (6) collagen-vascular disorders. Many occur in children with personal or family histories of allergies or asthma. These disorders may be related to hypersensitivity to migratory parasitic nematodes (*Ascaris, Strongyloides, Ancylostoma, Toxocara, Trichuris*), larval forms of filariae (*Wuchereria bancrofti*), or fungi (*Aspergillus, Candida*). Eosinophilic pneumonias also can be associated with drug hypersensitivity, sarcoidosis, Hodgkin's disease or other lymphomas, and bacterial infections, including brucellosis and those caused by *M tuberculosis* and atypical mycobacteria.

Clinical Findings

A. Symptoms and Signs: Patients may present asthma (Loffler's syndrome) or exacerbation of cystic fibrosis. In most cases, cough, wheezing, or dyspnea are presenting complaints. In Loffler's syndrome, fever, malaise, sputum production, and, rarely, hemoptysis may be present. In allergic bronchopulmonary aspergillosis, patients may present all of these findings and commonly produce brown mucus plugs. Anorexia, weight loss, night sweats, and clubbing can also occur.

B. Laboratory Findings and Imaging: Elevated absolute peripheral blood eosinophil counts ($3000/\mu L$ and often exceeding 50% of leukocytes) are present in Loffler's syndrome, tropical eosinophilia, and allergic bronchopulmonary aspergillosis. Serum IgE levels as high as 1000–10,000 IU/mL are common. In allergic bronchopulmonary aspergillosis, the serum IgE concentration appears to correlate with activity of the disease. Stools should be examined for ova and parasites, often several times, to clarify the diagnosis. Isohemagglutinin titers are often markedly elevated in Loffler's syndrome.

In allergic bronchopulmonary aspergillosis and related disorders, patients may have central bronchiectasis demonstrable by chest radiograph ("tramlines") or CT scan. Saccular proximal bronchiectasis of the upper lobes is pathognomonic. Although the chest radiograph may be normal, peribronchial haziness, focal or plate-like atelectasis, or patchy to massive consolidation can occur. Positive immediate skin tests, serum IgG precipitating antibodies, or IgE specific for the offending fungus are present.

Differential Diagnosis

These disorders must be differentiated from exacerbations of asthma, cystic fibrosis, or other underlying lung disorders that cause infiltrates on chest x-ray films.

Complications

Although Loffler's syndrome is usually self-limited, delayed recognition and treatment of allergic bronchopulmonary aspergillosis may cause progressive lung damage and bronchiectasis. Lesions of the conducting airways in bronchocentric granulomatosis can extend into adjacent lung parenchyma and pulmonary arteries, resulting in a secondary vasculitis.

Treatment

Therapy for parasites causing Loffler's syndrome should be given, and corticosteroids may be required when illness is severe. Treatment of disease due to microfilariae is both diagnostic and therapeutic. Allergic bronchopulmonary aspergillosis and related disorders are treated with prolonged courses of oral corticosteroids, bronchodilators, and chest physical therapy. Antifungal agents are not useful in these latter disorders.

Ahmad M et al: Thoracic aspergillosis: 2. Primary pulmonary aspergillosis, allergic bronchopulmonary aspergillosis, and related conditions. Cleve Clin Q 1984; 51:631.

Buchheit J et al: Acute eosinophilic pneumonia with respiratory failure: A new syndrome? Am Rev Respir Dis 1992;145:716.

Christensen WN, Hutchins GM: Hypereosinophilic mucoid impaction of bronchi in 2 children under 2 years of age. Pediatr Pulmonol 1985;1:278.

Howard WA: Pulmonary infiltrates with eosinophilia (Loffler syndrome). In: *Disorders of the Respiratory Tract in Children,* 5th ed. Chernick V, Kendig EL Jr (editors). Saunders, 1990.

Lee TM et al: Allergic bronchopulmonary candidiasis: Case report and suggested diagnostic criteria. J Allergy Clin Immunol 1987;80:816.

Vijayan V-K et al: Pulmonary eosinophilia in pulmonary tuberculosis. Chest 1992;101:1708.

LUNG ABSCESS

General Considerations

Lung abscesses are most likely to occur in immunocompromised patients, in those with severe infections elsewhere (embolic spread), or in those with recurrent aspiration, malnutrition, or blunt chest trauma. Although organisms such as *S aureus, H influenzae, Streptococcus viridans,* and *S pneumoniae* more commonly affect the previously normal host, anaerobic and gram-negative organisms as well as *Nocardia, Legionella* species, and fungi (*Candida, Aspergillus*) should also be considered in the immunocompromised host.

Clinical Findings

A. Symptoms and Signs: High fever, malaise, and weight loss are often present. Symptoms and signs referable to the chest may or may not be present. In infants, evidence of respiratory distress can be present.

B. Laboratory Findings and Imaging: Elevated peripheral white blood cell count with a neutrophil predominance or an elevated erythrocyte sedimentation rate may be present. Blood cultures are rarely positive except in the overwhelmed host.

Chest radiographs usually reveal single or multiple thick-walled lung cavities. Air-fluid levels can be present. Local compressive atelectasis, pleural thickening, or adenopathy may also occur. Chest CT scan may provide better localization of the lesions.

In patients producing sputum, stains and cultures may provide the diagnosis. Direct percutaneous aspiration of material for stains and cultures directed by fluoroscopy or ultrasonography should be considered in the severely compromised or ill.

Differential Diagnosis

Loculated pyopneumothorax, *Echinococcus* cyst, neoplasms, plasma cell granuloma, and infected congenital cysts and sequestrations should be considered in the differential diagnosis.

Complications

Although complications due to abscesses are now rare, mediastinal shift, tension pneumothorax, and spontaneous rupture can occur. Diagnostic maneuvers such as lung puncture may also cause complications (pneumothorax).

Treatment

Because of the risks of lung puncture, uncomplicated abscesses are frequently treated in the uncompromised host with appropriate broad-spectrum antibiotics directed at *S aureus, H influenzae,* and streptococci. Additional coverage for anaerobic and gram-negative organisms should be provided for others. Prolonged therapy (3 weeks or more) may be required. Attempts to drain abscesses via bronchoscopy have caused life-threatening airway compromise. Surgical drainage or lobectomy is occasionally required, primarily in immunocompromised patients. However, such procedures may themselves cause life-threatening complications.

Prognosis

Although radiographic resolution may be very slow, resolution occurs in most patients without propensity to lower respiratory tract infections or loss of pulmonary function. Nonetheless, in the immunocompromised host, the outlook depends on the underlying disorder.

Bruckheimer E et al: Primary lung abscess in infancy. Pediatr Pulmonol 1995;19(3):188.

Emanuel B, Shulman ST: Lung Abscess in infants and children. Clin Pediatr Pulmonol 1995;19(3):188.

Lewin S et al: Legionnaire's disease. A cause of severe abscess-forming pneumonia. Am J Med 1979;67:339.

Lui RC, Inculet RI: Job's syndrome: A rare cause of recurrent lung abscess in childhood. Ann Thoracic Surg 1990;50:992.

Shim C, Santos GH, Zelefsky M: Percutaneous drainage of lung abscess. Lung 1990;168:201.

Tan TQ, Seiheimer DK, Kaplan SL: Pediatric lung abscess: Clinical management and outcome. Pediatr Infect Dis J 1995;14(1):51.

PULMONARY TUMORS

Primary tumors of the airway and parenchyma of the lung are unusual in pediatrics. Most intrathoracic tumors occur in or close to the mediastinum (see Mediastinal Masses, p 469). Other pulmonary tumors may be classified as benign, malignant, or metastatic. Benign pulmonary tumors include plasma cell granulomas, hamartomas, adenomas, papillomas, angiomas, leiomyomas, lipomas, and neurogenic tumors. The most common malignant tumor in children is a bronchogenic carcinoma, but this is again very rare. Other malignant tumors include fibrosarcomas and leiomyosarcomas. Metastatic tumors in childhood include Wilms' tumor, hepatoblastoma, osteogenic sarcoma, chondrosarcoma, Ewing's tumor, reticulum cell sarcoma, and soft tissue sarcomas. Lung tumors in children are more often metastatic than primary.

Clinical Findings

A. Symptoms and Signs: When tumors produce symptoms, these may include pain, fever, cough, wheezing, weight loss, malaise, anemia, anorexia, and hemoptysis. On physical examination, signs of a pleural effusion, volume loss, or consolidation may be present if the tumor has led to significant airway obstruction.

B. Laboratory Findings and Imaging: In addition to frontal and lateral chest x-rays, fluoroscopy, CT scans, and angiography may be helpful in defining and delineating the tumor. Sputum cultures and cytology, as well as tuberculin and fungal skin tests plus fungal serology, may be needed to exclude other conditions.

Differential Diagnosis

The differential diagnosis includes acute, recurrent, or persistent viral and bacterial pneumonia, tuberculosis, and pulmonary infiltrates due to fungal infections. In infants, congenital malformations (pulmonary sequestration, cystic adenomatoid malformation) may also present as mass lesions.

Treatment & Prognosis

Both the appropriate therapy and the response to therapy depend on the type and location of the tumor. Benign lesions may be cured with surgical resection, but the prognosis is more guarded with both primary and metastatic malignant lesions.

Hammer J et al: Plasma cell granuloma of the lung: Associated laboratory findings and ultrastructural evidence of inflammatory origin. Pediatr Pulmonol 1991;10:299.

Hartman GE, Shochat SJ: Primary pulmonary neoplasms in childhood: A review. Ann Thorac Surg 1983;36:108.

Watterson J et al: Thoracopulmonary neoplasms and lung complications of childhood cancer. In: *Pediatric Respiratory Disease.* Hilman B (editor). Saunders, 1993.

DISEASES OF THE PULMONARY CIRCULATION

PULMONARY HEMORRHAGE

Acute pulmonary hemorrhage with or without hemoptysis, and is usually accompanied by filling alveolar infiltrates on chest x-ray. Hemosiderin-laden macrophages are found in the sputum and tracheal or gastric aspirate. Many cases are secondary to infection (bacterial, mycobacterial, parasitic, viral, or fungal), lung abscess, bronchiectasis (cystic fibrosis or other causes), foreign body, coagulopathy (often with overwhelming sepsis), or elevated pulmonary venous pressure (secondary to congestive heart failure or anatomic heart lesions). Other causes include lung contusion from trauma, arteriovenous fistula, multiple telangiectasia, pulmonary sequestration, agenesis of a single pulmonary artery, and esophageal duplication or bronchogenic cyst. Rarer causes are tumors, such as bronchial adenoma or left atrial myxoma, and pulmonary infarction secondary to pulmonary embolus.

Primary alveolar hemorrhage may be idiopathic, drug-related, or occur in Goodpasture's syndrome, rapidly progressive glomerulonephritis, and systemic vasculitides (often associated with such collagen-vascular diseases as systemic lupus erythematosus, rheumatoid arthritis, Wegener's granulomatosis, polyarteritis nodosa, Schönlein-Henoch purpura, and Behçet's disease). Idiopathic pulmonary hemosiderosis refers to the accumulation of hemosiderin in the lung, especially the alveolar macrophage, as a result of chronic or recurrent hemorrhage (usually from pulmonary capillaries) that is not associated with the causes listed above. Children and young adults are primarily affected, with the age at onset ranging between 6 months and 20 years. This group of disorders includes young infants with milk allergy (Heiner's syndrome).

Clinical Findings

A. Symptoms and Signs: Idiopathic pulmonary hemosiderosis usually presents with nonspecific respiratory symptoms (cough, tachypnea, retractions), with or without hemoptysis, poor growth, and fatigue. Some children or young adults may present with massive hemoptysis, marked respiratory distress, stridor, or a pneumonia-like syndrome. Fever, abdominal pain, digital clubbing, and chest pain may be reported. Jaundice and hepatosplenomegaly may be present with chronic bleeding. Physical examination often reveals decreased breath sounds, rales, rhonchi, or wheezing.

B. Laboratory Findings and Imaging: Laboratory studies demonstrate iron deficiency anemia and heme-positive sputum. Nonspecific findings may include lymphocytosis and an elevated erythrocyte sedimentation rate. Peripheral eosinophilia is present in up to 25% of patients. Chest x-ray findings include a range of findings, from transient perihilar infiltrates to large, fluffy alveolar infiltrates with or without atelectasis and mediastinal adenopathy. Pulmonary function testing generally reveals a restrictive impairment, with low lung volumes and poor compliance. Hemosiderin-laden macrophages are found in bronchial or gastric aspirates. The usefulness of lung biopsy in reaching the diagnosis is controversial. Suspected cases of cow's milk-induced pulmonary hemosiderosis can be confirmed by laboratory findings that include high titers of serum precipitins to multiple constituents of cow's milk and positive intradermal skin tests to various cow's milk proteins. Improvement after an empiric trial of a diet free of cow's milk also supports the diagnosis.

Differential Diagnosis

In contrast to idiopathic pulmonary hemosiderosis, Goodpasture's syndrome presents in a slightly older age group (15–35 years), tends to have a more aggressive pulmonary course, and has renal involvement (crescentic proliferative glomerulonephritis and circulating anti-glomerular basement membrane antibody). Wegener's granulomatosis also has renal involvement (granulomatous glomerulitis with necrotizing vasculitis, but renal biopsy may be nonspecific) and other systemic manifestations, especially with upper and lower respiratory tract inflammation. Upper tract involvement includes sinusitis, rhinitis, recurrent epistaxis, otitis media, saddle nose deformity, and subglottic stenosis. Wegener's granulomatosis may present without renal involvement early in the course of the disease. The diagnosis can be made by biopsy or an elevated antineutrophil cytoplasmic antibody titer.

Treatment

Therapy should be aimed at direct treatment of the underlying disease. Supportive measures, including iron therapy, supplemental oxygen, and blood transfusions, may be needed. A cow's milk-free diet should be tried in infants. The usefulness of corticosteroids or cytotoxic agents is unproved in idiopathic pulmonary hemosiderosis but appears to be beneficial in Wegener's granulomatosis and perhaps Goodpasture's syndrome.

Prognosis

The outcome of idiopathic pulmonary hemosiderosis is markedly variable, typically characterized by a waxing and waning course of intermittent intrapulmonary bleeds and the gradual development of chronic lung disease over time. The severity of the underlying renal disease contributes to the mortality rates associated with Goodpasture's syndrome and Wegener's granulomatosis.

Bradley JD: Pulmonary hemorrhage syndromes. Clin Chest Med 1982;3:593.

Hall SL et al: Wegener granulomatosis in pediatric patients. J Pediatr 1985;106:739.

Kjellman B et al: Idiopathic pulmonary hemosiderosis in Swedish children. Acta Paediatr Scand 1984;73:584.

Leatherman JW et al: Alveolar hemorrhage syndromes. Medicine (Baltimore) 1984;63:343.

Miller RW et al: Pulmonary hemorrhage in pediatric patients with systemic lupus erythematosus. J Pediatr 1986;108:576.

PULMONARY EMBOLISM

Although apparently rare in children, the incidence of pulmonary embolism is probably underestimated because it is often not considered in the differential diagnosis of respiratory distress. It occurs most commonly in children with sickle cell anemia as part of the "acute chest syndrome" and with rheumatic fever, infective endocarditis, schistosomiasis, bone fracture, dehydration, polycythemia, nephrotic syndrome, atrial fibrillation, "complicated" pneumonia, and other conditions. The emboli may be single or multiple, large or small, with the clinical signs and symptoms dependent on the severity of pulmonary vascular obstruction.

Clinical Findings

A. Symptoms and Signs: Most often, pulmonary embolism presents clinically as an acute onset of dyspnea and tachypnea. Heart palpitations or "a sense of impending doom" may be reported.

Pleuritic chest pain and hemoptysis may be present (but are not common), along with splinting, cyanosis, and tachycardia. Massive emboli may be present with syncope and cardiac arrhythmias. Physical examination is usually normal (except for tachycardia and tachypnea) unless the embolism is associated with an underlying disorder. Mild hypoxemia, rales, focal wheezing, or a pleural friction rub may be found.

B. Laboratory Findings and Imaging: Radiologic findings may be normal, but a peripheral infiltrate, small pleural effusion, or elevated hemidiaphragm can be present. If the emboli are massive, differential blood flow and pulmonary artery enlargement may be appreciated. The ECG is usually normal unless the pulmonary embolus is massive. Ventilation/perfusion scans show localized areas of ventilation without perfusion. If this study is normal, pulmonary embolus is virtually excluded. Further evaluation may include radiofibrinogen leg scanning and impedance plethysmography to search for deep venous thrombosis. Coagulation studies, including assessments of antithrombin III and protein C or S deficiencies, or defective fibrinolysis may be indicated. However, 90% of adult patients with venous thromboembolism have no identified coagulopathy.

Treatment

Acute treatment includes supplemental oxygen, sedation, and anticoagulation. Although controversial, current recommendations include heparin administration to maintain an activated partial thromboplastin time that is 1½ or more times the control value. Thrombolytic therapy with streptokinase and urokinase may be necessary if the pulmonary embolus is massive. In patients with identifiable deep venous thrombosis of the lower extremities and significant pulmonary emboli (with hemodynamic compromise despite anticoagulation), inferior vena caval interruption may be necessary. Long-term prospective data are lacking, however.

Malik AR, Johnson A: Role of humoral mediators in the pulmonary vascular response to pulmonary embolism. In: *Pulmonary Vascular Physiology and Pathophysiology.* Weir EK, Reeves JT (editors). Dekker, 1989.

Moser KM: Pulmonary embolism. In: *Textbook of Respiratory Medicine,* 2nd ed. Murray JF, Nadel JA (editors). Saunders, 1994.

PULMONARY EDEMA

Pulmonary edema is defined as the excessive accumulation of extravascular fluid in the lung. This occurs when fluid is filtered into the lungs faster than it can be removed, leading to detrimental changes in lung mechanics, such as decreased lung compliance, worsening hypoxemia from ventilation/perfusion mismatch, bronchial compression, and, if advanced, decreased surfactant function. There are two basic types of pulmonary edema: increased pressure (cardiogenic or hydrostatic) and increased permeability (noncardiogenic or "primary"). Hydrostatic pulmonary edema is usually due to excessive increases in pressure, which is most commonly due to congestive heart failure from multiple causes. In contrast, many lung diseases, especially ARDS; (see below) are characterized by the development of pulmonary edema secondary to changes in permeability due to injury to the alveolocapillary barrier. In these settings, pulmonary edema occurs independent of the elevations of pulmonary venous pressure.

Clinical Findings

A. Symptoms and Signs: Clinical findings depend on the underlying cause and clinical setting. In general, cyanosis, tachypnea, tachycardia, and respiratory distress are present. Physical findings include rales, diminished breath sounds, and (in young infants) expiratory wheezing. More severe disease is characterized by progressive respiratory distress with marked retractions, dyspnea, and severe hypoxemia.

B. Imaging: Chest x-ray findings depend on the cause of the edema. Typically, pulmonary vessels appear prominent, often with diffuse interstitial or alveolar infiltrates. Heart size is usually normal in permeability edema but enlarged in hydrostatic edema.

Treatment

Although specific therapy depends on the underlying cause of the pulmonary edema, supplemental oxygen therapy and, if needed, ventilator support for respiratory failure are instituted. Diuretics, digoxin, and vasodilators may be indicated for congestive heart failure, along with restriction of salt and water. Recommended interventions for permeability edema are reducing vascular volume and maintaining the lowest central venous or pulmonary arterial wedge pressure, without sacrificing cardiac output or causing hypotension (see below).

Malik AR: Mechanisms of neurogenic pulmonary edema. Circ Res 1985;57:1.
Staub NC: Pathogenesis of pulmonary edema. Prog Cardiovasc Dis 1980;23:53.

CONGENITAL PULMONARY LYMPHANGIECTASIA

Structurally, congenital pulmonary lymphangiectasia appears as dilated subpleural and interlobular lymphatic channels and may present as part of a generalized lymphangiectasis (in association with obstructive cardiovascular lesions, especially total anomalous pulmonary venous return) or as an isolated, idiopathic lesion. Pathologically, the lung appears firm, bulky, and noncompressible, with prominent cystic lymphatics visible beneath the pleura. On cut section, dilated lymphatics are present near the hilum, along interlobular septa, around bronchovascular bundles, and beneath the pleura. Histologically, dilated lymphatics have a thin endothelial cell lining overlying a delicate network of elastin and collagen.

Clinical Findings

Congenital pulmonary lymphangiectasia is a rare, usually fatal disease that generally presents as acute or persistent respiratory distress at birth. Although most patients do not survive the newborn period, some survive longer, and there are isolated case reports of its diagnosis later in childhood. It may be associated with features of Noonan's syndrome, asplenia, total anomalous pulmonary venous return, septal defects, atrioventricular canal, hypoplastic left heart, aortic arch malformations, and renal malformations. Chylothorax has been reported. Chest x-ray findings include a "ground glass" appearance, prominent interstitial markings suggesting lymphatic distention, diffuse hyperlucency of the pulmonary parenchyma, and hyperinflation with depression of the diaphragm.

Prognosis

The outcome is poor. Although the onset of symptoms may be delayed for as long as the first few months of life, prolonged survival is extremely rare. Most deaths occur within weeks after birth.

Gardner TW et al: Congenital pulmonary lymphangiectasis. Clin Pediatr 1983;22:75.

DISORDERS OF THE CHEST WALL

EVENTRATION OF THE DIAPHRAGM

Eventration of the diaphragm occurs where striated muscle is replaced with connective tissue and is demonstrated on x-ray film by elevation of part or all of the diaphragm. This congenital disorder is thought to represent incomplete formation of the diaphragm in utero. When defects are small, there is no paradoxic movement of the diaphragm and little symptomatology. Small eventrations may be detected on a chest x-ray film taken for another reason. When defects are large, there may or may not be paradoxic movement of the diaphragm, depending on the nature of the tissue replacing the normal diaphragm. The degree of respiratory distress depends in large part on the amount of paradoxic motion of the diaphragm. When the diaphragm moves upward during inspiration, instability of the inferior border of the chest wall increases the work of breathing and can lead to respiratory muscle fatigue. Treatment for respiratory distress is surgical plication, which stabilizes the diaphragm.

The differential diagnosis of eventration includes phrenic nerve injury and partial diaphragmatic hernia. The former can result from birth or other trauma and may also be seen following cardiac surgery. Usually, only one phrenic nerve is involved. An elevated hemidiaphragm is noted on chest x-ray film, and paradoxic motion of the diaphragm may be seen by fluoroscopy or ultrasonography. Often, patients cannot be extubated or have persistent respiratory compromise, particularly with feeding. If symptoms persist for 2–4 weeks, the diaphragm is surgically plicated as described previously. Function returns to the diaphragm in about 50% of cases of phrenic nerve injury whether or not plication was performed. Recovery periods of up to 100 days have been reported in these cases.

Ribet M, Linder JL: Plication of the diaphragm for unilateral eventration or paralysis. Eur J Cardiothorac Surg 1992;6:357.

SCOLIOSIS

Scoliosis—lateral curvature of the spine—can, if uncorrected, lead to severe restrictive lung disease and death from cor pulmonale. Most cases of idiopathic scoliosis occur in adolescent girls and are corrected before there is significant pulmonary impairment. Congenital scoliosis of a severe degree or with other major abnormalities carries a more guarded prognosis. Scoliosis may also occur in patients with progressive neuromuscular disease, such as Duchenne's muscular dystrophy, and can be a major contributor to respiratory failure.

Day GA et al: Pulmonary functions in congenital scoliosis. Spine 1994;19:1027.
Kearon C et al: Factors determining pulmonary function in adolescent idiopathic thoracic scoliosis. Am Rev Respir Dis 1993;148:288.

PECTUS EXCAVATUM

Pectus excavatum is an anterior depression of the chest wall that may be symmetric or asymmetric with respect to the midline. Reports of exercise testing and pulmonary function testing in patients with pectus excavatum have not clearly demonstrated any marked abnormalities. Therefore, the decision to repair the deformity is usually based on cosmetic considerations. Postoperative care of patients following pectus excavatum requires mechanical ventilation and careful respiratory monitoring because of the weak chest wall following surgery.

Morshius W et al: Pulmonary function before surgery for pectus excavatum and at long-term follow-up. Chest 1994;105:1646.

PECTUS CARINATUM

Pectus carinatum is a bowing out of the sternum, usually apparent at birth. The abnormality may be associated with some systemic diseases such as the mucopolysaccharidoses. As with pectus excavatum, abnormalities of pulmonary function tests are unusual in the absence of other disorders. The decision to repair this deformity is based primarily on cosmetic grounds. Postoperative care similarly requires careful monitoring because of chest wall instability produced by the repair.

Cahill JL, Lees GM, Robertson HT: A summary of preoperative and postoperative cardiorespiratory performance in patients undergoing pectus excavatum and carinatum repair. J Pediatr Surg 1984;19:430.

NEUROMUSCULAR DISORDERS

Weakness of the respiratory and pharyngeal muscles lead to chronic or recurrent pneumonia secondary to aspiration and infection, atelectasis, hypoventilation, and respiratory failure in severe cases. Scoliosis, which frequently accompanies long-standing neuromuscular disorders, may further compromise respiratory function. Typical physical findings are a weak cough, decreased air exchange, rales, wheezing, and dullness to percussion. Signs of cor pulmonale (loud pulmonary component to the second heart sound, hepatomegaly, elevated neck veins) may be evident in advanced cases. Chest films generally show small lung volumes. If chronic aspiration is present, increased interstitial infiltrates and areas of atelectasis or consolidation may be present. Arterial blood gases demonstrate hypoxemia in the early stages and compensated respiratory acidosis in the late stages. Typical pulmonary function abnormalities include low lung volumes and decreased inspiratory force generated against an occluded airway. Treatment is supportive and includes vigorous pulmonary toilet, antibiotics with infection, and oxygen to correct hypoxemia. Unfortunately, despite aggressive medical therapy, many neuromuscular conditions progress to respiratory failure and death. The decision to intubate and ventilate is a difficult one; it should be made only when there is real hope that deterioration, though acute, is potentially reversible or when chronic ventilation is wanted. Chronic mechanical ventilation using either noninvasive or invasive techniques is being used more frequently in patients with chronic respiratory insufficiency.

Fields AI et al: Outcome of home care for technology-dependent children: Success of an independent, community-based care management model. Pediatr Pulmonol 1991;11:310.

Shaffner DH, Gioia FR: Neuromuscular disease and respiratory failure. In: *Textbook of Pediatric Intensive Care,* 2nd ed. Rogers MC (editor). Williams & Wilkins, 1992.

DISORDERS OF THE PLEURA & PLEURAL CAVITY

The pleural membranes cover the outer surface of the lungs (visceral pleura) and the inner surface of the chest wall (parietal pleura). Disease processes can lead to accumulation of air or fluid in the pleural space. Pleural effusions are classified as transudates or exudates. Transudates occur when there is imbalance between hydrostatic and oncotic pressure, so that fluid filtration exceeds reabsorption (eg, congestive heart failure). Exudates form as a result of inflammation of the pleural surface leading to increased capillary permeability (eg, parapneumonic effusions). Other pleural effusions include chylothorax and hemothorax.

Thoracentesis is helpful in characterizing the fluid and providing definitive diagnosis. Recovered fluid is considered an exudate (as opposed to a transudate) if any of the following are found: a pleural fluid to serum protein ratio greater than 0.5, a pleural fluid to serum lactic dehydrogenase (LDH) ratio greater than 0.6, or a pleural fluid LDH greater than 200 IU/L. Important additional studies on pleural fluid include cell count; pH and glucose; Gram's, acid-fast, and fungal stains; cultures; counterimmunoelectrophoresis for specific organisms; cytology; and, occasionally, amylase concentration.

PARAPNEUMONIC EFFUSION & EMPYEMA

Bacterial pneumonia is often accompanied by pleural effusion. Some of these effusions harbor infection, and others represent inflammatory reactions to pneumonia. The nomenclature in this area is somewhat confusing. Some use the term empyema for grossly purulent fluid and parapneumonic effusion for nonpurulent fluid. It is clear, however, that some nonpurulent effusions will also contain organisms and represent either partially treated or early empyema. It is probably best to refer to all effusions associated with pneumonia as parapneumonic effusions, some of which are infected and some of which are not.

The most common organisms associated with empyema is *S pneumoniae*. Other common organisms include *H influenzae* and *S aureus*. Less common causes are group A streptococci, gram-negative organisms, and anaerobic organisms. Effusions associated with tuberculosis are almost always sterile and constitute an inflammatory reaction.

Clinical Findings

A. Symptoms and Signs: Patients usually present with typical signs of pneumonia, including fever, tachypnea, and cough. In addition, they may have chest pain, decreased breath sounds, and dullness to percussion on the affected side. They may prefer to lie on the affected side. With large effusions, there may be tracheal deviation to the contralateral side.

B. Laboratory Findings: The white blood count is often elevated, with left shift. Blood cultures are sometimes positive. The tuberculin skin test is positive in most cases of tuberculosis except when anergy is present or when the disease process is in a very early stage. Thoracentesis reveals findings consistent with an exudate. Cells in the pleural fluid are usually neutrophils in bacterial disease and lymphocytes in tuberculous effusions. In bacterial disease, the pleural fluid pH and glucose is often low. Although in adults the presence of low pH and glucose necessitates aggressive and thorough drainage procedures, the prognostic significance of these findings in children is not known. Gram's stain, cultures, or counterimmunoelectrophoresis is often positive for the offending organism.

C. Imaging: The presence of pleural fluid is suggested by a homogeneous density on chest x-ray that obscures the underlying lung. Large effusions may cause a shift of the mediastinum to the contralateral side. Small effusions may only blunt the costophrenic angle. Lateral decubitus films may help to detect freely movable fluid by demonstrating a "layering-out" effect. If the fluid is loculated, no such effect is perceived. Ultrasonography can be extremely valuable in localizing the fluid and detecting loculations, especially when thoracentesis is contemplated.

Treatment & Prognosis

Appropriate intravenous antibiotics for at least 14 days and adequate drainage of the fluid remain the mainstay of therapy. Although there is a trend toward managing smaller pneumococcal empyemas without a chest tube, most larger effusions require chest tube drainage. More aggressive procedures such as thoracotomy with open drainage or decortication are rarely indicated except for less common causes of this disorder such as infection with group A streptococci and gram-negative and anaerobic organisms. Early decortication using thoracoscopic techniques may reduce morbidity and the need for prolonged hospitalization.

The prognosis is related to the severity of disease but is generally excellent, with complete or nearly complete recovery expected in most instances.

Foglia RP, Randolph J: Current indications for decortication in the treatment of empyema in children. J Pediatr Surg 1987;22:28.

Heffner JE et al: Pleural fluid chemical analysis in parapneumonic effusions: A meta analysis. Am J Respir Crit Care Med 1995;151:1700.

Kennedy AS et al: Decortication for childhood empyema: The primary provider's peccadillo. Arch Surg 1991;126:1287.

McLaughlin FJ et al: Empyema in children: Clinical course and long-term follow-up. Pediatrics 1984;73:587.

HEMOTHORAX

Accumulation of blood in the pleural space can be caused by surgical or accidental trauma, coagulation defects, and pleural or pulmonary tumors. With blunt trauma, hemopneumothorax may be present. Symptoms are related to blood loss and compression of underlying lung parenchyma. There is some risk of secondary infection resulting in empyema. Drainage of a hemothorax is required when significant compromise of pulmonary function is present, as with hemopneumothorax. In uncomplicated cases, observation is indicated, because blood is readily absorbed spontaneously from the pleural space.

CHYLOTHORAX

The accumulation of chyle in the pleural space usually results from accidental or surgical trauma to the thoracic duct. In the newborn, chylothorax can be congenital or secondary to birth trauma. This condition also occurs as a result of superior vena cava obstruction secondary to central venous lines and following Fontan procedures for tricuspid atresia. Symptoms of chylothorax are related to the amount of fluid accumulation and degree of compromise of underlying pulmonary parenchyma. Thoracentesis reveals typical milky fluid (unless the patient has been fasting) containing predominantly T lymphocytes.

Treatment should be conservative because many chylothoraces resolve spontaneously. This includes the use of oral feedings with medium-chain triglycerides to reduce lymphatic flow through the thoracic duct. Drainage of chylous effusions should be performed only in the event of respiratory compromise, because the fluid often rapidly reaccumulates. Repeated or continuous drainage may lead to protein malnutrition and T-cell depression, rendering the patient relatively immunocompromised. If reaccumulation of fluid persists for a prolonged period, surgical ligation of the thoracic duct or sclerosis of the pleural space can be attempted, although the results may be less than satisfactory.

Puntis JWL, Roberts KD, Handy D: How should chylothorax be managed? Arch Dis Child 1987;62:593.

van Straaten HL, Gerards LJ, Krediet TG: Chylothorax in the neonatal period. Eur J Pediatr 1993;152:2.

PNEUMOTHORAX & RELATED AIR LEAK SYNDROMES

Pneumothorax can occur spontaneously in newborns and in older children or, more commonly, as a result of birth trauma, positive-pressure ventilation, underlying obstructive or restrictive lung disease, and rupture of a congenital or acquired lung cyst. Pneumothorax can also occur as an acute complication of tracheostomy. Usually, air dissects from the alveolar spaces into the interstitial spaces of the lung. Migration to the visceral pleura ultimately leads to rupture into the pleural space. Associated conditions include pneumomediastinum, pneumopericardium, pneumoperitoneum, and subcutaneous emphysema. These conditions are more commonly associated with dissection of air into the interstitial spaces of the lung with retrograde dissection along the bronchovascular bundles toward the hilum.

Clinical Findings

A. Symptoms and Signs: The clinical spectrum can vary from patients who are asymptomatic to those with severe respiratory distress. Associated symptoms include cyanosis, chest pain, and dyspnea. Physical examination may reveal decreased breath sounds and hyperresonance to percussion on the affected side with tracheal deviation to the opposite side. When the pneumothorax is under tension, cardiac function may be compromised, resulting in hypotension or narrowing of the pulse pressure. Pneumopericardium is a life-threatening condition that presents with muffled heart tones and shock. Pneumomediastinum rarely causes symptoms by itself.

B. Imaging: Chest films usually demonstrate the presence of free air in the pleural space. If the pneumothorax is large and under tension, compressive atelectasis of the underlying lung and shift of the mediastinum to the opposite side may be demonstrated. Cross-table lateral and lateral decubitus films can aid in the diagnosis of free air. Pneumopericardium is identified by the presence of air completely surrounding the heart, whereas in patients with pneumomediastinum, the heart and mediastinal structures may be outlined with air but the air does not involve the diaphragmatic cardiac border.

Differential Diagnosis

When a patient on a ventilator acutely deteriorates,

one must consider not only tension pneumothorax but also obstruction or dislodgment of the endotracheal tube and failure of the mechanical ventilator. Radiographically, pneumothorax must be distinguished from diaphragmatic hernia, lung cysts, congenital lobar emphysema, and cystic adenomatoid malformation, but this task is usually not difficult.

Treatment

Small or asymptomatic pneumothoraces usually do not require treatment and can be managed with close observation. Larger or symptomatic ones usually require drainage, though inhalation of 100% oxygen to wash out blood nitrogen can be tried.

Needle aspiration should be used to relieve tension acutely, followed by chest tube placement. Pneumopericardium requires immediate identification and needle aspiration to prevent death, followed by pericardial tube placement.

In older patients with spontaneous pneumothorax, recurrences are common; sclerosing and surgical procedures are often required.

Fan LL et al: Giant pulmonary cyst simulating a pneumothorax. Am J Dis Child 1988;142:189.

Fackler JC, Yaster M: Multiple trauma in the pediatric patient. In: *Textbook of Pediatric Intensive Care,* 2nd ed. Rogers MC (editor). Williams & Wilkins, 1992.

DISORDERS OF THE MEDIASTINUM

MEDIASTINITIS

Acute infection involving the mediastinum in pediatric patients is usually due to perforation of the esophagus secondary to trauma. The trauma may be self-induced (foreign body, puncture injury to the pharynx with a sharp object) or iatrogenic (endoscopy, attempted endotracheal intubation). Spontaneous esophageal perforation leading to mediastinitis can accompany vomiting, but this is rare. In addition, acute suppurative mediastinitis without trauma does occur but is unusual.

Clinical Findings

A. Symptoms and Signs: The early symptoms and signs of acute mediastinitis may be vague and include the gradual onset of fever, chills, and dysphagia with substernal pain. Dyspnea and cough may also be present. Inspiration may be accompanied by discomfort due to stretching of inflamed mediastinal structures, leading to a pattern of spasmodic or "halting" inspiration. On physical examination, evidence of obstruction of venous return may be present, with substernal pain elicited on palpation of the structures of the thorax. In addition, subcutaneous emphysema may be appreciated in the thoracic and cervical areas.

B. Laboratory Findings and Imaging: The white blood count of the patient with mediastinitis is usually high, with neutrophils and band forms prominent on the differential. The chest x-ray may reveal widening of the upper mediastinum; the lateral view shows anterior displacement of the trachea and the esophagus. Mediastinal emphysema, pleural effusions, and pyopneumothorax may also be present.

Differential Diagnosis

The differential diagnosis includes diseases that lead to the toxic appearance of an infant or child. A primary bacterial pneumonia as well as septicemia must be considered. Retropharyngeal abscesses may also lead to the pattern of respiratory distress seen with a suppurative mediastinitis.

Complications

If not recognized and rapidly treated, mediastinitis can progress rapidly and lead to death. Death may result from the infection or tracheal obstruction. The formation of a mediastinal abscess may also complicate the clinical course of the disease.

Treatment

As soon as the diagnosis is made, parenterally administered broad-spectrum antibiotics must be given. If significant tracheal obstruction is present, an airway must be provided. Drainage of abscesses in the mediastinum may also be indicated.

Templeton JM: Thoracic emergencies. In: *Textbook of Pediatric Emergency Medicine,* 3rd ed. Fleisher GR, Ludwig S (editors). Williams & Wilkins, 1993.

MEDIASTINAL MASSES

Mediastinal masses may come to a physician's attention because of symptoms produced by pressure on the esophagus, airways, nerves, or vessels within the mediastinum or may be discovered unexpectedly on a routine chest x-ray. Once the mass is identified, localization to one of four mediastinal compartments aids in the differential diagnosis (Figure 18–1). The superior mediastinum is the area above the pericardium that is bordered inferiorly by an imaginary line from the manubrium to the fourth thoracic vertebra. The anterior mediastinum is bordered by the sternum anteriorly and the pericardium posteriorly, whereas the posterior mediastinum is defined by the pericardium and diaphragm anteriorly and the lower eight thoracic vertebrae posteriorly. The middle mediastinum is surrounded by these three compartments.

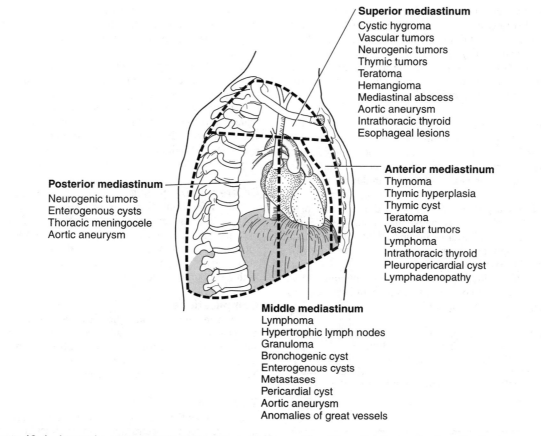

Superior mediastinum
Cystic hygroma
Vascular tumors
Neurogenic tumors
Thymic tumors
Teratoma
Hemangioma
Mediastinal abscess
Aortic aneurysm
Intrathoracic thyroid
Esophageal lesions

Posterior mediastinum
Neurogenic tumors
Enterogenous cysts
Thoracic meningocele
Aortic aneurysm

Anterior mediastinum
Thymoma
Thymic hyperplasia
Thymic cyst
Teratoma
Vascular tumors
Lymphoma
Intrathoracic thyroid
Pleuropericardial cyst
Lymphadenopathy

Middle mediastinum
Lymphoma
Hypertrophic lymph nodes
Granuloma
Bronchogenic cyst
Enterogenous cysts
Metastases
Pericardial cyst
Aortic aneurysm
Anomalies of great vessels

Figure 18–1. Anatomic compartments within the mediastinum. The differential diagnosis of mediastinal masses is based on location within these four compartments.

Clinical Findings

A. Symptoms and Signs: When present, respiratory symptoms are due to pressure on an airway and may include cough, wheezing, and complaints consistent with an infectious process caused by partial or complete obstruction of an airway (unresolving pneumonia in one area of lung). Hemoptysis can also occur but is an unusual presenting symptom. Dysphagia may occur secondary to compression of the esophagus. Encroachment of the mass on the recurrent laryngeal nerve can cause hoarseness due to paralysis of the left vocal cord. Superior vena caval obstruction can lead to dilatation of neck vessels as well as other signs and symptoms of obstruction of venous return from the upper part of the body (superior mediastinal syndrome).

B. Laboratory Findings and Imaging: The mass is initially defined by frontal and lateral chest x-rays together with thoracic CT scans and perhaps MRI. A barium swallow may also help define the extent of a mass. Other studies that may be required include angiography (to define the blood supply to large tumors), electrocardiography, echocardiogra-phy, ultrasound of the thorax, fungal and mycobacterial skin tests, and urinary catecholamine assays. An MR scan or myelogram may be necessary in children suspected of having a neurogenic tumor in the posterior mediastinum.

Differential Diagnosis

The differential diagnosis classified by the mediastinal compartment housing the mass is shown in Figure 18–1. Several general points should be kept in mind. In some series, more than 50% of mediastinal tumors occur in the posterior mediastinum and are mainly neurogenic tumors or enterogenous cysts. Most neurogenic tumors in children under 4 years of age are malignant (neuroblastoma, neuroganglioblastoma), whereas a benign ganglioneuroma is the most common histologic type in older children. In the mid and anterior mediastinum, tumors of lymphatic origin (lymphomas) are the primary concern. Bulky anterior mediastinal tumors that compress the trachea and the great vessels can lead to a superior mediastinal syndrome, and the children can present difficult diagnostic problems because of anesthesia hazards. Definitive diagnosis in most instances relies on surgery to obtain the mass or a part of the mass for a histologic assessment. In cases of lymphoma, the scalene nodes may also contain tumor and may be biopsied in an attempt to establish a diagnosis.

Treatment & Prognosis

Both the appropriate therapy and the response to therapy depend on the cause of the mediastinal mass.

Filler RM, Simpson HS, Ein SH: Mediastinal masses in infants and children. Pediatr Clin North Am 1979;26:677.

Halpern S et al: Anterior mediastinal masses: Anesthesia hazards and other problems. J Pediatr 1983;102:407.

Templeton JM: Thoracic emergencies. In: *Textbook of Pediatric Emergency Medicine,* 3rd ed. Fleisher GR, Ludwig S (editors). Williams & Wilkins, 1993.

Watterson J et al: Thoracopulmonary neoplasms and lung complications of childhood cancer. In: *Pediatric Respiratory Disease.* Hilman B (editor). Saunders, 1993.

DISORDERS OF THE CONTROL OF BREATHING

ACUTE LIFE-THREATENING EPISODES IN INFANCY

A substantial number of infants are brought to medical attention following apparently acute life-threatening episodes of cardiorespiratory instability involving cyanosis, pallor, or apnea. In 50% of cases, a well-recognized medical entity that accounts for the episode can be found. The infants in whom no explanation for the episode can be found are said to have apnea of infancy. Initial interest in these infants was sparked in part by the observation that some died suddenly, leading some to speculate that such events may provide a clue to the identification of infants at risk for the sudden infant death syndrome (SIDS). After almost 2 decades of study, the picture emerging is that of a weak relationship between apnea of infancy and SIDS, with only a small percentage of patients with apnea of infancy at risk for sudden death. In addition, only a small percentage of infants succumbing to SIDS have identifiable episodes of apnea beforehand.

The following section describes an approach to the patient who has undergone an acute life-threatening episode, taking note of the very broad differential diagnosis in this syndrome and uncertainties in both evaluation and treatment. The clinical features of acute life-threatening episodes are discussed in relationship to the differential diagnosis.

Differential Diagnosis

Table 18–2 lists a classification of disorders asso-

Table 18–2. Differential diagnosis of acute life-threatening episodes (ALTE).

Infectious	Viral: respiratory syncytial virus and other respiratory viruses Bacterial: sepsis, pertussis
Gastrointestinal	Gastroesophageal reflux with or without obstructive apnea
Respiratory	Airway abnormality; vascular rings, pulmonary slings, tracheomalacia Pneumonia
Neurologic	Seizure disorder CNS infection: meningitis, encephalitis Vasovagal response Leigh's encephalopathy Brain tumor
Cardiovascular	Congenital malformation Dysrhythmias Cardiomyopathy
Nonaccidental trauma	Battering Drug overdose Munchausen-by-proxy syndrome
No definable cause	Apnea of infancy

ciated with acute life-threatening events. A careful history is often the most helpful part of the evaluation. Attention must be focused on the details of episodes. It is useful to determine whether the infant has been chronically ill or essentially well. A report of several days of poor feeding, temperature instability, or respiratory or gastrointestinal symptoms suggests an infectious process. Reports of "struggling to breathe" or "trying to breathe" imply airway obstruction. Association of the episodes with feeding implies discoordinated swallowing, gastroesophageal reflux, or airway obstruction. Episodes that typically follow crying may be related to breath-holding. Association of episodes with sleeping may also suggest gastroesophageal reflux or apnea of infancy. Attempts should be made to determine the duration of the episode, but this is often difficult. It is helpful to role-play the episode with the family. Details regarding the measures taken to resuscitate the infant and the infant's recovery from the episode are often useful in determining the severity of the episode.

The physical examination provides further direction in pursuing the differential diagnosis. The presence of fever or hypothermia suggests infection. An altered state of consciousness implies a postictal state or drug overdose. Respiratory distress implies cardiac or pulmonary lesions.

Most patients are hospitalized for observation in order to reduce stress on the family and allow prompt completion of the evaluation. Laboratory evaluation includes a complete blood count for evidence of infection. Serum electrolytes are usually obtained. Elevations in serum bicarbonate suggest chronic hypoventilation, whereas decreases suggest acute acidosis, perhaps due to hypoxia during the episode. Chronic acidosis is suggestive of an inherited metabolic disorder. The chest x-ray film is examined for infiltrates suggesting acute infection or chronic aspiration and for cardiac size as a clue to intrinsic cardiac disease. Arterial blood gas studies provide an initial assessment of oxygenation and acid-base status, and low PaO_2 or elevated $PaCO_2$ (or both) implies cardiorespiratory disease. A significant base deficit suggests that the episode was accompanied by hypoxia or circulatory impairment. On-line oxygen saturation measurements in the hospital assess the infant's oxygenation status during different activities and are more comprehensive than a single blood gas sample.

Because apnea has been associated with respiratory infections, diagnostic studies for infection with respiratory syncytial virus in particular but also other viruses and B pertussis may contribute to the diagnostic process. The apnea seen with infection often precedes other physical findings. If there is any possibility that the episode involved airway obstruction, a barium swallow and air laryngotracheogram should be done. Vascular rings, pulmonary slings, and other intrathoracic lesions impinging upon the trachea are often best demonstrated on barium swallow. The air laryngotracheogram also aids in identifying structural lesions or tracheomalacia. Fiberoptic bronchoscopy may also be used to evaluate the airway. The barium swallow is not done to identify gastroesophageal reflux, because it is presumed that the majority of normal infants demonstrate reflux. If reflux is suspected to be the cause of the apnea, it should be documented by esophageal pH monitoring coupled with respiratory pattern recording. Most infants with reflux and apnea can be treated with medical antireflux measures. Infants with reflux and repeated episodes of apnea may benefit from a surgical antireflux procedure.

There are several neurologic causes of acute life-threatening episodes. Apnea as the sole manifestation of a seizure disorder is unusual but may occur. In cases of repeated episodes, 24-hour electroencephalographic monitoring may be helpful in detecting a seizure disorder. Leigh's disease, a brain stem disorder characterized pathologically by neuronal dropout, may present with apneic episodes.

Apneic episodes have been linked to child abuse in several ways. Head injury following nonaccidental trauma may be first brought to medical attention because of apnea. Other signs of abuse are usually immediately apparent in these cases. Drug overdose, either accidental (eg, mistakes in application of antecolic medications containing barbiturates) or intentional, may also present with apnea. Several series document that apneic episodes may be falsely reported by parents seeking attention—one of the instances of Munchausen-by-proxy syndrome. In addition, parents may physically interfere with respiratory efforts. Pinch marks on the nares are sometimes found in these cases.

Treatment

Therapy is directed at the underlying cause if one is found. After blood cultures are taken, antibiotics should be administered to infants who appear toxic. Seizure disorders are treated with anticonvulsants. Vascular rings and pulmonary slings must be corrected surgically because of severe morbidity and high mortality rates in uncorrected cases.

The approach to care in apnea of infancy is controversial. These are infants presenting with acute life-threatening episodes where no definable cause can be ascertained. Treatment in this group of patients has centered around the use of electronic monitors for the detection of apnea or bradycardia in the home. Parents are then taught cardiopulmonary resuscitation so that they may intervene in the event of a serious episode. The rationale for the use of monitors implies that infants who are at risk for subsequent severe episodes can be identified. Medical personnel have made a number of attempts to predict which infants are at risk for subsequent severe episodes. These attempts have included hypoxic and hypercapnic challenges and determinations of the frequency of periodic breathing or apnea, usually through the use of pneumograms. None of these techniques is sufficiently specific or selective to be useful in prediction. In addition, the efficacy of home monitoring has never been demonstrated in controlled trials.

The decision to monitor these infants involves the participation of the family as well as the physician. Infants with severe initial episodes or repeated severe episodes are now thought to be at significant increased risk for sudden death and should probably be monitored in the home despite the uncertainty of the effectiveness of this step. Episodes in these children are so severe that the parents want to know the infant's condition at all times. Monitoring is not indicated in patients who have isolated episodes of lesser severity unless the parents clearly express a wish for it. Pneumograms can be used to determine whether apnea is occurring if there is uncertainty. However, pneumograms are not predictive and play no role in the decision to monitor or when to stop monitoring. Discontinuing the monitor is usually based on the infant's ability to go several months without triggering the alarm. Aminophylline has been suggested as treatment for apnea of infancy, but controlled trials are lacking; at this point, this drug is not recommended.

Brooks JG: Apparent life-threatening events and apnea of infancy. Clin Perinatol 1992;19:809.

National Institutes of Health Consensus Development Conference Statement: Infantile apnea and home monitoring. Sept 29 to Oct 1, 1986. Pediatrics 1987;79:292.

SUDDEN INFANT DEATH SYNDROME

Essentials of Diagnosis

- Sudden and unexpected death in infancy.
- Adequate postmortem examination excluding known causes of death.

General Considerations

The sudden infant death syndrome (SIDS) is a poorly understood disorder encompassing cases of sudden and unexpected death of previously well or nearly well infants that remain unexplained after an adequate postmortem examination. The postmortem examination is an important feature of the definition because approximately 20% of cases of sudden death can be explained by autopsy findings. The incidence of SIDS in the United States (1–2:1000) makes it the leading cause of death in infancy after the neonatal period. The overall incidence of SIDS has steadily declined over the past few decades.

Epidemiologic and pathologic data constitute most of what is known about SIDS. The number of deaths peaks at age 2 months, and most deaths occur in infants a few weeks of age to 6 months of age. There is an increase in deaths during the peak respiratory virus season, and most deaths occur between midnight and 8:00 AM. The syndrome is more common among minorities and socioeconomically disadvantaged populations. There is a 3:2 male predominance in most series. Other risk factors include low birth weight, teenage or drug-addicted mothers, maternal smoking, and a family history of SIDS. Most of these risk factors are associated with a two- or threefold elevation of incidence but are not specific enough to be useful in predicting which infants will die unexpectedly. Recent immunization is not a risk factor.

The most consistent pathologic findings are intrathoracic petechiae and mild inflammation and congestion of the respiratory tract. Subtler pathologic findings include brain stem gliosis, extramedullary hematopoiesis, and increases in periadrenal brown fat. These latter findings suggest that infants who succumb to SIDS have had intermittent or chronic hypoxia before death.

The mechanism or mechanisms of death in SIDS are unknown. For example, it is not known whether the initiating event at the time of death is cessation of breathing or cardiac arrhythmia or asystole. Suggested hypotheses have included upper airway obstruction, catecholamine excess, brain stem immaturity or injury, and increased fetal hemoglobin. It has been recognized that some infants who presented with apneic episodes subsequently died from SIDS; however, study of these infants and prospective studies of large numbers of newborns have indicated that most infants with apnea do not die from SIDS and that most infants with SIDS have no identifiable episodes of apnea (see discussion of acute life-threatening episodes, above).

A history of mild symptoms of upper respiratory infection before death is not uncommon, and SIDS victims are sometimes seen by physicians a day or so before death. When infants are discovered blue, cold, and motionless by parents or caretakers, they are most commonly taken to the emergency room, where resuscitative efforts are almost uniformly of no avail. Families must then be supported following the death. The National Sudden Infant Death Syndrome Foundation provides information about psychosocial support groups and counseling for families of SIDS victims. The postmortem examination can be of value to the family; when the diagnosis of SIDS is established, lingering questions about other possible causes of death are resolved. For this reason, as well as for ascertaining causes of death in infancy, postmortem examination should always be recommended. Some recent reports have suggested that a death scene investigation may also be important in determining the cause of sudden unexpected deaths in infancy.

Positioning & SIDS

A variety of recent studies from other countries have presented evidence that the incidence of SIDS is significantly higher when infants are placed in their beds for sleeping in the prone position. A Task Force on Infant Positioning and SIDS of the American Academy of Pediatrics has reviewed these studies and has made the following summary statement:

Based on careful evaluation of existing data indicating an association between Sudden Infant Death Syndrome (SIDS) and prone sleeping position for infants, the Academy recommends that healthy infants, when being put down for sleep, be positioned on their side or back.

This statement has been made with full knowledge of the limitations of many of the studies that were reviewed and with concern for the still valid reasons why certain infants—such as preterm infants with respiratory distress, infants with gastroesophageal reflux, or certain airway anomalies—do better sleeping in the prone position. Nevertheless, the current evidence is compelling for recommending the side or back position for sleeping in healthy term infants.

Berry PJ: Pathological findings in SIDS. J Clin Pathol 1992;45:11.

Goldberg J: The counseling of SIDS parents. Clin Perinatol 1992;19:927.

Freed GE, Steinschneider A, Glassman M, Winn K: Sudden infant death syndrome prevention and an understanding of selected clinical issues. Pediatr Clin North Am 1994;41:967.

Willinger M, Hoffman HJ, Hartford RB: Infant sleep position and risk for sudden infant death syndrome. Pediatrics 1994;93:814.

19

Cardiovascular Diseases

Robert R. Wolfe, MD, Marc Boucek, MD, Michael S. Schaffer, MD, & James W. Wiggins, MD

Cardiovascular disease is a significant cause of death and chronic illness in children. In North America, more than 1% of newborn infants have congenital heart disease, usually resulting from multifactorial causes. Preventive medicine is the most important aspect of pediatrics, and it is becoming obvious that the prevention of adult heart disease must begin in childhood (eg, prevention of atherosclerosis by diet modification). But prevention requires an understanding of the causes of disease, and in this there are wide discrepancies, ranging from significant accomplishments in the case of rheumatic fever to the very tentative steps being taken to understand the causes of congenital heart disease, atherosclerosis, and essential hypertension.

CLUES TO THE PRESENCE OF HEART DISEASE

The most important clues to the presence of heart disease requiring prompt attention are congestive heart failure and cyanosis. These clinical conditions are discussed in more detail in subsequent sections. The presence of a heart murmur may suggest the possibility of heart disease in an infant, or the murmur may be a functional or innocent murmur. Not all serious cardiovascular disorders are accompanied by an easily detectable murmur.

DIAGNOSTIC EVALUATION

Sequence of Evaluation
  (1) History
  (2) Physical examination
  (3) Electrocardiogram
  (4) Chest x-ray
  (5) Echocardiogram
  (6) Cardiac catheterization (with angiography)

HISTORY

In obtaining the history from the family or the patient, one must keep in perspective the age and relative activity of that patient. A history of increasing feeding difficulties and diaphoresis is the most common feature of early congestive heart failure.

Family History
Most cardiac diseases are familial, so the history of heart disease in a first-degree relative should be sought. These details might suggest the need to evaluate the child for hyperlipidemia.

Pregnancy
The history of pregnancy should elicit information regarding first-trimester exposure to illness or medications that place infants at high risk for congenital heart disease. A history of significant problems related to labor and delivery, such as perinatal stress or asphyxia at birth, suggests causes of myocardial dysfunction and pulmonary hypertension in the neonate.

Growth & Development
Major cardiac problems frequently affect a child's ability to grow. There may be a history of poor feeding (early fatigue, vomiting, lethargy) or failure to thrive despite adequate caloric intake. Gross motor development may also be delayed in children with significant congestive heart failure or cyanosis, although other aspects of development are less frequently affected.

Tachypnea
Parents frequently notice rapid breathing in the child. Although infants at rest rarely breathe faster than 40 respirations per minute, infants in congestive heart failure usually have respiratory rates in excess of 60/min (and often as rapid as 80–100/min). Tachypnea may be considered the cardinal sign of left-sided heart failure in the pediatric patient.

Cyanosis

Cyanotic heart disease may go unrecognized because of lack of appreciation of the subtleties of diagnosing cyanosis. The infant with a cyanotic heart lesion may be more gray than blue (and may have no heart murmur).

Hypoxemic Spells

It is important to determine whether the patient with a cyanotic heart lesion such as tetralogy of Fallot is having hypoxemic spells, because prompt surgical intervention may be required. These spells usually occur on morning awakening or after a feeding or bowel movement; the infant begins breathing fast, becomes progressively more gray or blue, and cries as if having severe pain. Such a spell rarely may progress to unconsciousness, paresis, or even death.

Other Clinical Clues

Orthopnea, dyspnea, easy fatigability, growth failure, sweating, squatting, and pneumonia are common clues to the presence of heart disease.

PHYSICAL EXAMINATION

The examination should begin with a careful general inspection to note activity (agitation, lethargy) and skin perfusion and color. Vital signs, including temperature, pulse rate, respiratory rate, and particularly blood pressure (in all four extremities in symptomatic infants), can reflect the overall status of the patient. Auscultation of the heart and lungs should be performed early in the overall examination, because the infant's crying limits the physician's ability to hear even pronounced cardiac sounds. Abdominal examination for position and size of organs is also important. The presence of other congenital abnormalities, particularly chromosomal disorders, increases the probability of congenital heart disease.

1. CARDIOVASCULAR EXAMINATION

Inspection & Palpation

Conformation of the chest can give clues to past or present cardiomegaly. Prominence of the precordial chest wall is frequently seen in infants and children with cardiomegaly. Increased cardiac activity is often noted on inspection.

Palpation may reveal precordial activity, right ventricular lift, or left-sided heave; a diffuse point of maximal impulse; or the presence of a thrill caused by a loud murmur. Thrills are typically located where the murmur is most intense and can sometimes be felt at the point of radiation, as in a suprasternal notch or carotid thrill with aortic stenosis. In patients with severe pulmonary hypertension, palpable pulmonary closure is frequently noted, usually at the mid to upper left sternal border.

Auscultation

A. Normal Heart Sounds: S_1 (the first heart sound) is the sound of atrioventricular valve closure. It is best heard at the lower left sternal border and is usually medium-pitched. Although four components of S_1 can be detected by phonocardiography, only one or two of these are usually heard with a stethoscope.

S_2 (the second heart sound) is the sound of semilunar valve closure. It has a higher pitch than S_1 and is best heard along the lower and upper left sternal border. S_2 has two component sounds, A_2 and P_2 (aortic and pulmonary valve closure). A_2 is best appreciated at the mid and lower left sternal border, whereas P_2 is best heard at the upper left sternal border and is normally softer than A_2. Splitting of S_2 varies with respirations, widening with inspiration and narrowing with expiration. It is best heard at the second left intercostal space at the sternal border.

S_3 (the third heart sound) is the sound of rapid filling of the left ventricle. It occurs in early diastole and after S_2 and is a medium- to low-pitched thud. When heard in healthy children, the sound diminishes or disappears when the position changes from supine to sitting or standing; it is usually intermittent.

S_4 (the fourth heart sound) is associated with atrial contraction and increased atrial pressure and has a low pitch similar to that of S_3. It occurs just prior to S_1 and is not normally audible.

B. Abnormal Heart Sounds: Abnormalities in splitting or intensity of the component sounds of S_2 can be helpful in the diagnosis of major heart problems. With inspiration, there is a decrease in the intrathoracic pressure; this decrease causes increased filling of the right side of the heart, thereby prolonging the ejection time and delaying closure of the pulmonary valve. Normal intrathoracic pressure changes have little effect on the filling of the left side of the heart. Widening of splitting can be a clue to right-sided volume overload, whereas narrowing may indicate increased pulmonary artery pressure. A single S_2 is often heard in cases of malposition of the great vessels or severe pulmonary hypertension.

Ejection clicks are high-pitched and are usually related to dilated great vessels or valve abnormalities (or both). They can be heard throughout the ventricular systole and are classified as early, mid, or late. Early ejection clicks at the upper left sternal border are usually of pulmonary origin. Aortic clicks are heard in a wider distribution but best at the apex. Widespread clicks originating or loudest at the apex can be mitral or aortic in origin. The mid to late ejection click at the apex is most typically mitral valve prolapse. Early clicks may also be heard in spontaneous closure of ventricular septal defects.

S_3 can be a functional sound in childhood, although it often is associated with cardiac abnormalities.

S_4 is not normally audible; its finding on auscultation is almost always associated with cardiac abnormalities.

Opening snap is a relatively rare sound in pediatrics, occurring early in diastole and usually preceding a diastolic murmur of atrioventricular stenosis. It is medium-pitched in intensity.

C. Murmurs: Murmurs are the most common cardiovascular finding. The presence of a murmur in a child almost always causes alarm in the parents, who associate murmurs with major heart disease. However, most children have functional or innocent murmurs.

1. Characteristics–Murmurs can be evaluated on the basis of the following characteristics:

a. Location and radiation–Where the murmur is best heard and where the sound extends.

b. Relationship to cardiac cycle and duration–Systolic (with the pulse), diastolic, continuous, or to-and-fro.

c. Intensity–Classified as grade I, soft and heard with difficulty; grade II, soft but easily heard; grade III, loud but without a thrill; grade IV, loud and associated with a precordial thrill; grade V, loud, with thrill, and audible with the edge of the stethoscope; or grade VI, very loud and audible with the stethoscope off the chest or with the naked ear.

d. Quality–Harsh, musical, or rough; high, medium, or low in pitch.

e. Variation with position–Audible when the patient is supine, sitting, standing, or squatting.

2. Functional murmurs–The seven most common functional murmurs heard in childhood are as follows:

a. Newborn murmur–As the name implies, this murmur is frequently heard within the first few days of life. Typically, it is located at the lower left sternal border, without significant radiation. Newborn murmur is a soft, short, vibratory grade I–II/VI early systolic murmur that often subsides when mild pressure is applied to the abdomen. Newborn murmur usually disappears by 2–3 weeks of age.

b. Functional murmur of peripheral arterial pulmonary stenosis–This murmur is frequently heard in the premature infant, often after closure of a patent ductus arteriosus. It is secondary to mild narrowing of the branches of the pulmonary artery. Typically, the murmur is heard with equal intensity at the upper left sternal border, at the back, and in both axillas. It is a soft, short, high-pitched, grade I–II/VI systolic ejection murmur and usually disappears by 6 months of life. This murmur must be differentiated from true peripheral arterial pulmonary stenosis (rubella syndrome), coarctation of the thoracic aorta, valvular pulmonary stenosis, and atrial septal defect. These entities should, however, have other findings to suggest their organic nature.

c. Still's murmur–Probably the most common murmur of early childhood, this murmur can be heard in infancy, although it is most typically heard from the age of 2 years until adolescence. Classically, Still's murmur is loudest midway between the apex and the lower left sternal border, and often it may be transmitted (depending on loudness) to the remainder of the precordial area. Still's murmur is a musical or vibratory, short, high-pitched, grade I–III early systolic ejection murmur. It is loudest when the patient is in the supine position; it diminishes or disappears when the patient sits or stands or during Valsalva's maneuver. Still's murmur may be louder in patients with fever or tachycardia.

d. Pulmonary outflow ejection murmur–This murmur may be heard throughout childhood. It is usually a soft, short, systolic ejection murmur, grade I–II in intensity and well localized to the upper left sternal border. The murmur becomes louder when the patient is in the supine position or when cardiac output is increased and softens with standing or during Valsalva's maneuver. Pulmonary outflow ejection murmur must be differentiated from other murmurs, such as those associated with pulmonary stenosis, coarctation of the aorta, atrial septal defect, and peripheral pulmonary artery stenosis.

e. Venous hum–This very common murmur of childhood is usually heard after 3 years of age. The murmur is located at the upper right and left sternal borders and in the lower neck. It is described as a continuous musical hum of grade I–II intensity, and it may be accentuated in diastole and with inspiration. This murmur always disappears when the patient is placed in a supine position or when the jugular vein is compressed. Venous hum is thought to be produced by turbulence in the subclavian and jugular veins.

f. Innominate or carotid bruit–This murmur is more common in the older child and adolescent. It is heard in the right supraclavicular and neck areas. This is a long systolic ejection murmur, somewhat harsh and of grade II–III intensity. The bruit can be accentuated by light pressure on the carotid artery and must be differentiated from all types of aortic stenosis.

g. Hemic murmur–Hemic murmurs are heard whenever anemia, fever, stress, or any increase in cardiac output is present. Typically, they are heard best in the aortic and pulmonary areas. These systolic ejection murmurs are of grade I–II intensity and are high-pitched. They disappear with normalization of cardiac output.

When functional murmurs are found in a child, the physician should assure the parents that these are normal heart sounds of the developing child and that they represent no abnormality of the heart.

3. Organic murmurs–Organic murmurs are evaluated on the basis of the characteristics outlined above (eg, location, intensity). These murmurs are discussed in relation to specific lesions later in this chapter.

2. NONCARDIAC EXAMINATION

Arterial Pulse

A. Rate & Rhythm: Cardiac rate and rhythm are usually determined by palpation of the radial or brachial pulse. Throughout infancy and childhood, the rate is subject to great variation. Multiple determinations must be made under properly evaluated conditions before conclusions can be drawn about their significance. This cautious approach is particularly important in infants.

Marked variations in heart rate occur with activity; therefore, the resting heart rate may be most accurately determined during sleep. In older children, exercise and emotional factors have a marked effect on the heart rate. All of these factors should be taken into account when examining the child, because many children are apprehensive and may react emotionally to the initial phases of the examination. It is possible for normal infants to have heart rates of 180 or 190 during the activity associated with a physical or electrocardiographic examination. Average resting heart rates range from 120/min in infants to 80/min in older children.

In the pediatric age group, the rhythm may be regular, or there may be a phasic variation in the heart rate (sinus arrhythmia), which is normal. Variations occasionally occur without relation to the respiratory cycle.

B. Quality & Amplitude of Pulse: Examination of the cardiovascular system should always include comparison of the pulses of the upper and lower extremities. A bounding pulse is characteristic of patent ductus arteriosus or aortic regurgitation. Narrow or thready pulses are found in patients with congestive heart failure or severe aortic stenosis.

The suprasternal notch should be examined, where visible pulsation is usually abnormal, although it may be seen in patients who are emotionally excited. A prominent pulsation is found in aortic insufficiency, patent ductus arteriosus, and coarctation of the aorta. A palpable thrill in the suprasternal notch is characteristic of aortic stenosis and is occasionally found with valvular pulmonary stenosis, coarctation of the aorta, and patent ductus arteriosus.

Assessment of the femoral pulse is an essential part of the physical examination of every infant and child. The femoral pulse should be readily palpable and equal in amplitude and time of appearance with the brachial pulse. A femoral pulse that is absent or weak or one that is delayed in comparison with the brachial pulse suggests coarctation of the aorta. An absent or diminished femoral pulse may be the only clue to the cause of a life-threatening problem.

Arterial Blood Pressure

Blood pressures should be obtained in the upper and lower extremities. Systolic pressure in the lower extremities determined by the auscultatory technique is usually higher than that found in the upper extremities in patients *over age 1 year.* In normal infants, the pressure in the arms may be slightly higher. The cuff must cover the same relative area of the arm and leg; for this reason, a larger cuff usually must be used for the leg than for the arm.

A. Procedures: Because of variation of blood pressure with respiration and slower rhythmic variations (Mayer or Traube-Hering waves), pressure obtained by any method should be repeated several times.

1. Auscultatory method–Hearing Korotkoff sounds by stethoscope and sphygmomanometer is the most common measure of blood pressure in children and correlates well with direct intra-arterial measurements. However, many factors affect its accuracy. Among these are the dimensions of the inflatable bag within the cuff. The length of the bag should be 100% and the width 50% of the circumference of the limb. A cuff that is too narrow or too short will produce a blood pressure reading that is higher than the true pressure.

2. Doppler ultrasound or automated blood pressure method–The combination of a small ultrasound transducer and a sphygmomanometer has proved to be especially applicable to the small infant. Considerations of cuff dimensions are still critical, however.

B. Pulse Pressure: Pulse pressure is determined by subtracting the diastolic pressure from the systolic pressure. Normally, the pulse pressure is less than 50 mm Hg or less than half the systolic pressure. A widened pulse pressure (which is associated with a bounding pulse) is present in aorticopulmonary shunt (eg, patent ductus arteriosus), aortic insufficiency, fever, anemia, and complete heart block. A narrow pulse pressure is seen in congestive heart failure, severe aortic stenosis, and pericardial tamponade.

Venous Pressure & Pulse

The level of the distended jugular vein above the suprasternal notch when the patient is at a 45-degree angle is a measure of venous pressure in older children and adults. Normally, one may observe the level of the transition between collapse and distention of the jugular vein approximately 1–2 cm above the notch. In addition to the level of the pulse, the wave pattern should be observed. Two waves can frequently be seen: (1) The *a* wave, because of right atrial contraction, is a rather sharply rising wave and therefore occurs immediately before or with the first heart sound or point of maximum impulse. (2) The *v* wave, caused by filling of the right atrium during ventricular systole, is a more slowly rising wave and occurs toward the end of ventricular systole. The venous pulse is not too helpful in examining infants and young children, however, because their necks are short and fat.

Extremities

Cyanosis of the extremities usually indicates congenital heart disease, but severe pulmonary disease must be excluded. Cyanosis is characterized by a bluish discoloration of the nails and mucous membranes.

A. Clubbing of Fingers & Toes: Clubbing implies fairly severe cyanotic congenital heart disease. It usually does not appear until approximately age 1, although occasionally, in patients with severe cyanosis, it may occur earlier. The first sign of clubbing is softening of the nail beds, followed by rounding of the fingernails and then by thickening and shininess of the terminal phalanx, with loss of creases.

Hypoxemia producing cyanosis is by far the most common cause, but clubbing occurs also in patients with infective endocarditis, severe liver disease, and lung abscess.

B. Edema: Edema of the lower extremities is characteristic of right ventricular heart failure in older children and adults. However, in infants and younger children, peripheral edema is more likely to affect first the face, then the presacral region, and eventually the extremities.

Abdomen

Hepatomegaly is the cardinal sign of right heart failure in the infant and child. Presystolic pulsation of the liver may occur with right atrial hypertension and systolic pulsation with tricuspid insufficiency. Congestive splenomegaly may be present in patients who have had longstanding congestive heart failure. Enlargement of the spleen is one of the characteristic features of subacute infective endocarditis. Ascites is occasionally present in right heart failure.

Payne RM et al: Toward a molecular understanding of congenital heart disease. Circulation 1995;91:494.

Rosner B et al: Blood pressure nomograms for children and adolescents, by height, sex, and age, in the United States. J Pediatr 1993;123:871.

Van Oort A et al: The vibratory innocent heart murmur in schoolchildren: A case-control Doppler echocardiographic study. Pediatr Cardiol 1994;15:275.

ELECTROCARDIOGRAM & VECTORCARDIOGRAM

The electrocardiogram (ECG) is an essential part of the evaluation of the cardiovascular system. The ECG is the sine qua non for the diagnosis of dysrhythmias and may offer the best clue to the specific diagnosis of congenital lesions (eg, left axis deviation in a blue baby, suggesting tricuspid atresia).

Conversely, the ECG may provide little or no help (as in assessing right ventricular hypertrophy in the newborn or left ventricular hypertrophy in the child with congenital aortic stenosis).

It is not possible, within the limitations of this presentation, to teach the interpretation of the ECG, but a few basic facts and definitions should help to orient the student.

A. Propagation of Electrical Force: As shown in Figure 19–1, a wave of electrical force traveling toward an electrode inscribes a positive (upward) deflection; away from an electrode, a negative deflection; and perpendicular to an electrode, a low-voltage, isodiphasic complex. These forces are inscribed as loops on the vectorcardiogram (VCG), and abnormalities are manifested as alterations in direction and duration of force or as increased or decreased electrical force (amplitude of QRS complex on the ECG or loop on the VCG).

B. Age-Related Variations: The ECG and VCG evolve with the age of the patient. The rate gradually decreases and intervals generally increase with age. There is also progressive change in dominance of ventricles from right ventricular dominance in the young infant to left ventricular dominance in the older infant, child, and adult. The normal ECG of the 1-week-old would be highly abnormal for a 1-year-old, and the ECG of a 5-year-old would not be normal for an adult.

C. Electrocardiographic Interpretation: Figure 19–2 defines the events recorded on the ECG. The sequence of recording the findings of the ECG is usually as follows: rate, rhythm, P wave, PR interval, QRS complex (including axis, amplitude, and duration), QT interval, ST segment, and T wave.

1. Rate—The paper speed at which ECGs are usually taken is 25 mm/s. Each small square is 1 mm,

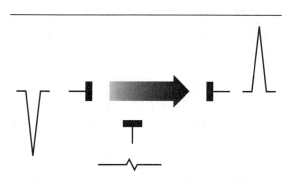

Figure 19–1. Depolarization of the myocardium. The arrow represents the wave of electrical force. As it travels toward the electrode, it inscribes a positive (upward) deflection; away from the electrode, a negative (downward) deflection; and perpendicular to the electrode, a low-voltage, isodiphasic deflection.

Figure 19–2. Complexes and intervals of the electrocardiogram.

and each large square, 5 mm. Therefore, five large squares represent 1 second, one large square 0.2 second, and one small square 0.04 second. A common method of estimating the ventricular rate is to count the number of large squares between two QRS complexes: If QRS complexes appear at a rate of one per large square (5/s), the ventricular rate is 300; if QRS complexes appear every two squares, the ventricular rate is 150, and so on. The formula is to divide the number of large squares between QRS complexes into 300 and roughly interpolate for fractions of large squares.

2. Rhythm–Normal sinus rhythm consists of a normal P wave followed by a normal PR interval and a normal QRS complex.

3. P wave–The P wave represents atrial depolarization. In the pediatric patient, it is normally not taller than 2.5 mm or more than 0.08 second in duration.

4. PR interval–This interval is measured from the beginning of the P wave to the beginning of the QRS complex. It increases with age and with slower rates. The PR interval ranges from a minimum of 0.11 second in infants to a maximum of 0.18 second in older children with slow rates. The PR interval is commonly prolonged in rheumatic heart disease and by digitalis.

5. QRS complex–This represents ventricular depolarization, and its amplitude and direction of force (axis) reveal the relative size of (viable) ventricular mass in hypertrophy, hypoplasia, and infarction. Abnormal ventricular conduction (eg, right bundle branch block, anterior fascicular block) is also revealed. Interpretation of the QRS complex is one of the most important aspects of cardiologic diagnosis. V.A.T. is the ventricular activation time.

6. QT interval–This interval is measured from the beginning of the QRS complex to the end of the T wave. The QT duration is affected by drugs such as digitalis and electrolyte imbalances such as hypocalcemia and hypokalemia (really QU interval prolongation). The normal duration is rate-related and must be corrected using the following formula:

$$QT_c = \frac{QT\ interval(s)}{\sqrt{R - R\ interval(s)}}$$

The normal QT_c is usually less than 0.44 second.

7. ST segment–This short segment lying between the end of the QRS complex and the beginning of the T wave is affected by drugs and electrolyte imbalances and reflects myocardial injury.

8. T wave–The T wave represents myocardial

repolarization and is altered by electrolytes, myocardial hypertrophy, and ischemia.

9. Impression–The ultimate impression of the ECG is derived from a systematic analysis of features such as those described above as compared with expected normal values for the age of the child.

Benson DW Jr: The normal electrocardiogram. In: *Moss and Adams Heart Disease in Infants, Children, and Adolescents,* 5th ed. Emmanouilides GC et al (editors). Williams & Wilkins, 1995.

Gillette PC, Garson A Jr: *Pediatric Arrhythmias: Electrophysiology and Pacing.* Saunders, 1990.

Liebman J, Plonsey R, Gillette PC: *Pediatric Electrocardiography.* Williams & Wilkins, 1982.

CHEST X-RAY

The chest x-ray requires systematic evaluation. Accurate conclusions about the presence or absence of congenital heart defects and bone abnormalities can be drawn only if the proper procedures were followed—for example, the penetration of x-ray was adequate, and the films were obtained on adequate inspiration (distortions resulting from inadequate inspiration may look like cardiomegaly and increased vascular markings). The size of the heart, as seen on the chest x-ray film, must be evaluated in relation to the age and size of the patient. Chest films of the normal newborn show a greater heart size and more pronounced vascular markings than those of the normal older child. These factors must all be taken into consideration in evaluating heart size and configuration and lung fields. The standard posteroanterior and left lateral chest films are usually adequate for this evaluation (Figure 19–3). If there is suspicion of vascular ring or mediastinal mass, multiple-view films with barium swallow are indicated.

Condon V: The heart and great vessels. In: *Caffey's Pediatric X-Ray Diagnosis: An Integrated Imaging Approach.* Silverman FN (editor). Year Book, 1985.

ECHOCARDIOGRAPHY & DOPPLER ULTRASONOGRAPHY

Echocardiography is now the major noninvasive method for diagnosis of congenital heart defects and is used to define anatomy, function, chamber and vessel size, and valve abnormalities. The use of M-mode and two-dimensional echocardiography will, in most instances, allow accurate diagnosis. These methods, along with Doppler ultrasonography (color, pulsed, or continuous-wave ultrasound measurements) can now be used to predict cardiac output, flow direction, valve gradients, and pulmonary artery pressure. New techniques of transesophageal and three-dimensional echocardiography are adding anatomic information that is particularly helpful in the surgical management of patients with congenital heart disease. Interpretation of the results of these studies requires the skill of the pediatric cardiologist. In cases of major heart disease, cardiac catheterization should also be performed.

Silverman NH: *Pediatric Echocardiography.* Williams & Wilkins, 1993.

Snider AR, Serwer GA: *Echocardiography in Pediatric Heart Disease.* Year Book, 1990.

Stümper O, Sutherland GR: *Transesophageal Echocardiography in Congenital Heart Disease.* Arnold, 1994.

NUCLEAR CARDIOLOGY

Use of radionuclide tracers in infants and children includes detection and quantification of left-to-right

Figure 19–3. Position of cardiovascular structures in principal x-ray views. Ao = aorta, IVC = inferior vena cava, LA = left atrium, LA APP = left atrial appendage, LV = left ventricle, PA = pulmonary artery, RA = right atrium, RV = right ventricle, SVC = superior vena cava.

and right-to-left intracardiac shunting, quantification of cardiac output at rest and during exercise using gated blood pool scintigraphy, and myocardial imaging with thallium 201 (^{201}Tl) and technetium 99m (^{99m}Tc) sestamibi for ischemia or infarction. In the older child, the latter method can be enhanced by exercise stress testing. These tests yield more objective data for evaluation of children with heart disease.

Hurwitz RA: Radionuclide methods. In: *Moss and Adams Heart Disease in Infants, Children, and Adolescents,* 5th ed. Emmanouilides GC et al (editors). Williams & Wilkins, 1995.

Wiles HB: Nuclear cardiology. In: *The Science and Practice of Pediatric Cardiology.* Garson A Jr, Bricker JT, McNamara DG (editors). Lea & Febiger, 1990.

MAGNETIC RESONANCE IMAGING

Magnetic resonance imaging (MRI) is now a valuable tool in the evaluation and noninvasive follow-up of many congenital heart defects. Particularly in the imaging of vascular structures of the thorax, MRI can be matched only by angiography. The addition of "gated" imaging or cine MRI now allows dynamic evaluation of the structure and blood flow patterns within the heart and great vessels. MRI is invaluable in the long-term follow-up of coarctation of the aorta after angioplasty.

Friedman BJ et al: Comparison of magnetic resonance imaging and echocardiography in determination of cardiac dimensions in normal subjects. J Am Coll Cardiol 1985;5:1369.

Higgins CB et al: *Congenital Heart Disease Echocardiography and Magnetic Resonance Imaging.* Raven, 1990.

Vick GW, Rohey R, Johnston DL: Nuclear magnetic resonance and positron emission tomography. In: *The Science and Practice of Pediatric Cardiology.* Garson A Jr, Bricker JT, McNamara DG (editors). Lea & Febiger, 1990.

ERGOMETRY

Pediatric ergometry is a newly evolving technique. It has long been hampered by lack of appreciation of its applications and availability of normal data. Most children with heart disease are capable of normal activity, and exercise data are essential to prevent overprotection. The response to exercise is valuable in determining the need for cardiovascular surgery and its timing. Bicycle ergometers or treadmills can often be used to test children as young as 6 years. Important exercise parameters include stress ECGs, conditioning, and performance data. Significant stress ischemia or dysrhythmias warrant physical restrictions or appropriate therapy. Children demonstrating poor performance with suboptimal conditioning benefit from an exercise prescription. The preoperative and

postoperative child can then be objectively guided into appropriate recreational and competitive activities and given prevocational guidance.

Driscoll DJ: Exercise testing. In: *Moss and Adams Heart Disease in Infants, Children, and Adolescents,* 5th ed. Emmanouilides GC et al (editors). Williams & Wilkins, 1995.

ARTERIAL BLOOD GASES (Arterial PO_2, Systemic O_2 Saturation)

Because cyanosis is difficult to measure (and sometimes to recognize) by inspection of the patient, objective laboratory determinations are required. The quantitative response of arterial PO_2 or O_2 saturation (eg, by pulse oximetry) to administration of 100% oxygen is one of the most useful methods of distinguishing cyanosis produced by heart disease from cyanosis related to lung disease in sick infants. In cyanotic heart disease, PaO_2 increases very little from values obtained while breathing ambient room air compared with values during 100% oxygen administration. However, there is usually a very significant increase in PaO_2 when oxygen is administered to a patient with lung disease. Continuous noninvasive methods for monitoring arterial PO_2 include the transcutaneous O_2 monitor and pulse oximetry. Inherent limitations have prevented the general substitution of these noninvasive methods for direct arterial sampling in this evaluation, but they are valuable in overall cardiopulmonary care of the sick infant. Table 19–1 illustrates the sort of response one might expect following at least 10 minutes of 100% oxygen administration to cyanotic infants with heart disease versus lung disease.

OTHER NONINVASIVE LABORATORY STUDIES

In children of all ages, but particularly in the infant and newborn, many metabolic abnormalities can have a major influence on the performance of the cardiovascular system. In evaluating the sympto-

Table 19–1. Examples of responses to 10 minutes of 100% oxygen in lung disease and heart disease.

	Lung Disease		Heart Disease	
	Room Air	100% O_2	Room Air	100% O_2
Color	Blue →	Pink	Blue →	Blue
Oximetry	60% →	99%	60% →	62%
PaO_2 (mm Hg)	35 →	120	35 →	38

matic infant, it is important to rule out infection, hypoglycemia, hypocalcemia, hypovolemia, hyperkalemia, inborn errors of metabolism, anemia, and so on. Likewise, severe cardiovascular problems may be accompanied by some of these abnormalities.

CARDIAC CATHETERIZATION & ANGIOCARDIOGRAPHY

The definitive anatomic and physiologic study of infants and children with heart disease is cardiac catheterization. It is essential for the primary physician to distinguish those infants and children who require the specialized diagnostic and therapeutic facilities of the pediatric cardiac center from those who may be safely managed without such facilities and consultation. On the basis of the preceding steps of diagnostic evaluation—history, physical examination, ECG, chest x-ray, and other noninvasive laboratory studies—the consulting pediatric cardiologist has a rather precise assessment of the anatomic and physiologic abnormalities in simple malformations and considerable useful information about complex malformations.

Indications & Objectives
A. Infants:
1. Indications–
a. Infants with cyanosis presumed to be cardiovascular in origin should be catheterized as soon as a reasonably stable clinical condition can be achieved. This should be performed for diagnosis of anatomic abnormalities not easily appreciated by echocardiography and for therapeutic interventions such as balloon atrial septostomy or valvuloplasty of a stenotic pulmonary or aortic valve.

b. Infants with severe congestive heart failure that does not respond promptly and satisfactorily to anticongestive measures.

c. Infants in whom early operation for congenital heart disease is contemplated.

d. Infants in whom the anatomic and physiologic abnormality is sufficiently vague that appropriate medical management is not possible.

e. Infants who have evidence of complicating or potentially progressive problems, such as pulmonary hypertension.

2. Objectives–(In descending order of importance.)

a. To perform the study with the lowest possible rate of death or serious complications. Pediatric cardiologists and pediatric cardiac catheterization laboratories with experience in studying infants are required so that these objectives can be met: to gain meaningful information promptly; to care for the critically ill infant with temperature and pH control, fluid management, and all essential pediatric treatment; and to anticipate and handle life-threatening crises.

b. To gain information which is not available by other methods and which will provide the basis for therapeutic decisions (medical or surgical).

c. To provide therapeutic intervention (eg, Rashkind septostomy, balloon valvuloplasty).

d. To obtain sufficient physiologic and anatomic data so that repeat catheterization to complete the study will not be necessary.

B. Children:
1. Indications–
a. All children for whom heart surgery is contemplated (with the exception of children with unequivocal patent ductus arteriosus or atrial septal defect [or both] or other uncomplicated anatomy or physiology).

b. All children in whom there is question about the anatomic or physiologic abnormality which would significantly influence management and which cannot be completely answered by noninvasive methods.

c. Children with progressive lesions that require careful physiologic monitoring (eg, pulmonary hypertension).

d. Children who have had cardiovascular surgery and require assessment of the adequacy of the repair.

e. Children with mild to moderate cardiovascular lesions when important information about the natural history is required. This procedure should be done only in the setting of a well-designed protocol and fully informed consent.

2. Objectives–Conducting the study with the lowest possible risk is the most important objective of cardiac catheterization of the child as well as the infant; and the risk to the child (<0.2%) is certainly much less than the risk to the sick infant (2%). Complete anatomic and physiologic data are important objectives of catheterization in children and infants. No physician or laboratory should undertake the catheterization of a child unless prepared to obtain a completely informative study and unless physicians and surgeons are available who are capable of proceeding with whatever medical or surgical therapy may be indicated.

Contraindications
Cardiac catheterization is contraindicated in infants and children who present with no clinical urgency and none of the indications listed above. It should not be done if personnel and facilities fail to meet high standards of patient safety and clinical diagnostic and therapeutic expertise.

Cardiac Catheterization Data
Figure 19–4 shows oxygen saturation (in percent) and pressure (in mm Hg) values obtained at cardiac catheterization from the chambers and great arteries of the heart. These values would be within the normal range for a child.

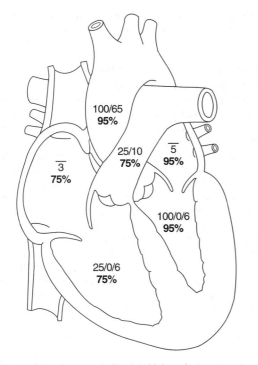

Figure 19–4. Pressures (in mm Hg) and oxygen saturation (in percent) obtained by cardiac catheterization in a healthy child. 3 = mean pressure of 3 mm Hg in the right atrium, 5 = mean pressure of 5 mm Hg in the left atrium.

A. Oxygen Content & Saturation; Pulmonary & Systemic Blood Flow (Cardiac Output): In most laboratories, evidence of left-to-right shunt is determined by changes of blood oxygen content or saturation during passage of the catheter through the right side of the heart. A significant increase in oxygen content or oxygen saturation from one chamber to another indicates the presence of a left-to-right shunt at the site of the increase. The oxygen saturation of the peripheral arterial blood should always be determined during cardiac catheterization. Normal arterial oxygen saturation is 91–97%. A decrease (at sea level) below 91% suggests the presence of a right-to-left shunt, underventilation, or pulmonary disease.

The size of a left-to-right shunt is usually expressed as a ratio of the pulmonary to systemic blood flow or as liters per minute as determined by the Fick principle:

$$\frac{\text{Cardiac output}}{\text{(L/min)}} = \frac{\text{Oxygen consumption (mL/min)}}{\text{Arteriovenous difference (mL/L)}}$$

B. Pressures: Pressures should be determined in all chambers and vessels entered. Pressures should always be recorded when a catheter is pulled back from a distal chamber or vessel into a more proximal chamber. It is not normal for systolic pressure in the ventricles to exceed systolic pressure in the great arteries or mean diastolic pressure in the atria to exceed end-diastolic pressure in the ventricles. If a "gradient" in pressure does exist, it means that there is obstruction, and the severity of the gradient is one criterion for the necessity of operative repair. A right ventricular systolic pressure of 100 mm Hg and a pulmonary artery systolic pressure of 20 mm Hg yield a gradient of 80 mm Hg. In this case, the patient would be classified as having severe pulmonary stenosis requiring repair.

C. Pulmonary & Systemic Vascular Resistance: The vascular resistance is calculated from the following formula and reported in units or in dynes • cm^{-5}/m^2:

$$\text{Resistance} = \frac{\text{Pressure}}{\text{Flow}}$$

Pulmonary vascular resistance equals mean pulmonary artery pressure minus the mean pulmonary artery wedge or left atrial pressure divided by pulmonary blood flow per square meter of body surface area. (Pulmonary blood flow is determined from the Fick principle, as noted previously.) **Systemic vascular resistance** equals mean systemic arterial pressure minus the mean central nervous pressure divided by systemic blood flow.

Normally, the pulmonary vascular resistance ranges from 1 to 3 units, or from 80 to 240 dynes • cm^{-5}/m^2. If pulmonary resistance is above 10 units or the pulmonary/systemic resistance ratio is above 0.7, all other diagnostic findings should be reviewed carefully to confirm the presence of pulmonary hypertension that is so severe as to render the patient inoperable.

D. Special Techniques: Special techniques used during cardiac catheterization include the following:

1. Hydrogen electrode catheter–Used to determine the presence of very small left-to-right shunts, this technique enables the operator to detect such shunts even in the absence of any increase in oxygen saturation.

2. Indicator dilution curves–This involves injection of an indicator, such as indocyanine green (Cardio-Green), at specific places in the heart and detection of the dye downstream, usually in a peripheral artery. This technique permits the detection of both right-to-left and left-to-right shunts at the specific points within the cardiovascular system. Cardiac output is frequently determined by this method.

3. Selective angiocardiography & cineangiocardiography–In this technique, contrast material is injected in a specific chamber or vessel and the course of the contrast material is followed by serial large-film x-rays (angiocardiography) or by motion pictures (cineangiocardiography).

4. Contrast echocardiography–Saline or indocyanine green is rapidly injected via the cardiac catheter, and downstream "clouding" is imaged with either M-mode or two-dimensional echocardiography. Dynamic spatial or structural relationships of chambers, valves, and vessels are visualized; this procedure may be done repetitively without the risk of radiation.

5. Interventional catheterization–Specially designed catheters are now used for dilatation of stenotic valves and vascular structures. Balloon valvuloplasty/angioplasty is now the treatment of choice for valve pulmonary stenosis, coarctation of the thoracic aorta, aortic valve stenosis, and pulmonary arterial stenoses. Other valve and vascular dilating techniques, such as intravascular stents, are now in use along with techniques for closure of patent ductus arteriosus and atrial septal defect (under study). Many simple defects are now treated effectively through these and other procedures.

Bridges ND, Freed MD: Cardiac catheterization, angiocardiography. In: *Moss and Adams Heart Disease in Infants, Children, and Adolescents,* 5th ed. Emmanouilides GC et al (editors). Williams & Wilkins, 1995.

Mullins CE, O'Laughlin MP: Therapeutic cardiac catheterization. In: *Moss and Adams Heart Disease in Infants, Children, and Adolescents,* 5th ed. Emmanouilides GC et al (editors). Williams & Wilkins, 1995.

PRENATAL & NEONATAL CIRCULATION

Fetal Circulation

In the fetus, the placenta is the organ of respiration and for exchange of waste products. Oxygenated blood (approximately 80% saturated) passes from the placenta through the umbilical vein to the heart. As it flows toward the heart, it mixes with blood from the inferior vena cava and the portal vein, so that blood entering the right atrium is approximately 65% saturated. A considerable amount of this blood is shunted immediately across the foramen ovale into the left atrium. The venous blood derived from the upper part of the body is much less saturated (approximately 30%), and most of it enters the right ventricle through the tricuspid valve. Thus, the blood in the right ventricle is a mixture of both relatively highly saturated blood from the umbilical vein and desaturated blood from the venae cavae. This mixture results in a blood oxygen saturation of approximately 50% in the right ventricle.

The blood in the left atrium is derived from the blood shunting across the foramen ovale and the blood returning from the pulmonary veins. A great deal of the left ventricular output goes to the head, whereas the lower portion of the body is supplied by blood both from the right ventricle, through the patent ductus arteriosus, and from the left ventricle.

Physiologic Changes at Birth & in the Neonatal Period

At birth, two dramatic events that affect the cardiovascular and pulmonary system occur: (1) the umbilical cord is clamped, removing the placenta from the circulation; and (2) breathing commences. As a result, marked changes in the circulation occur. During fetal life, the placenta offers little resistance to the flow of blood, so that the systemic circuit is a low-resistance one. On the other hand, the pulmonary arterioles are markedly constricted and offer strong resistance to the flow of blood into the lung. Clamping the cord causes a sudden increase in resistance to flow in the systemic circuit. As the lung becomes the organ of respiration, the oxygen tension (PO_2) increases in the vicinity of the small pulmonary arterioles, resulting in a release of the constriction and thus a significant decrease in the pulmonary arteriolar resistance. Indeed, the pulmonary vascular resistance shortly after birth is less than that of the systemic circuit.

Because of the changes in resistance, most of the right ventricular outflow now passes into the lung rather than through the ductus arteriosus into the descending aorta. In fact, functional closure of the ductus arteriosus begins to develop shortly after birth. Recent studies have demonstrated that the ductus arteriosus remains patent for a variable period, usually 24–48 hours. During the first hour after birth, there is a small right-to-left shunt (as in the fetus). However, after 1 hour, bidirectional shunting occurs, with the left-to-right direction predominating. In most cases, right-to-left shunting completely disappears by 8 hours. However, in patients with severe hypoxia (eg, in respiratory distress syndrome), the pulmonary vascular resistance remains elevated, resulting in a continued right-to-left shunt. The cause of the functional closure of the ductus arteriosus is not completely known. However, evidence indicates that the increased PO_2 of the arterial blood causes spasm of the ductus. Anatomically, however, the ductus arteriosus does not close until approximately age 3 months.

In fetal life, the foramen ovale serves as a one-way valve, permitting shunting of blood from the inferior vena cava through the right atrium into the left atrium. At birth, because of the changes in the pulmonary and systemic vascular resistance and the increase in the quantity of blood returning from the pulmonary veins to the left atrium, the left atrial pressure rises above that of the right atrium. This functionally closes the flap of the one-way valve, essentially preventing flow of blood across the septum. It has been shown, however, that a small right-to-left shunt does continue for the first week of life. Although the foramen ovale remains functionally closed throughout life, it remains patent in about 25% of patients.

A clinical syndrome has been recognized that is characterized in term infants by onset of tachypnea, cyanosis, and clinical evidence of pulmonary hypertension during the first 8 hours after delivery. These infants have massive right-to-left ductal or foramen shunting or both for 3–7 days because of the high pulmonary vascular resistance. The clinical course is generally one of progressive cor pulmonale, hypoxia, and acidosis, terminating in early death unless the pulmonary resistance can be lowered. The resistance can usually be reversed by instituting appropriate means to increase alveolar PO_2: high-frequency, low tidal volume hyperventilation (to produce respiratory alkalosis) and intravenous administration of vasoactive drugs. Recently, extracorporeal membrane oxygenation (ECMO) and inhaled nitric oxide have shown promise in selected cases. At postmortem, the findings include increased thickness of the pulmonary arteriolar media, which is believed to represent persistence of the fetal circulation.

Changes in the First Year of Life

The most significant changes occur at birth and within the neonatal period. However, pulmonary vascular resistance and the pulmonary arterial pressure continue to fall during the first year of life. This phenomenon results from the involution of the pulmonary arteriole from a relatively thick-walled, small-lumen vessel to a thin-walled, large-lumen vessel. Adult levels of resistance and pressure are usually achieved by age 6 months to 1 year.

Heymann MA: Fetal and postnatal circulation: Pulmonary circulation. In: *Moss and Adams Heart Disease in Infants, Children, and Adolescents,* 5th ed. Emmanouilides GC et al (editors). Williams & Wilkins, 1995.

Kanto WP: A decade of experience with neonatal extracorporeal membrane oxygenation. J Pediatr 1994;124:335.

Kinsella JP et al: Clinical responses to prolonged treatment of persistent pulmonary hypertension of the newborn with low doses of inhaled nitric oxide. J Pediatr 1993; 123:103.

MAJOR CLUES TO HEART DISEASE IN INFANTS & CHILDREN

CONGESTIVE HEART FAILURE

Congestive heart failure at the clinical level is the failure of the heart to meet the circulatory and metabolic needs of the body. Congestive heart failure is one of the two major clues to the presence of impor-

tant heart disease. (The other is cyanosis; see later in chapter.) It has been estimated that congestive heart failure begins before age 1 year in over 90% of infants and children who ever develop the disorder in the pediatric age period—and most of these patients are less than 6 months of age.

Congestive heart failure beginning in infancy may persist throughout childhood until operation relieves the underlying malformation (unless surgery is not possible). Other infants with moderately severe heart failure in the first few months of life may gradually compensate (for a variety of reasons) and not require medical intervention after age 12 or 18 months even though their congenital heart lesions are still unrepaired.

Clinical Findings

The three cardinal signs of congestive heart failure in the pediatric patient are cardiomegaly (the sine qua non), tachypnea (left side), and hepatomegaly (right side).

Cardiomegaly represents a homeostatic (compensatory) mechanism that maintains adequate cardiac output by enlarging the capacity of the pump. This mechanism is frequently referred to as Starling's law of the heart. Up to a point, the enlarging heart can deliver a greater stroke volume output, but limits are soon reached (the descending limb of Starling's curve). Figure 19–5 shows a family of ventricular performance curves. The curve at the right depicts a damaged myocardium; the curve in the center, a normal myocardium; and the curve at the left, a myocardium under inotropic stimulation. One should be very cautious about the diagnosis of congestive heart failure in the absence of an enlarged heart (an exception being a condition such as total anomalous ve-

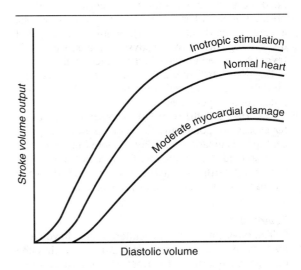

Figure 19–5. Ventricular performance curves.

nous return below the diaphragm, which will, for a short period of time, be characterized by other signs of congestive heart failure without an enlarged heart). Cardiomegaly without other signs of congestive failure may well be taken as early or homeostatically compensated congestive heart failure.

Tachypnea may be considered the cardinal sign of left-sided heart failure. It may be present for a short time before hepatomegaly occurs, although pure left-sided or pure right-sided heart failure does not commonly exist independently for long.

Hepatomegaly is the cardinal sign of right-sided heart failure. The liver is capable of trapping relatively large amounts of edema fluid in the infant that would be more evident as peripheral edema in the older child and adult. It is therefore common rather than unusual for the infant in moderately severe heart failure to have an enlarged liver with no pretibial or even presacral or facial edema. Peripheral edema is found in infants only in the most severe cases of congestive heart failure.

Additional signs and symptoms of congestive heart failure are feeding difficulties, dyspnea, restlessness, easy fatigability, weak pulses, pallor, rales, peripheral edema, weight gain from fluid accumulation, tachycardia, sweating, pneumonia, orthopnea, and growth failure.

Underlying Causes of Heart Failure in the Pediatric Age Group

By far the most common cause of congestive heart failure in the pediatric patient is congenital heart disease. Causes in infancy and childhood appear in the outline below:

A. Heart Failure in Infancy:

1. Cardiovascular causes–Congenital heart disease (producing volume overload, outflow obstruction, myocardial impairment), congenital vascular disease (eg, coarctation of the aorta, an outflow obstruction disorder; peripheral arteriovenous shunts, a volume overload disorder), acquired myocardial disease (eg, myocarditis), dysrhythmias, rheumatic fever (very rare in infants in the United States).

2. Noncardiovascular causes–Acidosis, respiratory disease, central nervous system disease, anemia, sepsis, hypoglycemia.

B. Heart Failure in Childhood: Cardiovascular causes are potentially the same as in infancy except that rheumatic fever plays a more important role in childhood. Noncardiovascular causes become less important with increasing age—especially such mechanisms as acidosis and hypoglycemia.

Treatment

The physician caring for children must have facility with routine measures and familiarity with some emergency measures for treating congestive heart failure.

A. Routine Measures:

1. Digitalis–Digitalis is the keystone of the treatment of congestive heart failure. The desired effect is improvement in myocardial performance (inotropic effect), shifting the patient to a more efficient ventricular performance in the family of curves shown in Figure 19–5. The preparation most widely used in pediatrics is digoxin, which may be administered (in order of rapidity of onset of effect) intravenously, intramuscularly, or orally. The clinical urgency of the individual case dictates how quickly digitalization should be accomplished. Although there are general guidelines, the ultimate dosage (on a milligram-per-kilogram basis) must be individualized for each patient.

a. Protocols for digitalization–

(1) In hospital–

Age	Parenteral	Oral
Premature	0.035 mg/kg	0.04 mg/kg
1 wk to 2 y	0.05 mg/kg	0.07 mg/kg
<2 wk or >2 y	0.04 mg/kg	0.06 mg/kg

Use of the elixir (0.05 mg/mL) is advisable even in older children because the bioavailability of the tablet preparations is unreliable.

The routine schedule consists of giving one-quarter of the digitalizing dose intramuscularly or orally every 6 hours for four doses. For rapid digitalization, give half the digitalizing dose intravenously or intramuscularly and repeat in 4–6 hours. For very rapid digitalization, give the full digitalizing dose intravenously with very close monitoring. For maintenance, give one-quarter to one-third of the oral digitalizing dose daily (divided into morning and evening doses).

(2) Digitalization of outpatients–Give the maintenance dose of digoxin (see above) divided into morning and evening doses. In less than 1 week, adequate digitalization is obtained without running the risk of a parent's inadvertently failing to revert to a maintenance dosage schedule and continuing a high digitalizing dose to the point of toxicity (even death).

b. Digitalis toxicity–Slowing of the heart rate below 100 in infants, below 80 in young children, and below 60 in older children is often taken as a guide to reducing the dosage of digoxin. Any dysrhythmia that occurs during digitalis therapy should be attributed to the drug until proved otherwise, although ventricular bigeminy and various degrees of atrioventricular block are characteristic of digitalis toxicity. Age-specific serum levels suggestive of toxicity during maintenance therapy are as follows: newborn, over 4 ng/mL; 1 month to 1 year, over 3 ng/mL; after 1 year, over 2 ng/mL.

c. Digitalis poisoning–*This is an acute emergency that must be treated without delay. The sooner* the stomach is emptied, the better the prognosis, but even if many hours have passed, the stomach should still be emptied. Attention must then be paid to maintaining an adequate cardiac rate and output and to controlling the dysrhythmia. A useful basic intravenous solution is 10% glucose in water to which KCl (3 meq/kg/d) and regular insulin (20 U/1000 mL) have been added. KCl must be used with caution in patients with electrocardiographic high-grade block. It should be given in amounts not to exceed the maintenance requirement per 24 hours for the weight or surface area of the patient. To this solution may be added isoproterenol (in the calibrated administration set) titrated in quantities appropriate to maintain adequate heart rate and output in the face of complete heart block. Phenytoin may be administered through the intravenous tubing to treat arrhythmias by beginning with a 1-mg/kg slow intravenous push followed every 5–10 minutes with doubling doses to a maximum total combined dose of 15 mg/kg. In severe cases, digoxin immune Fab (ovine) dosage is determined by total body load (TBL) of digoxin:

$$IV\ TBL = C\ (ng/mL) \times 5.6 \times body\ weight\ (kg)/1000$$
or
$$TBL = mg\ of\ digoxin\ ingested \times 0.8$$

where C = the postdistribution digoxin concentration (serum digoxin level). The dose of digoxin immune Fab (in mg) = TBL × 66.7. Fab is infused over 15–20 minutes. If this agent is not available, a temporary transvenous pacemaker may be required to control arrhythmias.

2. Diuretics–If digitalis alone is inadequate to achieve satisfactory compensation, diuretics may be required. For rapid inpatient diuresis, give furosemide intravenously or intramuscularly; for maintenance therapy, give thiazides or furosemide orally daily along with spironolactone.

The dosages are as follows:

a. Furosemide–
(1) Intravenously or intramuscularly, 1 mg/kg per dose, given two or three times daily while monitored in the hospital; monitor electrolytes.
(2) Orally, 2–5 mg/kg/d.
b. Thiazides–These drugs should be given daily with spironolactone (which helps to prevent excessive potassium loss). Do not give daily for prolonged periods unless spironolactone is being given also and serum electrolytes are being monitored periodically.
(1) Chlorothiazide suspension (250 mg/tsp), 20 mg/kg/d.
(2) Hydrochlorothiazide tablets, 2 mg/kg/d.
c. Spironolactone–Give 2–4 mg/kg/d in two divided doses.
3. Rest and sedation–The decompensated and mildly distressed patient requires rest; the severely distressed and anxious infant or child requires seda-

tion. Parenteral morphine, 0.1 mg/kg, is useful for sedation as well as for control of acute pulmonary edema, but it should be given only with good airway control.

4. Oxygen–Oxygen will not make a patient with cyanotic heart disease pink, but it will raise the systemic PaO_2 in patients with severe congestive heart failure, overcoming the capillary-alveolar block of pulmonary edema and alleviating the hypoxemic contribution to congestive failure.

5. Salt restriction–Salt restriction must be approached with caution in infants and children. Treatment of the disease entity known as low-salt congestive heart failure is one of the more hazardous undertakings in medical management. Our feeling is that there is no place for salt-free formulas in the treatment of congestive failure in infants. Standard SMA or Similac 60/40 has about the same sodium content as human milk and about half the sodium content of cow's milk and other prepared formulas. Most cases of "low-salt failure" are largely the result of overly vigorous salt restriction (sometimes combined with the other major factor, overly vigorous diuretic therapy). Clearly, salty foods such as potato chips and bacon should be avoided, and no salt should be used beyond what is normally used in cooking. It is important that food be palatable enough to eat for a child, who may already be undernourished as a consequence of chronic, poorly compensated heart failure.

B. Emergency & Heroic Measures: The acute emergencies of congestive heart failure are usually related to fluid retention with pulmonary edema and low cardiac output. Some emergency therapeutic measures that may be lifesaving include the following:

1. Morphine–For acute pulmonary edema, give 0.1 mg/kg intravenously or subcutaneously.
2. Diuretics–Furosemide or ethacrynic acid may be given intravenously in an initial dosage of 1 mg/kg to produce a rapid diuresis.
3. Positive-pressure breathing–Pulmonary edema may sometimes be managed by intubation or mask with bag-breathing or a respirator to raise the alveolar pressure above pulmonary capillary pressure.
4. Peritoneal dialysis–Although furosemide has largely met the need for the extremely rapid relief of fluid retention, there are three specific instances in which peritoneal dialysis with a hypertonic solution may be indicated: (1) when fluid retention (especially pulmonary edema) is life-threatening and diuretics are unsuccessful; (2) in low-salt congestive heart failure when both the fluid retention and the electrolyte imbalance require correction; and (3) in the early postoperative care of an infant who may have transient renal failure with both fluid retention and hyperkalemia.

The advantages of hypertonic peritoneal dialysis

are that the procedure promptly (within minutes) draws fluid into the peritoneal cavity, where it is subject to immediate removal, while simultaneously correcting the electrolyte imbalance, whether it is low-sodium, high-potassium, or both. For methods of dialysis, see Chapter 22. If the major problem is electrolyte imbalance, such as potassium retention, a hypertonic solution is not required and the usual "isotonic" dialyzing fluid is indicated.

5. Intravenous inotropic support–Use of agents such as dopamine (1–20 μg/kg/min), dobutamine (2–15 μg/kg/min), isoproterenol (0.1–1 μg/kg/min), and amrinone (0.75 mg/kg bolus then 5–10 μg/kg/min) may help in stabilizing patients with severe myocardial dysfunction, hypotension, or low cardiac output. These agents can be lifesaving in myocarditis and cardiogenic shock.

6. Afterload reduction–A relatively new form of therapy for "pump" failure is to effect afterload reduction by decreasing systemic vascular resistance with an intravenous infusion of vasodilators. Experience in children is limited. The procedure has been used largely in postoperative patients with reduced cardiac output and peripheral vasoconstriction. Agents such as nitroprusside have been lifesaving but must be used in a setting where central venous pressure, arterial pressure, cardiac output, and so on, can be carefully monitored.

Latson L: Captopril in children with cardiomyopathies. Circulation 1991;83:707.
Padbury JF et al: Dopamine pharmacokinetics in newborn infants. J Pediatrics 1990;117:472.
Wernovsky G, Chang AC, Wessel DL: Intensive care. In: *Moss and Adams Heart Disease in Infants, Children, and Adolescents,* 5th ed. Emmanouilides GC et al (editors). Williams & Wilkins, 1995.

CYANOSIS

One of the two major clues to the presence of heart disease in the infant and child is cyanosis. (The other is congestive heart failure; see previous section.)

Cyanosis represents an increased concentration (4–5 g/dL) of reduced hemoglobin in the blood. Bluish discoloration is usually, but not always, a sign. Patients with anemia and cyanosis may not appear blue; patients with polycythemia may appear cyanotic, even though inadequate blood oxygen content is not present. Visible cyanosis accompanies low cardiac output, hypothermia, and systemic venous congestion, even in the presence of adequate oxygenation.

In patients with true central cyanosis, the cause of cyanosis (cardiac, pulmonary, hematologic, or central nervous system disorder) must be determined. Most often, the physician is faced with differentiat-ing between cardiac and pulmonary problems. Evaluation of arterial blood gases (see above) is one of the easiest ways to differentiate between lung and heart disease. Cyanosis in heart disease is also related to pulmonary blood flow. In some "cyanotic" congenital heart defects, the decrease in pulmonary blood flow is minimal and results in minimal cyanosis. Presence of pulmonary hypertension also influences pulmonary blood flow, and thus oxygen therapy may cause a partial increase in oxygen saturation; the increase is usually much less in patients with heart disease than in those with pulmonary disease.

Evaluation for methemoglobinemia may be necessary to rule out hematologic causes of cyanosis. If the cause of cyanosis is a disease of the central nervous system, the patient usually responds to oxygen therapy.

Cyanotic heart disease is usually a medical emergency, most often requiring palliative or corrective surgery.

CONGENITAL HEART DISEASE

Congenital heart disease is present in about 1% of studied North American and British populations, making this the most common category of congenital structural malformation. Curative or palliative surgical correction is now available for over 90% of patients with congenital heart disease.

The customary division of congenital heart diseases into noncyanotic and cyanotic types is useful if one understands the basis for it. By convention, patients with right-to-left shunts fall into the cyanotic category whether they have readily recognizable cyanosis or not; patients who do not have right-to-left shunts—even if they are cyanotic for other reasons, such as low cardiac output—are placed in the noncyanotic category.

Etiologic Considerations

Only 8% of all congenital heart defects are known to be associated with single mutant gene or chromosome abnormalities, and the remainder are the result of various other causes. Multiple environmental factors, including diabetes, alcohol consumption, progesterone use, certain viruses, and other teratogens, are now associated with an increased incidence of malformations. These factors probably represent environmental triggers in persons susceptible or predisposed to congenital heart defects. The effect of rubella virus is probably independent of hereditary factors and consequently predisposes the patient to patent ductus arteriosus and pulmonary artery branch stenosis. Acquired heart diseases, such as rheumatic fever, appear to have much stronger environmental influence. Atherosclerosis clearly can have distinct familial patterns but in some circumstances can be influenced by diet, drugs, or lifestyle.

In dealing with families of children with congenital heart disease, the physician must often answer the question of risk to future pregnancies. Table 19–2 outlines the risk for certain lesions in patients with one affected first-degree relative. Studies indicate that the incidence in children of affected mothers may be as high as 10–15%. With more than one affected first- degree relative, recurrence is also much higher, and some families may have a hereditary predisposition to congenital heart disease.

Ferencz C, Villasenor AC: Epidemiology of cardiovascular malformations: The state of the art. Cardiol Young 1991; 1:264.

Nora JJ, Nora AH: Maternal transmission of congenital heart disease: New recurrence risk figures and the questions of cytoplasmic inheritance and vulnerability to teratogens. Am J Cardiol 1987;59:459.

Table 19–2. Observed and expected recurrence risks in siblings of 1478 probands with congenital heart lesion.[1]

Anomaly	Probands	Affected Siblings		
		No.	Percent	Exp. ($\sqrt{p}$)
Ventricular septal defect	212	24/543	4.4	5.0
Patent ductus arteriosus	204	17/505	3.4	3.5
Tetralogy of Fallot	157	9/338	2.7	3.2
Atrial septal defect	152	11/342	3.2	3.2
Pulmonary stenosis	146	10/345	2.9	2.9
Aortic stenosis	135	7/317	2.2	2.1
Coarctation of aorta	128	5/272	1.8	2.4
Transpositions of great vessels	103	4/209	1.9	2.2
Atrioventricular canal	73	4/151	2.6	2.0
Tricuspid atresia	51	1/96	1.1	1.4
Ebstein's anomaly	42	1/96	1.1	0.7
Truncus arteriosus	41	1/86	1.2	0.7
Pulmonary atresia	34	1/77	1.3	1.0
Total	1478	95/3377		

[1]Reproduced, with permission, from Nora JJ: Etiologic factors in congenital heart disease. Pediatr Clin North Am 1971;18:1059.

NONCYANOTIC HEART DISEASE

ATRIAL SEPTAL DEFECT OF THE OSTIUM SECUNDUM VARIETY

Essentials of Diagnosis

- S_2 widely split and usually fixed.
- Grade I–III/VI ejection systolic murmur at the pulmonary area.
- Widely radiating systolic murmur mimicking peripheral pulmonary artery stenosis (common in infancy).
- Diastolic flow murmur at the lower left sternal border (if the shunt is significant in size).
- ECG with rsR' in lead V_1.

General Considerations

An atrial septal defect is an opening in the atrial septum permitting the shunting of blood between the two atria. There are three major types: (1) The ostium secundum type (discussed here) is the most common and is in an intermediate position. (2) The sinus venosus type is positioned high in the atrial septum, is the least common, and is frequently associated with partial anomalous venous return. (3) The ostium primum type is low in position and is a form of atrioventricular septal defect; it is discussed in that section.

Atrial septal defect of the ostium secundum variety occurs in approximately 10% of patients with congenital heart disease and is twice as common in

females as in males. Diagnosis in infancy is becoming more common.

Pulmonary hypertension and growth failure are increasingly recognized in infancy and childhood. After the third decade, an increased pulmonary vascular resistance develops, the left-to-right shunting decreases, and right-to-left shunting begins.

Clinical Findings

A. Symptoms & Signs: Infants may present with congestive heart failure often unresponsive to medical management, necessitating early total corrective surgery. However, children with atrial septal defects often have no cardiovascular symptoms. Some patients remain asymptomatic throughout life; others develop easy fatigability as older children or adults. Cyanosis does not occur until pulmonary hypertension develops. This may never occur; if it does, it is not seen until after the third decade of life. Congestive heart failure is uncommon in infants and young children.

The arterial pulses are normal and equal throughout. In the usual case, the heart is hyperactive, with a heaving impulse felt best at the lower left sternal border and over the xiphoid process. There are usually no thrills. S_2 at the pulmonary area is widely split and sometimes fixed. The pulmonary component is normal in intensity. A grade I–III/VI ejection-type systolic murmur is heard best at the left sternal border in the second intercostal space. An additional murmur of relative peripheral pulmonary artery stenosis may be heard, more commonly in infants. A mid-diastolic murmur can often be heard in the fourth intercostal space at the left sternal border. This murmur is caused by increased blood flow across the tricuspid valve during diastole (tricuspid flow murmur). The presence of this murmur suggests a high flow (pulmonary to systemic blood flow ratio greater than 2:1).

B. Imaging: Chest x-ray films usually demonstrate cardiac enlargement. The main pulmonary artery may be dilated. The pulmonary vascular markings are increased as a result of increased pulmonary blood flow.

C. Electrocardiography & Vectorcardiography: The usual ECG shows right axis deviation with a clockwise loop in the frontal plane. In the right precordial leads, there is usually an rsR' pattern.

D. Echocardiography: M-mode echocardiography shows (1) paradoxic motion of the ventricular septal wall (moving in the same direction rather than the direction opposite that of the free left ventricular wall) and (2) dilated right ventricular cavity with increased tricuspid valve excursion. Direct visualization of the atrial septal defect by two-dimensional echocardiography, plus demonstration of a left-to-right shunt through the defect by color flow Doppler, confirms the diagnosis and may eliminate the need for cardiac catheterization.

E. Cardiac Catheterization: Oximetry reveals evidence of a significant increase in oxygen saturation at the atrial level. The pulmonary artery pressure is usually normal. The right ventricular pressure is occasionally greater than the pulmonary artery pressure, the increased right-sided "flow." Pulmonary vascular resistance is usually normal. The ratio of pulmonary to systemic blood flow may vary from 1.5:1 to 4:1. A catheter can easily be passed across the atrial septum into the left atrium.

Treatment

Surgical closure is generally recommended for ostium secundum–type atrial septal defects in which the ratio of pulmonary to systemic blood flow is greater than 2:1. Operation is usually performed electively in patients between ages 2 and 4 years. The death rate for surgical closure is less than 1%. When surgical intervention is early, late complications of right ventricular dysfunction and significant dysrhythmias may be avoided or diminished. Early surgery is also indicated in infants presenting with congestive heart failure or significant pulmonary hypertension. Double-umbrella closure devices to close selected atrial septal defects by interventional cardiac catheterization are in clinical trials.

Course & Prognosis

Patients with atrial septal defects usually tolerate them very well in the first 2 decades of life, and an occasional patient may live a completely normal life without symptoms. Frequently, however, pulmonary hypertension and reversal of the shunt develop by the third or fourth decade. Heart failure may also occur at this time. Subacute infective endocarditis is a very rare complication. Spontaneous closure occurs and is sometimes associated with an aneurysm of the atrial septum. Exercise tolerance and oxygen consumption in surgically corrected children are generally normal, and physical limitations are unnecessary.

Ettedgui J et al: Diagnostic echocardiographic features of the sinus venosus defect. Br Heart J 1990;64:329.

Fukazawa M, Fukushige J, Ueda K: Atrial septal defects in neonates with reference to spontaneous closure. Am Heart J 1988;116:123.

Mahoney LT et al: Atrial septal defects that present in infancy. Am J Dis Child 1986;140:1115.

Pollick C et al: Doppler color flow imaging assessment of shunt size in atrial septal defect. Circulation 1987;78:522.

Reybrouck T et al: Cardiorespiratory exercise capacity after surgical closure of atrial septal defect is influenced by the age at surgery. Am Heart J 1991;122:1073.

Rome JJ et al: Double umbrella closure of atrial defects. Circulation 1990;82:751.

VENTRICULAR SEPTAL DEFECTS

Essentials of Diagnosis

Small- to moderate-sized left-to-right shunt without pulmonary hypertension:
- Acyanotic, relatively asymptomatic.
- Grade II–IV/VI pansystolic murmur, maximal along the lower left sternal border.
- P_2 not accentuated.

Large left-to-right shunt:
- Acyanotic.
- Easy fatigability.
- Congestive heart failure in infancy (often).
- Hyperactive heart; biventricular enlargement.
- Grade II–V/VI pansystolic murmur, maximal at the lower left sternal border.
- P_2 usually accentuated.
- Diastolic flow murmur at the apex.

Insignificant left-to-right shunt or bidirectional shunt with pulmonary hypertension:
- Quiet precordium with right ventricular lift.
- Palpable P_2.
- Short ejection systolic murmur along the left sternal border; single accentuated S_2.
- Systemic arterial oxygen desaturation may be present; pulmonary arterial pressure and systemic arterial pressures are equal; little or no oxygen saturation increase at the right ventricular level by catheterization.

General Considerations

Simple ventricular septal defect (without other lesions) is the single most common congenital heart malformation, accounting for about 25% of all cases of congenital heart disease. Defects in the ventricular septum can occur both in the membranous portion of the septum (most common) and in the muscular portion.

There are five different courses that patients with ventricular septal defect may follow:

A. Spontaneous Closure: Thirty percent to 50% of all ventricular septal defects close spontaneously. The small defects close in 60–70% of cases. Larger defects may occasionally also close spontaneously, and there are many documented examples of spontaneous closure of ventricular septal defects in the second and third decades of life. Half of the defects that do not close become functionally or anatomically smaller.

B. Shunts Too Small to Justify Repair: Asymptomatic patients with hearts normal in size (as seen on x-ray film) and without pulmonary hypertension are generally not subjected to surgical repair. In those who have had cardiac catheterization, the ratio of pulmonary to systemic blood flow is usually found to be less than 2:1, and serial cardiac catheterizations demonstrate that the shunts get progressively smaller.

C. Disease Severe Enough to Require Surgery: The time of surgery depends on the nature of the disease. Patients may require surgery in infancy because of intractable congestive heart failure; surgery before 2 years of age because of progression of pulmonary hypertension; or surgery between 2 and 5 years of age as an elective procedure.

D. Defect Inoperable Because of Pulmonary Hypertension: The vast majority of patients with inoperable pulmonary hypertension develop this condition progressively. The combined data of the multicenter National History Study indicate that most cases of irreversible pulmonary hypertension can be prevented by surgical repair of the defect before 2 years of age.

E. Development of Infundibular Pulmonary Stenosis: Approximately 5% of infants with large left-to-right shunts will develop progressive infundibular obstruction effecting an outflow gradient and diminution of the shunt. A small proportion of these infants have precyanotic tetralogy of Fallot, as evidenced by coexistent right aortic arch or abnormal spatial orientation of the infundibulum.

Clinical Findings

A. Symptoms & Signs: Patients with small or moderate left-to-right shunts usually have no cardiovascular symptoms. There may be a history of frequent respiratory infections in infancy and early childhood. Patients with large left-to-right shunts frequently are sick early in infancy. Such patients have frequent respiratory infections, including bouts of pneumonitis. They grow slowly, with very poor weight gain. Dyspnea, exercise intolerance, and fatigue are quite common. Congestive heart failure may develop between 1 and 6 months of age. Pa-

tients who survive the first year usually improve, although easy fatigability may persist. With severe pulmonary hypertension (Eisenmenger's syndrome), cyanosis is present.

1. Small left-to-right shunt–There are usually no lifts, heaves, thrills, or shocks. The first sound at the apex is normal, and the second sound at the pulmonary area is split physiologically. The pulmonary component is normal. A grade II–IV/VI, medium- to high-pitched, blowing pansystolic murmur is heard best at the left sternal border in the third and fourth intercostal spaces. There is slight radiation over the entire precordium. No diastolic murmurs are heard.

2. Moderate left-to-right shunt–Slight prominence of the precordium is common. There is a moderate left ventricular thrust. A systolic thrill may be palpable at the lower left sternal border between the third and fourth intercostal spaces. The second sound at the pulmonary area is most often split but may be single. A grade IV/VI, harsh pansystolic murmur is heard best at the lower left sternal border in the fourth intercostal space. A diastolic flow murmur is heard and indicates that the pulmonary venous return across the mitral valve is large and that the pulmonary to systemic blood flow ratio is at least 2:1.

3. Very large ventricular septal defects with pulmonary hypertension–The precordium is prominent, and the sternum bulges. A left ventricular thrust and a right ventricular heave are palpable. A shock of the second sound can be felt at the pulmonary area. A thrill may or may not be present at the lower left sternal border. A second heart sound is usually single or narrowly split, with accentuation of the pulmonary component. The murmur ranges from grade II to grade V/VI and is usually harsh and pansystolic. Occasionally, when the defect is large, very little murmur can be heard. A diastolic flow murmur may or may not be heard, depending on the size of the shunt.

B. Imaging: X-ray findings of the chest vary, depending on the size of the shunt. In patients with small shunts, x-ray findings may be normal. The heart is normal in size, and the pulmonary vascular markings may be just beyond the upper limits of normal. Patients with large shunts usually show significant cardiac enlargement involving both the left and right ventricles and the left atrium. The aorta is usually small to normal in size, and the main pulmonary artery segment is dilated. The pulmonary vascular markings are significantly increased in patients with large shunts.

C. Electrocardiography: There is some correlation between the electrocardiographic and hemodynamic findings. The ECG is normal in patients with small left-to-right shunts and normal pulmonary arterial pressures. Left ventricular hypertrophy is usually found in patients with large left-to-right shunts and normal pulmonary vascular resistance. Combined ventricular hypertrophy (both right and left) is found in patients with pulmonary hypertension caused by increased flow, increased resistance, or both. Pure right ventricular hypertrophy is found in patients with pulmonary hypertension secondary to pulmonary vascular obstruction.

D. Echocardiography: Two-dimensional echocardiography provides visualization of defects that are 4 mm or larger in about 65–75% of cases and often can pinpoint the anatomic location. Addition of color flow Doppler, however, allows detection of virtually all defects, including the smaller defects.

E. Cardiac Catheterization & Angiocardiography: Oxygen saturation is increased at the right ventricular level. The pulmonary artery pressure may vary from normal to that in the systemic arteries. Left atrial pressure (pulmonary capillary pressure) may be normal to increased. Pulmonary vascular resistance varies from normal to markedly increased. The ratio of pulmonary to systemic blood flow may vary from 1.1:1 to 4:1. Hydrogen electrode curves and dye dilution curves may indicate a shunt at the ventricular level. Angiocardiographic examination defines the number, size, and location of the defects.

Treatment

A. Medical Management: Patients who develop congestive heart failure should be treated vigorously with anticongestive measures (see Congestive Heart Failure, above). If the patient does not respond to vigorous anticongestive measures or shows signs of progressive pulmonary hypertension, surgery is indicated without delay. Transcatheter closure of ventricular septal defects is being evaluated as an experimental procedure.

B. Surgical Treatment: The age for elective surgery is becoming progressively younger in most centers (range, <2 years to 5 years). Patients with cardiomegaly, poor growth, poor exercise tolerance, or other clinical abnormalities who have cardiac catheterization findings of significant shunt (≥2:1) without significant pulmonary hypertension (>10 units of resistance) are candidates for surgery. In general, patients with mean pulmonary artery pressures equal to systemic pressure who are unresponsive to oxygen administration, with little or no left-to-right shunt or bidirectional shunting, and pulmonary resistance calculated to be greater than 10 resistance units (or pulmonary/systemic resistance ratios >0.7) are considered inoperable. There are patients who have pulmonary hypertension of lesser degree who remain operable, but there is a progressively greater risk with increasing pulmonary hypertension (from 1% risk for patients without pulmonary hypertension to 25% for those at the upper limits of operability).

To prevent pulmonary hypertension from reaching inoperable levels, early surgical intervention is recommended for patients who have increased pulmonary vascular resistance. In centers with the capability of doing total correction on infants with or without deep hypothermia, complete repair before 2 years of age is recommended. The presence of multiple muscular defects in a tiny symptomatic infant is still considered to be an indication for pulmonary artery banding as an initial palliative procedure. Transcatheter closure of selected defects is in clinical trials.

Course & Prognosis

Significant late dysrhythmias are uncommon. Functional exercise capacity and oxygen consumption are usually normal, and physical restrictions are unnecessary. Adults with corrected defects have a normal quality of life. Definite congenital heart disease occurred in approximately 3% of probands of male and female patients with ventricular septal defect.

Driscoll DJ et al: Occurrence risk for congenital heart disease in relatives of patients with aortic stenosis, pulmonary stenosis, or ventricular septal defect. Circulation 1993;87(Suppl):I-121.

Hornberger LK et al: Elucidation of the natural history of ventricular septal defects by serial Doppler color flow mapping studies. J Am Coll Cardiol 1989;13:1111.

Lock JE et al: Transcatheter closure of ventricular septal defects. Circulation 1988;78:361.

Mehta AV et al: Ventricular septal defect in the first year of life. Am J Cardiol 1992;70:364.

Soto B, Ceballos R, Kirklen JW: Ventricular septal defects: A surgical viewpoint. J Am Coll Cardiol 1989;14:1291.

ATRIOVENTRICULAR SEPTAL DEFECT

Essentials of Diagnosis

- Murmur often inaudible in neonates.
- Loud pulmonary component of S_2.
- Common in infants with Down's syndrome.
- ECG with left axis deviation.

General Considerations

An atrioventricular septal defect is a congenital cardiac abnormality that results from incomplete fusion of the embryonic endocardial cushions. The endocardial cushions help to form the lower portion of the atrial septum, the membranous portion of the ventricular septum, and the septal leaflets of the tricuspid and mitral valves. These defects are not very common. They account for about 4% of all cases of congenital heart disease. The incidence of this abnormality is 20% in patients with Down syndrome.

Atrioventricular septal defects may be divided into incomplete and complete forms. The complete form, also known as persistent common atrioventricular canal, consists of a high ventricular septal defect, a low atrial septal defect of the ostium primum variety that is continuous with the ventricular septal defect, and a cleft in both the septal leaflet of the tricuspid valve and the anterior leaflet of the mitral valve. In the incomplete form, any one of these components may be present. The most common partial form of atrioventricular septal defect is the ostium primum type of atrial septal defect with a cleft in the mitral valve.

The complete form (persistent common atrioventricular canal) results in large left-to-right shunts at both the ventricular and atrial levels, tricuspid and mitral regurgitation, and marked pulmonary hypertension, usually with some increase in pulmonary vascular resistance. When the latter is present, the shunts may be bidirectional. The hemodynamics in the incomplete form are dependent on the lesions present.

Clinical Findings

A. Symptoms & Signs: The clinical picture varies depending on the severity of the defect. In the incomplete form, these patients may be indistinguishable from patients with the ostium secundum type of atrial septal defect. They are often asymptomatic. On the other hand, patients with atrioventricular canal usually are severely affected. Congestive heart failure often develops in infancy, and recurrent bouts of pneumonitis are common.

In the complete form, the murmur may be inaudible in the neonate. After 4–6 weeks, a nonspecific systolic murmur develops; the murmur is usually not as harsh as that of an isolated ventricular septal defect. The heart is significantly enlarged (both the right and left sides), and a systolic thrill may be palpated at the lower left sternal border. The second heart sound is split, with an accentuated pulmonary component. A pronounced diastolic flow murmur may be heard at the apex and the lower left sternal border.

When severe pulmonary vascular obstruction is present, there is evidence of dominant right ventricular enlargement. A shock of the second sound can be palpated at the pulmonary area. No thrill is felt. The second sound is markedly accentuated and single. A nonspecific short systolic murmur is heard at the lower left sternal border. No diastolic flow murmurs are heard. Cyanosis is detectable in severe cases with predominant right-to-left shunts.

The physical findings in the incomplete form depend on the lesions. In the most common variety (ostium primum atrial septal defect with mitral regurgitation), the findings are similar to those of the ostium secundum type of atrial septal defect with or without findings of mitral regurgitation.

B. Imaging: As indicated on x-ray film, cardiac enlargement is present depending on the degree of specific anatomic defect and the severity. In the complete (canal) form, there is enlargement of all four chambers. The pulmonary vascular markings are increased. In patients with pulmonary vascular obstruc-

tion, only the main pulmonary artery segment and its branches are prominent. The peripheral markings are usually decreased.

C. Electrocardiography: In all forms of atrioventricular septal defect, left axis deviation with a counterclockwise loop in the frontal plane is present. The mean axis varies from approximately −30 to −90 degrees. Since left axis deviation is present in all patients with this defect, the ECG is a very important diagnostic tool. First-degree heart block is present in over 50% of cases. Right, left, or combined ventricular hypertrophy is present depending on the particular type of defect and the presence or absence of pulmonary vascular obstruction.

D. Echocardiography: Echocardiography is the diagnostic technique of choice. On M-mode echocardiography, excursion of the atrioventricular valve through the plane of the interventricular septal defect is characteristic. The anatomy can be directly visualized by two-dimensional echocardiography; the sensitivity of this method is equal to that of selective cineangiography. Color flow mapping can indicate the location of septal defects and valve regurgitation.

E. Cardiac Catheterization & Angiocardiography: The results of cardiac catheterization vary depending on the type of defect present. When catheterization is performed from the leg, the catheter is easily passed across the atrial septum in its lowest portion and frequently enters the left ventricle directly. This catheter course is a result of the very low atrial septal defect and the cleft in the mitral valve. Increased oxygen saturation in the right ventricle or the right atrium identifies the level of the shunt. Angiocardiography reveals a characteristic "gooseneck" deformity in the complete canal form. Two-dimensional Doppler color flow echocardiography is extremely useful in identifying the subgroups of endocardial cushion defects.

Treatment

Treatment consists of anticongestive measures and eventual surgical correction. In the incomplete form, surgery is associated with a relatively low death rate (2–5%). The complete form is associated with a significantly higher death rate (about 15–25%), but complete correction in the first year of life, prior to the onset of irreversible pulmonary hypertension, is advisable.

Pulmonary artery banding procedures are contraindicated in infants with shunts predominantly at the atrial level. They are less effective in patients with predominantly ventricular level shunts than in patients with simple ventricular septal defect. At corrective surgery, transesophageal echo is useful in assessing the adequacy of repair.

Hawort SG: Pulmonary vascular bed in children with complete atrioventricular septal defect: Relation between structure and hemodynamic abnormalities. Am J Cardiol 1986;57:833.

Marino B et al: Atrioventricular canal in Down syndrome. Am J Dis Child 1990;144:1120.

Moscoso G: Developmental morphology of atrioventricular cushions and atrioventricular septal structures: A clue to understanding atrioventricular septal defects. J Perinatal Med 1991;19:215.

PATENT DUCTUS ARTERIOSUS

Essentials of Diagnosis

- Variable murmur, with active precordium and full pulses, in newborn premature infants.
- Continuous murmur and full pulses in older infants.

General Considerations

Patent ductus arteriosus is the persistence in extrauterine life of the normal fetal vessel that joins the pulmonary artery to the aorta. It closes spontaneously in normal term infants by 4 days of age. It is a common abnormality, accounting for about 12% of all cases of congenital heart disease. It is very common in children born to mothers who had rubella during the first trimester of pregnancy. There is a higher incidence of patent ductus arteriosus in infants born at high altitudes (over 10,000 ft). It is twice as common in females as in males. In preterm infants weighing less than 1500 g, the frequency of patent ductus arteriosus may be as high as 20–60%.

The defect occurs as an isolated abnormality, but associated lesions are not infrequent. Coarctation of the aorta, patent ductus arteriosus, and ventricular septal defect are commonly associated. Even more important to recognize are those patients with murmurs of patent ductus but without readily apparent findings of other associated lesions who are being kept alive by the patent ductus (eg, a patient with patent ductus with unsuspected pulmonary atresia).

Clinical Findings

A. Symptoms & Signs: The clinical findings and the clinical course depend on the size of the shunt and the degree of pulmonary hypertension.

1. Typical patent ductus arteriosus–The pulses are bounding, and pulse pressure is widened (pulse pressure is greater than half of the systolic pressure). The first heart sound is normal. The second heart sound is usually narrowly split and very rarely (when the shunt is maximal) paradoxically split (ie, the second sound closes on inspiration and splits on expiration). The paradoxic splitting is caused by the maximal overload of the left ventricle and the prolonged ejection of blood from this chamber.

The murmur is quite characteristic. It is a very rough "machinery" murmur that is maximal at the second intercostal space at the left sternal border and inferior to the left clavicle. It begins shortly after the first heart sound, rises to a peak at the second heart sound, and passes through the second heart sound into diastole, where it becomes a decrescendo murmur and fades or disappears before the first heart sound. The murmur tends to radiate fairly well over the lung fields anteriorly but relatively poorly over the lung fields posteriorly. A diastolic flow murmur is often heard at the apex. Depending on the pulmonary artery pressure, the murmur may be only systolic in time. This characteristic should be fully appreciated when trying to reach a diagnosis of patent ductus arteriosus in infants.

2. Patent ductus arteriosus with pulmonary hypertension–The physical findings depend on the cause of the pulmonary hypertension. If pulmonary hypertension is primarily the result of a marked increase in blood flow and only a slight increase in pulmonary vascular resistance, the physical findings are similar to those listed above. The significant difference is the presence of an accentuated pulmonary component of S_2. Bounding pulses and a loud continuous heart murmur are present. In patients with pulmonary vascular resistance and predominant right-to-left shunt, the findings are quite different. There may be evidence of cyanosis. The second heart sound is single and quite accentuated, and there is no significant heart murmur. The pulses are normal rather than bounding.

3. Patent ductus arteriosus in the premature neonate with associated respiratory distress syndrome–A preterm neonate during or after the clinical course of respiratory distress syndrome may have a significant associated patent ductus arteriosus that is paradoxically difficult to detect clinically but is often threatening in magnitude. A soft, nonspecific systolic murmur or no murmur is more common than the classic continuous murmur. The peripheral pulse and precordium are often bounding but typically are not characteristic for several days after the onset of a large left-to-right shunt. An early sign indicating the presence of a significant left-to-right shunt with concomitant congestive heart failure is increasing dependence on oxygen and respiratory support. In addition, increasing radiographic cardiomegaly and pulmonary edema plus increasing echocardiographic evidence of a left-to-right shunt differentiate this clinical and laboratory picture from bronchopulmonary dysplasia.

B. Imaging: In simple patent ductus arteriosus, the x-ray appearance depends on the size of the shunt. If the shunt is relatively small or moderate in size, the heart is not enlarged. If the shunt is large, there is evidence of both left atrial and left ventricular enlargement. In both cases, the aorta is prominent, as is the main pulmonary artery segment.

C. Electrocardiography: The ECG may be normal or may show left ventricular hypertrophy, depending on the size of the shunt. In patients with pulmonary hypertension caused by increased blood flow, there is usually biventricular hypertrophy. In those with pulmonary vascular obstruction, there is pure right ventricular hypertrophy. An anterior ST depression (V_1) of 2 mm suggests subendocardial ischemia as a result of a diastolic "steal" from the coronary arteries via the ductus; this finding indicates the need for closure.

D. Echocardiography: Enlargement of the left atrium as measured by M-mode echocardiography is an important clue to the presence of congestive heart failure and is especially useful in diagnosing patent ductus arteriosus in the preterm infant. A left atrial to ascending aorta ratio of greater than 1.2 or 1.3 is considered evidence of a sizable left-to-right ductal shunt. Preterm infants with patent ductus arteriosus who are undergoing medical or surgical therapy for closure should have a complete two-dimensional echocardiographic evaluation to rule out associated heart disease, especially ductus-dependent lesions. The use of color flow pulsed Doppler ultrasonography and two-dimensional echocardiography can provide visualization of the ductus and confirmation of the direction and degree of shunting and usually eliminates the need for a diagnostic cardiac catheterization.

E. Cardiac Catheterization & Angiocardiography: Cardiac catheterization will reveal increased oxygen content or saturation at the level of the pulmonary artery. Hydrogen electrode curves are positive in the pulmonary artery and negative in the right ventricle. The catheter can often be passed through the ductus from the pulmonary artery into the descending thoracic aorta. Arteriograms taken following injection of contrast material into the aortic arch show a shunt at the level of the ductus. If catheterization is not performed, the cardiologist must be completely satisfied that there is neither an associated lesion nor pulmonary hypertension. Transcatheter closure of patent ductus arteriosus is once again being evaluated in selected centers staffed by personnel with expertise in interventional cardiology in older children.

Patients with patent ductus arteriosus and pulmonary hypertension resulting from large left-to-right shunts show a marked increase in oxygen saturation at the pulmonary artery level and normal systemic arterial saturation. Those with marked pulmonary vascular obstruction show little or no increase in oxygen content at the pulmonary artery and a decrease in systemic arterial saturation. In both cases, a catheter may be passed through the ductus into the descending thoracic aorta.

Cardiac catheterization is rarely indicated in the premature infant with symptomatic ductus.

Treatment

Treatment consists of surgical correction, except in patients with pulmonary vascular obstruction. Patients with large left-to-right shunts and pulmonary hypertension should be operated on very early (even under the age of 1 year) to prevent the development of progressive pulmonary vascular obstruction. Simple patent ductus arteriosus should be corrected after the child reaches age 1, although the operation may be delayed until later without increasing the risk of death. Transcatheter closure with an occluder device is being evaluated as an experimental technique. Transcatheter closure of small defects with a coil is becoming standard therapy.

Patients with nonreactive pulmonary vascular obstruction who have resistance greater than 10 units and a pulmonary/systemic resistance ratio greater than 0.7 should not be operated on. These patients are made worse by closure of the ductus, because the ductus serves as an escape route and limits the degree of pulmonary hypertension.

The preterm infant with symptomatic ductus presents a special and controversial problem. At some institutions, it is customary to operate on virtually all preterm infants weighing under 1200 g. At other institutions, surgery is rarely done, and most infants receive a maximum of three doses of either oral indomethacin (0.1–0.3 mg/kg every 8–24 hours) or parenteral indomethacin (0.1–0.3 mg/kg every 12 hours) if adequate renal, hematologic, and hepatic function is demonstrated. Contraindications to indomethacin treatment include hyperbilirubinemia of 12 mg/dL or greater, renal failure, shock, necrotizing enterocolitis, intracranial hemorrhage, hemorrhagic disease, and evidence of a spontaneously closing ductus. Efficacy and safety of indomethacin use are enhanced by the careful monitoring of serum levels of indomethacin. A serum level of less than 250 ng/mL is associated with treatment failure. Conventional conservative management includes fluid restriction with or without diuretics and ligation only if these fail. Factors to be considered in making a rational decision on the modality of therapy include a high rate of spontaneous ductus closure without therapy and an extremely low surgical risk in experienced centers; the inability of a laboratory to monitor serum levels of indomethacin may influence the decision.

Course & Prognosis

Patients with simple patent ductus arteriosus and small to moderate shunts usually do quite well even without surgery. However, in the third or fourth decade of life, symptoms of easy fatigability, dyspnea on exertion, and exercise intolerance appear, usually as a consequence of the development of pulmonary hypertension or congestive heart failure.

Spontaneous closure of a patent ductus arteriosus may occur within the first 2 years of life or beyond. This is especially true in infants who were born preterm. After age 2, spontaneous closure is less common. Because subacute infective endocarditis is a potential complication, surgical ligation is recommended if the defect persists beyond age 2 years.

Patients with large shunts or pulmonary hypertension do not do as well. Poor growth and development, frequent episodes of pneumonitis, and the development of congestive heart failure are not uncommon in patients with large left-to-right shunts. If these patients do not succumb to congestive heart failure in early infancy, they frequently go on to develop pulmonary vascular obstruction in later childhood or adolescence. Life expectancy is markedly reduced, and these patients often die in their second or third decade. Those rare patients with pulmonary vascular obstruction from very early infancy are actually less symptomatic than those with pulmonary hypertension without obstruction.

Cambier PA et al: Percutaneous closure of the small patent ductus arteriosus using coil embolization. Am J Cardiol 1992;69:815.

Goldberg SJ: Response of the patent ductus arteriosus to indomethacin treatment. Am J Dis Child 1987;141:250.

Rashkind WJ et al: Nonsurgical closure of patent ductus arteriosus. Circulation 1987;75:583.

Reller MD et al: Duration of ductal shunting in healthy preterm infants: An echocardiographic color flow Doppler study. J Pediatr 1988;112:441.

Reller MD et al: The timing of spontaneous closure of the ductus arteriosus in infants with respiratory distress syndrome. Am J Cardiol 1990;66:75.

Valdez-Cruz M et al: Real-time Doppler color flow mapping for detection of patent ductus arteriosus. J Am Coll Cardiol 1986;8:1105.

MALFORMATIONS ASSOCIATED WITH OBSTRUCTION TO BLOOD FLOW ON THE RIGHT SIDE OF THE HEART

1. VALVULAR PULMONARY STENOSIS WITH INTACT VENTRICULAR SEPTUM

Essentials of Diagnosis

- No symptoms with mild and moderately severe cases.
- Cyanosis and a high incidence of right-sided congestive heart failure in very severe cases.
- Right ventricular lift; systolic ejection click at the pulmonary area in mild to moderately severe cases.
- S_2 widely split with soft to inaudible P_2; grade I–VI/VI obstructive systolic murmur, maximal at the pulmonary area.
- Dilated pulmonary artery on posteroanterior chest x-ray film.

General Considerations

Obstruction of right ventricular outflow at the pulmonary valve level accounts for about 10% of all cases of congenital heart disease. In the usual case, the cusps of the pulmonary valve are fused to form a membrane or diaphragm with a hole in the middle that varies from 2 mm to 1 cm in diameter. Occasionally, there may be a fusion of only two cusps, producing a bicuspid pulmonary valve. Very frequently, especially in the more severe cases, there is secondary infundibular stenosis. The pulmonary valve ring is usually small. There is usually moderate to marked poststenotic dilatation of both the main and left pulmonary arteries. Patent foramen ovale is fairly common.

Obstruction to blood flow across the pulmonary valve results in an increase in pressure developed by the right ventricle to maintain an adequate output across that valve. Pressures greater than systemic are potentially life-threatening and are associated with "critical" obstruction. As a consequence of the increased work required of the right ventricle, severe right ventricular hypertrophy and eventual right ventricular failure can occur. In contrast to patients with right ventricular outflow obstruction, patients with this obstruction who also have a large ventricular septal defect (ie, tetralogy of Fallot) are not at great risk for heart failure; because of the septal defect, there is communication between the ventricles, which limits the amount of pressure developed in the right ventricle (pressure is equal to systemic pressure) and thereby makes heart failure extremely uncommon.

When the obstruction is severe and the ventricular septum is intact, a right-to-left shunt will often occur at the atrial level through a patent foramen ovale. Accordingly, patients with this condition may have a varying degree of cyanosis. The presence of cyanosis indicates a relatively severe degree of valvular obstruction.

Clinical Findings

A. Symptoms & Signs: The history depends on the severity of the obstruction. Patients with a mild or even a moderate degree of valvular pulmonary stenosis are completely asymptomatic throughout infancy, childhood, and adolescence. Patients with a more severe type of valvular obstruction may develop cyanosis and congestive heart failure very early—even in the neonatal period. Hypoxemic spells characterized by a sudden onset of marked cyanosis and dyspnea are much less common than in tetralogy of Fallot.

Patients with mild to moderate obstruction are acyanotic. Patients with severe or critical stenosis usually show evidence of central cyanosis. These patients are usually well developed and well nourished. They often have a round face and widely spaced eyes. The pulses are normal and equal throughout. Clubbing may occur in severe cases in which cyanosis has persisted for a long time. On examination of the heart, there may be prominence of the precordium. A heaving impulse of the right ventricle can frequently be palpated. A systolic thrill is often palpated in the pulmonary area and occasionally in the suprasternal notch. The first heart sound is normal. In patients with mild to moderate stenosis, a prominent ejection click of pulmonary origin is heard best at the second left intercostal space. This click varies with respiration. It is much more prominent during expiration than inspiration. In patients with severe stenosis, the click tends to merge with the first heart sound. The second heart sound also varies with the degree of stenosis. In mild valvular stenosis, the second heart sound is normally split and the pulmonary component is normal in intensity. In moderate degrees of obstruction, the second heart sound is more widely split and the pulmonary component is softer. In severe pulmonary stenosis, the second heart sound is single, since the pulmonary component cannot be heard. An ejection-type, rough, obstructive systolic murmur is best heard at the second interspace at the left sternal border. It radiates very well to the back. No diastolic murmurs are audible. In older children, a prominent "A" wave is seen in the jugular venous pulse. If there is congestive heart failure, the liver is enlarged.

B. Imaging: In the mild form of pulmonary stenosis, the heart may be normal in size. Poststenotic dilatation of the main pulmonary artery segment and the left pulmonary artery is often present. In moderate to severe cases, there may be a slight right ventricular enlargement, and there may or may not be poststenotic dilatation of the main pulmonary artery. In patients who are cyanotic, the pulmonary vascular markings are decreased; otherwise, they are normal.

C. Electrocardiography: Electrocardiographic findings are usually normal in patients with mild obstruction. Right ventricular hypertrophy is present in patients with moderate to severe valvular obstruction. In severe obstruction, right ventricular hypertrophy and the right ventricular strain pattern (deep inversion of the T wave) are seen in the right precordial leads. In the most severe form, right atrial hypertrophy is also present. Right axis deviation is also seen in the moderate to severe forms. Occasionally, the axis is greater than +180 degrees.

D. Echocardiography: The pulmonary valve appears to be unusually echo-dense. The pulmonary valve image on two-dimensional echocardiography shows a thickened structure with less than normal excursion. The transvalvular pressure gradient can be noninvasively and accurately estimated by echo Doppler technique.

E. Cardiac Catheterization & Angiocardiography: There is no increase in oxygen saturation or oxygen content in the right side of the heart. In the more severe cases, there is a right-to-left shunt at the atrial level. Pulmonary artery pressure is normal in milder cases and quite low in moderately severe to severe cases. Right ventricular pressure is always higher than pulmonary artery pressure. The gradient across the pulmonary valve varies from 10 to 200

mm Hg. In severe cases, the right atrial pressure is often elevated, with a predominant "A" wave. Cineangiocardiography with injection of contrast material into the right ventricle shows thickening of the pulmonary valve and the very narrow opening of the pulmonary valve. This produces a "jet" of contrast from the right ventricle into the pulmonary artery. Infundibular hypertrophy may be present. Diagnostic catheterization is usually combined with a balloon pulmonary valvotomy.

Treatment

Elective valvotomy is recommended for children with right ventricular pressures of greater than 50 mm Hg or higher than two-thirds of systemic pressure. Immediate correction is indicated for patients with systemic or greater right ventricular pressure. Percutaneous balloon valvuloplasty has become the procedure of choice in most institutions. It appears to be as effective as surgery in relieving obstruction and causes less valve insufficiency.

The need for additional surgical resection of associated infundibular hypertrophy is controversial. Because additional surgery increases the risk and because the outflow obstruction usually regresses, many centers perform only the balloon valvotomy.

Course & Prognosis

Patients with mild pulmonary stenosis live a normal life and have a normal life span. Those with stenosis of moderate severity rarely are symptomatic. Those with severe valvular obstruction may develop severe cyanosis and congestive heart failure in early life.

Postoperative follow-up suggests that most patients with right ventricular pressure equal to or less than systemic pressure who were treated surgically early in life have good voluntary maximum exercise capacity. If relief of valvular obstruction occurs prior to 20 years of age, longevity is essentially the same as that of the general population. Physical restriction is unwarranted in these patients. The quality of life of adults with pulmonary stenosis is comparable to that of the normal population . The risk of coronary heart disease is 1.7% in the offspring of males and approximately 4% in probands of females.

Driscoll DJ et al: Occurrence risk for congenital heart defects in relatives of patients with aortic stenosis, pulmonary stenosis, or ventricular septal defect. Circulation 1993;87(Suppl):I-121.

Kopecky SL et al: Long term outcome of patients undergoing surgical repair of isolated pulmonary valve stenosis. Circulation 1988;78:1150.

Lloyd T, Donnerstein R: Rapid T-wave normalization after balloon pulmonary valvuloplasty in children. Am J Cardiol 1989;64:399.

Marantz PM et al: Results of balloon valvuloplasty in typical and dysplastic pulmonary valve stenosis: Doppler

echocardiographic follow up. J Am Coll Cardiol 1988;
12:476.

McCrindle B, Kan J: Long term results after balloon valvuloplasty. Circulation 1991;83:1915.

Rey C et al: Percutaneous transluminal balloon valvuloplasty of congenital pulmonary valve stenosis, with a special report on infants and neonates. J Am Coll Cardiol 1988;11:815.

2. INFUNDIBULAR PULMONARY STENOSIS WITHOUT VENTRICULAR SEPTAL DEFECT

Pure infundibular pulmonary stenosis is rare. One should suspect infundibular pulmonary stenosis where there is evidence of mild to moderate pulmonary stenosis and intact ventricular septum and (1) no pulmonary ejection click is audible and (2) the murmur is maximal in the third and fourth intercostal spaces rather than in the second intercostal space. The clinical picture is identical.

3. DISTAL PULMONARY STENOSIS

Supravalvular Pulmonary Stenosis

Supravalvular pulmonary stenosis, a relatively rare condition, is caused by coarctation of the body of the main pulmonary artery. The clinical picture may be identical to that of valvular pulmonary stenosis, although the murmur is maximal in the first intercostal space at the left sternal border and in the suprasternal notch. No ejection click is audible. A second heart sound is usually narrowly split, and the pulmonary component is quite loud as a result of closure of the pulmonary valve under high pressure. The murmur radiates extremely well into the neck and over the lung fields.

Peripheral Pulmonary Branch Stenosis

In peripheral pulmonary branch stenosis, there are multiple small coarctations of the branches of the pulmonary artery in the periphery of the lung. Systolic murmurs may be heard over both lung fields, both anteriorly and posteriorly. The transient pulmonary branch stenosis murmurs of infancy (previously described in the section on heart murmurs, under Diagnostic Evaluation) are innocent. Pulmonary artery branch stenosis murmurs may be the most audible murmurs in atrial septal defects in infancy and early childhood. The most common cause of significant pulmonary artery branch stenosis is maternal rubella. Several types of supravalvular aortic stenosis syndromes may be found in association with this condition.

Surgery is often unsuccessful. Transvenous angioplasty is currently being assessed but does not appear to be as efficacious in patients with peripheral pulmonary branch stenosis as in patients with pulmonary valvular stenosis.

Absence of a Pulmonary Artery

Absence of a pulmonary artery may be an isolated malformation or may occur in association with other congenital heart diseases. It is occasionally seen in patients with tetralogy of Fallot.

Dunkle LM, Rowe RD: Transient murmur simulating pulmonary artery stenosis in premature infants. Am J Dis Child 1972;124:666.

Rothma A et al: Early results and follow-up of balloon angioplasty for branch pulmonary artery stenosis. J Am Coll Cardiol 1990;15:1109.

MALFORMATIONS ASSOCIATED WITH OBSTRUCTION TO BLOOD FLOW ON THE LEFT SIDE OF THE HEART

1. COARCTATION OF THE AORTA

Essentials of Diagnosis

- Pulse lag in lower extremities.
- Blood pressure of 20 mm Hg or pressure greater in the upper than in the lower extremities.
- Blowing systolic murmur in the left axilla.

General Considerations

Coarctation is a common cardiac abnormality accounting for about 6% of all cases of congenital heart disease. Three times as many males as females are affected. In the vast majority of cases, coarctation occurs in the thoracic portion of the descending aorta. The abdominal aorta is very rarely involved. Coarctations are usually in the juxtaductal position rather than the preductal or postductal position. The term **coarctation of aorta syndrome** is a useful concept, because most symptomatic infants have associated patent ductus arteriosus, tubular hypoplasia of the aortic isthmus (frequently erroneously termed a coarctation), ventricular septal defect, and bicuspid aortic valve. The tubular hypoplasia of the aortic isthmus is probably related to paucity of blood flow in the fetus and often spontaneously enlarges with postnatal growth.

Clinical Findings

A. Symptoms & Signs: Patients with coarctation may or may not have cardiovascular symptoms in infancy, childhood, and adolescence. Congestive heart failure may develop in early infancy, and symptoms of decreased exercise tolerance and fatigability may appear in childhood.

The important physical finding is diminution or

absence of femoral pulses. However, a significant number of infants will initially have equal upper and lower extremity pulses until the coexistent patent ductus arteriosus closes. Normally, the blood pressure in the upper extremities is slightly higher than in the lower extremities during the first few months of life. After 1 year of age, blood pressure higher in the arms than in the legs is suggestive of coarctation of the aorta. The actual level of blood pressure in the arms may be only moderately elevated, even in severe coarctation, or it may be significantly elevated. In the presence of severe congestive heart failure, the differences in pulses in the upper and lower extremities may not be readily apparent, but with compensation, the pulses in the arms are palpably stronger than those of healthy infants; the pulses in the legs remain diminished or absent in affected infants. The left subclavian artery is occasionally involved in the coarctation, in which case the left brachial pulse is weak. If the coarctation is uncomplicated, the heart sounds are normal. The aortic component of the second heart sound is occasionally increased in intensity. An ejection systolic murmur of grade II/VI intensity is often heard at the aortic area and the lower left sternal border. The pathognomonic murmur of coarctation is heard in the left axilla. This murmur is usually systolic in timing but may spill into diastole. If the coarctation is complicated by other malformations, murmurs associated with these other abnormalities will be audible.

B. Imaging: In the older child, x-ray findings may indicate a heart normal in size, although there is usually some evidence of left ventricular enlargement. The ascending aorta is usually normal in size. On barium swallow, the esophagus has a characteristic ε shape. The first arc of the ε is caused by dilatation of the aorta just proximal to the coarctation. The second arc results from poststenotic dilatation of the aorta. The middle bar of the ε is due to the coarctation itself. In older children, notching or scalloping of the ribs caused by marked enlargement of the intercostal collaterals can be seen. Magnetic resonance imaging (MRI) has become extremely useful for determining noninvasively the anatomy of the coarctation.

In infants in congestive heart failure, there is evidence of marked cardiac enlargement and pulmonary venous congestion.

C. Electrocardiography: ECGs in children may be normal or may show evidence of slight left ventricular hypertrophy. In infants with or without congestive heart failure, the ECG usually demonstrates right ventricular hypertrophy.

D. Echocardiography: Real-time two-dimensional echocardiography may visualize the coarctation directly, and color flow Doppler may serve as a predictor of severity. However, if the ductus arteriosus is still patent, echocardiography may not detect the coarctation. Associated lesions such as a bicuspid

aortic valve or mitral abnormalities may suggest the presence of a coarctation.

E. Cardiac Catheterization & Angiocardiography: These studies demonstrate the position, anatomy, and severity of the coarctation and will assess the adequacy of the collateral circulation.

Treatment

Infants with coarctation of the aorta and congestive heart failure require vigorous anticongestive measures. Dilation of the associated patent ductus arteriosus with a constant infusion of prostaglandin E_1 (PGE_1) at 0.05–0.20 micrograms/kg/min may stabilize the critically ill infant until operation can be performed. Many with isolated coarctation and no associated lesions respond well and do not require surgery in infancy. In infants with striking congestive heart failure and without associated cardiovascular abnormalities, severe systemic hypertension is often a contributing factor.

Infants with associated intracardiac defects sometimes need immediate surgery but frequently require revision of the recoarctation later in life. Modification of the surgical technique utilizing a subclavian flap anastomosis reduces the likelihood of this late complication. This technique has been used successfully in infants weighing as little as 1000 g. Patients repaired with patch aortoplasty must be followed frequently (every 1–2 years) because of the potential for rapid progression of aortic aneurysms.

Percutaneous balloon angioplasty has been used successfully as a palliative procedure to stabilize critically ill infants with coarctation of aorta syndrome and as primary therapy in older children. Percutaneous balloon angioplasty is also being utilized to dilate recoarctations in postoperative patients.

Patients who do not require surgery early in life may be corrected electively at ages 3–5 years unless significant systemic hypertension develops.

Course & Prognosis

Children who survive the neonatal period without developing congestive heart failure do quite well throughout childhood and adolescence. Fatal complications (eg, hypertensive encephalopathy, intracranial bleeding) occur uncommonly. Subacute infective endocarditis is also rare before adolescence.

Children with coarctation corrected during school age are at significant risk for systemic hypertension and myocardial dysfunction. Careful exercise testing is mandatory prior to their participation in athletic activities.

Balderson S et al: Maximal voluntary exercise variables in children with postoperative coarctation of the aorta. J Am Coll Cardiol 1992;191:154.

Cohen M et al: Coarctation of the aorta: Long-term follow-up and prediction of outcome after surgical correction. Circulation 1989;80:840.

Mendelsohn AM et al: Rapid progression of aortic aneurysms after patch aortoplasty repair of coarctation of the aorta. J Am Coll Cardiol 1992;20:381.

Simpson IA et al: Color flow Doppler flow mapping in patients with coarctation of the aorta: New observations and improved evaluation with color flow diameter and proximal acceleration as predictors of severity. Circulation 1988;77:736.

Ward KE et al: Delayed detection of coarctation in infancy: Implications for timing newborn follow-up. Pediatrics 1990;86:972.

2. AORTIC STENOSIS

Essentials of Diagnosis

- Systolic ejection murmur at the upper right sternal border.
- Thrill in the carotid arteries.
- Systolic click at the apex.
- Dilatation of the ascending aorta on chest x-ray.

General Considerations

Aortic stenosis may be defined from the anatomic or physiologic point of view. Anatomically, it consists of an obstruction to the outflow from the left ventricle at or near the aortic valve. Physiologically, *aortic stenosis* may be defined as a condition in which a systolic pressure gradient of more than 10 mm Hg exists between the left ventricle and the aorta. Aortic stenosis accounts for approximately 5% of all cases of congenital heart disease. Anatomically, congenital aortic stenosis may be divided into four types:

A. Valvular Aortic Stenosis (75%): Critical aortic stenosis presenting in infancy usually consists of a unicuspid diaphragm-like structure without well-defined commissures. Preschool and school-age children more commonly present with a bicuspid valve. Teenagers and young adults characteristically present with tricuspid but partially fused leaflets. This lesion is more common in males than in females.

B. Discrete Membranous Subvalvular Aortic Stenosis (20%): This consists of a membranous or fibrous ring just below the aortic valve. The ring forms a diaphragm with a hole in the middle and results in obstruction to left ventricular outflow. The aortic valve itself and the anterior leaflet of the mitral valve are often deformed.

C. Supravalvular Aortic Stenosis: In this variety, there is a constriction of the ascending aorta just above the coronary arteries. This condition is often associated with a family history, abnormal facies, and mental retardation (Williams syndrome).

D. Idiopathic Hypertrophic Subaortic Stenosis (IHSS): In this case, there is a marked hypertrophy of the entire left ventricle and, predominantly, the ventricular septum. With contraction of the ventricle, the hypertrophic portion of the septum, together with the mitral valve, causes obstruction of left ventricular outflow. A family history is often present.

Obstruction to outflow from the left ventricle causes the left ventricle to work harder to maintain an adequate pressure and flow in the systemic arterial circuit, resulting in hypertrophy of the left ventricle and increased oxygen requirement. If the stenosis is severe, the oxygen requirements may exceed the capacity of the coronary arteries to supply oxygen, and relative coronary insufficiency may develop. In critical aortic stenosis, left ventricular failure may occur. The left ventricle is usually able to adapt to the increased pressure load for a considerable period before heart failure or coronary insufficiency develops.

Clinical Findings

A. Symptoms & Signs: Most patients with aortic stenosis have no cardiovascular symptoms. Except in the most severe cases, the patient may do well up until the third to fifth decades of life, although some patients have mild exercise intolerance and easy fatigability. A small percentage of patients have significant symptoms within the first decade, that is, dizziness and syncope. Sudden death, although uncommon, may occur in all forms of aortic stenosis, the greatest risk being IHSS.

Although isolated valvular aortic stenosis seldom causes symptoms in infancy, severe heart failure occasionally occurs when critical obstruction is present. The response to medical management is poor; therefore, an aggressive surgical approach is recommended.

The physical findings vary somewhat depending on the anatomic type of lesion:

1. Valvular aortic stenosis—Affected patients are well developed and well nourished. The pulses are usually normal and equal throughout. If the stenosis is severe and there is a gradient of greater than 80 mm Hg, the pulses are small with a slow upstroke. Examination of the heart reveals a left ventricular thrust at the apex. A systolic thrill at the right base, the suprasternal notch, and both carotid arteries accompanies moderate disease. If only one carotid artery manifests a thrill, it is the right carotid (usually seen in milder disease).

The first heart sound is normal. A prominent aortic-type ejection click or ejection sound is best heard at the apex. In infants, this click can be heard at the lower left sternal border and at the aortic area. It is separated from the first heart sound by a short but appreciable interval. It does not vary with respiration. The second heart sound at the pulmonary area is physiologically split. The aortic component of the second heart sound is of good intensity. There is a grade III–V/VI, rough, medium- to high-pitched ejection-type systolic murmur, loudest at the first and second intercostal spaces, which radiates well into the suprasternal notch and along the carotids. The murmur also radiates fairly well down the lower left sternal border and can be heard at the apex. The murmur transmits to the neck, and its grade correlates roughly with the severity of the stenosis.

2. Discrete membranous subvalvular aortic stenosis–The findings are essentially the same as those of valvular aortic stenosis. Absence of an aortic ejection click is an important differentiating point, and the thrill and murmur are usually somewhat more intense at the left sternal border in the third and fourth intercostal spaces than at the aortic area. Frequently, however, the murmur is equally intense at both areas. A diastolic murmur of aortic insufficiency is commonly heard after 5 years of age.

3. Supravalvular aortic stenosis–Affected patients often have abnormal facies and are mentally retarded. The thrill and murmur are characteristically best heard in the suprasternal notch and along the carotids, although they are well transmitted over the aortic area and near the mid left sternal border. A difference in pulses and blood pressure between the right and left arms may be found, with the more prominent pulse and pressure in the right arm.

4. Idiopathic hypertrophic subaortic stenosis–The murmur in this case is ejection in quality, grade II–III/VI, and heard from the left sternal border toward the apex and sometimes associated with a murmur of mitral insufficiency. There is often an atrial fourth heart sound with a diastolic murmur. No ejection click is audible. The arterial pulse wave has a rapid upstroke and frequently a bisferiens quality.

B. Imaging: In most cases, x-ray findings indicate that the heart is not enlarged. The left ventricle, however, is slightly prominent. In valvular and discrete subvalvular aortic stenosis, dilatation of the ascending aorta is frequently seen (more commonly in the former). The ascending aorta is usually normal in IHSS and in supravalvular aortic stenosis.

C. Electrocardiography: There is some correlation between the severity of the obstruction and the ECG. Patients with mild aortic stenosis have normal ECGs. Patients with severe obstruction frequently demonstrate evidence of left ventricular hypertrophy and left ventricular strain, but many do not. In about 25% of severe cases, the ECG is normal. Progressive increase in left ventricular hypertrophy on serial ECGs indicates a significant degree of obstruction. Left ventricular strain is taken as a potential indication for operation.

D. Echocardiography: This has become a reliable noninvasive technique for the initial diagnosis and follow-up evaluation of IHSS. It also provides clues to the progression of other forms of aortic stenosis. Doppler echocardiographic techniques can now predict transvalvular gradients quite accurately.

E. Cardiac Catheterization & Angiocardiography: Left heart catheterization demonstrates the pressure differential between the left ventricle and the aorta and the level at which the gradient exists. Patients with severe aortic stenosis may be asympto-

matic and have normal ECGs and chest x-rays. Serial cardiac catheterization is frequently the only reliable guide to the progression and severity of the lesion. In the case of valvular aortic stenosis, an asymptomatic patient with a resting gradient of 60–80 mm Hg is considered to require surgery. In the face of symptoms, patients with lesser gradients are surgical candidates. Cineangiocardiography is helpful in demonstrating the level of the obstruction.

Treatment

Because the results of surgery are frequently unsatisfactory, surgical repair should be considered only in patients with symptoms or a large resting gradient (60–80 mm Hg). In many cases, the gradient can be only moderately to minimally relieved without producing aortic insufficiency (which is potentially more harmful than the lesion for which surgery was undertaken). Percutaneous balloon valvuloplasty is now accepted as standard treatment. Discrete subvalvular aortic stenosis requires a lesser gradient for surgical intervention, because continued trauma to the aortic valve by the subvalvular jet may destroy the valve. Unfortunately, simple resection is followed by recurrence in more than 25% of patients with subvalvular aortic stenosis. Asymmetric septal hypertrophy has even less satisfactory results than muscle resection; therefore, medical management with propranolol should be tried initially.

All patients should have close follow-up, and those over age 6 years should undergo yearly exercise testing. If exercise testing is normal, restriction of physical activity may not be necessary in patients with mild to moderate aortic stenosis; in many cases, these patients may participate in competitive sports.

Course & Prognosis

All forms of left ventricular outflow tract obstruction tend to be progressive diseases. However, regression of the obstruction has been documented in a few patients with supravalvular obstruction. Pediatric patients with left ventricular outflow tract obstruction—with the exception of those with critical aortic stenosis of infancy—are usually asymptomatic. Symptoms accompanying severe unoperated obstruction (angina, syncope, congestive heart failure) are all rare currently because of detection and surgical intervention. The vast majority of children without asymmetric septal hypertrophy not only are asymptomatic but also tend to have the personality and capabilities to compete in sports. There is increasing evidence that preoperative or postoperative children whose obstruction is mild to moderate have above-average oxygen consumption and maximum voluntary working capacity. Children in this category with normal findings on resting and exercising ECG and normal heart size may safely participate in vigorous physical activity, including nonisometric competitive sports. Children with severe aortic stenosis tend to demonstrate ventricular dysrhythmias as adults.

Kasten-Sportas CH et al: Percutaneous balloon valvuloplasty in neonates with critical aortic stenosis. J Am Coll Cardiol 1991;13:1101.

Kennedy KD et al: Natural history of moderate aortic stenosis. J Am Coll Cardiol 1991;17:313.

Oh JK et al: Prediction of the severity of aortic stenosis by Doppler aortic valve area determination. J Am Coll Cardiol 1988;11:1227.

Shaddy RE et al: Gradient reduction aortic valve regurgitation and prolapse after balloon aortic valvuloplasty in 32 consecutive patients with congenital aortic stenosis. J Am Coll Cardiol 1990;16:451.

Witsenburg M et al: Short and midterm results of balloon valvuloplasty for valvar aortic stenosis in children. Am J Cardiol 1992;69:945.

Wolfe RR et al: Arrhythmias in patients with valvar aortic stenosis, valvar pulmonic stenosis, and ventricular septal defect. Circulation 1993;87(Suppl):I-89.

Zeevi B et al: Neonatal critical valvar aortic stenosis. Circulation 1989;80:831.

3. MITRAL VALVE PROLAPSE

Essentials of Diagnosis

- Midsystolic click best heard with the patient in the standing or squatting position.
- Occasional late systolic murmur.

General Considerations

Mitral valve prolapse is the most common entity to present with abnormal auscultatory findings in pediatric patients. It is secondary to redundant valve tissue or abnormal tissue comprising the mitral valve apparatus. The mitral valve prolapses, moving posteriorly or superiorly into the left atrium during ventricular systole. A systolic click occurs at the time of this movement and is the clinical hallmark of this entity. Mitral insufficiency may occur late in systole, causing an atypical, short, late systolic murmur with variable radiation. It is most commonly found in individuals with the following characteristics: over 6 years of age, female, slender habitus, and bony thoracic abnormalities. Its incidence is estimated to vary from 2% to 20%, with the higher part of the range representing incidence in slender teenage females.

Clinical Findings

A. Symptoms & Signs: The vast majority of patients with mitral valve prolapse are asymptomatic. Chest pain, palpitations, and dizziness are reported, but it is not clear whether or not these symptoms are more common in affected patients than in the normal population. Significant dysrhythmias are uncommon, and true exercise intolerance is rare. The standard approach to auscultation must be modified to diagnose mitral valve prolapse; that is, auscultation should be performed with the patient placed in various positions. Clicks with or without systolic murmur are more commonly elicited in the standing and squatting positions than in the supine and sitting positions. The systolic click occurs earlier in children than in adults; that is, it tends to be midsystolic rather than late systolic. Although it is usually heard at the apex, it may be audible at the left sternal border or even occasionally may be panthoracic. A midsystolic or systolic murmur following the click implies mitral insufficiency and is much less common than isolated prolapse. The murmur tends to be atypical for mitral insufficiency in that it is not pansystolic and radiates to the sternum rather than to the left axilla. A coexistent diastolic murmur of relative or real mitral stenosis is rare. Occasionally, a systolic "honk" is heard.

B. Imaging: In the rare case of significant mitral insufficiency, the left atrium may be enlarged; this is visualized best on lateral film x-ray. Most chest x-rays show normal findings, and their use is therefore largely unwarranted.

C. Electrocardiography: Despite the fact that flat or inverted T waves in precordial lead V_6 have been reported, almost all electrocardiographic findings are normal. Disabling chest pain is rare and should be assessed with ergometric electrocardiography.

D. Echocardiography: Significant posterior systolic movement of the anterior mitral valve leaflet is considered diagnostic. Many false-positive results are the result of multiple leaflet images (chevroning) or to the presence of insignificant (small duration and amplitude) posterior systolic valve movement. False-negative results are also common, partly because of performance of the procedure when the patient is in the supine position. If the physical findings are typical for isolated prolapse, echocardiography is not warranted.

E. Cardiac Catheterization & Angiography: Invasive procedures are very rarely indicated.

Treatment & Prognosis

Use of oral propranolol may be effective in rare cases of disabling chest pain. Prophylaxis for subacute infectious endocarditis is indicated only in individuals with associated mitral insufficiency.

The natural course of disease is largely unknown. Twenty years of observation indicate, however, that mitral valve prolapse in childhood is a largely benign entity. It merges with a common variation from normal in slender children and is associated with an asthenic body build that presumably results from altered geometry of the left ventricle and mitral valve.

Alpert MA et al: Frequency of isolated panic attacks and panic disorder in patients with mitral valve prolapse syndrome. Am J Cardiol 1992;69:1489.

Arfken CL et al: Mitral valve prolapse: Associations with symptoms and anxiety. Pediatrics 1990;85:311.

Barlow JB, Pocock WA: Billowing, floppy, prolapsed or flail valves? Am J Cardiol 1985;55:501.

Kessler KM: Prolapse paranoia. J Am Coll Cardiol 1988; 11:48.

Levine RA: Reconsideration of echocardiographic standards for mitral valve prolapse: Lack of association between leaf displacement isolated to the apical 4-chamber view and independent echocardiographic evidence of abnormality. J Am Coll Cardiol 1988;11:1010.

4. OTHER CONGENITAL VALVULAR LESIONS

Congenital Mitral Stenosis

In this rare disorder, the valve leaflets are thickened and fused to produce a diaphragm-like or funnel-like structure with an opening in the center. Frequent associated malformations include subaortic and aortic stenosis and coarctation of the aorta. This lesion complex is known as Shone syndrome. Most patients develop symptoms early in life. Early symptoms include tachypnea, dyspnea, and severe failure to thrive. Physical examination reveals a first heart sound that is accentuated, and the pulmonary closure sound is loud. No opening snap can be heard. In most cases, a presystolic crescendo murmur is heard at the apex. Occasionally, only a mid- diastolic murmur can be heard. Rarely, no murmur at all is heard. Electrocardiography shows right axis deviation, biatrial enlargement, and right ventricular hypertrophy. X-ray reveals evidence of left atrial enlargement and, frequently, pulmonary venous congestion. Echocardiography shows abnormal valve structures with reduced excursion and left atrial enlargement. Cardiac catheterization reveals an elevated pulmonary capillary pressure and wedge pressure and pulmonary hypertension.

Surgical treatment, including valve replacement with a prosthetic mitral valve, has become possible even in infants weighing 3–5 kg.

Cor Triatriatum

This is an extremely rare abnormality in which the pulmonary veins enter a separate chamber rather than pass directly into the left atrium. The chamber communicates with the left atrium through an opening of variable size. The physiologic consequences of this condition are very similar to those of mitral stenosis. The clinical findings depend on the size of the opening. If the opening is extremely small, symptoms develop very early in life. If the opening is large, patients may be asymptomatic for a considerable period of time. Echocardiography may reveal a dense shadow in the left atrium. Two-dimensional color flow Doppler echocardiographic techniques have greatly enhanced the noninvasive accuracy of the diagnosis. Cardiac catheterization may be diagnostic. Finding a high pulmonary capillary pressure (high pulmonary venous pressure) and a low left atrial pressure (if the catheter can be passed through the foramen ovale into the true left atrial chamber) makes the diagnosis certain. Angiocardiographic studies may identify two "left atrial" chambers.

Surgical repair is usually successful.

Congenital Mitral Regurgitation

This is a relatively rare abnormality that is usually associated with other congenital heart lesions, including corrected transposition of the great vessels, endocardial cushion defect, and endocardial fibroelastosis. Uncomplicated congenital mitral regurgitation is very rare. It is sometimes present in patients with Marfan syndrome. Occasionally, there is a congenital dilatation of the valve ring with an otherwise normal valve. In other cases, the chordae tendineae are malformed, resulting in mitral regurgitation.

Congenital Aortic Regurgitation

The most common causes of this disorder are bicuspid aortic valve, either uncomplicated or with coarctation of the aorta; ventricular septal defect and aortic insufficiency; and fenestration of the aortic valve cusp (one or more holes in the cusp).

Absence of the Pulmonary Valve

This rare abnormality is usually associated with ventricular septal defect. In about 50% of cases, pulmonary stenosis is present (tetralogy of Fallot).

Ebstein's Malformation of the Tricuspid Valve

This uncommon abnormality consists of downward displacement of the tricuspid valve such that the greater portion of the valve is attached to the ventricular wall rather than to the fibrous ring. As a result, the upper portion of the right ventricle is functionally within the right atrium. The portion of the ventricle below the apex of the tricuspid valve is very small and represents the true functioning right ventricle. Clinically, there is a wide spectrum of abnormalities ranging from relative absence of symptoms to death in early infancy. The severity depends on the degree of malattachment of the valve and the associated abnormalities. Echocardiography is useful in diagnosis.

Surgical repair consists of an annuloplasty procedure to modify the level of tricuspid orifice and diminish mitral insufficiency. The procedure's rate of success is highly variable. Late arrhythmias are common. Postoperative tolerance of exercise is significantly increased compared to preoperative status but decreased compared to healthy individuals.

Driscoll DJ, Mottram CD, Danielson GK: Spectrum of exercise intolerance in 45 patients with Ebstein's anomaly and observations on exercise tolerance in 11 patients after surgical repair. J Am Coll Cardiol 1988;11:831.

Lang D et al: Pathologic spectrum of malformations of the tricuspid valve in prenatal and neonatal life. J Am Coll Cardiol 1991;17:1161.

Quaegebeur JN et al: Surgery for Ebstein's anomaly. J Am Coll Cardiol 1991;17:722.

Saxena A et al: The left ventricular function in patients 20 years of age with Ebstein's anomaly of the tricuspid valve. Am J Cardiol 1991;67:217.

Spevak PJ et al: Balloon angioplasty for congenital mitral stenosis. Am J Cardiol 1990;66:472.

MYOCARDIAL DISEASES

Myocardial diseases are characterized by significant cardiac enlargement. Murmurs may or may not be present. Electrocardiographic changes include left ventricular hypertrophy, ST depression, and T-wave inversion.

1. GLYCOGEN STORAGE DISEASE OF THE HEART

At least 10 types of glycogen storage disease are recognized. The type that primarily involves the heart is known as Pompe disease. The deficient enzyme (acid maltase) is necessary for hydrolysis of the outer branches of glycogen, and its absence results in marked deposition of glycogen within the myocardium. Cardiac glycogenosis is a rare heritable (autosomal recessive) disorder.

Affected infants are usually normal at birth, but onset commonly begins by the sixth month of life. These children have a history of retardation of growth and development, feeding problems, poor weight gain, and then the findings of heart failure. Physical examination reveals generalized muscular weakness, a large tongue, cardiomegaly, no significant heart murmurs, and, occasionally, evidence of congestive heart failure. Chest x-rays reveal marked cardiomegaly with or without pulmonary venous congestion. The ECG shows a short PR interval with left ventricular hypertrophy and shows ST depression and T-wave inversion over the left precordial leads. Echocardiography shows extremely thick ventricular wall structures.

Children with this disease usually die within the first year of life. Death may be sudden or the result of progressive congestive heart failure.

2. ANOMALOUS ORIGIN OF THE LEFT CORONARY ARTERY

In this condition, the left coronary artery arises from the pulmonary artery rather than from the aorta. In the neonatal period, while the pulmonary arterial pressure is relatively high, blood is supplied to the left ventricle from the pulmonary artery. Accordingly, during this period the child is asymptomatic and does well. However, within the first 2 months of life, the pulmonary arterial pressure decreases to normal. This phenomenon results in a marked decrease of flow to the left coronary artery. Infarction of the heart usually occurs. If the patient survives, collateral channels appear that join the peripheral branches of the right with the branches of the left coronary artery. As a result, the direction of blood flow in the left coronary artery changes. Whereas previously there was some flow from the pulmonary artery into the myocardium through the left coronary, flow now occurs from the right coronary artery through the collateral into the left coronary artery and then into the pulmonary artery. In essence, then, an arteriovenous fistula is formed that further removes blood from the myocardium, resulting in further myocardial infarction and fibrosis. Death occurs eventually as a result of marked dilatation of the heart and congestive heart failure. At autopsy, the left ventricle is found to be markedly fibrosed and thin.

Clinical Findings

A. Symptoms & Signs: Patients appear to be healthy at birth. Growth and development are relatively normal for a few months, although detailed questioning of the parents often discloses a history of intermittent episodes of severe abdominal pain, pallor, and sweating, especially during or after feeding. These episodes are thought to be secondary to "colic," and attacks are similar to anginal attacks in adults.

On physical examination, the patients are usually well developed and well nourished. The pulses are usually weak but equal throughout. The heart is enlarged but not very active. A murmur of mitral regurgitation is frequently present, although no murmur may be heard.

B. Imaging: Chest x-ray films show significant cardiac enlargement with or without pulmonary venous congestion.

C. Electrocardiography: The ECG is usually diagnostic. There are T-wave inversions in leads I and aVL. The precordial leads show T-wave inversions from V_4 to V_7. Deep Q waves are often seen in leads I, aVL, and V_4 to V_6. These findings of myocardial infarction are similar to those in adults.

D. Echocardiography: The diagnosis can be made with two-dimensional techniques by visualizing a single large right coronary artery arising from the aorta.

E. Cardiac Catheterization & Angiocardiography: A small left-to-right shunt (a result of the flow of blood from the right through the left coronary artery into the pulmonary artery) can often be detected at the pulmonary artery level. Frequently, however, the shunt is very small and can be detected only by the most sensitive techniques, for example, by the use of a hydrogen electrode catheter. Cineangiocardiography following injection of contrast material into the root of the aorta shows absence of origin of the left coronary artery from the aorta. A huge right coronary artery fills directly from the aorta, and the contrast material will flow through the right coronary system into the left coronary arteries and finally into the pulmonary artery.

Treatment & Prognosis

Medical management with anticongestives and afterload reduction is advocated by some but fails to correct the anatomic defect. Operations requiring cardiopulmonary bypass to effect two functional coronary arteries from the aorta have a significant mortality rate in critically ill infants, but survival rates are improving with experience. Simple ligation of the left coronary artery or subclavian to coronary artery anastomosis (without cardiopulmonary bypass) should be considered for the most critically ill infants.

The prognosis is guarded. No therapeutic modality has been shown to be superior in follow-up studies of survivors.

Midgley A et al: Repair of anomalous origin of the left coronary artery in the infant and small child. J Am Coll Cardiol 1984;4:1231.

Sauer U et al: Risk factors for perioperative mortality in children with anomalous origin of the left coronary artery from the pulmonary artery. J Thorac Cardiovasc Surg 1991;102:566.

3. ENDOCARDIAL FIBROELASTOSIS

The incidence of endocardial fibroelastosis has decreased dramatically over the past 2 decades, and this entity is now uncommon. The cause is not known, although intrauterine infection with mumps or coxsackievirus B has been suggested.

Pathologic examination discloses a marked milky white thickening of the endocardium, the subendocardial layers of the left ventricle, and, usually, the left atrium. The mitral valve is frequently involved also. The myocardial fibers themselves are fibrotic and disorganized, and associated hypervascularization is common. Serial sections often show coexistent evidence of myocarditis. Thus, endocardial fibroelastosis appears to be part of a continuum of primary endomyocardial diseases and may be a sequela to myocarditis.

Clinical Findings

A. Symptoms & Signs: Patients appear normal at birth, and growth and development during early infancy are normal. About half develop symptoms within the first 5 months of life, and most are symptomatic by age 1 year. An occasional patient may have no symptoms until age 5 years.

The symptoms and signs that do develop are associated with left ventricular heart failure. These include dyspnea, easy fatigability, feeding difficulties, and, eventually, findings of left and right heart failure.

On physical examination, these children are often small and undernourished. The heart is usually enlarged, and the heart tones are poor (when there is evidence of decompensation). A murmur of mitral regurgitation may be present.

B. Imaging: Chest x-ray films show generalized cardiac enlargement with or without pulmonary venous congestion.

C. Electrocardiography: The ECG almost always shows evidence of left ventricular hypertrophy and, quite frequently, ST depression and T-wave inversion. If there has been pulmonary hypertension secondary to left heart failure, right ventricular hypertrophy may be present. Right atrial hypertrophy is sometimes present. Complete heart block is occasionally seen.

D. Echocardiography: M-mode and two-dimensional techniques reveal dilatation of cardiac chambers and echo-dense endocardial images. Myocardial systolic function is decreased.

E. Cardiac Catheterization & Angiocardiography: Catheterization reveals the absence of left-to-right shunts. Pulmonary hypertension may be present. Cineangiocardiography demonstrates diminished myocardial contractility. Transcatheter endomyocardial biopsy has become a more common technique in infants and children for primary myocardial disease but seldom reveals a cause.

Treatment & Prognosis

Treatment of endocardial fibroelastosis is medical and consists of adequate and prolonged use of digitalis afterload reduction and oral diuretics. If response to the usual dose is not satisfactory, the dosage of both digitalis and diuretics can be increased until a satisfactory response is noted or toxicity occurs. Infants who respond favorably to medical therapy should continue these agents for several years. Infants and children who fail to respond to medical therapy will require cardiac transplantation.

Some children appear to improve initially with treatment but then develop recurrent bouts of heart failure. Complete recovery in such patients is very infrequent, and unless receiving a transplant, most eventually die with intractable congestive heart failure. The prognosis is most favorable in patients who present between 6 months and 3 years of age and respond promptly to treatment.

Chan KY et al: Immunosuppressive therapy in the management of acute myocarditis in children: A clinical trial. J Am Coll Cardiol 1991;17:458.

CYANOTIC HEART DISEASE

TETRALOGY OF FALLOT

Essentials of Diagnosis

- Cyanosis after the neonatal period.
- Hypoxemic spells during infancy.
- Right-sided aortic arch in 25%.
- Systolic ejection murmur at the upper left sternal border.

General Considerations

In Fallot tetralogy, there is a ventricular septal defect and severe obstruction to right ventricular outflow such that the intracardiac shunt is predominantly from right to left. This is the most common type of cyanotic heart lesion, accounting for 10–15% of all cases of congenital heart disease. The ventricular defect is usually located in the membranous portion of the septum but may be totally surrounded by muscular tissue and is usually quite large. Obstruction to right ventricular outflow may be solely at the infundibular level (50–75%), at the valvular level alone (rarely), or at both levels (25% or more). The primary embryologic abnormality is in the septation of the conus and truncus arteriosus, resulting in an enlarged overriding aorta and hypoplasia of the pulmonary trunk. Experimental lesions in specific loci of ectodermal (neural crest) tissue which migrate to the conus can reproduce the defects seen in tetralogy of Fallot. The term *tetralogy* has been used to describe this combination of lesions, since there is always associated right ventricular hypertrophy and a varying degree of "overriding of the aorta." The overriding is present because of the position of the ventricular septal defect in relation to a dilated and often dextroposed aorta. These two factors (right ventricular hypertrophy, overriding aorta) plus the major lesions make up the tetralogy. A right-sided aortic arch is present in 25% of cases, and an atrial septal defect in 15%.

Severe obstruction to right ventricular outflow plus a large ventricular septal defect results in a right-to-left shunt at the ventricular level and desaturation of the arterial blood. The degree of desaturation and the extent of cyanosis depend on the size of the shunt. This in turn is dependent on the resistance to outflow from the right ventricle, the size of the ventricular septal defect, and the systemic vascular resistance. The greater the obstruction, the larger the ventricular septal defect, and the lower the systemic vascular resistance, the greater the right-to-left shunt. Although the patient may be deeply cyanotic, the amount of pressure the right ventricle can develop is limited to that of the systemic (aortic) pressure. In other words, right ventricular pressure cannot exceed left ventricular pressure. The right ventricle is usually able to maintain this level of pressure without developing heart failure.

Clinical Findings

A. Symptoms & Signs: The clinical findings vary depending on the degree of right ventricular outflow obstruction. Patients with a mild degree of obstruction are only minimally cyanotic or acyanotic and may even present initially with congestive heart failure. Those with maximal obstruction are deeply cyanotic from birth. However, few children are asymptomatic; most have cyanosis by 4 months of age, and the cyanosis usually is progressive. Growth and development are retarded, and easy fatigability and dyspnea on exertion are common. Squatting is seen when the children become old enough to walk.

Hypoxemic spells (cyanotic spells) are characterized by the following signs and symptoms: (1) sudden onset of cyanosis or deepening of cyanosis; (2) sudden onset of dyspnea; (3) alterations in consciousness, encompassing a spectrum from irritability to syncope; and (4) decrease in intensity or disappearance of the systolic murmur. These episodes may begin in the neonatal period and continue until nearly school age. It is unusual, however, for the initial episode to occur after 2 years of age. Acute treatment of cyanotic spells consists of giving oxygen and placing the patient in the knee-chest position. Acidosis, if present, should be corrected with intravenous sodium bicarbonate. Morphine sulfate should be administered cautiously by a parenteral route in a dosage of 0.1 mg/kg. Propranolol, 0.1–0.2 mg/kg intravenously, has been found to be useful. Chronic (daily) treatment of cyanotic spells with propranolol, 1 mg/kg orally every 4 hours while awake, remains controversial; however, in a significant number of patients, this regimen has prevented subsequent "spells" and made it possible to delay operation until total correction can be performed.

Patients with tetralogy are usually small and thin. The degree of cyanosis is variable. The fingers and toes show varying degrees of clubbing depending on the age of the child and the severity of the cyanosis.

On examination of the heart, a right ventricular lift is palpable. No thrills are present. The first sound is normal; occasionally, there is an ejection click at the apex that is aortic in origin. The second sound is predominantly aortic and single and best heard at the left sternal border between the third and fourth intercostal spaces. The second heart sound at the pulmonary area is soft. There is a grade I–III/VI, rough, ejection-type systolic murmur that is maximal at the left sternal border in the third intercostal space.

B. Laboratory Findings: The hemoglobin, hematocrit, and red blood cell count are usually mildly to markedly elevated, depending on the degree of arterial oxygen desaturation.

C. Imaging: Chest x-rays reveal the overall heart size to be normal, and indeed the x-ray film may sometimes be interpreted as being entirely normal. However, the right ventricle is hypertrophied, and this is often shown in the posteroanterior projection by an upturning of the apex (boot-shaped heart). The main pulmonary artery segment is usually concave, and the aorta in 25% of cases arches to the right. The pulmonary vascular markings are usually decreased.

D. Electrocardiography: The cardiac axis is to the right, ranging from +90 to +180 degrees. The P waves are usually normal, although there may be evidence of slight right atrial hypertrophy. Right ventricular hypertrophy is always present, but right ventricular strain patterns are rare.

E. Echocardiography: Two-dimensional imaging reveals thickening of the free right ventricular wall, with overriding of the aorta and a membranous ventricular septal defect, and is diagnostic. Furthermore, obstruction at the level of the infundibulum and pulmonary valve can be identified, and the size of the proximal pulmonary arteries can be measured. The anatomy of the coronary arteries may be visualized.

F. Cardiac Catheterization & Angiocardiography: Cardiac catheterization reveals the presence of a right-to-left shunt in most cases. There is arterial blood desaturation of varying degree. The right-to-left shunt exists at the ventricular level. The right ventricular pressure is at systemic levels, and the pressure contour in the right ventricle is identical to that of the left ventricle. The pulmonary artery pressure is extremely low (mean ranges of 5–10 mm Hg). The pressure gradients may be noted at the valvular level, the infundibular level, or both. The catheter frequently is passed from the right ventricle into the overriding ascending aorta but may cause a transient right bundle branch block.

Cineangiocardiography is diagnostic. Injection of contrast material into the right ventricle reveals the right ventricular outflow obstruction and the right-to-left shunt at the ventricular level. With improved echocardiographic techniques, the major indications for cardiac catheterization are to establish coronary artery and distal pulmonary artery anatomy. In addition, some patients may be palliated by balloon dilatation of the right ventricular outflow tract.

Treatment

A. Palliative Treatment: Palliative treatment is recommended for very small infants who are markedly symptomatic (severely cyanotic, frequent severe anoxic spells) and in whom complete correction would be difficult or impossible. Medical (chronic oral beta-blocking agents) or, more often, surgical (creation of a systemic arterial to pulmonary arterial anastomosis) palliation can be used.

The most common surgical palliation is the creation of a Gortex shunt from the subclavian artery to a branch pulmonary artery (modified Blalock-Taussig shunt).

B. Total Correction: The timing of total correction ranges from birth to 2 years, varying with the philosophies and results of each treatment center. It involves closing the ventricular septal defect and removing the obstruction to right ventricular outflow. The surgical death rate varies from 2% to 15%. The major limiting anatomic feature of total correction is the size of the pulmonary artery and its branches.

Course & Prognosis

Infants with the most severe form of the disease are usually deeply cyanotic at birth. Hypoxemic spells may occur during the neonatal period. Death is extremely rare during a severe hypoxemic spell. Many patients who survive the first year of life seem to improve. This may be because of the development of systemic-to-pulmonary collateral vessels. Although hypoxemic spells may decrease in severity, these children remain deeply cyanotic and markedly limited in their activity. They seldom survive the second decade of life without surgical treatment.

Complete repair prior to the school-age years usually results in fair to good function, although patients are occasionally subject to sudden death from dysrhythmias. A competent pulmonary valve without a dilated right ventricle appears to diminish arrhythmias and enhance exercise performance.

Garson A Jr, Gillette PC, McNamara DG: Propranolol: The preferred palliation for tetralogy of Fallot. Am J Cardiol 1981;47:1098.

Gatzoulig MA et al: Right ventricular diastolic function 15 to 35 years after repair of tetralogy of Fallot. Circulation 1995;91:1775.

Murphy JG et al: Long-term outcome in patients undergoing surgical repair of tetralogy of Fallot. N Engl J Med 1993;9:593.

Vaksmann G et al: Frequency and prognosis of arrhythmias after operative "correction" of tetralogy of Fallot. Am J Cardiol 1990;66:346.

Vobecky SJ et al: Survival analysis of infants under age 18 months with tetralogy of Fallot. Ann Thorac Surg 1993;56:944.

Warner KG et al: Restoration of the pulmonary valve reduces right ventricular volume overload after previous repair of tetralogy of Fallot. Circulation 1993;88(Suppl):II-189.

PULMONARY ATRESIA WITH VENTRICULAR SEPTAL DEFECT

This condition consists of complete atresia of the pulmonary valve in association with ventricular septal defect. Essentially, it is an extreme form of tetralogy of Fallot. Since there is no flow outward from the right ventricle into the pulmonary artery, the pulmonary blood flow must be derived either from a patent ductus arteriosus or from collateral channels.

The clinical picture depends entirely on the size of the ductus or the collateral channels (or both). If they are large, patients may do well and actually do better than those with severe tetralogy of Fallot. If effective pulmonary blood flow is small, death occurs secondary to severe anoxia early in life. This may occur suddenly with postnatal closure of a patent ductus arteriosus.

Echocardiography or cardiac catheterization and angiocardiography are diagnostic. If patent ductus arteriosus dependency is established, a PGE_1 infusion to dilate the patent ductus arteriosus may help stabilize the patient until surgery.

Infants who are severely hypoxemic require urgent systemic-to-pulmonary anastomosis in order to provide sufficient oxygenated blood to the body.

A corrective surgical procedure that has been successful in patients with adequate-sized pulmonary arteries consists of bypassing the obstructed right ventricular outflow and closing the ventricular septal defect. Success may depend on precise definition of pulmonary arterial and collateral blood supply to the lung and prior unifocalization of segments with dual arterial blood supply. More recently, an approach has been adopted to create initially a central connection between the right ventricle or aorta to the central pulmonary artery.

Hoffback KM et al: Analysis of survival in patients with pulmonic valve atresia and ventricular septal defect. Am J Cardiol 1991;67:737.

Marelli AJ et al: Pulmonary atresia with ventricular septal defect in adults. Circulation 1994;89:243.

PULMONARY ATRESIA WITH INTACT VENTRICULAR SEPTUM

Essentials of Diagnosis

- Cyanosis at birth.
- Chest x-ray film with a concave pulmonary artery segment and the apex tilted upward.

General Considerations

In this uncommon condition, the pulmonary valve is absent and is replaced by a small diaphragm consisting of the fused cusps. The ventricular septum is intact. The main pulmonary artery segment is somewhat hypoplastic but almost always patent. In type 1 deformity (80%), the cavity volume of the right ventricle is extremely small and the wall is thickened and fibrotic. In type 2, the right ventricular cavity is frequently of normal size.

During intrauterine life, if the tricuspid valve is intact and normal, very little blood enters the right ventricle, since there is no outlet for this chamber. Almost all of the blood passes through the foramen ovale directly into the left side of the heart. In type 2 deformity, there is usually an outlet for the right ventricle (tricuspid valve insufficiency), and the right ventricle receives a sufficient quantity of blood to permit it to develop in a relatively normal fashion.

Following birth, the pulmonary circulation is maintained primarily by a patent ductus arteriosus. Although a bronchial pulmonary collateral network is present, it is usually insufficient to maintain the pulmonary circulation. Accordingly, whether or not the patients live depends on the patency of the ductus arteriosus. The ductus usually remains open for only a short period. As it closes, hypoxia becomes progressively more severe, and death occurs within several hours.

Clinical Findings

A. Symptoms & Signs: Patients may be normal at birth, although they are usually cyanotic. Cyanosis becomes progressively more severe and is associated with severe dyspnea. A blowing systolic murmur resulting from the associated patent ductus arteriosus may be heard at the pulmonary area and under the left clavicle. In type 2 deformity, a loud pansystolic murmur caused by the tricuspid insufficiency is heard at the lower left sternal border. Not infrequently, the liver is pulsatile.

B. Imaging: Chest x-rays vary from a small to a markedly enlarged heart, depending on the presence or degree of tricuspid insufficiency. With striking tricuspid insufficiency, right atrial enlargement may be massive and the cardiac silhouette may virtually fill the chest.

C. Electrocardiography: Electrocardiography reveals an axis that is usually normal in the frontal plane. Evidence for right atrial enlargement is usually striking. Voltage criteria for other chamber enlargement are variable.

D. Echocardiography: M-mode and two-dimensional echocardiography shows absence of the pulmonary valve, with varying degrees of hypoplasia of the right ventricular cavity and tricuspid annulus. The severity of tricuspid regurgitation often correlates positively with right ventricular size.

E. Cardiac Catheterization & Angiocardiography: Right ventricular pressure is very high (greater than systemic). A cineangiocardiogram following injection of contrast material into the right ventricle reveals absence of filling of the pulmonary artery from the right ventricle. It also demonstrates the size of the right ventricular chamber, relative hypoplasia of the components of the tripartite right ventricle (inflow, trabecular, infundibulum), and the presence or absence of tricuspid regurgitation, and right ventricular sinusoids that anastomose with the coronary arteries may fill.

Treatment & Prognosis

As in pulmonary atresia with ventricular septal defect, a PGE_1 infusion is useful in stabilizing the patient and maintaining patency of the ductus until surgery can be performed. Surgery should be undertaken as soon as the diagnosis is made. A Rashkind atrial septostomy is performed, depending on right ventricular size, to open up the communication across the atrial septum. Occasionally, a balloon valvotomy can be done. Subsequent surgical approaches vary widely. In cases of type 1 deformity, it is necessary to immediately establish a surgical aorticopulmonary anastomosis (usually a Blalock-Taussig shunt). Later in infancy, a communication between the right ventricle and pulmonary artery should be created in an attempt to stimulate right ventricular cavity growth. In cases of type 2 deformity, a closed valvotomy may be all that is necessary initially, with a more definitive reconstruction of the right ventricular outflow tract accomplished at a later date.

The prognosis is unpredictable for patients with type 1 or type 2 deformity who survive the surgery. In type 1 patients, the dimensions of the right ventricle can increase significantly after the initial procedure. Overall, however, this disorder remains one of the least satisfactory forms of cyanotic congenital heart disease.

Giaglia TM et al: Diagnosis and management of right ventricle dependent coronary circulation in pulmonary atresia with intact ventricular septum. Circulation 1992; 86:1516.

Hanley FL et al: Outcomes in neonatal pulmonary atresia with intact ventricular septum: A multiinstitutional study. J Am Coll Cardiol 1993;21:1454.

TRICUSPID ATRESIA

Essential of Diagnosis

- Marked cyanosis present from birth.
- ECG with left axis deviation, right atrial enlargement, and left ventricular hypertrophy.

General Considerations

This relatively rare condition (<1% of cases of congenital heart disease) is characterized by complete atresia of the tricuspid valve. As a result, no direct communication exists between the right atrium and the right ventricle.

Tricuspid atresia may be divided into two types, depending on the relationship of the great vessels:

Type 1. Without transposition of the great arteries: (a) No ventricular septal defect. Hypoplasia or atresia of the pulmonary artery. Patent ductus arteriosus. (b) Small ventricular septal defect. Pulmonary stenosis. Hypoplastic pulmonary artery. (c) Large ventricular septal defect and no pulmonary stenosis. Normal-sized pulmonary artery.

Type 2. With transposition of the great arteries: (a) With ventricular septal defect and pulmonary stenosis. (b) With ventricular septal defect but without pulmonary stenosis.

Because there is no direct communication between the right atrium and the right ventricle, the entire systemic venous return must flow through the atrial septum (either an atrial septal defect or patent foramen ovale) into the left atrium. Accordingly, the left atrium receives both the systemic venous return and the pulmonary venous return. Complete mixing occurs in the left atrium, resulting in a greater or lesser degree of arterial desaturation.

As a result of this lack of direct communication, the development of the ventricle depends on the presence of a left-to-right shunt at the ventricular level. Therefore, severe hypoplasia of the right ventricle occurs in those forms in which there is no ventricular septal defect or in which the ventricular septal defect is very small.

Clinical Findings

A. Symptoms & Signs: In most patients with tricuspid atresia, symptoms develop very early in infancy. Except in patients whose pulmonary blood flow is great, cyanosis is present at birth. Growth and development are very poor, and there is usually easy fatigability on feeding, tachypnea, dyspnea, anoxic spells, and evidence of right heart failure. Patients with marked increase in pulmonary blood flow (types 1c and 2b) may develop evidence of left heart failure as well.

Clubbing is present if the child is old enough. On examination of the heart, a slight bulge on the right side of the sternum may occasionally be seen. The first heart sound is normal. The second heart sound is most often single (owing to aortic closure). A murmur is usually present, although it is variable. It ranges from grade I to grade III/VI in intensity and usually is a harsh blowing murmur heard best at the lower left sternal border.

B. Imaging: Chest x-ray findings are variable. The heart may be slightly to markedly enlarged. The main pulmonary artery segment is usually small or absent. The size of the right atrium varies from huge to only moderately enlarged, depending on the size of the communication at the atrial level. The pulmonary vascular markings are usually decreased, although in types 1c and 2b they are increased.

C. Electrocardiography: The ECG is usually helpful. It often shows a left axis deviation with a counterclockwise loop in the frontal plane. The P waves are tall and peaked, indicative of right atrial hypertrophy. The size of the P wave depends on the right atrial pressure, which in turn depends on the size of the interatrial communication (the taller the P wave, the smaller the communication). Left ventricular hypertrophy or left ventricular preponderance is found in almost all cases. Voltage over the right precordium is usually low.

D. Echocardiography: M-mode and two-dimensional methods are diagnostic and show absence of the tricuspid valve, the relationship of the great vessels, and the sources of pulmonary blood flow.

E. Cardiac Catheterization & Angiocardiography: This reveals the marked right-to-left shunt at the atrial level and desaturation of the left atrial blood. Because of the complete mixing in the left atrial chambers, oxygen saturation in the left ventricle, right ventricle, pulmonary artery, and aorta is identical to that in the left atrium. The right atrial pressure is increased. Left ventricular and systemic pressures are normal. The catheter cannot be passed through the tricuspid valve from the right atrium to the right ventricle. The course of the catheter is always from the right atrium into the left atrium and from there into the left ventricle. An atrial balloon septostomy is performed if a restrictive communication is present.

Treatment & Prognosis

In infants with high pulmonary artery flow, conventional anticongestive therapy should be given until the infant begins to outgrow the ventricular septal defect. Occasionally, a pulmonary artery band is needed to protect the pulmonary vascular bed in preparation for a Fontan procedure. A Fontan procedure (connection of the right atrium to the right ventricle or pulmonary artery) is performed when increasing cyanosis occurs.

In infants with extremely low pulmonary artery flow, PGE_1 should be infused until an aorticopulmonary shunt can be performed. The Fontan procedure is rapidly gaining acceptance as the palliative procedure of choice. The optimal timing is controversial, but the procedure has been performed successfully in infants under 1 year of age.

The prognosis for all patients with tricuspid atresia depends on achieving a balance of pulmonary blood flow that permits adequate oxygenation of the tissues without producing intractable congestive heart failure. For children treated by the Fontan procedure, the prognosis is as yet undefined; initial results are moderately encouraging.

Franklin RCG et al: Tricuspid atresia presenting in infancy: Survival and suitability for the Fontan operation. Circulation 1993;87:427.

HYPOPLASTIC LEFT HEART SYNDROME

Essentials of Diagnosis

- Mild cyanosis at birth. Minimal auscultatory findings.
- Rapid onset of shock with ductal closure.

General Considerations

Hypoplastic left heart syndrome includes a number of conditions in which there are either valvular or vascular lesions on the left side of the heart, resulting in hypoplasia of the left ventricle. The syndrome is found in 1.4–3.8% of infants with congenital heart disease.

The lesions that make up this syndrome are mitral atresia, aortic atresia, or both. In all of these conditions, there is severe obstruction to either filling or emptying of the left ventricle. As a result, during intrauterine life, the quantity of blood filling the left ventricle is extremely small, resulting in hypoplasia of this chamber. Following birth, survival depends on a patent ductus arteriosus. there is marked impairment of the circulation because of the very small size of the left ventricle and the presence of obstructing lesions. Congestive heart failure develops rapidly, in most cases within several days to 3 months of life.

Patients with aortic atresia develop congestive heart failure very early, usually within the first week. Death occurs earliest in this group. Patients with mitral atresia who have large atrial and ventricular communications may live longer. Some patients have lived beyond the first decade. Patients with involvement of the aortic arch usually die within 1 month or less.

Clinical Findings

A. Symptoms & Signs: The clinical picture depends on the type of obstructing lesion. Cyanosis is usually present early in life and is usually generalized. Patients with hypoplasia or atresia of the aortic arch may show differential cyanosis. Murmurs may or may not be present and are usually nondiagnostic. Congestive heart failure and shock accompany closure of the ductus arteriosus.

B. Imaging: Chest x-ray findings usually are relatively normal at birth. Rapid and progressive cardiac enlargement then occurs, frequently associated with pulmonary venous congestion. These changes occur earliest in patients with aortic atresia.

C. Electrocardiography: The ECG usually demonstrates right axis deviation, right atrial hypertrophy, and right ventricular hypertrophy with relative paucity of left ventricular forces and absence of a Q wave in V_6.

D. Echocardiography: Echocardiography is usually diagnostic and eliminates the need for cardiac catheterization. A diminutive aorta and left ventricle with a poorly defined mitral valve in the presence of a normal and easily definable tricuspid valve are diagnostic. The systemic circulation is dependent on the patent ductus arteriosus. There is retrograde flow in the aortic arch with color Doppler imaging.

Treatment & Prognosis

PGE_1 infusion is essential initial management, since systemic circulation depends on a patent ductus arteriosus. Further management depends on balancing pulmonary and systemic blood flow, because the right ventricle provides both. With increasing postnatal age, the pulmonary resistance falls, favoring pulmonary overcirculation and compromised systemic perfusion. Techniques to increase pulmonary vascular tone—such as hypoxia and hypercapnic ventilation, increased viscosity (hematocrit), and avoidance of pharmacologic pulmonary vasodilators—can improve systemic perfusion.

Definitive therapy at present is creation of single-ventricle physiology operatively, as with the Norwood procedure and its variants. An increasing number of infants are receiving orthotopic cardiac transplantation in infancy to replace the defective cardiac anatomy.

The prognosis for this once uniformly lethal syndrome is improving. Palliative operations can now be performed with survival rates of 50–75%. Many palliated infants may ultimately require transplantation. The 1-year survival rates with primary transplantation are over 80%. Further advances in surgery and immunology are likely to continue to improve the prognosis.

Bailey LL et al: One hundred fifteen late survivors of heart transplantation during the first year of life. J Thorac Cardiovasc Surg 1993;105:805.

Boucek MM, Bernstein D: Heart transplantation in infancy. Prog Pediatr Cardiol 1993;2:20.

Morris CD, Outcalt J, Menashe VD: Hypoplastic left heart syndrome: Natural history in a geographically defined population. Pediatrics 1990;85:977.

COMPLETE TRANSPOSITION OF THE GREAT ARTERIES

Essentials of Diagnosis

- Cyanotic newborn without respiratory distress.
- More common in males.

General Considerations

Complete transposition of the great vessels is the second most common variety of cyanotic congenital heart disease, accounting for about 16% of all cases. The male/female ratio is 3:1. The disorder is caused by an embryologic abnormality in the spiral division of the truncus arteriosus.

The aorta is located anterior to the pulmonary artery—either directly anterior or to the left or right. The pulmonary artery usually ascends parallel to the aorta rather than crosses it. In most cases, associated intracardiac abnormalities are present. These include ventricular septal defect, atrial septal defect, pulmonary stenosis, and patent ductus arteriosus. Obstructive changes within the pulmonary arteriolar bed are common in patients past infancy.

Transposition of the great vessels can be classified as follows:

Group 1. Transposition with intact ventricular septum: (a) Without pulmonary stenosis or (b) with pulmonary stenosis, subvalvular or valvular (or both).

Group 2. Transposition with ventricular septal defect: (a) With pulmonary stenosis, (b) with pulmonary vascular obstruction, or (c) without pulmonary vascular obstruction (normal pulmonary vascular resistance).

Since the aorta arises directly from the right ventricle, life would not be possible unless there were mixing between the systemic and pulmonary circulations; oxygenated blood from the pulmonary veins must, in some way, reach the systemic arterial circuit. In patients with intact ventricular septum (group 1), mixing occurs at the atrial and also at the ductal levels. However, in most patients, these communications are small, and the ductus arteriosus often closes shortly after birth. These patients are therefore severely cyanotic, and congestive heart failure occurs rapidly as a result of the marked increase in cardiac output. Patients with a ventricular septal defect show greater or lesser degrees of cyanosis, depending on the ratio of the pulmonary to systemic blood flow. Patients with ventricular septal defect and pulmonary stenosis (groups 2a and 2b) are usually severely cyanotic because of the limited blood flow to the lungs. Patients with ventricular septal defect and pulmonary vascular obstruction (group 2b) show a moderate degree of cyanosis. Patients with ventricular septal defect and normal pulmonary vascular resistance (group 2c) show the least cyanosis but often develop heart failure very early because of the enormous pulmonary blood flow.

Congestive heart failure develops not only because of the high cardiac output but also because of the poor oxygenation of the myocardium and the presence of systemic pressure in both ventricles.

Clinical Findings

A. Symptoms & Signs: Many of the neonates are large, some weighing 4 kg (9 lb) at birth, and most are cyanotic at birth, although cyanosis occasionally does not develop until later. Patients in groups 1 and 2a are most cyanotic. Retardation of growth and development after the neonatal period is common. Congestive heart failure occurs in patients in groups 1 and 2c. Patients in group 2a show no evidence of congestive heart failure but often have severe anoxic spells in early life.

Although these infants are usually large at birth, growth and development are retarded before definitive surgery. The findings on cardiovascular examination depend somewhat on the intracardiac defects. Group 1a patients have only soft murmurs or none at all. The first heart sound is usually normal. The second heart sound is single and accentuated and is best heard at the lower left sternal border. Patients in group 1b have loud obstructive systolic murmurs that are maximal at the second and third intercostal spaces and the left sternal border, radiating well to the first and second intercostal spaces. Group 2a patients have a murmur of pulmonary stenosis (obstructive systolic murmur at the base of the heart, best heard to the right of the sternum). Those in group 2c have a systolic murmur along the lower sternal border and a mitral diastolic flow murmur at the apex.

B. Imaging: In the sick, blue newborn, at a time when any diagnostic clues are greatly appreciated, the chest x-ray in transposition is often very nonspecific.

C. Electrocardiography: Early in infancy, the ECG is usually of little positive help. It reveals the usual amount of right ventricular hypertrophy expected for age.

D. Echocardiography: Two-dimensional imaging and Doppler evaluation can accurately describe the anatomy and physiology in infants with transposition. The abnormal relationship of the great vessels is the hallmark of transposition on echocardiography. Even the balloon septostomy may be performed with echo guidance.

E. Cardiac Catheterization & Angiocardiography: Cardiac catheterization has a dual purpose in this malformation: diagnosis and therapy. As soon as the cardiologist has confidently demonstrated that complete transposition of the great arteries exists and that there are two well-developed ventricles, a Rashkind septostomy may be performed. The coronary anatomy can be delineated by ascending aortography.

Treatment

It has become increasingly apparent at many pediatric cardiology centers throughout the world that survival of patients with transposition of the great arteries depends on early, aggressive management. Cardiac catheterization is no longer routine for all types of transposition. Complex variations such as 2a, 2b, and 2c may still require invasive evaluation. PGE$_1$ infusion may improve mixing of oxygenated blood by opening the ductus arteriosus.

All patients with favorable anatomic and hemodynamic criteria (type 1) should be offered corrective surgery by 1 month of age. Surgery traditionally involved insertion of an intra-atrial baffle (by either a Mustard or a Senning operation) to redirect systemic and pulmonary venous blood to the appropriate pulmonary and aortic ventricles. Since 1975, surgical techniques to "switch" the great vessels to their anatomically appropriate locations have undergone a slow evolution. A key feature in the development of techniques has been careful patient selection. The left ventricular musculature in this entity rapidly loses its muscle mass and potential to meet systemic afterload unless a large ventricular septal defect or left ventricular outflow obstruction occurs; consequently, newborns with either of these conditions are appropriate candidates.

The incidence of death from this type of surgery

has fallen from 25% to approximately 10%. Although the death rate following an intra-atrial baffling procedure may be lower, there is growing concern about the long-term ability of an anatomic right ventricle to function as a systemic circulation pump. During the past several years, most institutions have begun using anatomic correction techniques in almost all patients. As the use of anatomic correction (vessel switch) techniques has spread to more centers, postoperative complications such as supravalvular pulmonary stenosis and stenoses or kinking of coronary arteries have been noted. The long-term exercise capacity of patients after interatrial rerouting operations has, in some studies, turned out to be better than that projected by early studies. Long-term results for anatomic correction are yet to be determined. The intermediate-term results appear to be excellent for the arterial switch procedure.

Lupinetti FM et al: Intermediate-term survival and functional results after arterial repair for transposition of the great arteries. J Thorac Cardiovasc Surg 1992;103:421.

Serraf A et al: Anatomic correction of transposition of the great arteries in neonates. J Am Coll Cardiol 1993; 22:1933.

ORIGIN OF BOTH GREAT VESSELS FROM THE RIGHT VENTRICLE

In this rare malformation, the aorta is completely transposed, but the pulmonary artery occupies a relatively normal position. Accordingly, both great vessels arise from the right ventricle. Ventricular septal defect is present in all cases and provides the only outlet for the left ventricle.

This malformation may be divided into five types on the basis of the relationship of the ventricular septal defect to the great arteries and the presence or absence of pulmonary stenosis: (1) ventricular septal defect related to the aorta, (2) ventricular septal defect related to the pulmonary artery (Taussig-Bing type), (3) ventricular septal defect committed to both great vessels, (4) ventricular septal defect uncommitted to the great vessels, and (5) ventricular septal defect related to the aorta, with pulmonary stenosis (tetralogy of Fallot type).

The clinical and laboratory features depend on which of the five anatomic types occurs. Two-dimensional echocardiography has proved to be extremely important in the diagnosis and classification of this entity.

Surgical correction is most satisfactory in patients with ventricular septal defect related to the aorta and is effected by closing the defect and creating a tunnel from the left ventricle to the aorta via the patch. Correction of uncommitted defects or defects related to the pulmonary artery requires patch closure and directing the blood to the pulmonary artery, thereby creating a transposition of the great vessels and an associated interatrial rerouting procedure. The use of a valved external conduit may be necessary in the complex varieties.

Roberson DA, Silverman NH: Malaligned outlet septum with subpulmonary ventricular septal defect and abnormal ventriculoarterial connection: A morphologic spectrum defined echocardiographically. J Am Coll Cardiol 1990;16:459.
Serraf A et al: Subaortic obstruction in double outlet right ventricles. Circulation 1993;88(Suppl):II-177.

TOTAL ANOMALOUS PULMONARY VENOUS RETURN WITH OR WITHOUT OBSTRUCTION

Essentials of Diagnosis

- Cyanosis.
- Systolic ejection murmur with left sternal border flow rumble and accentuated P_2.
- Right atrial and right ventricular hypertrophy.
- Pulmonary venous connection.

General Considerations

This malformation accounts for approximately 2% of all congenital heart lesions. The pulmonary venous blood drains not into the left atrium but either directly or indirectly (via a systemic venous connection) into the right atrium. Thus, the entire venous drainage of the body drains into the right atrium.

This malformation may be classified according to the site of entry of the pulmonary veins into the right side of the heart.

Type 1 (55%): Entry into the left superior vena cava (persistent anterior cardinal vein) or right superior vena cava.

Type 2: Entry into the right atrium or into the coronary sinus.

Type 3: Entry below the diaphragm (usually into the portal vein).

Type 4: Multiple types of entry.

Since the entire venous drainage from the body drains into the right atrium, a right-to-left shunt is always present at the atrial level. This may take the form of either a large atrial septal defect or a patent foramen ovale. Relatively complete mixing of the systemic and pulmonary venous return occurs in the right atrium, so that the left atrial and hence the systemic arterial saturation levels approximately equal that of the right atrial saturation.

The degree of desaturation of the blood (and thus the degree of cyanosis present) is determined by the ratio of the quantity of pulmonary blood flow to that of the systemic blood flow.

Clinical Findings

A. With Normal Pulmonary Vascular Resistance: Most patients in this group have some eleva-

tion of the pulmonary artery pressure owing to the marked increase in pulmonary blood flow. In most cases, the pressure does not reach systemic levels.

1. Symptoms and signs–These patients may have a history of mild cyanosis in the neonatal period and during early infancy. Thereafter, they do relatively well except for frequent respiratory infections. They are usually rather small and thin and resemble patients with very large atrial septal defects.

Careful examination discloses duskiness of the nail beds and mucous membranes, but definite cyanosis and clubbing are usually not present. The arterial pulses are normal. The jugular venous pulses usually show a significant V wave. Examination of the heart shows left chest prominence. A right ventricular heaving impulse is palpable.

The pulmonary component of the second sound is usually increased in intensity. A grade II–IV/VI ejection-type systolic murmur is heard at the pulmonary area. It radiates very well over the lung fields anteriorly and posteriorly. An early to mid-diastolic flow murmur is often heard at the lower left sternal border in the third and fourth intercostal spaces (tricuspid flow murmur).

2. Imaging–Chest x-ray reveals evidence of cardiac enlargement primarily involving the right atrium, right ventricle, and pulmonary artery. There is a marked increase in pulmonary vascular markings. There is often a characteristic contour called a "snowman" or "figure of 8," which is seen where the anomalous veins drain into a persistent left superior vena cava.

3. Electrocardiography–Electrocardiography reveals right axis deviation and varying degrees of right atrial and right ventricular hypertrophy. There is often a QR pattern over the right precordial leads.

4. Echocardiography–Demonstration by echocardiography of a chamber posterior to the left atrium is strongly suggestive of the diagnosis. However, echocardiographic discrimination between anomalies of pulmonary venous return and persistence of pulmonary fetal circulation can still be challenging. The availability of two-dimensional echocardiography plus color flow Doppler has increased the diagnostic accuracy.

B. With Increased Pulmonary Vascular Resistance: This group includes patients in whom the pulmonary veins drain into a systemic venous structure below the diaphragm. It also includes a small number of patients in whom the venous drainage is into a systemic vein above the diaphragm.

1. Symptoms and signs–These infants are usually quite sick. Fifty percent die within the first 6 months; most are dead by age 1 year unless treated surgically. Cyanosis is common at birth and is evident by 1 week. Another common early symptom is severe tachypnea. Congestive heart failure develops later.

Cardiac examination discloses a striking right ventricular impulse. A shock of the second sound is palpable. The first heart sound is accentuated. The second heart sound is markedly accentuated and single. A grade I–II/VI ejection-type systolic murmur is frequently heard over the pulmonary area with radiation over the lung fields. Diastolic murmurs are uncommon. In many cases, no murmur is heard at all.

2. Imaging–In the most severe and classic cases, the heart is small and pulmonary venous congestion is marked. In less severe cases, the heart may be slightly enlarged or normal in size, with only slight pulmonary venous congestion.

3. Electrocardiography–The ECG shows right axis deviation, right atrial hypertrophy, and right ventricular hypertrophy.

4. Echocardiography–Echocardiography may demonstrate the combination of a small left atrium and a vessel lying parallel and anterior to the descending aorta and to the left of the inferior vena cava. Color flow Doppler echocardiographic patterns are useful in establishing the diagnosis and are often diagnostic.

5. Cardiac catheterization and angiocardiography–These procedures are diagnostic. Cardiac catheterization demonstrates the presence of total anomalous pulmonary venous return and (usually) the site of entry of the anomalous veins. It also demonstrates the ratio of the pulmonary to systemic blood flow and the degree of pulmonary hypertension and pulmonary vascular resistance.

Cineangiocardiography following injection of contrast material into the right ventricle or pulmonary artery demonstrates the presence of anomalous pulmonary venous return and the site of entry of the anomalous veins.

Treatment

If immediate surgical intervention is not contemplated, atrial balloon septostomy should be performed during the initial diagnostic cardiac catheterization. This procedure, combined with vigorous medical management, may sustain some infants for several months. Most centers have reported excellent surgical results using either cardiopulmonary bypass or deep hypothermia (cooling to 20 °C). A modification of the anastomosis allowing a larger communication has also greatly improved the surgical results. In such centers, the option of immediate surgical correction may be taken.

Course & Prognosis

Patients with normal pulmonary vascular resistance and only modest elevation of pulmonary artery pressures may do well through the first or second decade. Eventually, however, a progressive increase in pulmonary vascular resistance and pulmonary hypertension does occur. Patients with increased pulmonary vascular resistance and pulmonary hypertension do poorly, and most die unless treated before age 1 year.

Cobanoglu A, Menashe VD: Total anomalous pulmonary venous connection in neonates and young infants: Repair in the current era. Ann Thorac Surg 1993;55:43.

Wang JK et al: Obstructed total anomalous pulmonary venous connection. Pediatr Cardiol 1993;14:28.

PERSISTENT TRUNCUS ARTERIOSUS

Essentials of Diagnosis

- Neonatal cyanosis.
- Systolic ejection click.

General Considerations

Persistent truncus arteriosus probably accounts for less than 1% of all congenital heart malformations. Only one (huge) great vessel arises from the heart and supplies both the systemic and pulmonary arterial beds. It develops embryologically as a result of complete lack of formation of the spiral ridges that divide the fetal truncus arteriosus into the aorta and the pulmonary artery. A high ventricular septal defect is always present. The number of valve leaflets varies from two to 6, and the valve may be sufficient, insufficient, or stenotic.

The classification most commonly used is divided into four types:

Type 1: One pulmonary artery that arises from the base of the trunk just above the semilunar valve and runs parallel with the ascending aorta (48%).

Type 2: Two pulmonary arteries that arise side by side from the posterior aspect of the truncus (29%).

Type 3: Two pulmonary arteries that arise independently from either side of the trunk (11%).

Type 4: No demonstrable pulmonary artery (12%). Pulmonary circulation is derived from bronchials arising from the descending thoracic aorta. (The existence of this variety of truncus is controversial. Many authorities consider it an extreme form of tetralogy of Fallot with an atretic main pulmonary artery.)

In this condition, blood leaves the heart through a single common exit. Therefore, the saturation of the blood in the pulmonary artery is the same as that in the systemic arteries. The degree of systemic arterial oxygen saturation depends on the ratio of the pulmonary to systemic blood flow. If pulmonary vascular resistance is normal, the pulmonary blood flow is much greater than the systemic blood flow and the saturation is relatively high. If pulmonary vascular resistance is great, owing either to pulmonary vascular obstruction or to very small pulmonary arteries, pulmonary blood flow is reduced and oxygen saturation is low. The systolic pressures in both ventricles are identical to that in the aorta.

Clinical Findings

A. Symptoms & Signs: The clinical picture

varies depending on the degree of pulmonary blood flow.

1. Large pulmonary blood flow–Patients with large pulmonary blood flow do well and are usually acyanotic, although the nail beds are commonly dusky. They function similarly to patients with large ventricular septal defects and pulmonary hypertension. Examination of the heart reveals a hyperactive impulse, felt both at the apex and over the xiphoid process. A systolic thrill is common at the lower left sternal border. The first heart sound is normal. A loud early systolic ejection click is commonly heard. The second sound is single and accentuated. A grade IV/VI, completely pansystolic murmur is audible at the lower left sternal border. A diastolic flow murmur can often be heard at the apex (mitral flow murmur).

2. Decreased pulmonary blood flow–Patients with decreased pulmonary blood flow have marked cyanosis early and do very poorly. The most common manifestations include retardation of growth and development, easy fatigability, dyspnea on exertion, and congestive heart failure. The heart is not unduly active. The first and second heart sounds are loud. A systolic grade II–IV/VI murmur is heard at the lower left sternal border. No diastolic flow murmur is heard. A continuous heart murmur is very uncommon except in type 4, in which the continuous murmur is caused by the large bronchial collateral vessels. A very loud systolic ejection click is commonly heard.

B. Imaging: The most common x-ray findings are a boot-shaped heart, absence of the main pulmonary artery segment, and a large aorta that frequently arches to the right. The pulmonary vascular markings vary, depending on the degree of pulmonary blood flow.

C. Electrocardiography: The axis is usually normal, although left axis deviation occurs rarely. Evidence of right ventricular hypertrophy or combined ventricular hypertrophy is commonly present. Left ventricular hypertrophy as an isolated finding is rare.

D. Echocardiography: A characteristic image would exhibit override of a single great artery (similar to tetralogy of Fallot) without a demonstrable right ventricular infundibulum. The origin or the pulmonary arteries and the degree of truncal valve abnormality can be seen. Color flow Doppler can aid in the description of pulmonary flow.

E. Angiocardiography: This procedure is usually diagnostic. Injection of contrast material into the right ventricle demonstrates the presence of a ventricular septal defect and the single vessel arising from the heart. The exact type of truncus, however, may be somewhat difficult to determine even from angiocardiograms.

Treatment

Anticongestive measures are indicated for patients with high pulmonary blood flow and congestive failure. Aortic homografting for "total correction" of the truncus has been performed in selected patients. During the past several years, the number of severely symptomatic infants undergoing successful "total correction" in the first 3 months of life has increased. Operative repair requires placement of a conduit from right ventricle to the pulmonary artery, and as the child grows replacement will be necessary.

Course & Prognosis

The outcome depends to a great extent on the status of the pulmonary circulation and the competence of the truncal valve. Patients with a low pulmonary blood flow usually do very poorly and die within 1 year. Those with increased pulmonary blood flow can survive for a variable period. A few cases of survival without surgery into the third decade have been reported. Death is usually the result of congestive heart failure, hypoxia, subacute infective endocarditis, or brain abscess. Surgical repair has dramatically improved the prognosis.

Juanida E, Haworth SG: Pulmonary vascular disease in children with truncus arteriosus. Am J Cardiol 1984; 54:1315.

Pierpont MEM et al: Cardiac malformations in relatives of children with truncus arteriosus or interruption of the aortic arch. Am J Cardiol 1988;61:423.

Samanek M: Children with congenital heart disease: Probability of natural survival. Pediatr Cardiol 1992;13:152.

DEXTROCARDIA

This lesion consists of right-sided heart with or without reversal of position of other organs (situs inversus). If there is no reversal of other organs, the heart usually has other severe defects. With complete situs inversus, the heart is usually normal.

Apical pulse and sounds are heard on the right side of the chest. X-ray film shows the cardiac silhouette on the right side. On electrocardiography, the P waves are usually inverted in lead I; QRS is predominantly down in lead I; and lead II resembles normal lead III and vice versa. Two-dimensional echocardiography is extremely useful in defining the complex anatomy.

With situs inversus and no heart defects, the prognosis is excellent. If severe heart defects are present, definitive diagnosis is imperative, because corrective surgery is frequently beneficial.

Emmanouilides GC, Baylen BG: Dextrocardia and the cardiosplenic syndromes. In: *Neonatal Cardiopulmonary Distress.* Emmanouilides GC, Baylen BG (editors). Year Book, 1988.

Van Praagh R et al: Malposition of the heart. In: *Heart Disease in Infants, Children, and Adolescents,* 4th ed.

Adams FH, Emmanouilides GC, Riemenschneider TA (editors). Williams & Wilkins, 1989.

ACQUIRED HEART DISEASE

RHEUMATIC FEVER

Rheumatic fever is a disease in transition. Although it is still an important disease in the United States, its incidence has diminished significantly over the past half-century. Penicillin is largely responsible, but the decrease in rheumatic fever was already apparent before the antibiotic era. In the United States and other developed countries in the temperate zone, improvement in standards of living, general hygiene, and opportunities for medical care have greatly reduced the incidence of this disease. However, there has been a resurgence of acute rheumatic fever in several regions of the United States (the Midwest in 1984 and the intermountain West in 1987). In addition, the character of the illness is more malignant than that seen in the 1970s, with a high incidence of associated carditis and chorea. The reason for these regional epidemics is not as yet known, but it is clear that the disease has returned.

Until the recent epidemic, the symptomatic presentation of the disease had also changed significantly in the United States within the past 2 decades. The frequency with which one encounters severe, disabling carditis has greatly diminished, and the attack rate of acute rheumatic fever is considerably less than the original estimate of 0.3% in untreated children. Current manifestations of carditis are often mild and transient and require serial examinations by a skilled auscultator or echocardiography to confirm or rule out the diagnosis. The combination of chorea and carditis, previously noted to be rare, has been common during the recent epidemic. One can only speculate on the reasons for these changes in the epidemiologic characteristics of the disease in different communities.

Group A β-hemolytic streptococcal infection of the upper respiratory tract is the essential environmental trigger that acts on predisposed individuals. The latest attempts to define host susceptibility implicate immune response (Ir) genes, which are present in approximately 15% of the population. The immune response triggered by colonization of the pharynx with group A streptococci consists of (1) sensitization of B lymphocytes by streptococcal antigens, (2) formation of antistreptococcal antibody, (3) formation of immune complexes that cross-react with cardiac sarcolemma antigens, and (4) myocardial and valvular inflammatory response.

The peak period of risk in the United States is age 5–15 years. The disease is slightly more common in girls and is now more common in blacks, perhaps reflecting socioeconomic factors. The average annual attack rate in the total North American population is less than 1 per 10,000, and the presence of rheumatic heart disease in the school-age population is less than 1 per 1000. The annual death rate from rheumatic heart disease in school-age children (whites and nonwhites) recorded a decade ago was less than 1 per 100,000.

Jones Criteria (Revised) for Diagnosis of Rheumatic Fever

> Major manifestations
> > Carditis
> > Polyarthritis
> > Sydenham chorea
> > Erythema marginatum
> > Subcutaneous nodules
>
> Minor manifestations
> > Clinical
> > > Previous rheumatic fever or rheumatic heart disease
> > > Polyarthralgia
> > > Fever
> > Laboratory
> > > Acute phase reaction: elevated erythrocyte sedimentation rate, C-reactive protein, leukocytosis
> > > Prolonged PR interval

Plus

Supporting evidence of preceding streptococcal infection, that is, increased titers of antistreptolysin O or other streptococcal antibodies, positive throat culture for group A *Streptococcus.*

Traditionally, two major or one major and two minor criteria (plus supporting evidence of streptococcal infection) justified the presumptive diagnosis of rheumatic fever. However, the major modern dilemma regarding diagnosis is that the physical findings may be so subtle and transient that the criteria are marginal. Since improper diagnosis has lifelong and serious consequences, it is justified to hospitalize patients with marginal findings so that serial clinical studies of the patient, including multiple examinations by a pediatric cardiologist, can be performed. If rheumatic fever appears likely on the basis of appropriate and careful evaluation but does not fully meet the revised Jones criteria, the diagnosis of suspect acute rheumatic fever is appropriate. This diagnosis mandates anti-infective prophylaxis but attempts to avoid the social and economic sequelae of the full diagnosis.

Major Manifestations of Rheumatic Fever

A. Active Carditis: Any one of the following—

1. A significant *new* murmur that is clearly mitral insufficiency (with or without a transient apical diastolic Carey Coombs murmur) or aortic insufficiency. It should be remembered that mitral insufficiency, while commonly caused by rheumatic fever, has many other causes in childhood.

2. Pericarditis, manifested by a pericardial friction rub or evidence of pericardial effusion.

3. Evidence of congestive heart failure.

B. Polyarthritis: Two or more joints must be involved; involvement of one joint does not constitute a major manifestation. The joints may be involved simultaneously or (more diagnostically) in a migratory fashion. The most commonly involved joints are the ankles, knees, hips, wrists, elbows, and shoulders. Heat, redness, swelling, severe pain, and tenderness are usually all present. Arthralgia alone without the other signs of inflammation is not sufficient to meet the criterion of polyarthritis.

C. Sydenham Chorea: Sydenham chorea is characterized by emotional instability and involuntary movements. These findings become progressively more severe and are often followed by the development of ataxia and slurring of speech. Muscular weakness becomes apparent following the onset of the involuntary movements. The individual attack of chorea is self-limiting, although it may last up to 3 months. It is not uncommon to find involvement on only one side. Manifestations may not be apparent for months to years after the acute episode of rheumatic fever.

D. Erythema Marginatum: Although this is a specific and major manifestation of acute rheumatic fever, many physicians fail to distinguish it from other skin lesions. It usually occurs only in severe cases and is rarely an essential diagnostic clue. It consists of a macular erythematous rash with a circinate border and appears primarily on the trunk and the extremities. The face is usually not involved.

E. Subcutaneous Nodules: These are usually seen only in severe cases, and then most commonly over the joints, scalp, and spinal column. They vary from a few millimeters to 2 cm in diameter and are nontender and freely movable under the skin.

Minor Manifestations of Rheumatic Fever

A. Polyarthralgia: Pain in two or more joints without heat, swelling, and tenderness is a minor rather than a major manifestation.

B. Fever: The fever is usually low-grade, although occasionally it reaches 39.4–40 °C.

C. Acute Phase Reaction: The sedimentation rate is accelerated and, more specifically, the C-reactive protein is elevated. Congestive heart failure does not influence the C-reactive protein and usually does not affect the sedimentation rate. Leukocytosis is the rule.

D. Electrocardiographic Changes: Prolonga-tion of the PR interval represents only a minor manifestation and does not qualify as active carditis.

E. History: There is a prior history of acute rheumatic fever or the presence of inactive rheumatic heart disease.

Essential Manifestation

Except in cases of rheumatic fever presenting solely as Sydenham chorea or longstanding carditis, there should be clear supporting evidence of a streptococcal infection such as scarlet fever, a positive throat culture for group A β-hemolytic *Streptococcus,* and increased antistreptolysin O or other streptococcal antibody titers. The antistreptolysin O titer is significantly higher in rheumatic fever than in uncomplicated streptococcal infections.

Other Manifestations

Associated findings may include erythema multiforme; abdominal, back, and precordial pain; and nontraumatic epistaxis, vomiting, malaise, weight loss, and anemia. The abdominal pain may mimic a "surgical abdomen," and many negative laparotomies have been performed in patients with acute rheumatic fever.

Treatment & Prophylaxis

A. Treatment of the Acute Episode:

1. Anti-infective therapy–Eradication of the streptococcal infection is essential. Benzathine penicillin G is the drug of choice. Depending on the age and weight of the patient, give a single intramuscular injection of 0.6–1.2 million U, or 125–250 mg orally four times a day for 10 days. Erythromycin, 250 mg orally four times a day, may be substituted if the patient is allergic to penicillin.

2. Anti-inflammatory agents–

a. Aspirin–Patients with the contemporary form of the disease need significantly less aspirin than in the past. Currently, 30–60 mg/kg/d is given in four divided doses; this dosage is often more than sufficient to effect dramatic relief of the arthritis and fever. In general, higher dosages carry a greater risk of side effects, and there are no proved short-term or long-term benefits of giving high doses to effect salicylate blood levels of 20–30 mg/dL. The duration of therapy must be tailored to meet the needs of the patient, but use of aspirin for 2–6 weeks, with reduction in dosage toward the end of the course, is usually sufficient.

b. Corticosteroids–Corticosteroids are rarely indicated in current therapy. However, in the unusual patient with severe carditis and manifestations of congestive heart failure (as evidenced by radiographic findings of cardiomegaly or by cardiopulmonary symptoms or a gallop rhythm), therapy may be not only effective but lifesaving. Corticosteroid therapy may be given as follows: prednisone, 2 mg/kg/d orally for 2 weeks (or comparable doses of other corticosteroids); reduce prednisone to 1 mg/kg/d the third week, and begin aspirin, 50 mg/kg/d; stop prednisone at the end of 3 weeks, and continue aspirin for 8 weeks or until the C-reactive protein is negative and the sedimentation rate is falling.

3. Therapy of congestive heart failure–See Congestive Heart Failure, above.

4. Bed rest and ambulation–Strict bed rest is not required for patients with arthritis and mild carditis without congestive heart failure. It is preferable to maintain a regimen of bed-to-chair with bathroom privileges and meals at the table for patients who are relatively asymptomatic while on aspirin therapy. Asymptomatic patients can be kept in bed only under duress anyway. Patients with severe carditis (congestive heart failure) have no desire to get out of bed and should be at bed rest at least as long as corticosteroid therapy is required. *Gradual* indoor ambulation followed by modified outdoor activity may be ordered when symptoms have disappeared but there is still clinical and laboratory evidence of rheumatic activity. Modified bed rest for 2–6 weeks is generally adequate. Children should not return to school while there is clear evidence of rheumatic activity.

B. Treatment After the Acute Episode:

1. Prevention–The patient who has had rheumatic fever has a greatly increased risk of developing rheumatic fever following the next inadequately treated group A β-hemolytic streptococcal infection. *Prevention is thus the most important therapeutic course for the physician to emphasize.* The purpose of follow-up visits after the acute episode is not so much to evaluate the evolution of mitral insufficiency murmurs as to reinforce the physician's advice about the necessity for antibacterial prophylaxis with benzathine penicillin G. At such times, the physician should stress that greater protection is afforded by administration via the intramuscular route than via the oral route and that, in addition, failure to comply with regular oral medication programs increases the risk for recurrence of rheumatic fever. Thus, patients should be informed that the parenteral route will be favored until they are adults, at which time their internists may elect oral medication.

If myocardial or valvular disease persists, antibacterial prophylaxis is a lifelong commitment. More commonly with transient cardiac involvement, 3–5 years of therapy or discontinuance at adolescence is a practical and effective approach.

The following regimens are in current use:

a. Benzathine penicillin G, 1.2 million U intramuscularly every 21–28 days, is the drug of choice.

b. Sulfadiazine, 500 mg daily as a single oral dose for patients weighing over 27 kg (60 lb), is the drug of second choice. Blood dyscrasias and a lesser effectiveness in reducing streptococcal infections make this drug less satisfactory than benzathine penicillin G.

c. Penicillin G (buffered), 250,000 U orally twice daily, offers approximately the same protection afforded by sulfadiazine but is much less effective than intramuscular benzathine penicillin G (5.5 versus 0.4 streptococcal infections per 100 patient-years).

d. Erythromycin, 250 mg orally twice a day, may be given to those patients who may be allergic to both penicillin and sulfonamides.

2. Residual valvular damage–Chronic congestive heart failure may follow a single severe episode of acute rheumatic carditis or, more commonly, may follow repeated episodes. In children in the United States, the typical manifestations of residual valvular damage are heart murmurs of mitral and aortic insufficiency; murmurs are not accompanied by congestive heart failure during most of the pediatric age period *as long as repeated attacks are prevented.*

Methods of managing congestive heart failure have been discussed previously. Children with severe valvular damage who cannot be adequately managed on a medical regimen must be considered for valve replacement—and considered before the myocardium is irreversibly damaged.

Ayoub EM: Resurgence of rheumatic fever in the United States: The changing picture of a preventable illness. Postgrad Med 1992;92:139.

Dajani AS et al: Guidelines for the diagnosis of rheumatic fever: Jones criteria, updated 1992. Ciruclation 1993; 87:302.

Lue HC et al: Long term outcome of patients with rheumatic fever receiving benzathine penicillin G prophylaxis every three weeks versus every four weeks. J Pediatr 1994;125:812.

Veasy LG et al: Resurgence of acute rheumatic fever in the intermountain West of the United States. N Engl J Med 1987;316:421.

RHEUMATIC HEART DISEASE

Mitral Insufficiency

Mitral insufficiency, the most common valvular residual of acute rheumatic carditis, is characterized by a pansystolic murmur that is localized at the apex. In patients with mitral involvement, the murmur appears early in the course of rheumatic carditis, and, depending on the severity of the damage, may disappear over a period of days or months or may persist for life.

Among the many other causes of mitral insufficiency, the most common is the mitral dysfunction syndrome, characterized by a mid to late apical systolic murmur introduced by a click.* Other causes are myocarditis, endocardial fibroelastosis, anomalous left coronary artery, and congenital anomalies

---

*A word of caution about diagnosing the mitral dysfunction syndrome: The echocardiographic finding of prolapse (redundancy) of the mitral valve, which characterizes mitral dysfunction, may also be found in patients with acute rheumatic fever and recently acquired rheumatic heart disease.

of the mitral valve, which occur as isolated lesions or as part of a complex of anomalies (eg, endocardial cushion defects).

Mitral Stenosis

There are murmurs of mitral stenosis that are secondary to structural stenosis of the valve; those that result from relative excess of flow (in large volumes of regurgitation); and those that are present during acute valvulitis (Carey Coombs murmur). Mitral stenosis caused by structural stenosis is rarely encountered in the United States before 5–10 years following the first episode of acute rheumatic carditis and is much more commonly discovered in adults than in children. Early structural mitral stenosis murmurs, flow murmurs, and Carey Coombs murmurs are short and heard in mid diastole. Progressively more severe mitral stenosis murmurs become longer in duration until they attain the classic crescendo, presystolic configuration.

Aortic Insufficiency

This early decrescendo diastolic murmur is not commonly encountered as the sole valvular involvement of rheumatic carditis. It is the second most common valve affected in polyvalvular as well as in single valvular disease. It appears that the aortic valve is involved more often in males and in blacks. A short aortic systolic murmur resulting from excess flow may accompany the aortic insufficiency murmur.

Aortic Stenosis

Dominant aortic stenosis of rheumatic origin does not occur in pediatric patients. Aortic stenosis in children is congenital. In one large series, the shortest length of time observed for a patient to develop dominant aortic stenosis secondary to rheumatic heart disease was 20 years.

Edwards BS, Edwards JE: Congestive heart failure in rheumatic carditis: Valvular or myocardial origin? J Am Coll Cardiol 1993;22:830.

Horstkotte D et al: Pathomorphologic aspects, etiology, and natural history of acquired mitral stenosis. Eur Heart J 1991;12(Suppl B):55.

MYOCARDITIS

In most cases, the cause of myocarditis is not determined. Coxsackievirus B is the most common infectious agent isolated. Coxsackievirus A, rubella virus, cytomegalovirus, mumps virus, herpesvirus, adenovirus, and many other viral agents have been implicated. Virtually every other infectious agent, including bacteria, fungi, rickettsiae, chlamydiae, spirochetes, parasites, and human immunodeficiency virus, has been suggested as a cause of myocarditis,

but laboratory confirmation is seldom possible. It is important to emphasize that myocarditis is part of a spectrum of primary endomyocardial diseases and may be one of the causes of endocardial fibroelastosis.

Clinical Findings

A. Symptoms & Signs: The clinical picture usually falls into two separate patterns: (1) Onset of congestive heart failure is sudden in a newborn who has been in relatively good health 12–24 hours previously. This is a malignant form of the disease and is thought to be solely secondary to overwhelming viremia and tissue invasion of multiple organ systems, including the heart. (2) In the older child, the onset of cardiac findings tends to be much more gradual. There is often a history of an upper respiratory tract infection or gastroenteritis within the month prior to the development of cardiac findings. This is a more insidious form of the disease and may have a late postinfectious or autoimmune component. Recovery from the initial infection is followed by gradual and progressive development of easy fatigability, dyspnea on exertion, and malaise.

In the newborn infant, the signs of congestive heart failure are usually apparent. The skin is pale and gray, and peripheral cyanosis may be present. The pulses are rapid, weak, and thready. Edema of the face and extremities may be seen. Significant cardiomegaly is present, and the left and right ventricular impulses are weak. On auscultation, the heart sounds may be muffled and distant. Third and fourth heart sounds are common, resulting in a gallop rhythm. Murmurs are usually absent, although a murmur of tricuspid or mitral insufficiency can occasionally be heard. Moist rales are usually present at both lung bases. The liver is enlarged and frequently tender. The level of the jugular venous pulse is elevated.

B. Imaging: Generalized cardiomegaly can be seen on x-ray. There is evidence of moderate to marked pulmonary venous congestion. Pneumonitis is commonly present.

C. Electrocardiography: The ECG is variable. Classically, there is evidence of low voltage of the QRS throughout all frontal and precordial leads and depression of the ST segment and inversion of the T waves in leads I, III, and aVF and in the left precordial leads during the acute malignant stage. Dysrhythmias are common, and atrioventricular and intraventricular conduction disturbances may be present. With the more benign form—or during the recovery phase of the malignant form—high-voltage QRS complexes are commonly seen and are indicative of left ventricular hypertrophy.

D. Echocardiography: Echocardiography demonstrates four-chamber dilation with poor ventricular function and atrioventricular valve regurgitation.

Treatment

A. Digitalis: The use of digitalis in a rapidly deteriorating child with myocarditis is dangerous and should be undertaken with great caution. Because the inflamed myocardium is markedly sensitive to digitalis, only about two-thirds of the usual total digitalizing dose should be used. During the initial phase of therapy, ECGs should be taken frequently. If serious dysrhythmias or other evidence of digitalis intoxication develops, the drug should be stopped and not reinstituted until all evidence of digitalis toxicity has disappeared. If toxicity is not evident and there is no clinical response, digitalis doses should be increased until one or the other is noted.

B. Diuretics: Diuretics should be administered with caution, since they may potentiate digitalis toxicity.

C. Corticosteroids: The administration of corticosteroids is controversial but seems more rational when used in the treatment of the more benign postinfectious autoimmune cases. If the patient's condition continues to deteriorate despite anticongestive measures, corticosteroids are commonly used.

D. Systemic Vasodilators: The use of systemic vasodilators such as nitroprusside in a hypotensive deteriorating critically ill patient is risky but may be lifesaving.

Prognosis

The prognosis for a patient with myocarditis is related to the age at onset, the response to therapy, and the presence or absence of recurrences. If the patient is less than 6 months of age or older than 3 years, responds poorly to therapy, and manifests multiple recurrences of congestive heart failure, the prognosis is poor. Many patients recover clinically but have persistent cardiomegaly. It is possible that subclinical myocarditis in childhood is the pathophysiologic basis for some of the idiopathic myocardiopathies seen later in life.

Chan KY et al: Immunosuppressive therapy in the management of acute myocarditis in children. J Am Coll Cardiol 1991;17:458.

Hilton DA, Variend S, Pringle JH: Demonstration of coxsackie virus RNA in formalin-fixed tissue sections from childhood myocarditis cases by in situ hybridization and polymerase chain reaction. J Pathol 1993;170:45.

INFECTIVE ENDOCARDITIS

Essentials of Diagnosis

- Pre-existing organic heart murmur.
- Persistent fever.
- Increasing symptoms of heart disease (ranging from easy fatigability to heart failure).
- Splenomegaly (70%).
- Embolic phenomena (50%).
- Leukocytosis, elevated erythrocyte sedimentation rate, hematuria, positive blood culture.

General Considerations

Bacterial infection of the endocardial surface of the heart or the intimal surface of certain arterial vessels (coarcted segment of aorta and ductus arteriosus) is a rare condition that usually occurs when an abnormality of the heart or great vessels exists. It may develop in a normal heart during the course of septicemia.

The incidence of infective endocarditis appears to be increasing owing to many factors, including (1) increased survival rates for children with congenital heart disease, (2) greater long-term use of central venous catheters, and (3) increased use of prosthetic material and valves. Pediatric patients without pre-existing heart disease also are at increased risk for infective endocarditis owing to (1) increased survival rates for children with immune deficiencies, (2) greater long-term use of indwelling lines in critically ill newborns, and (3) increased incidence of intravenous drug abuse.

Patients at greatest risk include those with aortico-pulmonary shunts, left-sided outflow obstruction, and ventricular septal defects. Predisposing factors can be identified approximately 30% of the time and include dental procedures, nonsterile surgical procedures, and cardiovascular surgery.

Organisms causing endocarditis include *Streptococcus viridans* (about 50% of cases), *Staphylococcus aureus* (about 30%), and fungal agents (about 10%).

Clinical Findings

A. History: Almost all patients with infective endocarditis have a history of heart disease. There may or may not be a history of infection or a surgical procedure (tooth extraction, tonsillectomy).

B. Symptoms, Signs, & Laboratory Findings: In one large study, the following symptoms, signs, and laboratory findings were reported (in order of decreasing frequency): changing murmurs, fever, positive blood culture, weight loss, cardiomegaly, elevated sedimentation rate, splenomegaly, petechiae, embolism, and leukocytosis. Other findings are hematuria, signs of congestive heart failure, clubbing, joint pains, and hepatomegaly. Echocardiography has become a valuable tool in diagnosing large vegetations.

Prevention

It is recommended that patients at risk for infective endocarditis be given appropriate antibiotics before any type of dental work (tooth extraction, cleaning) and before operations within the oropharynx, gastrointestinal tract, and genitourinary tract. Continuous antibiotic prophylaxis (as in the treatment of rheumatic fever) is *not* recommended in patients with congenital heart disease.

The following schedule is recommended: under 15 kg, 750 mg of oral amoxicillin; 15–30 kg, 1500 mg; over 30 kg, 3000 mg. This dose is to be given 1 hour prior to dental procedures and followed by one-half the initial dose 6 hours later.

Treatment

In a patient with known heart disease, the presence of an otherwise unexplained fever should alert the physician to the possibility of infective endocarditis. A positive blood culture or other major findings of infective endocarditis confirm the diagnosis. If a positive blood culture is obtained and the organism is identified, specific treatment should be begun immediately. Even if blood cultures are negative after 48 hours, it is advisable to begin penicillin therapy (if there is other evidence of infective endocarditis), because most positive cultures are obtained within the first 48 hours. Naficillin parenterally or dichoxacillin enterally are the drugs of choice in most cases. Other antibiotics may be added (see Chapter 34). If congestive heart failure occurs and progresses unremittingly in the face of adequate antibiotic therapy, surgical excision of the infected area and prosthetic valve replacement should be considered.

Course & Prognosis

The prognosis depends on how early in the course of the infectious process treatment is instituted. The prognosis is better in patients in whom blood culture is positive. If congestive heart failure develops, the prognosis is usually poor.

Even though bacteriologic cure of the infectious process is achieved, death may occur as a result of congestive heart failure secondary to severe valvular destruction. Intractable congestive heart failure may occur weeks or months following bacteriologic cure. Embolization may occur following bacteriologic cure when vegetations tear off from the involved area.

The death rate for infective endocarditis is still about 20%.

Awadallah SM et al: The changing pattern of infective endocarditis in childhood. Am J Cardiol 1991;68:90.

Biancaniello TM, Romero JR: Bacterial endocarditis after adjustment of orthodontic appliances. J Pediatr 1991; 118:248.

Dajani AS et al: Prevention of bacterial endocarditis: Recommendations by the American Heart Association. JAMA 1990;264:2919.

Saiman L, Prince A, Gerony WM: Pediatric infective endocarditis in the modern era. J Pediatr 1993;122:847.

PERICARDITIS

Essentials of Diagnosis

- Retrosternal pain made worse by deep inspiration and decreased by leaning forward.
- Fever.
- Shortness of breath and grunting respirations are common.
- Pericardial friction rub.
- Tachycardia.
- Hepatomegaly and distention of the jugular veins.
- ECG with elevated ST segment.

General Considerations

Involvement of the pericardium rarely occurs as an isolated event. In most cases, pericardial disease occurs in association with a more generalized process. Important causes include rheumatic fever, viral pericarditis, purulent pericarditis, rheumatoid arthritis, uremia, and tuberculosis.

In the pediatric age group, pericardial disease usually takes the form of acute pericarditis. In most cases, there is effusion of fluid into the pericardial cavity. The consequences of such effusion depend on the amount, type, and speed of fluid accumulation. Under certain circumstances, serious compression of the heart occurs. The direct compression and the body's attempt to correct it result in cardiac tamponade. Unless the pericardial fluid is evacuated, death occurs very rapidly.

Clinical Findings

A. Symptoms & Signs: The symptoms depend to a great extent on the cause of the pericarditis. Pain is common. It is usually sharp and stabbing, located in the mid chest and in the shoulder and neck, made worse by deep inspiration, and considerably decreased by sitting up and leaning forward. Shortness of breath and grunting respirations are common findings in all patients.

The physical findings depend on whether or not a significant amount of effusion is present: (1) In the absence of significant accumulation of fluid, the pulses are normal and the level of the jugular venous pulse is normal. On examination of the heart, a characteristic scratchy, high-pitched friction rub may be heard. It is often systolic and diastolic and can be located at any point between the apex and the left sternal border. The location and timing vary considerably from time to time. The heart sounds are usually normal, and the heart is not enlarged to percussion. (2) If there is a considerable accumulation of pericardial fluid, the cardiovascular findings are different. The heart is enlarged to percussion, but on inspection of the precordium, it seems to be very quiet. Auscultation reveals distant and muffled heart tones. Friction rub is usually not present. In the absence of cardiac tamponade, the peripheral, venous, and arterial pulses are normal.

Cardiac tamponade is characterized by distention of the jugular veins, tachycardia, enlargement of the liver, peripheral edema, and "paradoxic pulse," in which the systolic pressure drops by more than 10 mm Hg during inspiration. The term *paradoxic pulse* is a misnomer, since the drop is only an accentuation of a normal event. (Normally, the systolic pressure drops by no more than 5 mm Hg.) This finding is best determined with the use of a blood pressure cuff. At this point, the patient is critically ill and has all the symptoms and signs suggestive of right-sided congestive heart failure.

Not all patients with marked cardiac compression demonstrate all the findings listed above. If the patient appears critically ill and has evidence of pericarditis and effusion, treatment should be instituted even though all the clinical signs of cardiac tamponade are not present.

B. Imaging: In pericarditis without effusion, chest x-ray findings are normal. With pericardial effusion, the cardiac silhouette is enlarged, often in the shape of a water bottle, with blunting of the cardiodiaphragmatic borders. When there is evidence of cardiac tamponade, the lung fields are clear. This is in contrast to patients with myocardial dilatation, who show evidence of pulmonary congestion.

C. Electrocardiography: A number of electrocardiographic abnormalities occur in patients with pericarditis. Low voltage is commonly seen in patients with significant pericardial effusion, although the voltage may be normal. The ST segment is commonly elevated during the first week of involvement. The T wave is usually upright during this time. Following this, the ST segment is normal and the T wave becomes flattened. After about 2 weeks, the T wave inverts and remains inverted for several weeks or months. In contrast to findings in patients with myocardial infarction, there is no reciprocal relationship between the findings in lead I and lead III in the frontal plane and the right and left precordial leads.

D. Echocardiography: Echocardiography has become a most reliable form of noninvasive diagnosis of pericardial effusion. The results must be considered in light of the clinical picture in deciding whether or not to remove the fluid.

Treatment

Treatment of the patient with pericarditis depends on the cause of the pericarditis. Cardiac tamponade resulting from any cause must be treated by evacuation of the fluid. It is usually desirable to perform a wide resection of the pericardium through a surgical incision. However, needle insertion into the pericardial sac may be lifesaving in an emergency situation.

Prognosis

The prognosis depends to a great extent on the cause of the pericardial disease. Cardiac tamponade from any cause results in death unless the fluid is evacuated.

SPECIFIC DISEASES INVOLVING THE PERICARDIUM

Acute Rheumatic Fever

When pericarditis occurs during the course of acute rheumatic fever, it is almost always associated with involvement of the myocardium and the endocardium (pancarditis). Thus, heart murmurs are almost always present. The pericarditis is usually of the serofibrinous variety and usually not associated with significant pericardial effusion.

Patients with acute rheumatic fever and pericarditis are usually very ill, with severe cardiac involvement. They respond extremely well to corticosteroid therapy. Pericarditis usually disappears rapidly (1 week) after corticosteroid therapy is started. Constrictive pericarditis almost never occurs secondary to this disease.

Viral Pericarditis

Viral pericarditis is uncommon in children and young adults. The most common cause is coxsackievirus B4. Influenza virus has also been implicated. There is usually a history of a protracted upper respiratory tract infection.

The pericardial effusion usually lasts for several weeks. Cardiac tamponade is rare. Recurrences of pericardial effusion are common even months or years after the initial episode. Constrictive pericarditis has been reported in this disease.

Purulent Pericarditis

The most common causes of purulent pericarditis are pneumococci, streptococci, staphylococci, *Escherichia coli,* and *Haemophilus influenzae.* This disorder is always secondary to infection elsewhere, although occasionally the primary site is not obvious. In addition to demonstrating signs of cardiac compression, patients are septic and run extremely high fevers. The purulent fluid accumulating within the pericardial sac is usually quite thick and filled with polymorphonuclear leukocytes. Although antibiotics will sterilize the pericardial fluid, pericardial tamponade commonly develops, and evacuation of the pericardial sac is usually necessary. Wide resection of the pericardium through a surgical incision performed in the operating room is most desirable, but pericardiocentesis is often dramatically effective and lifesaving. Drainage of the purulent fluid is followed by marked improvement of symptoms.

Postpericardiotomy Syndrome

Postpericardiotomy syndrome is characterized by fever, chest pain, friction rub, and elevation of ST segment noted on ECG 1–2 weeks after open heart surgery. It appears to be an autoimmune disease with high titers of antiheart antibody and with detectable evidence of fresh or reactivated viral illness. The syndrome is often self-limited and responds well to short courses of aspirin or corticosteroid therapy. Occasionally, it lasts for months to years and may require pericardiocentesis or pericardiectomy.

Dupuis C et al: Bacterial pericarditis in infancy and childhood. Am J Cardiol 1994;74:807.

Guindo J et al: Recurrent pericarditis: Relief with colchicine. Circulation 1990;82:1117.

Mason TG, Neal WA, DiBartolomeo AG: Elevated antinuclear antibody titers and the postpericardiotomy syndrome. J Pediatr 1990;116:403.

HYPERTENSION*

Blood pressure determinations are being more routinely obtained in the examination of infants and children; as a result, systemic hypertension has become more widely recognized as a pediatric problem. Pediatric standards for blood pressure have been published, but the studies from which these standards were derived suffered from three methodologic problems. The first and most important is that the widest cuff that would fit between the axilla and the antecubital fossa was not routinely used. The use of a wide cuff either has no effect on blood pressure or decreases blood pressure by a maximum of 5 mm Hg. Use of a narrow cuff, however, routinely increases blood pressure by 10–50 mm Hg. The second methodologic problem was lack of an ethnic cross section. Third, the fact that systemic blood pressure decreases with increasing altitude of residence was not taken into consideration.

These three problems were addressed in a study of a triracial population at sea level and at an altitude of 10,000 ft. The widest cuff that would fit between the axilla and the antecubital fossa was used in each case. Most children 10–11 years of age needed a standard adult-size cuff (bladder width of 12 cm), and many high school students needed a large adult-size cuff (width of 16 cm) or leg cuff (width of 18 cm). Results of the study are shown in Table 19–3. The 95th percentile value for blood pressure was similar for both sexes and all three ethnic groups. Blood pressure varied more with altitude and body weight than with sex or ethnic origin. If the blood pressure taken in a quiet atmosphere and sitting position exceeds the 95th percentile for systolic, diastolic muffle, or diastolic disappearance pressures, it should be repeated twice in 1- to 2-week intervals. If it is abnormal all three times, a pediatric hypertension diagnostic center should be consulted.

Essential hypertension is the most common form of pediatric hypertension. Coarctation of the thoracic

---

*The diagnostic evaluation of renal hypertension and the treatment of hypertensive emergencies, as well as the ambulatory treatment of chronic hypertension, are discussed in Chapter 22.

Table 19–3. The 95th percentile value for blood pressure (mm Hg) taken in the sitting position.[1]

Age (y)	Sea Level			10,000 ft		
	S	Dm	Dd	S	Dm	Dd
5				92	72	62
6	106	64	60	96	74	66
7	108	72	66	98	76	70
8	110	76	70	104	80	70
9	114	80	76	106	80	70
10	118	82	76	108	80	70
11	124	82	78	108	80	72
12	128	84	78	108	80	72
13	132	84	80	116	84	76
14	136	86	80	120	84	76
15	140	88	80	120	84	80
16	140	90	80	120	84	80
17	140	92	80	122	84	80
18	140	92	80	130	84	80

[1]Blood pressures: S = systolic (Korotkoff's sound 1; onset of tapping), Dm = diastolic muffling (Korotkoff's sound 4), Dd = diastolic disappearance (Korotkoff's sound 5).

or abdominal aorta, renal artery stenosis, renal disease, and pheochromocytoma should be ruled out.

Patients with essential hypertension often show improvement with reduction of obesity, reduction of excessive salt intake, institution of an exercise program, avoidance of cigarette smoking, and avoidance of oral contraceptives. The use of antihypertensive drugs in pediatric hypertension is controversial, but thiazide diuretics and propranolol are useful in selected cases.

Badenhop RF, Wang XL, Wilcken DEL: Angiotensin-converting enzyme genotype in children and coronary events in their grandparents. Circulation 1995;91:1655.

Gifford RW et al: The fifth report of the Joint National Committee on detection, evaluation, and treatment of high blood pressure. Arch Intern Med 1993;153:154.

Gillman MW et al: Identifying children at high risk for the development of essential hypertension. J Pediatr 1993;122:837.

Heggi T et al: Blood pressure ranges in premature infants. J Pediatr 1994;124:627.

Steinfeld L et al: Sphygmomanometry in pediatric patients. J Pediatr 1978;92:934.

Task force on blood pressure control in children. Pediatrics 1987;79:1.

ATHEROSCLEROSIS AS A PEDIATRIC PROBLEM

Awareness of the importance of coronary artery risk factors in general—and atherosclerosis in particular—has risen dramatically in the general population during the past 25 years. In adults, the incidence of death from ischemic heart disease has been decreasing over the last decade, presumably as a result of modifying the diet or lifestyle to avoid known risks for heart disease. During this same decade, a large number of serum samples from the pediatric population have been collected and analyzed for lipids, and epidemiologic studies have been performed to determine the relationship of lipid levels to coronary heart disease. The level of serum lipids in childhood usually remains the same through adolescence. Biochemical abnormalities in the lipid profile appear early in childhood and correlate with higher risk for coronary artery disease in adulthood. High-density lipoprotein has been identified as an antiatherogenic agent through these studies.

The concept of pediatric screening for hyperlipidemia has been evaluated carefully. Currently, only children at high risk—that is, children with a family history of early myocardial infarction (prior to 50–55 years) in parents or grandparents or with known familial hyperlipidemia or adopted children—are screened routinely. In addition, some researchers consider adolescents with total cholesterol levels of greater than 180 mg/dL or low-density lipoprotein levels of greater than 110 mg/dL to be at risk for coronary artery disease in adulthood.

In most cases, treatment consists of dietary restrictions, exercise, abstinence from smoking, and avoidance of other ischemic heart disease risk factors. In patients with life-threatening familial hyperlipidemia, pharmacologic and surgical intervention (ileal bypass, portacaval shunt) may be considered.

Lauer RM, Clark WR: Use of cholesterol measurements in childhood for the prediction of adult hypercholesterolemia: The Muscatine Study. JAMA 1990;264:3034.

Lauer RM et al: National cholesterol education program (NCEP): Highlights of report. Pediatrics 1992;89:495.

Muhonen LE et al: Coronary risk factors in adolescents related to their knowledge of familial coronary heart disease and hypercholesterolemia: The Muscatine Study. Pediatrics 1994;93:444.

MUCOCUTANEOUS LYMPH NODE SYNDROME

Mucocutaneous lymph node syndrome, also known as Kawasaki disease, was first described in Japan in 1967. The acute illness is characterized by (1) prolonged fever (over 5 days) that is unresponsive to antibiotics; (2) conjunctivitis; (3) cracking and fissuring of the lips, with inflammation of mucous membranes; (4) cervical lymphadenopathy; (5) rash involving the trunk and the extremities, with reddened palms and soles of the hands and feet and subsequent desquamation of tips of the toes and fingers; and (6) edema. Patients may also have associated arthritis. Thrombocytosis and increased sedimentation rate are seen on laboratory examination.

Cardiovascular complications during the acute illness include myocarditis, pericarditis, and arteritis that predisposes the patient to aneurysm formation in the coronary arteries in approximately 20% of patients. Aneurysm formation may occur 7–45 days after the onset of illness. Acute myocardial infarction may occur during the acute illness secondary to thrombosis of these aneurysms. Death occurs in 1–2% of patients during this phase of the illness. Long-term follow-up of patients with aneurysms shows some resolution of aneurysms in 50% of those affected; the remainder may continue to have aneurysms, may develop stenosis, and, possibly later, may develop myocardial ischemia.

During the acute illness and for 2–3 months after, patients should be monitored closely by serial electrocardiography, chest x-ray, and M-mode and two-dimensional echocardiography. Selective coronary angiography is recommended in those patients with coronary abnormalities detected by echocardiography.

The acute illness is now treated with high doses of intravenous immune globulin (IGIV), 2 g/kg as a single dose given over 10–12 hours. If fever recurs within 48–72 hours and no other source of the fever is detected, a repeat dose is recommended, and high doses of aspirin, 20 mg/kg per dose given four times a day until day 14 of illness, then 3–5 mg/kg/d for 2–3 months from the onset of illness if the echocardiogram is normal or indefinitely if coronary abnormalities are present. Evidence of myocardial ischemia or infarction warrants early cardiac catheterization and bypass surgery if obstruction exists.

American Heart Association Committee on Rheumatic Fever, Endocarditis, Kawasaki Disease: Guidelines for long term management of patients with Kawasaki disease. Circulation 1994;89:916.

Gersony WM: Diagnosis and management of Kawasaki disease. JAMA 1991;265:2699.

Management of Kawasaki syndrome: A consensus statement prepared by North American participants of the third international Kawasaki disease symposium, Tokyo, Japan, December 1988. Pediatr Infect Dis J 1989;8:663.

DISORDERS OF RATE & RHYTHM & ELECTROLYTE IMBALANCE

The recognition and treatment of cardiac arrhythmias have markedly increased in the recent past. Better monitoring (electrocardiography, bedside monitors, Holter monitors, etc) has increased the awareness and detection of rhythm disturbances. There is also a true rise in the incidence of arrhythmias. More children are now surviving cardiac surgery and acute carditis and live chronically with altered hemodynamics, physiology, and structural changes. These changes over time will create altered conduction and new arrhythmias.

The advent of invasive electrophysiology with recordings from the endocardium has greatly improved our understanding of the conduction system. And now, with cardiac ablation techniques, we can offer these children a "cure" rather than lifelong antiarrhythmia treatment.

Sinus Arrhythmia

It is normal to have phasic variation in the heart rate (sinus arrhythmia). Typically, the sinus rate varies with the respiratory cycle, while P-QRS-T intervals remain normal. "Marked" sinus arrhythmia is defined as a greater than 100% variation in heart rate. It may be found in association with respiratory distress or increased intracranial pressure, or it may be pressure in normal children. It alone virtually never requires treatment. However, it may be associated with sinus node dysfunction (see below).

Sinus Bradycardia

Depending on the age of the patient, *sinus brady-cardia* is defined as either (1) a heart rate below the normal limit for age (neonates to 6 years, 60 beats/min; 7–11 years, 45 beats/min; >12 years, 40 beats/min) or (2) a heart rate inappropriately slow for the functional status of the patient (chronotropic incompetence). In critically ill patients, common causes of sinus bradycardia include hypoxia, central nervous system damage, and iatrogenic medication side effects. Only symptomatic bradycardia (syncope, low cardiac output, or exercise intolerance) requires treatment (atropine or artificial cardiac pacing).

Sinus Tachycardia

The heart rate normally accelerates in response to stress (eg, fever, hypovolemia, anemia, congestive heart failure). Tachycardia with decreased cardiac output is more ominous and warrants evaluation for shock or tachyarrhythmia. Treatment may be indicated for correction of the underlying cause of tachycardia (eg, transfusion for anemia, correction of hypovolemia or fever).

Gillette PC, Garson A Jr: *Pediatric Arrhythmias: Electrophysiology and Pacing.* Saunders, 1990.

PREMATURE ATRIAL CONTRACTIONS

Premature atrial contractions are triggered by an ectopic focus in the atrium. They are one of the most common premature beats seen in the pediatric population, particularly during the fetal and newborn periods. They may be conducted (with associated QRS) or nonconducted (without associated QRS) (Figure

19–6). There is usually some delay until the next normal sinus beat. Depending on the ectopic focus of the premature contraction, the frontal plane vector of the P wave may be normal (+60 degrees) or abnormal. As an isolated finding, premature atrial contractions are benign and require no treatment. They may need to be suppressed with antiarrhythmic agents when they trigger tachyarrhythmias or produce bradycardia secondary to nonconduction.

PREMATURE JUNCTIONAL CONTRACTIONS

Premature junctional contractions arise within the atrioventricular node or the bundle of His. Most often, they induce a normal QRS complex with no preceding P wave. When conducted aberrantly to the ventricles, they cannot be distinguished from premature ventricular contractions except by invasive electrophysiologic study. Premature junctional contractions are usually benign and require no specific therapy.

PREMATURE VENTRICULAR CONTRACTIONS

Premature ventricular contractions may originate in either ventricle and are characterized by a bizarre QRS of over 80 ms duration in newborns and 120 ms in children (Figure 19–7). Premature ventricular contractions originating from a single ectopic focus all have the same configuration; those of multifocal origin show varying configurations. The consecutive occurrence of more than one beat can result in coupling (Figure 19–7) or ventricular tachycardia (three or more consecutive ventricular beats).

Most unifocal premature ventricular contractions in otherwise normal patients are benign. The nature of contractions can be confirmed by having the patient exercise. As the heart rate increases, benign premature contractions disappear. If exercise results in an increase or coupling of contractions, there may be underlying disease. Multifocal premature ventricular contractions are always abnormal and may be more dangerous. They may be associated with drug overdose (tricyclic antidepressants, digoxin toxicity), electrolyte imbalance, or hypoxia. Treatment is directed at correcting the underlying disorder.

SINUS NODE DYSFUNCTION

Sinus node dysfunction (SND), or sick sinus syndrome (SSS), is a clinical syndrome of inappropriate sinus nodal function and rate. The abnormality may be a true anatomic defect of the sinus node or its surrounding tissue, or it may be an abnormality of the

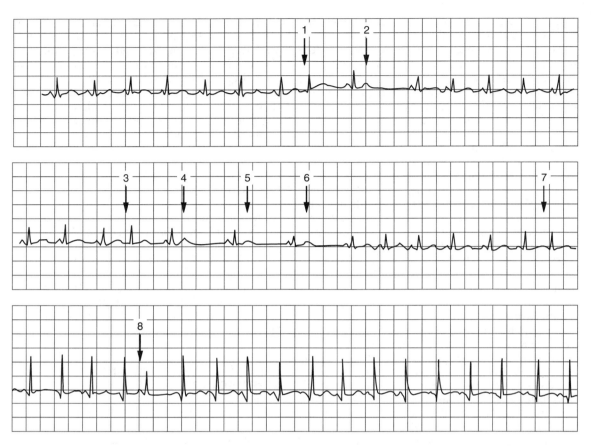

Figure 19–6. Lead II rhythm strip with premature atrial contractions. Beats 1, 3, 7, and 8 are conducted to the ventricles, whereas beats 2, 4, 5, and 6 are not.

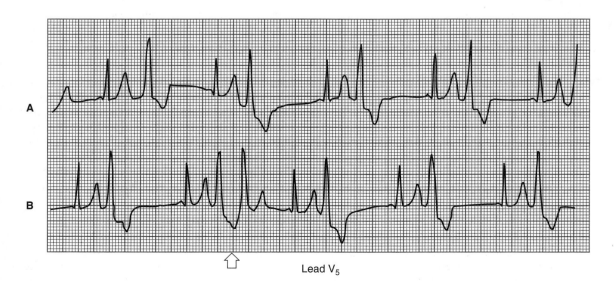

Lead V$_5$

Figure 19–7. Lead V$_5$ rhythm strip with unifocal premature ventricular contractions in a bigeminy pattern. The arrow shows a ventricular couplet.

autonomic input. It is defined as one or more of the following: (1) sinus bradycardia, (2) marked sinus arrhythmia, (3) sinus pause or arrest, (4) sinoatrial exit block, (5) combined brady- and tachyarrhythmias, (6) sinus node reentry, and (7) atrial muscle reentry tachycardia. It is usually associated with postoperative repair of congenital heart disease (most commonly the Mustard or Senning repair for transposition of the great arteries), but it is also seen in unoperated congenital heart disease, in acquired heart diseases, and in normal hearts. Sometimes SND is inherited. Symptoms usually manifest between 2 and 17 years and consist of syncope, presyncope, or disorientation. Some patients may experience palpitations, pallor, or exercise intolerance.

The evaluation of sinus node dysfunction involves both external electrocardiography and electrophysiologic recordings. Resting ECGs, exercise testing, and ambulatory monitoring help define the arrhythmia and correlate rhythm changes with symptoms. Invasive electrophysiologic recordings measure sinus node automaticity, sinoatrial conduction, and intrinsic heart rate with and without autonomic nervous system blockade. The correction of SND during autonomic blockade with atropine and propranolol implies that the dysfunction is secondary to abnormal autonomic tone rather than an anatomic abnormality of the sinus node.

Treatment of SND is usually reserved for symptomatic patients. Asymptomatic patients can just be observed, since there is little chance of sudden death. Bradyarrhythmias are treated with vagolytic (scopolamine) or adrenergic (aminophylline) agents or permanent cardiac pacemakers. Antiarrhythmic treatment of tachyarrhythmias often produces or enhances bradycardia, thus requiring permanent pacing. In selected cases, permanent cardiac pacing is performed prophylactically prior to the initiation of antiarrhythmic medications. The prognosis for SND is excellent when appropriate treatment is provided, with total morbidity and mortality rates nearly equal to those of the underlying heart disease. However, if left untreated, SND may lead to chronic dysfunction and even sudden death.

SUPRAVENTRICULAR TACHYCARDIA

Supraventricular tachycardia, also known as paroxysmal supraventricular tachycardia or paroxysmal atrial tachycardia, is defined as an abnormal arrhythmia mechanism arising above or within the bundle of His (thus excluding sinus tachycardia). The mode of presentation is dependent on the interaction of the rate of the tachycardia, the cardiovascular system, and the patient in general. A tachycardia may be poorly tolerated in a child with pre-existing congestive heart failure or an underlying systemic disease such as anemia or sepsis or may go unnoticed in an otherwise healthy child. Incessant tachycardia in an otherwise healthy individual, albeit slow (120–150 beats/min), may cause myocardial dysfunction and congestive heart failure if left untreated.

Tachycardia mechanisms can be divided into three groups: reentry, enhanced automaticity, and triggered dysrhythmias.

Reentry is conduction through two or more pathways, creating a sustained repetitive circular loop. The circuit can be confined to the atrium (intra-atrial reentry, a form of atrial flutter) (Figure 19–8). It may be confined within the atrioventricular node (atrioventricular nodal reentrant tachycardia) or it may encompass an atrioventricular accessory connection, producing orthodromic reciprocating tachycardia, in which the electrical impulse travels anterograde down the atrioventricular node and then retrograde up the accessory connection and then back down the atrioventricular node to complete the reentrant loop (Figure 19–9). Wolff-Parkinson-White syndrome is a subclass of these in which, during sinus rhythm, the

Figure 19–8. Leads aVF (F) and V$_1$, showing atrial flutter with "sawtooth" atrial flutter waves.

impulse travels anterograde down the accessory connection, bypassing the atrioventricular node and creating ventricular pre-excitation (early eccentric activation of the ventricle with a short PR interval and slurred upstroke of the QRS, a delta wave (Figure 19–10). Reentrant tachycardia represents approximately 80% of pediatric arrhythmias, has a wide range of rates, and may or may not demonstrate P waves and initiate and terminate abruptly.

Enhanced automaticity (also known as automatic or ectopic tachycardia) is created when a focus of cardiac tissue develops an abnormally fast spontaneous rate of depolarization. These arrhythmias represent approximately 20% of childhood arrhythmias

Figure 19–9. Supraventricular tachycardia. **A:** Twelve-lead ECG showing orthodromic reciprocating tachycardia (see text). **B:** Lead II rhythm strip showing spontaneous conversion to normal sinus rhythm with ventricular pre-excitation (Wolff-Parkinson-White syndrome) and then spontaneous resolution with loss of the delta wave and a normal PR interval at the end of the tracing.

Figure 19–10. Leads I and II with spontaneous intermittent ventricular pre-excitation (Wolff-Parkinson-White syndrome).

and are usually under autonomic influence. Electrocardiography demonstrates a normal QRS complex preceded by an abnormal P wave (Figure 19–11). Junctional ectopic tachycardia may show atrioventricular dissociation or 1:1 retrograde conduction (Figure 19–12). These tachycardias demonstrate a gradual onset and offset and may be paroxysmal or incessant. When they are incessant, they usually present with congestive heart failure and a clinical picture of dilated cardiomyopathy.

Triggered dysrhythmia is extremely rare. It is caused by enhanced afterdepolarizations of the action potential that reach the takeoff potential. It is one of the side effects of digitalis toxicity.

Clinical Findings

A. Symptoms & Signs: Clinical presentation varies with the age of the patient. Infants tend to turn pale and mottled with onset of tachycardia and may become irritable. With long duration of tachycardia, symptoms of congestive heart failure develop. Heart rates can be from 240 to 300 beats/min. Older children may complain of dizziness, palpitations, fatigue, and chest pain. Heart rates usually range from 240/min in the younger child to 150–180/min in the teenager. Congestive heart failure is less common in children than in infants. Tachycardia may be associated with either congenital heart defects such as Ebstein's anomaly or acquired conditions such as cardiomyopathies and myocarditis.

B. Imaging: Findings on chest x-ray are normal during the early course of tachycardia. If congestive heart failure is present, the heart is enlarged and there is evidence of pulmonary venous congestion.

C. Electrocardiography: Electrocardiography is the most important tool in the diagnosis of supraventricular tachycardia.

1. The heart rate is rapid and out of proportion

Figure 19–11. Lead II rhythm strip of ectopic atrial tachycardia. The tracing demonstrates a variable rate with a maximum of 260 beats/min, an abnormal P wave, and a gradual termination.

Figure 19–12. Three-lead rhythm strip of junctional ectopic tachycardia. Lead I is an atrial electrogram showing atrial (a)–ventricular (v) dissociation.

to the patient's physical status (ie, a rate of 140/min with an abnormal P wave while quiet and asleep).

2. The rhythm is extremely regular. There is little variation in the rate throughout the entire tracing.

3. P waves may or may not be present. If they are present, there is no variation in the appearance or in the PR interval. P waves may be difficult to find because they are superimposed on the preceding T wave. Furthermore, if the abnormal focus is located within the atrioventricular node, the P waves will not be seen (Figure 19–9).

4. The QRS complex is usually the same as during normal sinus rhythm. However, the QRS complex is occasionally widened (supraventricular tachycardia with aberrant ventricular conduction), in which case the condition may be difficult to differentiate from ventricular tachycardia.

Treatment

A. Acute Treatment: During initial episodes of supraventricular tachycardia, patients require close monitoring. Correction of acidosis and electrolyte abnormalities is also indicated.

1. Vagal maneuvers–The "diving reflex," an icebag placed on the nasal bridge for 20 seconds (for infants) or facial immersion in ice water (for children or adolescents), will increase parasympathetic tone and terminate some tachycardias. The Valsalva maneuver, which can be performed by older compliant children, may also terminate supraventricular tachycardia.

2. Adenosine–Adenosine transiently blocks atrioventricular conduction and terminates tachycardias that incorporate the atrioventricular node. It does not convert tachycardias whose mechanism is confined to the atria (atrial ectopic tachycardia, intra-atrial reentry).

Adenosine does not convert tachycardias whose mechanism is confined to the atria (atrial ectopic tachycardia, intra-atrial reentry). However, it serves as a diagnostic tool in these arrhythmias by demonstrating continuation of the tachycardia during atrioventricular block, implying that atrioventricular node conduction is not a crucial element of the tachycardia circuit. The dose is 50–250 µg/kg by rapid intravenous bolus. It is antagonized by aminophylline and should be used with caution in patients with asthma.

3. Transesophageal atrial pacing–Atrial overdrive pacing and termination can be performed from a bipolar electrode-tipped catheter positioned in the esophagus adjacent to the left atrium. Overdrive pacing at rates approximately 30% faster than the tachycardia rate will interrupt the tachycardia circuit and restore sinus rhythm.

4. DC cardioversion–Direct current (DC) cardioversion (0.5–2 synchronized J/kg) should be used immediately when a patient presents in cardiovascular collapse.

B. Chronic Treatment:

1. Digitalis–Digitalis is the drug of choice for long-term therapy. Conversion should be accomplished within 8–12 hours. Doses used are the same as those for congestive heart failure.

2. Beta-adrenergic blocking agents–Propranolol decreases sinus heart rate and atrioventricular nodal conduction. It is effective in the treatment of both reentrant and ectopic arrhythmias in doses ranging from 1 to 4 mg/kg/d. Newer beta-blockers such as atenolol and nadolol have recently become popular because they have fewer central nervous system side effects than propranolol and may be given only once or twice a day.

3. Calcium channel antagonists–Verapamil and other calcium channel blockers markedly prolong conduction through the atrioventricular node and are effective in interrupting and preventing reentrant tachycardias that incorporate the atrioventricular node. They are ineffective in terminating atrial tachycardias but may be useful to control the ventricular response by producing atrioventricular blockade. Verapamil comes in short- and long-acting preparations; the dose is 4–17 mg/kg/d. In well-tolerated, infrequent tachycardias, it can be taken on an as-needed basis to terminate individual episodes.

4. Other drugs–Recently introduced antiarrhythmic medications (eg, flecainide, propafenone, sotalol, amiodarone) have increased pharmacologic actions and are extremely effective. However, these drugs also have serious side effects, including proarrhythmia (production of arrhythmias) and sudden death, and should be used only under the direction of a pediatric cardiologist.

5. Radiofrequency ablation–This is a nonsurgical transvenous catheter technique that will desiccate an arrhythmia focus or accessory pathway and permanently "cure" an arrhythmia. The immediate success rate is approximately 85%, with a low rate of recurrence of 10%. The risk of developing complete heart block is about 1%. The procedure can be performed in infants and adults. In younger children, it should be reserved for those whose arrhythmias are refractory to medical management.

Prognosis

Supraventricular tachycardia has an excellent prognosis. When it presents in early infancy, 90% will respond to initial treatment. Approximately 30% will recur at an average age of 8 years.

Kugler JD et al: Radiofrequency catheter ablation for tachyarrhythmias in children and adolescents. N Engl J Med 1994;330:1481.

Munger TM et al: A population study of the natural history of Wolff-Parkinson-White syndrome in Olmsted County, Minnesota, 1953–1989. Circulation 1993;87:866.

ATRIAL FLUTTER & FIBRILLATION

Atrial flutter and fibrillation are rare in children and are most often associated with organic heart disease—particularly postoperative congenital heart disease and SND. Atrial flutter (Figure 19–8) can present in infancy and can mimic supraventricular tachycardia. The atrial rate is usually greater than 240/min and often more than 300/min. The ventricular rate depends on the rate of atrioventricular conduction and is usually slower than the atrial rate.

Treatment & Prognosis

Transesophageal atrial pacing is the treatment of choice to terminate atrial flutter. When it is not successful, antiarrhythmic medications (eg, digoxin, sotalol, amiodarone) may succeed; however, DC cardioversion is frequently necessary. Recently, radiofrequency ablation has been successful in selective refractory cases.

The prognosis in neonates without structural heart disease is excellent, and following conversion these patients may need no medications, whereas postoperative atrial flutter and fibrillation are often refractory to medical management. In extreme cases, creation of complete heart block and permanent pacing may be necessary.

VENTRICULAR TACHYCARDIA

Ventricular tachycardia is uncommon in childhood (Figure 19–13). It is usually associated with underlying abnormalities of the myocardium (myocarditis, cardiomyopathy, myocardial tumors, postoperative congenital heart disease) or toxicity (hypoxia, electrolyte imbalance, drug toxicity). Sustained tachycardia is generally an unstable situation and, if left untreated, will usually degenerate into ventricular fibrillation.

Accelerated idioventricular rhythm is a sustained ventricular tachycardia seen in neonates with normal hearts. The rate is within 10% of the preceding sinus rate, and it is a self-limiting arrhythmia that requires no treatment.

Acute termination of ventricular tachycardia involves restoration of the normal myocardium when possible (correct electrolyte imbalance, drug toxicity, etc) and DC cardioversion (1–4 J/kg), cardioversion with lidocaine (1 mg/kg), or both. Chronic suppression of ventricular arrhythmias with antiarrhythmic drugs has many side effects (including proarrhythmia and death), and it must be initiated in the hospital under the direction of a pediatric cardiologist.

MacLelland-Tobert SG, Porter CJ: Accelerated idioventricular rhythm: A benign arrhythmia in childhood. Pediatrics 1995;96:122.

LONG QT SYNDROME

The long QT syndrome in children is an arrhythmic disorder in which ventricular repolarization is irregular and prolonged (QT_c >0.44 s). It presents as

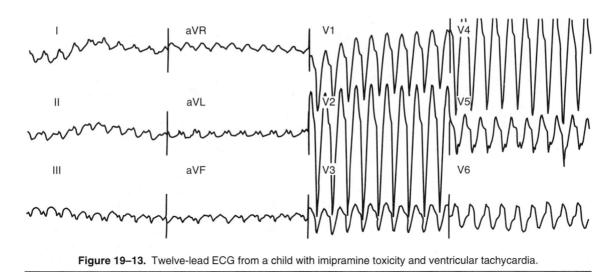

Figure 19–13. Twelve-lead ECG from a child with imipramine toxicity and ventricular tachycardia.

syncope or seizures in response to exercise or sudden death, and if untreated, it has a very high mortality rate (5% per year). It is transmitted genetically in an autosomal dominant or recessive pattern (the latter associated with congenital deafness), or it may be sporadic. Treatment is with beta blockade and exercise limitation and is only partially successful.

Garson A Jr et al: The long QT syndrome in children: An international study of 287 patients. Circulation 1993; 87:1866.

HEART BLOCK

1. FIRST-DEGREE HEART BLOCK

First-degree heart block is an electrocardiographic diagnosis of prolongation of the PR interval. The block does not in itself cause problems, but it is frequently seen in association with such congenital heart defects as atrial septal defect and with diseases such as rheumatic carditis. The PR interval may also be prolonged as a result of digoxin therapy.

2. SECOND-DEGREE HEART BLOCK

Mobitz type I (**Wenckebach**) heart block is recognized by progressive prolongation of the PR interval until there is no QRS following a P wave (Figure 19–14). Mobitz type I heart block occurs in normal hearts at rest and is usually benign. In **Mobitz type II** heart block, there is no progressive lengthening of the PR interval before the dropped beat (Figure 19–15). Mobitz type II heart block is frequently associated with organic heart disease, and a complete evaluation is necessary.

3. COMPLETE HEART BLOCK

In complete heart block, the atria and ventricles beat independently. Ventricular rates can range from 40 to 80 beats/min, whereas atrial rates may be faster (Figure 19–16).

Congenital complete heart block, the most common form of complete heart block, has a very high association with maternal systemic lupus erythematosus (80% at our institution). Serologic screening should be performed in the mother of an infant with complete heart block even if she has no symptoms of collagen vascular disease. Congenital complete heart block is also associated with congenitally corrected transposition of the great vessels and endocardial cushion defect. Acquired complete heart block may be secondary to acute myocarditis, drug toxicity, electrolyte imbalance, hypoxia, and cardiac surgery.

Clinical Findings

Prenatal bradycardia is frequently noted in infants with congenital complete heart block, and emergent delivery is required if hydrops fetalis develops. Postnatal adaptation is largely dependent on the heart rate; infants with heart rates lower than 55 beats/min are at significantly greater risk for low cardiac output, congestive heart failure, and death. Wide QRS complexes and a rapid atrial rate are also poor prognostic signs. Most patients have an innocent flow murmur from increased stroke volume. In symptomatic patients, the heart can be quite enlarged and pulmonary edema may be present. In older patients, Stokes-Adams syncope can be the presenting symptom, or heart block may be found unexpectedly on routine physical examination. Complete cardiac evaluation, including echocardiography and Holter monitoring, is necessary to assess the patient for ventricu-

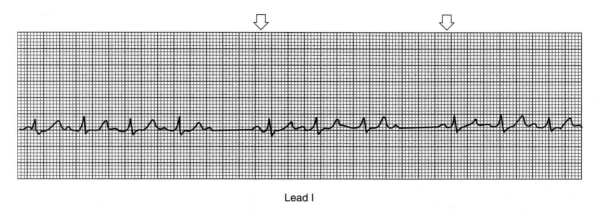

Lead I

Figure 19–14. Lead I rhythm strip with Mobitz type I (Wenckebach) second-degree heart block. There is progressive lengthening of the PR interval prior to the nonconducted P wave.

lar dysfunction and to relate any symptoms to concurrent arrhythmias.

Treatment

In patients thought to be at risk for Stokes-Adams attacks or congestive heart failure, the treatment of choice for complete heart block is surgical insertion of a permanent pacemaker. Until permanent pacing can be instituted, patients can be temporarily assisted by infusions of isoproterenol or by temporary transcutaneous pacemakers.

Friedman RA: Congenital AV block Pace Me Now or Pace Me Later? Circulation 1995;92:283.

SYNCOPE
(Fainting)

Syncope is a sudden transient loss of consciousness that resolves spontaneously. The common form

of syncope (simple fainting) occurs in 15% of children and is a disorder of control of heart rate and blood pressure by the autonomic nervous system that causes hypotension or bradycardia. It is often associated with rapid rising and postural hypotension, prolonged standing, or hypovolemia. Patients exhibit "vagal" symptoms such as pallor, nausea, or diaphoresis. Syncope, also known as autonomic dysfunction, can be evaluated with head-up tilt table testing. The patient is placed supine on a tilt table, and then—under constant heart rate and blood pressure monitoring—is tilted to the upright position. If symptoms develop, they can be classified as vasodepressor (hypotension), cardioinhibitory (bradycardia), or mixed. Treatment can then be directed accordingly. Syncope is usually self-limited and can be controlled with dietary salt and volume loading to prevent hypovolemia. Syncope that occurs during exercise or stress or is associated with a positive family history is a warning sign that there may be a serious

Lead III

Figure 19–15. Lead III rhythm strip with Mobitz type II second-degree heart block. There is a consistent PR interval with occasional loss of atrioventricular conduction (arrow).

Figure 19–16. Twelve-lead ECG and lead II rhythm strip of complete heart block. The atrial rate is 150/min and the ventricular rate is 60/min.

A

B

Figure 19–17. Rhythm strips of hyperkalemia, beginning with tall, peaked T waves and progressing to sinusoidal ventricular tachycardia.

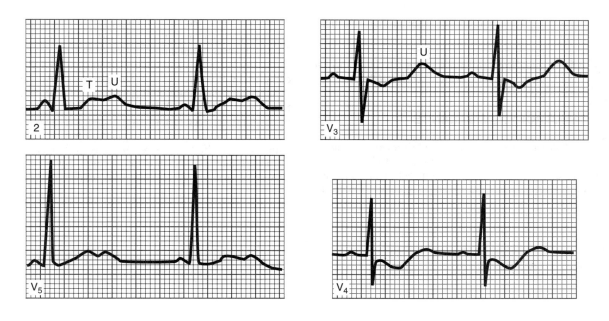

Figure 19–18. ECGs of hypokalemia, showing ST-segment depression and prominent U waves.

Figure 19–19. ECGs of hypocalcemia, demonstrating QT-interval prolongation and T-wave inversion.

underlying dysrhythmia calling for further investigation.

Balaji S et al: Neurocardiogenic syncope in children with a normal heart. J Am Coll Cardiol 1994;23:779.

ELECTROLYTE IMBALANCE

Potassium, calcium, and, to a lesser extent, magnesium imbalances are reflected on the ECG. Electrolyte disturbances resulting from potassium and calcium excess or deficiency are of greatest concern to the pediatrician, and some familiarity with these abnormal tracings is essential. In hyperkalemia (Figure 19–17), there is gradual progression from tall, peaked T waves (5–7 meq/L) through widening of the QRS complex (8–9 meq/L) to a broad, almost sinusoidal ventricular tachycardia configuration (>10 meq/L). Hypokalemia (Figure 19–18) is characterized by progressive prominence of the U wave and prolongation of the QT interval with ST-segment depression. In hypocalcemia (Figure 19–19), there is prolongation of the QT interval, and in extreme cases T-wave inversion occurs.

Gastrointestinal Tract

20

Judith M. Sondheimer, MD

GASTROESOPHAGEAL REFLUX & CHALASIA

Clinical Findings

Postprandial regurgitation is the most common symptom of gastroesophageal reflux in young infants. Regurgitation ranges from effortless spitting to forceful vomiting. Although usually harmless, severe gastroesophageal reflux may cause failure to thrive, esophagitis with hematemesis, occult blood loss, anemia, esophageal stricture, and inflammatory esophageal polyps. Aspiration pneumonia, chronic cough, wheezing, and asthma-like attacks are reported. Dysphagia, colic after feedings, and neck contortions (Sandifer's syndrome) may occur. Ruminative behavior is sometimes a symptom. Apneic spells in young infants, especially occurring with position change after feeding, may be caused by gastroesophageal reflux. Gastroesophageal reflux is common in neurologically impaired children (Table 20–1).

Gastroesophageal reflux is usually diagnosed clinically in thriving infants under 6 months of age. It can be diagnosed on barium swallow by observing free regurgitation of barium from stomach to esophagus. However, both false-positive and false-negative tests are common. An upper GI series is important to rule out anatomic causes of vomiting. Prolonged monitoring of esophageal pH is a more sensitive test. Esophageal and gastric scintiscanning is sometimes helpful in identifying pulmonary aspiration. Esophagoscopy is not diagnostic, but esophagitis can be identified.

Treatment & Prognosis

In 85% of patients, gastroesophageal reflux is self-limited, disappearing between 6 and 12 months, often coincident with assumption of erect posture and initiation of solid feedings. Regurgitation is reduced by conservative measures such as small, frequent feedings thickened with rice cereal (2–3 tsp per ounce of formula) and placing the child in a prone position. H_2 receptor antagonists (ranitidine 5.0 mg/kg/d in two doses) or proton pump inhibitors (omeprazole) are effective in controlling esophagitis. Use of the latter agents promotes hypergastrinemia, whose long-term effects in infants are not defined. Prokinetic agents such as metoclopramide (0.1 mg/kg before meals), or cisapride (0.2 mg/kg/dose three or four times daily) hasten gastric emptying and improve esophageal motor function.

Surgery is indicated if reflux causes: (1) persistent vomiting with failure to thrive; (2) esophagitis or esophageal stricture; and (3) apneic spells or chronic pulmonary disease unresponsive to 2–3 months of medical therapy. Children over 18 months, children with large hiatus hernias, and neurologically handicapped children respond less well to medical therapy.

Gunasekaran TS, Hassall EG: Efficacy and safety of omeprazole for severe gastrointestinal reflux in children. J Pediatr 1993;123:148.

Orenstein SR et al: Gastroesophageal reflux and respiratory disease in children. J Pediatr 1988;112:847.

Sondheimer JM: Gastroesophageal reflux in children: Clinical presentation and diagnostic evaluation. Gastrointest Endosc Clin North Am 1994;4:55.

ACHALASIA OF THE ESOPHAGUS

Esophageal achalasia is characterized by failure of relaxation of the lower esophageal sphincter and lack of propulsive peristalsis in the esophageal body.

Clinical Findings

A. Symptoms and Signs: Achalasia occurs at any age but is uncommon under the age of 5 years. Typical symptoms include retrosternal pain and episodes of food "sticking" in the throat or upper chest. Patients eat slowly and often drink large amounts of fluid with meals. Dysphagia is relieved by repeated forceful swallowing or by vomiting. Familial cases have been described. Chronic cough, wheezing, recurrent pneumonitis, anemia, and weight loss may occur.

B. Imaging and Manometric Studies: The barium swallow shows a dilated esophagus with a

Table 20–1. Causes of vomiting and regurgitation.

GASTROINTESTINAL TRACT DISORDERS

Esophagus
Achalasia
Gastroesophageal
  reflux (chalasia)
Hiatal hernia
Esophagitis
Atresia with or without
  fistula
Congenital vascular or
  mucosal rings, webs
Stenosis
Duplication and divertic-
  ulum
Foreign body
Periesophageal mass

Stomach
Hypertrophic pyloric
  stenosis
Pylorospasm
Diaphragmatic hernia
Peptic disease and
  gastritis
Antral web

Duodenum
Atresia, diaphragm
Annular pancreas
Duodenitis and ulcer
Malrotation
Mesenteric bands
Superior mesenteric
  artery syndrome

Intestine & Colon
Atresia and stenosis
Meconium ileus
Malrotation, volvulus
Duplication
Intussusception
Foreign body
Polyposis
Soy or cow's milk protein
  intolerance
Gluten enteropathy
Food allergy
Hirschsprung's disease
Chronic intestinal pseudo-
  obstruction
Appendicitis
Inflammatory bowel disease
Gastroenteritis, infections

Other abdominal organs
Hepatitis
Gallstones
Pancreatitis
Peritonitis

EXTRAGASTROINTESTINAL TRACT DISORDERS

Sepsis
Pneumonia
Otitis media
Urinary tract infection
Meningitis
Subdural effusion
Hydrocephalus
Brain tumor
Reye's syndrome
Rumination
Intoxications
  Alcohol
  Aspirin
  Acetaminophen

Adrenal insufficiency
Renal tubular acidosis
Inborn errors
  Urea cycle disorders
  Phenylketonuria
  Maple syrup urine
    disease
  Organic acidemia
  Galactosemia
  Fructose intolerance
  Tyrosinosis
  Scleroderma
  Epidermolysis bullosa

short, tapered stricture at the distal end. In infants, esophageal dilation may not be present. Cinefluoroscopy may show absence of normal peristalsis. Esophageal manometry may show high resting pressure in the lower esophageal sphincter, failure of the sphincter to relax with swallowing and abnormal or absent peristalsis.

Differential Diagnosis

Congenital esophageal stricture, esophageal webs, peptic stricture secondary to chronic reflux, and esophageal masses may mimic esophageal achalasia.

Treatment & Prognosis

Pneumatic dilation of the lower esophageal sphincter is of value in most cases and can be re-peated if symptoms recur. More definitive results can be achieved by surgically splitting the lower esophageal sphincter muscle (Heller myotomy). Because of the shorter duration of the illness in pediatric patients, the prognosis for return of the esophagus to normal caliber after surgical treatment is better than in adults.

Berquist WE et al: Achalasia: Diagnosis, management and clinical course in 16 children. Pediatrics 1983;71:798.
Nakayama DK et al: Pneumatic dilation and operative treatment of achalasia in children. J Pediatr Surg 1987;22: 619.

CAUSTIC BURNS OF THE ESOPHAGUS

Ingestion of caustic solids or liquids (pH > 12) may produce esophageal lesions ranging from superficial inflammation to coagulative necrosis with ulceration, perforation, and mediastinitis (or peritonitis if the stomach is involved). The severity of the accompanying oral or laryngeal lesions does not correlate well with the degree of esophageal injury. Esophageal or laryngeal obstruction secondary to edema and exudate occurs within 24 hours. Pain may be severe. Strictures of the esophagus may develop quickly or gradually over several months. Esophageal strictures develop in areas of anatomic narrowing, such as the cervical region, at the point at which the left bronchus crosses the esophagus and at the gastroesophageal junction. Stricture occurs only with full-thickness esophageal necrosis. Short, circumferential strictures may occur, or the entire esophagus may become twisted and narrowed. Shortening of the esophagus may lead to a hiatal hernia.

The child with a history of alkali ingestion should have a careful examination of the lips and mouth and airway. Drooling is common. Oral lesions are especially common with solid agents. Vomiting should not be induced. Hospitalization is recommended even if ingestion is only suspected. Intravenous corticosteroids (eg, methylprednisolone), 1–2 mg/kg/d, are started immediately if oral cavity swelling is severe and laryngeal edema is suspected. Intravenous fluids may be necessary if dysphagia is present. Esophagoscopy should be done within 24–48 hours after ingestion. Treatment may be stopped if there are only first-degree burns. Corticosteroids may be beneficial in first- and second-degree burns, but are not likely to prevent stricture formation from third-degree burns. Repeated esophageal dilations may be necessary as a stricture develops but are not performed acutely. When x-rays show erosion into the mediastinum or peritoneum, antibiotics are mandatory. Intraluminal esophageal stenting may be beneficial during early management. Surgical replacement of the esophagus with a segment of colon may be necessary if dilation fails to control stricture.

Although other ingestants may cause esophageal irritation (eg, bleach, detergents, or acids), it is rare for any but the strongest acids and detergents to result in full-thickness necrosis and stricture.

Anderson KD, Rouse TM, Randolph JG: A controlled trial of corticosteroids in children with corrosive injury of the esophagus. N Engl J Med 1990;323:637.

Crain FC, Gershel JC, Mezey AP: Symptoms as predictors of esophageal injury. Am J Dis Child 1984;138:863.

Gaudreault P et al: Predictability of esophageal injury from signs and symptoms. A study of caustic ingestion in 378 children. Pediatrics 1983;71:767.

HIATAL HERNIA

Hiatal hernias are classified as (1) paraesophageal, in which the esophagus and gastroesophageal junction are normally placed with the gastric cardia herniated beside the esophagus through the esophageal hiatus; and (2) sliding, in which the gastroesophageal junction and a portion of the proximal stomach are herniated through the esophageal hiatus. Paraesophageal hernia is rare in childhood and presents with pain, esophageal obstruction, or respiratory compromise. Sliding hernia is common in children. Gastroesophageal reflux may accompany sliding hiatal hernia, though many, even those of large size, cause no symptoms.

PYLORIC STENOSIS

The cause of postnatal pyloric circular muscle hypertrophy causing gastric outlet obstruction is not known. The incidence is from 1 to 8 per 1000 births with a 4:1 male predominance and a positive family history in 13%.

Clinical Findings

A. Symptoms and Signs: Vomiting usually begins between 2 and 4 weeks of age and rapidly becomes projectile after every feeding; it starts at birth in about 10% of cases. Onset of symptoms may be delayed in premature infants. The vomitus is rarely bilious but may be blood-streaked. The infant is hungry and nurses avidly. Constipation, dehydration, weight loss, fretfulness, and finally apathy occur. The upper abdomen may be distended after feeding, and prominent gastric peristaltic waves from left to right may be seen. An olive-sized mass can often be felt on deep palpation in the right upper abdomen, especially after the child has vomited.

B. Laboratory Findings: There is hypochloremic alkalosis with potassium depletion. Hemoconcentration is reflected by elevated hemoglobin and hematocrit values. Elevated unconjugated bilirubin occurs in 2–5% of cases.

C. Imaging: An upper gastrointestinal series reveals delay in gastric emptying and an elongated narrowed pyloric channel with a double tract of barium. The enlarged pyloric muscle causes characteristic semilunar impressions on the gastric antrum. Ultrasonography shows a hypoechoic ring with a hyperdense center. thickness of circular muscle is greater than 4 mm in pyloric stenosis.

Differential Diagnosis

Other causes of vomiting in young infants must be ruled out. (See Table 20–1.) In esophageal stenosis or achalasia, the emesis contains no gastric contents, and metabolic alkalosis is rare. With annular pancreas, malrotation, volvulus, and lesions causing small bowel obstruction, the emesis is bilious. The absence of virilization and hyperkalemia generally rules out congenital adrenal hyperplasia with adrenal insufficiency. Seizures, irritability, and metabolic acidosis are often associated with other metabolic disorders. Sepsis and urinary tract infections should be checked by culture. Pylorospasm during barium x-ray may cause delay in gastric emptying, but the elongated narrow pyloric canal is not seen and no mass is palpable. Antral webs or diaphragms, duplications, cysts, and ulcers of the pyloric canal are rare causes of gastric outlet obstruction.

Treatment & Prognosis

Pyloromyotomy is the treatment of choice and consists of incision down to the mucosa along the pyloric length. Prior to surgery, it is imperative to repair dehydration and electrolyte abnormalities even if it takes 24–48 hours.

The outlook is excellent following surgery. Sometimes there is vomiting postoperatively in cases with a long preoperative history. The postoperative barium x-ray remains abnormal despite relief of symptoms.

Moazam F, Kolts BE, Rodgers B: In pursuit of the etiology of congenital hypertrophic pyloric stenosis. J Pediatr Gastroenterol Nutr 1982;1:97.

Stunden RJ, LeQuense GW, Little KET: The improved ultrasound diagnosis of pyloric stenosis. Pediatr Radiol 1986;16:200.

EVALUATION OF THE CHILD WITH VOMITING

Assessment of the child with vomiting should start with a complete history, physical examination, and description of the vomitus. Emesis of gastric contents is characteristic of gastric outlet obstruction, central nervous system masses or infection, peptic disease, urinary tract infection, otitis or sinusitis, metabolic diseases (especially those causing acidosis), rumination, or psychogenic vomiting. Gastroesophageal reflux should be suspected in a healthy child with effortless postprandial spitting. An upper gastrointestinal series is essential to rule out anatomic causes. Further evaluations may include serum electrolytes, calcium, magnesium, urea nitrogen, urinalysis, and culture. The decision to obtain x-rays and scans of the central nervous system, chest, or sinuses requires specific indication from history or physical examination.

The child who vomits bile-stained material may have small intestinal obstruction and should be investigated urgently. Bile staining may be gold or green in color. The history and physical examination are the essential starting points and should include duration of vomiting, the presence of blood in the vomitus, the presence of abdominal pain or distention, the character of the stools, and the presence of fever. Pain localized to the right lower quadrant suggests appendicitis. Midline or diffuse abdominal pain suggests pancreatitis or generalized peritonitis. Abdominal distention suggests intestinal obstruction. Viral and bacterial gastroenteritis associated with diarrhea and may produce a generalized ileus with bilious emesis. Gallbladder disease is uncommon in childhood but should be suspected in children with a positive family history or primary medical conditions promoting gallstones. The presence of mucus and blood in the stool should raise the suspicion of intestinal intussusception or bacterial or toxic colitis. Three-way radiographs of the abdomen are a first diagnostic step in localizing the site of intestinal obstruction.

The evaluation of bloody vomitus should start with confirmation that the material vomited is indeed blood. Numerous causes must be considered including swallowed maternal blood in newborns, oropharyngeal lesions, nosebleed, peptic disease, bleeding disorders, foreign bodies, and esophageal varices. Mallory-Weiss tear of the gastroesophageal junction is common after prolonged vomiting. Careful assessment of the cardiovascular stability of the child is essential before extensive evaluation is initiated. Passage of a nasogastric tube will help determine whether bleeding is ongoing. Hematocrit should be measured. The history and physical examination will provide specific clues to diagnosis which may make further testing unnecessary. If further diagnostic testing is desired, the most productive test is upper intestinal endoscopy.

PEPTIC DISEASE

Peptic ulcers may occur at any age but are more common between 12 and 18 years. Boys are affected more frequently than girls. Up to age 6, most ulcers are secondary to an underlying illness, toxin, or drug.

A positive family history is present in about 30% of cases of primary duodenal ulcer.

Commonly, primary or secondary peptic disease is caused by breakdown in the normal mucosal defense, which permits acid peptic digestion of gastric or duodenal mucosa. Causes include (1) reduced mucous protective layer (aspirin, nonsteroidal anti-inflammatory drugs, hypoxia); (2) reduced metabolic activity of the mucosal cell, which allows for the diffusion of hydrogen ions into the cell (hypoxia, hypotension); (3) increased secretion of acid or pepsin (increased parietal cell mass, increased postprandial secretion of gastrin, increased vagal tone); (4) reflux of bile from duodenum to stomach; and (5) decreased neutralizing activity in duodenal secretions. The most common causes of secondary ulcer are toxins (alcohol, aspirin, and nonsteroidal anti-inflammatory medications), sepsis, hypotension, burns, and injury of the central nervous system.

There is a close association between *Helicobacter pylori* infection of the gastric antrum and the primary peptic conditions—antral gastritis, duodenal ulcer, and gastric ulcer. The incidence of *H pylori* infection is low in North American children but increases with age (50% of blood donors in the United States have *H pylori* antibodies). There is no evidence that *H pylori* infection causes recurrent abdominal pain of childhood or dyspepsia without gastritis.

Clinical Findings

A. Symptoms and Signs:

1. At 0–3 years of age—Symptoms of primary ulcers include anorexia, vomiting, crying after meals, and melena or hematemesis. Secondary ulcers are more acute, and hemorrhage or perforation may be the first signs.

2. At 3–6 years of age—Vomiting related to eating is usually present. Gastric outlet obstruction may cause protracted vomiting. Periumbilical or generalized pain is common. Melena and hematemesis are common symptoms of secondary ulcers.

3. At 6–18 years of age—Fewer than 50% of patients have "typical" ulcer symptoms. Melena or hematemesis is noted in over 50%; occult bleeding and anemia may occur without other symptoms. Acute illnesses responsible for secondary ulcers include central nervous system disease, burns, sepsis, and chronic multiple organ failure. Chronic conditions such as pulmonary insufficiency, Crohn's disease, hepatic cirrhosis, and rheumatoid arthritis are associated with peptic disease. *H pylori* infection may be found with increased frequency.

B. Gastric Analysis: Gastric analysis is rarely performed. It may be useful in identifying extreme hypersecretion such as that associated with the Zollinger-Ellison syndrome, but a secretin stimulation test is much less cumbersome.

C. Imaging: Radiologic signs of ulceration or a

deformity may be present. Duodenal spasticity and irregularity are found in normal infants, making this finding unreliable. In patients with severe duodenal irritability, a crater may not be demonstrated, because the barium is moved out of the bulb very rapidly.

D. Panendoscopy: Upper intestinal endoscopy should be performed if x-ray is negative or equivocal. If upper gastrointestinal bleeding (hematemesis or melena) is present, endoscopy should be the first diagnostic test if it can be done within 48 hours of the episode. Endoscopy permits gastric biopsy necessary for the identification of *H pylori* by culture, histology and urease activity. The presence of serum anti-*H pylori* antibody appears to correlate with infection; titers fall with eradication of the organism.

Differential Diagnosis

Secondary ulcers should be suspected in any child with a severe underlying disease who suddenly presents with hematemesis, or melena. The differential diagnosis of primary peptic ulcer includes recurrent abdominal pain, irritable bowel syndrome, esophagitis, pancreatitis, cholelithiasis, and recurrent midgut volvulus. Suspicion should increase when there is a family history of primary peptic ulcer disease, even if the gastrointestinal complaints are vague.

Treatment

Peptic ulcer disease may be treated with liquid antacids, 0.5–2.5 mL/kg given every 1–2 hours. For mild to moderate symptoms, antacids are given 1 and 3 hours after meals and before bed. Cimetidine (5 mg/kg/dose given orally before meals and at bedtime) or ranitidine (2.5 mg/kg/dose given orally every 12 hours) produces effective healing of peptic ulceration in 4–8 weeks. Famotidine, another H_2 receptor antagonist, can be used, but the dosage in children is not determined. Proton pump inhibitors (omeprazole) are powerful inhibitors of gastric acid secretion. Appropriate dosage for children is not determined. The effects of prolonged hypergastrinemia seen with these agents are not known.

Strict "ulcer diet" is not indicated. Foods that cause pain should be avoided. Caffeine should be avoided because it increases gastric secretion. Three regular meals are recommended; snacks are to be avoided, especially at bedtime. Aspirin and nonsteroidal anti-inflammatory drugs should be avoided.

Surgical treatment is reserved for the complications, such as perforation, hemorrhage, obstruction, or incapacitating, intractable pain.

Cure of peptic disease associated with *H pylori* requires eradication of the organism. The optimal therapeutic regimen is still undetermined. A recent National Institutes of Health consensus conference recommends "triple therapy" with amoxicillin, metronidazole, and bismuth subsalicylate for 10–14 days. Double therapy with omeprazole and amoxicillin may be equally effective.

George DE, Glassman M: Peptic ulcer disease in children. Gastrointest Endosc Clin North Am 1994;4:23.
Peterson WL: *Helocobacter pylori* and peptic ulcer disease. N Engl J Med 1991;324:1043.
Tadataka Y et al: *H pylori* in peptic ulcer disease. NIH Consensus Statement 1994;12:1.

CONGENITAL DIAPHRAGMATIC HERNIA

Diaphragmatic hernia may be secondary to a posterolateral defect in the diaphragm (foramen of Bochdalek) or, in about 5% of cases, to a retrosternal defect (foramen of Morgagni). It represents failure of division of the thoracic and abdominal cavities at the eighth to tenth weeks of fetal life. All degrees of protrusion of the abdominal viscera through the diaphragmatic opening may occur. Eighty percent of posterolateral defects involve the left diaphragm. In eventration of the diaphragm, a leaf of the diaphragm with hypoplastic muscular elements balloons into the chest and leads to similar, milder symptoms.

Mild to severe respiratory distress are usually present at birth. The abdomen may be scaphoid because of the displacement of the viscera. Breath sounds in the affected hemithorax are absent, with displacement of the point of maximal cardiac impulse. Occasionally, a diaphragmatic hernia may be found on incidental chest x-ray. Thirty percent of infants with diaphragmatic hernia die, mostly from pulmonary insufficiency. The lung on the affected side is hypoplastic, with decreased generations of airways and pulmonary arteries, and pulmonary hypertension. Other complications include mediastinal shift with vascular kinking, pulmonary infection, prematurity, cardiac anomalies, and intestinal malrotation. Extracorporeal membrane oxygenation may decrease the early postoperative mortality rate in patients with poor lung compliance. There is growing enthusiasm for the use of nitric oxide for treatment of pulmonary vascular hypertension in these patients.

Adzick NS et al: Diaphragmatic hernia in the fetus: Prenatal diagnosis and outcome in 94 cases. J Pediatr Surg 1985;20:357.
Kinsella JP et al: Clinical responses to prolonged treatment of persistent pulmonary hypertension of the newborn with low doses of inhaled nitric oxide. J Pediatr 1993;123:103.
Van Meurs KP et al: Congenital diaphragmatic hernia: Long-term outcome in neonates treated with extracorporeal membrane oxygenation. J Pediatr 1993;122:893.

CONGENITAL DUODENAL OBSTRUCTION

Extrinsic duodenal obstruction is usually due to congenital peritoneal bands associated with intestinal malrotation, annular pancreas, or duodenal duplication. Intrinsic obstruction is a result of stenosis, mucosal diaphragm ("wind-sock" deformity), or duodenal atresia. The duodenal lumen may be obliterated by a membrane or completely interrupted with a fibrous cord between the two segments. Atresia may be proximal or distal to the ampulla of Vater.

Clinical Findings

A. Atresia: A history of polyhydramnios is common. Vomiting (usually bile-stained) begins within a few hours after birth, with epigastric distention. Meconium may be normally passed. Duodenal atresia is commonly associated with other congenital anomalies (30%), including esophageal atresia, other intestinal atresias, and cardiac and renal anomalies. Prematurity (25–50%) and Down's syndrome (20–30%) are associated conditions. Abdominal x-rays show distention of the stomach and proximal duodenum ("double bubble"). With protracted vomiting, there may be little air in the stomach. Absence of gas distal to the obstruction suggests atresia or an extrinsic obstruction severe enough to completely occlude the lumen, whereas air scattered over the lower abdomen may indicate a partial duodenal obstruction. A barium enema may be helpful in determining the presence of incomitant malrotation or atresia lower in the gastrointestinal tract.

B. Duodenal Stenosis: Obvious symptoms of duodenal obstruction may be delayed for weeks or years. Although the stenotic area is usually postampullary, the vomitus does not always contain bile.

Treatment & Prognosis

Duodenoduodenostomy is performed to bypass stenosis or atresia. Thorough exploration is necessary to ensure that no additional anomalies are present lower in the gastrointestinal tract. The mortality rate (35–40%) is significantly affected by prematurity, Down's syndrome, and associated congenital anomalies. Postoperative duodenal dilation and hypomotility may cause continued symptoms.

CONGENITAL INTESTINAL ATRESIAS & STENOSIS

Excluding anal anomalies, intestinal atresia and stenosis account for one-third of all neonatal intestinal obstruction. Polyhydramnios occurs in most infants and can be diagnosed before birth by ultrasonography. Neonates present with a clinical triad of abdominal distention, bilious vomiting, and obstipation or failure to pass meconium. Prematurity and other congenital anomalies may be present. The localization and relative incidence of atresias and stenoses are given in Table 20–2.

Bile-stained vomiting with abdominal distention usually begins in the first 48 hours of life. Small

Table 20–2. Localization and incidence of congenital gastrointestinal atresias and stenoses.

	Area Involved	Type of Lesion	Relative Frequency
Pylorus		Atresia Web or diaphragm	1%
Duodenum	80% are distal to the ampulla of Vater	Atresia, stenosis Web or diaphragm	45%
Jejunoileal	Proximal jejunum and distal ileum	Atresia (multiple in 6–29%) Stenosis	50%
Colon	Left colon and rectum	Atresia (usually associated with atresias of the small bowel)	5–9%

amounts of meconium may be passed. Prematurity and severe congenital anomalies often coexist. Atresias, stenoses, and obstructing membranes may affect multiple sites. The small intestine may be significantly shortened. X-ray features include dilated loops of small bowel and absence of colonic gas. Barium enema will reveal a narrow-caliber microcolon if the atresia is in the lower small bowel. In more than 10% of cases of intestinal atresia, there is absence of the mesentery, and the superior mesenteric artery cannot be identified beyond the origin of the right colic and ileocolic arteries. The ileum coils around one of these two arteries, giving rise to the "Christmas tree" deformity. The tenuous blood supply often compromises surgical anastomoses. Multiple intestinal atresias may be associated with immunodeficiency. The differential diagnosis includes Hirschsprung's disease, paralytic ileus secondary to sepsis, gastroenteritis or pneumonia, midgut volvulus, and meconium ileus. Surgery is mandatory in newborn infants with small bowel atresia. Postoperative complications include short bowel syndrome and hypomotility.

Walker MW et al: Multiple areas of intestinal atresia associated with immunodeficiency and post transfusion graft versus host disease. J Pediatr 1993;123:93.

ANNULAR PANCREAS

Annular pancreas is a result of incomplete rotation and fusion of the dorsal and ventral pancreatic anlagen. The symptoms are those of partial or complete duodenal obstruction. Down's syndrome and congenital anomalies of the gastrointestinal tract occur frequently. As with other gastrointestinal obstructive lesions of the neonate, polyhydramnios is common. Clinical manifestations can develop late in childhood. Treatment consists of duodenoduodenostomy or duodenojejunostomy without operative dissection or division of the pancreatic annulus.

Kiernan PD et al: Annular pancreas: Mayo Clinic experience from 1957 to 1976 with review of the literature. Arch Surg 1980;115:46.

Merrill JR, Raffensperger JG: Pediatric annular pancreas: Twenty years' experience. J Pediatr Surg 1976;11:921.

INTESTINAL MALROTATION WITH OR WITHOUT VOLVULUS

Normally, the midgut (which extends from the duodenojejunal junction to the mid transverse colon and which is supplied by the superior mesenteric artery) returns to the intra-abdominal position during the tenth week of embryonic life. The root of the mesentery rotates in a counterclockwise direction during retraction. This causes the colon to cross ventrally; the cecum moves from the left to the right lower quadrant, and the duodenum crosses dorsally to become partly retroperitoneal. When this rotation is incomplete, the posterior fixation of the mesentery is defective, so that the bowel from the ligament of Treitz to the mid transverse colon may twist, causing a volvulus around the narrow mesenteric root.

Clinical Findings

A. Symptoms and Signs: Malrotation and its complications account for 10% of neonatal intestinal obstruction. Most infants present with recurrent bile-stained vomiting or acute small bowel obstruction in the first 3 weeks of life. The first signs may occur later in life, with symptoms of intermittent intestinal obstruction or, rarely, with malabsorption, protein-losing enteropathy, or intermittent diarrhea. Associated congenital anomalies, especially cardiac, occur in over 25% of symptomatic cases.

B. Imaging: An upper gastrointestinal series may show partial or complete small bowel obstruction. The duodenojejunal junction may lie to the right of the spine along with the jejunal loops. The diagnosis of malrotation can be further confirmed by barium enema, which may demonstrate a mobile cecum located in the midline.

Treatment & Prognosis

Midgut volvulus is a surgical emergency, Bowel necrosis results from occlusion of the superior mesenteric artery. When necrosis is extensive, it is recommended that a first operation include only reduction of the volvulus with lysis of mesenteric bands. Intestinal resection should be delayed if possible until a second-look operation 24–48 hours later can be undertaken in the hope that some bowel can be salvaged. The prognosis is guarded if there is perforation, peritonitis, or extensive intestinal necrosis.

Janik JS, Ein SH: Normal intestinal rotation with nonfixation: A cause of chronic abdominal pain. J Pediatr Surg 1979;14:670.

Millar AJW et al: The deadly vomit: Malrotation and midgut volvulus. Pediatr Surg Int 1987;2:172.

Stewart DR et al: Malrotation of the bowel in infants and children: A 15 year experience. Surgery 1976;79:716.

MECKEL'S DIVERTICULUM & OMPHALOMESENTERIC DUCT REMNANTS

Meckel's diverticulum is the most common of the omphalomesenteric duct remnants. It is usually found on the antimesenteric border of the mid to distal ileum. It is present in 1.5% of the population but rarely causes symptoms. In addition to the ileal mucosa, diverticula may contain gastric, pancreatic, jejunal, or colonic mucosa. Familial cases have been reported. Complications occur three times more frequently in males than in females, and in 50–60% of cases within the first 2 years of life. Acid secreted by heterotopic gastric tissue causes ulceration and bleeding from adjacent ileal mucosa.

Clinical Findings

A. Symptoms and Signs: In 40–60% of symptomatic cases, painless rectal bleeding of maroon or melanotic blood occurs. Acute bleeding may cause shock. Occult bleeding is less common but may cause anemia. Intestinal obstruction occurs in 25% of symptomatic cases as a result of ileocolonic intussusception. Intestinal volvulus may occur around a fibrous remnant of the vitelline duct extending from the tip of the diverticulum to the abdominal wall. In some cases, entrapment of a bowel loop under a band running between the diverticulum and the base of the mesentery occurs. The diverticulum may be trapped in an inguinal hernia (Littre's hernia). Diverticulitis occurs in 10–20% of symptomatic cases and is clinically indistinguishable from acute appendicitis. Perforation and generalized peritonitis may occur. There may be chronic recurrent abdominal pain.

B. Imaging: Diagnosis of Meckel's diverticulum is seldom made on barium x-ray. Radionuclide imaging with ^{99m}Tc pertechnetate taken up by the diverticulum lined with heterotopic gastric mucosa. Stimulation of ^{99m}Tc uptake by both pentagastrin and cimetidine can reduce the number of false-negative results. Angiography may be useful when bleeding is brisk.

Treatment

Treatment is surgical. At laparoscopy or laparoscopy, close inspection of the ileum proximal and distal to the diverticulum may reveal ulcerations and heterotopic tissue adjacent to the neck of the diverticulum.

Other Remnants of the Omphalomesenteric Duct

Fecal discharge from the umbilicus is evidence of a patent omphalomesenteric duct. The duct may be completely closed, causing a fibrous cord joining ileum and umbilicus and potentially the origin of a volvulus. A mucoid umbilical discharge may be indicative of a mucocele, which can protrude through the umbilicus and be mistaken for an umbilical granuloma, since it is firm and bright red. In all cases, surgical excision of the omphalomesenteric remnant is indicated.

Prognosis

The prognosis for Meckel's diverticulum is good. Marked hemorrhage may occur but is rarely exsanguinating.

Mackey WC, Dineen P: A fifty-year experience with Meckel's diverticulum. Surg Gynecol Obstet 1983;156:56.

DUPLICATIONS OF THE GASTROINTESTINAL TRACT

Duplications are congenital anomalies of the gastrointestinal tract. They are fluid-filled, spherical, or tubular structures found anywhere along the gastrointestinal tract, most commonly in the ileum. Duplications usually contain fluid and sometimes blood, if necrosis has taken place. Most duplications do not communicate with the intestinal lumen; they are attached to the mesenteric side of the gut and share a common muscular coat. The epithelial lining of the duplication is usually of the same type as that from which it originates. Some duplications (neuroenteric cysts) are attached to the spinal cord and are associated with hemivertebrae, and anterior or posterior spina bifida.

Symptoms of vomiting, abdominal distention, colicky pain, rectal bleeding, partial or total intestinal obstruction, or an abdominal mass may start in infancy. Physical examination reveals a rounded, smooth, freely movable mass, and x-ray films of the abdomen show a noncalcified mass displacing the intestines or stomach. Scanning with ^{99m}Tc pertechnetate is useful in duplications containing gastric mucosa. Involvement of the terminal small bowel can give rise to an intussusception. Prompt surgical treatment is indicated.

Bissler JJ, Klein RL: Alimentary tract duplications in children. Clin Pediatr 1988;27:152.

PERITONITIS

Primary bacterial peritonitis is rare. The most common organisms responsible include *Escherichia coli* and other enteric organisms, hemolytic streptococci, and pneumococci. Primary peritonitis occurs in patients with splenectomy, splenic dysfunction, or ascites (nephrotic syndrome, advanced liver disease, kwashiorkor). It also occurs in infants with pyelonephritis or pneumonia. Secondary peritonitis is associated with peritoneal dialysis, penetrating abdominal trauma, or ruptured viscus. (Appendicitis, perforated peptic ulcer, cholecystitis, pancreatitis, inflammatory bowel disease, midgut volvulus, intussusception, and strangulated hernia are some primary events.) Intra-abdominal abscesses may form in pelvic, subhepatic, or subphrenic areas, but localization of infection is less common in young infants than it is in adults.

Symptoms include severe abdominal pain, fever, nausea, and vomiting. Respirations are shallow. The abdomen is tender, rigid, and distended, with involuntary guarding. Bowel sounds may be absent. Diarrhea is fairly common in primary peritonitis and less so in secondary peritonitis.

The leukocyte count is initially high (greater than $20,000/\mu L$) with a predominance of immature forms, and later may fall to neutropenic levels, especially in primary peritonitis. Bacterial peritonitis should be suspected if paracentesis fluid contains more than 500 leukocytes/μL or more than 32 mg/dL of lactate, has a pH less than 7.34, or if the pH of ascites is more than 0.1 pH unit less than arterial pH. Etiologic diagnosis is made by Gram's stain and culture, preferably of 5–10 mL of fluid for optimal yield.

Antibiotic treatment and supportive therapy for dehydration, shock, and acidosis are indicated. Surgical treatment of the underlying cause of secondary peritonitis is critical. Drainage of localized abscess is often required.

Bell MJ: Peritonitis in the newborn: Current concepts. Pediatr Clin North Am 1985;32:1181.

Clark JH et al: Spontaneous bacterial peritonitis. J Pediatr 1984;104:495.

Garcia-Tsau G, Conn HO, Lerner E: The diagnosis of bacterial peritonitis: Comparison of pH, lactate concentration and leukocyte count. Hepatology 1985;5:91.

CONGENITAL AGANGLIONIC MEGACOLON (Hirschsprung's Disease)

General Considerations

Hirschsprung's disease results from an absence of ganglion cells in the mucosal and muscular layers of the colon. There is a failure of neural crest cells to migrate to the mesodermal layers, possibly mediated by abnormalities in end-organ cell surface receptors or local deficiency of nitric oxide synthesis. The rectum alone (30%) or the rectosigmoid (44%) is usually affected. The entire colon is aganglionic in 8%

of cases. Segmental aganglionosis is very rare and may be an acquired lesion. The aganglionic segment is narrowed, with dilation of the proximal normal colon. In the mucosa of the dilated colonic segment may become thin and inflamed (enterocolitis) resulting in diarrhea, bleeding, and protein loss.

A familial pattern has been described, particularly in total colonic aganglionosis. The disease is four times more common in boys than in girls, and 10–15% of patients have Down's syndrome.

Clinical Findings

A. Symptoms and Signs: Failure of the newborn to pass meconium—followed by vomiting, abdominal distention, and reluctance to feed—suggests the diagnosis of Hirschsprung's disease. In some cases, symptoms appear later and are those of partial intestinal obstruction, with abdominal distention and bilious vomiting. Bouts of enterocolitis manifested by fever, explosive diarrhea, and prostration are reported in about 50% of newborns with this disease. These episodes may lead to acute inflammatory and ischemic changes in the colon, with perforation (especially cecal) and sepsis. In later infancy, alternating obstipation and diarrhea predominate. The older child is more likely to present with constipation. The stools are offensive and ribbon-like, the abdomen enlarged, and the veins prominent; peristaltic patterns are readily visible, and fecal masses are palpable. Intermittent bouts of intestinal obstruction due to fecal impaction, hypochromic anemia, hypoproteinemia, and failure to thrive are common. Encopresis is rarely seen.

On digital examination, the anal canal and rectum are devoid of fecal material despite fecal impaction obvious on abdominal examination or x-ray. If the aganglionic segment is short, there may be a gush of flatus and stool as the finger is withdrawn.

B. Laboratory Findings: Ganglion cells are absent in both the submucosal and muscular layers of the involved bowel. Special stains may show nerve trunk hypertrophy and increased acetylcholinesterase activity.

C. Imaging: X-ray examination of the abdomen may reveal dilated proximal colon and absence of gas in the pelvic colon. A barium enema using a catheter with the tip inserted barely beyond the anal sphincter, usually demonstrates the narrowed segment distally with a sharp transition to proximal dilated colon. However, in neonates a "transition zone" may not be seen. Retention of barium for 24–48 hours is not diagnostic of Hirschsprung's disease but can be seen in retentive constipation as well.

D. Special Examinations: Failure of reflex relaxation of the internal sphincter muscle after balloon distention of the rectum is seen in all patients with Hirschsprung's disease, regardless of the length of the aganglionic segment.

Differential Diagnosis

Hirschsprung's disease accounts for 15–20% of cases of neonatal intestinal obstruction. In childhood, this disease must be differentiated from retentive constipation. It can also be confused with celiac disease because of the striking abdominal distention and failure to thrive.

Treatment

Treatment is surgical. Initially, diverting colostomy (or ileostomy) is performed proximal to the aganglionic segment. Resection of the aganglionic segment is usually delayed until the infant is at least 6 months of age. During operation, location of the transition between ganglionated and nonganglionated bowel is identified. Aganglionic bowel is resected. The Soave procedure, in which the ganglionated proximal bowel is pulled through seromuscular cuff of the distal rectum, is the surgical procedure most commonly performed in the United States for treatment of Hirschsprung's disease.

Prognosis

Complications following surgery include chronic constipation, fecal incontinence, anastomotic breakdown, or stricture. Postoperative obstruction may result from inadvertent retention of a distal aganglionic segment or postoperative destruction of ganglion cells secondary to vascular impairment. Neuronal dysplasia of the remaining bowel may result in a pseudo-obstruction syndrome. Enterocolitis may occur postoperatively in 15% of procedures.

Bealer J et al: Nitric oxide synthase is deficient in the aganglionic colon of patients with Hirschprung's disease. Pediatrics 1994;93:647.

Klein MD et al: Hirschsprung's disease in the newborn. J Pediatr Surg 1984;19:370.

Romeo G et al: Point mutations affecting the tyrosine kinase domain of the RET proto-oncogene in Hirschprung's disease. Nature 1994;367:377.

CHYLOUS ASCITES

Chylous ascites due to congenital infection or developmental abnormality of the lymphatic system may be observed at birth. If the thoracic duct is involved, chylothorax may be present. Later in life, chylous ascites may result from congenital lymphatic abnormality, tumors, peritoneal bands, or trauma to major lymphatics.

Clinical Findings

A. Symptoms and Signs: In both congenital and acquired forms, diarrhea and failure to thrive are noted. The abdomen is distended, with a fluid wave and shifting dullness. Unilateral or generalized peripheral edema may be present.

B. Laboratory Findings: Laboratory findings include hypoalbuminemia, hypogammaglobulinemia, and lymphopenia. Ascitic fluid contains lymphocytes and has the biochemical composition of chyle if the patient has just been fed; otherwise it is indistinguishable from ascites secondary to cirrhosis.

Differential Diagnosis

Chylous ascites must be differentiated from ascites due to liver failure and, in the older child, from constrictive pericarditis and neoplastic, infectious, or inflammatory diseases causing lymphatic obstruction.

Complications & Sequelae

Severe chylous ascites can be fatal. Chronic loss of albumin and gamma globulin through the gastrointestinal tract may lead to edema and increase the risk of infection. Rapidly accumulating chylous ascites may cause respiratory complications.

Treatment & Prognosis

If there is a congenital abnormality due to hypoplasia, aplasia, or ectasia of the lymphatics, little can be done for the patient. Shunting of peritoneal fluid into the venous system is sometimes effective. A fat-free diet supplemented with medium-chain triglycerides decreases the formation of chylous ascitic fluid. Total parenteral nutrition may be necessary. The congenital form of chylous ascites may spontaneously disappear following paracentesis and a medium-chain triglyceride diet. The prognosis is guarded, although spontaneous cures have been reported.

Cochran WJ et al: Chylous ascites in infants and children: A case report and literature review. J Pediatr Gastroenterol Nutr 1985;4:668.

Guttman FM, Montupet P, Bloss RS: Experience with peritoneovenous shunting for congenital chylous ascites in infants and children. J Pediatr Surg 1982;17:368.

CONGENITAL ANORECTAL ANOMALIES

Anorectal anomalies occur once in every 3000–4000 births, and most types are more common in males. Inspection of the perianal area is essential in all newborns.

Classification

A. Anterior Displacement of the Anal Opening: This condition is more common in girls than in boys. It may be associated with a posterior rectal shelf and usually is characterized by constipation that responds poorly to medical management.

B. Anal Stenosis: The anal aperture is very small and filled with a dot of meconium. Defecation is difficult, and there may be ribbon-like stools, fecal impaction, and abdominal distention. This malformation accounts for about 10% of cases of anorectal anomalies.

C. Imperforate Anal Membrane: The infant fails to pass meconium, and a greenish bulging membrane is seen. After excision, bowel and sphincter function are normal.

D. Anal Agenesis: An anal dimple is present, and stimulation of the perianal area leads to puckering indicative of the presence of the external sphincter. If there is no associated rectoperineal fistula, intestinal obstruction occurs. Fistulas may also be vulvar in the female and urethral in the male.

E. Anorectal Agenesis: Anorectal agenesis accounts for 75% of total anorectal anomalies. Fistulas are almost invariably present. In the female, they may be vaginal or may enter a urogenital sinus, which is a common passageway for the urethra and vagina. In the male, fistulas are rectovesical or rectourethral. Associated major congenital malformations are common. Sacral defects and absence of internal and external anal sphincters are common.

Radiologic Findings

Careful radiologic evaluation is indicated immediately so that the anal anomaly and the extent of associated anomalies of the bowel and the urogenital tract can be fully appraised.

Treatment & Prognosis

Dilation of the anus should be undertaken in cases of anal stenosis. Treatment for imperforate anal membrane consists of excision of the membrane and dilation. Colostomy is advocated for all cases of anorectal agenesis. In patients with anal agenesis and a visible fistula of sufficient size to pass meconium, surgery can be deferred. Males without a visible fistula may have a urethral fistula; therefore, colostomy is recommended.

Of the patients with "low" defects, 80–90% are continent after surgery; with "high" defects, only 30% achieve continence. Gracilis muscle transplants may improve continence. Levatorplasty may also be used as a secondary operation following surgery for anorectal agenesis. Antegrade continence enema procedures may allow for continence in children without anal sphincter function.

Bar-Maor JA, Eiten A: Determination of the normal location of the anus. J Pediatr Gastro Nutr 1987;6:559.

Koyle MA et al: The Malone antegrade continence enema for neurogenic and structural fecal incontinence and constipation. J Urol 1995;154:759.

Smith ED: The bathwater needs changing, but don't throw out the baby: An overview of anorectal anomalies. J Pediatr Surg 1987;22:335.

ACUTE ABDOMEN

Many disorders must be considered in the differential diagnosis of acute abdomen. Emergency surgery should not be considered until the differential diagnosis has been completed. The patient may be too young to describe symptoms, and the parent's description is a subjective interpretation of what he or she thinks is wrong. A classification of acute abdomen is shown in Table 20–3. Some of the specific entities are discussed in subsequent sections. Reaching a speedy and accurate diagnosis in the patient with an acute abdomen is critical and requires skill in physical diagnosis, intimate acquaintance with the characteristic symptoms of a large number of conditions, and the judicious selection of laboratory and radiologic tests.

Hatch EI: The acute abdomen in children. Pediatr Clin North Am 1985;32:1151.

ACUTE APPENDICITIS

General Considerations

Acute appendicitis is the most common cause of emergency abdominal surgery in childhood. The frequency increases with age and peaks between 15 and 30 years. Obstruction of the appendix by fecaliths (25%) or parasites is a predisposing factor.

The incidence of perforation is high (40%) in infants and children. In order to avoid delay in diagnosis, it is important to maintain close communication with parents, perform a thorough physical examination and sequential examinations of the abdomen over a period of several hours, and interpret correctly the evolving symptoms and signs.

Clinical Findings

A. Symptoms and Signs: The typical child with appendicitis has low-grade fever and periumbilical abdominal pain, which then localizes to the right lower quadrant, accompanied by signs of peritoneal irritation. Anorexia, vomiting, constipation, and diarrhea also occur. The clinical picture is often atypical and includes generalized pain, tenderness around the umbilicus, and no leukocytosis. Rectal examination should always be done and may reveal localized mass or tenderness. Because many conditions give rise to symptoms mimicking appendicitis and because physical findings are often inconclusive, it is important to repeat examinations of the abdomen. In children under 2 years old, the pain of appendicitis is poorly localized, and perforation before surgery is common.

B. Laboratory Findings: White blood cell counts are seldom higher than 15,000/μL. Fecal leukocytes and blood are rare.

C. Imaging: A radiopaque fecalith is reportedly present in two-thirds of cases of ruptured appendix. A barium enema examination showing a normal appendix and cecum usually rules out appendicitis. However, a positive diagnosis of nonperforated appendicitis cannot be made by barium enema. Ultrasonography of the acutely inflamed appendix shows a noncompressible, thickened appendix in 93% of cases. A localized fluid collection adjacent to or surrounding the appendix may also be seen. Enlarged mesenteric lymph nodes are a nondiagnostic finding.

Differential Diagnosis

The presence of intrathoracic infection (eg, pneumonia) or urinary tract infection should be kept in mind, along with other medical and surgical condi-

Table 20–3. Etiologic classification of acute abdomen.

Mechanical Obstruction		Inflammatory Diseases and Infections			
Intraluminal Obstruction	Extraluminal Obstruction	Gastrointestinal Disease	Paralytic Ileus	Blunt Trauma	Miscellaneous

Foreign body
Bezoar
Fecalith
Gallstone
Parasites
Meconium ileus
  equivalent
Tumor
Fecaloma
	Hernia
	Intussusception
	Volvulus
	Duplication
	Stenosis
	Tumor
	Mesenteric cyst
	Superior mesenteric
	  artery syndrome
	Pyloric stenosis
		Appendicitis
		Crohn's disease
		Ulcerative colitis
		Henoch-Schönlein
		  purpura and other
		  causes of vasculitis
		Peptic ulcer
		Meckel's diverticulitis
		Acute gastroenteritis
		Pseudomembranous
		  enterocolitis
			Sepsis
			Pneumonia
			Pyelonephritis
			Peritonitis
			Pancreatitis
			Cholecystitis
			Renal and gall-
			  bladder stones
			Pelvic inflammation
			Lymphadenitis due
			  to viral or bacterial
			  infection
				Accident
				Battered child
				  syndrome
					Lead poisoning
					Sickle cell crisis
					Familial Mediterra-
					  nean fever
					Porphyria
					Diabetic acidosis
					Addisonian crisis
					Torsion of testis
					Torsion of ovarian
					  pedicle

Reproduced, with permission, from Roy CC, Morin CL, Weber AM: Gastrointestinal emergency problems in paediatric practice. Clin Gastroenterol 1981;10:225.

tions leading to acute abdomen (see previous section).

Treatment & Prognosis

Exploratory laparotomy or laparoscopy is indicated whenever the diagnosis of appendicitis cannot be ruled out after a period of close observation. Postoperative antibiotic therapy directed to the treatment of anaerobes and coliforms is reserved for cases with gangrenous or perforated appendix. A single intraoperative dose of cefoxitin or cefotetan is recommended for all cases, to prevent postoperative complications. The mortality rate is less than 1% during childhood, despite the high incidence of perforation. Laparoscopic removal of a nonruptured appendix is associated with a shortened hospital stay.

Antimicrobial prophylaxis in surgery. Med Lett Drugs Ther 1995;37:79.

Gilbert SR: Appendicitis in children. Surg Gynecol Obstet 1985;161:261.

Harrison MW et al: Acute appendicitis in children: Factors affecting morbidity. Am J Surg 1984;147:605.

INTUSSUSCEPTION

General Considerations

Intussusception is the most frequent cause of intestinal obstruction in the first 2 years of life. It is three times more common in males than in females. In most cases (85%) the cause is not apparent, although polyps, Meckel's diverticulum, Schönlein-Henoch purpura, lymphomas, lipomas, parasites, foreign bodies, or adenovirus or rotavirus infections with hypertrophy of Peyer's patches are predisposing factors. Intussusception of the small intestine occurs in patients with celiac disease and cystic fibrosis, usually related to the bulk of stool in the terminal ileum. In children older than 6 years of age, lymphoma is the most common lesion. Intermittent small bowel intussusception is a rare cause of recurrent abdominal pain.

The intussusception usually starts just proximal to the ileocecal valve, so that invagination is ileocolic. Other forms include ileoileal and colocolic. Swelling, hemorrhage, incarceration with necrosis of the intussuscepted bowel, and eventual perforation and peritonitis occur as a result of impairment of venous return.

Clinical Findings

Characteristically, a thriving infant 3–12 months of age develops paroxysmal abdominal pain with screaming and drawing up of the knees. Vomiting and diarrhea occur soon afterward (90% of cases), and bloody bowel movements with mucus appear within the next 12 hours (50%). Prostration and fever supervene. The abdomen is tender and becomes distended. On palpation, a sausage-shaped mass may be found usually in the upper mid abdomen. Some patients show signs of altered consciousness, particularly lethargy between spasms of pain, or may have seizures.

The intussusception can persist for several days when obstruction is not complete, and such cases may present as separate attacks of enterocolitis. In older children, sudden attacks of abdominal pain may be related to chronic recurrent intussusception with spontaneous reduction.

Treatment

A. Conservative Measures: A barium enema is both diagnostic and therapeutic. It is a safe procedure in experienced hands if the following recommendations are observed:

1. No attempt should be made at hydrostatic reduction if there are signs of strangulated bowel, perforation, or severe toxicity.

2. The barium solution should be allowed to drip by gravity through a Foley catheter inserted in the rectum from a height not more than 1 meter (3½ feet) above the fluoroscopy table.

3. There should be no manipulation of the abdomen during hydrostatic reduction under fluoroscopic examination, because this may increase intraluminal pressure and thus the risk of perforation.

4. Upon reduction, there should be free reflux of barium for a distance of 24–30 cm into the ileum; this is best demonstrated in a postevacuation film.

5. Careful insufflation of the colon with air is a safe and effective alternative to hydrostatic reduction.

B. Surgical Measures: For patients not suitable for hydrostatic or pneumatic reduction or in whom these procedures are unsuccessful (25%), surgery is required. This has the advantages of demonstrating any lead point (such as Meckel's diverticulum) and of a lower recurrence rate.

Prognosis

The prognosis relates directly to the duration of the intussusception before reduction. The mortality rate with treatment is 1–2%. The patient should be observed carefully after hydrostatic or pneumatic reduction because intussusception recurs in 3–4% of patients within 24 hours.

Bruce J et al: Intussusception: Evolution of current management. J Pediatr Gastroenterol Nutr 1987;6:663.

Palder SB et al: Intussusception: Barium or air? J Pediatr Surg 1991;26:271.

FOREIGN BODIES IN THE ALIMENTARY TRACT

Most foreign bodies pass through the gastrointestinal tract without difficulty, although objects longer than 5 cm may have difficulty negotiating the ligament of Treitz. Ingested foreign bodies tend to lodge in areas of natural constriction—valleculae, thoracic inlet, gastroesophageal junction, pylorus, ligament of Treitz, and ileocecal junction. Foreign bodies lodged in the esophagus for more than 24 hours require removal. Smooth foreign bodies in the stomach, such as buttons or coins, may be watched without attempting removal for up to several months if the child is free of symptoms. Straight pins, screws, and nails generally pass without incident. Removal of open safety pins or wooden toothpicks is recommended. Camera batteries that contain 45% potassium hydroxide are hazardous and should be removed endoscopically if present in the esophagus or in the stomach after 24 hours. The use of balanced electrolyte lavage solutions containing polyethylene glycol (eg, GoLYTELY) may help the passage of small, smooth foreign bodies lodged in the stomach or intestine. Lavage is especially useful in hastening the passage of button batteries or ingested tablets that may be toxic. Failure of a smooth foreign body to exit the stomach suggests the possibility of gastric outlet obstruction.

Esophagogastroscopy will permit the removal of most foreign bodies lodged in the esophagus and stomach. A Foley catheter may be used to dislodge smooth, round esophageal foreign bodies in healthy children with no previous esophageal disease. It is introduced into the esophagus, and the balloon at the distal end is inflated below the foreign body. Careful withdrawal of the catheter under fluoroscopic observation will bring the foreign body into the mouth, where it can be extracted. Only an experienced radiologist should attempt this maneuver.

Bertoni G et al: A new protector device for safe endoscopic removal of sharp gastroesophageal foreign bodies in infants. J Pediatr Gastroenterol Nutr 1993;16:393.

Bloom RR et al: Foreign bodies of the gastrointestinal tract. Am Surg 1986;52:618.

Campbell JB, Foley LC: A safe alternative to endoscopic removal of blunt esophageal foreign bodies. Arch Otolaryngol 1983;109:323.

ANAL FISSURE

Anal fissure consists of a slit-like tear in the anal canal, usually secondary to the passage of large, hard, fecal masses. Anal stenosis, anal crypt abscess, and trauma can be contributory factors. Sexual abuse must be considered in any child with large, irregular, or multiple anal fissures. Anal fissures may be the presenting symptoms of Crohn's disease in older children.

The infant or child with anal fissure typically cries with defecation and will try to hold back stools. Sparse, bright red bleeding is seen on the outside of

the stool or on the toilet tissue following defecation. The fissure can often be seen if the patient is examined in a knee-chest position with the buttocks spread apart.

When a fissure cannot be identified, it is essential to rule out other causes of rectal bleeding such as juvenile polyp, perianal inflammation (due to group A streptococcal infection), or inflammatory bowel disease.

Anal fissures should be treated promptly, to break the constipation-fissure-retention-constipation cycle. A stool softener should be given. Anal dilation relieves sphincter spasm. Warm sitz baths after defecation may be helpful. In rare cases, silver nitrate cauterization or surgery is indicated. Anal surgery should be avoided in Crohn's disease.

INGUINAL HERNIA

A peritoneal sac precedes the testicle as it descends from the genital ridge to the scrotum. The lower portion of this sac envelops the testis to form the tunica vaginalis, and the remainder normally atrophies by the time of birth. In some cases, peritoneal fluid may become trapped in the tunica vaginalis of the testis (noncommunicating hydrocele). If the processus vaginalis remains open, peritoneal fluid or an abdominal structure may be forced into it (indirect inguinal hernia).

Most inguinal hernias are of the indirect type and occur much more frequently in boys than in girls (9:1). Hernias may be present at birth or may appear at any age thereafter. The incidence in premature infants is close to 5%. In those weighing 1000 g or less, inguinal hernia is reported in 30%.

Clinical Findings

There are no symptoms associated with an empty processus vaginalis. In most cases, a hernia is a painless inguinal swelling of variable size. There may be a history of inguinal fullness associated with coughing or long periods of standing; or there may be a firm, globular, and tender swelling, sometimes associated with vomiting and abdominal distention.

Spontaneous reduction frequently occurs during sleep or with mild external pressure. In some instances, a herniated loop of intestine may become partially obstructed, leading to pain and partial intestinal obstruction. Rarely, bowel becomes trapped in the hernia sac, and complete intestinal obstruction occurs. Gangrene of the hernia contents or testis may occur; in the female, the ovary may prolapse into the hernial sac.

Inspection of the two inguinal areas may reveal a characteristic bulging or mass. Infants should be observed for evidence of swelling after crying and older children after bearing down.

A suggestive history is often the only criterion for

diagnosis, along with the "silk glove" feel of the rubbing together of the two walls of the empty hernial sac.

Differential Diagnosis

An inguinal mass may represent lymph nodes. They are usually multiple and more discrete. Hydrocele of the cord transilluminates. An undescended testis may be moved along the canal and is associated with absence of the testicle in the scrotum.

Treatment

Manual reduction of incarcerated inguinal hernia can be attempted after placing the sedated infant in the Trendelenburg position with an ice bag on the affected side. This is contraindicated if incarceration has been present for more than 12 hours or if bloody stools are noted. Surgery is usually indicated if a hernia has once incarcerated. Hydroceles frequently resolve by the age of 2 years. There is still controversy about exploring the opposite side. Exploration of the unaffected groin can document the patency of the processus vaginalis, but patency does not always mean herniation will occur, especially in patients over 1 year of age, in whom risk of contralateral hernia is about 10%.

Incarcerated inguinal hernias occur most often in the first 10 months of life and are more common in girls than in boys.

McGregor DB et al: The unilateral pediatric inguinal hernia: Should the contralateral side be explored? J Pediatr Surg 1980;15:313.
Viidik T, Marshall DG: Direct inguinal hernias in infancy and early childhood. J Pediatr Surg 1980;15:646.

UMBILICAL HERNIA

Umbilical hernias are more common in premature than in full-term infants, and more common in black infants than in white.

Small bowel may incarcerate in small-diameter umbilical hernias. Most umbilical hernias regress spontaneously if the fascial defect has a diameter of less than 1 cm. Large defects and smaller hernias persisting after 4 years of age should be treated surgically. Reducing the hernia and strapping the skin do not accelerate the healing process.

TUMORS OF THE GASTROINTESTINAL TRACT

1. JUVENILE POLYPS

Juvenile polyps are usually pedunculated and solitary, with a stalk covered in part by colonic mucosa. The head of the polyp is composed of hyperplastic glandular and vascular elements, often with cystic transformation. Juvenile polyps are benign, and 80% occur in the rectosigmoid. They are rare before age 1. Their incidence is highest between 3 and 5 years of age, and they are rare after age 15 years because of autoamputation. They are more frequent in boys. The painless passage of small amounts of bright red blood on a normal or constipated stool is the most frequent manifestation. Abdominal pain is infrequent, but a juvenile polyp can be the lead point for an intussusception. Low-lying polyps may prolapse during defecation.

Rarely, there are many juvenile polyps in the colon, causing anemia, diarrhea, and protein loss. A few cases of generalized juvenile polyposis involving the stomach and the small and large bowel have been reported. These cases are associated with a slightly increased risk of cancer.

Colonoscopy is both diagnostic and therapeutic when polyps are suspected. After removal of the polyp by electrocautery, nothing further should be done if histologic findings confirm the diagnosis. There is a slight risk of developing further juvenile polyps.

Other polyposis syndromes are summarized in Table 20–4.

Erbe RW: Inherited gastrointestinal polyposis syndromes. N Engl J Med 1976;294:1101.
Haggitt RC, Reid BJ: Hereditary polyposis syndromes. Am J Surg Pathol 1986;10:871.

2. CANCER OF THE ESOPHAGUS & SMALL & LARGE INTESTINE

Esophageal cancer is rare in childhood. Cysts, leiomyomas, and hamartomas predominate. Caustic injury of the esophagus increases the risk of squamous cell carcinoma, and chronic peptic esophagitis is associated with Barrett's esophagus, a precancerous lesion.

The most common gastric or small bowel cancer in children is lymphoma or lymphosarcoma. Intermittent abdominal pain, abdominal mass, intussusception, or a celiac-like picture may be present. Long-term survivals are reported in patients without lymph node involvement at surgery.

Carcinoid tumors are usually benign, discovered incidentally following appendectomy. Metastasis is rare, as are symptoms associated with serotonin secretion.

Adenocarcinoma of the colon is rare in the pediatric age group. The transverse colon and rectosigmoid are the two most commonly affected sites. The low 5-year survival relates to the nonspecificity of presenting complaints and the large percentage of undifferentiated types. Children with a family history of

Table 20–4. Gastrointestinal polyposis syndromes.

	Location	Number	Histology	Extraintestinal Findings	Malignant Potential
Juvenile polyps	Colon	Single (70%) Several (30%)	Hyperplastic, hamartomatous	None	None
Familial juvenile polyposis coli[1]	Colon	Multiple	Hyperplastic with focal adenomatous change	None	10–25%
Generalized juvenile polyposis[1]	Stomach, small bowel, colon	Multiple	Hyperplastic with focal adenomatous change	Hydrocephaly, cardiac lesions, mesenteric lymphangioma, malrotation	10–25%
Familial polyposis adenomatous[1]	Colon; less commonly, stomach and small bowel	Multiple	Adenomatous	None	95–100%
Peutz-Jeghers syndrome[1]	Small bowel, stomach, colon	Multiple	Hamartomatous	Pigmented cutaneous and oral macules; ovarian cysts and tumors; bony exostoses	2–3%
Gardner's syndrome[1]	Colon; less commonly, stomach and small bowel	Multiple	Adenomatous	Cysts, tumors, and desmoids of skin and bone; other tumors, retinal pigmentation can be a screening tool in families.	95–100%
Cronkhite-Canada syndrome	Stomach, colon; less commonly, esophagus and small bowel	Multiple	Hamartomatous	Alopecia; onychodystrophy; hyperpigmentation	Rare
Turcot syndrome[2]	Colon	Multiple	Adenomatous	Thyroid and brain tumors	Possible

[1]Autosomal dominant.
[2]Autosomal recessive.

colon cancer, chronic ulcerative colitis or familial polyposis syndromes are at greater risk.

Aiges HW et al: Adenocarcinoma of the colon in an adolescent with the family cancer syndrome. J Pediatr 1979; 94:632.
Collins RH et al: Colon cancer, dysplasia and surveillance in patients with ulcerative colitis: A critical review. N Engl J Med 1987;316:1654.
Gray GM et al: Lymphomas involving the gastrointestinal tract. Gastroenterology 1982;82:143.
Hassall E: Barrett's esophagus: New definitions and approaches in children. J Pediatr Gastroenterol Nutr 1993; 16:345.

3. MESENTERIC CYSTS

These rare tumors may be small or large, single or multiloculated. Invariably thin-walled, they contain either serous, chylous, or hemorrhagic fluid. They are commonly located in the mesentery of the small intestine but may also be seen in the mesocolon. Most mesenteric cysts are asymptomatic. Traction on the mesentery eventually leads to colicky abdominal pain, which can be mild and recurrent but may present acutely with vomiting. Volvulus is reported, as is hemorrhage into the cyst. A rounded mass can occasionally be palpated or can be seen on x-ray film to displace adjacent intestine. Abdominal ultrasonography is usually diagnostic. Surgical removal is indicated.

Christensen JA et al: Mesenteric cysts. Am Surg 1975;41: 352.

4. INTESTINAL HEMANGIOMA

Hemangiomas of the bowel may cause acute or chronic blood loss. They may also cause intestinal obstruction by triggering intussusception, by local stricture, or by intramural hematoma formation. Thrombocytopenia and consumptive coagulopathy are occasional complications. Some lesions are telangiectasias (Rendu-Osler-Weber syndrome), and others are capillary hemangiomas. However, the largest group consists of cavernous hemangiomas, which are large, thin-walled vessels arising from the submucosal vascular plexus. They may protrude into the lumen as polypoid lesions or may invade the intestine from mucosa to serosa.

Abrahamson J, Shandling B: Intestinal hemangiomata in childhood and a syndrome for diagnosis: A collective review. J Pediatr Surg 1973;8:487.

Mestre JR, Andres JM: Hereditary hemorrhagic telangiectasia causing hematemesis in an infant. J Pediatr 1982; 101:577.

ACUTE INFECTIOUS DIARRHEA
(Gastroenteritis)

Viruses are the most common cause of acute gastroenteritis in developing and developed countries. Bacterial and parasitic enteric infections are discussed in Chapters 37 and 38. Of the viral agents proved to cause enteric infection, rotavirus, a 67-nM double-stranded RNA virus with at least eight serotypic variants, is the most common. As with most viral pathogens, rotavirus affects the small intestine, causing voluminous watery diarrhea without leukocytes or blood. In the United States, rotavirus predominantly affects infants between 3 and 15 months. Peak incidence in the United States is in the winter months. Sporadic cases occur at other times. The virus is transmitted via the fecal-oral route and survives for hours on hands and for days on environmental fomites.

Diagnosis & Treatment
of Rotavirus Infections

The incubation period for rotavirus is 24–48 hours. Vomiting is the first symptom in 80–90% of cases, followed within 24 hours by low-grade fever and profuse watery diarrhea. Diarrhea usually lasts 4–8 days, but may last longer in young infants or immunocompromised patients. The white cell count is rarely elevated. The stool sodium is usually less than 40 mEq/L. Thus, as patients become dehydrated from unreplaced stool losses, they may become hypernatremic. The stool does not contain blood or white cells. Metabolic acidosis results from bicarbonate loss in the stool, ketosis from poor intake, and lactic acidemia from hypotension and hypoperfusion.

Appropriate fluid and replacement of electrolyte deficits and ongoing losses is critical, especially in small infants. (Oral and intravenous therapy is discussed in Chapter 40.) The use of oral rehydration fluid is appropriate in most cases, but clear liquid and hypocaloric (dilute formula) diets for more than 48 hours are not advisable in uncomplicated viral gastroenteritis, because starvation depresses digestive function and prolongs the diarrhea.

Intestinal lactase levels are reduced during rotavirus infection. Brief use of a lactose-free diet is associated with a shorter period of diarrhea, but is not critical to successful recovery in most healthy infants. Reduced fat intake during recovery may reduce nausea and emesis.

Antidiarrheal medications are ineffective (kaolin-pectin combinations) or even dangerous (loperamide, tincture of opium, diphenoxylate-atropine). Bismuth subsalicylate preparations may reduce stool volume, but are not critical to recovery. Oral immunoglobulin has occasionally been useful in limiting duration of disease in immunocompromised patients.

Specific identification of rotavirus is not required in every case, especially in epidemic outbreaks. Rotavirus antigens can be identified in stool. False-positives (which may actually be nonpathogenic rotavirus) are seen in neonates. Electron microscopy of the stool will also reveal the virus, but is less sensitive.

Some immunity is imparted by the first episode of rotavirus. Serum antibodies are present, but their role in prevention of subsequent attacks is not clear. Repeat infections occur, but are usually less severe. Prevention of rotavirus is mainly by good hygiene and prevention of fecal-oral contamination. A quadrivalent oral vaccine that incorporates attenuated viruses of the four major pathogenic serotypes is under investigation, with protection ranging from 57–77%.

Diagnosis & Treatment
of Other Viruses

Other viral pathogens in stool have been identified by electron microscopy, special viral cultures, or enzyme-linked immunoassays in infants with diarrhea. Enteric adenoviruses (serotypes 40 and 41) are the second most common viral pathogens in infants. The symptoms of enteric adenovirus infection are similar to those produced from rotavirus, but infection is not seasonal and duration of illness may be longer. The Norwalk agent is a small RNA virus that predominantly causes vomiting, but also some diarrhea in older children and adults, usually in common source outbreaks (perhaps water-borne). The duration of symptoms is short, usually 24–48 hours. Other potentially pathogenic viruses include astroviruses, caliciviruses, corona-like viruses, and other small round viruses. Cytomegalovirus (CMV) and herpesvirus rarely cause diarrhea, but may cause colitis or enteritis in immunocompromised hosts. CMV enteritis is particularly common after bone marrow transplantation and in late stages of HIV infection.

Kapikian AZ: Viral gastroenteritis. JAMA 1993;269:627.

Leiberman JM: Rotavirus and other viral causes of gastroenteritis. Pediatr Ann 1994;23:529.

CHRONIC DIARRHEA

It is difficult to define chronic diarrhea because there are wide variations in normal bowel habit. Some infants pass one firm stool every second to third day, whereas others may have 5–8 soft small stools daily. A gradual or sudden increase in the number and volume of stools (>15 g/kg/d), combined with an increase in fluidity should raise a suspicion that an organic cause of chronic diarrhea is present.

Diarrhea may result from any of the following pathogenetic mechanisms: (1) interruption of normal cell transport processes for water, electrolytes, or nutrients; (2) decrease in the surface area available for absorption, which may be due to shortening of the bowel or mucosal disease; (3) increase in intestinal motility; (4) increase in unabsorbable osmotically active molecules in the intestinal lumen; and (5) increase in intestinal permeability, leading to increased loss of water and electrolytes.

The differential diagnosis of chronic diarrhea is lengthy. Table 20–5 lists some disease categories and specific conditions in which diarrhea is a prominent feature.

Noninfectious Causes of Diarrhea

A. Antibiotic Therapy: Diarrhea accompanies antibiotic therapy in up to 30% of cases. Some antibiotics decrease carbohydrate transport and intestinal lactase levels. Eradication of normal gut flora and overgrowth of other organisms may cause diarrhea. Most antibiotic-associated diarrhea is watery in nature, is unassociated with systemic symptoms, and decreases when antibiotic therapy is stopped. Pseudomembranous colitis, caused by the toxins produced by *Clostridium difficile,* occurs in 0.2–10% of patients treated with antibiotics, especially clindamycin, cephalosporins, and amoxicillin. Patients develop fever, tenesmus, and abdominal pain with diarrhea, which contains leukocytes and sometimes gross blood up to 8 weeks after antibiotic exposure. Treatment with oral vancomycin (30–50 mg/kg/d) or metronidazole (30 mg/kg/d) for 7 days is recommended. Relapse occurs after treatment in up to 10% of cases.

B. Parenteral Infections: Infections of the urinary tract and upper respiratory tract (especially otitis media) are at times associated with diarrhea. The mechanism remains obscure. Antibiotic treatment of the primary infection, toxins released by infective agents, and local irritation of the rectum (in patients with bladder infections) may play a role.

C. Malnutrition: Malnutrition is associated with an increased occurrence of enteral infections, decreased bile acid synthesis, decreased pancreatic enzyme output, decreased disaccharidase activity, altered motility, and changes in the intestinal flora, all of which may produce diarrhea.

D. Diet: Overfeeding may cause diarrhea, especially in young infants. Relative deficiency of pancreatic amylase in young infants may produce diarrhea after starchy foods. Fruit juices, especially those high in fructose or sorbitol, produce osmotic diarrhea. Intestinal irritants (spices and foods high in roughage) and histamine-containing or -releasing foods (eg, citrus, tomatoes, certain cheeses, red wines, and fish) also cause diarrhea.

E. Allergic Diarrhea: Diarrhea caused by allergy to dietary proteins is a frequently entertained but rarely documented entity. Protein allergy is more common in infants under 12 months of age, who may experience mild to severe colitis. A personal or family history of atopy is common in infants with protein allergy. Older children may develop a celiac-like syndrome with a flat mucosal lesion, steatorrhea, hypoproteinemia, and occult blood loss. Skin testing is not reliable. Double-blind oral challenge with the suspected food under careful observation is necessary to confirm intestinal protein allergy. In infants, the condition usually disappears after 12 months. Allergies to fish, peanuts, and eggs are more likely to be lifelong. Multiple food allergy (more than three) is rare.

F. Chronic, Nonspecific Diarrhea: Chronic, nonspecific diarrhea is the most common cause of loose stools in thriving children. The typical patient is a healthy toddler 6–20 months of age who was a colicky baby and who has 3–6 loose, mucoid stools per day during the waking hours. The diarrhea worsens with a low-residue, low-fat, or high-carbohydrate diet and during periods of stress and infection. It clears spontaneously at about 3½ years of age (usually coincident with toilet training). No organic disease is discoverable. Possible causes include abnormalities of bile acid absorption in the terminal ileum, incomplete carbohydrate absorption (excessive fruit juice ingestion seems to worsen the condition), and abnormal motor function. A high familial incidence of functional bowel disease is observed. Stool tests for blood, fat, parasites, and ova are negative.

The following measures are helpful: institution of a high-fat, low-carbohydrate, high-fiber diet; avoidance of between-meal snacks; and avoidance of chilled fluids, especially fruit juices. It may be helpful to give loperamide, 0.1–0.2 mg/kg/d in two or three divided doses; cholestyramine, 2–4 g in divided doses; or psyllium agents, 1–2 tsp twice daily.

Greene HL, Ghishan FK: Excessive fluid intake as a cause of chronic diarrhea in young children. J Pediatr 1983; 102:836.

Hoekstra JH et al: Apple juice malabsorption: Fructose or sorbitol? J Pediatr Gastroenterol Nutr 1993;16:39.

Hyams JS et al: Carbohydrate malabsorption following fruit juice ingestion in young children. Pediatrics 1988;82:64.

Jonas A, Diver-Haber A: Stool output and composition in the chronic non-specific diarrhoea syndrome. Arch Dis Child 1982;57:35.

Kelly CP et al: Clostridium difficile colitis. N Engl J Med 1994;330:257.

THE MALABSORPTION SYNDROMES

Malabsorption of ingested food has many causes. Shortening of the small bowel (usually via surgical

Table 20–5. Guide to differential diagnosis of chronic diarrhea.

Disease	Age	Type of Diarrhea	Associated Features
Bacterial infections	Any age	Mucoid, bloody stool with poly-morphonuclear leukocytes.	Rarely chronic except in immunocom-promised hosts; *Salmonella, Yersinia, Campylobacter* most likely.
Viral infections	Any age	Watery.	Rarely chronic except in immunocom-promised hosts; cytomegalovirus, adenovirus, rotavirus.
Parasitic infections	Any age	Depends on organism.	*Entamoeba, Giardia, Cryptosporidium.*
Dietary factors Overfeeding (especially starches)	< 6 mo	Watery.	Colicky behavior without weight loss.
Protein allergy	< 2 mo	Watery with or without malabsorp-tion of fat; at times, blood and mu-cus.	Colic, vomiting (anemia, hypoprotein-emia).
Acrodermatitis enteropathica	< 12 mo	Voluminous with steatorrhea.	Malnutrition, skin rash; low serum zinc; usually genetic; sometimes secondary to severe dietary zinc deficiency.
Primary bile acid malabsorption	< 1 mo	Voluminous with steatorrhea.	Malnutrition; defective ilea transport of bile acids.
Irritable colon/chronic, nonspecific diarrhea	6–36 mo	Watery, frequent, with mucus, un-digested food: no steatorrhea.	Healthy child; often starts with bout of gastroenteritis.
Toxic diarrhea (antibiotics, cancer chemotherapy, radiation)	Any age	Loose; sometimes steatorrhea, with occult blood or pus.	Vomiting; anorexia.
Functional tumors (neuroblastoma, carcinoid, pancreatic cholera, Zollinger-Ellison syndrome)	Any age	Secretory diarrhea, watery; per-sists when patient fasts.	Hypokalemia; other symptoms depend upon tumor.
Carbohydrate malabsorption Congenital deficiencies Sucrase-isomaltase	 < 6 mo	 Watery; low pH; reducing substance-positive after acid hydrolysis; volume varies with sucrose intake.	 Abdominal distention; poor growth; defi-ciency present in 0.8% of North Ameri-cans, 10% of Alaskan natives.
Glucose-galactose malabsorption	< 1 mo	Intractable diarrhea with feeding; stool pH low; watery; reducing substances present.	Poor growth; defect in glucose transport.
Genetic deficiencies Lactase	> 4 y	Watery diarrhea with lactose; low pH; reducing substances present.	Deficiency develops in 100% of Asians, 80% of African-Americans, 15% of Ameri-can whites.
Acquired deficiencies Lactase and sucrase	Any age	Watery; low pH; reducing sub-stances present.	Follows intestinal injury or infection.
Monosaccharide intolerance	< 6 mo	Watery; low pH; reducing sub-stances present.	Rare; follows infection, made worse by malnutrition.
Pancreatic disorders Cystic fibrosis	< 6 mo	Steatorrhea; bulky, foul, pale.	Respiratory infection; poor weight gain.
Shwachman syndrome	< 2 y	Steatorrhea; bulky, foul, pale.	Neutropenia; short stature, bacterial in-fections; metaphyseal dysostosis.
Chronic pancreatitis	Any age	Steatorrhea; bulky, foul, pale.	Rare in children; usually associated with alcoholism.
Celiac disease	> 12 mo	Steatorrhea; bulky, foul, pale.	Vomiting, distention, irritability, anorexia.
Intestinal lymphangiectasia	3 mo	Voluminous; steatorrhea.	Lymphedema, lymphopenia, hypoalbu-minemia.

(*continued*)

Table 20–5. Guide to differential diagnosis of chronic diarrhea. (continued)

Disease	Age	Type of Diarrhea	Associated Features
Immune defects Hypogammaglobulinemia; IgA deficiency	Any age	Watery; sometimes steatorrhea.	Recurrent cutaneous and respiratory infection.
Combined immunodeficiency	< 1 mo	Severe; watery.	Stomatitis, skin rash, recurrent infection, opportunistic infection.
HIV infection	Any age	Steatorrhea.	Other opportunistic infections.
Defective cellular immunity	< 2 y		
Genetic-metabolic disorders Chloride-losing diarrhea	< 1 mo	Watery.	Alkalosis; growth failure.
Abeta- and hypobetalipo-proteinenemia	< 3 mo	Profuse; steatorrhea.	Progressive neurologic symptoms; low serum cholesterol; acanthocytosis.
Wolman's disease	< 1 mo	Profuse; steatorrhea.	Vomiting; severe growth failure; adrenal calcification; hypercholesterolemia.
Folate malabsorption	< 1 mo	Watery.	Megaloblastic anemia, stomatitis, seizures, retardation.
Anatomic abnormalities Blind (stagnant) loop/bacterial overgrowth	Any age	Watery; fat and carbohydrate malabsorption.	Caused by surgical adhesions, intestinal duplication, abnormal gastrointestinal motility, partial obstruction.
Short bowel	Any age	Watery; malabsorption of all nutrients.	Rarely congenital; usually secondary to surgical resection.
Intestinal pseudo-obstruction	Any age	Watery; malabsorption of all nutrients.	Distention; may be acquired or congenital; diarrhea secondary to bacterial overgrowth.
Inflammatory bowel disease Crohn's disease	Usually > 10 y	Loose with or without steatorrhea.	Pain, fever, abdominal mass, growth failure; joint pain, perianal disease.
Ulcerative colitis	Usually > 10 y	Bloody stools with polymorphonuclear leukocytes.	Tenesmus, anemia, abdominal pain, fever, joint pain; less severe growth failure.
Eosinophilic gastroenteritis	Any age	Watery or bloody, depending upon site of disease.	Intestinal or gastric obstruction, eczema, asthma.
Hirschsprung's disease with enterocolitis	< 1 y	Foul, liquid with white and red blood cells.	Abdominal distention, fever, history of constipation.
Malnutrition	< 1 y	Loose, steatorrhea; sometimes with carbohydrate malabsorption.	Becomes temporarily worse with refeeding.
Endocrine disorders Hyperthyroidism	Any age	Frequent, loose stool without malabsorption.	Other signs of hyperthyroidism.

resection) or mucosal damage (celiac disease) both reduce surface area. Impaired motility of the small intestine may interfere with normal propulsive movements and mixing of food with pancreatic and biliary secretions. Anaerobic bacteria proliferate under these conditions and impair fat absorption by deconjugation of bile acids, (intestinal pseudo-obstruction, postoperative blind loop syndrome). Impaired intestinal lymphatic (congenital lymphangiectasis) or venous drainage also cause malabsorption. Diseases reducing pancreatic exocrine function (cystic fibrosis, Shwachman syndrome) or the production and flow of biliary secretions cause nutrient malabsorption. Malabsorption may be genetically determined—disaccharidase deficiency, glucose–galactose malabsorption, and abetalipoproteinemia.

Clinical Findings

Gastrointestinal symptoms such as diarrhea, vomiting, anorexia, abdominal pain, and bloating are common but not universal. Certain physical features such as potbelly and wasted buttocks may indicate celiac disease. Observation of the stools for abnormal color, consistency, bulkiness, odor, mucus, and blood is important. Microscopic examination of stools for neutral and split fat (fatty acids) is helpful because most malabsorption syndromes involve some fat malabsorption.

Quantitative assessment of fat absorption requires measurement of fat excreted in the feces as a proportion of fat intake for defined period. Five percent excretion is normal for an infant over 1 year of age; 10–15% in a younger infant. Prothrombin time, serum carotene, vitamin E and vitamin D levels may be depressed by fat malabsorption. Accurate assessment of protein absorption is difficult and requires isotopic labeling of amino acids. Loss of serum proteins across the intestinal mucosa can be estimated by measurement of fecal α_1 antitrypsin. Malabsorption of complex carbohydrate is rarely measured. Disaccharide or monosaccharide malabsorption is estimated by reduction in stool pH, increased breath hydrogen, or decreased intestinal mucosal disaccharidase activity.

Other tests that may be helpful in suggesting a cause in a child with malabsorption include sweat chloride concentration (cystic fibrosis), intestinal mucosal biopsy (eg, celiac disease, intestinal lymphangiectasia, giardiasis, inflammatory bowel disease), liver function tests, and pancreatic secretion of enzymes after stimulation with secretin and cholecystokinin.

Differential Diagnosis

The pathophysiologic classification set forth in Table 20–6 may be helpful in view of the considerable variety of disorders giving rise to malabsorption.

Treatment & Prognosis

See specific syndromes (eg, celiac disease, disaccharidase deficiency).

Anderson CM: Malabsorption in children. Clin Gastroenterol 1977;6:355.
Friedman HI, Nylund B: Intestinal fat digestion, absorption, and transport: A review. Am J Clin Nutr 1980;33:1108.

CONSTIPATION

Constipation refers to the passage of bulky or hard stool at infrequent intervals (two per week). Retention of feces in the rectum results in encopresis in 60% of affected children. Organic causes of constipation are listed in Table 20–7. Most constipation in childhood is not organic, but a result of voluntary or involuntary retentive behavior.

Clinical Findings

Normal infants under 3 months of age often grunt, strain, and turn red in the face while passing normal stools. This pattern may be erroneously viewed as constipation. Failure to appreciate this normal developmental pattern may lead to the unwise use of laxatives or enemas. As children become older, they may gradually develop the ability to ignore the sensation of rectal fullness and retain stool. Many factors (painful defecation; skeletal muscle weakness; psychological issues, especially those relating to control and authority, modesty, and distaste for school bathrooms; medications, and others listed in Table 20–7) promote and reinforce this behavior, which finally results in impaction of the rectum and overflow incontinence or encopresis. The dilated rectum becomes less sensitive to dilation, thus perpetuating the problem, regardless of the original cause. As many as 1–2% of healthy primary school children have retentive constipation. The ratio of males to females is 4:1 in some studies.

Differential Diagnosis

Features distinguishing retentive constipation from Hirschsprung's disease are summarized in Table 20–8.

Treatment

Increased intake of fluids and high-residue foods such as bran, whole wheat, fruits, and vegetables may be sufficient therapy in cases of mild constipation. The use of a barley malt extract such as Maltsupex, 1–2 tsp added to feedings two or three times daily, is helpful in small infants. Stool softeners such as dioctyl sodium sulfosuccinate, 5–10 mg/kg/d, prevent excessive drying of the stool and are effective unless there is voluntary stool retention. Cathartics such as standardized extract of senna fruit (eg, Senokot syrup), 1–2 tsp twice daily depending on age, can be used for short periods of time.

If encopresis is present, treatment should start with relieving fecal impaction. An effective stool softener should be given in amounts sufficient to induce 3–4 loose stools per day (2–5 mL/kg/d of mineral oil in two doses). After several weeks to months of regular loose stools, the dosage of mineral oil can be tapered and stopped. Mineral oil should not be given to nonambulatory infants, retarded children, or those with gastroesophageal reflux. Aspiration of mineral oil may cause severe lipid pneumonia.

The prevention of stool holding and the establishment of a regular bowel habit are accomplished by "toileting" the child at regular times each day and by the daily administration of mineral oil over a period of several months in a reduced dosage. Recurrence of encopresis should be treated promptly with a short course of laxatives or enemas. A multiple vitamin is recommended while mineral oil is administered.

Psychiatric consultation may be indicated for patients with resistant symptoms or overt, severe emotional disturbances.

Table 20–6. Malabsorption syndromes.

Intraluminal phase abnormalities	**Intestinal phase abnormalities (cont'd)**
Acid hypersecretion; Zollinger-Ellison syndrome	Circulatory disturbances
Gastric resection	Cirrhosis
Exocrine pancreatic insufficiency	Congestive heart failure
Cystic fibrosis	Abnormal structure of gastrointestinal tract
Chronic pancreatitis	Dumping syndrome after gastrectomy
Pancreatic pseudocysts	Malrotation
Schwachman syndrome	Stenosis of jejunum or ileum
Enterokinase deficiency	Small bowel resection; short bowel syndrome
Lipase and colipase deficiency	Polyposis
Malnutrition	Selective inborn absorptive defects
Decreased conjugated bile acids	Congenital malabsorption of folic acid
Liver production and excretion	Selective malabsorption of vitamin B_{12}
Neonatal hepatitis	Cystinuria, methionine malabsorption
Biliary atresia: intrahepatic and extrahepatic	Hartnup disease, blue diaper syndrome
Acute and chronic active hepatitis	Glucose-galactose malabsorption
Disease of the biliary tract	Primary disaccharidase deficiency
Cirrhosis	Acrodermatitis enteropathica
Fat malabsorption in the premature infant	Abetalipoproteinemia
Intestinal malabsorption of bile acids	Congenital chloridorrhea
Short bowel syndrome	Primary hypomagnesemia
Bacterial growth	Hereditary fructose intolerance
Blind loop	Familial hypophosphatemic rickets
Fistula	Endocrine diseases
Strictures, regional enteritis	Diabetes
Scleroderma, intestinal pseudo-obstruction	Addison's disease
Intestinal phase abnormalities	Hyperthyroidism
Mucosal diseases	Hypoparathyroidism, pseudohypoparathyroidism
Infections, bacterial or viral	Neuroblastoma, ganglioneuroma
Infections, parasitic	**Vascular and lymphatic disorders**
Giardia lamblia	Whipple's disease
Fish tapeworm	Intestinal lymphangiectasis
Hookworm	Congestive heart failure
Cryptosporidium	Regional enteritis with lymphangiectasis
Malnutrition	Lymphoma
Marasmus	Abetalipoproteinemia
Kwashiorkor	**Miscellaneous**
Dermatitis herpetiformis	Renal insufficiency
Folic acid deficiency	Carcinoid, mastocytosis
Drugs: methotrexate, antibiotics	Immunity defects
Crohn's disease	Familial dysautonomia
Cow's milk and soy protein intolerance	Collagen disease
Secondary disaccharidase deficiency	Wolman's disease
Secondary monosaccharide intolerance	Histiocytosis X
Hirschsprung's disease with enterocoitis	
Tropical sprue	
Celiac disease	
Radiation enteritis, chemotherapy	
Lymphoma	

Loening-Baucke V: Chronic constipation in children. Gastroenterology 1993;105:1557.

GASTROINTESTINAL BLEEDING

Vomiting blood or passing blood per rectum are alarming symptoms. The history is the key to identifying the bleeding source and should provide detailed answers to the following questions:

1. Is it really blood and is it coming from the gastrointestinal tract? A number of substances simulate hematochezia or melena. The presence of blood should be confirmed chemically. A history of genitourinary problems, coughing, tonsillitis, lost teeth, or epistaxis may identify an extraintestinal bleeding source.

2. How much blood is there and what is its color and character? Table 20–9 lists the sites of gastrointestinal bleeding in relationship to the amount and the appearance of the blood in the stools. Table 20–10 lists causes of rectal bleeding.

3. Is the child acutely or chronically ill? The physical examination should be thorough. Physical signs of portal hypertension, intestinal obstruction, or coagulopathy are particularly important. The nasal passages should be inspected for signs of recent epistaxis; the vagina for menstrual blood; and the anus for fissures and hemorrhoids.

Table 20–7. Causes of constipation.

Functional or retentive causes	Abnormalities of myenteric ganglion cells
Dietary causes	Hirschsprung's disease
Undernutrition, dehydration	Waardenburg's syndrome
Excessive milk intake	Multiple endocrine neoplasia IIA
Lack of bulk	Hypo- and hyperganglionosis
Cathartic abuse	von Recklinghausen's disease
Drugs	Multiple endocrine neoplasia IIB
Narcotics	Intestinal neuronal dysplasia
Antihistamines	Chronic intestinal pseudo-obstruction
Some antidepressants	Spinal cord defects
Vincristine	Metabolic and endocrine disorders
Structural defects of gastrointestinal tract	Hypothyroidism
Anus and rectum	Hyperparathyroidism
Fissure, hemorrhoids, abscess	Renal tubular acidosis
Anterior ectopic anus	Diabetes insipidus (dehydration)
Anal and rectal stenosis	Vitamin D intoxication (hypercalcemia)
Presacral teratoma	Idiopathic hypercalcemia
Small bowel and colon	Skeletal muscle weakness/incoordination
Tumor, stricture	Cerebral palsy
Chronic volvulus	Muscular dystrophy/myotonia
Intussusception	
Smooth muscle diseases	
Scleroderma and dermatomyositis	
Systemic lupus erythematosus	
Chronic intestinal pseudo-obstruction	

Modified and reproduced, with permission, from Silverman A, Roy CC: *Pediatric Clinical Gastroenterology,* 3rd ed. Mosby, 1983.

A systolic blood pressure below 100 mm Hg and a pulse rate above 100/min in an older child suggest at least a 20% reduction of blood volume. A pulse rate increase of 20/min or a drop in systolic blood pressure greater than 10 mm Hg when the patient sits up is also a sensitive index of significant volume depletion.

4. Is the child still bleeding? Serial determination of vital signs and hematocrit are essential to assess ongoing bleeding. Detection of blood in the gastric aspirate confirms a bleeding site proximal to the ligament of Treitz. However, its absence does not rule out the duodenum as the source.

Table 20–8. Differentiation of retentive constipation and Hirschsprung's disease.

	Retentive Constipation	Hirschsprung's Disease
Onset	2–3 years	At birth
Abdominal distention	Rare	Present
Nutrition/growth	Normal	Poor
Soiling & retentive behavior	Intermittent or constant	Rare
Rectal examination	Ampulla full	Ampulla may be empty
Rectal biopsy	Ganglion cells present	Ganglion cells absent
Rectal manometry	Normal rectoanal reflex	Nonrelaxation of internal anal sphincter after rectal distention
Barium enema	Distended rectum	Narrow distal segment with proximal megacolon

Table 20–9. Identification of sites of gastrointestinal bleeding.

Symptom or Sign	Location of Bleeding Lesion
Effortless bright red blood from the mouth	Nasopharyngeal or oral lesions; tonsillitis; esophageal varices; lacerations of esophageal or gastric mucosa (Mallory-Weiss syndrome).
Vomiting of bright red blood or of "coffee grounds"	Lesion proximal to ligament of Treitz.
Melanotic stool	Lesion proximal to ligament of Treitz, upper small bowel. Blood loss in excess of 50–100 mL/24 h.
Bright red or dark red blood in stools	Lesion in the ileum or colon. (Massive upper gastrointestinal bleeding may also be associated with bright red blood in stool.)
Streak of blood on outside of a stool	Lesion in the rectal ampulla or anal canal.

Table 20–10. Differential diagnosis of rectal bleeding in infants and children.

Cause	Usual Age Group	Additional Complaints	Amount of Blood	Color of Blood
Swallowed foreign body	Any age	Rarely, perforation and abscess Hematemesis	Usually small	Melena
Systemic bleeding	Any age	Other evidence of bleeding	Variable	Dark or bright red
Milk intolerance	Infants	Colicky abdominal pain, diarrhea	Moderate to large	Red Blood streaks with diarrhea
Esophageal varices	> 4 years	Signs of portal hypertension Hematemesis	Variable	Usually dark; bright with massive bleed
Hemangioma or familial telangiectasia	Any age	Telangiectasia elsewhere	Variable	Dark or bright
Peptic ulcer, gastritis	Any age	Abdominal pain Coffee ground emesis	Usually small; can be massive	Melena
Duplication of bowel	Any age	Pain, obstruction, mass	Usually small	Usually dark
Meckel's diverticulum	Any age; rare under 2 months	Anemia, painless bleeding	Small to large; usually large	Maroon, brick red, occasionally melena
Volvulus	Infant or young child	Abdominal pain, intestinal obstruction, bilious emesis	Small to large	Dark or bright
Intussusception	< 18 months	Abdominal pain, mass, bilious emesis	Small to large	Dark or bright with "currant jelly" mucus
Ulcerative colitis & Crohn's colitis	> 4 years	Diarrhea, cramps	Small to large	Red blood with diarrhea
Bacterial enteritis	Any age	Diarrhea, cramps, fever	Small to large	Red blood with diarrhea
Juvenile polyp	2–8 years	None	Small to large	Red blood with normal stool
Inserted foreign body	Child	Rectal pain	Small	Red with mucus
Anal fissure or proctitis	< 2 years	Pain with defecation	Small	Red with mucus
Swallowed maternal blood	Newborn	None	Variable	Dark, occasionally bright red; check Apt test
Esophagitis	Any age	Dysphagia, hematemesis	Usually small	Dark
Schönlein-Henoch purpura	3–10 years	Purpuric rash, arthritis, abdominal pain, hematuria	Variable	Dark or bright
Lymphoid nodular hyperplasia	3–24 months	Loose stools	Small	Bright red

Management

If a hemorrhagic diathesis is detected, vitamin K should be given intravenously. In severe bleeding, needs for volume replacement are monitored by measurement of central venous pressure. In less severe cases, vital signs, serial hematocrits, and gastric aspirates are sufficient.

If blood is recovered from the gastric aspirate, gastric lavage with saline should be performed for 30–60 minutes, until only a blood-tinged return is obtained. Panendoscopy is then done to identify the bleeding site. Endoscopy is superior to barium contrast study for lesions such as esophageal varices, stress ulcers, and gastritis. Colonoscopy may identify the source of bright red rectal bleeding and should be performed if the extent of bleeding warrants immediate investigation and if plain x-ray films show no signs of intestinal obstruction.

Small or large bowel lesions that bleed briskly (> 0.5 mL/min) may be localized by angiography or radionuclide scanning following injection of labeled red cells.

Persistent vascular bleeding (varices, vascular anomalies) may be temporarily relieved using vasopressin (20 units/1.73 m^2 intravenously over a 20-minute period). Thereafter it may be necessary to sustain the infusion for 24 hours at a rate of 0.2–0.4 units/1.73 m/min. Bleeding from esophageal varices may be stopped by temporary compression with a pediatric Sengstaken-Blakemore tube. Sclerotherapy or banding of uncontrolled bleeding variees is the treatment of choice.

If gastric decompression, antacid therapy, and transfusion are ineffective in stopping ulcer bleeding, laser therapy, local injection of epinephrine, electrocautery, or emergency surgery may be necessary.

Treem WR: Gastrointestinal bleeding in children. Gastrointest Endosc Clin North Am 1994;4:75.

RECURRENT ABDOMINAL PAIN

About 10% of healthy school children between 5 and 15 years of age will at some time experience recurrent episodes of abdominal pain severe enough to affect activity. An organic cause can be found in fewer than 10% of cases.

Clinical Findings

A. Symptoms and Signs: Attacks of abdominal pain are characteristically of variable duration and intensity. Although the pain is usually located in the periumbilical area, location far from the umbilicus does not rule out recurrent abdominal pain. Pain may occur both day and night. Weight loss is rare. Pain may be associated with dramatic reactions; patients may clutch the abdomen, double over, or even throw themselves to the ground. School attendance may suffer. Indeed, reluctance to attend school (school phobia) may be an important etiologic factor. The pain may be associated with pallor, nausea, vomiting, and slight temperature elevation.

The pain usually bears little relationship to bowel habits and activity. At times, pain may occur during meals or before the child leaves for school. A precipitating or stressful situation in the child's life at the time the pains began can sometimes be elicited. A history of functional gastrointestinal complaints is often found in family members.

A thorough physical examination is essential and usually normal. Complaints of abdominal tenderness elicited during palpation sometimes seem out of proportion to visible signs of distress.

B. Laboratory Findings: Complete blood count, sedimentation rate, urinalysis, and stool test for occult blood usually suffice. If the pain is atypical, further testing suggested by symptoms should be done.

Differential Diagnosis

Abdominal pain secondary to disorders of the urinary tract and extraabdominal sources are listed in Table 20–3. Pinworms, mesenteric lymphadenitis, and chronic appendicitis are improbable causes of recurrent abdominal pain. Lactose intolerance usually causes pain, gas, and diarrhea. At times, however, abdominal discomfort may be the only symptom. Abdominal migraine and abdominal epilepsy are rare conditions. The incidence of peptic gastritis, esophagitis, duodenitis, and ulcer disease is probably underappreciated. Upper intestinal endoscopy may be useful.

Treatment & Prognosis

Treatment consists of reassurance based on a thorough physical appraisal and a sympathetic explanation of the functional nature of the complaint. Therapy for emotional problems is sometimes required, but drugs should be avoided. The prognosis is good.

Antonson DL: Abdominal pain. Gastrointest Endosc Clin North Am 1994;4:1.

Appley J: The Child With Abdominal Pain, 2nd ed. Blackwell, 1975.

PROTEIN-LOSING ENTEROPATHIES

Excessive loss of plasma proteins into the gastrointestinal tract occurs in association with a number of disorders.

Clinical Findings

Signs and symptoms include edema, chylous ascites, poor weight gain, and sometimes deficiencies of fat-soluble vitamins, and anemia. Serum albumin is usually less than 2.5 g/dL. Serum globulins may also be decreased. Fecal α_1-antitrypsin, a marker for protein loss, is elevated (> 3mg/g dry weight stool; slightly higher in breast-fed infants).

Disorders Associated With Protein-Losing Enteropathy

A. Vascular Obstruction: Congestive heart failure, constrictive pericarditis, atrial septal defect, primary myocardial disease, increased right atrial pressure. Children with Fontan procedure for tricuspid atresia are particularly prone.

B. Gastric: Giant hypertrophic gastritis, or Menetrier's disease (may be a result of CMV infection); polyps.

C. Small Intestine: Celiac disease, intestinal lymphangiectasia, regional enteritis, Whipple's disease, lymphosarcoma, acute gastrointestinal infection, allergic gastroenteropathy, blind loop syndrome, abetalipoproteinemia, chronic mucosal ischemia (eg, from chronic volvulus or radiation enteritis).

D. Colon: Ulcerative colitis, Hirschsprung's disease, pseudomembranous colitis, polyposis syndromes, villous adenoma, solitary rectal ulcer.

Differential Diagnosis

Hypoalbuminemia may be due to an increased catabolic rate or may be associated with poor protein intake, impaired hepatic protein synthesis, congenital malformations of lymphatics outside the gastrointestinal tract. It is especially important to rule out proteinuria, from such conditions as urinary infection, nephritis and nephrotic syndrome, as causes of protein loss.

Treatment

Albumin infusions in conjunction with diuretics may relieve symptoms temporarily. Treatment must be directed toward the primary underlying cause.

Magazzu G et al: Reliability and usefulness of random fecal alpha-1-antitrypsin concentration: Further simplification of the method. J Pediatr Gastroenterol Nutr 1985; 4:402.

Thomas DW et al: Random fecal alpha-1-antitrypsin concentration in children with gastrointestinal disease. Gastroenterology 1981;80:776.

CELIAC DISEASE
(Gluten Enteropathy)

General Considerations

Celiac disease results from intestinal sensitivity to the gliadin fraction of gluten from wheat, rye, barley, and oats. Most cases present during the second year of life, but the age at onset and the severity are both variable. The disease is more common in Europe and Canada than in the United States and is uncommon in blacks and Asians.

The underlying pathologic process is not yet clearly understood, but it is thought that intestinal damage and villous atrophy result from a cell-mediated immune response to gliadin, the alcohol-soluble fraction of gluten. Ten percent of first-degree relatives may be affected. The inheritance is probably polygenic, but it might result from a single gene in combination with an environmental precipitant such as intestinal adenovirus infection. The increased incidence of celiac disease in children with type I diabetes mellitus, IgA deficiency, and Down's syndrome suggests possible immunologic factors in the development of celiac disease.

Clinical Findings

A. Symptoms and Signs:

1. Diarrhea–Affected children present with a history of digestive disturbances starting at 6–12 months of age—the age at which wheat, rye, or oat glutens are first fed. Initially, the diarrhea may be intermittent. Subsequently, it is continuous, with bulky, pale, frothy, greasy, foul-smelling stools. During celiac crises, dehydration, shock, and acidosis are seen. Diarrhea is absent in 10% of cases, in which anorexia is severe.

2. Constipation, vomiting, and abdominal pain–This triad of symptoms may in a small number of cases dominate the clinical picture and suggest a diagnosis of intestinal obstruction. Constipation generally results from a combination of anorexia, dehydration, muscle weakness, and bulky, fatty stools.

3. Failure to thrive–The onset of diarrhea is usually accompanied by loss of appetite, failure to gain weight, and irritability in infants. In established cases, there is a loss of weight, which is most marked in the limbs and buttocks. The abdomen becomes distended secondary to gas and fluid in the intestinal tract. Short stature and delayed puberty are characteristic in older children.

4. Anemia and vitamin deficiencies–Anemia usually responds to iron and is rarely megaloblastic. Deficiencies in fat-soluble vitamins are common. Rickets can be seen when growth has not been completely halted by the disease. Osteomalacia is more common, however, and pathologic fractures may occur. Hypoprothrombinemia secondary to vitamin K malabsorption can cause easy bleeding.

B. Laboratory Findings:

1. Fat content of stools–A 3-day collection of stools usually reveals excessive fecal fat. A normal child will excrete 5–10% of ingested fats. The untreated celiac patient will excrete more than 15% of daily fat intake. Anorexia may be so severe that steatorrhea may not be present in 10–25% of cases until normal intake is established.

2. Impaired carbohydrate absorption–A low oral glucose tolerance curve is seen. Absorption of D-xylose is impaired, with blood levels lower than 20 mg/dL 60 minutes after ingestion.

3. Hypoproteinemia–Hypoalbuminemia can be severe enough to lead to edema. There is evidence of increased protein loss in the gut lumen and poor hepatic synthesis secondary to malnutrition.

C. Imaging: A small bowel series shows a malabsorptive pattern characterized by segmentation, clumping of the barium column, and hypersecretion. These changes are nonspecific, and can be found in other malabsorptive conditions (Table 20–6).

D. Biopsy Findings: Intestinal biopsy is the most reliable test for celiac disease. It is a safe and simple procedure even in infants. Under the dissecting microscope, the jejunal mucosa lacks the slender, finger-like projections that characterize normal villi. Under the light microscope, the celiac mucosa has shortened or absent villi, lengthened crypts of Lieberkuhn, and intense plasma cell infiltration of the lamina propria.

E. Serologic Tests: Anti-gliadin, anti-reticulin, and anti-endomysial antibodies are useful screening tests. IgG antibodies to gliadin are present in 10% of normal children. IgA antibodies are more specific to celiac patients. Antibody titers may be a good monitor of compliance with diet.

Differential Diagnosis

The differential diagnosis for celiac disease includes disorders that cause malabsorption. Strict adherence to two diagnostic criteria—the characteristic small bowel microscopic changes and clinical improvement on a gluten-free diet—is essential. Repeated mucosal biopsies to prove histologic recovery on gluten-free diet and relapse on gluten challenge are not critical to the diagnosis in typical patients.

Treatment

A. Diet: Treatment consists of dietary gluten restriction for life. All sources of wheat, rye, barley, and oat gluten must be eliminated during the initial treatment. Some patients may be able to tolerate oats in the diet, but this should be tested only after recovery has occurred. Initially, the diet should provide 25% more calories than calculated for expected weight. Lactose is poorly tolerated in the acute stage because the extensive mucosal damage causes disaccharidase deficiency. Normal amounts of fat are advisable. Supplemental vitamins and minerals are indicated in the acute phase.

In severely affected children, the diet should be tailored to the child's appetite and capacity to absorb. A full gluten-free diet can usually be given after 2–3 weeks. Clinical improvement is usually evident within a week, and histologic repair is complete after 3–12 months.

B. Corticosteroids: Corticosteroids can hasten clinical improvement but are indicated only in very ill patients with signs and symptoms of celiac crisis.

Prognosis

Clinical and histologic recovery is the rule but may be slow. Malignant lymphoma of the small bowel occurs with increased frequency in older adults with long-standing disease. Dietary treatment seems to decrease the risk of this complication.

Cacciari E et al: Short stature and celiac disease: A relationship to consider even in patients with no gastrointestinal tract symptoms. J Pediatr 1983;103:708.

Cooper BT et al: Celiac disease and malignancy. Medicine 1980;59:249.

Misra S, Ament ME: Diagnosis of coeliac sprue in 1994. Gastroenterol Clin North Am 1995;1:133.

DISACCHARIDASE DEFICIENCY

General Considerations

Starches and the disaccharides sucrose and lactose are quantitatively the most important dietary carbohydrates. The dietary disaccharides and oligosaccharides products of pancreatic amylase action on starch require hydrolysis by intestinal brush border disaccharidases before significant absorption can take place. Disaccharidase levels are higher in the jejunum and in the proximal ileum than in the distal ileum and duodenum.

In primary disaccharidase deficiency, a single enzyme is affected, disaccharide intolerance is likely to persist, intestinal histologic findings are normal, and a family history is common.

Because disaccharidases are confined to the outer cell layer of the intestinal epithelium, they are susceptible to mucosal damage. Many conditions cause secondary disaccharidase deficiency, which affects mucosal enzymes with lactase usually most severely depressed. Histologic examination reveals changes compatible with the underlying disorder. A familial incidence is uncommon.

Clinical Findings

A. Primary (Congenital):

1. Lactase deficiency–Congenital lactase deficiency is a rare condition leading to diarrhea after lactose is ingested. The stools are frothy and acid; their pH may fall below 4.5 owing to the presence of organic acids. The osmotic action of unhydrolyzed lactose leads to catharsis. Vomiting is common. Severe malnutrition may occur. Reducing substances are present in the stools, and lactosuria may occur. Infants with lactosuria, aminoaciduria, proteinuria, acidosis, and elevated blood urea nitrogen have been described. An oral lactose tolerance test (2 g/kg) is likely to result in within 8 hours; the blood glucose levels show no appreciable rise. A rise in breath hydrogen after oral administration of lactose is also diagnostic.

Patients respond to the reduction of lactose in their diets. Tolerance for dietary starch and sucrose is normal. Lactase extracted from *Aspergillus* and *Kluyvera* spp can be added to milk products or taken with meals to enhance lactose hydrolysis.

2. Sucrase and isomaltase deficiency–This is a combined defect that is inherited as an autosomal recessive trait. Ten percent of Alaskan natives are affected. The condition is rare in other groups. Abdominal distention, failure to thrive, and chronic diarrhea may be the presenting symptoms. Distaste for and avoidance of sucrose occurs even in young infants.

Because sucrose is not a reducing sugar, tests for reducing substances in the stool will be negative unless the sucrose in the stool is hydrolyzed. A sucrose tolerance test (2 g/kg) is likely to be flat. Breath hydrogen will be elevated after ingestion of sucrose. Diarrhea and dehydration may occur during oral disaccharide tolerance tests in patients with lactase or sucrase-isomaltase deficiency. Treatment of primary sucrase-isomaltase deficiency requires elimination of most sucrose. A preparation of yeast sucrase taken with meals is also effective. Starch intolerance is rarely a problem, because the 1–6 linkages of starch hydrolyzed by isomaltase constitute only a small part of the molecule.

B. Secondary (Acquired):

1. Secondary lactase deficiency—Diarrhea may be produced in normal individuals if a large dose of lactose is ingested. The threshold for lactose tolerance is much lower than that for sucrose. There is a high prevalence genetically determined lactase deficiency in certain racial groups (70% in North American blacks and nearly 100% in Asian populations) after 3–5 years of age. It is estimated that 30–60% of North American whites become lactase-deficient after 3–5 years. Neomycin and kanamycin administration can reduce lactase activity. Celiac disease, giardiasis, malnutrition, viral or bacterial gastroenteritis, abetalipoproteinemia, immunoglobulin deficiencies, and intestinal mucosal injury secondary to radiation and cancer chemotherapy all can decrease intestinal lactase activity.

2. Secondary sucrase deficiency—Intestinal mucosal damage tends to lower the levels of all disaccharidases. Signs of sucrose intolerance are usually masked by the more striking symptoms of lactose intolerance. Infectious diarrhea is the most common cause of secondary sucrose intolerance.

Treatment

A. Lactose-Free Diet: Many commercially available infant formulas are lactose-free. Foods containing whey, dry milk solids, and curds should be excluded. It is important to see if labels indicate any lactose content. Cheeses (cottage, cheddar, cream), ice cream, sherbet, yogurt, and chocolate milk powders contain variable amounts of lactose, small amounts of which may be well tolerated.

B. Sucrose-Restricted Diet: Glucose, fructose, or dietetic sugar substitutes may be used as sweeteners in cooking and baking. A small amount of sucrose in grapes, cherries, strawberries, and blackberries may be tolerated. Other fruits contain significant sucrose and may cause diarrhea. Most green vegetables are sucrose-free, but peas, beans, and lentils should be avoided.

Prognosis

Primary disaccharidase deficiency is a lifelong defect. However, in both lactase and sucrase deficiencies, tolerance for the disaccharide may increase with age. The prognosis in the secondary or acquired forms of disaccharidase deficiency depends on the underlying illness. Normal tolerance for lactose may not be regained for many months after an acute mucosal injury.

Heitlinger LA, Lebenthal E: Disorders of carbohydrate digestion and absorption. Pediatr Clin North Am 1988;35:239.

GLUCOSE-GALACTOSE MALABSORPTION

Glucose-galactose malabsorption is a rare disorder in which the transport protein for glucose is defec-

tive. Severe diarrhea begins with the first feedings. Small bowel histologic findings are normal. Glycosuria and aminoaciduria may occur. The glucose tolerance test is flat. Fructose is well tolerated. The diarrhea promptly subsides on withdrawal of glucose and galactose from the diet. Reducing substances are consistently found in the stool. The acquired form of glucose-galactose malabsorption is mainly seen in infants under 6 months of age, usually following an acute viral or bacterial enteritis. Both disaccharides and monosaccharides, including fructose, are malabsorbed.

In the congenital disease, total exclusion of glucose and galactose from the diet is mandatory. A satisfactory formula consists of a carbohydrate-free formula base with added fructose. The prognosis is good if the disease is diagnosed early, because tolerance for glucose and galactose improves with age. In the secondary form, prolonged parenteral nutrition may be required until intestinal transport mechanisms for monosaccharides return.

Fairclough PD et al: Absorption of glucose and maltose in congenital glucose-galactose malabsorption. Pediatr Res 1978;12:1112.

Nichols VN et al: Acquired monosaccharide intolerance in infants. J Pediatr Gastroenterol Nutr 1989;8:51.

INTESTINAL LYMPHANGIECTASIA

This form of protein-losing enteropathy results from a congenital abnormality of the bowel lymphatic system, often associated with abnormalities of the lymphatics in the extremities. Obstruction of lymphatic drainage of the intestine leads to rupture of the intestinal lacteals with leakage of lymph into the lumen of the bowel. Fat loss may be significant and lead to steatorrhea. Chronic loss of lymphocytes and immunoglobulins increases the susceptibility to infections.

Clinical Findings

Peripheral edema, diarrhea, abdominal distention, lymphedematous extremities, chylous effusions, and repeated infections are common. Laboratory findings are low serum albumin, decreased immunoglobulin levels, lymphocytopenia, and anemia. Serum calcium is frequently depressed, and stool fat may be elevated. Lymphocytes may be seen in large numbers on a stool smear. Fecal α_1-antitrypsin is elevated. X-ray studies reveal an edematous small bowel mucosal pattern, and biopsy reveals dilated lacteals in the villi and lamina propria. If only the lymphatics of the deeper layers of bowel or intestinal mesenterics are involved, laparotomy may be necessary to establish the diagnosis.

Differential Diagnosis

Other causes of protein-losing enteropathy must

be considered, although an associated lymphedematous extremity strongly favors this diagnosis.

Treatment & Prognosis

Medium chain triglycerides as a fat source are effective only in mucosal lymphangiectasia. Vitamin and calcium supplements should be given. Antibiotics are used for specific infections. Total parenteral nutrition is helpful on a temporary basis. Surgery is needed when the lesion is localized to a small area of the bowel or in cases of constrictive pericarditis or obstructing tumors. Intravenous albumin and gamma-globulin may also be used to control symptoms.

The prognosis at present is not favorable, although there may be remission with age.

Tift WL, Lloyd JK: Intestinal lymphangiectasia: Long-term results with MCT diet. Arch Dis Child 1975;50:269.

Vardy PA, Lebenthal E, Shwachman H: Intestinal lymphangiectasia: A reappraisal. Pediatrics 1975;55:842.

COW'S MILK PROTEIN INTOLERANCE

Milk protein intolerance is more common in males and in young infants with a family history of atopy. The estimated prevalence is 0.5–1%. Colic, vomiting, and diarrhea are the major symptoms. Stools often contain blood and mucus. Sigmoidoscopic examination reveals a superficial colitis, often with an eosinophilic infiltrate. Pneumatosis intestinalis may be present on x-ray. Viral gastroenteritis sometimes precedes the onset of symptoms. Less commonly, milk protein may induce eosinophilic gastroenteritis with protein-losing enteropathy, hypoalbuminemia, and hypogammaglobulinemia. A celiac-like syndrome with villous atrophy, malabsorption, hypoalbuminemia, occult blood in the stool, and anemia can occur in older children. IgE-mediated anaphylactic shock is a rare manifestation of milk protein sensitivity in infancy.

Breast-fed infants under 6 months of age can also develop blood-streaked stools and a sigmoidoscopic picture similar to that of infants with milk protein sensitivity. Tiny amounts of intact allergen passed in breast milk may be the cause. Elimination of whole cow's milk from the mother's diet sometimes causes resolution of bloody diarrhea. A switch to semielemental diet almost always results in improvement. Because the blood loss and diarrhea in these breast-fed infants are rarely severe, it is not essential that breast feeding be stopped. If symptoms are severe or prolonged, however, a trial of semielemental formula is recommended. The colitic pattern of milk protein sensitivity and colitis in breast-fed infants usually clears spontaneously by 6–12 months of age.

Patients with milk protein allergy have a 30% incidence of sensitivity to soy protein, with similar symptoms. It is therefore best to use a casein hydrolysate formula as an elimination diet.

Estaban MM (editor): Adverse reactions to foods in infancy and childhood. J Pediatr 1992;121(Suppl):S1.

IMMUNOLOGIC DEFICIENCY STATES WITH DIARRHEA OR MALABSORPTION

Diarrhea is a frequent finding in immune deficiency states, but the cause is often obscure. Fifty to 60 percent of patients with idiopathic acquired hypogammaglobulinemia have steatorrhea and intestinal villous atrophy. Lymphonodular hyperplasia is a common feature in this group of patients. Patients with congenital or Bruton type agammaglobulinemia uniformly have diarrhea and abnormal intestinal morphology. Patients with isolated IgA deficiency may also present with chronic diarrhea, a celiac-like picture, lymphoid nodular hyperplasia, and giardiasis. Patients with isolated cellular immunity defects, combined cellular and humoral immune incompetence, and HIV infection may have severe chronic diarrhea leading to malnutrition. The cause of diarrhea may be common bacterial, viral, or parasitic pathogens, organisms usually considered nonpathogenic *(Blastocystis hominis, Candida),* or unusual organisms (cytomegalovirus, *Cryptosporidium, Isospora belli, Mycobacterium* species, Microsporidia, and algal organisms such as Cyanobacteria). Often, the cause is not found. There is a high incidence of disaccharidase deficiency. Chronic granulomatous disease may be associated with intestinal symptoms suggestive of chronic inflammatory bowel disease. A rectal biopsy may reveal the presence of typical macrophages.

Treatment must be directed toward correction of the immunologic defect. Specific treatments are available or being developed for many of the unusual pathogens causing diarrhea in the immunocompromised host. Thus, a vigorous diagnostic search for specific pathogens is warranted in these individuals.

Deveikis A: Gastrointestinal disease in immunocompromised children. Pediatr Ann 1994;23:562.

INFLAMMATORY BOWEL DISEASE

Crohn's disease and ulcerative colitis are the two major idiopathic inflammatory bowel diseases of children. They share many features resulting from bowel inflammation, such as diarrhea, pain, fever, and blood loss, but they differ in important aspects, such as distribution of disease, histologic findings, incidence and type of extraintestinal symptoms, response to medications and surgery, and prognosis. A

Table 20–11. Features of Crohn's disease and ulcerative colitis.

	Crohn's Disease	Ulcerative Colitis
Age of onset	10–20 years	10–20 years
Incidence	4–6 per 100,000	3–15 per 100,000
Area of bowel affected	Oropharynx, esophagus, and stomach, rare; small bowel only, 25–30%, colon and anus only, 25%; ileocolitis, 40%; diffuse disease, 5%	Total colon, 90%; proctitis, 10%
Distribution	Segmental; disease-free skip areas common.	Continuous; distal to proximal.
Pathology	Full-thickness, acute, and chronic inflammation; noncaseating granulomas (50%), extraintestinal fistulas, abscesses, stricture, and fibrosis may be present.	Superficial, acute inflammation of mucosa with microscopic crypt abscess.
X-ray findings	Segmental lesions; thickened, circular folds, cobblestone appearance of bowel wall secondary to longitudinal ulcers and transverse fissures; fixation and separation of loops; narrowed lumen; "string sign"; fistulas.	Superficial colitis; loss of haustra; shortened colon and pseudopolyps (islands of normal tissue surrounded by denuded mucosa) are late findings.
Intestinal symptoms	Abdominal pain, diarrhea (usually loose with blood if colon involved), perianal disease, enteroenteric/enterocutaneous fistula, abscess, anorexia.	Abdominal pain, bloody diarrhea, urgency, and tenesmus.
Extraintestinal symptoms Arthritis/arthralgia	15%	9%
Fever	40–50%	40–50%
Stomatitis	9%	2%
Weight loss	90% (mean 5.7 kg)	68% (mean 4.1 kg)
Delayed growth and sexual development	30%	5–10%
Uveitis/conjunctivitis	15% (in Crohn's colitis)	4%
Sclerosing cholangitis	—	4%
Renal stones	6% (oxalate)	6% (urate)
Pyoderma gangrenosum	1–3%	5%
Erythema nodosum	8–15%	4%
Laboratory findings	High erythrocyte sedimentation rate; microcytic anemia; low serum iron and total iron-binding capacity; increased fecal protein loss; low serum albumin; antineutrophil cytoplasmic antibodies present in 10–20%.	High erythrocyte sedimentation rate; microcytic anemia, high white blood cell count with left shift; antineutrophil cytoplasmic antibodies present in 80%.

Source: Kirschner BS: Inflammatory bowel disease in children. Pediatr Clin North Am 1988;35:189.

comparison of these two conditions is shown in Table 20–11. The cause is unknown but is probably an abnormal or uncontrolled, genetically determined immunologic or inflammatory response to an environmental antigenic trigger, possibly a virus or bacterium. There is no indication that emotional factors are a primary cause of these diseases.

Differential Diagnosis

A. Crohn's Disease: When extraintestinal symptoms predominate, Crohn's disease can be mistaken for rheumatoid arthritis, systemic lupus erythematosus, or hypopituitarism. Frequently, the acute onset of ileocolitis is mistaken for acute appendicitis. Symptoms sometimes suggest celiac disease, peptic ulcer, intestinal obstruction, or intestinal lymphoma.

B. Ulcerative Colitis: In the acute stage, bacterial pathogens and toxins causing colitis must be ruled out. These include *Shigella, Salmonella, Yersinia, Campylobacter, Entamoeba histolytica,* invasive *Escherichia coli, Aeromonas hydrophila,* and the toxin-producing *E coli* and *Clostridium difficile.*

Mild ulcerative colitis sometimes mimics irritable bowel symptoms. Crohn's disease of the colon is an important differential possibility.

Complications
(See Table 20–11.)

A. Crohn's Disease: Intestinal obstruction, fistula, and abscess formation are common. Perforation and hemorrhage are rare. Malnutrition is caused by anorexia and compounded by malabsorption, protein-losing enteropathy, disaccharidase deficiency, and diarrhea induced by bile salts. Systemic complications include perianal disease, pyoderma gangrenosum, arthritis, amyloidosis, and growth retardation.

B. Ulcerative Colitis: Arthritis, uveitis, pyoderma gangrenosum, and malnutrition all occur. Growth failure and delayed puberty are less common than in Crohn's disease. Liver disease (chronic active hepatitis, sclerosing cholangitis) is more common. In patients with pancolitis, carcinoma of the colon occurs with an incidence of 1–2% per year after the first 10 years of disease. Cancer risk is a function of disease duration and not age of onset. Mortality with colon cancer is high, because the usual screening tests (occult blood in stool, pain, and abnormal x-ray findings) are not specific, may be ignored in a patient with colitis, and diagnosis may be delayed.

Treatment

Medical treatment for Crohn's disease and ulcerative colitis is similar and includes anti-inflammatory, antidiarrheal, and antibiotic medication. No medical therapy has proved uniformly effective.

A. Diet: A high-protein, high-carbohydrate diet with normal amounts of fat is recommended. Decreased amounts of roughage may help decrease symptoms in those with colitis or with partial intestinal obstruction. Lactose is poorly tolerated when disease is active. The main concern should be ensuring adequate caloric intake. Restrictive or "bland" diets are counterproductive because they usually result in poor intake. Vitamin and iron supplements are recommended. Zinc levels are often low in patients with Crohn's disease and should be repleted. Supplemental calories in the form of liquid diets are well tolerated. Total parenteral nutrition for periods of 4–6 weeks may induce remission of symptoms and stimulate linear growth and sexual development. Enteral administration of low-residue or elemental liquid diets may also be associated with rapid nutritional repletion and temporary remission of symptoms, perhaps because of reduced enteral antigen load. Home programs of both enteral and parenteral nutritional support have been used in many patients with intractable symptoms or growth failure.

B. Sulfasalazine: This drug is effective in mild cases of ulcerative colitis and possibly in cases of Crohn's disease of the colon. It prevents relapse of ulcerative colitis once remission is induced. The drug is not absorbed in the small intestine. It is hydrolyzed by colon flora into sulfapyridine and 5-aminosalicylate. The sulfa moiety is probably inactive but is responsible for the allergic side effects of the drug. The salicylate moiety probably has a local anti-inflammatory activity in the colon. Side effects are common, including skin rash, nausea, headache, and abdominal pain. More rarely, serum sickness, hemolytic anemia, aplastic anemia, and pancreatitis occur. Response to therapy may be slow. Sulfasalazine inhibits folic acid absorption, and supplemental folic acid is recommended.

Two to 3 grams per day in three divided doses are recommended for children over 10, or 50 mg/kg/d for those under 10. Half of this dose is used as a maintenance medication for well-controlled ulcerative colitis. Salicylate polymers for both oral and rectal use (olsalazine, mesalamine) are available. They are no more effective than sulfasalazine but can be tolerated by sulfonamide-sensitive patients and have fewer side effects.

C. Corticosteroids: With more severe inflammatory bowel disease, corticosteroids are used.

1. Intravenous steroids–Methylprednisolone, 2 mg/kg/d, or hydrocortisone, 10 mg/kg/d, may be given when disease is severe. Adrenocorticotropic hormone (ACTH) has more side effects and is no more effective.

2. Prednisone-Prednisone–1–2 mg/kg/d orally in two or three divided doses, is given for 6–8 weeks, followed by a gradual tapering. Alternate-day steroids are associated with fewer side effects as the dosage of drug is tapered. There is no evidence that corticosteroids prevent relapses. Prednisone is often given in conjunction with sulfasalazine. The patient or the parents should be warned about the risk of varicella infection and the other numerous side effects of high-dose steroids.

Hydrocortisone in the form of enema or foam can be instilled into the rectum in patients with severe tenesmus or ulcerative proctitis.

D. Azathioprine: Azathioprine, 1–2 mg/kg/d orally, is used only when a high maintenance dose of corticosteroids is necessary to keep the disease under control and there are serious risks of steroid-induced complications. Positive results of this therapy may be delayed weeks to months. Similarly, GMP is now under evaluation as a steroid-sparing maintenance medication for severe Crohn's disease in childhood.

E. Metronidazole: This drug is now used routinely in Crohn's disease patients with perianal disease. Disease tends to recur when the drug is discontinued. It may also be effective in Crohn's disease of the colon. The dose of metronidazole is 15–30 mg/kg/d in three divided doses. Peripheral neuropathy may be a side effect with prolonged use.

F. Cyclosporine: This powerful immunosuppressant is effective in severe, steroid-resistant ulcerative colitis, but because of side effects and rapid relapse after discontinuation, it is usually used to "buy time" in severely affected patients in whom surgical treatment is planned.

G. Surgery:

1. Crohn's disease–Crohn's disease is not cured by surgery. However, 70% of patients eventually require surgery to relieve obstruction, drain abscess, relieve intractable symptoms, or encourage growth and sexual maturation. The relapse rate 6 years after surgery is 60%. The recurrence usually occurs at the site of anastomosis. Recurrence of disease is most likely in the first 2 years after surgery. The rate of recurrence may be less in disease limited to the colon. Surgery performed for the alleviation of growth retardation must be performed before puberty.

2. Ulcerative colitis–Surgery is curative in this disease. It is reserved for those with uncontrolled hemorrhage, toxic megacolon, unrelenting pain and diarrhea, high-grade mucosal dysplasia, or malignant growths. There are now several surgical approaches (ileoanal anastomosis, Koch-type continent ileostomy) that allow a near normal lifestyle after colectomy. Liver disease may not be improved by the removal of the colon.

Prognosis

A. Crohn's Disease: Although mortality is low (2% in the first 7 years), morbidity is high. The disease is progressive in most cases, and its course is interspersed with acute and chronic complications, leading to variable degrees of disability. Over 50% of patients experience symptoms affect the quality of life. About 20% have severe disabling disease, and 20% have so few symptoms that they describe themselves as healthy.

B. Ulcerative Colitis: The prognosis for ulcerative colitis is good. About 5% of patients present with toxic megacolon and require immediate colectomy. Seventy-five percent have a relapsing remitting course. Twenty-five to 40% require colectomy, especially those with pancolitis, anemia, and hypoalbuminemia at the time of presentation.

Fonkalsrud EW, Loar N: Long term results after colectomy and endorectal ileal pullthrough procedure in children. Ann Surg 1991;215:57.

Hyams JS: Extraintestinal manifestations of inflammatory bowel disease in children. J Pediatr Gastroenterol Nutr 1994;19:7.

Kirschner BS: Inflammatory bowel disease in children. Pediatr Clin North Am 1988;35:189.

Noel RA, Ferry GD: Pediatric inflammatory bowel disease. Curr Opin Gastroenterol 1992;8:676.

REFERENCES

Silverman A, Roy CC: *Pediatric Clinical Gastroenterology,* 4th ed. Mosby, 1995.

Suchy FJ (editor): *Liver Disease in Children,* Mosby, 1994.

Walker WA et al (editors): *Pediatric Gastrointestinal Disease.* Decker, 1995.

Wyllie R, Hyams JS (editors): *Pediatric Gastrointestinal Disease.* Saunders, 1993.

21

Liver & Pancreas

Ronald J. Sokol, MD, & Michael R. Narkewicz, MD

LIVER

PROLONGED NEONATAL CHOLESTATIC JAUNDICE

The main clinical features of disorders causing prolonged neonatal cholestasis are (1) elevated direct-reacting bilirubin fraction (>2 mg/dL or >20% of total bilirubin), (2) elevated serum bile acids (>10 μmol/L), (3) variably acholic stools, (4) dark urine, and (5) hepatomegaly.

Prolonged neonatal cholestasis (decreased bile flow) may be the result of intrahepatic or extrahepatic causes. Although many specific causes of intrahepatic cholestasis have been identified, a specific cause is found only in about 25% of cases. With rare exceptions, extrahepatic cholestasis is caused by anatomic defects that may be congenital or acquired.

Attention to specific clinical clues distinguishes these two major categories of jaundice in 85% of cases. Histologic examination of tissue obtained by percutaneous liver biopsy increases the accuracy of differentiation to 95% (Table 21–1).

INTRAHEPATIC CHOLESTASIS

Intrahepatic cholestasis is characterized by patency of the extrahepatic biliary system—despite cholestasis—and abnormalities of liver function tests. A specific cause can be identified in about 25% of cases. Patency of the extrahepatic biliary tract can least invasively be confirmed by hepatobiliary scintigraphy using ^{99m}Tc-diethyliminodiacetic acid (diethyl-IDA, DIDA). Radioactivity in the bowel within 4–24 hours is evidence of patency. Patency of the extrahepatic biliary system can also be determined by cholangiography carried out intraoperatively, percutaneously by transhepatic cholecystogra-

phy, or by utilizing the newly designed pediatric-sized side-viewing endoscope.

1. PERINATAL OR NEONATAL HEPATITIS RESULTING FROM INFECTION

This diagnosis is considered in infants with jaundice, hepatomegaly, vomiting, lethargy, and other systemic signs. A perinatally acquired viral, bacterial, or protozoal infection must be identified. Infection may occur by transplacental spread, via the ascending route from vaginal or cervical structures into amniotic fluid; from swallowed contaminated fluids (maternal blood, urine) during delivery; or from breast milk, contaminated hands, etc. The infectious agents most often associated with neonatal intrahepatic cholestasis include herpes simplex virus, varicella virus, coxsackieviruses, cytomegalovirus, rubella virus, echoviruses, adenovirus, hepatitis B virus, human immunodeficiency virus, *Treponema pallidum,* and *Toxoplasma gondii.* The degree of liver cell injury caused by these agents is variable, ranging from massive hepatic necrosis (herpes simplex) to focal necrosis and mild inflammation (cytomegalovirus, hepatitis B virus). Serum bilirubin, bile acids, ALT, AST, and alkaline phosphatase are elevated. The infant is jaundiced and generally appears ill.

Clinical Findings

A. Symptoms & Signs: Clinical symptoms usually appear in the first 2 weeks of life but may appear as late as 2–3 months. Jaundice may be noted in the first 24 hours or may develop later. Loss of appetite, poor sucking reflex, lethargy, and vomiting are frequent. Stools may be normal to pale in color but are seldom acholic. Dark urine stains the diaper. Hepatomegaly is present, and the liver has a uniform firm consistency. Splenomegaly is variably present. Macular, papular, or petechial rashes may occur. In less severe cases, failure to thrive may be the major complaint. Unusual presentations include liver fail-

Table 21–1. Differentiating clinical and histologic features of intrahepatic and extrahepatic neonatal cholestasis.

	Intrahepatic	Extrahepatic
Clinical features	Preterm, small for gestational age, appears ill; hepatosplenomegaly, other organ or system involvement; incomplete cholestasis (stools with some color); associated cause identified (infections, metabolic, familial, etc)	Full-term, seems well; hepatomegaly (firm to hard); complete cholestasis (acholic stools); polysplenia syndrome, equal right and left hepatic lobes
Histologic features	Cholestasis, lobular disarray, giant cells, portal inflammation, minimal fibrosis, rare neoductular formation, steatosis, extramedullary hematopoiesis	Cholestasis, neoductular proliferation, portal fibrosis, bile lakes, normal lobular architecture, rare giant cells

ure, hypoproteinemia, and anasarca (nonhemolytic hydrops) and hemorrhagic disease of the newborn.

B. Laboratory Findings: The blood count often shows neutropenia, thrombocytopenia, and signs of mild hemolysis. Mixed hyperbilirubinemia, elevated aminotransferases with near-normal alkaline phosphatase, prolongation of clotting studies, mild acidosis, and elevated cord serum IgM suggest congenital infection. Nasopharyngeal washings, urine, stool, and cerebrospinal fluid should be cultured for virus. Specific serologic tests may be useful, as are long-bone x-rays to determine the presence of "celery stalking" in the metaphyseal regions of the humeri, femurs, and tibias. When indicated, CT and MRI can identify intracranial calcifications. Nuclear hepatobiliary imaging shows decreased hepatic clearance of the circulating isotope with excretion into the gut.

Histologic examination of liver biopsy tissue obtained by the percutaneous route is performed to distinguish intrahepatic from extrahepatic cholestasis, rather than to identify a specific infectious agent within the liver tissue. Exceptions to this generalization include the finding of intracytoplasmic and intranuclear inclusions of cytomegalovirus in hepatocytes or bile duct epithelial cells and the finding of intranuclear acidophilic inclusions of herpes simplex. Variable degrees of lobular disarray characterized by focal necrosis, multinucleated giant cell transformation, and ballooned pale hepatocytes with loss of cord-like arrangement of liver cells are usual. Intrahepatocytic and canalicular cholestasis may be prominent. Portal changes are not striking, but modest neoductular proliferation and mild fibrosis may occur.

Differential Diagnosis

Great care must be taken to distinguish infectious causes of intrahepatic cholestasis from genetic or metabolic causes (inborn errors), because the clinical presentations are very similar. Galactosemia, congenital fructose intolerance, and tyrosinemia must be investigated promptly, because specific dietary therapy is available. Alpha$_1$-antitrypsin deficiency, cystic fibrosis, and neonatal iron storage disease must also be considered. Specific physical features may be helpful when considering Alagille's or Zellweger's syndrome.

Unless the extrahepatic bile duct has spontaneously perforated, infants with extrahepatic cholestasis do not appear ill; stools are usually completely acholic, and the liver is enlarged and firm. Histologic findings are shown in Table 21–1.

Treatment

Most forms of viral neonatal hepatitis are treated symptomatically. Infants with herpes simplex or varicella infections are treated with acyclovir. Fluids and adequate calories are encouraged. Intravenous dextrose may be needed if feedings are not well tolerated. The consequences of cholestasis are treated as indicated (Table 21–2). Vitamin K orally or by injection and vitamins D and E orally should be provided. Choleretics (cholestyramine, phenobarbital, ursodeoxycholic acid) are used if cholestasis persists. Corticosteroids are contraindicated. Penicillin for suspected syphilis or specific antibiotics for bacterial hepatitis need to be administered promptly.

Prognosis

Multiple organ involvement is commonly associated with neonatal infectious hepatitis and has a poor outcome. Death from hepatic or cardiac failure, intractable acidosis, or intracranial hemorrhage is seen, especially in herpesvirus or echovirus infection and occasionally in cytomegalovirus or rubella infection. Hepatitis B virus may rarely cause fulminant neonatal viral hepatitis; most infected infants become asymptomatic carriers of hepatitis B. On the other hand, infants with transplacental diseases may recover completely or suffer sequelae, especially neurologic ones. Persistent liver disease results in mild chronic hepatitis, portal fibrosis, or cirrhosis. Chronic cholestasis may lead to dental enamel hypoplasia, failure to thrive, biliary rickets, severe pruritus, and xanthoma.

Specific Infectious Agents

A. Neonatal Hepatitis B Virus Disease: Infection with hepatitis B virus (HBV) may occur at any time during perinatal life, but the risk is higher when acute maternal disease occurs during the last trimester of pregnancy. However, most cases of neonatal disease are acquired from mothers who are asymptomatic carriers of hepatitis B. HBV has been found in most body fluids, including breast milk, but it is not present in feces. In chronic HBsAg carrier

Table 21–2. Treatment of complications of chronic cholestatic liver disease.

Indication	Treatment	Dose	Toxicity
Intrahepatic cholestasis	Phenobarbital	3–10 mg/kg/d	Drowsiness, irritability, interference with vitamin D metabolism
	Cholestyramine/colestipol hydro-chloride	250–500 mg/kg/d	Constipation, acidosis, binding of drugs, increased steatorrhea
	Ursodeoxycholic acid	10–20 mg/kg/d	Transient increase in pruritus
Pruritus	Phenobarbital or cholestyramine/ colestipol (or both)	Same as above	
	Antihistamines: Diphenhydramine hydrochloride Hydroxyzine	5–10 mg/kg/d 2–5 mg/kg/d	Drowsiness
	Ultraviolet light B	Exposure as needed	Skin burn
	Carbamazepine	20–40 mg/kg/d	Hepatotoxicity, marrow suppression, fluid retention
	Rifampin	10 mg/kg/d	Hepatotoxicity, marrow suppression
	Ursodeoxycholic acid	10–20 mg/kg/d	Transient increase in pruritus
Steatorrhea	Formula containing medium-chain triglycerides (eg, Pregestimil)	120–150 calories/kg/d for infants	Expensive
	Oil supplement containing medium-chain triglycerides	1–2 mL/kg/d	Diarrhea, aspiration
Malabsorption of fat-soluble vitamins	Vitamin A	10,000–25,000 U/d	Hepatitis, pseudotumor cerebri, bone lesions
	Vitamin D	800–5000 U/d	Hypercalcemia, hypercalciuria
	25-Hydroxycholecalciferol (vitamin D)	3–5 µg/kg/d	Hypercalcemia, hypercalciuria
	1,25-Dihydroxycholecalciferol (vitamin D)	0.05–0.2 µg/kg/d	Hypercalcemia, hypercalciuria
	Vitamin E (oral)	25–200 IU/kg/d TPGS,[1] 15–25 IU/kg/d	Potentiation of vitamin K deficiency
	Vitamin E (intramuscular)	1–2 mg/kg/d	Muscle calcifications
	Vitamin K (oral)	2.5 mg twice per week to 5.0 mg per day	
	Vitamin K (intramuscular)	2–5 mg each 4 wk	
Malabsorption of other nutrients	Multiple vitamin	1–2 times the standard dose	
	Calcium	25–100 mg/kg/d	Hypercalcemia, hypercalciuria
	Phosphorus	25–50 mg/kg/d	Gastrointestinal intolerance
	Zinc	1 mg/kg/d	Interference with copper absorption

[1]Tocopheryl polyethylene glycol–1000 succinate (water-soluble vitamin E).

mothers, fetal and infant acquisition risk is greatest if the mother (1) is also HBeAg-positive and HBeAb-negative, (2) has detectable levels of serum-specific hepatitis B DNA polymerase, or (3) has high serum levels of HBcAb. These findings are markers of high infectivity; however, hepatitis B can be transmitted even if HBsAg is the only marker present.

Neonatal liver disease resulting from HBV is extremely variable. The infant has a 70–90% chance of acquiring HBV at birth from HBsAg-positive mothers if nothing is done to prevent infection (ie, administration of hepatitis B immune globulin [HBIG] or vaccine). Most infected infants become asymptomatic carriers of HBV, usually for life. Fulminant hepatic necrosis has rarely been reported, especially in association with intrapartum or postpartum transfusions of infected blood. However, it also can occur from maternally transmitted virus. In such cases, progressive jaundice, stupor, shrinking liver size, and coagulation abnormalities dominate the clinical picture. Respiratory, circulatory, and renal failure usually follow. Histologically, the liver shows massive hepatocyte necrosis, collapse of the reticulum framework, minimal inflammation, and occasional pseudoacinar structures. Rare survivors are reported with reasonable restitution of liver architecture toward normal.

In less severe cases, focal hepatocyte necrosis is seen with a mild portal inflammatory response. Cholestasis is intracellular and canalicular. Chronic persistent and chronic active hepatitis may be present for many years, with serologic evidence of persisting antigenemia (HBsAg) and mildly elevated serum aminotransferases. Chronic active hepatitis may rarely progress to cirrhosis within 1–2 years.

To prevent perinatal transmission, all infants of mothers who are HBsAg-positive (regardless of HBeAg status) should receive HBIG and hepatitis B vaccine within the first 24 hours after birth and vaccine again at 1 and 6 months of age (see Chapter 10).

B. Neonatal Bacterial Hepatitis: Most bacterial liver infections in newborns are acquired by transplacental invasion from amnionitis with ascending spread from maternal vaginal or cervical infection. Onset is abrupt, usually within 48–72 hours after delivery, with signs of sepsis and often shock. Jaundice, seen in less than 25% of cases, appears early and is of the mixed type. The liver enlarges rapidly, and the histologic picture is that of diffuse hepatitis with or without micro- or macroabscess. The most common organisms are *Escherichia coli, Listeria monocytogenes,* and group B streptococci and, rarely, *Mycobacterium tuberculosis.* Isolated neonatal liver abscess caused by *E coli* or *Staphylococcus aureus* is often associated with omphalitis or umbilical vein catheterization. Bacterial hepatitis and neonatal liver abscesses require specific antibiotics in large doses and, rarely, surgical drainage. Deaths are common, but survivors show no long-term consequences of liver disease.

C. Neonatal Jaundice With Urinary Tract Infection: Jaundice in affected infants—usually males—typically appears between the second and fourth weeks of life. The manifestations of this disorder are lethargy, fever, poor appetite, jaundice, and hepatomegaly. Except for mixed hyperbilirubinemia, other liver function tests are not remarkable. Leukocytosis is present, and infection is confirmed by culture techniques. The mechanism for the liver impairment is unknown, although toxic action of bacterial products (endotoxins) and the inflammatory response have been incriminated.

Treatment of the infection leads to prompt resolu-

tion of the cholestasis without hepatic sequelae. Metabolic liver diseases may present with gram-negative bacterial urinary tract infection and should be considered.

Krugman S: Viral hepatitis: A, B, C, D, and E: Prevention. Pediatr Rev 1992;13:245.

Pickering LK: Management of the infant of a mother with viral hepatitis. Pediatr Rev 1988;9:315.

Rosenthal P: Neonatal hepatitis and congenital infections. In: *Liver Disease in Children.* Suchy FJ (editor). Mosby–Year Book, 1994.

Spivak WF: Diagnostic utility of hepatobiliary scintigraphy with ^{99m}Tc-DISIDA in neonatal cholestasis. J Pediatr 1987;110:885.

Stevens CE et al: Perinatal hepatitis B virus transmission in the United States. JAMA 1985;253:1740.

2. INTRAHEPATIC CHOLESTASIS RESULTING FROM INBORN ERRORS OF METABOLISM, FAMILIAL CAUSES, & "TOXIC" CAUSES

These cholestatic syndromes are caused by specific enzyme deficiencies or other inherited disorders; a positive history of certain precipitants associated with neonatal liver disease; and features of intrahepatic cholestasis—that is, jaundice, hepatomegaly, and normal to completely acholic stools. Some of the specific clinical conditions have characteristic clinical signs.

Enzyme Deficiencies & Other Inherited Disorders

Early specific diagnosis is important because dietary treatment may be available (Table 21–3). Reversal of liver disease and clinical symptoms is prompt and permanent in several disorders as long as the diet is maintained. As with other genetically inherited inborn errors of metabolism, genetic counseling for parents of the affected infant should be done as soon as possible.

Cholestasis caused by metabolic diseases such as galactosemia, fructose intolerance, and tyrosinemia may be accompanied by vomiting, lethargy, poor feeding, and irritability. Hepatomegaly is a constant finding. The infants often appear septic; gram-negative bacteria can be cultured from blood in 25–50% of cases, especially in patients with galactosemia.

Other inherited conditions that present with neonatal intrahepatic cholestasis are outlined in Table 21–3. Treatment of these disorders is outlined in Chapter 34.

"Toxic" Causes of Neonatal Cholestasis

A. Neonatal Ischemic/Hypoxic Conditions: Perinatal events that result in hypoperfusion of the gastrointestinal system are sometimes followed in

Table 21–3. Metabolic and genetic causes of neonatal cholestasis.[1]

Disease	Inborn Error	Hepatic Pathology	Diagnostic Studies
Galactosemia	Galactose-1-phosphate uridylyltransferase	Cholestasis, steatosis, necrosis, pseudoacini, fibrosis	Galactose-1-phosphate uridylyltransferase assay of red blood cells
Fructose intolerance	Fructose-1-phosphate aldolase	Steatosis, necrosis, pseudoacini, fibrosis	Liver fructose-1-phosphate aldolase assay or leukocyte DNA analysis
Tyrosinemia	Fumarylacetoacetase	Necrosis, steatosis, pseudoacini, portal fibrosis	Urinary succinylacetone, fumarylacetoacetase assay of red blood cells
Cystic fibrosis	Cystic fibrosis transmembrane regular gene abnormality	Cholestasis, neoductular proliferation, excess bile duct mucus, portal fibrosis	Sweat test and leukocyte DNA analysis
Hypopituitarism	Deficient production of pituitary hormones	Cholestasis, giant cells	Thyroxine, TSH, cortisol levels
α_1-Antitrypsin deficiency	Abnormal α_1-antitrypsin molecule (Pi ZZ phenotype)	Giant cells, cholestasis, steatosis, neoductular proliferation, fibrosis, PAS-diastase–resistant cytoplasmic granules	Serum α_1-antitrypsin phenotype
Gaucher's disease	β-Glucosidase	Cholestasis, cytoplasmic inclusions in Kupffer's cells (foam cells)	β-Glucosidase assay in leukocytes
Niemann-Pick disease	Lysosomal sphingomyelinase	Cholestasis, cytoplasmic inclusions in Kupffer's cells	Sphingomyelinase assay of leukocytes or liver
Glycogen storage disease type IV	Branching enzyme	Fibrosis, cirrhosis, PAS-diastase–resistant cytoplasmic inclusions	Brancher enzyme analysis of leukocytes or liver
Neonatal hemochromatosis	Unknown	Giant cells, portal fibrosis, hemosiderosis, cirrhosis	Histology, iron stains
Peroxisomal disorders (eg, Zellweger's syndrome)	Deficient peroxisomal enzymes or assembly	Cholestasis, necrosis, fibrosis, cirrhosis, hemosiderosis	Plasma very long chain fatty acids, qualitative bile acids, plasmalogen, pipecolic acid, liver electron microscopy
Abnormalities in bile acid metabolism	Several enzyme deficiencies defined	Cholestasis, necrosis, giant cells	Urine, serum, duodenal fluid analyzed for bile acids by fast atom bombardment–mass spectroscopy
Byler's disease (familial progressive intrahepatic cholestasis)	Unknown	Cholestasis, necrosis, giant cells, fibrosis	Histology, family history, normal cholesterol, low or normal γ-glutamyl transpeptidase
Alagille's syndrome (syndromic paucity of interlobular bile ducts)	Unknown	Cholestasis, paucity of interlobular bile ducts, increased copper levels	Three or more clinical features, liver histology

[1]TSH = thyroid-stimulating hormone, PAS = periodic acid–Schiff.

1–2 weeks by cholestasis. This is seen in premature infants with respiratory distress, severe hypoxia, hypoglycemia, shock, and acidosis. When these perinatal conditions develop in association with gastrointestinal lesions such as ruptured omphalocele, gastroschisis, or necrotizing enterocolitis, a subsequent cholestatic picture is common (25–50% of cases).

Liver function studies reveal mixed hyperbilirubinemia, elevated alkaline phosphatase and γ-glutamyl transpeptidase values, and variable elevation of the aminotransferases. Stools are seldom persistently acholic.

Choleretics (cholestyramine, phenobarbital, ursodeoxycholic acid), introduction of enteral feedings as soon as possible, and nutritional support are the mainstays of treatment until the cholestasis resolves (see Table 21–2). In some cases, this resolution may take 3–6 months. Complete resolution of the hepatic abnormalities is the rule, but portal fibrosis with periportal scarring is occasionally seen on follow-up biopsy.

B. Prolonged Parenteral Nutrition: Cholestasis may develop after 1–2 weeks in premature newborns receiving total parenteral nutrition. The mechanism is multifactorial, including possible toxicity of intravenous amino acids, diminished stimulation of bile flow from prolonged absence of feedings, translocation of intestinal bacteria and their cell wall products, missing nutrients or antioxidants, photo-oxidation of amino acids, and the "physiologic cholestatic" propensity of the premature infant. Histology of the liver may resemble that of extrahepatic biliary atresia.

Early introduction of feedings has reduced the frequency of this disorder. The prognosis is generally good. Rare cases of portal fibrosis, cirrhosis, and hepatoma may develop, particularly in infants with intestinal resections or anomalies.

C. "Inspissated Bile Syndrome": This is the result of accumulation of bile in canaliculi and in the small and medium-sized bile ducts in hemolytic disease of the newborn (Rh, ABO) and in some infants receiving total parenteral nutrition. The same mechanisms may cause intrinsic obstruction of the common duct. An ischemia-reperfusion injury may also contribute to cholestasis in Rh incompatibility. In extreme hemolysis, the cholestasis may be seemingly complete, with acholic stools. Levels of bilirubin may reach 40 mg/dL, primarily direct-reacting. If inspissation of bile occurs within the extrahepatic biliary tree, differentiation from biliary atresia may be difficult. A trial of choleretics is indicated. Once stools show a return to normal color or ^{99m}Tc-DIDA scanning shows biliary excretion into the duodenum, patency of the extrahepatic biliary tree is ensured. Small bile-colored plugs in the stools are sometimes reported by parents at the time stool color becomes normal. Although most cases slowly improve over 2–6 months, persistence of complete cholestasis for more than 2 weeks requires further studies (ultrasonography, DIDA scanning, liver biopsy) with possible examination of the extrahepatic biliary tree. Irrigation of the common bile duct is sometimes necessary to dislodge the obstructing inspissated biliary material.

Balistreri WF, Bove KE: Hepatobiliary consequences of parenteral alimentation. Prog Liver Dis 1990;9:567.

Bhatia J et al: Total parenteral nutrition–associated alterations in hepatobiliary function and histology in rats: Is light exposure a clue? Pediatr Res 1993;33:487.

Dunn L et al: Beneficial effects of early hypocaloric enteral feedings on neonatal gastrointestinal function: Preliminary report of a randomized trial. J Pediatr 1988; 112:622.

Enzenauer RW et al: Total parenteral nutrition cholestasis: A cause of mechanical biliary obstruction. Pediatrics 1985;76:905.

Odievre M et al: Hereditary fructose intolerance in childhood. Am J Dis Child 1978;132:605.

Singh I et al: Peroxisomal disorders: Biochemical and clinical diagnostic considerations. Am J Dis Child 1988;142:1297.

Sokol RJ et al: Hepatic oxidant injury associated with glutathione depletion during total parenteral nutrition in weanling rats. Am J Physiol 1995;270:G691.

3. IDIOPATHIC NEONATAL HEPATITIS (Giant Cell Hepatitis)

This type of cholestatic jaundice of unknown cause presents with features of cholestasis and a typical appearance on examination of biopsied liver tissue; it accounts for up to 75% of cases of neonatal intrahepatic cholestasis. The degree of cholestasis is variable, and the disorder may be indistinguishable from extrahepatic causes in 10% of cases. Alpha$_1$-antitrypsin deficiency, Alagille's syndrome, and Byler's disease may present in a similar clinical and histologic manner.

Intrauterine growth retardation, prematurity, poor feeding, emesis, poor growth, and partially or intermittently acholic stools are typical clinical characteristics of intrahepatic cholestasis. Neonatal lupus erythematosus may present with giant cell hepatitis; however, thrombocytopenia, skin rash, or congenital heart block is usually also present.

In cases of suspected idiopathic neonatal hepatitis (absence of infectious, metabolic, and toxic causes), patency of the biliary tree should be verified to exclude extrahepatic "surgical" disorders. DIDA scanning and ultrasonography may be helpful in this regard. Some have used the enteral string test during DIDA scanning to confirm bile duct patency. Liver biopsy findings are usually diagnostic after 6–8 weeks of age (see Table 21–1) but may be misleading before 4 weeks of age. Failure to detect patency of the biliary tree, nondiagnostic liver biopsy findings, or persisting complete cholestasis (acholic stools) are indications for minilaparotomy and intraoperative cholangiography by an experienced surgeon. Occasionally, a small but patent (hypoplastic) extrahepatic biliary tree is demonstrated and is probably the result rather than the cause of diminished bile flow; reconstruction of hypoplastic biliary trees should not be attempted.

Once a patent extrahepatic tree is confirmed, therapy should include choleretics, a special formula with medium-chain triglycerides (Pregestimil, Alimentum), and supplemental fat-soluble vitamins in water-miscible form. (See Table 21–2.) These are continued as long as significant cholestasis remains (conjugated bilirubin >1 mg/dL). Fat-soluble vitamin levels should be monitored while supplements are given.

Eighty percent of patients recover without significant hepatic fibrosis. However, if a relative previously had neonatal hepatitis, there is a 70–80% probability of progression to cirrhosis (Byler's disease).

Long-term consequences correlate best with the duration of the cholestasis. In general, failure to resolve the cholestatic picture by 6–12 months is associated with progressive liver disease and evolving cirrhosis. This may occur either with normal numbers of interlobular bile ducts or when diminished numbers of ducts (paucity of interlobular ducts) result. Perilobular and intralobular fibrosis both progress, and portal hypertension eventually ensues, with splenomegaly and esophageal varices. Finally, ascites with rising bilirubin levels heralds the onset of hepatic failure. Liver transplantation has been successful when signs of hepatic decompensation are noted (rising bilirubin, intractable ascites).

Dick MC, Mowat AP: Hepatitis syndrome in infancy: An epidemiological survey with 10 year follow-up. Arch Dis Child 1985;60:512.

Laxer RM et al: Liver disease in neonatal lupus erythematosus. J Pediatr 1990;116:238.

Odievre M et al: Long-term prognosis for infants with intrahepatic cholestasis and patent extrahepatic biliary tract. Arch Dis Child 1981;56:373.

Ramierez RO, Sokol RJ: Medical management of cholestasis. In: *Liver Disease in Children.* Suchy FJ (editor). Mosby–Year Book, 1994.

Rosenthal P et al: Hepatobiliary scintigraphy and the string test in the evaluation of neonatal cholestasis. J Pediatr Gastroenterol Nutr 1989;8:292.

4. PAUCITY OF INTERLOBULAR BILE DUCTS

Forms of intrahepatic cholestasis caused by decreased numbers of interlobular bile ducts may be classified according to whether or not they are associated with other malformations. The syndromic form, Alagille's syndrome (arteriohepatic dysplasia), is sometimes recognized by identification of the characteristic facies, which becomes more obvious with age. The forehead is prominent, as is the nasal bridge. The eyes are set deep and sometimes widely apart (hypertelorism). Often the chin is small and slightly pointed and projects forward. Ears are prominent. The severity of cholestasis is variable; thus, stool color varies. Pruritus begins by 3–6 months of age. Firm, smooth hepatomegaly is present, and cardiac murmurs are frequent. Xanthomas develop later in the disease. Occasionally, early cholestasis is mild and not recognized.

Direct hyperbilirubinemia may be mild to severe (2–15 mg/dL). Serum alkaline phosphatase, γ-glutamyl transpeptidase, and cholesterol are markedly elevated, especially early in life. Serum bile acids are always elevated. Aminotransferases are slightly increased, but clotting factors and other liver proteins are usually normal.

The cardiovascular abnormalities include peripheral and valvular pulmonary stenoses (most common), atrial septal defect, coarctation of the aorta, and tetralogy of Fallot.

Vertebral arch defects are common, including incomplete fusion of the vertebral body or anterior arch (butterfly deformity) and diminished interpedicle distance in the thoracolumbar spine. Eye abnormalities (posterior embryotoxon) and renal abnormalities (dysplastic kidneys, renal tubular ectasia, single kidney, hematuria) are also associated with this disorder. Growth retardation with normal to increased levels of growth hormone is common. Although variable, the IQ is frequently low. Hypogonadism with micropenis may be present. A weak, high-pitched voice may develop. Neurologic disorders resulting from vitamin E deficiency (areflexia, ataxia, ophthalmoplegia) eventually develop in many children.

In the nonsyndromic form, paucity of interlobular bile ducts is seen in the absence of the extrahepatic malformations. Paucity may also be seen in α_1-antitrypsin deficiency, in Zellweger's syndrome and in association with lymphedema (Aagenaes' syndrome), in Byler's disease, in cystic fibrosis, in cytomegalovirus or rubella infection, and in inborn errors of bile acid metabolism.

High doses (250 mg/kg/d) of cholestyramine may control pruritus, lower cholesterol, and clear xanthomas. Phenobarbital may lower serum bilirubin. Ursodeoxycholic therapy (10–20 mg/kg/d) appears to be more effective and less toxic than cholestyramine or phenobarbital. Nutritional therapy to prevent wasting and deficiencies of fat-soluble vitamins is of particular importance because of the severity of cholestasis (see Table 21–2).

Prognosis is more favorable in the syndromic than in the nonsyndromic varieties. In the former, only 30–40% of patients have severe complications of disease, whereas over 70% of patients suffering from the latter progress to cirrhosis. In Alagille's syndrome, cholestasis may improve by age 2–4 years, with minimal residual hepatic fibrosis. Survival into adulthood despite raised serum bile acids, aminotransferases, and alkaline phosphatase is common. Several patients have developed hepatocellular carcinoma. Hypogonadism has been noted; however, fertility is not obviously affected. Cardiovascular anomalies may shorten life expectancy. Some patients have persistent, severe cholestasis, rendering their quality of life poor; liver transplantation has been performed under these circumstances.

The gene for Alagille's syndrome is located on chromosome 20p, although it has not yet been isolated and cloned. The biochemical cause is unknown.

Alagille D et al: Syndromic paucity of interlobular bile ducts (Alagille syndrome or arteriohepatic dysplasia): Review of 80 cases. J Pediatr 1987;110:195.

Balistreri WF et al: Biochemical and clinical response to

ursodeoxycholic acid administration in pediatric patients with chronic cholestasis. In: *Bile Acids as Therapeutic Agents.* Paumgartner G, Stiehl A, Gerok W (editors). Kluwer, 1991.

Hoffenberg EJ et al: Outcome of syndromic paucity of interlobular bile ducts (Alagille syndrome) with onset of cholestasis in infancy. J Pediatr 1995;127:220.

Schnittger S: Molecular and cytogenic analysis of an interstitial 20p depletion associated with syndromic intrahepatic ductular hypoplasia (Alagille syndrome). Hum Genet 1989;83:239.

Schwarzenberg SJ et al: Long-term complications of arteriohepatic dysplasia. Am J Med 1992;93:171.

Sokol RJ et al: Multicenter trial of d-alpha tocopheryl polyethylene glycol–1000 succinate for treatment of vitamin E deficiency in children with chronic cholestasis. Gastroenterology 1993;104:1727.

EXTRAHEPATIC NEONATAL CHOLESTASIS

Extrahepatic neonatal cholestasis is characterized by complete and persistent cholestasis (acholic stools) in the first 1–4 weeks of life, lack of patency of the extrahepatic biliary tree proved by intraoperative, percutaneous, or endoscopic cholangiography, firm to hard hepatomegaly, and typical features on histologic examination of liver biopsy tissue. (See Table 21–1.) Causes include extrahepatic biliary atresia, choledochal cyst, intrinsic obstruction of the common duct, and spontaneous perforation of the extrahepatic ducts.

Extrahepatic Biliary Atresia

In whites, extrahepatic biliary atresia occurs in 1:13,000–1:8000 births, and the incidence in both sexes is equal. In Asians, the incidence is higher, and the disorder is twice as common in girls. The abnormality found most commonly is complete atresia of all extrahepatic biliary structures. The specific cause is not known, although evidence supports an insult to the biliary structures in the perinatal period that progresses in postnatal life. Extrahepatic atresia has not been found in stillborn fetuses and is rarely seen in premature infants. Meconium and first-passed stools are usually normal in color, suggesting early patency of the ducts. Furthermore, the presence of patent intrahepatic bile ducts near the porta hepatis is not consistent with congenital absence of the primitive bile duct. Evidence obtained from surgically removed remnants of the extrahepatic biliary tree suggests an inflammatory or sclerosing cholangiopathy. Although an infectious cause seems reasonable, no agent has been consistently found in such cases. A role for reovirus type 3 and rotavirus group C in biliary atresia has been suggested but recently disputed. Although other congenital malformations, especially vascular ones, occur in 20–30% of cases of extrahepatic biliary atresia, only polysplenia syndrome (situs inversus, preduodenal portal vein, interruption of the inferior vena cava, polysplenia, midline liver) is consistently associated with extrahepatic biliary atresia.

Jaundice may be noted in the newborn period but is more often delayed until 2–3 weeks of age. The urine stains the diaper, and the stools are often pale yellow, buff-colored, gray, or acholic. Seepage of bilirubin products across the intestinal mucosa gives some yellow coloration to the stools. Hepatomegaly is common, and the liver may feel firm to hard; splenomegaly develops later. Pruritus, digital clubbing, xanthomas, and a rachitic rosary may be noted in slightly older patients. Murmurs reflecting increasing cardiovascular output or shunting through bronchial arteries may be heard over the entire precordium and back. By 2–6 months, the growth curves reveal poor weight gain. Late in the course, ascites and bleeding complications occur.

No single laboratory test will consistently differentiate this entity from other causes of "complete" obstructive jaundice. A DIDA excretion study performed early in the course of disease and after pretreatment with phenobarbital (3–5 mg/kg/d for 5–7 days) helps to distinguish intrahepatic from extrahepatic causes of cholestasis. Although biliary atresia is suggested by persistent elevation of serum γ-glutamyl transpeptidase or alkaline phosphatase levels, high cholesterol levels, and prolonged prothrombin times, these findings have also been reported in severe neonatal hepatitis, α_1-antitrypsin deficiency, and bile duct paucity. Furthermore, these tests will not differentiate the location of the obstruction within the extrahepatic system. Generally, the aminotransferases are only modestly elevated in biliary atresia. Serum proteins and blood clotting factors are not affected early in the disease. Routine chest x-ray may reveal abnormalities suggestive of polysplenia syndrome. Ultrasonography of the biliary system should be performed to ascertain the presence of choledochal cyst and intra-abdominal anomalies. Liver biopsy specimens can differentiate intrahepatic causes of cholestasis from biliary atresia in over 90% of cases.

The major diagnostic dilemma is between this entity and neonatal hepatitis, bile duct paucity, choledochal cyst, or intrinsic bile duct obstruction (stones, bile plugs). Although spontaneous perforation of extrahepatic bile ducts leads to jaundice and acholic stools, the infants are usually quite ill with chemical peritonitis from biliary ascites, and hepatomegaly is not found.

If the diagnosis of biliary atresia cannot be excluded by the diagnostic evaluation before 60 days of life, surgical exploration is necessary. Laparotomy must include liver biopsy and an operative cholangiogram if a gallbladder is present. The presence of yellow bile in the gallbladder implies patency of the proximal extrahepatic duct system. Radiographic visualization of dye in the duodenum excludes obstruction to the distal extrahepatic ducts.

In the absence of surgical correction, the following eventually develop: failure to thrive, marked pruritus, portal hypertension, hypersplenism, bleeding diathesis, rickets, ascites, and cyanosis. Bronchitis and pneumonia are common. Eventually, hepatic failure and death occur, almost always by age 18–24 months.

Except for the occasional example of "correctable" biliary atresia where choledochojejunostomy is feasible, the standard procedure is hepatoportoenterostomy (Kasai procedure). Occasionally, portocholecystostomy (gallbladder Kasai procedure) may be performed if the gallbladder is present and the passage from it to the duodenum is patent. These procedures are best done in specialized centers where experienced surgical, pediatric, and nursing personnel are available. It is recommended that surgery be performed as early as possible (age 6–10 weeks); the Kasai procedure should generally not be undertaken in infants over 4 months of age, because the likelihood of bile drainage at this age is very low.

Orthotopic liver transplantation is now indicated for patients who fail to drain bile after the Kasai procedure or who progress to end-stage biliary cirrhosis despite surgical treatment. The 5-year survival rate following transplantation is 60–80%.

Whether or not the Kasai procedure is performed, supportive medical treatment measures consist of vitamin and caloric support (using water-miscible forms of vitamins A, D, K, and E and formulas containing medium-chain triglycerides [Pregestimil or Alimentum]). (See Table 21–2.) Bacterial infections (eg, ascending cholangitis) should be treated promptly with broad-spectrum antibiotics, and signs of bleeding tendency should be corrected with intramuscular vitamin K. Ascites can be managed with reduced sodium intake and spironolactone. Choleretics and bile acid–binding products (cholestyramine, aluminum hydroxide gel) are of little use. The value of ursodeoxycholic acid remains to be determined.

When bile flow is sustained, the 5-year survival rate is 35–50%. Complete surgical failures have the same outcome as nonoperated cases, but patients die sooner (age 8–15 months versus age 18–36 months). Death is usually caused by liver failure, sepsis, acidosis, or respiratory failure secondary to intractable ascites. Surprisingly, terminal hemorrhage is unusual. Liver transplantation has dramatically changed the outlook for these patients.

Butler SN, Smith D: Living with chronic pediatric liver disease: The parent's experience. Pediatr Nurs 1992; 18:453.

Karrer FM et al: Biliary atresia registry, 1976 to 1989. J Pediatr Surg 1990;25:1076.

Kaufman SS et al: Nutritional support for the infant with extrahepatic biliary atresia. J Pediatr 1987;100:679.

Laurent J: Long-term outcome after surgery for biliary atresia: Study of 40 patients surviving for more than 10 years. Gastroenterology 1990;99:1793.

Lilly JR et al: The surgery of biliary atresia. Ann Surg 1989;210:289.

Ohtomo Y et al: Glomerular alterations in children with biliary atresia. J Pediatr 1992;120:404.

Riepenhoff-Talty M et al: Group A rotaviruses produce extrahepatic biliary obstruction in orally inoculated newborn mice. Pediatr Res 1993;33:394.

Ryckman F et al: Improved survival in biliary atresia patients in the present era of liver transplantation. J Pediatr Surg 1993;28:382.

Silveira TR et al: Association between HLA and extrahepatic biliary atresia. J Pediatr Gastroenterol Nutr 1993;16:114.

Choledochal Cyst

Choledochal cysts cause 2–5% of cases of extrahepatic neonatal cholestasis; the incidence is higher in Asians. In most cases, the clinical manifestations, basic laboratory findings, and histopathologic features on liver biopsy are indistinguishable from those seen in biliary atresia. Neonatal symptomatic cysts are usually associated with atresia of the distal common duct—accounting for the diagnostic dilemma—and may simply be part of the spectrum of biliary atresia. However, a palpable subhepatic mass, positive ultrasound scan, or pressure deformity on the first and second portions of duodenum seen on upper gastrointestinal series promptly resolves the question. Immediate operation is indicated once abnormalities in clotting factors have been corrected and bacterial cholangitis, if present, has been treated with intravenous antibiotics. Discovery of such a mass eliminates the need for other studies. In older children, choledochal cyst presents as recurrent episodes of obstructive jaundice or abdominal pain or as a right abdominal mass.

Excision of the cyst and choledochojejunal anastomosis are recommended. In some cases, because of technical problems, only the mucosa of the cyst can be removed with jejunal anastomosis to the proximal bile duct. Anastomosis of cyst to jejunum or duodenum is not recommended.

The prognosis depends on the presence or absence of associated evidence of atresia and the appearance of the intrahepatic ducts. If atresia is found, the prognosis is similar to that described above. If an isolated extrahepatic cyst is encountered, the outcome is generally excellent, with resolution of the jaundice and return to normal liver cellular architecture the rule. However, bouts of ascending cholangitis, particularly if intrahepatic cysts are present, or obstruction of the anastomotic site may occur. The risk of biliary carcinoma developing within the cyst is about 5–15% at adulthood; therefore, cystectomy should be done whenever possible.

Bancroft JD et al: Antenatal diagnosis of choledochal cyst. J Pediatr Gastroenterol Nutr 1994;18:142.

Lilly JR et al: Forme fruste choledochal cyst. J Pediatr Surg 1985;20:449.

Saing H et al: Surgical management of choledochal cysts: A review of 60 cases. J Pediatr Surg 1985;20:443.

Voyles CR et al: Carcinoma in choledochal cysts: Age-related incidence. Arch Surg 1983;118:986.

Spontaneous Perforation of the Extrahepatic Ducts

The sudden appearance of obstructive jaundice, acholic stools, and abdominal enlargement with ascites in a sick newborn is suggestive of this condition. The liver is usually normal in size, and a yellow-green discoloration can often be discerned under the umbilicus or in the scrotum. In 24% of cases, stones or sludge is found obstructing the common bile duct. DIDA scan shows leakage from the biliary tree, and ultrasonography confirms ascites or fluid around the bile duct.

Treatment is surgical. Simple drainage, without attempt at oversewing the perforation, is sufficient in primary perforations. A diversion anastomosis is constructed in cases associated with choledochal cyst or stenosis.

The prognosis is generally good.

Haller JO et al: Spontaneous perforation of the common bile duct in children. Radiology 1989;172:621.

Megison SM et al: Management of common bile duct obstruction associated with spontaneous perforation of the biliary tree. Surgery 1992;111:237.

OTHER NEONATAL HYPERBILIRUBINEMIC CONDITIONS (Noncholestatic Nonhemolytic)

This group of disorders associated with hyperbilirubinemia is of two types: (1) unconjugated hyperbilirubinemia, consisting of breast milk jaundice, Lucey-Driscoll syndrome, congenital hypothyroidism, upper intestinal obstruction, Gilbert's syndrome, Crigler-Najjar syndrome, and drug-induced hyperbilirubinemia; and (2) conjugated noncholestatic hyperbilirubinemia, consisting of Dubin-Johnson syndrome and Rotor's syndrome.

1. UNCONJUGATED HYPERBILIRUBINEMIA

Breast Milk Jaundice

Persistent elevation of the indirect bilirubin fraction may occur in up to 36% of breast-fed infants. Recent studies implicate an enhancer of intestinal absorption of unconjugated bilirubin in jaundice-causing human milk rather than an inhibitor of bilirubin conjugation acting on hepatocytes. The increased enterohepatic shunting of unconjugated bilirubin exceeds the normal conjugating capacity in the liver of these infants.

Hyperbilirubinemia does not usually exceed 20 mg/dL, with most in the range of 10–15 mg/dL. In those whose bilirubin levels are above 4–5 mg/dL, the jaundice is noticeable by the fifth to seventh days of breast-feeding. It may accentuate the underlying physiologic jaundice—especially early, when total fluid intake may be less than optimal. Except for jaundice, the physical examination is usually normal; urine does not stain the diaper, and the stools are golden yellow.

The jaundice peaks by the third week and clears before 3 months in almost all infants, even when breast feedings are continued.

Kernicterus has never been reported in this condition. In special situations, breast-feeding may be temporarily discontinued and replaced by formula feedings for 2–3 days until serum bilirubin decreases by 2–8 mg/dL. Cow's milk formulas inhibit the intestinal reabsorption of unconjugated bilirubin. When breast-feeding is reinstituted, the serum bilirubin may increase slightly but not to the previous level. Phototherapy is not indicated in the healthy term infant with this condition.

Alonso EM et al: Enterohepatic circulation of nonconjugated bilirubin in rats fed with human milk. J Pediatr 1991;118:425.

Gourley GR, Aren RA: β-Glucuronidase and hyperbilirubinemia in breast-fed and formula-fed babies. Lancet 1986;1:644.

Gourley GR: Bilirubin metabolism and neonatal jaundice. In: *Liver Disease in Children.* Suchy FJ (editor). Mosby–Year Book, 1994.

Newman TB, Maisels MJ: Evaluation and treatment of jaundice in the term newborn: A kinder, gentler approach. Pediatrics 1992;89:809.

Congenital Hypothyroidism

Although the differential diagnosis should always include consideration of congenital hypothyroidism as a cause of indirect hyperbilirubinemia, the diagnosis may be obvious from other clinical and physical clues or from the newborn screening results. The jaundice quickly clears with replacement thyroid hormone therapy, although the mechanism is unclear.

Labrune P et al: Bilirubin uridine diphosphate glucuronosyltransferase hepatic activity in jaundice associated with congenital hypothyroidism. J Pediatr Gastroenterol Nutr 1992;14:79.

Upper Intestinal Obstruction

The association of indirect hyperbilirubinemia with high intestinal obstruction—for example, duodenal atresia, annular pancreas, pyloric stenosis—in the newborn has been observed repeatedly; the mechanism is unknown. Diminished levels of hepatic glucuronyl transferase have been found on liver biopsy in pyloric stenosis.

Treatment is that of the underlying obstructive

condition (usually surgical). Jaundice disappears once adequate nutrition is achieved.

Wolley MM et al: Jaundice, hypertrophic pyloric stenosis and hepatic glucuronyl transferase. J Pediatr Surg 1974;9:359.

Gilbert's Syndrome

This is a common form (3–7% of the population) of familial hyperbilirubinemia associated with a partial reduction of hepatic bilirubin uridine diphosphate glucuronyl transferase activity and perhaps an abnormality in the function or amount of one or more hepatocyte membrane protein carriers. Mild fluctuating jaundice, especially with illness, and vague constitutional symptoms are common. Jaundice is first recognized after puberty. Shortened red blood cell survival time in some patients is thought to be caused by reduced activity of enzymes involved in heme biosynthesis (protoporphyrinogen oxidase). Subsidence of hyperbilirubinemia has been achieved in patients by administration of phenobarbital (5–8 mg/kg/d), although this therapy is not justified.

The disease is inherited as an autosomal dominant with incomplete penetrance. Males are affected more often than females (4:1). Serum unconjugated bilirubin is less than 3–6 mg/dL. The findings on liver biopsy and most other liver function tests are normal except for prolonged indocyanine green and sulfobromophthalein (BSP) retention. An increase in the level of unconjugated bilirubin after a 2-day fast (300 kcal/d) of 1.4 mg/dL or more is consistent with the diagnosis of Gilbert's syndrome. The nicotinic acid provocation test is seldom used in pediatric patients.

Gentile S et al: Dose dependence of nicotinic acid–induced hyperbilirubinemia and its dissociation from hemolysis in Gilbert's syndrome. J Lab Clin Med 1986;107:166.

Crigler-Najjar Syndrome

Patients with type I disease usually develop rapid severe elevation of unconjugated bilirubin, with neurologic consequences (kernicterus). Prompt recognition of this entity and treatment with exchange transfusions are required, followed by phototherapy. Some survive without neurologic signs until adolescence or early adulthood, at which time deterioration may suddenly occur. The bile is colorless and contains a predominance of unconjugated bilirubin, small amounts of monoconjugates, and only traces of conjugated bilirubin. Phenobarbital administration in these patients does not significantly alter these findings, nor does it lower serum bilirubin levels. The glucuronyl transferase deficiency is inherited in an autosomal recessive pattern. A combination of phototherapy and cholestyramine may keep bilirubin levels below 25 mg/dL. The use of tin protoporphyrin or tin mesoporphyrin remains experimental. Liver transplantation is curative and may prevent kernicterus if

performed early. An auxiliary orthotopic transplantation also relieves the jaundice while the patient retains native liver.

A milder form (type II) with both autosomal dominant and recessive inheritance is rarely associated with neurologic complications. Hyperbilirubinemia is less severe, and the bile is pigmented and contains bilirubin mono- and diglucuronide. Patients with this form respond to phenobarbital with lowering of serum bilirubin levels. An increased proportion of monoconjugated and diconjugated bilirubin in the bile follows phenobarbital treatment.

Liver biopsy findings and liver function tests are consistently normal in both types.

Galbraith RA et al: Suppression of bilirubin production in the Crigler-Najjar type I syndrome: Studies with the heme oxygenase inhibitor tin mesoporphyrin. Pediatrics 1992;89:175.
Shevell MI et al: Crigler-Najjar syndrome type I: Treatment by home phototherapy followed by orthotopic liver transplantation. J Pediatr 1987;110:429.
Whitington PF et al: Orthotopic auxiliary liver transplantation for Crigler-Najjar syndrome type I. Lancet 1993;342:779.

Drug-Induced Hyperbilirubinemia

Vitamin K_3 (menadiol) may elevate indirect bilirubin levels by causing hemolysis. Vitamin K_1 (phytonadione) can be safely used in neonates. Rifampin may cause unconjugated hyperbilirubinemia. Other drugs (eg, ceftriaxone, sulfonamides) may displace bilirubin from albumin, potentially increasing the risk of kernicterus—especially in the sick premature infant.

Fink S, Karp W, Robertson A: Ceftriaxone effect on bilirubin- albumin binding. Pediatrics 1987;80:873.

2. CONJUGATED NONCHOLESTATIC HYPERBILIRUBINEMIA (Dubin-Johnson Syndrome & Rotor's Syndrome)

The diagnosis is aided by a positive family history (autosomal recessive inheritance) and jaundice that persists or recurs.

The basic defect in Dubin-Johnson syndrome is impaired hepatocyte excretion of conjugated bilirubin into bile, with a variable degree of impairment in uptake and conjugation complicating the picture. In Rotor's syndrome, the defect lies in hepatic uptake and storage of bilirubin. Bile acids are normally handled so that cholestasis does not occur. Bilirubin values range from 2 to 5 mg/dL, and other liver function tests are normal. In Rotor's syndrome, the liver is normal; in Dubin-Johnson syndrome, it is darkly pigmented on gross inspection. Microscopic examination reveals numerous dark-brown pigment granules consisting of polymers of epinephrine metabolites, especially in the centrilobular regions. However, the amount of pigment varies within families, and some jaundiced members may have no demonstrable pigmentation in the liver. Otherwise, the liver is histologically normal. Oral cholecystography fails to visualize the gallbladder in Dubin-Johnson syndrome but is normal in Rotor's syndrome. Differences in the excretion patterns of BSP, in results of DIDA cholescintigraphy, in urinary coproporphyrin I and III levels, and in the serum pattern of monoglucuronide and diglucuronide conjugates of bilirubin can help distinguish between these two conditions.

The prognosis is excellent, and no treatment is needed.

Crawford JM, Gollan JL: Bilirubin metabolism and the pathophysiology of jaundice. In: *Diseases of the Liver,* 7th ed. Schiff L, Schiff ER (editors). Lippincott, 1993.

Rosenthal P et al: The distribution of serum bilirubin conjugates in pediatric hepatobiliary diseases. J Pediatr 1987;110:201.

Shieh CC et al: Dubin-Johnson syndrome presenting with neonatal cholestasis. Arch Dis Child 1990;65:898.

Sotelo-Avila C et al: Cholecystitis in a 17-year-old boy with recurrent jaundice since childhood. J Pediatr 1988;112:668.

HEPATITIS A

Essentials of Diagnosis

- Gastrointestinal upset (anorexia, vomiting, diarrhea).
- Jaundice.
- Liver tenderness.
- Abnormal liver function tests.
- Local epidemic of the disease.
- Specific antibody rise.

HEPATITIS VIRUS ABBREVIATIONS	
HAV	Hepatitis A virus
Anti-HAV IgM	IgM antibody to HAV
HBV	Hepatitis B virus
HBsAg	HBV surface antigen
HBcAg	HBV core antigen
HBeAg	HBV e antigen
Anti-HBs	Antibody to HBsAg
Anti-HBc	Antibody to HBcAg
Anti-HBc IgM	IgM antibody to HBcAg
Anti-HBe	Antibody to HBeAg
HCV	Hepatitis C virus
Anti-HCV	Antibody to HCV
HDV	Hepatitis D (delta) virus
Anti-HDV	Antibody to HDV
HEV	Hepatitis E virus
Anti-HEV	Antibody to HEV
NANBNC	Non-A, non-B, non-C hepatitis virus

General Considerations (See Table 21–4.)

Hepatitis A viral (HAV) disease is caused by a virus that occurs in both epidemic and sporadic fashion. Transmission by the fecal-oral route explains epidemic outbreaks from contaminated food or water supplies, particularly by food handlers. Particles 27 nm in diameter have been found in stools during the acute phase of type A hepatitis and are similar in appearance to the enteroviruses. Sporadic cases usually result from contact with an affected individual. Transmission through blood products obtained during the viremic phase has occurred, though very rarely. The overt form of the disease is easily recognized by the clinical manifestations, but two-thirds of affected individuals have an anicteric and unrecognized form of the disease. This has been especially true in outbreaks of hepatitis A reported in day care centers accepting children younger than 3 years of age. Lifelong immunity to HAV is conferred follow-

Table 21–4. Hepatitis viruses.

	HAV	HBV	HCV	HDV	HEV
Type of virus	Enterovirus (RNA)	Hepadnavirus (DNA)	Flavivirus (RNA)	Incomplete (RNA)	Calicivirus (RNA)
Transmission routes	Fecal-oral	Parenteral, sexual, vertical	Parenteral, sexual	Parenteral, sexual	Fecal-oral
Incubation period	15–40 d	50–150 d	1–5 mo	20–90 d	2–9 wk
Diagnostic test	Anti-HAV IgM	HBsAg, anti-HBc IgM	Anti-HCV	Anti-HDV	Anti-HEV
Mortality rate (acute)	0.1–0.2%	0.5–2%	1–2%	2–20%	1–2% (in pregnant women, 20%)
Carrier state	No	Yes	Yes	Yes	No
Vaccine available	Yes	Yes	No	Yes (HBV)	No
Treatment	None	Interferon-α	Interferon-α	Interferon-α	None

ing infection. In developing countries, most children are exposed to HAV by age 10 years, whereas only 20% are exposed by age 20 years in developed countries.

Antibody to HAV appears within 1–4 weeks of clinical symptoms. While the great majority of children with infectious hepatitis are asymptomatic or have mild disease and recover completely, some will develop fulminant hepatitis. Children who die during the initial attack of the disease do so from massive hepatic necrosis secondary to overwhelming viremia, an immunologic deficiency state, or perhaps exposure to a mutant strain of virus.

Clinical Findings

A. History: A history of direct exposure to a previously jaundiced individual or of eating seafood or drinking contaminated water in the recent past should be sought. Following an incubation period of 15–40 days, the initial nonspecific symptoms usually precede the development of jaundice by 5–10 days.

B. Symptoms & Signs: Fever, anorexia, vomiting, headache, and abdominal pain are the usual symptoms. Darkening of the urine precedes jaundice, which peaks in 1–2 weeks and then begins to subside. The stools may become light or clay-colored during this time. Clinical improvement can be noted as jaundice develops. Tender hepatomegaly and jaundice are typically present; splenomegaly is variable.

C. Laboratory Findings: Aminotransferases and conjugated and unconjugated bilirubin levels are elevated. The leukocyte count is normal to low; the sedimentation rate is elevated. Serum proteins are generally normal, but an elevation of the gamma globulin fraction (>2.5 g/dL) can occur and indicates a worse prognosis. Hypoalbuminemia, hypoglycemia, and marked prolongation of prothrombin time are serious prognostic findings. Urine bile and urobilinogen are increased. Diagnosis is made by serology. A positive anti-HAV IgM indicates acute disease, whereas the IgG remains elevated after recovery.

Percutaneous liver biopsy is rarely indicated but may be safely performed in most children—provided the partial thromboplastin time, platelet count, and bleeding time are normal and the prothrombin time is prolonged no more than 4–5 seconds. The presence of ascites may increase the risk of percutaneous liver biopsy. "Balloon cells" and acidophilic bodies are characteristic histologic findings. Liver cell necrosis may be diffuse or focal, with accompanying infiltration of inflammatory cells containing polymorphonuclear leukocytes, lymphocytes, macrophages, and plasma cells, particularly in portal areas. Some bile duct proliferation may be seen in the perilobular portal areas alongside areas of bile stasis. Regenerative liver cells and proliferation of reticuloendothelial cells are present. Occasionally, massive hepatocyte necrosis is seen, portending a bad prognosis.

Differential Diagnosis

Before jaundice appears, the symptoms are those of a nonspecific viral enteritis. Other diseases with somewhat similar onset include pancreatitis, infectious mononucleosis, leptospirosis, drug-induced hepatitis, Wilson's disease, autoimmune hepatitis, and, most often, type B, C, E, or NANBNC hepatitis. Acquired cytomegalovirus disease may also mimic HAV, although lymphadenopathy is usually present in the former.

Prevention

Some attempt at isolation of the patient is indicated, although most patients with type A hepatitis are noninfectious by the time the disease becomes overt. Stool, diapers, and other fecally stained clothing should be handled with care for 1 month after the appearance of jaundice.

Passive-active immunization of exposed susceptibles can be achieved by giving standard immune globulin, 0.02–0.04 mL/kg intramuscularly. Illness is prevented in 80–90% of individuals if immune globulin is given within 1–2 weeks of exposure. Individuals traveling to endemic disease areas should receive 0.02–0.06 mL/kg as prophylaxis or the new HAV vaccine, depending on length of stay. HAV vaccines are now available for those at high risk, during epidemics, or for travel to endemic areas.

Treatment

There are no specific measures. Sedatives and corticosteroids should be avoided.

At the start of the illness, a light diet is preferable. During the icteric phase, lower-fat foods may diminish gastrointestinal symptoms but do not affect overall outcome. Drugs and elective surgery should be avoided.

Prognosis

Ninety-five percent of children recover without sequelae. In rare cases of fulminant hepatitis, the patient may die in 5 days or may survive as long as 1–2 months. The prognosis is poor if the signs and symptoms of hepatic coma develop, with deepening of jaundice and development of ascites; orthotopic liver transplantation is indicated under these circumstances. Incomplete resolution leads to prolonged hepatitis or chronic cholestatic hepatitis but not to cirrhosis. Rare cases of aplastic anemia following acute infectious hepatitis have also been reported. A benign relapse of symptoms may occur in 10–15% of cases after 6–10 weeks of apparent resolution.

Balistreri WF: Acute and chronic viral hepatitis. In: *Liver Disease in Children.* Suchy FJ (editor). Mosby–Year Book, 1994.

Hoofnagle JH, DiBisceglie AM: Serologic diagnosis of acute and chronic viral hepatitis. Semin Liver Dis 1991;11:73.

Katkov WN, Dienstag JL: Hepatitis vaccines. Gastroenterol Clin North Am 1995;24:147.

Krugman S: Viral hepatitis A, B, C, D, and E: Infection and prevention. Pediatr Rev 1992;13:203, 245.

Noble RC et al: Post transfusion hepatitis A in a neonatal intensive care unit. JAMA 1984;252:2711.

Werzberger A et al: A controlled trial of a formalin-inactivated hepatitis A vaccine in healthy children. N Engl J Med 1992;327:453.

HEPATITIS B

Essentials of Diagnosis

- Gastrointestinal upset, anorexia, vomiting, diarrhea.
- Jaundice, tender hepatomegaly, abnormal liver function tests.
- Serologic evidence of hepatitis B disease: HBsAg, HBeAg, anti-HBc IgM.
- History of parenteral, sexual, or household exposure or maternal HBsAg carriage.

General Considerations
(See Table 21–4.)

In contrast to hepatitis A, hepatitis B has a later onset with an incubation period of 21–135 days. The disease is caused by a DNA virus (42-nm Dane particle) that is usually acquired perinatally from a carrier mother; from blood products, shared needles, needle sticks, or tattoos; or through sexual transmission. Breast milk, urine, and saliva have been shown to contain viral antigen. Transmission via blood products has been almost eliminated by HBsAg donor-screening protocols. Mutant viruses predispose the patient to fulminant hepatitis.

The complete Dane particle is composed of a core (28-nm particle) that is found in the nucleus of infected liver cells and a double outer shell (surface antigen). The Dane particle is found in the cytoplasm where the completed virus particle is synthesized. The surface antigen in blood is termed HBsAg. This is found as a 22-nm spherical particle in the serum but occasionally occurs as a filamentous structure as well. The antibody to it is anti-HBs. The core antigen is termed HBcAg and its antibody is anti-HBc. A specific anti-HBc IgM occurs during primary viral replication.

Another important antigen-antibody system associated with HBV disease is the "e" antigen system. HBeAg, a truncated soluble form of HBcAg, appears in the serum of infected patients early and correlates with active virus replication. Persistence of HBeAg is a marker of infectivity, whereas the appearance of anti-HBe generally implies termination of viral replication. Other serologic markers indicating viral replication include the presence of DNA polymerase and circulating HBV DNA.

Clinical Findings

A. Symptoms & Signs: The symptoms are nonspecific, consisting only of slight fever (which may be absent) and mild gastrointestinal upset. Visible jaundice is usually the first significant finding. It is accompanied by darkening of the urine and pale or clay-colored stools. Hepatomegaly is present. Occasionally, a symptom complex of macular rash, urticarial lesions, and arthritis antedates the appearance of icterus. When acquired vertically at birth, chronic disease is frequently asymptomatic despite ongoing liver injury.

B. Laboratory Findings: To diagnose acute HBV infection, the HBsAg and anti-HBc IgM are the only tests needed. To document recovery, immunity, or response to the HBV vaccine, the anti-HBs is useful. If HBsAg persists after 8 weeks in acute infections, it may signify a chronic infection. Vertical transmission to newborns is documented by positive HBsAg.

Liver function test results are similar to those discussed previously for hepatitis A. Liver biopsy seldom differentiates HAV and HBV disease, although specific stains may detect HBcAg or HBsAg in the liver.

Renal involvement may be suspected on the basis of urinary findings suggesting glomerulonephritis.

Differential Diagnosis

The differentiation between HAV and HBV disease is made easier by a history of parenteral exposure, a parent who is HBsAg-positive, and an unusually long period of incubation. HBV and hepatitis C infection are differentiated serologically. The history may suggest a drug-induced hepatitis, especially if a serum sickness prodrome is reported. Autoimmune hepatitis and Wilson's disease should also be considered.

NANBNC hepatitis is diagnosed in the absence of serologic markers of hepatitis type A, B, or C.

Prevention

Control of the incidence of hepatitis B in the population is based on screening of blood donors and pregnant women, use of properly sterilized needles and surgical equipment, avoidance of sexual contact with carriers, and vaccination of household contacts, sexual partners, medical personnel, and those at high risk. Universal immunization of all infants born in the United States and of adolescents is now recommended. When acquired vertically at birth, chronic disease is frequently asymptomatic despite ongoing liver injury. The vaccine is highly effective for pre-exposure prophylaxis (see Chapter 10). Postexposure administration of hepatitis B immune globulin (0.06 mL/kg intramuscularly, given as soon as possible after exposure, up to 7 days) and initiation of vaccination are also effective.

Treatment

Supportive measures such as bed rest and a nutritious diet are used during the active stage of disease. Corticosteroids are contraindicated. For patients with progressive disease (chronic active hepatitis), treatment with interferon alfa (5–6 million U/m^2 body surface area three times a week for 4–6 months) inhibits viral replication in 40% of patients, although relapses may occur after completion of therapy. Side effects are common. Younger children may respond better. Asymptomatic HBsAg carriers do not respond. Liver transplantation is successful in acute fulminant hepatitis B; however, reinfection is common following liver transplantation performed as treatment for chronic hepatitis B. Chronic HBIG therapy reduces recurrence after transplantation.

Prognosis

The prognosis is good, although fulminant hepatitis, chronic persistent hepatitis, or chronic active hepatitis and cirrhosis may supervene in 10% of patients. The course of the disease is variable, but jaundice seldom persists for more than 2 weeks. HBsAg disappears in 95% of cases at the time of clinical recovery. Persistent asymptomatic antigenemia may occur, particularly in children with Down's syndrome or leukemia and those undergoing chronic hemodialysis. Persistence of neonatally acquired HBsAg occurs in 70–90% of infants, and the presence of e antigen in the HBsAg carrier patient seems to imply a poorer prognosis. Chronic hepatitis B disease predisposes the patient to development of hepatocellular carcinoma. After 8–10 years of HBV infection, surveillance for development of hepatocellular carcinoma with hepatic ultrasonography and serum alpha-fetoprotein is performed annually.

Bortolotti F et al: Long-term outcome of chronic hepatitis type B in patients who acquired hepatitis B infection in childhood. Gastroenterology 1990;99:805.

Chang MH et al: Factors affecting clearance of hepatitis B e antigen in hepatitis B surface antigen carrier children. J Pediatr 1989;115:385.

Hepatitis B virus: A comprehensive strategy for eliminating transmission in the United States through universal childhood vaccination. Recommendations of the Immunization Practices Advisory Committee. MMWR 1991;40:1.

Narkewicz MR et al: Clearance of chronic hepatitis B virus infection in young children after alpha interferon treatment. J Pediatr 1995;127:815.

Ruiz-Moreno M et al: Prospective, randomized controlled trial of interferon-α in children with chronic hepatitis B. Hepatology 1991;13:1035.

Shapiro CN et al: Hepatitis B virus transmission between children in day care. Pediatr Infect Dis J 1989;8:870.

Xu Z-Y et al: Prevention of perinatal acquisition of hepatitis B virus carriage using vaccine: Preliminary report of a randomized, double-blind placebo-controlled and comparative trial. Pediatrics 1985;76:713.

HEPATITIS C

Hepatitis C virus (HCV) causes the chronic form of non-A, non-B hepatitis (90% of post-transfusion hepatitis cases). Risk factors include illicit use of intravenous drugs (40%), occupational or sexual exposure (10%), and transfusions (10%); 40% of cases have no known risk factors. Children with hemophilia or on chronic hemodialysis are particularly at risk. The risk from transfused blood products has greatly diminished (from 1–2:100 to 1:1000 units of blood) since the advent of blood testing for ALT and anti-HCV. Vertical transmission from HCV-infected mothers appears to occur more commonly in mothers who are HIV-positive (10–20%) compared to HIV-negative (0–6%) and is of unknown significance. Transmission from breast milk is probably quite rare. HCV rarely causes fulminant hepatitis in children or adults in Western countries, but different serotypes do so in Asia.

HCV is a single-stranded RNA virus in the flavivirus family. Several well-defined HCV antigens are the basis for serologic antibody tests. The second-generation ELISA test for anti-HCV is highly accurate; anti-HCV is generally present when symptoms occur. HCV RNA, which can be detected in serum by polymerase chain reaction and the new branched-DNA test, indicates active infection.

A history of intravenous drug use, previous transfusions, chronic use of blood products, or hemodialysis is obtained in most pediatric cases. Cases have been caused by contaminated immune serum globulin preparations.

Clinical Findings

A. Symptoms & Signs: The incubation period is 1–5 months, but the onset of symptoms is insidious. Many childhood cases are asymptomatic despite development of chronic hepatitis. More typical flu-like prodromal symptoms and jaundice occur in less than 25% of cases. Hepatosplenomegaly is evident in chronic hepatitis. Ascites, clubbing, palmar erythema, or spider angiomas indicate progression to cirrhosis.

B. Laboratory Findings: Fluctuating mild to moderate elevations of aminotransferases over long periods are characteristic of chronic HCV infection. Diagnosis is established by the presence of anti-HCV (second-generation ELISA) confirmed by the radioimmunoblot assay (RIBA) or HCV RNA by polymerase chain reaction. Anti-HCV is acquired passively at birth and does not indicate disease for the first 6–12 months.

Percutaneous liver biopsy is indicated in chronic cases. Histologic examination shows portal triaditis with chronic inflammatory cells, occasional lymphocyte nodules in portal tracts, mild macrovesicular steatosis, and variable bridging necrosis, fibrosis, and cirrhosis.

Differential Diagnosis

HCV hepatitis should be distinguished from HAV, HBV, and NANBNC cases by serologic testing. Other causes of childhood cirrhosis should be considered in chronic cases (eg, Wilson's disease, α_1-antitrypsin deficiency), or chronic hepatitis may be caused by drug or autoimmune reactions.

Treatment

Treatment of acute hepatitis is supportive. Chronic HCV infection responds to interferon alfa (3 million U/m² three times a week for 6 months) in 40–50% of cases. Relapses are common. Treatment for 12–15 months appears to be more durable. End-stage liver disease secondary to HCV responds well to liver transplantation, although reinfection is common but indolent. There appears to be no benefit (or harm) from using immune globulin in infants born to infected mothers.

Prognosis

In adults, 80% of HCV cases develop chronic hepatitis, and cirrhosis develops in 20% of those with chronic disease in 10 to more than 30 years. A strong association exists between chronic HCV disease and the development of hepatocellular carcinoma as little as 15 years after infection. The outcome of infected children is less well defined, although cirrhosis may develop rapidly or after decades. Infants infected at birth generally have concomitant HIV infection; their outcome is unknown at present. In adults, chronic HCV infection has been associated with mixed cryoglobulinemia, polyarteritis nodosa, a sicca-like syndrome, and membranoproliferative glomerulonephritis.

Choo Q-L et al: Isolation of a cDNA clone derived from a blood-borne non-A, non-B hepatitis genome. Science 1989;244:359.

Clemente MG et al: Effect of iron overload on the response to recombinant interferon-alfa treatment in transfusion-dependent patients with thalassemia major and chronic hepatitis C. J Pediatr 1994;125:123.

Ohto H et al: Transmission of hepatitis C virus from mothers to infants. N Engl J Med 1994;330:744.

Tonas MM et al: Hepatitis C infection in a pediatric dialysis population. Pediatrics 1992;89:707.

Ruis-Moreno et al: Treatment of children with chronic hepatitis C with recombinant interferon-α: A pilot study. Hepatology 1992;16:882.

Zanetti AR et al: Mother-to-infant transmission of hepatitis C virus. Lancet 1995;345:289.

HEPATITIS D
(Delta Agent)

The hepatitis D virus (HDV) is a 35-nm defective virus that requires a coat of HBsAg to be infectious. HDV infection thus can occur only in the presence of HBV infection. In developing countries, transmission is by intimate contact; in Western countries, by parenteral exposure. HDV is rare in North America. HDV can coinfect simultaneously with HBV, causing acute hepatitis, or can superinfect a patient with chronic HBV infection, predisposing the individual to chronic hepatitis or fulminant hepatitis. In children, there is a strong association between chronic HDV coinfection with HBV and chronic active hepatitis and cirrhosis. Vertical HDV transmission is rare. The diagnosis of HDV is made by anti-HDV IgM. Treatment is directed at therapy for HBV infection (eg, interferon alfa) or for fulminant hepatic failure.

Bortolotti F et al: Long-term evaluation of chronic delta hepatitis in children. J Pediatr 1993;122:736.

HEPATITIS E

Hepatitis E virus (HEV) is the cause of enterically transmitted, epidemic non-A, non-B hepatitis. It is rare in the United States. HEV is a calicivirus-like agent that is transmitted via the fecal-oral route. It occurs predominantly in developing countries, is associated with water-borne epidemics, and has only a 3% secondary attack rate in household contacts. Areas reporting epidemics include southeast Asia, China, the Indian subcontinent, the Middle East, northern and western Africa, Mexico, and Central America. Its clinical manifestations are similar to those of HAV except that symptomatic disease is rare in children but more common in adolescents and adults and is associated with a high mortality rate (10–20%) in pregnant women, particularly in the third trimester of pregnancy. Diagnosis is established by anti-HEV. The outcome in nonpregnant individuals is benign, with no chronic hepatitis or chronic carrier state reported. There is no effective treatment or vaccine.

Hyams KC et al: Acute sporadic hepatitis E in Sudanese children: Analysis based on a new Western blot assay. J Infect Dis 1992;165:1001.

Krawczynski K: Hepatitis E. Hepatology 1993;17:932.

FULMINANT HEPATITIS
(Acute Massive Hepatic Necrosis, Acute Yellow Atrophy)

Fulminant hepatitis is defined as acute hepatitis resulting in hepatic coma and coagulopathy within 6 weeks of onset and has a mortality rate of 80–90% in children (without liver transplantation). An unusual virulence of the infectious agent or peculiar host susceptibility is postulated in these cases. In the first few weeks of life, fulminant hepatic necrosis can be caused by herpes simplex, echovirus, or adenovirus. Metabolic diseases that may be responsible include galactosemia, fructose intolerance, tyrosinemia, neonatal iron storage disease, respiratory chain defects, bile acid synthesis defects, and peroxisomal diseases. Later, HBV, NANBNC hepatitis viruses, and HEV are sometimes causative. HAV rarely is responsible. Patients with immunologic deficiency diseases and those receiving immunosuppressive drugs are especially vulnerable. In the older child, Wilson's disease, autoimmune hepatitis, and drugs (eg, acetaminophen, anesthetic agents) or toxins (eg, poisonous mushrooms) must also be considered.

Clinical Findings

In a number of patients, the disease proceeds in a rapidly fulminant course with deepening jaundice, coagulopathy, hyperammonemia, ascites, a rapidly shrinking liver, and progressive coma. Terminally, AST and ALT, which were exceptionally elevated (2000–10,000 IU/L), may improve at the time when the liver is getting smaller and undergoing massive necrosis and collapse. Another group of patients start with a course typical of "benign" hepatitis and then suddenly become ill once again during the second week of the disease. Fever, anorexia, vomiting, and abdominal pain may be noted, and worsening of liver function tests parallels changes in sensorium or impending coma. Hyper-reflexia and a positive extensor plantar response are seen. A characteristic breath odor (fetor hepaticus) is present. A generalized bleeding tendency occurs at this time. Impairment of renal function, manifested by either oliguria or anuria, is an ominous sign. The striking laboratory findings include elevated serum bilirubin levels (usually >20 mg/dL), high AST and ALT (>5000 IU/L) that may decrease terminally, low serum albumin, hypoglycemia, and prolonged prothrombin time. Blood ammonia levels may be elevated, whereas blood urea nitrogen is often very low. Hyperpnea is frequent, and a mixed respiratory alkalosis and metabolic acidosis is present. A rise in the polymorphonuclear white blood cell count often presages acute liver failure.

Differential Diagnosis

Other known causes of fulminant hepatitis, such as drugs and other chemical poisons or naturally occurring plant toxins, may be difficult to exclude. Patients with Reye's syndrome are typically anicteric. A liver biopsy may be helpful. Wilson's disease, autoimmune chronic active hepatitis, acute leukemia, cardiomyopathy, and Budd-Chiari syndrome should be considered.

Complications

The development and depth of hepatic coma determine the prognosis. Patients in grade 3 or 4 coma (combativeness, unresponsive to verbal stimuli,

decorticate function) rarely survive without transplantation. Cerebral edema, which usually accompanies coma, is frequently the cause of death. Sepsis, hemorrhage, renal failure, or cardiorespiratory arrest is a common terminal event. Thus, when patients enter grade 3 coma, liver transplantation should be performed. The rare survivor without transplantation may have degrees of residual fibrosis or even cirrhosis.

Treatment

Many regimens have been tried, but controlled evaluation of therapy remains difficult. Exchange transfusion (with fresh heparinized blood) temporarily repairs both the chemical and hematologic abnormalities. Response may be delayed, and repeated exchange transfusions may become necessary. Plasmapheresis with plasma exchange, total body washout, charcoal hemoperfusion, and hemodialysis using a special high-permeability membrane have been used in the treatment of fulminant hepatic failure. Removal of circulating toxins may be of greater benefit to extrahepatic organ function (brain) than to the liver itself. Reversal of hepatic encephalopathy may follow any of these therapeutic modalities but without improvement in the final prognosis. Survival in adults is not improved over the control group (about 20%). Orthotopic liver transplantation has met with success in approximately 60–85% of cases; however, patients in grade 4 coma may not always recover cerebral function. Therefore, patients in hepatic failure should be transferred early to centers where liver transplantation can be performed. Criteria for deciding when to perform transplantation on these patients are not firmly established; however, serum bilirubin over 20 mg/dL, prothrombin time over 30 seconds, and factor V levels less than 20% are ominous signs.

Corticosteroids may actually be harmful. Sterilization of the colon with oral antibiotics such as metronidazole, neomycin, or gentamicin is recommended. An alternative is acidification of the colon with lactulose, 1–2 mL/kg three or four times daily, which reduces blood ammonia levels and traps ammonia in the colon. Intravenous infusions of prostaglandin E are of questionable benefit.

Close monitoring of fluid and electrolytes is mandatory and requires a central venous line. Ten percent dextrose solutions should be infused (6–8 mg/kg/min) to maintain normal blood glucose. Diuretics, sedatives, and tranquilizers are to be used sparingly. Early signs of cerebral edema are treated with infusions of mannitol (0.5–1 g/kg).

Comatose patients are intubated, given mechanical ventilatory support, and monitored for signs of infection. Coagulopathy is treated with fresh-frozen plasma, other clotting factor concentrates, platelet infusions, or exchange transfusion. Plasmapheresis and hemodialysis may help maintain a patient while awaiting liver transplantation. Epidural monitoring for increased intracranial pressure in patients awaiting liver transplantation is advocated. Artificial hepatic support devices are being developed and tested to "bridge" patients to transplantation. Prophylactic immune globulin, 0.02 mL/kg intramuscularly, should be given to close contacts of the patient with HAV and, perhaps, NANBNC hepatitis.

Prognosis

The overall prognosis remains grave. Exchange transfusions or other modes of heroic therapy do not improve survival figures. The presence of nests of liver cells seen on liver biopsy amounting to more than 25% of the total cells and rising levels of clotting factors V and VII coupled with rising levels of serum alpha-fetoprotein may signify a more favorable prognosis for early survival. Only the rare survivor escapes postnecrotic cirrhosis. Results of liver transplantation (60–85% survival) exceed survival in nontransplanted patients (20–25%).

Alonso E et al: Fulminant hepatitis associated with centrilobular necrosis in young children. J Pediatr 1995; 127:888.

Devictor D et al: Emergency liver transplantation for fulminant liver failure in infants and children. Hepatology 1992;16:1156.

Emond JC et al: Liver transplantation in the management of fulminant hepatic failure. Gastroenterology 1989;96: 1583.

Fraser CL, Arieff AI: Hepatic encephalopathy. N Engl J Med 1985;313:865.

O'Grady JG et al: Early indicators of prognosis in fulminant hepatic failure. Gastroenterology 1989;97:439.

Psacharopoulos HT et al: Fulminant hepatic failure in childhood. Arch Dis Child 1980;55:252.

Sokol RJ: Fulminant hepatic failure and hepatic coma. In: *Pediatric Clinical Gastroenterology,* 4th ed. Roy CC, Silverman A, Alagille D (editors). Mosby–Year Book, 1995.

AUTOIMMUNE HEPATITIS
(Lupoid Hepatitis)

Autoimmune hepatitis is most common in teenage girls, although it occurs at all ages and in either sex. Chronic active hepatitis may also follow HBV, HCV, and delta hepatitis infections. Rarely, chronic active hepatitis evolves from drug-induced hepatitis (eg, pemoline) or may develop in conjunction with such diseases as ulcerative colitis, Sjögren's syndrome, or autoimmune hemolytic anemia. Wilson's disease and α_1-antitrypsin deficiency may also present as chronic active hepatitis. A positive HBsAg test indicates chronic active hepatitis caused by HBV, and anti-HCV and anti-HDV indicate HCV and delta hepatitis, respectively. Positive antinuclear antibodies, smooth muscle antibodies or liver-kidney microso-

mal antibodies, and systemic manifestations (eg, arthralgia, acne, amenorrhea) are characteristic of autoimmune hepatitis.

A genetic susceptibility to development of this entity is suggested by the increased incidence of the histocompatibility antigens HLA-A1 and HLA-B8. These histocompatibility antigens may code for the defect in suppressor T-cell function noted in patients with chronic active hepatitis. Increased autoimmune disease in families of patients and a high prevalence of seroimmunologic abnormalities in relatives have been noted.

Clinical Findings

Fever, malaise, recurrent or persistent jaundice, skin rash, arthritis, amenorrhea, gynecomastia, acne, pleurisy, pericarditis, or ulcerative colitis may be found in the history of these patients, or asymptomatic hepatomegaly or splenomegaly may be found on examination. Cutaneous signs of chronic liver disease may be noted (eg, spider angiomas, liver palms, digital clubbing). Hepatosplenomegaly is frequently present.

Liver function tests reveal moderate elevations of serum bilirubin, AST, ALT, and serum alkaline phosphatase. Serum albumin may be low. Serum IgG levels are strikingly elevated (in the range of 2–6 g/dL), with reports of values as high as 11 g/dL. Low levels of C3 complement have been seen. Three subtypes have been described based on autoantibodies present: anti–smooth muscle (anti-actin), anti–liver-kidney microsome, and anti–soluble liver antigen.

Histologic examination of liver biopsy specimens shows loss of the lobular limiting plate, "piecemeal" necrosis, portal fibrosis, an inflammatory reaction of lymphocytes and plasma cells in the portal areas and perivascularly, and some bile duct and Kupffer cell proliferation and pseudolobule formation. Cirrhosis may be present at diagnosis in up to 50% of patients.

Differential Diagnosis

Laboratory and histologic findings differentiate other types of chronic hepatitis (eg, HBV, HCV, and delta infection; Wilson's disease; chronic persistent hepatitis; α_1-antitrypsin disease; primary sclerosing cholangitis). Wilson's disease and α_1-antitrypsin deficiency must be excluded if HBV and HCV studies are negative. Drug-induced (isoniazid, methyldopa, pemoline) chronic active hepatitis should be ruled out. In acute, severe viral hepatitis, histologic examination may also show an "aggressive" lesion early in the disease (<3 months).

Complications

Untreated disease that continues for months to years eventually results in postnecrotic cirrhosis. Persistent malaise, fatigue, and anorexia parallel disease activity. Bleeding from esophageal varices and development of ascites usually usher in hepatic failure.

Treatment

Corticosteroids (prednisone, 2 mg/kg/d) decrease the mortality rate during the early active phase of the disease. Azathioprine, 1 mg/kg/d, is of value in decreasing the side effects of long-term corticosteroid therapy but should not be used alone during the "induction" phase of treatment. Steroids are reduced over a 6- to 12-month period, and azathioprine is continued for 1–2 years. Relapses are treated similarly. Ursodeoxycholic acid or cyclosporine may be helpful in poorly responsive cases. Liver transplantation is indicated when disease progresses to decompensated cirrhosis despite therapy.

Prognosis

The overall prognosis for chronic active hepatitis has been significantly improved by early therapy. Some report cures (normal histologic findings) in 15–20% of cases. Relapses (seen clinically and histologically) occur in 40–50% of cases after cessation of therapy; remissions follow repeat treatment. Survival for 10 years is common despite residual cirrhosis. Progressive portal hypertension is seen, and complications (bleeding varices, ascites) require specific therapy. Liver transplantation is successful 70–90% of the time. Disease recurrence after transplantation is rare.

Johnson PJ et al: Meeting report: International Autoimmune Hepatitis Group. Hepatology 1993;18:998.

Maddrey WC: Subdivisions of idiopathic autoimmune chronic active hepatitis. Hepatology 1987;7:1372.

Maggiore G et al: Liver disease associated with anti–liver-kidney microsome antibody in children. J Pediatr 1986;108:399.

Maggiore G et al: Treatment of autoimmune chronic active hepatitis in childhood. J Pediatr 1984;104:839.

Odievre M et al: Seroimmunologic classification of chronic hepatitis in 57 children. Hepatology 1983;3:407.

CIRRHOSIS

General Considerations

Cirrhosis is a histologically defined condition of the liver, characterized by diffuse hepatocyte injury and regeneration, an increase in connective tissue (fibrosis), and disorganization of the lobular and vascular architecture. It may be micronodular or macronodular in appearance and may vary from one area of the liver to the next, but the entire liver is typically involved. It is the vasculature distortion that leads to increased resistance to blood flow, producing portal hypertension and its consequences.

Many liver diseases may progress to cirrhosis. In children, the two most common forms of cirrhosis are postnecrotic and biliary—with different causes, symptomatology, and treatment requirements. Both forms can eventually lead to liver failure and death.

In the pediatric population, postnecrotic cirrhosis is often a result of acute or chronic liver disease (eg, idiopathic neonatal giant cell hepatitis; viral HBV, HCV, or NANBNC; drug-induced hepatitis) or certain inborn errors of metabolism (Table 21–3). Cirrhosis is an exceptional outcome of HAV infection and only follows massive hepatic necrosis. The evolution to cirrhosis may be insidious, with no recognized icteric phase, as in some cases of hepatitis B, Wilson's disease, or α_1-antitrypsin deficiency. At the time of diagnosis of cirrhosis, the underlying liver disease may be active, with abnormal liver function test results; or it may be quiescent, with only minimal derangement of liver tests. Most cases of biliary cirrhosis result from congenital abnormalities of the bile ducts (biliary atresia, choledochal cyst, common duct stenosis), tumors of the bile duct, Caroli's disease, Byler's disease, primary sclerosing cholangitis, hypoplasia of the intrahepatic bile ducts, and cystic fibrosis.

Occasionally, cirrhosis may follow a hypersensitivity reaction to certain drugs, such as phenytoin. Parasites (*Clonorchis sinensis, Fasciola, Ascaris*) may be causative in children living in endemic areas.

Clinical Findings

A. Symptoms & Signs: General malaise, loss of appetite, failure to thrive, and nausea are frequent complaints, especially in anicteric varieties. Easy bruising may be reported. Jaundice may or may not be present. The first indication of underlying liver disease may be ascites, gastrointestinal hemorrhage, or even signs of hepatic encephalopathy. There may be variable hepatosplenomegaly, spider angiomas, warm skin, and red "liver" palms. A small, shrunken liver may be detected by percussion over the right chest wall that reveals resonance rather than expected dullness. Most often, the liver is slightly enlarged, especially in the subxiphoid region, where it has a firm to hard quality and an irregular edge. Ascites may be detected as shifting dullness or a fluid wave. Gynecomastia may be noted in males. Digital clubbing is found in 10–15% of cases. Pretibial edema is often seen, reflecting underlying hypoproteinemia. In adolescent girls, irregularities of menstruation and amenorrhea may be early complaints.

In biliary cirrhosis, patients often have jaundice, dark urine, pruritus, hepatomegaly, and sometimes xanthoma in addition to the above clinical findings. Undernutrition and failure to thrive because of steatorrhea may be more apparent in this form of cirrhosis.

B. Laboratory Findings: Mild abnormalities of aminotransferases (AST, ALT) are often present, with a decreased level of albumin and a variable increase in the level of gamma globulins. Prothrombin time is prolonged and may be unresponsive to vitamin K administration. Burr red cells may be noted on the peripheral blood smear. Anemia, thrombocytopenia, and leukopenia are present if hypersplenism exists.

In biliary cirrhosis, elevated conjugated bilirubin, bile acids, γ-glutamyl transpeptidase, alkaline phosphatase, and cholesterol are commonly found.

C. Imaging: Hepatic ultrasound or CT examination may demonstrate abnormal hepatic texture and nodules. In biliary cirrhosis, abnormalities of the biliary tree may be apparent by ultrasonography, CT, hepatobiliary scintigraphy, or cholangiography.

D. Pathologic Findings: Liver biopsy findings of regenerating nodules and surrounding fibrosis are hallmarks of cirrhosis. Pathologic features of biliary cirrhosis also include canalicular and hepatocyte cholestasis, as well as plugging of bile ducts. The interlobular bile ducts may be increased or decreased, depending on the cause and the stage of the disease process.

Complications & Treatment

Major complications of cirrhosis in childhood include progressive nutritional disturbances, hormonal disturbances, the evolution of portal hypertension and its complications (see Tables 21–2 and 21–6). Hepatocarcinoma occurs with increased frequency in the cirrhotic liver, especially in patients with the chronic form of hereditary tyrosinemia. At present, there is no proven medical treatment for cirrhosis, but wherever a treatable condition is identified (eg, Wilson's disease, galactosemia, congenital fructose intolerance) or an offending agent eliminated (drugs, toxins), the disease's progression can be altered; in occasional cases, regression of fibrosis has been noted. Immunosuppressive treatment in autoimmune chronic liver disease also halts the progression of cirrhosis in most cases. Surgical correction of biliary tree abnormalities can stabilize the disease process or lead to a reversal in some situations. Liver transplantation may be appropriate in patients with cirrhosis whose disease is continuing to progress or in whom the complications of cirrhosis are no longer manageable.

Prognosis

Postnecrotic cirrhosis follows an unpredictable pattern. Prior to the development of liver transplantation, death occurred in the majority of patients within 10–15 years after diagnosis, usually from liver failure. A rising bilirubin or vitamin K–unresponsive coagulopathy coupled with diuretic-refractory ascites in a cirrhotic patient portends demise from hepatic decompensation within 6–12 months or less. The terminal event in some patients may be generalized hemorrhage, sepsis, or cardiorespiratory arrest. For patients with biliary cirrhosis, the prognosis is similar, except for those with surgically corrected lesions that result in regression or stabilization of the underlying liver condition. With liver transplantation, survival is 70–80%.

Conn HO, Atterbury CE: Cirrhosis. In: *Diseases of the Liver,* 7th ed. Schiff L, Schiff ER (editors). Lippincott, 1993.

Hardy SC, Kleinman RE: Cirrhosis and chronic liver failure. In: *Liver Disease in Children.* Suchy FJ (editor). Mosby–Year Book, 1994.

Zironi G et al: Value of measurement of mean portal flow velocity by Doppler flowmetry in the diagnosis of portal hypertension. J Hepatol 1992;16:298.

ALPHA₁-ANTITRYPSIN DEFICIENCY LIVER DISEASE

Essentials of Diagnosis

- Serum α_1-antitrypsin level less than 50–80 mg/dL.
- Identification of a specific phenotype (Pi ZZ, SZ).
- Detection of diastase-resistant glycoprotein deposits in periportal hepatocytes.
- Histologic evidence of liver disease.
- Family history of early-onset pulmonary disease or liver disease.

General Considerations

The disease is caused by a deficiency in the protease inhibitor system (Pi), predisposing patients to chronic liver disease and an early onset of pulmonary emphysema. It is most often associated with the Pi phenotype ZZ. With the intermediate serum levels of α_1-antitrypsin present in the heterozygote phenotype (MZ), the incidence of liver disease in adults is only slightly greater than that in the general population, despite the presence of glycoprotein deposits in hepatocytes. The exact relationship between low levels of serum α_1-antitrypsin and the development of liver disease is unclear. Emphysema develops because of a lack of inhibition of elastase, which destroys pulmonary connective tissue. Inclusion bodies in the liver contain a protein component immunologically cross-reactive with serum α_1-antitrypsin, containing excess mannose but lacking sialic acid. This structural abnormality leads to aggregation in the endoplasmic reticulum and is resistant to sialization by sialyltransferase. Although all patients with the ZZ genotype have antitrypsin inclusions in hepatocytes, that may be the only histologic evidence of liver disease. A second defective protein involved in microsomal disposal of accumulated aggregates may be necessary for the liver disease phenotype.

About 20% of affected individuals present with neonatal cholestasis. From 30% to 50% of adults with α_1-antitrypsin deficiency develop cirrhosis. A few children will have only pulmonary or pulmonary and hepatic involvement. Most children are asymptomatic, without any evidence of liver disease.

Clinical Findings

A. Symptoms & Signs: α_1-Antitrypsin deficiency should be suspected in all small–for–gestational age newborns with neonatal cholestasis. Poor appetite, lethargy, slight irritability, and jaundice suggest neonatal hepatitis but are not pathognomonic of any one cause. Hepatosplenomegaly is present. Family history may be positive for emphysema or cirrhosis.

In the older child, hepatomegaly or physical findings suggestive of cirrhosis, especially in the face of a negative history of liver disease, should always lead one to suspect α_1-antitrypsin deficiency. Recurrent pulmonary disease (bronchitis, pneumonia) may be present in a few children.

B. Laboratory Findings: Low levels (<0.2 mg/dL) of the α_1-globulin fraction may be noted on serum protein fractionation. Specific quantitation of α_1-antitrypsin reveals levels of less than 50–80 mg/dL in homozygotes (ZZ) deficient in this glycoprotein. Specific Pi phenotyping should be done to confirm the diagnosis. Liver function tests often reflect underlying hepatic pathologic changes. Hyperbilirubinemia (mixed) and elevated aminotransferases, alkaline phosphatase, and γ-glutamyl transpeptidase are present early. Hyperbilirubinemia generally resolves, while aminotransferase elevation may persist. Signs of cirrhosis and portal hypertension may develop.

Liver biopsy after 2–6 months of age shows diastase-resistant intracellular granules positive to periodic acid–Schiff staining, with hyaline masses, particularly in periportal zones.

Differential Diagnosis

In the newborn, other specific causes of neonatal cholestasis need to be considered. In the older child, other causes of insidious cirrhosis (eg, viral hepatitis type B or C, autoimmune hepatitis, Wilson's disease, cystic fibrosis, glycogen storage disease) should be considered.

Complications

Of all infants with Pi ZZ α_1-antitrypsin deficiency, only 20% develop liver disease in childhood. The complications of portal hypertension, cirrhosis, and chronic cholestasis predominate in affected children.

Early-onset pulmonary emphysema occurs in young adults (aged 30–40 years), particularly in smokers. An increased susceptibility to hepatocarcinoma has been noted in cirrhosis with α_1-antitrypsin deficiency.

Treatment

There is no specific treatment for the liver disease of this deficiency disorder. Affected infants who are breast-fed may have less severe liver disease. Replacement of the protein by transfusion therapy is successful in preventing pulmonary disease in affected adults. The neonatal cholestatic condition is treated with choleretics, medium-chain triglyceride-

containing formula, and water-miscible vitamins (see Table 21–2). Portal hypertension, esophageal bleeding, ascites, and other complications are treated as described elsewhere. Genetic counseling is indicated whenever the diagnosis is made. Diagnosis by prenatal screening is possible. Liver transplantation has been shown to cure the deficiency.

Prognosis

Thirty percent to 50% of patients with liver injury either die from progressive liver disease or develop cirrhosis. A correlation between histologic patterns and clinical course has been documented in the infantile form of the disease. Liver failure can be expected 5–15 years after development of cirrhosis. Recurrence or persistence of hyperbilirubinemia along with worsening coagulation studies indicates the need for evaluation for possible liver transplantation. Decompensated cirrhosis caused by this disease is an excellent indication for liver transplantation; the survival rate is 70–90%.

Ibarguen E: Liver disease in alpha-1–antitrypsin deficiency: Prognostic indicators. J Pediatr 1990;117:864.

Schwarzenberg SJ, Sharp HL: Pathogenesis of alpha-1–antitrypsin deficiency–associated liver disease, 1990. J Pediatr Gastroenterol Nutr 1990;10:5.

Sveger T: Prospective study of children with α_1-antitrypsin deficiency: Eight-year old follow-up. J Pediatr 1984;104:91.

Sveger T, Eriksson S: The liver in adolescents with α_1-antitrypsin deficiency. Hepatology 1995;22:514.

Wewers MD et al: Replacement therapy for alpha$_1$-antitrypsin deficiency associated with emphysema. N Engl J Med 1987;316:1055.

Wu Y et al: A lag in intracellular degradation of mutant α_1-antitrypsin correlated with the liver disease phenotype in homozygous Pi ZZ α_1-antitrypsin deficiency. Proc Natl Acad Sci USA 1995;91:9014.

BILIARY TRACT DISEASE

1. CHOLELITHIASIS

Gallstones may develop at all ages in the pediatric population and in utero. Gallstones may be divided into cholesterol stones, which contain more than 50% cholesterol, and pigment stones, black (sterile bile) and brown (infected bile). Pigment stones predominate in the first decade of life, while cholesterol stones account for up to 90% of gallstones in adolescence. For some patients, gallbladder dysfunction is associated with biliary sludge formation, which may evolve into "sludge balls" or tumefaction bile and thence into gallstones. The process may be reversible in many patients.

Clinical Findings

A. History: Most symptomatic gallstones present with acute and recurrent episodes of moderate to severe, sharp right upper quadrant or epigastric pain. The pain may radiate substernally or to the right shoulder. On rare occasions, the presentation may include a history of jaundice, back pain, or generalized abdominal discomfort, where it is associated with pancreatitis, suggesting stone impaction in the common duct or ampulla hepatopancreatica. Nausea and vomiting may occur during attacks. Pain episodes often occur postprandially, especially with ingestion of fatty foods. The groups at risk for gallstones include the following: patients with known or suspected hemolytic disease; females; teenagers with prior pregnancy; obese individuals; certain racial or ethnic groups, particularly Native Americans (Pima Indians); Hispanics; and infants and children with ileal disease (Crohn's disease) or prior ileal resection. Fasting premature infants on prolonged parenteral hyperalimentation (with or without chronic furosemide therapy) are at particular risk for gallstone formation. Patients with cystic fibrosis or Wilson's disease also have an increased incidence of gallstones. Other, less certain risk factors include a positive family history, use of birth control pills, and diabetes mellitus.

B. Symptoms & Signs: During acute episodes of pain, tenderness is present in the right upper quadrant or epigastrium, usually without peritoneal signs. If present, scleral icterus is helpful. Evidence of underlying hemolytic disease in addition to icterus may include pallor (anemia), splenomegaly, tachycardia, and high-output cardiac murmur. Fever is unusual in uncomplicated cases.

C. Laboratory Findings: Laboratory tests are usually normal unless calculi have lodged in the extrahepatic biliary system, in which case elevated serum bilirubin and γ-glutamyl transpeptidase (or alkaline phosphatase) are noted. Serum pancreatic amylase may be increased if stone obstruction occurs at the ampulla hepatopancreatica.

D. Imaging: Ultrasound evaluation is the diagnostic procedure of choice and reveals the presence of abnormal intraluminal contents (stones, sludge) as well as anatomic alterations of the gallbladder or dilation of the biliary ductal system. The presence of an anechoic acoustic shadow differentiates calculi from intraluminal sludge or sludge balls. Plain abdominal x-rays will show calculi with a high calcium content in the region of the gallbladder in up to 15% of cases. Lack of visualization of the gallbladder with hepatobiliary scintigraphy may suggest chronic cholecystitis. In selected cases, endoscopic retrograde cholangiopancreatography (ERCP) may be helpful in defining subtle abnormalities of the bile ducts and locating intraductal stones.

Differential Diagnosis

Other abnormal conditions of the biliary system with similar presentation are summarized in Table 21–5. Liver disease (hepatitis, abscess, tumor) can cause similar symptoms or signs. Peptic disease, reflux esophagitis, paraesophageal hiatal hernia, cardiac disease, and pneumomediastinum must be considered when the pain is epigastric or substernal in location. Renal or pancreatic disease is a possible explanation if the pain is localized to the right flank or mid back. Subcapsular or supracapsular lesions of the liver (abscess, tumor, hematoma) or right lower lobe infiltrate may also be a cause of nontraumatic right shoulder pain.

Complications

Major problems are related to stone impaction in either the cystic or common duct and lead to stricture formation or perforation. Acute distention and subsequent perforation of the gallbladder may occur when gallstones cause obstruction of the cystic duct. Stones impacted at the level of the ampulla hepatopancreatica often cause "gallstone pancreatitis."

Treatment

Symptomatic cholelithiasis is best treated by either open or laparoscopic cholecystectomy. Intraoperative cholangiography via the cystic duct is required so that the physician can be certain the ductal system is free of retained stones. Calculi in the extrahepatic bile ducts may be removed by ERCP, sphincterotomy, and balloon extraction or by surgical exploration and removal, often with T-tube drainage. There is an increased risk of cholangitis and bile duct stricture with the latter procedure.

Gallstones developing in premature infants on total parenteral nutrition can be followed by ultrasound examination. Most of the infants are asymptomatic, and the stones will resolve in 3–12 months. Gallstone dissolution using modalities such as cholelitholytics (ursodeoxycholic acid) or mechanical means (lithotripsy) has not been approved for use in children. Asymptomatic gallstones can be followed expectantly, as only 20% will eventually cause problems.

Prognosis

The prognosis is excellent in uncomplicated cases that come to surgery not requiring exploration and T-tube drainage of the common bile duct. Cystic duct "stump pain" is not reported to occur in the pediatric population.

Bowen JC et al: Gallstone disease: Pathophysiology, epidemiology, natural history, and treatment options. Med Clin North Am 1992;76:1143.

Debray D et al: Cholelithiasis in infancy: A study of 40 cases. J Pediatr 1993;122:385.

Sloven DG, Lebenthal E: Gallstones in children. Am J Dis Child 1991;145:105.

Ware RE et al: Laparoscopic cholecystectomy in young patients with sickle hemoglobinopathies. J Pediatr 1992;120:58.

Table 21–5. Biliary tract abnormalities.

	Acute Hydrops Transient Dilatation of Gallbladder[1,2]	Choledochal Cyst[3,4] (See Figure 21–1.)	Acalculous Cholecystitis[5]	Primary Sclerosing Cholangitis[6-8]	Caroli's Disease[9] (Idiopathic Intrahepatic Bile Duct Dilatation)	Congenital Hepatic Fibrosis[10]
Predisposing or associated conditions	Premature infants with prolonged fasting or systemic illness. Hepatitis. Abnormalities of cystic duct. Kawasaki disease. Bacterial sepsis.	Congenital lesion. Female sex. Asians. Rarely with Caroli's disease or congenital hepatic fibrosis.	Systemic illness, sepsis (*Streptococcus, Salmonella, Klebsiella,* etc). HIV infection. Gallbladder stasis, obstruction of cystic duct (stones, nodes, tumor).	Most have chronic ulcerative colitis (70%); 75% are males. Increased incidence of HLA-B8. Sicca syndrome, fibroinflammatory conditions, familial immunodeficiency syndrome.	Congenital lesion. Also found in congenital hepatic fibrosis or with choledochal cyst. Female sex. Autosomal recessive polycystic kidney disease.	Familial (autosomal recessive) 25% with autosomal recessive polycystic kidney disease. Choledochal cyst. Caroli's disease. Meckel-Gruber, Ivemark's, or Jeune's syndrome.
Symptoms	Absent in premature infants. Vomiting, abdominal pain in older children.	Abdominal pain, vomiting, jaundice	Acute severe abdominal pain, vomiting, fever	Pruritus, jaundice, abdominal pain, fatigue	Recurrent abdominal pain, vomiting. Fever, jaundice when cholangitis occurs.	Hematemesis, melena from bleeding esophageal varices
Signs	Right upper quadrant abdominal mass. Tenderness in some.	Icterus, acholic stools, dark urine in neonatal period. Right upper quadrant abdominal mass or tenderness in older child.	Tenderness in mid abdomen and right upper abdomen. Occasional palpable mass in right upper quadrant.	Icterus, hepatomegaly, splenomegaly	Icterus, hepatomegaly	Hepatosplenomegaly
Laboratory abnormalities	Most are normal. Increased WBC count in sepsis (may be decreased in premature infants). Abnormal LFTs in hepatitis.	Conjugated hyperbilirubinemia, elevated GGTP, slightly increased AST. Elevated pancreatic serum amylase if ampulla hepatopancreatica is involved.	Elevated WBC count, normal or slight abnormality of LFTs.	Elevated serum bile acids, bilirubin, GGTP. Slight elevation of AST. Perinuclear antinuclear cytoplasmic antibodies (pANCA) often positive.	Abnormal LFTs. Increased WBC count with cholangitis. Urine abnormalities if associated with CHF.	Low platelet and WBC count (hypersplenism), slight elevation of AST, GGTP. Inability to concentrate urine.
Diagnostic studies most useful	Gallbladder ultrasonography	Gallbladder ultrasonography hepatobiliary scintigraphy, and ERCP	Scintigraphy to confirm nonfunction of gallbladder. Ultrasonography or abdominal CT scan to rule out other neighboring disease.	Ultrasonography of the biliary tree, ERCP, hepatobiliary scintigraphy	Transhepatic cholangiography, ERCP, scintigraphy, ultrasonography, intravenous pyelography	Liver biopsy. Ultrasonography of the liver and kidneys. Upper endoscopy, splenoportography
Treatment	Treatment of associated condition. Needle or tube cystostomy rarely required. Cholecystectomy seldom indicated.	Surgical resection and choledochoenterostomy rather than simple drainage	Broad-spectrum antibiotic coverage, then cholecystectomy or cholecystostomy drainage and definitive surgery 3–4 wk later	Ursodeoxycholic acid, cholestyramine. Liver transplantation. Balloon dilation, stenting of extrahepatic bile ducts.	Antibiotics and surgical or endoscopic drainage for cholangitis. Liver transplantation for some. Lobectomy for localized disease.	Treatment of portal hypertension. Liver and/or kidney transplantation for some.

Complications	Perforation with bile peritonitis rare	Progressive biliary cirrhosis. Increased incidence of cholangiocarcinoma. Cholangitis in some.	Perforation and bile peritonitis, sepsis, abscess or fistula formation. Pancreatitis.	Progressive biliary cirrhosis, portal hypertension, fat malabsorption, vitamin deficiencies, cholangiocarcinoma, liver failure	Sepsis with episodes of cholangitis, biliary cirrhosis, portal hypertension. Intraductal stones. Cholangiocarcinoma.	Bleeding from varices. Splenic rupture, severe thrombocytopenia. Progressive renal failure.
Prognosis	Excellent with resolution of underlying condition. Consider cystic duct obstruction if disorder fails to resolve.	Depends on anatomic type of cyst, associated condition, and success of surgery. Liver transplantation required in some.	Good with early diagnosis and treatment	Guarded; disease progression is expected even with medical treatment. Course not changed by colectomy.	Poor, with gradual deterioration of liver function. Multiple surgical drainage procedures expected. Liver transplantation should alter long-term prognosis.	Good in absence of serious renal involvement and with control of portal hypertension. Slightly increased risk of cholangiocarcinoma.

Ultrasonography = liver and biliary tract scanning; scintigraphy = hepatobiliary scan using radiolabeled ^{99m}technetium; AST = aspartate aminotransferase (SGOT); CHF = congenital hepatic fibrosis; CT = computed tomography; ERCP = endoscopic retrograde cholangiopancreatography; LFT = liver function test; GGTP = γ-glutamyl transpeptidase; WBC = white blood count.

[1]Crankson S et al: Acute hydrops of the gallbladder in childhood. Eur J Pediatr 1992;151:318.
[2]Suddleson E et al: Hydrops of the gallbladder associated with Kawasaki syndrome. J Pediatr Surg 1987;22:956.
[3]Shian WJ et al: Choledochal cysts: A nine year review. Acta Paediatr 1993;82:383.
[4]Altman RP: Choledochal cyst. Semin Pediatr Surg 1992;1:130.
[5]Babb RR: Acute acalculous cholecystitis. A review. J Clin Gastroenterol 1992;15:238.
[6]El-Shabrawi M et al: Primary sclerosing cholangitis in childhood. Gastroenterology 1987;92:1226.
[7]Lo SK et al: Antineutrophil antibody: A test for autoimmune primary sclerosing cholangitis in childhood? Gut 1993;34:199.
[8]Beuers U et al: Ursodeoxycholic acid for treatment of primary sclerosing cholangitis: A placebo-controlled trial. Hepatology 1992;16:707.
[9]Inui A et at: A case of Caroli's disease with special reference to hepatic CT and US finding. J Pediatr Gastroenterol Nutr 1992;14:463.
[10]Alvarez F et al: Congenital hepatic fibrosis in children. J Pediatr 1981;99:370.

2. ACUTE HYDROPS, CHOLEDOCHAL CYST, ACALCULOUS CHOLECYSTITIS, PRIMARY SCLEROSING CHOLANGITIS, CAROLI'S DISEASE, CONGENITAL HEPATIC FIBROSIS
(See Table 21–5.)

For a schematic representation of the various types of choledochal cysts, see Figure 21–1. See also the references associated with Table 21–5.

PYOGENIC & AMEBIC LIVER ABSCESS

Pyogenic liver abscesses are usually secondary to bacterial seeding via the portal vein from infected viscera and occasionally from ascending cholangitis or gangrenous cholecystitis. Solitary or mixed flora of intestinal origin (aerobes and anaerobes) are usually grown from aspirated material. Blood cultures are positive in up to 60% of cases. The resulting lesion tends to be solitary and located in the right hepatic lobe. Bacterial seeding may also occur from infected burns, pyodermas, and osteomyelitis. Unusual causes include omphalitis, subacute bacterial endocarditis, pyelonephritis, Crohn's disease, and perinephric abscess. Multiple pyogenic liver abscesses are associated with severe sepsis. Children receiving anti-inflammatory and immunosuppressive agents and children with defects in white blood cell function (chronic granulomatous disease) are more prone to pyogenic hepatic abscesses, especially those caused by *Staphylococcus aureus*.

Amebic liver abscess is rare in children. An increased risk is associated with travel through endemic areas (Mexico, Southeast Asia). *Entamoeba histolytica* invasion occurs via the large bowel, although a history of diarrhea (colitis-like picture) is not always obtained.

Clinical Findings

With pyogenic liver abscess, nonspecific complaints of fever, chills, malaise, and abdominal pain are frequent. Weight loss is very common, especially in delayed diagnosis. A few patients have shaking chills and jaundice. The dominant complaint is a constant dull pain over an enlarged liver that is tender to palpation. An elevated hemidiaphragm with reduced or absent respiratory excursion may be demonstrated on physical examination and confirmed by fluoroscopy. Laboratory studies show leukocytosis and, at times, anemia. Liver function tests may be normal or reveal mild elevation of transaminases and alkaline phosphatase. Elevated vitamin B_{12} levels are reported. Amebic liver abscesses are usually heralded by an acute illness with high fever, chills, and leukocytosis. Early in the course, liver tests may suggest mild hepatitis. An occasional prodrome may include cough, dyspnea, and shoulder pain as rupture of the abscess into the right chest occurs. Consolidation of the right lower lobe is common (30%).

Ultrasound liver scan is the most useful diagnostic aid in evaluating pyogenic and amebic abscesses, detecting lesions as small as 1–2 cm. Nuclear scanning with gallium or technetium sulfur colloid or CT imaging may be useful to differentiate tumor or hydatid cyst.

The distinction between pyogenic and amebic abscesses is best made by indirect hemagglutination test (which is positive in more than 95% of patients with amebic liver disease) and the prompt response of the latter to antiamebic therapy (metronidazole). Examination of material obtained by needle aspiration of the abscess using ultrasound guidance is often diagnostic.

Differential Diagnosis

Hepatitis, hepatoma, hydatid cyst, gallbladder disease, or biliary tract infections can mimic liver abscess. Subphrenic abscesses, empyema, and pneumonia may give a similar picture. Inflammatory disease of the intestines or of the biliary system may be complicated by liver abscess.

Complications

Spontaneous rupture of the abscess may occur with extension of infection into the subphrenic space, thorax, peritoneal cavity, and, occasionally, the peri-

TYPE		FINDINGS
I	GB CBD	Spherical dilatation of the common duct
II		Congenital diverticulum of the common bile duct
III		Intraduodenal diverticulum of the common bile duct (choledochocele)
IVa		Multiple intrahepatic communicating cysts (Caroli's)
IVb		Mixed extrahepatic and intrahepatic fusiform or cystic dilation (possibly variants of Caroli's, congenital hepatic fibrosis)

Figure 21–1. Classification of cystic dilation of the bile ducts. Types I, II, and III are extrahepatic. Type IVa is solely intrahepatic, and type IVb is both intrahepatic and extrahepatic.

cardium. Bronchopleural fistula with large sputum production and hemoptysis can develop in severe cases. Simultaneously, the amebic liver abscess may be secondarily infected with bacteria (10–20% of cases). Metastatic hematogenous spread to the lungs and the brain has been reported.

Treatment

Ultrasound- or CT-guided percutaneous needle aspiration for aerobic and anaerobic culture with simultaneous placement of a catheter for drainage, combined with appropriate antibiotic therapy, is the treatment of choice for solitary pyogenic liver abscess. Multiple liver abscesses may also be treated successfully by this method. Surgical intervention may be indicated if there is rupture outside the capsule of the liver or if enterohepatic fistulae are suspected.

Amebic abscesses should be treated promptly. Only those that are sufficiently large and threaten to rupture need to be aspirated. Uncomplicated cases can be treated with oral metronidazole, 35–50 mg/kg/d in three divided doses for 10 days. Intravenous metronidazole can be used in patients unable to take oral medication. In severe cases, give dehydroemetine, 1–1.5 mg/kg/d intramuscularly for 5 days, and chloroquine, 10 mg/kg/d in one or two divided doses for 21 days. Failure to improve after 72 hours of drug therapy indicates superimposed bacterial infection or an incorrect diagnosis. At this point, needle aspiration or surgical drainage is indicated. Once oral feedings can be tolerated, a 20-day course of iodoquinol (30 mg/kg/d in three doses) is started as a luminal amebicide. Resolution of the abscess cavity occurs over 3–6 months.

Prognosis

An unrecognized and untreated pyogenic liver abscess is universally fatal. With drainage and antibiotics, the cure rate is about 90%. Most amebic abscesses are cured with conservative medical management; the mortality rate is less than 3%. If extrahepatic complications occur (empyema, bronchopleural fistula, pericardial complications), 10–15% of patients will succumb.

Moore SW et al: Conservative initial treatment for liver abscesses in children. Br J Surg 1994;81:872.

Nazir Z, Moazam F: Amebic liver abscess in children. Pediatr Infect Dis J 1993;12:929.

Norvak DA, Dolson DJ: Bacterial, parasitic and fungal infections of the liver. In: *Liver Disease in Children.* Suchy FJ (editor). Mosby–Year Book, 1994.

PORTAL HYPERTENSION

General Considerations

Portal hypertension is defined as an increase in the portal venous pressure to more than 5–10 mm Hg. Portal hypertension is most commonly a result of cirrhosis. However, portal hypertension without cirrhosis may be divided into prehepatic, suprahepatic, and intrahepatic causes. Although the specific lesions vary somewhat in clinical signs and symptoms, the end result of portal hypertension is common to all.

A. Prehepatic Portal Hypertension: Prehepatic portal hypertension from acquired abnormalities of the portal and splenic veins accounts for 5–8% of cases of gastrointestinal bleeding in children. A history of neonatal omphalitis, sepsis, dehydration, and umbilical vein catheterization is present in 30–50% of cases. Less common known causes in older children include local trauma, peritonitis (pylephlebitis), hypercoagulable states, and pancreatitis. Symptoms may occur before 1 year of age, but in most cases the diagnosis is not made until 3–5 years of age. Those with a positive neonatal history tend to become symptomatic earlier.

A variety of portal or splenic vein malformations, some of which may be congenital, have been described, including valves and atretic segments. "Cavernous" transformation is probably the result of attempted collateralization about the thrombosed portal vein rather than a congenital malformation. The site of the venous obstruction may be anywhere from the hilum of the liver to the hilum of the spleen.

B. Suprahepatic Vein Occlusion or Thrombosis (Budd-Chiari Syndrome): In most instances, no cause can be demonstrated. Endothelial injury to hepatic veins by bacterial endotoxins has been demonstrated experimentally. The occasional association of hepatic vein thrombosis in inflammatory bowel disease favors the presence of endogenous toxins traversing the liver. Allergic vasculitis leading to endophlebitis of the hepatic veins has been described occasionally. In addition, hepatic vein obstruction may be secondary to tumor, abdominal trauma, hyperthermia, or sepsis, or it may occur following the repair of an omphalocele or gastroschisis. Congenital vena caval bands, webs, a membrane, or strictures above the hepatic veins are sometimes causative. Hepatic vein thrombosis may be a complication of oral contraceptive medications. Underlying thrombotic conditions (antithrombin III, protein C, or protein S deficiency) should be considered.

C. Intrahepatic Veno-occlusive Disease (Acute Stage): This entity now occurs most frequently in patients who have undergone bone marrow transplantation. The disorder may also develop after chemotherapy for acute leukemia, particularly with 6-thioguanine. Additional causes include the ingestion of pyrrolizidine alkaloids ("bush tea") or other herbal teas, and a familial form of the disease seen in congenital immunodeficiency states.

The acute form of the disease generally occurs in the first month after bone marrow transplantation and is heralded by the triad of weight gain (ascites), hepatomegaly, and jaundice. The disease may be rapidly fatal, although about 50% of patients recover. Subacute and chronic forms also exist.

D. Congenital Hepatic Fibrosis: This is an autosomal recessive, rare cause of intrahepatic presinusoidal portal hypertension (Table 21–5). Splenoportography reveals patency of the portal venous system even though splenic pulp pressure is increased. The intrahepatic branches of the portal vein may be abnormal (duplicated). Renal abnormalities (microcystic disease) are often associated with the hepatic lesion; therefore, renal ultrasonography and urography should be routinely performed.

E. Hepatoportal Sclerosis (Idiopathic Portal Hypertension, Noncirrhotic Portal Fibrosis), Noncirrhotic Nodular Transformation of the Liver, & Schistosomal Hepatic Fibrosis: These are also rare causes of intrahepatic presinusoidal portal hypertension.

Clinical Findings

A. Symptoms & Signs: Splenomegaly in an otherwise well child is the most constant physical sign. Recurrent episodes of abdominal distention resulting from ascites may also be noted. The usual presenting symptoms are hematemesis and melena.

The presence of prehepatic portal hypertension is suggested by the following: (1) an episode of severe infection in the newborn period or early infancy—especially omphalitis, sepsis, gastroenteritis, severe dehydration, or prolonged or difficult umbilical vein catheterizations; (2) no previous evidence of liver disease; and (3) a history of well-being prior to onset or recognition of symptoms.

Most patients with suprahepatic portal hypertension present with abdominal enlargement caused by ascites and with hepatomegaly of acute onset. Abdominal pain and tender hepatosplenomegaly are frequent, whereas jaundice is present in only 25% of cases. Vomiting, hematemesis, and diarrhea are less common. Cutaneous signs of chronic liver disease are often absent, as the obstruction is usually acute. The presence of distended superficial veins on the back and the anterior abdomen, along with dependent edema, is seen with inferior vena cava obstruction affecting hepatic vein outflow. Absence of hepatojugular reflux (jugular distention when pressure is applied to the liver) is a helpful clinical sign.

B. Laboratory Findings & Imaging: Most other common causes of splenomegaly or hepatosplenomegaly may be excluded by proper laboratory tests. Cultures, Epstein-Barr virus titers, hepatitis serologies, blood smear examination, bone marrow studies, and liver function tests may be necessary. Liver function tests are generally not helpful. In prehepatic portal hypertension, they are generally normal. In Budd-Chiari syndrome and veno-occlusive disease, mild to moderate hyperbilirubinemia with modest elevations of aminotransferases is often present. Hypersplenism with mild leukopenia and thrombocytopenia is present in most cases. Fiberoptic esophagoscopy will reveal varices in symptomatic patients. When possible, confirmation of a normal liver is best obtained directly by liver biopsy.

Doppler-assisted ultrasound scanning of the liver, portal vein, splenic vein, inferior vena cava, and hepatic veins may assist in localizing the defect. In prehepatic portal hypertension, abnormalities of the portal or splenic vein may be apparent, whereas the hepatic veins are normal. When noncirrhotic portal hypertension is suspected, angiography often is diagnostic. The finding of an elevated splenic pulp pressure (normal, 8–12 mm Hg) and demonstration of the block by simultaneous splenic portography confirm the diagnosis of prehepatic portal hypertension. Filling of collateral vessels to stomach and esophagus by the dye is frequently demonstrated. Selective arteriography using the superior mesenteric artery is recommended prior to definitive surgery to determine the patency of the superior mesenteric vein.

For suprahepatic portal hypertension, an inferior venacavogram using catheters from above or below the suspected obstruction may reveal an intrinsic filling defect, an infiltrating tumor, or extrinsic pressure and obstruction of the inferior vena cava by an adjacent lesion. A large caudate lobe of the liver suggests Budd-Chiari syndrome. Care must be taken in interpreting extrinsic pressure defects of the subdiaphragmatic inferior vena cava in the face of significant ascites.

Simultaneous wedge hepatic vein pressure and hepatic venography are also useful procedures. Obstruction to major hepatic vein ostia and smaller vessels may be demonstrated by this procedure. In the absence of obstruction, reflux across the sinusoids into the portal vein branches can be accomplished. Pressures should also be taken from the right heart and supradiaphragmatic portion of the inferior vena cava. These should eliminate constrictive pericarditis and pulmonary hypertension from the differential diagnosis. Hepatic vein pressure is elevated to a greater degree than portal vein and splenic pulp pressures.

Differential Diagnosis

All causes of splenomegaly must be included in the differential diagnosis, the most common ones being infections, immune thrombocytopenic purpura, blood dyscrasias, lipidosis, reticuloendotheliosis, cirrhosis of the liver, and cysts or hemangiomas of the spleen. When hematemesis or melena occurs, other causes of gastrointestinal bleeding are possible, that is, gastric or duodenal ulcers, tumors, duplications, or inflammatory bowel disease.

As ascites is almost always present in suprahepatic portal hypertension, cirrhosis resulting from any cause must be excluded. Other suprahepatic (cardiac, pulmonary) causes of portal hypertension must also be ruled out. Although ascites may occur in prehepatic portal hypertension, it is not common.

Complications

The major manifestation and complication of portal hypertension is bleeding esophageal varices. Fatal exsanguination appears to be uncommon, but hypovolemic shock or resulting anemia may require prompt treatment. Congestive splenomegaly with granulocytopenia and thrombocytopenia occurs but seldom causes major symptoms. Rupture of the enlarged spleen secondary to trauma is always a threat. Retroperitoneal edema has been reported (Clatworthy's sign).

Without treatment, complete and persistent hepatic vein obstruction leads to liver failure, coma, and death. A nonportal type of cirrhosis may develop in the chronic form of hepatic veno-occlusive disease in which small and medium-sized hepatic veins are affected. Death from renal failure may occur in rare cases of congenital hepatic fibrosis.

Treatment

Definitive treatment of noncirrhotic portal hypertension is generally lacking. In prehepatic portal hypertension, the experience with surgical portosystemic shunts is complicated by a lack of sustained patency in most children less than 10 years old. Therefore, aggressive medical treatment of the complications of prehepatic portal hypertension is the preferred option. Veno-occlusive disease may be prevented with the prophylactic use of ursodeoxycholic acid prior to conditioning for bone marrow transplantation. Withdrawal of the suspected offending agent, if possible, may increase the chance of recovery. For suprahepatic portal hypertension, efforts should be directed at determining the underlying cause and correction, if possible. Either surgical or angiographic relief of obstruction should be attempted if a defined obstruction of the vessels is apparent. Liver transplantation should be considered early in the course if direct correction is not possible.

However, in most cases, management of portal hypertension is directed at management of the complications (Table 21–6).

Prognosis

For prehepatic portal hypertension, the prognosis depends on the site of the block, the effectiveness of sclerotherapy, the availability of suitable vessels for shunting procedures, and the experience of the surgeon. Each unsuccessful surgical procedure worsens the prognosis. In patients managed by medical means, bleeding episodes seem to diminish with adolescence.

The prognosis in patients managed by medical and supportive therapy may be better than in the surgically treated group, especially when surgery is performed at an early age. Portacaval encephalopathy is unusual in the postshunted child except when protein intake is excessive.

The mortality rate of hepatic vein obstruction is very high—95%. In veno-occlusive disease, the prognosis is better, with complete recovery possible in 50% of acute forms and 5–10% of subacute forms.

Carreras E et al: Hepatic veno-occlusive disease after bone marrow transplant. Blood Rev 1993;7:43.

Dilawari JB et al: Hepatic outflow obstruction (Budd-Chiari syndrome). Experience with 177 patients and a review of the literature. Medicine 1994;73:21.

Gentil-Kocher S et al: Budd-Chiari syndrome in children: Report of 22 cases. J Pediatr 1988;113:30.

Hassall E: Nonsurgical treatments for portal hypertension in children. Gastrointest Endosc Clin North Am 1994;4:223.

McCormick PA et al: Review article: The transjugular intrahepatic portosystemic shunt (TIPS) in the treatment of

Table 21–6. Treatment of complications of portal hypertension.

Complication	Diagnosis	Treatment[1]
Bleeding esophageal varices	Endoscopic verification of variceal bleeding	Endosclerosis or variceal ligation. Vasopressin 0.1–0.3 U/min IV. Pediatric Sengstaken-Blakemore tube. Surgical variceal ligation, selective venous embolization, TIPS, OLT. Propranolol may be useful to prevent recurrent bleeding.
Ascites	Clinical examination (fluid wave, shifting dullness), abdominal ultrasonography	Sodium restriction (1–2 meq/kg/d), spironolactone (3–5 mg/kg/d), furosemide (1–2 mg/kg/d), IV albumin (0.5–1 g/kg per dose), paracentesis, peritoneovenous (LeVeen) shunt, TIPS, surgical portosystemic shunt, OLT.[2]
Hepatic encephalopathy	Abnormal neurologic examination, elevated plasma ammonia	Protein restriction (0.5–1 g/kg/d), IV glucose (6–8 mg/kg/min), neomycin (2–4 g/m^2 BSA PO in 4 doses), lactulose (1 mL/kg per dose [up to 30 mL] every 4–6 h PO), plasmapheresis, hemodialysis, OLT.[2]
Hypersplenism	Low WBC count, platelets, and/or hemoglobin. Splenomegaly.	No intervention, partial splenic embolization, TIPS, surgical portosystemic shunt, OLT. Splenectomy may worsen variceal bleeding.

[1]TIPS = transjugular, intrahepatic portosystemic shunt, OLT = orthotopic liver transplantation, BSA = body surface area.
[2]In order of sequential management.

portal hypertension. Aliment Pharmacol Ther 1994;8:273.

Stiegmann GV et al: Endoscopic variceal ligation: An alternative of sclerotherapy. Gastrointest Endosc 1989;35:431.

HEPATOMAS

Essentials of Diagnosis

- Abdominal enlargement and pain, weight loss, anemia.
- Hepatomegaly with or without a definable mass.
- Laparotomy and tissue biopsy.

General Considerations

Primary epithelial neoplasms of the liver represent 0.2–5.8% of all malignant conditions in the pediatric age group. After Wilms' tumor and neuroblastoma, hepatomas are the third most common intra-abdominal cancer. The incidence is higher in Southeast Asia, where childhood cirrhosis is more common. There are two basic morphologic types with certain clinical and prognostic differences. Hepatoblastoma predominates in male infants and children, with most cases appearing before age 3. Most lesions are found in the right lobe of the liver. Pathologic differentiation from hepatocarcinoma may be difficult.

Hepatocarcinoma, the other major malignant tumor of the liver, occurs more frequently after age 3. This type of neoplasm carries a poorer prognosis than hepatoblastoma and causes more abdominal discomfort. Patients with chronic hepatitis B, cirrhosis, glycogen storage disease type I, tyrosinemia, or α_1-antitrypsin deficiency have an increased risk for hepatic adenoma and carcinoma. The late development of hepatoma in patients treated with androgens for de Toni–Fanconi syndrome and aplastic anemia must also be kept in mind. The increased use of anabolic steroids by body-conscious adolescents poses a risk of hepatic neoplasia. An interesting aspect of primary epithelial neoplasms of the liver has been the increased incidence of associated anomalies and unusual conditions found in these children. Virilization has been reported as a consequence of gonadotropin activity of the tumor. Feminization with bilateral gynecomastia may occur in association with high estradiol levels in blood, the latter a consequence of increased aromatization of circulating androgens by the liver. Leydig cell hyperplasia without spermatogenesis is found on testicular biopsy. Hemihypertrophy, congenital absence of the kidney, macroglossia, and Meckel's diverticulum have been found in association with hepatocarcinoma.

Clinical Findings

A. History: A noticeable increase in abdominal girth with or without pain is the most constant feature of the history. A parent may note a "bulge" in the upper abdomen or report feeling a hard mass. Constitutional symptoms (anorexia, fatigue, fever, chills, etc) may be present. A teenage male may complain of gynecomastia.

B. Symptoms & Signs: Weight loss, pallor, and abdominal pain associated with a large abdomen are common. Physical examination reveals hepatomegaly with or without a definite tumor mass, usually to the right of the midline. In the absence of cirrhosis, signs of chronic liver disease are usually absent. However, evidence of virilization or feminization in prepubertal children may be noted.

C. Laboratory Findings: Normal to slightly distorted liver function tests are the rule. Anemia is frequently seen, especially in cases of hepatoblastoma. Cystathioninuria has been reported. Alpha-fetoprotein levels are often elevated, especially in hepatoblastoma. Elevated estradiol levels are sometimes seen. Final tissue diagnosis is best obtained at laparotomy, although some physicians utilize ultrasound- or CT-guided needle biopsy of the liver mass.

D. Imaging: Ultrasonography, CT, and MRI are useful for diagnosis and for following tumor response to therapy. A scintigraphic study of bone and lung and selective angiography are generally part of the preoperative workup to evaluate metastatic disease.

Differential Diagnosis

In the absence of a palpable mass, the differential diagnosis is that of hepatomegaly with or without anemia or jaundice. Hematologic and nutritional conditions should be ruled out, as well as HBV infection, α_1-antitrypsin deficiency disease, lipid storage diseases, histiocytosis X, glycogen storage disease, tyrosinemia, congenital hepatic fibrosis, hepatic abscess (pyogenic or amebic), cysts, adenoma, focal nodular hyperplasia, inflammatory pseudotumor, and hemangiomas. If fever is present, hepatic abscess (pyogenic or amebic) must be considered. Veno-occlusive disease and hepatic vein thrombosis are also rare possibilities. Tumors in the left lobe may be mistaken for pancreatic pseudocysts.

Complications

Progressive enlargement of the tumor, abdominal discomfort, ascites, respiratory difficulty, and widespread metastases (especially to the lungs and the abdominal lymph nodes) are the rule. Rupture of the neoplastic liver and intraperitoneal hemorrhage have been reported. Progressive anemia and emaciation predispose the patient to an early septic death.

Treatment

An energetic surgical approach has resulted in the only long-term survivals. Complete resection of the lesion offers the only chance for cure. It appears that every isolated lung metastasis should also be surgically resected. Radiotherapy and chemotherapy have been disappointing in the treatment of primary liver neoplasms, although new combinations of drugs are continually being evaluated. These modalities are also used for initial cytoreduction of tumors found to be unresectable at the time of primary surgery. Second-look celiotomy has, in some cases, allowed resection of the tumor, resulting in a reduced mortality rate. Organ transplantation has been disappointing but continues to be performed in selected patients. The survival rate may be better for those patients in whom the tumor is incidental to another disorder (tyrosinemia, biliary atresia, cirrhosis).

Prognosis

The survival rate if the tumor is completely removed is 60% for hepatoblastoma and 33% for hepatocellular carcinoma. Fibrolamellar oncocytic hepatocarcinoma has a more favorable prognosis. The overall survival and cure rate is less than 20%.

Ni YH et al: Hepatocellular cancer in children: Clinical manifestations and prognosis. Cancer 1991;68:1737.

Stocker JT: Hepatic tumors in children. In: *Liver Disease in Children.* Suchy FJ (editor). Mosby–Year Book, 1994.

WILSON'S DISEASE
(Hepatolenticular Degeneration)

Essentials of Diagnosis

- Acute or chronic liver disease.
- Deteriorating neurologic status.
- Kayser-Fleischer rings.
- Elevated liver copper.
- Abnormalities in levels of ceruloplasmin and serum and urine copper.

General Considerations

In Wilson's disease, the increased hepatic copper is caused by a mutation in the gene on chromosome 13 coding for a specific P-type ATPase involved in copper transport. This results in impaired bile excretion of copper and incorporation of copper into ceruloplasmin by the liver. The accumulated copper causes oxidant (free radical) damage to the liver. The disease should be considered in all children with evidence of liver disease or with suggestive neurologic signs. A family history is often present, and 25% of cases are identified by screening asymptomatic homozygous family members. The disease is autosomal recessive and occurs in 1:30,000 live births in all populations.

Clinical Findings

A. Symptoms & Signs: Hepatic involvement may be fulminant, may masquerade as chronic active liver disease, or may progress insidiously to postnecrotic cirrhosis. Findings include jaundice, hepatomegaly early in childhood, splenomegaly, Kayser-Fleischer rings, and neurologic manifestations such as tremor, dysarthria, and drooling beginning after 10 years of age. Deterioration in school performance is often the earliest neurologic expression of disease. Psychiatric symptoms may also occur. The Kayser-Fleischer rings can sometimes be detected by unaided visual inspection as a brown band at the junction of the iris and cornea, but slit-lamp examination is always necessary. Absence of Kayser-Fleischer rings does not exclude this diagnosis unless neurologic signs are present.

B. Laboratory Findings: The laboratory diagnosis is sometimes difficult. Serum ceruloplasmin levels (measured by the oxidase method) are usually less than 20 mg/dL. (Normal values are 23–43 mg/dL.) Low values, however, are seen normally in infants under 3 months of age, and in 3–5% of homozygotes the levels may be toward the lower end of the normal range (20–30 mg/dL). Serum copper levels are low, but the overlap with normal is too great for satisfactory discrimination. In acute fulminant Wilson's disease, serum copper levels are markedly elevated owing to hepatic necrosis and release of copper. The presence of anemia, hemolysis, very high serum bilirubin (>20–30 mg/dL), and low alkaline phosphatase are characteristic of acute Wilson's disease. Urine copper excretion in children over 3 years of age is normally less than 30 µg/d; in Wilson's disease, it is greater than 190 µg/d. Finally, the tissue content of copper from a liver biopsy, normally less than 20 µg/g wet tissue, is greater than 250 µg/g in Wilson's disease.

Glycosuria, aminoaciduria, and depressed serum uric acid levels have been reported. Hemolysis and gallstones may be present; bone lesions simulating those of osteochondritis dissecans have also been found.

The coarse nodular cirrhosis and glycogen nuclei seen on liver biopsy may distinguish Wilson's disease from other types of cirrhosis. Early in the disease, vacuolation of liver cells, steatosis, and lipofuscin granules can be seen, as well as Mallory bodies. The presence of the latter in a child is strongly suggestive of Wilson's disease. Stains for copper may sometimes be negative despite high copper content in the liver. Therefore, liver copper levels must be determined on biopsy specimens.

Differential Diagnosis

During the icteric phase, acute viral hepatitis, α_1-antitrypsin deficiency, chronic active hepatitis, Indian childhood cirrhosis, and drug-induced hepatitis are the usual diagnostic possibilities. Later, other causes of cirrhosis and portal hypertension require consideration. Laboratory testing for serum ceruloplasmin, urine copper excretion, and liver copper concentration will differentiate Wilson's disease from the others. The radiocopper ceruloplasmin incorporation test is sometimes needed to differentiate Wilson's disease with a normal ceruloplasmin level from other liver disease with increased liver and urine copper values. Urinary copper excretion during penicillamine challenge may help differentiate Wilson's disease from other causes.

Complications

Progressive liver disease, postnecrotic cirrhosis, hepatic coma, and death are not uncommon in the untreated patient. The complications of portal hypertension (variceal hemorrhage, ascites) are poorly tolerated by these patients. Progressive degenerating central nervous system disease and terminal aspiration pneumonia are common in untreated older people. Acute hemolytic disease may result in renal impairment and profound jaundice as part of the presentation of fulminant hepatitis.

Treatment

Penicillamine, 1000–2000 mg/d orally, is the drug of choice in all cases, whether or not the patient is symptomatic. It is best to begin with 250 mg/d and increase the dose weekly by 250-mg increments. The target dose is 20 mg/kg/d. Dietary restriction of copper intake is not practical. Supplementation with zinc sulfate may reduce copper absorption. Penicillamine is continued for life, although doses may be transiently reduced at the time of surgery or early in pregnancy. Vitamin B_6 (25 mg) is given daily while on penicillamine to prevent optic neuritis. For patients who cannot tolerate penicillamine, trientine hydrochloride is effective at a dose of 1–1.5 g/d. Noncompliance with the drug regimen can lead to fulminant liver failure and death.

General treatment measures for acute hepatitis are as outlined for infectious hepatitis. Liver transplantation is indicated for all cases of acute fulminant disease, progressive hepatic decompensation despite several months of penicillamine, and severe progressive hepatic insufficiency in patients who unadvisably discontinue penicillamine therapy.

Prognosis

The prognosis of untreated Wilson's disease is poor. Without transplantation, all patients with the fulminant presentation succumb. Copper chelation reduces hepatic copper content and reverses many of the liver lesions, but it does not have a profound effect on established cirrhosis. Neurologic symptoms generally respond to therapy. All siblings should be immediately screened and homozygotes treated with copper chelation even if asymptomatic. Genetic testing is now available for family members.

DaCosta CM et al: Value of urinary copper excretion after penicillamine challenge in the diagnosis of Wilson's disease. Hepatology 1992;15:609.

Scheinberg IH, Sternlieb I: *Wilson's Disease*. Saunders, 1984.
Sokol RJ: Wilson's disease and Indian childhood cirrhosis. In: *Liver Disease in Children*. Suchy FJ (editor). Mosby–Year Book, 1994.
Sternlieb I: Perspectives on Wilson's disease. Hepatology 1990;12:1234.
Tanzi RE et al: The Wilson disease gene is a copper transporting ATPase with homology to the Menkes disease gene. Nature Genet 1993;5:344.

REYE'S SYNDROME (Encephalopathy With Fatty Degeneration of the Viscera)

Essentials of Diagnosis

- Prodromal upper respiratory tract infection, influenza A or B illness, or chickenpox.
- Vomiting.
- Lethargy, drowsiness progressing to semicoma.
- Elevated AST, hyperammonemia, normal or slightly elevated bilirubin, prolonged prothrombin time.
- Variable hypoglycemia.
- Microvesicular steatosis of the liver, kidneys, brain, etc.

General Considerations

The number of reported cases of Reye's syndrome is decreasing, perhaps because of a decline in the use of salicylates among younger children, who seem to be at greater risk. Varicella, influenzas A and B, echovirus 2, coxsackievirus A, and Epstein-Barr virus have been isolated from some patients. Epidemics of Reye's syndrome seem to cluster during influenza B epidemics. Salicylate use is associated with Reye's syndrome. Many apparent cases are actually caused by defects in fatty acid oxidation. The mode of onset may lead to confusion with other causes of coma, particularly toxic encephalopathy and hepatic coma.

The mechanism is thought to be damage to mitochondria caused by salicylate metabolites or some other toxin or chemical in the milieu of a viral infection. Mitochondrial dysfunction leads to elevated short-chain fatty acids and hyperammonemia as well as directly to cerebral edema.

Clinical Findings

A. Symptoms & Signs: Chickenpox or minor upper respiratory tract illness precedes the development of vomiting, irrational behavior, progressive stupor, and coma. Restlessness and convulsions may also occur. Striking physical findings are hyperpnea, irregular respirations, and dilated, sluggishly reacting pupils. Jaundice is minimal or absent. The liver may be normal or slightly enlarged. Splenomegaly is absent. A positive Babinski sign, hyper-reflexia, and decorticate and decerebrate posturing are consistent with cerebral edema.

B. Laboratory Findings: Cerebrospinal fluid is acellular, and cerebrospinal fluid glucose may be low in younger patients. Cerebrospinal fluid pressure is variably elevated. The serum glucose is proportionately decreased. Moderate to severe elevations of AST, ALT, and lactate dehydrogenase are found. Serum bilirubin and alkaline phosphatase values are normal to slightly elevated. The prothrombin time is usually prolonged, and the blood ammonia is usually elevated. A mixed respiratory alkalosis and metabolic acidosis is seen. In a few cases, the blood urea nitrogen has been elevated. Hyperaminoacidemia (glutamine, alanine, lysine) and hypocitrullinemia are present.

Histopathologic changes in Reye's syndrome are most striking in the brain, liver, and kidneys, less so in the heart and pancreas. The brain shows gross cerebral edema, occasionally with evidence of herniation. Histologically, loss of neurons and fatty vacuolation around small vessels have been noted. The liver shows diffuse microvesicular steatosis with minimal inflammatory changes. Glycogen is virtually absent from the hepatocytes in biopsy specimens taken before administration of hypertonic glucose. Ultrastructural changes are mitochondrial.

The kidney changes include swelling and fatty degeneration of the proximal lobules.

C. Electroencephalography: The EEG shows diffuse slow wave activity.

Differential Diagnosis

Differentiation of Reye's syndrome from encephalitis, acute toxic encephalopathy, hepatic coma, or fulminant hepatitis can be made on clinical and laboratory grounds. A negative history and urine screen for ingestion of poisons and drugs, absence of cells in the cerebrospinal fluid, and absence of jaundice favor a diagnosis of Reye's syndrome. The fatty acid oxidation defects (eg, medium-chain acyl-CoA dehydrogenase deficiency) and other metabolic disorders may resemble Reye's syndrome; urine gas chromatographic analysis will help differentiate them. Liver biopsy and electron microscopy can be diagnostic, and the procedure is indicated in atypical cases.

Complications

Aspiration pneumonitis and respiratory failure are common, as with any comatose patient. Most patients die of cerebral edema rather than hepatic or renal failure. Cardiac dysrhythmias may develop, as may inappropriate vasopressin excretion, diabetes insipidus, and acute pancreatitis.

Treatment

Treatment is supportive. A nasogastric tube, Foley catheter, and arterial and central venous pressure lines should be inserted immediately. Mechanical ventilation may become necessary if the patient reaches grade 3 (Lovejoy). Intracranial pressure should be monitored directly and kept below 15–20 mm Hg, and systemic blood pressure should be kept sufficiently high to maintain cerebral perfusion pressure above 45–50 mm Hg. Hyperventilation, mannitol infusions (0.5–1 g/kg every 4 hours), barbiturates, or ventricular drainage is used to lower intracranial pressure. Maintenance fluids using 10% glucose should be given at a rate sufficient to produce a urine flow of 1–1.5 mL/kg/h. Careful attention to central venous pressure is needed when using hyperosmolar agents. Vitamin K_1, 3–5 mg intramuscularly, should be administered. Hypothermia (30–33 °C) and pharmacologic doses of pentobarbital (10–50 mg/kg/d) have been used to decrease body (brain) metabolic needs during the period of uncontrolled intracranial pressure.

Prognosis

At least 70% of these patients survive. The prognosis is related to the depth of coma and the peak ammonia level on admission. Because Reye's syndrome is less common now, many patients are diagnosed only when comatose. Severe neurologic residuals are common in younger children (<2 years) who recover from prolonged grade 3–4 coma (Lovejoy). All patients should be screened for fatty acid oxidation and other metabolic defects.

Heubi JE et al: Grade I Reye's syndrome: Outcome and predictors of progression to deeper coma grades. N Engl J Med 1984;311:1539.

Heubi JE et al: Reye's syndrome: Current concepts. Hepatology 1987;7:155.

Partin JC: Reye's syndrome. In: *Liver Disease in Children.* Suchy FJ (editor). Mosby–Year Book, 1994.

Shaywitz BA, Rothstein P, Venes JL: Monitoring and management of increased intracranial pressure in Reye's syndrome: Results in 29 patients. Pediatrics 1980; 66:198.

LIVER TRANSPLANTATION

Orthotopic liver transplantation is no longer experimental. Children with end-stage liver disease, acute fulminant hepatic failure, or complications from metabolic liver disorders should be considered for liver transplantation. Recent advances in immunosuppression (eg, introduction of cyclosporine and tacrolimus, use of monoclonal antibodies against T cells), better candidate selection, improvements in surgical techniques, and experience in postoperative management have contributed to improved results.

The major indications for childhood transplantation are (1) a failed Kasai operation or decompensated cirrhosis caused by extrahepatic biliary atresia,

(2) α_1-antitrypsin deficiency, (3) posthepatitic (autoimmune chronic active hepatitis, hepatitis B or C disease) cirrhosis, (4) tyrosinemia, (5) Crigler-Najjar syndrome type I, (6) Wilson's disease, (7) acute fulminant hepatic failure when recovery is unlikely, (8) primary sclerosing cholangitis, and (9) cases in which the consequences of chronic cholestasis severely impair the patient's quality of life. Children should be referred early for evaluation because the limiting factor for success is the small donor pool. Pared-down adult livers are being used in children in many centers, and living related donors are used in several centers. In general, 75–85% of children survive at least 2–5 years after transplantation, with long-term survival expected to be comparable. Lifetime immunosuppression therapy using combinations of cyclosporine, tacrolimus, prednisone, or azathioprine, with its incumbent risks, appears necessary to prevent rejection. The overall quality of life for children with a transplanted liver appears to be excellent. The lifelong risk of Epstein-Barr virus–induced lymphoproliferative disease is increased.

Broelsch CE et al: Application of reduced-size liver transplants as split grafts, auxiliary orthotopic grafts, and living related segmental transplants. Ann Surg 1990; 212:368.

de Ville de Goyet J: Split liver transplantation in Europe—1988 to 1993. Transplantation 1995;59:1371.

Emond JC et al: Improved results of living-related liver transplantation with routine application in a pediatric program. Transplantation 1993;55:835.

Rand EB et al: Measles vaccination after orthotopic liver transplantation. J Pediatr 1993;123:87.

Ryckman FC et al: Liver transplantation in children. In: *Liver Disease in children.* Suchy FJ (editor). Mosby–Year Book, 1994.

Whitington PF, Balistreri WF: Liver transplantation in pediatrics: Indications, contraindications, and pretransplant management. J Pediatr 1991;118:169.

Zitelli BJ et al: Changes in life-style after liver transplantation. Pediatrics 1988;82:173.

PANCREAS

ACUTE PANCREATITIS

Most cases of acute pancreatitis are the result of drugs, viral infections, systemic diseases, or accidental or nonaccidental abdominal trauma, although more than 20% are idiopathic. Other causes of obstruction of pancreatic flow include stones, choledochal cyst, tumors of the duodenum, pancreas divisum, and ascariasis. Acute pancreatitis has been seen with high-dosage corticosteroid therapy and adminis-

tration of sulfasalazine, thiazides, valproic acid, azathioprine, mercaptopurine, asparaginase, antiretroviral drugs (especially ddI), and other drugs. It may also occur in cystic fibrosis, systemic lupus erythematosus, α_1-antitrypsin deficiency, diabetes, Crohn's disease, glycogen storage disease type I, hyperlipidemia types I and V, hyperparathyroidism, Schönlein-Henoch purpura, Reye's syndrome, organic acidopathies, Kawasaki disease, or chronic renal failure; during rapid refeeding in cases of malnutrition; and in familial cases. Alcohol-induced pancreatitis should be considered in the teenage patient.

Clinical Findings

A. Symptoms & Signs: An acute onset of persistent (hours to days), moderate to severe upper abdominal and midabdominal pain occasionally referred to the back, with vomiting and fever, is the common presenting picture. The abdomen is tender but not rigid, and bowel sounds are diminished, suggesting peritoneal irritation. Abdominal distention is common in infants and younger children. Jaundice is unusual. Ascites may be noted, and a left-sided pleural effusion is present in some. Cullen's and Grey Turner's signs indicate hemorrhagic pancreatitis.

B. Laboratory Findings: Leukocytosis and an elevated serum ($>1\frac{1}{2}-2$ times normal) amylase should be expected early, except in infants under 6 months of age who may have hypoamylasemia. Serum lipase is elevated and persists longer than serum amylase. The immunoreactive trypsinogen test may also be of value. Pancreatic amylase isoenzyme determination can help differentiate nonpancreatic causes (salivary, intestinal, tubo-ovarian, etc) of serum amylase elevation. Hyperglycemia (serum glucose >300 mg/dL), hypocalcemia, falling hematocrit, rising blood urea nitrogen, hypoxemia, and acidosis may all occur in severe cases and impart a poor prognosis.

C. Imaging: Plain x-ray films of the abdomen may show a localized ileus (sentinel loop). Ultrasonography shows decreased echodensity of the gland in comparison to the left lobe of the liver. Pseudocyst formation can also be seen early in the course. CT scanning is better for detecting pancreatic phlegmon or abscess formation. Endoscopic retrograde pancreatography may be useful in confirming patency of the main pancreatic duct in cases of abdominal trauma, in recurrent acute pancreatitis, or in revealing stones, ductal strictures, and pancreas divisum.

Differential Diagnosis

Other causes of acute upper abdominal pain include lesions of the stomach, duodenum, liver, and biliary system; acute gastroenteritis or atypical appendicitis; pneumonia; volvulus; intussusception; and nonaccidental trauma.

Complications

Complications early in the disease include shock caused by fluid and electrolyte disturbances, ileus, acute respiratory distress syndrome, and hypocalcemic tetany. Hypervolemia is seen between the third and fifth days, at which time renal tubular necrosis may occur. The gastrointestinal, neurologic, musculoskeletal, hepatobiliary, dermatologic, and hematologic systems may also be involved.

Later, 5–20% of patients develop a pseudocyst heralded by recurrence of abdominal pain and rise in the serum amylase. Up to 60–70% of these will resolve spontaneously. Infection, hemorrhage, rupture, fistulization, or obstruction may occur. Phlegmon formation is frequently seen (30–50%) and may extend from the gland into the retroperitoneum or into the lesser sac. Most regress, but some require drainage. Infection in this inflammatory mass is a constant threat. Pancreatic abscess formation is rare (3–5%) and develops 2–3 weeks after the initial insult. Fever, leukocytosis, and pain occur; diagnosis is by ultrasound or CT scanning.

Chronic pancreatitis, exocrine or endocrine pancreatic insufficiency, and pancreatic lithiasis are rare sequelae of acute pancreatitis.

Treatment

Medical management includes rest, gastric suction, fluids, electrolyte replacement, and blood or colloid as needed. Pain should be controlled with meperidine. Oxygen may be required if desaturation occurs. An H_2 blocker helps to maintain gastric neutrality at a pH greater than 4.5. Nutrition is provided by the parenteral route. Broad-spectrum antibiotic coverage is used only in severe hemorrhagic pancreatitis. Drugs known to produce acute pancreatitis should be discontinued. Recurrence of pain after oral feedings may be prevented by giving pancreatic enzymes with the meal.

Surgical treatment is reserved for traumatic disruption of the gland, intraductal stone, other anatomic obstructive lesions, and unresolved or infected pseudocysts or abscesses. Early endoscopic decompression of the biliary system reduces the morbidity associated with biliary pancreatitis.

Prognosis

In the pediatric age group, the prognosis is surprisingly good with conservative management. The mortality rate is 5–10% in patients treated by operation and 1% in those treated medically. The morbidity rate is high with surgery as a result of fistula formation.

Fan ST et al: Early treatment of acute biliary pancreatitis by endoscopic papillotomy. N Engl J Med 1993;328:228.
Steinberg W, Tenner S: Acute pancreatitis. N Engl J Med 1994;330:1198.

Weizman Z, Durie PR: Acute pancreatitis in childhood. J Pediatr 1988;113:24.

CHRONIC PANCREATITIS

Chronic pancreatitis is differentiated from acute pancreatitis in that the pancreas is structurally or functionally abnormal before and after an attack.

The causes include stenotic lesions of the ampulla hepatopancreatica, strictures of the pancreatic ducts, intraductal stones, or persisting pseudocyst following acute pancreatitis. The role of pancreas divisum in chronic pancreatitis remains controversial. Chronic disease rarely follows acute nontraumatic pancreatitis. Choledochal and duplication cysts can be an unrecognized cause of chronic pancreatitis. Hyperlipidemias (types I and V), hyperparathyroidism, familial chronic relapsing pancreatitis, and cystic fibrosis should be considered. Alcohol abuse is the leading cause in adults in the United States.

Clinical Findings

The diagnosis often is delayed by the nonspecific symptoms and the lack of persistent laboratory abnormalities.

A. Symptoms & Signs: There is usually a history of recurrent upper abdominal pain of variable severity but prolonged (1–6 days) duration. Radiation of the pain into the back is a frequent complaint. Fever and vomiting are not common in the chronic form. Steatorrhea and symptoms of diabetes may develop later in the course of this disease, and malnutrition secondary to failure of pancreatic exocrine secretions may also occur.

B. Laboratory Findings: The serum amylase and lipase are usually elevated during early acute attacks but are often normal later. Pancreatic insufficiency and reduced volume and bicarbonate response may be found at duodenal intubation after intravenous administration of synthetic cholecystokinin (0.02 µg/kg) and secretin (2 U/kg). A threefold increase above normal serum amylase is considered a positive test for obstruction. An indirect screening test for pancreatic insufficiency with bentiromide, a synthetic peptide, measures urine excretion of the chymotrypsin cleaved marker p-aminobenzoic acid (PABA). Healthy subjects excrete over 50% of the ingested dose, with some overlap occurring in normal and diseased patients who have mild pancreatic insufficiency.

Blood lipids and urinary amino acids are elevated in familial forms of the disease associated with hyperlipoproteinemia and should be studied in all cases. Elevated blood glucose and glycohemoglobin levels and glycosuria are frequently found in protracted disease. Sweat chloride should be checked for cystic fibrosis and serum calcium for hyperparathyroidism.

C. Imaging: X-rays of the abdomen may show

pancreatic calcifications in up to 30%. Ultrasound or CT examination demonstrates pancreatic enlargement, ductal dilation, and calculi in up to 80%. ERCP is the procedure of choice to establish the diagnosis. Pancreatograms show ductal dilation, stones, strictures, or stenotic segments.

Differential Diagnosis

Other causes of recurrent abdominal pain must be considered. Specific causes such as hyperparathyroidism, systemic lupus erythematosus, infectious disease, and ductal obstruction by tumors, stones, or helminths must be excluded by appropriate tests.

Complications

Disabling abdominal pain, steatorrhea, nutritional deprivation, pancreatic pseudocysts, and diabetes are the most frequent long-term complications. Pancreatic carcinoma occurs in 4% of patients within 20 years of their diagnosis.

Treatment

Medical management of acute attacks is indicated (see Acute Pancreatitis, above). If ductal obstruction is strongly suspected, endoscopic therapy (balloon dilation, stenting, stone removal, sphincterotomy) should be pursued. Biliary sphincterotomy and biopsy are recommended even when obvious obstruction is not found. Relapses seem to occur in most patients. Orally ingested pancreatic enzymes at mealtime may reduce pain episodes in some patients. The daily injection of a somatostatin analogue (octreotide acetate) has shown promise in relieving pain episodes and decreasing the serum amylase of some patients. Antioxidant therapy is being investigated. Pseudocysts may be marsupialized to the surface or drained into the stomach or into a loop of jejunum in those failing to regress spontaneously. Recent experience in pediatric patients indicates that lateral pancreaticojejunostomy can reduce pain in appropriately selected patients.

Prognosis

In the absence of a correctable lesion, the prognosis is not good. Disabling episodes of pain, pancreatic insufficiency, and diabetes may ensue. Narcotic addiction and suicide are risks in teenagers with disabling disease.

Crombleholme TM et al: The modified Puestow procedure for chronic relapsing pancreatitis in childhood. J Pediatr Surg 1990;25:749.
Little JM et al: Chronic pancreatitis beginning in childhood and adolescence. Arch Surg 1992;127:90.
Steer ML et al: Chronic pancreatitis. N Engl J Med 1995;332:1482.

GASTROINTESTINAL & HEPATOBILIARY MANIFESTATIONS OF CYSTIC FIBROSIS

Cystic fibrosis is a disease with protean manifestations. Although pulmonary and pancreatic involvement dominates the clinical picture for most patients (see Chapter 20), a variety of other organs can be involved. Table 21–7 lists the important gastrointestinal, pancreatic, and hepatobiliary conditions that may affect cystic fibrosis patients along with their clinical findings, incidence, most useful diagnostic studies, and preferred treatment.

Colombo C et al: Hepatobiliary disease in cystic fibrosis. Semin Liver Dis 1994;14:259.
Dodge JA, Macpherson C: Colonic strictures in cystic fibrosis. J R Soc Med 1995;88S25:3.
Littlewood JM: Cystic fibrosis: Gastrointestinal complications. Br Med Bull 1992;48:847.

SYNDROMES WITH PANCREATIC EXOCRINE INSUFFICIENCY

Several syndromes are associated with exocrine pancreatic insufficiency. Clinically, the patients present with a history of failure to thrive, diarrhea, fatty stools, and an absence of respiratory symptoms. Laboratory findings include a normal sweat chloride, with low to absent pancreatic lipase, amylase, and trypsin on duodenal intubation. Each disorder has several associated clinical features that aid in the differential diagnosis. In Schwachman's syndrome, pancreatic exocrine hypoplasia with widespread fatty replacement of the glandular acinar tissue is associated with neutropenia because of maturational arrest of the granulocyte series. Metaphyseal dysostosis and an elevated fetal hemoglobin are common, while immunoglobulin deficiency and hepatic dysfunction are also reported. CT examination of the pancreas demonstrates the widespread fatty replacement.

Other causes of exocrine pancreatic insufficiency include (1) exocrine pancreatic insufficiency with aplastic alae, aplasia cutis, deafness (Johanson-Blizzard syndrome); (2) exocrine pancreatic insufficiency with aplastic anemia, developmental delay, seizures (Pearson bone marrow pancreas syndrome); (3) exocrine pancreatic insufficiency associated with duodenal atresia or stenosis; (4) exocrine pancreatic insufficiency associated with malnutrition; and (5) exocrine pancreatic insufficiency associated with pancreatic hypoplasia or agenesis.

The complications and sequelae of deficient pancreatic enzyme secretion are malnutrition, diarrhea, and growth failure. The degree of steatorrhea may lessen with age. Intragastric lipolysis primarily caused by lingual lipase may compensate in patients

Organ	Condition	Symptoms	Age at Presentation	Incidence	Diagnostic Evaluation	Management
Esophagus	Gastroesophageal reflux, esophagitis	Pyrosis, dysphagia, epigastric pain, hematemesis	All ages	10–20%	Endoscopy and biopsy, overnight pH study	H$_2$ blockers, antacids, carafate, omeprazole, cisapride, surgical antireflux procedure
	Varices	Hematemesis, melena	Childhood and adolescents	3–10%	Endoscopy, barium swallow	Endosclerosis, drugs (see p 595), portacaval shunt, liver transplantation
Stomach	Gastritis	Upper abdominal pain, vomiting, hematemesis	School age and older	10–25%	Endoscopy and biopsy	H$_2$ blockers, antacids, carafate, omeprazole, cisapride
	Hiatal hernia	Reflux symptoms (see above), epigastric pain	School age and older	3–5%	Endoscopy; barium swallow	As above. Surgery in some.
Intestine	Meconium ileus	Abdominal distention, bilious emesis	Neonate	10–15%	X-ray studies, plain abdominal films; contrast enema shows microcolon.	Dislodgement of obstruction with gastrografin enema. Surgery if unsuccessful or if case complicated by atresia, perforation, or volvulus.
	Distal intestinal obstruction syndrome	Abdominal pain, acute and recurrent; distention; occasional vomiting	Any age, usually school age through adolescence	10–15%	Palpable mass in right lower quadrant, x-ray studies	Gastrografin enema, intestinal lavage solution, diet, bulk laxatives, adjustment of pancreatic enzyme intake
	Fibrosing colonopathy	As above. History of high enzyme dosage.	≥3 y	<1%	Barium enema or UGI/SBFT, abdominal ultrasound, or CT	Reduce pancreatic enzyme dose to <2000 U of lipase/kg per dose if indicated. Surgical resection may be necessary.
	Intussusception	Acute, intermittent abdominal pain; distention; emesis	Infants through adolescence	1–3%	X-ray studies, barium enema	Reduction by barium or air enema or surgery if needed, diet, bulk laxatives. Adjustment of pancreatic enzyme intake.
	Rectal prolapse	Anal discomfort, rectal bleeding	Infants and children to age 4–5 y	15–25%	Visual mass protruding from anus	Manual reduction, adjustment of pancreatic enzyme dosage, reassurance as problem resolves by age 3–5 y
	Carbohydrate intolerance	Abdominal pain, flatulence, continued diarrhea with adequate replacement therapy	Any age	10–25%	Intestinal mucosal biopsy and disaccharidase analysis. Breath hydrogen after lactose load.	Reduce lactose intake; reduction of gastric hyperacidity if mucosa shows partial villous atrophy. Beware concurrent celiac disease or *Giardia* infection.
Pancreas	Total exocrine insufficiency	Diarrhea, steatorrhea, malnutrition, failure to thrive. Specific fat-soluble vitamin deficiency states.	Neonate through infancy	80–90%	72-h fecal fat evaluation	Pancreatic enzyme replacement, may need elemental formula, fat-soluble vitamin and vitamin E supplements.

(continued)

Table 21–7. Gastrointestinal and hepatobiliary manifestations of cystic fibrosis. (continued)

Organ	Condition	Symptoms	Age at Presentation	Incidence	Diagnostic Evaluation	Management
Pancreas cont'd	Partial exocrine insufficiency (pancreatic sufficiency)	Occasional diarrhea, mild growth delay	Any age	10–15%	72-h fecal fat evaluation, direct pancreatic function tests	Pancreatic enzyme replacement in selected patients. Fat-soluble vitamin supplements as indicated by biochemical evaluation.
	Pancreatitis	Recurrent abdominal pain, vomiting	Older children through adolescence. Primarily in patients with pancreatic sufficiency.	0.1%	Increased serum lipase and amylase, pancreatic provocative test, endoscopic pancreatogram	Addition of pancreatic enzymes to feeds, endoscopic removal of sludge or stone(s) if present, endoscopic papillotomy
	Diabetes	Weight loss, polyuria, polydipsia	Older children through adolescence	5–7%	Glucose tolerance test and insulin levels	Diet, insulin
Liver	Steatosis	Hepatomegaly	Neonates and infants, but can be seen at all ages	15–30%	Liver biopsy	Improved nutrition, replacement of pancreatic enzymes and vitamins
	Focal biliary cirrhosis	Hepatomegaly	Infants and older patients	20–25%	Liver biopsy	As above. Taurine supplements (still experimental), ursodeoxycholic acid (unproved benefit).
	Multilobular biliary cirrhosis	Hepatosplenomegaly, hematemesis from esophageal varices; hypersplenism, jaundice, ascites late in course	School age through adolescence	1–3%	Liver biopsy, endoscopy	Improved nutrition, ursodeoxycholic acid (unproved benefit), endosclerosis of varices, splenic embolization, liver transplantation
	Neonatal jaundice	Cholestatic jaundice hepatomegaly; often seen with meconium ileus	Neonates	0.1–1%	Sweat chloride test, liver biopsy	Nutritional support, special formula with medium-chain triglyceride-containing oil, pancreatic enzyme replacement
Gallbladder	Microgallbladder	None	Congenital—present at any age	15–20%	Ultrasound or hepatobiliary scintigraphy	None needed
	Cholelithiasis	Recurrent abdominal pain, rarely jaundice	School age through adolescence	3–5%	Ultrasound	Surgery if symptomatic and low risk, trial of cholelitholytics in others
Extrahepatic bile ducts	Intraluminal obstruction (sludge, stones, tumor)	Jaundice, hepatomegaly, abdominal pain	Neonates, then older children through adolescence	Rare in neonates (<0.1%)	Ultrasound and hepatobiliary scintigraphy, endoscopic cholangiography	Surgery in neonates, endoscopic intervention in older patients or surgery
	Extraluminal obstruction (intrapancreatic compression, tumor)	As above	As above	Rare (<1%)	As above	Surgical biliary drainage procedure or biliary stent placement endoscopically
	Stenosis	As above	As above	1–40%	As above	Endoscopic balloon dilatation, surgical drainage

with low or absent pancreatic function. In Schwachman's syndrome, the major sequela seems to be short stature. Increased numbers of infections may be the result of chronic neutropenia. Neutrophil mobility is also impaired in many patients. In addition, an increased incidence of leukemia has been noted in these patients.

Pancreatic enzyme replacement therapy and fat-soluble vitamin replacement are required in most patients. The prognosis appears to be good for those able to survive the increased number of bacterial infections early in life and those patients without severe associated defects.

Cleghorn GJ et al: Exocrine pancreatic dysfunction in malnourished Australian aboriginal children. Med J Aust 1991;154:45.

Dupont C et al: Pancreatic lipomatosis and duodenal stenosis or atresia in children. J Pediatr 1990;115:603.

McShane MA et al: Pearson syndrome and mitochondrial encephalomyopathy in a patient with a deletion of mtDNA. Am J Hum Genet 1991;48:39.

Roberts IM: Disorders of the pancreas in children. Gastroenterol Clin North Am 1990;19:963.

Sarles J, Guys JM, Sauniere JF: Pancreatic function and congenital duodenal abnormalities. J Pediatr Gastroenterol Nutr 1993;16:284.

Winter WE et al: Congenital pancreatic hypoplasia: A syndrome of exocrine and endocrine pancreatic insufficiency. J Pediatr 1986;109:465.

Wright NM et al: Permanent neonatal diabetes mellitus and pancreatic exocrine insufficiency resulting from congenital pancreatic agenesis. Am J Dis Child 1993;47:607.

ISOLATED EXOCRINE PANCREATIC ENZYME DEFECT

Normal premature infants and most newborns produce little, if any, pancreatic amylase following meals or exogenous hormonal stimulation. This temporary physiologic insufficiency may persist for the first 3–6 months of life and be responsible for diarrhea when complex carbohydrates (cereals) are introduced into their diet.

Congenital pancreatic lipase deficiency and congenital colipase deficiency are extremely rare disorders, causing diarrhea and variable malnutrition with malabsorption of dietary fat and fat-soluble vitamins. The sweat chloride iontophoresis test is normal, and neutropenia is absent. Treatment involves use of oral replacement of pancreatic enzymes and a low-fat diet or formula containing medium-chain triglycerides.

Exocrine pancreatic insufficiency of proteolytic enzymes (trypsinogen, trypsin, chymotrypsin, etc) is caused by enterokinase deficiency, a duodenal mucosal enzyme required for activation of the pancreatic proenzymes. These patients present with malnutrition associated with hypoproteinemia and edema but are free of respiratory symptoms and have a normal sweat test. They respond to pancreatic enzyme replacement therapy and feeding formulas that contain a casein hydrolysate (eg, Nutramigen, Pregestimil).

Gaskin KJ: Hereditary disorders of the pancreas. In: *Pediatric Gastrointestinal Disease: Pathophysiology, Diag-*

Table 21–8. Pancreatic tumors.

	Age	Major Findings	Diagnosis[1]	Treatment	Associated Conditions
Insulinoma	Any age	Hypoglycemia, seizures; high serum insulin; abdominal pain and mass infrequent	Ultrasound, CT scan, MRI	Surgery	
Adenocarcinoma	Any age	Epigastric pain, mass weight loss, anemia, biliary obstruction	Ultrasound, CT scan, MRI	Surgery	Hereditary (calcific) pancreatitis
Gastrinoma	Over age 5–8 y	Male sex, gastric hypersecretion, peptic symptoms, multiple ulcers, gastrointestinal bleeding, anemia, diarrhea	Elevated fasting gastrin and postsecretin suppression test (>300 pg/mL), CT scan, MRI, laparotomy	H$_2$ blockers, omeprazole, surgical resection, total gastrectomy	Zollinger-Ellison syndrome, multiple endocrine neoplasia syndrome type I, neurofibromatosis
VIPoma	Any age	Secretory diarrhea, hypokalemia, weight loss	Elevated vasoactive intestinal polypeptide (VIP) levels; sometimes, elevated serum gastrin and pancreatic polypeptide	Surgery, octreotide	
Glucagonoma	Older patients	Necrolytic rash, diarrhea, anemia, thrombotic events	Elevated glucagon, gastrin, VIP	Surgery	

[1]CT = computed tomography, MRI = magnetic resonance imaging.

nosis, Management, 2nd ed. Walker WA et al (editors). Mosby–Year Book, 1996.

Mann NS, Mann SK: Enterokinase. Proc Soc Exp Biol Med 1994;206:114.

PANCREATIC TUMORS

Pancreatic tumors, whether benign or malignant, are rare lesions. They most often arise from ductal or acinar epithelium (malignant adenocarcinoma) or from islet (endocrine) components within the gland, such as the benign insulinoma (adenoma) derived from β cells. Other pancreatic tumors also originate from these pluripotential endocrine cells (gastrinoma, VIPoma, glucagonoma). These malignant lesions produce diverse symptoms, because they release bio-logically active polypeptides from this ectopic location. The clinical features of these tumors are summarized in Table 21–8. The differential diagnosis of these abdominal tumors includes Wilms' tumor, neuroblastoma, and malignant lymphoma. In older children, endoscopic ultrasonography can aid in localizing these tumors.

Jaksic T et al: A 20-year review of pediatric pancreatic tumors. J Pediatr Surg 1992;27:1315.

Weber HC et al: Diagnosis and management of Zollinger-Ellison syndrome. Semin Gastrointest Dis 1995;6:79.

Wynick D, Williams SJ, Bloom SR: Symptomatic secondary hormone syndromes in patients with established malignant pancreatic endocrine tumors. N Engl J Med 1988;319:605.

REFERENCES

Lebenthal E (editor): Pediatric gastroenterology. (Two parts.) Pediatr Clin North Am 1996;43:1.

Roy CC, Silverman A, Alagille D (editors): *Pediatric Clinical Gastroenterology,* 4th ed. Mosby–Year Book, 1995.

Schiff L, Schiff ER (editors): *Diseases of the Liver,* 7th ed. Lippincott, 1993.

Suchy FJ (editor): *Liver Disease in Children.* Mosby–Year Book, 1994.

Walker WA et al (editors): *Pediatric Gastrointestinal Disease: Pathophysiology, Diagnosis, Management,* 2nd ed. Mosby–Year Book, 1996.

Kidney & Urinary Tract

22

Gary M. Lum, MD

EVALUATION OF THE KIDNEY & URINARY TRACT

HISTORY

When renal disease is suspected, a history should include (1) family history of cystic disease, hereditary nephritis, deafness, dialysis, or renal transplantation; (2) preceding acute or chronic illnesses (eg, urinary tract infection, pharyngitis, impetigo, or endocarditis); (3) rashes or joint pains; (4) growth delay or failure to thrive; (5) polyuria, polydipsia, enuresis, frequency, or dysuria; (6) hematuria or discolored urine; (7) pain (abdominal, costovertebral angle, or flank) or trauma; (8) sudden weight gain or edema; and (9) drug or toxin exposure. In the newborn or small infant, obtain birth history and information regarding prenatal ultrasonographic studies, birth asphyxia, Apgar scores, oligohydramnios, dysmorphic features, abdominal masses, voiding patterns, anomalous development, and umbilical artery catheterization.

PHYSICAL EXAMINATION

Important aspects of the physical examination include the height, weight, skin lesions (café-au-lait or ash leaf spots), pallor, edema, or skeletal deformities. Anomalies of the ears, eyes or external genitalia may be associated with renal disease. The blood pressure should be measured in a quiet setting. The cuff should cover two-thirds of the child's upper arm, and peripheral pulses should be noted. An ultrasonic device is useful for measurements in infants. The abdomen should be palpated, with attention to the kidneys, abdominal masses, musculature, and the presence of ascites.

LABORATORY EVALUATION OF RENAL FUNCTION

Urinalysis

Commercially available dipsticks can be used to screen for the presence of red blood cells, hemoglobin, leukocytes, nitrites, and protein; and to approximate pH. The urinary sediment must be examined by microscope. The use of low illumination and a urine stain facilitates the examination. Casts should be sought at the periphery of the coverslip. Bacteria and cells are studied with the high-power objective. Crystals should be carefully described. The urine, collected properly, can be sent for culture when indicated.

Serum Analysis

The standard indicators of renal function are serum levels of creatinine and urea nitrogen. The ratio of serum urea nitrogen to creatinine is normally about 10:1. The ratio may increase in cases where renal perfusion or urine flow is decreased, because serum urea nitrogen levels are more affected by these and other factors (eg, nitrogen intake, catabolism, use of tetracyclines) than are creatinine levels or in urinary tract obstruction. Therefore, the most reliable, easily assessed blood indicator of glomerular function is the serum level of creatinine.

For example, serum creatinine increasing from 0.5 mg/dL to 1 mg/dL represents a 50% decrease in glomerular filtration rate (GFR). Small children should have serum creatinine levels well under 0.8 mg/dL, and only the larger adolescents should have levels exceeding 1 mg/dL. Laboratory results should be compared with age-matched control values.

Less precise but nonetheless important indicators of the presence of renal disease are abnormalities of serum electrolytes, pH, calcium, phosphorus, magnesium, albumin, or complement.

Measurement of Glomerular Filtration Rate (GFR)

The determination of GFR is of paramount importance in the evaluation of suspected renal disease or in the serial follow-up of the child with established renal insufficiency.

The endogenous creatinine clearance (C_{Cr}) in milliliters per minute gives an estimate of the GFR. A 24-hour urine collection is usually obtained; however, in small children from whom collection is difficult, a 12-hour daytime specimen, collected when urine flow rate is greatest, is acceptable. The procedure for collecting a quantitative urine specimen should be carefully explained so that the parent or patient understands fully the rationale of (1) first emptying the bladder (discarding that urine) and noting the time; and (2) putting all urine subsequently voided into the collection receptacle, including the last void, 12 or 24 hours later. Reliability of the 24-hour collection can be approximated by measurement of the total 24-hour creatinine excretion in the specimen. Total daily creatinine excretion (creatinine index) should be in the range of 14–20 mg/kg. If the creatinine index does not fall within this range, collections may be either inadequate or excessive. Calculation by the following formula requires measurements of plasma creatinine (P_{Cr}) in mg/mL, urine creatinine (U_{Cr}) in mg/mL, and urine volume (V) expressed as mL/min.

$$C_{Cr} = \frac{U_{Cr} \, V}{P_{Cr}}$$

Creatinine is a reflection of body muscle mass. Because accepted ranges of normal creatinine clearance are based on adult parameters, "correction" for size is needed to determine normal ranges in children. Clearance is "corrected" to a standard body surface area of 1.73 m^2, in the formula:

$$\text{"Corrected" } C_{Cr} = \frac{\text{Patient's } C_{Cr} \times 1.73 \text{ m}^2}{\text{Patient's body surface area}}$$

Although 80–125 mL/min/1.73 m^2 is the normal range for creatinine clearance, estimates at the lower end of this range may indicate problems.

A simple and tested formula for quick approximation of creatinine clearance incorporates use of the plasma creatinine level and the child's length in centimeters:

$$C_{Cr} \text{ (mL/min/1.73 m}^2) = \frac{0.55 \times \text{Height in cm}}{P_{Cr} \text{ in mg/dL}}$$

Note: This formula takes into consideration an expression of body surface area; thus, further correction is not necessary. Use 0.45 × length in centimeters in newborns less than 1 year old. This method of calculation is not meant to detract from the importance of clearance determinations but is of great help to the clinician who desires a quick estimate of the appropriateness of a suspect level of plasma creatinine.

Urine Concentrating Ability

Inability to concentrate urine is associated with polyuria, polydipsia, or enuresis and is often the first sign of chronic renal failure. The first morning void should be concentrated. Evaluation of other abnormalities of urinary concentration or dilution is discussed under specific disease entities, such as diabetes insipidus.

Microhematuria or Isolated Proteinuria

Hematuria and proteinuria occur with glomerular lesions. In children with *asymptomatic* hematuria or proteinuria, the search for *renal* origins will yield the most results. Dipstick detection of microhematuria should be followed by microscopic analysis. The presence of red cell casts supports the diagnosis of glomerulonephritis, but the absence of casts does not rule out the disease.

The diagnosis of benign hematuria, including benign familial hematuria, is by exclusion. In this group are children whose hematuria is caused by asymptomatic hypercalciuria. Figure 22–1 suggests an approach to the renal workup of hematuria. Further discussion of glomerulonephritis follows.

The association of proteinuria with hematuria is characteristic of more significant glomerular disease. Proteinuria alone, however, indicates the presence of either a benign or more serious entity.

A positive dipstick test for proteinuria should be followed by quantitation of urinary protein excretion. Significant proteinuria exceeds 150 mg/d. A spot urine sample which reveals a protein:creatinine ratio of more than 0.1 is abnormal.

A timed (usually 24-hour) urine collection is useful, especially to demonstrate orthostatic or "postural" proteinuria. Urine voided upon arising in the morning is collected in one container, and urine formed in the upright position during the rest of the day is collected in a separate container which is completed with a void just before going to bed. The two quantities can then be used to calculate total protein excretion, and the amount of protein can be compared in upright versus recumbent specimens to determine an orthostatic component. If the upright collection contains 80–100% of the measured protein and does not exceed a total of 1.5 g, the diagnosis of orthostatic (benign) proteinuria is acceptable. Measuring the creatinine in the specimen and calculating the creatinine index confirms specimen reliability.

An approach to the workup of isolated proteinuria is shown in Figure 22–2. Note that corticosteroid therapy is indicated in the algorithm because this may be initiated prior to referral. Discussion of other renal lesions with proteinuric presentations follows.

Special Tests of Renal Function

Measurements of urinary sodium, creatinine, and osmolality are useful in differentiating prerenal

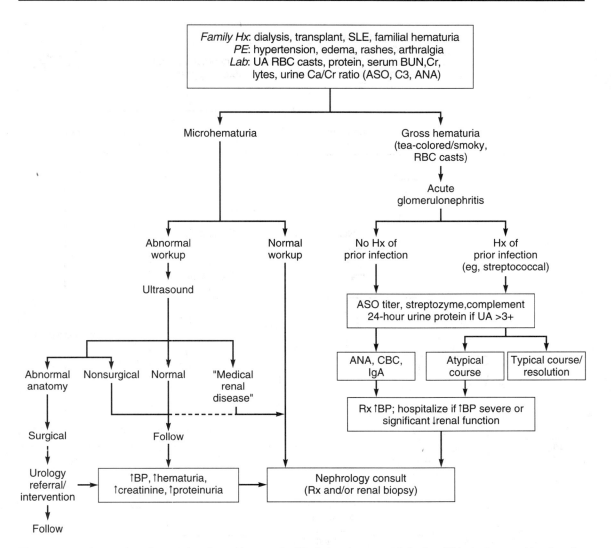

Figure 22–1. Approach to the renal workup of hematuria. (Exclude urinary tract infection, lithiasis, trauma, bleeding disorders, sickle cell disease, etc.)

causes of renal insufficiency from renal causes when the possibility of acute tubular necrosis is raised.

The physiologic response to decreased renal perfusion is an increase in urine concentration (osmolality usually more than 800 mosm/L), a rise in urinary solutes, and a decrease in urinary sodium (usually less than 20 meq/L). Therefore, when an increase in serum creatinine or blood urea nitrogen concentration or a decrease in urinary output suggests the possibility of renal failure, appropriate steps can be taken to assess the status of renal function by qualitative and quantitative urinalysis. (See Acute Renal Failure.)

The presence of some substances in urine suggests tubular dysfunction. For example, urine glucose should be less than 5 mg/dL. Hyperphosphaturia occurs with significant tubular abnormalities (eg, Fan-

coni's syndrome). Measurement of the phosphate concentration of a 24-hour urine specimen and evaluation of tubular reabsorption of phosphorus (TRP) will help document renal tubular diseases as well as hyperparathyroid states. TRP (expressed as percentage of reabsorption) is calculated as follows:

$$\text{TRP} = 100\left[1 - \frac{S_{Cr} \times U_{PO_4}}{S_{PO_4} \times U_{Cr}}\right]$$

where S_{Cr} = serum creatinine; U_{Cr} = urine creatinine; S_{PO4} = serum phosphate; and U_{PO4} = urine phosphate. All values for creatinine and phosphate are expressed in milligrams per deciliter for purposes of calculation. A TRP value of 80% or more is considered normal, though it depends somewhat on the S_{PO4}.

Figure 22–2. Approach to the workup of isolated proteinuria.

The urinary excretion of amino acids in generalized tubular disease reflects a quantitative increase rather than a qualitative change.

The ability of the proximal tubule to reabsorb bicarbonate is affected in several disease states—including isolated renal tubular acidosis, Fanconi's syndrome (which is present in such diseases as cystinosis), and chronic renal failure—and is discussed later under specific entities.

LABORATORY EVALUATION OF IMMUNOLOGIC FUNCTION

Much of parenchymal renal disease is mediated by immune mechanisms, many of which are not well de-

fined or known. Examples of mechanisms in the kidney include (1) deposition of circulating antigen-antibody complexes that are themselves injurious or incite injurious responses and (2) formation of antibody directed against the glomerular basement membrane itself (rare in children).

Total serum complement, the C3 and C4 complement components, and serum immunoglobulins should be measured when immune-mediated renal injury or chronic glomerulonephritis is suspected. Abnormal serum protein levels are often associated with immune complex deposition; in such cases, tests should be performed to detect antinuclear antibodies, hepatitis-associated antigen, rheumatoid factor, and cold-precipitable proteins (cryoglobulins). Where indicated, special studies to measure circulating immune complexes, C3 "nephritic" factor, and anti-glomerular basement membrane (anti-GBM) antibody may be performed. Very often, the diagnosis rests on the description of renal histology.

RADIOGRAPHIC EVALUATION

Renal ultrasonography is a useful noninvasive tool in the evaluation of renal parenchymal disease, urinary tract abnormalities, or renal blood flow. Excretory urography is useful in assessing the anatomy and function of the kidney, collecting system, and bladder. Radioisotope studies provide valuable information concerning renal anatomy, blood flow, and glomerular, tubular, and collecting system function.

Evaluation of the lower urinary tract (voiding cystourethrography or cystoscopy) is indicated when vesicoureteral reflux or bladder outlet obstruction is suspected. Cystoscopy is rarely useful in the evaluation of asymptomatic hematuria or proteinuria in children.

Renal arteriography or venography is indicated in children only to define vascular abnormalities (eg, renal artery stenosis) prior to surgical intervention. Less invasive measures such as ultrasonography and Doppler studies can demonstrate renal blood flow or thromboses.

Gusmano R et al: Natural history of reflux nephropathy in children. Contrib Nephrol 1988;61:200.

RENAL BIOPSY

Histologic information is valuable for diagnosis, treatment, and prognosis. Satisfactory evaluation of renal tissue requires examination by light microscopy, immunofluorescence microscopy, and electron microscopy.

When a biopsy is anticipated, a pediatric nephrologist should be consulted. In children, percutaneous renal biopsy is an acceptable low-risk procedure when performed by an experienced physician; it avoids the risks of general anesthesia. An experienced surgeon should perform the biopsy if operative exposure of the kidney is necessary, if an increased risk factor (eg, bleeding disorder) is present, or if a wedge biopsy is preferred.

CONGENITAL ANOMALIES OF THE URINARY TRACT

RENAL PARENCHYMAL ANOMALIES

About 10% of children have congenital anomalies of the genitourinary tract. Severity ranges from abnormalities which remain asymptomatic through adult life to malformations incompatible with intrauterine or extrauterine life.

Some asymptomatic abnormalities have significant complications. For example, patients with horseshoe kidney (kidneys fused in their lower poles) have a higher incidence of renal calculi. Unilateral agenesis is usually accompanied by compensatory hypertrophy of the contralateral kidney and thus should be compatible with normal renal function. Supernumerary and ectopic kidneys are usually of no significance. Abnormal genitourinary development can result in varying degrees of renal maldevelopment and function, of which complete renal agenesis is the most severe. When the agenesis is bilateral it causes early death. Oligohydramnios is present and can result in pulmonary hypoplasia and peculiar (Potter) facies.

Renal Hypoplasia & Dysplasia

Renal hypoplasia and dysplasia represent a spectrum of anomalies. In simple hypoplasia, which may be unilateral or bilateral, the affected organs are smaller than normal. In the various forms of dysplasia, immature, undifferentiated renal tissue persists. In some of the dysplasias, the number of normal nephrons is insufficient to sustain life once the child reaches a critical body size. Such lack of renal tissue may not be readily discernible in the newborn period because the infant's urine production, although poor in concentration, may be adequate in volume. Often, the search for renal insufficiency is initiated only when growth fails or chronic renal failure develops.

Other forms of renal dysplasia include oligomeganephronia (characterized by the presence of only a few large glomeruli) and the cystic dysplasias (characterized by the presence of renal cysts). This group includes microcystic disease (congenital nephrosis). A simple cyst within a kidney may be clinically unimportant because it does not predispose to progressive polycystic development. An entire kidney lost to multicystic development with concomitant hypertrophy and normal function of the contralateral side may also be of little clinical consequence. Nonetheless, even a simple cyst could pose problems if it becomes a site for lithiasis, infection, or hematuria.

Polycystic Kidney Disease

The autosomal recessive form of polycystic kidney disease ("infantile" polycystic kidney disease) is characterized by large cystic kidneys, often associated with multiple organ systems affected by cystic malformations. Some children with this type die in the newborn period, but many progress to end-stage renal failure. When autosomal recessive polycystic kidney disease is diagnosed at a later age, it may be predominantly manifested by liver rather than renal involvement. Autosomal dominant disease ("adult" form), though rarely of clinical significance (if at all) before the fourth decade, may also be detected in the newborn period and, depending on degree of severity, could be fatal. Although renal insufficiency and hypertension usually occur late in this type, there are exceptions. Careful documentation (usually by ultrasonography), close monitoring and management of the complications of renal insufficiency, and strict attention to hypertension control—as well as genetic counseling—are suggested. Management of end-stage renal failure is by dialysis or renal transplantation.

Medullary Cystic Disease (Juvenile Nephronophthisis)

Medullary cystic disease is characterized by varying sizes of cysts in the renal medulla and is associated with tubular and interstitial nephritis. Children present with renal failure and signs of tubular dysfunction (decreased concentrating ability, Fanconi's syndrome). This lesion should not be confused with medullary sponge kidney (renal tubular ectasia), a frequently asymptomatic disease usually found in adults.

Gabow PA: Autosomal dominant polycystic kidney disease. N Engl J Med 1993;329:332.

Kissane JM: Renal cysts in pediatric patients. Pediatr Nephrol 1990;4:69.

Pretorius DH et al: Diagnosis of autosomal dominant polycystic kidney disease in utero and in the young infant. J Ultrasound Med 1987;6:249.

DISTAL URINARY TRACT ANOMALIES

Obstruction at the ureteropelvic junction may be the result of intrinsic muscle abnormalities, aberrant vessels, or fibrous bands. The lesion can cause hydronephrosis and usually presents as an abdominal mass in the newborn. Obstruction can occur in other parts of the ureter, especially at its entrance into the bladder, with resulting proximal hydroureter and hydronephrosis. Whether impediments to normal flow of urine are intrinsic or extrinsic, steps should immediately be taken to rectify the problem and minimize damage to the renal parenchyma.

Severe bladder malformations such as exstrophy are clinically obvious and provide a surgical challenge. More subtle—but urgent in terms of diagnosis—is obstruction of urine flow from aberrant posterior urethral valves. This anomaly, almost invariably confined to males, usually presents as anuria or a poor voiding stream in the newborn period, with severe obstruction of urine flow. Ascites may occur and the kidneys and bladder may be easily palpable. Provided that severe, irreversible damage to renal development has not occurred in utero, prompt intervention must be taken to avert further renal damage. The same can be said of many such complex genitourinary anomalies, including those of the external genitalia.

Complex Anomalies

Prune-belly syndrome is an association of urinary tract anomalies with cryptorchidism and absent abdominal musculature. Although complex anomalies, especially renal dysplasia, usually cause early death or the need for dialysis or transplantation, some patients have lived into the third decade with varying degrees of renal insufficiency. Early urinary diversion is essential to sustain renal function. A renal biopsy at the time of this surgery may predict subsequent renal function.

Other complex malformations and such external genitalia anomalies as hypospadias are beyond the scope of this text. Overall, urologic abnormalities resulting in severe compromise and destruction of renal tissue provide therapeutic and management challenges aimed at preserving all remaining function and treating the complications of progressive chronic renal failure.

Fernbach SK: The dilated urinary tract in children. Urol Radiol 1992;14:34.

Tripp BM, Honsy YL: Neonatal hydronephrosis: The controversy and the management. Pediatr Nephrol 1995;9:503.

HEMATURIA & GLOMERULAR DISEASE

Children with painful hematuria should be investigated for causes of direct injury to the urinary tract whether the pain is dysuria, associated with cystitis or urethritis; back pain secondary to pyelonephritis; or colicky flank pain accompanying the passage of a stone. "Bright red" blood or clots in the urine occur with bleeding disorders, trauma, and arteriovenous malformations. Abdominal masses suggest the presence of urinary tract obstruction, cystic disease, or tumors involving the renal or perirenal structures.

Asymptomatic hematuria is a challenge because clinical and diagnostic data must be obtained to determine whether the problem is transient or whether the child should be referred to a nephrologist. Figure 22–1 suggests the outpatient approach to renal hematuria. The concern regarding the differential diagnosis is the possible presence of glomerular disease.

Acute poststreptococcal glomerulonephritis is the most common form of postinfectious glomerulonephritis. The epidemiologic relationship between certain strains of streptococci and glomerulonephritis is well recognized. Antigen-antibody complexes induced by the infection are formed in the bloodstream and deposited in the glomeruli. These deposited complexes may cause glomerular inflammation and activate the complement system.

The diagnosis of poststreptococcal disease may be supported by a recent history (7–14 days previously) of group A β-hemolytic streptococcal infection. Recent streptococcal infection is demonstrated by an elevated antistreptolysin titer or by elevation of one or more antibody titers in the streptozyme panel. Other infections have been shown to cause similar glomerular injury; thus, postinfection glomerulonephritis is the better term for this type of acute glomerulonephritis. Patients whose renal function deteriorates rapidly should be biopsied.

The clinical presentation of glomerulonephritis is usually with gross hematuria ("coffee"- or "tea-colored" urine), with or without some (eg, periorbital) edema. Symptoms are usually nonspecific; in cases of severe hypertension, there may be headache. Fever is not expected. Severe glomerular injury (which usually occurs in severe, acute presentations of the more chronic or destructive forms of glomerulonephritis) may be accompanied by massive proteinuria (nephrotic syndrome), anasarca or ascites, and severe compromise in renal function.

There is no specific treatment for the nephritis. Appropriate antibiotic therapy is indicated for infection, if still present. The disturbances in renal function and resulting hypertension may require dietary management, diuretics, or antihypertensive drugs. In severe cases, hemodialysis or peritoneal dialysis may be necessary; corticosteroids may also be administered in an attempt to influence the course.

The acute abnormalities generally resolve in 2–3 weeks; serum complement may be normal as early as 3 days or as late as 30 days. Although microscopic hematuria may persist for 1–2 years, most children recover completely. Persistent deterioration in renal function, urinary abnormalities beyond 18 months, persistent hypocomplementemia, and nephrotic syndrome are ominous signs and are indications for renal biopsy.

The various types of glomerulonephritis present similarly. Their severity and course are useful guides to the diagnosis. The most commonly encountered entities in childhood and their clinical and histopathologic descriptions are listed in Table 22–1. Severe glomerular histopathologic and clinical entities, such as anti-glomerular basement membrane

(anti-GBM) antibody disease (Goodpasture's syndrome) and idiopathic, rapidly progressive glomerulonephritis, may be considered in the differential diagnosis of acute glomerulonephritis, but these disorders are exceedingly rare in children.

Couser WG: Pathogenesis of glomerulonephritis. Kidney Int 1991;44:5.

Ford DM et al: Childhood membranoproliferative glomerulonephritis type I: Limited steroid therapy. Kidney Int 1992;41:1606.

Jennetti JC, Falk RJ: Diagnosis and management of glomerulonephritis and vasculitis presenting as acute renal failure. Med Clin North Am 1990;74:893.

Oliviera DBG, Peters DK: Autoimmunity and the pathogenesis of glomerulonephritis. Pediatr Nephrol 1990; 4:185.

Williams DG: Pathogenesis of idiopathic IgA nephropathy. Pediatr Nephrol 1993;7:303.

ACUTE INTERSTITIAL NEPHRITIS

Acute interstitial nephritis is characterized by diffuse or focal inflammation and edema of the renal interstitium and secondary involvement of the tubules but little or no secondary glomerular damage unless a combined or chronic picture is encountered. It seems to be related most often to drugs (eg, antibiotics, especially methicillin).

Fever, rigor, abdominal or flank pain, and rashes may occur in drug-associated cases. Urinalysis should reveal leukocyturia and hematuria. Hansel's staining of the urinary sediment is helpful in demonstrating the presence of eosinophils. The inflammation can be severe enough to cause rapid deterioration of renal function. Histologic demonstration of tubular and interstitial inflammation of the kidneys is helpful for diagnosis. Immediate identification and removal of the causative agent is imperative. A relentless course with progressive renal insufficiency or nephrotic syndrome may require supportive dialysis and treatment with corticosteroids.

PROTEINURIA & RENAL DISEASE

Urine is not normally completely protein-free, but the average excretion is well below 150 mg/24 h. Small increases in urinary protein can accompany febrile illnesses or exertion and in some cases are produced while in the upright posture.

Table 22–1. Glomerular diseases encountered in childhood.

Entity	Clinical Course	Prognosis
Postinfection glomerulonephritis (GN). Onset occurs 10–14 days after acute illness, commonly streptococcal. Characteristics include acute onset, tea-colored urine, mild to severe renal insufficiency and edema.	Acute phase is usually over in 2 weeks. There is complete resolution in 95% of cases. Severity of renal failure and hypertension varies. Microhematuria may persist to 18 months. Hypocomplementemia resolves in 1–30 days.	Excellent. Chronic disease is rare. Severe proteinuria, atypical presentation/course, or persistent hypocomplementemia suggest another entity is likely.
Membranoproliferative glomerulonephritis. Presentation ranges from mild microhematuria to acute GN syndrome. Diagnosis is made by renal biopsy. Etiologic origin is unknown. Type I and Type II are most common. Lesion is chronic.	Course can be mild to severe (rapid deterioration in renal function); may mimic postinfection GN. Proteinuria can be severe. Complement depression is intermittent to persistent. Hypertension is usually significant.	Type I may respond to corticosteroids. Type II (dense deposit disease) is less treatable; functions decrease immediately to as long as 15 years later in 30–50% of untreated cases.
IgA Nephropathy. Classic presentation consists of asymptomatic gross hematuria during acute unrelated illness, with microhematuria between episodes. There are occasional instances of acute GN syndrome. Etiologic origin is unknown. Diagnosis is made by biopsy.	90% of cases resolve in 1–5 years. Gross hematuric episodes resolve with recovery from acute illness. Severity of renal insufficiency and hypertension varies. Proteinuria occurs in more severe, atypical cases.	Generally good. Small percentage develops chronic renal failure. Proteinuria in the nephrotic range is a poor sign. There is no universally accepted medication. (Corticosteroids may be useful in severe cases.)
Schönlein-Henoch purpura glomerulonephritis. Degree of renal involvement varies. Asymptomatic microhematuria is most common, but GN syndrome can occur. Renal biopsy is recommended in severe cases; it can provide prognostic information.	Presentation varies with severity of renal lesion. In rare cases, course may progress rapidly to serious renal failure. Hypertension varies. Proteinuria in the nephrotic range and severe decline in function can occur.	Overall, prognosis is good. Cases presenting with greater than 50% reduction in function or proteinuria exceeding 1 g/24 h may develop chronic renal failure. Severity of renal biopsy picture can best guide approach in such cases. There is no universally accepted medication.
Glomerulonephritis of systemic lupus erythematosus (SLE). Microhematuria and proteinuria are rarely first signs of this systemic disease. Renal involvement varies. GN often causes the most concern.	Renal involvement is mild to severe. Clinical complexity depends on degree of renal insufficiency and other systems involved. Hypertension is significant. Manifestations of the severity of the renal lesion guide therapeutic intervention.	Renal involvement accounts for most of significant morbidity in SLE. Control of hypertension affects renal prognosis. Medication is guided by symptoms, serology, and renal lesion. End-stage renal failure can occur.
Hereditary glomerulonephritis (eg, Alport's syndrome). Transmission is autosomal dominant/X-linked, with family history marked by end-stage renal failure, especially in young males. Deafness and eye abnormalities are associated.	There is no acute syndrome. Females are generally less affected but are carriers. Hypertension and increasing proteinuria occur with advancing renal failure. There is no known treatment.	Progressive proteinuria and hypertension occur early, with gradual decline in renal function in those most severely affected. Disease progresses to end-stage renal failure in most males.

An algorithm to investigate isolated proteinuria is shown in Figure 22–2. In idiopathic nephrotic syndrome without associated features of glomerulonephritis, treatment with corticosteroids may be initiated as described below. Nephrologic advice or follow-up should be pursued, especially in difficult or frequently relapsing cases.

CONGENITAL NEPHROSIS

Congenital nephrosis is a rare autosomal recessive disorder. The kidneys are pale and large and may show microcystic dilations (microcystic disease) of the proximal tubules and glomerular changes. The latter consist of proliferation, crescent formation, and thickening of capillary walls. The pathogenesis is not well understood.

Infants with congenital nephrosis commonly have low birth weight, a large placenta, wide cranial sutures, delayed ossification, and mild edema. The edema may become apparent after the first few weeks or months of life. Anasarca follows, and the abdomen can become greatly distended by ascites. Massive proteinuria associated with typically appearing nephrotic syndrome and hyperlipidemia is the rule. Hematuria is common. If the patient lives long enough, progressive renal failure occurs. Most affected infants succumb to infections at the age of a few months.

Treatment has little to offer other than nutrition support and management of the chronic renal failure.

IDIOPATHIC NEPHROTIC SYNDROME OF CHILDHOOD
("Nil" Disease, Lipoid Nephrosis, Minimal Change Disease)

Nephrotic syndrome is characterized by proteinuria, hypoproteinemia, edema, and hyperlipidemia. It may occur as a result of any form of glomerular disease and may be associated with a variety of extrarenal conditions. In children under 5 years of age, the disease usually takes the form of idiopathic nephrotic syndrome of childhood ("nil" disease, lipoid nephrosis), which has characteristic clinical and laboratory findings.

Clinical Findings

Affected patients are generally under 5 years of age at the time of their first episode. Often following an influenza-like syndrome, the child is noted to have periorbital swelling and perhaps oliguria. Within a few days, increasing edema—even anasarca—becomes evident. Other than vague malaise and occasionally abdominal pain, complaints are few. With significant "third spacing" of plasma volume, however, some children may even present with shock. With marked edema, there may also be dyspnea due to pleural effusions.

Despite heavy proteinuria, the urine sediment is usually normal. Microscopic hematuria (> 20 RBCs/high-power field) should raise the suspicion of a glomerular lesion (eg, focal glomerular sclerosis). Plasma albumin is low and lipids are raised. Immunoglobulin M may be raised and IgG may be low. Serum complement is normal and there are no cryoglobulins. Humoral immunity does not appear to cause this nephrotic syndrome. When azotemia occurs it is secondary to intravascular volume depletion rather than to impairment of function.

Glomerular morphology is unremarkable except for fusion of foot processes of the visceral epithelium of the glomerular basement membrane. This finding, however, is nonspecific and is seen in many proteinuric states. There may be "minimal changes" in the glomerular mesangium, with unremarkable findings on immunofluorescence and electron microscopic examination.

Complications

Infectious complications (eg, peritonitis) are occasionally encountered, and pneumococci are frequently responsible. Immunization with pneumococcal vaccine is helpful. Hypercoagulability may be present, and thromboembolic phenomena are commonly reported.

Treatment & Prognosis

As soon as the diagnosis of idiopathic nephrotic syndrome is made, corticosteroid treatment should be started. Prednisone, 2 mg/kg/d (maximum of 60 mg), is given daily until the urine protein falls to "trace" or "negative" for a maximum of 8 weeks. The same dose is then administered on an alternate-day schedule for 1–2 months; thereafter, the dose is very gradually tapered and discontinued over an ensuing month. If remission is achieved only to be followed by another relapse, the treatment course may be repeated. If at any time the nephrosis becomes refractory to treatment or if there are three relapses within a year's time, renal biopsy should be considered. If the histologic findings are consistent with "minimal change disease," other cytotoxic agents can be considered; however, these agents are generally most helpful when there is corticosteroid dependence and not resistance. If corticosteroid treatment gives little or no response, then the nephrotic syndrome is probably secondary to glomerulonephritis.

Other therapeutic measures may be directed to the complications of the nephrotic syndrome itself. Unless the edema is symptomatic (eg, respiratory compromise due to ascites), diuretics should be used with extreme care; the patients are expected to have a decreased circulating volume and are also at risk for intravenous thrombosis. However, careful restoration of compromised circulating volume with intravenous albumin infusion and administration of diuretics is helpful in mobilizing edema. Immediate attention to infections (eg, acute peritonitis) is important to reduce morbidity.

Prognosis is often suggested by the initial response to corticosteroids. A prompt remission lasting for 3 years is almost always permanent. Failure to respond or early relapse usually heralds a prolonged series of relapses, which may indicate the presence of more serious nephropathy. Chlorambucil or other cytotoxic drug therapy is predictably successful only in children who respond to corticosteroids. As previously mentioned, renal biopsy is recommended in atypical cases. Patients who do not respond to corticosteroids or who relapse frequently should be referred to a pediatric nephrologist.

Gregory MJ et al: Long-term cyclosporine therapy for pediatric nephrotic syndrome: A clinical and histologic analysis. J Am Soc Nephrol 1996;7:543.

Mendosa SA, Tune BM: Treatment of childhood nephrotic syndrome. J Am Soc Nephrol 1992;3:889.

FOCAL GLOMERULAR SCLEROSIS

Focal glomerular sclerosis is one cause of corticosteroid-resistant or frequent-relapsing nephrotic syndrome. The diagnosis is made by renal biopsy, which shows normal-appearing glomeruli as well as some partially or completely sclerosed glomeruli. The lesion has serious prognostic implications; as many as 15–20% of cases can progress to end-stage renal failure. The clinical response to treatment is variable; experience with cyclosporine shows some promise.

Ingulli E et al: Aggressive long-term cyclosporine therapy for steroid-resistant focal segmental glomerulosclerosis. J Am Soc Nephrol 1995;5:1820.

Ponticelli C et al: A randomized trial of cyclosporine in steroid-resistant idiopathic nephrotic syndrome. Kidney Int 1993;43:1377.

Wyszynska T et al: Evaluation of prednisolone pulse therapy in steroid-resistant nephrotic syndrome: A multicenter collaborative study. Contrib Nephrol 1988;67:183.

MESANGIAL NEPHROPATHY
(Mesangial Glomerulonephritis)

Mesangial nephropathy is another cause of corticosteroid-resistant nephrotic syndrome. The renal biopsy shows a distinct increase in the mesangial matrix of the glomeruli. Very often the expanded mesangium contains deposits of IgM demonstrated on immunofluorescent staining.

MEMBRANOUS NEPHROPATHY
(Membranous Glomerulonephritis)

Although largely idiopathic in nature, membranous nephropathy can be found in association with diseases such as hepatitis B antigenemia, systemic lupus erythematosus, congenital and secondary syphilis, and renal vein thrombosis; with immunologic disorders such as autoimmune thyroiditis; and with administration of drugs such as penicillamine. The pathogenesis is unknown, but it is thought that the glomerular lesion is the result of prolonged deposition of circulating antigen-antibody complexes.

The onset of membranous nephropathy may be insidious or may resemble that of idiopathic nephrotic syndrome of childhood (see previous text). It occurs more often in older children. The proteinuria of membranous nephropathy responds little if at all to corticosteroid therapy. Low-dose corticosteroid therapy, however, has been shown to reduce or delay development of chronic renal insufficiency. The diagnosis is made by renal biopsy.

Cameron JS: Membranous nephropathy in childhood and its treatment. Pediatr Nephrol 1990;4:193.

DISEASES OF THE RENAL VESSELS

RENAL VEIN THROMBOSIS

In the newborn period, renal vein thrombosis may suddenly complicate sepsis or dehydration. It may be observed in an infant of a diabetic mother, or it may be the result of umbilical vein catheterization. Renal vein thrombosis is less common in older children and adolescents; it may develop following trauma or without any apparent predisposing factors. Nephrotic syndrome may either cause or result from renal vein thrombosis. There may also be an underlying membranous glomerulonephropathy.

Clinical Findings

Renal vein thrombosis in newborns generally presents with the sudden development of an abdominal mass. If the thrombosis is bilateral, oliguria may be present; urine output may be normal with a unilateral thrombus. In older children, flank pain, sometimes with a palpable mass, is a common presentation.

No single laboratory test is diagnostic of renal vein thrombosis. Hematuria usually is present and occasionally is gross. Proteinuria is less constant. In the newborn, thrombocytopenia may be found; this is rare in older children. The diagnosis is made by ultrasonography and Doppler-flow studies.

Treatment

Anticoagulation with heparin is the treatment of choice both in newborns and in older children. In the newborn, a course of heparin combined with treatment of the underlying problem is usually all that is required. Management in other cases is less straightforward. The tendency for recurrence and embolization has led some workers in this field to recommend long-term anticoagulation. If an underlying membranous glomerulonephritis is suspected, biopsy should be performed.

Course & Prognosis

The mortality in newborns from renal vein thrombosis depends on the underlying cause. If the child survives the acute phase, the prognosis for adequate renal function is good. Renal vein thrombosis may recur in the same kidney or occur in the other kidney years after the original episode of thrombus formation. Extension into the vena cava, with fatal pulmonary emboli, is possible.

RENAL ARTERIAL DISEASE

Children may develop renovascular hypertension due to fibromuscular hyperplasia, congenital stenosis, or other renal arterial lesions. The proportion of children whose hypertension is due to these lesions is small. Unfortunately, there are few clinical clues to underlying arterial lesions. Nonetheless, arterial lesions should be suspected in children whose hypertension is severe, with onset at or below 10 years, or associated with delayed visualization on excretory urogram. The diagnosis is established by renal arteriography with selective renal vein renin measurements. Some of these lesions may be repaired surgically (see Hypertension in the following text) but repair may be technically impossible in many small children. Although thrombosis of renal arteries is rare, it should be considered in a patient with acute onset of hypertension and hematuria in an appropriate setting (eg, in association with hyperviscosity or umbilical artery catheterization). Early diagnosis and treatment (eg, heparin) provides the best chance of reestablishing renal blood flow.

HEMOLYTIC-UREMIC SYNDROME

Hemolytic-uremic syndrome is the commonest single cause of renal failure due to glomerular vascular injury in childhood. The glomerular damage is exacerbated by severe fluid imbalances during the gastrointestinal prodrome.

The cause of hemolytic-uremic syndrome is not well established, but epidemiologic studies have suggested both a genetic and an infectious or immunologic component. The primary lesion seems to be one of the endothelium of arterioles, especially in the kidney, with formation of platelet thrombi and resulting microangiopathic hemolysis. Recent data suggest that hemolytic-uremic syndrome involves a disorder of immunoregulation and that a unique class of anti-endothelial cell antibodies which may take part in the pathogenesis of the vascular injury is produced. However, the epidemic form of the disease in most cases is precipitated by *E coli* O157.

Clinical Findings
Hemolytic-uremic syndrome is most common under 2 years of age but is more severe in older children. It usually begins with a prodromal phase characterized by gastrointestinal symptoms, including abdominal pain, diarrhea, and vomiting. Oliguria, pallor, and bleeding manifestations, principally cutaneous and gastrointestinal, occur next. Hypertension and seizures develop in some infants, especially those who develop severe renal failure and fluid overload.

The triad of anemia, thrombocytopenia, and renal failure characterizes the syndrome. Anemia is pro-

found and is associated with red blood cell fragments on smear. A high reticulocyte count confirms the hemolytic nature of the anemia. The platelet count is almost invariably below 100,000/μL. Other coagulation abnormalities are less consistent. Serum fibrin split products are often present, but fulminant disseminated intravascular coagulation is rare. Hematuria is often present. The serum complement level is normal.

Complications
The complications of hemolytic-uremic syndrome usually result from renal failure. Neurologic problems, particularly seizures, may result from electrolyte abnormalities such as hyponatremia, hypertension, or central nervous system vascular disease. Severe bleeding, transfusion requirements, and complicating infections must be anticipated.

Treatment
Meticulous attention to fluid and electrolyte status is crucial. Early dialysis improves the prognosis; the size of the patient and the bleeding tendency will usually dictate peritoneal dialysis as the technique of choice. Seizures usually respond to control of hypertension and electrolyte abnormalities. It has been suggested that the plasma in some cases lacks a prostacyclin-stimulating factor, which is a potent inhibitor of platelet aggregation. Therefore, plasma infusion or plasmapheresis has been advocated in severe cases. Platelet inhibitors have also been tried, but the results have not been impressive, especially late in the disease. Nonetheless, it appears beneficial to use a platelet inhibitor early in the disease, which may obviate the need for platelet transfusion and has been observed to reduce, in some cases, the progression of renal failure. Red cell and platelet transfusions may be necessary; although the risk of volume overload is significant, it can be minimized by dialysis. Erythropoietin treatment may reduce red cell transfusion needs. While there is no universally accepted therapy for patients with this syndrome, the strict control of hypertension and nutrition and the use of dialysis appear to affect the long-term outcome. Renal failure may mandate dialysis.

Course & Prognosis
Geographic factors may determine the severity of hemolytic-uremic syndrome. Most commonly, children recover from the acute episode within 2–3 weeks, and follow-up reveals no residual renal insufficiency. However, some patients who recover from the acute episode have severe and occasionally progressive renal dysfunction or hypertension. Thus, follow-up of children recovering from hemolytic-uremic syndrome should include serial determinations of renal function for 1–2 years and meticulous attention to blood pressure for 5 years. Mortality in the

early phase from the complications of central nervous system disease or acute renal failure is low.

Kaplan BS et al: Recent advances in understanding the pathogenesis of the hemolytic uremic syndromes. Pediatr Nephrol 1990;4:276.

Rizzoni G et al: Plasma infusion for hemolytic-uremic syndrome in children: Results of a multicenter controlled trial. J Pediatr 1988;112:284.

Southwest Pediatric Nephrology Study Group: A clinicopathologic study of 24 children with hemolytic uremic syndrome. Pediatr Nephrol 1990;4:52.

Van Damme-Lombaerts J et al: Heparin plus dipyridamole in childhood hemolytic-uremic syndrome: A prospective, randomized study. J Pediatr 1988;113:913.

RENAL FAILURE

ACUTE RENAL FAILURE

Acute renal failure is the sudden inability to excrete urine of sufficient quantity or adequate composition to maintain body fluid homeostasis. It has many causes, including impaired renal perfusion, acute renal disease, renal ischemia, renal vascular compromise, or obstructive uropathy. Pre-renal, renal, and postrenal causes are shown in Table 22–2.

Table 22–2. Classifications of renal failure.

Prerenal
  Dehydration due to gastroenteritis, malnutrition, or diarrhea
  Hemorrhage, aortic or renal vessel injury, trauma, surgery, cardiac surgery, renal arterial thrombosis
  Diabetic acidosis
  Hypovolemia associated with capillary leak or nephrotic syndrome
  Shock
  Heart failure
Renal
  Hemolytic-uremic syndrome
  Acute glomerulonephritis
  Extension of prerenal hypoperfusion
  Nephrotoxins
  Acute tubular necrosis or vascular nephropathy
  Renal (cortical) necrosis
  Intravascular coagulation—septic shock, hemorrhage
  Diseases of the kidney and vessels
  Iatrogenic disorders
  Severe infections
  Drowning, especially fresh water
  Hyperuricacidemia from cancer treatment
Postrenal
  Obstruction due to tumor, hematoma, or the presence of posterior urethral valves or ureteropelvic junction stricture, ureterovesical junction stricture, ureterocele
  Crystaluria: sulfonamide or uric acid
  Stones
  Trauma to a solitary kidney or collecting system
  Renal vein thrombosis

Clinical Findings

The hallmark of early renal failure is oliguria. The initial approach to an oliguric child should be aimed at classifying the problem in one of the categories outlined in Table 22–2. Although an exact etiologic diagnosis is not necessary, accurate classification is helpful before initiating appropriate therapy.

If the cause of renal failure or oliguria is not clear, entities that can be treated (eg, volume depletion) should be considered first. After treatable problems or glomerular diseases are ruled out, a diagnosis of acute tubular necrosis (eg, vasomotor nephropathy, ischemic injury) may be entertained.

A. Postrenal Causes: Postrenal failure is found in newborns with anatomic abnormalities. Obstruction of the bladder outlet should be relieved by insertion of a urethral catheter, followed by surgical correction. Timely intervention may prevent irreversible renal injury and chronic renal failure. Delayed voiding in the newborn period, anuria, or poor urinary stream usually suggests obstruction. Ureteropelvic junctional obstruction usually presents as an abdominal mass. Obstructive uropathy is accompanied by variable degrees of renal insufficiency.

B. Prerenal Causes: The commonest cause of decreased renal function in children is compromised renal perfusion. It is usually secondary to dehydration, although abnormalities of renal vasculature and poor cardiac performance may also be considered. Possible secondary causes should be addressed and, if possible, eliminated in order to determine if true renal functional disturbances are present.

C. Renal Causes: The various acute glomerulonephritides, hemolytic-uremic syndrome, acute interstitial nephritis, and nephrotoxic injury are examples of "renal" entities that produce varying degrees of acute renal failure. The diagnosis of acute tubular necrosis or vasomotor nephropathy is considered in clinical situations where—with no evidence of specific renal parenchymal diseases—the elimination of any prerenal or postrenal factors produces no improvement in renal performance.

Table 22–3 lists the urinary indices that are helpful in distinguishing prerenal conditions from acute tubular necrosis.

Complications

The clinical severity of the complications depends on the degree of renal functional impairment and oliguria. Common complications include (1) fluid overload (hypertension, congestive heart failure, pulmonary edema), (2) electrolyte disturbances (hyperkalemia), (3) metabolic acidosis, (4) hyperphosphatemia, and (5) uremia.

Treatment

An indwelling catheter is inserted to monitor urine output. If urine volume is insignificant and renal failure is established, the catheter should be removed, as

Table 22–3. Urine studies.

Prerenal Failure	Acute Tubular Necrosis
Urine osmolality 50 mOsm/kg greater than plasma osmolality	Urine osmolality equal to or less than plasma osmolality
Urine sodium < 10 meq/L	Urinary sodium > 20 meq/L
Ratio of urine creatinine to plasma creatinine > 14:1	Ratio of urine creatinine to plasma creatinine < 14:1
Specific gravity > 1.020	Specific gravity 1.012–1.018

it will be more of a hazard than an aid. Prerenal or postrenal factors should be excluded or rectified and the circulating volume maintained with appropriate fluids. The patient's response is assessed by physical examination and observed urinary output. Measurement of central venous pressure may be indicated. If diuresis does not occur in response to the above measures, give furosemide, 1–5 mg/kg intravenously, the dose being higher with higher serum creatinine levels. Allow 1 hour for a response to occur. If the urine output remains low (< 200–250 mL/m^2/24 h), repeat the furosemide (up to 5 mg/kg). If no diuresis occurs, the further administration of diuretics will not be helpful.

If these maneuvers produce return of urine flow but biochemical evidence of acute renal failure persists, the resulting "nonoliguric" acute renal failure or acute tubular necrosis should be more manageable. Fluid overload and dialysis may be averted. However, if the medications and nutrients required exceed the urinary output, dialysis is indicated. Institution of dialysis before the early complications of acute renal failure develop is likely to improve clinical management and outcome.

A. Indications for Dialysis: The need for dialysis is determined on the basis of individuals' clinical findings. There are, however, some immediate indications for dialysis: (1) severe hyperkalemia; (2) unrelenting metabolic acidosis (usually in a situation where fluid overload prevents sodium bicarbonate administration); (3) fluid overload with or without severe hypertension or congestive heart failure (a situation that would seriously compromise caloric or drug administration); and (4) symptoms of uremia, usually manifested in children by central nervous system depression. The rate of rise of both blood urea nitrogen and serum creatinine levels may indicate the need for dialysis; it is generally accepted that the blood urea nitrogen level should not be allowed to exceed 100 mg/dL in small children.

B. Methods of Dialysis: The choice between peritoneal dialysis and hemodialysis may be dictated by their availability. Peritoneal dialysis is generally preferred in children because of the ease of performance and patient tolerance. Although peritoneal dialysis is technically less efficient than hemodialy-sis, hemodynamic stability and metabolic control can be better sustained because this technique can be applied on a relatively continuous basis. However, hemodialysis should be considered if: (1) rapid removal of toxins is desired; (2) the size of the patient makes hemodialysis less technically cumbersome and hemodynamically well-tolerated; or (3) impediments to efficient peritoneal dialysis are present (eg, ileus).

C. Complications of Dialysis: Complications of peritoneal dialysis include peritonitis, volume depletion, and such technical complications as dialysate leakage or respiratory compromise from intra-abdominal dialysate fluid. Peritonitis can be avoided by strict adherence to aseptic technique. Peritoneal fluid cultures are obtained as clinically indicated. Dialysate can leak around the dialysis catheter or through tissue planes, causing dissection. Leakage is reduced by good catheter placement technique and appropriate intra-abdominal dialysate volumes. Any technical problems that result in abnormal flow of dialysate in and out of the peritoneal cavity require the attention of the nephrology consultant. Dialysis is useful in maintaining electrolyte balance; because potassium is absent from standard dialysate solutions, potassium may be added to the dialysate as clinically indicated. Phosphate is also absent because hyperphosphatemia is an expected problem in renal failure. Nonetheless, if phosphate intake is inadequate, it is important not to cause hypophosphatemia by dialysis. High dextrose concentrations (maximum 4.25%) can correct fluid overload rapidly at the risk of causing hyperglycemia. Fluid removal may be increased with more frequent exchanges of the dialysate but rapid osmotic transfer of water may result in hypernatremia.

Even in small infants, hemodialysis can rapidly correct major metabolic and electrolyte disturbances, as well as volume overload. The process is highly efficient, but the speed of the changes can cause such problems as hemodynamic instability. Anticoagulation is usually required, but may entail minimal exposure to the risks of heparin administration. Careful monitoring by experienced personnel of the appropriate biochemical parameters is important. Note that during or immediately following the procedure, blood sampling will produce misleading results because equilibration between extravascular compartments and the blood will not yet have been completed.

Continuous arteriovenous devices (eg, subclavian catheters) must be inspected for thrombotic or infectious complications. Continuous ambulatory peritoneal dialysis (CAPD) and continuous cycling peritoneal dialysis (CCPD) are both extremely useful for children. These methods carry the advantages of simple application in the home setting and avoidance of the vascular access problems inherent with chronic hemodialysis. Although renal transplantation is the ultimate goal for most children with end-stage renal failure, improvement in dialysis has greatly simplified their long-term management.

Course & Prognosis

The period of severe oliguria, if it occurs, usually lasts about 10 days. Oliguria lasting longer than 3 weeks, or complete anuria, makes a diagnosis of acute tubular necrosis very unlikely; vascular injury, severe ischemia (cortical necrosis), glomerulonephritis, or obstruction is more probable. The diuretic phase begins with an increase in urinary output to the passage of large volumes of isosthenuric urine containing sodium levels of 80–150 meq/L. During the recovery phase, signs and symptoms subside rapidly, although polyuria may persist for several days or weeks. Urinary abnormalities usually disappear completely within a few months.

CHRONIC RENAL FAILURE

Chronic renal failure in children most commonly results from developmental abnormalities of the kidneys or urinary tract. The kidneys may develop poorly (hypoplasia, dysplasia) or not at all (aplasia). Cystic development may result in immediate or progressive insufficiency. Abnormal development of the urinary tract may not permit normal renal development. Depending, however, on the degree of interference with normal renal parenchymal development, timely surgery may minimize parenchymal injury and perhaps even achieve totally normal function. In older children, the chronic glomerulonephritides and nephropathies, irreversible nephrotoxic injury, or hemolytic-uremic syndrome may also result in chronic renal failure.

When chronic renal failure is the result of an inadequate amount of normally functioning renal tissue, the clinical presentation is with polyuria, polydipsia, or enuresis. Depending on the degree of renal insufficiency, failure to thrive may be the chief concern. Renal failure due to abnormalities of the collecting system may follow unrecognized urinary tract infection. Progressive deterioration of renal function may occur in the absence of infection. Without appropriate health maintenance children may present with overt complications of long-standing chronic renal failure, such as rickets or growth delay.

Chronic renal failure resulting from glomerulonephritis usually presents as progressive oliguria. Growth failure depends on age at presentation and the rapidity of functional decline. Some of the chronic glomerulonephritides (eg, membranoproliferative glomerulonephritis) can progress unnoticed if subtle abnormalities of the urinary sediment are undetected or ignored. Any child with a history of chronic glomerulonephritis or significant renal injury needs close follow-up and monitoring of renal function. The use of angiotensin-converting enzyme (ACE) inhibitors has been shown to be useful in decreasing the glomerulosclerosis that occurs after glomerular injury.

Complications

Despite the kidney's ability to compensate for gradual loss of functioning nephrons in chronic renal failure progression, there are resulting complications that are expected early as well as those that occur toward end-stage renal disease (GFR < 15 mL/min/1.73 m^2); at this point, the compensatory capability is exhausted. In children who have developmentally reduced function but who are unable to concentrate the urine, polyuria and thus dehydration is more likely to be a problem than fluid overload. As renal homeostatic capability approaches end-stage, there may be a reduction in output; however, many such children can continue to produce generous quantities of urine (but not of "good quality"), even when renal replacement therapies are initiated. Moreover, a "salt-wasting" state can occur. On the other hand, children who develop chronic renal failure due to the glomerular disease will characteristically have difficulty with sodium and water retention and hypertension relatively early in the course of chronic renal failure.

Other early manifestations of chronic renal failure include metabolic acidosis and growth retardation. Disturbances in calcium, phosphorus, and vitamin D metabolism leading to renal osteodystrophy require prompt attention. Although renal compensation and increased parathyroid hormone can maintain a normal serum phosphate early in the course, this is offset by tertiary hyperparathyroidism with resulting skeletal abnormalities. This can be reflected early by an increase in serum alkaline phosphatase.

Overt uremic symptoms are late manifestations of chronic renal failure. If left unchecked, chronic renal failure eventually adversely affects every organ system. The subjective symptoms of uremia are anorexia, nausea, and lethargy. Children display failure to thrive. Central nervous system manifestations of the condition range from subtle changes to confusion, apathy, and lethargy. These symptoms usually occur late in the course of disease and may be unsuspected clinically until the patient is carefully evaluated. With advancing uremia, stupor and coma may be present. Associated electrolyte abnormalities (eg, hyponatremia) may precipitate seizures (more commonly, a result of untreated hypertension).

Anemia is usual in chronic renal failure. It is usually normochromic and normocytic and results from decreased renal erythropoietin synthesis as renal parenchyma atrophies. Platelet dysfunction and other abnormalities of the coagulation system may be present. Bleeding phenomena, especially gastrointestinal bleeding, may be a problem.

Cardiovascular manifestations may be life-threatening. Uremic pericarditis may develop. Congestive heart failure or hypertension may be seen with volume overload, excessive renin excretion, or both. Patients with chronic renal failure tend to be more susceptible to infections.

Treatment

The aim of treatment in chronic renal failure prior to dialysis is to preserve any remaining renal function and to minimize the aforementioned complications.

Controlling hypertension (see Treatment of Hypertension), hyperphosphatemia, and urinary tract infection contribute greatly toward this endeavor. Acidosis may be treated with sodium citrate solutions, provided the added sodium will not aggravate hypertension. Hyperphosphatemia is controlled by dietary restriction and the use of dietary phosphate binders (eg, calcium carbonate). Vitamin D should be administered to maintain normal serum calcium. When the blood urea nitrogen exceeds approximately 50 mg/dL, or if the child is lethargic or anorexic, dietary protein restriction should be initiated. Sodium restriction is advisable when hypertension is present. Potassium restriction will be necessary as the GFR falls to a level where urinary output decreases sharply. Meanwhile, the diet must continue to meet the child's specific daily requirements.

Renal function must be regularly monitored (creatinine and blood urea nitrogen), as well as serum electrolytes, calcium, phosphorus, and alkaline phosphatase. Results guide changes in dietary management as well as adjustment in phosphate binder, citrate buffer, vitamin D, fluid intake, and blood pressure medications. Anemia may be treated with erythropoietin. All of these areas require careful monitoring to minimize symptomatology while continuing to assess the need for chronic dialysis and transplantation.

Caution must be taken to avoid medications that (1) aggravate the uremic condition (eg, tetracyclines, which increase blood urea); (2) depend on renal excretion (eg, compounds containing magnesium); (3) raise blood pressure (eg, over-the-counter cold preparations containing vasoconstrictive agents); or (4) contain high amounts of substances of particular concern in the management of chronic renal failure (eg, sodium, potassium, and phosphate). Successful management relies greatly upon the education of patient and family.

Attention must also be directed to the psychosocial needs of the patient and family during adjustment to chronic illness. The strategy for patient management, and the need for family education and adjustment, changes when a plan for chronic dialysis and possible renal transplantation is initiated. These changes may include a reduction in medications or dietary limitations, with the potential for improving growth. Significant growth acceleration has been of concern with the use of human recombinant growth hormone in some uremic children.

Dialysis & Transplantation

The method of treatment of end-stage renal disease best tolerated by the child is a successful and uncomplicated renal transplant. The North American Pediatric Renal Transplant Collaborative Study reports a 1-year graft survival of living-related kidney transplants of 90% with 85% at 2 years and 75% at 5 years. With cadaveric transplantation, percentages of graft survivals are 76, 71, and 62 respectively. Overall, mortality is 4% for recipients of living-related donors, and 6.8% for recipients of cadaver donors. These percentages are affected by the increased mortality, which has been reported to be as high as 75%, in infants under 1 year of age. Most transplantation centers are waiting until infants reach about 15 kg. This appears to be associated with a significantly improved survival rate. Adequate growth and well-being are directly related to acceptance of the graft, the degree of normal function, and the side effects of medications employed.

Great advances have also been made in peritoneal dialysis and hemodialysis, both in technique and in our understanding of the specialized approach required. Hemodialysis is now performed in major centers that devote their entire effort to the management of pediatric patients, and is regarded as a reasonable long-range method of treating the child with end-stage renal disease. The demonstrated feasibility of chronic peritoneal dialysis in children, however, has made it the primary choice of dialysis therapy for children. It is well accepted and can be performed in the home.

The best measure of the success of chronic dialysis in children is the level of physical and psychosocial rehabilitation achieved. Patients continue to participate in day-to-day activities and attend school. Although catch-up growth rarely occurs, patients can grow at an acceptable rate even though they may remain in the lower percentiles. Use of erythropoietin, growth hormone, and better control of renal osteodystrophy contribute to improved outcome.

Fine RN et al: Recombinant human growth hormone in infants and young children with chronic renal insufficiency. Pediatr Nephrol 1995;9:451.

McEnery PT et al: Renal transplantation in children: A report of the North American Pediatric Renal Transplant Cooperative study. N Engl J Med 1992;326:1721.

Maschio G et al: Effect of the angiotensin-converting enzyme of chronic renal insufficiency. N Engl J Med 1996;334:939.

Nakano M et al: Protein intake and renal function in children. Am J Dis Child 1989;143:160.

RENAL HYPERTENSION

Hypertension in children is commonly of renal origin. It is anticipated as a complication of known renal parenchymal disease, but it may be found on routine physical examination in an otherwise normal child. Increased understanding of the roles of water and salt retention on the one hand and overactivity of the renin-angiotensin system on the other has done much to guide therapy; it is nevertheless clear that not all forms of hypertension can be explained by these two mechanisms.

The causes of hypertension in the newborn period include (1) congenital anomalies of the kidneys or renal vasculature; (2) obstruction of the urinary tract; (3) thrombosis of renal vasculature or kidneys; and (4) volume overload. There are also reported instances of apparent paradoxical elevations of blood pressure in clinical situations in which chronic diuretic therapy is used, such as in bronchopulmonary dysplasia. Hypertensive infants should also be examined for renal, vascular, or aortic abnormalities (eg, thrombosis, neurofibromatosis, coarctation), as well as some endocrine disorders.

Diagnosis

A child is normotensive if the average recorded systolic and diastolic blood pressures are lower than the 90th percentile for age and sex. The 90th percentile in the newborn period is approximately 85–90/55–65 mm Hg for both sexes. In the first year of life, the acceptable levels are 90–100/60–67 mm Hg. Incremental increases with growth occur, gradually approaching young adult ranges of 100–120/65–75 mm Hg in the late teens. Careful measurement of the blood pressure includes ensuring correct cuff size and reliable equipment. The cuff should be wide enough to cover two-thirds of the upper arm and should encircle the arm completely without causing an overlap in the inflatable bladder. Although an anxious child may have an elevation in blood pressure, abnormal readings must not be too hastily attributed to this cause. Repeat measurement is helpful, especially after the child has been consoled.

Routine laboratory studies include a complete blood count, urinalysis, and urine culture. Radiography and ultrasonography are used to study the anatomy of the urinary tract, the blood flow to the kidneys, and their function. A renal biopsy (which rarely reveals the cause of hypertension unless there is clinical evidence of renal disease) should always be undertaken with special care in the hypertensive patient and preferably after pressures have been controlled by therapy. A suggested approach to the outpatient work-up is shown in Figure 22–3.

Treatment

A. Treatment of Acute Emergent Hypertension: A hypertensive emergency may be said to exist when central nervous system signs of hypertension appear, such as papilledema or encephalopathy. Retinal hemorrhages or exudates indicate a need for prompt and effective control. It is common in children, however, to see no end-organ abnormalities secondary to hypertension. Treatment varies with the clinical presentation. The primary classes of useful antihypertensive drugs are (1) diuretics, (2) alpha- and beta-adrenergic blockers, (3) angiotensin-converting enzyme (ACE) inhibitors, (4) calcium channel blockers, and (5) vasodilators.

1. Sublingual nifedipine, a calcium channel blocker, is rapid-acting and in appropriate doses should not result in hypotensive blood pressure levels. The liquid from a 10-mg capsule can be withdrawn with a syringe, and dosage approximated. The exact dosage for children who weigh less than 10–30 kg is difficult to ascertain by this method, but 5 mg is a safe starting point. Because the treatment is directed at emergent levels of blood pressure, it is unlikely that the effects will be greater than desired. Larger children with malignant hypertension require 10 mg. In such cases, the capsule may simply be pierced and the medication squeezed under the patient's tongue.

2. Intravenous hydralazine can be effective in some cases. Dosage varies according to the severity of the hypertension and should begin at around 0.15 mg/kg.

3. Sodium nitroprusside is also effective in an intensive care setting for reducing severely elevated blood pressure. Intravenous administration of 0.5–10 μg/kg/min will reduce blood pressure in seconds, but the dose must be carefully monitored.

4. Furosemide, 1–5 mg/kg intravenously, will reduce blood volume and enhance the effectiveness of other drugs.

Whatever method is used to control emergent hypertension, medications for sustained control should also be initiated so that the effect will be maintained when the emergent measures are discontinued (Table 22–4).

Acute elevations of blood pressure not exceeding the 95th percentile for age may be approached with oral medication, and measures should be aimed at progressive improvement and control within 48 hours.

B. Treatment of Sustained Hypertension: There are several choices in antihypertensive medication (Table 22–5). A single drug such as a beta-blocker may be adequate in mild hypertension, unless this is contraindicated (eg, in reactive airway disease). Diuretics are useful in renal insufficiency, but disadvantages of possible electrolyte imbalance must be considered. Single-drug therapy with an ACE inhibitor is useful, especially since most hyper-

Figure 22–3. Approach to the outpatient workup of hypertension.

tension in children has renal causes. Specialist advice is recommended when drug combinations are needed.

The use of the vasodilator type of antihypertensive drug requires concomitant administration of a diuretic to counter the effect of vasodilation on increasing renal sodium and water retention and a beta-blocker to counter reflex tachycardia. Minoxidil, considered the most powerful of the orally administered vasodilators, can be extremely efficacious in the treatment of severe, sustained hypertension, but its effect is greatly offset by the other effects described. Hirsutism is a significant side effect. Hydralazine hydrochloride may still be the most common vasodilator in pediatric use, but, again, the

necessity of using two additional drugs for maximum benefit keeps vasodilators in reserve for those severe situations that mandate the intervention of three or four drugs.

Bandel-Stenzel M, Najarian JS, Sinaiko AR: Renal artery stenosis in infants: Long-term medical treatment before surgery. Pediatr Nephrol 1996;10:147.

Hanna JD, Chan JCM, Gill JR Jr: Hypertension and the kidney. J Pediatr 1991;118:327.

Ingelfinger JR: Investigating hypertension in children. Nephrol News Issues (Feb) 1989;3:29.

Sinaiko AR: Treatment of hypertension in children. Pediatr Nephrol 1994;8:603.

Table 22–4. Antihypertensive drugs for emergent treatment.

Drug	Oral Dose	Major Side Effects[1]
Nifedipine	0.25–0.5 mg/kg/ SL	Flushing, tachycardia
Labetalol	1–3 mg/kg/h IV	Secondary to beta-blocking activity
Sodium nitroprusside	0.5–10 mg/kg/min IV drip	Cyanide toxicity, sodium and water retention
Furosemide	1–5 mg/kg IV	Secondary to severe volume contraction, hypokalemia
Diazoxide	2–10 mg/kg IV bolus	Hyperglycemia, hyperuricemia, sodium and water retention
Hydralazine	0.1–0.2 mg/kg IV	Sodium and water retention, tachycardia, flushing

[1]Many more side effects than those listed have been reported.

Table 22–5. Antihypertensive drugs for ambulatory treatment.

Drug	Oral Dose	Major Side Effects[1]
Hydrochloro-thiazide	2–4 mg/kg/24 h as single dose or in 2 individual doses	Potassium depletion, hyperuricemia.
Furosemide	1–5 mg/kg/dose, 2–3 doses per day	Potassium and volume depletion.
Hydralazine	0.75 mg/kg/24 h in 4–6 divided doses	Lupus erythematosus, tachycardia, headache.
Methyldopa	10–40 mg/kg/24 h in 3 divided doses	False-positive Coombs test, hemolytic anemia, fever, leukopenia, abnormal liver function tests.
Propranolol	0.2–5 mg/kg/dose, 2–3 doses per day	Syncope, cardiac failure, hypoglycemia.
Minoxidil	0.15 mg/kg/dose, 2–3 doses per day	Tachycardia, angina, fluid retention, hirsutism.
Captopril	0.3–2 mg/kg/dose, 2–3 doses per day	Rash, hyperkalemia, glomerulopathy.
Enalapril	0.2–0.5 mg/kg/d in 2 divided doses	Proteinuria, cough, hyperkalemia.
Nifedipine	0.5–1 mg/kg/d, 3 doses per day	Flushing, tachycardia.
Verapamil	3–7 mg/kg/d in 2 or 3 divided doses	AV conduction disturbance.

[1]Many more side effects than those listed have been reported.

INHERITED OR DEVELOPMENTAL DEFECTS OF THE URINARY TRACT

There are many developmental, hereditary, or metabolic abnormalities of the kidneys and collecting system. Their clinical consequences include metabolic abnormalities, failure to thrive, nephrolithiasis, renal glomerular or tubular dysfunction, and chronic renal failure. Table 22–6 lists some of the major entities by etiology; discussion of the rarer conditions is beyond the scope of this book.

DISORDERS OF THE RENAL TUBULES

Three subtypes of renal tubular acidosis are well recognized: (1) the "classic" form, called type I or distal renal tubular acidosis; (2) the bicarbonate "wasting" form, designated as type II or proximal renal tubular acidosis; and (3) type IV, or hyperkalemic renal tubular acidosis (rare in children), which is associated with hyporeninemic hypoaldosteronism. Type I and type II and their variants are encountered most frequently in children.

Primary tubular disorders in childhood, such as glycinuria, hypouricemia, or renal glycosuria, may result from a defect in a single tubular transport pathway (Table 22–6).

DISTAL RENAL TUBULAR ACIDOSIS (TYPE I)

The most common form of distal renal tubular acidosis in childhood is the hereditary form. The clinical presentation is one of failure to thrive, anorexia, vomiting, and dehydration. Hyperchloremic metabolic acidosis occurs, with hypokalemia and a urinary pH exceeding 6.5. The acidosis is more severe in the presence of a bicarbonate "leak." This variant of distal renal tubular acidosis with bicarbonate wasting has been called type III but for clinical purposes need not be considered as a distinct entity. Concomitant hypercalciuria may lead to rickets, nephrocalcinosis, nephrolithiasis, and renal failure.

Other situations that may be responsible for distal renal tubular acidosis are listed in Table 22–6.

Table 22–6. Inherited or developmental defects of the urinary tract.

Cystic diseases of genetic origin
Polycystic disease
  Autosomal recessive form (infantile)
  Autosomal dominant form (adult)
  Other syndromes that include either form
Cortical cysts
  Several syndromes are known to have various renal cystic manifestations, including "simple" cysts; may not have significant effect on renal functional status nor be associated with progressive disease
Medullary cysts
  Medullary sponge kidney
  Medullary cystic disease (nephronophthisis)
Hereditary and familial cystic dysplasia
  Congenital nephrosis
  "Finnish" disease
Dysplastic renal diseases
Renal aplasia (unilateral, bilateral)
Renal hypoplasia (unilateral, bilateral, total, segmental)
Multicystic renal dysplasia (eg, unilateral, bilateral, multiocular, postobstructive)
Familial and hereditary renal dysplasias
Oligomeganephronia
Hereditary diseases associated with nephritis
Hereditary nephritis with deafness and ocular defects (Alport's syndrome)
Nail-patella syndrome
Familial hyperprolinemia
Hereditary nephrotic syndrome
Hereditary osteolysis with nephropathy
Hereditary nephritis with thoracic asphyxiant dystrophy syndrome
Hereditary diseases associated with intrarenal deposition of metabolites
Angiokeratoma corporis diffusum (Fabry's disease)
Heredopathia atactica polyneuritiformis (Refsum's disease)
Various storage diseases (eg, G_{M1} monosialogangliosidosis, Hurler's syndrome, Niemann-Pick disease, familial metachromatic leukodystrophy, glycogenosis type I [von Gierke's disease], glycogenosis type II [Pompe's disease])
Hereditary amyloidosis (familial Mediterranean fever; heredofamilial urticaria with deafness and neuropathy; primary familial amyloidosis with polyneuropathy)
Hereditary renal diseases associated with tubular transport defects
Hartnup disease
Immunoglycinuria
Fanconi's syndrome
Oculocerebrorenal syndrome of Lowe
Cystinosis (infantile, adolescent, adult types)
Wilson's disease
Galactosemia
Hereditary fructose intolerance
Renal tubular acidosis (many types)
Hereditary tyrosinemia
Renal glycosuria
Vitamin D-resistant rickets
Pseudohypoparathyroidism
Vasopressin-resistant diabetes insipidus
Hypouricemia
Hereditary diseases associated with lithiasis
Hyperoxaluria
L-Glyceric aciduria
Xanthinuria
Lesch-Nyhan syndrome and variants, gout
Nephropathy due to familial hyperparathyroidism
Cystinuria (types I, II, III)
Glycinuria
Miscellaneous
Hereditary intestinal vitamin B_{12} malabsorption
Total and partial lipodystrophy
Sickle cell anemia
Bartter's syndrome

Distal renal tubular acidosis appears to result from a defect in the distal nephron, in the tubular transport of hydrogen ion, or in the maintenance of a steep enough gradient for proper excretion of hydrogen ion. This defect can be accompanied by degrees of bicarbonate wasting, or the defect may not be severe enough to lead to frank acidosis.

The classic method for determining the ability to handle an acid load in suspected distal renal tubular acidosis is the administration of NH_4Cl.

Acid load testing is cumbersome to perform and could produce severe acidosis. A clinical trial of alkali administration should be used to rule out proximal (type II) renal tubular acidosis. The dose of alkali required to achieve a normal plasma HCO_3^- concentration in patients with distal renal tubular acidosis is low (seldom exceeds 2–3 meq/kg/24 h) in contrast to that required in proximal renal tubular acidosis (> 10 meq/kg/24 h). Higher doses are, however, needed if distal renal tubular acidosis is accompanied by bicarbonate wasting. Alkali therapy can result in reduced complications and improved growth.

Distal renal tubular acidosis is usually a permanent disorder, although it sometimes occurs as a secondary complication. If renal damage is prevented, the prognosis is good.

PROXIMAL RENAL TUBULAR ACIDOSIS (TYPE II)

Proximal renal tubular acidosis is characterized by an alkaline urine pH, loss of bicarbonate in the urine, and mildly reduced serum bicarbonate concentrations. About 85–90% of bicarbonate reabsorption occurs in the proximal tubules. The lesion in proximal renal tubular acidosis is a lowering of the renal bicarbonate threshold, ie, the concentration of serum bicarbonate above which bicarbonate appears in the urine. With more severe acidosis, the concentration of serum bicarbonate drops and bicarbonate disappears from the urine; this reflects normal distal tubular acidification.

The proximal type is the most common type of renal tubular acidosis encountered in children. It is often an isolated defect, and in the newborn infant, it can be considered an aspect of renal immaturity. Onset in infants is accompanied by failure to thrive, hyperchloremic acidosis, hypokalemia, and, rarely, nephrocalcinosis. Secondary forms result from reflux or obstructive uropathy and are seen in association with other tubular disorders (Table 22–6).

As previously described, the amount of alkali required to correct acidosis may aid in distinguishing the proximal (requires > 3 meq/kg of alkali per day) from the distal type. Monitor serum bicarbonate weekly until a level of at least 20 meq/L is attained.

The available forms of bicarbonate therapy that are somewhat more easily tolerated than sodium bicarbonate are the citrate solutions (eg, Bicitra, Poly-citra). Bicitra contains 1 meq of Na^+ and citrate per milliliter. Polycitra contains 2 meq per milliliter of citrate and 1 each of Na^+ and K^+. The required daily dosage is given in three divided doses. Potassium supplementation may be required, because the added sodium load presenting to the distal tubule may exaggerate potassium losses.

In cases of isolated defects, especially where the problem is related to renal immaturity, the prognosis is excellent. Alkali therapy can usually be discontinued after several months to 2 years. Growth should be normal, and the gradual increase in the serum bicarbonate level to above 22 meq/L heralds the presence of a raised bicarbonate threshold in the tubules. If the defect is part of a more complex tubular abnormality (Fanconi's syndrome with attendant phosphaturia, glycosuria, and amino aciduria), the prognosis depends on the underlying disorder or syndrome.

OCULOCEREBRORENAL SYNDROME
(Lowe's Syndrome)

Lowe's syndrome has been described in males only and is therefore thought to be transmitted as an X-linked recessive gene leading to anomalies involving the eyes, brain, and kidneys. The physical stigmas and the degree of mental retardation are variable. In addition to congenital cataracts and buphthalmos, the typical facies includes prominent epicanthal folds, frontal prominence, and a tendency to scaphocephaly. Muscle hypotonia is a prominent finding. The incidence of hypophosphatemic rickets is variable; it is characterized by low serum phosphorus levels, low to normal serum calcium levels, elevated serum alkaline phosphatase levels, renal tubular acidosis, and aminoaciduria. Treatment includes alkali therapy, phosphate replacement, and vitamin D. Mothers of affected males have punctate lens opacities.

CONGENITAL HYPOKALEMIC ALKALOSIS
(Bartter's Syndrome)

Bartter's syndrome is characterized by severe hypokalemic, hypochloremic metabolic alkalosis; extremely high levels of circulating renin and aldosterone; and a paradoxic absence of hypertension. On renal biopsy, there is a striking juxtaglomerular hyperplasia. Most patients present in early infancy with severe failure to thrive.

The cause and pathogenesis are not known. The pathogenesis is thought to be related to sodium reabsorption defects in the proximal or distal tubule. Studies have associated elevated levels of prostaglandins with the syndrome, and treatment with in-

hibitors of prostaglandin (eg, indomethacin) has been advocated. A prostaglandin-independent chloride-reabsorptive defect has been proposed.

Treatment with prostaglandin inhibitors and potassium-conserving diuretics (eg, amiloride combined with magnesium supplements) and potassium may be beneficial. Although the prognosis is guarded, a few patients seem to have less severe forms of the disease that are compatible with long survival.

CYSTINOSIS

Three types of cystinosis have been identified: adult, adolescent, and infantile. The adult type is a relatively benign condition characterized by cystine deposition in the corneas, granulocytes, and fibroblasts but no renal disease. The adolescent type is also characterized by cystine deposition but is accompanied by the development of mild renal failure with Fanconi's syndrome during adolescence; growth is normal. The infantile type is both the most common and the most severe. Characteristically, children present in the first or second year of life with Fanconi's syndrome.

Cystinosis is an autosomal recessive condition. The exact biochemical nature of the disease remains obscure. Cystine is stored in cellular lysosomes in virtually all tissues—the consequence of a now-recognized lysosomal cystine afflux transport system. Eventually, cystine accumulation results in cell damage and cell death, particularly in the renal tubules. Renal failure between ages 6 and 12 is common.

Whenever the diagnosis of cystinosis is suspected, slit-lamp examination of the corneas should be performed, since cystine crystal deposition causes an almost pathognomonic ground-glass "dazzle" appearance. Increased white cell cystine levels are diagnostic. Hypothyroidism is common.

Phosphocysteamine therapy is giving good results in the treatment of cystinosis. Depending on the progression of chronic renal failure, management is directed toward all side effects of renal failure with particular attention being paid to the control of renal osteodystrophy. Dialysis and transplantation may be needed.

Markello TC, Bernadini IM, Gahl WA: Improved renal function in children with cystinosis treated with cysteamine. N Engl J Med 1993;328:1157.

PHOSPHATE-LOSING RENAL TUBULAR SYNDROMES & OTHER FORMS OF RICKETS

Recent investigation of the metabolic products of vitamin D_3 has done much to clarify the causes of various forms of rickets. Those forms due primarily to a lack of available calcium are described in Chapter 11. They include idiopathic hypercalciuria, in which there is low calcium intake or excessive urinary calcium loss; lack of vitamin D_3 because of low dietary intake or from steatorrhea; and vitamin D dependency and azotemic rickets. In vitamin D_3 dependency, there is an inborn or acquired inability to synthesize 1,25-dihydroxycholecalciferol (the calcium transport stimulating factor, type I), or there may be end-organ insensitivity to this factor (type II). Treatment consists of giving supplementary calcium or vitamin D in appropriate doses.

Diseases associated with decreased availability of phosphorus also cause rickets. Excessive use of antacids may be responsible. Most commonly, the defect is an inherited or acquired one in which a defect of phosphorus reabsorption is variably associated with other transport defects (eg, Fanconi's syndrome). Certain generalized metabolic diseases—notably Wilson's disease, galactosemia, fructose intolerance, and cystinosis—may cause similar tubular damage. Treatment of the primary type is to give extra phosphorus. Treatment of the acquired forms is that of the basic disease.

Familial hypophosphatemic vitamin D-resistant rickets is an example of a tubular nephropathy in which only phosphorus transport is affected. Most patients present during the second year of life, but some conditions occur in the first 6 months.

Clinical features vary. Changes may be only biochemical, with a strikingly low serum phosphorus level and an elevated alkaline phosphatase level. Muscle hypotonia may be severe; growth failure, bowing of the legs, and enlargement of the wrists, knees, and costochondral junctions are often associated with spinal deformities. Craniosynostosis has been described in infants with this disease. Pathologic fractures may be seen on x-ray, as well as certain unique findings consisting of an irregular mosaic formation of the haversian system and trabecular "halos" of low-density bone.

In most cases, the serum phosphorus level is less than 2 mg/dL. The urinary calcium level is low, and the serum calcium level may be normal or slightly low. Serum levels of 1,25-dihydroxycholecalciferol are low, probably because high levels of phosphate in the tubule cell shut off the 1α-hydroxylase activity. Aminoaciduria is rare.

Treatment consists of giving 1–3 g of phosphorus daily either as a buffered monosodium and disodium hydrogen phosphate solution at pH 7.4 or as Fleet's Phospho-Soda. Magnesium oxide, 10–15 mg/kg/d by mouth, may be of value. Supplementary calcitriol, up to 40 mg/kg/d, should be given if the serum calcium levels remain below normal.

Normal growth is never achieved unless every effort is made to keep the serum phosphorus level over 3 mg/dL.

NEPHROLITHIASIS

Renal calculi in children may result from certain inborn errors of metabolism, such as cystine in cystinosis, glycine in hyperglycinuria, urates in Lesch-Nyhan syndrome, and oxalates in oxalosis. Stones may occur secondary to hypercalciuria in distal tubular acidosis, and large stones are quite often seen in children with spina bifida who have paralyzed lower limbs. Treatment is limited to that of the primary condition, if possible. Surgical removal of stones should be considered only for obstruction, intractable severe pain, and chronic infection.

Cystinuria

Cystinuria, like Hartnup's disease and a number of other disorders, is primarily an abnormality of amino acid transport across both the enteric and proximal renal tubular epithelium. There appear to be at least three biochemical types. In the first type, the bowel transport of basic amino acids and cystine is impaired, but transport of cysteine is not impaired. In the renal tubule, basic amino acids are again rejected by the tubule, but cystine absorption into kidney slices in vitro seems to be normal. The reasons for the cystinuria are, therefore, still obscure. Heterozygotes have no aminoaciduria. The second type is similar to the first, except that the heterozygotes excrete excess cystine and lysine in the urine, and cystine transport in the bowel is normal. In the third type, only the nephron is involved.

The only clinical manifestations relate to stone formation. These include ureteral colic, dysuria, hematuria, proteinuria, and secondary urinary tract infection. The urinary excretion of cystine, lysine, arginine, and ornithine is increased.

The most reliable way to prevent stone formation is to maintain a constantly high free water clearance. This involves a water intake of about 400 mL/m^2 every 4 hours night and day. If this is not effective, treatment with sodium bicarbonate, 6 g/m^2/d, should also be given. Such measures will certainly prevent increases in stone formation and very often lead to dissolution.

Operative removal of the stone may occasionally be required. Penicillamine in doses of 1000–1500 mg/m^2/d will also decrease cystine excretion and bring about partial or complete dissolution of stones.

Primary Hyperoxaluria

Oxalate production in humans is derived from the oxidative deamination of glycine to glyoxalate (about 40%), from the serine-glycolate pathway (about 50%), and from ascorbic acid. At least two enzymatic blocks have been described. Type 1 is a deficiency of liver-specific peroxisomal alanine:glyoxylate aminotransferase. Type 2 is glyoxalate reductase deficiency.

Excess oxalate combines with calcium to form insoluble deposits in the kidneys, lungs, and other tissues. The onset is during childhood. The joints are occasionally involved, but the main impact is on the kidneys, where progressive oxalate deposition leads to fibrosis and eventual renal failure.

Pyridoxine supplementation and a low-oxalate diet have been tried as therapy, but the overall prognosis is poor, and most patients succumb to uremia by early adulthood. Renal transplantation is not very successful, due to the destruction of the transplant kidney. However, there are encouraging results with concomitant liver transplantation correcting the metabolic defect. Calcium carbamide, 1 mg/kg/24 h, has been tried as an inhibitor of the serine-glycolate pathway of oxalate production and was shown to substantially diminish oxalate excretion in type 1 oxalosis. The use of methylene blue has also been reported.

Hyperoxaluria may also occur secondary to ileal disease or after ileal resection.

Coe FL, Parks JH, Asplin JR: The pathogenesis and treatment of kidney stones. N Engl J Med 1992;327:1721.

Leumann E, Hoppe B, Neuhaus T: Management of primary hyperoxaluria: Efficacy of oral citrate administration. Pediatr Nephrol 1993;7:207.

NEPHROGENIC DIABETES INSIPIDUS

In the normal kidney, the interstitial fluid of the papilla is hyperosmolar to the fluid in the collecting duct. The luminal cells have a specific receptor for antidiuretic hormone (ADH), which, acting via cAMP, permits water to move across the cell membrane in response to the osmotic gradient. In the common X-linked recessive form (type I) of nephrogenic diabetes insipidus, there is a disorder of the ADH:adenylyl cyclase receptor, and urinary adenylyl cyclase is not increased after administration of vasopressin. In the type II variety, cAMP is formed by ADH action but has no effect on water transport. There are probably many variants of this complex mechanism, which is also influenced by prostaglandin E_1 and by its inhibitor, indomethacin.

The symptoms are limited to polyuria, polydipsia, and failure to thrive. In some children, particularly if the solute intake is unrestricted, some acclimatization to an elevated serum osmolality may develop. However, these children are particularly liable to episodes of dehydration, fever, vomiting, and convulsions.

Clinically, the diagnosis can be made on the basis of a history of polydipsia and polyuria that are not sensitive to the administration of vasopressin, desmopressin acetate (DDAVP), or lypressin. It is wise to confirm this in all cases by performing a vasopressin test. Carefully monitored water restriction does not increase the tubular reabsorption of water (T^cH_2O) to above 3 mL/min/m^2. Urine osmolality will remain lower than 450 mosm/kg, whereas serum osmolality rises and total body weight falls. Before greater than 5% weight reduction occurs or before serum osmolality exceeds 320 mosm/kg, administer vasopressin. Urine concentrating ability is impaired in a number of conditions—sickle cell anemia, pyelonephritis, potassium depletion, hypercalcemia, cystinosis and other renal tubular disorders, and obstructive uropathy—and as a result of nephrotoxic drugs.

In infants, it is usually best to allow water as demanded and to restrict salt. Serum sodium levels should be evaluated at intervals to ensure against hyperosmolality from inadvertent water restriction. In later childhood, sodium intake should continue to be restricted to 2–2.5 meq/kg/24 h. Studies have suggested that water clearance is decreased by chlorothiazide, 60 mg/m^2/24 h orally; and indomethacin, 3 mg/kg/24 h.

Roth KS, Diagnosis of renal tubular disorders: A guide for the clinician. Clin Pediatr (Phila) 1988;27:463.

URINARY TRACT INFECTIONS

Predisposing Factors

Urinary tract infections occur in approximately 1% of premature infants and newborns. Many of these infections are hematogenously spread; however, outside the clinical setting of perinatal acute illness and prematurity, urinary tract infections raise the possibility of urinary tract abnormalities. Within the first year of life, males are more likely to have an anatomic basis for developing urinary tract infection; nevertheless, the initial infection in a small child should alert the physician to the possibility of abnormal anatomy regardless of the patient's sex.

Older boys with a first infection should be examined for urinary tract abnormalities, whereas a more conservative, watchful approach may be taken with older girls, especially if sexual activity or poor personal hygiene is a possible cause. Such an approach, of course, assumes there are no other clinical abnormalities present that raise the suspicion of significant urinary tract disease (eg, enuresis or short stature).

The most common causes of urinary tract infections are *Escherichia coli, Klebsiella, Staphylococcus*, and the enteric streptococci (all present in normal rectal and perineal flora). Unless there is reason to suspect that bacteremia is responsible for the development of the urinary tract infection, bacteria usually are presumed to gain access to the urinary tract via the urethra. The problem is greatly aggravated by poor hygiene, perineal infection (eg, pinworms), sexual activity, and instrumentation. Despite the fact that voiding provides some safeguard against such contamination developing into infection, abnormalities of the collecting system contribute to clinical infection and may lead to upper tract disease and renal parenchymal damage.

Clinical Findings

A. Symptoms & Signs: Newborns may present with fever, hypothermia, poor feeding, jaundice, failure to thrive, or sepsis. Infants may have strong-smelling urine and irritability. Preschool children may have abdominal pain, vomiting, strong-smelling urine, fever, enuresis, increased frequency of urination, dysuria, or urgency. School-age children may develop the "classic" signs of urinary tract infection, including enuresis, increased frequency of urination, dysuria, urgency, fever, and costovertebral angle tenderness (flank pain). Occasionally, children with bacterial urinary tract infection will present with hemorrhagic cystitis.

Not all symptoms suggestive of urinary tract infection will actually prove to be related to bacterial infection. Anatomic abnormalities producing voiding discomfort, irritation of the external genitalia, or viral hemorrhagic cystitis are examples of such problems. On the other hand, some infections may actually be relatively asymptomatic. In either case, the presence of a urinary tract infection should be documented through the performance of a urinalysis and urine culture.

B. Laboratory Tests: The clean-catch, midstream method may be satisfactory for children who can void upon request and who can be assisted in obtaining a proper specimen or be relied upon to obtain one unassisted. A bladder catheterization or suprapubic bladder tap may be performed when necessary (eg, highly suspicious clinical picture with the inability to obtain a satisfactory clean-catch specimen). Any procedure, however, carries the risk of contamination; for this reason, the more invasive procedures demand appropriate indication as well as the proper technique.

After the specimen is obtained care must be taken to decant an aliquot for urinalysis prior to sending the specimen for culture and sensitivity. The aliquot is then spun and prepared for microscopic analysis. The presence of bacteria in the specimen is highly suggestive of a urinary tract infection, provided that the specimen is clean-catch and midstream. The presence of pyuria (more than five white blood cells per high-power field) is also consistent with infection, but, again, specimen reliability is important because the perineal region, vagina, or external genitalia may be responsible for the presence of white or red blood cells in urine specimens. Nonetheless, such findings in the face of highly suspicious clinical symptoms should prompt the initiation of antibiotic treatment until the culture results are obtained.

The presence of multiple organisms suggests specimen contamination; however, this possibility must be evaluated in light of the method used in obtaining the specimen, as well as the level of confidence in the technical performance of the procedure used. If the child is not already receiving the appropriate antibiotic as indicated by the sensitivities, a change should be made accordingly.

Nonculture methods, such as nitrite sticks, for early detection of a urinary tract infection may be useful in following the child with recurrent infection or being treated prophylactically with antibiotic suppression therapy.

Treatment

A. Initial Treatment: After urinary tract infection is confirmed, initial therapy should be based on the patient's history of antibiotic use, the location of the infection, and the subsequent drug sensitivities of the organism.

For uncomplicated cases of urethritis or cystitis, a single oral antibiotic (eg, ampicillin, a sulfonamide, nitrofurantoin) that the patient has not used recently can be administered for 10 days. The choice of antibiotic therapy must be verified by prior culture and sensitivity. A patient with suspected pyelonephritis need not always be admitted to the hospital but antibiotic coverage should be broad (ampicillin, a sulfonamide, or a cephalosporin plus gentamicin). This regimen ensures adequate coverage until the patient improves and the results of antibiotic sensitivity tests are available, allowing selection of a single effective oral antibiotic. Antibiotic dosages (depending on choice of drug) are appropriately modified in patients with acute or chronic renal failure.

Most urinary tract infections can be successfully treated with inexpensive drugs given orally. Follow-up urinalysis or use of nitrite sticks within 2–3 days can confirm therapeutic success. If symptoms persist, reexamination and repeat urine culture are necessary.

B. Treatment of Refractory Infection: Persistent bacteriuria indicates superinfection with a different organism or with the same organism due to obstruction, the presence of a foreign body, or conversion of the organism to a variant form.

C. Urologic Intervention: Voiding cystourethrography should be obtained with proved infection. Renal ultrasonography is a helpful, noninvasive tool for evaluating the anatomy of the urinary tract.

Obvious structural ureteral reflux or obstructive anomalies require referral to a urologist experienced in dealing with children. Vesicoureteral reflux is common in younger children. Mild reflux does not cause renal damage and will disappear in time if repeated infections can be prevented. Stages 3–5 reflux generally require ureteral reimplantation.

In patients without structural or functional urinary tract abnormalities, possible causes of recurrent infection include infrequent or incomplete voiding, poor perineal hygiene, pinworms, constipation, and the use of bubble bath. If attempts to deal with these problems are unsuccessful, single-dose prophylaxis at bedtime with agents such as nitrofurantoin or trimethoprim-sulfamethoxazole may be useful in combination with a program of frequent voiding.

D. Follow-Up of Patients With Urinary Tract Infection: All patients with urinary tract infection should be checked for recurrence every 1–2 months until they have remained free of infection for 1 year. Home testing of first morning concentrated urine specimens by nitrite stick may reduce the cost of follow-up without compromising accuracy.

Prognosis

As long as urinary tract infections can be confined to the lower urinary tract (bladder and below), the prognosis is excellent. Once an infectious process has entered the kidney, the prognosis becomes more guarded. Hence, every diagnostic and therapeutic effort should be made to prevent recurrences.

Bailey RR: Vesico-ureteric reflux and reflux nephropathy. Kidney Int 1991;44:5.

Smellie JM, Rigden SP, Prescod NP: Urinary tract infection: A comparison of four methods of investigation. Arch Dis Child 1995;72:247.

REFERENCES

Edelmann CM Jr et al (editors): *Pediatric Kidney Disease,* 2nd ed. Little, Brown, 1992.

Holliday MA, Barratt TM, Avner ED: *Pediatric Nephrology,* 4th ed. Williams & Wilkins, 1994.

Neurologic & Muscular Disorders

23

Paul G. Moe, MD, & Alan R. Seay, MD

NEUROLOGIC ASSESSMENT & NEURODIAGNOSTIC PROCEDURES

NEUROLOGIC HISTORY & EXAMINATION

The history is usually taken with the child and parents together. Questions can be addressed directly to the older child with further details supplemented by the parent. If time permits, a teenager should be interviewed alone. If strong psychosocial factors become evident by the end of the joint interview, the parent may be asked to leave. Sensitive issues (eg, drug use, sexual activity) can then be reexplored with the older child.

A patient data form filled out by the parent in advance of the visit or in the physician's waiting room is helpful. The form should include the chief complaint, the patient's strengths and talents, birth and family history, medical history, and school and behavioral history. A checklist of behavioral issues such as hyperactivity, depression, short attention span, and so on, can bring attention to areas that need to be more carefully explored during the interview. Developmental delays suspected in the infant or older child can also be addressed in a checklist. A physician interviewing a child aged 5–7 can begin with neutral questions regarding age and birthday. It is often informative to see whether these children know their birthday or even year of birth.

The core of the history is the present illness. What the parent or child sees as important should be the initial focus. In recurrent conditions (eg, seizures or headaches), it is important to find out what happened during the first as well as the most recent episode. Details of recurrent episodes should be thoroughly discussed, including frequency, duration, change in character over time, and precipitating and alleviating factors. The effect of emotions, medications, and environmental manipulations such as diet change

should be reviewed. The physician should ascertain, if possible, whether the disease is congenital or age-acquired and whether it is progressive.

As the interview progresses, the clinician begins to form ideas about a possible diagnosis; these can be explored with searching questions. Occasionally, the patient and parent see things from different viewpoints. The child, for instance, may consider the headaches a trivial matter that does not interfere with activity; the mother may feel differently. It may be helpful to observe the emotional interchange between parent and child and to note each one's opinions regarding the severity of disease, the degree of interference with peer group and school activities, side effects and efficacy of medications, and the like.

Depending on the nature of the complaint, the past medical history may or may not be extremely detailed. For example, in the case of a teenager with headaches, the mother's history of pregnancy and birth is of little importance. In the case of a 2-month-old child with hypotonia, detailed information about these events is essential. The family and genetic history may be important. A strong family history of migraine or a history of myotonic dystrophy in an uncle might be the key to diagnosis in the examples cited. The parents may have to do some searching with inquiries to relatives or hospitals to assemble family history details.

Available health records, roentgenograms, electroencephalograms (EEGs), and school records may complement the interview. Developmental history is essential in the assessment of any infant. The Denver Developmental Screening Test (DDST) is one helpful tool for reviewing each major area of behavior in infancy, that is, gross motor, fine motor, personal/social, and language. Some developmental expectations and landmarks are listed in Table 23–1.

In the older child, the developmental history can be explored with questions concerning school progress. The clinician should ask how the patient is getting along with the peer group, in physical activities, and in the family setting. Open-ended questions (eg, "What is she like? What is an average day in her

Table 23–1. Neurologic developmental landmarks.

	Birth	3 Months	6 Months	9 Months	12–15 Months	24 Months
Motor	Flexor posture, lifts head prone, hands grasped	Sits: head forward, bobbing, lifts head supine, hands open, retains briefly	Rolls both ways, begins to sit alone, supports (erect), bounces	Creeps, pulls up standing, pincer grasp, sits well	Walks with 1 or 2 hands held, stands alone briefly, releases on command	Walks and runs well, walks downstairs, turns pages singly
Special senses	Regards (vision), may follow 45 degrees	Looks at hands, follows 90–180 degrees	Discriminates voices, localizes sounds	Picks up raisin, "bye-bye"	Localizes noises, localizes pain	Towers 6–7 cubes, imitates scribble
Adaptive	Startles to sound, delayed nociceptive response	Smiles socially, vocalizes socially, follows vertically	Holds cube, palmar grasp, retrieves toy, transfers and rakes raisin	Bangs toys together, pat-a-cake	Assists in dressing, attempts spoon feeding, tries 2-cube tower	Asks for toilet, pulls on garments, spoon-feeds well, parallel play
Language	Throaty noises	Coos, chuckles, vocal social response	Babbles (polysyllables), "mmm-mmm"	"Ma-ma, Da-da," one other "word"	Understands simple command, speaks 1–3 words	Speaks in phrases, names 3–5 pictures, pronouns: "I, me, you"
Reflex	Tonic neck, palmar grasp	Disappearing tonic neck, Moro reflex	Begins voluntary stepping	Parachute response		
Automatisms	Moro reflex, sucks, roots, stepping, supporting, traction: head lag	Landau response, traction: no head lag	Neck righting, blinks to threat			

life? What does she do?") can help the clinician assess the child's social functioning.

During examination, the infant or toddler is often held in the mother's lap. Much information can be obtained by observing a child carefully and noting spontaneous movements, curiosity, ability to understand directions, and alertness to visual and auditory cues (eg, a tinkling bell).

Part of the neurologic examination includes a brief **general physical examination** with emphasis on the skin (birth marks), spine, neck, and skull (including palpation of the fontanelle and measurement of head circumference). At some point in the examination, the baby should be inspected virtually unclothed. In an older child, asking about birthmarks and inspecting the spine with the shirt pulled up and the child bent over for evaluation of scoliosis may be sufficient.

Developmental assessment should be included in the neurologic examination of the infant. At an appropriate age (eg, 6–18 months), the physician may start with handing blocks to the baby, offering a raisin, and evaluating reach and type of grasp. A younger baby often enjoys a bell, the older child a reflex hammer. Using the block and the raisin, the clinician can assess the items on the DDST that have not been elucidated by the history.

Having the child run around the room and retrieve a ball allows testing of his or her **station and gait**.

Children usually enjoy having their **reflexes** tested. Be sure reflexes are present proximally and distally, such as knee jerk/ankle jerk, triceps/brachial radialis. Sometimes, a subtle case of hemiparesis can be suggested by a unilateral absence of abdominal or cremasteric cutaneous reflexes. Occasionally, tapping one's finger over a hamstring or biceps reflex can show an absent reflex or asymmetry in a lumbosacral plexus or brachial plexus injury.

Infantile automatisms—their presence, absence, or asymmetry—are important in examination of the newborn and very young infant (Table 23–1).

Running around the room, squatting, jumping, etc, are tests of the child's **motor functions**. In infants, tone—the examiner's subjective feeling while manipulating the limb—is important. (See the section on hypotonic infants.) Occasionally, formal muscle testing is necessary, such as abduction at the shoulder and hand grasp, rising from a squat, and dorsiflexion of the foot to test proximal and distal strength. **Sensory testing** is rarely contributory, but touch, tickle, and pinprick testing can be used in small children.

At this point, the infant's **cranial nerves** have usually been satisfactorily assessed by observation (eg, extraocular movements, vision, and hearing). If there is concern about swallowing or tongue size or function, these areas can be examined with a flashlight and tongue blade. Lastly, the fundi should be assessed by having the infant look at a distant object or by having the parent attract the child's attention with a pinwheel or bell. The physician can approach from the side to observe the disk before light on the macula causes miosis. Sometimes, mydriatics to dilate the pupil are necessary.

In the older child, formal examination of **mental status** is rarely necessary. Simple assessment of cognition can be achieved by having the child obey right-and-left commands (eg, "Put your right hand on your left ear"), do simple arithmetic problems, and read paragraphs appropriate for grade level (Table 23–2).

In the older child, the **Romberg test** (standing with eyes closed, feet together, and hands straight out), tandem walking, and standing and hopping on each foot are tests of **station and gait. Limb coordination** can be tested by finger pursuit, that is, having children touch the clinician's moving finger with their own. Finger-nose alternating movements and patting the palm and the back of the hand alternately on the lap are other tests of **lateral coordination**. In the older child, tests for **sense of position, vibration**, and even **cortical sensory status** (eg, position of the limb in space and finger writing) are occasionally important.

Because children can be uncooperative and findings uncertain, serial examinations are sometimes necessary. Reasons for a follow-up examination should be explained in detail to the parent. No neurologic examination is a complete failure. The clinician has the opportunity to observe the child during the interview and during play; these observations may give a reasonable assessment of neurologic function.

Finally, it must be emphasized that a complete examination should be performed and results told to the parents in plain language, even when the complaint seems trivial.

LUMBAR PUNCTURE

The principal purpose of lumbar puncture is to obtain an aliquot of cerebrospinal fluid (CSF) for the diagnosis of infectious and inflammatory conditions of the central nervous system (Table 23–3). The uses of CSF specimens in cytologic studies, bioassays of enzymes and neurotransmitters, and specific rapid tests for viruses are widening the clinical (and research) applicability of lumbar puncture. However, lumbar puncture for manometric determinations, cellular content, and protein levels in many conditions—including head injuries, brain and spinal cord tumors, and seizure disorders— has been superseded by the use of brain imaging and biochemical techniques that are far more specific.

Therapeutically, lumbar puncture may be used to drain CSF to reduce its hematotoxic effects in hemorrhagic conditions (eg, intraventricular hemorrhage in newborns, ruptured berry aneurysm) and to lower intracranial pressure in pseudotumor cerebri. Symptoms may be improved in viral meningitis.

Lumbar puncture is usually performed with the patient in the lateral recumbent or decubitus position. Entry is at the level of the iliac crest or the L3–L4 interspace, with the patient's head initially flexed and then extended. In small infants—especially premature infants and neonates in the first months of life–lumbar puncture is more safely and satisfactorily performed with the infant in the sitting position and the head only slightly flexed or supported with a pillow propped between the outstretched arms and legs resting against the infant's chest and abdomen. The wrists and ankles should be held by an assisting nurse, and the needle should be pointed slightly cephalad.

Note: Before lumbar puncture is performed, the fundi should always be checked for papilledema. Lumbar puncture is contraindicated in the presence of elevated intracranial pressure, especially when there are focal neurologic deficits, because of the risk of tentorial or tonsillar herniation. This risk is less likely when there is diffuse cerebral swelling than when elevated pressure is due to a mass lesion. Therefore, if equipment for computed tomographic (CT) brain scanning is readily available, lumbar puncture should usually be delayed until a scan can be done; it should not be delayed, however, if examination of cerebrospinal fluid is indispensable for diagnosis and vital therapeutic intervention.

Lumbar puncture must be performed promptly when a diffuse central nervous system infection (meningitis, meningoencephalitis, encephalitis, cerebritis) is suspected. Only a small-gauge needle should be used, and only enough fluid should be withdrawn to permit cell count, protein and glucose determination, and such stains and cultures (bacterial, fungal, and viral) and other studies as may be needed. A specimen of 2–3 mL is usually adequate for microchemical determinations.

It is occasionally important to obtain opening and closing CSF pressures. To obtain valid pressure readings, the child's head, neck, and legs should be gently brought into a straight line. Pressure in the sitting

---

Table 23–2. Mental status examination.

Orientation: Time, place, situation, name, date, year.
Memory: Recent and remote, eg, "What did you have for lunch?" "What did you do on your birthday?" Remember (for 10 minutes): "Red flag, Washington's birthday, Christmas presents."
Calculation: Depends on educational background. Example: Subtract serial sevens.
Proverbs: Interpret: "Too many cooks spoil the broth." "A rolling stone gathers no moss."
Situation: "What would you do if you saw a fire?"
Aphasia: "What's this?" (chalk). "Stick out your tongue." "Put your right finger on your left ear." Sample speech, reading, and writing.

Table 23–3. Characteristics of cerebrospinal fluid (CSF) in the normal child and in central nervous system infections and inflammatory conditions.

Condition	Initial Pressure (mm H$_2$O)	Appearance	Cells/μL	Protein (mg/dL)	Glucose (mg/dL)	Other Tests	Comments
Normal	< 180	Clear	0–5 lymphocytes. First 3 months, 1–3 PMNs. Neonates, up to 30 lymphocytes, 20–50 RBCs.	15–35 (lumbar), 5–15 (ventricular). Up to 150 (lumbar) for short time after birth; to 6 months, up to 65	50–80 (two-thirds of blood glucose); may be increased after seizure	CSF IgG index; < 0.7 units = CSF IgG/Serum IgG. CSF albumin/Serum albumin Lactate dehydrogenase (LDH), 2–27 IU/L.	CSF protein in first month may be up to 170 mg/dL in small-for-dates or premature infants. No increase in WBCs due to seizure.
Bloody tap	Normal or low	Bloody (sometimes with clot)	One additional WBC/700 RBCs.[1] RBCs not crenated.	One additional mg/800 RBCs[1]	Normal	RBC number should fall between first and third tube; wait 5 minutes between tubes.	Spin down fluid; supernatant will be clear and colorless.
Bacterial meningitis, acute	200–750 +	Opalescent to purulent	Up to 1000s, mostly PMNs. Early, few cells.	Up to 100s	Decreased; may be none	Smear and culture mandatory. LDH > 24 IU/L. Bacterial antigen tests if Gram's stain and culture are negative.	Very early, glucose may be normal. Immunofluorescence tests.
Bacterial meningitis, partially treated	Usually increased	Clear or opalescent	Usually increased. PMNs usually predominate.	Elevated	Normal or decreased	LDH usually > 24 IU/L. Bacterial antigen tests.	Smear and culture often negative. Prior antibiotic therapy.
Tuberculous meningitis	150–750 +	Opalescent; fibrin web or pellicle	250–500, mostly lymphocytes. Early, more PMNs.	45–500; parallels cell count; increases over time	Decreased; may be none	Smear for acid-fast organism; CSF culture and inoculation; PCR.[2]	Note: Bacterial meningitis may be superimposed.
Fungal meningitis	Increased	Variable; often clear	10–500. Early, mostly PMNs; then mostly lymphocytes.	Elevated and increasing.	Decreased	India ink preparations, cryptococcal antigen, culture, inoculations, immunofluorescence tests.	Often superimposed in patients who are debilitated or on immunosuppressive therapy.
Aseptic meningoencephalitides (viral meningitis, or parameningeal disease)	Normal or slightly increased	Clear unless cell count > 300	0 to few hundred, mostly lymphocytes; PMNs predominate early.	20–125	Normal; may be low in mumps, herpes, or other viral infections	CSF, blood stool, throat wash for viral cultures. LDH < 28 IU/L (90% < 24 IU/L). PCR for herpes, CMV, EBV, enterovirus, etc.	Acute and convalescent antibody titers for some viruses. In mumps, up to 1000 lymphocytes; serum amylase often elevated. Rarely, several thousand cells present in enteroviral infection.
Neurosyphilis	Normal to 400	Clear unless protein is very high	10–100, mostly lymphocytes.	25–150; higher in meningitis	Normal	Positive CSF serology CSF IgG index increased.	Blood serology positive in untreated cases; *Treponema pallidum* immobilization test positive.
Parainfectious encephalomyelitis	80–450, usually increased	Usually clear	0–50, mostly lymphocytes.	15–75	Normal	CSF IgG index may be increased. Oligoclonal bands variable.	No organisms. Fulminant cases resemble bacterial meningitis.
Polyneuritis Early	Normal and occasionally increased	Normal	Normal; occasionally slight increase.	Normal	Normal	Bacterial cultures negative; gamma globulin may be elevated.	Try to find cause (viral infections, toxins, lupus, diabetes, etc).
Late		Xanthochromic if protein high		45–1500			
Meningeal carcinomatosis	Often elevated	Clear to opalescent	Cytologic identification of tumor cells.	Often mildly to moderately elevated	Often depressed	Cytology.	Seen with leukemia, medulloblastoma, meningeal melanosis, histiocytosis X. Note: May mimic meningitis.
Brain abscess	Normal or increased	Usually clear	5–500 in 80%; mostly PMNs.	Usually slightly increased	Normal; occasionally decreased	Imaging study of brain (MRI).	Cell count related to proximity to meninges; findings as in purulent meningitis if abscess perforates.

[1] Many studies document pitfalls in using these ratios due to WBC lysis. Clinical judgment and repeat taps may be necessary to rule out meningitis in this situation. (See references.)
[2] Polymerase chain reaction.

position should be measured with the level of the foramen magnum as "zero"; the length of the fluid column above that level is the pressure in millimeters of water.

Many other CSF components have useful clinical applications.

Anbar R: Pitfalls in interpretation of traumatic lumbar puncture formula. (Letter.) Am J Dis Child 1986; 140:638.

Carraccio C, Blotny K, Fisher MC: CSF analysis in systemically ill children without CNS disease. Pediatrics 1995;96:48.

Chow G, Schmidley JW: Lysis of erythrocytes and leukocytes in traumatic lumbar puncture. Arch Neurol 1984; 41:1984.

Jaffe M et al: The ameliorating effect of lumbar puncture in viral meningitis. Am J Dis Child 1989;143:682.

Markowitz H, Kokmen E: Neurologic diseases and the cerebrospinal fluid immunoglobin profile. Mayo Clin Proc 1983;58:273.

Novak RW: Lack of validity of standard corrections for white blood cell counts of blood-contaminated cerebrospinal fluid in infants. Am J Clin Pathol 1984;82:95.

Portnoy J, Olson L: Normal cerebrospinal fluid values in children: Another look. Pediatrics 1985;75:484.

Ricevuti G: Meningeal leukemia diagnosed by cytocentrifuge study of cerebrospinal fluid. Arch Neurol 1986; 43:466.

Rubenstein S, Yager R: What represents pleocytosis in blood-contaminated ("traumatic tap") CSF in childhood? J Pediatr 1985;107:249.

Ward EM, Gushurst D: Uses and techniques of pediatric lumbar puncture. Am J Dis Child 1992;196:1160.

Wood J (editor): *Neurology of CSF*. Plenum Press, 1982.

ELECTROENCEPHALOGRAPHY

This widely used, noninvasive electrophysiologic method for recording cerebral activity has its greatest clinical applicability in the study of seizure disorders. "Activation" techniques to accentuate abnormalities or disclose latent abnormalities include photic stimulation, well-sustained hyperventilation for 3 minutes, and depriving the patient of sleep from about midnight until after breakfast, at which time the EEG is recorded. The latter is an excellent though less widely used "activation" method.

Electroencephalography is also used in the evaluation of tumors, cerebrovascular accidents, neurodegenerative diseases, and other neurologic disorders causing brain dysfunction; but with some notable exceptions, it is nonspecific. Recordings over a 24-hour period or all-night recordings are invaluable in the diagnosis of sleep disturbances and narcolepsy. Electroencephalography with telemetry or simultaneous monitoring of behavior on videotape, has great usefulness in selected cases. The EEG can be helpful in determining a possible cause or mechanism of coma and is frequently used to help determine whether coma is irreversible and brain death has occurred.

The limitations of electroencephalography are considerable: In most cases, the duration of the actual tracing is about 45 minutes and reflects only surface cortical function. Many drugs—especially barbiturates and benzodiazepines—have considerable effects on the EEG and may confuse interpretation. Moreover, about 15% of nonepileptic individuals, especially children, may have an abnormal EEG. Electroencephalographic findings such as those seen in migraine, learning disabilities, or behavior disorders do not reflect permanent "brain damage." A major usefulness of EEG is to show epileptiform activity in children with seizure disorders; sometimes the findings are virtually diagnostic, as in the hypsarhythmia EEG of infantile spasms or the prolonged 3-second spike wave of absence seizures.

At present, use of CT scans, evoked potentials, positron emission tomography, regional cerebral blood flow studies, single-photon emission computed tomography (SPECT), and magnetic resonance imaging (MRI) supplements the use of EEGs as a diagnostic and prognostic tool.

EVOKED POTENTIALS

Cortical auditory, visual, or somatosensory evoked potentials (evoked responses) may be recorded from the scalp surface over the temporal, occipital, or frontoparietal cortex after repetitive stimulation of the retina by light flashes, of the cochlea by sounds, or of a nerve by galvanic stimuli of varying frequency and intensity, respectively. Computer averaging is used to recognize and enhance these responses while subtracting or suppressing the asynchronous background electroencephalographic activity. The presence or absence of evoked potential waves and their latencies (time from stimulus to wave peak or time between peaks) figure in the clinical interpretation.

The reproducible and quantifiable results obtained from brain stem auditory, pattern-shift visual, and short-latency somatosensory evoked potentials (see below) indicate the level of function of the relevant sensory pathway or system and identify the site of anatomic disruption. Although results of these tests alone are usually not diagnostic, the tests are noninvasive, sensitive, objective, and relatively inexpensive extensions of the clinical neurologic examination. Because the auditory and somatosensory tests and one type of visual test are completely passive, requiring only that the patient remain still, they are particularly useful in the evaluation of neonates and small children as well as in patients unable to cooperate (eg, as a result of mental retardation, degenerative disorder, anesthesia, or coma). Knowledge of normal values and experience in testing of the applicable patient group are mandatory.

Brain Stem Auditory Evoked Potentials

A brief auditory stimulus (click) of varying intensity and frequency is delivered to the ear to activate the auditory nerve (nerve VIII) and sequentially activate the cochlear nucleus, tracts and nuclei of the lateral lemniscus, and inferior colliculus. Thus, this technique assesses hearing and function of the brain stem auditory tracts.

Hearing in the neonate or uncooperative (but sedated) patient can be objectively assessed, making the technique particularly useful in high-risk infants—especially those in intensive care nurseries—and in retarded and autistic patients. Brain stem auditory evoked potentials are used to judge brain stem dysfunction in sleep apnea, in Arnold-Chiari malformation, and achondroplasia. Because high doses of anesthetic agents or barbiturates do not seriously affect results, the test is used to assess and monitor brain stem function of surgical patients (in the operating room) and those in hypoxic-ischemic coma or coma following head injury. Absence of evoked potential waves beyond the first wave from the auditory nerve usually signifies brain death. Brain stem auditory evoked potentials are also useful in the early evaluation of diseases affecting myelin—the various leukodystrophies and multiple sclerosis (although auditory evoked potentials are less valuable than visual evoked potentials in the latter)—and in intrinsic brain stem gliomas. They are sometimes useful in evaluation of hereditary ataxias, Wilson's disease (hepatolenticular degeneration), and other degenerative disorders affecting the brain stem.

Pattern-Shift Visual Evoked Potentials

The preferred stimulus is a shift (reversal) of a checkerboard pattern, and the response is a single wave (called P100) generated in the striate and parastriate visual cortex. The absolute latency of P100 (time from stimulus to wave peak) and the difference in latency between the two eyes are sensitive indicators of disease. The amplitude of response is affected by any process resulting in poor fixation on the stimulus screen or affecting visual acuity. Ability to focus on a checkerboard pattern is necessary. An LED (light-emitting diode), goggles, or bright flash stimulus can be used in younger and uncooperative children, but the norms are less standardized. Evoked potentials suggest that visual acuity may be 20/20 in infants by 6–7 months of age.

Clinical application of the test includes detection and monitoring of strabismus (ie, in amblyopia ex anopsia), optic neuritis, and lesions near the optic nerve and chiasm such as optic gliomas and craniopharyngiomas. Degenerative and immunologic diseases that affect visual transmission may be detected early and followed by serial evaluations by this technique, including adrenoleukodystrophy, Pelizaeus-Merzbacher disease, some spinocerebellar degenerations, sarcoidosis, and even multiple sclerosis. Flash visual evoked potentials are used to monitor function during surgery involving the eyes and optic nerve; to assess cortical or hysterical blindness; and to evaluate patients with photosensitive epilepsy, who may have exaggerated responses.

Short-Latency Somatosensory Evoked Potentials

Responses are commonly produced by electrical stimulation of peripheral sensory nerves, since this evokes potentials of greatest amplitude and clarity; finger tapping and muscle stretching may also be used. The function of this test is similar to that of the auditory test in closely correlating wave forms with function of the sensory pathways and permitting localization of conduction defects.

Short-latency somatosensory evoked potentials are used in the assessment of a wide variety of lesions of the peripheral nerve, root, spinal cord, and central nervous system following trauma, neuropathies (eg, in diabetes mellitus or Guillain-Barré syndrome), myelodysplasias, cerebral palsy, and many other disorders. The procedure is often performed on an outpatient basis. One method is stimulation of the median nerve at the wrist with small (nonpainful) electrical shocks and recording of responses from the brachial plexus above the clavicle, the neck (cervical cord), and the opposite scalp area overlying the sensorimotor cortex. After stimulation from the knee (peroneal nerve) or ankle (tibial nerve), impulses are recorded from the lower lumbar spinal cord, cervical cord, and sensorimotor cortex. Such potentials are used to monitor spinal cord sensory functioning during surgery for disorders including scoliosis, myelodysplasias, and tumors and other lesions of the spinal cord or blood vessels supplying the cord. The technique is also used in leukodystrophies involving peripheral nerves, in multiple sclerosis, and in the differential diagnosis of hysteria and malingering (anesthetic limbs). In the diagnosis of coma and brain death, somatosensory evoked potentials supplement the results of auditory evoked potentials.

Aldrich MS, Jahnke B: Diagnostic value of video EEG polysomnography. Neurology 1991;41:1060.

Chiappa KH, Ropper AH: Evoked potentials in clinical medicine. (Two parts.) N Engl J Med 1982;306:1140, 1205.

Cohen BA, Schenk VA, Sweeney DB: Meningitis-related hearing loss evaluated with evoked potentials. Pediatr Neurol 1988;4:18.

DeMeirleir LJ, Taylor MJ: Prognostic utility of SEPs in comatose children. Pediatr Neurol 1987;3:78.

Eyre JA (editor): The neurophysiologic examination of the

newborn infant. *Clinics in Developmental Medicine,* No. 120. MacKeith Press, 1992.

Fagan ER, Taylor MJ, Logan WJ: Somatosensory evoked potentials. P2. A review of the clinical applications in pediatric neurology. Pediatr Neurol 1987;3:189.

Goldie WD et al: Brain stem auditory evoked potentials as a tool in the clinical assessment of children with posterior fossa tumors. J Child Neurol 1987;2:272.

Hecox KE, Cone B, Blaw ME: Brain stem auditory evoked response in the diagnosis of pediatric neurologic disease. Neurology 1981;31:832.

Kamimura N et al: Spinal somatosensory evoked potentials in infants and children with spinal cord lesions. Brain Dev 1988;10:355.

Mutoh K et al: Maturation of somatosensory evoked potentials upon posterior tibial nerve stimulation. Pediatr Neurol 1988;4:342.

Rotteveel JJ et al: The applications of evoked potentials in the diagnosis and follow-up of children with intracranial tumors. Childs Nerv Syst 1985;1:172.

Taylor MJ, McCullough D: Prognostic value of VEPs in young children with acute-onset cortical blindness. Pediatr Neurol 1992;7:111.

Whyte HE et al: Prognostic utility of visual evoked potentials in term asphyxiated neonates. Pediatr Neurol 1986; 2:220.

BRAIN ELECTRICAL ACTIVITY MAPPING (BEAM)

Brain electrical activity mapping is a relatively new technique in which electroencephalographic and evoked potential data recorded from multiple scalp electrodes are graphically displayed in color on a computer-driven video screen. Values between electrodes are obtained by interpolation. Learning-disabled, dyslexic, and epileptic children are being studied in research protocols. Expense, lack of normative data, and lack of numbers of homogeneous clinical patients preclude current use of this modality in pediatric practice.

Duffy FH: The BEAM method for neurophysiological diagnosis. Ann N Y Acad Sci 1985;457:19.

Nuwer M: Quantitative EEG. 1. Techniques and problems of frequency, analysis, and topographic mapping. Neurol Clin 1988;5:1.

Nuwer M, Sharbrough F: American EEG Society statement on clinical use of quantitative EEG. Neurology 1987; 37:28A.

PEDIATRIC NEURORADIOLOGIC PROCEDURES

Sedation for Procedures

Radiologic procedures in infants and children are usually performed by pediatric radiologists, but sedation for these procedures remains largely the responsibility of the physician caring for the child. The choice of sedation must take into account the patient's age and physical condition, the type of neurologic disorder, the effect and duration of the procedure, and whether immediate neurosurgery is anticipated. The prescribing physician should be familiar with the agent used.

Oral or rectal chloral hydrate, 30–60 mg/kg/dose, is safest. Many radiology departments, however, use only nonoral administration because of the risks of vomiting and aspiration. One favorite is pentobarbital, 6 mg/kg for children weighing less than 15 kg and 5 mg/kg for larger children (up to a maximum of 200 mg) given intramuscularly or rectally (at least 20 minutes before a procedure) or 2–4 mg/kg given intravenously. Equipment to support blood pressure and respiration must be available. This dosage usually achieves sedation for up to 2 hours. If, however, sedation is inadequate 30 minutes after injection—and if the condition of the child permits—a second dose of pentobarbital, 2 mg/kg, is given. A "cardiac cocktail," usually of intramuscularly administered meperidine hydrochloride, secobarbital, and promethazine hydrochloride or chlorpromazine, may be used by pediatricians familiar with it. General anesthesia may be indicated, especially if the child is to undergo surgery immediately on completion of a radiologic examination.

Computed Tomography (CT Scanning)

CT scanning consists of a series of cross-sectional (axial) roentgenograms and can be performed on an outpatient basis. Radiation exposure is approximately the same as that from a skull roentgenogram series. The images can be viewed on an oscilloscope as the scan is being done and later examined on printed-out films; both oscilloscope views and films record variations in tissue densities. CT scanning is of high sensitivity (88–96% of lesions larger than 1–2 cm can be seen) but low specificity (a tumor, focus of infection, or infarct may have the same appearance).

The CT scan is often repeated after intravenous injection of iodized contrast for enhancement, which reflects the vascularity of a lesion or its surrounding tissues. Precautions should be taken to ensure that the patient is not hypersensitive to iodinated dyes and that allergic reactions can be managed promptly. Sufficient information is often obtained from a nonenhanced scan; in these cases, cost and risk are minimized.

Sedation may be required for CT scanning. For positioning the head of children up to 8 years of age, a specially shaped headrest may be needed. The indications for CT scanning and the findings in specific conditions are discussed below in the sections on specific disorders.

Magnetic Resonance Imaging

Magnetic resonance imaging (MRI) is a noninvasive technique that uses the magnetic properties of certain nuclei to produce diagnostically useful signals. Currently, the technique is based on detecting the response (resonance) of hydrogen proton nuclei to applied radiofrequency electromagnetic radiation; these nuclei are abundant in the body and more sensitive to magnetic resonance imaging than other nuclei. The strength of MRI signals varies with the relationship of water to protein and the amount of lipids present. The image displayed, which is made up of a mixture of signals and is similar to the CT film, provides high-resolution contrast of soft tissues. MRI can, in fact, provide information about the histologic, physiologic, and biochemical status of tissues in addition to gross anatomic data.

MRI has been used to delineate brain tumors, edema, ischemic and hemorrhagic lesions, hydrocephalus, vascular disorders, inflammatory and infectious lesions, and degenerative processes. MRI can be used to study myelination and demyelination and, through the demonstration of changes in relaxation time, metabolic disorders of the brain, muscles, and glands. Because bone causes no artifact in the images, the posterior fossa and its contents can be studied far better using MRI than with CT scans; even blood vessels and the cranial nerves can be imaged. On the other hand, the inability of MRI to detect calcification limits its usefulness in the investigation of calcified lesions such as craniopharyngioma or leptomeningeal angiomatosis.

It is believed that the strong magnetic fields used in this procedure do not cause molecular or cellular damage. Work is progressing on imaging from nuclei other than hydrogen, such as phosphorus and sodium.

The cost of MRI is two or three times that of a contrast-enhanced CT scan. The procedure can be frightening and requires sedated sleep or light anesthesia for the child to ensure complete immobility. Magnetic resonance angiography (MRA) is a noninvasive (no arterial or venous puncture or dye injection) technique to show large extra- and intracranial blood vessels; it often now replaces the more hazardous intra-arterial injection angiogram.

Positron Emission Tomography

Positron emission tomography (PET) is an imaging technique that measures the metabolic rate at a given site by CT scanning to detect positron (proton) emission. For measurement of local cerebral metabolism, the radiolabeled substrate most frequently used has been fluorodeoxyglucose ^{18}F by injection. Gray matter and white matter are clearly distinguishable; the skull and air- or fluid-filled cavities are least active metabolically.

PET has been used to study the cerebral metabolism of neonates and brain activation by visual or auditory stimuli. Pathologic states that have been studied include epilepsy (during and between seizures), brain infarcts and tumors, and dementias. This functional test of brain metabolism is clinically useful in

preoperative evaluation for epilepsy surgery. The "epileptogenic zone" will often be hypermetabolic during ictal events and hypoactive during the time between seizures. The information complements electrical (EEG) and imaging (MRI) findings to aid in the decision about tissue removal.

With PET, infants with infantile spasms have occasionally been found to have a focal lesion, sometimes leading to successful surgical removal.

Clinical application is limited by the cost of the procedure and the clinician's need for access to a nearby cyclotron for preparation of the radiopharmaceuticals.

Ultrasonography

Ultrasonography offers a pictorial display (eg, echoencephalogram, echocardiogram) of the varying densities of tissues in a given anatomic region or structure by recording the echoes of ultrasonic waves reflected from it. These waves, modulated by pulsations, are introduced into the tissue by means of a piezoelectric transducer. The many advantages of ultrasonography include the ability to assess a structure and its positioning quickly by means of portable equipment, without ionizing radiation and at about one fourth the cost of CT scanning. Sedation is usually not necessary, and the procedure can be repeated as often as indicated. In brain imaging, B-mode and real-time sector scanners are usually used, permitting excellent detail in the coronal and sagittal planes. Contiguous structures can be studied by a continuous sweep and reviewed on videotape.

Ultrasonography has been used for in utero diagnosis of hydrocephalus and other anomalies. In neonates, the thin skull and the open anterior fontanelle have facilitated imaging of the brain, and ultrasonography is now used in many nurseries to screen and follow all infants of less than 32 weeks' gestation or under 1500 g for intracranial hemorrhage. Other uses in neonates include detection of hydrocephalus, major brain and spine malformations, and even calcifications from intrauterine infection with cytomegalovirus or *Toxoplasma*.

Cerebral Angiography

Arteriography remains a useful procedure in the diagnosis of many cerebrovascular disorders, particularly vascular malformations, and is sometimes used when a potentially operable lesion is suspected. In some instances of brain tumor, arteriography may be necessary to define the precise location or vascular bed, to differentiate among tumors, or to distinguish tumor from abscess or infarction. Noninvasive CTs, MRIs, and MRAs are often satisfactory in cases of static or flowing blood disorders (eg, sinus thromboses). Thus, invasive arteriography is used infrequently.

Myelography

X-ray examination of the spine following injection

of a dye, water-soluble contrast medium, or air into the subarachnoid space via the lumbar or, rarely, the cervical route may be indicated in cases of spinal cord tumors or various forms of spinal dysraphism and in rare instances of herniated disks in children. However, in most institutions, MRI or CT metrizamide myelography is employed instead.

Adams C et al: Comparison of SPECT, EEG, CT, MRI, and pathology in partial epilepsy. Pediatr Neurol 1992;8:97.

Altman NR, Purser RK, Post MJ: Tuberous sclerosis: Characteristics at CT and MR imaging. Radiology 1988; 167:527.

Barkovich AJ: *Pediatric Neuroimaging*. Raven Press, 1989.

Chugani K: The role of positron emission tomography in childhood epilepsy. Int Pediatr 1992;7:260.

Doyle LW et al: Regional cerebral glucose metabolism of newborn infants measured by positron emission tomography. Dev Med Child Neurol 1983;25:143.

Edelman RR, Warach S: Magnetic resonance imaging. (Two parts.) N Engl J Med 1993;11:708, 785.

Faerber EN (editor): CNS magnetic resonance imaging in infants & children. *Clinics in Developmental Medicine.* No. 134. MacKeith Press, 1995.

Harvey AS: Functional neuro-imaging with SPECT & PET in childhood developmental disabilities. Int Pediatr 1995;10:177.

Jackson SD et al: Functional magnetic resonance imaging of focal seizure. Neurology 1989;44:850.

Koelfen W et al: Magnetic resonance angiography in 140 patients. Pediatr Neurol 1995;12:31.

Shields WD: Anatomic & functional imaging in epilepsy. Int Pediatr 1995;10:72.

DISORDERS AFFECTING THE NERVOUS SYSTEM IN INFANTS & CHILDREN

ALTERED STATES OF CONSCIOUSNESS

Essentials of Diagnosis

- Reduction or alteration in cognitive and affective mental functioning and in arousability or attentiveness.
- Acute onset.

General Considerations

Coma and other states of unconsciousness are imprecisely defined. Many terms are used to describe the continuum from full alertness and attentiveness to complete unresponsiveness and deep coma, including clouding, obtundation, somnolence or stupor, semicoma or light coma, and deep coma. Several scales have been used to grade the depth of unconsciousness (Tables 23–4 and 23–5). Physicians should use one of these tables and provide further descriptions in case narratives. These descriptions help subsequent observers quantify unconsciousness and evaluate changes in the patient's condition.

The neurologic substrate for consciousness is the reticular activating system in the brain stem, up to and including the thalamus and paraventricular hypothalamus. Large lesions of the cortex, especially of the left hemisphere, can also cause coma. "**Locked-in syndrome**" is a term used for patients who are conscious but have no access to motor or verbal expression because of massive loss of motor function of the brain stem. "**Coma vigil**" is the term used for patients who seem to be comatose but have some

Table 23–4. Gradation of coma.

| | "Deep Coma" | | "Light Coma" | | |
	Grade 4	Grade 3	Grade 2	Grade 1	Stupor
Response to pain	0	+	Avoidance	Avoidance	Arousal unsustained
Tone/posture	Flaccid	Decerebrate	Variable	Variable	Normal
Tendon reflexes	0	+/–	+	+	+
Pupil response	0	+	+	+	+
Response to verbal stimuli	0	0	0	0	+
Other corneal reflex	0	+	+	+	+
Gag reflex	0	+	+	+	+

Table 23–5. "Glasgow Coma Scale" for recording assessment of consciousness.[1]

		Date				
		Time	Time	Time	Time	etc
Best motor response	6 Obeys commands 5 Localizes pain 4 Withdraws 3 Abnormal flexing 2 Extensor response 1 None					
Best verbal response	5 Oriented 4 Confused conversation (words) 3 Inappropriate words (vocal sounds) 2 Incomprehensible sounds (cries) 1 None					
Eye opening	4 Spontaneous 3 To speech 2 To pain 1 None					
	Total Score					

Modified and reproduced, with permission, from Jennett B, Teasdale G: Aspects of coma after severe head injury. Lancet 1977;1:878.

[1]The scale can also be modified for infants. The sections regarding motor response and eye opening remain unchanged; items in parentheses in verbal response section are to be applied to infants. Under 6 months of age, the best verbal response is a cry (score 2) and the best motor response is usually flexion (score 3), for a total maximal score of 9. Adjusted maximal scores are as follows:

Birth–6 months:	9	2–5 years:	13
6–12 months:	11	Over 5 years:	14–15
1–2 years:	12		

spontaneous motor behavior, such as eye opening or eye tracking, almost always at a reflex level. **"Persistent vegetative state"** denotes a chronic condition in which there is preservation of the sleep-wake cycle but no awareness and no recovery of mental function; this has been documented in infants.

Emergency Measures

The clinician's first response is to ensure that the patient will survive the initial examination. The "ABCs" of resuscitation are pertinent: **A**irway must be kept open with positioning or even endotracheal intubation. **B**reathing and adequate air exchange can be assessed by auscultation; hand bag respiratory assistance with oxygen may be needed. **C**irculation must be ensured by assessing pulse and blood pressure. *An intravenous line is always necessary.* Fluids, plasma, blood, or even a dopamine drip (5–20 μg/kg/min) may be required in cases of hypotension. An extremely hypothermic or febrile child may require vigorous cooling or warming to save life. The assessment of vital signs may signal the diagnosis. Slow, insufficient respirations suggest poisoning by hypnotic drugs; apnea may indicate diphenoxylate hydrochloride poisoning. Rapid, deep respirations suggest acidosis, possibly metabolic, as with diabetic coma; toxic, such as that due to aspirin; or neurogenic, as in Reye's syndrome. Hyperthermia may indicate infection or heat stroke; hypothermia may in-

dicate cold exposure, ethanol poisoning, or hypoglycemia (especially in infancy).

The signs of impending brain herniation are another priority of the initial assessment. Bradycardia, high blood pressure, irregular breathing, increased extensor tone, and third nerve palsy with the eye deviated outward and the pupil dilated are possible signs of impending temporal lobe or brain stem herniation. These signs suggest a need for hyperventilation, reducing cerebral edema, prompt neurosurgical consultation, and possibly, in an infant with a bulging fontanelle, subdural or ventricular tap (or both).

Initial intravenous fluids should contain glucose until further assessment disproves hypoglycemia as a cause.

A history obtained from parents or witnesses is desirable. Sometimes the only history will be obtained from ambulance attendants. An important point is whether the child is known to have a chronic illness, such as diabetes, hemophilia, epilepsy, or cystic fibrosis. Recent acute illness raises the possibility of coma caused by Reye's syndrome, viral or bacterial meningitis, or the much rarer hemolytic-uremic syndrome. A combination of viral illness with 1–3 days of sudden and intractable vomiting invariably precedes the coma of Reye's syndrome. (The illness is usually respiratory, sometimes varicella.)

Trauma is a common cause of coma. Lack of a

history of trauma, especially in infants, does not rule it out; nonaccidental trauma or a fall unwitnessed by caretakers may have occurred.

In coma of unknown cause, poisoning is always a possibility. Absence of a history of ingestion of a toxic substance or of medication in the home does not rule out poisoning as a cause.

Often the history is obtained concurrently with a brief pediatric and neurologic screening examination. After the assessment of vital signs and their meaning, the general examination proceeds with a trauma assessment. Palpation of the head and fontanelle, inspection of the ears for infection or hemorrhage, and a careful examination for neck stiffness are indicated. If circumstances suggest head or neck trauma, the head and neck must be immobilized so that any fracture or dislocation will not be aggravated. The skin must be inspected for petechiae or purpura that might suggest bacteremia, infection, bleeding disorder, or traumatic bruising. Examination of the chest, abdomen, and limbs is important to exclude enclosed hemorrhage, traumatic fractures, and the like.

Neurologic examination quantifies the stimulus response and depth of coma, such as responsiveness to verbal or painful stimuli. Examination of the eyes in reference to pupils, fundi, and eye movements is important. Are the eye movements spontaneous, or is it necessary to do the doll's-eye maneuver (rotating the head rapidly to see whether the eyes follow)? Motor and sensory examinations assess reflex asymmetries, Babinski's sign, and evidence of spontaneous posturing or posturing induced by noxious stimuli (eg, decorticate or decerebrate posturing).

If the cause of the coma is not obvious, emergency laboratory tests must be obtained. Table 23–6 lists some of the causes of coma in children and mnemonics for its investigation. An immediate blood glucose (or Dextrostix), complete blood count, urine obtained by catheterization if necessary, pH and electrolytes (including bicarbonate), serum urea nitrogen, and AST are initial screens. Urine, blood, and even gastric contents must be saved for toxin screen if the underlying cause is not obvious. Spinal tap is often necessary to rule out central nervous system infection. Papilledema is a relative contraindication to lumbar puncture. Occasionally, blood culture is obtained, antibiotics started, and imaging study of the brain done prior to a diagnostic spinal tap. If meningitis is suspected and a tap is believed to be hazardous, antibiotics should be started and the diagnostic spinal puncture done later. Tests that are less readily available but helpful in obscure cases of coma include PO_2, PCO_2, ammonia levels, serum and urine osmolality, porphyrins, lead levels, and, in the newborn, urine and serum amino acids and urine organic acids.

If there is any suspicion of head trauma or increased pressure, an emergency CT scan or MRI is necessary. Bone windows on the former study or skull x-rays can be done at the same sitting. The absence of skull fracture, of course, does not rule out coma caused by life-threatening closed head trauma; injury that results from shaking a child is one example. In a child with an open fontanelle, a real-time ultrasound may be substituted for the other, more definitive imaging studies if there is good local expertise.

Rarely, an emergency EEG aids in diagnosing the cause of coma. A nonconvulsive status epilepticus or focal finding seen with herpes encephalitis (periodic lateralized epileptiform discharges) or focal slowing as seen with stroke or cerebritis are cases in which the EEG might be helpful. The EEG also may correlate with the stage of coma (eg, in Reye's syndrome) and add prognostic information. An improving (or deteriorating) EEG may herald clinical improvement, aid in predicting outcome, and suggest the need for more (or less) heroic therapy.

Treatment

A. General Measures: Vital signs must be monitored and maintained. Most emergency rooms and intensive care units have flow sheets that provide space for repeated monitoring of the coma; one of the coma scales can be a useful tool for this purpose. The patient's response to vocal or painful stimuli and orientation to time, place, and situation when coming out of the coma are monitored. Posture and movements of the limbs, either spontaneously or in response to pain, are serially noted. Pupillary size, equality, and reaction to light and movement of the eyes to the doll's-eye maneuver or ice-water calorics should be recorded. Intravenous fluids can be tailored to the situation, as for treatment of acidosis, shock, or hypovolemia. Nasogastric suction is initially important; when the coma is prolonged, nasogastric feedings are sometimes part of treatment. The patient needs to be catheterized for monitoring urine output and for urinalysis. The child should be protected from decubiti with frequent turning and, if necessary, by providing a foam mattress. The eyes should be protected with pads and artificial tears.

B. Seizures: An EEG should be ordered if there is a question of ongoing seizures. If there are obvious motor seizures, treatment for status epilepticus is given with intravenous drugs (see below). If there is suggestion of brain stem herniation or increased pressure, an intracranial monitor may be necessary. This procedure is described in more detail in Chapter 13. Initial treatment of this possible complication includes keeping the patient's head up (15–30 degrees) and hyperventilation. Mannitol, diuretics, corticosteroids, and drainage of CSF are more heroic measures covered in detail elsewhere.

Prognosis

About 50% of children with nontraumatic causes of coma have a good outcome. In studies of adults assessed on admission or within the first days after

Table 23–6. Some causes of coma in childhood.

Mechanism of Coma	Likely Cause	
	Newborn, Infant	Older Child
Anoxia		
Asphyxia	Birth asphyxia	CO poisoning
Respiratory obstruction	Meconium aspiration, infection (especially respiratory syncytial virus)	Croup, epiglottitis
Severe anemia	Hydrops fetalis	Hemolysis, blood loss
Ischemia		
Cardiac	Shunting lesions, hypoplastic left heart	Shunting lesions, aortic stenosis
Shock	Asphyxia (cardiac), sepsis	Blood loss, infection
Trauma	Birth contusion, hemorrhage, nonaccidental trauma	Falls, auto accidents
Infection	Gram-negative meningitis, herpes encephalitis, postimmunization encephalitis	Bacterial meningitis, viral encephalitis, postinfectious encephalitis
Vascular	Intraventricular hemorrhage (premature), sinus thrombosis	Arterial, venous occlusion with congenital heart disease
Neoplasm	Rare; variety, medulloblastoma	Brain stem glioma, increased pressure with posterior fossa tumors
Drugs	Maternal sedatives, injected analgesics	"Any" drugs
Epilepsy	Constant minor motor seizures	Constant minor motor seizures, petit mal status, postictal state
Toxins	Lead	Arsenic, alcohol, drugs, pesticides
Hypoglycemia	Birth injury, diabetic progeny, toxemic progeny	Diabetes, "prediabetes," "idiopathic," hypoglycemic agents
Increased intracranial pressure	Anoxic brain damage, hydrocephalus, unusual metabolic disorders (urea cycle; amino, organic acidurias)	Toxic encephalopathy, Reye's syndrome, head trauma, tumor of posterior fossa
Hepatic causes	Hepatitis, fulminant (rare), bile duct atresia, inborn metabolic errors in bilirubin conjugation	Acute hepatitis, chronic aggressive hepatitis
Renal causes	Hypoplastic kidneys	Nephritis, acute and chronic
Hypertensive encephalopathy		Acute nephritis, vasculitis
Hypercapnia	Congenital lung anomalies, bronchopulmonary dysplasia	Cystic fibrosis
Electrolyte abnormalities		
Hypernatremia	Iatrogenic ($NaHCO_3$ use), salt poisoning	Diarrhea, dehydration
Hyponatremia	Inappropriate antidiuretic hormone, adrenogenital syndrome, dialysis (iatrogenic)	Diarrhea, dehydration, gastroenteritis
Severe acidosis	Septicemia, cold injury, metabolic errors	Infection, diabetic coma, poisoning (eg, aspirin)
Hyperkalemia	Renal failure, adrenogenital syndrome	Poisoning (aspirin)
Purpuric	Disseminated intravascular coagulation (many causes), hemolytic-uremic syndrome	Disseminated intravascular coagulation (many causes), leukemia, thrombotic purpura (rare)

Modified and reproduced, with permission, from Lewis J, Moe PG: The unconscious child. In: *Current Diagnosis,* 5th ed. Conn H, Conn R (editors). WB Saunders, 1977.

the onset of coma, an analysis of multiple variables was most helpful in assessing prognosis. Abnormal neuro-ophthalmologic signs (eg, the absence of pupillary movement or of movement in response to the doll's-eye maneuver or ice-water calorics and the absence of corneal responses) were unfavorable. Delay in the return of motor responses, tone, or eye opening was also unfavorable. In children, the assessment done on admission is about as predictive as one done in succeeding days. Approximately two

thirds of outcomes can be successfully predicted at an early stage on the basis of coma severity, extraocular movements, pupillary reactions, motor patterns, blood pressure, temperature, and seizure type. Other characteristics, such as the need for assisted respiration, the presence of increased intracranial pressure, and the duration of coma, were not significantly predictive.

Published reports suggest that an anoxic (in contrast to traumatic, metabolic, toxic, and so on) cause of coma, such as that caused by near drowning, has a much grimmer outlook.

BRAIN DEATH

Many medical and law associations have endorsed the following definition of death: "An individual who has sustained either (1) irreversible cessation of circulatory and respiratory functions, or (2) irreversible cessation of all functions of the entire brain, including the brain stem, is dead. A determination of death must be made in accordance with accepted medical standards." Representatives from several pediatric and neurologic associations have endorsed the Guidelines for the Determination of Brain Death in Children. The criteria in term infants (older than 38 weeks) were applicable 1 week after the neurologic insult. Difficulties in assessing premature infants and term infants shortly after birth were acknowledged.

Prerequisites

In assessment of brain death, the history is important. The physician must determine proximate causes to make sure there are no remediable or reversible conditions. Examples of such causes are metabolic conditions, toxic agents, sedative-hypnotic drugs, surgically remediable conditions, hypothermia, and paralytic agents.

Physical Examination Criteria (Chapter 13)

The following criteria are those established by the Task Force on Brain Death in Children.

  1. **Coexistence of coma and apnea.** The patient must exhibit complete loss of consciousness, vocalization, and volitional activity.

  2. **Absence of brain stem function** as defined by the following: (a) Midposition or fully dilated pupils that do not respond to light. Drugs may influence and invalidate pupillary assessment. (b) Absence of spontaneous eye movements and those induced by oculocephalic and caloric (oculovestibular) testing. (c) Absence of movement of bulbar musculature, including facial and oropharyngeal muscles. The corneal, gag, cough, sucking, and rooting reflexes are absent. (d) Absence of respiratory movements when the patient is off the respirator. Apnea testing using standardized methods can be performed but is done after other criteria are met.

  3. **Temperature and blood pressure:** The patient must not be significantly hypothermic or hypotensive for age.

  4. **Tone is flaccid,** and spontaneous or induced movements, excluding spinal cord events such as reflex withdrawal or spinal myoclonus, are absent.

  5. **The examination should remain consistent with brain death** throughout the observation and testing period.

Confirmation

Details of apnea testing suggest documentation of a PCO_2 level greater than 60 mm Hg, with oxygenation maintained throughout; this level may be reached 3–15 minutes after taking the patient off the respirator. The recommended observation period to confirm brain death (repeated examinations) is 12–24 hours (longer in infants); *reversible causes must be ruled out.*

If an irreversible cause is documented, laboratory testing is not essential. Helpful tests to support the clinical contention of brain death include the following:

  1. **Electroencephalography:** Electrocerebral silence should persist for 30 minutes. Drug concentrations must be insufficient to suppress EEG activity.

  2. **Angiography:** Failure of arterial intracerebral blood flow confirms brain death. Carotid arteriography and cerebral radionuclide angiography are two methods. Dural sinus flow may persist and not invalidate the diagnosis of brain death.

Other laboratory studies have not been sufficiently documented to be considered definitive; cerebral evoked potentials and ultrasound blood pulsations are two common examples. Xenon-enhanced computer tomography is a more elaborate method.

In rare cases, preserved intracranial perfusion in the presence of electroencephalographic silence has been documented, and the converse has also been reported. Controversy attends the definition and criteria of brain death in the newborn. This debate inevitably acknowledges the issue of withdrawing support from the infant with a hopeless prognosis who is not brain dead.

Ashwal S, Schneider S: Brain death in the newborn. Pediatrics 1989;84:427.

Ashwal S, Schneider S, Thompson J: Xenon computed tomography measuring cerebral blood flow in the determination of brain death in children. Ann Neurol 1989; 25:539.

Childs NL, Mercer WN, Childs HW: Accuracy of diagnosis of persistent vegetative state. Neurology 1993;43:1465.

Fishman MA: Validity of brain death criteria in infants. Pediatrics 1995;96:513.

Goldie WD: Physiologic parameters for evaluating severe brain injury in infants and young children. Am J EEG Technol 1988;28:153.

Jones KM, Barnes PD: MR diagnosis of brain death. AJNR Am J Neuroradiol 199 2;13:65.

Lang CJG: Apnea testing by artificial CO_2 augmentation. Neurology 1995;45:966.

Lewis J, Moe PG: The unconscious child. In: *Current Diagnosis*, 5th ed. Conn H, Conn R (editors). Saunders, 1977.

Mizrahi EM, Pollack MA, Kellaway P: Neocortical death in infants: Behavioral, neurologic, and electroencephalographic characteristics. Pediatr Neurol 1985;1:302.

Shewmon DA: Commentary on guidelines for the determination of brain death in children. Ann Neurol 1988; 24:789.

Task Force on Brain Death in Children: Guidelines for the determination of brain death in children. Ann Neurol 1987;21:616. [Also Arch Neurol 1987;44:587. Neurology 1987;37:1077. Pediatr Neurol 1987;3:242. Pediatrics 1987;80:298.]

Teasdale G, Jennett B: Assessment of coma and impaired consciousness: A practical scale. Lancet 1974;2:81.

Vegetative state: Report of the American Neurological Association Committee on Ethical Affairs. Ann Neurol 1993;33:386.

Yager JY, Johnston B, Seshia SS: Coma scales in pediatric practice. Am J Dis Child 1990;144:1088.

SEIZURE DISORDERS (Epilepsies)

Essentials of Diagnosis

- Recurrent nonfebrile seizures.
- Often, interictal electroencephalographic changes.

General Considerations

A **seizure** is a sudden, transient disturbance of brain function, manifested by involuntary motor, sensory, autonomic, or psychic phenomena, alone or in any combination, often accompanied by alteration or loss of consciousness. A seizure may occur after a transient metabolic, traumatic, anoxic, or infectious insult to the brain.

Repeated seizures without evident time-limited cause justify the label of **epilepsy**. Seizures and epilepsy occur most commonly at the extremes of life. The incidence is highest in the newborn and higher in childhood than in later life. Epilepsy in childhood often remits. Prevalence flattens out after age 10–15. The chance of having a second seizure after an initial unprovoked episode is 30%. The chance of remission from epilepsy in childhood is 50%. The recurrence rate after the withdrawal of drugs is about 30%. Factors adversely influencing recurrence include (1) difficulty in getting the seizures under control (ie, the number of seizures occurring before control is achieved); (2) neurologic dysfunction or mental retardation; (3) age at onset under 2 years; and (4) abnormal EEG at the time of discontinuing medication. The type of seizures also often determines prognosis.

Seizures are caused by any factor that can disturb brain function. Seizures and epilepsy are often classified as **symptomatic** (the cause is strongly identified or presumed) or **idiopathic** (the cause is unknown, or genetic influences are strongly etiologic). The younger the infant or child, the more likely that the cause can be identified. Idiopathic or genetic epilepsy most often appears between ages 4 and 16. A seizure disorder or epilepsy should not be considered idiopathic unless a searching history, examination, and appropriate laboratory tests have turned up no apparent cause.

Clinical Findings

A. Symptoms & Signs: The key to the diagnosis of epilepsy is the history. The initial symptom often identifies the aura to the seizure itself. A feeling of fear, numbness or tingling in the fingers, or bright lights in one visual field might be examples of an aura (really the onset of the seizure). Sometimes the patient recalls nothing because there has been no aura or warning. The parent might report that the patient's eyes went off to one side or that extreme pallor, trismus, or overall body stiffening occurred first. Occasionally there is a prodrome; for example, a feeling of "unwellness," of something about to happen, or a recurrent thought over minutes or hours prior to the aura and seizure itself.

Minute details of the seizure can help determine the site of onset and aid in classification. Did the patient become extremely pale before falling? Was the patient able to respond to queries during the episode? Did the patient become completely unconscious? Did the patient fall stiffly or gradually slump to the floor? Was there an injury? How long did the stiffening or jerking last? Where were the sites of jerking?

Events after the seizure can be helpful in diagnosis. Was there loss of speech? Was the patient able to respond accurately before going to sleep?

All these events prior to, during, and after the seizure can help to classify the seizure and, indeed, may help to determine if the event actually was a probable epileptic seizure or a pseudoseizure (a nonepileptic phenomenon mimicking a seizure). Classifying the seizure may aid in diagnosis or prognosis and suggest desirable or necessary laboratory tests and medications (Tables 23–7 and 23–8).

B. Status Epilepticus: Status epilepticus is a clinical or electrical seizure lasting at least 30 minutes, or a series of seizures without complete recovery over the same period of time. After 30 minutes, the brain begins to suffer from hypoxia and acidosis, with depletion of local energy stores, cerebral edema, and structural damage. Eventually, high fever, hypotension, respiratory depression, and even death may occur. Thus, *status epilepticus is a relative medical emergency.*

Status epilepticus is classified as (1) convulsive—the common tonic-clonic, or "grand mal" status epilepticus; or (2) nonconvulsive, such as simple motor status without loss of consciousness. Other nonconvulsive types include absence status, or "spike-wave stupor," and (very rare) partial complex status epilepticus.

An EEG may be necessary to aid in diagnosing the less common variants, such as a patient with known absence who now is in a partially-in-contact, stuporous state.

A child with status epilepticus often has a high

Table 23–7. Clinical seizure correlation with electroencephalographic patterns.[1]

Clinical Seizure Type	EEG Ictal	EEG Interictal
Focal (partial) Simple partial (focal) Motor, sensory	Local contralateral discharge (eg, spike, slow wave)	Same
Complex partial (psychomotor)	Focal or bilateral frontal, temporal discharge	Temporofrontal local or asynchronous discharge
Partial seizures with generalization	Above discharges become lateralized	
Generalized Absence (petit mal) Simple (impairment of consciousness only) Complex (with tonic, clonic, autonomic component)	3/sec spike wave	Normal
Atypical absence	Irregular 1–4/s spike-wave	Abnormal, often slow spike wave, asymmetric
Myoclonic seizures	Multiple spike-wave	Same
Tonic-clonic (grand mal)	10/s spike/slowing, then spike/slow wave	Multiple spikes, spike wave sharp, slow
Atonic (astatic, akinetic)	Multiple spike-wave	Same

[1]According to the International Classification of Epileptic Seizures. Some subtypes are not listed. Some age-limited syndromes occurring in childhood are not easily incorporated into this scheme.

fever with or without intracranial infection, such as viral encephalitis or bacterial meningitis. Status epilepticus may be the initial seizure; various studies show that 25–75% of children experience status epilepticus as the initial seizure. Often, it is a reflection of a remote insult (eg, anoxic or traumatic). Tumor, vascular disease (strokes), or head trauma, which are common causes of status epilepticus in adults, are uncommon causes in childhood. Fifty percent of cases are symptomatic of acute (25%) or chronic (25%) CNS disorders. Infection or metabolic disorders are the most common symptomatic causes in children. The cause is unknown in 50% of cases, but many of these will be febrile.

Status epilepticus is more common in children under 1 year of age, with 37% of cases occurring under that age and 85% under age 5. Thus, the pediatrician sees status epilepticus most commonly in infants and preschoolers. For treatment, see Table 23–9.

C. Febrile Seizures: Criteria for febrile seizures are (1) age of 3 months to 5 years (most occur between the ages of 6–18 months), (2) fever of 38.8 °C, and (3) non-central nervous system infection. Most (greater than 90%) are generalized and brief (less than 5 minutes) and occur early in an OMPA (otitis media, pharyngitis, adenitis) illness. Febrile seizures occur in 2–3% of children. Gastroenteritis, especially when caused by *Shigella* or *Campylobacter*, and urinary tract infections are less common causes. Roseola infantum is a rare but classic cause. One study implicated viral causes in 86% of cases. Immunizations may be a cause.

Rarely, status epilepticus may occur; fever is a common cause of status epilepticus in early childhood. Febrile seizures rarely (2– 4%) lead to epilepsy or recurrent nonfebrile seizures in later childhood and adult life. The chance of later epilepsy is higher if the febrile seizures have complex features, such as a duration of over 15 minutes, more than one seizure in the same day, or focal features. Other adverse factors are an abnormal neurologic status preceding the seizures (eg, cerebral palsy or mental retardation); early onset of febrile seizure (before 1 year of age); and a family history of epilepsy. Even with adverse factors, the risk of epilepsy in later life is low, in the range of 15–20%.

Recurrent febrile seizures occur in 20–40% of cases but, in general, do not worsen the long-term outlook.

The child with a febrile seizure must be examined. Routine studies such as serum electrolytes, glucose, calcium, skull x-rays, or brain imaging studies are seldom helpful. A white count above 20,000/μL or with an extreme left shift may correlate with bacteremia; complete blood count and blood cultures may be appropriate studies. Serum sodium is often slightly low but not low enough to require treatment or to cause the seizure. *Meningitis must be ruled out.* Bacterial meningitis can present with a fever and seizure. Signs of meningitis (eg, bulging fontanelle, stiff neck, stupor, and irritability) may all be absent, especially in a child under 18 months of age.

After controlling the fever and stopping an ongoing seizure, the physician must decide whether to do a spinal tap. The fact that the child has had a previous febrile seizure does not rule out meningitis as the cause of the current episode. The younger the child, the more important the tap, because physical findings are less reliable in diagnosing meningitis. Although the yield is low, a tap should probably be done if the child is under age 2, if recovery is slow, if no other cause for the fever is found, or if close follow-up will not be possible. Occasionally, observation in the emergency room for several hours obviates the need for a tap. A negative tap does not rule out the emergence of meningitis during the same febrile illness; sometimes a second tap needs to be done.

Table 23–8. Seizures by age at onset, pattern, and preferred treatment.

Age Group and Seizure Type	Age at Onset	Clinical Manifestations	Causative Factors	Electroencephalographic Pattern	Other Diagnostic Studies	Treatment and Comments (Anticonvulsants by Order of Choice)
Neonatal seizures	Birth to 2 weeks	Often "atypical"; sudden limpness or tonic posturing, brief apnea, and cyanosis; odd cry; eyes "rolling up"; blinking or mouthing or chewing movements; nystagmus, twitchiness or clonic movements—focal, multifocal, or generalized. Some seizures are nonepileptic–decerebrate, or other posturings; release from forebrain inhibition; poor response to drugs.	Neurologic insults (hypoxia/ischemia; intracranial hemorrhage) present more in first 3 days or after eighth day; metabolic disturbances alone between third and eighth days; hypoglycemia, hypocalcemia, hyper- and hyponatremia. Drug withdrawal. Pyridoxine deficiency and other metabolic causes. CNS infections and structural abnormalities.	May correlate poorly with clinical seizures. Focal spikes or slow rhythms; multifocal discharges. "Electroclinical dissociation" may occur: EEG-electrical seizure without clinical manifestations and vice versa.	Lumbar puncture; serum Ca^{2+}, PO_4^{3-}, glucose Mg^{2+}; BUN, amino acid screen, blood ammonia, organic acid screen, TORCHES[1] screen. Ultrasound or CT scan for suspected intracranial hemorrhage and structural abnormalities.	Phenobarbital, IV or IM; if seizures not controlled, add phenytoin IV (loading dose 20 mg/kg each). Diazepam 0.3 mg/kg. Treat underlying disorder. Seizures due to brain damage often resistant to anticonvulsants. When cause in doubt, stop protein feedings until enzyme deficiencies of urea cycle or amino acid metabolism ruled out.
West's syndrome "infantile spasms." (See also Lennox-Gastaut syndrome, below.)	3–18 months; occasionally up to 4 years	Sudden, usually symmetric adduction and flexion of limbs with concomitant flexion of head and trunk; less often abduction and extensor movements like Moro reflex. Tendency for spasms to occur in clusters, on waking or falling asleep, or when fatigued, or may be noted particularly when the infant is being handled, is ill, or is otherwise irritable. Tendency for each patient to have own stereotyped pattern.	Pre- or perinatal brain damage or malformation in approximately one-third; biochemical, infectious, degenerative causes in approximately one-third; unknown in approximately one-third. With early onset, pyridoxine deficiency, aminoi or organic aciduria. Tuberous sclerosis in 5–10%. Chronic inflammatory disease and toxoplasmosis. Aicardi syndrome (females with mental retardation, agenesis of corpus callosum, ocular and vertebral anomalies).	Hypsarrhythmia; chaotic high-voltage slow waves, random spikes, all leads (90%), other abnormalities in rest. Rarely "normal." EEG normalization usually correlates with reduction of seizures; not helpful prognostically regarding mental development.	Funduscopic and skin examination, trial of pyridoxine. Amino- and organic acid screen. Chronic inflammatory disease. TORCHES[1] screen, CT or MRI scan shall be done to (1) establish definite diagnosis, (2) aid in genetic counseling. SPECT or PET scan may identify focal lesion.	ACTM preferred (2–4 units/kg/d IM Acthar gel 1/d, then slow withdrawal). Some prefer oral corticosteroids. Clonazepam, valproic acid. In resistant cases, ketogenic or medium-chain triglyceride diet (see text). Retardation of varying degree in approximately 90% of cases. Occasionally, surgical extirpation of focal lesion may be curative.
Febrile convulsions	3 months to 5 years (maximum 6–18 mo)	Usually generalized seizures, less than 15 minutes; rarely focal in onset. May lead to status epilepticus. Latter usually benign. Recurrence risk of second febrile seizure 30%; 50% if under 1 year of age.	Nonneurologic febrile illness (temperature rises to 102.5°F or higher); family history frequently positive for febrile convulsions.	Normal interictal EEG, especially when obtained 8–10 days after seizure. In older infants, 3/s spikes often seen.	Lumbar puncture in infants or whenever suspicion of meningitis exists.	Treat underlying illness, fever. Diazepam orally or rectally as needed 0.3–0.5 mg/kg 3 times daily during illness. Prophylaxis with phenobarbital (valproic acid if phenobarbital not tolerated), with neurologic deficits, prolonged seizure, family history of epilepsy.
Myoclonic-astatic (akinetic, atonic) seizures, formerly atypical absence. When mental retardation is presented, this is called Lennox-Gastaut syndrome	Any time in childhood; normally 2–7 years	Shocklike violent contractions of one or more muscle groups, singly or irregularly repetitive; may fling patient suddenly to side, forward, or backward. Usually no or only brief loss of consciousness. Half of patients or more also have generalized grand mal seizures.	Multiple causes, usually resulting in diffuse neuronal damage. History of West's syndrome; prenatal or perinatal brain damage; viral meningoencephalitides; subacute sclerosing panencephalitis; CNS degenerative disorders; lead or other encephalopathies; structural cerebral abnormalities, eg, porencephaly.	Atypical slow (1–2.5 Hz) spike-wave complexes ("petit mal variant") and bursts of high-voltage generalized spikes, often with diffusely slow background frequencies. See text.	As dictated by index of suspicion. Lumbar puncture with measles antibody titer and CSF IgG index. Nerve conduction studies. Skin biopsy for electron microscopy. MRI scan, WBC lysosomal enzymes if metabolic degeneration disease suspected.	Difficult to treat. Valproic acid, clonazepam, or ethosuximide. Felbamate. Imipramine as adjunct. Diazepam. Ketogenic or medium-chain triglyceride diet. ACTH or corticosteroids as in West's syndrome. Protect head with helmet and chin padding.
Absence ("petit mal"). Also juvenile and myoclonic absence.	3–15 years	Lapses of consciousness or vacant stares, lasting about 10 seconds, often in "clusters." Automatisms of face and hands; clonic activity in 30–45%. Often confused with complex partial seizures but no aura or postictal confusion.	Unknown. Genetic component: probably an autosomal dominant gene.	3/s bilaterally synchronous, symmetric, high-voltage spikes and waves. EEG "normalization" correlates closely with control of seizures.	Hyperventilation when patient on inadequate or no medication often provokes attacks. CT scan is rarely of value.	Valproic acid or ethosuximide; with latter, add phenobarbital or valproate if major motor seizures. In resistant cases, ketogenic or medium-chain triglyceride diet. Also, in resistant cases, valproic acid and ethosuximide together.

	Age	Clinical Features	Etiology/Genetics	EEG	Diagnostic Studies	Treatment
Simple partial or focal seizures (motor/sensory/jacksonian). (Complex partial or psychomotor seizures, below.)	Any age	Seizure may involve any part of body; may spread in fixed pattern (jacksonian march), becoming generalized. In children, epileptogenic focus often "shifts," and epileptic manifestations may change concomitantly.	Often secondary to birth trauma, inflammatory process, vascular accidents, meningoencephalitis, etc. If seizures are coupled with new or progressive neurologic deficits, a structural lesion (eg, brain tumor) is likely	Focal spikes or slow waves in appropriate cortical region; sometimes diffusely abnormal or even normal.	If seizures are difficult to control or progressive deficits occur, neuroradiodiagnostic studies, particularly CT brain scan, imperative (see text).	Carbamazepine, phenytoin, phenobarbital or primidone. Valproic acid useful adjunct.
Complex partial seizures (psychomotor, temporal lobe, or limbic seizures).	Any age	Aura may be a sensation of fear, epigastric discomfort, odd smell or taste (usually unpleasant), visual or auditory hallucination (either vague and "unformed" or well-formed image, words, music). Aura and seizure stereotyped for each patient. Seizure may consist of vague stare; facial, tongue, or swallowing movements and throaty sounds; or various complex automatisms. Unlike absences, complex partial seizures tend not to occur in clusters but singly and to last longer (1 minute or more), followed by confusion. History of aura (or child running to adult from "vague fear") and of automatisms involving more than face and hands establishes diagnosis.	As above. Temporal lobes especially sensitive to hypoxia; thus, this seizure type may be sequela of birth trauma, febrile convulsions, etc. Also especially vulnerable to certain viral infections, especially herpes simplex. Remediable other causes are small cryptic tumors or vascular malformations.	As above, but occurring in temporal lobe and its connections, eg, frontotemporal, temporoparietal, temporo-occipital regions.	MRI when structural lesions suspected. PCR of cerebrospinal fluid in acute febrile situation for herpes; rarely temporal lobe biopsy. Carotid amobarbital injection when lateralization of speech dominance in quesiton, and surgical extirpation of epileptogenic area is contemplated.	Carbamazepine, phenytoin, phenobarbital, or primidone. More than one drug may be necessary. Valproic acid may be useful. Phenacemide in seizures difficult to control. In cases uncontrolled by drugs and where a primary epileptogenic focus is identifiable, excision of anterior third of temporal lobe. Adjunctive psychotherapy required frequently. Gabapentin, and lamotrigine (for > 16 year olds).
"Benign epilepsy of childhood" (with "centrotemporal" or "rotandic" foci).	5–16 years	Partial motor or generalized seizures. Similar seizure patterns may be observed in patients with focal cortical lesions.	Seizure history of abnormal EEG findings in relatives of 40% of affected probands and 18- to 20% of parents and siblings, suggesting transmission by a single autosomal dominant gene, possibly with age-dependent penetrance.	Centrotemporal spikes or sharp waves ("rolandic discharges") appearing paroxysmally against a normal EEG background.	Seldom need CT or MRI scan.	Carbamazepine or phenytoin. Primidone or phenobarbital.
Juvenile myoclonic epilepsy (of Janz).	Late childhood and adolescence, peaking at 13 years	Mild myoclonic jerks of neck and shoulder flexor muscles after waking up or "awakening" grand mal seizures. Intelligence usually normal.	40% of relatives have myoclonias, especially in females; 15% have the abnormal EEG pattern with clinical attacks.	Interictal EEG shows fast variety of spike-and-wave sequences or 4- to 6-Hz multispike and wave complexes.	Differentiate from progressive myoclonic encephalopathy of Unverricht-Lafora and other degenerative disorders by appropriate biopsies (muscle, liver, etc).	Valproic acid. Phenobarbital. Primidone.
Generalized tonic-clonic seizures (grand mal).	Any age	Loss of consciousness; tonic-clonic movements, often preceded by vague aura or cry. Bladder and bowel incontinence in approximately 15%. Postictal confusion; sleep. Often mixed with or masking other seizure patterns.	Often unknown. Genetic component. May be seen with metabolic disturbances, trauma, infection, intoxication, degenerative disorders, brain tumors.	Bilaterally synchronous, symmetric multiple high-voltage spikes, spikes and waves, mixed patterns. Often normal under age 4.	As above.	Phenobarbital in first 12 months; carbamazepine or valproic acid; phenytoin; primidone. Combinations may be necessary.

[1]TORCHES is a mnemonic formula for toxoplasmosis, rubella, cytomegalovirus, herpes simplex, and syphilis.

Table 23–9. Status epilepticus treatment.

1. ABCs
   a. Airway: Maintain oral airway; intubation may be necessary.
   b. Breathing: Oxygen by mouth (if available).
   c. Circulation: Assess pulse, blood pressure; support with IV fluids, drugs. Monitor vital signs.
2. Start glucose-containing IV; draw Dextrostix/blood glucose; evaluate electrolytes, HCO_3^-, CBC, BUN, anticonvulsant levels.
3. Arterial blood gases, pH.
4. Give 50% glucose if dextrose low (1–2 mL/kg).
5. Begin IV drug therapy; goal is to control status in 20–60 minutes.
   a. Diazepam 0.1–0.3 mg/kg over 1–5 minutes (20 mg maximum); may repeat in 5–20 minutes (short action: 20 minutes; watch for respiratory depression), **or,** lorazepam 0.05–0.2 mg/kg, less effective with repeated doses, longer-acting than diazepam. Midazolam hydrochloride; ICU use only IM, IV; intubation desirable.
   b. Phenytoin 10–20 mg/kg over 5–20 minutes (*not* IM) 1000 mg maximum); monitor with blood pressure and ECG if available.
   c. Phenobarbital 5–20 mg/kg (sometimes higher for newborns, refractory status in intubated patients in hospital and with monitored blood levels.)
6. Correct metabolic perturbations (eg, low-sodium, acidosis).
7. Other drug approaches in refractory status:
   a. Repeat phenytoin, phenobarbital (5–10 mg/kg); monitor blood levels. Support respiration, BP as necessary.
   b. IV paraldehyde 4% solution or rectal paraldehyde 0.1–0.3 mL/kg diluted 1:1 in olive oil.
   c. Valproic acid suspension 50 mg/mL diluted 1:1, 30–60 mg/kg orally or rectally.
8. General anesthetic.
9. Consider underlying causes:
   a. Structural disorders or trauma (even nonaccidental trauma). Consider CT scan.
   b. Infection: Spinal tap, blood culture, antibiotics.
   c. Metabolic disorders: Lactic acidosis, toxins, uremia. May need HCO_3^-, medication, toxin screen, judicious fluid administration.
10. Give maintenance drug (if diazepam only was sufficient to halt status epilepticus): phenytoin 10 mg/kg, phenobarbital 5–10 mg/kg, daily dose IV (or by mouth) divided every 12 hours.

Treatment after the seizure is problematic. Many clinicians choose to treat the child with maintenance dosage of anticonvulsant medication during the course of that febrile illness. Diazepam, 0.5 mg/kg two or three times a day orally or rectally, has been used in Europe and Japan with success both for prophylaxis and for prevention of subsequent seizures. (Suppositories are not currently available in the United States.) Phenobarbital and valproate sodium are other choices; however, the somnolence due to the phenobarbital load (about 5–10 mg/kg) is often disquieting to both the doctor and parent and sometimes confuses follow-up assessments. Valproic acid imposes greater risks and should not be given if there is vomiting or acidosis.

Most clinicians choose to follow up the patient without administering anticonvulsant medication. Measures to control fever (sponging, antipyretics, and appropriate antibiotics if a bacterial illness is suspected or found) are the mainstays of treatment. The family can be reassured that simple febrile seizures are not thought to have any long-term adverse consequences. An EEG should be ordered if the febrile seizure is complicated or unusual; in the uncomplicated febrile seizure, the EEG is most often normal. About 10% will have slowing or other occipital abnormalities. Ideally, the study should be done at least a week after the illness to avoid transient findings due to the fever or seizure itself. In older children, 3 per second spike-wave discharge, suggestive of a genetic propensity to epilepsy, may occur. In the young infant, electroencephalographic findings seldom aid in assessing the chance of recurrence of febrile or nonfebrile seizures.

Prophylactic anticonvulsants are not indicated in the uncomplicated febrile seizure patient. If febrile seizures are complicated or prolonged, or if medical reassurance fails to relieve family anxiety, anticonvulsant prophylaxis may be indicated and can reduce the incidence of recurrent febrile or nonfebrile seizures. One remedy is to use diazepam at the first onset of fever for the duration of the febrile illness as noted above. Phenobarbital, 3–5 mg/kg/d as a single bedtime dose, is an inexpensive and safe alternative. Often, increasing the dose gradually (eg, starting with 2 mg/kg/d the first week and increasing to 3 mg/kg/d the second week, and so on) decreases side effects and noncompliance. A plasma phenobarbital level in the range of 15–40 μg/mL is desirable.

Valproate sodium is more hazardous. In infants, the liquid suspension must often be used but has a short half-life and causes more gastrointestinal upset than the coated capsules used in older children. The dose is 15–60 mg/kg/d in three or four divided doses. Precautionary laboratory studies are necessary.

Phenytoin and carbamazepine have not shown effectiveness in the prophylaxis of febrile seizures.

D. Laboratory Findings & Imaging: Ordering of laboratory tests depends on the age of the child, the severity and type of the seizure, whether the child is ill or injured, and the clinician's suspicion about the underlying cause. *Every case of suspected seizure disorder warrants an EEG.* Other studies are used selectively. Seizures in early infancy are often symptomatic. Therefore, the younger the child, the more careful must be the laboratory assessment (Table 23–10).

Metabolic abnormalities are seldom found in the well child with seizures; unless there is a high clinical suspicion of uremia, hyponatremia, or other serious condition, laboratory tests are not necessary. Special studies may be necessary in unusual circumstances, as when hemolytic-uremic syndrome or lead poisoning is a suspected cause. CT scans are

Table 23–10. Laboratory studies in first seizure of epilepsy (nonneonatal).

Well infant: EEG. Calcium, BUN, or urinalysis, and perhaps CT or MRI (abnormal examination or focally abnormal EEG may prompt an imaging study).
Well older child: EEG. Consider CT or MRI.
Ill infant: Calcium, magnesium, CBC, BUN, electrolytes, blood culture, LP, EEG, possibly CT or MRI.
Ill older child: CBC, BUN, LP, EEG, CT, or MRI.
Generalized tonic-clonic seizure: As above.
Generalized absence: EEG only.
Atypical absence: EEG, CT, MRI: Consider studies for mental retardation: serum and urine amino and organic acids, and chromosomes, including fragile X. If there is progressive worsening, consider lysosomal enzymes, LP (protein, enzymes, IgG), perhaps long-chain fatty acids, skin/conjunctival biopsies.
Infantile spasms: See Atypical absence.
Myoclonic, progressive seizure with mental retardation: See Atypical absence.
Focal: EEG. In cases of mental retardation, positive neurologic examination, EEG focal slow wave, or poorly controlled seizures, do CT or MRI. In refractory cases, consider surgical evaluation.

overused in patients with seizures. The youngster with a routine febrile seizure, a nonfebrile generalized seizure with normal examination and normal EEG, or an absence seizure does not need a CT or MRI scan. The yield in a child with normal neurologic examination and EEG is less than 5%. Conversely, in children with symptomatic epileptic syndromes, the yield of positive results is as high as 60–80%. Examples include infantile spasms, Lennox-Gastaut syndrome, and progressive myoclonic epilepsy.

In focal seizures, children with benign rolandic epilepsy do not need a CT scan; it will invariably be normal. The yield with other focal seizures is 15–30%, with most of the findings unimportant in relation to diagnosis and prognosis (eg, a mildly dilated single ventricle, superficial atrophy). Nonetheless, an imaging study eases anxiety and rules out the remote possibility of tumor or vascular malformation. Other indications for CT or MRI scan include difficulty in controlling seizures, progressive neurologic findings on serial examinations, worsening focal findings on the EEG, suspicion of increased pressure, and, of course, any case in which surgery is being considered. A previous normal scan does not rule out an emerging tumor; if the course is unsatisfactory, repeating the scan may be necessary. A neoplasm or other unexpected treatable lesion is found in a small number, perhaps 2–3%, of CT scans.

E. Electroencephalography: The limitations of electroencephalography—even in epilepsy, where it is most useful—are considerable. *A seizure is a clinical phenomenon*; an EEG showing epileptiform activity may confirm and even extend the clinical diagnosis, but it cannot make the diagnosis.

The EEG need not be abnormal in the presence of a definite seizure disorder. Normal EEGs are seen following a first generalized seizure in one third of children under 4 years of age; the initial EEG is normal in about 20% of older epileptic children and in about 10% of adults with epilepsy. These percentages are reduced when serial tracings are obtained. On the other hand, various grades of "arrhythmias" are frequently observed in children; focal spikes and generalized spike-wave discharges are seen in 30% of close nonepileptic relatives of patients with centrencephalic epilepsy.

1. Diagnostic value: The greatest value of the EEG in convulsive disorders is to help classify seizure types and thus to select appropriate therapy (Table 23–7). Petit mal absences and partial complex or psychomotor seizures are sometimes difficult to distinguish, especially when the physician must rely on the history and cannot observe one; their differing electroencephalographic patterns will then prove most helpful. Another frequent illustration of the role of the EEG in guiding therapy is the finding of mixed seizure patterns in a child who clinically has only grand mal or only petit mal absences, since some anticonvulsants efficacious for one seizure type may provoke the other. The EEG may often help in diagnosing neonatal seizures with minimal and "atypical" clinical manifestations; it may show "hypsarhythmia" in infantile spasms or the pattern associated with the Lennox-Gastaut syndrome, both expressions of diffuse brain dysfunctioning of multiple causes and generally of grave significance. The EEG may help differentiate "convulsive equivalents" from somatic complaints of psychogenic origin.

The EEG may show focal slowing that, if constant—particularly when there are corresponding focal seizure manifestations and abnormal neurologic findings—will alert the physician to the presence of a structural lesion, in which case brain imaging may establish the cause and help determine further investigation and treatment.

2. Prognostic value: A normal EEG following a first convulsion suggests (but does not guarantee) a favorable prognosis. Markedly abnormal EEGs may become normal with treatment (1) immediately following intravenous injection of 50 mg of vitamin B_6 in pyridoxine dependency or deficiency; (2) in infantile spasms and sometimes the Lennox-Gastaut syndrome (ACTH or corticosteroids); (3) in petit mal absences (anticonvulsants); and (4) in petit mal and other minor motor seizures, including the Lennox-Gastaut syndrome (ketogenic diet). If so, it is likely that seizure control will be achieved (though this offers no clues to the mental status of the patient).

Electroencephalography should be repeated when there is an increase in the severity and frequency of seizures despite exhaustive and adequate anticonvulsant therapy; when there is a significant change in the clinical seizure pattern; or when there are progressive neurologic deficits. Focal or diffuse slowing may indicate a progressive lesion.

The EEG may be helpful in determining when to discontinue anticonvulsant therapy. The presence or absence of epileptiform activity on the EEG prior to withdrawal of anticonvulsants after a seizure-free period of several years on the medications has been shown to be correlated with the degree of risk of recurrence of seizures.

Differential Diagnosis

It is extremely important that a nonepileptic condition be accurately labeled. To the lay person, epilepsy often has connotations of brain damage and limitation of activity; a person so diagnosed may be precluded from certain occupations in later life. It is often very difficult to change an inaccurate diagnosis of many years' standing.

Some of the common nonepileptic events that mimic seizure disorder are listed in Table 23–11.

Complications

Emotional disturbances—notably anxiety, depression, anger, feelings of guilt and inadequacy—often occur in the parents of the affected child as a reaction to the seizures, as well as in the child old enough to understand. The seizures, particularly the hallucinatory auras and psychomotor attacks, frequently set off in the prepubescent and adolescent patient fantasies (and sometimes obsessive ruminations) about dying and death that may become so strong that they lead to suicidal behavior and attempts. The limitations many school systems place on epileptic children add to the problem. Commonly, the child expresses painful feelings by "acting out."

Pseudoretardation may occur in poorly controlled epileptic children because their seizures (or the subclinical paroxysms sustained) may interfere with their learning ability. Anticonvulsants are less likely to "slow the child down" but may do so when given in toxic amounts; phenobarbital is particularly implicated.

True mental retardation is most commonly part of the same pathologic process that causes the seizures but may occasionally occur when seizures are frequent, prolonged, and accompanied by hypoxia.

Physical injuries, especially lacerations of the forehead and chin, are frequent in astatic or akinetic seizures ("drop attacks"). In all other seizure disorders in childhood, injuries as a direct result of an attack are impressively rare.

Treatment

The ideal treatment of seizures is the correction of specific causes. However, even when a biochemical disorder (eg, leucine hypoglycemia), a tumor, or septic meningitis is being treated, anticonvulsant drugs are often still required.

A. Precautionary Management of Individual Brief Seizures: Protect the patient against self-injury and aspiration of vomitus. Beyond that, no specific therapy is necessary. The less done to the patient during a relatively brief seizure (up to 10 or 15 minutes), the better. Thrusting a spoon handle or tongue depressor into the clenched mouth of a convulsing patient or trying to restrain tonic-clonic movements may cause worse injuries than a bitten tongue or bruised limb. Mouth-to-mouth resuscitation is rarely necessary.

B. General Management of the Young Epileptic:

1. Education: The patient and parents must be helped to understand the problem of seizures and their management. Many children—some even as young as 3 years of age—are capable of cooperating with the physician in problems of seizure control.

All bottles containing antiepileptic drugs should bear a label. The parents should know the names and dosage of the anticonvulsants being administered.

Materials on epilepsy—including pamphlets (some in Spanish), monographs, films, and videotapes suitable for children and teenagers, parents, teachers, and medical professionals—may be purchased through the Epilepsy Foundation of America, Materials Service Center, 4351 Garden City Drive, Landover, MD 20785. The Foundation's local chapter and other community organizations are eager to provide guidance and other services. In many cities, there are support groups for older children and adolescents and for their parents and others concerned.

2. Privileges and precautions in daily life: Encourage normal living within reasonable bounds. Children should engage in physical activities appropriate to their age and social group. After seizure control is established, swimming is generally permissible with a "buddy system" or adequate lifeguard coverage. High diving and high climbing should not be permitted. Physical training and sports (other than contact sports) are usually to be welcomed rather than restricted. Driving is discussed below.

Loss of sleep should be avoided. Emotional disturbances may need to be treated. Alcohol intake—a serious problem usually beginning in adolescence—should be avoided because it may precipitate seizures. Prompt attention should be given to infections. Further neurologic disturbances should be brought to the physician's attention promptly.

Although every effort should be made to control seizures, this must not interfere with a child's ability to function. Sometimes a child is better off having an occasional mild seizure than being so heavily sedated that function at home, in school, or at play is impaired. Therapy and medication adjustment often require much art and fortitude on the physician's part. Indeed, some pediatricians and pediatric neurologists, after discussion with the parents, are now not instituting anticonvulsant therapy after up to three nonfebrile convulsions in an otherwise neurologically intact child.

3. Driving: Driving becomes important to most

Table 23–11. Nonepileptic paroxysmal events.

Breath-holding attacks: Age 6 months to 3 years. Always precipitated by trauma and fright. Cyanosis; sometimes stiffening, tonic (or jerking-clonic) convulsion (anoxic seizure). Patient may sleep following attack. Family history positive in 30%. EEG is normal. Treatment is interpretation and reassurance.

Infantile syncope (pallid breath holding): No external precipitant (perhaps internal pain, cramp, or fear?). Pallor may be followed by seizure (anoxic/ischemic). Vagally (heart-slowing) mediated, like adult syncope. EEG normal; may get cardiac slowing with vagal stimulation (eyeball pressure, cold cloth on face) during EEG.

Tics or Tourette's syndrome: Simple or complex stereotyped (the same time after time) jerks or movements, coughs, grunts, sniffs. Worse at repose or with stress. May be suppressed during physician visit. Family history often positive. EEG negative. Nonanticonvulsant drugs may benefit.

Night terrors, sleep talking, walking, "sit-ups": Age 3–10. Usually occur in first sleep cycle (30–90 minutes after going to sleep), with crying, screaming, and "automatic discharge" (pupils dilatated, perspiring, etc). Lasts minutes. Child goes back to sleep and has no recall of event the next day. Sleep studies (polysomnogram and EEG) are normal. Disappears with maturation. Sleep talking and walking and short "sit-ups" in bed are fragmentary arousals. If a spell is recorded, EEG shows arousal from deep sleep, but the behavior seems wakeful. The youngster needs to be protected from injury and gradually settled down and taken back to bed.

Nightmares: Nightmares or vivid dreams occur in subsequent cycles of sleep, often in the early morning hours, and generally are partially recalled the next day. The bizarre and frightening behavior may sometimes be confused with complex partial seizures. These occur during REM (rapid eye movement) sleep; epilepsy usually does not occur during that phase of sleep. In extreme or difficult cases, an all-night sleep EEG may help to differentiate seizures from nightmares.

Migraine: One variant of migraine can be associated with an acute confusional state. There may be the usual migraine prodrome with spots before the eyes, dizziness, visual field defects, and then agitated confusion. A history of other, more typical migraine with severe headache and vomiting but without confusion may aid in the diagnosis. The severe headache with vomiting as the youngster comes out of the migraine may aid in distinguishing the attack from epilepsy. Other seizure manifestations are practically never seen, eg, tonic-clonic movements, falling, and complete loss of consciousness. The EEG in migraine is usually normal and seldom has epileptiform abnormalities often seen in patients with epilepsy. Lastly, migraine and epilepsy are sometimes linked: migraine-caused ischemia on the brain surface sometimes leads to later epilepsy.

Syncope: Syncope often has a precipitant. The patient may remember feeling dizzy, lightheaded, and nauseated or ill, and sensing the room going dark. Observers will often notice extreme pallor at the onset. The fall is often but not necessarily gradual; injury may occur. Heart rate is often very slow. Patient may often have memory of beginning to fall. Occasionally, a tonic or tonic-clonic seizure due to anoxia may occur, especially if the patient is held upright and circulation to the head is not restored. An EEG is invariably normal. The family history is often positive for syncope.

Shuddering: Shuddering or shivering attacks can occur in infancy and be a forerunner of essential tremor in later life. Often, the family history is positive for tremor. The shivering may be very frequent. EEG is normal. There is no clouding or loss of consciousness.

Gastroesophageal reflux: Seen more commonly in children with cerebral palsy or brain damage, reflux of acid gastric contents may cause pain that cannot be described by the child. At times, there may be unusual posturings (dystonic or other) of the head and neck or trunk, an apparent attempt to stretch the esophagus or close the opening. There is no loss of consciousness, but there may be eye rolling, apnea, occasional vomiting that may simulate a seizure. An upper GI series, cine of swallowing, sometimes even an EEG (which is always normal), may be necessary to distinguish this from seizures.

Masturbation: Rarely in infants, repetitive rocking or rubbing motions may simulate seizures. The youngster may look out of contact, be poorly responsive to the environment, and have autonomic expressions (eg, perspiration, dilated pupils) that may be confused with seizures. Observation by a skilled individual, sometimes even in a hospital situation, may be necessary to distinguish this from seizures. EEG is of course normal between or during attacks. Interpretation and reassurance are the only necessary treatment.

Conversion reaction/pseudoseizures: As many as 50% of patients with pseudoseizures are epileptic. As episodes may be writhing, intercourselike movements, tonic episodes, bizarre jerking and thrashing around, or even apparently sudden unresponsiveness. Often, there is ongoing psychological trauma. Often, but not invariably, the patients are developmentally delayed. The spells must often be seen or recorded on videotape in a controlled situation to distinguish them from epilepsy. A normal EEG during a spell is a key diagnostic feature. Often the spells are so bizarre that they are easily distinguished. Sometimes, pseudoseizures can be precipitated by suggestion with injection of normal saline in a controlled situation. Combativeness is common, self-injury and incontinence rare.

Temper tantrums and rage attacks: These are sometimes confused with epilepsy. The youngster is often amnesic or at least claims amnesia for events during the spell. The attacks are usually precipitated by frustration or anger and are often directed either verbally or physically and subside with behavior modification and isolation. EEGs are generally normal but unfortunately seldom obtained during an attack. Anterior temporal leads may be helpful in ruling out temporal or lateral frontal abnormalities, the latter sometimes seen in partial complex seizures. Improvement of the attacks with psychotherapy, milieu therapy, or behavioral modification helps rule out epilepsy.

Benign paroxysmal vertigo: These are brief attacks of vertigo in which the youngster often appears frightened and pale and clutches the parent. The attacks last 5–30 seconds. Sometimes, nystagmus is identified. There is no loss of consciousness. Usually, the child is well and returns to play immediately afterward. The attacks may occur in clusters, then disappear for months. Attacks are usually seen in infants and preschoolers aged 2–5. EEG is normal. If caloric tests can be obtained (often very difficult in this age group), abnormalities with hypofunction of one side are sometimes seen. Medications are usually not desirable or necessary.

Staring spells: Teachers often make referral for absence or petit mal seizures in youngsters who stare or seem preoccupied at school. Helpful in the history is the lack of these spells at home, eg, in the early morning hours prior to breakfast, as might be seen with absence seizures. A lack of other epilepsy in the child or family history often is helpful. Sometimes, these children have difficulties with school and a cognitive or learning disability. The child can generally be brought out of this spell by a firm command. An EEG is sometimes necessary to confirm that absence seizures are not occurring. A 24-hour ambulatory EEG to record attacks during the child's everyday school activities is occasionally necessary.

young people at age 15 or 16. Restrictions vary from state to state; in most, a learner's permit or driver's license will be issued if the patient has been under a physician's care and free of seizures for at least 2 years, provided that the treatment or basic neurologic problem does not interfere with the ability to drive. A guide to this and other legal matters pertaining to persons with epilepsy is published by the Epilepsy Foundation of America, whose legal department may be able to provide additional information (see reference below).

4. Pregnancy: In the pregnant teenager with epilepsy, the possibility of teratogenic effects of anticonvulsants, such as facial clefts (about 5%), must be weighed against the risks from seizures. Such malformations occur in the infants of about 2.5% of untreated epileptic mothers.

C. Principles of Anticonvulsant Therapy:

1. Treat with the drug appropriate to the clinical situation, as outlined in Table 23–12.

2. Start with one drug in conventional dosage, and increase the dosage until seizures are controlled. If seizures are not controlled on the tolerated maximal dosage of one major anticonvulsant, gradually switch over to another before adding a second anticonvulsant. The dosages and usually effective blood levels listed in Table 23–12 are guides. Individual variations must be expected. The "therapeutic range" may also vary somewhat with the method used to determine levels.

3. Advise the parents and the patient that the prolonged use of anticonvulsant drugs will not produce significant or permanent "mental slowing" (although the underlying cause of the seizures might) and that prevention of seizures for 2–4 years substantially reduces the chances of recurrence. Advise them also that anticonvulsants are given to prevent further seizures and that they should be taken as prescribed. Changes in medications or dosages should not be made without the physician's knowledge. Unsupervised sudden withdrawal of anticonvulsant drugs may precipitate severe seizures or even status epilepticus.

Anticonvulsants must be kept where they cannot be ingested by small children or suicidal patients.

4. Check the patient at intervals, depending on the underlying cause of the seizures, the degree of control, and the toxic properties of the anticonvulsant drug or drugs used. Blood counts, urinalyses, and liver function or other biologic tests must be obtained periodically in the case of some anticonvulsants, as indicated in Table 23–12.

Periodic neurologic reevaluation is important. CT scanning may be indicated. Repeat EEGs are not needed to achieve seizure control. Indications for repeat EEGs are discussed above.

5. Continue anticonvulsant treatment until the patient is free of seizures for 2 or more years or, in some cases, through adolescence. In about 75% of

cases, seizures may not recur. Such variables as younger age at onset, normal EEG, and ease of controlling seizures carry a favorable prognosis, whereas later onset, slowing or spikes on EEG, a history of atypical febrile convulsions, and possibly an abnormal neurologic examination carry a higher risk of recurrence.

6. In general, there is no need to withdraw anticonvulsants before taking an EEG.

7. Discontinue anticonvulsants gradually. If it becomes necessary to withdraw anticonvulsants abruptly, the patient should be under close medical surveillance. If seizures recur during or after withdrawal, anticonvulsant therapy should be reinstituted and again maintained for at least 2 or more years.

D. Blood Levels of Antiepileptic Drugs:

1. General comments: Most anticonvulsants take two or three times the length of their half-life to reach the "steady states" indicated in Table 23–12. This must be considered when blood levels are assessed after anticonvulsants are started or dosages are changed.

Individuals vary in their metabolism and their particular pharmacokinetic characteristics. These and external factors, including, for example, food intake or illness, also affect the blood level. Thus, the level reached on a milligram per kilogram or surface area basis varies among patients.

Experience and clinical research in the determination of antiepileptic blood levels have shown that there is some correlation between (1) drug dose and blood level, (2) blood level and therapeutic effect, and (3) blood level and some toxic effects.

2. Effective levels: The ranges given in Table 23–12 are those within which seizure control without toxicity will be achieved in most patients. The level for any given individual will vary not only with metabolic makeup (including biochemical defects) but also with the nature and severity of the seizures and their underlying cause, with other medications being taken, and other factors. Seizure control may be achieved at lower levels in some, and higher levels may be reached without toxicity in others. When control is achieved at a lower level, the dose should not be increased merely to get the level into the "therapeutic range." Likewise, toxic side effects will be experienced at different levels even within the "therapeutic range"; lowering the dose usually resolves the problem, but sometimes the drug must be withdrawn or another added (or both). Some serious toxic effects, including allergic reactions, LE phenomenon, and bone marrow or liver toxicity, are independent of dosage; liver toxicity especially may be the effect not just of a particular drug but also of its use in a patient who is or has been on several—and often a whole gamut—of other drugs.

3. Interaction of antiepileptic drugs: Blood levels of anticonvulsants may be affected by other

Table 23–12. Guide to pediatric anticonvulsant drug therapy.

Drug	Average Total (mg/kg/d)	In	Divided Doses	Steady State: Days	Effective Blood Levels (µg/mL)[1]	Side Effects and Precautions	Usage and Remarks
Primary anticonvulsant							
Carbamaze-pine (Tegretol)	15–25	:	2–4	3–6	4–12 (> 15)	Dizziness, ataxia, diplopia. Thrombocytopenia, leukopenia, rash. Rare: hepatotoxicity; bone marrow depression; dystonia; inappropriate ADH secretion; bizarre behaviors; tics.	Monitor CBC, platelet count, liver functions first 6 months closely; then periodically. Blood effects usually early and transient.
Valproic acid (Depakene, Depakote)	15–60	:	2–4	2–4	50–120 (> 140)	Weight gain. Occasional gastric discomfort, constipation. Rare: hepatotoxicity; hyperammonemia, leukopenia. Tremor, hair loss in 5%.	For prophylaxis in febrile convulsion, see text. Monitor CBC, platelets, liver functions first 6 months closely; then periodically. Can be given rectally (suspension: 250 mg/5 mL).
Phenytoin (Dilantin)	5–10	:	1–2	5–10	5–20 (> 25)	Gum hypertrophy, hirsutism, ataxia, nystagmus, diplopia, rash, anorexia, nausea, osteomalacia. Severe toxicity may cause pseudodementia and liver damage. Rare: macrocytic anemia, lymph node involvement, exfoliative dermatitis, peripheral neuropathy.	Generally very effective and safe effect on behavior. Good dental hygiene reduces gum hyperplasia. May aggravate absence and myoclonic seizures. Consider supplemental vitamin D. Poorly absorbed by neonatal gut. Absorption after intramuscular injection erratic. Useful (IV) in neonatal seizures and status epilepticus. *Note:* Suspension not recommended.
Phenobarbital	3–8	:	1	10–21	15–40 (> 45)	Irritability and overactivity in many children; sedative effects in others. Mild ataxia, nystagmus, skin rash. May interfere with learning.	Safest overall drug. Bitter taste. Higher blood levels sometimes required and tolerated in severe chronic epileptics. Consider supplemental vitamin D. Useful in neonatal seizures and status epilepticus.
Primidone (Mysoline)	10–25	:	3–4	1–5	4–12 (> 15)	Drowsiness, ataxia, vertigo, anorexia, nausea, vomiting, rash.	Start slowly with 25–35% of expected maintenance dose; increase every 2 days until full dose reached.
Ethosuximide (Zarontin)	10–40	:	1–2	5–6	40–100 (> 150)	Nausea, gastric discomfort. Rare: bone marrow depression; hepatotoxicity, lupus.	May aggravate generalized seizures. Combine with valproic acid in refractory absence seizures.
Clonazepam (Klonopin)	0.1–0.2	:	2–3	5–10	15–80 ng/mL (> 80)	Drowsiness (>50%): soporific effects greatest drawback. Behavior problems (25%). Slurred speech, ataxia, salivation.	Start slowly with 25% of expected maintenance dose; increase every 2–3 days. Useful with difficult to treat minor motor seizures (astatic, myoclonic, infantile spasms; absences). Tolerance often occurs after a few months, but drug may be restarted after period of withdrawal.
Adjunctive or secondary drug							
Acetazolamide (Diamox)	5–20	:	2–3	1–2	10–14	Anorexia; numbness and tingling. Increase in urinary frequency; hence, do not give in evening. Renal stones.	Supplement to other medications, especially in absence and complex partial seizures. Also in females 4 days prior to and in the first 2–3 days of menstrual periods.
Methsuximide (Celontin)	15–30	:	3–4	(Not known) 14	10–40 (Normethsuximide)	Drowsiness, ataxia, headache, diplopia. Skin rash (15%).	Useful in complex partial and myoclonic-astatic seizures.
Clorazepate (Tranxene)	0.3–1	:	2–3	(Not known) 21	0.2–1.5 (> 2)	Lethargy.	May be useful adjunct in generalized tonic-clonic, partial, and astatic seizures.

(continued)

Table 23–12. Guide to pediatric anticonvulsant drug therapy. (continued)

Drug	Average Total (mg/kg/d)	In	Divided Doses	Steady State: Days	Effective Blood Levels (µg/mL)[1]	Side Effects and Precautions	Usage and Remarks
Felbamate (Felbatol)	15–45	:	3–4	(Not known)	...	Anorexia, vomiting, insomnia, headache, somnolence, rash (1%). Aplastic anemia and hepatic failure significant hazards.	Dangerous. In children with Lennox-Gastaut syndrome. (Adults: complex partial seizures.) May interact with other anticonvulsants. Get informed consent.
Phenacemide (Phenurone)	25–50	:	2–4	(Not known)	...	Rash, anorexia, nausea. *Warning:* Hepatitis, psychosis, blood dyscrasias.	Especially effective in complex partial seizures when all other drugs fail. Frequent CBC, liver function tests initial 3–4 months, then 2–4/yr.
Gabapentin (Neurontin) > 12 years	900–1800 (total daily dose)	:	3	1–2	...	Drowsiness, dizziness, ataxia.	Add-on drug for partial seizures; no effect on other anticonvulsant levels.
Dextroamphetamine (Dexedrine)	0.25–0.75	:	Breakfast and noon	(Not known)	...	Nervousness, palpitations, anorexia, insomnia.	To counteract sedative effect of other drugs. Narcolepsy. ADHD (attention deficit hyperactivity disorder).
Trimethadione (Tridione)	20–50	:	3–4	(Not known)	470–1200 (dimethadione)	Rash, photophobia, irritability. *Warning:* Leukopenia, agranulocytosis, nephrosis. LE phenomenon.	Useful primary in absences if ethosuximide and valproic acid fail. May aggravate generalized seizures; if so, add phenobarbital. Monthly CBC, urinalysis.
Mephobarbital (Mebaral)	4–10	:	1–2	(Not known)	15–40 (phenobarbital)	As with phenobarbital.	Twice the quantity of phenobarbital required for comparable effect.
Lamotrigine (Lamictol) > 16 years	50–300 (total daily dose)	:	2–4	(Not known)	...	Dizziness, headaches, diplopia, ataxia, nausea, rash (5–10%).	Add-on drug for > 10 year olds with complex partial epilepsy; slow incremented dose over 2 mo (see package insert) may effect other drug levels.

Treatment of status epilepticus

Drug	Dose	Side Effects and Precautions	Usage and Remarks
Diazepam (Valium)	0.3 mg/kg IV initially. Repeat dose 0.1–0.3.	Administer slowly IV. Monitor pulse and blood pressure. May cause respiratory depression in presence of phenobarbital.	May need to be repeated every 3–4 hours. Follow with phenytoin or phenobarbital for long-range control. ***Note:*** Administration IM for status epilepticus ineffective.
Lorazepam	0.05–0.2 mg/kg IV. May repeat.	Mild respiratory depression.	May be more effective than diazepam. Longer-acting.
Phenobarbital	5–20 mg/kg IV initially. Repeat dose 5–10 mg/kg IV.	See above.	Rule out pyridoxine deficiency. In neonatal seizures, load with 15–30 mg/kg IV (IM if IV impossible).
Phenytoin (Dilantin)	10–20 mg/kg IV initially. Repeat dose 5–10 mg/kg IV.	Administer IV over a 5-minute period. IM absorption uncertain. Monitor blood levels.	Adjunct in neonatal seizures (20 mg/kg IV) if phenobarbital alone fails.
Paraldehyde	0.1–0.15 mL/kg IV; 0.2–0.3 mL/kg rectally.	Administer slowly IV mixed in saline; rectal dose in vegetable oil 1:1. Avoid in patient with pulmonary disease or in croupette.	Avoid IM administration if possible: may cause fat necrosis. Do not use plastic syringes. (No longer manufactured in United States.)
Lidocaine (Xylocaine)	2 mg/kg IV.	Administer slowly.	Useful especially when reluctant to give more diazepam, barbiturates, or paraldehyde. Effect brief (about 30 min).

General anesthesia if other measures fail.

Treatment of infantile spasms

See text regarding use of corticotropin or corticosteroids. Also, clonazepam, or valproic acid, especially with recurrences.

[1] In monotherapy, level at which clinical toxicity becomes manifest.

drugs. Individual variations occur; adjustment of doses may be required.

4. Indications for determination of blood levels: Drug blood levels should be measured in a new patient or after a new drug is introduced and seizure control without toxicity is achieved to determine the effective level for that patient. Blood level monitoring is useful also when expected control on a "usual" dosage has not been achieved, either with a single drug or after adding another; when seizures recur in a previously well-controlled patient; or when control is poor in a patient taking anticonvulsants being seen for the first time. A low level may indicate inadequate dosage, drug interaction, or noncompliance with the prescribed regimen. A high level may indicate refractoriness, drug interaction, or a worsening neurologic process.

Note: Brief and limited "breakthroughs" are common in children (particularly younger ones) with intercurrent infections or significant excitement or other stresses, and they do not necessitate blood levels.

Blood levels are mandatory when there are signs and symptoms of toxicity—particularly where there is polydrug therapy, the dosage of a drug has been raised, or another drug has been added. Blood levels may be the only means of detecting intoxication in a comatose patient or very young child. Toxic levels also occur with drug abuse or liver disease.

Finally, when the patient is well controlled (or is controlled as well as one may hope for in a patient refractory to antiepileptics or one with difficult-to-control seizures) and free of toxic signs, blood levels are desirable once or twice a year.

E. Side Effects of Antiepileptic Drugs: (See also Table 23–12.)

1. Serious allergic reactions usually necessitate discontinuance of a drug. However, not every rash in a child receiving an anticonvulsant is due to the drug. If a useful antiepileptic drug is discontinued for this reason and the rash disappears, restarting the drug in a smaller dosage is often warranted to see if the reaction recurs.

2. Signs of drug toxicity often disappear when the daily dosage is reduced by 25–30%.

3. The sedative effect of many of the anticonvulsants is often easily counteracted by the judicious use of coffee or dextroamphetamine sulfate, 2.5–5 mg at breakfast and 2.5 mg at noon.

4. Gingival hyperplasia secondary to phenytoin is best minimized through good dental hygiene but occasionally requires gingivectomy. This condition (but not hypertrichosis) usually disappears within about 6 months after the drug is discontinued.

F. ACTH & Corticosteroids:

1. Indications: These drugs are indicated for infantile spasms not due to causes amenable to specific therapy and in the Lennox-Gastaut syndrome which cannot be controlled by anticonvulsant drugs.

Duration of therapy is guided by cessation of clinical seizures and normalization of the EEG. ACTH or oral corticosteroids are usually continued in full doses for 2 weeks and then, if seizures have ceased, tapered over 1 week. Others use a total treatment period of about 2 months. If seizures recur, the dosage is increased to the last effective level and repeated for 2–4 weeks, or switching to or from prednisone is tried. Some clinicians maintain the patient for up to 6 months on this dosage before attempting withdrawal. There is no strong evidence, however, that longer courses of treatment are more beneficial.

2. Dosages:

a. ACTH gel, starting with 2–4 units/kg/d intramuscularly in a single morning dose. Parents can be taught to give injections.

b. Prednisone, starting with 2–4 mg/kg/d orally in two or three divided doses.

3. Precautions: Give additional potassium, guard against infections, and discuss the cushingoid appearance and its disappearance. Do not withdraw oral corticosteroids suddenly. Side effects in some series occur in up to 40% of cases, especially with higher doses than those listed here (used by some authorities).

G. Ketogenic or Medium-Chain Triglyceride Diet in Treatment of Epilepsy: A ketogenic diet should be recommended in astatic and myoclonic seizures and absence seizures not responsive to drug therapy; it is occasionally recommended for infantile spasms that do not respond to corticotropin or the corticosteroids. Ketosis is induced by a diet high in fats and very limited in carbohydrates with sufficient protein for body maintenance and growth; by the feeding of medium-chain triglycerides (MCT); or by a combination of these methods. The MCT diet induces ketosis more readily than does a high level of dietary fats and thus requires less carbohydrate restriction. The mechanism for the anticonvulsant action of the ketogenic diet is not understood. It is, however, the ketosis, not the acidosis, that raises the seizure threshold.

The diet is usually most effective in young children under the age of 8 years, but when all other measures fail, it should be tried even in adolescents.

As ketosis is achieved, a repeat EEG may be helpful; seizure control by the diet is more likely to occur if the EEG shows improvement.

The ketogenic diet is difficult and expensive, tends to be monotonous, and depends on the caregiver's ability to weigh out the foods as well as on absolute adherence to the diet prescribed. Whether the ketosis is achieved by high-fat meals or an MCT diet is often a matter of the physician's, the dietitian's, or the patient's preference. The result may also depend on which form of the diet is better tolerated. Full cooperation of all family members is required, including the patient if old enough. However, when seizure control is achieved by this method, the child is alert, often needs no anticonvulsants or only small amounts, and parental and patient satisfaction is most gratifying.

H. Surgery: In seizure disorders intractable to anticonvulsant therapy and primarily of focal origin, neurosurgery should be considered. Useful procedures, depending on the lesion, include corticectomy, hemispherectomy, anterior temporal lobectomy (for complex partial seizures), callosotomy (or commissurotomy), and stereotactic ablation.

Annegars J: Factors prognostic of unprovoked seizures after febrile convulsions. N Engl J Med 1987;316:493.

Bobele GB, Bodensteiner JB: Infantile spasms. Neurol Clin 1990;8:633.

Camfield CS, Camfield PR: Febrile seizures: An Rx for parent fears and anxieties. Contemp Pediatr 1993;10:26.

Camfield P et al: A randomized study of carbamazepine versus no medication after a first unprovoked seizure in childhood. Neurology 1989;39:851.

Chugani HT et al: Infantile spasms: I. PET identifies focal cortical dysgenesis in cryptogenic cases for surgical treatment. Ann Neurol 1990;27:406.

Committee on Drugs, American Academy of Pediatrics: Behavioral and cognitive effects of anticonvulsant therapy. Pediatrics 1985;76:644.

Crawford TO et al: Lorazepam in childhood status epilepticus and serial seizures. Neurology 1987;37:190.

Dieckmann RA: Rectal diazepam for prehospital pediatric status epilepticus. Ann Emerg Med 1994;23(2):216.

Duchowny MS: Surgery for intractable epilepsy, issues and outcomes. Pediatrics 1989;84:886.

Dulac O, Chugani M, Dalla Bernardina B: *Infantile Spasms and West Syndrome.* Saunders, 1994.

Farwell JR et al: Phenobarbital for febrile seizures: Effects on intelligence and on seizure recurrence. N Engl J Med 1990;322:364.

First Seizure Trial Group: Randomized clinical trial on the efficacy of antiepileptic drugs in reducing the risk of relapse after a first unprovoked tonic-clonic seizure. Neurology 1993;43:478.

Gross-Tsur V, Shinnar S: Convulsive status epilepticus in children. Epilepsia 1993;34(Suppl 1):S12.

Haines ST, Casto DR: Treatment of infantile spasms. Ann Pharmacother 1994;28(6):779.

Hrachovy R, Glaze DG, Frost JD: A retrospective study of spontaneous remission and long term outcome in patients with infantile spasms. Epilepsia 1991;32:212.

Jayakar P: The role of EEG in management of childhood epilepsy. Int Pediatr 1993;8:253.

Krumholz A et al: Driving and epilepsy. JAMA 1991;265:622.

Mahahito M et al: Infantile spasms localized cerebral lesions on SPECT. Epilepsia 1994;35:988.

Maytal J, Moshe S, Shinnar S: Status epilepticus. Pediatrics 1990;84:939.

Maytal J, Shinnar S: Febrile status epilepticus. Pediatrics 1990;86:611.

McAbee GN, Barasch ES, Kurfist LA: Results of computed tomography in "neurologically normal" children after initial onset of seizures. Pediatr Neurol 1989;5:102.

Painter MJ, Gaines L: Neonatal seizures: Diagnosis and treatment. J Child Neurol 1991;6:101.

Pellock JM: The classification of childhood seizures and epilepsy syndromes. Neurol Clin 1990;8:619.

Phillips S, Shanohan R: Etiology and morbidity of status epilepticus in children. Ann Neurol 1989;46:74.

Prats JM et al: Infantile spasms treated with high doses of sodium valproate: Initial response and follow-up. Dev Med Child Neurol 1991;33:617.

Rivera R et al: Midazolam in the treatment of status epilepticus in children. Crit Care Med 1993;21:991.

Rosman NP et al: A controlled trial of diazepam administered during febrile illnesses to prevent recurrence of febrile seizures. N Engl J Med 1993;328:79.

Shinnar S et al: Discontinuing antiepileptic medication in children with epilepsy after two years without seizures: A prospective study. N Engl J Med 1985;313:976.

Shinnar S et al: Sleep state and the risk of seizure recurrence following a first unprovoked seizure in childhood. Neurology 1993;43:701.

Snead OC: Treatment of infantile spasms. Pediatr Neurol 1990;6:147.

Taylor DC, McKinlay I: When not to treat epilepsy with drugs: Annotations. Dev Med Child Neurol 1984;26:822.

Wallace SJ: Anti-epileptic drug monitoring: An overview. Dev Med Child Neurol 1990;32:923.

Watanabe K: Medical treatment of West syndrome in Japan. J Child Neurol 1995;10(2):143.

Working Group on Status Epilepticus: Treatment of convulsive status epilepticus. Bone RC (editor). JAMA 1992; 270:854.

Wyllie E: Temporal lobe epilepsy in children. Int Pediatr 1993;8:267.

HEADACHES

Headache is not usually a psychosomatic symptom in very young children, whereas it is more apt to be so in older children and adolescents. Headaches occur in 37% and migraine in 2.7% of children by 7 years of age; by 14 years, the rates are 69% and 10.9%, respectively. A careful description of the headaches, associated circumstances, and other neurologic and systemic symptoms should be obtained. The family history and emotional problems should be discussed in detail. Systemic and neurologic examination, including blood pressure, ophthalmoscopic examination, and station and gait, will usually distinguish organic from psychogenic headaches. Differential features are given in Table 23–13.

If there is evidence of a specific intracranial cause or systemic disorder (eg, renal disease), diagnosis and treatment should be directed at the primary disorder.

The most common headache with onset in adolescence is tension headache. Unlike vascular headache of migraine, the typical tension headache is variable in location, frontal, generalized ("hatband-like"), or occipital, not accompanied by visual, gastrointestinal, neurologic (eg, dizziness) symptoms. Unless accompanied by depression (a linkage common in adults, less common in children), markedly de-

Table 23–13. Differential features of headaches in children.

	Muscle Contraction (Tension/Psychogenic)	Vascular (Migraine)	Traction and Inflammatory (Increased Intracranial Pressure)
Time course	Chronic, recurrent	Acute, paroxysmal, recurrent	Chronic or intermittent but increasingly frequent; progressive severity
Prodromes	No	Yes	No
Description	Diffuse, bandlike, tight	Intense, pulsatile, unilateral in older child (70%)	Diffuse; more occipital with infratentorial mass, more frontal with supratentorial mass
Characteristic findings	Feelings of inadequacy, depression, or anxiety	Neurologic symptoms and signs usually transient	Positive neurologic signs, especially papilledema
Predisposing factors	Problems at home or school or socially (sexually)	Positive family history (75%); trivial head trauma may precipitate	No

creased school attendance or diminished athletic prowess seldom occurs. Adolescents with tension headaches usually, in spite of head pain, continue to function well. If there is fall-off in peer group or family relationships or schoolwork, more extensive interviewing in reference to adverse events or stress in those areas is needed.

Physical and neurologic examination in tension headaches is normal. Underlying depression must be ruled out. Laboratory studies are unnecessary. Treatment includes searching out and avoiding precipitants (eg, stress, noise) and use of minor analgesics, relaxation techniques, even biofeedback. Prophylactic medication (eg, amitriptyline) may be helpful.

The prognosis is guarded. Minor morbidity and decreased school and work efficiency may persist. Psychogenic etiology or enmeshment may be sought out in the especially difficult headache patient; psychiatric consultation may be needed.

A chronic progressive headache may represent brain tumor causing headache because of its midline location, obstructing spinal fluid flow, resulting in a painful, progressive hydrocephalus. Or, the tumor mass may distort pain-sensitive structures, such as blood vessels, meninges, or dura.

Although brain tumor headache may initially mimic migraine, tension, or sinus headaches, certain history and physical findings alert the clinician.

Headache of recent onset in a child in the age group from 3 to 10, the peak age for brain tumors, is worrisome. A progressive headache with worsening frequency (eg, from weekly to daily) and severity (eg, from mild to prostrating) suggests tumor.

Headache in the morning, perhaps due to change of position and change in intracranial dynamics, with vomiting (often without nausea) is ominous.

A child with headache who is deteriorating in social, school and athletic (coordination) prowess causes concern.

Even more important are positive neurologic findings. *The typical headache patient has a normal physical and neurological examination.* Strabismus, weakness of extraocular muscles, visual loss, poor pupillary response, and papilledema or optic atrophy must be ruled out. Coordination and gait must be assessed with finger-nose-finger pursuit, balancing on each leg, hopping, and tandem walking forward and backward on a straight line.

If suspicion remains high in spite of a normal neurologic examination, a follow-up examination is essential. An imaging study should be strongly considered.

The preferred study is MRI, which is superior to CT scan for posterior fossa tumors and for visualization around bony structures such as the sella and foramen magnum. However, if suspicion for tumor is low, the more available and less expensive CT scan is a sensible alternative.

To summarize, a reasonable history with the key points listed above and a good physical and neurological examination usually picks up the rare headache with brain tumor. A recent study of 104 children with onset of headaches prior to 7 years of age, seen by age 9, found mostly (75%) migraines. A pertinent quote from that article: "No child who presented for evaluation of headaches with a normal neurologic exam was found to have a brain tumor."

Migraine attacks are usually paroxysmal, throbbing, pulsating, or pounding in character (initial vasoconstriction of intracranial vessels followed by vasodilation of extracranial vessels). The pain in children is as often bilateral as unilateral, frontal or retro-orbital as hemicranial. Between attacks, the child is asymptomatic. Migraine in children is associated (in order of frequency) with nausea, gastric discomfort, or vomiting; dizziness or vertigo; photophobia, visual auras, and, less frequently, visual loss; sensory and motor disturbances, especially involving the face and arms; speech disturbances; and, occasionally, hemiplegia (sometimes alternating), acute confusional states, or impairment of space, time, and body image perceptions (termed the "Alice-in-Wonderland syndrome"). The child frequently seeks rest in a dark, quiet room.

Migraine of varying severity may occur in up to 6.6% of children between 7 and 14 years of age. Onset by age 4 is not uncommon. After 10 years of age, it is twice as common in girls as in boys. The family history is positive for migraine in up to 75% of patients and not infrequently also for epilepsy. School stresses (headache often occurs after school) and foods occasionally precipitate migraine. Head trauma may precipitate onset. In most instances, the migraine attack is brief (hours, not days), and sleep gives relief. Motion sickness is an associated feature in 45% of cases.

EEG may be abnormally slow to mildly or moderately dysrhythmic in up to 80% of patients soon after an attack of complicated migraine (emphasizing the relationship between migraine and epilepsy). Neuroradiologic studies, such as CT scanning, are usually not warranted unless there are definite neurologic or progressive abnormalities.

Acetaminophen or ibuprofen is often effective in children. The patient should be allowed to remain quiet in a darkened room. In children over 12 years of age, severe migraine may often be controlled by Fiorinal, Fioricet, or Midrin, one or two capsules every 4 hours. If these measures are ineffective, especially in the older child, and when anxiety and nausea are prominent symptoms, Cafergot is often useful.*

In the prevention of severe, frequent, and disabling migraine—especially in children too young to alert an adult to their symptoms or to follow the above regimen—prophylaxis is recommended as follows: propranolol, 10–40 mg three times daily depending on weight (contraindications are respiratory and cardiac disorders); cyproheptadine, 2–4 mg every 8–12 hours; or calcium channel blockers (in varying forms and dosages; they may have anticonvulsant action as well). Antidepressants such as imipramine or amitriptyline may be useful (25–50 mg at bedtime). Methysergide maleate is not recommended in children.

Operant conditioning and biofeedback are lengthy and expensive options, studied almost exclusively in children in conjunction with vascular, not tension, headaches. Biofeedback was studied and reported in a position paper of the American College of Physicians in 1985 and was thought unproved. A recent

pediatric study suggested utility of these therapies in vascular headaches in children.

Chu ML, Shinnar S: Headaches in children younger than 7 years of age. Arch Neurol 1992;49:79.

Honig PJ, Charney EB: Children with brain tumor headaches: Distinguishing features. Am J Dis Child 1982;136:121.

Igarashi M et al: Pharmacologic treatment of childhood migraine. J Pediatr 1992;120:653.

Jensen R, Brinck T, Olesen J: Sodium valproate has a prophylactic effect in migraine without aura: A triple-blind, placebo-controlled crossover study. Neurology 1994; 44:647.

Larson B et al: Therapist-assisted self-help relaxation treatment of chronic headaches in adolescents: A school-based intervention. J Child Psychol Psychiatry 1987;28: 127.

Linet MS et al: An epidemiologic study of headache among adolescents and young adults. JAMA 1989;261:2211.

Maytal J et al: The value of brain imaging in children with headaches. Pediatrics 1995;96:413.

Rapoport AM et al: Oral sumatriptan in preventing headache recurrence after treatment of migraine attacks with subcutaneous sumatriptan. Neurology 1995;45: 1505.

Rothner AD: Classification, pathogenesis, evaluation, and management of headaches in children and adolescents. Curr Opin Pediatr 1992;4:949.

Singer HS: Migraine headaches in children. Pediatr Rev 1994;15:94.

Singer HS et al: Chronic recurrent headaches in children. Pediatr Ann 1992;21:369.

The Childhood Brain Tumor Consortium: The epidemiology of headache among children with brain tumor: Headache in children with brain tumors. J Neurooncol 1991;10:31.

SLEEP DISORDERS

Sleep Apnea Syndrome in Older Children

Sleep apnea syndrome should be considered if there is a history of restless sleep with snoring or respiratory noise during sleep and frequent awakenings in an older child who shows poor school performance associated with excessive daytime sleepiness or irritability and hyperactivity. Children with these problems frequently have hypertrophied tonsils or adenoids, causing partial airway obstruction. Occasionally, they have facial dysmorphism; neuromuscular disorders with muscle hypotonia and poor pharyngeal muscle control; and hyperplastic tissues, as seen in myxedema, Hodgkin's disease, or pickwickian syndrome. Evaluation includes soft tissue x-rays of the lateral neck; chest x-ray; electrocardiography to rule out cardiomegaly, sinus dysrhythmias, and incipient or actual right-sided heart failure; arterial blood gas determinations while awake and during sleep; and polysomnography. Therapy is generally surgical, ranging from tonsillectomy and adenoidec-

---

*One capsule of Fiorinal or Lanorinal contains butalbital, 50 mg; aspirin, 325 mg; and caffeine, 40 mg. One capsule of Fioricet contains butalbital, 50 mg; acetaminophen, 325 mg; and caffeine, 40 mg. Midrin contains isometheptene mucate, 65 mg; dichloralphenazone, 100 mg; and acetaminophen, 325 mg. Cafergot contains ergotamine tartrate, 1 mg, and caffeine, 100 mg.

tomy when appropriate, to tracheostomy when medical measures fail.

Narcolepsy

Narcolepsy, a primary disorder of sleep and wakefulness, is characterized by chronic, excessive daytime sleeping that occurs regardless of activity or surroundings and is not relieved by increased sleep at night. Onset occurs as early as 3 years of age; about 18% of patients are 10 years or younger. Sixty percent are between puberty and their late teens. Narcolepsy usually interferes severely with normal living. Often months to years after onset, there may also be cataplexy (transient partial or total loss of muscle tone, often triggered by laughter, anger, or other emotional upsurge); hypnagogic hallucinations (visual or auditory); and sensations of paralysis on falling asleep. Studies have shown that rapid eye movement (REM) sleep, with loss of muscle tone and an electroencephalographic low-amplitude mixed frequency pattern, occurs soon after sleep onset in patients with cataplexy, whereas normal subjects experience 80–100 minutes or longer of non-REM (NREM) sleep before the initial REM period.

Narcolepsy is treated with a CNS stimulant (dextroamphetamine or long-acting methylphenidate is preferred); occasionally, a tricyclic antidepressant, in low doses titrated to the need of the patient, is added to the treatment regimen. The condition persists throughout life.

Somnambulism

Somnambulism has been assigned to a group of sleep disturbances known as disorders of arousal. It is characterized by abrupt onset early in the night of an episode of veiled consciousness and coordinated activity (eg, walking, sometimes moving objects without seeming purpose). The episode is relatively brief and ceases spontaneously. There is poor recall of the event on waking in the morning. Somnambulism may be related to mental activities occurring in stages 3 and 4 of NREM sleep. Incidence has been estimated at only 2–3%, but up to 15% of cases are reported in children 6–16 years of age, with boys affected more often than girls and many having recurrent episodes. No psychopathologic features can usually be demonstrated, but a strong association (30%) between childhood migraine and somnambulism has been noted. Episodes of somnambulism may be triggered in predisposed children by stresses, including febrile illnesses. No treatment of somnambulism is required, and it is not necessary to seek psychiatric consultation.

Night Terrors

Night terrors (pavor nocturnus) are a disorder of arousal from NREM sleep. Most cases occur in children 3–8 years of age, and the disorder rarely occurs after adolescence. It is characterized by sudden (but only partial) waking, with the severely frightened child unable to be fully roused or comforted. Concomitant autonomic symptoms include rapid breathing, tachycardia, and perspiring. The next morning, the child has no recall of any nightmare. Psychopathologic mechanisms are unclear, but falling asleep after watching scenes of violence on television or hearing frightening stories may play a role. Elimination of such causes and administration of a mild antianxiety agent such as chlordiazepoxide may be helpful. It is important to differentiate these episodes from complex partial (psychomotor) seizures.

Aldrich MS: Narcolepsy. Neurology 1992;42(Suppl 6):34.

Barabas G, Ferrari M, Matthews WS: Childhood migraine and somnambulism. Neurology 1983;33:948.

Guilleminault C: Obstructive sleep apnea syndrome and its treatment in children. Pediatr Pulmonol 1987;3:429.

Kotagal S, Hartse KM, Walsh JK: Characteristics of narcolepsy in preteenaged children. Pediatrics 1990;85:205.

Sheldon S, Spire JP, Levy H: *Pediatric Sleep Medicine.* Saunders, 1992.

HEAD & SPINAL INJURIES

Serious accidental injury constitutes one of the most common causes of childhood hospitalization and death in the United States.

Injury of the brain can result from sudden acceleration-deceleration movements or from sudden rotational or torsional movements of the head. Direct impact of the brain against the inner table of the skull, together with blood vessel rupture and dural tears, leads to parenchymal damage.

Closed head injury includes injuries in which the skull remains intact or in which there is only a small linear fracture. **Open head injury** consists of injuries involving major scalp lacerations and compound or depressed skull fractures. Brain parenchymal injury can occur in either closed or open head injuries but is more frequent and often more severe with open head injury.

The clinical severity of head injury is classified as mild, moderate, or severe, depending on the type and extent of brain damage, the presence of brain edema, and the presence or absence of intracranial hemorrhage. Intracranial hemorrhages can occupy a variety of potential spaces within the cranial vault, including epidural, subdural, and subarachnoid spaces. Cerebral contusions consist of a localized region of petechial hemorrhage and edema. Intraparenchymal hemorrhages can be small or massive, rapidly expanding to produce markedly elevated intracranial pressure and cerebral herniation.

Clinical Findings

A. Symptoms & Signs: In mild head injuries, loss of consciousness may not occur or may be only momentary. Frequently, patients experience mild to moderate headache, nausea, vomiting, vertigo, and light-headedness. Although tachycardia may be present, blood pressure and other vital signs are normal. There is rapid resolution of all symptoms. Occasionally, a brief, generalized clonic seizure may occur shortly after the head injury, but post-traumatic epilepsy is rare.

Moderately severe head injuries are associated with loss of consciousness for several minutes to 1 hour. Headache may be severe, and the patient may experience severe irritability, drowsiness, emotional lability, and signs of mild to moderate delirium. Nausea and vomiting can be prominent. Vertigo, tinnitus, and light-headedness may be moderately severe for a short period. Symptoms resolve in 1–2 days, though vertigo and some alteration in behavior, mood, and concentration persist for several days. Some children also experience relatively protracted problems regarding attention, concentration, and school performance after seemingly mild or moderate head injury.

Severe head injury is associated with prolonged loss of consciousness, usually longer than 1 hour. Headache, nausea, vomiting, and tinnitus are severe and at times incapacitating. Marked behavioral changes and seizures can develop immediately after the head injury. Post-traumatic epilepsy occurs in approximately 10% of children. Symptoms usually persist for several days or weeks, in some patients for months.

When intracranial hemorrhages occur, symptoms of progressively increasing intracranial pressure may develop. Patients have progressive loss of consciousness and severe nausea and vomiting. Seizures occur in about 50–70% of children with subdural hematomas. Fever and nuchal rigidity are often present with subdural hematomas, and meningitis may be suspected. Epidural and acute subdural hematomas may be acute and require emergency surgical drainage. These forms of intracranial hemorrhage can rapidly lead to death, particularly if they occur in the posterior fossa. Subarachnoid hemorrhages are unusual in childhood unless they are associated with an underlying cerebrovascular malformation. Intracerebral hematomas, particularly in the frontal and temporal regions, can occur after either a closed or open head injury. When intracerebral hemorrhages occur, an underlying bleeding diathesis should be excluded by appropriate laboratory testing.

B. Physical Examination: Initial assessment of patients who have suffered head injury includes frequent monitoring of heart rate, blood pressure, and temperature. Sudden changes in blood pressure, particularly hypotension, may be an indication of intrathoracic, intra-abdominal, or other systemic injury associated with bleeding.

Head circumference should be measured in infants after head injury; size and tension of the fontanelle should be carefully documented. Evaluation of the head and neck region is important in the search for signs of CSF leakage from the ear and nose. Care should be taken to move the head as little as possible because injury to the spinal cord and cervical vertebrae may not be initially apparent. The patient should be examined thoroughly for signs of injury to extremities, abdomen, back, and chest. The skin should also be carefully examined for evidence of recent or remote injury. The possibility of nonaccidental trauma should be suspected when multiple sites of injury or injuries of different ages are present.

Neurologic examination includes assessment of pupillary size, symmetry, and light reflexes. Evidence of ocular and orbital injury may be associated with basilar skull fracture. Funduscopic examination may disclose retinal flame-shaped hemorrhages that can be indicative of subdural or subarachnoid hemorrhages. Increased intracranial pressure related to intracranial hemorrhages or cerebral edema may result in dilated, nonpulsating retinal veins and swelling of the optic disk. Assessment of muscle tone, strength, and reflexes may provide evidence of focal or lateralized neurologic dysfunction.

C. Laboratory Studies & Imaging: A sudden or progressive decrease in hematocrit may suggest rapidly evolving acute subdural hematoma. Injury may result in fluid and electrolyte abnormalities as a consequence of inappropriate secretion of antidiuretic hormone or diabetes insipidus.

Radiographic studies, particularly CT scanning, should be conducted to search for skull fracture, intracranial hemorrhage, and intracranial foreign bodies. Skull films in general are not as helpful as CT scanning; however, in certain situations when CT scanning is not available, skull films may demonstrate clinically significant depressed or comminuted skull fractures. In addition, plain radiographs of the neck, chest, abdomen, and extremities are important in searching for more generalized evidence of injury. X-ray films of the neck should be obtained on all patients with head injury because unsuspected spinal injury can be present and require immediate stabilization. MRI can also demonstrate intracranial hemorrhage and some types of foreign bodies. MRI is not, however, as helpful as CT scanning at defining bony abnormalities. Cerebral angiography may be required at times when major vascular damage is suspected or when the patient develops clinical signs suggesting arterial dissection.

Lumbar puncture is rarely needed in the evaluation of patients with head injury and in most instances is contraindicated. Infants with tense fontanelles and fever may be suspected initially of having bacterial meningitis; in this situation lumbar puncture may be necessary.

Subdural tap is an important immediate diagnostic as well as therapeutic maneuver in acute and rapidly progressing subdural or epidural hematomas. When an acute subdural hematoma is suspected and the patient is deteriorating rapidly, a subdural tap should be performed as an emergency procedure. *The tap should not be delayed in order to obtain a CT scan.* With posterior fossa subdural and epidural hematomas, a cisternal tap can also be life-saving.

EEGs after acute head injury are frequently abnormal but nonspecific, and their role is quite limited in initial evaluation and management of head injury. EEGs may be useful in monitoring seizure activity and may complement serial neurologic examinations and assessments of a patient's progress after head injury.

Differential Diagnosis

Whenever the cause for the head injury is not readily apparent, nonaccidental trauma should be suspected. Intracranial hemorrhage may occur with relatively minor injuries in patients with bleeding diatheses. Some metabolic disorders, such as scurvy, rickets, and Menkes' disease, may predispose the patient to pathologic fractures and intracranial hemorrhage.

Complications

Seizures, either focal or generalized, have been reported in 5–15% of children with head injury. Usually the seizures are brief, but a few patients experience status epilepticus. Chronic post-traumatic epilepsy develops in 10% of children who have suffered brain lacerations or who have experienced prolonged loss of consciousness immediately after head injury. When post-traumatic seizures develop, approximately 50% occur in the first 6 months after the injury, and 80% will have developed within 2 years. Antiepileptic medications may be started when patients have one or more immediate post-traumatic seizures and continued for up to 6 months. If seizures develop later, chronic antiepileptic medication is continued for 2–4 years.

Massive cerebral swelling, cerebral edema, and intracranial hematomas may lead to herniation of the temporal lobe through the tentorial notch with subsequent brain stem compression and rapid deterioration of the patient's mental status and neurologic function. Cerebellar tonsillar herniation results from posterior fossa hematomas and leads to clinical evidence of lower brain stem dysfunction, progressive loss of consciousness, and impaired cardiorespiratory functions.

Cerebrospinal fluid leakage through basilar skull fractures predisposes the patient to chronic, recurrent bacterial meningitis with organisms that normally inhabit the upper airway, such as *Streptococcus pneumoniae* and *Haemophilus influenzae*. Most CSF leaks stop spontaneously, but chronic leaks require surgical closure. If the patient develops signs of fever, nuchal rigidity, or other evidence of possible meningitis, antibiotics are necessary.

Hydrocephalus can develop after head injury, particularly when subarachnoid hemorrhage leads to basilar arachnoiditis or impairment of the cerebrospinal fluid absorption through the arachnoid villi.

Some patients develop pseudotumor cerebri shortly after head injury. The mechanism is not clear.

Patients with diastatic linear fractures develop leptomeningeal cysts. This type of cyst develops when a tear in the dura and arachnoid is followed by entrapment of the arachnoid between the margins of the diastatic fracture. CSF accumulates within the cyst and produces a progressively enlarging, fluid-filled mass over the fracture line. Removal of the cyst and closure of the dural tear requires surgical repair.

Postconcussion syndrome is seen in children, adolescents, and adults, but its pathogenesis is not clear. Principal manifestations are changes in behavior, personality, and sleep pattern, headache, vertigo, tinnitus, and various head and neck pains. School or job performance deteriorates, and the ability to concentrate is impaired. Hyperactivity can impair the child's normal daily function. Treatment is symptomatic, and postconcussion syndrome usually abates gradually over a period of days to weeks.

Treatment

Immediate treatment of a patient with serious head injury consists of securing the airway and supporting the cardiovascular system. Seizures, particularly status epilepticus, may require acute anticonvulsant medication. Subdural or cisternal taps are required if the patient is rapidly deteriorating because of an acute subdural or epidural hematoma.

After initial assessment, the patient must be observed carefully for several hours after head injury, whether in the emergency room, in an ambulatory clinic setting, or at home. The patient's arousability, pupillary light reflexes, extraocular movements, and extremity movements must be serially documented. Hospitalization of patients after head injury is necessary when the patient has focal or asymmetric neurologic deficits that do not rapidly resolve or when loss of consciousness is prolonged. It is important to admit and monitor carefully patients who show signs of deterioration and to initiate rapid treatment to relieve intracranial pressure.

Severe headache, nausea, vomiting, and restlessness can usually be treated symptomatically. Tetanus prophylaxis (0.5 mL tetanus toxoid) may be required for patients with scalp lacerations or open head injuries. Most patients do not require antibiotics. However, patients with CSF leakage from the nose or ears should be monitored carefully and antibiotics started if meningitis is suspected. Cerebral edema may be treated with diuretics, osmotic agents, or glucocorticoids or by lowering the patient's PCO_2. If acute obstructive hydrocephalus occurs, a ventricular drain aids in controlling increased intracranial pressure.

Patients with depressed or displaced fractures, epidural hematomas, progressive acute subdural hematomas, and some chronic subdural hematomas require operation. Evacuation of intracerebral hematomas is usually not indicated, though superficial intracerebral hematomas occasionally may be evacuated in an attempt to relieve severe and rapidly increasing mass effect.

Prognosis

Ninety percent or more of children who suffer from mild to moderate head injuries become free of symptoms and do not develop serious, long-term complications. Severe head injury is associated with a mortality rate of 5–10%. From 3% to 5% of children with severe head injury have severe, long-term neurologic deficits, and another 5–6% have moderate long-term deficits. Over 80% of children with severe head injury, however, enjoy good functional recovery.

SPINAL CORD INJURY

Spinal cord injury can occur at any age and often coexists with head injury. A high degree of suspicion is required to promptly diagnose and treat spinal injuries in infants and children. In neonates, spinal cord injury results from traction and hyperextension during difficult delivery. Generalized flaccidity and respiratory failure are frequently the predominant acute clinical manifestations, with spasticity and hyperreflexia developing later. In older children, the clinical signs of spinal cord injury depend on the level at which the injury occurs. Cervical cord injury results in respiratory weakness, flaccid weakness, and areflexia in the upper extremities; loss of bowel and bladder control; and spasticity and hyperreflexia in the lower extremities. A sensory level may be detectable in older children with low cervical, thoracic, and lumbosacral cord injury.

Diagnosis is based on the clinical history, pattern of neurologic deficits, and MRI. Plain films can be useful in the initial evaluation if fractures and bone displacements are present, but a normal plain x-ray of the spinal column does not exclude spinal cord injury or replace the need for MRI if a spinal cord injury is suspected. Initial management of suspected spinal cord injury involves stabilizing the neck, minimizing movement of the patient, and supporting respiratory and cardiovascular functions. Additional measures include use of osmotic agents and corticosteroids to reduce edema, surgery to remove epidural or subdural hematoma, and surgery to stabilize bone fractures and displacements. Long-term management of residual neurologic dysfunction requires intensive rehabilitation; bowel and bladder care; treatment of spasticity with baclofen, diazepam, or dantrolene sodium; and psychologic counseling.

The prognosis varies with the severity of the injury. Children with complete cord transections have a poor prognosis for recovery. Late complications include progressive spinal deformity, contractures, dysesthetic pain syndromes, recurrent infections, and decubitus ulcers.

Davis PC et al: Spinal injuries in children: Role of MR. AJNR Am J Neuroradiol 199 1993;14:607.

Edwards MSB, Cogen PH: Craniospinal trauma in children. In: *Neurologic Aspects of Pediatrics.* Berg BO (editor). Butterworth-Heinemann, 1992.

Ghajar J, Hariri RJ: Management of pediatric head injury. Pediatr Clin North Am 1992;39:1093.

PERINATAL HEAD INJURY

Injury to the scalp and skull occurs during the perinatal period in association with prolonged pressure on the infant's skull, breech presentation, shoulder dystocia, or malpositioned forceps. Several types of head and scalp injury may be visibly apparent at the time of birth. **Caput succedaneum** is characterized by hemorrhagic edema of the scalp skin and muscles. **Cephalhematoma** is a localized subperiosteal hemorrhage; this type of hemorrhage is limited in extent by the periosteum that attaches at suture margins. Caput and cephalhematomas resolve spontaneously and require no specific treatment. Cephalhematomas occasionally prolong neonatal jaundice, and approximately 25% of them overlie linear skull fractures. **Subgaleal hemorrhage** represents the most dangerous extracranial hemorrhage in the neonate. The blood of this hemorrhage dissects underneath the fascia of muscles of the head and neck. Blood may dissect and extend into the face, down the neck, and over the chest and back. Massive blood loss can take place, and subgaleal hemorrhage can result in exsanguination. Subgaleal hemorrhage usually occurs in association with an underlying bleeding disorder or after severe head trauma that results in tears of the dura that form the dural sinuses.

Skull fractures in the perinatal period involving the skull base and occipital region can be associated with dural tears and massive intracranial hemorrhage. Hemorrhage secondary to dural tear often results in catastrophic, rapid clinical deterioration and death.

Intracranial hemorrhage is the most serious consequence of head injury during the perinatal period. Epidural hematomas are usually associated with depressed skull fractures. *Emergency surgical removal is mandatory.* Subarachnoid hemorrhage is relatively frequent in the perinatal period and is often asymptomatic. However, hydrocephalus may develop after subarachnoid hemorrhage and may require ventriculoperitoneal shunting. Subdural hematomas are occasionally seen in the perinatal period and are often associated with cerebral laceration or contusion. Acute subdural hematomas may progress rapidly, and the patient may require emergency surgery for evacuation of the hematoma. Chronic subdural hematomas are manifested by increasing head circumference and the gradual appearance of neurologic deficits, anemia, poor weight gain, irritability, and somnolence.

Intracerebral hematomas usually indicate severe head trauma in the perinatal period and are frequently associated with dural lacerations or with bleeding disorders.

Intracranial Hemorrhage in the Premature

Approximately 25–40% of all newborns weighing less than 2000 g develop periventricular-interventricular hemorrhage. This type of hemorrhage originates in the germinal matrix and is related to immature blood vessel structure, poor blood vessel support by the germinal matrix, and the unusual tortuous course of veins in the region of the germinal matrix in the premature brain. Germinal matrix hemorrhages are classified as grade I, II, or III. Grade I indicates a hemorrhage limited to the subependymal, germinal matrix region with little or no intraventricular extension. Grade II represents the germinal matrix hemorrhage with moderate extension into the ventricular system. Grade III represents germinal matrix hemorrhage with massive intraventricular extension and usually ventriculomegaly. Furthermore, intraventricular hemorrhage may be associated with hemorrhagic infarction of the white matter dorsal and lateral to the anterior lateral ventricle.

Clinical symptoms of intraventricular-periventricular hemorrhage are related to the size of the hemorrhage and its degree of extension into the ventricular system. In addition, symptoms are modified by the degree of the infant's systemic illness. Small grade I hemorrhages limited to the germinal matrix can be asymptomatic and are often diagnosed by ultrasonography but not suspected clinically. Some patients develop a waxing and waning course with a gradual, stuttering evolution of neurologic deficits. The most dramatic presentation of intraventricular-periventricular hemorrhage, however, is the sudden catastrophic onset of seizures, anemia, and cardiovascular instability. Acute grade III hemorrhages combined with periventricular hemorrhagic infarction are associated with a mortality rate of more than 60% (Table 23–14).

Laboratory evaluation of infants with periventricular-intraventricular hemorrhage includes assessment of the hematocrit, electrolytes, calcium, magnesium, blood glucose concentration, coagulation system, and acid-base status. Examination of CSF after intraventricular hemorrhage is usually not necessary but reveals grossly bloody spinal fluid with elevated protein and decreased glucose concentration.

The primary diagnostic test in neonates suspected of having periventricular-intraventricular hemorrhage is cranial ultrasonography. This test is excellent for displaying germinal matrix hemorrhage with or with-

Table 23–14. Prognosis of periventricular-intraventricular hemorrhage (IVH) in premature infants.

	Acute		Long-Term
	Mortality (%)	Hydrocephalus (%)	Neurologic Impairment (%)
Grade I	5	5	5
Grade II	10	25	15
Grade III	20	55	40
IVH and periventricular hemorrhagic infarction (grade IV)	50	80	90

out intraventricular extension and can be used for serial monitoring of ventricular size. However, ultrasonography is not an adequate method for evaluating cerebral hemispheres or structures of the posterior fossa. CT or MRI scanning is necessary for full evaluation of the cerebral parenchyma, the posterior fossa, and the subarachnoid, subdural, and epidural spaces.

Treatment

Treatment of infants with periventricular-intraventricular hemorrhage is directed at stabilizing and supporting the cardiovascular system. Abnormalities of the cardiovascular, renal, gastrointestinal, and other organ systems require specific monitoring and management. Fluid, electrolyte, and acid-base disturbances should be identified and corrected. Secondary infections and seizures should be treated with antibiotics and anticonvulsant medications. Any underlying bleeding diathesis should be corrected, and vitamin K_1 should be given to infants to ensure that a bleeding diathesis secondary to vitamin K deficiency does not contribute to the patient's problems.

For patients with progressive ventriculomegaly and hydrocephalus, ventricular drains and subsequent ventriculoperitoneal shunting are often required. The value of serial lumbar punctures is controversial, but this procedure can be useful in some patients if ventriculostomy is not readily available to relieve acute posthemorrhagic ventriculomegaly.

Prognosis

The outcome of intracranial hemorrhage is related to the extent of underlying brain injury. Brain lacerations and contusions predispose to the development of posttraumatic epilepsy and focal or multifocal areas of cerebral atrophy.

The outcome of neonatal intraventricular-periventricular hemorrhage is related to the size and extent of the hemorrhage and associated factors such as the presence of hemorrhagic infarction and systemic complications secondary to cardiovascular, renal, gastrointestinal, and other systemic abnormalities. Table 23–14 displays the mortality and morbidity rates with regard to neurologic deficits and hydrocephalus.

Lescohier I, DiScala C: Blunt trauma in children: Causes and outcomes of head versus extracranial injury. Pediatrics 1993;91:721.

Volpe JJ: Intraventricular hemorrhage in the premature infant: Current concepts. Parts I and II. Ann Neurol 1989;25:3, 109.

NEOPLASMS OF THE CENTRAL NERVOUS SYSTEM

1. INTRACRANIAL TUMORS

Neoplasms of the central nervous system (CNS) account for approximately 20% of all malignant neoplasms of childhood and are second only to leukemia in frequency. The incidence of primary CNS tumors in people under 20 years of age is 20–25 per million per year, or about one third to one half of the incidence of childhood leukemia. The incidence of CNS tumors in children under age 2 is approximately 10% of that in older children, or approximately 2–2.5 per million per year. Approximately 1500 new cases of brain tumor occur each year in the United States, including 150–200 cases in children under 2 years old. The peak incidence of brain tumors occurs between the ages of 5 and 10 years, and the male:female ratio is approximately 1.2:1. Primary brain tumors can be classified generally by their cell of origin (Table 23–15). In children over the age of 2, approximately

65% of brain tumors are infratentorial and 35% supratentorial. Secondary involvement of the nervous system is common in the early stages of acute leukemia, and the brain may be invaded directly by tumors that involve extraneural tissue in the head and neck region. Hematogenous metastatic spread from solid malignant tumors outside the nervous system is rare in childhood, but the true incidence of this phenomenon is unknown. Some highly aggressive and malignant intracranial tumors in childhood, such as medulloblastoma, commonly spread throughout the subarachnoid spaces within the central nervous system. Rarely, primary CNS tumors may metastasize to extraneural sites such as bone marrow, lung, and viscera.

Clinical Manifestations

Manifestations of intracranial tumors consist of nonspecific signs due to increased intracranial pressure (Table 23–16). Infratentorial tumors, regardless of histologic type, frequently present with gait disturbance, incoordination, multiple and often asymmetric cranial nerve deficits, and nystagmus. The patient may tilt the head in an attempt to relieve discomfort at the base of the skull due to cerebellar tonsillar herniation, or head tilt may be a compensatory adjustment to correct double vision.

Specific neurologic manifestations of supratentorial tumors are dictated by the location of the tumor. Focal motor and sensory abnormalities and focal seizures occur frequently in the more common types of hemispheric tumors. Abnormalities of eye movements and vision are also common. Endocrine and autonomic disturbances may indicate the presence of a hypothalamic or thalamic tumor.

Diagnosis

When the clinical history and the findings of physical examination suggest the presence of an intracranial mass, a CT or MRI scan of the head should be obtained to define the precise anatomic site and ex-

Table 23–15. Classification of primary brain tumors of childhood.

Tumor Type	Incidence (%)	Common Examples
Glial cell tumors	50–60	Astrocytoma Optic nerve glioma Brain stem glioma Ependymoma
Neuroectodermal tumors	25–35	Medulloblastoma Pinealoblastoma
Craniopharyngioma	5–10	
Germ cell tumors	< 10	Teratoma Dermoid Germinoma
Meningeal tumors	< 5	Meningioma Meningeal sarcoma
Lymphoma (non-Hodgkin's)	< 1	

Table 23–16. Signs of increased intracranial pressure.

Acute
Macrocephaly
Excessive rate of head growth
Altered behavior
Decreased level of consciousness
Vomiting
Blurred vision
Double vision
Optic disk swelling
Abducens nerve paresis
Chronic
Macrocephaly
Growth impairment
Developmental delay
Optic atrophy
Visual field loss

tent of the tumor. Skull x-rays may show scalloping of the inner table of the skull, truncation of the sella turcica, or widening of the suture lines as evidence of increased intracranial pressure. Electroencephalographic findings in brain tumors are nonspecific, and EEGs are rarely necessary in the initial diagnostic evaluation of brain tumor. However, EEGs done on patients who have focal or generalized seizures as a manifestation of their tumor may show localized epileptiform discharges. An EEG done before initiation of treatment for the brain tumor may provide a useful baseline assessment of electrocerebral activity for future reference. Examination of CSF is usually not necessary in the diagnosis of localized mass lesions within the nervous system. However, examination of spinal fluid, particularly cytopathologic examination, may be helpful when tumors are disseminated throughout the subarachnoid space.

Treatment

Some tumors, such as cerebellar astrocytomas, may be completely removed by surgery and require no additional treatment. Most primary CNS tumors, however, are currently treated by a combination of surgery, radiation, and chemotherapy. Surgery is frequently used to reduce the mass of tumor and is followed by localized radiation to the tumor bed. Some tumors with a propensity for subarachnoid seeding and spread (eg, medulloblastoma) are also treated with prophylactic total craniocerebral radiation. Given the many chemotherapeutic agents available, it is recommended that children with brain tumors be enrolled in multicenter protocols that use combinations of surgery, radiation, and chemotherapy.

2. PSEUDOTUMOR CEREBRI

Pseudotumor cerebri is a condition characterized by increased intracranial pressure in the absence of an identifiable intracranial mass or hydrocephalus. Clinical manifestations of pseudotumor cerebri are those of increased intracranial pressure as outlined in Table 23–16. The precise cause is usually not known, but pseudotumor cerebri has been described in association with a variety of inflammatory, metabolic, toxic, and connective tissue disorders (Table 23–17). The diagnosis of pseudotumor cerebri is one of exclusion. CT or MRI scans of the head are needed to exclude hydrocephalus and intracranial masses; these studies demonstrate ventricles of small or normal size but no other structural abnormalities. Lumbar puncture should be performed to document elevated CSF pressure. Examination of cerebrospinal fluid reveals a normal cell count, a normal glucose concentration, and a normal or low protein concentration. In some inflammatory and connective tissue diseases, however, the CSF protein may be increased.

Specific treatment of pseudotumor cerebri is aimed

Table 23–17. Conditions associated with pseudotumor cerebri.

Metabolic-toxic disorders
Hypervitaminosis A
Hypovitaminosis A
Prolonged steroid therapy
Steroid withdrawal
Tetracycline therapy
Nalidixic acid therapy
Iron deficiency
Plumbism
Hypocalcemia
Hyperparathyroidism
Adrenal insufficiency
Lupus erythematosus
Chronic CO_2 retention
Infectious and parainfectious disorders
Chronic otitis media
Poliomyelitis
Guillain-Barré syndrome
Dural sinus thrombosis
Minor head injury

at correcting any identifiable underlying predisposing condition. In addition, some patients may benefit from the use of furosemide or acetazolamide to decrease the volume and pressure of cerebrospinal fluid within the central nervous system. These drugs may be used in combination with repeated lumbar punctures to remove CSF. If a program of repeated spinal fluid removal and medical management is not successful or if visual field loss is detected despite these measures, lumboperitoneal shunt or another surgical decompression procedure may be necessary to prevent irreparable visual loss and damage to the optic nerves.

3. SPINAL CORD TUMORS

The incidence of tumors within the spinal canal is one sixth to one fifth that of tumors within the intracranial compartment. The peak age at occurrence is approximately 4 years. Spinal tumors can be classified as intradural or extradural. Intradural tumors within the substance of the spinal cord are referred to as intramedullary and those outside as extramedullary. Recent reports suggest that approximately one third of intraspinal tumors are intramedullary, approximately one third are intradural extramedullary, and approximately one-third are extradural. About 10% of intraspinal tumors arise in the sacral region, and the remainder are distributed equally in the cervical, thoracic, and lumbar regions. Neurofibromas, meningiomas, dermoid cysts, teratomas, and metastatic tumors constitute the most frequent tumors that are extradural or intradural extramedullary. Astrocytomas and ependymomas are the most common intramedullary tumors.

Clinical manifestations of spinal cord tumors result from direct invasion of the tumor into neural tissue as well as from compression of neural tissue. Symptoms of gait disturbance, pain, and bowel and bladder dysfunction occur in association with abnormal muscle stretch reflexes, weakness, and sensory loss. The specific patterns of neurologic deficits are determined by the location and size of tumor mass.

When the clinical course and physical examination suggest the presence of an intraspinal mass, neuroimaging procedures are required. Spinal CT scan, metrizamide myelography, and spinal MRI scans are used to define tumors. The use of gadolinium with MRI scanning enhances the definition of tumors within the spinal cord and within the spinal subarachnoid and extradural spaces. Although examination of CSF may demonstrate the presence of neoplastic cells and markedly elevated protein concentrations, this test is not required for the diagnosis of intraspinal tumors and is contraindicated when significant cord compression is suspected clinically.

Primary intraspinal tumors may be totally removed by surgery, but many intramedullary tumors require a combination of surgery, radiation, and chemotherapy similar to the treatment of intracranial tumors discussed in the preceding section.

In addition to primary intraspinal tumors, the spinal cord and intraspinal compartment may be the site of direct invasion or hematogenous metastatic spread of tumors that arise outside the nervous system. Important examples include spinal neuroblastoma that may be an extension of paraspinous retroperitoneal neuroblastoma. Lymphoma, sarcoma, and leukemia may involve paraspinous tissue and spread to the intraspinal compartment through neural foramina. Treatment of these secondary neoplasms usually requires some combination of surgical excision, radiation, and chemotherapy.

Albright AL: Pediatric brain tumors. CA Cancer J Clin 1993;43:272.

Allen ED et al: The clinical and radiological evaluation of primary brain tumors in children. Part I: Clinical evaluation. J Natl Med Assoc 1993;85:445.

Baker RS, Baumann RJ, Buncic JR: Idiopathic intracranial hypertension (pseudotumor cerebri) in pediatric patients. Pediatr Neurol 1989;5:5.

Maria BL et al: Brainstem glioma: I. Pathology, clinical features, and therapy. J Child Neurol 1993;8:112.

Murovic J, Sundaresen N: Pediatric spinal axis tumors. Neurosurg Clin North Am 1992;3:947.

Packer RJ: Brain tumors in children. Curr Opin Pediatr 1995;7:64.

Weisberg LA, Chutorian AM: Pseudotumor cerebri of childhood. Am J Dis Child 1977;131:1243.

CEREBROVASCULAR DISEASE

Cerebrovascular disease, or stroke, occurs with an incidence in the pediatric population of approxi-

mately 1.2–2.5:100,000 per year. Although stroke occurs most frequently between the ages of 1 and 5 years, it may occur at any age during infancy and childhood. Congenital cyanotic heart disease is the most common underlying systemic disorder predisposing to stroke.

The initial approach to the patient should take into account the patient's age and any underlying systemic or neurologic illness. A systematic search for evidence of cardiac, vascular, or hematologic disease and intracranial disorders should be undertaken (Table 23–18).

Clinical Findings

A. Symptoms & Signs: Clinical manifesta-

Table 23–18. Etiologic risk factors for stroke in children.

Cardiac disorders
  Cyanotic heart disease
  Valvular disease
    Rheumatic
    Endocarditis
  Cardiomyopathy
  Cardiac dysrhythmia
Vascular occlusive disorders
  Arterial trauma (carotid dissections)
  Homocystinuria
  Mitochondrial encephalomyopathy
  Vasculitis
    Meningitis
    Polyarteritis nodosa
    Systemic lupus erythematosus
    Drug abuse (amphetamines)
  Fibromuscular dysplasia
  Moya-Moya syndrome
  Diabetes
  Nephrotic syndrome
  Systemic hypertension
  Dural sinus and cerebral venous thrombosis
    Meningitis
    Hyperviscosity
    Hypovolemia
  Cortical venous thrombosis
  Carotid-cavernous fistula
Hematologic disorders
  Polycythemia
  Thrombotic thrombocytopenia
  Thrombocytopenic purpura
  Thrombocythemia
  Hemoglobinopathies
    Sickle cell disease
    S-C disease
  Coagulation defects
    Hemophilia
    Vitamin K deficiency
  Hypercoagulable states
    Pregnancy
    Systemic lupus erythematosus
    Use of oral contraceptives
    Antithrombin III deficiency
    Protein C and S deficiencies
  Leukemia
Intracranial vascular anomalies
  Arteriovenous malformation
  Arterial aneurysm
  Carotid-cavernous fistula

tions of stroke in childhood vary according to the vascular distribution to the brain that is involved. Because many conditions leading to childhood stroke result in emboli, multifocal neurologic involvement is common. Children may present with acute hemiplegia similar to stroke in adults. Symptoms of unilateral weakness, sensory disturbance, dysarthria, and dysphasia may develop over a period of minutes, but at times progressive worsening of symptoms may evolve over several hours. Bilateral hemispheric involvement may lead to a depressed level of consciousness. The patient may also demonstrate disturbances of mood and behavior and experience focal or multifocal seizures. Physical examination of the patient is aimed not only at identifying the specific deficits related to impaired cerebral blood flow but also at seeking evidence for any predisposing disorder. Retinal hemorrhages, splinter hemorrhages in the nail beds, cardiac murmurs, and signs of trauma are especially important findings.

When stroke is ushered in by a focal hemiconvulsion followed by hemiplegia, a chronic epilepsy syndrome may persist for years in association with hemiplegia. This combination of hemiconvulsion, hemiplegia, and chronic epilepsy has been referred to as the **HHE syndrome.**

B. Laboratory Findings: Laboratory investigation can be carried out systemically, with particular attention to disorders involving the heart, blood vessels, platelets, red cells, hemoglobin, and coagulation proteins. Additional laboratory tests for systemic disorders such as systemic lupus erythematosus and polyarteritis nodosa are usually indicated.

Examination of spinal fluid is indicated in patients with fever, nuchal rigidity, or marked obtundation when the diagnosis of intracranial infection requires exclusion. Lumbar puncture, however, may be deferred until a neuroimage excluding brain abscess or a space-occupying lesion that might contraindicate lumbar puncture has been obtained. In the absence of infection and frank intracranial subarachnoid hemorrhage, CSF examination is rarely helpful in defining the cause of the cerebrovascular disorder.

C. Imaging: CT and MRI scans of the brain are often helpful in defining the extent of cerebral involvement with ischemia or hemorrhage. CT scans, however, may be normal within the first few hours of an ischemic stroke and may need to be repeated several hours later. A CT scan early after the onset of neurologic deficits is valuable in excluding significant intracranial hemorrhage. This information may be helpful in the early stages of management and in the decision to treat with anticoagulants.

Cerebral angiography is usually not urgently needed but may be needed to confirm such disorders as fibromuscular dysplasia and cerebral arteritis. If angiography is done, all major vessels should be studied. If evidence of fibromuscular dysplasia is present in the intracranial or extracranial vessels, re-

nal arteriography is indicated. With additional technical advances, MRA will soon replace conventional contrast angiography for most cases of childhood stroke.

When seizures are prominent, an EEG may be used as an adjunct in the patient's evaluation. An EEG and sequential electroencephalographic monitoring may help in patients with severely depressed consciousness.

Electrocardiography and echocardiography are useful both in the diagnostic approach to the patient and in ongoing monitoring and management, particularly when hypotension or cardiac arrhythmias complicate the clinical course.

Differential Diagnosis

Patients with an acute onset of neurologic deficits must be evaluated not only for cerebrovascular disease but also for other disorders that can cause focal neurologic deficits. Hypoglycemia, prolonged focal seizures, a prolonged postictal paresis (Todd's paralysis), meningitis, encephalitis, and brain abscess should all be considered. Migraine with focal neurologic deficits may be difficult to differentiate initially from ischemic stroke. Occasionally, the onset of a neurodegenerative disorder (eg, adrenoleukodystrophy) may begin with the abrupt onset of seizures and focal neurologic deficits. The possibility of drug abuse (particularly cocaine) and other toxic exposures must be investigated diligently.

Treatment

The initial management of children with stroke is aimed at providing support for pulmonary, cardiovascular, and renal function. Appropriate fluid and electrolyte infusions should be started, and careful monitoring of heart rate and rhythm and blood pressure are required. Specific treatment of stroke depends in part upon the underlying pathogenesis and the specific predisposing disorder. In some situations, heparinization for emboli and consumption coagulopathies is indicated. In other disorders, such as fibromuscular dysplasia, treatment to decrease platelet adhesiveness may be an acceptable alternative to anticoagulation.

Long-term management requires intensive rehabilitation efforts, anticonvulsant treatment, and therapy aimed at improving the child's language, educational, and psychologic performance.

Prognosis

The outcome of stroke in infants and children is variable. Underlying predisposing conditions and the vascular territory involved all play a role in dictating the outcome for an individual patient. When the stroke involves extremely large portions of one hemisphere or large portions of both hemispheres and cerebral edema develops, the patient's level of consciousness may deteriorate rapidly, and death may occur within the first few days. Some patients may achieve almost complete recovery of neurologic function within several days if the cerebral territory is small. Seizures, either focal or generalized, may occur in 30–50% of patients at some point in the course of their cerebrovascular disorder. Chronic problems with learning, behavior, and activity are common.

Broderick J et al: Stroke in children within a major metropolitan area: The surprising importance of intracerebral hemorrhage. J Child Neurol 1993;8:250.

Edwards MSB, Hoffman B: *Cerebral Vascular Disease in Children and Adolescents*. Williams & Wilkins, 1989.

Kerr LM et al: Ischemic stroke in the young: Evaluation and age comparison of patients six months to thirty-nine years. J Child Neurol 1993;8:266.

Reila AR, Roach ES: Etiology of stroke in children. J Child Neurol 1993;8:201.

Yang JS, Park YD, Hartlage PL: Seizures associated with stroke in childhood. Pediatr Neurol 1995;12:136.

Young RSK: Neurologic aspects of cardiovascular disease. In: *Neurologic Aspects of Pediatrics*. Berg BO (editor). Butterworth-Heinemann, 1992.

CONGENITAL MALFORMATIONS OF THE NERVOUS SYSTEM

Malformations of the nervous system occur in 1–3% of living neonates and are present in 40% of infants who die. Developmental anomalies of the central nervous system may result from a variety of causes, including infectious, toxic, metabolic, and vascular insults that affect the fetus. The specific type of malformation that results from such insults, however, may depend more upon the gestational period during which the insult occurs than on the specific cause. The period of induction, days 0–28 of gestation, is the period during which the neural plate appears and the neural tube forms and closes. Insults during this phase can result in a major absence of neural structures, such as anencephaly, or in a defect of neural tube closure, such as spina bifida, meningomyelocele, or encephalocele. Cellular proliferation and migration characterize neural development that occurs after 28 days of gestation. Lissencephaly, pachygyria, agyria, and agenesis of the corpus callosum are caused by insults that occur during the period of cellular proliferation and migration.

1. ABNORMALITIES OF NEURAL TUBE CLOSURE

Defects of neural tube closure constitute some of the most common congenital malformations affecting the nervous system. Spina bifida with associated meningomyelocele or meningocele is commonly found in the lumbosacral region. Depending on the extent and severity of the involvement of the spinal cord and peripheral nerves, clinical findings include lower extremity weakness, bowel and bladder dysfunction, and hip dislocation. Operation to close meningoceles and meningomyeloceles is usually indicated. Additional treatment is necessary to manage chronic abnormalities of the urinary tract, orthopedic abnormalities such as kyphosis and scoliosis, and paresis of the lower extremities. Hydrocephalus associated with meningomyelocele usually requires ventriculoperitoneal shunting.

Arnold-Chiari Malformations

Arnold-Chiari malformation type I consists of elongation and displacement of the caudal end of the brain stem into the spinal canal with protrusion of the cerebellar tonsils through the foramen magnum. In association with this hindbrain malformation, there are often minor to moderate abnormalities of the base of the skull, including basilar impression (platybasia) and small foramen magnum. Arnold-Chiari malformation type I may remain asymptomatic for years, but in older children and young adults it may cause progressive ataxia, paresis of the lower cranial nerves, and progressive vertigo. Posterior cervical laminectomy may be necessary to provide relief from cervical cord compression. Ventriculoperitoneal shunting is required for hydrocephalus.

Arnold-Chiari malformation type II consists of the malformations found in Arnold-Chiari type I plus an associated lumbosacral meningomyelocele. Hydrocephalus is present in approximately 90% of children with Arnold-Chiari type II. These patients may also have aqueductal stenosis, hydromyelia, or syringomyelia. The clinical manifestations of Arnold-Chiari type II are most commonly caused by the associated hydrocephalus and meningomyelocele. In addition, dysfunction of the lower cranial nerves may be present.

Arnold-Chiari malformation type III is characterized by occipital encephalocele, a closure defect of the rostral end of the neural tube. Hydrocephalus is extremely common with this malformation.

In general, the diagnosis of neural tube defects is obvious at the time of birth. Diagnosis may be strongly suspected prenatally on the basis of ultrasonographic findings and the presence of elevated alpha-fetoprotein in the amniotic fluid. Folate deficiency in pregnant women has been associated with an increased incidence of neural tube defects in their infants.

2. DISORDERS OF CELLULAR PROLIFERATION AND MIGRATION

Lissencephaly

Lissencephaly is a severe malformation of brain characterized by an extremely smooth cortical surface with minimal sulcal and gyral development. Such a smooth surface is characteristic of fetal brain at the end of the first trimester. In addition, many lissencephalic brains have a primitive cytoarchitectural construction with a four-layered cerebral mantle instead of the mature six-layered mantle. **Pachygyria** (thick gyri) and **agyria** (absence of gyri) are closely associated with lissencephaly but represent more restricted forms of migrational abnormalities. Patients with lissencephaly usually suffer from severe neurodevelopmental delay, microcephaly, and seizures (including infantile spasms) and frequently have additional associated malformations and dysmorphic features. Walker-Warburg syndrome or Miller-Dieker syndrome can often be identified in some of these patients. Walker-Warburg syndrome is an autosomal recessive disorder, and Miller-Dieker syndrome is associated with defects of chromosome 17; it is particularly important to identify these syndromes because of their genetic importance. In addition to these two syndromes, lissencephaly may be a component of Zellweger's syndrome, a metabolic peroxisomal abnormality associated with the presence of elevated concentrations of very long-chain fatty acids in plasma. A peroxisomal defect in fatty acid degradation in cultured skin fibroblasts confirms the diagnosis. No specific treatment for lissencephaly is available. Seizures may be controlled by the use of phenobarbital, phenytoin, or clonazepam.

MRI scans have helped to define a number of presumed migrational defects that are similar to but anatomically more restricted than lissencephaly. A distinctive example is bilateral perisylvian cortical dysplasia. Patients with this disorder have pseudobulbar palsy, variable cognitive deficits, facial diplegia, dysarthria, developmental delay, and epilepsy. Seizures are often difficult to control with antiepileptic drugs; some patients have benefited from corpus callosotomy. The cause of this syndrome is as yet unknown, though intrauterine cerebral ischemic injury has been postulated. Therapy is aimed at improving speech and oromotor functions and controlling seizures.

Agenesis of the Corpus Callosum

Agenesis of the corpus callosum, once thought to be a relatively rare cerebral malformation, has been seen frequently with modern neuroimaging techniques such as CT and MRI. The cause of this malformation is unknown. Occasionally, it appears to be inherited in an autosomal dominant or autosomal recessive pattern. X-linked recessive patterns have also been described. Agenesis of the corpus callosum has been found in some patients with pyruvate dehydrogenase deficiency and in others with nonketotic hyperglycinemia. Most cases, however, are sporadic. Maldevelopment of the corpus callosum may be partial or complete. No specific syndrome is typical of agenesis of the corpus callosum, although many pa-

tients have seizures, developmental delay, microcephaly, or mental retardation. Neurologic abnormalities may be related to microscopic cytoarchitectural abnormalities of the brain that occur in association with agenesis of the corpus callosum. The malformation may be found coincidentally by neuroimaging studies in otherwise normal patients, and has been described as a coincidental finding at autopsy in neurologically normal individuals. A special form of agenesis of the corpus callosum occurs in Aicardi's syndrome. In this X-linked disorder, agenesis of the corpus callosum is associated with infantile spasms, mental retardation, lacunar chorioretinopathy, and vertebral body abnormalities.

Dandy-Walker Malformation

Dandy-Walker malformation is characterized by aplasia of the vermis, cystic enlargement of the fourth ventricle, rostral displacement of the tentorium, and absence or atresia of the foramina of Magendie and Luschka. Although hydrocephalus is usually not present congenitally, it develops within the first few months of life; 90% of patients who develop hydrocephalus do so by the age of 1 year. On physical examination, there is often a rounded protuberance or exaggeration of the cranial occiput. In the absence of hydrocephalus and increased intracranial pressure, there may be few physical findings to suggest neurologic dysfunction. An ataxic syndrome occurs in fewer than 20% of patients and is usually late in appearing. Many long-term neurologic deficits result directly from hydrocephalus. Diagnosis of Dandy-Walker malformation is confirmed by CT or MRI scanning of the head. Treatment is directed at the management of hydrocephalus.

3. CRANIOSYNOSTOSIS

Craniosynostosis, or premature closure of cranial sutures, is usually sporadic and idiopathic. However, some patients have hereditary disorders, such as Apert's syndrome and Crouzon's disease, that are associated with abnormalities of the digits, extremities, and heart. Occasionally, craniosynostosis may be associated with an underlying metabolic disturbance such as hyperthyroidism and hypophosphatasia. The most common form of craniosynostosis involves the sagittal suture and results in scaphocephaly, an elongation of the head in the anterior to posterior direction. Premature closure of the coronal sutures causes brachycephaly, an increase in cranial diameter from left to right. Unless many or all cranial sutures close prematurely, intracranial volume will not be compromised, and the brain's growth will not be impaired. Closure of only one or a few sutures will not cause impaired brain growth or neurologic dysfunction. Management of craniosynostosis is directed at preserving normal skull shape and consists of excising the fused suture and applying material to the edge of the craniectomy to prevent reossification of the bone edges. The best cosmetic effect on the skull is achieved when surgery is done during the first 6 months of life.

4. HYDROCEPHALUS

Hydrocephalus is characterized by an increased volume of cerebrospinal fluid in association with progressive ventricular dilation. In communicating hydrocephalus, CSF circulates through the ventricular system and into the subarachnoid space without obstruction. In noncommunicating hydrocephalus, an obstruction blocks the flow of spinal fluid within the ventricular system or blocks the egress of spinal fluid from the ventricular system into the subarachnoid space. A wide variety of disorders, such as hemorrhage, infection, tumors, and congenital malformations, may play an etiologic role in development of hydrocephalus.

Clinical features of hydrocephalus include macrocephaly, an excessive rate of head growth, irritability, vomiting, loss of appetite, impaired upgaze, impaired extraocular movements, hypertonia of the lower extremities, and generalized hyperreflexia. Without treatment, optic atrophy may occur. In infants, papilledema may not be present, whereas older children with closed cranial sutures can eventually develop swelling of the optic disk.

Hydrocephalus can be diagnosed on the basis of the clinical course, findings on physical examination, and CT or MRI scan.

Treatment of hydrocephalus is directed at providing an alternative outlet for CSF from the intracranial compartment. The most common method is ventriculoperitoneal shunting. Other treatment should be directed, if possible, at the underlying cause of the hydrocephalus.

Dobyns WB, Trumit CL: Lissencephaly and other malformations of cortical development: 1995 update. Neuropediatrics 1995;26:132.

Hirsch JF et al: The Dandy-Walker malformation. J Neurosurg 1984;61:515.

Hoffman HJ, Epstein F (editors): *Disorders of the Developing Nervous System: Diagnosis and Treatment.* Blackwell, 1986.

Kuzniecky R et al: Congenital bilateral perisylvian syndrome: Study of 31 patients. Lancet 1993;341:608.

ABNORMAL HEAD SIZE

Bone plates of the skull have almost no intrinsic capacity to enlarge or grow, unlike long bones. They depend on extrinsic forces to stimulate new bone formation at the suture lines. Although gravity and traction on bone by muscle and scalp probably stimulate some growth, the single most important stimulus for head growth during infancy and childhood is brain growth. Therefore, accurate assessment of head growth is one of the most important aspects of the neurologic examination of young children. A head circumference that is 2 SD above or below the mean for age requires investigation and explanation.

1. MICROCEPHALY

A head circumference more than 2 SD below the mean for age and sex is by definition microcephaly. More important, however, than a single head circumference measurement is the rate or pattern of head growth through time. Head circumference measurements that progressively drop to lower percentiles with increasing age are indicative of a process or condition that has impaired the brain's capacity to grow. The causes of microcephaly are numerous. Some examples are listed in Table 23–19.

Clinical Findings

A. Symptoms & Signs: Microcephaly may be suspected in the full-term newborn and in infants up

Table 23–19. Microcephaly.

Causes	Examples
Prenatal chromosomal	Trisomy 13, 18, 21
Malformation	Lissencephaly schizencephaly
Syndromes	Rubenstein-Taybi, Cornelia de Lange
Toxins	Alcohol, anticonvulsants (?), maternal phenylketonuria
Infections (intrauterine)	TORCHES[1]
Radiation	Maternal pelvis, 1st and 2nd trimester
Placental insufficiency	Toxemia, infection
Familial	Autosomal dominant, autosomal recessive
Perinatal hypoxia, trauma	Birth asphyxia, injury
Infections (perinatal)	Bacterial meningitis (especially group B streptococci) Viral encephalitis (coxsackie B, herpes simplex)
Metabolic	Hypoglycemia, phenylketonuria, maple syrup urine disease
Postnatal sequela from earlier insult	As above
Degenerative disease	Tay-Sachs, Krabbe's

[1]A mnemonic formula for *to*xoplasmosis, *r*ubella, *cy*tomegalovirus, *her*pes simplex, and *s*yphilis.

to 6 months of age whose chest circumference exceeds the head circumference (unless the child is very obese). Microcephaly may be discovered when the child is examined because of delayed developmental milestones or neurologic problems, such as seizures or spasticity. There may be a marked backward slope of the forehead (as in familial microcephaly) with narrowing of the bitemporal diameter. The fontanelle may close earlier than expected, and sutures may be prominent.

B. Laboratory Findings: These vary with the cause. Abnormal dermatoglyphics may be present when the injury occurred before the 19th week of gestation. In the newborn, IgM, antibody titers for toxoplasmosis, rubella, cytomegalovirus, herpes simplex virus, and syphilis must be assessed. Elevated specific IgM titer is indicative of congenital infection. The urine culture for cytomegalovirus (CMV) will be positive at birth when this virus is the cause of microcephaly. Eye, cardiac, and bone abnormalities may also be clues to congenital infection. The child's serum and urine amino and organic acid determination are occasionally diagnostic. The mother may require screening for phenylketonuria. Karyotyping, including fragile X, should be considered.

C. Imaging: CT or MRI scans may aid in diagnosis and prognosis. These studies may demonstrate calcifications, malformations, or atrophic patterns that suggest specific congenital infections or genetic syndromes. Plain skull x-rays may show closed sutures, but these studies are of limited value in diagnosis and have been replaced by more sensitive and more informative scanning procedures. Genetic counseling should be done in any infant with significant microcephaly.

Differential Diagnosis

Congenital craniosynostosis involving multiple sutures is easily differentiated by inspection (head shape), history, identification of syndromes, hereditary pattern, and sometimes signs and symptoms of increased intracranial pressure. Common forms of craniosynostosis involving sagittal, coronal, and lambdoidal sutures are associated with abnormally shaped heads but do not cause microcephaly. Treatable undergrowth of the brain due to hypopituitarism, hypothyroidism, or severe protein-calorie undernutrition is recognized by the history and clinical findings.

Treatment & Prognosis

Except for the treatable disorders noted above, treatment is usually supportive and directed at the multiple neurologic and sensory deficits, endocrine disturbances (eg, diabetes insipidus) and seizures. Many children with head circumferences more than 2 SD below the mean show variable degrees of mental retardation. The notable exceptions are found in

cases of hypopituitarism (rare) or familial autosomal dominant microcephaly.

Ishihara T et al: Growth and achievement of large and small headed children in a normal population. Brain Dev 1988;10:295.

Jaffe M et al: The dilemma in prenatal diagnosis of idiopathic microcephaly. Dev Med Child Neurol 1987;29: 187.

2. MACROCEPHALY

A head circumference more than 2 SD above the mean for age and sex denotes macrocephaly. Excessive head growth rate through time suggests increased intracranial pressure most likely caused by hydrocephalus, extra-axial fluid collections, or neoplasms. Macrocephaly with normal head growth rate suggests familial macrocephaly or true megalencephaly, as might occur in neurofibromatosis. Other example of causes of macrocephaly are listed in Table 23–20.

Clinical Findings

Clinical and laboratory findings vary with the underlying process. In infants, transillumination of the

Table 23–20. Macrocephaly.

Causes	Examples
"Pseudomacrocephaly," "pseudohydrocephalus," "catch-up growth" crossing percentiles	Premature "grower," cystic fibrosis treatment, congenital heart disease recovery, parenteral alimentation.

Increased intracranial pressure
  With dilated ventricles
 	
  With other mass
	Progressive hydrocephalus, subdural effusion.
	Arachnoid cyst, porencephalic cyst, brain tumor.

Benign familial macrocephaly (idiopathic external hydrocephalus)	"External hydrocephalus," "benign enlargement of the subarachnoid spaces," "congenital communicating hydrocephalus," "benign subdural collections of infancy."

Megalencephaly (large brain)
  With neurocutaneous disorder
  With gigantism
  With dwarfism
  Metabolic
  Lysosomal
  Other leukodystrophy
	Benign familial (see above).
	Neurofibromatosis, tuberous sclerosis, etc.
	Soto's syndrome.
	Achondroplasia.
	Mucopolysaccharidoses.
	Metachromatic leukodystrophy.
	Canavan's spongy degeneration.

Thickened skull	Fibrous dysplasia (bone), hemolytic anemia (marrow), sicklemia, thalassemia.

skull with an intensely bright light in a completely darkened room may disclose chronic subdural effusions, hydrocephalus, hydranencephaly, and large cystic defects.

A surgically or medically treatable condition must be ruled out. Thus, the first decision is whether and when to perform an imaging study.

A. Imaging Study Deferred:

1. "Catch-up growth," as in the thriving, neurologically intact premature infant whose rapid head enlargement is most marked in the first weeks of life, or the infant in the early phase of recovery from deprivation dwarfism. As the expected "normal" is reached, head growth slows down, then resumes a normal growth pattern. If the fontanelle is open, cranial ultrasonography can assess ventricular size and diagnose or exclude hydrocephalus.

2. Familial macrocephaly, in which another family member may have an unusually large head with no signs or symptoms referable to such disorders as neurocutaneous dysplasias (especially neurofibromatosis) or cerebral gigantism (Soto's syndrome) nor significant mental or neurologic abnormalities in the child.

B. Imaging Study: CT or MRI scans (or ultrasonography, if the anterior fontanelle is open) are used to define any structural cause of macrocephaly and to determine an operable disorder. Even when the condition is not treatable (or is benign), the information gained may permit more accurate diagnosis and prognosis, guide management and genetic counseling, and serve as a basis for comparison should future abnormal cranial growth or neurologic changes necessitate a repeat study. An imaging study is necessary if there are any signs or symptoms of increased intracranial pressure (Table 23–16).

Gooskens RHJM et al: Megalencephaly: Definition and classification. Brain Dev 1988;10:1.

Wilms G et al: CT and MR in infants with pericerebral collections and macrocephaly: Benign enlargement of the subarachnoid spaces versus subdural collections. AJNR Am J Neuroradiol 1993;14:855.

NEUROCUTANEOUS DYSPLASIAS

Neurocutaneous dysplasias are diseases of the neuroectoderm and sometimes involve endoderm and mesoderm. Birthmarks and skin growths appearing later often suggest a need to look for brain, spinal cord, and eye disease. **Hamartomas** (histologically normal tissue growing abnormally rapidly or in aberrant sites) are common. The most common dysplasias are dominantly inherited. Benign and even malignant tumors may develop.

1. NEUROFIBROMATOSIS (Recklinghausen's Disease)

Essentials of Diagnosis

- More than six café-au-lait spots 5 mm in greatest diameter in prepubertal individuals and over 15 mm of greatest diameter in postpubertal individuals.
- Two or more neurofibromas of any type or one plexiform neurofibroma.
- Freckling in the axillary or inguinal regions.
- Optic glioma.
- Two or more Lisch nodules (iris hamartomas).
- Distinctive osseous lesions, such as sphenoid dysplasia or thinning of long bone with or without pseudarthroses.
- First-degree relative (parent, sibling, offspring) with neurofibromatosis type 1 by above criteria.

Clinical Findings

A. Symptoms & Signs: The most common presenting symptoms are cognitive or psychomotor problems such as school difficulties; 40% of patients have learning disabilities, and mental retardation is seen in 8%. The family history is important in identifying dominant gene manifestations in parents; they should be examined in detail. The history should focus on lumps or masses causing disfigurement, functional problems, or pain. The clinician should ask about visual problems; strabismus or amblyopia dictates a search for optic glioma, a common tumor in neurofibromatosis. Any progressive neurologic deficit might call for studies to rule out tumor of the spinal cord or central nervous system. Tumors of the eighth nerve are virtually never seen in common neurofibromatosis type 1.

The physician should check blood pressure and examine the spine for scoliosis and the limbs for pseudarthroses. Head measurement often shows macrocephaly. Hearing and vision need to be assessed. The eye examination should include a check for proptosis and iris Lisch nodules; the optic disk should be examined for atrophy or papilledema. Short stature and precocious puberty are occasional findings. An examination for neurologic manifestations of tumors (eg, asymmetric reflexes, spasticity) is important.

B. Laboratory Findings: Laboratory tests are not likely to be of any value in asymptomatic patients. Selected patients require brain MRI or CT scans with special cuts through the optic nerves to rule out optic glioma. Hypertension necessitates a look at renal arteries for dysplasia and stenosis as a cause. Cognitive and school achievement testing may be indicated. Scoliosis or limb abnormalities should be studied by appropriate roentgenograms such as an MRI scan of the spinal cord and roots.

Differential Diagnosis

Patients with Albright's syndrome often have

larger café-au-lait spots with precocious puberty. Many normal individuals have one or two café-au-lait spots.

Treatment

Genetic counseling is important. The risk to siblings is up to 50%. The disease may be progressive, with serious complications rarely seen. Patients sometimes worsen during puberty or pregnancy. Family members need to be evaluated for the presence of the gene. Annual or semiannual visits are important in the early detection of school problems or bony or neurologic abnormalities.

Multidisciplinary clinics at medical centers around the United States are often an excellent resource. Prenatal diagnosis is probably on the horizon, but the variability of manifestations (trivial to severe) will make therapeutic abortion an unlikely option. Chromosomal linkage studies are underway (chromosome 17).

Information for lay people and physicians is available from the National Neurofibromatosis Foundation, Inc., 70 West 40th Street, New York, NY 10018.

Committee on Genetics: Health supervision for children with neurofibromatosis. Pediatrics 1995;96:368.

Gomez MR (editor): *Neurocutaneous Diseases*. Butterworths, 1987.

Hoffman KJ, Boehm CD: Familial neurofibromatosis type 1: Clinical experience with DNA testing. J Pediatr 1992; 120:394.

Korf BR, Carranza E, Holmes GL: Patterns of seizures observed in association with neurofibromatosis I. Epilepsia 1993;34:616.

Listernick R, Charrow J, Greenwald M: Emergence of optic pathway gliomas in children with neurofibromatosis is type I after neuroimaging results. J Pediatr 1992;121: 584.

Riccardi VM: Neurofibromatosis: Past, present, and future. N Engl J Med 1991;324:1283.

Sevick RJ et al: Evolution of white matter lesions in neurofibromatosis type I: MR findings. AJR Am J Roentgenol 1992;159:171.

2. TUBEROUS SCLEROSIS (Bourneville's Disease)

Essentials of Diagnosis

- Facial angiofibromas or subungual fibromas.
- Often hypomelanotic macules, gingival fibromas.
- Retinal hamartomas.
- Cortical tubers or subependymal glial nodules, often calcified.
- Renal angiomyolipomas.

General Considerations

Tuberous sclerosis, a disease of unknown cause, is of autosomal dominant inheritance. A triad of seizures, mental retardation, and adenoma sebaceum is seen in only 33% of patients. The disease was earlier thought to have a high rate of mutation. As a result of more sophisticated techniques such as MRI, parents formerly thought not to harbor the gene are now being diagnosed as asymptomatic carriers.

Like neurofibromatosis, tuberous sclerosis may present with a wide variety of symptoms. The patient may be asymptomatic but for skin findings or may be devastated by severe infantile spasms in early infancy, by continuing epilepsy, and by mental retardation. Seizures in early infancy correlate with later mental retardation.

Clinical Findings
A. Symptoms & Signs:
1. Dermatologic features: Skin findings bring most cases to the physician's attention. Ninety-six percent have one or more hypomelanotic macules, facial angiofibromas, ungual fibromas, or shagreen patches. Adenoma sebaceum, the facial skin hamartomas, may first appear in early childhood, often on the cheek, chin, and dry sites of the skin where acne is not usually seen. They often have a reddish hue. The off-white hypomelanotic macules are more easily seen in tanned or dark-skinned individuals. They often are oval or "ash leaf" in shape and follow dermatomes. A Wood lamp (ultraviolet light) shows the macules more clearly—a great help in the light-skinned patient. In the scalp, poliosis (whitened hair) is the equivalent. In infancy, the presence of these macules accompanied by seizures is virtually diagnostic of the disease. Subungual or periungual fibromas are more common in the toes. Leathery, orange peel-like shagreen patches support the diagnosis. Café-au-lait spots are occasionally seen. Fibrous or raised plaques may resemble coalescent angiofibromas.

2. Neurologic features: Seizures are the most common presenting symptom. Five percent of cases of infantile spasm (a serious epileptic syndrome) occur in patients with tuberous sclerosis. Thus, any patient presenting with infantile spasms (and the parents as well) should be carefully examined for this disorder. An imaging study of the central nervous system, such as a CT scan, may show calcified subependymal nodules; MRI may show dysmyelinating white matter lesions or cortical tubers. Virtually any kind of symptomatic seizure (eg, atypical absence, partial complex, and generalized tonic-clonic seizures) may occur.

3. Mental retardation: Mental retardation is seen in up to 50% of patients referred to centers; the incidence is probably much lower in randomly selected patients. Patients with seizures are more prone to retardation or learning disabilities.

4. Renal lesions: Renal cysts or angiomyolipomas may be asymptomatic. Hematuria or obstruction of urine flow sometimes occurs; the latter requires operation. Ultrasonography of the kidneys should be done in any patient suspected of tuberous sclerosis, both to aid in diagnosis if lesions are found and to rule out renal obstructive disease.

5. Cardiopulmonary involvement: Rarely, cystic lung disease may occur. Rhabdomyomas of the heart may be asymptomatic but can lead to outflow obstruction, conduction difficulties, and death. Chest x-rays and echocardiograms can detect these rare manifestations.

6. Eye involvement: Retinal hamartomas are often near the disk.

7. Skeletal involvement: Findings sometimes helpful in diagnosis are cystic rarefactions of the bones of the fingers or toes.

B. Diagnostic Studies: Plain radiographs may detect areas of thickening within the skull, spine, and pelvis; and cystic lesions in the hands and feet. Chest x-rays may show lung honeycombing. More helpful is CT scanning, which can show the virtually pathognomonic subependymal nodular calcifications and sometimes widened gyri or tubers and brain tumors. Contrast material may show the often classically located tumors near the foramen interventriculare. Hypomyelinated lesions may be seen with magnetic resonance imaging.

EEG is helpful in delineating the presence of seizure discharges.

Treatment

Therapy is as indicated by underlying disease (eg, seizures and tumors of the brain, kidney, and heart). Skin lesions on the face may need dermabrasion or other removal. Genetic counseling emphasizes identification of the carrier. There is a 50% risk of appearance in offspring if either parent is a carrier. The patient should be seen annually for counseling and reexamination in childhood. Identification of the chromosome and gene marker may in the future make intrauterine diagnosis possible.

Aicardi J: Tuberous sclerosis. Int Pediatr 1993;8:171.
Martin N et al: Gadolinium-DTPA enhanced MR imaging in tuberous sclerosis. Neuroradiology 1990;31:492.
Oppenheimer EY et al: Late appearance of hypopigmented maculae in tuberous sclerosis. Am J Dis Child 1985; 139:408.
Stefanson K: Tuberous sclerosis. Mayo Clin Proc 1991;66: 868.

3. ENCEPHALOFACIAL ANGIOMATOSIS (Sturge-Weber Disease)

Sturge-Weber disease consists of a facial port wine nevus involving the upper part of the face (in the first division of the fifth nerve), a venous angioma of the meninges in the occipitoparietal re-

gions, and choroidal angioma. The syndrome has been described without the facial nevus.

Clinical Findings

In infancy, the eye may show congenital glaucoma, or buphthalmos, with a cloudy, enlarged cornea. In early stages, the facial nevus may be the only indication, with no findings in the brain even on radiologic studies. The characteristic atrophy and calcifications of the cortex and meningoangiomatosis may appear with time, solidifying the diagnosis.

Physical examination may show focal seizures or hemiparesis on the side opposite the cerebral lesion. The facial nevus may be much more extensive than the first division of the fifth nerve; it can involve the lower face, mouth, lip, neck, and even torso. Hemiatrophy of the opposite limbs may occur. Mental handicap may result from poorly controlled seizures. Late-appearing glaucoma and, rarely, CNS hemorrhage occur.

Radiologic studies may show calcification of the cortex; CT scanning may show this much earlier than plain film studies. MRI scans often show underlying brain involvement.

The EEG often shows depression of voltage over the involved area in early stages; later, epileptiform abnormalities may be present focally.

Treatment

Sturge-Weber disease is sporadic. Early control of seizures is important to avoid consequent developmental setback. If seizures do not occur, normal development can be anticipated. Careful examination of the newborn, with ophthalmologic assessment to detect early glaucoma, is indicated. Rarely, surgical removal of the involved meninges and the involved portion of the brain may be indicated, even hemispherectomy.

Strauss RP, Resnick SD: Pulsed dye laser therapy for portwine stains in children: Psychosocial and ethical issues. J Pediatr 1993;122:505.
Tallman B et al: Location of port-wine stains and the likelihood of ophthalmic and/or central nervous system complications. Pediatrics 1991;87:323.
Taly AB et al: Sturge-Weber-Dimitri disease without facial nevus. Neurology 1987;37:1063.

4. VON HIPPEL-LINDAU DISEASE (Retinocerebellar Angiomatosis)

Von Hippel-Lindau disease is a rare, dominantly inherited condition with retinal and cerebellar hemangioblastomas; cysts of the kidneys, pancreas, and epididymis; and sometimes renal cancers. The patient may present with ataxia, slurred speech, and nystagmus due to a hemangioblastoma of the cerebellum or with a medullary spinal cord cystic hemangioblastoma. Retinal detachment may occur from hemorrhage or exudate in the retinal vascular malformation. Rarely, a pancreatic cyst or renal tumor may be the presenting symptom.

The diagnostic criteria for the disease are a retinal or cerebellar hemangioblastoma with or without a positive family history, intra- abdominal cyst, or renal cancer.

Choyke PL et al: von Hippel-Lindau disease: Genetic, clinical, and imaging features. Radiology 1995;194:629.

CENTRAL NERVOUS SYSTEM DEGENERATIVE DISORDERS OF INFANCY & CHILDHOOD

Essentials of Diagnosis

- Arrest of psychomotor development.
- Loss, usually progressive but at variable rates, of mental and motor functioning and often vision.
- Seizures are common in some disorders.
- Symptoms and signs vary with age at onset and primary sites of involvement of specific types.

General Considerations

The CNS degenerative disorders of infancy and childhood are fortunately rare. An early clinical pattern of decline often follows normal early development. Referral for sophisticated biochemical testing is usually necessary before definitive diagnosis can be made. (See Tables 23–21 and 23–22.)

Aubourg P et al: Brain MRI and electrophysiologic abnormalities in preclinical and clinical adrenomyeloneuropathy. Neurology 1992;42:85.

Brown FR et al: Peroxisomal disorders: Neurodevelopmental and biochemical aspects. Am J Dis Child 1993;147: 617.

Dyken PR: The neuronal ceroid lipofuscinoses. J Child Neurol 1989;4:165.

Goebel HH: Neuronal ceroid-lipofuscinoses: The current status. Brain Dev 1992;14:203.

Jaeken J, Carchon H: The carbohydrate-deficient glycoprotein syndromes: Recent developments. Int Pediatr 1993; 8:60.

Jaeken J, Stibler H, Hagberg B: The carbohydrate-deficient glycoprotein syndrome. Acta Paediatr Scand Suppl 1991; 375:1.

Mehler M, Rabinowich L: Inflammatory myeloclastic diffuse sclerosis. Ann Neurol 1988;23:413.

Menkes J: Huntington disease: Finding the gene and after. Pediatr Neurol 1988;4:73.

ATAXIAS OF CHILDHOOD

1. ACUTE CEREBELLAR ATAXIA

Acute cerebellar ataxia occurs most commonly in children 2–6 years of age. The onset is abrupt, and the evolution of symptoms is rapid. In about 50% of cases, there is a prodromal illness with fever, respiratory or gastrointestinal symptoms, or an exanthem within 3 weeks of onset. Associated viral infections include varicella, rubeola, mumps, rubella, echovirus infections, poliomyelitis, infectious mononucleosis, and influenza. Bacterial infections such as scarlet fever and salmonellosis have also been incriminated.

Clinical Findings

A. Symptoms & Signs: Ataxia of the trunk and extremities may be severe, so that the child exhibits a staggering, reeling gait and inability to sit without support or to reach for objects; or there may be only mild unsteadiness. Hypotonia, tremor of the extremities, and horizontal nystagmus may be present. Speech may be slurred. The child is frequently irritable, and vomiting may occur.

There are no clinical signs of increased intracranial pressure. Sensory and reflex testing usually shows no abnormalities.

B. Laboratory Findings: CSF pressure and protein and glucose levels are normal; slight lymphocytosis (up to about 30/μL) may be present. Attempts should be made to identify the etiologic viral agent.

C. Imaging: CT scans are normal; MRI may show cerebellar postinfectious demyelinating lesions. The EEG may be normal or may show nonspecific slowing.

Differential Diagnosis

Acute cerebellar ataxia must be differentiated from acute cerebellar syndromes due to phenytoin, phenobarbital, primidone, or lead intoxication. For phenytoin, the toxic level in serum is usually above 25 μg/mL; for phenobarbital, above 50 μg/mL; for primidone, above 14 μg/mL. (See Seizure Disorders.) With lead intoxication, papilledema, anemia, basophilic stippling of erythrocytes, proteinuria, typical x-rays, and elevated CSF protein are clinical clues, confirmed by serum, urine, or hair lead levels. An occult neuroblastoma, usually seen with the polymyoclonus-opsoclonus syndrome (see below) occasionally begins as acute cerebellar ataxia.

In rare cases, acute cerebellar ataxia may be the presenting sign of acute bacterial meningitis or may be mimicked by corticosteroid withdrawal, vasculitides such as in polyarteritis nodosa, trauma, the first attack of ataxia in a metabolic disorder such as Hartnup's disease, or the onset of acute disseminated encephalomyelitis or of multiple sclerosis. The history and physical findings may differentiate these disturbances, but appropriate laboratory studies are often necessary. For ataxias with more chronic onset and course, see the sections on spinocerebellar degeneration (below) and the other degenerative disorders.

Treatment & Prognosis

Treatment is supportive. The use of corticosteroids has no rational justification.

Table 23–21. Central nervous system degenerative disorders of infancy.

Disease	Enzyme Defect and Genetics	Onset	Early Manifestations	Vision and Hearing	Somatic Findings	Motor System	Seizures	Laboratory and Tissue Studies	Course
WHITE MATTER									
Globoid (Krabbe's) leukodystrophy	Recessive Galactocerebrosidase and lactosylceramidase 1 deficiency.	First 6 months; "late-onset forms."	Feeding difficulties. Shrill cry. Irritability. Arching of back.	Optic atrophy, mid-course to late. Hyperacusis occasionally.	Head often small. Often underweight.	Early spasticity, occasionally preceded by hypotonia. Prolonged nerve conduction.	Early. Myoclonic and generalized, decerebrate posturing.	CSF protein elevated; usually normal in late-onset forms. Sural nerve; nonspecific myelin breakdown. Enzyme deficiency in leukocytes, cultured skin fibroblasts. Demyelination, gliosis; low-signal CT scan, high-signal T$_2$-weighted MRI.	Rapid. Death usually by 1½–2 years. Late-onset cases may live 5–10 years.
Metachromatic leukodystrophy	Recessive. Arylsulfatase A deficiency.	Second year. Less often, later in childhood, or adult.	Incoordination, especially gait disturbance; then general regression. Reverse in juveniles.	Optic atrophy, usually late. Hearing normal.	Head enlarged late. None in juvenile form.	Combined upper and lower motor neuron signs. Ataxia. Prolonged nerve conduction.	Infrequent, usually late and generalized	Metachromatic cells in urine: negative sulfatase A test. CSF protein elevated: occasionally normal early. Sural nerve biopsy: metachromasia. Enzyme deficiency in leukocytes, cultured skin fibroblasts. Imaging: Same as globoid leukodystrophy.	Moderately slow. Death in infantile form by 3–8 years, in "juvenile" form by 10–15 years.
Neuroaxonal degeneration (Seitelberger's disease). Same as, or resembling, Hallervorden-Spatz disease	Familial, (?) recessive. More common in girls than boys; defect unknown.	1–3 years	Arrest of development and dementia. Loss of motor functions. Occasionally hypesthesia over trunk and legs.	Nystagmus frequent; optic atrophy, hearing impairment.		Combined upper and lower motor neuron lesions. Early, may lie in "frog" position.	Variable, but usually not a prominent feature	Denervation on EMG; elevated serum LDH and transaminase. Increased iron uptake in region of basal ganglia by scintillation counter probes over the temples. Brain and sural nerve: axonal swellings or "spheroids." Iron deposition in globus pallidus.	Very slowly progressive, with death early in second decade or earlier.
Pelizaeus-Merzbacher disease	X-linked recessive; rare female.	(?) Birth to 2 years.	"Eye rolling" often shortly after birth. Head bobbing. Slow loss of intellect.	Slowly developing optic atrophy. Hearing normal.	Head and body normal.	Cerebellar signs early, hyperactive deep reflexes. Spasticity usually only very late.	Usually only late	None specific. Brain biopsy: extensive demyelination with small perivascular islands of intact myelin.	Exceedingly slow, often seemingly stationary. Many survive well into adult life.
DIFFUSE, BUT PRIMARILY GRAY MATTER									
Poliodystrophy (Alpers' disease)	Occasionally familial, recessive. Possibly viral. Metabolic forms.	Infancy to adolescence.	Variable: loss of intellect, seizures, incoordination. Vomiting, hepatic failure.	"Cortical blindness and deafness.	Head normal initially; may fail to grow.	Variable: incoordination, spasticity.	Often initial manifestation: myoclonic, akinetic, and generalized	Nonspecific. CSF protein normal or slightly elevated. Extensive neuronal loss in cortex: may occur very late. Variably increased serum pyruvate, lactate; liver steatosis, cirrhosis late. Increased serum pyruvate, lactate.	Usually rapid, with death within 1–3 years after onset.
Tay-Sachs disease and G$_{M2}$ gangliosidosis variants: Sandhoff disease; juvenile; chronic-adult.	Recessive. Hexosaminidase deficiencies. Tay-Sachs 93% East European Jewish, hexosaminidase A deficiency. Others panethnic. Sandhoff hexosaminidase A and B deficiency.	Tay-Sachs, Sandhoff similar: 3–6 months. Others 2–6 years or later. Juvenile: partial hexosaminidase A.	Variable: shrill cry, loss of vision, infantile spasms, arrest of development. In juvenile and chronic forms: motor difficulties; later, mental difficulties.	Cherry-red macula, early blindness. Hyperacusis early. Strabismus in juvenile form, blindness late.	Head enlarged late. Liver occasionally enlarged. None in juvenile or chronic forms.	Initially floppy. Eventual decerebrate rigidity. In juvenile and chronic forms: dysarthria, ataxia, spasticity.	Frequent, in mid-course and late. Infantile spasms and generalized	Blood smears: vacuolated lymphocytes; basophilic hypergranulation. Enzyme deficiencies in serum, leukocytes, culture skin fibroblasts. High-density thalami on CT scan, low-density white matter.	Moderately rapid. Death usually by 2–5 years. In juvenile form, 5–15 years.

Disease	Genetics	Age of Onset	Early Symptoms	Eyes	Head/Organs	Motor Signs	Seizures	Laboratory Findings	Course
Niemann-Pick disease and variants	50% Jewish. Recessive. Sphingomyelinase deficiency in types A and C involving the CNS.	First 6 months. In variants, later onset; often non-Jewish.	Slow development. Protruding belly.	Cherry-red macula in 35–50%. Blindness late. Deafness occasionally.	Head usually normal. Spleen enlarged more than liver. Occasional xanthomas of skin.	Initially floppy. Eventually spastic. Occasionally extrapyramidal signs.	Rare and late	Blood: vacuolated lymphocytes; increased lipids. X-rays: "mottled" lungs, decalcified bones. "Foam cells" in bone marrow, spleen, lymph nodes	Moderately slow. Death usually by 3–5 years.
Infantile Gaucher's disease (glucosyl ceramide lipidosis)	Recessive. Glucocerebrosidase deficiency.	First 6 months; rarely, late infancy.	Stridor or hoarse cry; retraction; feeding difficulties.	Occasional cherry-red macula. Convergent squint. Deafness occasionally.	Head usually normal. Liver and spleen equally enlarged.	Opisthotonos early, followed rapidly by decerebrate rigidity.	Rare and late	Anemia. Increased acid phosphatase. X-rays: thinned cortex, trabeculation of bones. "Gaucher cells" in bone marrow, spleen. Enzyme deficiency in leukocytes or cultured skin fibroblasts	Very rapid.
Lipogranulomatosis (Farber's disease)	Ceramidase deficiency	Early in infancy.	Hoarseness, irritability, restricted joint movements.	Usually normal.	Painful nodular swelling of joints; subcutaneous nodules.	Psychomotor retardation and progressive paralysis.	Usually none	Chest x-rays may show pulmonary infiltrates. Nodules: granulomatous lesions, resembling those in reticuloendotheliosis. Multiple infarcts on CNS imaging	Rapid: death usually in 1–2 years.
Generalized gangliosidosis and juvenile type (G_{M1} gangliosidoses)	Recessive; β-galactosidase deficiency.	First year; less often, second year.	Arrest of development. Protruding belly. Coarse facies in infantile (generalized) form.	50% "cherry-red spot." Hearing usually normal. In juvenile type, occasionally retinitis pigmentosa.	Head enlarged early; liver enlarged more than spleen	Initially floppy, eventually spastic.	Usually late	Blood: vacuolated lymphocytes. X-rays: dorsolumbar kyphosis, "beaking" of vertebrae. "Foam cells" similar to those in Niemann-Pick disease	Very rapid. Death within a few years. Slower in juvenile type (to 10 years).
Subacute necrotizing encephalomyelopathy (Leigh's disease)	Recessive or variable. May have deficiency of pyruvate carboxylase, pyruvate dehydrogenase, cytochrome enzymes.	Infancy to late childhood.	Difficulties in feeding; feeble or absent cry; floppiness.	Optic atrophy, often early. Roving eye movements. Ophthalmoplegia.	Head usually normal, occasionally small; cardiac and renal tubular dysfunction occasionally	Flaccid and immobile; may become spastic. Spinocerebellar forms; ataxia.	Rare and late	Increased CSF and blood lactate and pyruvate. High-signal MRI T_2 foci in thalami; globus pallidus, subthalamic nuclei	Usually rapid in infants, but may be slow with death after several years. Central hypoventilation a frequent cause of death.
"Steel wool," or kinky hair," disease (Menkes')	X-linked recessive; defect in copper absorption	Infancy.	Peculiar facies; secondary hair white, twisted, split; hypothermia.	May show optic disk pallor and microcysts of pigment epithelium.	Normal to small.	Variable: floppy to spastic.	Myoclonic infantile spasms; status epilepticus	Defective absorption of copper. Cerebral angiography shows elongated arteries. Hair shows pili torti, split shafts. CT scan may show diffuse multifocal areas of low density.	Moderately rapid. Death usually by 3–4 years.
Carbohydrate-deficient glycoprotein syndrome	Recessive glycoprotein abnormality	Infancy	Failure to thrive, retardation.	Strabismus.		Variable.	Rare	Transferrin decreased. Liver steatosis. Cerebellar hypoplasia.	Cardiomyopathy, thrombosis
Bassen-Kornzweig disease	Recessive; primary defect unknown.	Early childhood.	Diarrhea in infancy.	Retinitis pigmentosa; late ophthalmoplegia.	None.	Ataxia, late extrapyramidal movement disorder.	None	Abetalipoproteinemia: acanthocytosis, low serum vitamin E; cerebellar atrophy on imaging.	Progression arrested with vitamin E.

Table 23–22. Central nervous system degenerative disorders of childhood.[1]

Disease	Enzyme Defect and Genetics	Onset	Early Manifestations	Vision and Hearing	Motor System	Seizures	Laboratory and Tissue Studies	Course
Adrenoleukodystrophy and variants	X-linked recessive. Neonatal form recessive. Acyl CoA synthetase deficiency	5–10 years. Newborn.	Impaired intellect, behavioral problems.	"Cortical blindness and deafness."	Ataxia, spasticity. Motor deficits may be asymmetric, or one-sided initially.	Occasionally	Hyperpigmentation and adrenocortical insufficiency. ACTH elevated. Accumulation of very long chain fatty acids: Plasma test available.	Fairly rapid, death usually within 2–3 years after onset.
Neuronal ceroid lipofuscinosis (cerebromacular degeneration): Late infantile cerebral sphingolipidosis (Bielschowsky-Jansky disease)	Recessive; defect unknown	2–4 years	Ataxia. Visual difficulties. Arrested intellectual development.	Pigmentary degeneration of macula. Optic atrophy. Hearing may be impaired.	Ataxia, spasticity progressing to decerebrate rigidity.	Often early; myoclonic and later generalized; difficult to control	Blood: vacuolated lymphocytes, azurophilic dispersed hypergranulation of polymorphonuclear cells. Electroretinography helpful. Bone marrow: sea-blue histiocytes. In skin, skeletal muscle, peripheral nerves, brain: "curvilinear bodies" and "fingerprint profiles" autofluorescent lipopigments.	Moderately slow. Death in 3–8 years.
Subacute sclerosing panencephalitis (Dawson's disease, SSPE)	None. Measles "slow virus" infection; also reported as result of rubella	3–22 years; rarely earlier or later	Impaired intellect, emotional lability, incoordination.	Occasionally chorioretinitis or optic atrophy. Hearing normal.	Ataxia, slurred speech, occasionally involuntary movements, spasticity progressing to decerebrate rigidity.	Myoclonic and akinetic seizures relatively early; later, focal and generalized	CSF protein normal to moderately elevated. High CSF gamma globulin,[2] oligoclonal bands. Elevated CSF and serum measles (or rubella) antibody titers. Characteristic EEG. Brain biopsy: inclusion body encephalitis; culturing of measles virus, possibly rubella virus.	Variable, death in months to years. Remissions of variable duration may occur.
Multiple sclerosis (See also Chapter 29.)	None; diagnosis difficult in childhood; defect unknown	Adolescent; rare in childhood	Highly variable: may strike one or more sites of CNS. Paresthesias common.	Optic neuritis; diplopia, nystagmus at some time. Vestibulocochlear nerves occasionally affected.	Motor weakness, spasticity, ataxia, sphincter disturbances, slurred speech, mental difficulties.	Rare: focal or generalized	CSF may show slight pleocytosis, elevation of protein and gamma globulin,[2] oligoclonal bands present. CT scan may show areas of demyelination. Auditory, visual, and somatosensory evoked responses often show lesions in respective pathways. Changes in T cell subsets.	Variable: complete remission possible. Recurrent attacks and involvement of multiple sites are prerequisites for diagnosis.
Cerebrotendinous xanthomatosis	?Recessive; abnormal accumulation of cholesterol	Late childhood to adolescence	Xanthomas in tendons. Mental deterioration.	Cataracts; xanthelasma.	Cerebellar deficits. Late: bulbar paralysis.	Myoclonus	Xanthomas may appear in lungs. Xanthomas in tendons (especially Achilles).	Very slowly progressive into middle life. Replace deficient bile acid.
Huntington's disease	Dominant; genetic marker on chromosome 4.	10% childhood onset.	Rigidity, dementia.	Ophthalmoplegia late.	Rigidity; chorea frequently absent in children.	50% with major motor seizures	CT Scan may show "butterfly" atrophy of caudate and putamen.	Moderately rapid with death in 5–15 years.
Refsum's disease	Recessive. Phytanic acid oxidase deficiency	5–10 years	Ataxia, ichthyosis, cardiomyopathy.	Retinitis pigmentosa.	Ataxia.	None	Serum phytanic acid elevated; slow nerve conduction velocity; elevated CSF protein. Peroxisomal disease.	Treat with low phytanic acid diet.

[1]For late infantile metachromatic leukodystrophy, Pelizaeus-Merzbacher disease, poliodystrophy, Gaucher's disease of later onset, and subacute necrotizing encephalomyelopathy, see Table 23–21.
[2]CSF gamma globulin (IgG) is considered elevated in children when > 9% of total protein (possibly even > 8.3%); definitively elevated when > 14%.

Between 80% and 90% of children with acute cerebellar ataxia not secondary to drug toxicity recover without sequelae within 6–8 weeks. In the remainder, neurologic disturbances, including disorders of behavior and of learning, ataxia, abnormal eye movements, and speech impairment, may persist for months or years, and recovery may remain incomplete.

Cohen HA et al: Mumps-associated acute cerebellar ataxia. Am J Dis Child 1992;146:930.

Dunn DW, Patel H: Ataxia: From the benign to the ominous. Contemp Pediatr 1991;88:82.

Swaimen K: Ataxia in childhood. Int Pediatr 1990;5:153.

2. POLYMYOCLONIA-OPSOCLONUS SYNDROME OF CHILDHOOD (Infantile Myoclonic Encephalopathy, "Dancing Eyes– Dancing Feet" Syndrome)

The symptoms and signs of this syndrome are at first similar to those of acute cerebellar ataxia. Often of sudden onset, polymyoclonia- opsoclonus syndrome is characterized by severe incoordination of the trunk and extremities with lightning-like jerking or flinging movements of a group of muscles, causing the child to be in constant motion while awake. Extraocular muscle involvement results in sudden irregular eye movements (opsoclonus). Irritability and vomiting are often present, but there is no depression of level of consciousness. This syndrome occurs in association with viral infections, tumors of neural crest origin, and many other disorders. Immunologic mechanisms have been postulated. There are usually no signs of increased intracranial pressure. Cerebrospinal fluid may show normal or mildly increased protein levels. Special techniques show increased CSF levels of plasmacytes and abnormal immunoglobulins. The EEG may be slightly slow, but when performed together with electromyography, it shows no evidence of association between cortical discharges and the muscle movements. An assiduous search must be made to rule out tumor of neural crest origin by x-rays of the chest and CT scan or ultrasound (or both) of the adrenal area as well as by assays of urinary catecholamine metabolites (vanillylmandelic acid, etc) and cystathionine.

The symptoms respond (often dramatically) to large doses of corticotropin. Otherwise, treatment is as for specific entities. When a neural crest (or other) tumor is found, surgical excision should be followed by irradiation and chemotherapy. Life span is determined by the biologic behavior of the tumor.

The syndrome is usually self-limited but may be characterized by exacerbations and remissions. However, even after removal of a neural crest tumor and without other evidence of its recurrence, symptoms may reappear. Mild mental retardation may be a sequela.

Boltshauser E, Deonna TH, Hirt HR: Myoclonic encephalopathy of infants or "dancing eyes syndrome": Report of seven cases with long-term follow-up and review of the literature (cases with and without neuroblastoma). Helv Paediatr Acta 1979;34:119.

Mitchell WG, Snodgrass SR: Opsoclonus-ataxia due to childhood neural crest tumors: A chronic neurologic syndrome. J Child Neurol 1990;5:153.

Pranzatelli MR: The neurobiology of the opsoclonus-myoclonus syndrome. Clin Neuropharmacol 1992;15:186.

3. SPINOCEREBELLAR DEGENERATION DISORDERS

Spinocerebellar degeneration disorders may be hereditary or may occur in sporadic distribution. Hereditary disorders include Friedreich's ataxia, dominant hereditary ataxia, and a group of miscellaneous diseases.

Friedreich's Ataxia

This is a recessive disorder characterized by onset of gait ataxia or scoliosis before puberty, becoming progressively worse. Reflexes, light touch, and position sensation are reduced. Dysarthria becomes progressively more severe. Cardiomyopathy usually develops, and diabetes mellitus is found in 40% of patients, with half of these requiring insulin. Pes cavus typically is found.

Treatment includes surgery for scoliosis and intervention as needed for cardiac disease and diabetes. Patients are usually confined to a wheelchair after age 20 years. Death occurs, usually from heart failure or dysrhythmias, in the third or fourth decade; some patients survive longer.

Dominant Ataxia

This disease (also known as olivopontocerebellar atrophy, Holmes's ataxia, Marie's ataxia, etc) occurs with varying manifestations, even among members of the same family. Ataxia occurs at onset, and progression continues with ophthalmoplegias, extrapyramidal tract and motor neuron degeneration, and later dementia. One type has been found to be caused by a CAG trinucleotide repeat. Levodopa may ameliorate rigidity and bradykinesia, but no other therapy is available. Only 10% of cases have onset in childhood, and their course is often more rapid.

Miscellaneous Hereditary Ataxias

Associated findings permit identification of these recessive disorders. These include ataxia-telangiectasia (telangiectasia, immune defects; see below), Wilson's disease (Kayser-Fleischer rings), Refsum's disease (ichthyosis, cardiomyopathy, retinitis pigmentosa, large nerves), Rett's syndrome (regression to autism at 7–18 months in girls, loss of use of hands, progressive failure of brain growth), and abetalipoproteinemia (infantile diarrhea, acanthocytosis, retinitis pigmentosa). Patients with juvenile and chronic gangliosidoses and some hemolytic anemias and long-term survivors of Chédiak-Higashi disease may develop spinocerebellar degeneration. Idiopathic familial ataxia is called Behr's syndrome. Neuropathies such as Charcot-Marie-Tooth disease produce ataxia.

Dubourg O et al: Analysis of the SCA1 CAG Repeat in a large number of families with dominant ataxia: Clinical and molecular correlations. Ann Neurol 1995;37:176.
Haas R, Rapin I, Moser H: Rett syndrome and autism. J Child Neurol 1988;3(Suppl):52.
Kameya T et al: Analysis of spinocerebellar ataxia type 1 (SCA1)-related in CAG trinucleotide expansion in Japan. Neurology 1995;45:1587.
Sheu KFR et al: Mitochondrial enzymes in hereditary ataxias. Metab Brain Dis 1988;3:151.
Stumpf DA: The inherited ataxias. Neurol Clin 1985;3:47.

ATAXIA-TELANGIECTASIA (Louis-Bar Syndrome)

Ataxia-telangiectasia is a multisystem disorder inherited as an autosomal recessive trait. It is characterized by progressive ataxia; telangiectasia of the bulbar conjunctiva, external ears, nares, and (later) other body surfaces, appearing in the third to sixth year; and recurrent respiratory, sinus, and ear infections. Ocular dyspraxia, slurred speech, choreoathetosis, hypotonia and areflexia, and psychomotor and growth retardation may be present. Endocrinopathies are common. Nerve conduction velocities may be reduced. The entire nervous system may be affected in late stages of the disease. A spectrum of involvement may be seen in the same family. Immunodeficiencies of IgA and IgE are common (see Chapter 28), and the incidence of certain cancers is high.

Ataxia-telangiectasia: A multisystem hereditary disease with immunodeficiency, impaired organ maturation, x-ray hypersensitivity, and a high incidence of neoplasia. (NIH Conference.) Ann Intern Med 1983;99:367.
Swift M et al: Incidence of cancer in 161 families affected by ataxia-telangiectasia. N Engl J Med 1991;325:1831.

EXTRAPYRAMIDAL DISORDERS

Extrapyramidal disorders are characterized by the presence in the waking state of one or more of the following features: dyskinesias, athetosis, ballismus, tremors, rigidity, and dystonias.

For the most part, precise pathologic and anatomic localization is not understood. Motor pathways synapsing in the striatum (putamen and caudate nu-

cleus), globus pallidus, red nucleus, substantia nigra, and the body of Luys are involved; this "system" is modulated by pathways originating in the thalamus, cerebellum, and reticular formation.

1. SYDENHAM'S POSTRHEUMATIC CHOREA

Sydenham's chorea is characterized by an acute onset of choreiform movements and variable degrees of psychologic disturbance. It is frequently associated with rheumatic endocarditis and arthritis. Although the disorder follows infections with group A β-hemolytic streptococci, the interval between infection and chorea may be greatly prolonged; throat cultures and antistreptolysin O (ASO) titers may therefore be negative. Chorea has also been associated with hypocalcemia; with vascular lupus erythematosus; and with toxic, viral, infectious and parainfectious, and degenerative encephalopathies.

Clinical Findings

A. Symptoms & Signs: Chorea, or rapid involuntary movements of the limbs and face, is the hallmark physical finding. In addition to the jerky incoordinate movements, the following are noted: emotional lability, waxing and waning ("milkmaid's") grip, darting tongue, "spooning" of the extended hands and their tendency to pronate, and knee jerks slow to return from the extended to their prestimulus position ("hung up"). Seizures, while uncommon, may be masked by choreic jerks.

B. Laboratory Findings: Anemia, leukocytosis, and an increased erythrocyte sedimentation rate (ESR) may be present. The ASO titer may be elevated and C-reactive protein (CRP) present. Throat culture is sometimes positive for group A β-hemolytic streptococci.

Electrocardiography and echocardiography are often essential to detect cardiac involvement. Antineuronal antibodies are present in most patients but are not specific. Electroencephalography may show nonspecific slowing or seizure activity.

Differential Diagnosis

The diagnosis of Sydenham's chorea is usually not difficult. Tics, drug-induced extrapyramidal syndromes, Huntington's chorea, and hepatolenticular degeneration (Wilson's disease), as well as other rare movement disorders, can usually be ruled out on historical and clinical grounds.

Other causes of chorea can be ruled out by laboratory tests, such as ANA (antinuclear antibody) for lupus, TSH, T_4 for thyroid disease, serum calcium for hypocalcemia, Monospot for mononucleosis.

Treatment

There is no specific treatment. Dopaminergic

blockers such as haloperidol, 0.5 mg to 3–6 mg/d, or pimozide, 4–12 mg /d, have been used. Parkinsonian side effects such as rigidity and masked facies and, with high doses, tardive dyskinesia rarely occur in childhood. A variety of other drugs have been used with success in individual cases, such as the anticonvulsant sodium valproate, 50–60 mg/kg/d in divided doses; or prednisone, 0.5–2 mg/kg in divided doses. Emotional lability and depression sometimes warrant antidepressants such as amitriptyline, 25 or 50 mg/d.

All patients should be given antistreptococcal rheumatic fever prophylaxis.

Prognosis

Sydenham's chorea is a self-limiting disease that may last from a few weeks to months. Two thirds of patients relapse one or more times, but the ultimate outcome does not appear to be worse in those with recurrences. Valvular heart disease occurs in about one third of patients, particularly if other rheumatic manifestations appear. Psychoneurotic disturbances, if not already present at the onset of illness, occur in a significant percentage of patients.

Dhanaraj M et al: Sodium valproate in Sydenham's chorea. Neurology 1985;35:114.

Kiessling LS, Marcotte AC, Culpepper L: Antineuronal antibodies in movement disorders. Pediatrics 1993;92:39.

Peters ACB et al: ECHO 25 focal encephalitis and subacute hemichorea. Neurology 1979;29:676.

Pranzatelli MR: An approach to movement disorders in childhood. Pediatr Ann 1993;22:13.

Swedo SE: Sydenham's chorea. JAMA 1994;272:1788.

Swedo SE et al: Sydenham's chorea: Physical and psychological symptoms of St. Vitus' dance. Pediatrics 1993; 91:706.

2. TICS
(Habit Spasms)

Tics, or habit spasms, are quick repetitive but irregular movements, often stereotyped, and briefly suppressible. Coordination and muscle tone are not affected. A psychogenic basis is seldom discernible.

Transient tics of childhood (12–24% incidence in school-age children) last from 1 month to 1 year and seldom need treatment. Many children with tics have a history of encephalopathic past events, "soft signs" on neurologic examination, and school problems.

Facial tics such as grimaces, twitches, and blinking predominate, but the trunk and extremities are often involved and there are twisting or flinging movements. Vocal tics are less common.

Gilles de la Tourette's syndrome is a chronic disorder of multiple fluctuating motor and vocal tics, with onset in childhood, lasting more than a year, with absence of other recognizable causes for tics. Tics evolve slowly, new ones being added to or replacing old ones. Coprolalia and echolalia are rela-

tively infrequent. Partial forms are common. The usual age at onset is 2–15 years, and the familial incidence is 35–50%; the disorder is now reported in almost all ethnic groups. Gilles de la Tourette's syndrome may be triggered by stimulants such as methylphenidate and dextroamphetamine. An imbalance of neurotransmitters, especially dopamine and serotonin, has been hypothesized.

In relatively mild cases, tics are self-limited and, when disregarded, disappear. When attention is paid to one tic, it may disappear only to be replaced by another that is often worse. If the tic and its underlying anxiety or compulsive neurosis are severe, psychiatric evaluation and treatment are needed.

Important comorbidities are attention deficit hyperactivity disorder (ADHD) and obsessive-compulsive disorder (OCD). Medications such as methylphenidate and dextroamphetamine should be carefully titrated to treat ADHD and avoid worsening tics. Fluoxetine and clomipramine may be useful for OCD in patients with tics.

When medication is required to treat Tourette's syndrome, the most effective agents are dopamine blockers. However, many pediatric patients can manage without drug treatment. Generally, medications are reserved for patients with disabling symptoms; treatment may be relaxed or discontinued when the symptoms abate.

Nonpharmacologic treatment of Tourette's syndrome includes education of patients, family members, and school personnel. In some cases, restructuring the school environment to prevent tension and teasing may be necessary; supportive counseling, either at or outside school, should be provided.

Usually, medications will not eradicate the tics. Accordingly, the goal of treatment should be to reduce the tics to tolerable levels without inducing undesirable side effects. Dosage should be increased at weekly intervals until a satisfactory response is obtained. Often, a single dose at bedtime is sufficient. The two neuroleptic agents used most often are haloperidol and fluphenazine; side effects to be avoided include akathisia and tardive dyskinesia. The newest neuroleptic agent in use is pimozide; motor side effects of this drug are the same as those encountered with the use of other dopamine blockers.

Clonidine, clonazepam, and calcium channel blockers have been used in individual patients with some success; sometimes these agents are used for combined therapy (eg, haloperidol with nifedipine).

Barbas G (editor): [Many articles on Tourette's syndrome.] Psychiatr Ann (July) 1988;18:393.

Calderone-Gonzales R, Calderone-Sepulveda R: Tourette syndrome: Current concepts. Int Pediatr 1993;8:176.

Como PG, Kurlan R: An open-label trial of fluoxetine for obsessive-compulsive disorder in Gilles de la Tourette's syndrome. Neurology 1991;41:872.

Harlan R et al: Transient tic disorder and the spectrum of Tourette syndrome. Arch Neurol 1988;45:1200.

Singer H: Neurobiological issues in Tourette syndrome. Brain Develop 1994;16:353.

Singer H: Tic disorders. Pediatr Ann 1993;33:33.

Stokes A et al: Peer problems in Tourette's disorder. Pediatrics 1991;87:936.

INFECTIONS & INFLAMMATORY DISORDERS OF THE CENTRAL NERVOUS SYSTEM

Infections of the central nervous system are among the most common neurologic disorders encountered by pediatricians. Although infections are among the CNS disorders most amenable to treatment, they also have a very high potential for causing catastrophic destruction of the nervous system. It is imperative for the clinician to recognize such infections early, in order to treat as early as possible to prevent massive tissue destruction.

Clinical Manifestations

Patients with central nervous system infections, whether caused by bacteria, viruses, or other microorganisms, present with similar manifestations. Systemic signs of infection include fever, generalized malaise, or impaired heart, lung, liver, or kidney function. General features suggesting CNS infection include headache, stiff neck, fever or hypothermia, changes in mental status (including hyperirritability evolving into lethargy and coma), seizures, and focal sensory and motor deficits. On examination, meningeal irritation is manifested by the presence of Kernig's and Brudzinski's signs. In very young infants, signs of meningeal irritation may be absent, and temperature instability and hypothermia are often more prominent than fever. In young infants, a bulging fontanelle and an increased head circumference are common. Papilledema may eventually develop, particularly in older children and adolescents. Cranial nerve palsies may develop acutely or gradually during the course of neurologic infections. No specific clinical sign or symptom is reliable in distinguishing bacterial infections from infections caused by other microbes.

During the initial clinical assessment, conditions that predispose the patient to infection of the central nervous system should be sought. Infections involving the sinuses or other structures in the head and neck region can result in direct extension of infection into the intracranial compartment. Open head injuries, recent neurosurgical procedures, immunodeficiencies, and the presence of a mechanical shunt may predispose to intracranial infection.

Laboratory Investigation

When CNS infections are suspected, blood should be obtained for a complete blood count (CBC), general chemistry panel, and culture. Most important, however, is obtaining cerebrospinal fluid. In the absence of focal neurologic deficits or signs of increased intracranial pressure, CSF should be obtained immediately from any patient in whom serious CNS infection is suspected. When papilledema or focal motor signs are present, a lumbar puncture may be delayed until a neuroimaging procedure has been done to exclude brain abscess or other space-occupying lesion. It is generally safe to obtain spinal fluid from infants with nonfocal neurologic examination even if the fontanelle is bulging. Spinal fluid should be examined for the presence of red and white blood cells, protein concentration, glucose concentration, bacteria and other microorganisms; a sample should be cultured. In addition, serologic, immunologic, and nucleic acid detection (PCR) tests may be performed on the spinal fluid in an attempt to identify the specific organism. As a general rule, spinal fluid that contains a high proportion of polymorphonuclear leukocytes, a high protein concentration, and a low glucose concentration strongly suggests bacterial infection. CSF containing predominantly lymphocytes, a high protein concentration, and a low glucose concentration suggests infection with mycobacteria, fungi, uncommon bacteria, and some viruses such as lymphocytic choriomeningitis virus, herpes simplex virus, mumps virus, and arboviruses. Cerebrospinal fluid that contains a high proportion of lymphocytes, normal or only slightly elevated protein concentration, and a normal glucose concentration is most suggestive of viral infections, although partially treated bacterial meningitis and parameningeal infections may also result in this type of CSF formula. Typical spinal fluid findings in a variety of infectious and inflammatory disorders are shown in Table 23–3.

Neuroimaging with CT and MRI scans may be helpful in demonstrating the presence of brain abscess, meningeal inflammation, or secondary problems such as venous and arterial infarctions, hemorrhages, and subdural effusions when these are expected. In addition, these procedures may identify sinus or other focal infections in the head or neck region that are related to the central nervous system infection. CT scanning may demonstrate bony abnormalities, such as basilar fractures.

EEGs may be helpful in the assessment of patients who have had seizures at the time of presentation. The changes are often nonspecific and characterized by generalized slowing. In some instances, such as herpes simplex virus infection, focal electronegative activity may be seen early in the course and may be one of the earliest laboratory abnormalities to suggest the diagnosis. EEGs may also show focal slowing over regions of abscesses. Unusual but characteristic electroencephalographic patterns are seen in some patients with subacute sclerosing panencephalitis.

In some cases, brain biopsy may be needed to identify the presence of specific organisms and clarify the diagnosis. Herpes simplex virus infections can be confirmed using the PCR to assay for herpes DNA in spinal fluid. This test has a 95% sensitivity and 99% specificity.

Brain biopsy may be needed to detect the rare PCR-negative case of herpes simplex and various parasitic infections, brain tumors, and other structural abnormalities.

BACTERIAL MENINGITIS

Bacterial infections of the central nervous system may present acutely (symptoms evolving rapidly over 1–24 hours), subacutely (symptoms evolving over 1–7 days), or chronically (symptoms evolving over more than 1 week). Diffuse bacterial infections involve the leptomeninges, superficial cortical structures, and blood vessels. Although the term "meningitis" is used to describe these infections, it should not be forgotten that the brain parenchyma is also inflamed and that blood vessel walls may be infiltrated by inflammatory cells that result in endothelial cell injury, vessel stenosis, and secondary ischemia and infarction.

Pathologically, the inflammatory process involves all intracranial structures to some degree. Acutely, this inflammatory process may result in cerebral edema or impaired cerebrospinal fluid flow through and out of the ventricular system resulting in hydrocephalus.

Treatment

A. Specific Measures: (See also Chapter 37, *Haemophilus influenzae* type B infections, and Chapter 34.)

While awaiting results of diagnostic tests, the physician should start broad-spectrum antibiotic coverage as noted below. After specific organisms are identified, antibiotic therapy can be tailored based on antibiotic sensitivity patterns. Children under 3 months of age are treated initially with cefotaxime (or ceftriaxone if over 1 month of age) and ampicillin; the latter agent is used to treat *Listeria* and enterococci, agents that rarely affect older children. Children older than 3 months are treated with ceftriaxone, cefotaxime, or ampicillin plus chloramphenicol. If *S pneumoniae* cannot be ruled out by the initial Gram's stain, vancomycin or rifampin are added until cultures are reported, since penicillin-resistant pneumococci are common in the United States. Therapy may be narrowed when organism sensitivity allows. Duration of therapy is 7 days for meningococcal infections, 10 days for *H influenzae* or pneumococcal infection, and 14–21 days for other organisms. Slow clinical response or the occurrence of complications may prolong the need for therapy. Although therapy for 7 days has proved successful in many children with *Haemophilus* infection, it cannot be recommended if steroids are also used (see below) without further study.

B. General & Supportive Measures: Children with bacterial meningitis are often systemically ill. The following complications should be looked for and treated aggressively: hypovolemia, hypoglycemia, hyponatremia, acidosis, septic shock, increased intracranial pressure, seizures, disseminated intravascular coagulation, and metastatic infection (eg, pericarditis, arthritis, and pneumonia). Children should initially be monitored closely (cardiorespiratory monitor, strict fluid balance and frequent urine specific gravity assessment, daily weights, neurologic assessment every few hours), not fed until neurologically very stable, isolated until the organism is known, rehydrated with isotonic solutions until euvolemic, and then given intravenous fluids containing dextrose and sodium at no more than maintenance rate (assuming no unusual losses occur).

Complications

Abnormalities of water and electrolyte balance result from either excessive or insufficient production of antidiuretic hormone and require careful monitoring and appropriate adjustments in fluid administration. Monitoring serum sodium every 8–12 hours during the first 1 or 2 days, and urine sodium if the inappropriate secretion of antidiuretic hormone is suspected, usually uncovers significant problems.

Seizures occur in up to 30% of children with bacterial meningitis. Seizures tend to be most common in neonates and less common in older children. Persistent focal seizures or focal seizures associated with focal neurologic deficits strongly suggest subdural effusion, abscess, or vascular lesions such as arterial infarct, cortical venous infarcts, or dural sinus thrombosis. Because generalized seizures in a metabolically compromised child may have severe sequelae, early recognition and therapy are critical; some practitioners prefer phenytoin for acute management because it is less sedating than phenobarbital.

Subdural effusions occur in as many as 50% of young children with *H influenzae* meningitis. Subdural effusions are often seen on CT scans of the head during the course of meningitis. They do not require treatment unless they are producing increased intracranial pressure or progressive mass effect. Although subdural effusions may be detected in children with persistent fever, such effusions do not usually have to be sampled or drained if the infecting organism is *Haemophilus*, meningococcus, or pneumococcus. These are usually sterilized with the standard treatment duration, and slowly waning fever during an otherwise uncomplicated recovery may be followed clinically. Under any other circumstance, however, aspiration of the fluid for documentation of sterilization or relief of pressure should be considered.

Cerebral edema can participate in the production of increased intracranial pressure, requiring treatment with dexamethasone, osmotic agents, diuretics, or hyperventilation; continuous pressure monitoring may be needed.

Long-term sequelae of meningitis result from direct inflammatory destruction of brain cells, vascular injuries, or secondary gliosis. Focal motor and sensory deficits, visual impairment, hearing loss, seizures, hydrocephalus, and a variety of cranial nerve deficits can result from meningitis. Sensorineural hearing loss in *H influenzae* meningitis occurs in approximately 5–10% of cases during long-term follow-up. Recent studies have suggested that early addition of dexamethasone to the antibiotic regimen may modestly decrease the risk of hearing loss in some children with *H influenzae* meningitis (Chapter 37).

In addition to the variety of disorders mentioned above, some patients with meningitis suffer from mental retardation and severe behavioral disorders that limit their function at school and later performance in life. Table 23–23 lists the overall mortality and morbidity figures for the most common organisms associated with acute bacterial meningitis in childhood.

BRAIN ABSCESS

Patients with brain abscess often appear to have systemic illness similar to patients with bacterial meningitis, but in addition they show signs of focal neurologic deficits, papilledema, and other evidence of increased intracranial pressure or a mass lesion. Symptoms may be present for a week or more; children with bacterial meningitis usually present within a few days. Conditions predisposing to development of brain abscess include penetrating head trauma;

chronic infection of the middle ear, mastoid, or sinuses (especially the frontal sinus); chronic dental or pulmonary infection; cardiovascular lesions allowing right-to-left shunting of blood (including arteriovenous malformations); and endocarditis.

When brain abscess is strongly suspected, a neuroimaging procedure such as CT or MRI scans should be done prior to lumbar puncture. If a brain abscess is identified, lumbar puncture may be dangerous and rarely alters the choice of antibiotic or clinical management since the CSF abnormalities usually reflect only parameningeal inflammation. With spread from contagious septic foci, streptococci and anaerobic bacteria are most common. Staphylococci most often enter from trauma or from infections. Enteric organisms may form an abscess from chronic otitis. Unfortunately, cultures from a large number of brain abscesses remain negative.

The diagnosis of brain abscess is based primarily on a strong clinical suspicion and confirmed by a neuroimaging procedure. Electroencephalographic changes are nonspecific but frequently demonstrate focal slowing in the region of brain abscess. Initial therapy for infection from presumed contagious foci uses penicillin and metronidazole. Cefotaxime is a good alternative to penicillin, especially if enteric organisms are suspected. Enteric organisms are also often susceptible to trimethoprim-sulfamethoxazole. Suspicion of staphylococci, or their recovery from an aspirate, should be treated with nafcillin or vancomycin. Treatment may include neurologic consultation and anticonvulsant and edema therapy if necessary. In their early stages, brain abscesses are areas of focal cerebritis and can be "cured" with antibiotic treatment alone. Well-developed abscesses require surgical drainage.

Differential diagnosis of brain abscess includes any condition that produces focal neurologic deficits and increased intracranial pressure, such as neoplasms, subdural effusions, cerebral infarctions, and certain infections (herpes simplex, cysticercosis, and toxocariasis).

Table 23–23. Outcome of acute bacterial meningitis by organism.

Organism	Mortality (%)	Motor Handicap (%)		Intellect (%)	
		None	Severe	Normal	Severe Mental Retardation
Escherichia coli gram-negative organisms	20–50	62	25	75	25
Haemophilus influenzae	5–10	87	3	82	5
Streptococcus pneumoniae	10–30	96	0	83	0
Neisseria meningitidis	5–10	100	0	93	0
Group B streptococci	20	85	10–15	100	0
Overall total	10–25	85	5	82	6

The surgical mortality rate in the treatment of brain abscess is lower than 5%. Untreated cerebral abscesses lead to irreversible tissue destruction and may rupture into the ventricle, producing catastrophic deterioration in neurologic function and death. Because brain abscesses are often associated with systemic illness and systemic infections, the death rate is frequently high in these patients.

VIRAL INFECTIONS

Viral infections of the central nervous system can involve primarily meninges (meningitis) (see Chapter 35) or cerebral parenchyma (encephalitis). All patients, however, have some degree of involvement of both the meninges and cerebral parenchyma (meningoencephalitis). Many viral infections are generalized and diffuse, but some viruses, notably herpes simplex and some arboviruses, characteristically cause prominent focal disease. Focal cerebral involvement is clearly evident on neuroimaging procedures. Some viruses have an affinity for specific CNS cell populations. Poliovirus and other enteroviruses can selectively infect anterior horn cells (poliomyelitis) and some intracranial motor neurons.

Although most viral infections of the nervous system present with an acute or subacute course in childhood, chronic infections can occur. Subacute sclerosing panencephalitis, for example, represents a chronic indolent infection caused by measles virus and is characterized clinically by progressive neurodegeneration and seizures.

Inflammatory reactions within the nervous system may occur during the convalescent stage of systemic viral infections. Parainfectious or postinfectious inflammation of the central nervous system results in several well-recognized disorders: acute disseminated encephalomyelitis, transverse myelitis, optic neuritis, polyneuritis, and Guillain-Barré syndrome.

Congenital viral infections can also affect the central nervous system. Cytomegalovirus, herpes simplex virus, and rubella virus are the most notable causes of viral brain injury in utero.

Treatment of CNS viral infections is usually limited to symptomatic and supportive measures, except for herpes simplex virus. Acyclovir is the treatment in suspected or proven cases of herpes simplex virus encephalitis. Acyclovir is also useful in some patients with varicella-zoster virus infections of the central nervous system.

Encephalopathy of HIV Infection

Neurologic syndromes associated directly with HIV infection include subacute encephalitis, meningitis, myelopathy, polyneuropathy, and myositis. In addition, secondary opportunistic infections of the central nervous system occur in patients with HIV-induced immunosuppression; toxoplasmal and cy-

tomegaloviral infections are particularly common. Progressive multifocal leukoencephalopathy, a secondary papillomavirus infection, herpes simplex virus, and herpes zoster virus infections also occur frequently in patients with HIV infection. A variety of fungal (especially cryptococcal), mycobacterial, and bacterial infections have been described.

Neurologic abnormalities in these patients can also be the result of noninfectious neoplastic disorders. Primary CNS lymphoma and metastatic lymphoma to the nervous system are the most frequent neoplasms involving the nervous system in these patients. See Chapters 28 and 35 for diagnosis and management of HIV infection.

OTHER INFECTIONS

A wide variety of other microorganisms, including *Toxoplasma*, mycobacteria, spirochetes, rickettsiae, amebas, and mycoplasmas, can cause CNS infections. Central nervous system involvement in these infections is usually secondary to systemic infection or other predisposing factors. Appropriate cultures and serologic testing are required to confirm infections by these organisms. Parenteral antimicrobial treatment for these infections is discussed elsewhere in this text.

NONINFECTIOUS INFLAMMATORY DISORDERS OF THE CENTRAL NERVOUS SYSTEM

The differential diagnosis of bacterial, viral, and other microbial infections of the central nervous system includes disorders that cause inflammation but for which no specific etiologic organism has been identified. Sarcoidosis, Behçet's syndrome, systemic lupus erythematosus (SLE), other collagen-vascular disorders, and Kawasaki disease are examples. In these disorders, CNS inflammation usually occurs in association with characteristic systemic manifestations that allow proper diagnosis. Management of central nervous system involvement in these disorders is the same as the treatment of the systemic illness.

OTHER PARAINFECTIOUS ENCEPHALOPATHIES

In association with systemic infections or other illnesses, CNS dysfunction may occur in the absence of direct central nervous system inflammation or infection. **Reye's syndrome** is a prominent example of this type of encephalopathy that often occurs in association with varicella virus or other respiratory or systemic viral infections. In Reye's syndrome, cerebral edema and cerebral dysfunction occur, but there is no evidence of any direct involvement of the nervous system by the associated microorganism or inflammation. Cerebral edema in Reye's syndrome is accompanied by liver dysfunction and fatty infiltration of the liver. As a result of efforts to discourage use of aspirin in childhood febrile illnesses, there has been a marked decrease in the number of patients with Reye's syndrome. The precise relationship, however, between aspirin and Reye's syndrome is not clear.

Aebi C, Kaufmann F, Schaad UB: Brain abscess in childhood: Long-term experience. Eur J Pediatr 1991;2:662.

Ashwal S et al: Bacterial meningitis in children. Neurology 1992;42:739.

Burns D: The neuropathology of pediatric acquired immunodeficiency syndrome. J Child Neurol 1992;7:332.

DeCarli C et al: The prevalence of computed tomographic abnormalities of the cerebrum in 100 consecutive children symptomatic with the human immune deficiency virus. Ann Neurol 1993;34:198.

Epstein LG, Gendelman HE: Human immunodeficiency virus type 1 infection of the nervous system: Pathogenetic mechanisms. Ann Neurol 1993;33:429.

Kimura H et al: Detection of viral DNA in neonatal herpes simplex virus infections: Frequent and prolonged presence in serum and cerebrospinal fluid. J Infect Dis 1991;164:289.

Kohl S: Herpes simplex virus encephalitis in children. Pediatr Clin North Am 1988;35:465.

Lebel MH et al: Dexamethasone therapy for bacterial meningitis. N Engl J Med 1988;319:964.

McCracken GH: Current management of bacterial meningitis in infants and children. Pediatr Infect Dis 1992;11:169.

Patrick CC, Kaplan SL: Current concepts in the pathogenesis and management of brain abscesses in children. Pediatr Clin North Am 1988;35:625.

Quagliarello V, Scheld WM: Bacterial meningitis: Pathogenesis, pathophysiology, and progress. N Engl J Med 1992;327:864.

Schaad UB et al: Dexamethasone therapy for bacterial meningitis in children. Lancet 1993;342:457.

Troendle-Atkins J, Gemmler G, Buffone J: Rapid diagnosis of herpes simplex virus encephalitis by using the polymerase chain reaction. J Pediatr 1993;123:376.

Whitley RJ: Viral encephalitis. N Engl J Med 1990;323:242.

SYNDROMES PRESENTING AS ACUTE FLACCID PARALYSIS

Flaccid paralysis evolving over hours or a few days suggests involvement of the lower motor neuron complex (see Floppy Infant Syndrome). **Anterior horn cells** (spinal cord) may be involved by viral infection (paralytic poliomyelitis) or by paraviral or postviral immunologically mediated disease (acute transverse myelitis). The **nerve trunks** (polyneuritis) may be diseased as in Guillain-Barré syndrome or af-

fected by toxins (diphtheria, porphyria). The **neuromuscular junction** may be blocked by tick toxin or botulinum toxin. The paralysis rarely will be due to metabolic (periodic paralysis) or inflammatory muscle disease (myositis). *A lesion compressing the spinal cord must be ruled out.*

Clinical Findings

A. Symptoms & Signs: (Table 23–24.) Features assisting diagnosis are age, a history of preceding or waning illness, the presence (at time of paralysis) of fever, rapidity of progression, cranial nerve findings, and sensory findings. The examination may show "long tract" findings (pyramidal tract), causing increased reflexes and positive Babinski sign. The spinothalamic tract may be interrupted, causing loss of pain and temperature. Back pain, even tenderness to percussion, may occur, as well as bowel and bladder incontinence. Often, the paralysis is ascending, symmetric, and painful (muscle tenderness or myalgia). Laboratory findings occasionally are diagnostic.

B. Laboratory Findings: (See Table 23–24.) The examination of spinal fluid is most helpful. Imaging studies of the spinal column (plain films) and spinal cord (MRI, myelogram) are occasionally essential. Viral cultures (spinal fluid, throat, stool) and titers aid in diagnosing poliomyelitis. A high sedimentation rate may suggest tumor or abscess; antinuclear antibody (ANA) may suggest lupus arteritis.

Electromyography and nerve conduction velocity can be helpful in diagnosing polyneuropathy. Nerve conduction is usually slowed after 7–10 days. Findings in botulism and tick-bite paralysis can be specific and diagnostic. Rarely, elevation of muscle enzymes—or even myoglobinuria—may aid in diagnosis of myopathic paralysis. Porphyrin urine studies and heavy metal assays (arsenic, thallium, lead) can reveal those rare toxic causes of polyneuropathic paralysis.

Differential Diagnosis

The child who has been well and becomes paralyzed often has polyneuritis. Acute transverse myelitis sometimes occurs in an afebrile child. The child who is ill and febrile at the time of paralysis often has acute transverse myelitis (or poliomyelitis); *acute* epidural spinal cord abscess (or other compressive lesion) must be ruled out. Poliomyelitis is very rare in our immunized population. Paralysis due to tick bites occurs seasonally (spring and summer). The tick is usually found in the occipital hair. Removal is curative.

Paralysis due to botulism occurs most commonly under age 1; food-borne and wound botulism are very rare. An investigative history and laboratory studies are diagnostic. Intravenous drug abuse can lead to myelitis and paralysis. Furthermore, *chronic* myelopathy occurs with two human immunodefi-

Table 23–24. Acute flaccid paralysis in children.

	Poliomyelitis (Paralytic, Spinal, and Bulbar), With or Without Encephalitis	Landry-Guillain-Barré Syndrome ("Acute Idiopathic Polyneuritis")	Botulism	Tick-Bite Paralysis	Transverse Myelitis and Neuromyelitis Optica
Etiology	Poliovirus types I, II, and III; other enteroviruses; vaccine strain poliovirus (rare)	Likely delayed hypersensitivity-immunologic. Mycoplasmal and viral infections (including infectious mononucleosis) and various systemic or toxic disorders may be underlying cause. *Campylobacter* enteritis. Hepatitis B.	*Clostridium botulinum* toxin. Block at neuromuscular junction. Under age 1, toxin forms in bowel from ingested dust or honey in formula. At older ages, contaminated food (preformed toxin). Rarely from wound infection.	Probable interference with transmission of nerve impulse caused by toxin in tick saliva.	Usually unknown; multiple viruses (herpes, EBV, varicella, hepatitis A) often postviral (see Guillain-Barré syndrome).
History	None, or inadequate polio immunization. Upper respiratory or gastrointestinal symptoms followed by brief respite. Bulbar paralysis more frequent after tonsillectomy. Often in epidemics, in summer and early fall	Nonspecific respiratory or gastrointestinal symptoms in preceding 5–14 days common. Any season, though slightly lower incidence in summer.	Infancy: dusty environment (eg, construction area), suburbs; honey. Older: "food poisoning." Multiple cases hours to days after ingesting contaminated food.	Exposure to ticks (dog tick in eastern United States; wood ticks). Irritability 12–24 hours before onset of a rapidly progressive ascending paralysis.	Rarely symptoms compatible with multiple sclerosis or optic neuritis. Progression from onset to paraplegia often rapid, usually without a history of bacterial infection.
Presenting complaints	Febrile at time of paralysis. Meningeal signs, muscle tenderness, and spasm. Asymmetric weakness widespread or segmental (cervical, thoracic, lumbar). Bulbar symptoms early or before extremity weakness; anxiety; delirium	Symmetric weakness of lower extremities, which may ascend rapidly to arms, trunk, and face. Verbal child may complain of paresthesias. Fever uncommon. Facial weakness early. Miller-Fisher variant presents as ataxia and ophthalmoplegia.	Infancy: constipation, poor suck and cry. "Floppy." Apnea. Lethargy. Choking (cause of SIDS?). Older: blurred vision, diplopia, ptosis, choking, weakness.	Rapid onset and progression of ascending flaccid paralysis; often accompanied by pain and paresthesias. Paralysis of upper extremities usually occurs on second day after onset.	Root and back pain in about one-third to one-half of cases. Sensory loss below level of lesion accompanying rapidly developing paralysis. Sphincter difficulties common.
Findings	Flaccid weakness, usually asymmetric. Cord level: Lumbar: legs, lower abdomen Cervical: shoulder, arm, neck, diaphragm Thoracic: intercostals, spine, upper abdomen Bulbar: respiratory lower cranial nerves Fever in first days	Flaccid weakness, symmetric, usually greater proximally, but may be more distal or equal in distribution. Facial diplegia in about 85%, rarely IX–XI, III–VI. Bulbar involvement may occur. Slight distal impairment of position, vibration, touch; difficult to assess in young children.	Infants: flaccid weakness. Alert. Eye, pupil, facial weakness. Deep tendon reflexes (DTR) decreased to 0? Absent suck, gag. Constipation. Older: paralysis accommodation, eye movements. Weak swallow. Respiratory paralysis.	Flaccid, symmetric paralysis. Cranial nerve and bulbar (respiratory) paralysis, ataxia, sphincter disturbances, and sensory deficits may occur. Some fever. Diagnosis rests on finding tick, which is especially likely to be on occipital scalp.	Paraplegia with areflexia below level of lesion early; later, may have hyperreflexia. Sensory loss below and hyperesthesia or normal sensation above level of lesion. Paralysis of bladder and rectum. Optic neuritis rarely may be present.
CSF	Pleocytosis (20–500+ cells) with PMN predominance in first few days, followed by rapid decrease and monocytic preponderance. Glucose normal. Protein frequently elevated (50–150 mg/dL).	Cytoalbuminologic dissociation; 10 or fewer mononuclear cells with high protein after first week. Normal glucose. Gamma globulin may be elevated.	Normal.	Normal.	Usually no manometric block; CSF may show increased protein, pleocytosis with predominantly mononuclear cells, increased gamma globulin.

(*continued*)

Table 23–24. Acute flaccid paralysis in children. (continued)

	Poliomyelitis (Paralytic, Spinal, and Bulbar), With or Without Encephalitis	Landry-Guillain-Barré Syndrome ("Acute Idiopathic Polyneuritis")	Botulism	Tick-Bite Paralysis	Transverse Myelitis and Neuromyelitis Optica
EMG	Denervation after 10–21 days. Nerve conduction normal.	Nerve conduction velocities markedly decreased; may be normal early, or in axonal-only damage.	EMG distinctive: BSAP ("brief small abundant potentials").	Nerve conduction slowed; returns rapidly to normal after removal of tick.	Normal early. Denervation at level of lesion after 10–21 days.
Other studies	Initially, leukocytosis. Virus in stool and throat. Serologic titers.	Search for specific cause such as infection, intoxication, metabolic or endocrine disease, allergic phenomena, neoplasm. Lymphocyte transformation demonstrated. *Mycoplasma pneumoniae* implicated in some cases.	Infancy: stool culture, toxin. Rare serum toxin +. Older: serum (or wound) toxin.	Leukocytosis, often with moderate eosinophilia.	Normal spine x-rays do not exclude spinal epidural abscess. MRI has largely replaced myelography to rule out cord-compressive lesions. Cord may be swollen myelitis.
Course and prognosis	Paralysis usually maximal 3–5 days after onset. Transient bladder paralysis may occur. Outlook varies with extent and severity of involvement. **Note:** Mortality greatest from respiratory failure and superinfection. Early muscle atrophy common.	Course progressive over a few days to about 2 weeks. Transient bladder paralysis may occur. **Note:** Threat greatest from respiratory failure, autonomic crises (eg, BP, arrhythmia) and superinfection. Majority recover completely. Plasmapheresis may have a role. Intravenous IgG (IGIV) a new therapy; relapses occasionally occur.	Infancy: supportive. Penicillin ? Purge stool ? Antitoxin unnecessary. Respiratory support (prolonged often), gavage feeding. Avoid aminoglycosides. Older: penicillin, antitoxin, prolonged respiratory support. Prognosis: excellent with good quality intensive care. Fatality 3%.	Total removal of tick is followed by rapid improvement and recovery. Otherwise, mortality rate due to respiratory paralysis is very high.	Large degree of functional recovery possible. Corticosteroids are of controversial benefit in shortening duration of acute attack or altering the overall course.

ciency virus infections, HTLV-I and HTLV-III (now called HIV-1).

Complications

A. Respiratory Paralysis: Early and careful attention to oxygenation is essential; administration of oxygen, intubation, mechanical respiratory assistance, and careful suctioning of secretions may be required. Increasing anxiety and a rise in diastolic and systolic blood pressures are early signs of hypoxia. Cyanosis is a late sign. Deteriorating spirometric findings (forced expiratory volume in 1 second [FEV_1] and total vital capacity) may indicate the need for controlled intubation and respiratory support.

B. Infections: Pneumonia is common, especially in cases of respiratory paralysis. Prophylactic antibiotic administration is generally contraindicated. Antibiotic therapy is best guided by results of cultures. Bladder infections occur when an indwelling catheter is required because of bladder paralysis. Recovery from myelitis may be delayed by urinary tract infection.

C. Autonomic Crisis: This may be a cause of death in Guillain-Barré syndrome; strict attention to vital signs to detect and treat hypotension or hypertension and cardiac arrhythmias in an intensive care setting is advisable, at least early in the course in severely ill patients.

Treatment

There is no specific treatment in most of these syndromes; however, ticks causing paralysis must be removed. Other therapies include the use of erythromycin in *Mycoplasma* infections and botulism equine antitoxin in wound botulism. Recognized associated disorders (eg, endocrine, neoplastic, toxic) should be treated by appropriate means. Supportive care also involves pulmonary toilet, adequate fluids and nutrition, bladder and bowel care, prevention of decubiti, and, in many cases, psychiatric support.

A. Corticosteroids: These agents are believed by most to be of no benefit in Guillain-Barré syndrome. Autonomic symptoms (eg, hypertension) in polyneuritis may require treatment.

B. Plasmapheresis: Plasma exchange or intravenous immunoglobulin G (IgG) has been beneficial in severe cases of Guillain-Barré syndrome.

C. Physical Therapy: Rehabilitative measures are best instituted when acute symptoms have subsided and the patient is stable.

D. Antibiotics: Appropriate antibiotics and drainage are required for epidermal abscess.

Prognosis

Prognosis varies greatly with the extent of involvement, duration of the inflammatory process, complications, and other factors.

Bleck TP: IVIg for GBS: Potential problems in the alphabet soup. Neurology 1993;43:857.

Bolton CF: The changing concepts of Guillain-Barré syndrome. (Editorial.) N Engl J Med 1995;333:1415.

Briscoe DM et al: Prognosis in Guillain-Barré syndrome. Arch Dis Child 1987;62:733.

Dunne K et al: Acute transverse myelopathy in childhood. Dev Med Child Neurol 1986;28:198.

Freeman JM: Diagnosis and evaluation of acute paraplegia. Pediatr Rev 1983;4:328.

Griffen JW, Ho T: The Guillain-Barré syndrome at 75. Ann Neurol 1993;34:125.

Irani DN et al: Relapse in Guillain-Barré syndrome after treatment with human immune globulin. Neurology 1993;43:872.

Johnson RT, McArthur J: Myelopathic and retrovirus infections. Ann Neurol 1987;21:113.

Khatri BO et al: Plasmapheresis with acute inflammatory polyneuropathy. Pediatr Neurol 1990;6:17.

McKhahn G, Griffin JW: Plasmapheresis and GB syndrome. (Editorial.) Ann Neurol 1987;22:762.

Novak RW, Jones G, Chi'ien LT: Acute transverse myelopathy in childhood: A study of four cases. Clin Pediatr 1978;17:894.

Packer RJ et al: Magnetic resonance imaging of spinal cord disease in childhood. Pediatrics 1986;78:251.

Ropper AH, Wijdicks EFM, Truax BT: *Guillain-Barré Syndrome.* Davis, 1993.

Vriesendorp FJ et al: Serum antibodies to GM1, GD1b, peripheral nerve myelin, and *Campylobacter jejuni* in patients with Guillain-Barré syndrome and controls: Correlation and prognosis. Ann Neurol 1993;34:130.

DISORDERS OF CHILDHOOD AFFECTING MUSCLES

This section is concerned with specific muscle and neuromuscular disorders, including the muscular dystrophies, myasthenia gravis, and miscellaneous congenital neuromuscular disorders (Table 23–25).

Certain studies that are commonly used in the diagnosis of muscle diseases merit special consideration.

Serum Enzymes

CPK (creatine phosphokinase) reflects muscle damage or "leak" from muscle into plasma. Blood should be drawn before electromyography or muscle biopsy, which may lead to release of the enzyme. Corticosteroids may suppress levels despite very active muscle disease.

Muscle Imaging

MRI scans are used in research studies to assist the diagnosis and assessment of muscular dystrophies, congenital myopathies and myotonias, and spinal muscular atrophies.

Electromyography (EMG)

Electromyography is often helpful in grossly differentiating **myopathic** from **neurogenic** processes. Fibrillations occur in both. In the myopathies, very low spikes are more typical, and the motor unit action potentials seen during contraction characteristically are of short duration, polyphasic, and increased in number for the strength of the contraction (increased interference pattern). Neurogenic findings include decreased numbers of motor units, which may be polyphasic, larger than normal, or both. The interference pattern is decreased. In myotonic dystrophy, the EMG is characterized by prolonged discharge of electrical activity on movement of the probing needle ("dive bomber" sound).

Muscle Biopsy

Properly executed (by "open" biopsy or by using the Bergstrom muscle biopsy needle), this procedure is usually most helpful. Histochemical techniques, histogram analysis of muscle fiber types and sizes, and electron microscopy are offering new classifications of the myopathies. Findings common to the dystrophies include variation in the size and shape of muscle fibers, increase in connective tissue, interstitial infiltration of fatty tissue, degenerative changes in muscle fibers, and central location of nuclei.

Dystrophin is a normal intracellular plasma membrane protein in muscle, the gene product missing in Duchenne's (and Becker's) dystrophy. Staining the muscle for dystrophin aids in differentiating Duchenne's from Becker's dystrophy; dystrophin is absent in Duchenne's, reduced in Becker's dystrophy. Electrophoresis can confirm whether the dystrophin is absent or present in small amounts and whether there is a qualitative difference from normal dystrophin, the latter two patterns being characteristic of Becker's dystrophy.

Genetic Testing & Carrier Detection

To date, detection of carriers for Duchenne's dystrophy (mothers and sisters of affected boys) has rested on CPK enzyme elevations (two thirds will have this finding); physical findings of mild dystro-

Table 23–25. Muscular dystrophies and myotonias of childhood.

Disease	Genetic Pattern	Age at Onset	Early Manifestations	Involved Muscles	Reflexes
Muscular dystrophies Duchenne's muscular dystrophy (pseudohypertrophic infantile)	X-linked recessive; autosomal recessive unusual. Thirty to 50% have no family history.	2–6 years; rarely in infancy	Clumsiness, easy fatigability on walking, running, and climbing stairs. Walking on toes; waddling gait. Lordosis. (Climbing up on legs rising from supine position—Gower's maneuver.)	Axial and proximal before distal. Pelvic girdle; pseudohypertrophy of gastrocnemius (90%), triceps brachii, and vastus lateralis. Shoulder girdle usually later, also articulation difficulties. Eventually cardiomyopathy (50%).	Knee jerks ± or 0; ankle jerks + to ++
Becker's muscular dystrophy (late onset)	X-linked recessive. (Allele at Xp21)	Childhood (usually later than in Duchenne's)	Similar to Duchenne's	Similar to Duchenne's	Similar to Duchenne's
Limb-girdle muscular dystrophy A. Pelvifemoral (Leyden-Möbius) B. Scapulohumeral (Erb's juvenile) (Chromosome 15)	Autosomal recessive in 60%; high sporadic incidence. A. Relatively common B. Rare	Variable; early childhood to adulthood.	Weakness, with distribution according to type. Waddling gait, difficulty climbing stairs. Lordosis.	A. Pelvic girdle usually involved first and to greater extent. B. Shoulder girdle often asymmetric. Quadriceps and hamstrings may be weakest. Pseudohypertrophy of calves uncommon.	Usually present
Facioscapulohumeral muscular dystrophy (Landouzy-Déjérine) Scapuloperoneal variant (Chromosome 4)	Autosomal dominant; sporadic cases not uncommon.	Usually late in childhood and adolescence; rare in infancy; not uncommon in twenties.	Diminished facial movements with inability to close eyes, smile, or whistle. Face may be flat; unlined. Difficulty in raising arms over head. Lordosis. Tripping in scapuloperoneal type.	Facial muscles followed by shoulder girdle, with occasional spread to hips or distal legs (scapuloperoneal variant).	Present
Spinal muscular atrophy (SMA) Infantile SMA (Werdnig-Hoffman disease)	Autosomal recessive.	0–2 years	Floppy infant	Big muscles: shoulder, hip. Tongue. Intercostals. Fingerstoes spared.	0 or nearly so
Juvenile SMA (Kugelburg-Welander disease)	Autosomal recessive.	Onset after age 2 usually (age 5–15 typical).	Weakness. "Fasciculations" 50%. Rarely a cause of "floppy infant."	Same	Same
Metabolic myopathies Carnitine deficiency (lipid sortage myopathy) Primary (rare) Secondary: multiple forms	Genetics variable.	Infancy to adolescence	Fasting hypoglycemia and coma; less ketosis than expected. Myopathy. Cardiomyopathy. Fatty liver. Don't confuse with Reye's, SIDS.	Weakness variable; may be precipitated by exercise (with resultant myoglobulinuria) or fasting.	Normal to decreased
"Oculocraniosomatic syndrome" (ophthalmoplegia and "ragged reds"; progressive external ophthalmoplegia) Kearns-Sayer	(?) Acquired; 80% female; other hereditary neurologic disorders may be found in patient or family.	Variable; from infancy to adult life; most at about 10 years of age.	Ptosis and limitation of eye movements; hearing and visual loss (retinitis pigmentosa); intellectual loss; cerebellar disturbance (ataxia).	Extraocular muscles, often asymmetric. Variable involvement of axial muscles; cardiac muscles, with conduction defect.	Depressed to ± or 0
Myasthenia gravis Transient neonatal	Variable	At birth	Difficulty sucking, swallowing; trouble with secretions.	Somatic and cranial muscles.	Normal to decreased

(continued)

Table 23–25. Muscular dystrophies and myotonias of childhood. (continued)

Muscle Biopsy Findings	Other Diagnostic Tests	Treatment	Prognosis
Degeneration and variation in fiber size; proliferation of connective tissue. Basophilia, phagocytosis. Poor differentiation of fiber types on ATPase reaction; deficiency of type 2B fibers. Dystrophin absent.	EMG myopathic. CK (4000–5000 IU) very high with decrease toward normal over the years. ECG. Chest x-ray. Cloned dystrophin cDNA probes to detect deletions on Xp21 chromosome from blood,amniotic fluid, chorionic villi.	Physical therapy, braces, wheelchair eventually, weight control.	Ten percent show nonprogressive mental retardation. Death from pneumonia 10–15 years after dignosis with 75% of patients dead by age 20.
Similar to above, except type 2B fibers present. Reduced or abnormal size dystrophin.	Similar to above, although muscle enzymes may not be as elevated.	As above. Wheelchair in late childhood or early adult life.	Slower progression than Duchenne's, with death usually in adulthood.
Variation in muscle fiber size with many very large fibers. Fiber splitting and internal nuclei common. Many "moth-eaten" whorled fibers. Dystrophin normal.	EMG myopathic. CK variable; often normal but may be elevated ECG.	Physical therapy, weight control.	Mildly progressive: spread from lower to upper limbs may take 15–20 years. Life expectancy mid to late adulthood.
Predominantly large fibers with scattered tiny atrophic fibers, "moth-eaten" and whorled fibers. Inflammatory response. Little or no fiber splitting, fibrosis, or type 1 fiber predominance.	EMG myopathic. Muscle enzymes usually normal.	Physical therapy where indicated. Wheelchair in old age. ? steroids in inflammatory infant variant.	Very slowly progressive, often with plateaus, except in infantile form where there may be difficulties in walking by adolescence. Usually normal life span.
Small, group atrophy. Twin peak fiber size. Fiber type grouping. Minimal fibrosis.	EMG "neuropathic." Nerve conduction, CSF, muscle enzymes normal. Chromosome 5; linkage studies for prenatal diagnosis.	Supportive: respiratory care, positioning, secretion management. Genetic counseling.	80–95% of patients 0–4 years die of pneumonia and respiratory failure.
Same	Same. CK ("enzymes") may be mildly elevated.	Physical therapy, wheelchair positioning to avoid scoliosis. May walk, usually later lose this.	Fairly normal life expectancy. 4–40+ years.
Normal or lipid droplets ("Ragged red" fibers with lipid stain, eg, oil red O).	Muscle biochemistry (carnitine, CPT enzyme). Urine organic acids (at time of illness). Plasma carnitine. WBC, fibroblast enzyme studies.	Avoid fasting and mitochondrial toxins, eg, ASA, valproic acid. Carbohydrate. Treat acidosis. Carnitine orally.	Variable: occasionally fatal in infants. Progressive weakness, developmental delay, cardiomyopathy may occur.
Mitochondrial abnormalities. "Ragged red" fibers. Changes in fiber size, usually due to type 2 fiber atrophy.	CK usually normal. ECG with conduction block. CSF protein elevated. Nerve conduction slowed. CT, brain scan, and brain stem auditory evoked response may be abnormal. Mitochondrial deletions.	Plastic retraction of eyelids. Cardiac support. Anticipate diabetes mellitus. Coenzyme Q?	Dysphagia may develop (50%) as well as generalized muscle weakness. Prognosis fail if disease is confined to ocular muscles. In severe cases, spongy vacuolization of brain and brain stem.
Unnecessary	Edrophonium or neostigmine tests. Acetylcholine receptor (AChR) antibodies. Repetitive nerve stimulation, EMG.	Supportive. Anticholinergic drugs.	Usually transient (< 2 months).

(continued)

Table 23–25. Muscular dystrophies and myotonias of childhood. (continued)

Disease	Genetic Pattern	Age at Onset	Early Manifestations	Involved Muscles	Reflexes
Persistent neonatal	Variable	Variable: birth, neonatal, infancy.	Same	Same	Same
Congenital myopathies Myotonic dystrophy (Neonatal onset)	Autosomal dominant	At birth	Same as myasthenia. Ptosis. Facial diplegia. Arthrogyposis, club feet, thin ribs.	Cranial and somatic, pharyngeal.	Decreased to 0
"Other" Central core Nemaline (rod body) Myotubular (centronuclear) Congenital fiber type disproportion	Variable, often autosomal recessive	Severe variants present at birth; milder variants (more common) infancy, childhood	Severe variant, as in myasthenia, myotonic dystrophy. Later presentation—facial weakness, mild to moderate weakness, even "toe walking" only.	Similar to myotonic dystrophy.	Decreased to 0
Congenital muscular dystrophy (Fukayama)	? Genetic ? Infectious	Birth	Hypotonia. Facial weakness, joint contractures, mental retardation. Ocular abnormalities	Heterogenous. Facial (cranial) and somatic. Contracture common.	Variable
Congenital muscular dystrophy ("occidental")	Unknown; usually not familial	Birth (or early infancy)	As above. Normal IQ.	Same	Same
Benign congenital hypotonia (Oppenheim)	Variable	Variable	Hypotonia only. Deep tendon reflexes +. Laboratory tests, biopsy normal.	Somatic muscles (respiratory muscles spared).	Normal to decreased
Myotonias Myotonia congenita (Thomsen)	Autosomal dominant (autosomal recessive cases reported)	Early infancy to late childhood	Difficulty in relaxing muscles after contracting them, especially after sleep; agravated by cold, excitement.	Hands especially; muscles may be diffusely enlarged, giving patient herculean appearance.	Normal
Myotonic dystrophy (Steinert) (childhood and adult form)	Autosomal dominant	Late childhood to adolescence; neonatal and infantile forms increasingly recognized (see above)	Myotonia of grasp, tongue; worsened by cold, emotions. "Hatchet-face." Nasal voice. Weakness and easy fatigability. Mild to moderate mental retardation noted.	Wasting and weakness of facial muscles, including muscles of mastication; sternocleidomastoids, hands. Myotonic phenomena: "bunching up" of muscles of tongue, thenar eminance, finger extensors after tapping with percussion hammer.	In infantile form, marked hyporeflexia

(continued)

phy (large calves, muscle weakness); abnormal muscle EMGs; or biopsy results. All are unreliable for diagnostic purposes.

DNA probes are now available for carrier detection and prenatal diagnosis of Duchenne's and Becker's dystrophy. Deletions are often found on the short arm of the X chromosome; it is postulated that all patients and most mothers will show deletions when sufficient probes are developed to search the whole Duchenne genome (perhaps 4000 kb in length).

Amplification of DNA by the polymerase chain reactions (PCR) can detect the deletion. Moreover, this technique plus Southern blot analysis can detect abnormal DNA base repeats. For example, in myotonic dystrophy, a GCT triplet excess is currently the most sensitive test for that disease. The tests can be used for intrauterine diagnosis and prediction of whether the triplet is within the normal or mutant range. Thus, in many cases, the greater the number of repeats, the more severely involved the fetus or patient.

Table 23–25. Muscular dystrophies and myotonias of childhood. (continued)

Muscle Biopsy Findings	Other Diagnostic Tests	Treatment	Prognosis
Sophisticated end plate, nerve terminal ultrastructural studies may be necessary.	May be similar to above. AChR antibodies negative.	May not respond to ACh-ase drugs, steroids, or immunosuppressants.	Variable, may have long-term severe course.
Generalized fiber hypertrophy, delay in maturation. Type I atrophy. Internal nuclei.	EMG "myotonic" in some (waning amplitude and pitch). Test mother. CK often normal. DNA testing (chromosome 19) for GCT repeat.	Supportive, even respiratory support. Genetic counseling.	Severely involved infant may improve dramatically over months; expect mental retardation in this same variant.
Distinctive diagnostic histochemistry, eg, "central cores," "nemaline rods," myotubes type II–I fibers of unequal size.	Myopathic EMG.	Supportive. Genetic counseling.	Variable. May shorten life. Death in infancy or severe handicap. Scoliosis prominent.
"Dystrophic" changes. Fibrosis. Necrotic fibers. Internal nuclei. ? regenerative fibers.	Myopathic EMG. CK increased or normal. Positive CT, MRI scans: white matter low density, polymicrogyria, lissencephaly, etc.	Supportive.	Physical and mental handicap lifelong.
Same	As above, CT, MRI variably low density; may have absent dystrophin-associated protein (DAP).		May improve, walk. Scoliosis.
Normal with sophisticated studies (histochemistry, electron microscopy, even metabolic studies).	Use of this diagnosis is shrinking with increasingly sophisticated biochemical (eg, cytochrome oxidase) studies.	Supportive.	Good (by definition). (Few documented long-term studies.)
Nonspecific and minor changes; type 2B fibers may be absent.	EMG "myotonic."	Usually none. Phenytoin, especially in cold weather, may improve muscle functioning.	Normal life expectancy, with only mild disability.
Type I fiber atrophy, type 2 hypertrophy, sarcoplasmic masses, internal nuclei, phagocytosis, fibrosis, and cellular reaction.	EMG markedly "myotonic." Glucose tolerance test, thyroid tests. ECG. Chest x-ray and pulmonary function tests. Immunoglobulins. PCR amplification of GCT repeat on chromosome 19q13 to distinguish normal from mutant alleles.	Procainamide, 250 mg 3 times daily orally, increased to tolerance; phenytoin 5–7 mg/kg/d orally. (Drugs usually little role.)	Frontal baldness, cataracts (85%), gonadal atrophy (85% of males), thyroid dysfunction, diabetes mellitus (20%). Cardiac conduction defects; impaired pulmonary function. Low IgG. Life expectancy decreased.

DNA linkage analysis on chromosome 5 is used to predict the risk of recurrence for infantile spinal muscular atrophy.

Lastly, Kearns-Sayer progressive external ophthalmoplegia with retinopathy is inherited via maternal cytoplasmic mitochondria. Assay of mutations and deletions from blood or muscle samples are now commercially available.

Therapy for Duchenne's muscular dystrophy continues to be frustrating. Prednisone in low doses has increased muscle strength and prolonged ambulation. Research emphasis is on gene therapy, but there is great difficulty in finding viral vectors able to carry the very large dystrophin gene into muscle cells.

Engel A: Gene therapy for Duchenne dystrophy. Ann Neurol 1993;34:3.

Fenichel GM et al: Long-term benefit from prednisone therapy in Duchenne muscular dystrophy. Neurology 1991;14:1874.

Hilton T et al: End of life care in Duchenne muscular dystrophy. Pediatr Neurol 1993;9:165.

Hoffman EP: Characterization of dystrophin in muscle biopsy specimens from patients with Duchenne's or Becker's muscular dystrophy. N Engl J Med 1988;318:1363.

Holt IF et al: Mitochondrial myopathies: Clinical and biochemical features of 30 patients with major deletions of muscle mitochondrial DNA. Ann Neurol 1989;26:699.

Karpati G et al: Myoblast transfer in muscular dystrophy. Ann Neurol 1993;34:8.

Mendell JR, Sahenk Z, Prior TW: The childhood muscular dystrophies: Diseases sharing a common pathogenesis of membrane instability. J Child Neurol 1995;10:150.

Miller G, Wessel HB: Diagnosis of dystrophinopathies: Review for the clinician. Pediatr Neurol 1993;9(1):3.

Miller RG, Hoffman EP: Molecular diagnosis and modern management of Duchenne muscular dystrophy. Neurol Clin 1994;12:699.

Milu JM, Gilbert-Barnes E: Type I spinal muscular atrophy (Werdnig- Hoffman disease). Am J Dis Child 1993;147:908.

Parano E et al: Congenital muscular dystrophy: Clinical review and proposed classification. Pediatr Neurol 1995;13:97.

Redman JB et al: Relationship between parental trinucleotide GTC repeat length and severity of myotonic dystrophy in offspring. JAMA 1993;269:1960.

Roland EM: Neuromuscular diseases in childhood. Curr Opin Pediatr 1994;6:636.

Russman BS: Rehabilitation of the pediatric patient with a neuromuscular disease. Neurol Clin 1990;8:727.

Russman BS, Schwartz RC: Neuromuscular diseases of childhood. Curr Opin Pediatr 1993;5:669.

Tritschler HJ, Medori R: Mitochondrial DNA alterations as a source of human disorders. Neurology 1993;43:280.

Wolff JA: Gene therapy for neuromuscular disorders. Int Pediatr 1993;8:14.

BENIGN ACUTE CHILDHOOD MYOSITIS

Benign acute childhood myositis (myalgia cruris epidemica) is characterized by transient severe muscle pain and weakness affecting mainly the calves and occurring 1–2 days following an upper respiratory tract infection. Though symptoms involve mainly the gastrocnemius muscles, all skeletal muscles appear to be invaded directly by virus; recurrent episodes are due to different viral types. By seroconversion or isolation of the virus, acute myositis has been shown to be largely due to influenza types B and A and occasionally due to parainfluenza and adenovirus.

Ruff RL, Secrist D: Viral studies in benign acute childhood myositis. Arch Neurol 1982;39:261.

MYASTHENIA GRAVIS

Essentials of Diagnosis

- Weakness, chiefly of muscles innervated by the brain stem, usually coming on or increasing with use (fatigue).
- Positive response to neostigmine and edrophonium.
- Acetylcholine receptor antibodies in serum (except in congenital form).

General Considerations

Myasthenia gravis is characterized by easy fatigability of muscles, particularly the extraocular muscles and those of mastication, swallowing, and respiration. In the neonatal period, however, or in early infancy, the weakness may be so constant and general that an affected infant may present nonspecifically as a "floppy infant." Girls are affected more frequently than boys. The age at onset is over 10 years in 75% of cases, often shortly after menarche. If diagnosed before age 10, congenital myasthenia should be considered in retrospect. Thyrotoxicosis is found in almost 10% of affected female patients. The essential abnormality is a circulating antibody that binds to the acetylcholine receptor protein and thus reduces the number of motor end plates for binding by acetylcholine.

Clinical Findings

A. Symptoms & Signs:

1. Neonatal (transient) myasthenia gravis: This disorder occurs in 12% of infants born to myasthenic mothers. The condition is due to maternal acetylcholine receptor antibody transferred across the placenta; a thymic factor in the infant may also be involved. A sibling may have died in the neonatal period with similar symptoms and nondiagnostic autopsy.

2. Congenital (persistent) myasthenia gravis: In this form of the disease, the mothers of the affected infants rarely have myasthenia gravis, but other relatives may. Sex distribution is equal. Symptoms are often subtle and not recognized initially. Differential diagnosis includes many other causes of the "floppy infant" syndrome, such as infant botulism, ocular myopathy, congenital ptosis, and Möbius' syndrome (facial nuclear aplasia and other anomalies). Congenital myasthenia gravis is not caused by receptor antibodies and often responds poorly to therapy. It may result from a genetic abnormality of the acetylcholine receptor protein or other neurotransmitter vagaries.

3. Juvenile myasthenia gravis: In this autoimmune form, the symptoms and signs are similar to those in adults. Receptor antibodies are usually present. The patient may be first seen by an otolaryngologist or psychiatrist. The more prominent signs are difficulty in chewing, dysphagia, a nasal voice, ptosis, and ophthalmoplegia. Pathologic fatigability of limbs, chiefly involving the proximal limb and neck muscles, may be more prominent than the bulbar signs and may lead to an initial diagnosis of conversion hysteria, muscular dystrophy, or polymyositis. Weakness may be limited to ocular muscles only. Associated disorders include autoimmune conditions, especially thyroid disease.

An acute fulminant form of myasthenia gravis has been reported in children of age 2–10 years and presents with rapidly progressive respiratory difficulties. Bulbar paralysis may evolve within 24 hours. There is no history of myasthenia. The differential diagnosis includes Guillain-Barré syndrome and bulbar poliomyelitis. Administration of anticholinesterase agents establishes the diagnosis and is lifesaving.

B. Laboratory Findings:

1. Neostigmine test: In newborns and very young infants, the neostigmine test may be preferable to the edrophonium (Tensilon) test because the longer duration of its response permits better observation, especially of sucking and swallowing movements. The test dose of neostigmine is 0.02 mg/kg subcutaneously, usually given with atropine, 0.01 mg/kg subcutaneously. There is a delay of about 10 minutes before the effect may be manifest. The physician should be prepared to suction secretions.

2. Edrophonium test: Testing with edrophonium is used in older children who are capable of cooperating in certain tasks, such as raising and lowering their eyelids and squeezing a sphygmomanometer bulb or the examiner's hands. The test dose is 0.1–1 mL intravenously, depending on the size of the child. Maximum improvement occurs within 2 minutes.

3. Other laboratory tests: Serum acetylcholine receptor antibodies are often found in the neonatal and juvenile forms. Ophthalmologic tests of ocular motility with edrophonium are often positive in patients able to cooperate. In juveniles, thyroid studies are appropriate.

C. Electrical Studies of Muscle: Repetitive stimulation of a motor nerve at slow rates (3/s) with recording over the appropriate muscle reveals a progressive fall in amplitude of the muscle potential in myasthenic patients. A maximal stimulus must be given. At higher rates of stimulation (50/s), there may be a transient repair of this defect before the progressive decline is seen.

If this study is negative, single-fiber electromyography is now employed to determine if "mean jitter" exceeds the normal rate.

D. Imaging: Chest x-ray and CT scanning in older children may disclose benign thymus enlargement. Thymus tumors are rare in children.

Treatment

A. General & Supportive Care: In the newborn or in a child in myasthenic or cholinergic crisis

(see following text), suctioning of secretions is essential. Respiratory assistance may be required.

Treatment should be conducted by physicians with experience in this disorder.

B. Anticholinesterase Drug Therapy:

1. Pyridostigmine bromide: The dose must be adjusted for each patient. A frequent starting dose is 15–30 mg orally every 6 hours.

2. Neostigmine: Fifteen milligrams of neostigmine are roughly equivalent to 60 mg of pyridostigmine bromide. Neostigmine often causes gastric hypermotility with diarrhea, but it is the drug of choice in newborns, in whom prompt treatment may be lifesaving. It may be given parenterally.

3. Atropine: Atropine may be added on a maintenance basis to control mild cholinergic side effects such as hypersecretion, abdominal cramps, and nausea and vomiting.

4. Immunologic intervention: This is primarily with prednisone. Plasmapheresis is effective in removing acetylcholine receptor antibody in severely affected patients.

5. Myasthenic crisis: Relatively sudden difficulties in swallowing and respiration may be observed in myasthenic patients. Edrophonium results in dramatic but brief improvement; this may make evaluation of the condition of the small child difficult. Suctioning, tracheostomy, respiratory assistance, and fluid and electrolyte maintenance may be required.

6. Cholinergic crisis: Cholinergic crisis may result from overdosage of anticholinesterase drugs. The resulting weakness may be similar to that of myasthenia, and the muscarinic effects (diarrhea, sweating, lacrimation, miosis, bradycardia, hypotension) are often absent or difficult to evaluate. The edrophonium test may help to determine whether the patient is receiving too little of the drug or is manifesting toxic symptoms due to overdosage. Improvement after the drugs are withdrawn suggests cholinergic crisis. A respirator should be available. The patient may require atropine and tracheostomy.

C. Surgical Measures: Early thymectomy is beneficial in many patients whose disease is not confined to ocular symptoms; the effects may be delayed. Experienced surgical and postsurgical care are prerequisites.

Prognosis

Neonatal (transient) myasthenia presents a great threat to life, primarily due to aspiration of secretions. With proper treatment, the symptoms usually begin to disappear within a few days to 2–3 weeks, after which the child usually requires no further treatment.

In the congenital (persistent) form, the symptoms may initially be as acute as in the transient variety; more commonly, however, they are relatively benign and constant, with gradual worsening as the child grows older. Fatal cases occur.

In the juvenile form, patients may become resistant or unresponsive to anticholinesterase compounds and require corticosteroids or treatment in a hospital, where respiratory assistance can be given. The overall prognosis for survival, for remission, and for improvement after therapy with prednisone and thymectomy is favorable.

Death in myasthenic or cholinergic crisis may occur unless prompt treatment is given.

Engel AG: Myasthenia gravis and myasthenic syndromes: Neurologic progress. Ann Neurol 1984;16:519.

Gordon N: Congenital myasthenia. Dev Med Child Neurol 1986;28:810.

Lefvert AK, Osterman PO: Newborn infants to myasthenic mothers: A clinical study and investigation of acetylcholine receptor antibodies in 17 children. Neurology 1983;33:133.

Morel E et al: Neonatal myasthenia gravis: A new clinical and immunologic appraisal in 30 cases. Neurology 1988;38:138.

Pascuzzi RM, Coslett HB, Johns TR: Long-term corticosteroid treatment of myasthenia gravis: Report of 116 patients. Ann Neurol 1984;15:291.

Rodriguez M et al: Myasthenia gravis in children: Long-term follow-up. Ann Neurol 1983;13:504.

Snead OC et al: Juvenile myasthenia gravis. Neurology 1980;30:732.

PERIPHERAL NERVE PALSIES

1. FACIAL WEAKNESS

Facial asymmetry may be present at birth or may develop later, either suddenly or gradually, unilaterally or bilaterally. Nuclear or peripheral involvement of the facial nerves results in sagging or drooping of the mouth and inability to close one or both eyes, particularly when newborns and infants cry. Inability to wrinkle the forehead may be demonstrated in infants and young children by getting them to follow an object (light) moved vertically above the forehead. Loss of taste of the anterior two-thirds of the tongue on the involved side may be demonstrated in intelligent, cooperative children by age 4 or 5; playing with a younger child and the judicious use of a tongue blade may enable the physician to note whether the child's face puckers up when something sour (eg, lemon juice) is applied with a swab to the anterior tongue. Ability to wrinkle the forehead is preserved, owing to bilateral innervation, in supranuclear facial paralysis.

Injuries to the facial nerve at birth occur in 0.25–6.5% of consecutive live births. Forceps delivery is the cause in some cases; in others, the side of the face affected may have abutted in utero against the sacral prominence. Often, no cause can be established.

Acquired peripheral facial weakness (Bell's palsy) of sudden onset and unknown cause is common in children. It often follows a viral illness (postinfectious) or physical trauma (eg, cold). It may be a presenting sign of a disorder such as tumor, hypertension, infectious mononucleosis, or Guillain-Barré syndrome, usually diagnosable by the history, physical examination, and appropriate laboratory tests.

Bilateral facial weakness in early life may be due to agenesis of the affected muscles or to nuclear causes (part of Möbius' syndrome) or may even be familial. Myasthenia gravis, polyneuritis, and myotonic dystrophy must be considered.

"Asymmetric crying facies," in which one side of the lower lip depresses with crying (this is the normal side) and the other does not, is a common innocent congenital malformation inherited as an autosomal dominant. The defect in the parent (the asymmetry often improves with age) may be almost inapparent. Electromyography suggests congenital absence of the depressor anguli oris muscle of the lower lip. Forceps pressure is often erroneously incriminated as a cause of this innocent congenital anomaly. Occasionally, other major (eg, cardiac septal) congenital defects accompany the palsy.

In the vast majority of cases of isolated peripheral facial palsy—both those present at birth and those acquired later—improvement begins within 1–2 weeks, and near or total recovery of function is observed within 2 months. Methylcellulose drops, 1%, should be instilled into the eyes to protect the cornea during the day; at night, the lid should be taped down with cellophane tape. Upward massage of the face for 5–10 minutes three or four times a day may help maintain muscle tone. Prednisone therapy reduces the pain of Bell's palsy and promotes recovery of facial strength and reduction of motor synkinesis ("crocodile tears").

Faradic or galvanic stimulation of facial muscles is not advised.

In the few children with permanent and cosmetically disfiguring facial weakness, plastic surgical intervention at 6 years of age or older may be of benefit. New procedures, such as attachment of facial muscles to the temporal muscle or transplantation of cranial nerve XI, are being developed.

Adour KK: Current concepts in neurology: Diagnosis and management of facial paralysis. N Engl J Med 1982; 307:348.

Miller M, Hall J: Familial asymmetric crying facies. Am J Dis Child 1979;133:743.

Painter ML, Bergman I: Obstetrical trauma to the neonatal central and peripheral nervous system. Semin Perinatol 1982;6:89.

Reroque H et al: Möbius' syndrome and transposition of the great vessels. Neurology 1988;38:1894.

Sudarshan A, Goldie WD: The spectrum of congenital facial diplegia (Moebius syndrome). Pediatr Neurol 1985; 1:180.

CHRONIC POLYNEUROPATHY

Polyneuropathy, usually insidious in onset and slowly progressive, occurs in children of any age. The presenting complaints are chiefly disturbances of gait and easy fatigability in walking or running and, slightly less often, weakness or clumsiness of the hands. Pain, tenderness, or paresthesias are less frequently mentioned. Neurologic examination discloses muscular weakness, greatest in the distal portions of the extremities, with steppage gait and depressed or absent deep tendon reflexes. Cranial nerves are sometimes affected. Sensory deficits (difficult to demonstrate in fearful children or those under 5 years of age) occur in a stocking and glove distribution. The muscles may be tender, and trophic changes such as glassy or "parchment" skin and absent sweating may occur. Thickening of the ulnar and peroneal nerves may be felt. Pure sensory neuropathies show up as chronic trauma; that is, the patient does not feel minor trauma and burns to the fingers and toes.

Known causes include (1) toxins (lead, arsenic, mercurials, vincristine, and benzene); (2) systemic disorders (diabetes mellitus, chronic uremia, recurrent hypoglycemia, porphyria, polyarteritis nodosa, and lupus erythematosus); (3) "inflammatory" states (chronic or recurrent Guillain-Barré syndrome and neuritis associated with mumps or diphtheria); (4) hereditary, often degenerative conditions, which in some classifications include certain storage diseases, leukodystrophies, spinocerebellar degenerations with neurogenic components, and Bassen-Kornzweig syndrome (Table 23–25); and (5) hereditary sensory or combined motor and sensory neuropathies. Polyneuropathies associated with carcinomas, beriberi or other vitamin deficiencies, or excessive vitamin B_6 intake are not reported or are exceedingly rare in children.

The most common chronic neuropathy of insidious onset often has no identifiable cause. This "chronic idiopathic neuropathy" is assumed to be immunologically mediated and may have a relapsing course. Sometimes there is facial weakness. Spinal fluid protein is elevated. Nerve conduction is slowed, and nerve biopsies are abnormal. Immunologic abnormalities are seldom demonstrated, although nerve biopsies may show round cell infiltration. Corticosteroids and other immunosuppressants may give long-term benefit.

Of the four defined hereditary sensory neuropathies, the prototype is **familial dysautonomia**, also called Riley-Day syndrome and hereditary sensory neuropathy type III. Transmitted as an autosomal recessive trait and seen mostly in Jewish children, this disorder has its onset in infancy. It is characterized by vomiting and difficulties in feeding that are due to abnormal esophageal motility, pulmonary infections, decreased or absent tearing, indifference to pain, diminished or absent tendon reflexes, absence of fungiform papillae of the tongue, emotional lability, abnormal temperature control with excessive sweating, labile blood pressure, abnormal intradermal histamine responses, and other evidences of autonomic dysfunction.

A careful genetic history (pedigree) and examination and electrical testing (motor and sensory nerve conduction, electromyography) of relatives are keys to diagnosis of hereditary neuropathy. This is the most common cause of chronic neuropathy in children.

Other hereditary neuropathies may have ataxia as a prominent finding often overshadowing the neuropathy. Examples are Friedreich's ataxia, dominant cerebellar ataxia, and Marinesco-Sjögren's syndrome. Finally, some hereditary neuropathies are associated with identifiable and occasionally treatable metabolic errors (Table 23–26). These disorders are described in more detail in other sections.

Laboratory diagnosis of chronic polyneuropathy is made by measurement of motor and sensory nerve conduction velocities; electromyography may show a neurogenic polyphasic pattern. Cerebrospinal fluid protein levels are often elevated, sometimes with an increased IgG index as well. Nerve biopsy, with teasing of the fibers as well as staining for metachromasia, may demonstrate loss of myelin and (to a lesser degree) loss of axons and increased connective tissue or concentric lamellas ("onion skin" appearance) around the nerve fiber. Muscle biopsy may show the pattern associated with denervation. Other laboratory studies directed toward specific causes mentioned above include screening for heavy metals and for metabolic, renal, or vascular disorders. Chronic lead intoxication, which rarely causes neuropathy in childhood, may escape detection until the child is given edetate calcium disodium (EDTA) and lead levels are determined in timed urines.

Therapy is directed at specific disorders whenever possible. Occasionally, the weakness is profound and involves bulbar nerves, in which case tracheostomy and respiratory assistance are required. Corticosteroid therapy may be of considerable benefit in cases where the cause is unknown or neuropathy is considered to be due to "chronic inflammation" (this is not the case in acute Guillain-Barré syndrome). Prednisone, 1-2.5 mg/kg/d orally, with tapering to the lowest effective dose—discontinued if the process seems to be arresting and reinstituted when symptoms recur—is recommended. Prednisone should probably not be used for treatment of hereditary neuropathy (HMSN). In all cases considered for corticosteroid therapy, the risks and benefits should be carefully weighed. When treatment is available, symptoms regress and may disappear altogether over a period of months.

The long-term prognosis varies with the cause and

Table 23–26. Hereditary motor and sensory neuropathies; metabolic error unknown.

Name	Prototype Unknown	Inheritance	Clinical Features	Nerve Biopsy
Sensory and autonomic neuropathy	(1) Familial dysautonomia (2) Other	Autosomal recessive (AR) AR, ? autosomal dominant (AD)	See text Rare (see references)	(1) Decreased unmyelinated fibers posterior column and cord (2) Variable (see references)
HMSN I (if tremor is present, Roussy-Lévy syndrome) (60–90% of HMSN are type I)	"Classic" Charcot-Marie-Tooth (CMT) disease (1) CMT 1A (2) CMT 1B (3) CMT 1C	AD (1) Chromosome 17p11.2–12 duplication (2) Rare. Chromosome 1—linkage to Duffy blood group (3) No linkage yet	Onset 0–15 y. Weakness, atrophy of feet, calves (pes cavus, "stork legs"), hands. Sensory loss 0 or variable. Deep tendon reflexes (DTR) 0. MNCV slowed. Often hypertrophic (palpable) nerves. Linked to Duffy blood group.	Segmental demyelination.
HMSN II (10–30% of cases)	Neuronal/axonal Charcot-Marie-Tooth disease	AD	Less severe; onset 10–20. Leg cramps, numbness, MNCV normal or slightly slow. CSF protein often normal.	Axonal loss, secondary demyelination
HMSN III	Hypertrophic Charcot-Marie-Tooth disease; Déjérine-Sottas disease	AR	Onset in infancy. Severe. CSF protein increased. Very slow MNCV. Slowly progressive.	Hypertrophic ("onion bulb") interstitial changes
HMSN IV	Refsum disease		Severe sensory, mild motor. Thick nerves. CSF protein elevated. Ichthyosis, retinitis pigmentosa, ataxia, deafness. Urine phytanic acid.	See HMSN III
HMSN V	Charcot-Marie-Tooth disease with spastic paraparesis		Abnormal pyramidal tract findings. Rule out adrenomyelopathy.	Defined in pedigrees. Rule out adrenomyelopathy with LCFA.
HMSN VI, VII	Optic atrophy, retinitis pigmentosa, etc.		Poorly defined. Multiple systems involved.	See HMSN V

HMSN = hereditary motor and sensory neuropathy.
LCFA = long-chain fatty acids.
MNCV = motor nerve conduction velocities.

the ability to offer specific therapy. In the "corticosteroid-dependent" group, residual deficits and deaths within a few years are more frequent.

Axelrod FB, Pearson J: Congenital sensory neuropathies: Diagnostic distinction from familial dysautonomia. Am J Dis Child 1984;138:947.

Bird SJ, Slodky JT: Corticosteroid responsive dominant neuropathy in childhood. Neurology 1991;41:437.

Chance PF, Pleasure D: Charcot-Marie-Tooth syndrome. Arch Neurol 1993;50:1180.

Chatorian, AM: Chronic polyneuropathy in childhood. Int Pediatr 1988;3:125.

Dyck PJ et al: The 10 P's: A mnemonic helpful in characterization and differential diagnosis of peripheral neuropathy. Neurology 1992;42:14.

Evans OB: Polyneuropathy in childhood. Pediatrics 1979; 64:96.

Hagberg B: Polyneuropathies in paediatrics. Eur J Pediatr 1990;149:296.

Prensky AL, Dodson WE: The steroid treatment of hereditary motor and sensory neuropathy. Neuropediatrics 1984;15:203.

MISCELLANEOUS NEUROMUSCULAR DISORDERS

FLOPPY INFANT SYNDROME

Essentials of Diagnosis

- In early infancy, decreased muscular activity, both spontaneous and in response to postural reflex testing and to passive motion.

- In young infants, "frog posture" or other unusual positions at rest.
- In older infants, delay in motor milestones.

General Considerations

In the young infant, ventral suspension, ie, supporting the infant with a hand under the chest, normally results in the infant's holding its head slightly up (45 degrees or less), the back straight or nearly so, the arms flexed at the elbows and slightly abducted, and the knees partly flexed. The "floppy" infant droops over the hand like an inverted U. The normal newborn attempts to keep the head in the same plane as the body when pulled up from supine to sitting by the hands (traction response). Marked head lag is characteristic of the floppy infant. Hyperextensibility of the joints is not a dependable criterion.

The usual reasons for seeking medical evaluation in older infants are delays in walking, running, or climbing stairs or motor difficulties and lack of endurance.

Hypotonia or decreased motor activity is a frequent presenting complaint in neuromuscular disorders but may also accompany a variety of systemic conditions or may be due to certain disorders of connective tissue.

Clinical Types

A. Paralytic Group: There is significant lack of movement against gravity (eg, failure to kick the legs, hold up the arms, or attempt to stand when held) or in response to stimuli such as tickling or slight pain.

B. Nonparalytic Group: There is floppiness without significant paralysis.

Note: Deep tendon reflexes may be depressed or absent in the nonparalytic group also. Brisk reflexes with hypotonia point to suprasegmental or general cerebral dysfunction.

1. PARALYTIC GROUP

The hypotonic infant who is weak ("paralyzed") usually has a lesion of the lower motor neuron complex (Table 23–27). Infantile progressive spinal muscular atrophy (Werdnig-Hoffman disease) is the most common cause. Neuropathy is rare. Botulism and myasthenia gravis (rare) are neuromuscular junction causes. Myotonic dystrophy and rare myopathies (eg, central core myopathy) are muscle disease entities.

In anterior horn cell or muscle disease, weakness is proximal (shoulder and hips); finger movement is preserved. Tendon reflexes are absent or depressed; strength (to noxious stimuli) is decreased (paralytic). Intelligence is preserved. Fine motor, personal/social, and language milestones are normal, such as on a Denver Developmental Screening Test (DDST).

Table 23–27. Floppy infant: paralytic causes.

Disease	Genetic	Early Manifestations
IPSMA (Infantile Progressive Spinal Muscular Atrophy) "Malignant" form	Autosomal recessive (AR)	In utero movements decreased by one-third. Gradual weakness, delay in gross motor milestones. Weak cry. Abdominal breathing. Poor limb motion ("no kicking"). Deep tendon reflexes (DTR)—0. Fasciculations of tongue. Normal personal-social behavior.
"Intermediate" form	AR	Onset under age 1 usual. *Progression slower:* may be impossible to predict early course of IPSMA. Hand tremors common.
Infantile botulism	Acquired under age 1 (mostly under 6 months); botulism spore in stool makes toxin	Poor feeding. Constipation. Weak cry. Failure to thrive. Lethargy. Facial weakness, ptosis, ocular muscle palsy. Inability to suck, swallow. Apnea. Source: soil dust (outdoor construction workers may bring it home on clothes), honey.
Myasthenia gravis Neonatal transient	12% of infants born from a myasthenia mother	Floppiness. Poor sucking and feeding; choking. Respiratory distress. Weak cry.
Congenital persistent	Mother normal. Rare AR (AD)	As above; may improve and later exacerbate.
Myotonic dystrophy	Autosomal dominant (AD) (almost always *mother* transmits gene in neonatal/infant severe form)	Polyhydramnios; failure of suck, respirations. Facial diplegia. Ptosis. Arthrogryposis. Thin ribs. Later, developmental delay.
Neonatal "rare myopathy," severe variant Nemaline, central core, "minimal change," myotubular (centronuclear), reducing body	AR, AD	Virtually all of the rare myopathies may have a severe (even fatal) neonatal or early infant form. Clinical features similar in infancy to infantile myotonic dystrophy.
Congenital muscular dystrophy Fukayama	? Genetic ? infectious	Early onset. Facial weakness. Joint contractures. Severe mental retardation. Ill-defined.
Other		Severe or benign (improve). No mental retardation.
Essential hypotonia ("benign congenital hypotonia")	Unknown cause	Diagnosis of exclusion. Family history variable. Mild to moderate hypotonia with weakness.

Myopathies

The congenital, relatively nonprogressive myopathies, muscular dystrophy, myotonic dystrophy, polymyositis, and periodic paralysis are discussed elsewhere. Most cases of congenital or early infantile muscular dystrophy reported in the past probably represented congenital myopathies (Table 23–25). Congenital muscular dystrophy, diagnosed by muscle biopsy, occurs in two forms: (1) a benign form, with gradual improvement in strength; and (2) a severe form, in which there is either rapid progression of weakness and death in the first months or year of life or severe disability with little or no progression but lifelong marked limitation of activity.

Glycogenosis With Muscle Involvement

Glycogen storage diseases are described in Chapter 31. Patients with type II (Pompe's disease, due to a deficiency of acid maltase) are most likely to present as floppy infants. The weakness in type III (limit dextrinosis) is less marked than in type II, while the rare instances of type IV (amylopectinosis) are severely hypotonic. Muscle cramps on exertion or easy fatigability, rather than floppiness in infancy, is the presenting complaint in type V (McArdle's phosphorylase deficiency) or the glycogenosis due to phosphofructokinase deficiency or phosphohexose isomerase inhibition.

Myasthenia Gravis

Neonatal transient and congenital persistent myasthenia gravis, with patients presenting as "paralytic" floppy infants, is described elsewhere in this chapter.

Arthrogryposis Multiplex (Congenital Deformities About Multiple Joints)

This symptom complex, sometimes associated with hypotonia, may be of "neurogenic" or "myopathic" origin (or both) and may be associated with a wide variety of other anomalies. Orthopedic aspects are discussed in Chapter 24.

Spinal Cord Lesions

Severe limpness in newborns following breech extraction with stretching or actual tearing of the lower cervical to upper thoracic spinal cord is rarely seen today, owing to improved obstetric delivery. Klumpke's lower brachial plexus paralysis may be present; the abdomen is usually exceedingly soft, and the lower extremities are flaccid. Urinary retention is present initially; later, the bladder may function autonomously. Myelography or MRI scanning may define the lesion. After a few weeks, spasticity of the lower limbs becomes obvious. Treatment is symptomatic and consists of bladder and skin care and eventual mobilization on crutches or in a wheelchair.

2. NONPARALYTIC GROUP

The nonparalytic group often has "brain damage" (Table 23–28). Intrauterine or perinatal insults to brain or spinal cord, while sometimes difficult to document, are major causes. (Occasionally, severe congenital myopathies presenting in the newborn period cause confusion.) Persisting severe hypotonia is ominous. Tone will often vary. Spasticity and other forms of cerebral palsy may emerge; hypertonia and hypotonia may occur at varying times in the same infant. Choreoathetoid or ataxic movements and developmental delay can clarify the diagnosis. Reflexes are often increased; pathologic reflexes (Babinski, tonic neck) may persist or worsen.

The creatine kinase level and the EMG are usually normal. Prolonged nerve conduction velocities point to polyneuritis or leukodystrophy. Muscle biopsies, utilizing special stains and histographic analysis, often show a remarkable reduction in size of type II fibers associated with decreased voluntary motor activity.

Limpness in the neonatal period and early infancy and subsequent delay in achieving motor milestones are the presenting features in a large number of children with a variety of CNS disorders, including mental retardation, as in trisomy 21. In many such cases, no specific diagnosis can be made. Close observation and scoring of motor patterns and adaptive behavior, as by the DDST, are most helpful.

Crawford TO: Clinical evaluation of the floppy infant. Pediatr Ann 1992;21:348.

Dobyns WB: Classification of the cerebro-oculo-muscular syndrome(s). Brain Dev 1993;15:242.

Gay CT, Bodensteiner JB: The floppy infant: Recent advances in the understanding of disorders affecting the neuromuscular junction. Neurol Clin 1990;8:715.

Long SS: Botulism in infancy. Pediatr Infect Dis J 1984; 3:266.

Milu JM, Gilbert-Barnes E: Myotubular myopathy. Am J Dis Child 1993;147:905.

Thilo EK, Townsend SF, Deacon J: Infant botulism at 1 week of age: Report of two cases. Pediatrics 1993;92:151.

CEREBRAL PALSY

Essentials of Diagnosis

- Impairment of movement and posture since birth or early infancy.
- Nonprogressive and nonhereditary.

General Considerations

Cerebral palsy is a term of clinical convenience for disorders of impaired motor functioning and posture with onset before or at birth or during the first year of life, basically nonprogressive, and varying widely in their causes, manifestations, and prognosis.

Table 23–28. Floppy infant: nonparalytic causes.

	Causes	Manifestations
Central nervous system disorders		
Atonic diplegia ("prespastic diplegia")	Intrauterine, perinatal asphyxia, cord injury	Limpness, stupor; poor suck, cry, Moro reflex, grasp; later, irritability, increased tone and reflexes
Choreoathetosis	As above; kernicterus	Hypotonic early; movement disorder emerges later (6–18 months)
Ataxic cerebral palsy	Same	Same
Syndromes with hypotonia (CNS origin)		
Trisomy 21	Genetic	100% have hypotonia early
Prader-Willi syndrome	Genetic deletion 15q11	Hypotonia, hypomentia, hypogonadism, obesity
Marfan syndrome	AD[1]	Arachnodactyly
Dysautonomia	AR[1]	Respiratory, corneal anesthesia
Turner's syndrome	45 X, or mosaic	Somatic stigmata (Chapter 32)
Degenerative disorders		
Tay-Sachs	AR	Macular cherry-red spot
Metachromatic leukodystrophy	AR	Deep tendon reflexes increased early, polyneuropathy late; mental retardation
Systemic diseases		
Malnutrition	Deprivation, cystic fibrosis, celiac disease	See underlying disease elsewhere in text
Chronic illness	Congenital heart disease; chronic pulmonary disease (eg, bronchopulmonary dysplasia); uremic, renal acidosis	
Metabolic	Hypercalcemia, Lowe's disease	
Endocrine	Hypothyroid	

[1]AD = autosomal dominant
AR = autosomal recessive

The most obvious manifestation is impaired function of voluntary muscles. In the United States, cerebral palsy affects about 0.2% of neonatal survivors.

Classification

Classification is commonly based on the predominant motor deficit.

A. Spastic Forms: About 75% of cases. Often associated with other forms.

1. Quadriplegia (tetraplegia): The four extremities may be involved about equally, or upper limbs may show more severe involvement. The main lesion is in the cerebral white matter. Quadriplegia due to perinatal damage often shows symptoms earlier than that due to fetal undernutrition or prematurity. Nearly 90% of patients are profoundly retarded.

2. Diplegia: Legs involved more than arms.

3. Hemiplegia: One side involved primarily.

4. Paraplegia: Legs only involved.

5. Monoplegia: One extremity only involved.

6. Triplegia: Three extremities involved.

B. Ataxia: About 15% of cases. Pure and in combination with other forms.

C. Dyskinesia (Choreoathetosis): About 5% of cases. Often associated with rigidity or spastic quadriplegia or diplegia.

D. Hypotonic Form: Fewer than 1% of cases. Persistent hypotonia with variable degrees of weakness.

Etiology

The cause is often obscure or multifactorial. No definite etiologic diagnosis is possible in over one-third of cases. The incidence is high among infants small for gestational age. Intrauterine hypoxia is a frequent cause. Other known causes are intrauterine bleeding, infections, toxins, congenital malformations, obstetric complications (including birth hypoxia), neonatal infections, kernicterus, neonatal hypoglycemia, acidosis, and a small number of genetic syndromes (about 2%).

Associated Deficits

A. Seizures: Seizures afflict about 50% of all children with cerebral palsy and are more prevalent in those with severe involvement.

B. Mental Retardation: Mild to moderate retardation is seen in 26% of patients and profound retardation in 27%. The incidence is correlated with the severity of cerebral palsy.

C. Sensory & Speech Deficits: Impairment of speech, vision, hearing, and perceptual functions is found often in varying degrees and combinations.

Clinical Findings

A. Symptoms & Signs: The typical spastic child exhibits muscular hypertonicity of the clasp-knife type that may eventually end in contractures. In the limb or limbs involved, tendon reflexes, if sufficient muscle relaxation can be achieved, are hyperactive; clonus may be present, and the plantar responses are often extensor. Although voluntary control, especially of fine movements, is decreased, there is spread or overflow of associated movements. In extreme cases, the child may lie with elbows flexed and fists clenched ("straphanger's posture") and legs crossed or scissored. In early infancy, the child may appear floppy, although tendon jerks are abnormally increased (hypotonic, atonic, or prespastic diplegia). Rigidity often accompanies cerebral palsy.

Ataxia may be difficult to delineate in the presence of spasticity or hyperkinetic movements.

Microcephaly (head circumference 2 SD below the mean for age and sex and decreasing) is present in about 25% of spastic quadriplegics and diplegics. Partial atrophy of the cranium on the involved side or of involved extremities is observed frequently.

A smaller hand or foot, when combined with mild weakness on muscle testing or hyperreflexia, often justifies a diagnosis of mild cerebral palsy of which the patient or the family may not even have been aware. Occasionally, multiple minor malformations suggest an intrauterine origin.

B. Laboratory & Other Findings: No routine workup can be outlined. The clinical findings, the presence or absence of seizures, and the overall outlook for the child—particularly with respect to intelligence and the ability to carry on activities of daily living—determine what studies should be performed. Hip films in abduction are indicated to rule out dislocations secondary to spasticity. Electroencephalography is indicated when seizures are present or suspected. MRI scans may be helpful in determining timing of insult or malformation, eg, prenatal-intrauterine or perinatal.

Urine screening tests for amino and organic acidurias are indicated. In choreoathetosis with self-injury, serum uric acid determinations should be considered to rule out Lesch-Nyhan syndrome. Macrocephaly and dystonia suggest glutaricaciduria (organic acid).

Differential Diagnosis

The diagnosis is usually not difficult. Progressive deterioration in the first 3 months is more likely to denote a metabolic disorder; subsequently, it denotes one of the CNS degenerative disorders (Tables 23–21 and 23–22). In the ataxic form, cerebellar dysgenesis (sometimes familial) or a spinocerebellar degeneration may have to be ruled out.

Prevention

Obstetric advances in late third-trimester management and delivery have resulted in less cerebral palsy. Much more needs to be done in prenatal care, especially during the second and early third trimester. Examples are maternal counseling to avoid cocaine and alcohol abuse and earlier detection of hypertensive disorders of pregnancy. The number of cases in which cerebral palsy is associated with aggressive efforts to salvage premature infants has decreased as a result of advances in neonatal care.

Treatment

Realistically, a child with cerebral palsy should be helped to achieve maximum potential rather than "normality." Special educational programming depends on the physical and mental potential of the child. The degree of improvement with physical therapy correlates positively with better intelligence. Treat seizures in the same way as those occurring in other children. The orthopedic aspects of cerebral palsy are discussed in Chapter 24.

Spasticity occasionally is reduced by diazepam or baclofen. Optimal doses vary according to the degree of spasticity, the size and age of the child, and other medications taken. Surgical amelioration of moderate to severe spasticity in cerebral palsy has been attempted by various procedures over many years; dorsal rhizotomy is the newest procedure.

Management of "hyperactivity" is dealt with in Chapter 6 in connection with attention deficit hyperactivity disorder.

Psychologic counseling and support of the child and family are of paramount importance.

Prognosis

In patients with severe cerebral palsy, especially spastics with profound retardation and seizures that are difficult to control, death due to intercurrent infections is not uncommon; nearly 50% die by 10 years of age. In nearly 30% of patients, chiefly in those with mild involvement, motor deficits resolve by the seventh birthday. Many children with cerebral palsy and average or near-average intelligence lead fairly normal, satisfying, and productive lives.

Bhushan V, Paneth N, Kiely JL: Impact of improved survival of very low birth weight infants on recent secular trends in the prevalence of cerebral palsy. Pediatrics 1993;96:1094.

Coorssen EA, Msall ME, Duffy LC: Multiple minor malformations as a marker for prenatal etiology of cerebral palsy. Dev Med Child Neurol 1991;33:730.

Freeman JM, Nelson BL: Intrapartum asphyxia and cerebral palsy. Pediatrics 1988;82:240.

Hendricks-Ferguson VL, Ortman MR: Selective dorsal rhizotomy to decrease spasticity in cerebral palsy. AORN J 1995;61(3):514, 521, 525.

Hughes I, Newton R: Genetic aspects of cerebral palsy. Dev Med Child Neurol 1992;34:80.

Kuban KCK, Leviton A: Cerebral palsy. N Engl J Med 1994;330:1888.

Molnar GE: Rehabilitation medicine, adding life to years: Rehabilitation in cerebral palsy. West J Med 1991;154:569.

Nelson KB: What proportion of cerebral palsy is related to birth asphyxia? (Editorial.) J Pediatr 1988;112:572.

Palmer FB et al: The effects of physical therapy on cerebral palsy: A controlled trial in infants with spastic diplegia. N Engl J Med 1988;318:803.

Rosenbloom L: Diagnosis and management of cerebral palsy. Arch Dis Childhood 1995;72(4):350.

Scheuerle AE et al: Arginase deficiency presenting as cerebral palsy. Pediatrics 1993;91:995.

Volpe JJ: Brain injury in the premature infant: Current concepts of pathogenesis and prevention. Biol Neonate 1992;62:231.

Volpe JJ: Value of MR in definition of the neuropathology of cerebral palsy in vivo. AJNR Am J Neuroradiol 199 1992;13:79.

REFERENCES

Aicardi J: *Diseases of the Nervous System in Childhood.* MacKeith Press, 1992.

Dodson WE, Pellock JM: *Pediatric Epilepsy: Diagnosis and Therapy.* Demos, Inc., 1993.

Guilleminault C: *Sleep and Its Disorders in Children.* Raven Press, 1987.

Holmes GL: *Diagnosis and Management of Seizures in Childhood.* Saunders, 1987.

Illingworth RS: *The Development of the Infant and Young Child: Normal and Abnormal,* 8th ed. Churchill Livingstone, 1983.

Menkes JH: *Textbook of Child Neurology,* 5th ed. Williams & Wilkins, 1995.

Plum F, Posner J: *The Diagnosis of Stupor and Coma,* 3rd ed. Davis, 1980.

Shinnar S, Amir N, Branski D: *Childhood Seizures: Pediatric and Adolescent Medicine,* vol. 6. S Karger, 1995.

Swaiman KF: *Pediatric Neurology: Principles and Practice,* vols 1 and 2. Mosby, 1994.

Volpe JJ: *Neurology of the Newborn,* 3rd ed. Saunders, 1995.

24

Orthopedics

Robert E. Eilert, MD, & Gaia Georgopoulos, MD

Orthopedics is the medical discipline that deals with disorders of neuromuscular and skeletal systems. Patients with orthopedic problems usually present with pain, loss of function, or deformity. Their symptoms must be considered not only in terms of the bones and joints but also in a more general sense relating to the anatomy, particularly of the extremities, and the blood vessels, skin, nerves, tendons, and muscles. The physical examination is the most important feature of orthopedic diagnosis and depends upon an intimate knowledge of human anatomy.

DISTURBANCES OF PRENATAL ORIGIN

CONGENITAL AMPUTATIONS

Congenital amputations may be due to teratogens (eg, drugs or viruses), amniotic bands, or metabolic diseases (eg, diabetes in the mother). Rarely, they are genetically determined. The history of the pregnancy must be reviewed in a search for possible teratogenic factors. There is a 30% incidence of multiple limb involvement, and children with congenital limb deficiencies also have a high incidence of associated congenital anomalies, including genitourinary and cardiac defects and cleft palates. According to the currently accepted international classification, amputations are either terminal or longitudinal. In terminal amputation, all parts are missing distal to the level of involvement—such as absence of the forearm, wrist, and hand in the case of a terminal below-the-elbow amputation. A longitudinal amputation consists of partial absence of structures in the extremity along one side or the other. In radial clubhand, the entire radius is absent, but the thumb may be either hypoplastic or completely absent; that is, the effect on structures distal to the amputation may vary. Complex tissue defects are nearly always associated with longitudinal amputations in that the associated nerves and muscles are usually not completely represented when a bone is absent.

Terminal amputations are treated by prosthesis, such as to compensate for shortness of one leg. With longitudinal deficiencies, reconstructive surgery may reduce deformity and stabilize joints. In certain types of severe anomalies, operative treatment is indicated to remove a portion of the malformed foot so that a prosthesis can be fitted early. This applies to such anomalies as congenital absence of the fibula, which is the lower extremity bone most commonly congenitally absent. Fortunately, there is rarely a problem with tenting of the skin by relative overgrowth of bone within the stump in congenital amputations.

Lower extremity prostheses are best fitted between 12 and 15 months of age when walking starts. They are consistently well accepted, since they are necessary for balancing and walking. Upper extremity prostheses are not as well accepted. Fitting the child with a dummy-type prosthesis as early as 6 months of age has the advantage of instilling an accustomed pattern of proper length and bimanual manipulation. Children fitted later than age 2 years nearly always reject upper extremity prostheses.

Children quickly learn how to function with their prostheses and can lead active lives, participating in sports with peers.

Choi DH, Kumar SJ, Bowen JR: Amputation or limb lengthening for partial or total absence of the fibula. J Bone Joint Surg [Am] 1990;72:1391.

Miller LS, Bell DF: Management of congenital fibular deficiency by Slizarov techniques. J Pediatr Orthop 1992;12:651.

Swanson AB, Swanson GD, Tada K: A classification of congenital limb malformation. J Hand Surg [Am] 1983; 8:693.

DEFORMITIES OF THE EXTREMITIES

1. METATARSUS VARUS

Metatarsus varus is a common congenital foot deformity characterized by inward deviation of the forepart of the foot. The longitudinal arch is often creased vertically when the deformity is more rigid. The lateral border of the foot demonstrates sharp angulation at the level of the base of the fifth metatarsal, and this bone will be especially prominent. The deformity varies from flexible to rigid. Most flexible deformities are secondary to intrauterine posture and usually resolve spontaneously. Several investigators have noticed a relationship between metatarsus varus and hip dysplasia, an incidence of 10–15%. The hips in these children should be very carefully checked.

If the deformity is rigid and cannot be manipulated past the midline, it is worthwhile to use a plaster cast changed at intervals of 2 weeks to correct the deformity. "Corrective" shoes do not live up to their name, although they can be used to maintain correction obtained by casting.

The prognosis for this common deformity of the foot is excellent, and few long-term problems are reported. If the deformity persists, the child will exhibit an in-toed gait and may have some problems with shoe wear secondary to the prominence of the base of the fifth metatarsal.

Bleck EE: Metatarsus adductus: Classification and relationship to outcomes of treatment. J Pediatr Orthop 1983; 3:2.

Rushforth GF: The natural history of the hooked forefoot. J Bone Joint Surg [Br] 1978;60:530.

2. CLUBFOOT
(Talipes Equinovarus)

The diagnosis of classic talipes equinovarus, or clubfoot, requires three features: (1) equinus or plantar flexion of the foot at the ankle joint, (2) varus or inversion deformity of the heel, and (3) forefoot varus. The incidence of talipes equinovarus is approximately 1:1000 live births. There are three major categories of clubfoot: (1) idiopathic; (2) neurogenic; and (3) those associated with syndromes, such as arthrogryposis and Larsen's syndrome. Any infant with a clubfoot should be examined carefully for associated anomalies, especially of the spine. Idiopathic clubfeet are hereditary in some families.

Treatment consists of manipulation of the foot to stretch the contracted tissues on the medial and posterior aspects, followed by splinting to hold the correction. When this treatment is instituted shortly after birth, correction is rapid. When treatment is delayed, the foot tends to become more rigid within a matter of days. Treatment in the nursery by strapping and splinting is often effective. As the child gets older, casting following manipulation and stretching is necessary. The casts are applied sequentially, correcting first the forefoot adduction, then the inversion of the heel, and finally the equinus of the ankle. After full correction is obtained, a night brace is often prescribed for long-term maintenance of correction. Treatment by means of casting requires patience and experience; if it is not done properly in sequence, iatrogenic deformities of the foot may result, such as rocker-bottom foot.

About 50% of children with clubfoot eventually need an operative procedure to lengthen the tightened structures about the foot. A supple foot that is easily corrected by strapping and casting has a more favorable prognosis. If the foot is rigid and requires prolonged treatment to obtain correction, perhaps combined with surgery, the prognosis must be guarded.

Howard CB: Clubfoot: Its pathological anatomy. J Pediatr Orthop 1993;13:654.

Ikeda K: Conservative treatment of idiopathic clubfoot. J Pediatr Orthop 1992;12:217.

3. CONGENITAL DYSPLASIA OF THE HIP JOINT (Developmental Dislocation of the Hip)

Developmental dysplasia of the hip encompasses a spectrum of conditions in which there is an abnormal relationship between the proximal femur and the acetabulum. In the most severe condition, the femoral head is located completely outside the acetabulum; the hip may be either reducible or irreducible. This most severe condition is termed a dislocated hip. A dislocatable hip is one in which the hip is within the socket but can be dislocated with a provocative (Barley) maneuver. A subluxatable hip is one in which the femoral head comes partially out of the joint with a provocative maneuver. In acetabular dysplasia, the acetabulum is shallower than normal.

Developmental dysplasia of the hip occurs in approximately 1:1000 live births. At birth, there is lack of the development of both the acetabulum and the femur in cases of congenital hip dysplasia. The dysplasia becomes progressive with growth unless the dislocation is corrected. If the dislocation is corrected in the first few days or weeks of life, the dysplasia is completely reversible and a normal hip will develop. As the child becomes older and the dislocation or subluxation persists, the deformity will worsen to the point where it will not be completely reversible, especially after the walking age. For this reason, it is important to diagnose the deformity in the nursery or, at the latest, the 6-week checkup.

Clinical Findings

The diagnosis of developmental hip dislocation in

the newborn depends upon demonstrating instability of the joint by placing the infant on the back and obtaining complete relaxation by feeding with a bottle if necessary. The examiner's long finger is then placed over the greater trochanter and the thumb over the inner side of the thigh. Both hips are flexed 90 degrees and then slowly abducted from the midline, one hip at a time. With gentle pressure, an attempt is made to lift the greater trochanter forward. A feeling of slipping as the head relocates is a sign of instability (as first described by Ortolani). In other infants, the joint is more stable, and the deformity must be provoked by applying slight pressure with the thumb on the medial side of the thigh as the thigh is adducted, thus slipping the hip posteriorly and eliciting a jerk as the hip dislocates. This sign was first described by Barlow. The signs of instability are the most reliable criteria for diagnosing congenital dislocation of the hip in the newborn. X-rays of the pelvis are notoriously unreliable until about 6 weeks of age; however, ultrasonography has recently been used in both screening for and confirmation of developmental dysplasia. Asymmetric skinfolds are present in about 40% of newborns and therefore are not particularly helpful.

After the first month of life, the signs of instability as demonstrated by Ortolani's test or Barlow's test become less evident. Contractures begin to develop about the hip joint, causing limitation of abduction. Normally, the hip should abduct fully to 90 degrees on either side during the first few months of life. It is important that the pelvis be held level to detect asymmetry of abduction. When the hips and knees are flexed, the knees are at unequal heights, with the dislocated side lower (Allis's sign). After the first few weeks of life, x-ray examination becomes more valuable, with lateral displacement of the femoral head being the most reliable sign. In mild cases, the only abnormality may be increased steepness of acetabular alignment, so that the acetabular angle is greater than 35 degrees.

If congenital dislocation of the hip has not been diagnosed during the first year of life and the child begins to walk, there will be a painless limp and a lurch to the affected side. When the child stands on the affected leg, there is a dip of the pelvis on the opposite side owing to weakness of the gluteus medius muscle. This is called Trendelenburg's sign and accounts for the unusual swaying gait. In children with bilateral dislocations, the loss of abduction is almost symmetric and may be deceiving. Abduction, however, is never complete, and x-ray of the pelvis is indicated in children with incomplete abduction in the first few months of life. As a child with bilateral dislocation of the hips begins to walk, the gait is waddling. The perineum is widened as a result of lateral displacement of the hips, and there is flexion contracture as a result of posterior displacement of the hips. This flexion contracture contributes to marked lumbar lordosis, and the greater trochanters are easily palpable in their elevated position. Treatment is still possible in the first 2 years of life, but the results are not nearly as effective as in children treated in the nursery.

Treatment

Dislocation or dysplasia diagnosed in the first few weeks or months of life can easily be treated by splinting, with the hip maintained in flexion and abduction. Full abduction is contraindicated, since this often leads to avascular necrosis of the femoral head. The use of double or triple diapers is never indicated for medical reasons, because diapers are not adequate to obtain proper positioning of the hip. In cases of joint laxity without true dislocation, improvement will be spontaneous; diapers are excessive treatment.

Various splints to maintain flexion and abduction of the hip, such as the ones designed by Pavlik, Ilfeld, or von Rosen, are available. Treatment of children requiring splints is best supervised by an orthopedic surgeon with a special interest in the problem.

In the first 4 months of life, reduction can be obtained by simply flexing and abducting the hip; no other manipulation is usually necessary. If force is used to reduce the hip, the excessive pressure may cause avascular necrosis. In such cases, preoperative traction for 2–3 weeks is important to relax soft tissues about the hip. Following traction in which the femur is brought down opposite the acetabulum, reduction can be easily achieved without force under general anesthesia. It is then necessary to place the child in a plaster cast for approximately 6 months. The position in the cast should be carefully adjusted in order to avoid stretching of the delicate blood supply to the femoral head. The hip is flexed slightly more than 90 degrees and abducted only 45–60 degrees. Internal rotation is avoided, because this tends to "wring out" the blood vessels in the capsule of the joint. If the reduction is not stable within a reasonable range following closed reduction, open reduction, combined with tightening of the lax capsule in order to maintain reduction, may be necessary.

If reduction is done at an older age, operations to correct the deformities of the acetabulum and femur may be necessary during growth.

Anderson JE, Funnemark P: Neonatal hip instability: Screening with anterior dynamic ultrasound method. J Pediatr Orthop 1995;15:322.

Ando A, Gotoh E: Significance of inguinal folds for diagnosis of congenital dislocation of the hip in infants aged three to four months. J Pediatr Orthop 1990;10:331.

Forlin E et al: Prognostic factors in congenital dislocation of the hip treated with closed reduction: The importance of arthrographic evaluation. J Bone Joint Surg [Am] 1992;74:1140.

Hensinger RN: Congenital dislocation of the hip: Treatment in infancy to walking age. Orthop Clin North Am 1987;18:597.

Viere RG, Birch JG, Herring JA: Use of the Pavlik harness in congenital dislocation of the hip: An analysis of failure of treatment. J Bone Joint Surg [Am] 1990;72:238.

Yngve D, Gross R: Late diagnosis of hip dislocation in infants. J Pediatr Orthop 1990;10:777.

4. TORTICOLLIS

Wryneck deformities in infancy may be due either to injury to the sternocleidomastoid muscle during delivery or to disease affecting the cervical spine. In the case of muscular deformity, the chin is rotated to the side opposite to the affected sternocleidomastoid muscle contracture, and the head is tilted toward the side of the contracture. A mass felt in the midportion of the sternocleidomastoid muscle is not a true tumor but fibrous transformation within the muscle.

In mild cases, passive stretching is usually effective. If the deformity has not been corrected by passive stretching within the first year of life, surgical division of the muscle will correct it. It is not necessary to excise the "tumor" of the sternocleidomastoid muscle, because this tends to resolve spontaneously. If the deformity is left untreated, an unsightly facial asymmetry will result.

Torticollis is occasionally associated with congenital deformities of the cervical spine, and x-rays of the spine are indicated in all cases. In addition, there is a 20% incidence of hip dysplasia.

Acute torticollis may follow upper respiratory infection or mild trauma in children. Rotatory subluxation of the upper cervical spine should be sought by appropriate x-ray views. Traction or a cervical collar usually results in resolution of the symptoms within 1 or 2 days. Other causes of torticollis include spinal cord or cerebellar tumors, syringomyelia, and rheumatoid arthritis.

Davids JR, Wenger DR, Meebarek SJ: Congenital muscular torticollis: Sequela of intrauterine or perinatal compartment syndrome. J Pediatr Orthop 1993;13:141.

Phillips WA, Hensiger RN: The management of rotary atlanto-axial subluxation in children. J Bone Joint Surg [Am] 1989;71:664.

GENERALIZED AFFECTIONS OF SKELETAL OR MESODERMAL TISSUES

1. ARTHROGRYPOSIS MULTIPLEX CONGENITA
(Amyoplasia Congenita)

Arthrogryposis multiplex congenita consists of incomplete fibrous ankylosis (usually symmetric) of many or all joints of the body. There may be contractures either in flexion or extension. Upper extremity deformities usually consist of adduction of the shoulders, extension of the elbows, flexion of the wrists, and stiff, straight fingers with poor muscle control of the thumbs. In the lower extremities, common deformities are dislocation of the hips, extension of the knees, and severe clubfoot. The joints are fusiform and the joint capsules decreased in volume, producing contractures. Various investigations have attributed the basic defect to an abnormality of muscle or of the lower motor neuron. Muscular development is poor, and muscles may be represented only by fibrous bands. The joint deformities appear to be secondary to a lack of active motion during intrauterine development.

Passive mobilization of joints should be done early. Because of poor muscle control, however, joint mobility cannot be maintained by active motion. Prolonged casting for correction of deformities is contraindicated in these children because further stiffness is often produced. Use of removable splints combined with vigorous therapy is the most effective conservative treatment. Surgical release of the affected joints is often necessary. The clubfoot associated with arthrogryposis is very stiff and nearly always requires an operation. Surgery about the knees, including capsulotomy, osteotomy, and tendon lengthening, is used to correct deformity. In the young child, a single vigorous attempt at reduction of the dislocated hip is worthwhile. Multiple operative procedures about the hip are contraindicated because further stiffness may be produced with consequent impairment of motion. The dislocation of the hip that occurs in arthrogryposis is associated with severe dysplasia of the bones and does not respond to treatment as ordinary congenital hip dislocation does. Affected children are often able to walk with bilateral dislocation of the hips, and in cases of severe rigidity it is better to leave the hips out of joint. The long-term disability is not as severe as it would be in a person with normal mobility and strength.

The long-term prognosis for physical and vocational independence is poor. Patients usually have normal intelligence, but they have such severe physical restrictions that gainful employment is hard to find.

Sarwark JF et al: Amyoplasia: A common form of arthrogryposis. J Bone Joint Surg [Am] 1990;72:465.

Shapiro F et al: The diagnosis and orthopaedic treatment of childhood muscular atrophy, peripheral neuropathy, Friedreich's ataxia and arthrogryposis. J Bone Joint Surg (Am) 1993;75:1699.

2. MARFAN'S SYNDROME

Marfan's syndrome is a connective tissue disorder characterized by unusually long fingers and toes (arachnodactyly); hypermobility of the joints; subluxation of the ocular lenses; other eye abnormalities including cataract, coloboma, megalocornea, strabismus, and nystagmus; a high-arched palate; a strong tendency to scoliosis; pectus carinatum; and thoracic aortic aneurysms due to weakness of the media of the vessels. Serum mucoproteins may be decreased and urinary excretion of hydroxyproline increased. The condition is easily confused with homocystinuria, since the phenotypic presentation is identical. The two diseases may be differentiated by the presence of homocystine in the urine in homocystinuria.

Treatment is usually supportive for associated problems such as flatfoot. Scoliosis may involve more vigorous treatment by bracing or spine fusion. The long-term prognosis has improved for patients because better treatment for their aortic aneurysms has been devised.

Joseph KN et al: Orthopaedic aspects of the Marfan phenotype. Clin Orthop 1992;277:251.

3. KLIPPEL-FEIL SYNDROME

Klippel-Feil syndrome is characterized by fusion of some or all of the cervical vertebrae. Multiple spinal anomalies may be present, with hemivertebrae and scoliosis. The neck is short and stiff, the hairline is low, and the ears are often low-set. Common associated defects include congenital scoliosis, cervical rib, spina bifida, torticollis, web neck, high scapula, renal anomalies, and deafness. Examination of the urinary tract by urinalysis, and renal ultrasound is indicated as well as a hearing test.

Scoliotic deformities, if progressive, may require treatment. Occasionally, it is necessary to correct the high scapula, also called **Sprengel's deformity.**

Guilde JT et al: The natural history of Klippel-Feil syndrome: Clinical roentgenographic and magnetic resonance imaging findings at adulthood. J Pediatr Orthop 1995;15:617.

4. SPRENGEL'S DEFORMITY

Sprengel's deformity is a congenital condition in which one or both scapulas are elevated and small. The child cannot raise the arm completely on the affected side, and torticollis may be present. The deformity occurs alone or may be associated with Klippel-Feil syndrome.

If the deformity is functionally limiting, the scapula may be surgically relocated lower in the thorax. Excision of the upper portion of the scapula improves cosmetic appearance but has little effect on function.

Leibovic SJ et al: Sprengel deformity. J Bone Joint Surg [Am] 1990;72:192.

5. OSTEOGENESIS IMPERFECTA

Osteogenesis imperfecta is a rare, mainly dominantly inherited connective tissue disease characterized by multiple and recurrent fractures. The severe fetal type (osteogenesis imperfecta congenita) is characterized by multiple intrauterine or perinatal fractures. Affected children continue to have fractures and are dwarfed as a result of bony deformities and growth retardation. Intelligence is not affected. The shafts of the long bones are reduced in cortical thickness, and wormian bones are present in the skull. Other features include blue sclerae, thin skin, hyperextensibility of ligaments, "otosclerosis" with significant hearing loss, and hypoplastic and deformed teeth. Recurrent epistaxis, easy bruisability, mild hyperpyrexia (which may increase significantly during anesthesia), and excessive diaphoresis are common. In the tarda type, fractures begin to occur at variable times after the perinatal period, resulting in relatively fewer fractures and deformities in these cases. Affected patients are sometimes suspected of having suffered induced fractures, and the condition should be ruled out in any case of nonaccidental trauma.

Metabolic defects include elevated serum pyrophosphate, decreased platelet aggregation, and decreased incorporation of sulfate into acid mucopolysaccharides by skin fibroblasts. Normal parents can be counseled that the likelihood of a second affected child is negligible.

There is no effective treatment by medication. Surgical treatment involves correction of deformity of the long bones. Multiple intramedullary rods have been used to prevent deformity from poor healing of fractures.

The overall prognosis is poor, and patients are often confined to wheelchairs during adulthood.

Cole WG: Etiology and pathogenesis of heritable connective tissue diseases. J Pediatr Orthop 1993;13:392.
Dent JA, Patterson CR: Fractures in early childhood: Osteogenesis imperfecta or child abuse. J Pediatr Orthop 1991;11:184.
Hanscom DA et al: Osteogenesis imperfecta. J Bone Joint Surg [Am] 1992;74:598.

6. OSTEOPETROSIS (Osteitis Condensans Generalisata; Marble Bone Disease; Albers-Schönberg Disease)

Osteopetrosis is an unusual disorder of osteoclastic resorption of bone resulting in abnormally dense bones. The marrow spaces are smaller, resulting in anemia. There are two types—a milder autosomal dominant type and a more malignant type inherited as an autosomal recessive trait. The findings may appear at any age. On x-ray examination, the bones show increased density, transverse bands in the shafts, clubbing of ends, and vertical striations of long bones. There is thickening about the cranial foramina, and there may be heterotopic calcification of soft tissues. Treatment with corticosteroids to ameliorate the hematologic abnormalities should be tried.

The autosomal recessive form of osteopetrosis has recently been successfully treated by allogeneic bone marrow transplantation.

Kaplan FS, August CS, Fallon MD: Successful treatment of infantile malignant osteopetrosis by bone marrow transplantation: A case report. J Bone Joint Surg [Am] 1988;70:617.

7. ACHONDROPLASIA
(Classic Chondrodystrophy)

Achondroplasia is the most common form of short-limbed dwarfism. The upper arms and thighs are proportionately shorter than the forearms and legs. Findings frequently include bowing of the extremities, a waddling gait, limitation of motion of major joints, relaxation of the ligaments, short stubby fingers of almost equal length, frontal bossing, moderate hydrocephalus, depressed nasal bridge, and lumbar lordosis. Mentality and sexual function are normal. The disorder is transmitted as an autosomal dominant trait, but 80% of cases result from a random mutation. X-rays demonstrate short, thick tubular bones and irregular epiphysial plates. The ends of the bones are thick, with broadening and cupping. Epiphysial ossification may be delayed.

Osteotomies of the long bones are occasionally necessary if deformities are severe.

The spinal canal is narrowed, so that herniated disk in adulthood may lead to acute paraplegia.

Beals RK, Horton W: Skeletal dysplasias: An approach to diagnosis. J Am Acad Orthop Surg 1995;3:174.

8. OSTEOCHONDRODYSTROPHY
(Morquio's Disease)

Morquio's disease is an autosomal recessive disorder of mucopolysaccharide storage. Skeletal abnormalities include shortening of the spine, kyphosis, scoliosis, shortened extremities, pectus carinatum, genu valgum, and a hypoplastic odontoid with atlantoaxial instability. The child may appear normal at birth but begins to develop deformities between 1 and 4 years of age as a result of abnormal deposition of mucopolysaccharides.

X-rays demonstrate wedge-shaped flattened vertebrae and irregular, malformed epiphyses. The ribs are broad and have been likened to canoe paddles. The lower extremities are more severely involved than the upper ones.

There is no treatment, and the prognosis is poor, although many individuals survive into adulthood. Progressive clouding of the cornea leads to increasing visual impairment.

GROWTH DISTURBANCES OF THE MUSCULOSKELETAL SYSTEM

SCOLIOSIS

The term **scoliosis** denotes lateral curvature of the spine, which is always associated with some rotation of the involved vertebrae. Scoliosis is classified by its anatomic location, in either the thoracic or lumbar spine, with rare involvement of the cervical spine. The convexity of the curve is designated right or left. Thus, a right thoracic scoliosis would denote a thoracic curve in which the convexity is to the right; this is the most common type of idiopathic curve. Posterior curvature of the spine (kyphosis) is normal in the thoracic area, although excessive curvature may become pathologic. Anterior curvature is called **lordosis** and is normal in the lumbar and cervical spines. Idiopathic scoliosis generally begins at about 8 or 10 years of age and progresses during growth. In rare instances, infantile scoliosis may be seen in children 2 years of age or less.

Idiopathic scoliosis is about four or five times more common in girls than in boys. The disorder is usually asymptomatic in the adolescent years, but severe curvature may lead to impairment of pulmonary function in later years. It is important to examine the back of any adolescent coming in for a routine physical examination in order to identify scoliosis early. The examination is performed by having the patient bend forward 90 degrees with the hands joined in the midline. An abnormal finding consists of asymmetry of the height of the ribs or paravertebral muscles on one side, indicating rotation of the trunk associated with lateral curvature.

Diseases that may be associated with scoliosis include neurofibromatosis, Marfan's syndrome, cerebral palsy, muscular dystrophy, poliomyelitis, and myelodysplasia. Neurologic examination should be performed in all children with scoliosis to determine whether these disorders are present.

Five to 7% of cases of scoliosis are due to congenital vertebral anomalies such as a hemivertebral or unilateral vertebral bridge. These curves are more rigid than the more common idiopathic curve (see below) and will often increase with growth, especially during adolescence.

Eighty percent of scoliosis is idiopathic. Since 30% of family members are also affected, siblings of an affected child should be examined.

Idiopathic infantile scoliosis, occurring in children 2–4 years of age, is quite uncommon in the United States; it is more common in Great Britain. If the curvature is less than 30 degrees, the prognosis is excellent, as 70% resolve spontaneously. If the curvature is more than 30 degrees, there may be progression, and the prognosis is therefore guarded.

Postural compensation of the spine may lead to lateral curvature from such causes as unequal length of the lower extremities. Sciatic scoliosis may result from pressure on the spinal cord or roots by infectious processes or herniation of the nucleus pulposus; the underlying cause must be sought. The curvature will resolve as the primary problem is treated.

Clinical Findings

A. Symptoms & Signs: Scoliosis in adolescents is classically asymptomatic. It is imperative to seek the underlying cause in any case where there is pain, since in these instances the scoliosis is almost always secondary to some other disorder such as a bone or spinal cord tumor. Deformity of the rib cage and asymmetry of the waistline are evident with curvatures of 30 degrees or more. A lesser curvature may be detected by the forward bending test as described above, which is designed to detect early abnormalities of rotation that are not apparent when the patient is standing erect.

B. Imaging: The most valuable x-rays are those taken of the entire spine in the standing position in both the anteroposterior and lateral planes. Usually, there is one primary curvature with a compensatory curvature that develops to balance the body. At times there may be two primary curvatures, usually in the right thoracic and left lumbar regions. Any left thoracic curvature should be suspected of being secondary to neurologic or muscular disease, prompting a more meticulous neurologic examination. If the curvatures of the spine are balanced (compensated), the head is centered over the center of the pelvis and the patient is "in balance." If the spinal alignment is uncompensated, the head will be displaced to one side, which produces an unsightly deformity. Rotation of the spine may be measured by scoliometer as described by Bunnell (1984). This rotation is associated with a marked rib hump as the lateral curvature increases in severity. Deformity of the rib cage causes long-term problems when lung volumes are reduced.

Treatment

Treatment of scoliosis depends on curve magnitude, skeletal maturity, and risk of progression. Curvatures of less than 20 degrees usually do not require treatment unless they show progression. Bracing is indicated for curvature of 20–40 degrees in a skeletally immature child. Treatment is indicated for any curvature that demonstrates progression on serial x-ray examination. Curvatures greater than 40 degrees are resistant to treatment by bracing. Thoracic curvatures greater than 60 degrees have been correlated with poor pulmonary function in adult life. Curvatures of such severity are an indication for surgical correction of the deformity and posterior spinal fusion to maintain the correction. Curvatures between 40 and 60 degrees may also require spinal fusion if they appear to be progressive or are causing decompensation of the spine or are cosmetically unacceptable.

Surgical fusion involves decortication of the bone over the laminas and spinous processes, with the addition of autogenous bone graft from the iliac crest. Postoperative correction is usually maintained by rods and hooks, with activity restriction for several months until the fusion is solid.

Treatment is prolonged and difficult and is best done in centers where full support facilities are available.

Prognosis

Compensated small curvatures that do not progress may be well tolerated throughout life, with very little cosmetic concern. The patients should be counseled regarding the genetic transmission of scoliosis and cautioned that their children should be examined at regular intervals during growth. Large thoracic curvatures greater than 60 degrees are associated with shortened life span and may progress even during adult life. Large lumbar curvatures may lead to subluxation of the vertebrae and premature arthritic degeneration of the spine, producing disabling pain in adulthood. Early detection allows for simple brace treatment. In patients so treated, the long-term prognosis is excellent, and surgery is not necessary. For this reason, school screening programs for scoliosis have gained popular support.

Bunnell WP: An objective criterion for scoliosis screening. J Bone Joint Surg [Am] 1984;66:1381.

Nachemson AL et al: Effectiveness of treatment with a brace in girls who have adolescent idiopathic scoliosis. J Bone Joint Surg 1995;77:815.

Peterson LE et al: Prediction of progression of the curve in girls who have adolescent idiopathic scoliosis of moderate severity. J Bone Joint Surg 1995;77:823.

Weinstein SL: Idiopathic scoliosis: Natural history. Spine 1986;11:780.

SLIPPED CAPITAL FEMORAL EPIPHYSIS

Slipped capital femoral epiphysis is separation of the proximal femoral epiphysis through the growth plate. The head of the femur is usually displaced medially and posteriorly relative to the femoral neck. The condition occurs in adolescence and is most common in obese males. The cause is not clear, although some authorities have shown experimentally that the strength of the perichondrial ring stabilizing the epiphysial area is sufficiently weakened by hormonal changes during the adolescent years that the simple overload of excessive body weight can produce a pathologic fracture through the growth plate. Hormonal studies in these children have not demonstrated any abnormality. The histology of the area of separation is identical with that seen with traumatic separation. The condition occasionally occurs acutely following a fall or direct trauma to the hip.

More commonly there are vague symptoms over a protracted period of time in an otherwise healthy child who presents with pain and limp. The pain is often referred into the thigh or the medial side of the knee. It is important to examine the hip joint in any child complaining of knee pain, particularly in adolescents. The consistent finding on physical examination is limitation of internal rotation and abduction of the hip. There usually is also an associated hip flexion contracture as well as local tenderness about the hip. X-rays should be taken in both the anteroposterior and lateral planes and should include both hips.

Treatment is based on the same principles that govern treatment of fracture of the femoral neck in adults in that the head of the femur is fixed to the neck of the femur and the fracture line allowed to heal. Unfortunately, the severe complication of avascular necrosis occurs in 30% of these patients. There has been a positive correlation between forceful reduction of the slip and avascular necrosis. In cases of acute slip, as evidenced by the absence of any callus formation about the growth plate, it may be possible to reduce the hip by gentle traction. In more chronic cases, a more expeditious procedure is to pin the slip as it lies. Remodeling of the fracture site often improves the position of the hip without further surgery.

The long-term prognosis is guarded because most of these patients continue to be overweight and overstress their hip joints. Follow-up studies have shown a high incidence of premature degenerative arthritis in this group of patients—even those who do not develop avascular necrosis. The development of avascular necrosis almost always guarantees a poor prognosis, because new bone does not replace the femoral head at this late stage of skeletal growth.

About 30% of patients have bilateral involvement, and patients should be followed up for slipping of the opposite side, which may occur as long as 1 or 2 years after the primary episode.

Aronson DD, Carlson WE: Slipped capital femoral epiphysis: A prospective study of fixation with a single screw. J Bone Joint Surg [Am] 1992;74:810.

Loder RT et al: Slipped capital femoral epiphysis associated with endocrine disorders. J Pediatr Orthop 1995; 15:349.

Stanitski CL: Acute slipped capital femoral epiphysis: Treatment alternatives. J Am Acad Orthop Surg 1994; 2:96.

GENU VARUM & GENU VALGUM

Genu varum (bowleg) is normal from infancy through 2 years of life. The alignment then changes to **genu valgum** (knock-knee) until about 8 years of age, at which time adult alignment is attained. Criteria for referral to an orthopedist include persistent bowing beyond age 2, bowing that is increasing rather than decreasing, bowing of one leg only, and knock-knee associated with short stature.

Bracing may be appropriate, or, rarely, an osteotomy is necessary for a severe problem such as Blount's disease (proximal tibial epiphysial dysplasia).

Health CH, Staheli LT: Normal limits of knee angle in white children: Genu varum and genu valgum. J Pediatr Orthop 1993;13:259.

Stricker SJ et al: Langenskïold classification of tibia vara: An assessment of interobserver variability. J Pediatr Orthop 1994;14:152.

TIBIAL TORSION

The physician is often asked about "toeing in" in small children. The disorder is routinely asymptomatic. Tibial torsion is rotation of the leg between the knee and the ankle. Internal rotation amounts to about 20 degrees at birth but decreases to neutral rotation by 16 months of age. The deformity is sometimes accentuated by laxity of the knee ligaments, allowing excessive internal rotation of the leg in small children. In children who have a persistent internal rotation of the tibia beyond 16–18 months of age, the condition is often due to sleeping with feet turned in and can be reversed with an external rotation splint worn only at night.

FEMORAL ANTEVERSION

"Toeing in" beyond 2 or 3 years of age is usually secondary to femoral anteversion, which produces excessive internal rotation of the femur rather than external rotation. This femoral alignment follows a natural history of progressive decrease toward neutral up to 8 years of age, with slower change to 16 years of age. Studies comparing the results of treatment with shoes or braces to the natural history have shown that little is gained by active treatment. Active external rotation exercises such as ballet, skating, or bicycle riding may be worthwhile. Osteotomy for rotational correction is rarely required. Refer those who have no external rotation of hip in extension.

Fabry G, MacEwen GD, Shands AR Jr: Torsion of the femur. J Bone Joint Surg [Am] 1973;55:1726.

Wedge JH, Munkacsi I, Loback D: Anteversion of the femur and idiopathic osteoarthritis of the hip. J Bone Joint Surg [Am] 1989;71:1040.

COMMON FOOT PROBLEMS

When a child begins to stand and walk, the long arch of the foot is flat with a medial bulge over the inner border of the foot. The forefeet are mildly pronated or rotated inward, with a slight valgus alignment of the knees. As the child grows and muscle power improves, the long arch is better supported and more normal relationships occur in the lower extremities. (See also Metatarsus Varus and Talipes Equinovarus.)

1. FLATFOOT

Flatfoot is a normal condition in infants. Children presenting for examination should be checked to determine that the heel cord is of normal length when the heel is aligned in the neutral position, allowing complete dorsiflexion and plantar flexion. As long as the foot is supple and the presence of a longitudinal arch is noted when the child is sitting in a non-weight-bearing position, the parents can be assured that a normal arch will probably develop. There is usually a familial incidence of relaxed flatfeet in children who have prolonged loss of the arch. In any child with a shortened heel cord or stiffness of the foot, other causes of flatfoot such as tarsal coalition or vertical talus should be ruled out by a complete orthopedic examination and x-ray.

In the child with an ordinary relaxed flatfoot, no active treatment is indicated unless there is calf or leg pain. In children who have leg pains attributable to flatfoot, an orthopedic shoe with Thomas heel or an orthotic that holds the heel in neutral and supports the arch may relieve discomfort. An arch insert should not be prescribed unless passive correction of the arch is easily accomplished; otherwise, there will be irritation of the skin over the medial side of the foot.

Any child with a painful or rigid flatfoot should be referred to an orthopedist.

Gonzalez PK, Kumar SJ: Calcaneonavicular coalition treated by resection and interposition of the extensor digitorum brevis muscle. J Bone Joint Surg [Am] 1990; 72:71.

Wenger DR et al: Corrective shoes and inserts as treatment for a flexible flatfoot in infants and children. J Bone Joint Surg [Am] 1989;71A:800.

2. TALIPES CALCANEOVALGUS

Talipes calcaneovalgus is characterized by excessive dorsiflexion at the ankle and eversion of the foot. It is often present at birth and almost always corrects spontaneously. The deformity is due to intrauterine position.

Treatment consists of passive exercises by the mother, stretching the foot into plantar flexion. In rare instances, it may be necessary to use plaster casts to help with manipulation and positioning. Complete correction is the rule.

3. CAVUS FOOT

In cavus foot, the deformity consists of an unusually high longitudinal arch of the foot. It may be hereditary or associated with neurologic conditions such as poliomyelitis, Charcot-Marie-Tooth disease, Friedreich's ataxia, or diastematomyelia. There is usually an associated contracture of the toe extensor, producing a claw toe deformity in which the metatarsal phalangeal joints are hyperextended and the interphalangeal joints acutely flexed. Any child presenting with cavus feet should have a careful neurologic examination including x-rays of the spine.

Stretching exercises for the heel cord and arch of the foot are indicated for conservative therapy. In resistant cases that do not respond to shoe adjustments (metatarsal bars and supports), operation may be necessary to lengthen the contracted extensor and flexor tendons and to release the plantar fascia and other tight plantar structures. Arthrodesis of the foot may be necessary later. If these feet are left untreated, they are often painful and limit walking. The overall prognosis is much poorer than with low arch or pes planus.

4. BUNIONS
(Hallux Valgus)

Girls may present in adolescence with lateral deviation of the great toe associated with a prominence over the head of the first metatarsal. This deformity is painful only with shoe wear and almost always can be relieved by fitting shoes that are wide enough. Surgery should be avoided in the adolescent age group, because the results are much less successful than in adult patients with the same condition.

Groiso J: Juvenile hallux: A conservative approach to treatment. J Bone Joint Surg [Am] 1992;74:1375.

Peterson HA et al: Adolescent bunion deformity treated with double osteotomy and longitudinal pin fixation of the first ray. J Pediatr Orthop 1993;13:80.

DEGENERATIVE PROBLEMS
(Arthritis, Bursitis, & Tenosynovitis)

Degenerative arthritis may follow childhood skeletal problems such as infection, slipped capital femoral epiphysis, avascular necrosis, trauma, or it may occur in association with hemophilia. Early effective treatment of these disorders will prevent arthritis. Late treatment is often unsatisfactory.

Degenerative changes in the soft tissues around joints may occur as a result of overuse syndrome in adolescent athletes. Young boys throwing excessive numbers of pitches, especially curve balls, may develop "little leaguer's elbow," consisting of degenerative changes around the humeral condyles associated with pain, swelling, and limitation of motion. In order to enforce the rest necessary for healing, a plaster cast may be necessary. A more reasonable preventive measure is to limit the number of pitches thrown by children.

Acute bursitis is uncommon in childhood, and other causes should be ruled out before this diagnosis is accepted.

Tenosynovitis is most common in the region of the knees and feet. Children taking dancing lessons, particularly toe dancing, may have pain around the flexor tendon sheaths in the toes or ankles. Rest is effective treatment. At the knee level, there may be irritation of the patellar ligament, with associated swelling in the infrapatellar fat pad. Synovitis in this area is usually due to overuse and is also treated by rest. Corticosteroid injections are contraindicated.

Kunnamo I et al: Clinical signs and laboratory tests in the differential diagnosis of arthritis in children. Am J Dis Child 1987;141:34.

TRAUMA

SOFT TISSUE TRAUMA
(Sprains, Strains, & Contusions)

A **sprain** is the stretching of a ligament, and a **strain** is a stretch of a muscle or tendon. In either of these injuries, there may be some degree of tissue tearing. Contusions are generally due to tissue compression, with damage to blood vessels within the tissue and the formation of hematoma.

A severe sprain is one in which the ligament is completely divided, resulting in instability of the joint. A mild or moderate sprain is one in which incomplete tearing of the ligament occurs, but in which there is associated local pain and swelling.

Mild or moderate sprains are treated by rest of the affected joint, with ice and elevation to prevent prolonged symptoms. By definition, mild or moderate sprain is not associated with instability of the joint.

If there is more severe trauma resulting in tearing of a ligament, instability of the joint may be demonstrated by gross examination or by stress testing with x-ray documentation. Such deformity of the joint may cause persistent instability resulting from inaccurate apposition of the ligament ends during healing. If instability is evident, surgical repair of the torn ligament may be indicated. If a muscle is torn at its tendinous insertion, it should be repaired.

The initial treatment of any sprain consists of ice, compression, and elevation. The purpose of the treatment is to decrease local edema and residual stiffness resulting from gelling of blood proteins in the interstitial space. Splinting of the affected joint protects against further injury and relieves swelling and pain.

1. ANKLE SPRAINS

The history will indicate that the injury was by either forceful inversion or eversion. The more common inversion injury results in tearing or injury to the lateral ligaments, whereas an eversion injury will injure the medial ligaments of the ankle. The injured ligaments may be identified by means of careful palpation for point tenderness around the ankle. The joint should be supported or immobilized at a right angle, which is the functional position. Adhesive taping may be effective to maintain this position but should be applied by one skilled in the use of tape and changed frequently to prevent the formation of blisters and skin damage. A posterior plaster splint is more easily applied and gives good joint rest if the extremity is protected by using crutches for weight bearing. Prolonged use of a plaster cast is usually not necessary, but the sprained ankle should be rested sufficiently to allow complete healing. This may take 3–6 weeks. Because fractures usually receive more attention and adequate follow-up, the results are often better. A properly treated ankle sprain should not be the source of prolonged and repeated disability.

2. KNEE SPRAINS

Sprains of the collateral and cruciate ligaments are uncommon in children. These ligaments are so strong that it is more common to injure the epiphysial growth plates, which are the weakest structures in the region of the knees of children. In adolescence, however, the physes have started to close, and the knee joint is more like that of an adult, so that rupture of the anterior cruciate ligament can result from a twisting injury. If the injury produces avulsion of the tibial spine, open anatomic reduction is often required.

Effusion of the knee after trauma deserves referral to an orthopedic specialist. The differential diagnosis includes torn ligament, torn meniscus, and osteochondral fracture. Nontraumatic effusion should be evaluated for inflammatory conditions (such as juvenile rheumatoid arthritis) or patellar malalignment.

3. INTERNAL DERANGEMENTS OF THE KNEE

Meniscal injuries are uncommon under age 12. Clicking or locking of the knee may occur in young children as a result of a discoid lateral meniscus, which is a rare type of congenital anomaly. As the child approaches adolescence, internal damage to the knee from a torsion weight-bearing injury may result in locking of the knee if tearing and displacement of the meniscus occur. Osteochondral fractures secondary to osteochondritis dissecans may also present as internal derangements of the knee in adolescence. Post-traumatic synovitis may mimic a meniscal lesion as well. In any severe injury to the knee, epiphysial injury should be suspected; stress films will sometimes demonstrate separation of the distal femoral epiphysis in such cases. Epiphysial injury should be suspected whenever there is tenderness on both sides of the metaphysis of the femur after injury.

Cahill B: Osteochondritis dissecans of the knee: Treatment of juvenile and adult forms. J Am Acad Orthop Surg 1995;3:237.

Stanitski CL et al: Observations on acute knee hemarthrosis in children and adolescents. J Pediatr Orthop 1993; 13:506.

4. BACK SPRAINS

Sprains of the ligaments and muscles of the back are unusual in children but may occur as a result of violent trauma from automobile accidents or athletic injuries. A child with back pain should not be presumed to have had trauma to the spine unless the history warrants that conclusion. The reason for back pain should be carefully sought by x-ray and physical examination. Inflammation, infection, and tumors are more common causes of back pain in children than sprains.

5. CONTUSIONS

Contusion of muscle with hematoma formation produces the familiar "charley horse" injury. Treatment of such injuries is by application of ice, compression, and rest. Exercise should be avoided for 5–7 days. Local heat may hasten healing once the acute phase of tenderness and swelling is past.

6. MYOSITIS OSSIFICANS

Ossification within muscle occurs when there is sufficient trauma to cause a hematoma that later heals in the manner of a fracture. The injury is usually a contusion and occurs most commonly in the quadriceps of the thigh or the triceps of the arm. When such a severe injury with hematoma is recognized, it is important to splint the extremity and avoid activity. If further activity is allowed, ossification may reach spectacular proportions and resemble an osteosarcoma.

Disability is great, with local swelling and heat and extreme pain upon the slightest motion of the adjacent joint. The limb should be rested, with the knee in extension or the elbow in 90 degrees of flexion, until the local reaction has subsided. After local heat and tenderness have decreased, gentle active exercises may be initiated. Passive stretching exercises are not indicated, because they may stimulate the ossification reaction. It is occasionally necessary to excise excessive bony tissue if it interferes with muscle function once the reaction is mature. Surgery should not be attempted before 9 months to 1 year after injury, because it may restart the process and lead to an even more severe reaction.

Micheli LJ (editor): Injuries in the young athlete. Clin Sports Med 1988;7:459.

TRAUMATIC SUBLUXATIONS & DISLOCATIONS

Dislocation of a joint is always associated with severe damage to the ligaments and joint capsule. In contrast to fracture treatment, which may be safely postponed, dislocations must be reduced immediately. Dislocations can usually be reduced by gentle sustained traction. It often happens that no anesthetic is necessary for several hours after the injury, because of the protective anesthesia produced by the injury. Following reduction, the joint should be splinted for transportation of the patient.

The dislocated joint should be treated by immobilization for at least 3 weeks, followed by graduated active exercises through a full range of motion. Physical therapy is usually not indicated for children with injuries. As a matter of fact, vigorous manipulation of the joint by a therapist may be harmful. The child should be permitted to perform therapy alone. No stretching should be permitted.

1. SUBLUXATION OF THE RADIAL HEAD (Nursemaid's Elbow)

Infants frequently sustain subluxation of the radial head as a result of being lifted or pulled by the hand. The child appears with the elbow fully pronated and painful. The usual complaint is that the child's elbow will not bend. X-ray findings are normal, but there is point tenderness over the radial head. When the elbow is placed in full supination and slowly moved from full flexion to full extension, a click may be palpated at the level of the radial head. The relief of pain is remarkable, as the child usually stops crying immediately. The elbow may be immobilized in a sling for comfort for a day. Occasionally, symptoms last for several days, requiring more prolonged immobilization.

Pulled elbow may be a clue to battering. This should be remembered during examination, especially if the problem is recurrent.

2. RECURRENT DISLOCATION OF THE PATELLA

Recurrent dislocation of the patella is more common in loose-jointed individuals, especially adolescent girls. If the patella completely dislocates, it nearly always goes laterally. Pain is severe, and the patient is brought to the doctor with the knee slightly flexed and an obvious bony mass lateral to the knee joint and a flat area over the usual location of the patella anteriorly. X-ray findings confirm the diagnosis. The patella may be reduced by extending the knee and placing slight pressure on the patella while gentle traction is exerted on the leg. In subluxation of the patella, the symptoms may be more subtle, and the patient may say that the knee "gives out" or "jumps out of place."

In the case of complete dislocation, the knee should be immobilized for 3–4 weeks, followed by a physical therapy program for strengthening the quadriceps muscle. Operation may be necessary to tighten the knee joint capsule if dislocation or subluxation is recurrent. In such instances, if the patella is not stabilized, repeated dislocation produces damage to the articular cartilage of the patellofemoral joint and premature degenerative arthritis.

Vähäsarja V et al: Operative realignment of patellar malalignment in children. J Pediatr Orthop 1995;15:281.

EPIPHYSIAL SEPARATIONS

In children, epiphysial separations and fractures are more common than ligamentous injuries. This finding is based on the fact that the ligaments of the joints are generally stronger than the associated growth plates.

In instances in which dislocation is suspected, an x-ray should be taken in order to rule out epiphysial fracture. Films of the opposite extremity, especially around the elbow, may be valuable for comparison. Reduction of a fractured epiphysis should be done under anesthesia to align the growth plate with the least amount of force necessary. Fractures across the growth plate may produce bony bridges that will cause premature cessation of growth or angular deformities in the growth plate. Epiphysial fractures around the shoulder, wrist, and fingers can usually be treated by closed reduction, but fractures of the epiphyses around the elbow often require open reduction. In the lower extremity, accurate reduction of the epiphysial plate is necessary to prevent joint deformity if a joint surface is involved. Unfortunately, some of the most severe injuries to the epiphysial plate occur from compression injuries, where the amount of force is not immediately apparent. If angular deformities result, corrective osteotomy may be necessary.

Mizuta T et al: Statistical analysis of the incidence of physical injuries. J Pediatr Orthop 1987;7:518.

TORUS FRACTURES

Torus fractures consist of "buckling" of the cortex as a result of minimal trauma. They usually occur in the distal radius or ulna. Alignment is satisfactory, and simple immobilization for 3–5 weeks is sufficient.

GREENSTICK FRACTURES

With greenstick fractures there is frank disruption of the cortex on one side of the bone but no discernible cleavage plane on the opposite side. These fractures are angulated but not displaced, since the bone ends are not separated. Reduction is achieved by straightening the arm into normal alignment, and reduction is maintained by a snugly fitting plaster cast. It is necessary to x-ray children with greenstick fractures again in a week to 10 days to make certain that the reduction has been maintained in plaster. A slight angular deformity can be corrected by remodeling of the bone. The farther the fracture is from the growing end of the bone, the longer the time required for healing. The fracture can be considered healed when there are no findings of tenderness and local swelling or heat and when adequate bony callus is seen on x-ray.

FRACTURE OF THE CLAVICLE

Clavicular fractures are very common injuries in infants and children. They can be immobilized by a figure-of-eight dressing that retracts the shoulders and brings the clavicle to normal length. The healing callus will be apparent when the fracture has consolidated, but this unsightly lump will generally resolve over a period of months to a year.

SUPRACONDYLAR FRACTURES OF THE HUMERUS

Supracondylar fractures tend to occur in the age group from 3 to 6 years and are potentially dangerous because of the proximity to the brachial artery in the distal arm. They are usually associated with a significant amount of trauma, so that swelling may be severe. **Volkmann's ischemic contracture** of the forearm may occur as a result of vascular embarrassment. When severe swelling is present, the safest course is to place the arm in traction and carefully observe nerve function and the vascular supply to the hand. In these cases, the children should be hospitalized and followed up carefully by experienced nurses. If the blood supply is compromised, exposure of the brachial artery may be necessary, although this is rarely needed when satisfactory reduction and traction are employed. Most often, these fractures are treated by closed reduction and percutaneous pinning. Complications associated with supracondylar fractures also include a resultant cubitus varus secondary to poor reduction. It is often difficult to ascertain adequacy of the reduction because a flexed position is necessary to maintain normal alignment. Such a "gunstock" deformity of the elbow may be somewhat unsightly but does not usually interfere with joint function.

Kurer MH, Regan MW: Completely displaced supracondylar fracture of the humerus in children: A review of 1708 comparable cases. Clin Orthop 1990;256:205.

Topping RE et al: Clinical evaluation of crossed pin versus lateral pin fixation in displaced supracondylar humerus fractures. J Pediatr Orthop 1995;15:435.

GENERAL COMMENTS ON OTHER FRACTURES IN CHILDREN

Reduction of fractures in children is usually accomplished by simple traction and manipulation; open reduction is rarely indicated. Remodeling of the fracture callus usually produces an almost normal appearance of the bone over a matter of months. The younger the child, the more remodeling is possible. Angular deformities remodel with ease. Rotatory deformities do not remodel, and this produces the cubitus varus deformity sometimes seen after supracondylar fractures.

The physician should be suspicious of child abuse whenever the age of a fracture does not match the history given or when the severity of the injury is more than the alleged accident would have produced. In suspected cases of battering where no fracture is present on the initial x-ray film, a repeat film 10 days later is in order. Bleeding beneath the periosteum will be calcified by 7–10 days, and the x-ray appearance is almost diagnostic of severe closed trauma characteristic of a battered child.

Cumming WA: Neonatal skeletal fractures: Birth trauma or child abuse? J Can Assoc Radiol 1979;30:30.

Dent JA, Patterson CR: Fractures in early childhood: Osteogenesis imperfecta or child abuse? J Pediatr Orthop 1991;11:184.

Ogden JA: *Skeletal Injury in the Child.* Lea & Febiger, 1982.

Rang M: *Children's Fractures,* 2nd ed. Lippincott, 1983.

Weber BG, Brunner C, Freuler F (editors): *Treatment of Fractures in Children and Adolescents.* Springer-Verlag, 1980.

INFECTIONS OF THE BONES & JOINTS

OSTEOMYELITIS

Osteomyelitis is an infectious process that usually starts in the spongy or medullary bone and then extends to involve compact or cortical bone. The lower extremities are most often affected, and there is commonly a history of trauma. Osteomyelitis may occur as a result of direct invasion from the outside through a penetrating wound (nail) or open fracture, but hematogenous spread of infection (eg, pyoderma or upper respiratory tract infection) from other infected areas is more common. The most common infecting organism is *Staphylococcus aureus*, which seems to have a special tendency to infect the metaphyses of growing bones. Anatomically, circulation in the long bones is such that the arterial supply to the metaphysis just below the growth plate is by end arteries, which turn sharply to end in venous sinusoids, causing a relative stasis. In the infant under 1 year of age, there is direct vascular communication with the epiphysis across the growth plate, so that direct spread may occur from the metaphysis to the epiphysis and subsequently into the joint. In the older child, the growth plate provides an effective barrier and the epiphysis is usually not involved, although the infection spreads retrograde from the metaphysis into the diaphysis and, by rupture through the cortical bone, down along the diaphysis beneath the periosteum.

1. EXOGENOUS OSTEOMYELITIS

To avoid osteomyelitis by direct extension, all wounds must be carefully examined and cleansed. Puncture wounds are especially liable to lead to osteomyelitis if not carefully debrided. Cultures of the wound made at the time of exploration and debridement may be useful if signs of inflammation and infection develop subsequently. Copious irrigation is necessary, and all nonviable skin, subcutaneous tissue, fascia, and muscle must be excised. In extensive or contaminated wounds, antibiotic coverage is indicated. Contaminated wounds should be left open and secondary closure performed 3–5 days later. If at the time of delayed closure further necrotic tissue is present, it should be excised. Leaving the wound open allows the infection to stay at the surface rather than extend inward to the bone.

Initially, broad-spectrum antibiotics should be used; after cultures have been read, an appropriate alternative antibiotic can be chosen if there is lingering inflammation. A tetanus toxoid booster is indicated for any questionable wound. Gas gangrene is better prevented by adequate debridement than by antitoxin.

After exogenous osteomyelitis has become established, treatment becomes more complicated, requiring extensive surgical debridement and drainage in hospital with intravenous antibiotics.

2. HEMATOGENOUS OSTEOMYELITIS

Hematogenous osteomyelitis is usually caused by pyogenic bacteria; 85% of cases are due to staphylococci. Streptococci are rare causes of osteomyelitis today, but *Pseudomonas* organisms have often been documented in cases of nail puncture wounds. Children with sickle cell anemia are especially prone to osteomyelitis caused by salmonellae.

Clinical Findings

A. Symptoms & Signs: In infants, the manifestations of osteomyelitis may be subtle, presenting as irritability, diarrhea, or failure to feed properly; the temperature may be normal or slightly low; and the white blood count may be normal or only slightly elevated. There may be pseudoparalysis of the involved limb. In older children, the manifestations are more striking, with severe local tenderness and pain, high fever, rapid pulse, and elevated white blood count and sedimentation rate. Osteomyelitis of a lower extremity often presents around the knee in a child 7–10 years of age. Tenderness is most marked over the metaphysis of the bone where the process has its origin. The child may limp or refuse to bear weight.

B. Laboratory Findings: Blood cultures are often positive early. The most significant test in in-

fancy is the aspiration of pus when suspicion arises because of lack of movement in a painful extremity. It is useful to needle the bone in the area of suspected infection and aspirate any fluid present. This fluid should be stained for organisms as well as cultured. Even edema fluid may be useful for determining the causative organism. The white blood cell count is usually elevated, as is the sedimentation rate.

C. Imaging: Nonspecific local swelling is the first x-ray finding. This is followed by elevation of the periosteum, with formation of new bone from the cambium layer of the periosteum occurring after 3–6 days. As the infection becomes chronic, areas of cortical bone are isolated by pus spreading down the medullary canal, causing rarefaction and demineralization of the bone. Such isolated pieces of cortex become ischemic and form sequestra (dead bone fragments). These x-ray findings are late, and osteomyelitis should be diagnosed clinically before significant x-ray findings are present. Bone scan is valuable in suspected cases before x-ray findings become positive. Magnetic resonance imaging (MRI) can be used for diagnosis, especially for infections of the pelvis or spine, which may have a false-negative bone scan.

Treatment

A. Specific Measures: Antibiotics should be started intravenously as soon as the diagnosis of osteomyelitis is made. Agents that cover *Staphylococcus aureus* and *Streptococcus pyogenes* (eg, oxacillin, nafcillin, or cefazolin) are appropriate for most cases. For specific recommendations and for possible *Pseudomonas* infection, see Chapter 37.

Chronic infections are treated for months. Following surgical debridement, *Pseudomonas* foot infections usually respond to 1–2 weeks of treatment.

B. General Measures: Splinting of the limb minimizes pain and decreases spread of the infection by lymphatic channels through the soft tissue. The splint should be removed periodically to allow active use of adjacent joints and prevent stiffening and muscle atrophy. In chronic osteomyelitis, splinting may be necessary to guard against fracture of the weakened bone.

C. Surgical Measures: Aspiration of the metaphysis is a useful diagnostic measure in any case of suspected osteomyelitis. In the first 24–72 hours, it may be possible to treat osteomyelitis by antibiotics alone. If frank pus is aspirated from the bone, however, surgical drainage is indicated. If the infection has not shown a dramatic response within 24 hours, surgical drainage is also indicated. It is important that all devitalized soft tissue be removed and adequate exposure of the bone obtained to permit free drainage. Excessive amounts of bone should not be removed when draining acute osteomyelitis, because they may not be completely replaced by the normal healing process.

Little damage is done by surgical drainage, but failure to drain the pus in acute cases may lead to more severe damage.

Prognosis

When osteomyelitis is diagnosed in the early clinical stages and prompt antibiotic therapy is begun, the prognosis is excellent. If the process has been unattended for a week to 10 days, there is almost always some permanent loss of bone structure, as well as the possibility of growth abnormality.

Dormans JP, Drummond DS: Pediatric hematogenous osteomyelitis: New trends in presentation, diagnosis and treatment. J Am Acad Orthop Surg 1994;2:333.

Jacobs RF et al: Management of *Pseudomonas* osteochondritis complicating puncture wounds of the foot. Pediatrics 1982;69:432.

Mazur JM et al: Usefulness of magnetic resonance imaging for diagnosis of acute musculoskeletal infections in children. J Pediatr Orthop 1995;15:144.

PYOGENIC ARTHRITIS

The source of pyogenic arthritis varies according to the age of the child. In the infant, pyogenic arthritis often develops by spread from adjacent osteomyelitis. In the older child, it presents as an isolated infection, usually without bony involvement. In teenagers with pyogenic arthritis, an underlying systemic disease is usually the cause, such as an obvious generalized infection or an organism (eg, the gonococcus) that has an affinity for joints.

The infecting organism varies with age: group B streptococcus and *Staphylococcus aureus* in those under 4 months; *Haemophilus influenzae* and *Staphylococcus* in those 4 months to 4 years old; and *Staphylococcus* and *Streptococcus pyogenes* in older children.

The initial effusion of the joint rapidly becomes purulent. An effusion of the joint may accompany osteomyelitis in the adjacent bone. A white blood cell count exceeding 100,000/μL in the joint fluid indicates a definite purulent infection. Generally, spread of infection is from the bone into the joint, but unattended pyogenic arthritis may also affect adjacent bone. The sedimentation rate is elevated.

Clinical Findings

A. Symptoms & Signs: In older children, the signs are striking, with fever, malaise, vomiting, and restriction of motion. In infants, paralysis of the limb due to inflammatory neuritis may be evident. Infection of the hip joint in infants can be diagnosed if suspicion is aroused by decreased abduction of the hip in an infant who is irritable or feeding poorly. A history of umbilical catheter treatment in the newborn nursery should alert the physician to the possibility of pyogenic arthritis of the hip.

B. Imaging: Early distention of the joint capsule is nonspecific and difficult to measure by x-ray. In the infant with unrecognized pyogenic arthritis, dislocation of the joint may follow within a few days as a result of distention of the capsule by pus. Later changes include destruction of the joint space, resorption of epiphysial cartilage, and erosion of the adjacent bone of the metaphysis. The bone scan shows increased flow and increased uptake about the joint.

Treatment

Diagnosis may be made by aspiration of the joint. In the hip joint, pyogenic arthritis is most easily treated by surgical drainage because the joint is deep and difficult to aspirate as well as being inaccessible to thorough cleaning through needle aspiration. In more superficial joints, such as the knee, aspiration of the joint at least twice daily may maintain adequate drainage. More recently, arthroscopic irrigation and debridement have been successful in treating pyogenic arthritis of the knee. If fever and clinical symptoms do not subside within 24 hours after treatment is begun, open surgical drainage is indicated. Antibiotics can be selected based on age, Gram's stains, and cultures of the aspirated pus. Reasonable empiric therapy in infants includes cefuroxime (200 mg/kg/d in four divided doses) or oxacillin (150 mg/kg/d) plus a third-generation cephalosporin. An antistaphylococcal alone is usually adequate for children over 5 years. For staphylococcal infections, 3 weeks of therapy is recommended; for other organisms, 2 weeks is usually sufficient. Oral therapy may be begun when clinical signs have markedly improved. It is not necessary to give intra-articular antibiotics, since good levels are achieved in the synovial fluid.

Prognosis

The prognosis for the patient with pyogenic arthritis is excellent if the joint is drained early, before damage to the articular cartilage has occurred. If infection is present for more than 24 hours, there is dissolution of the proteoglycans in the articular cartilage, with subsequent arthrosis and fibrosis of the joint. Damage to the growth plate may also occur, especially within the hip joint, where the epiphysial plate is intracapsular.

Betz RR et al: Late sequelae of septic arthritis of the hip in infancy and childhood. J Pediatr Orthop 1990;10:365.

Shaw BA, Kasser JR: Acute septic arthritis in infancy and childhood. Clin Orthop 1990;257:212.

TUBERCULOUS ARTHRITIS

Tuberculous arthritis is now a rare disease in the United States. It must be considered, however, in children with resistant infections of the joints, especially those with a history of tuberculosis in family members. Generally, the infection may be ruled out by skin testing. The joints most commonly affected in children are the intervertebral disks, resulting in gibbus or dorsal angular deformity at the site of involvement.

Treatment is by local drainage of the "cold abscess," followed by antituberculosis therapy with isoniazid, rifampin, and ethambutol. Prolonged immobilization in a plaster cast or prolonged bed rest is necessary to promote healing. Spinal fusion may be required to preserve stability of the vertebral column.

TRANSIENT SYNOVITIS OF THE HIP

The most common cause of limping and pain in the hip of children in the United States is transitory synovitis, an acute inflammatory reaction that often follows an upper respiratory infection and is generally self-limited. In questionable cases, aspiration of the hip yields only yellowish fluid, ruling out pyogenic arthritis. Generally, however, toxic synovitis of the hip is not associated with elevation of the erythrocyte sedimentation rate, the white blood count or a temperature above 38.3 °C. It classically affects children 3–10 years of age and is more common in boys. There is limitation of motion of the hip joint, particularly internal rotation, and x-ray changes are nonspecific, with some swelling apparent in the soft tissues around the joint.

Treatment consists of bed rest and the use of traction with slight flexion of the hip. Nonsteroidal anti-inflammatory medications may shorten the course of the disease, although even with no treatment the disease usually is self-limited to a matter of days. It is important to maintain x-ray follow-up because toxic synovitis may be the precursor of avascular necrosis of the femoral head (next section) in a small percentage of patients. X-ray films can be obtained at 1 month and 3 months, or earlier if there is persistent limp or pain.

Hodges DL, McGuire TJ: Hip pain in children: An anatomic approach. Orthop Rev 1988;17:251.

Terjesen T, Osthus P: Ultrasound in the diagnosis and follow-up of transient synovitis of the hip. J Pediatr Orthop 1991;11:608.

VASCULAR LESIONS & AVASCULAR NECROSIS (Osteochondroses)

AVASCULAR NECROSIS OF THE PROXIMAL FEMUR (Legg-Calvé-Perthes Disease)

The vascular supply of bone is generally precarious, and when it is interrupted, necrosis results. In contrast to other body tissues that undergo infarction, bone removes necrotic tissue and replaces it with living bone in a process called "creeping substitution." This replacement of necrotic bone may be so complete and so perfect that a completely normal bone results. Adequacy of replacement depends on the age of the patient, the presence or absence of associated infection, the congruity of the involved joint, and other physiologic and mechanical factors.

Because of their rapid growth in relation to their blood supply, the secondary ossification centers in the epiphyses are subject to avascular necrosis. Despite the number of different names referring to avascular necrosis of the epiphyses, the process is identical, necrosis of bone followed by replacement (Table 24–1).

Even though the pathologic and radiologic features of avascular necrosis of the epiphyses are well known, the cause is not generally agreed upon. Necrosis may follow known causes such as trauma or infection, but idiopathic lesions usually develop during periods of rapid growth of the epiphyses. Thus, the highest incidence of Legg-Calvé-Perthes disease is between 4 and 8 years of age.

Clinical Findings

A. Symptoms & Signs: Persistent pain is the most common symptom, and the patient may present with limp or limitation of motion.

Table 24–1. The osteochondroses.

Ossification Center	Eponym	Typical Age
Capital femoral	Legg-Calvé-Perthes disease	3–5
Tarsal navicular	Köhler's bone disease	6
Second metatarsal head	Freiberg's disease	12–14
Vertebral ring	Scheuemann's disease	13–16
Capitellum	Panner's disease	9–11
Tibial tubercle	Osgood-Schlatter disease	11–13
Calcaneus	Sever's disease	8–9

B. Laboratory Findings: Laboratory findings, including studies of joint aspirates, are normal.

C. Imaging: X-ray findings correlate with the progression of the process and the extent of necrosis. The early finding is effusion of the joint associated with slight widening of the joint space and periarticular swelling. Decreased bone density in and around the joint is apparent after a few weeks. The necrotic ossification center appears more dense than the surrounding viable structures, and there is collapse or narrowing of the femoral head.

As replacement of the necrotic ossification center occurs, there is rarefaction of the bone in a patchwork fashion, producing alternating areas of rarefaction and relative density or "fragmentation" of the epiphysis.

In the hip, there may be widening of the femoral head associated with flattening, giving rise to the term **coxa plana.** If infarction has extended across the growth plate, there will be a radiolucent lesion within the metaphysis. If the growth center of the femoral head has been damaged so that normal growth does not occur, varus deformity of the femoral neck will occur as a result of overgrowth of the greater trochanteric apophysis.

Eventually, complete replacement of the epiphysis will become apparent as new bone replaces necrotic bone. The final shape of the head depends on the extent of the necrosis and collapse that has been allowed to occur.

Differential Diagnosis

Differential diagnosis must include inflammatory and infectious lesions of the joints or apophyses. Transient synovitis of the hip may be distinguished from Legg-Calvé-Perthes disease by serial x-rays.

Treatment

Treatment consists simply of protection of the joint. If the joint is deeply seated within the acetabulum and normal joint motion is maintained, a reasonably good result can be expected. Bracing is no longer believed to be of benefit.

Prognosis

The prognosis for complete replacement of the necrotic femoral head in a child is excellent, but the functional result depends on the amount of deformity that develops during the time the softened structure exists. In Legg-Calvé-Perthes disease, the prognosis depends on the completeness of involvement of the epiphysial center. In general, patients with metaphyseal defects, those in whom the disease develops late in childhood, and those who have more complete involvement of the femoral head have a poorer prognosis.

Osteochondrosis due to vascular lesion may affect various growth centers. Table 24–1 indicates the common sites and the typical ages at presentation.

Fulford GE et al: A prospective study of non-operative and operative management for Perthes disease. J Pediatr Orthop 1993;13:281.

Martinez AG, Weinstein SL, Dietz FR: Weight bearing abduction brace treatment of Legg-Calvé-Perthes disease. J Bone Joint Surg [Am] 1992;74:12.

McAndrew MP, Weinstein SL: A long-term follow-up of Legg-Calvé-Perthes disease. J Bone Joint Surg [Am] 1984;66:860.

OSTEOCHONDRITIS DISSECANS

In osteochondritis dissecans, there is a pie-shaped necrotic area of bone and cartilage adjacent to the articular surface. The fragment of bone may be broken off from the host bone and displaced into the joint as a loose body. If it remains attached, the necrotic fragment may be completely replaced by creeping substitution.

The pathologic process is precisely the same as that described previously for avascular necrosing lesions of ossification centers. Because these lesions are adjacent to articular cartilage, however, there may be joint damage.

The most common sites of these lesions are the knee (medial femoral condyle), the elbow joint (capitellum), and the talus (superior lateral dome).

Joint pain is the usual presenting complaint. However, local swelling or locking may be present, particularly if there is a fragment free in the joint. Laboratory studies are normal.

Treatment consists of protection of the involved area from mechanical damage. If there is a fragment free within the joint as a loose body, it must be arthroscopically removed. For some marginal lesions, it may be worthwhile to drill the necrotic fragment to encourage more rapid vascular ingrowth and replacement. If large areas of a weight-bearing joint are involved, secondary degenerative arthritis may result.

NEUROLOGIC DISORDERS INVOLVING THE MUSCULOSKELETAL SYSTEM

ORTHOPEDIC ASPECTS OF CEREBRAL PALSY

Early physical therapy to encourage completion of the normal developmental patterns may be of benefit in patients with cerebral palsy. The greatest gains from this type of therapy are obtained during the first few years of life, and therapy should not be continued when no improvement is apparent.

Bracing and splinting are of questionable benefit, although night splints may be useful in preventing equinus deformity of the feet or adduction contractures of the hips. Orthopedic surgery can offer procedures to weaken hyperactive spastic muscles, to transfer function of deforming spastic muscles, or to stabilize joints. In general, muscle transfers are unpredictable in cerebral palsy, and most orthopedic procedures are directed at weakening deforming forces or bony stabilization by osteotomy or arthrodesis. Recently, selective dorsal rhizotomy has been used in select cases.

Flexion and adduction of the hip due to hyperactivity of the adductors and flexors may produce a progressive paralytic dislocation of the hip, which can lead to pain and dysfunction. Treatment of the dislocation once it has occurred is difficult and unsatisfactory. The principal preventive measure is abduction bracing, but this must often be supplemented by release of the adductors or hip flexors in order to prevent dislocation. In severe cases, osteotomy of the femur may also be necessary to correct the bony deformities of femoral anteversion and coxa valga that are invariably present.

Patients with a predominantly athetotic pattern are poor candidates for any surgical procedure or bracing. Neurosurgical procedures may be of some help.

Because it is difficult to predict the outcome of surgical procedures in cerebral palsy, the surgeon must examine patients on several occasions before any operative procedure is undertaken. Follow-up care by a physical therapist to maximize the anticipated long-term gains should be arranged before the operation.

Bleck EE: *Orthopaedic Management of Cerebral Palsy.* MacKeith, 1987.

Boscarino LF et al: Effects of selective dorsal rhizotomy on gait in children with cerebral palsy. J Pediatr Orthop 1993;13:174.

Little DG et al: Late hip subluxation in spastic diplegia associated with unrecognized hydrocephalus. J Pediatr Orthop 1995;15:368.

Moreau M et al: Adductor and psoas release for subluxation of the hip in children with spastic cerebral palsy. J Pediatr Orthop 1995;15:672.

ORTHOPEDIC ASPECTS OF MYELODYSPLASIA

Patients born with spina bifida cystica (aperta) should be examined early by an orthopedic surgeon. The level of neurologic involvement determines the muscle imbalance that will be present and apt to produce deformity with growth. The involvement is often asymmetric and tends to change during the first 12–18 months of life. Early closure of the sac is the rule, although there has been some hesitancy to treat all of these patients because of the extremely poor prognosis associated with congenital hydrocephalus, high levels of paralysis, and associated congenital anomalies. Associated musculoskeletal problems may include clubfoot, congenital dislocation of the hip, arthrogryposis type changes of the lower extremities, and congenital scoliosis, among others. The most common lesions are at the level of L3–4 and tend to affect the hip joint, with progressive dislocation occurring during growth. Foot deformities may be in any direction and are complicated by the fact that sensation is generally absent. Spinal deformities develop in a high percentage of these children, with scoliosis present in approximately 40%. Ambulation is impossible without braces or splints, and careful urologic follow-up must be obtained to prevent complications from incontinence. A high percentage of these children have hydrocephalus, which may be evident at birth or shortly thereafter, requiring shunting. The shunts are sources of infection and may require frequent replacement.

In children who have a reasonable likelihood of walking, operative treatment consists of reduction of the hip and alignment of the feet in the weight-bearing position as well as stabilization of the scoliosis. In children who do not have extension power of the knee, that is, those who lack active quadriceps function, the likelihood of ambulation is greatly decreased. In such patients, aggressive surgery in the hip region may result in stiffening of the joints, thus preventing sitting. Multiple foot operations are also contraindicated in these children.

The overall management of the child with spina bifida should be coordinated in a multidiscipline clinic where all doctors working in cooperation with each other can also work with therapists, social workers, and teachers to provide the best possible care.

Charney EB, Melchianni JB, Smith DR: Community ambulation by children with myelomeningocele and high level paralysis. J Pediatr Orthop 1991;11:579.

Menelaus MB: *The Orthopaedic Management of Spina Bifida Cystica,* 2nd ed. Churchill Livingstone, 1980.

MISCELLANEOUS DISEASES OF BONE

FIBROUS DYSPLASIA

Dysplastic fibrous tissue replacement of the medullary canal is accompanied by the formation of metaplastic bone in fibrous dysplasia. Three forms of the disease are recognized: monostotic, polyostotic, and polyostotic with endocrine disturbances (precocious puberty in females, hyperthyroidism, and hyperadrenalism [Albright's syndrome]).

Clinical Findings

A. Symptoms & Signs: The lesion or lesions may be asymptomatic. Pain, if present, is probably due to pathologic fractures. In females, endocrine disturbances may be present in the polyostotic variety and associated with café-au-lait spots.

B. Laboratory Findings: Laboratory findings are normal unless endocrine disturbances are present, in which case there may be increased secretion of gonadotropic, thyroid, or adrenal hormones.

C. Imaging: The lesion begins centrally within the medullary canal, usually of a long bone, and expands slowly. Pathologic fracture may occur. If metaplastic bone predominates, the contents of the lesion will be of the density of bone. Marked deformity of the bone may result, and a shepherd's crook deformity of the upper femur is a classic feature of the disease. The disease is often asymmetric, and limb length disturbances may occur as a result of stimulation of epiphysial cartilage growth.

Differential Diagnosis

The differential diagnosis may include other fibrous lesions of bone as well as destructive lesions such as bone cyst, eosinophilic granuloma, aneurysmal bone cyst, nonossifying fibroma, enchondroma, and chondromyxoid fibroma.

Treatment

If the lesion is small and asymptomatic, no treatment is needed. If the lesion is large and produces or threatens pathologic fracture, curettage and bone grafting are indicated.

Prognosis

Unless the lesions impair epiphysial growth, the prognosis for patients with fibrous dysplasia is good. Lesions tend to enlarge during the growth period but are stable during adult life. Malignant transformation has not been recorded.

UNICAMERAL BONE CYST

Unicameral bone cyst appears in the metaphysis of a long bone, usually in the femur or humerus. It begins within the medullary canal adjacent to the epiphysial cartilage. It probably results from some fault in enchondral ossification. The cyst is "active" as long as it abuts onto the metaphyseal side of the epiphysial cartilage and "inactive" when a border of normal bone exists between the cyst and the epiphysial cartilage. The lesion is usually identified when a pathologic fracture occurs, producing pain. Laboratory findings are normal. On x-ray films, the

cyst is identified centrally within the medullary canal, producing expansion of the cortex and thinning over the widest portion of the cyst.

Treatment consists of injection with corticosteroid. Several injections may be required. If injection fails, then curettage and bone grafting may be required. The cyst may heal after a fracture and not require treatment. The prognosis is excellent.

ANEURYSMAL BONE CYST

Aneurysmal bone cyst is similar to unicameral bone cyst, but it contains blood rather than clear fluid. It usually occurs in a slightly eccentric position in the long bone, expanding the cortex of the bone but not breaking the cortex, although some extraosseous mass may be produced. On x-ray films, the lesion appears somewhat larger than the width of the epiphysial cartilage, and this feature distinguishes it from unicameral bone cyst.

The aneurysmal bone cyst is filled by large vascular lakes, and the stoma of the cyst contains fibrous tissue and areas of metaplastic ossification.

The lesion may appear aggressive histologically, and it is important to differentiate it from osteosarcoma or hemangioma. Treatment is by curettage and bone grafting, and the prognosis is excellent.

INFANTILE CORTICAL HYPEROSTOSIS
(Caffey's Syndrome)

Infantile cortical hyperostosis is a benign disease of unknown cause that has its onset before 6 months of age and is characterized by irritability, fever, and nonsuppurating, tender, painful swellings. Swellings may involve almost any bone of the body and are frequently widespread. Classically, there are swellings of the mandible and clavicle in 50% of cases as well as of the ulna, humerus, and ribs. The disease is limited to the shafts of bones and does not involve subcutaneous tissues or joints. It is self-limited but may persist for weeks or months. Anemia, leukocytosis, an increased sedimentation rate, and elevation of the serum alkaline phosphatase are usually present. Cortical hyperostosis is demonstrable by a typical x-ray appearance and may be diagnosed on physical examination by an experienced pediatrician.

Fortunately, the disease appears to be decreasing in frequency. Corticosteroids are effective in severe cases. The prognosis is good, and the disease usually terminates without deformity.

GANGLION

A ganglion is a smooth, small cystic mass connected by a pedicle to the joint capsule, usually on the dorsum of the wrist. It may also be seen in the tendon sheath over the flexor surfaces of the fingers. These ganglia can be excised if they interfere with function or cause persistent pain.

BAKER'S CYST

Baker's cyst is a herniation of the synovium in the knee joint into the popliteal region. In children, the diagnosis may be made by aspiration of mucinous fluid, but the cyst nearly always disappears with time. Whereas Baker's cysts may be indicative of intra-articular disease in the adult, they usually are of no clinical significance in children and rarely require excision.

Dinham JM: Popliteal cysts in children: The case against surgery. J Bone Joint Surg [Br] 1975;57:69.

25

Rheumatic Diseases

J. Roger Hollister, MD

JUVENILE RHEUMATOID ARTHRITIS
(Juvenile Chronic Arthritis)

Essentials of Diagnosis
- Nonmigratory monarticular or polyarticular arthropathy, with a tendency to involve large joints or proximal interphalangeal joints and lasting more than 3 months.
- Systemic manifestations with fever, erythematous rashes, nodules, leukocytosis, and, occasionally, iridocyclitis, pleuritis, pericarditis, anemia, fatigue, and growth failure.

General Considerations

Juvenile rheumatoid arthritis (JRA) patients exhibit different immunogenetic traits from adult rheumatoid arthritis patients. In juvenile rheumatoid arthritis, HLA-DR5 is associated with iritis and the production of antinuclear antibodies, whereas HLA-DR4 is found in seropositive, polyarticular disease. These traits may be important in the formation of anti-suppressor cell antibodies, immune complex generation, and consequent chronic inflammatory disease.

Clinical Findings

A. Symptoms & Signs: There are three major patterns of presentation in JRA that provide clues to the prognosis and possible sequelae of the disease. In the **acute febrile** form, an evanescent salmon-pink macular rash, arthritis, hepatosplenomegaly, leukocytosis, and polyserositis characterize the constellation described by George Still. These patients have episodic illness, and remission of the systemic features can be expected within 1 year. They do not develop iridocyclitis.

The **polyarticular** pattern resembles the adult disease, with chronic pain and swelling of many joints in a symmetric fashion. Both large and small joints are usually involved. Systemic features are less prominent, although low-grade fever, fatigue, rheumatoid nodules, and anemia may be present. These patients tend to have long-standing arthritis, although the disease may wax and wane. Iridocyclitis

is occasionally seen in this group. Older children may have a positive latex fixation test.

The third pattern consists of **pauciarticular** disease characterized by chronic arthritis of a few joints—often the large weight-bearing joints—in asymmetric distribution. The synovitis is usually mild and may be painless. Systemic features are uncommon, but there is severe extra-articular involvement with inflammation in the eye. Up to 30% of children with pauciarticular juvenile rheumatoid arthritis develop insidious, asymptomatic iridocyclitis, which may cause blindness if untreated. The activity of the eye disease does not correlate with that of the arthritis. Therefore, routine ophthalmologic screening with slit-lamp examination must be performed every 6 months for 4 years, after which the risk is much lower.

B. Laboratory Findings: There is no diagnostic test for JRA. Rheumatoid factor is positive by the latex fixation test in about 15% of cases, usually when onset of polyarticular disease occurs after age 8 years. Antinuclear antibodies are most often present in pauciarticular disease with iridocyclitis and may serve as an indication of this complication; they are also fairly common in the late-onset rheumatoid factor-positive group. A normal erythrocyte sedimentation rate does not exclude the diagnosis.

In Table 25–1 are listed the general characteristics of joint fluid in various conditions. A positive Gram's stain or culture is the only definitive test. A leukocyte count over 2000/μL suggests inflammation; this may be due to infection, any of the collagen-vascular diseases, leukemia, or reactive arthritis. A very low glucose concentration (< 40 mg/dL) or very high polymorphonuclear leukocyte count (> 60,000/μL) is highly suggestive of bacterial arthritis in a child. Chemical analysis of synovial fluid is otherwise of little diagnostic benefit.

C. Imaging: In the early stages of the disease, only soft tissue swelling and regional osteoporosis are seen. MRI of involved joints may show joint damage earlier in the course of the disease than with other imaging modalities.

Table 25–1. Joint fluid analysis.

Disorder	Cells/μL	Glucose[1]
Trauma	More red cells than white cells; usually < 2000 white cells	Normal
Reactive arthritis	3000–10,000 white cells, mostly mono-nuclears	Normal
Juvenile rheumatoid arthritis and other inflammatory arthritides	5000–60,000 white cells, mostly neutrophils	Usually normal or slightly low
Septic arthritis	> 60,000 white cells, > 90% neutrophils	Low to normal

[1]Normal value is 75% or more of serum glucose value.

Table 25–2. Differential diagnosis of limb pain in children.

Orthopedic
  Stress fracture
  Overuse syndrome
  Chondromalacia patellae
  Osgood-Schlatter disease
  Slipped capital femoral epiphysis
  Legg-Calvé-Perthes disease
  Hypermobility syndrome
Reactive arthritis
  Schönlein-Henoch purpura
  Reactive arthritis following diarrhea
  Toxic synovitis of the hip
  Transient synovitis following viral infection
  Rheumatic fever
Infections
  Bacterial
    Lyme arthritis
    Osteomyelitis
    Septic arthritis
    Discitis
  Viral
    Parvovirus (in adolescents)
    Rubella
    Hepatitis B arthritis
Collagen-vascular
  Juvenile rheumatoid arthritis
  Spondyloarthropathy
  Systemic lupus erythematosus
  Dermatomyositis
Neoplastic
  Leukemia
  Lymphoma
  Neuroblastoma
  Reticuloendotheliosis
  Osteoid osteoma
  Bone tumors (benign or malignant)
Syndromes of psycho-organic origin
  Growing pains
  Fibromyalgia
  Reflex neurovascular dystrophy

Differential Diagnosis

Table 25–2 lists the most common causes of limb pain in childhood. A few points of information may indicate the most likely diagnosis. For instance, orthopedic causes are due to increased physical activity, not major trauma. Reactive arthritides are suggested by a preceding viral infection, strep throat, or purpuric rash, and their course is waxing and waning over several days. The characteristics of collagen-vascular and psycho-organic pain are not covered in this chapter.

Monarticular arthritis is the most important differential disorder to establish. Pain in the hip or lower extremity is a frequent symptom with childhood cancer, especially leukemia, neuroblastoma, and rhabdomyosarcoma. Infiltration of bone by tumor and actual joint effusion may be seen. X-rays of the affected site and a careful examination of the blood smear for unusual cells and thrombocytopenia are necessary. In doubtful cases, bone marrow examination is indicated.

Bacterial arthritis is usually acute and monarticular except for arthritis associated with *Haemophilus influenzae* infection and gonorrhea, both of which may be associated with a migratory pattern. Fever, leukocytosis, and increased sedimentation rate with an acute process in a single joint demand synovial fluid examination and culture to identify the pathogen. An elevated synovial fluid white count and low glucose (relative to plasma glucose) suggest sepsis.

The arthritis of rheumatic fever is migratory, transient, and often more painful than that of juvenile rheumatoid arthritis. Rheumatic fever is very rare under the age of 5 years. Evidence of rheumatic carditis should be carefully sought. Evidence of recent streptococcal infection is essential to the diagnosis. The fever pattern in rheumatic fever is low grade and persistent compared with the intermittent fever in the systemic form of JRA. Lyme arthritis resembles pauciarticular juvenile rheumatoid arthritis, but it occurs as discrete, recurrent episodes of arthritis lasting 2–6 weeks. A negative test for antibodies to *Borrelia burgdorferi* argues strongly against this diagnosis.

Treatment

The objectives of therapy are to restore function, relieve pain, and maintain joint motion. In recent years, other nonsteroidal anti-inflammatory drugs (NSAIDs) have replaced salicylates in the medical treatment of juvenile rheumatoid arthritis. Although their anti-inflammatory potency is not different from that of aspirin, their liquid form, decreased frequency of dosing, and diminished side effects appear to enhance compliance, cause fewer side effects, and justify their increased cost. Naproxen, 7.5 mg/kg twice daily; ibuprofen, 10 mg/kg four times daily; and tolmetin sodium, 10 mg/kg three times daily, may be used. If benefit occurs in the first 2 days, there will be continued improvement, with the maximum effect at 6 weeks. Aspirin, 75–100 mg/kg/d in three divided doses, is equally effective. Salicylates are withheld if the patient is exposed to chickenpox or Asian flu. Range-of-motion and muscle-strengthening exercises should be taught and supervised by a therapist, and a home program should be instituted. Bed rest is to be avoided except in the most acute stages. Joint casting is almost never indicated.

In JRA patients who fail to respond to aspirin, there are a number of alternatives. Methotrexate has replaced injectable gold salt therapy as a second-line medication. Symptomatic response usually occurs within 3–4 weeks. The low doses used (5–10 $mg/m^2/wk$ as a single dose) have been associated with few side effects. Stomatitis usually resolves with continued administration. Nausea may be prevented by splitting the dose. Hepatotoxicity, including fibrosis, is a concern. A CBC and liver function test should be obtained at 2-month intervals. Liver biopsy may be performed if there are recurrent elevations of aminotransferases. Injectable gold salts are an alternative in refractory cases.

Iridocyclitis should be treated by an ophthalmologist, and methotrexate may be used in difficult cases. Local corticosteroid injections into joints, synovectomy, or joint replacement may be indicated in selected patients.

Prognosis

In the primarily articular forms of JRA, disease activity progressively diminishes with age and ceases in about 95% of cases by puberty. In a few instances, this will persist into adult life. Problems after puberty therefore relate primarily to residual joint damage. Cases presenting in the teen years usually presage adult disease. The children most liable to be permanently handicapped are those with unremitting synovitis, hip involvement, or positive rheumatoid factor tests.

Foster CS, Barrett F: Cataract development and cataract surgery in patients with juvenile rheumatoid arthritis-associated iridocyclitis. Ophthalmology 1993;100:810.

Giannini EH et al: Methotrexate in resistant juvenile rheumatoid arthritis: Results of the U.S.A.-U.S.S.R. double-blind, placebo-controlled trial. New Engl J Med 1992;326:1043.

Kugathasan S et al: Liver biopsy findings in patients with juvenile rheumatoid arthritis receiving long-term weekly methotrexate therapy. J Pediatr 1996;128:149.

Ostrov BE et al: Differentiation of systemic juvenile rheumatoid arthritis from acute leukemia near the onset of disease. J Pediatr 1993;122:595.

Schneider R et al: Prognostic indicators of joint destruction in systemic onset juvenile rheumatoid arthritis. J Pediatr 1992;120:200.

Steele RW et al: Usefulness of scanning procedures for diagnosis of fever of unknown origin in children. J Pediatr 1991;119:526.

Szer IS et al: Long term course of Lyme arthritis in children. N Engl J Med 1991;325:159.

Tibbitts G: Juvenile rheumatoid arthritis: Old challenges, new insights. Postgrad Med 1994;96:75.

Wallace CA et al: Increased risk of facial scars in children taking nonsteroidal anti-inflammatory drugs. J Pediatr 1994;125:819.

SPONDYLOARTHROPATHY

Lower-extremity arthritis, particularly in males over 10 years of age, suggests a form of spondyloarthropathy. Inflammation of tendinous insertions (enthesopathy) such as the tibial tubercle or the heel occurs in these diseases and not in juvenile rheumatoid arthritis. Low back pain and sacroiliitis are quite specific for this form of arthritis. Carriage of HLA-B27 antigen occurs in 80% of these individuals. Specific syndromes of Reiter's disease, inflammatory bowel disease, psoriasis, or postdiarrheal reactive arthritis are suggested by the associated clinical findings and epidemiology. No autoantibodies are found, but inflammatory indicators such as an elevated erythrocyte sedimentation rate or C-reactive protein are usually present. The episodes are usually intermittent, in contrast to the more chronic symptoms of juvenile rheumatoid arthritis. Acute, not chronic, uveitis may occur.

The nonsteroidal medications, particularly indomethacin (2–4 mg/kg/d) and naproxen (15 mg/kg/d), are more effective than salicylates in the spondyloarthropathies. Refractory cases may respond to sulfasalazine. Local corticosteroid injections are contraindicated in Achilles tendinitis.

The arthritis is usually episodic. Unlike adults, children do not frequently progress to joint destruction or ankylosis.

Buxbaum J: Therapy for seronegative spondyloarthropathies. Curr Opin Rheumatol 1992;4:500.

SYSTEMIC LUPUS ERYTHEMATOSUS

Essentials of Diagnosis

- Multisystem inflammatory disease of joints, serous linings, skin, kidneys, and central nervous system.
- Antinuclear antibodies must be present in active, untreated disease.

General Considerations

Systemic lupus erythematosus (SLE) is the prototype of immune complex diseases; its pathogenesis is related to deposition in the tissue of soluble immune complexes existing in the circulation. The spectrum of symptoms appears to be due not to tissue-specific autoantibodies but rather to damage to the tissue by lymphocytes, neutrophils, and complement evoked by the deposition of antigen-antibody complexes. Many such antigen-antibody systems are present in this disorder, but the best correlation exists between

DNA-anti-DNA complexes and the activity of the disease. Laboratory tests of these antibodies and complement components give an objective assessment of disease pathogenesis and response to therapy. Autoreactive T lymphocytes that have escaped clonal deletion and unregulated B lymphocyte production of autoantibodies may initiate the disease.

Clinical Findings

A. Symptoms & Signs: The onset of systemic lupus erythematosus is most common in girls (8:1) between the ages of 9 and 15 years. The symptoms depend on what organ is involved with immune complex deposition.

1. Joint symptoms are the most common presenting feature. Nondeforming arthritis may involve any joint, often in a symmetric manner. Myositis may also occur and is more painful than the inflammation in dermatomyositis.

2. Systemic manifestations of SLE include weakness, anorexia, fever, fatigue, and loss of weight.

3. Skin lesions include butterfly erythema and induration, small ulcerations in skin and mucous membranes, purpura, alopecia, and Raynaud's phenomenon. The sun sensitivity of the dermal lesions may be striking.

4. Polyserositis may include pleurisy with effusions, peritonitis, and pericarditis. Libman-Sacks endocarditis may be seen in patients with anti-phospholipid antibodies.

5. Hepatosplenomegaly and lymphadenopathy may occur.

6. Renal systemic lupus erythematosus produces few symptoms at onset but is often progressive and is the leading cause of death. Renal biopsy is indicated in patients who do not respond to corticosteroids or who cannot have corticosteroids tapered to a less toxic alternate-day regimen. The histologic pattern of diffuse proliferative nephritis requires the most aggressive treatment. Late complications are nephrosis and uremia.

7. Central nervous system involvement produces a variety of symptoms such as seizures, coma, hemiplegia, focal neuropathies, and behavior disturbances, including psychosis.

B. Laboratory Findings: Leukopenia and anemia are frequently found with a low incidence of Coombs positivity. Thrombocytopenia and purpura may be early manifestations even in the absence of other organ involvement. The erythrocyte sedimentation rate (ESR) is elevated, and hypergammaglobulinemia is often present. Renal involvement is indicated by the presence in the urine of red cells, white cells, red cell casts, and proteinuria.

The antinuclear antibody (ANA) test is invariably positive in patients with active untreated SLE, and a negative ANA test effectively excludes the diagnosis. For patients with a positive antinuclear antibody test, a profile identifying individual disease-specific antibodies should be ordered. Anticardiolipin antibody and the lupus anticoagulant are two recently described autoantibodies that identify lupus patients at risk for thrombotic events.

In managing the disease, elevated titers of anti-DNA antibody and depressed levels of serum complement (hemolytic, C3, or C4) accurately reflect active disease, especially renal, central nervous system, and skin disease. A CT or MRI scan may identify pathologic conditions of the brain in lupus cerebritis, such as infarction, vasculitis, or atrophy.

Differential Diagnosis

Systemic lupus erythematosus may simulate many inflammatory diseases such as rheumatic fever, rheumatoid arthritis, and viral infections. It is essential to review all organ systems carefully to establish a clinical pattern. Renal and central nervous system involvement is unique to SLE. A negative ANA test excludes the diagnosis of systemic lupus erythematosus. Tests yielding false-positive results are usually of low titer (< 1:320).

An overlap syndrome known as **mixed connective tissue disease**, with features of several collagen-vascular diseases, has recently been described in adults and children. The symptom complex is diverse and does not readily fit previous classifications. Arthritis, fever, skin tightening, Raynaud's phenomenon, muscle weakness, and rashes are most commonly present. Important factors in recognition of this disease entity are the relative infrequency of renal disease, which implies a better prognosis than systemic lupus erythematosus, and the corticosteroid responsiveness of symptoms, which distinguishes mixed connective tissue disease from scleroderma. The definition of the disease includes the presence of serum antibody to a ribonuclear protein (RNP). The initial antinuclear antibody test is positive in very high titers. The ANA profile demonstrates the antibody to RNP. Pulmonary disease in childhood produces major morbidity.

Treatment

The treatment of systemic lupus erythematosus should be tailored to the organ system involved so that toxicities may be minimized. Prednisone, 0.5–1 mg/kg/d orally, has significantly lowered the mortality rate in SLE and should be used in all cases with renal, cardiac, or central nervous system involvement. The dose should be varied using clinical and laboratory parameters of disease activity, and the minimum amount of corticosteroid to control the disease should be used. Alternate-day regimens of corticosteroid are frequently possible. Skin manifestations may frequently be treated with antimalarials such as hydroxychloroquine, 5–7 mg/kg/d orally. Pleuritic pain or arthritis can often be managed with salicylates alone.

If disease control is inadequate with prednisone or if the dose required produces intolerable side effects, an immunosuppressant should be added. Either azathioprine, 2–3 mg/kg/d orally, or cyclophosphamide, $0.5–1$ g/m^2, administered intravenously once a month, has been most widely used. These drugs are ineffective during acute crises such as seizures.

The toxicities of the regimens must be carefully considered. In life-threatening disease, the choices are easier. Growth failure, osteoporosis, Cushing's syndrome, adrenal suppression, and aseptic necrosis are serious side effects of chronic use of prednisone. When high doses of corticosteroids are used (> 2 mg/kg/d), the risk of sepsis is very real. Cyclophosphamide causes bladder epithelial dysplasia, hemorrhagic cystitis, and sterility. Azathioprine has been associated with liver damage and bone marrow suppression. Immunosuppressant treatment should be withheld if the total white count falls below 3000/µL or the neutrophil count below 1000/µL. Retinal damage from chloroquine derivatives has not been observed with recommended dosages. Intravenous pulse steroid therapy and plasmapheresis are treatments that may be useful in selected cases.

Amenorrhea may result from uncontrolled systemic lupus erythematosus but may also be a consequence of prednisone, cyclophosphamide, or azathioprine administration.

Course & Prognosis

The prognosis in SLE relates to the presence of renal involvement or infectious complications of treatment. With improved diagnosis, milder cases are now identified. Nonetheless, the survival rate has improved from 51% at 5 years in 1954 to 90% today. The disease has a natural waxing and waning cycle, and periods of complete remission are not unusual.

Cervera R et al: Systemic lupus erythematosus: Clinical and immunologic patterns of disease expression in a cohort of 1000 patients. Medicine 1993;72:113.

Khamashta MA et al: The management of thrombosis in the antiphospholipid-antibody syndrome. N Engl J Med 1995;332:993.

Lindsley CB: Lupus: A brighter outlook, a continuing challenge. Contemporary Pediatr 1992;9:19.

Thomas C, Robinson JA: The antinuclear antibody test: When is a positive test clinically relevant. Postgrad Med 1993;94:191.

Tiddens HAWM et al: Juvenile-onset mixed connective tissue disease: Longitudinal follow-up. J Pediatr 1993;94:55.

West SG et al: Neuropsychiatric lupus erythematosus: A 10-year prospective study on the value of diagnostic tests. Am J Med 1995;99:153.

DERMATOMYOSITIS
(Polymyositis)

Essentials of Diagnosis

- Pathognomonic skin rash.
- Weakness of proximal muscles and occasionally of pharyngeal and laryngeal groups.
- Pathogenesis related to vasculitis.

General Considerations

Dermatomyositis, a rare inflammatory disease of muscle and skin in childhood, is uniquely responsive to corticosteroid treatment. The vasculitis observed in childhood dermatomyositis differs pathologically from the adult disease. Small arteries and veins are involved, with an exudate of neutrophils, lymphocytes, plasma cells, and histiocytes. The lesion progresses to intimal proliferation and thrombus formation. These vascular changes are found in the skin, muscle, kidney, retina, and gastrointestinal tract. Postinflammatory calcinosis is frequent.

The autoimmune pathogenesis of dermatomyositis has been difficult to prove. Recent studies have shown that both cellular and humoral mechanisms may be involved. Lymphocytes from patients are stimulated to undergo blastogenesis in the presence of muscle tissue and will release lymphotoxin, which destroys cultured fetal muscle cells. Biopsies studied with immunofluorescence techniques demonstrate immunoglobulin and complement in perivascular distribution. The putative antigen has not been identified and results of viral studies have been negative.

Clinical Findings

A. Symptoms & Signs: The predominant symptom is muscular weakness in proximal distribution affecting pelvic and shoulder girdles. Tenderness, stiffness, and swelling may be found but are not striking. Neurologic findings such as absence of tendon reflexes are not seen until late in the disease. Pharyngeal and respiratory involvement can be life-threatening. Flexion contractures and muscle atrophy produce significant residual deformities. Calcinosis may follow the inflammation in muscle and skin.

The rash of dermatomyositis is very helpful in the diagnosis of unknown muscle disease. Characteristically, the rash involves the upper eyelids and extensor surfaces of the knuckles, elbows, and knees with a distinctive heliotrope color that progresses to a scaling and atrophic appearance. Periorbital edema is not uncommon. Nail-fold capillary abnormalities may identify patients with a poorer prognosis. None of the rashes associated with other childhood rheumatic diseases have these features of distribution. The activity of the rash frequently does not parallel the muscle disease.

B. Laboratory Findings: Determination of muscle enzyme levels is the most helpful tool in diagnosis and treatment. All enzymes, including serum aldolase, should be screened to detect an abnormality that reflects activity of the disease. In later years of the illness, magnetic resonance imaging (MRI) of weak muscles may show disease activity when the enzymes are normal. No autoantibodies are found. Electromyography is useful to distinguish myopathic from neuropathic causes of muscle weakness. Muscle biopsy is indicated in doubtful cases of myositis without the pathognomonic rash.

Treatment

Prednisone in high doses (1–2 mg/kg/d orally) has been shown to speed recovery. The dose should be maintained or increased until muscle enzymes have returned to normal. Functional recovery will lag somewhat behind laboratory improvement. With improvement, the dose may be cut to that level which maintains disease control and normal muscle enzymes. Treatment must be continued for an average of 2 years. Immunosuppressant agents are occasionally required in childhood dermatomyositis. Intravenous immune globulin or cyclosporine therapy may be tried in refractory cases. Physical therapy is critical to prevent or allay contractures.

Course & Prognosis

Most children will recover and discontinue medications in 1–3 years. Relapses may occur. Functional ability is very good in most patients. Myositis in childhood is not associated with an increased risk of cancer.

Dalakas MC et al: A controlled trial of high-dose intravenous immune globulin infusions as treatment for dermatomyositis. N Engl J Med 1993;329:1993.

Hattori H et al: Benign acute myositis associated with rotavirus gastroenteritis. J Pediatr 1992;121:748.

Martin A et al: Recurrent juvenile dermatomyositis and cutaneous necrotizing arteritis with molecular mimicry between streptococcal type 5 M protein and human skeletal myosin. J Pediatr 1992;121:739.

Miller LC et al: Methotrexate treatment of recalcitrant childhood dermatomyositis. Arthritis Rheum 1992; 35:1143.

Sigurgeirsson B et al: Risk of cancer in patients with dermatomyositis or polymyositis. N Engl J Med 1992; 326:363.

POLYARTERITIS NODOSA

Polyarteritis nodosa is a rare disease, but a significant number of cases have been reported in childhood and infancy. No single cause has been found, but evidence of a streptococcal trigger and poorly controlled parvovirus infection have been found in some series.

Pathologically, the disease is a vasculitis of medium-sized arteries with fibrinoid degeneration in the media extending to the intima and adventitia.

Neutrophils and eosinophils comprise the inflammatory reaction. Aneurysms may be palpated or seen radiographically. Thrombosis of diseased arteries may cause infarction in many organs. Fibrosis of vessels and surrounding tissues accompanies the healing stages.

Symptomatology involves many tissues, and diagnosis is difficult. In childhood, unexplained fever, conjunctivitis, central nervous system involvement, and cardiac disease are more prominent than is the case in adult disease. Many cases appear as acute myocarditis, and the peripheral neuropathy so common in the adult is unusual. Diagnosis depends on biopsy-proved vasculitis or characteristic aneurysms on angiography.

The mortality rate is high, especially with cardiac involvement. Treatment consists of prednisone, 1–1.5 mg/kg/d orally, immunosuppressants, and intravenous gammaglobulin, but controlled studies of the efficacy of therapy of this rare disease are not yet available.

Corman LC, Dolson DJ: Polyarteritis nodosa and parvovirus B19 infection. Lancet 1992;339:491.

Finkel TH et al: Chronic parvovirus B19 infection and systemic necrotizing vasculitides: Opportunistic pathogen or etiologic agent. Lancet 1994;343:1255.

Ozen S et al: Diagnostic criteria for polyarteritis nodosa in childhood. J Pediatr 1992;120:206.

DIFFUSE SCLERODERMA (Progressive Systemic Sclerosis)

Scleroderma is a rare disease in childhood. Both the generalized systemic type and **morphea** (the more localized benign form) have been described. The diagnosis is made on a clinical basis with the finding of a skin disease that progresses from an edematous phase to an atrophic, taut, immobile dermis involving some or all of the skin. Systemic involvement may include Raynaud's phenomenon, arthralgias, pulmonary fibrosis, and renal disease. Involvement of the lungs and kidneys leads to rapid demise. Histologically, the diagnosis may not be specific but includes dermal atrophy with increased fibrosis and collagen content. The pathogenesis remains obscure, but studies indicate an increased synthesis of immature collagen by cultured scleroderma fibroblasts.

Effective therapy still awaits a better understanding of disease pathogenesis. Physical therapy is sometimes helpful in reducing debilitation from contractures and muscle wasting.

Birdi N et al: Localized scleroderma progressing to systemic disease. Arthritis Rheum 1993;36:410.

Miller JJ: The fasciitis-morphea complex in children. Am J Dis Child 1992;146:733.

NONRHEUMATIC PAIN SYNDROMES

Reflex Sympathetic Dystrophy

Reflex sympathetic dystrophy is a painful condition that is frequently confused with arthritis. There appears to be both an increased prevalence and an increased recognition of the condition. Severe extremity pain leading to nearly complete loss of function is the hallmark of the condition. Evidence of autonomic dysfunction is demonstrated by color changes, temperature differences, and dyshidrosis in the affected extremity. Foot involvement is more common than hand involvement. A puffy swelling of the entire hand or foot is common. On examination, there is marked cutaneous hyperesthesia to even the slightest touch. Results of laboratory tests are negative. X-ray findings are normal except for late development of osteoporosis. Bone scans are very helpful and demonstrate either increased or decreased blood supply to the painful extremity.

The cause of this condition remains elusive. Unlike adults, children only occasionally have a history of significant physical trauma at onset. How the autonomic dysfunction causes severe somatic pain is not known, but the feedback cycle does provide the basis for treatment. In mild cases, a program of rehabilitative physical therapy in combination with desensitization techniques will restore function and relieve pain. Refractory cases need family counseling and may respond to steroids or ganglionic blocks by local anesthesia. Long-term prognosis is good if recovery is rapid; recurrent episodes imply a less favorable prognosis.

Wilder RT et al: Reflex sympathetic dystrophy in children. J Bone Joint Surg [Am] 1992;74:910.

Fibromyalgia

Fibromyalgia is a diffuse pain syndrome in which patients experience pain all over their bodies without objective swelling. Weather changes and fatigue exacerbate symptoms. A sleep disturbance, such as insomnia or prolonged waking periods in the night, is an almost universal symptom; therefore, patients should be carefully questioned in this regard. On examination, patients are normal except for characteristic trigger points at the insertion of muscles, especially along the neck, spine, and pelvis.

Treatment consists of physical therapy and relieving the sleep disorder. Low-dose antidepressant medication (amitriptyline, 25 mg) taken before sleep may produce remarkable benefit in reduction of pain. Physical therapy should emphasize a graded rehabilitative approach to stretching and exercise. Analgesic medications provide poor pain relief and should be avoided because their use leads to escalation of medication, including narcotics.

The prognosis for young patients is not clear, and long-term strategies may be necessary to enable them to cope with the condition.

Malleson PN et al: Idiopathic musculoskeletal pain syndromes in children. J Rheumatol 1992;19:1786.
Sigal LH, Patella SJ: Lyme arthritis as the incorrect diagnosis in pediatric and adolescent fibromyalgia. Pediatrics 1992;90:523.

Chronic Fatigue Syndrome

Since 1985, chronic fatigue syndrome has become an increasingly common diagnosis. The distinction between this apparent organic fatigue and emotional causes of fatigue is not easily made. Criteria have been developed by NIH to assist in classification. The fatigue should have a defined date of onset, and there is a long list of excludable diagnoses. Other clinical manifestations include low-grade fevers, sore throat, painful lymph nodes, and neuropsychiatric problems. Epstein-Barr virus (EBV) infection does not account for all the patients described. Treatment is symptomatic and somewhat unsatisfactory.

Goldenburg DL: Fibromyalgia, chronic fatigue syndrome and myofascial pain syndrome. Curr Opin Rheumatol 1994;6:223.
Wessely S et al: Postinfectious fatigue: Prospective cohort study in primary care. Lancet 1995;345:1333.
Wilson A et al: The treatment of chronic fatigue syndrome: Science and speculation. Am J Med 1994;96:544.

HYPERMOBILITY SYNDROME

Ligamentous laxity, which previously was thought to occur only in Ehlers-Danlos syndrome or Down syndrome, is now recognized as a common cause of joint pain in our physically competitive society.

Children are now participating in a wide range of physically demanding sports and activities. Patients with hypermobility present with episodic joint pain and occasionally with swelling that lasts a few days after increased physical activity. Depending on the activity, almost any joint may be affected.

Physical examination may reveal joint swelling and tenderness, but the key to diagnosis is the demonstration of ligamentous laxity. Five criteria have been established: (1) passive opposition of the thumb to the flexor surface of the forearm; (2) passive hyperextension of the fingers so that they are parallel to the extensor surface of the forearm; (3) hyperextension of the elbow; (4) hyperextension of the knee (genu recurvatum); and (5) palms on floor with knees extended. Results of laboratory tests are normal. The pain associated with the syndrome is produced by improper joint alignment caused by the laxity during exercise.

Treatment consists of a graded conditioning program designed to provide muscular support of the joints to compensate for the loose ligaments. The prognosis is good provided conditioning before activities is adequate.

Gedalia A, Press J: Articular symptoms in hypermobile schoolchildren: A prospective study. J Pediatr 1991; 119:944.

REFERENCES

Cassidy JT, Petty RE: *Textbook of Pediatric Rheumatology,* 3rd ed. Saunders, 1995.

Jacobs JC: *Pediatric Rheumatology for the Practitioner,* 2nd ed. Springer-Verlag, 1993.

Pediatric rheumatology. Pediatr Clin North Am 1995;42:5. Entire issue.

26

Hematologic Disorders

Peter A. Lane, MD, Rachelle Nuss, MD, & Daniel R. Ambruso, MD

NORMAL VALUES

The normal ranges for peripheral blood counts vary significantly with age. Normal neonates show a relative polycythemia with a hematocrit of 45–65%. The reticulocyte count at birth is relatively high at 2–8%. Within the first few days of life, erythrocyte production decreases, and the levels of hemoglobin and hematocrit fall to a nadir at about 2–3 months. During this period, known as *physiologic anemia of infancy,* normal infants have hemoglobins as low as 10 g/dL and hematocrits as low as 30%. (Premature infants can reach a nadir hemoglobin of 7–8 g/dL at 8–10 weeks.) Thereafter, the normal values for hemoglobin and hematocrit gradually increase until adult values are reached after puberty.

Newborns have larger red cells than children and adults, with a mean corpuscular volume (MCV) at birth of more than 94 fL. The MCV subsequently falls to a nadir of 70–84 fL at about 6 months of age. Thereafter, the MCV gradually increases until it reaches adult normal values after puberty.

The normal number of white blood cells is higher in infancy and early childhood than later in life. Neutrophils predominate in the differential white count at birth and in the older child. There is a predominance of lymphocytes (up to 80%) between about 1 month and 6 years of age.

Normal values for the platelet count are 150,000–400,000/μL and vary little with age.

BONE MARROW FAILURE

Failure of the marrow to produce adequate numbers of circulating blood cells may be congenital or acquired and may cause pancytopenia (aplastic anemia) or involve only one cell line (single cytopenia). Constitutional and acquired aplastic anemia will be discussed in detail here, whereas the more common single cytopenias (Table 26–1) will be dealt with in subsequent sections. Bone marrow failure caused by malignancy or other infiltrative disease is discussed in Chapter 27. It is also important to remember that many drugs and toxins may affect the marrow and cause single or multiple cytopenias.

Suspicion of bone marrow failure should be high in children with pancytopenia and in children with single cytopenias and without evidence of peripheral red cell, white cell, or platelet destruction. Macrocytosis often accompanies bone marrow failure, and many of the constitutional bone marrow disorders are associated with a variety of congenital anomalies.

Alter DP, Young NS: The bone marrow failure syndromes. In: *Hematology of Infancy and Childhood,* 4th ed. Nathan DG, Oski FA (editors). WB Saunders, 1993.

Young NS, Alter BP: *Aplastic Anemia Acquired and Inherited.* WB Saunders, 1994.

CONSTITUTIONAL APLASTIC ANEMIA (Fanconi's Anemia)

Essentials of Diagnosis

- Thrombocytopenia or neutropenia progressing to pancytopenia.
- Macrocytosis.
- Multiple congenital anomalies.
- Increased chromosome breakage in peripheral blood lymphocytes.

General Considerations

Fanconi's anemia is a syndrome characterized by DNA instability caused by different gene defects which map to C9q22. Inheritance is autosomal recessive and the disease occurs in all ethnic groups. Hematologic manifestations usually begin with thrombocytopenia or neutropenia and subsequently progress over the course of months to years to pancytopenia. Typically, the diagnosis is made between the ages of 2 and 15 years.

Table 26–1. Important single cytopenias.

Red cell aplasia
    Congenital hypoplastic anemia (Diamond-Blackfan
      anemia)
    Transient erythroblastopenia of childhood
    Transient aplasia with chronic hemolysis
Neutropenia
    Kostmann's syndrome
    Shwachman-Diamond syndrome
    Cyclic neutropenia
Thrombocytopenia
    Thrombocytopenia with absent radii
    Amegakaryocytic thrombocytopenia

Clinical Findings

A. Symptoms and Signs: Symptoms are due principally to the degree of hematologic abnormality. Thrombocytopenia may cause purpura, petechiae, and bleeding; neutropenia may cause severe or recurrent infections; and anemia may cause weakness, fatigue, and pallor. Congenital anomalies are present in at least 50% of patients. The most common include abnormal pigmentation of the skin (generalized hyperpigmentation, café au lait or hypopigmented spots), short stature with delicate features, and skeletal malformations (hypoplasia, anomalies, or absence of the thumb and radius). More subtle anomalies include hypoplasia of thenar eminence or weakness of the radial pulse. Associated renal anomalies include aplasia, horseshoe kidney, and duplication of the collecting system. Other anomalies are microcephaly, microphthalmia, strabismus, ear anomalies, and hypogenitalism.

B. Laboratory Findings: Thrombocytopenia or leukopenia typically occur first, followed over the course of months to years by anemia and progression to severe aplastic anemia. Macrocytosis is virtually always present, is usually associated with anisocytosis and an elevation in fetal hemoglobin, and is an important diagnostic clue. The bone marrow reveals hypoplasia or aplasia consistent with the degree of peripheral cytopenias. The diagnosis is confirmed by the demonstration of an increased number of chromosome breaks and rearrangements in peripheral blood lymphocytes. The use of diepoxybutane to stimulate these breaks and rearrangements provides for a sensitive assay that is virtually always positive in children with Fanconi's anemia, even before the onset of hematologic abnormalities. Such testing is sometimes used for prenatal diagnosis as well.

Differential Diagnosis

Because patients with Fanconi's anemia frequently present with thrombocytopenia, the disorder must be differentiated from idiopathic thrombocytopenic purpura (ITP) and other more common causes of decreased platelets. In contrast to those with ITP, patients with thrombocytopenia of Fanconi's anemia usually present with a gradual fall in the platelet count, and counts less than 20,000/µL are often accompanied by neutropenia or anemia. Furthermore, children with ITP do not have macrocytosis and would not typically have short stature, microcephaly, or other congenital anomalies. Fanconi's anemia may also present initially with pancytopenia and must be differentiated from acquired aplastic anemia and from diseases associated with bone marrow infiltration such as acute leukemia. Examination of the bone marrow in conjunction with chromosome studies of lymphocytes will usually distinguish between these disorders.

Complications

The most important complications of Fanconi's anemia are those related to thrombocytopenia and neutropenia. In addition, persons with Fanconi's anemia have a significantly increased risk of developing malignancies, especially acute nonlymphocytic leukemia. Death is usually the result of thrombocytopenic hemorrhage, overwhelming infection, or malignancy.

Treatment

Attentive supportive care is a critical feature of management. Patients with neutropenia who develop fever require prompt evaluation and parenteral broad-spectrum antibiotics. Transfusions are important but should be used judiciously, especially in the management of thrombocytopenic patients, who frequently become refractory to platelet transfusions as a consequence of alloimmunization. Transfusions from family members should be discouraged because of the negative impact on the outcome of bone marrow transplantation. At least 50% of patients with Fanconi's aplastic anemia respond, albeit incompletely, to androgen therapy with or without corticosteroids, and many recommend institution of androgens before transfusions are needed. However, such treatments are associated with hepatotoxicity, and masculinization is particularly troublesome in females.

Successful bone marrow transplantation cures the aplastic anemia and this is an important treatment option for children with Fanconi's anemia who are fortunate enough to have an HLA-identical sibling donor. First, it is important to exclude the possibility of Fanconi's anemia in the donor by testing lymphocytes for chromosome breakage.

Prognosis

Many patients succumb to bleeding, infection, or malignancy in adolescence or early adulthood. The long-term outlook for those undergoing successful bone marrow transplantation is uncertain, particularly with regard to the risk of developing leukemia or other malignancies.

Alter BP: Clinical features of Fanconi's anemia. In: *Aplastic Anemia: Acquired and Inherited.* Young NS, Alter BP (editors). WB Saunders, 1994:275.

Butturini A et al: Hematologic abnormalities in Fanconi anemia: An international Fanconi anemia registry study. Blood 1994;84:1650.

Gluckman E, et al: Bone marrow transplantation for Fanconi anemia. Blood 1995;86:2856.

ACQUIRED APLASTIC ANEMIA

Essentials of Diagnosis

- Weakness and pallor.
- Petechiae, purpura, and bleeding.
- Frequent or severe infections.
- Pancytopenia with empty bone marrow.

General Considerations

Acquired aplastic anemia is characterized by peripheral pancytopenia with a hypocellular bone marrow. Approximately 50% of the cases in childhood are idiopathic, without evidence of any etiologic agent or associated abnormality. Other cases appear to be secondary to idiosyncratic reactions to drugs such as chloramphenicol, phenylbutazone, sulfonamides, nonsteroidal anti-inflammatories, and anticonvulsants. Toxic causes include exposure to benzene, insecticides, and heavy metals. Infectious causes include viral hepatitis, infectious mononucleosis, and HIV. In immunocompromised children, aplastic anemia has been associated with human parvovirus.

Clinical Findings

A. Symptoms and Signs: Weakness, fatigue, and pallor are the result of anemia; petechiae, purpura, and bleeding occur because of thrombocytopenia; and fevers due to generalized or localized infections are the result of neutropenia. Hepatosplenomegaly and significant lymphadenopathy are unusual.

Anemia is usually normocytic, with a low reticulocyte count. The white blood cell count is low, with a marked neutropenia. The platelet count is typically below 50,000/μL and frequently below 20,000/μL. Bone marrow aspiration and biopsy are essential to the diagnosis and show hypocellularity, often marked, with the marrow space replaced with fat.

Differential Diagnosis

Examination of the bone marrow usually excludes pancytopenia caused by peripheral destruction of blood cells or by infiltrative processes such as acute leukemia, storage diseases, and myelofibrosis. Many of these other conditions are associated with hepatosplenomegaly. Occasionally, children with pancytopenia and hypocellular bone marrows ultimately prove to have preleukemic conditions. In this regard, cytogenetic analysis of the marrow is helpful, since the presence of a clonal abnormality may predict the subsequent development of leukemia. Some children with Fanconi's anemia do not have congenital anomalies, and for that reason all children with newly diagnosed aplastic anemia should be studied for the presence of chromosome breaks and rearrangements in peripheral blood lymphocytes.

Complications

Acquired aplastic anemia is characteristically complicated by overwhelming infection and severe hemorrhage, and these two complications are the leading causes of death. Other complications are those associated with therapy.

Treatment

Comprehensive supportive care is most important in the management of children with acute acquired aplastic anemia. All febrile illnesses require prompt evaluation and usually parenteral antibiotics. Packed red blood cells should be transfused to alleviate symptoms of anemia. Platelet transfusions may be lifesaving, but they should be used sparingly since many patients eventually develop platelet alloantibodies.

Bone marrow transplantation is the treatment of choice for patients with severe aplastic anemia when an HLA-compatible sibling donor is available. Because the likelihood of success with transplantation is adversely influenced by multiple transfusions, HLA typing of family members should be undertaken as soon as the diagnosis of aplastic anemia is made. An increasing number of patients who lack HLA-matched siblings are able to find unrelated but matched donors through the National Bone Marrow Registry.

The best alternative to bone marrow transplantation for patients without an HLA-identical sibling is immunosuppression with antithymocyte globulin (ATG), cyclosporine, or corticosteroids, singly or in combination. Hematologic improvement occurs in over 50% of children treated with ATG, but remissions are often incomplete or not sustained. Recent studies suggest that a combination of ATG and cyclosporine are more effective than either therapy alone, especially for patients with severe disease.

Prognosis

The prognosis for patients with severe aplastic anemia is extremely poor if bone marrow transplantation is not available and if immunosuppression is not effective. In such cases, patients usually die of infection or hemorrhage within 6–12 months after diagnosis. Children treated early with bone marrow transplantation from an HLA-identical sibling have a long-term survival rate of greater than 80%.

Matloub YH et al: Antithymocyte globulin, cyclosporin, and prednisone for the treatment of severe aplastic anemia in children. Am J Pediatr Hematol Oncol 1994; 16:104.

Rosenfeld SJ et al:Intensive immunosuppression with antithymocyte globulin and cyclosporin as treatment for severe aplastic anemia. Blood 1995;85:3058.

Sanders JE et al: Marrow transplant experience for children with severe aplastic anemia. Am J Pediatr Hematol Oncol 1994;16:43.

Young NS, Barrett AJ:The treatment of severe acquired aplastic anemia. Blood 1995;85:3367.

ANEMIAS

APPROACH TO THE CHILD WITH ANEMIA

Anemia is a relatively common finding, and finding the cause is always important. Even thouhg anemia in childhood has many causes, the correct diagnosis can usually be established with relatively little laboratory cost.

Frequently, the cause is suggested by a careful history. The possibility of nutritional causes should be addressed by inquiry about dietary intake, growth and development, and symptoms of chronic disease, malabsorption, or blood loss. Hemolytic disease may be suggested by a history of jaundice (including neonatal jaundice) or by a family history of anemia, jaundice, gallbladder disease, splenomegaly, or splenectomy. The child's ethnic background may suggest the possibility of certain hemoglobinopathies or of deficiencies of red cell enzymes such as glucose-6-phosphate dehydrogenase (G6PD). The review of systems may reveal clues to a previously unsuspected systemic disease with which anemia may be associated. The age of the patient is important because some causes of anemia are age-related. For example, iron deficiency anemia and β-globin disorders present more commonly between 6 and 24 months of age than at other times in life.

The physical examination may also reveal clues to the cause of anemia. Poor growth may suggest chronic disease or hypothyroidism. Congenital anomalies may be associated with constitutional aplastic anemia (Fanconi's anemia) or with constitutional hypoplastic anemia (Diamond-Blackfan anemia). Other disorders may be suggested by the findings of petechiae or purpura (leukemia, aplastic anemia, hemolytic uremic syndrome), jaundice (hemolysis or liver disease), generalized lymphadenopathy (leukemia, juvenile rheumatoid arthritis, HIV infection), splenomegaly (leukemia, sickle syndromes, hereditary spherocytosis, liver disease, hypersplenism), or evidence of chronic or recurrent infections.

The initial laboratory evaluation of the anemic child generally consists of a complete blood count (CBC) with differential and platelet count, review of the peripheral blood smear, and usually a reticulocyte count. The algorithm in Figure 26–1 shows how this limited laboratory information, together with the history and physical examination, may lead to a specific diagnosis or focus additional laboratory investigations to a limited diagnostic category (eg, microcytic anemia, bone marrow failure, pure red cell aplasia, or hemolytic disease). This diagnostic scheme depends principally on the MCV to determine whether the anemia is microcytic, normocytic, or macrocytic, according to the percentile curves of Dallman and Siimes (Figure 26–2).

With regard to microcytic anemias, the incidence of iron deficiency in the United States has decreased significantly with improvements in infant nutrition. Still, iron deficiency is an important cause of microcytic anemia, especially between 6 and 24 months of age. A trial of therapeutic iron is appropriate in such children, provided the dietary history is compatible with the development of iron deficiency and the physical examination or CBC results do not suggest an alternative cause for the anemia. If this is not the case—or if a trial of therapeutic iron fails to correct the anemia and microcytosis—then further laboratory evaluation is warranted.

Another key element of Figure 26–1 is the use of both the reticulocyte count and the peripheral blood smear to determine whether a normocytic or macrocytic anemia is due to hemolysis. Typically, hemolytic disease is associated with an elevated reticulocyte count, but some children with chronic hemolysis initially present during a period of virus-induced aplasia when the reticulocyte count is not elevated. Thus, review of the peripheral smear for evidence of hemolysis (eg, spherocytes, red cell fragmentation, sickle forms) is important in the evaluation of children with normocytic anemias and low reticulocyte counts. When hemolysis is suggested, the correct diagnosis may be suspected by specific abnormalities of red cell morphology or by clues from the history or physical examination. Autoimmune hemolysis can be excluded by Coombs' testing. Review of blood counts and the peripheral smears of the mother and father may suggest congenital disorders such as hereditary spherocytosis. Children with normocytic or macrocytic anemias, with relatively low reticulocyte counts and no evidence of hemolysis on the blood smear, usually have anemias caused by inadequate erythropoiesis in the bone marrow. The presence of neutropenia or thrombocytopenia in such children suggests bone marrow failure and the possibility of aplastic anemia or malignancy and usually dictates examination of the bone marrow. Pure red cell aplasia may be constitutional (Diamond-Blackfan anemia), acquired and transient (transient erythroblastopenia of childhood), a mani-

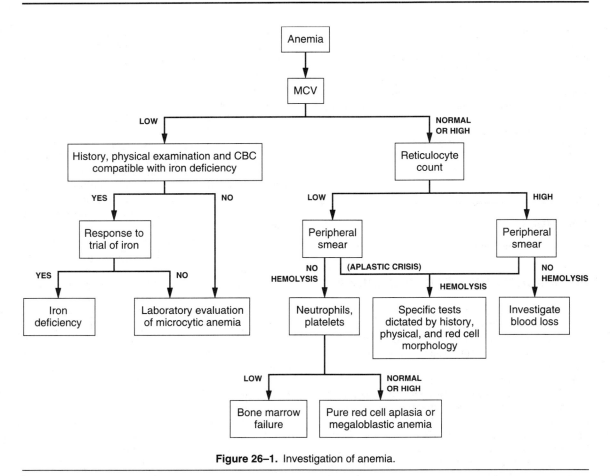

Figure 26–1. Investigation of anemia.

festation of a systemic disease such as renal disease or hypothyroidism, or due to malnutrition or deficiencies of folate or cobalamin.

Dallman PR et al: Percentile curves for hemoglobin and red cell volume in infancy and childhood. J Pediatr 1979; 94:26.

Oski FA: Differential diagnosis of anemia. In: *Hematology of Infancy and Childhood,* 4th ed. Nathan DG, Oski FA (editors). WB Saunders, 1993.

PURE RED CELL APLASIA

Infants and children with normocytic or macrocytic anemia, a low reticulocyte count, and normal or elevated numbers of neutrophils and platelets should be suspected of having pure red cell aplasia. Examination of the peripheral smear in such cases is important because signs of hemolytic disease suggest the possibility of chronic hemolysis complicated by an aplastic crisis due to parvovirus infection. Appreciation of this phenomenon is important because children with chronic hemolytic disease may not be diagnosed until the anemia is exacerbated by an episode

of red cell aplasia that results in a rapidly falling hemoglobin. In such cases, cardiovascular compromise and congestive heart failure are imminent threats.

1. CONGENITAL HYPOPLASTIC ANEMIA (Diamond-Blackfan Anemia)

Essentials of Diagnosis
- Age: birth to 1 year.
- Macrocytic anemia with reticulocytopenia.
- Bone marrow with erythroid hypoplasia.
- Short stature or congenital anomalies in one third.

General Considerations

Diamond-Blackfan anemia is a relatively rare cause of anemia that usually presents in infancy or early childhood. Early diagnosis is important because prompt treatment with corticosteroids results in increased erythropoiesis in about two thirds of patients, thus avoiding the difficulties and complications of long-term chronic transfusion therapy. The cause of the disorder is unclear, and both autosomal dominant

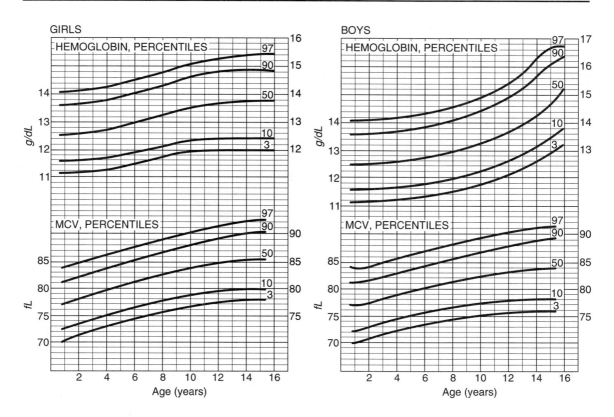

Figure 26–2. Hemoglobin and red cell volume in infancy and childhood. (From Dallman PR, Siimes MA: Percentile curves for hemoglobin and red cell volume in infancy and childhood. J Pediatr 1979;94:26.)

and autosomal recessive modes of inheritance have been suggested.

Clinical Findings

A. Symptoms and Signs: Signs and symptoms are generally those of chronic anemia, such as pallor, and congestive heart failure sometimes follows. Jaundice, splenomegaly, or other evidence of hemolysis is usually absent. Short stature or other congenital anomalies are present in one third of patients. A wide variety of anomalies have been described, and those affecting the head, face, and thumbs are probably the most common.

B. Laboratory Findings: Diamond-Blackfan anemia is characterized by severe anemia and marked reticulocytopenia. The neutrophil count is usually normal or slightly decreased, and the platelet count is normal or elevated. The bone marrow usually shows a marked decrease in erythroid precursors but is otherwise normal. In older children, levels of fetal hemoglobin are usually increased and there is evidence of persistent fetal erythropoiesis such as the presence of the i antigen on erythrocytes. In addition, the level of adenosine deaminase in erythrocytes is elevated.

Differential Diagnosis

The principal disorder from which Diamond-Blackfan anemia must be differentiated is transient erythroblastopenia of childhood. In contrast to that condition, patients with Diamond-Blackfan anemia generally present at an earlier age, often have macrocytosis, and have evidence of fetal erythropoiesis and an elevated level of red cell adenosine deaminase. In addition, short stature and congenital anomalies, which occur in one third of patients with Diamond-Blackfan anemia, are not associated with transient erythroblastopenia. Lastly, transient erythroblastopenia of childhood usually resolves within 6–8 weeks of diagnosis, whereas Diamond-Blackfan anemia is generally a lifelong affliction. Other disorders associated with decreased red cell production such as renal failure, hypothyroidism, and the anemia of chronic disease need to be considered.

Treatment

Oral corticosteroids should be initiated as soon as the diagnosis of Diamond-Blackfan anemia is made. Two thirds of patients will respond to prednisone, 2 mg/kg/d, and many of those who respond subsequently tolerate significant tapering of the dose. Patients who are unresponsive to prednisone generally require chronic red cell transfusion therapy, which inevitably causes transfusion-induced hemosiderosis and the need for chelation with parenteral deferoxamine. Bone marrow transplantation is an alternative therapy that should be considered for transfusion-dependent patients who have HLA-matched siblings. Hematopoietic growth factors have been used in some cases with limited success. Unpredictable, spontaneous remissions occasionally occur.

Prognosis

The prognosis for patients responsive to corticosteroids is generally good, particularly if remission is maintained with low doses of alternate-day prednisone. Patients dependent upon transfusion are at risk for the complications of hemosiderosis, including death from congestive heart failure, cardiac arrhythmias, or hepatic failure. This remains a significant threat, particularly during adolescence, when compliance with nightly subcutaneous infusions of deferoxamine is often a difficult issue.

Alter BP: Diamond-Blackfan anemia. In: *Aplastic Anemia: Acquired and Inherited.* Young NS, Alter BP. WB Saunders, 1994:361.

Dunbar CE et al: Treatment of Diamond-Blackfan anaemia with haematopoietic growth factors, granulocyte-macrophage colony stimulating factor and interleukin 3: Sustained remissions following IL-3. Br J Haematol 1991;79:316.

Greinix HT et al: Long-term survival and cure after marrow transplantation for congenital hypoplastic anaemia (Diamond-Blackfan syndrome). Br J Haematol 1993;84:515.

Olivieri NF et al: Failure of recombinant human interleukin-3 therapy to induce erythropoiesis in patients with refractory Diamond-Blackfan anemia. Blood 1994;83:2444.

2. TRANSIENT ERYTHROBLASTOPENIA OF CHILDHOOD

Essentials of Diagnosis

- Age 6 months to 4 years.
- Normocytic anemia with reticulocytopenia.
- Absence of hepatosplenomegaly or lymphadenopathy.
- Erythroid precursors initially lacking from bone marrow.

General Considerations

Transient erythroblastopenia of childhood is a relatively common cause of acquired anemia in early childhood. The disorder is generally suspected when a normocytic anemia is discovered during evaluation of pallor or when a CBC is obtained for another reason. Because the anemia is due to decreased red cell production and thus develops slowly, the cardiovascular system has time to compensate. Therefore, chil-

dren with hemoglobins as low as 4 or 5 g/dL may look remarkably well. The disorder is thought to be autoimmune in most cases, since IgG from some patients has been shown to suppress erythropoiesis in vitro.

Clinical Findings

Pallor is the most common sign, and hepatosplenomegaly and lymphadenopathy are absent. The anemia is normocytic, and the smear shows no evidence of hemolysis. The platelet count is normal or elevated, and the neutrophil count is normal or, in some cases, somewhat decreased. The Coombs' test is negative, and there is no evidence of chronic renal disease, hypothyroidism, or other systemic disorder. Bone marrow examination shows severe erythroid hypoplasia initially; subsequently, erythroid hyperplasia develops along with reticulocytosis and the anemia resolves.

Differential Diagnosis

Transient erythroblastopenia of childhood must be differentiated from Diamond-Blackfan anemia, particularly in infants less than 1 year of age. In contrast to Diamond-Blackfan anemia, transient erythroblastopenia is not associated with macrocytosis, short stature, or congenital anomalies, or with evidence of fetal erythropoiesis prior to the phase of recovery. Also in contrast to Diamond-Blackfan anemia, levels of red cell adenosine deaminase are normal. Transient erythroblastopenia of childhood must also be differentiated from chronic disorders associated with decreased red cell production, such as renal failure, hypothyroidism, and other chronic states of infection or inflammation. As with other single cytopenias, the possibility of malignancy (ie, leukemia) should always be considered, particularly if fever, bone pain, hepatosplenomegaly, or lymphadenopathy is present. In such cases, examination of the bone marrow is generally diagnostic. Confusion may sometimes arise when the anemia of transient erythroblastopenia is first identified during the early phase of recovery when the reticulocyte count is high. In such cases, the disorder may be confused with the anemia of acute blood loss or with hemolytic disease. In contrast to hemolytic disorders, however, there is no jaundice and no evidence of hemolysis on the blood smear.

Treatment & Prognosis

By definition, transient erythroblastopenia of childhood is a transient disorder. Some children require red cell transfusions if signs of cardiovascular compromise are present. Resolution of the anemia is heralded by an increase in the reticulocyte count, which generally occurs within 4–8 weeks of diagnosis. In contrast to other autoimmune disorders of childhood (eg, ITP, autoimmune hemolytic anemia), the use of corticosteroids is of no proven benefit and is not indicated.

Alter BP: Transient erythroblastopenia of childhood. In: *Aplastic Anemia: Acquired and Inherited.* Young NS, Alter BP. WB Saunders, 1994:384.

Cherrick I, Karayakin G, Lanzkowsky P: Transient erythroblastopenia of childhood: Prospective study of fifty patients. Am J Pediatr Hematol Oncol 1994;15:320.

Miller R, Berman B. Transient erythroblastopenia of childhood in infants <6 months of age. Am J Pediatr Hematol Oncol 1994;16:246.

NUTRITIONAL ANEMIAS

1. IRON DEFICIENCY ANEMIA

Essentials of Diagnosis

- Pallor and fatigue.
- Poor dietary intake of iron (age 6–24 months).
- Chronic blood loss (age >2 years).
- Microcytic, hypochromic anemia.

General Considerations

Long considered the most common cause of anemia in pediatrics, iron deficiency has seen a dramatic decrease in incidence during the past two decades. This is the direct result of improved nutrition and the increased availability of iron-fortified infant formulas and cereals. Thus, the current approach to anemia in childhood must take into consideration a relatively greater chance of other causes than was formerly the case.

Normal term infants are born with sufficient iron stores to prevent iron deficiency for the first 4 months of life. Thereafter, enough iron needs to be absorbed to keep pace with the needs of rapid growth. For this reason, nutritional iron deficiency is most common between 6 and 24 months of life. A deficiency earlier than 6 months of age may occur if iron stores at birth are reduced by prematurity, small birth weight, neonatal anemia, or perinatal blood loss or if there is subsequent iron loss due to hemorrhage. Iron-deficient children older than 24 months of age should be investigated for blood loss.

A significant body of evidence indicates that iron deficiency, in addition to causing anemia, has adverse effects on behavior and cognitive function. Thus, the importance of the identification of iron deficiency and of its treatment extends past the resolution of any symptoms directly attributable to a lowered hemoglobin concentration.

Clinical Findings

A. Symptoms and Signs: Symptoms and signs vary with the severity of the deficiency. Mild iron deficiency is usually asymptomatic. In infants with more severe iron deficiency, pallor, fatigue, irritability, and delayed motor development are common. Children whose iron deficiency is due in part to ingestion of unfortified cow's milk may be fat and flabby, with poor muscle tone. A history of pica is common.

B. Laboratory Findings: The severity of anemia depends on the degree of iron deficiency, and the hemoglobin may be as low as 3–4 g/dL in severe cases. Red cells are microcytic and hypochromic, with a low MCV and low MCH. The red blood cell distribution width (RDW) is typically elevated, even with mild iron deficiency. The reticulocyte count is usually normal but may be slightly elevated in severe cases. Iron studies show a decreased serum ferritin as well as a low serum iron, elevated total iron-binding capacity, and decreased transferrin saturation. Free erythrocyte protoporphyrin is elevated. All of these laboratory abnormalities are usually present with moderate to severe iron deficiency, but mild cases may show variable laboratory results.

The bone marrow examination is not helpful in the diagnosis of iron deficiency in infants and small children because little or no iron is stored as marrow hemosiderin at these ages.

Differential Diagnosis

The differential diagnosis is that of microcytic, hypochromic anemia. The possibility of thalassemia (α-thalassemia, β-thalassemia, hemoglobin E disorders) should be considered, especially in infants of African, Mediterranean, or Asian ethnic background. In contrast to those with iron deficiency, infants with thalassemia generally have an elevated number of erythrocytes (the index of the MCV divided by the red cell number is usually <13) and are less likely, in mild cases, to have an elevated RDW. Thalassemias are associated with normal or increased levels of serum iron and ferritin and with normal iron-binding capacity and free erythrocyte protoporphyrin levels. The hemoglobin electrophoresis in β-thalassemia trait typically shows an elevation of hemoglobin A_2, but coexistent iron deficiency may lower the percentage of hemoglobin A_2 into the normal range. Hemoglobin electrophoresis will also identify children with hemoglobin E, a cause of microcytosis common in Southeast Asians. In contrast, the hemoglobin electrophoresis in α-thalassemia trait is normal. Lead poisoning has also been associated with microcytic anemia, but anemia with lead levels less than 40 μg/dL is usually due to coexistent iron deficiency.

The anemia of chronic inflammation or infection may also be microcytic. This anemia is usually suspected because of the presence of a chronic systemic disorder. The level of serum iron is low, but serum ferritin is elevated. Finally, it should be appreciated that relatively mild infections, particularly during infancy, may cause transient anemia. For this reason, caution should be exercised when the diagnosis of mild iron deficiency is entertained in infants and young children who have had recent viral or bacterial infections. Ideally, screening tests for anemia should not be obtained within 3–4 weeks of such infections.

Treatment

The recommended oral dose of elemental iron is 4–6 mg/kg/d in three divided daily doses. Mild cases may be treated with 3 mg/kg/d given once daily before breakfast. Parenteral administration of iron is rarely necessary. Iron therapy results in an increased reticulocyte count within 3–5 days, which is maximal between 5 and 7 days. The hemoglobin level begins to increase thereafter. The rate of hemoglobin rise is inversely related to the hemoglobin level at diagnosis. In moderate to severe cases, an elevated reticulocyte count 1 week after initiation of therapy confirms the diagnosis and documents compliance and response to therapy. When iron deficiency is the only cause of anemia, adequate treatment usually results in a resolution of the anemia within 4–6 weeks. Treatment is generally continued for a few additional months to replenish iron stores.

Lozoff B: Iron deficiency and infant development. J Pediatr 1994;125:577.

Moffatt MEK et al: Prevention of iron deficiency and psychomotor decline in high-risk infants through use of iron-fortified infant formula: A randomized clinical trial. J Pediatr 1994;125:527.

Oski FA: Iron deficiency in infancy and childhood. N Engl J Med 1993;329:190.

Piscane A et al: Iron status of breast-fed infants. J Pediatr 1995;127:429.

2. MEGALOBLASTIC ANEMIAS

Essentials of Diagnosis

- Pallor and fatigue.
- Nutritional deficiency or intestinal malabsorption.
- Macrocytic anemia.
- Megaloblastic bone marrow changes.

General Considerations

Megaloblastic anemia is a macrocytic anemia caused by deficiency of cobalamin (vitamin B_{12}), folic acid, or both. Cobalamin deficiency due to dietary insufficiency may occur in infants who are breast-fed by mothers who are strict vegetarians or who have pernicious anemia. Intestinal malabsorption is the usual cause of cobalamin deficiency in pediatrics and occurs with Crohn's disease, chronic pancreatitis, bacterial overgrowth of the small bowel, infection with the fish tapeworm (*Diphyllobothrium latum*), or after surgical resection of the terminal ileum. Deficiencies due to inborn errors of metabolism (transcobalamin II deficiency, methylmalonic aciduria) have also been described. Malabsorption of cobalamin due to deficiency of intrinsic factor (pernicious anemia) is rare in childhood.

Folic acid deficiency may be caused by inadequate dietary intake, malabsorption, increased folate requirements, or some combination of the three. Folate deficiency due to dietary deficiency alone is rare but occurs in severely malnourished infants and has been reported in infants fed goat's milk not fortified with folic acid. Folic acid is absorbed in the proximal small bowel, and deficiencies are encountered in malabsorptive syndromes such as celiac disease. Anticonvulsant medications (eg, phenytoin and phenobarbital) and cytotoxic drugs (eg, methotrexate) have also been associated with folate deficiency, caused by interference with folate absorption or metabolism. Finally, folic acid deficiency is more likely to develop in infants and children with increased requirements. This occurs during infancy because of rapid growth and also in children with chronic hemolytic anemia. Premature infants are particularly susceptible to the development of the deficiency because of low body stores of folate.

Clinical Findings

A. Symptoms and Signs: Infants with megaloblastic anemia may show pallor and mild jaundice due to ineffective erythropoiesis. Classically, the tongue is smooth and beefy red. Infants with cobalamin deficiency may be irritable and may be poor feeders. Older children with cobalamin deficiency may complain of paresthesias, weakness, or an unsteady gait and may show decreased vibratory sensation and proprioception on neurologic examination.

B. Laboratory Findings: The laboratory findings of megaloblastic anemia include an elevated MCV and mean corpuscular hemoglobin (MCH). The blood smear shows numerous macro-ovalocytes with anisocytosis and poikilocytosis. Neutrophils are large and have hypersegmented nuclei. The white cell count and the platelet count are normal with mild deficiencies, but may be decreased in more severe cases. Examination of the bone marrow typically shows erythroid hyperplasia with large erythroid and myeloid precursors. There is nuclear-cytoplasmic dissociation and ineffective erythropoiesis. The serum indirect bilirubin concentration may be slightly elevated.

Children with cobalamin deficiency have a low serum vitamin B_{12} level. In addition, the urinary concentration of methylmalonic acid is significantly elevated. The latter test is useful in the diagnosis because decreased levels of serum vitamin B_{12} may also be seen in about 30% of patients with folic acid deficiency. Assessment of folate stores is best done by measuring the level of red cell folate rather than the serum folic acid.

Differential Diagnosis

It is important to recognize that most macrocytic anemias in pediatrics are not megaloblastic. Other causes of an increased MCV include an elevated reticulocyte count (hemolytic anemias), bone marrow failure syndromes (Fanconi's anemia, Diamond-Blackfan anemia), liver disease, and hypothyroidism.

Treatment

Treatment of cobalamin deficiency due to inadequate dietary intake is readily accomplished with oral supplementation. Most cases, however, are due to intestinal malabsorption and require parenteral treatment. In severe cases, parenteral therapy may induce life-threatening hypokalemia and require supplemental potassium. Folic acid deficiency is effectively treated with oral folic acid in most cases. Children at risk for the development of folic acid deficiencies such as premature infants and those with chronic hemolysis are usually given supplementary folic acid prophylactically.

Graham SM et al: Long-term neurologic consequences of nutritional vitamin B_{12} deficiency in infants. J Pediatr 1992;121:710.

Pappo AS, Fields BW, Buchanan GR: Etiology of red blood cell macrocytosis during childhood: Impact of new diseases and therapies. Pediatrics 1992;89:1063.

ANEMIA OF CHRONIC DISORDERS

Anemia is a common manifestation of many chronic illnesses in children. In some instances, causes may be mixed. For example, children with chronic disorders involving intestinal malabsorption or blood loss may have anemia of chronic inflammation in combination with nutritional deficiencies of iron, folate, or cobalamin. In other settings, the anemia is due to dysfunction of a single organ (eg, renal failure, hypothyroidism), and correction of the underlying abnormality causes resolution of the anemia.

1. ANEMIA OF CHRONIC INFLAMMATION

Anemia is frequently associated with chronic illness, particularly those with a significant inflammatory component. The anemia is usually mild to moderate in severity, with a hemoglobin of 8–12 g/dL. In general, the severity of the anemia corresponds to the severity of the underlying disorder. The reticulocyte count is low, and the anemia is thought to be due to inflammatory cytokines that inhibit erythropoiesis and impair iron release by reticuloendothelial cells. The serum iron concentration is low, but in contrast to iron deficiency, the iron-binding capacity is not elevated and the serum ferritin is elevated. Treatment consists of correction of the underlying disorder, which, if controlled, generally results in improvement in hemoglobin level.

Means RT Jr, Krantz SB: Progress in understanding the pathogenesis of the anemia of chronic disease. Blood 1992;80:1639.

2. ANEMIA OF CHRONIC RENAL FAILURE

Severe normocytic anemia occurs in most forms of renal disease that have progressed to renal insufficiency. Although white cell and platelet production remain normal, the bone marrow shows significant hypoplasia of the erythroid series and the reticulocyte count is low. The principal mechanism responsible for this anemia is deficiency of erythropoietin, a hormone normally produced in the kidney. In the presence of significant uremia, there may also be a component of hemolysis. In the past, treatment of the anemia of chronic renal failure depended on transfusions of packed red blood cells. However, recombinant human erythropoietin (epoetin alfa) has been shown to correct the anemia, and its use has largely eliminated the need for transfusions.

Montini G et al: Pharmacokinetics and hematologic response to subcutaneous administration of recombinant human erythropoietin in children undergoing long-term peritoneal dialysis: A multicenter study. J Pediatr 1993; 122:297.

Morris KP et al: Non-cardiac benefits of human recombinant erythropoietin in end stage renal failure and anaemia. Arch Dis Child 1993;69:580.

Siimes MA et al: Factors limiting the erythropoietin response in rapidly growing infants with congenital nephrosis on a peritoneal dialysis regimen after nephrectomy. J Pediatr 1992;120:44.

3. ANEMIA OF HYPOTHYROIDISM

Some patients with hypothyroidism develop significant anemia. Occasionally, anemia is detected before the diagnosis of the underlying disorder. A decreased growth velocity in an anemic child suggests hypothyroidism. The anemia is usually normocytic or macrocytic, but it is not megaloblastic and hence not due to deficiencies of cobalamin or folate. Replacement therapy with thyroid hormone is usually effective in correcting the anemia.

Cheu J-Y et al: Anemia in children and adolescents with hypothyroidism. Clin Pediatr 1981;20:696.

CONGENITAL HEMOLYTIC ANEMIAS: RED CELL MEMBRANE DEFECTS

The congenital hemolytic anemias are usually divided into three categories: defects of the red cell membrane, hemoglobinopathies, and disorders of red cell metabolism. Hereditary spherocytosis and elliptocytosis are the most common red cell membrane disorders and are described here. The diagnosis is suggested by the peripheral blood smear, which shows characteristic red cell morphology (eg, spherocytes, elliptocytes). These disorders usually have an autosomal dominant inheritance, and the diagnosis may be suggested by a family history. The hemolysis is usually due to the deleterious effect of the membrane abnormality on red cell deformability. Decreased cell deformability leads to entrapment of the abnormally shaped red cells in the spleen. Many patients have splenomegaly, and the hemolysis is often alleviated by splenectomy.

Becker PS, Lux SE: Disorders of the red cell membrane. In: *Hematology of Infancy and Childhood,* 4th ed. Nathan DG, Oski FA (editors). WB Saunders, 1993.

Clark MR, Wagner GM: Disorders of the erythrocyte membrane. In: *The Hereditary Hemolytic Anemias.* Mentzer WC, Wagner GM (editors). Churchill Livingstone, 1989.

1. HEREDITARY SPHEROCYTOSIS

Essentials of Diagnosis

- Anemia and jaundice.
- Splenomegaly.
- Positive family history of anemia, jaundice, or gallstones.
- Spherocytosis with increased reticulocytes.
- Increased osmotic fragility.
- Negative Coombs' test.

General Considerations

Hereditary spherocytosis is a relatively common inherited hemolytic anemia that occurs in all ethnic groups but is most common in persons of Northern European ancestry, in whom the incidence is about 1:5000. The disorder is a heterogeneous one, marked by variable degrees of anemia, jaundice, and splenomegaly. In some persons, the disorder is mild and there is no anemia because erythroid hyperplasia fully compensates for hemolysis. Severe cases are transfusion-dependent prior to splenectomy. The hallmark of hereditary spherocytosis is the presence of microspherocytes in the peripheral blood. The disease is inherited in an autosomal dominant fashion in about 80% of cases; the remainder are thought to be autosomal recessive or to be caused by new mutations.

Hereditary spherocytosis is the result of a partial deficiency of *spectrin,* an important structural protein of the red cell membrane skeleton. Spectrin deficiency weakens the attachment of the cell membrane to the underlying membrane skeleton and causes the red cell to lose membrane surface area. This process creates spherocytes that are poorly deformable and have a shortened life span because they are trapped in the microcirculation of the spleen and engulfed by splenic macrophages. The extreme heterogeneity of hereditary spherocytosis is directly related to variable degrees of spectrin deficiency. In general, children who inherit hereditary spherocytosis in an autosomal

dominant fashion have lesser degrees of spectrin deficiency and mild or moderate hemolysis. In contrast, those with nondominant forms of spherocytosis tend to have greater deficiencies of spectrin and a more severe anemia.

Clinical Findings

A. Symptoms and Signs: Symptoms and signs of hereditary spherocytosis are those related to hemolytic anemia. Fifty percent of affected children have significant hyperbilirubinemia in the newborn period. Splenomegaly subsequently develops in the majority and is usually present by the age of 5 years. Jaundice is variably present and in many patients may only be noted during infection. Patients with significant chronic anemia may complain of pallor, fatigue, or malaise. Intermittent exacerbations of the anemia are caused by increased hemolysis or by aplastic crises and may be associated with severe weakness, fatigue, fever, abdominal pain, or even congestive heart failure.

B. Laboratory Findings: Most patients have mild chronic hemolysis with hemoglobin values between 9 and 12 g/dL. In some cases, the hemolysis is fully compensated and the hemoglobin is in the normal range. Rare cases of severe disease require frequent transfusions. The anemia is usually normocytic and hyperchromic, and many patients have an elevated MCHC. The blood smear shows numerous microspherocytes and polychromasia. The reticulocyte count is elevated and is often higher than might be expected for the degree of anemia. White blood cells and platelets are usually normal. The osmotic fragility is increased, particularly after incubation at 37 °C for 24 hours. Serum bilirubin usually shows an elevation in the unconjugated fraction. Coombs' testing is negative.

Differential Diagnosis

Spherocytes are frequently present in persons with immune hemolysis. Thus, in the newborn, hereditary spherocytosis must be distinguished from hemolytic disease caused by ABO or Rh incompatibilities. In older patients, autoimmune hemolytic anemia frequently presents with jaundice and splenomegaly and with spherocytes on the blood smear. The direct Coombs' test is positive in most cases of immune hemolysis and negative in hereditary spherocytosis. Occasionally, the diagnosis is confused in patients with splenomegaly from other causes, especially when hypersplenism increases red cell destruction and when some spherocytes are noted on the blood smear. In such cases, the true cause of the splenomegaly is frequently suggested by signs or symptoms of portal hypertension or by laboratory evidence of chronic liver disease. In contrast to children with hereditary spherocytosis, those with hypersplenism typically have some degree of thrombocytopenia or neutropenia.

Complications

Severe jaundice may occur in the neonatal period and, if not controlled by phototherapy, may occasionally require exchange transfusion. Splenectomy is associated with an increased risk of overwhelming bacterial infections, particularly with pneumococci. Gallstones occur in 60–70% of adults who have not undergone splenectomy and may form as early as 8–10 years of age.

Treatment

Supportive measures include the administration of folic acid to prevent the development of red cell hypoplasia due to folate deficiency. Acute exacerbations of anemia due to increased rates of hemolysis or to aplastic crises due to infection with human parvovirus may be severe enough to require red cell transfusions. Splenectomy is performed in many cases and always results in significant improvement. The procedure increases the survival of the spherocytic red cells and leads to complete correction of the anemia in most cases. Patients with more severe disease may show some degree of hemolysis after splenectomy. Except in unusually severe cases, the procedure should be postponed until the child is at least 5 or 6 years of age because of the greater risk of postsplenectomy sepsis prior to this age. Alternatively, partial splenectomy may be considered for young children with severe hemolysis. All patients scheduled for splenectomy should be immunized with pneumococcal vaccine prior to the procedure, and some recommend prophylactic penicillin afterward. The need for splenectomy in mild cases is somewhat controversial. Splenectomy in the middle childhood years prevents the subsequent development of cholelithiasis and eliminates the need for the activity restrictions recommended for children with splenomegaly. However, these benefits must be weighed against the risks of the surgical procedure and the subsequent lifelong risk of postsplenectomy sepsis.

Prognosis

Splenectomy eliminates signs and symptoms in all but the most severe cases and prevents the development of cholelithiasis. The abnormal red cell morphology and increased osmotic fragility persist without clinical consequence.

Eber SW et al: Variable clinical severity of hereditary spherocytosis: Relation to erythrocytic spectrin concentration, osmotic fragility, and autohemolysis. J Pediatr 1990;117:409.

Manno CS et al: Splenectomy in mild hereditary spherocytosis: Is it worth the risk? Am J Pediatr Hematol Oncol 1989;11:300.

Savvides P et al: Combined spectrin and ankyrin deficiency is common in autosomal dominant hereditary spherocytosis. Blood 1993;82:2953.

Tchernia G et al: Initial assessment of the beneficial effect of partial splenectomy in hereditary spherocytosis. Blood 1993;81:2014.

2. HEREDITARY ELLIPTOCYTOSIS

Hereditary elliptocytosis is a heterogeneous disorder whose severity ranges from an asymptomatic carrier state with normal red cell morphology to severe hemolytic anemia. Most affected persons have numerous elliptocytes on the blood smear but mild or no hemolysis. Those with hemolysis have an elevated reticulocyte count and may have jaundice and splenomegaly. These disorders are caused by mutations of red cell membrane skeletal proteins, and most have an autosomal dominant inheritance. Because most cases are asymptomatic, no treatment is indicated. Patients with significant degrees of hemolytic anemia may benefit from folate supplementation or from splenectomy.

Some infants with hereditary elliptocytosis present in the neonatal period with moderate to marked hemolysis and significant hyperbilirubinemia. This disorder has been termed *transient infantile poikilocytosis* because such infants exhibit bizarre erythrocyte morphology with elliptocytes, budding red cells, and small misshapen cells that defy description. The MCV is low, and the anemia may be severe enough to require red cell transfusions. Typically, one parent has hereditary elliptocytosis, usually mild or asymptomatic. The infant's hemolysis gradually abates during the first year of life, and the erythrocyte morphology subsequently becomes more typical of hereditary elliptocytosis.

Mentzer WC et al: Modulation of erythrocyte membrane mechanical stability by 2,3-diphosphoglycerate in the neonatal poikilocytosis/elliptocytosis syndrome. J Clin Invest 1987;79:943.

Palek J, Sahr KE: Mutations of the red cell membrane proteins: From clinical evaluation to detection of the underlying genetic defect. Blood 1992;8:308.

CONGENITAL HEMOLYTIC ANEMIAS: HEMOGLOBINOPATHIES

The hemoglobinopathies are an extremely heterogeneous group of congenital disorders that occur in many different ethnic groups. The relatively high frequency of these genetic variants is thought to be related to the protection afforded heterozygotes from malaria. The hemoglobinopathies are generally classified into two major groups. The first, the thalassemias, are caused by quantitative deficiencies in the production of globin chains. These quantitative defects in globin synthesis result in a microcytic and hypochromic anemia. The second group of hemoglobinopathies are those caused by structural abnormalities of globin chains. The most important of these, hemoglobins S, C, and E, are all the result of point mutations and single amino acid substitutions in the β globin.

Figure 26–3 shows the normal developmental changes that occur in globin-chain production during gestation and the first year of life. At birth, the predominant hemoglobin is fetal hemoglobin, which is composed of two α-globin chains and two γ-globin chains. Subsequently, the production of γ globin decreases and the production of β globin increases so that adult hemoglobin (two α chains and two β chains) predominates after 4–6 months. Because α-globin chains are present in both fetal and adult hemoglobin, disorders of α-globin synthesis (α-thalassemia) are clinically manifest in the newborn as well as later in life. In contrast, β-globin disorders such as β-thalassemia and sickle cell disease are generally asymptomatic during the first 3–4 months of age and present clinically after γ-chain production—and hence fetal hemoglobin levels—have decreased substantially.

1. ALPHA-THALASSEMIA

Essentials of Diagnosis
- African, Mediterranean, Middle Eastern, Chinese, or Southeast Asian ancestry.
- Microcytic, hypochromic anemia of variable severity.

General Considerations
Most of the α-thalassemia syndromes are the result of deletions of one or more of the α-globin genes on chromosome 16. Normal diploid cells have four α-globin genes, and thus the variable severity of the α-thalassemia syndromes is related to the number of gene deletions. Persons with one α-globin gene deletion (silent carrier) are asymptomatic and have normal blood findings. Persons with two α-globin gene deletions (α-thalassemia trait) have microcytosis and hypochromia with a normal or slightly decreased hemoglobin level. Persons with three α-globin gene deletions (hemoglobin H disease) have a moderately severe anemia. The deletion of all four α-globin genes results in fetal demise due to hydrops fetalis.

The severity of the α-thalassemia syndromes varies among affected ethnic groups, depending on the genetic abnormalities prevalent in the population. In persons of African descent, α-thalassemia is usually caused by the deletion of only one of the two α-globin genes on each chromosome. Thus, heterozygotes in the African population are silent carriers, and homozygotes have α-thalassemia trait. In Asians, however, deletions of one or of both α-globin genes on the same chromosome are common. Thus, heterozygotes are either silent carriers or have α-thalassemia trait and homozygotes or compound heterozygotes have α-thalassemia trait, hemoglobin H disease, or hydrops fetalis. Thus, the presence of α-thalassemia in a child of Asian ancestry may have important implications for genetic counseling, whereas this is not usually the case in families of African ancestry.

Clinical Findings
The clinical findings depend upon the number of α-globin genes deleted. The thalassemia syndromes and associated laboratory findings in newborns are shown in Table 26–2.

Persons with three α-globin genes (one-gene deletion) are asymptomatic and have no hematologic abnormalities. Hemoglobin levels and MCV are nor-

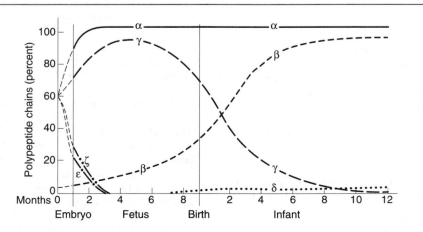

Figure 26–3. Changes in hemoglobin polypeptide chains during human development. (From Miller DR, Baehner RL: *Blood Diseases of Infancy and Childhood,* 6th ed. CV Mosby, 1989.)

Table 26–2. Clinical and laboratory findings in newborns with α-thalassemia.

Syndrome (Clinical Features)	Usual Genotype	α Gene Number	Hb (g/dL)	MCV (fL)	Hb Barts (%)
Normal	αα/αα	4	14–22	> 100	None
Silent carrier (no clinical abnormalities)	–α/αα	3	13.6–21	87–116	0–5.8
Alpha thalassemia trait (mild anemia)	- -/αα or –α/–α	2	14.3–19.3	84–101	2–10
Hemoglobin H disease (hemolytic anemia)	- -/–α	1	12.4–14.2	80–93	19–27
Homozygous alpha thalassemia (stillborn—hydrops fetalis)	- -/- -	0	3–10	110–119	> 75

From Embury SH, Mentzer WC: The thalassemia syndromes. In: *The Hereditary Hemolytic Anemias.* Mentzer WC, Wagner GM (editors). Churchill Livingstone, 1989.
MCV = mean corpuscular volume.

mal. Hemoglobin electrophoresis in the neonatal period shows 1–3% Barts hemoglobin, a variant hemoglobin composed of four γ-globin chains. Hemoglobin electrophoresis after the first few months of life is normal. Thus, this condition is usually suspected only in the context of family studies or when a small amount of Barts hemoglobin is detected by neonatal screening for hemoglobinopathies.

Persons with two α-globin genes (two-gene deletion) are typically asymptomatic. The MCV is usually less than 100 fL at birth. Hematologic studies in older infants and children show a normal or slightly decreased hemoglobin level with a low MCV and a slightly hypochromic blood smear with some target cells. The hemoglobin electrophoresis typically shows 5–10% Barts hemoglobin in the neonatal period but is normal in older children and adults.

Persons with one α-globin gene (three-gene deletion) have a moderately severe microcytic hemolytic anemia (Hb 7–10 g/dL), which is often accompanied by hepatosplenomegaly and some bony abnormalities caused by the expanded medullary space. The reticulocyte count is elevated, and the red cells show marked hypochromia and microcytosis with significant poikilocytosis and some basophilic stippling. Hemoglobin electrophoresis in the neonatal period typically shows 15–25% Barts hemoglobin. Later in life, hemoglobin H (composed of four β-globin chains) is detected and may make up as much as 20–30% of the hemoglobin. Incubation of red cells with brilliant cresyl blue (hemoglobin H preparation) shows inclusion bodies formed by denatured hemoglobin H.

The deletion of all four α-globin genes causes severe intrauterine anemia and asphyxia and results in hydrops fetalis and fetal demise or neonatal death shortly following delivery. There is extreme pallor and massive hepatosplenomegaly. Hemoglobin electrophoresis reveals a predominance of Barts hemoglobin with a complete absence of normal fetal or adult hemoglobin.

Differential Diagnosis

α-Thalassemia trait (two-gene deletion) must be differentiated from other mild microcytic anemias including iron deficiency and β-thalassemia trait. In contrast to children with iron deficiency, those with α-thalassemia trait show normal or increased levels of ferritin and serum iron, and the free erythrocyte protoporphyrin is not elevated. In contrast to children with β-thalassemia trait, those with α-thalassemia trait have a normal hemoglobin electrophoresis after 4–6 months of age. Finally, the history of a low MCV (96 fL) at birth or the presence of Barts hemoglobin on the neonatal hemoglobinopathy screening test suggests α-thalassemia.

Children with hemoglobin H disease may have jaundice and splenomegaly, and the disorder must be differentiated from other hemolytic anemias. The key to the diagnosis is the decreased MCV and the marked hypochromia on the blood smear. With the exception of β-thalassemia, most other significant hemolytic disorders have a normal or elevated MCV and are not hypochromic. Infants with hydrops fetalis due to severe α-thalassemia must be distinguished from those with hydrops due to other causes of anemia such as isoimmunization.

Complications

The principal complication of α-thalassemia trait is the needless administration of iron, given in the belief that a mild microcytic anemia is due to iron deficiency. Persons with hemoglobin H disease may have intermittent exacerbations of their anemia, which require blood transfusions. Splenomegaly may become a significant problem, may exacerbate the anemia, and may require splenectomy. Women pregnant with hydropic α-thalassemia infants are subject to increased complications of pregnancy, particularly toxemia and postpartum hemorrhage.

Treatment

Persons with α-thalassemia trait require no treatment. Those with hemoglobin H disease should receive supplemental folic acid and avoid the same oxidant drugs that cause hemolysis in persons with G6PD deficiency, because exposure to these drugs may exacerbate their anemia. The anemia may also be exacerbated during periods of infection, and transfusions may be required. Occasionally, infants with hemoglobin H disease may show failure-to-thrive without red cell transfusions. Hypersplenism may develop later in childhood and require surgical splenectomy. Genetic counseling and prenatal diagnosis should be offered to families at risk for children with hemoglobin H disease or fetal hydrops.

Embury SH et al: The thalassemia syndromes. In: *The Hereditary Hemolytic Anemias.* Mentzer WC, Wagner GM (editors). Churchill Livingstone, 1989.

Giardina P, Hilgartner MW: Update on thalassemia. Pediatr Rev 1992;13:55.

2. BETA-THALASSEMIA

Essentials of Diagnosis

Beta-thalassemia minor:
- African, Mediterranean, Middle Eastern, or Asian ancestry.
- Mild microcytic, hypochromic anemia.
- No response to iron therapy.
- Elevated level of hemoglobin A_2.

Beta-thalassemia major:
- African, Mediterranean, Middle Eastern, or Asian ancestry.
- Moderate to very severe microcytic, hypochromic anemia with marked hepatosplenomegaly.
- Elevated fetal and A_2 hemoglobin.

General Considerations

In contrast to the four α-globin genes, only two β-globin genes are present in diploid cells, one on each chromosome 11. Some β-thalassemia genes produce no β-globin chains and are termed β^0-*thalassemia.* Other β-globin genes produce some β-globin but in diminished quantities and are termed β^+-*thalassemia.* Persons affected by β-thalassemia may be heterozygous or homozygous. Heterozygotes for most β-thalassemia genes have β-thalassemia minor. Most homozygotes have β-thalassemia major (Cooley's anemia), which is a severe transfusion-dependent anemia. Other homozygotes have a condition known as *thalassemia intermedia* that is more severe than thalassemia minor but not generally transfusion-dependent.

The worldwide importance of β-thalassemia can-

not be overstated. β-Thalassemia major is the most common cause of transfusion-dependent anemia in childhood. In addition, β-thalassemia interacts with structural β-globin variants such as hemoglobin S and hemoglobin E to cause serious disease in compound heterozygotes. These disorders are discussed further in the sections dealing with sickle hemoglobinopathies and with hemoglobin E disorders.

Clinical Findings

A. Symptoms and Signs: Persons with β-thalassemia minor are usually asymptomatic with a normal physical examination. Those with β-thalassemia major are normal at birth but develop a significant anemia during the first year of life as fetal hemoglobin production decreases. If the disorder is not identified and treated with blood transfusions, such children develop massive hepatosplenomegaly and enlargement of the medullary space with thinning of the bony cortex. The skeletal changes cause characteristic facial deformities (prominent forehead and maxilla) and predispose the child to pathologic fractures. Inadequate treatment causes poor growth and development in these children.

B. Laboratory Findings: Laboratory findings in β-thalassemia minor include a normal or modestly decreased hemoglobin level. The MCV is almost always decreased. The blood smear typically shows hypochromia, target cells, and sometimes basophilic stippling. Hemoglobin electrophoresis is usually diagnostic when hemoglobin A_2 or hemoglobin F or both is elevated. Infants with β-thalassemia major are hematologically normal at birth but develop severe anemia after the first few months of life. The blood smear typically shows a severe hypochromic, microcytic anemia with marked anisocytosis and poikilocytosis. Target cells are prominent, and nucleated red blood cells often exceed the number of circulating white blood cells. The hemoglobin usually falls to 5–6 g/dL or less, and the reticulocyte count is significantly elevated. Platelet and white blood cell counts may be increased, and the serum bilirubin is elevated. The bone marrow shows marked erythroid hyperplasia but is rarely needed for diagnosis. Hemoglobin electrophoresis shows only fetal and A_2 hemoglobin in children with homozygous β^0-thalassemia. Those with β^+-thalassemia genes make some hemoglobin A_1 but have a marked increase in fetal and in A_2 hemoglobin. The diagnosis of homozygous β-thalassemia may also be suggested by the finding of β-thalassemia minor in both parents.

Differential Diagnosis

β-Thalassemia minor must be differentiated from other causes of mild microcytic, hypochromic anemias, principally iron deficiency and α-thalassemia. In contrast to those with iron deficiency anemia, persons with β-thalassemia minor typically have an elevated number of red blood cells, and the index of the

MCV divided by the red cell count is under 13. Generally, the finding of an elevated hemoglobin A_2 is diagnostic; however, the A_2 level is lowered by co-existent iron deficiency, and this may lead to some confusion. Thus, in children thought to be iron-deficient, hemoglobin electrophoresis with quantitation of hemoglobin A_2 is best performed after a course of iron therapy.

β-Thalassemia major is rarely confused with other disorders. Hemoglobin electrophoresis and family studies readily distinguish it from hemoglobin E–β-thalassemia, which is the other important cause of transfusion-dependent thalassemia.

Complications

The principal complication of β-thalassemia minor is the unnecessary use of iron therapy in a futile attempt to correct the microcytic anemia. Children with β-thalassemia major who are inadequately transfused suffer from poor growth and recurrent infections and may have massive hepatosplenomegaly, thinning of the cortical bone, and pathologic fractures. Without treatment, most children die within the first decade of life. The principal complications of β-thalassemia major in transfused children are hemosiderosis, splenomegaly and hypersplenism, and viral infections (especially hepatitis). Transfusional hemosiderosis requires chelation therapy with deferoxamine to prevent cardiac, hepatic, and endocrine dysfunction. Noncompliance with chelation in adolescents and young adults may lead to death from congestive heart failure, cardiac arrhythmias, or hepatic failure. Even with adequate transfusions, most patients develop splenomegaly and some degree of hypersplenism. This necessitates splenectomy because of the increasing transfusion requirements, usually between ages 5 and 10 years. Unfortunately, this procedure leaves the child at risk for overwhelming septicemia.

Treatment

β-Thalassemia minor requires no specific therapy but has important implications for genetic counseling. For those with β-thalassemia major, two approaches to treatment are now available: chronic transfusion with iron chelation or bone marrow transplantation. Programs of blood transfusion are generally targeted to maintain a nadir hemoglobin level above 11 g/dL. This gives increased vigor and well-being, improved growth, and fewer overall complications. However, maintenance of good health currently requires iron chelation with nightly subcutaneous infusion of deferoxamine. Small doses of supplemental ascorbic acid may enhance the efficacy of iron chelation. Newly developed oral iron chelators are under study. Patients on chronic transfusion programs generally develop hypersplenism and require splenectomy when their yearly transfusion requirement of packed red cells exceeds 200–250

mL/kg. Splenectomy results in a decrease in the transfusion requirement and hence a lesser rate of iron loading but is associated with a high risk of postsplenectomy sepsis. For this reason, thalassemic patients should receive pneumococcal vaccine prior to the procedure and prophylactic penicillin afterward.

Bone marrow transplantation is an important therapeutic option for children with β-thalassemia major who have an HLA-identical sibling donor. In a large series from Italy, the probability of 3-year event-free survival was 94% when transplantation was performed prior to the development of hepatomegaly or portal fibrosis.

Lucarelli G et al: Marrow transplantation in patients with thalassemia responsive to iron chelation therapy. N Engl J Med 1993;329:840.

Olivieri NF et al: Survival in medically treated patients with homozygous β-thalassemia. N Engl J Med 1994;331:574.

Weatherall DJ: The treatment of thalassemia: Slow progress and new dilemmas. N Engl J Med 1993; 329:877.

3. SICKLE CELL DISEASE

Essentials of Diagnosis

- African, Mediterranean, Middle Eastern, or Indian ancestry.
- Anemia, elevated reticulocyte count, jaundice.
- Recurrent episodes of musculoskeletal or abdominal pain.
- Hemoglobin electrophoresis with hemoglobins S and F, hemoglobins S and C, or hemoglobins S, F, and A with S > A.
- Splenomegaly in early childhood with later disappearance.
- High risk of overwhelming bacterial sepsis.

General Considerations

A high incidence of sickle hemoglobin is found in persons of central African origin. It also occurs in other ethnic groups in Sicily, Italy, Greece, Turkey, Saudi Arabia, and India. Sickle cell anemia is caused by homozygosity for the sickle gene and is the most common form of sickle cell disease. Other clinically important sickling disorders are caused by compound heterozygous conditions in which the sickle gene interacts with genes for hemoglobin C, D_{Punjab}, O_{Arab}, C_{Harlem}, or β-thalassemia.

Overall, sickle cell disease occurs in about one of every 400 African-American infants. Eight percent of African-Americans are heterozygous carriers of the sickle gene and are said to have sickle cell trait.

The protean clinical manifestations of sickle hemoglobinopathies all can be linked directly or indirectly to the propensity of deoxygenated hemoglobin

S to polymerize. Polymerization of sickle hemoglobin distorts erythrocyte morphology, decreases red cell deformability, causes a marked reduction in red cell life span, increases blood viscosity, and predisposes to episodes of vaso-occlusion.

During the past decade, neonatal screening for sickle hemoglobinopathies has been established in many regions of the United States. The identification of affected infants during the first few months of life, when combined with follow-up programs of parental education, comprehensive medical care, and prophylactic penicillin, markedly reduces the morbidity and mortality rate in early childhood.

Clinical Findings

A. Symptoms and Signs: The symptoms and signs of sickle cell disease are related to the hemolytic anemia and to tissue ischemia caused by vaso-occlusion. Children are normal at birth, and onset of symptoms is unusual before 3–4 months of age because high levels of fetal hemoglobin inhibit sickling. A moderately severe hemolytic anemia is often present by 1 year of age, causes pallor, fatigue, and jaundice, and predisposes to the development of gallstones during adolescence and early adulthood. Intense congestion of the spleen with sickled cells may cause splenomegaly in early childhood and results in functional asplenia as early as 3 months of age. This places children at great risk for overwhelming infection with encapsulated bacteria, particularly pneumococci. Up to 30% of patients experience one or more episodes of acute splenic sequestration, characterized by sudden enlargement of the spleen with pooling of red cells, acute exacerbation of anemia, and, in severe cases, shock and death. Acute exacerbation of anemia also occurs with aplastic crises, usually caused by infection with human parvovirus.

Recurrent episodes of vaso-occlusion and tissue ischemia cause a myriad of acute and chronic problems. Dactylitis, or hand-and-foot syndrome, is the most common initial symptom of the disease and occurs in up to 50% of children before the age of 3 years. Recurrent episodes of ischemic pain—particularly abdominal and musculoskeletal pain—occur throughout life. Strokes occur in about 8% of children and tend to be recurrent. The acute chest syndrome, characterized by fever, pleuritic chest pain, and acute pulmonary infiltrates with hypoxemia, is caused by pulmonary infection, infarction, or fat embolism from ischemic bone marrow. All tissues are susceptible to damage from vaso-occlusion, and multiple organ dysfunction is common by adulthood. Table 26–3 lists the common manifestations of sickle cell disease in children and adults.

B. Laboratory Findings: Children with sickle cell anemia (Hb SS) generally show a baseline hemoglobin level between 7 and 10 g/dL. This value may fall to life-threatening levels at the time of a sequestration or aplastic crisis. The baseline reticulocyte

Table 26–3. Common clinical manifestations of sickle cell disease.

	Acute	Chronic

Children	Bacterial sepsis or meningitis[1]
	Splenic sequestration[1]
	Aplastic crisis
	Vaso-occlusive events
	  Dactylitis
	  Bone infarction
	  Acute chest syndrome[1]
	  Stroke[1]
	  Priapism
		Functional asplenia
		Delayed growth and development
		Aseptic necrosis of the hip
		Hyposthenuria
		Cholelithiasis

Adults	Bacterial sepsis[1]
	Aplastic crisis
	Vaso-occlusive events
	  Bone infarction
	  Acute chest syndrome[1]
	  Stroke[1]
	  Priapism
	  Acute multi-organ failure syndrome[1]
		Leg ulcers
		Proliferative retinopathy
		Aseptic necrosis of the hip
		Cholecystitis
		Chronic organ failure[1]
		  Liver
		  Lung
		  Kidney
		Decreased fertility

[1]Associated with significant mortality rate.

count is markedly elevated. The anemia is normocytic or macrocytic, and the blood smear typically shows the characteristic sickle cells as well as numerous target cells. Patients with sickle β-thalassemia generally have a low MCV and hypochromia as well. Those with sickle β+-thalassemia tend to have lesser degrees of hemolysis and anemia. Persons with sickle hemoglobin C (Hb SC) disease have fewer sickle forms and more target cells, and the hemoglobin level may be normal or only slightly decreased as the rate of hemolysis is much less than in sickle cell anemia.

Most infants with sickle hemoglobinopathies born in the United States are now identified by neonatal screening. Results indicative of possible sickle cell disease require prompt confirmation with hemoglobin electrophoresis. Children with sickle cell anemia and with sickle β0-thalassemia have only hemoglobins S and F. Persons with sickle β+-thalassemia have a preponderance of hemoglobin S with a lesser amount of hemoglobin A1. Persons with sickle hemoglobin C disease have equal amounts of hemoglobin S and hemoglobin C. The use of solubility tests to screen for the presence of sickle hemoglobin should be avoided because a negative result is frequently encountered in infants with sickle cell disease, and because a positive result an older child does not differentiate sickle cell trait from sickle cell disease. Thus, hemoglobin electrophoresis is always necessary to accurately identify a sickle disorder.

Serum chemistries are often abnormal, depending on the severity of the hemolysis and on the presence of hepatic or renal dysfunction. X-rays of the skull and spine reveal cortical thinning, enlargement of the marrow spaces, and increased trabecular markings.

Differential Diagnosis

Hemoglobin electrophoresis and sometimes hematologic studies of the parents are usually sufficient to confirm the correct diagnosis of a sickle cell disorder. Infants whose neonatal screening test shows only hemoglobin S and F occasionally have disorders other than sickle cell anemia or sickle β^0-thalassemia. The most important of these is a compound heterozygous condition of sickle hemoglobin and pancellular high persistence of fetal hemoglobin. Such children, when older, typically have 30% fetal hemoglobin and 70% hemoglobin S, but they do not have significant anemia nor are they subject to vaso-occlusive episodes.

Complications

Repeated tissue ischemia and infarction causes damage to virtually every organ system. The most important complications are listed in Table 26–3. Patients who require multiple transfusions are at risk for transfusional hemosiderosis and the development of red cell alloantibodies, as well as transmission of infectious agents.

Treatment

The cornerstone of treatment is enrollment in a program that provides for patient and family education, comprehensive outpatient care, and appropriate treatment of acute complications. Important to the success of such a program are psychosocial services, blood bank services, and the ready availability of baseline patient information in the setting where acute problems are handled. Treatment of children with sickle cell anemia and sickle β^0-thalassemia includes prophylactic penicillin, which should be initiated by 3 months of age and continued at least until 5 years of age. Some recommend the continuation of prophylactic penicillin past this age, but conclusive evidence of benefit in older patients is lacking. The routine use of penicillin prophylaxis in hemoglobin SC disease and sickle β^+-thalassemia is controversial. Pneumococcal vaccine should be administered to all children with sickle cell disease at 2 years of age and again 3 years later. Other routine immunizations, including yearly vaccination against influenza, should be provided. All illnesses associated with fever greater than 38.5 °C should be evaluated promptly with bacterial cultures, administration of parenteral broad-spectrum antibiotics, and careful inpatient or outpatient observation.

Treatment of painful vaso-occlusive episodes includes the maintenance of adequate hydration (with avoidance of over hydration), correction of acidosis if present, administration of adequate analgesia, maintenance of normal oxygen saturation, and the treatment of any associated infections.

Red cell transfusions play an important role in management. Transfusions are indicated to improve oxygen-carrying capacity during acute exacerbations of anemia, as occurs during episodes of splenic sequestration or aplastic crisis. Red cell transfusions are not indicated for the treatment of chronic steady-state anemia, which is usually well tolerated, or for uncomplicated episodes of vaso-occlusive pain. Partial exchange transfusion to reduce the percentage of circulating sickle cells is indicated for a number of severe acute vaso-occlusive events and may be life-saving. These events include stroke or transient ischemic attack, severe acute chest syndrome, and acute life-threatening failure of other organs. Transfusions may also be used prior to high-risk procedures such as surgery with general anesthesia or arteriograms with ionic contrast materials. A subset of patients are treated with chronic transfusion programs. The most common indication for this type of transfusion is stroke. Without transfusions, children with stroke have a 70% chance of recurrent stroke within a 2-year period. This risk of recurrent neurologic events is markedly reduced by the transfusion therapy.

Successful bone marrow transplantation cures sickle cell disease, but to date its use has been limited because of the risks associated with the procedure, the inability to predict in young children the severity of future complications, and the paucity of HLA-identical sibling donors. Experimental therapy using chemotherapeutic agents such as hydroxyurea to ameliorate the disease in children by increasing levels of fetal hemoglobin is under study.

Prognosis

Early identification by neonatal screening of infants with sickle cell disease, combined with comprehensive care that includes prophylactic penicillin, has markedly reduced the mortality rate in childhood. Most patients are now expected to live well into adulthood, but they eventually succumb to complications.

Dampier CD et al: Intravenous morphine pharmokinetics in pediatric patients with sickle cell disease. J Pediatr 1995;126:461.

Gill FM et al: Clinical events in the first decade in a cohort of infants with sickle cell disease. Blood 1995;86:776.

Platt OS et al: Mortality in sickle cell disease: Life expectancy and risk factors for early death. N Engl J Med 1994;330:1639.

Styles LA, Vichinsky E: Effects of long-term transfusion regimen on sickle cell-related illness. J Pediatr 1994;125:909.

Wayne AS, Kevy SV, Nathan DG: Transfusion management of sickle cell disease. Blood 1993;81:1109.

Wilimas JA et al: A randomized study of outpatient treatment with ceftriaxone for selected febrile children with sickle cell disease. N Engl J Med 1993;329:472.

4. SICKLE CELL TRAIT

Individuals who are heterozygous for the sickle gene are said to have sickle cell trait. This genetic carrier state occurs in 8% of African-Americans and is even more common in some areas of Africa and the Middle East. Accurate identification of persons with sickle cell trait depends on hemoglobin electrophoresis, which typically shows about 60% hemoglobin A_1 and about 40% hemoglobin S with normal levels of hemoglobin A_2 and F. There is no anemia or hemolysis, and the physical examination is normal. Persons with sickle cell trait are generally healthy, and most experience no illness attributable to the presence of sickle hemoglobin in their red cells. Life expectancy is normal.

Sickle trait erythrocytes are capable of sickling, particularly under conditions of significant hypoxemia, and a number of clinical abnormalities have been linked to this genetic carrier state. Exposure to environmental hypoxia (altitude 10,000 feet above sea level) may precipitate splenic infarction or splenic sequestration. However, most persons with sickle cell trait who choose to visit such altitudes for skiing, hiking, or climbing do so without difficulty. Many develop some degree of hyposthenuria, and about 4% experience painless hematuria, usually microscopic but occasionally macroscopic. For the most part, these renal abnormalities are subclinical, and they do not progress to significant renal dysfunction. The incidence of bacteriuria and pyelonephritis may be increased during pregnancy, but overall rates of maternal and infant morbidity and mortality are not affected by the presence of sickle cell trait in the pregnant woman.

An epidemiologic study of army recruits in military basic training found a higher risk of sudden unexplained death following strenuous exertion in recruits with sickle cell trait than in those with normal hemoglobin. This study has raised concerns about exercise and exertion for persons with the trait. However, considerable evidence suggests that exercise is generally safe and that athletic performance is not adversely affected by sickle cell trait. Exercise tolerance is normal, and the incidence of sickle cell trait in African-American professional football players is similar to that of the general African-American population, suggesting no barrier to achievement in such a physically demanding profession. Thus, restrictions on athletic competition for children with sickle cell trait are not warranted. Sickle cell trait continues to be most significant for its implications regarding genetic counseling, not for any associated health risks.

Committee on Sports Medicine, American Academy of Pediatrics: Recommendations for participation in competitive sports. Pediatrics 1988;81:737.

Kark JA et al: Sickle cell trait as a risk factor for sudden death in physical training. N Engl J Med 1987;317:781.

Nuss R et al: Cardiopulmonary function in men with sickle cell disease who reside at moderately high altitude. J Lab Clin Med 1993;122:382.

Pearson HA: Sickle cell trait in competitive athletics: Is there a risk? Pediatrics 1989;83:613.

5. HEMOGLOBIN C DISORDERS

Two percent of African-Americans are heterozygous for hemoglobin C and are said to have hemoglobin C trait. Such individuals have no symptoms, anemia, or hemolysis, but the blood smear may show some target cells. Identification of persons with hemoglobin C trait is important for genetic counseling, particularly with regard to the possibility of hemoglobin SC disease in offspring.

Persons with homozygous hemoglobin C have a mild microcytic hemolytic anemia and may develops splenomegaly. The blood smear shows prominent target cells. As with other hemolytic anemias, complications of homozygous hemoglobin C include gallstones and aplastic crises.

Olson JF et al: Hemoglobin C disease in infancy and childhood. J Pediatr 1994;125:745.

6. HEMOGLOBIN E DISORDERS

Hemoglobin E is the second most common hemoglobin variant worldwide, with a gene frequency greater than 10% in some areas of Thailand and Cambodia. In Southeast Asia, an estimated 30 million people have hemoglobin E trait. Persons heterozygous for hemoglobin E are asymptomatic and usually not anemic but there may be mild microcytosis. Persons homozygous for hemoglobin E are also asymptomatic but may have a mild anemia and have microcytosis and some target cells on the blood smear.

Hemoglobin E is most important because of its interaction with β-thalassemia. Compound heterozygotes for hemoglobin E and $β^0$-thalassemia are normal at birth but subsequently develop a moderate to severe hemolytic anemia that resembles homozygous β-thalassemia. Such children may show jaundice, hepatosplenomegaly, and poor growth if the disorder is not recognized and treated appropriately. In about 50%, the anemia becomes severe enough to require lifelong transfusion therapy. In some areas of the United States, hemoglobin E–$β^0$-thalassemia has become a more common cause of transfusion-dependent anemia than homozygous β-thalassemia.

Johnson JP et al: Differentiation of homozygous hemoglobin E from compound heterozygous hemoglobin E-β-thalassemia by hemoglobin E mutation analysis. J Pediatr 1992;120:775.

7. UNSTABLE HEMOGLOBIN DISORDERS (Congenital Heinz Body Anemias)

Unstable hemoglobin disorders differ from most other structural hemoglobin variants because heterozygotes have hemolytic anemia and often jaundice. The anemia may be exacerbated during hemolytic crises precipitated by fever or by the ingestion of oxidant drugs. Splenomegaly is variably present, and patients are susceptible to the development of gallstones later in life. Patients with more severe hemolysis may have dark brown urine.

Laboratory findings include a variable hemolytic anemia with elevated reticulocyte count. The blood smear may show basophilic stippling. Inclusion bodies of precipitated denatured hemoglobin called Heinz bodies are demonstrated by special stains. Some unstable hemoglobins may be detected by hemoglobin electrophoresis, but many are electrophoretically silent. Thus, the diagnosis depends on the demonstration of hemoglobin instability, usually with the isopropanol precipitation test.

The differential diagnosis includes most other causes of congenital hemolytic anemias. The autosomal dominant genetic transmission may arouse suspicion of a red cell membrane defect, but abnormalities on the peripheral smear are not typical of either spherocytosis or elliptocytosis. The exacerbation of hemolysis during infection or with ingestion of oxidant drugs and the presence of Heinz bodies may suggest a G6PD deficiency, but normal or elevated levels of G6PD and the increased hemoglobin precipitation with isopropanol are usually sufficient to differentiate unstable hemoglobin disorders from G6PD deficiency.

Treatment of children with unstable hemoglobin disorders generally depends on the severity of the hemolysis. Folic acid may prevent the development of a folate deficiency. The avoidance of oxidant drugs is important for some of these disorders, since their use may precipitate hemolytic crises. The role of splenectomy is unclear.

Vichinsky EP, Lubin PH: Unstable hemoglobins, hemoglobins with altered oxygen affinity, and M-hemoglobins. Pediatr Clin North Am 1980;27:421.

Wagner GM et al: Sickling syndromes and unstable hemoglobin disease. In: *The Hereditary Hemolytic Anemias.* Mentzer WC, Wagner GM (editors). Churchill Livingstone, 1989.

8. OTHER HEMOGLOBINOPATHIES

Hundreds of other human globin-chain variants have been identified and described. Some, such as hemoglobins D and G, are relatively common. Heterozygotes, who are frequently detected during the course of neonatal screening programs for hemoglobinopathies, are generally asymptomatic and usually have no anemia or hemolysis. The principal significance of most hemoglobin variants is the potential for disease in compound heterozygotes who also inherit a gene for β-thalassemia or sickle hemoglobin. For example, children compound heterozygous for hemoglobins S and D_{Punjab} ($D_{Los\ Angeles}$) have a severe hemolytic anemia with a peripheral blood smear and clinical problems virtually identical with those of children with sickle cell anemia.

CONGENITAL HEMOLYTIC ANEMIAS: DISORDERS OF RED CELL METABOLISM

Erythrocytes are dependent on the anaerobic metabolism of glucose for the maintenance of adenosine triphosphate (ATP) levels sufficient for normal homeostasis. Glycolysis also produces the 2,3-DPG levels needed to modulate the oxygen affinity of adult hemoglobin. In addition, glucose metabolism via the hexosemonophosphate shunt is necessary to generate sufficient reduced nicotinamide adenine dinucleotide phosphate (NADPH) and reduced glutathione to protect the red cell against oxidant damage. Congenital deficiencies of many (not all) glycolytic pathway enzymes have been associated with hemolytic anemias. In general, the morphologic abnormalities present on the blood smear are nonspecific, and the inheritance of these disorders is autosomal recessive or X-linked. Thus, the possibility of a red cell enzyme defect should be considered during the evaluation of a congenital hemolytic anemia when the blood smear does not show red cell morphology typical of membrane or hemoglobin defects (eg, spherocytes, sickle forms, target cells), when hemoglobin disorders are excluded by hemoglobin electrophoresis and by isopropanol precipitation tests, and when family studies do not suggest an autosomal dominant disorder. The diagnosis is confirmed by finding a low level of the deficient enzyme.

The following section focuses on the two most common disorders of erythrocyte metabolism: G6PD deficiency and pyruvate kinase deficiency.

1. GLUCOSE-6-PHOSPHATE DEHYDROGENASE (G6PD) DEFICIENCY

Essentials of Diagnosis

- African, Mediterranean, or Asian ancestry.
- Neonatal hyperbilirubinemia.
- Sporadic hemolysis associated with infection or with ingestion of oxidant drugs or fava beans.
- X-linked inheritance.

General Considerations

Deficiency of G6PD is easily the most common

red cell enzyme defect that causes hemolytic anemia. The disorder has X-linked recessive inheritance and occurs with high frequency among persons of African, Mediterranean, and Asian ancestry. Hundreds of different G6PD variants have now been identified and characterized. In most instances, enzyme deficiency is due to the instability of the abnormal enzyme, and older red cells are thus more deficient than younger ones. The consequence of the deficiency is the inability of erythrocytes to generate the sufficient amounts of NADPH to maintain the levels of reduced glutathione necessary to protect the red cell against oxidant stress. Thus, most persons with G6PD deficiency do not have a chronic hemolytic anemia, but they do have episodic hemolysis at times of exposure to the oxidant stress of infection or of certain drugs or food substances. The severity of the disorder varies among ethnic groups; G6PD deficiency in persons of African ancestry usually is less severe than in other ethnic groups.

Clinical Findings

A. Symptoms and Signs: Infants with G6PD deficiency may have significant hyperbilirubinemia and may require the use of phototherapy or exchange transfusion to prevent kernicterus. The deficiency is an important cause of neonatal hyperbilirubinemia in Mediterranean and Chinese infants but less so in black infants. Older children with G6PD deficiency are asymptomatic and appear normal between episodes of hemolysis. Hemolytic episodes are often triggered by infection or by the ingestion of oxidant drugs, most importantly antimalarial compounds and sulfonamide antibiotics (Table 26–4). Ingestion of fava beans may trigger hemolysis in Mediterranean and Asian children but not in African children. Episodes of hemolysis are associated with pallor, jaundice, hemoglobinuria, and sometimes cardiovascular compromise.

B. Laboratory Findings: The hemoglobin, reticulocyte count, and blood smear are usually normal in the absence of oxidant-induced hemolysis. Episodes of hemolysis are associated with a variable fall in hemoglobin. "Bite" cells or blister cells may be seen, along with a few spherocytes. Hemoglobinuria is common, and the reticulocyte count increases within a few days. Heinz bodies may be demonstrated with appropriate stains. The diagnosis is con-

Table 26–4. Some common drugs and chemicals that can induce hemolytic anemia in persons with G6PD deficiency.

Acetanilid	Niridazole
Doxorubicin	Nitrofurantoin
Furazolidone	Phenazopyridine
Methylene blue	Primaquine
Nalidixic acid	Sulfamethoxazole

From Beutler E: Glucose-6-phosphate dehydrogenase deficiency. N Engl J Med 1991;324:171.

firmed by the finding of reduced levels of G6PD in erythrocytes. Because this enzyme is present in increased quantities in reticulocytes, the test is best performed at a time when the reticulocyte count is normal or near normal.

Complications

Kernicterus is a risk for infants with significant neonatal hyperbilirubinemia. Episodes of acute hemolysis in older children may be life-threatening if severe enough to cause cardiovascular collapse. Rare G6PD variants that are associated with chronic hemolytic anemia may be complicated by splenomegaly and by the formation of gallstones.

Treatment

The most important issue is avoidance of drugs known to be associated with hemolysis (see Table 26–4). For some Mediterranean and Asian patients, the consumption of fava beans must also be avoided. Infections should be treated promptly and antibiotics given when appropriate. Most episodes of hemolysis are self-limiting, but red cell transfusions may be lifesaving when signs and symptoms indicate cardiovascular compromise.

Beutler E: G6PD deficiency. Blood 1994;84:3613.
Kaplan M, Abramov A: Neonatal hyperbilirubinemia associated with glucose-6-phosphate dehydrogenase deficiency in Sephardic-Jewish neonates: Incidence, severity, and effect of phototherapy. Pediatrics 1992;90:401.
Seidman DS et al: Role of hemolysis in neonatal jaundice associated with glucose-6-phosphate dehydrogenase deficiency. J Pediatr 1995;127:804
Slusher TM et al: Glucose-6-phosphate dehydrogenase deficiency and carboxyhemoglobin concentrations associated with bilirubin-related morbidity and death in Nigerian infants. J Pediatr 1995;126:102.

2. PYRUVATE KINASE DEFICIENCY

Pyruvate kinase deficiency is an autosomal recessive disorder that has been described in all ethnic groups but is most common in northern Europeans. The deficiency is associated with a chronic hemolytic anemia of varying severity. Approximately one third of those affected present in the neonatal period with jaundice and hemolysis that require phototherapy or exchange transfusion. Occasionally, the disorder causes hydrops fetalis and neonatal death. In older children, the hemolysis may require intermittent support with red cell transfusions or may be mild enough to go unnoticed for many years. Jaundice and splenomegaly are frequently present in the more severe cases. The diagnosis of pyruvate kinase deficiency may occasionally be suggested by the presence of echinocytes on the blood smear, but these may be absent prior to splenectomy. Measurement of 2,3-DPG and ATP levels in red cells may suggest the diagnosis of pyruvate kinase deficiency if 2,3-DPG levels are elevated and ATP levels are reduced. The diagnosis depends on the demonstration of low levels of pyruvate kinase activity in red cells.

Treatment of pyruvate kinase depends on the severity of the hemolysis. Blood transfusions may be required for significant anemia, and splenectomy may be beneficial. The procedure does not cure the disorder but does ameliorate the anemia and its symptoms. Characteristically, the reticulocyte count *increases* after splenectomy, despite the decreased hemolysis and increased hemoglobin level. In addition, echinocytes frequently become more prevalent.

Gilsanz F et al: Fetal anaemia due to pyruvate kinase deficiency. Arch Dis Child 1993;69:523.

Mentzer WC Jr: Pyruvate kinase deficiency and disorders of glycolysis. In: *Hematology of Infancy and Childhood,* 4th ed. Nathan DG, Oski FA (editors). WB Saunders, 1993.

ACQUIRED HEMOLYTIC ANEMIA

1. AUTOIMMUNE HEMOLYTIC ANEMIA

Essentials of Diagnosis

- Pallor, fatigue, and jaundice.
- Splenomegaly common.
- Positive Coombs' test.
- Reticulocytosis and spherocytosis.

General Considerations

Acquired autoimmune hemolytic anemia is rare during the first 4 months of life but is one of the more common causes of acute anemia after the first year. It may arise as an isolated problem or may complicate an infection (hepatitis, upper respiratory tract infections, mononucleosis, cytomegalovirus infection), systemic lupus erythematosus and other autoimmune syndromes or immunodeficiency states.

Clinical Findings

A. Symptoms and Signs: The disease usually has an acute onset, presenting with weakness, pallor, and fatigue. Jaundice is a prominent finding, and splenomegaly is often present. Some cases are chronic and insidious in onset. Clinical evidence of the underlying disease may be present.

B. Laboratory Findings: The anemia is normochromic and normocytic and may vary from mild to severe (hemoglobin concentration <5 g/dL). The reticulocyte count is usually increased but occasionally may be normal or low. Spherocytes and nucleated red cells may be seen on the peripheral smear. Although leukocytosis and elevated platelet counts are a common finding, thrombocytopenia is occasionally seen. Other laboratory data consistent with hemolysis are present such as increased indirect and total bilirubin, lactic dehydrogenase (LDH), aspartate

transaminase (AST), and urinary urobilinogen. The hemolysis is intravascular if there is hemoglobinemia or hemoglobinuria. Examination of bone marrow shows a marked erythroid hyperplasia.

Serologic studies provide important information about the disease, which is helpful in defining the pathophysiology, planning therapeutic strategies, and assessing prognosis (Table 26–5). In almost all cases, the direct and indirect antiglobulin (Coombs') tests are positive. Further evaluation allows distinction of three syndromes. The presence of IgG, maximal in vitro activity at 37 °C, and either no antigen specificity or an Rh-like specificity constitute warm autoimmune hemolytic anemia with extravascular destruction by the reticuloendothelial system. In contrast, the detection of complement alone and optimal reactivity in vitro at 4 °C with I or i antigen specificity are diagnostic of cold autoimmune hemolytic anemia with intravascular hemolysis. Paroxysmal cold hemoglobinuria appears identical with cold autoimmune hemolytic anemia but has a different antigen specificity and exhibits hemolysis as well as agglutination in vitro.

Differential Diagnosis

Autoimmune hemolytic anemia must be differentiated from other forms of congenital or acquired hemolytic anemias. The Coombs' test discriminates antibody-mediated hemolysis from other causes such as hereditary spherocytosis.

Complications

The anemia may be very severe and result in cardiovascular collapse requiring emergency management. The complications of the underlying disease such as disseminated lupus erythematosus or lymphoma may be present.

Treatment

Medical management of the underlying disease is important in symptomatic cases. Defining the clinical syndrome provides a useful guide to treatment. Most patients with warm autoimmune hemolytic anemia (in which hemolysis is extravascular) respond to prednisone. After the initial treatment, the dose of corticosteroids may be decreased slowly. Patients may respond to 2 g of intravenous immune globulin (IGIV) per kilogram for 1–3 days, but fewer patients respond to IGIV than to prednisone. Although the rate of remission with splenectomy may be as high as 50%, particularly in warm autoimmune hemolytic anemia, this approach should be withheld until other treatments have been tried. In severe cases unresponsive to more conventional therapy, immunosuppressive agents such as cyclophosphamide, azathioprine, or busulfan may be tried alone or in combination with corticosteroids.

Patients with cold autoimmune hemolytic anemia and paroxysmal cold hemoglobinuria are less likely to

Table 26–5. Classification of autoimmune hemolytic anemia (AIHA) in children.

Syndrome	Warm AIHA	Cold AIHA	Paroxysmal Cold Hematuria
Specific antiglobulin test IgG Complement	Strongly positive Negative or mildly positive	Negative Strongly positive	Negative Strongly positive
Temperature at maximal reactivity	37 °C	4 °C	4 °C
Antigen specificity	May be panagglutinin or may have an Rh-like specificity	I or i	P
Other	. . .	. . .	Positive biphasic hemolysin test
Pathophysiology	Extravascular hemolysis, destruction by the RES (eg, spleen)	Intravascular hemolysis	Intravascular hemolysis
Prognosis	May be more chronic (>3 months) with significant morbidity and mortality. May be associated with a primary disorder (lupus, immunodeficiency, etc)	Generally acute (<3 months). Good outlook: Often associated with infection.	Acute, self-limited. Associated with infection.
Therapy	Respond to RES blockade, including steroids (prednisone, 2 mg/kg/d), IGIV (1 g/kg/d for 3 days), or splenectomy	May not respond to RES blockade. Severe cases may benefit from plasmapheresis.	Usually self-limited. Symptomatic management.

RES = reticuloendothelial system.

respond to corticosteroids or IGIV. Since both of these syndromes are most apt to be associated with infections and have an acute, self-limited course, supportive care may be all that is required. Plasma exchange is effective in cold autoimmune (IgM) hemolytic anemia (and may be helpful in severe cases) because the offending antibody has only an intravascular distribution.

Supportive therapy is crucial. Patients with cold-reacting antibodies, particularly paroxysmal cold hemoglobinuria, should be kept in a warm environment. Transfusion may be necessary because of the complications of severe anemia but should be used only when there is no alternative. In most patients, crossmatch–compatible blood will not be found, and the least incompatible unit should be identified. Transfusion must be conducted carefully, beginning with a test dose (see Transfusion Medicine later in this chapter). Identification of the patient's phenotype for minor red cell alloantigens may be helpful in avoiding alloimmunization or providing appropriate transfusions if alloantibodies arise after initial transfusions during the period of supportive care. Patients with severe intravascular hemolysis may have associated disseminated intravascular coagulation (DIC), and heparin therapy should be considered in such cases.

Prognosis

The outlook for autoimmune hemolytic anemia in childhood is usually good unless there are associated diseases (congenital immunodeficiency, AIDS, lupus erythematosus, malignancy), in which case the he-

molysis is likely to persist for more than 3 months. In general, children with warm autoimmune hemolytic anemia are at greater risk for more severe and chronic disease with higher morbidity and mortality rates. Hemolysis and positive antiglobulin tests may continue for months or years. Patients with cold autoimmune hemolytic anemia or paroxysmal cold hemoglobinuria are more likely to have acute, self-limited disease (<3 months). Paroxysmal cold hemoglobinuria is almost always associated with infection (eg, with *Mycoplasma* infection, cytomegalovirus, Epstein-Barr virus).

Bussel JB et al: Intravenous treatment of autoimmune hemolytic anemia with gammaglobulin. Pediatr Res 1984;12:237.

Heidemann SM et al: Exchange transfusion for autoimmune hemolytic anemia. Am J Pediatr Hematol Oncol 1988;9:302.

Petz LD, Garratty G: Unusual problems regarding autoimmune hemolytic anemias. In: *Acquired Immune Hemolytic Anemias.* Churchill Livingstone, 1980.

Salama A, Mueller-Eckhardt C: Autoimmune haemolytic anaemia in childhood associated with noncomplement binding IgM autoantibodies. Br J Haematol 1987;65:67.

2. NONIMMUNE ACQUIRED HEMOLYTIC ANEMIA

Hepatic disease may alter the lipid composition of the red cell membrane. This usually results in the formation of target cells and is not associated with significant hemolysis. Occasionally, however, severe hepatocellular damage is associated with the formation of "spur" cells and brisk hemolytic anemia. Renal disease may also be associated with significant hemolysis; hemolytic uremic syndrome is the best-known example. In this disorder, hemolysis is associated with the presence on the blood smear of echinocytes, fragmented red cells, and spherocytes.

A microangiopathic hemolytic anemia with fragmented red cells and some spherocytes may be observed in a number of conditions associated with intravascular coagulation and fibrin deposition within vessels. This occurs with DIC such as may complicate overwhelming infection, but it may also occur when the intravascular coagulation is localized, as with giant cavernous hemangiomas (Kasabach-Merritt syndrome).

POLYCYTHEMIA & METHEMOGLOBINEMIA

CONGENITAL ERYTHROCYTOSIS (Familial Polycythemia)

In pediatrics, polycythemia is usually secondary to some hypoxemic disorder. However, a number of families with congenital erythrocytosis have been described. The disorder differs from polycythemia vera in that it affects only the erythroid series; the white cell count and platelet count are normal. It frequently occurs as an autosomal dominant, although it can also occur as an autosomal recessive. There are usually no physical findings except for plethora and splenomegaly. The hemoglobin may be as high as 27 g/dL, with a hematocrit of 80% and a red cell count of 10 million/μL. There are usually no symptoms other than headache and lethargy. Recent studies in a number of families have revealed (1) an abnormal hemoglobin with increased oxygen affinity, (2) reduced red cell diphosphoglycerate, (3) autonomous increase in erythropoietin production, or (4) hypersensitivity of erythroid precursors to erythropoietin.

Treatment is not indicated unless symptoms are marked. Phlebotomy is the treatment of choice.

Juvonen E et al: Autosomal dominant erythrocytosis caused by increased sensitivity to erythropoietin. Blood 1991;78:3066.

Sokol L et al: Primary familial polycythemia: A frameshift mutation in the erythropoietin receptor gene and increased sensitivity of erythroid progenitors to erythropoietin. Blood 1995;86:15.

SECONDARY POLYCYTHEMIA

Secondary polycythemia occurs in response to hypoxemia. The most common cause of secondary polycythemia in children is cyanotic congenital heart disease. It also occurs in chronic pulmonary disease such as cystic fibrosis and in pulmonary arteriovenous shunts. Persons living at extremely high altitudes, as well as some with methemoglobinemia and sulfhemoglobinemia, develop polycythemia. It has on rare occasions been described without hypoxemia in association with renal tumors, brain tumors, Cushing's disease, or hydronephrosis.

Polycythemia occurs normally in the neonatal period; it is particularly exaggerated in infants who are preterm or small for gestational age. In these infants, polycythemia is sometimes associated with other symptoms. It may occur in infants of diabetic mothers, and it has been described as a manifestation of Down's syndrome in the newborn and as a complication of congenital adrenal hyperplasia.

Iron deficiency may complicate polycythemia and aggravate the hyperviscosity. This complication should always be suspected when the MCV falls below the normal range. Multiple coagulation and bleeding abnormalities have also been described in severely polycythemic cardiac patients, including thrombocytopenia, mild consumption coagulopathy, and elevated fibrinolytic activity. Bleeding at surgery may be severe.

The ideal treatment of secondary polycythemia is correction of the underlying disorder. When this cannot be done, phlebotomy is often necessary to control the symptoms. Iron sufficiency should be maintained. Adequate hydration of the patient and phlebotomy with plasma replacement may be indicated prior to major surgical procedures; these measures prevent the complications of thrombosis and hemorrhage. Isovolumetric exchange transfusion is the treatment of choice in severe cases.

Balcerzak SP, Bromberg PA: Secondary polycythemia. Semin Hematol 1975;12:353.

METHEMOGLOBINEMIA

Methemoglobin is continuously formed at a slow rate by the oxidation of heme iron to the ferric state. Normally, it is enzymatically reduced back to hemoglobin. Methemoglobin is unable to transport oxygen and causes a shift in the dissociation curve of the residual oxyhemoglobin. Cyanosis is produced with methemoglobin levels of approximately 15% or greater. There are several mechanisms for the excess production of methemoglobin, which occurs as a congenital or acquired disorder.

1. HEMOGLOBIN M

The designation M is given to several abnormal hemoglobins associated with methemoglobinemia. Affected individuals are heterozygous for the gene, and it is transmitted as an autosomal dominant. The different types of hemoglobin M result from different amino acid substitutions in the α-globin or β-globin. Hemoglobin electrophoresis at the usual pH will not always demonstrate the abnormal hemoglobin, and isoelectric focussing or spectroscopy may be needed. The patient has marked and persistent cyanosis but is otherwise usually asymptomatic. Exercise tolerance may be normal, and life expectancy is not affected. This type of methemoglobinemia does not respond to any form of therapy.

Vichinsky EP, Lubin BH: Unstable hemoglobins, hemoglobins with altered oxygen affinity, and M-hemoglobins. Pediatr Clin North Am 1980;27:421.

2. CONGENITAL METHEMOGLOBINEMIA DUE TO ENZYME DEFICIENCIES

Congenital methemoglobinemia is most frequently caused by congenital deficiency of the reducing enzyme diaphorase I (coenzyme factor I). It is transmitted as an autosomal recessive trait. Affected patients may have as high as 40% methemoglobin but usually have no symptoms, although a mild compensatory polycythemia may be present. Patients with methemoglobinemia associated with a deficiency of diaphorase I respond readily to treatment with ascorbic acid and with methylene blue (see below). However, treatment is not usually indicated.

3. ACQUIRED METHEMOGLOBINEMIA

A number of compounds activate the oxidation of hemoglobin from the ferrous to the ferric state, forming methemoglobin. These include the nitrites and nitrates (contaminated water), chlorates, and quinones. Drugs in this group are the aniline dyes, sulfonamides, acetanilid, phenacetin, bismuth subnitrate, and potassium chlorate. Poisoning with a drug or chemical containing one of these substances should be suspected in any infant or child who presents with sudden cyanosis. Methemoglobin levels in such cases may be extremely high and can produce severe anoxia and dyspnea with unconsciousness, circulatory failure, and death. Young infants and newborns are more susceptible to poisoning because their red cells have difficulty reducing hemoglobin, probably because their NADH methemoglobin reductase is transiently deficient. Infants with metabolic acidosis from diarrhea and dehydration or other causes may also develop methemoglobinemia.

Patients with the acquired form of methemoglobinemia respond dramatically to methylene blue in a dosage of 1–2 mg/kg given intravenously. For infants and young children, a smaller dose (1–1.5 mg/kg) is recommended. Ascorbic acid administered orally or intravenously also reduces methemoglobin, but it acts more slowly.

Mansouri A, Lurie AA: Concise review: Methemoglobinemia. Am J Hematol 1993;42:7.
Murray KF, Christie DL: Dietary protein intolerance in infants with transient methemoglobinemia and diarrhea. J Pediatr 1993;122:90.
Osterhoudt KC et al: Rebound severe methemoglobinemia from ingestion of a nitroethane artificial-fingernail remover. J Pediatr 1995;126:819.
Sager S et al: Methemoglobinemia associated with acidosis of probable renal origin. J Pediatr 1995;126:59.

DISORDERS OF LEUKOCYTES

NEUTROPENIA

Essentials of Diagnosis

- Increased frequency of infections.
- Ulceration of oral mucosa and gingivitis.
- Normal numbers of red cells and platelets.

General Considerations

Neutropenia is an absolute neutrophil (granulocyte) count of less than 1500/μL in infancy and childhood, or below 1000/μL between 1 week and 2 years of age. During the first few days of life, an absolute neutrophil count of less than 3500 cells/μL may be considered neutropenia. Neutropenias result from absent or defective granulocyte stem cells, ineffective or suppressed myeloid maturation, decreased production of hematopoietic cytokines (eg, granulocyte colony-stimulating factor [G-CSF], granulocyte-macrophage colony-stimulating factor [GM-CSF]), decreased marrow release, increased neutrophil destruction or consumption, or, in pseudoneutropenia, from an increased neutrophil "marginating pool" (Table 26–6).

The most severe types of congenital neutropenias include reticular dysgenesis (congenital aleukocytosis), Kostmann's syndrome (severe neutropenia with maturation defect in the marrow progenitor cells), Shwachman's syndrome (neutropenia with pancreatic insufficiency), neutropenia with immune deficiency states, cyclic neutropenia, and myelocathexis or dysgranulopoiesis. Neutropenia may also be associated with storage and metabolic diseases and immunodeficiency states. The most common causes of neutropenia are viral infection or drugs resulting ei-

Table 26–6. Classification of neutropenia of childhood.

Congenital neutropenia with stem cell abnormalities
    Reticular dysgenesis
    Cyclic neutropenia
Congenital neutropenia with abnormalities of committed myeloid progenitor cells
    Neutropenia with immunodeficiency disorders (T cells and B cells)
    Severe congenital neutropenia (Kostmann)
    Chronic benign neutropenia of childhood
    Myelokathexis of dysmyelopoiesis
    Shwachman's syndrome
    Cartilage-hair hypoplasia
    Dyskeratosis congenita
    Fanconi's syndrome
    Hyperglycinemia and isovaleric, propionic, and methylmalonic acidemia
    Glycogenosis Ib
    Osteopetrosis
Acquired neutropenias affecting stem cells
    Malignancies (leukemia, lymphoma) and preleukemic disorders
    Drugs or toxic substances
    Ionizing radiation
    Aplastic anemia
Acquired neutropenias affecting committed myeloid progenitors or survival of mature neutrophils
    Ineffective granulopoiesis (vitamin B_{12}, folate, and copper deficiency)
    Infection
    Immune (neonatal alloimmune or autoimmune; autoimmune neutropenia of childhood)
    Hypersplenism

ther in decreased production in the marrow or increased destruction. Severe bacterial infections may be associated with neutropenia. Although rare, neonatal alloimmune neutropenia can be severe and associated with increased risk for infection. Autoimmune neutropenia in the mother can result in passive transfer of antibody and neutropenia in the neonate. Malignancies, osteopetrosis, marrow failure syndromes, and hypersplenism are not usually associated with isolated neutropenia.

Clinical Findings

A. Symptoms and Signs: Acute severe bacterial or fungal infection is the most significant complication of neutropenia. Although the risk is increased when the absolute neutrophil count is less than $500/\mu L$, the actual susceptibility is variable and depends on the cause of neutropenia, marrow reserves, and other factors. The most common types of infection include septicemia, cellulitis, abscesses, pneumonia, and perirectal abscesses. Aphthous ulcers, gingivitis, and periodontal disease also cause significant problems for these patients. In addition to local signs and symptoms, patients may have chills, fever, and malaise. In most cases, the spleen and liver are not enlarged. *Staphylococcus aureus* and gram-negative bacteria are the most significant causes of infections.

B. Laboratory Findings: Neutrophils are absent or markedly reduced in the peripheral blood. In most forms of neutropenia or agranulocytosis, the monocytes and lymphocytes are normal and the red cells and platelets are not affected. The bone marrow

usually shows a normal erythroid series, with adequate megakaryocytes but a marked reduction in the myeloid cells or a significant delay in maturation of this series.

In the evaluation of neutropenia, careful attention should be paid to the duration and pattern of neutropenia, the types of infections and their frequency, and phenotypic abnormalities on physical examination. A careful family history as well as blood counts from the parents is useful. If there is no obvious acquired cause such as viral infection or drug ingestion and no other primary disease, white blood cell counts should be done once or twice weekly for 2 months to evaluate the possibility of cyclic neutropenia. Bone marrow aspiration and biopsy are most important to characterize the morphologic features of myelopoiesis. Measuring the neutrophil counts in response to steroid infusion will document the marrow reserves. Elevated urinary muramidase levels and elevated serum lactoferrin may be found if increased neutrophil destruction is the cause of neutropenia. Tests for specific causes of neutropenia include measurement of neutrophil antibodies, immunoglobulin levels, antinuclear antibodies, and lymphocyte phenotyping. Cultures of bone marrow are important for defining the numbers of stem cells and progenitors committed to the myeloid series or the presence of cytotoxic lymphocytes or humoral inhibitory factors. Cytokine levels in plasma can be measured directly.

Treatment

Identifiable toxic agents should be eliminated, or associated diseases (such as infections) treated. Prophylactic antimicrobial therapy is not indicated. Recombinant G-CSF and GM-CSF will increase neutrophil counts in most patients. Patients may be started on 5 μg/kg/d of G-CSF (filgrastim) given subcutaneously or intravenously once a day. Depending on the response, the dose may be escalated to 10 μg/kg. For patients with congenital neutropenia, the dose should be regulated to keep the absolute neutrophil count less than 10,000/μL. Some patients maintain adequate counts with G-CSF given on alternate days.

Prognosis

The prognosis varies greatly with the cause and severity of the neutropenia. In severe cases with persistent agranulocytosis, the prognosis is poor in spite of antibiotic therapy; in mild or cyclic forms of neutropenia, symptoms may be minimal and the prognosis for normal life expectancy excellent. Recombinant hematopoietic hormones hold hope in the future for treatment of the more severe syndromes. However, recent studies in Kostmann's syndrome raises the question of malignant potential secondary to cytokine-induced proliferation of progenitor cells.

Ambruso DR et al: Infectious and bleeding complications in patents with glycogenesis Ib. Am J Dis Child 1985;139:691.

Bussel J, Lalezari P, Fikrig S: Intravenous treatment with γ-globulin of autoimmune neutropenia of infancy. J Pediatr 1988;112:298.

Dale DC et al: A randomized controlled phase III trial of recombinant human granulocyte colony-stimulating factor (filgrastim) for treatment of severe chronic neutropenia. Blood 1993;81:2496.

Lalezari P et al: Autoimmune neutropenia of infancy. J Pediatr 1986;109:764.

Logue GL et al: Idiopathic neutropenia: Antineutrophil antibodies and clinical correlations. Am J Med 1991; 90:211.

Weetman RM, Boxer LA: Childhood neutropenia. Pediatr Clin North Am 1980;27:361.

NEUTROPHILIA

Neutrophilia is an increase in the peripheral blood absolute neutrophil count greater than 7500–8500 cells/μL for infants, children, and adults. To support the increased peripheral count, neutrophils may be mobilized from bone marrow storage or peripheral marginating pools. Acutely, neutrophilia is seen with bacterial or viral infections, inflammatory diseases (eg, juvenile rheumatoid arthritis, inflammatory bowel disease, Kawasaki disease), surgical or functional asplenia, liver failure, diabetic ketoacidosis, azotemia, and patients with congenital disorders of neutrophil function (eg, chronic granulomatous disease and leukocyte adherence deficiency) and hemolysis. Drugs such as corticosteroids, lithium, and epi-

nephrine increase the blood neutrophil count. Corticosteroids cause release of neutrophils from the marrow pool and inhibit egress from capillary beds and postpone apoptotic cell death. Epinephrine causes release of the marginating pool. Acute neutrophilia has been reported after stress such as electric shock, trauma, burns, surgery, and emotional upset. Tumors involving the bone marrow such as lymphomas, neuroblastomas, and rhabdomyosarcoma may be associated with leukocytosis and the presence of immature myeloid cells in the peripheral blood. Infants with Down's syndrome have defective regulation of proliferation and maturation of the myeloid series and may develop neutrophilia. At times this process may affect other cell lines and mimic myeloproliferative disorders or acute myelogenous leukemia.

The neutrophilias must be distinguished from myeloproliferative disorders such as chronic myelogenous leukemia and juvenile chronic myelogenous leukemia. In general, abnormalities involving other cell lines, the appearance of immature cells on the blood smear, and the presence of hepatosplenomegaly are important differentiating characteristics.

DISORDERS OF NEUTROPHIL FUNCTION

Neutrophils play a key role in host defenses. Circulating in capillary beds, they adhere to the vascular endothelium adjacent to sites of infection and inflammation. Moving between endothelial cells, the neutrophil migrates toward the offending agent. Contact with a microbe that is properly opsonized with complement or antibodies triggers ingestion, a process in which cytoplasmic streaming results in the formation of pseudopods that fuse around the invader, encasing it in a phagosome. During the ingestion phase, there is assembly and activation of the oxidase enzyme system, which takes oxygen from the surrounding medium and reduces it to form toxic oxygen metabolites critical to microbicidal activity. Concurrently, granules from the two main classes (azurophil and specific) fuse and release their contents into the phagolysosome. The concentration of toxic oxygen metabolites (hydrogen peroxide, hypochlorous acid, hydroxyl radical, and others) as well as other compounds (proteases, cationic proteins, cathepsins, defensins, and others) increases dramatically, resulting in the death and dissolution of the microbe. Complex physiologic and biochemical processes subserve and control these functions. Defects in any of these may lead to inadequate cell function and an increased risk of infection.

Classification

Congenital defects in neutrophil function are summarized in Table 26–7. Other congenital or acquired

Table 26–7. Classification of congenital neutrophil function deficits.

Disorder	Clinical Manifestations	Functional Defect	Biochemical Defect	Inheritance
Chédiak-Higashi syndrome	Oculocutaneous albinism, photophobia, nystagmus, ataxia. Recurrent infections of skin, respiratory tract, and mucous membranes caused by gram-positive and gram-negative organisms. Many die from lymphoproliferative phase with hepatomegaly, fever. This may be a viral associated hemophagocytic syndrome secondary to Epstein-Barr virus infection.	Neutropenia. Neutrophils, monocytes, lymphocytes, platelets, and all granule-containing cells have giant granules. Most significant defect is in chemotaxis. Also milder defects in microbicidal activity and degranulation.	Unknown. Alterations in membrane fusion with formation of giant granules. Other biochemical abnormalities in cAMP and cGMP, microtubule assembly.	Autosomal recessive.
Leukocyte adherence deficiency I	Recurrent soft tissue infections, including gingivitis, otitis, mucositis, periodontitis, skin infections. Delayed separation of the cord in newborn and problems with wound healing.	Neutrophilia. Diminished adherence to surfaces, leading to decreased chemotaxis.	Absence or partial deficiency of CD11/CD18 cell surface adhesive glycoproteins.	Autosomal recessive.
Leukocyte adherence deficiency II	Recurrent infections, mental retardation, craniofacial abnormalities, short stature. Red cells have Bombay phenotype.	Neutrophilia. Deficient "rolling" interaction with endothelial cells.	Deficient fucosyl transferase results in deficient sialyl Lewis X antigen, which interacts with P selection on endothelial cell to establish neutrophil rolling, a prerequisite for adherence and diapedesis.	Autosomal recessive.
Chronic granulomatous disease	Recurrent purulent infections with catalase-positive bacteria and fungi. May involve skin, mucous membranes. Also develop deep infections (lymph nodes, liver, bones).	Neutrophilia. Neutrophils demonstrate deficient bactericidal activity in the presence of normal chemotaxis and ingestion. Defect in the oxidase, resulting in absence or diminished production of toxic oxygen metabolites.	A number of molecular defects in oxidase components. Absent cytochrome b558 with decreased mRNA for either (1) or (2): 　(1) gp91-phox 　(2) p22-phox Absent p47-phox or p67-phox (cytosolic components).	(1) X-linked (60–65% of cases). (2) Autosomal recessive (<5% of cases). Autosomal recessive (30% of cases).
Myeloperoxidase deficiency	Generally healthy.	Diminished capacity to enhance hydrogen peroxide-mediated microbicidal activity.	Diminished or absent myeloperoxidase; posttranslational defect in processing protein.	Autosomal recessive.
Specific granule deficiency	Recurrent skin and deep tissue infections.	Decreased chemotaxis and bactericidal activity.	Failure to produce specific granules or their contents during myelopoiesis.	Autosomal recessive.

causes of mild to moderate neutrophil dysfunction include metabolic defects (glycogen storage disease, diabetes mellitus, renal disease, hypophosphatemia), viral infections and certain drugs. Neutrophils from newborn infants have abnormal adherence, chemotaxis, and bactericidal activity due to maturation-dependent differences in regulation of adhesion glycoproteins, oxidative metabolism, and a deficiency of specific granules and their contents. Cells from patients with thermal injury, trauma, and overwhelming infection have defects in cell motility and bactericidal activity and exhibit similar biochemical abnormalities with neutrophils from newborn infants.

Clinical Findings

Recurrent bacterial or fungal infections are the hallmark of neutrophil dysfunction. Although many patients will have infection-free periods, episodes of pneumonia, sinusitis, cellulitis, cutaneous and mucosal infections (including perianal or peritonsillar abscesses), and lymphadenitis are frequent. As with neutropenia, aphthous ulcers of mucous membranes, severe gingivitis, and periodontal disease are also major complications. In general, *S aureus,* along with gram-negative organisms, are commonly isolated from infected sites; other organisms may be specifically associated with a defined neutrophil function defect. In some disorders, fungi account for an increasing number of infections. Deep or generalized infections such as osteomyelitis, liver abscesses, sepsis, meningitis, and necrotic or even gangrenous soft tissue lesions occur in specific syndromes (eg, leukocyte adherence deficiency or chronic granulomatous disease). Patients with severe neutrophil dysfunction may die in childhood from severe infections or associated complications. Pertinent laboratory findings are summarized in Table 26–7.

Treatment

The mainstays of management of these patients remain the anticipation of infections and aggressive attempts to identify the foci and the causative agents. Surgical procedures to achieve these goals may be both diagnostic and therapeutic. Broad-spectrum antibiotics covering the range of possible organisms should be initiated without delay, switching to specific antimicrobial agents when the appropriate microbiologic diagnosis is made. When infections are unresponsive or when they recur, granulocyte transfusions may be helpful.

Chronic management includes prophylactic antibiotics. Trimethoprim-sulfamethoxazole and other antibiotic compounds enhance the bactericidal activity of neutrophils from patients with chronic granulomatous disease. Some patients with Chédiak-Higashi syndrome improve clinically when given ascorbic acid. Recently, recombinant γ-interferon has been shown to decrease the number and severity of infections in patients with chronic granulomatous disease. Demonstration of this activity with one patient group raises the possibility that cytokines, growth factors, and other biologic response modifiers may be helpful in other conditions in preventing recurrent infections. Bone marrow transplantation has been attempted in most major congenital neutrophil dysfunction syndromes, and reconstitution with normal cells and cell function has been documented. Combining genetic engineering with autologous bone marrow transplant may provide a future strategy for curing these disorders.

Prognosis

For mild to moderate defects, anticipation and conservative medical management ensure a reasonable outlook. For severe defects, excessive morbidity and significant mortality still exist. In some diseases, the development of noninfectious complications, such as the lymphoproliferative phase of Chédiak-

Higashi syndrome, may be of significant prognostic importance.

Ambruso DR, Johnston RB Jr: Chronic granulomatous disease. In: *Pediatric Respiratory Disease: Diagnosis and Treatment.* Hilman BC (editor). WB Saunders, 1993.

Curnutte JT, Orkin SH, Dinauer MC: Genetic disorders of phagocyte function. In: *The Molecular Basis of Blood Diseases.* Stamatoyannopoulos G, Neinhuis AW, Majerus PW, Varmus H (editors). WB Saunders, 1994.

Etzioni A et al: Brief report: Recurrent severe infections caused by a novel leukocyte adhesion deficiency. N Engl J Med 1992;327:1789.

Roos D et al: Mutations in the X-linked and autosomal recessive forms of chronic granulomatous disease. Blood 1996;87:1663.

LYMPHOCYTOSIS

From the first week up to the fifth year of life, lymphocytes are the most numerous leukocytes in blood. The ratio then reverses gradually to reach the adult pattern of neutrophil predominance. An absolute lymphocytosis in childhood is seen with acute or chronic viral infections, pertussis, syphilis, tuberculosis, and hyperthyroidism. Other noninfectious conditions, drugs, and hypersensitivity and serum sickness–like reactions cause lymphocytosis.

Clinical features, including fever, upper respiratory symptoms, gastrointestinal complaints, and rashes, are clues in distinguishing infectious from noninfectious causes. The presence of enlarged liver, spleen, or lymph nodes is crucial to the differential diagnosis, which includes acute leukemia and lymphoma. Most cases of infectious mononucleosis present with hepatosplenomegaly or adenopathy. The absence of anemia and thrombocytopenia helps to differentiate these disorders. Evaluation of the morphology of lymphocytes on peripheral blood smear is also crucial. Infectious causes—particularly infectious mononucleosis—are associated with atypical features in the lymphocytes such as basophilic cytoplasm, vacuoles, finer and less dense chromatin, and an indented nucleus. These features are distinct from the characteristic morphology seen in lymphoblastic leukemia. Lymphocytosis in childhood is most commonly associated with infections and resolves with recovery from the primary disease.

EOSINOPHILIA

Eosinophilia in infants and children is an absolute eosinophil count greater than 300/μL. Marrow eosinophil production is stimulated by the cytokine interleukin-5 (IL-5). In children, allergies, and particularly eczema, are the most common primary causes of eosinophilia. Eosinophilia also occurs in drug reactions, with tumors (Hodgkin's and non-Hodgkin's lymphomas and brain tumors), with immunodeficiency and histiocytosis syndromes. Increased eosinophil counts are a prominent feature of parasitic infections. Gastrointestinal disorders such as chronic hepatitis, ulcerative colitis, Crohn's disease, and milk precipitin disease may have eosinophilia. Increased blood eosinophil counts have been identified in several families without association with any specific illness. Rare causes of eosinophilia include the hypereosinophilic syndrome, characterized by counts greater than 1500/μL and organ involvement and damage (hepatosplenomegaly, cardiopathy, pulmonary fibrosis, and central nervous system injury). This is a disorder of middle-aged adults and is rare in children.

Eosinophils are sometimes the last type of mature myeloid cell to disappear after marrow ablative chemotherapy. Increased eosinophil counts are seen with graft versus host disease after bone marrow transplantation, and elevations are sometimes documented during rejection episodes in patients who have solid organ grafts.

Eosinophilic leukemia has been described, but its existence as a distinct entity is controversial.

BLEEDING DISORDERS

Bleeding disorders may occur as a result of (1) quantitative or qualitative abnormalities of platelets, (2) quantitative or qualitative abnormalities in plasma coagulation factors, or (3) vascular abnormalities. The coagulation cascade is shown in Figure 26–4.

Screening tests to investigate patients for possible bleeding disorders should include:

1. Prothrombin time (PT) to screen the tissue thromboplastin system of coagulation (factors VII, X, II, V, and fibrinogen).
2. Partial thromboplastin time (PTT) to measure clotting activity of the following factors: high-molecular-weight kininogen (HMWK), prekallikrein (PK), XII, XI, IX, VIII, X, V, II, and fibrinogen.
3. Platelet count.
4. Bleeding time to test small vessel integrity, von Willebrand and platelet function.
5. Thrombin time (TT) to measure the generation of fibrin following conversion of prothrombin to thrombin as well as the antithrombin effect of fibrin-split products or heparin.
6. Fibrinogen level.

Hathaway W, Goodnight Jr S: *Disorders of Hemostasis and Thrombosis.* McGraw-Hill 1993:50.
Sham R, Francis C: Evaluation of mild bleeding disorders and easy bruising. Blood Rev 1994;8:98.

ABNORMALITIES OF PLATELET NUMBER OR FUNCTION

1. IDIOPATHIC THROMBOCYTOPENIC PURPURA (ITP)

Essentials of Diagnosis
- Otherwise healthy child.
- Decreased platelet count.
- Petechiae, ecchymoses.

General Considerations
Acute ITP is the most common bleeding disorder of childhood. It most frequently occurs in children 2–5 years of age and follows infection with viruses such as rubella, varicella, measles, or Epstein-Barr virus. Most patients recover spontaneously within a few months. Chronic ITP (>6 months' duration) occurs in just 10–20%. The thrombocytopenia results from immune clearance of platelets, which have IgM or IgG on their surface. The spleen plays a major role by forming antibodies and by sequestering damaged platelets.

Clinical Findings
A. Symptoms and Signs: Onset of ITP is usually acute, with the appearance of multiple ecchymoses. Petechiae are often present, especially on the lips and buccal mucosa, and epistaxis is common. There are generally no other physical findings. Rarely, concurrent infection with Epstein-Barr virus or cytomegalovirus may cause hepatosplenomegaly or lymphadenopathy simulating acute leukemia.

B. Laboratory Findings:

1. Blood–The platelet count is markedly reduced (usually 50,000/μL and often 10,000/μL), and platelets frequently are of larger size on peripheral blood smear. The white blood count and differential count are normal. Anemia is not present unless hemorrhage has occurred.

2. Bone marrow–An increased number of megakaryocytes (which may be larger than normal) is present. Erythroid and myeloid cellularity is normal.

3. Other laboratory tests–The bleeding time is generally prolonged if the platelet count is less than 40,000/μL. PTT and PT are normal. Platelet-associated IgG or IgM or both may be demonstrated on the platelets or in the serum.

Differential Diagnosis
Causes of thrombocytopenia are shown in Table 26–8. ITP is a diagnosis of exclusion. Bone marrow

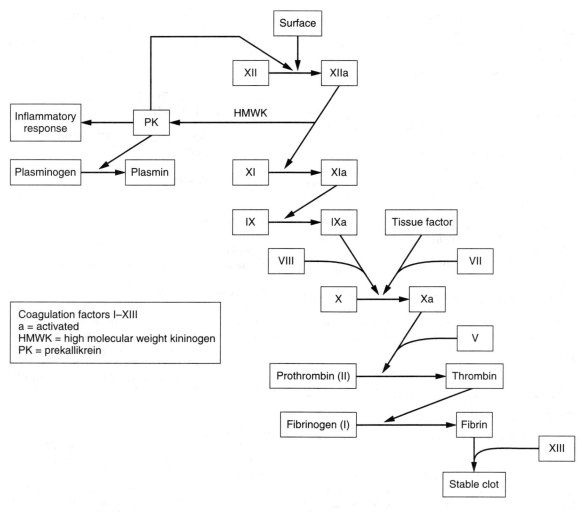

Figure 26–4. Blood coagulation cascade and terminology of coagulation factors.

examination may be indicated to exclude leukemia and aplastic anemia. Bone marrow examination should be performed if the history is atypical, if abnormalities other than purpura and petechiae are present on physical examination, if other cell lines are affected on the CBC, or possibly if corticosteroid therapy is to be administered. Family history should

be helpful in determining whether thrombocytopenia is hereditary.

Complications

Severe hemorrhage and bleeding into vital organs are the feared complications of ITP. Intracranial hemorrhage is the most serious but rarely seen com-

Table 26–8. Common causes of thrombocytopenia.

Destruction			Decreased Production	
Antibody-Mediated	**Coagulopathy**	**Other**	**Congenital**	**Acquired**
Idiopathic thrombocytic purpura Infection Immunologic diseases	Disseminated intravascular coagulopathy Sepsis Necrotizing enterocolitis Thrombosis Cavernous hemangioma	Hemolytic uremic syndrome Thrombotic thrombocytopenic purpura Hypersplenism Respiratory distress syndrome	Falconi's syndrome Wiskott-Aldrich syndrome Thrombocytopenia with absent radii Metabolic disorders Osteopetrosis	Aplastic anemia Leukemia and other malignancies Vitamin B_{12} and folate deficiencies

plication. The most important risk factor for hemorrhage is a platelet count less than 20,000/μL.

Treatment

A. General Measures: Many children require no therapy. Aspirin and aspirin-containing drugs should not be administered. Trauma should be avoided.

B. Corticosteroids: Patients with significant bleeding (ie, hematuria, hematochezia, epistaxis) or those with a platelet count of less than 10,000/μL are often treated with prednisone (2 mg/kg orally in divided daily doses) for a period of 2–4 weeks. The dosage is then tapered and stopped. No further prednisone is given regardless of the platelet count unless significant bleeding recurs, at which time prednisone in the smallest dose that will give symptomatic relief (usually 2.5–5 mg twice daily is administered). The patient is then followed until spontaneous remission occurs or until the patient is a candidate for further therapy.

C. Intravenous Immune Globulin (IVIG): As an alternative or adjunct to corticosteroid treatment, IVIG may raise the platelet count in acute and chronic ITP of childhood. IVIG may be effective even when the patient is resistant to corticosteroids; responses are prompt and may last for several weeks. Most patients respond to 1 g/kg/d for 1–3 days.

D. Splenectomy: Splenectomy produces permanent remission in 70–90% of children with ITP. It is usually reserved for those who fail to remit over a period of 6 months to 1 year. Although platelet transfusions are usually ineffective and bleeding is rarely a complication of splenectomy, platelet concentrates should be available for surgery. If the patient has been receiving corticosteroid therapy, the dose should be appropriately increased during and after surgery. Anticoagulant therapy is not indicated postoperatively even though the platelet count may rise to 1 million/μL.

The risk of overwhelming infection is increased after splenectomy, particularly in the young child. Therefore, the procedure should be postponed, if possible, until the child is at least 5 years of age. Administration of pneumococcal vaccine, meningococcal, and *Haemophilus influenzae* b vaccines prior to splenectomy is recommended. Prophylactic penicillin following splenectomy should be considered.

E. Other: $Rh_o(D)$ immune globulin (RhoGAM) intravenously appears equally as safe and as effective as IVIG in Rh-positive patients who have not been splenectomized. In addition, RhoGAM is substantially less expensive than IVIG. Ninety percent of children respond within 7 days to a single dose of 50 μg/kg. The median duration of response is 5 weeks. During treatment, Coombs'-positive hemolysis may transiently occur with subsequent anemia. Responses to cyclosporine and interferon have been reported in persons with chronic ITP.

Prognosis

Ninety percent of children with ITP will have a spontaneous remission. Features associated with the development of chronic ITP include female sex, age over 10 years at presentation, a more insidious onset of bruising, and the presence of other autoantibodies.

Andrew M et al: A multicenter study of the treatment of childhood chronic idiopathic thrombocytopenic purpura with anti-D. J Pediatr 1992;120:522.

Imbach P: Immune thrombocytopenia in children: The immune character of destructive thrombocytopenia and the treatment of bleeding. Semin Thromb Hemost 1995; 21:305.

2. THROMBOCYTOPENIA IN THE NEWBORN

Thrombocytopenia is one of the most common causes of purpura in the newborn and should be considered and investigated in any newborn with petechiae or a significant bleeding tendency. A platelet count less than 150,000/μL establishes a diagnosis of thrombocytopenia. A number of specific entities may be responsible (see Table 26–8). Infection and intravascular coagulation syndromes are the most common causes of thrombocytopenia in both sick term and preterm newborns. In the well-appearing newborn, antibody-mediated thrombocytopenia (alloimmune or maternal autoimmune), viral syndrome, hyperviscosity, or major vessel thrombosis are important causes. Management is directed toward alleviation of the specific cause.

Thrombocytopenia Associated With Platelet Alloimmunization

Platelet alloimmunization occurs in one of 2000 pregnancies. Alloimmunization occurs when a platelet antigen of the infant differs from that of the mother and when the mother is sensitized by platelets that cross from the fetal to the maternal circulation. Severe intracranial bleeding occurs in 10–30% of affected neonates either in utero or after delivery. Petechiae or other bleeding manifestations are usually present shortly after birth. The disease is self-limited with the platelet count normalizing within 2 weeks.

If severe alloimmunization occurs, platelet concentrate from the mother will be more effective in raising the platelet count than random donor platelets. Maternal platelets should be washed and irradiated. IVIG infusions have also been used successfully to raise the platelet count. If less severe, observation alone may be all that is required.

If alloimmunization has occurred with a previous pregnancy, ultrasound examination of the fetal brain to detect hemorrhage should be obtained at 20 weeks gestation and repeated regularly. Percutaneous umbilical blood sampling can be performed at midgestation with concentrated washed maternal platelets available to protect against fetal hemorrhage. If the fetal platelet count is low, IVIG with or without concomitant corticosteroids should be administered to the mother for 4–6 weeks. Delivery by elective cesarean section is recommended, if the fetal platelet count is less than 50,000/µL.

Thrombocytopenia Associated With Idiopathic Thrombocytopenic Purpura in the Mother

Infants born to mothers with ITP or antiphospholipid antibodies may develop thrombocytopenia as a result of transfer of antibody from the mother to the infant. Unfortunately, maternal platelet count, maternal antiplatelet antibody levels, and fetal scalp platelet counts are unreliable predictors of bleeding risk. Antenatal administration of either prednisone or IVIG to the mother has been advocated, but there are no controlled trials to support this approach.

Most neonates with thrombocytopenia secondary to passive transfer of maternal antibody do not bleed, and thus no specific treatment is indicated. The risk for intracranial hemorrhage is 0.2–2%. However, if petechiae or puncture wound bleeding ensues, a 1- to 2-week course of oral prednisone, 2 mg/kg/d, may be administered. If the platelet count remains consistently less than 25,000/µL or if severe hemorrhage is present, IVIG should be considered. Platelet transfusions may not be helpful without prior removal of antibody by exchange transfusion.

Neonatal Thrombocytopenia Associated With Infections

Thrombocytopenia is commonly associated with severe generalized infections during the newborn period. Fifty to seventy-five percent of neonates with bacterial sepsis are thrombocytopenic. Intrauterine infections such as rubella, syphilis, toxoplasmosis, cytomegalic inclusion disease, herpes simplex, and parvovirus are often associated with thrombocytopenia.

In addition to specific treatment for the underlying disease, platelet transfusions may be indicated in severe cases. Platelet concentrates in the dosage of 10 mL/kg will raise the platelet count by about 75,000/µL.

Thrombocytopenia Associated With Giant Hemangiomas (Kasabach-Merritt Syndrome)

A rare but important cause of thrombocytopenic purpura in the newborn is giant hemangioma. Platelet sequestration in the lesion results in peripheral depletion of platelets. The bone marrow usually shows megakaryocytic hyperplasia. In the presence of massive hemangiomas, the thrombocytopenia may be associated with DIC and result in fatal hemorrhage. Treatment is indicated if a serious coagulopathy is present or if the lesion exerts pressure on a vital structure or is cosmetically unacceptable. Surgery is usually contraindicated because of the risk of hemorrhage. Prednisone therapy has been associated with marked regression. If DIC is present, heparin or aminocaproic acid may be useful. Interferon-α has also been shown to be efficacious.

Burrows R, Kelton J: Fetal thrombocytopenia and its relation to maternal thrombocytopenia. N Engl J Med 1993;329:1463.

Bussell J et al: Recommendations for the evaluation and treatment of neonatal autoimmune and alloimmune thrombocytopenia. Thromb Haemost 1991;65:631.

George D, Bussel J: Neonatal thrombocytopenia. Semin Thromb Hemost 1995;21:276.

White CW et al: Treatment of childhood angiomatous diseases with recombinant interferon alfa-2a. J Pediatr 1991;118:59.

3. DISORDERS OF PLATELET FUNCTION

Platelet function is studied by assessing aggregation of platelets with agonists such as adenosine diphosphate (ADP), collagen, arachidonic acid, and ristocetin. Persons with platelet function defects have skin and mucosal bleeding similar to that seen in persons with thrombocytopenia.

The **hereditary** disorders of platelet function are characterized by a bleeding diathesis, usually associated with a prolonged bleeding time in spite of usually normal numbers of platelets. The findings in these diseases are summarized in Table 26–9.

Acquired disorders of platelet function may occur secondary to uremia, cirrhosis, sepsis, myeloproliferative disorders, acyanotic congenital heart disease, and viral infections. Many pharmacologic agents decrease platelet function. The most common agents are aspirin, nonsteroidal anti-inflammatory agents, and synthetic penicillins.

Treatment

Many individuals with hereditary and acquired platelet function defects will respond to therapy with desmopressin acetate (DDAVP) at a dose of 0.3 µg/kg intravenously. If this is not effective, treatment with random donor platelets at a dose of one bag per 6 kg is indicated. Alternatively, calculations may be based on surface area, where one unit of platelet concentrate per meter squared is expected to raise the platelet count by 20,000/µL.

Hathaway W, Goodnight S: *Disorders of Hemostasis and Thrombosis.* McGraw-Hill, 1993.

INHERITED ABNORMALITIES OF COAGULATION FACTORS

Normal values for coagulation factors are shown in Table 26–10. The more common factor deficiencies are discussed here.

Table 26–9. Hereditary platelet function disorders.[1]

Category	Heredity	Morphology	Platelet-Rich Plasma Aggregation to:				Specific Defects
			ADP	Colla-gen	AA	Risto-cetin	
Glanzmann's thrombasthenia[2]	AR	Normal	–	–	–	+	Decreased membrane glycoprotein IIb-IIIa; platelet fibrogen and abnormal adhesion to subendothelium
Bernard-Soulier syndrome[2]	AR	Giant platelets	+	+	+	–	Decreased membrane glycoprotein Ib IX complex
Storage pool deficiency syndromes:[2] Dense body deficiency, Hermansky-Pudlak syndrome	AR	Electron microscopy: decreased to absent dense bodies	±	–	±	±	Decreased ADP-ATP, Ca^{2+}, serotonin storage and release
Dense body with α-granule deficiency[2]	AD	Electron microscopy: decreased dense bodies and α-granules	±	–	±	±	Decreased ADP, Ca^{2+}, serotonin, PF_4, fibrinogen, βTG storage and release, decreased PDGF
α-Granule deficiency, gray platelet syndrome[2]	AR	Light gray platelets. Electron microscopy: decreased α-granules	±	±	+	+	Decreased PF_4, βTG, fibrinogen, decreased PDGF storage and release
Wiskott-Aldrich syndrome[2]	X-linked	Tiny platelets; decreased organelles	±	–	+	+	
Failure to release (aspirin-like defect)	Variable	Normal	±	–	–	±	Deficiency of cyclooxygenase or thromboxane synthetase
Isolated platelet factor V deficiency 2, factor Quebec	AD	Normal	?	?	?	?	Decreased platelet factor V function; decreased prothrombinase
Pseudo-von Willebrand's disease[2]	AD	Normal	+	+	+	Incr	Intrinsic platelet abnormality of increased reaction of GPIb with vWF

[1]Modified and reproduced, with permission, from Hathaway WE, Bonnar J: *Hemostatic Disorders of the Pregnant Woman and Newborn Infant.* Elsevier, 1987. © 1987 by Elsevier Science Publishing Co., Inc.
[2]Thrombocytopenia may be seen.

+ = yes: – = no; ± = partial or slight.
AA = arachidonic acid; AD = autosomal dominant; AR = autosomal recessive; PF_4 = platelet factor 4; βTG = β-thromboglobulin; PDGF = platelet-derived growth factor; GPLb = glycoprotein/b.

1. FACTOR VIII DEFICIENCY (Hemophilia A, Classic Hemophilia)

Essentials of Diagnosis

- Bruising, bleeding, and hemarthroses.
- Prolonged PTT.
- Reduced factor VIII activity.

General Considerations

Factor VIII deficiency is a bleeding disorder characterized by decreased activity of factor VIII. The disease occurs predominantly in males and is either inherited in an X-linked manner or is the result of a new mutation. One third of cases are due to a new mutation.

Clinical Findings

A. Symptoms and Signs: Patients with severe factor VIII deficiency, characterized by frequent spontaneous bleeding episodes involving skin, mucous membranes, joints, muscles, and viscera, have less than 1% circulating factor VIII activity. In con-

Table 26–10. Coagulation factor values.[1]

	Fetus (20 wk)	Preterm (25–32 wk)	Term Infant	Infant (6 mo)	Normal Adult
Fibrinogen (mg/dL)	96 (40)	250 (100)	240 (150)	251 (160)	278 (61)
II	16 (10)	32 (18)	52 (25)	88 (60)	100 (70)
V	70 (40)	80 (43)	100 (54)	91 (55)	100 (60)
VII	21 (12)	37 (24)	57 (35)	87 (50)	100 (60)
VIII	50 (23)	75 (40)	150 (55)	90 (50)	100 (60)
vWf	65 (40)	150 (90)	160 (84)	107 (60)	100 (60)
IX	10 (5)	22 (17)	35 (15)	86 (36)	100 (50)
X	19 (15)	38 (20)	45 (30)	78 (38)	100 (60)
XI	–	20 (12)	42 (20)	86 (38)	100 (60)
XII	30	22 (9)	44 (16)	77 (39)	100 (60)

[1]Expressed as mean % activity unless otherwise indicated.
Values in parentheses are -2SD.
Modified and reproduced, with permission, from Hathaway W, Goodnight S Jr: *Disorders of hemostasis and thrombosis.* McGraw-Hill, 1993:31.

trast, patients with mild factor VIII deficiency, 5–40% factor VIII activity, bleed only at times of trauma or surgery. Those with moderate factor VIII deficiency, 1–5% factor VIII activity, have intermediate bleeding manifestations. The most crippling aspect of factor VIII deficiency is the tendency to develop chronic hemarthroses, which incite joint destruction.

B. Laboratory Findings: Persons with factor VIII deficiency have a prolonged partial thromboplastin time (PTT). The bleeding time and PT are usually normal. The diagnosis is confirmed by finding decreased factor VIII activity with normal von Willebrand factor (vWF) activity.

In two thirds of families, the females are carriers and occasionally are mildly symptomatic. Carriers of hemophilia can be detected by determination of the ratio of factor VIII activity to vWF antigen and by molecular genetic techniques.

Complications

A serious complication of hemophilia is the development of an acquired circulating antibody to factor VIII after treatment with factor VIII. Inhibitors or antibodies to factor VIII develop in 15–25% of factor VIII–deficient persons with hemophilia. The inhibitor is an antibody that may be amenable to immunosuppressive therapy. Factor IX concentrate or activated prothrombin complex concentrates may be of help in stopping hemorrhage. Recombinant factor VIIa is an alternative.

Complications related to therapy included infection with HIV and hepatitis B (up until about 1985 in the United States) and hepatitis C (removed from most US preparations by 1990). By selecting donors seronegative for these infections and by heat- or chemically treating the factor concentrates to inactivate viruses, the risks of these infections seem to have been eliminated. Safe concentrates are expensive and unobtainable in many parts of the world. Transmission of parvovirus and hepatitis A remains a problem, even with concentrates that have had viral inactivation. Immunization with the killed hepatitis A vaccine may help. Recombinant factor VIII concentrates are available and have yet to be associated with any infectious complications.

Treatment

The aim is to raise the factor VIII activity. Some mild factor VIII–deficient persons may respond to DDAVP. Most factor VIII–deficient patients require administration of factor VIII concentrates to achieve hemostasis. Factor VIII is available as concentrates from human plasma or as a recombinant (and somewhat truncated) protein. The in vivo half-life of factor VIII is about 12 hours. There is no standard vial size for factor VIII concentrates. Factor VIII must be prescribed in units (U) rather than vials. Non–life-threatening hemorrhages are treated with about 20 U/kg body weight factor VIII concentrate. This will increase factor VIII activity to 40%. Life-threatening hemorrhage is initially treated with approximately 50 U/kg factor VIII concentrate; this will increase factor VIII activity by 100%. Subsequent doses are determined according to the situation. The dose given should be as close as possible to the desired dose as determined by vial size. Excess factor VIII concentrate should always be infused rather than discarded. Monitoring the factor VIII activity achieved may be warranted, depending on the situation.

Hemarthroses are common in persons with hemophilia. Initial therapy is with 20–40 U/kg factor VIII concentrate with subsequent doses in accordance with joint status. Prophylaxis with every other day infusions is likely to prevent the development of arthropathy. A prospective study of this is underway.

Prognosis

When care is coordinated through a hemophilia center, and attention is given to the emotional, social, and educational status of the child, the prognosis for a normal life is good.

Furie B, Limentani S, Rosenfield C: A practical guide to the evaluation and treatment of hemophilia. Blood 1994;84:3.

Gill J: Therapy of factor VIII deficiency. Semin Thromb Hemost 1993;19:1.

Nilsson I et al: Twenty-five years experience of prophylactic treatment in severe hemophilia A and B. J Intern Med 1992;232:25.

2. FACTOR IX DEFICIENCY
(Hemophilia B, Christmas Disease)

The mode of inheritance and clinical manifestations of factor IX deficiency are the same as those of factor VIII deficiency. Factor IX deficiency is 15–20% as prevalent as factor VIII deficiency. As in factor VIII deficiency, the PTT in factor IX deficiency is prolonged, but PT and thrombin time are normal. Diagnosis is made by assaying factor IX activity.

Factor IX concentrate is the treatment of choice. Unlike factor VIII, about 50% of the administered dose of factor IX diffuses into the extravascular space. One unit of factor IX per kilogram is expected to increase the factor IX level by 1%. Factor IX has a half-life of 20–22 hours in vivo. Cryoprecipitates and factor VIII concentrates do not contain factor IX. Virus-inactivating techniques for factor IX concentrates appear effective in eradicating HIV and hepatitis C. As with factor VIII, monoclonally derived factor IX concentrate is available, but in contrast to factor VIII, a recombinant concentrate is not yet commercially available. Persons with factor IX deficiency are less likely to form an inhibitor. The prognosis for persons with factor IX deficiency is comparable to those with factor VIII deficiency.

Thompson A: Factor IX concentrates for clinical use. Semin Thromb Hemost 1993;19:25.

3. FACTOR XI DEFICIENCY
(Hemophilia C)

Factor XI deficiency is a bleeding diathesis of mild to moderate severity. Heterozygotes may bleed at surgery or following severe trauma. Homozygous patients may have spontaneous hemorrhage into skin or mucosa but rarely have spontaneous hemarthroses. Hemophilia C accounts for less than 5% of all hemophilia diseases.

The defect may be mild, and a sensitive activated partial thromboplastin time (APTT) is required to identify the deficiency. The level of factor XI activity is not predictive of risk for bleeding. Intervention is usually only at the time of surgery or trauma. Treatment is with fresh frozen plasma (FFP) to the extent volume expansion is tolerated. Factor XI concentrate is in clinical trials.

The prognosis for an average life span is excellent.

Bolton-Maggs PHB et al: Definition of the bleeding tendency in factor XI-deficient kindreds: A clinical and laboratory study. Thromb Haemost 1995;73:194.

4. OTHER INHERITED COAGULATION FACTOR DEFECTS

Other hereditary single clotting factor deficiencies are rare. Transmission is generally autosomal. Homozygous individuals with a deficiency or structural abnormality of prothrombin, factor V, factor VII, or factor X have excessive bleeding.

Persons with dysfibrinogenemia (abnormal fibrinogen) are usually asymptomatic but may develop recurrent venous thromboembolic episodes or have a bleeding tendency. Immunologic determinations of fibrinogen are normal, but the thrombin time and PT are often prolonged. Treatment is similar to that outlined for afibrinogenemia (absence of fibrinogen).

Afibrinogenemia resembles hemophilia clinically but has an autosomal recessive inheritance. The patients have persistent bleeding from small injuries, hematomas, ecchymoses, and hemarthroses. Fatal bleeding from the umbilical cord has been reported. The principal laboratory finding in afibrinogenemia is complete absence of a fibrin clot by any of the usual clotting tests. Hypofibrinogenemia (fibrinogen level less than 100 mg/dL) is also rarely seen.

Treatment of rare single clotting factor deficient persons is usually with FFP. Cryoprecipitate generally controls the acute bleeding episodes in persons with fibrinogen abnormalities.

Galanakis KK: Fibrinogen anomalies and disease: A clinical update. Hematol Oncol Clin North Am 1992;5:1171.

VON WILLEBRAND'S DISEASE

Essentials of Diagnosis

- History of easy bruising and epistaxis from early childhood.
- Bleeding time usually prolonged, with a normal platelet count.
- Reduced activity or abnormal structure of von Willebrand factor.

General Considerations

Von Willebrand's disease and its variants are due to abnormalities of von Willebrand factor (vWF), a plasma protein which forms a multimeric complex that carries factor VIII. In classic von Willebrand's disease (type I), there is a partial quantitative deficiency of vWF. In von Willebrand's disease type II, there is a qualitative abnormality of vWF. Persons with type III disease have virtually complete deficiency of vWF. Von Willebrand's disease is the most common inherited bleeding disorder; 1% of persons are affected, but only 10% are symptomatic. It is usually transmitted as an autosomal dominant trait.

Clinical Findings
A. Symptoms and Signs: There is usually a

history of increased bruising and excessive epistaxis. Increased bleeding will also occur with lacerations or at surgery. Menorrhagia is often a problem.

B. Laboratory Findings: The PTT is usually prolonged but may be normal. A prolonged bleeding time is generally present because vWF is involved in platelet binding to the blood vessel. Platelet number is normal. Factor VIII and vWF antigen are decreased in types I and III but may be normal in type II von Willebrand's disease.

Treatment

The treatment for many is 0.3 μg/kg of desmopressin acetate (DDAVP) intravenously in at least 20–30 mL of normal saline given over 20–30 minutes. A twofold to threefold rise in vWF is expected. Efficacy is variable from patient to patient; bleeding time should be measured before and 30 minutes after infusion to assess response. A high concentration nasal DDAVP is an alternative, but the effect varies and response to intravenous DDAVP does *not* predict response to the nasal preparation. Since stored vWF release is limited, tachyphylaxis is often seen with DDAVP. If further therapy is indicated, vWF-rich concentrate is recommended.

For persons with type III or IIB von Willebrand's disease, the treatment of choice is with vWF-enriched concentrate. DDAVP is ineffective in patients with type III von Willebrand's disease, and in those with type IIB disease may evoke thrombocytopenia.

Antifibrinolytic drugs (aminocaproic acid or tranexamic acid) may be indicated for oral, nasal, or vaginal bleeding.

Prognosis

Life expectancy is normal.

Holmberg L, Nilsson IM: von Willebrand's disease. Eur J Haematol 1992;48:127.

Rose E, Aledort L: Nasal spray desmopressin (DDAVP) for mild hemophilia A and von Willebrand disease. Am Intern Med 1991;1214:563.

Sadler JE, Grainick HR: Commentary: A new classification for von Willebrand disease. Blood 1994;84:676.

ACQUIRED ABNORMALITIES OF COAGULATION FACTORS

1. DISSEMINATED INTRAVASCULAR COAGULATION

Essentials of Diagnosis

- Presence of disorder known to trigger disseminated intravascular coagulation.
- Evidence for activation of coagulation (prolonged PTT, PT, or thrombin time; decreased fibrinogen or platelets).

General Considerations

Disseminated intravascular coagulation (DIC) is an acquired pathologic process characterized by activation of the coagulation system. It may lead to thrombin generation, intravascular fibrin deposition, and platelet consumption. Microthrombi, composed of fibrin and platelets, may produce ischemic tissue damage. The fibrinolytic system is also frequently activated, producing plasmin-mediated destruction of fibrin, fibrinogen, and other clotting factors (factor V, factor VIII). Degradation or split products of fibrin-fibrinogen are formed and function as anticoagulants and inhibitors of platelet function. DIC commonly accompanies disorders seen in critically ill infants and children. Conditions known to trigger DIC include endothelial cell damage (endotoxin, virus), tissue destruction (necrosis, physical injuries), hypoxia (acidosis), ischemic and vascular changes (shock, hemangiomas), and release of tissue procoagulants (cancer, placental disorders).

Clinical Findings

A. Symptoms and Signs: Physical signs of DIC may include (1) evidence of a diffuse bleeding tendency (hematuria, melena, purpura, petechiae, persistent oozing from needle punctures or other invasive procedures); (2) circulatory collapse, poor skin perfusion, early ischemic changes; and (3) evidence of thrombotic lesions (major vessel thrombosis, gangrene, purpura fulminans).

B. Laboratory Findings: Tests that are most sensitive, easiest to perform, and best reflect the hemostatic capacity of the patient are the PT, PTT, platelet count, fibrinogen level, and a test for fibrin-fibrinogen split products. A test that measures the cross-linked fibrin degradation by-products called d-dimers may also be helpful in demonstrating activation of both coagulation and fibrinolysis. Often, the PT and PTT are prolonged and the platelet count and fibrinogen level are decreased. Levels of fibrin-fibrinogen split products and d-dimers are elevated.

The abnormalities associated with DIC may vary depending on the triggering event. Patients with infections may have primarily thrombocytopenia, with only slight prolongation of the PTT and PT and mild elevation of fibrin-fibrinogen split products; only platelets may be consumed in bacterial sepsis without any other evidence of activated coagulation. In contrast, asphyxia may produce significant consumption of fibrinogen and elevated fibrin-fibrinogen split products without depression of platelets.

Differential Diagnosis

Bleeding with liver disease, vitamin K deficiency, or uremia can mimic DIC. Patients with fulminant hepatitis or advanced cirrhosis often have evidence of both decreased production of liver-dependent coagulation factors and increased consumption of platelets and fibrinogen. Generally, factor VII levels is markedly decreased in liver disease compared with mild to moderate decreases in DIC. Factor VIII levels may be normal or even increased in liver disease compared with decreased levels in DIC.

Treatment

A. Therapy for Underlying Disorder: The most important aspect of therapy is identification and treatment of the triggering event. If this can be treated (eg, hypoxia, shock), often no other therapy is needed for the coagulopathy. Serial coagulation tests help in determining whether specific therapy is indicated.

B. Replacement Therapy: Replacement of depleted coagulation factors and platelets may be necessary in severe DIC. FFP replaces depleted coagulation factors; 10–15 mL/kg will raise clotting factor activities by about 20%. Fibrinogen (and factor VIII) can be given as cryoprecipitate also; one bag of cryoprecipitate per 3 kg in infants or one bag of cryoprecipitate per 6 kg in older children will raise the fibrinogen level by 75–100 mg/dL. Platelets are replaced with platelet concentrate; in the neonate, 10 mL of platelet concentrate per kilogram will raise the platelet count by 75,000–100,000/μL. In older children, one bag of platelet concentrate per 5–6 kg is the usual dose. An alternative formula is as follows: 1 U/m^2 of platelet concentrate will increase the platelet count by about 20,000/μL. The minimal hemostatic goals are a platelet count greater than 40,000/μL, PT of less than 16 seconds, and fibrinogen over 100 mg/dL.

C. Anticoagulant Therapy: Heparin is often given to interrupt the clotting process, particularly when consumption coagulopathy is problematic (eg, acute promyelocytic or monocytic leukemia, giant hemangioma, impending tissue necrosis or gangrene in septic shock, large vessel thrombosis, or purpura fulminans). The rationale for heparin therapy is to allow for more effective replacement therapy while the primary disease is being specifically treated, but there is no formal trial to show that heparin is beneficial. The most effective and safest method of giving heparin is by continuous intravenous administration. A loading dose of 50–100 U/kg is followed by 15–25 U/kg/h by continuous intravenous infusion. Heparin should be administered to achieve a therapeutic level between 0.3 and 0.6 U/mL.

D. Management of DIC in Neonates: Premature and full-term neonates frequently develop generalized bleeding tendencies associated with illnesses such as respiratory distress syndrome, cyanotic congenital heart disease, cerebral anoxia, and severe sepsis. Often present are hypoxia, acidosis, vascular fragility, decreased platelet number and function, and increased fibrinolytic activity. Laboratory tests of bleeding and coagulation are difficult to interpret because results in affected patients overlap with those in normal infants. The values for these tests seen in

"normal" full-term and premature neonates are shown in Table 26–10. The pathophysiologic mechanisms of these secondary bleeding syndromes are related to increased consumption or decreased production of clotting factors and platelets.

Treatment consists of correcting the associated conditions and replacing clotting factors and platelets with doses of FFP and platelets. Occasionally, exchange transfusion or heparinization is indicated.

2. LIVER DISEASE

The liver is the major synthesis site of high-molecular-weight kininogen (HMWK), XIII, XII, XI, X, IX, VII, V, prothrombin, and fibrinogen. It also produces plasminogen and three physiologic anticoagulants, antithrombin III, protein C, and protein S. α$_2$-Antiplasmin, which regulates fibrinolysis, is also produced in the liver. Deficiency of factor V and the vitamin K–dependent factors (II, VII, IX, and X) is most often a problem as a result of decreased hepatic synthesis. Prolongation of the PT and PTT is usually seen. Extravascular loss and increased consumption of clotting factors may also contribute to prolongation of the PT and PTT. The amount of fibrinogen may be decreased, or an abnormal fibrinogen (dysfibrinogen) containing excess sialic acid residues may be synthesized. Dysfibrinogenemia is associated with prolongation of thrombin time and reptilase time. Fibrin-fibrinogen degradation products and d-dimers may be present. Thrombocytopenia secondary to hypersplenism and platelet aggregation abnormalities may be seen. Treatment consists of replacement with FFP and platelets as needed. In cases in which liver disease is associated with fat malabsorption, vitamin K (1–5 mg) should be given. DDAVP may shorten the bleeding time and PTT in patients with chronic liver disease.

3. VITAMIN K DEFICIENCY

All newborns have physiologically depressed activity of the vitamin K–dependent factors (II, VII, IX, and X). If vitamin K is not administered at birth, a bleeding diathesis called *hemorrhagic disease of the newborn* may develop. One of three patterns is seen:

1. Early hemorrhagic disease of the newborn occurs within 24 hours of birth and is most often manifested by cephalhematoma, intracranial hemorrhage, or intra-abdominal bleeding. Although occasionally idiopathic, it is most often associated with maternal ingestion of drugs that interfere with vitamin K metabolism, eg, warfarin, phenytoin, isoniazid, and rifampin. This is often life-threatening.

2. Classic hemorrhagic disease of the newborn occurs at 24 hours to 7 days of age and usually is mani-

fested as gastrointestinal, skin, or mucosal bleeding. Bleeding after circumcision may occur. Although occasionally associated with maternal drug usage, it most often occurs in well babies that do not receive vitamin K at birth and are solely breast-fed.

3. Late hemorrhagic disease occurs in infants 1–6 months of age. Manifestations are intracranial, gastrointestinal, or skin bleeding. Usually, it is secondary to chronic diarrhea, malabsorption syndromes, obstructive jaundice, or prolonged antibiotic therapy.

The diagnosis of vitamin K deficiency is based on the history, physical examination, and laboratory results. The PT is markedly prolonged. The PTT may be prolonged. The thrombin time does not prolong until late in the course. Platelet counts are normal. The diagnosis is confirmed by a demonstration of noncarboxlyated vitamin K–dependent factors (PIVKA) in the plasma and by an improvement following treatment with vitamin K. Treatment with vitamin K should be given immediately and not withheld awaiting test results.

4. UREMIA

Bleeding occurs in approximately 50% of patients with chronic renal failure. It is most often manifested as purpura, menorrhagia, or gastrointestinal bleeding. Decreased activity of factors XII, XI, IX and prothrombin secondary to increased urinary losses result in prolongation of the PTT. An abnormality of von Willebrand factor may also occur, prolonging the bleeding time. Qualitative and quantitative platelet abnormalities may develop. Free protein S, protein C, and antithrombin III may be decreased. Bleeding may be managed with infusion of DDAVP, red blood cells, and FFP.

Bell B: Bleeding associated with hepatocellular disease. Int J Pediatr Hematol Oncol 1994;1:53.

Carvalho A: Acquired platelet dysfunction in patients with uremia. Hematol Oncol Clin North Am 1990;4:129.

Huysman M, Sauer P: The vitamin K controversy. Curr Opin Pediatr 1994;6:129.

Manco-Johnson M: Disseminated intravascular coagulation and other hypercoagulable syndromes. Int J Pediatr Hematol Oncol 1994;1:1.

VASCULAR ABNORMALITIES ASSOCIATED WITH BLEEDING

1. HENOCH-SCHÖNLEIN PURPURA (Anaphylactoid Purpura)

Essentials of Diagnosis
- Purpuric cutaneous rash.
- Migratory polyarthritis or polyarthralgias.
- Colicky abdominal pain.
- Nephritis.

General Considerations

Henoch-Schönlein purpura occurs primarily in males 2–7 years of age. Occurrence is highest in the spring and fall. Two thirds of affected children have a history of upper respiratory infection in the preceding 1–3 weeks.

Henoch-Schönlein purpura is characterized by vasculitis of the small vessels, particularly those of the skin, gastrointestinal tract, and kidney. Immune complexes are found in the kidney, intestine, and skin. Suspected though not proved inciting antigens include group A β-hemolytic streptococci and other bacteria, viruses, drugs, foods, and insect bites.

Clinical Findings

A. Symptoms and Signs: The skin rash is often urticarial initially and progresses to a macular-papular appearance, which transforms into a diagnostic symmetric purpuric rash distributed on the ankles, buttocks, and elbows. Purpuric areas of a few millimeters in diameter are present and may progress to form larger hemorrhages (palpable purpura). Petechial lesions may occur, but most hemorrhages are slightly larger. The rash usually begins on the lower extremities, but the entire body may be involved. New lesions can continue to appear for 2–4 weeks. Approximately two thirds of patients develop migratory polyarthralgias or polyarthritis, primarily of the ankles and knees. Edema of the hands, feet, scalp, and periorbital regions may occur. Abdominal colic—due to hemorrhage and edema primarily of the small intestine—occurs in about 50% of those affected. Twenty-five to fifty percent of those affected develop renal involvement, with hematuria, proteinuria, or nephrotic syndrome. Hematuria alone is never the presenting complaint for Henoch-Schönlein purpura, but usually manifests in the second to third week of illness. Renal involvement occurs more commonly in males and in older patients. Testicular torsion may occur. Neurologic symptoms are possible.

B. Laboratory Findings: The platelet count, platelet function tests, and bleeding time are usually normal, although the platelet count may even be elevated. Blood coagulation is normal. Urinalysis frequently reveals hematuria. Proteinuria may also be noted, but casts are uncommon. Stool analysis may be positive for blood even though melena is not observed. The ASO titer is frequently elevated and the throat culture positive for group A β-hemolytic streptococci. Serum IgA may be elevated.

Differential Diagnosis

Henoch-Schönlein purpura is differentiated from thrombocytopenic purpura in that the rash is palpable and the platelet count is normal. The rash of septicemia (especially meningococcemia) may be similar to that of Henoch-Schönlein purpura, although the distribution tends to be more generalized with meningococcemia. Blood culture may be necessary for final diagnosis. The possibility of child abuse should be considered in any child presenting with purpura.

Complications

Intussusception of the small bowel may occur. About 15% of patients develop renal failure as a result of advancing proliferative glomerulonephritis with an associated mortality rate of 3%.

Treatment

Generally treatment is unwarranted. Corticosteroid therapy may provide symptomatic relief for severe gastrointestinal or joint manifestations but does not alter skin or renal manifestations. Aspirin is useful for the arthritis. If culture for group A β-hemolytic streptococci is positive or if the ASO titer is elevated, penicillin should be given in full therapeutic doses for 10 days.

Prognosis

The prognosis for recovery is generally good, although symptoms frequently (25–50%) recur over a period of several months. In patients who develop renal manifestations, microscopic hematuria may persist for years. Progressive renal failure occurs in less than 5% of patients with Henoch-Schönlein purpura.

Lanzkowsky S, Lanzkowsky L, Lanzkowsky P: Henoch-Schönlein purpura. Pediatr Rev 1992;13:130.

2. OTHER VASCULAR DISORDERS

Mild to life-threatening bleeding may occur with some types of Ehlers-Danlos syndrome—the most common connective tissue disorder. Easy bruising is common. Coagulation findings are variable. Spontaneous rupture and dissection of aortic aneurysms have been reported in persons with type IV.

Hausser I, Anton-Lamprecht I: Differential ultrastructural aberrations of collagen fibrils in Ehlers-Danlos syndrome types I-IV as a means of diagnostics and classification. Hum Genet 1994;3:394.

THROMBOTIC DISORDERS

Conditions commonly associated with thrombosis during childhood are: venous access devices and other implanted foreign bodies, malignancy, infection, trauma, collagen vascular disease, surgery, renal disease, sickle cell anemia, cardiac disease, and immobilization. Initial evaluation of the child with a thrombosis must include a family history and definitive imaging study to delineate the type (venous versus arterial) and extent of the thrombosis. Laboratory evaluation is indicated to determine the presence of an underlying congenital or acquired hemostatic abnormality. A deficiency of the anticoagulant proteins, protein C, protein S, or antithrombin III may be congenital or acquired. Activated protein C resistance due to the factor V Leiden mutation is the most common inherited hypercoagulable condition.

1. PROTEIN C DEFICIENCY

Protein C is a vitamin K–dependent protein that is normally activated by thrombin bound to thrombomodulin and inactivates activated factors V and VIII. In addition, it stimulates fibrinolysis. Two phenotypes of hereditary protein C deficiency are seen. Heterozygotes with autosomal dominant protein C deficiency typically present with venous thromboembolism as young adults but may manifest during childhood.

Anticoagulation/fibrinolytic therapy is indicated for thrombosis. Homozygous or doubly heterozygous individuals generally present within the first 12 hours of life with purpura fulminans. Associated findings may include cerebral thrombosis or blindness. Immediate treatment to administer protein C by infusion of FFP about every 6 hours. Heparin is generally administered simultaneously. Subsequent management requires chronic anticoagulation with warfarin compounds or infusion of protein C concentrate. The long-term outlook is unknown.

2. PROTEIN S DEFICIENCY

Protein S is a cofactor for protein C. Persons with protein S deficiency have a course similar to those with protein C deficiency. Management for acute thrombotic events is with anticoagulation or fibrinolytic therapy or both. Lifelong coumadin may be indicated.

3. ANTITHROMBIN III DEFICIENCY

Antithrombin III is the most important physiologic inhibitor of thrombin. In addition, it inhibits activated factors IX, X, XI, and XII. Antithrombin III deficiency is transmitted in an autosomal dominant pattern and is associated with venous thromboembolism. Symptoms before puberty are rare.

Initial management of a patient with thrombosis is with anticoagulant therapy. Antithrombin III concentrate is available for replacement. Patients with recurrent venous thrombosis are maintained lifelong on oral anticoagulants. Asymptomatic persons are generally not anticoagulated except at times of increased risk for thrombosis.

4. FACTOR V LEIDEN MUTATION

An amino acid substitution in the gene coding for factor V results in the production of factor V Leiden, a factor V variant that is resistant to inactivation by activated protein C. About 20% of unselected consecutive adults with deep vein thrombosis and 40–60% of adults from families with unexplained thrombophilia have been identified with this mutation. Venous thrombosis has been reported in children heterozygous and homozygous for this mutation. Screening is with an assay for activated protein C resistance, which is based on the APTT. Confirmation is by molecular analysis.

5. OTHER CONGENITAL THROMBOTIC DISORDERS

Qualitative abnormalities of fibrinogen (dysfibrinogenemias) are usually inherited in an autosomal dominant manner. Most individuals with dysfibrinogenemia are asymptomatic. Some have problems with bleeding, and others develop venous or arterial thrombosis. This diagnosis is suggested by a prolonged thrombin time with a normal fibrinogen level. Dysfunction of the fibrinolytic system may play a role in the development of thrombosis, but the association between defects in this system and thrombosis is less well documented than that between deficiencies of the physiologic anticoagulants and thrombosis.

6. LUPUS ANTICOAGULANT

Lupus anticoagulants are immunoglobulins that interfere with phospholipid-dependent coagulation tests. They can occur in individuals without lupus following drug exposure, infection, or lymphoproliferative disorders. These anticoagulants may also be detected in persons who are well. The presence of a lupus anticoagulant is often first suspected following detection of a prolonged PTT. Mixing patient plasma 1:1 with normal plasma does not correct the PTT into the normal range if a lupus inhibitor is present. Other tests used to diagnose a lupus inhibitor include the Russell's viper venom time and the platelet neutralization procedure. Whether a lupus anticoagulant causes thrombosis or occurs following thrombosis is unclear. Anticoagulation or fibrinolytic therapy or both is indicated for a child with thrombosis and a lupus anticoagulant. Therapy is generally not indicated for an asymptomatic child with a lupus anticoagulant.

Andrew M et al: Venous thromboembolic complications (VTE) in children: First analyses of the Canadian Registry of VTE. Blood 1994;83:1251.

Dahlback B: Inherited thrombophilia: Resistance to activated protein C as a pathogenic factor of venous thromboembolism. Blood 1995;85:607.

Manco-Johnson M, Nuss R: Lupus anticoagulant in children with thrombosis. Am J Hematol 1995;48:243.

Nuss R, Hays T, Manco-Johnson M: Childhood thrombosis. Pediatrics 1995;96:291.

7. THE SPLEEN

SPLENOMEGALY & HYPERSPLENISM

The differential diagnosis of splenomegaly in children includes the general categories of congestive splenomegaly, chronic infections, leukemia and lymphomas, hemolytic anemias, reticuloendothelioses, and storage diseases (Table 26–11).

Splenomegaly due to any cause may be associated with hypersplenism and the excessive destruction of circulating red cells, white cells, and platelets. The degree of cytopenias is variable and, when mild, requires no specific therapy. In other cases, the thrombocytopenia may cause life-threatening bleeding, particularly when the splenomegaly is secondary to portal hypertension and associated with esophageal varices or the consequence of a storage disease. In such cases, treatment with surgical splenectomy or with splenic embolization may be warranted.

Israel DM et al: Partial splenic embolization in children with hypersplenism. J Pediatr 1994;124:95.

ASPLENIA & SPLENECTOMY

There is overwhelming evidence that children who lack normal splenic function are at risk for sepsis, meningitis, and pneumonia due to encapsulated bacteria such as pneumococci and *Haemophilus influenzae*. Such infections are often fulminant and fatal because of inadequate antibody production and impaired phagocytosis of hematogenous bacteria.

Congenital asplenia is usually suspected in an infant born with abnormalities of abdominal viscera and complex cyanotic congenital heart disease. Howell-Jolly bodies are usually present on the peripheral blood smear, and the absence of splenic tissue is confirmed by technetium radionuclide scanning. The prognosis depends on the underlying cardiac lesions, and many children die during the first few months. Prophylactic antibiotics, usually penicillin, and pneumococcal vaccine are recommended for those who survive.

The risk of overwhelming sepsis following surgical splenectomy is related to the child's age and to the underlying disorder. The risk is highest when the

Table 26–11. Causes of chronic splenomegaly in children.

Cause	Associated Clinical Findings	Diagnostic Investigation
Congestive splenomegaly	History of umbilical vein catheter or neonatal omphalitis. Signs of portal hypertension (varices, hemorrhoids, dilated abdominal wall veins); pancytopenia, history of hepatitis or jaundice.	Complete blood count, paltelet count, liver function tests, untrasonography.
Chronic infections	History of exposure to tuberculosis, histoplasmosis, coccidioidomycosis, other fungal disease; chonic sepsis (foreign body in bloodstream; subacute infective endocarditis).	Appropriate cultures and skin tests, ie, blood cultures; PPD, histoplasmin, coccidioidin skin tests; chest film; HIV serology.
Infectious mononucleosis	Fever, fatigue, pharyngitis, rash, adenopathy, hepatomegaly.	Heterophil antibodies.
Leukemia, lymphoma, Hodgkin's disease	Evidence of systemic involvement with fever, bleeding tendencies, hepatomegaly, and lymphadenopathy; pancytopenia.	Blood smear, bone marrow examination, chest film, gallium scan, LDH, uric acid.
Hemolytic anemias	Anemia, jaundice; family history of anemia, jaundice, and gallbladder disease in young adults.	Reticulocyte count, Coombs' test, blood smear, osmotic fragility test, hemoglobin electrophoresis.
Reticuloendothelioses (histiocytosis X)	Chronic otitis media, seborrheic or petechial skin rashes, anemia, infections, lymphadenopathy, hepatomegaly, bone lesions.	Skeletal x-rays for bone lesions; biopsy of bone, liver, bone marrow, or lymph node.
Storage diseases	Family history of similar disorders, neurologic involvement, evidence of macular degeneration, hepatomegaly.	Biopsy of rectal mucosa, liver, bone marrow, spleen, or brain in search for storage cells.
Splenic cyst	Evidence of other infections (postinfectious cyst) or congenital anomalies; peculiar shape of spleen.	Radionuclide scan, ultrasonography.
Splenic hemangioma	Other hemangiomas, consumptive coagulopathy.	Radionuclide scan, arteriography, platelet count, coagulation screen.

LDH = lactic dehydrogenase; PPD = purified protein derivative.

procedure is performed earlier in life, so splenectomy is usually postponed until after 5 years. The risk of postsplenectomy sepsis is also greater in children with malignancies, thalassemias, and reticuloendothelioses than in children whose splenectomy is performed for ITP, hereditary spherocytosis, or trauma.

Children with sickle cell anemia develop functional asplenia during the first year of life, and overwhelming sepsis is the leading cause of early deaths in this disease. Prophylactic penicillin has been shown to reduce the incidence of sepsis by 84%.

Lortan JE: Clinical annotation: Management of asplenic patients. Br J Haematol 1993;84:566.

Phoon CK, Neill CA: Asplenia syndrome: Insight into embryology through an analysis of cardiac and extracardiac anomalies. Am J Cardiol 1994;73:581.

TRANSFUSION MEDICINE

DONOR SCREENING & BLOOD PROCESSING: RISK MANAGEMENT

Minimizing the risks of transfusion begins with the donor interview. Questions are asked that will protect the recipient from transmission of infectious agents as well as other risks of transfusions. In addition, information defining high-risk groups whose behavior increases the possible transmission of AIDS, hepatitis, and other diseases is provided, with the request that these persons not donate blood. After completion of the phlebotomy, the donor is given a final opportunity to acknowledge previously undisclosed risk factors by confidentially indicating that his or her blood should not be used for transfusion.

Before blood components can be released for

transfusion, donor blood is screened for antibodies to hepatitis B, hepatitis C, HIV 1 and 2 (AIDS), human T-cell lymphocytotropic virus (HTLV) I and II and syphilis. In addition, testing for hepatitis B surface antigen and HIV p24 antigen is completed. The transaminases are measured as surrogate tests for hepatitis (Table 26–12). For special clinical conditions, serologic screening for cytomegalovirus may also be completed to identify seronegative units for transfusion. Positive tests are repeated, and upon their confirmation the unit in question is destroyed and the donor placed in a deferral category. Many of the screening tests used are very sensitive and have a high rate of false-positive results. Because of this, confirmatory tests have been developed to check the initial screening results and separate the false-positives from the true-positives.

With these techniques, the risk of an infectious complication from blood components has been minimized, with the greatest risk being post-transfusion hepatitis (see sections on hepatitis C virus and non-A, non-B hepatitis elsewhere in this book). Because

Table 26–12. Transmission risks of infectious agents for which screening of blood products is routinely performed.

Disease Entity	Transmission	Screening and Processing Procedures	Approximate Risk of Transmission
Syphilis	Low risk that fresh blood drawn during spirochetemia can transmit infection. Organism not able to survive behond 72 hours during storage at 4 °C.	Donor history. RPR or VDRL.	<1:100,000
Hepatitis A	Units drawn during prodrome could transmit virus. Because of brief viremia during acute phase, absence of asymptomatic carrier phase, and failure to detect transmission in multiple transfused individuals, infection by this agent is unlikely.	Donor history.	<1:1,000,000
Hepatitis B	Prolonged viremia during various phases of the disease and asymptomatic carrier state make HBV infection a significant risk of transfusion. Incidence has markedly decreased with screening strategies.	Donor history, education, and self-exclusion. Hepatitis B surface antigen (HBsAg). Surrogate tests for non-A, non-B hepatitis and screen for hepatitis C and retroviruses have helped screen out population at risk for transmitting hepatitis B virus.	1:200,000–1:5000
Hepatitis C	Over two-thirds of cases of non-A, non-B posttransfusion hepatitis may be due to this cause. The agent has characteristics similar to those of HBV which are responsible for the risk from transfusion. Infection may lead to a significant incidence of cirrhosis and end-stage liver disease.	Donor history. Surrogate tests: ALT and hepatitis B core antibody (anti-HBc), anti-HCV.	1:6000
Non-A, non-B, non-C hepatitis	Not a specific cause but a classification of agents other than HAV, HBV, HCV, Epstein-Barr virus, and cytomegalovirus, which can cause posttransfusion hepatitis.	Donor history. Surrogate tests: ALT and anti-HBc.	Undefined 1:6000
Human immunodeficiency virus (HIV-I) infection	Cytotoxic retrovirus spread by sexual contact, parenteral (including transfusion) and vertical routes. Resultant destruction of CD4-positive cells results in clinical manifestations of AIDS.	Donor history, education, and self-exclusion. Anti-HIV by EIA, screening test. Western blot confirmatory.	1:500,000
Human T cell lymphotropic virus I and II (HTLV-I and -II) infection	Transforming retroviruses spread by sexual contact, parenteral (including transfusion) and vertical. Over years to decades, infection with HTLV-I may cause lymphoid malignancies or myelopathy.	Donor history. Anti-HTLV-I and -II by enzyme immunoassay screening test. Western blot confirmatory.	<1:10,000

ALT = alanine transaminase; HAV, HBV, HCV = hepatitis A virus, hepatitis B virus, hepatitis C virus; HTLV = human T-cell lymphotrophic virus; RPR = rapid plasma reagin; VDRL = syphilis test.

there is no absolute way to completely eliminate the risk of infection from homologous blood, the safest type of blood is obtained from autologous donation. Issues of donor size make the techniques of autologous donation difficult to apply to the pediatric population. Whenever possible, however, autologous donation should be considered.

Primary cytomegalovirus infections are important complications of blood transfusion in transplant recipients, neonates, and those with immunodeficiency. Transmission of cytomegalovirus can be avoided by using seronegative donors or by using a leukocyte-depleting filter (to reduce white cell numbers to $< 5 \times 10^6$ per unit of red cells).

STORAGE & PRESERVATION OF BLOOD & BLOOD COMPONENTS

Blood is routinely fractionated into packed red cells, platelets, and FFP or cryoprecipitate for most efficient use. The storage conditions and biologic characteristics of the fractions are summarized in Table 26–13. The conditions provide the optimal environment to maintain appropriate recovery, survival, and function and are different for each blood component. For example, red cells undergo dramatic metabolic changes during their 35-day storage, with a decrease in 2,3-diphosphoglycerate (2,3-DPG) during the second week of storage, a decrease in ATP, and a gradual loss of intracellular potassium into the plasma. Fortunately, these changes are readily reversed within hours to days after the red cells are transfused. However, in certain clinical conditions, these effects may define the type of components used. For example, blood less than 7–10 days old would be preferred for exchange transfusion or replacement of red cells in persons with cardiopulmonary disease to ensure adequate oxygen carrying capacity. However, storage time is not an issue when administering transfusions to those with chronic anemia.

Under certain conditions, where excessive potassium load is a problem, one has the option of using blood less than 10 days old, making packed cells out of an older unit of whole blood, or washing blood stored as packed cells. No matter what the age of the blood, over 70% of the red cells will circulate after transfusion and approximate a normal survival.

Platelets can be stored at 22 °C for a maximum of 3–5 days. At the extremes of storage, there should be at least a 60% recovery, a survival time that approximates turnover of fresh autologous platelets, and normalization of the bleeding time in proportion to the peak platelet count. Frozen components, red cells, FFP, and cryoprecipitate are outdated at 3 years, 1 year, and 1 year, respectively. Frozen red cells retain the same biochemical and functional characteristics as the day they were frozen. FFP contains 80% or more of all of the clotting factors of fresh plasma. Factor VIII and fibrinogen are concentrated in cryoprecipitate.

PRETRANSFUSION TESTING

Both the donated blood and the recipient are tested for ABO and Rh(D) antigens and for autoantibodies or alloantibodies. The cross-match is required on any component that contains red cells. In the major cross-match, washed donor red cells are incubated with the serum from the patient, and agglutination is detected and graded. The antiglobulin phase of the test is then performed; Coombs reagent, which will detect the presence of IgG or complement on the surface of the red cells, is added to the mixture, and any possible reaction is evaluated. In the presence of a negative antibody screen in the recipient, a negative immediate spin or antiglobulin phase cross-match confirms the compatibility of the blood. Further testing is required if the antibody screen or the cross-match is positive, and blood should not be given until the nature of the reactivity is delineated. An incompatible cross-match is evaluated first with a direct antiglobulin or Coombs' test to detect IgG or complement on the surfaces of the recipient's red cells. The indirect antiglobulin test is also used to determine the presence of antibodies that will coat or activate complement on the surface of normal red cells.

TRANSFUSION PRACTICE

General Rules

Several general rules should be followed in administering any blood component.

1. In final preparation of the component, no solutions should be added to the bag or tubing set except for normal saline (0.9% sodium chloride for injection, USP), ABO-compatible plasma, or other specifically approved expanders. Hypotonic solutions cause hemolysis of red cells and, if transfused, result in a severe reaction in the recipient.

2. Transfusion products should be protected from contact with any calcium-containing solution (such as lactated Ringer's); recalcification and reversal of the citrate effect cause clotting of the blood component.

3. Blood components should not be warmed to a temperature greater than 37 °C. If a component is incubated in a water bath, it should be enclosed in a watertight bag to prevent contamination of entry ports.

4. Whenever a blood bag is entered, the sterile integrity of the system is violated, and that unit should be discarded within 4 hours if left at room tempera-

ture or within 24 hours if the temperature is between 1 ° and 4 °C.

5. In general, transfusions of red cell–containing products should not exceed 4 hours. Blood components in excess of what can be infused during this time period should be stored in the blood bank until needed.

6. Before transfusion, the blood component should be visually inspected for any unusual characteristics—such as the presence of flocculent material, hemolysis, or clumping of cells—and mixed thoroughly.

7. The unit and the recipient should be properly identified.

8. The administration set includes a standard 170–260 μm clot filter. Under certain clinical circumstances, an additional microaggregate filter may be used to eliminate small aggregates of fibrin, white cells, and platelets that will not be removed by the standard filter.

9. The patient should be observed during the entire transfusion, but especially during the first 15 minutes. Any adverse symptoms or signs should be evaluated immediately and reactions to the transfusion reported promptly to the transfusion service.

10. When cross-match incompatible red cells or whole blood must be given to the patient (as with autoimmune hemolytic anemia), a test dose of 10% of the total volume (not to exceed 75 mL) should be administered over 15–20 minutes; the transfusion is then stopped and the patient evaluated for reaction. If no adverse effects are noted, the remainder of the volume can be carefully infused.

11. Blood for exchange transfusion in the newborn period may be cross-matched with either infant's or mother's serum. If the exchange is for hemolysis, 500 mL of whole blood stored for less than 7 days will be adequate. If replacement of clotting factors is a key issue, packed red cells (7 days old) reconstituted with FFP may be considered. Based on posttransfusion platelet counts, platelet transfusion may be considered. Additional problems to anticipate are acid-base derangements, hyponatremia, hyperkalemia, hypocalcemia, hypoglycemia, hypothermia, and hypervolemia or hypovolemia.

Choice of Blood Component

In deciding on the need for blood transfusion, several principles should be considered. Indications for blood or blood components must be well defined, and the patient's medical condition and not just the laboratory numbers should be the basis for the decision. Specific deficiencies exhibited by the patient (eg, oxygen carrying capacity, thrombocytopenia) should be treated with appropriate blood components and the use of whole blood minimized. Information about specific blood components is summarized in Table 26–13.

A. Whole Blood: Whole blood may be used in patients who require replacement of oxygen carrying capacity and volume. In particular, it may be considered when more than 15% of blood volume is lost. Doses vary depending on volume considerations (see Table 26–13). In acute situations, the transfusion may be completed rapidly to support blood volume.

B. Packed Red Cells: Packed red cells (which include leukocyte-poor, filtered, or frozen deglycerolized products) prepared from whole blood by centrifugal techniques are the appropriate choice for almost all patients with deficient oxygen carrying capacity. Exact indications will be defined by the clinical setting, the severity of the anemia, the acuity of the condition, and any other factors affecting oxygen transport.

C. Platelets: The decision to transfuse platelets depends on the clinical condition of the patient, the status of plasma phase coagulation, the platelet count, the cause of the thrombocytopenia, and the functional ability of the patient's own platelets. With platelet counts less than 10,000–20,000/μL, the risk of severe, spontaneous bleeding is markedly increased, and—in the absence of antibody-mediated disease—transfusion should be considered. Under certain circumstances, especially with platelet dysfunction or treatment that inhibits the procoagulant system, transfusions at higher platelet counts may be necessary.

Transfused platelets are temporarily sequestered in the lungs and spleen before reaching their peak concentrations, 45–60 minutes after transfusion. A significant proportion of the transfused platelets never circulate but remain sequestered in the spleen. This phenomenon results in reduced recovery studies in which only 60–70% of the transfused platelets are counted when peripheral platelet count increments are used as a measure of response.

In addition to cessation of bleeding, two variables indicate the effectiveness of platelet transfusions. The first is platelet recovery, the measure of the maximum number of platelets circulating in response to transfusion. The practical measure is the platelet count at 1 hour after transfusion. In the absence of immune or nonimmune factors that markedly decrease platelet recovery, one would expect a 7000/μL increment for each random donor unit and a 40,000–70,000/μL increment for each single-donor apheresis unit in a large child or adolescent. For infants and small children, 10 mL/kg will increase the platelet count by at least 50,000/μL. The second variable is the survival of transfused platelets. Normally, transfused platelets have a half-life of 3–5 days. In the presence of immune or nonimmune destruction, the life span may be shortened to a few days or a few hours. Frequent platelet transfusions may be required to maintain adequate hemostasis.

A particularly troublesome outcome in patients receiving long-term platelet transfusions is the development of a refractory state characterized by poor

Table 26–13. Characteristic of blood and blood components.

Component	Storage Conditions	Composition and Transfusion Characteristics	Indications	Risks and Precautions	Administration
Whole blood	4 °C for 35 days. RBC characteristics: • **Survival:** Recovery decreases during storage but is always > 70%. Cells that circulate approximate normal survival. • **Function:** 2,3-DPG levels fall to undetectable after second week of storage. This defect repaired within 24 hours of transfusion. • **Electrolytes:** With storage, potassium increases in plasma. This rises to high levels after 2 weeks of storage.	Contains RBCs and many plasma compounds of whole blood. Leukocytes and platelets lose activity or viability after a few days under these conditions. Procoagulant clotting factors (particularly VIII and V) deteriorate rapidly during storage. Each unit has about 500 mL volume and Hct 36–40%.	Oxygen carrying capacity (anemia). Volume replacement (> 15–20%) for blood loss or severe shock.	Must be ABO-identical and crossmatch-compatible. Infectious diseases (see Table 28–12). Febrile or hemolytic transfusion reactions. Allo-immunization to red cell, white cell, or platelet antigens.	During acute blood loss, as rapidly as tolerated. In other settings, 2–4 hours. 10 mL/kg will raise Hct by 5% and support volume.
Packed red cells	Same as for whole blood.	Contains RBCs; plasma removed in preparation. Status of leukocytes, clotting factors, and platelets same as for whole blood. Hct about 70%, volume 200–250 mL. May request tighter pack to give Hct 80–90%.	Oxygen carrying capacity. Acute trauma or bleeding, or situations requiring intensive cardiopulmonary support (Hct < 25–30%). Chronic anemia (Hct < 20%).	Same as for whole blood.	May be given as patient will tolerate based on cardiovascular status over 2–4 hours. Dose of 3 mL packed RBC/kg will raise the Hct by 3%. If cardiovascular status stable, give 10 mL/kg over 2–4 hours. If unstable, use smaller volume or do packed RBC exchange.
Washed or filtered red cells	When cells are washed, there is a 24-hour outdate. Up to that time, they have the same characteristics as packed red cells.	Same as packed red cells.	Same as packed red cells. Depending on technique used and extent of reduction of white blood cells, washed red cells may achieve the following: • Avoid febrile reactions. • Decreased the transmission of CMV. • Decreased the incidence of allo-immunization to white cell antigens.	Same as whole blood. Removal of white cells dimishes the risk of febrile reactions. Filtration with white cell filters may decrease rate of allo-immunization to white cell antigens and transmission of CMV.	Same as packed red cells.
Frozen red cells	Packed red cells frozen in 40% glycerol solution at under –65 °C. Can be stored 3 years. Retain the same biochemical characteristics, function, and capacity for survival as the day in storage they were frozen; when thawed, 24-hour outdate.	Same as packed red cells.	Same as packed red cells. Useful for avoiding febrile reactions, decreasing transmission of CMV, autologous blood donation, and developing an inventory of rare red cell blood groups.	Same as for whole blood. Risk of CMV transmission is less.	Same as packed red cells.

(continued)

777

Table 26–13. Characteristic of blood and blood components. (*continued*)

Component	Storage Conditions	Composition and Transfusion Characteristics	Indications	Risks and Precautions	Administration
Fresh frozen plasma	Plasma from whole blood stored at under −18 °C for up to 1 year.	Contains > 80% of all procoagulant and anticoagulant plasma proteins.	Replacement of plasma procoagulant and anticoagulant plasma proteins. May provide "other" factors, eg, treatment of TTP.	Need not be crossmatched; should be type-compatible. Volume overload, infectious diseases, allergic reactions.	As rapidly as tolerated by patient but not > 4 hours. Dose: 10–15 mL/kg will increase level of all clotting factors by 10–20%.
Cryoprecipitate	Produced by freezing fresh plasma to under −65 °C, then allowing to thaw 18 hours at 4 °C. After centrifugation, cryoprecipitable proteins are separated. May be stored at under −18 °C for up to 1 year.	Contains factor VIII, fibrinogen, and fibronectin at concentrations greater than those of plasma. Also contains factor XIII. VIII > 80 IU/pack, fibrinogen 100–350 mg/pack.	Treatment of acquired or congenital deficiencies of VIII, von Willebrand factor, and fibrinogen. Useful in making biologic glues that contain fibrinogen.	Same as for fresh frozen plasma. ABO agglutinogens may also be concentrated and can give positive direct agglutination test if not type-specific.	Cryoprecipitate can be given as a rapid infusion. Dose: ½ pack per kg body weight will increase factor VIII level by 80–100% and fibrinogen by 200–250 mg/dL.
Platelet concentrates (whole blood donation)	Separated from platelet-rich plasma and stored with gentle agitation at 22 °C for 3–5 days. Containers currently in use are plastic and allow for gas exchange, diffusion of CO_2 helps keep pH > 6.00, a major factor in keeping platelets viable and functional.	Each unit contains about 5 × 10^{10} platelets. Survival: Although there may be some loss with storage, 60–70% recovery should be achieved, with stored platelets correcting the bleeding time in proportion to the peak counts reached.	Treatment of thrombocytopenia or platelet function defects.	No crossmatch necessary. Should be type-specific. Other risks as for whole blood.	Can be given as rapid transfusion or as defined by cardiovascular status, not more than 4 hours. Dose: 10 mL/kg should increase platelet count by at least 50,000/μL.
Platelet concentrates by aphersis techniques	Same as random donor units.	Platelet content is equivalent to 6–10 units of random donor concentrates. Depending on technique used, these may be relatively free of leukocytes, a product useful in avoiding alloimmunization.	As above, particularly useful in treating patients who have insufficient production in whom alloisoimmunization is a potential problem.	Same as above.	As above.
Granulocytes	Although they may be stored stationary at 20–24 °C, transfuse as soon as possible after collection.	Contains at least 1 × 10^{10} granulocytes but also platelets and red cells.	Severely neutropenic individuals (< 500/μL) with poor marrow reserves and suspected bacterial or fungal infections not responding to 48–72 hours of parenteral antibiotics. Also in patients with neutrophil dysfunction.	Same as for platelets. Pulmonary leukostasis reactions. Severe febrile reactions.	Given in an infusion over 2–4 hours. Dose: 1 unit daily for newborns and infants, 1 × 10^9 granulocytes per kg.

CMV = cytomegalovirus.

(< 30%) recovery or no response to platelet transfusion (as measured at 1 hour). Most (70–90%) of these refractory states result from the development of alloantibodies directed against HLA antigens on the platelet. Platelets have class I HLA antigens and the antibodies are primarily against HLA A or B determinants. A smaller proportion of these alloantibodies (10–30%) are directed against platelet-specific alloantigens. The most effective approach is probably to prevent HLA sensitization by leukocyte-depleting any cellular blood component. For the alloimmu-nized patient, the best approach is to provide HLA A- and HLA B-matched platelets for transfusion. Recent reports have suggested that platelet cross-matching procedures using HLA-matched and unmatched donors may be helpful in quickly identifying platelet concentrates with the highest probability of resulting in a successful transfusion.

D. Fresh Frozen Plasma (FFP): The indication for FFP is the replacement of plasma coagulation factors in clinical situations in which a deficiency of one or more clotting factors exists and

Table 26–14. Noninfectious complications of transfusions.

Event	Pathophysiology	Signs and Symptoms	Management
Acute hemolytic transfusion reaction	Preformed alloantibodies (most commonly to ABO) and occasionally autoantibodies cause rapid intravascular hemolysis of transfused cells with activation of clotting (DIC), activation of inflammatory mediators, and acute renal failure.	Fever, chills, nausea, chest pain, back pain, pain at transfusion site, hypotension, dyspnea, oliguria, dark urine.	The risk of this type of reaction overall is low (1:30,000), but the mortality rate is high (up to 40%). **Treatment:** Stop the transfusion; maintain renal output with intravenous fluids and diuretics (furosemide or mannitol); treat DIC with heparin; and institute other appropriate supportive measures.
Delayed hemolytic transfusion reaction	Formation of alloantibodies after transfusion and resultant destruction of transfused red cells, usually by extravascular hemolysis.	Fever, jaundice, anemia.	Detection, definition, and documentation (for future transfusions). Supportive care. Risk, 1:2500.
Bacterial contamination	Contamination of units results in growth of bacteria or production of clinically significant levels of endotoxin.	Chills, high fever, hypotension, other symptoms of sepsis or endotoxemia.	Stop transfusion; aggressive attempts to identify organism; vigorous supportive medical care.
Graft-versus-host disease	Lymphocytes from donor transfused in an immunoincompetent host.	Syndrome can present with a variety of organs involved, usually skin, liver, and bone marrow.	Preventive management: Irradiation (> 1500 cGy) of cellular blood components transfused to individuals with congenital or acquired immunodeficiency syndromes, intrauterine transfusion, severely premature infants, and when donors are relatives of the recipient.
Febrile reactions	Usually caused by leukoagglutinins in recipient cytokines or other biologically active compounds	Fever. May also have chills.	Supportive. Consider leukocyte-poor products for future. Risk, 1:200.
Allergic reactions	Most causes not identified. In IgA-deficient individuals, reaction occurs as a result of antibodies to IgA.	Itching, hives, occasionally chills and fever. In severe reactions, may see signs of anaphylaxis: dyspnea, pulmonary edema.	Mild to moderate reactions: diphenhydramine. More severe reactions: epinephrine SC and steroids IV. Risk for mild to moderate allergic reactions, 1:1000; severe anaphylactic reactions, 1:150,000.
Iron overload	There is no physiologic mechanism to excrete excess iron. Target organs include liver, heart, and endocrine organs. In patients receiving red cell transfusions over long periods of time, there is an increase in iron burden.	Signs and symptoms of dysfunctional organs affected by the iron.	Chronic administration of iron chelator such as deferoxamine.
Dilutional coagulopathy	Massive blood loss and transfusion with replacement with fluids or blood components and deficient clotting factors.	Bleeding.	Replacement of clotting factors or platelets with appropriate blood components.

there are associated bleeding manifestations. In some hereditary factor deficiencies such as factor VIII deficiency, commercially prepared concentrates contain these factors in higher concentrations and, because of viral inactivation, impose less infectious risk and are more appropriate than plasma.

E. Cryoprecipitate: This component may be used for acquired or congenital disorders of hypofibrinogenemia or afibrinogenemia. The dose given depends on the protein to be replaced. Cryoprecipitate can be given in a rapid transfusion over 30–60 minutes.

F. Granulocytes: With better supportive care over the past 10 years, the need for granulocytes in neutropenic patients with severe bacterial infections has decreased. Indications still remain for severe bacterial infections unresponsive to vigorous medical therapy in either newborns or older children with the presence of bone marrow failure.

G. Apheresis Products and Procedures: Apheresis equipment allows one or more blood components to be collected from a donor while the rest are returned. Platelet units are one example; granulocytes another. Apheresis techniques can also be used to collect hematopoietic stem cells that have been mobilized into the blood by cytokines (G-CSF or GM-CSF) given alone or after chemotherapy. These stem cells are used for autologous bone marrow transplantation. Blood cell separators can be used for the collection of single source plasma or removal of a component that is causing disease. Examples include red cell exchange in sickle cell disease and plasmapheresis in Goodpasture's syndrome or in myasthenia gravis.

Adverse Effects

The noninfectious complications of blood transfusions are outlined in Table 26–14. Most present a small but still significant risk to the recipient.

National Institutes of Health Consensus Conference: Fresh frozen plasma: Indications and risks. JAMA 1985;253:551.

National Institutes of Health Consensus Conference: Platelet transfusion therapy. JAMA 1987;257:1777.

Rossi EC, Simon TL, Moss GS (editors): *Principles of Transfusion Medicine.* Williams & Wilkins, 1991.

Stehling L et al: Guidelines for blood utilization review. Transfusion 1994;34:438.

Walker RH (editor): *Technical Manual of the American Association of Blood Banks.* American Association of Blood Banks, 1990.

REFERENCES

Buchanan GR (editor): Pediatric hematology. Pediatr Clin North Am 1996.

Bunn HF, Forget BG: *Hemoglobin: Molecular, Genetic and Clinical Aspects.* WB Saunders, 1986.

Embury SH, Hebbel RP, Mohandas N, Steinberg MH (editors): *Sickle Cell Disease: Basic Principles and Clinical Practice.* Raven Press, 1994.

Hathaway WE, Bonnar J: *Hemostatic Disorders of the Pregnant Woman and Newborn Infant.* Elsevier, 1987.

Hathaway WE, Goodnight SH: *Disorders of Hemostasis and Thrombosis: A Clinical Guide.* McGraw-Hill, 1993.

Mentzer WC, Wagner GM: *The Hereditary Hemolytic Anemias.* Churchill Livingstone, 1989.

Miller DR, Baehner RL: *Blood Diseases of Infancy and Childhood,* 6th ed. CV Mosby, 1989.

Nathan DG, Oski FA: *Hematology of Infancy and Childhood,* 4th ed. WB Saunders, 1993.

Oski FA, Naiman JL: *Hematologic Problems in the Newborn,* 3rd ed. WB Saunders, 1982.

Petz LD, Garratty G: *Acquired Immune Hemolytic Anemias.* Churchill Livingstone, 1980.

Rossi EC, Simon TL, Moss GS: *Principles of Transfusion Medicine.* Williams & Wilkins, 1991.

Serjeant GR: *Sickle Cell Disease,* 2nd ed. Oxford University Press, 1993.

Stamatoyannopoulos G, Neinhuis AW, Majerus PW, Varmus H (editors): *The Molecular Basis of Blood Diseases.* WB Saunders, 1994.

Young NS, Alter BP: *Aplastic Anemia: Acquired and Inherited.* WB Saunders, 1994.

Neoplastic Disease

27

Edythe A. Albano, MD, Linda C. Stork, MD, Brian S. Greffe, MD, Lorrie F. Odom, MD,
& Nicholas Foreman, MD

Cure of cancer in children is occurring with ever-increasing numbers. Combined-modality therapy (surgery, chemotherapy, radiation therapy) has improved survival dramatically, with the result that the overall cure rate of pediatric malignancies is now 60%. It is estimated that by the year 2000, one in 1000 adults will be a survivor of childhood cancer.

Therapeutic advances continue to be made. Pediatric malignancies are rare so the cooperative clinical trial has become the mainstay of treatment planning. The Children's Cancer Group (CCG) and Pediatric Oncology Group (POG) offer the most current therapeutic options and protocols and answer important the treatment questions in a timely manner. For progress to continue, a newly diagnosed child with cancer should be enrolled in a cooperative clinical trial whenever possible. Because many protocols are associated with significant toxicities, morbidity, and potential mortality, supervision of pediatric patients should be by a pediatric oncologist familiar with all the inherent hazards of treatment.

Advances in molecular genetics, cell biology, and tumor immunology contribute to our understanding of pediatric malignancies and their treatment. It is important that biopsies of suspected malignancies be handled by a pathologist who is familiar with these ancillary studies and will be able to arrive at a timely and accurate diagnosis.

No longer is formalin-fixed tissue adequate for the diagnosis of pediatric malignancy, particularly for tumors characterized as "little, round blue cells" on light microscopy. For example, fresh unfixed tissue is essential for metaphase chromosome analysis as well as molecular genetic analysis. The applicability can be seen in patients with chronic myeloid leukemia most of whom have a t(9;22) on cytogenetic analysis. However, not all patients have an obvious karyotype abnormality. In this smaller group of patients, molecular techniques can detect the aberrant gene product that results from the translocation, censuring greater diagnostic accuracy and appropriate therapy. The polymerase chain reaction (PCR) which amplifies minutes DNA fragments in an exponential fashion to yield easily detectable and manipulated amounts of DNA of interest, has wide applicability in diagnosis and detection of minimal residual disease.

Similar techniques can be used to determine whether a pathologic process is monoclonal (arising from a single cell and generally considered malignant) or polyclonal (arising from multiple cells and usually nonmalignant). Detecting rearrangements of DNA in antigen receptor gene as a clonal marker for the diagnosis of lymphoma is an example of this. Cells in a benign process have diverse rearrangements of antigen receptor genes, whereas clonal cells that make up a neoplasm have uniform rearrangements.

Similar molecular techniques have also led to the characterization of oncogene and tumor suppressor genes in human malignancies. An oncogene is a gene that causes malignant transformation or deregulated cell growth. For example, the proto-oncogene C–*myc* plays an important role in hematopoietic cell proliferation. It has been recognized at the site of three different translocations in Burkitt's lymphomas: t(8;14), t(8;22), and t(2;8). A tumor suppressor gene (anti-oncogene) constrains cell proliferation; its absence can lead to unchecked cell growth. The retinoblastoma gene is the prototypic tumor suppressor gene. Inactivation of both copies of this gene in a cell leads to tumor formation, first recognized in children with retinoblastoma.

Research in supportive care areas such as management of pain, emesis, and infection has improved the survival and quality of life for children undergoing cancer treatment. Long-term follow-up of childhood cancer survivors is yielding information that will provide a rational for modifying future treatment regimens to decrease morbidity.

ACUTE LYMPHOBLASTIC LEUKEMIA

Essentials of Diagnosis

- Pallor, petechiae, purpura (50%), bone pain (25%).
- Hepatosplenomegaly (60%), lymphadenopathy (50%).

- Single or multiple cytopenias: neutropenia, thrombocytopenia, anemia.
- Leukopenia or leukocytosis, often with leukemic leukocytes identifiable on blood smear.
- Diagnosis confirmed by bone marrow examination.

General Considerations

Acute lymphoblastic leukemia (ALL) is the most common malignancy of childhood, accounting for about 25% of all cancer diagnoses under the age of 15 years. The worldwide incidence of ALL is about 1:25,000 children per year, including 2500 children per year in the United States. The peak age at onset is 4 years, with 85% of patients diagnosed between the ages of 2 and 10 years. Before the advent of chemotherapy, this disease was fatal, usually within 3–4 months, with virtually no survivors 1 year after diagnosis. ALL results from uncontrolled proliferation of immature lymphocytes; its cause is unknown, and genetic factors may play a role. Leukemia is defined by the presence of more than 25% malignant hematopoietic cells (blasts) on bone marrow aspirate. Leukemic blasts from the majority of cases of childhood ALL have an antigen on the cell surface called the common ALL antigen (CALLA). These blasts derive from B cell precursors early in their development. Less commonly, lymphoblasts are of T-cell origin or of mature B-cell origin. Current estimates are that over 70% of children receiving aggressive combination chemotherapy and early presymptomatic treatment to the central nervous system (CNS) are cured of ALL.

Clinical Findings

A. Symptoms and Signs: Presenting complaints of patients with ALL include those related to decreased bone marrow production of red cells, white cells, and platelets and to leukemic infiltration of extramedullary (outside bone marrow) sites. Intermittent fevers are common, either as a result of cytokines induced by the leukemia itself or of infections secondary to leukopenia. About 25% of patients experience bone pain, especially in the pelvis, vertebral bodies, and legs. Physical examination at diagnosis ranges from virtually normal to highly abnormal. Signs related to bone marrow infiltration by leukemia include pallor, petechiae, and purpura. Hepatomegaly or splenomegaly occurs in over 60% of cases. Lymphadenopathy is common, either localized or generalized to cervical, axillary, and inguinal regions. The testes may be unilaterally or bilaterally enlarged secondary to leukemic infiltration. Superior vena caval syndrome is manifested by a prominent venous pattern over the upper chest resulting from collateral vein enlargement. The neck may feel full owing to venous engorgement. The face may appear plethoric, and the periorbital area may be edematous. Tachypnea, orthopnea, and respiratory distress

from a mediastinal mass may be apparent. Leukemic infiltration of cranial nerves may result in cranial nerve palsies along with mild nuchal rigidity. Funduscopic examination may show exudates of leukemic infiltration and hemorrhage from thrombocytopenia. The cardiac examination often reveals a flow murmur and tachycardia due to anemia; rarely, signs of congestive heart failure are present. Bone and joint pain may be appreciated on examination, particularly in the pelvis, lower spine, and femurs. In addition, signs of infection may be found on physical examination.

B. Laboratory Findings: The complete blood count (CBC) with differential is the most useful initial laboratory test in the diagnosis of ALL. Ninety-five percent of patients have a decrease in at least one cell type (single cytopenia): neutropenia, thrombocytopenia, or anemia. Most patients have decreases in at least two blood cell lines. The white count is low or normal ($< 10,000/\mu L$) in 50% of patients, but the differential often shows neutropenia (absolute neutrophil count $< 1000/\mu L$) along with a small percentage of blasts amid normal lymphocytes. In 30% of patients, the white count is between 10,000 and $50,000/\mu L$, and in 20% of cases it is $> 50,000/\mu L$, occasionally higher than $300,000/\mu L$. Blasts are usually readily identifiable on peripheral smears in patients with elevated white counts. Most patients with ALL have decreased platelet counts ($< 150,000/\mu L$) and decreased hemoglobin (< 11 g/dL) at diagnosis, although cases with normal platelet counts and hemoglobin do occur. Less than 1% of patients diagnosed with ALL have entirely normal CBCs and blood smears but have symptoms of bone marrow that lead to bone marrow examination. Serum chemistries—particularly uric acid and lactate dehydrogenase (LDH)—are often elevated at diagnosis as a result of cell breakdown. Serum phosphorus is occasionally elevated at diagnosis as well. Liver function tests may also be mildly abnormal.

The diagnosis of ALL is established by bone marrow examination, which shows a homogeneous infiltration of leukemic blasts replacing normal marrow elements. The morphology of blasts on bone marrow aspirate can usually distinguish ALL from acute nonlymphocytic leukemia (ANLL). Lymphoblasts are typically small, with cell diameters of approximately two erythrocytes. Lymphoblasts have scant cytoplasm, usually without granules. The nucleus typically contains no nucleoli or one small indistinct nucleolus. Immunophenotyping of ALL blasts helps distinguish precursor B-cell ALL from T-cell ALL. Histochemical stains specific for myeloblastic and monoblastic leukemias (myeloperoxidase and nonspecific esterase) distinguish ALL from ANLL. Between 5% and 10% of patients present with central nervous system leukemia, which is defined as a cerebrospinal fluid white cell count $> 5/\mu L$ with blasts apparent on cytocentrifuged specimen.

C. Imaging: Chest x-ray may show mediastinal widening or mediastinal mass and tracheal compression secondary to lymphadenopathy. Abdominal ultrasound may show kidney enlargement from leukemic infiltration or uric acid nephropathy and intra-abdominal adenopathy. Plain films of the long bones and spine may show demineralization and compression of vertebral bodies.

Differential Diagnosis

The differential diagnosis, based on the history and physical examination, includes chronic infections such as those caused by Epstein-Barr virus and cytomegalovirus, giving rise to lymphadenopathy, hepatosplenomegaly, fevers, and anemia. Prominent petechiae and purpura suggest a diagnosis of immune thrombocytopenic purpura. Significant pallor brings to mind diagnoses such as transient erythroblastopenia of childhood, autoimmune hemolytic anemias, and aplastic anemia. Fevers and joint pains, with or without hepatosplenomegaly and lymphadenopathy, suggest juvenile rheumatoid arthritis. The diagnosis of leukemia usually becomes straightforward once the CBC reveals multiple cytopenias and leukemic blasts. Serum LDH levels may help in distinguishing juvenile rheumatoid arthritis (JRA) from leukemia. LDH is usually normal in JRA but often elevated in ALL patients presenting with bone pain. An elevated white count with lymphocytosis is typical of pertussis infection; however, the lymphocytes are mature, and neutropenia is rarely associated.

Treatment & Prognosis

Specific treatment is determined by prognostic features present at diagnosis. The first month of therapy consists of **induction,** at the end of which over 95% of patients exhibit remission on bone marrow aspirates. The drugs most commonly used in induction include oral prednisone, intravenous vincristine, intramuscular asparaginase, intrathecal methotrexate, and intravenous daunorubicin. For T-cell ALL, intravenous cyclophosphamide is often given during induction as well.

Consolidation is the second phase of treatment, during which intrathecal chemotherapy and sometimes cranial radiation therapy are given to treat lymphoblasts that may be present in the meninges.

Maintenance therapy includes daily oral mercaptopurine, weekly oral or intramuscular methotrexate, and, often, monthly pulses of intravenous vincristine and oral prednisone. Intrathecal chemotherapy, either with methotrexate alone or combined with cytarabine and hydrocortisone, is usually administered every 2–3 months. Several months of intensive chemotherapy, termed **delayed intensification,** may be posed within the maintenance chemotherapy phase of treatment.

All these drugs have significant potential side effects. Patients need to be closely monitored to prevent drug toxicities and to ensure early treatment of complications. Most patients are treated on protocols designed by the national Children's Cancer Group or Pediatric Oncology Group. The duration of treatment is between 2 and 3½ years.

The chance of cure depends on specific prognostic features present at diagnosis of ALL. The two most important features are white count and age. Children from ages 2 through 9 years whose diagnostic white count was less than 50,000/μL, have a better chance of cure than other patients. Certain chromosomal abnormalities present in the leukemic blasts at diagnosis also have affect the prognosis. Patients with a translocation between chromosomes 9 and 22— t(9;22)—have a very poor chance of cure even with intensive therapy. Infants with a translocation between chromosomes 4 and 11—t(4;11)—have a poor chance of cure. On the other hand, patients whose blasts are hyperdiploid (contain over 50 chromosomes instead of the normal 46) have a better chance of cure than children without hyperdiploidy.

Treatment for ALL currently is tailored to prognostic groups. A child 1 through 9 years with a white count under 50,000/μL at diagnosis and without t(9;22) or t(4;11), or hypodiploidy (≤ 44 chromosomes) would be treated with less intensive therapy than a patient with a white count over 50,000/μL or older than 10 years. This treatment approach has significantly increased the cure rate among patients with less favorable prognostic features while minimizing treatment-related toxicities in those with favorable prognostic features. The overall chance of cure for ALL is now at least 70%. Bone marrow relapse is usually heralded by an abnormal CBC. After a patient has completed the entire course of chemotherapy, the chance of relapse is about 10% in the next 2 years and much less after that time.

The CNS and testes are sanctuary sites of extramedullary leukemia. Systemic chemotherapy does not penetrate these tissues as well as it penetrates other organs. "Presymptomatic" intrathecal chemotherapy is a critical part of ALL treatment to prevent CNS relapse. Before the institution of such therapy in the 1970s, the CNS was a major site of initial leukemic relapse. Relapses isolated to the central nervous system now occur in about 5–8% of patients. Symptoms suggestive of CNS disease include headache, nausea and vomiting, irritability, nuchal rigidity, photophobia, and cranial nerve palsies. Previously, up to 15% of boys relapsed in their testes following completion of chemotherapy. The presentation of testicular relapse is usually unilateral painless testicular enlargement. The incidence of testicular relapse has decreased significantly as treatment for ALL has intensified. Routine follow-up of boys both on and off treatment includes examination of the testes.

Bone marrow transplant is rarely used as initial treatment following induction of remission for ALL since most patients are cured with chemotherapy alone. However, patients with certain chromosomal abnormalities in their leukemic blasts, such as t(9;22), appear to have a much better cure rate with early bone marrow transplant from an HLA-DR-matched sibling donor than with intensive chemotherapy alone. Bone marrow transplantation offers virtually the only chance for cure for patients who have relapsed with ALL, particularly if the relapse is during the course of treatment or within about 6 months after completion of chemotherapy.

Supportive Care

Tumor lysis syndrome should be anticipated when treatment is started. Hydration, alkalinization of uric acid urine, and oral allopurinol should be given. If superior vena caval syndrome is present, general anesthesia may be temporarily contraindicated to tracheal and airway compression. If hyperleukocytosis (> 100,000/μL) is present along with mental status changes, leukapheresis may be indicated to rapidly reduce the number of circulating blasts and minimize the potential thrombotic or hemorrhagic CNS complications. Severe anemia at diagnosis can usually be corrected with a number of small red blood cell transfusions and intravenous furosemide. During induction and throughout the course of treatment, all transfused blood and platelet products should be irradiated in order to prevent graft-versus-host disease from the transfused lymphocytes. Whenever possible, blood products should be leukodepleted to minimize cytomegalovirus (CMV) transmission, transfusion reactions, and sensitization to platelets.

During the course of treatment, fever (temperature > 38.3 °C) and neutropenia (absolute neutrophil count < 500/μL) need to be treated with empiric broad-spectrum antibiotics. All patients receiving ALL treatment must receive prophylaxis against Pneumocystis carinii. Trimethoprim-sulfamethoxazole is the drug of choice, currently recommended to be given on 2–3 consecutive days per week, twice each day. Patients, nonimmune to varicella, are at risk for very serious, even fatal, infection if exposed to varicella. Such patients should receive varicella-zoster immune globulin (VZIG) within 72 hours after exposure. The management of a patient on chemotherapy and treatment with intravenous acyclovir for active infection for ALL is very complex because of the infectious complications and potential toxicities of chemotherapy. Treatment of patients with ALL should be guided by physicians and nurses who are specifically trained in pediatric oncology.

Ablin AR (editor): Supportive care of children with cancer. Johns Hopkins University Press, 1993.

Pui CH: Childhood leukemia. N Engl J Med 1995; 332:1618.

Rivera GK et al: Treatment of ALL: 30 years' experience at St. Jude's Research Hospital. N Engl J Med 1993; 329:1289.

Tubergen DG, et al: Improved outcome with delayed intensification for children with ALL and intermediate presenting features: A CCG phase III trial. J Clin Oncol 1993;11:527.

ACUTE NONLYMPHOCYTIC LEUKEMIA

Acute nonlymphocytic leukemia (ANLL) is one-fifth as common in childhood as acute lymphoblastic leukemia (ALL). There are 500 new cases per year in the United States. Ionizing radiation, cytotoxic chemotherapeutic agents, benzene exposure, Down's syndrome, and chromosomal instability syndromes are known to be predisposing factors, but most children have none. Cytogenetic clonal abnormalities occur in 80% of patients with ANLL and are often predictive of outcome.

ANLL is subdivided primarily by morphology and histochemical staining of the leukemic cells (French-American-British [FAB] classification). These subsets have different cytogenetic abnormalities, clinical features and responses to treatment (Table 27–1).

Clinical presentation is usually with anemia (44%) thrombocytopenia (33%), and neutropenia (69%). Symptoms can be few and innocuous or may be life-threatening. The median hemoglobin at diagnosis is 7 g/dL; platelets are usually less than 50,000/μL; and the absolute neutrophil count is under 1000/μL. The total white blood cell count is over 100,000/μL in 25% of children diagnosed with ANLL. Hyperleukocytosis is associated with life-threatening complications from venous stasis and sludging of blasts in small vessels causing hypoxia, hemorrhage, and infarction, most notably in the lung and CNS. This is a medical emergency requiring rapid intervention to decrease the leukocyte count. CNS leukemia is present in 5–15% of patients at diagnosis, which is a much higher rate of involvement than in ALL.

Treatment is more difficult than in ALL and requires more intensive chemotherapy, particularly anthracyclines and cytarabine. Toxicities from therapy are common and likely to be life-threatening. Only 70–85% of children achieve remission (vs 98% in ALL); the long-term disease-free survival is 33–49%. Retinoic acid (all-*trans*) can cause differentiation of promyelocytic leukemia cells and induce remission. Its role in the treatment of acute promyelocytic leukemia (M_3) is under investigation. Allogeneic bone marrow transplantation during first remission may offer a survival advantage over chemotherapy alone. Published results from various centers show a 55–70% survival at 5 years. For patients relapsing following conventional chemotherapy, bone marrow transplantation is a potentially curative option.

Bovlad F, Kernanna: Treatment of childhood acute non-lymphoblastic leukemia: A review. Cancer Invest 1995; 11:534.

Table 27–1. FAB subtypes of ANLL.

FAB Classification	Common Name	Distribution in Childhood		Cytogenetic Associations	Clinical Features
		< 2 Years	> 2 Years		
M₁	Acute myeloblastic leukemia without maturation	17%	25%	16q abnormalities	
M₂	Acute myeloblastic leukemia with maturation		26%	18;21, inv 16, del 16q	Myeloblastomas
M₃	Acute promyelocytic leukemia		4%	t15;17	DIC
M₄	Acute myelomonocytic leukemia	30%	26%	t3;3, inv 3, inv 16, del 16q, t11/del 11q	Hyperleukocytosis, CNS involvement, skin and gum infiltration
M₅	Acute monocytic leukemia	52%	16%	t9;11	Hyperleukocytosis, CNS involvement, skin and gum infiltration
M₆	Erythroleukemia		2%		
M₇	Acute megakaryocytic leukemia		5%	t1;21, t3;3, inv 3	Down syndrome

Grier HE et al: Acute myelogenous leukemia. In: *Principles and Practice of Pediatric Oncology.* Pizzo PA, Poplack DG (editors). Lippincott, 1993.

Sartori PCE et al: Treatment of childhood acute myeloid leukemia using the BFM-83 protocol. Med Pediatr Oncol 1993;21:8.

Warrell RP et al: Acute promyelocytic leukemia. N. Engl J Med 1993;329:177.

CHRONIC MYELOCYTIC LEUKEMIA

Chronic myelocytic leukemia (CML) accounts for less than 5% of the childhood leukemias. Two childhood variants are recognized: the Philadelphia chromosome t(9;22)-positive form, which is essentially identical with that occurring in adults, and the juvenile form (Table 27–2).

Adult CML can be palliated with single-drug chemotherapy (hydroxyurea or busulfan). The disease inexorably progresses from the chronic phase, usually within 3 years, to an accelerated phase and then to a blast crisis. The accelerated and blast phases are refractory to therapy. Bone marrow transplantation is the only known cure. The 4-year survival for patients under 20 years of age transplanted in the chronic phase is 75%. Unfortunately, only one third of patients have related, matched donors available. Consequently related mismatched, unrelated matched, autologous, and peripheral stem cell bone marrow transplantations are being investigated. Alpha interferon has shown promising results in clinical trials by reducing or eliminating the Philadelphia chromosome-positive malignant clone. The long-term results are not yet known.

Juvenile CML accounts for one third of chronic leukemias in childhood. Compared with the adult form it is a much more fulminant disease that occurs in infants and very young children. Survival is less than 9 months. Bone marrow transplant has been used successfully.

Altman A: Chronic leukemias of childhood. In: *Principles and Practice of Pediatric Oncology.* Pizzo PA, Poplack DG (editors). Lippincott, 1993.

Table 27–2. Comparison of juvenile and adult chronic myelogenous leukemia.

	Juvenile CML	Adult CML
Age at onset	< 2 years old	> 3 years old
Clinical presentation	Abrupt onset; eczematoid skin rash, markedly lymphadenopathy, bleeding tendency, moderate hepatosplenomegaly.	Nonspecific constitutional complaints, massive splenomegaly, variable hepatomegaly.
Chromosomal alterations	Absent.	t(9;22) present in 90% of cases.
Laboratory features	Moderate leukocytosis (<100,000/mL), thrombocytopenia, monocytosis, elevated fetal hemoglobin, normal to diminished leukocyte alkaline phosphatase, elevated muramidase, elevated immunoglobulins.	Marked leukocytosis (> 100,000/µL), normal to elevated platelet count, decreased to absent leukocyte alkaline phosphatase, usually normal muramidase.

Goldman JM et al: Choice of pretransplant treatment and timing of transplant for chronic myelogenous leukemia in chronic phase. Blood 1993;82:2235.

Kantarjian HM et al: Treatment of chronic myelogenous leukemia: Current status and investigational options. Blood 1996;87:3069.

The Italian Cooperative Study Group on Chronic Myeloid Leukemia: Interferon Alfa–2A as compared with conventional chemotherapy for the treatment of chronic myeloid leukemia. N Engl J Med 1994;330:820.

BRAIN TUMORS

Essentials of Diagnosis

- Cranial nerve palsies, dysarthria, ataxia, hemiplegia, papilledema, hyperreflexia, macrocephaly, cracked pot sign.
- Headache, vomiting, personality change, seizures, blurred vision, diplopia, weakness, decreased coordination, precocious or delayed puberty.

General Considerations

Brain tumors are the most common solid tumor of childhood, accounting for 1500–2000 new malignancies in children each year in the United States and for 25–30% of all childhood cancers. In general, children with brain tumors have a better prognosis than adults. Favorable outcome occurs most commonly with low-grade and fully resectable tumors. Unfortunately, cranial irradiation in young children can have significant neuropsychologic, intellectual, and endocrinologic sequelae.

Brain tumors in childhood are biologically and histologically heterogeneous, ranging from low-grade, localized lesions to high-grade tumors with neuraxis dissemination. High-dose systemic chemotherapy is being used more frequently, especially in young children with high-grade tumors, in an effort to delay, decrease or to completely avoid cranial irradiation. Such intensive treatment may be accompanied by autologous bone marrow transplantation or peripheral stem cell reconstitution.

The causes of pediatric brain tumors remain unknown. The risk of developing astrocytomas is increased in children with neurofibromatosis or tuberous sclerosis. Several studies show that some childhood brain tumors occur in families with increased genetic susceptibility to childhood cancers in general, brain tumors, or leukemia and lymphoma. An excess of seizures in relatives of children with astrocytoma has been observed. Certain pediatric brain tumors such as ependymoma have been linked to polyomavirus, but the exact relationship remains to be elucidated. The risk of developing a brain tumor is increased also in children who received cranial irradiation at a young age for treatment of presymptomatic meningeal leukemia.

Because pediatric brain tumors are rare, they are often misdiagnosed or diagnosed late; most pediatricians see no more than two children with brain tumors during their careers.

Clinical Findings

A. Symptoms and Signs: Clinical findings at presentation vary depending on the age of the child and the location of the tumor. Children under 2 years of age more commonly have infratentorial tumors. They usually present with nonspecific symptoms such as vomiting, unsteadiness, lethargy, and irritability and signs such as macrocephaly, ataxia, hyperreflexia, and cranial nerve palsies. Eye findings and apparent visual disturbances such as difficulty tracking can be seen in optic pathway tumors such as optic glioma. Optic glioma occurring in a young child is usually associated with neurofibromatosis.

Older children more commonly have supratentorial tumors, which present with headache, visual symptoms, seizures, and focal neurologic deficits. Seizures secondary to frontal lobe tumors may begin with a focal motor onset or may be generalized. Seizures secondary to temporal lobe tumors are typically associated with behaviors such as staring spells and automatic movements. Frontal lobe tumors also affect personality and movement; parietal lobe tumors may affect reading and awareness of the contralateral extremities; temporal lobe tumors may cause fluent aphasias; and occipital lobe tumors may cause visual field deficits. Suprasellar midline tumors such as craniopharyngiomas may cause short stature, delayed onset of puberty or hormonal insufficiencies, and visual field deficits.

Infratentorial tumors in older children characteristically present with symptoms and signs of hydrocephalus, which include progressively worsening morning headache and vomiting, gait unsteadiness, double vision, and papilledema. Cerebellar astrocytomas enlarge slowly, and symptoms may worsen over several months. Morning vomiting may be the only symptom of posterior fossa ependymomas, which originate in the floor of the fourth ventricle near the vomiting center. Brain stem tumors may present with facial and extraocular muscle palsies, ataxia, and hemiparesis; hydrocephalus occurs in approximately 25% of these patients at diagnosis.

B. Staging: In addition to the tumor biopsy, neuraxis imaging studies are obtained to determine whether dissemination has occurred. It is unusual for brain tumors in children and adolescents to disseminate outside of the CNS. However, it is generally recommended that bone marrow aspirates and biopsies be analyzed in a patient with newly diagnosed medulloblastoma or primitive neuroectodermal tumor, particularly if neuraxis spread is present.

MRI has become the preferred diagnostic study for pediatric brain tumors. MRI provides better definition of the tumor and delineates indolent gliomas that may not be seen on CT scan. On the other hand, a CT scan can be done in 15 minutes as opposed to 45 minutes for MRI and is still useful if an urgent diagnostic study is necessary or if there is a desire to demonstrate calcium. Both scans are generally done with and without contrast enhancement. Contrast enhances regions where the blood-brain barrier is disrupted. Postoperative scans to document the extent of tumor resection should be obtained within 48 hours after surgery to avoid postsurgical enhancement.

Imaging of the entire neuraxis and cerebrospinal fluid cytologic examination should be part of the diagnostic evaluation for patients with tumors such as medulloblastoma, ependymoma, and pineal region tumors. Diagnosis of neuraxis "drop metastases" can be accomplished by conventional myelography or, more recently and less invasively, by gadolinium-enhanced MRI incorporating sagittal and axial views. Levels of biomarkers in the blood and cerebrospinal fluid such as human chorionic gonadotropin (hCG) and alpha-fetoprotein (AFP) may be helpful at diagnosis and in follow-up.

C. Classification: About 50% of the common pediatric brain tumors occur above the tentorium and 50% in the posterior fossa. Most childhood brain tumors can be divided by the cell of origin into glial tumors (astrocytomas and ependymomas) or nonglial tumors such as medulloblastoma and other primitive neuroectodermal tumors. Some tumors contain both glial and neural elements (eg, ganglioglioma). There are also a group of less common CNS tumors that do not fit into this classification (craniopharyngiomas, germ cell tumors, choroid plexus tumors, and meningiomas). Low-grade and high-grade tumors are found in most categories. Table 27–3 sets forth the location and frequency of the common pediatric brain tumors.

Astrocytoma is the most common brain tumor of childhood. Most are low-grade tumors found in the posterior fossa with a bland cellular morphology, and few or no mitotic figures. Low-grade astrocytomas are in many cases curable by complete surgical excision alone.

Table 27–3. Location and frequency of common pediatric brain tumors.

Location	Frequency of Occurrence
Hemispheric	**37%**
Low-grade astrocytoma	23%
High-grade astrocytoma	11%
Other	3%
Posterior fossa	**49%**
Medulloblastoma	15%
Cerebellar astrocytoma	15%
Brain stem glioma	15%
Ependymoma	4%
Midline	**14%**
Craniopharyngioma	8%
Chiasmal glioma	4%
Pineal region tumor	2%

Medulloblastoma and related primitive neuroectodermal tumors are the most common high-grade brain tumors in children. These tumors usually occur in the first decade of life, with a peak incidence between 5 and 10 years of age and a 2.1:1.3 female-to-male ratio. These tumors typically arise in the midline cerebellar vermis, with variable extension into the fourth ventricle. Reports of neuraxis dissemination at diagnosis range from 10% to 46% of patients. Hyperdiploidy in medulloblastoma cells may be a favorable prognostic indicator, whereas the presence of an isochromosome for the long arm of chromosome 17 appears to be unfavorable. Other more traditional prognostic factors are outlined in Table 27–4.

Brain stem tumors are third in frequency of occurrence in children. This tumor is frequently of astrocytic origin and is often high-grade. The tumors that diffusely infiltrate the brain stem and primarily involve the pons have a long-term survival rate of less than 15%. Brain stem tumors that occur above or below the pons and grow in an eccentric or cystic manner have a somewhat better outcome. Exophytic tumors in this location may be amenable to surgery. Generally, brain stem tumors are treated without a tissue diagnosis.

Other brain tumors such as ependymomas, germ cell tumors, choroid plexus tumors, and craniopharyngiomas are less common and each is associated with unique diagnostic and therapeutic challenges.

Treatment

A. Supportive Care: Dexamethasone should be started prior to initial surgery (0.5–1 mg/kg initially, then 0.25–0.5 mg/kg/d in four divided doses). Anticonvulsants (usually phenytoin, 4–8 mg/kg/d) should be started if the child has had a seizure or if the surgical approach is likely to induce seizures. As postoperative treatment of young children with high-grade brain tumors incorporates increasingly more intensive systemic chemotherapy, consideration should also be given to the use of prophylaxis for prevention of oral candidiasis and *Pneumocystis* infection.

Table 27–4. Prognostic factors in children with medulloblastoma.

Factor	Favorable	Unfavorable
Extent of disease	Nondisseminated	Disseminated
Size of primary tumor after surgery	≤ 3 cm (completely resected)	> 3 cm
Histologic features	Undifferentiated	Foci of glial, ependymal, or neuronal differentiation
Age	≥ 4 years	< 4 years

Optimum care for the pediatric brain tumor patient requires a multidisciplinary team including subspecialists in pediatric neurosurgery, neuro-oncology, neurology, endocrinology, neuropsychology, radiation therapy, and rehabilitation medicine as well as highly specialized nurses, social workers, and staff in physical therapy, occupational therapy, and speech and language science.

B. Specific Therapy: The goal of treatment is to eradicate the tumor with the least short- and long-term morbidity. Long-term neuropsychologic morbidity becomes an especially important issue related to deficits caused by the tumor itself and the sequelae of treatment. Meticulous surgical removal of as much tumor as possible is generally the preferred initial approach. Technologic advances in the operating microscope, the ultrasonic tissue aspirator and CO_2 laser (the latter less commonly used in pediatric brain tumor surgery), the accuracy of computerized stereotactic resection, and intraoperative monitoring techniques such as evoked potentials and electrocorticography have increased the feasibility and safety of surgical resection of many pediatric brain tumors. Second look surgery after chemotherapy is increasingly being used when tumors are incompletely resected at initial surgery.

Radiation therapy for pediatric brain tumors is in a state of evolution. Radiation therapy portals are made as small as possible (eg, to the tumor as localized on MRI plus a margin of 1–2 cm). Approaches to the delivery of radiation to minimize the adverse effects on normal brain are being explored and include hyperfractionation, stereotactic radiation such as the "gamma knife," implantation of interstitial seeds, and use of three-dimensional treatment planning.

Chemotherapy is effective in treating malignant astrocytomas, medulloblastomas, and ependymomas. There is now general agreement that brain tumors in children under 5 years of age should be treated by extensive surgical resection and followed by intensive chemotherapy to eliminate irradiation. Unfortunately, the survival rate for those with some tumors, such as supratentorial primitive neuroectodermal tumors, treated with radiation therapy has proved poor.

In the older child with malignant glioma, the present approach would be surgical resection of the tumor and combined modality treatment with irradiation and intensive chemotherapy. In patients with glioblastoma, the use of high-dose chemotherapy and autologous bone marrow or peripheral stem cell reconstitution is being studied. Surgery is not indicated for diffuse brain stem gliomas. Traditional treatment of these tumors has been local irradiation. Hyperfractionation to increase the dose from the conventional 54 Gy to 72 to 78 Gy unfortunately shows no apparent benefit in a recent Children's Cancer Group study. New approaches are needed for this prognostically poor tumor.

The treatment of low-grade astrocytomas is also evolving. Increasing numbers of young children are treated with antitumor chemotherapeutic agents such as carboplatin and vincristine after incomplete resection of these tumors. The role of irradiation after subtotal resection even in the older child is being questioned. A combined CCG/POG study is currently evaluating the efficacy of irradiation and the natural history of this disease following subtotal resection. Management of axial low-grade astrocytomas presents a particular challenge. In part related to the technologic advances, near-total resection of these lesions is often possible.

Prognosis

Despite improvements in surgery and radiation therapy, the outlook for cure remains poor for children with high-grade brain tumors. For children with high-grade gliomas, an early CCG study showed a 45% progression-free survival rate for children who received radiation therapy and chemotherapy. A follow-up CCG study in which all patients had chemotherapy and radiation therapy showed a 5-year progression-free survival rate of 36%. There is a possibility of effective salvage therapy with high-dose chemotherapy for children who relapse. In addition, extent of resection appeared to correlate positively with prognosis, with a 3 year progression-free survival rate of 17% for biopsy-only patients, 29–32% for partially or subtotally resected patients, and 54% for those with 90% resections.

The 5- and even 10-year survival rate for low-grade astrocytomas of childhood is 60–90%. However, prognosis depends on both site and grade. A child with a pilocytic astrocytoma of the cerebellum has a considerably better prognosis than a child with a fibrillary astrocytoma of the cerebral cortex. For recurrent or progressive low-grade astrocytoma of childhood, relatively moderate chemotherapy may improve survival.

Conventional craniospinal irradiation for children with low-stage medulloblastoma results in survival rates of 60–90%. Ten-year survival rates are lower (40–60%). Chemotherapy may allow a reduction in the craniospinal radiation dose while preserving survival rates. Five-year survival rates for "poor risk" medulloblastoma have been 25–40%, but a recent publication reported an 87% survival rate for those treated with chemotherapy and radiation therapy. Children with supratentorial primitive neuroectodermal tumors may also have benefited from the addition of chemotherapy to craniospinal radiation.

Finlay JL et al: Randomized phase III trial in childhood high-grade astrocytoma comparing vincristine, lomustine, and prednisone with the eight-drugs-in-1-day regiment. J Clin Oncol 1995;13:112.

Finlay JL et al: A pilot study of high-dose thiotepa and etoposide with autologous bone marrow rescue in children and young adults with recurrent central nervous system tumors. J Clin Oncol 1996.

Goldwein JW et al: Update results of a pilot study for low dose craniospinal irradiation plus chemotherapy for children under five with cerebellar primitive neuroectodermal tumors (medulloblastoma). Int J Radiat Oncol Biol Phys 1996;34:899.

Packer RJ et al: Carboplatin and vincristine for recurrent and newly diagnosed low-grade gliomas of childhood. J Clin Oncol 1993;11:850.

Packer RJ et al: Outcome for children with medulloblastoma treated with radiation and cisplatin, CCNU, and vincristine chemotherapy. J Neurosurg 1994;81:690.

LYMPHOMAS

1. HODGKIN'S DISEASE

Essentials of Diagnosis

- Painless cervical (70–80%) or supraclavicular (25%) adenopathy; mediastinal mass (50%).
- Fatigue, anorexia, weight loss, fever, night sweats, pruritus, cough.

General Considerations

Children with Hodgkin's disease have a better response to treatment than do adults, with a 75% overall survival at more than 20 years' follow-up. While "adult" therapies are applicable, the management of Hodgkin's disease in children under 16 years of age frequently differs. Because excellent disease control can result from several different therapeutic approaches, selection of staging procedures and treatment are often based on the potential long-term toxicity associated with the intervention.

Although Hodgkin's disease represents 50% of the lymphomas of childhood, only 15% of all cases occur in children 16 years of age or younger. Children less than 5 years of age account for 3% of childhood cases, while 60% occur in the age group from 10 to 16 years of age. There is a 4:1 male predominance in the first decade.

Hodgkin's disease is a histologic diagnosis requiring Reed-Sternberg cell or variant. The presence of Hodgkin's disease is unique in that the bulk of the tumor is composed of normal cells while the malignant Reed-Sternberg cells are relatively scanty. The origin of the malignant cell remains elusive.

Hodgkin's disease is subdivided into four histologic groups, and the distribution parallels that of adults: lymphocyte-predominant in children (10–20%); nodular sclerosing (40–60%) (increases with age); mixed cellularity (20–40%); and lymphocyte-depleted (5–10%). Prognosis is independent of subclassification, with appropriate therapy based on stage.

Clinical Findings

A. Symptoms and Signs: Painless cervical adenopathy is the usual presentation of Hodgkin's disease. The lymph nodes often feel firmer than inflammatory nodes and have a rubbery texture. They may be discrete or matted together and are not fixed to surrounding tissue. The growth rate is variable, and involved nodes may wax and wane in size over weeks to months.

As Hodgkin's disease nearly always arises in lymph nodes and spreads to contiguous nodal groups, a detailed examination of all nodal sites is mandatory. Lymphadenopathy is common in children so the decision to biopsy is often difficult or delayed for a prolonged period. Indications for early lymph node biopsy include lack of identifiable infection in the region drained by the enlarged node, a node greater than 2 cm in size, supraclavicular adenopathy or abnormal chest x-ray, and lymphadenopathy increasing in size after 2 weeks or failing to resolve within 4–8 weeks.

Constitutional symptoms occur in about one-third of children at presentation. Symptoms of fever over 38 °C, weight loss of 10%, and drenching night sweats are defined by the Ann Arbor staging criteria as "B" symptoms. The "A" designation refers to the absence of these symptoms. "B" symptoms are of prognostic value, and more aggressive therapy is usually required for cure. Generalized pruritus and pain with alcohol ingestion may also occur.

Half of patients have asymptomatic mediastinal disease (adenopathy or anterior mediastinal mass), though symptoms due to compression of vital structures in the thorax may occur. A chest radiograph should be obtained when Hodgkin's disease is considered. Airway competency must be thoroughly evaluated before any surgical procedure is undertaken to avoid airway obstruction during anesthesia and possible death.

Splenomegaly and hepatomegaly (either or both) are generally associated with advanced disease.

B. Laboratory Findings: The blood count is usually normal, though anemia, neutrophilia, eosinophilia, and thrombocytosis may be present. The erythrocyte sedimentation rate and other acute-phase reactants are often elevated and can serve as markers of disease activity. Immunologic abnormalities occur, particularly in cell-mediated immunity, and anergy is common in advanced-stage disease at diagnosis. Autoantibody phenomenon such as hemolytic anemia and an idiopathic thrombocytopenic purpura-like picture have been reported.

C. Staging: Staging involves a systematic search for detectable disease using a variety of techniques. Imaging studies for thoracic disease include chest radiography and computed tomography (important to identify mediastinal disease). Assessment of abdominal and pelvic disease is usually accomplished by CT, though lymphangiography may be more accurate. The lack of retroperitoneal fat in young children compromises the adequacy of CT imaging. Lymphangiography in children is variably successful depending on the skill and tenacity of the examiner.

Bilateral bone marrow aspirates and biopsies are performed. Technetium bone scanning may show bony involvement and is usually reserved for patients with bone pain, since bone involvement is rare. Gallium scanning defines gallium-avid tumors and is most useful in evaluating residual mediastinal disease at the completion of treatment.

Clinical staging may be followed by laparotomy with multiple lymph node samplings, liver biopsy, and splenectomy. Although controversial, the staging laparotomy is less important now than it once was. It is performed only if radiation therapy is the preferred treatment and the detection of abdominal disease would alter therapy. Excellent disease control with radiation therapy can be achieved in laparotomy-staged children, but this option must be weighed against the toxicities of high-dose, extended-field radiation in prepubertal children and the complications of laparotomy, including postsplenectomy sepsis. Reports linking splenectomy with secondary acute myelogenous leukemia following Hodgkin's disease therapy are particularly disturbing.

Treatment & Prognosis

Both radiation therapy and combination chemotherapy are effective in treating Hodgkin's disease. The principles of therapy are to achieve long-term disease-free survival while minimizing the toxicities of therapy. Consequently, treatment of childhood Hodgkin's disease is evolving toward increased use of chemotherapy, even in stage I and stage II disease, with a corresponding reduction in radiation therapy.

Several combinations of chemotherapeutic agents are effective, but the most commonly used are MOPP (mechlorethamine, Oncovin [vincristine], procarbazine, and prednisone) and ABVD (Adriamycin [doxorubicin], bleomycin, vinblastine, and dacarbazine). These regimens are non–cross-resistant. When these schedules are alternated, exposure to an individual drug is decreased, and the toxicities associated with cumulative doses are in this way minimized.

Radiation continues to play a role in the treatment of childhood Hodgkin's disease, particularly in the control of residual disease following chemotherapy. Combined-modality therapy appears to increase the cure rate. The most efficacious chemotherapy regimen and radiation schema with the least long-term toxicities await further clinical trials.

With current therapeutic approaches, it is expected that children with stage I and stage II Hodgkin's disease will have at least a 90% disease-free survival 5 years from diagnosis. Since two thirds of all relapses occur within 2 years after diagnosis and since relapse rarely occurs beyond 4 years, 5-year disease-free survival generally equates with cure. In more advanced disease (stage III and stage IV), 5-year event-free survival ranges from over 60% to 90%.

Treatment of relapsed Hodgkin's disease involves radiation therapy in combination with chemotherapy. An alternative is autologous or allogeneic bone marrow transplantation. Although salvage therapy for Hodgkin's disease is relatively successful, this should not be a consideration in planning primary treatment.

Bierman PJ et al: Autologous transplantation for Hodgkin's disease: Coming of age? Blood 1994;83:1161.
De Vita VT et al: Hodgkin's disease. N Engl J Med 1993;328:560.
Leventhal BG et al: Hodgkin's disease. In: *Principles and Practice of Pediatric Oncology.* Pizzo PA, Poplack DG (editors). Lippincott, 1993.
Mauch PM: Controversies in the management of early stage Hodgkin's disease. Blood 1994;83:318.
Tura S et al: Splenectomy and the increasing risk of secondary acute leukemia in Hodgkin's disease. J Clin Oncol 1993;11:925.

2. NON-HODGKIN'S LYMPHOMA

Essentials of Diagnosis

- Cough, dyspnea, swelling of the face; abdominal pain, abdominal distention, vomiting, constipation.
- Lymphadenopathy, mediastinal mass, pleural effusion, abdominal mass, ascites, hepatosplenomegaly.

General Considerations

Non-Hodgkin's lymphomas are a diverse group accounting for 7–13% of malignancies in children less than 15 years of age (about 390 new cases per year in the United States). In equatorial Africa, non-Hodgkin's lymphoma represents almost 50% of pediatric malignancies. The incidence of non-Hodgkin's lymphoma increases with age. Children 15 years of age or younger account for only 3% of all cases of non-Hodgkin's lymphoma; it is uncommon before 5 years of age. There is a marked male predominance, with the male:female ratio of approximately 3:1.

Children with congenital or acquired immune deficiencies (eg, Wiscott-Aldrich syndrome, severe combined immunodeficiency syndrome, X-linked lymphoproliferative syndrome, HIV infection, immunosuppressive therapy following solid organ or marrow transplantation) have an increased risk of developing non-Hodgkin's lymphoma. It has been estimated that the risk is 100–10,000 times that of age-matched controls.

Most children who develop non-Hodgkin's lymphoma have no underlying immune defect. Animal models for non-Hodgkin's lymphoma support a viral contribution to their pathogenesis. In equatorial Africa, 95% of Burkitt's lymphomas contain Epstein-Barr viral (EBV) DNA. But, in North America, less than 20% of Burkitt's tumors contain the EBV genome. Disturbances in host immunologic defenses, perhaps as a consequence of viral infection, chronic immunostimulation, and specific chromosomal rearrangements, are all under investigation as potential triggers in the development of non-Hodgkin's lymphoma.

Pediatric non-Hodgkin's lymphomas are classified by histology into three main groups: lymphoblastic lymphoma, small non-cleaved cell lymphoma (endemic or sporadic Burkitt's lymphoma), and large cell lymphoma (Table 27–5). Malignant lymphoma cells retain features similar to those of the lymphoid lineage cell from which they are derived. Cell membrane markers can therefore help clarify the origins of these cancers and serve as an adjunct to histologic classification. Typically, lymphoblastic lymphoma is associated with T-cell surface markers, whereas small non-cleaved cell lymphomas have B-cell phenotype such as surface immunoglobulins. The large cell lymphomas, which make up less than 15% of pediatric non-Hodgkin's lymphomas, may show T-cell, B-cell, or histiocytic lineage.

Unlike adult non-Hodgkin's lymphoma, virtually all childhood non-Hodgkin's lymphomas are rapidly proliferating, diffuse malignancies arising from extranodal tissue. These tumors exhibit aggressive behavior but are responsive to treatment.

Clinical Findings

A. Symptoms and Signs: Childhood non-Hodgkin's lymphomas can arise in any site of lymphoid tissue. including lymph nodes, Waldeyer's ring, Peyer's patches, thymus, liver, and spleen. Common extralymphatic sites include bone, bone marrow, the CNS, skin, and testis. Signs and symptoms at presentation are determined by the location of lesions and the degree of dissemination. Because non-Hodgkin's lymphoma usually progresses very rapidly, the duration of symptoms is quite brief— from days to a few weeks. Nevertheless, children present with a limited number of syndromes, most of which correlate well with cell type.

Lymphoblastic lymphoma typically presents with symptoms of airway compression (cough, dyspnea, orthopnea) or superior venal caval obstruction (facial edema, chemosis, plethora, venous engorgement) which are a result of mediastinal disease. These symptoms are a true emergency necessitating rapid diagnosis and treatment. Pleural effusions may further compromise the patient's respiratory status. CNS and bone marrow involvement are not common at diagnosis. When bone marrow contains more than 25% lymphoblasts, patients are considered to have acute lymphoblastic leukemia.

Ninety percent of small non-cleaved cell lymphomas present with abdominal disease. Abdominal pain, distention, a right lower quadrant mass, or intussusception in a child older than 5 years of age all suggest the diagnosis of small non-cleaved cell lymphoma (Burkitt's lymphoma). Bone marrow involvement is common (up to 65% of patients). Burkitt's lymphoma is the most rapidly proliferating tumor known and has a high rate of spontaneous cell death as it outgrows its blood supply. Consequently, children with massive abdominal disease frequently have metabolic abnormalities at presentation (hyper-

Table 27–5. Comparison of pediatric non-Hodgkin's lymphomas.

	Lymphoblastic Lymphoma	Small Non-Cleaved Cell Lymphoma	Large Cell Lymphoma
Incidence	30–40%	40–50%	≤ 15%
Histopathologic features	Indistinguishable from ALL lymphoblasts.	Large nucleus with prominent nucleoli surrounded by very basophilic cytoplasm that contains lipid vacuoles.	Large cells with cleaved or noncleaved nuclei.
Immunophenotype	Immature T cell	B cell	B cell, T cell, or histiocyte
Cytogenetic markers	Translocations involving chromosome 14q11 and chromosome 7; interstitial deletions of chromosome 1.	t(8;14), t(8;22), t(2;8)	t(2;5)
Clinical presentation	Intrathoracic tumor, mediastinal mass (50–70%), lymphadenopathy above diaphragm (50–80%).	Intra-abdominal tumor (90%), jaw involvement (10–20% sporadic Burkitt's, 70% epidemic Burkitt's). Bone marrow involvement.	Abdominal tumor most common; unusual sites: lung, face, brain, skin, testes, muscle.
Treatment	Similar to therapy for ALL; 15–18 months' duration	Intensive administration of alkylating agents and intermediate- to high-dose methotrexate; intensive CNS prophylaxis; 6–9 months' duration.	Similar to therapy for small non-cleaved cell lymphomas.

ALL = acute lymphoblastic leukemia.

uricemia, hyperphosphatemia, and hyperkalemia). Impaired renal function because of tumor infiltration, urinary obstruction by tumor, or urate nephropathy further worsen the biochemical derangements of this life-threatening syndrome of acute tumor lysis. Although similar histologically, there are numerous differences between cases of Burkitt's lymphoma occurring in endemic areas of equatorial Africa and the sporadic cases of North America (Table 27–6).

Large cell lymphomas are similar clinically to the small non-cleaved cell lymphomas, though unusual sites of involvement are more common.

B. Diagnostic Evaluation: Diagnosis is by biopsy with histology, immunophenotyping, and cytogenetic studies. If mediastinal disease is present, anesthesia must be avoided if the airway is compromised by tumor. Samples of pleural or ascitic fluid, bone marrow, or peripheral nodes obtained under local anesthesia may provide the diagnosis. Following the diagnosis of non-Hodgkin's lymphoma, studies should be obtained to determine the extent of disease. The rapid growth of these tumors and the life-threatening complications demand that studies be done expeditiously so that specific therapy is not delayed.

After a thorough physical examination, a CBC and liver and renal function tests plus a biochemical profile (electrolytes, calcium, phosphorus, uric acid) should be obtained. The LDH concentration reflects tumor burden and can serve as a marker of disease activity. Imaging studies should include a chest radiograph and chest CT scan if the plain films are abnormal, an abdominal ultrasound or CT scan, and a radionuclide bone scan. Bone marrow and cerebrospinal fluid examinations are also essential.

Treatment

A. Supportive Care: The management of life-threatening problems at presentation is critical. The most common complications are the superior mediastinal syndrome and the acute tumor lysis syndrome. Patients with airway compromise require

prompt initiation of specific therapy. Because of the risk of general anesthesia in these patients—and if a specific diagnosis cannot be made from peripheral studies—it is occasionally necessary to initiate steroids or, rarely, low-dose radiation until the mass is small enough for a biopsy to be undertaken safely. Response to steroids is usually prompt (12–24 hours).

The tumor lysis syndrome should be anticipated in all non-Hodgkin's lymphoma patients with extensive disease. Maintaining a brisk urine output (> 3 mL/kg/h) with intravenous fluids and diuretics is the key to management. Allopurinol will reduce serum uric acid, and alkalinization of urine will increase its solubility. Because phosphate precipitates in an alkaline urine, alkali administration should be discontinued if hyperphosphatemia occurs. Renal dialysis may be necessary to control metabolic abnormalities. Every attempt should be made to correct or minimize metabolic abnormalities before initiating chemotherapy. However, this period of stabilization should not exceed 24–48 hours.

B. Specific Therapy: Chemotherapy is the bulwark of therapy for non-Hodgkin's lymphomas. Surgery has little to offer unless the entire tumor can be resected. There is no role for partial resection or debulking surgery. Radiation therapy also has little to offer. Its use is confined to exceptional circumstances.

Therapy for lymphoblastic lymphoma is generally based on treatment protocols designed for ALL. Anthracyclines are usually an integral agent in effective treatment regimens for lymphoblastic lymphoma; cytarabine and podophyllotoxin derivatives (etoposide, teniposide) are emerging as promising agents. Duration of therapy is determined by disease extent. Localized disease is treated for 6 months, whereas extensive disease is treated for 15 months.

Small non-cleaved cell lymphomas do not respond well to therapy based on ALL protocols even when bone marrow is involved. Protocols using alkylating agents and intermediate- to high-dose methotrexate administered on an intensive schedule produce the highest cure rates. Large cell lymphomas are treated similarly.

All non-Hodgkin's lymphoma patients require intensive CNA intrathecal chemotherapy for prophylaxis.

Prognosis

A major predictor of outcome in non-Hodgkin's lymphoma is the extent of disease at diagnosis. Ninety percent of patients with localized disease can expect long-term disease-free survival, while patients with extensive disease on both sides of the diaphragm, CNS involvement, or bone marrow involvement in addition to a primary site have a 70–80% failure-free survival. Relapses occur early in non-Hodgkin's lymphoma; patients with lym-

Table 27–6. Comparison of endemic and sporadic Burkitt's lymphoma.

	Endemic	Sporadic
Incidence	10 per 100,000	0.9 per 100,000
Cytogenetics	Chromosome 8 breakpoint upstream of c-*myc* locus	Chromosome 8 breakpoint within c-*myc* locus
EBV association	≥ 95%	≤ 20%
Disease sites at presentation	Jaw (58%), abdomen (58%), CNS (19%), orbit (11%), marrow (7%)	Jaw (7%), abdomen (91%), CNS (14%), orbit (1%), marrow (20%)

EBV = Epstein-Barr virus.

phoblastic lymphoma rarely have recurrences after 30 months from diagnosis, whereas patients with small non-cleaved cell lymphomas essentially never have recurrences beyond 1 year.

Patients who experience relapse may have a chance for cure by autologous or allogeneic bone marrow transplantation.

Magrath I: Malignant non-Hodgkin's lymphomas in children. In: *Principles and Practice of Pediatric Oncology.* Pizzo PA, Poplack DG (editors). Lippincott, 1993.

Sandlund JT et al: Non-Hodgkin's lymphoma in childhood. N Engl J Med 1996;334:1238.

Toogood IRG et al: Effective multi-agent chemotherapy for advanced abdominal lymphoma and FAB L3 leukemia of childhood. Pediatr Oncol 1993;21:103.

NEUROBLASTOMA

Essentials of Diagnosis

- Bone pain, abdominal pain, anorexia, weight loss, fatigue, fever, irritability.
- Abdominal mass (65%), adenopathy, proptosis, periorbital ecchymosis, skull masses, subcutaneous nodules, hepatomegaly, spinal cord compression.

General Considerations

Neuroblastoma arises from neural crest tissue of the sympathetic ganglia or adrenal medulla. It is composed of small, fairly uniform cells with little cytoplasm and hyperchromatic nuclei that may form rosette patterns. Pathologic diagnosis is not always easy, and neuroblastoma must be differentiated from the other "small, round, blue cell" malignancies of childhood (Ewing's sarcoma, rhabdomyosarcoma, peripheral neuroepithelioma, lymphoma).

Neuroblastoma accounts for 7–10% of pediatric malignancies and is the most common solid neoplasm outside the CNS. Fifty percent of neuroblastomas are diagnosed in the first 2 years of life and 90% before age 5.

The biologic diversity of neuroblastoma makes this a fascinating tumor for study. Spontaneous regression in stage IV-S disease and spontaneous or induced differentiation to a benign neoplasm are examples of the unique behavior of this tumor. Unfortunately, neuroblastoma is also an extremely malignant neoplasm, and the overall survival in advanced disease has changed little in 20 years despite significant advances in our understanding of this tumor at a cellular and molecular level.

Clinical Findings

A. Symptoms and Signs: Clinical manifestations vary with the primary site of metastatic disease and the neuroendocrine function of the tumor. Many children present with constitutional symptoms such as fever, weight loss, and irritability. Bone pain suggests metastatic disease, which is present in 70% of children older than 1 year at diagnosis. Physical examination may reveal a firm, fixed, irregularly shaped mass that extends beyond the midline. The margins are often poorly defined. Although most children have an abdominal primary (40% adrenal gland, 25% paraspinal ganglion), neuroblastoma can arise wherever there is sympathetic tissue. In the posterior mediastinum, it is usually asymptomatic and discovered on a chest x-ray obtained for other reasons. Cervical neuroblastoma presents with a neck mass, often misdiagnosed as infection. Horner's syndrome or heterochromia iridis may accompany cervical neuroblastoma. Paraspinal tumors can extend through the spinal foramina, causing cord compression. Patients may present with paresis, paralysis, and bowel or bladder dysfunction.

The most common sites of metastases are bone, bone marrow, lymph nodes (regional as well as disseminated), liver, and subcutaneous tissue. Neuroblastoma has a predilection for metastasis to the skull, in particular the sphenoid bone and retrobulbar tissue. This causes orbital ecchymosis and proptosis. Liver metastasis, particularly in the newborn, can be massive. Subcutaneous nodules are bluish in color and associated with an erythematous flush followed by blanching when compressed, probably secondary to catecholamine release.

Neuroblastoma may also have unusual paraneoplastic manifestations. Examples include chronic watery diarrhea associated with tumor secretion of vasoactive intestinal peptides and opsoclonus-myoclonus (dancing eyes and dancing feet). It is postulated that the neurologic manifestations are secondary to cross-reacting antibodies.

B. Laboratory Findings: Anemia is present in 60% of children with neuroblastoma and can be due to "chronic disease" or marrow infiltration. Thrombocytopenia may be present, but thrombocytosis is more common, even with metastatic disease in the marrow.

Measures of tumor markers have prognostic significance and provides parameters for follow-up. LDH and ferritin can be elevated at diagnosis. Urinary catecholamines (vanilmandelic acid, homovanillic acid) are elevated in at least 90% of patients at diagnosis and should be measured prior to surgery. Screening of infants is accomplished using this technique, although the cost-effectiveness remains to be established.

C. Imaging: Plain films or CT of the primary tumor may show stippled calcifications. CT scanning can evaluate the extent of the primary tumor, its effects on surrounding structures, and the presence of liver and lymph node metastases. Classically, in primary tumors originating from the adrenal, the kidney is displaced inferolaterally, which helps to differentiate neuroblastoma from Wilms' tumor. MRI is useful to evaluate for the presence of spinal cord involvement in tumors that appear to invade neural foramina.

Both skeletal survey and radionuclide bone scanning are obtained in the evaluation of bone metastases. On plain films, lesions are usually symmetric and appear irregular and lytic. Periosteal reaction and pathologic fractures may also be seen.

D. Staging: First a tissue diagnosis must be established and then the disease extent determined. In addition to the previously mentioned studies, bilateral bone marrow aspirates and biopsies are essential in evaluating for metastatic disease, even if the CBC is normal. The appearance of neuroblastoma in the bone marrow may simulate the appearance of acute lymphoblastic leukemia; differentiation is by monoclonal antibody phenotyping.

Molecular parameters are essential to supplement clinical staging and aid in treatment planning. Amplification of the N-*myc* proto-oncogene or its gene product can be detected in tumor tissue. Rapid disease progression is associated with N-*myc* amplification and necessitates aggressive therapy. Tumor DNA content is determined by flow cytometry. Hyperdiploidy is a favorable finding, whereas near-diploid DNA content is associated with advanced disease and a poor outcome. Double-minute chromosomes and homogenous staining regions of DNA, manifestations of gene amplification, along with deletion of the short arm of chromosome 1, are cytogenetic characteristics of neuroblastoma.

Treatment & Prognosis

As prognosis is independently influenced by age at diagnosis and stage of disease, both factors are taken into consideration when deciding a treatment plan. Infants less than 1 year of age with stage 4S disease may need little if any therapy to effect a cure, although treatment may be initiated because of bulky disease causing mechanical complications.

Therapy is usually multimodal and involves surgery, radiation therapy and chemotherapy. Bone marrow transplantation is being investigated as a treatment to improve the currently poor outcome for advanced neuroblastoma. Initial surgical efforts are aimed at resecting the primary tumor when feasible. The usually massive size of the tumor makes primary resection impossible. Under these circumstances, only a biopsy may be performed. Following chemotherapy, a second surgical procedure may allow for resection of the primary tumor. Radiation may be given intraoperatively at the time of resection or postoperatively by external-beam radiation therapy.

Active chemotherapeutic agents in the treatment of neuroblastoma include cyclophosphamide, doxorubicin, etoposide, cisplatin, and vincristine. There is a clear dose-response relationship in neuroblastoma. About 80% of patients achieve complete or partial remission, although in advanced disease this is seldom durable. A current Children's Cancer Study Group (CCSG) treatment protocol compares aggressive conventional chemotherapy with chemotherapy plus autologous bone marrow transplantation. Clinical trials using radioactive monoclonal antibodies against neuroblastoma cells such as ^{131}I-meta-iodobenzylguanidine (MIBG) and [131]I-3F8 (a murine IgG antibody specific for ganglioside GD2, the predominant antigen on neuroblastoma cells) are also under way. In another promising area of research, attempts are being made to manipulate the patient's immune system to eradicate residual disease.

For children with stage 1, 2, or 4S disease, the 5-year survival is 70–90%. Infants under 1 year of age who have stage 4 disease have a greater than 60% likelihood of long-term survival. Children over 1 year of age with stage 3 disease have an intermediate prognosis (approximately 40–70%), and those with stage 4 disease have a poor prognosis (5–20% survival 5 years from diagnosis).

Bonilla MA, Cheumng N-KV: Clinical progress in neuroblastoma. Cancer Invest 1994;12:644.

Brodeur GM et al: Molecular basis of clinical heterogeneity in neuroblastoma. Am J Pediatr Hematol Oncol 1992;14:111.

Brodeur GM et al: Neuroblastoma. In: *Principles and Practice of Pediatric Oncology*. Pizzo PA, Poplack DG: (editors). JB Lippincott, 1993.

Mattay KK et al: Allogenic versus autologous purge and bone marrow transplantation for neuroblastoma: A report from the Children's Cancer Study Group. J Clin Oncol 1994;12:2382.

WILMS' TUMOR
(Nephroblastoma)

Essentials of Diagnosis

- Asymptomatic abdominal mass or swelling (83%).
- Fever (23%), hematuria (21%).
- Hypertension (25%), genitourinary malformations (6%), aniridia, hemihypertrophy.

General Considerations

Approximately 460 new cases of Wilms' tumor occur annually in the United States, representing 5–6% of cancers in children under 15 years of age. This is the second most common abdominal tumor in children following neuroblastoma. The tumor arises from kidney and is usually composed of three elements: blastema, epithelium, and stroma. The majority of Wilms' tumor are sporadically occurring malignancies. There are several important malformations, syndromes, and cytogenetic associations, including aniridia, hemihypertrophy, genitourinary malformations (eg, cryptorchidism, hypospadias, gonadal dysgenesis, pseudohermaphroditism, horseshoe kidney), Beckwith-Wiedemann syndrome, Drash syndrome, and WAGR (Wilms', aniridia, ambiguous genitalia, mental retardation) syndrome. Although most patients with Wilms' tumor are karyotypically normal, those with sporadic aniridia frequently have a constitutional deletion at the 11p13 locus. This deletion has also been found in the tumor cells of Wilms' patients without aniridia and who are karyotypically normal.

The median age at diagnosis is related both to gender and laterality, with bilateral tumors presenting at a younger age than unilateral tumors and males being diagnosed earlier than females. Wilms' tumor occurs most commonly between 2 and 5 years of age; it is unusual after 6 years of age. The mean age at diagnosis is 3 years.

Clinical Findings

A. Symptoms and Signs: Most children with Wilms' tumor present with an increasing size of the abdomen or an abdominal mass incidentally discovered by a parent. The mass is usually smooth and firm, well demarcated, and rarely crosses the midline, although it can extend inferiorly into the pelvis. Gross hematuria is an uncommon presentation, although microscopic hematuria is found in approximately 25% of cases.

B. Laboratory Findings: The CBC is usually normal, but some patients have anemia secondary to hemorrhage into the tumor. BUN and serum creatinine are usually normal. Urinalysis may show some blood or leukocytes.

C. Staging: Ultrasonography or CT of the abdomen should establish the presence of an intrarenal mass. It is also essential to evaluate the contralateral kidney for presence and function as well as synchronous Wilms' tumor. The inferior vena cava needs to be evaluated for the presence and extent of tumor propagation. The liver should be imaged for the presence or absence of metastatic disease. A plain chest radiograph (four views) should be obtained to determine whether pulmonary metastases are present. Approximately 10% of patients will have metastatic disease at diagnosis. Of these, 80% will have pulmonary disease, and 15% will have liver metastases. Bone and brain metastases are very unusual and associated with certain unfavorable histologic types; hence, bone and brain scans are not routinely performed. The clinical stage is ultimately decided at surgery and confirmed by the pathologist.

Treatment & Prognosis

In the United States, treatment begins with surgical exploration of the abdomen. The contralateral kidney is inspected and palpated for tumor involvement (one third of patients with bilateral disease have no evidence of this on preoperative studies). The liver and lymph nodes are inspected and suspicious

areas biopsied or excised. An en bloc resection of tumor is performed. Every attempt is made to avoid tumor spillage at surgery. Because therapy is tailored to tumor stage, it is imperative that operation be done by a surgeon familiar with the staging requirements.

In addition to the staging, the histologic type has implications for therapy and prognosis. Favorable histology (FH; see below) refers to the class triphasic Wilms tumor and its variants. Unfavorable histology (UH) refers to anaplasia, clear cell sarcoma of the kidney, and rhabdoid tumor of the kidney and is present in 10–12% of cases. Although clear cell sarcoma and rhabdoid tumor are no longer felt to be Wilms' tumor variants, these histologic types were identified in early Wilms' tumor studies as being associated with a worse outcome when compared with favorable histology tumors. Anaplasia is defined by extreme nuclear atypia. Only a few small foci of anaplasia in a Wilms' tumor is sufficient to impart a worse prognosis to stage II, III, or IV patients. Following excision and pathologic examination, the patient is assigned a stage that defines further therapy.

The progress and success in the treatment of Wilms' tumor is a result of the cooperative clinical trials of the National Wilms' Tumor Study (NWTS). Clinical trials that began in 1969 have resulted in an overall cure rate of approximately 90%. The current NWTS-IV seeks to further improve survival rate by intensifying therapy during the initial treatment phase while shortening treatment duration (6 versus 15 months of treatment). It is the first study of a pediatric population to evaluate the economic impact of two different treatment approaches.

Vincristine and dactinomycin are used in the treatment of all Wilms' tumor patients; doxorubicin is also administered to stage III and stage IV patients. NWTS-III showed that stage II Wilms' tumor patients did not benefit from flank irradiation whereas stage III children had similar outcomes whether they received 10 or 20 Gy. Chemotherapy is optimally begun within 5 days after surgery, whereas radiation therapy should be started within 10 days.

Using these approaches, survival at 4 years from diagnosis for patients treated on NWTS-III are as follows: stage I FH, 96.5%; stage II FH, 92.2%; stage III FH, 86.9%; and stage IV FH, 82.5%. Patients with unfavorable histology (UH) have only a 55–68% 4-year survival, depending on stage. Patients with recurrent Wilms' tumor have approximately a 50% salvage rate with surgery, radiation therapy, and chemotherapy (singly or in combination).

Future Considerations

Although progress in the treatment of Wilms' tumor has been extraordinary, important questions remain to be answered. Results of previous NWTS and International Society of Pediatric Oncology (SIOP) trials suggest that not all stage I Wilms' tumor patients need chemotherapy and that some might be adequately treated with surgery alone. Many questions are being raised about the role of prenephrectomy chemotherapy in the treatment of Wilms' tumor. Presurgical chemotherapy seems to decrease tumor rupture at resection but may unfavorably affect outcome by changing staging. Whether pulmonary radiation can be eliminated in metastatic pulmonary disease is also being investigated.

Coppes MJ et al: Genetic events in the development of Wilms' tumor. N Engl J Med 1994;331:586.

Green DM et al: Wilms' tumor (nephroblastoma, renal embryoma). In: *Principles and Practice of Pediatric Oncology.* Pizzo PA, Poplack DG (editors). JB Lippincott, 1993.

BONE TUMORS

Primary malignant bone tumors are uncommon in childhood. Osteosarcoma accounts for 60% of cases and is seen primarily in adolescents and young adults. Ewing's sarcoma is the second most common malignant tumor of bony origin. Both tumors have a male predominance.

The cardinal signs of bone tumor are pain at the site of involvement, often following slight trauma; mass formation; and fracture through an area of cortical bone destruction.

1. OSTEOSARCOMA

Although osteosarcoma is the sixth most common malignancy in childhood, it ranks third among adolescents and young adults. This peak occurrence during the adolescent growth spurt suggests a causal relationship between rapid bone growth and malignant transformation. Further evidence for this relationship is found in epidemiologic data showing patients with osteosarcoma to be taller than their peers, osteosarcoma occurring most frequently at sites where the greatest increase in length and size of bone occurs, and osteosarcoma occurring at an earlier age in girls than boys, corresponding to their earlier growth spurt. Long tubular bones are primarily affected. The distal femur accounts for more than 40% of cases, with the proximal tibia, proximal humerus, and mid and proximal femur following in frequency. Typically, osteosarcoma arises in a metaphysial location.

Radiographic findings show a permeative destruction of the normal bony trabecular pattern with indistinct margins. In addition, periosteal new bone formation and lifting of the bony cortex may create a Codman triangle. A soft tissue mass plus calcifications in a radial or "sunburst" pattern are frequently noted. Despite this rather characteristic radiographic appearance, a tissue sample is needed to confirm the diagnosis. Further radiographic studies to better define the extent of the primary tumor include CT scan or MRI (or both). A bone scan is useful for detecting "skip" lesions as well as distant bony metastasis (present in 10% of newly diagnosed patients). A chest CT scan is essential to asses the lung for metastatic nodules. Pulmonary metastasis is present in as many as 20% of patients at diagnosis and implies a poor prognosis.

Placement of the incision for biopsy of a bone tumor is of critical importance. A misplaced incision could preclude a limb salvage procedure and necessitate amputation. Biopsy is best performed by the surgeon who would carry out the definitive surgical procedure. Histologically, osteosarcoma is characterized by the presence of malignant sarcomatous stroma associated with the production of tumor osteoid.

Once the diagnosis of osteosarcoma is established, treatment can begin. Over 70% of patients treated with surgery alone develop pulmonary metastases within 6 months after surgery. This suggests that micrometastatic disease is present at diagnosis though not detectable radiographically. Adjuvant chemotherapy trials have shown disease-free survival of 55–85% after 3–10 years of follow-up.

Chemotherapy is often administered prior to definitive surgery (neoadjuvant chemotherapy). This allows for an early attack on micrometastatic disease. Presurgical chemotherapy may also shrink the tumor, facilitating a limb salvage procedure. Preoperative chemotherapy allows for detailed histologic evaluation of tumor response to the preoperative chemotherapeutic agents. If there is a poor histologic response, postoperative chemotherapy can be changed on a more rational basis. Chemotherapy may be administered intra-arterially or intravenously. Agents having efficacy in the treatment of osteosarcoma include doxorubicin, cisplatin, high-dose methotrexate, and ifosfamide. A multi-agent regimen is most frequently employed.

Amputation and limb salvage are equally effective in achieving local control of osteosarcoma. Contraindications to limb-sparing surgery include major involvement of the neurovascular bundle by tumor; immature skeletal age, particularly for lower extremity tumors; infection in the region of the tumor; inappropriate biopsy site; and extensive muscle involvement that would result in a poor functional outcome.

Postsurgical chemotherapy is generally continued until the patient has received 1 year of treatment. Relapses are rare beyond 3 years. Histologic response to neoadjuvant chemotherapy is an excellent predictor of outcome. Patients having 90% tumor necrosis have a 70–90% long-term disease free survival.

2. EWING'S SARCOMA

Ewing's sarcoma accounts for only 10% of primary malignant bone tumors; there are fewer than

200 new cases a year in the United States. It is a disease primarily of white males and almost never affects blacks.

The radiographic appearance of Ewing's sarcoma overlaps with osteosarcoma, although Ewing's sarcoma usually involves the diaphyses of long bones. The central axial skeleton gives rise to 40% of Ewing tumors.

Ewing's sarcoma is a "small, round, blue cell" malignancy. Although most commonly a tumor of bone, it may also occur in soft tissue (extraosseous Ewing's sarcoma or peripheral neuroepithelioma). Histologically, it consists of sheets of undifferentiated cells with hyperchromatic nuclei, well-defined cell borders, and scanty cytoplasm. Necrosis is common. The differential diagnosis includes rhabdomyosarcoma, lymphoma, and neuroblastoma. Electron microscopy, immunocytochemistry, and cytogenetics may be necessary to confirm the diagnosis. A generous tissue biopsy is often necessary for diagnosis but should not delay starting chemotherapy.

A consistent cytogenetic abnormality (t11;22) has been identified in Ewing's sarcoma and in peripheral neuroepitheliomas. These tumors also express the proto-oncogene c-*myc*. Research suggests that these tumors arise from postganglionic parasympathetic cholinergic neurons.

Evaluation of a patient diagnosed with Ewing's sarcoma should include CT or MRI (or both) of the primary lesion to define the extent of local disease as precisely as possible. This is imperative for planning future surgical procedures or radiation therapy. Metastatic disease is present in 25% of patients at diagnosis. The lung (38%), bone (particularly the spine) (31%), and the bone marrow (11%) are the most common sites for metastasis. CT of the chest, bone scanning, and bilateral bone marrow aspirates and biopsies are all essential to the staging work-up.

Therapy usually commences with the administration of chemotherapy and is followed by local control measures. Depending on many factors, including the primary site of the tumor and response to chemotherapy, local control could be achieved by surgery, radiation therapy, or a combination of these methods. Following local control, chemotherapy continues for 1 year. Agents that have been shown to have efficacy in the treatment of Ewing's sarcoma include dactinomycin, vincristine, doxorubicin, cyclophosphamide, etoposide and ifosfamide. Modern therapy uses combinations of these drugs.

Patients with small localized primaries can expect a 50–70% long-term disease-free survival. For patients with metastatic disease and large pelvic primaries, survival is poor. Autologous bone marrow transplantation is being investigated for the management of these high-risk patients.

Davis AM et al: Prognostic factors in osteosarcoma: A critical review. J Clin Oncol 1994;12:423.

Horowitz ME et al: Ewing's sarcoma family of tumors: Ewing's sarcoma of bone and soft tissue and the peripheral primitive neuroectodermal tumors. In: *Principles and Practice of Pediatric Oncology.* Pizzo PA, Poplack DG (editors). Lippincott, 1993.

Link MP et al: Osteosarcoma. In: *Principles and Practice of Pediatric Oncology.* Pizzo PA, Poplack DG (editors). Lippincott, 1993.

RHABDOMYOSARCOMA

Essentials of Diagnosis

- Painless, progressively enlarging mass; proptosis; chronic drainage (nasal, aural, sinus, vaginal); cranial nerve palsies.
- Urinary obstruction, constipation, hematuria.

General Considerations

Rhabdomyosarcoma is the most common soft tissue sarcoma occurring in pediatrics and accounts for 10% of solid tumors in childhood. The peak incidence occurs between 2 and 5 years of age, with 70% of children diagnosed before 10 years of age. A second smaller peak is seen in adolescents with extremity tumors. Males are affected more commonly than females (1.4:1).

Arising from embryonic mesenchymal cells, rhabdomyosarcoma can occur anywhere in the body. When rhabdomyosarcoma imitates striated muscle, and cross-striations are seen by light microscopy, the diagnosis is straightforward. Sometimes immunocytochemistry, electron microscopy, or chromosomal analysis are necessary to make the diagnosis. Rhabdomyosarcoma is further classified into subtypes based on pathologic features: embryonal (63%), of which botryoid is a variant; alveolar (19%); pleomorphic, which is seen in adults (1%); undifferentiated sarcoma (10%); and other (7%). These subtypes occur in characteristic locations and have different metastatic potentials and outcomes (Table 27–7).

Although the pathogenesis of rhabdomyosarcoma is unknown, in rare cases a genetic predisposition has been determined. The Li-Fraumeni syndrome is an inherited mutation of the p53 tumor suppressor gene that results in a high risk of bone and soft tissue sarcomas in childhood plus breast cancer and other malignant neoplasms before age 45. A characteristic chromosomal translocation (t2;13) has been described in alveolar rhabdomyosarcoma, which may also shed light on the biology of this tumor.

Clinical Findings

A. Symptoms and Signs: The presenting signs and symptoms of rhabdomyosarcoma result from disturbances of normal body function due to tumor growth (Table 27–7). For example, orbital rhabdomyosarcoma presents as proptosis, while rhab-

Table 27–7. Characteristics of rhabdomyosarcoma.

Primary Site	Frequency	Symptoms and Signs	Three-Year Disease-Free Survival (Based on IRS-II)	Predominant Pathologic Subtype
Head and neck	**40%**			Embryonal
Orbit	10%	Proptosis	93%	
Parameningeal	20%	Cranial nerve palsies; aural or sinus obstruction with or without drainage	71%	
Other	10%	Painless, progressively enlarging mass	69%	
Genitourinary	**20%**			Embryonal (botryoid variant in bladder and vagina)
Bladder and prostate	12%	Hematuria, urinary obstruction	64–80%	
Vagina and uterus	2%	Pelvic mass, vaginal discharge	60–80%	
Paratesticular	6%	Painless mass	64–80%	
Extremities	**20%**	Adolescents, swelling of affected body part	56%	Alveolar (50%), undifferentiated
Trunk	**10%**	Mass	57%	Alveolar, undifferentiated

IRS = Intergroup Rhabdomyosarcoma Study.

domyosarcoma of the bladder can present with hematuria, urinary frequency, or a pelvic mass.

B. Imaging: A plain film as well as a CT scan or MRI should be obtained to determine the exact extent of the primary tumor and to assess regional lymph nodes. A lung CT is obtained to rule out pulmonary metastasis, the most common site of metastatic disease at diagnosis. A skeletal survey and a bone scan are obtained to determine whether bony metastasis is present. Bilateral bone marrow biopsies and aspirates are obtained to rule out bone marrow infiltration. Additional studies may be warranted in certain sites. For example, in parameningeal primaries, a lumbar puncture is performed to evaluate cerebrospinal fluid for tumor cells.

Treatment

Optimal management and treatment of children with rhabdomyosarcoma is complex and requires combined-modality therapy. When feasible, the tumor should be excised but, because of site of origin and size of tumor, this is seldom possible. When only partial tumor resection is feasible, the operative procedure is usually limited to biopsy and sampling of lymph nodes. The role of debulking of unresectable tumor is unclear. Chemotherapy can often convert an inoperable tumor to a resectable one. A second-look procedure to remove residual disease and confirm the clinical response to chemotherapy and radiation therapy is generally performed around week 20 of therapy.

Radiation therapy is an effective method of local

tumor control for both microscopic and gross residual disease. It is generally administered to all patients, the only exception being group I nonalveolar rhabdomyosarcoma.

Chemotherapy is administered to all patients with rhabdomyosarcoma, even when their tumor is fully resected at diagnosis. The exact regimen and duration of chemotherapy is determined by primary site, group, and TNM classification. Vincristine, dactinomycin, and cyclophosphamide have shown the greatest efficacy in the treatment of rhabdomyosarcoma.

Prognosis

The extent of the rhabdomyosarcoma at diagnosis, the primary site, pathologic subtype, and response to treatment all influence long-term disease-free survival from the time of diagnosis. Children with localized disease in a favorable site have a 93% 3-year disease-free survival rate, whereas children with metastatic disease at presentation (group IV) have a poor outcome (Table 27–7).

Newer treatment strategies for high-risk patients include different drug combinations and dosing schedules, hematopoietic growth factor support, hyperfractionated radiation therapy, and autologous bone marrow transplantation.

Crist W et al: The Third Intergroup Rhabdomyosarcoma Study. J Clin Oncol 1995;13:610.
Mandell LR: Ongoing progress in the treatment of childhood rhabdomyosarcoma. Oncology 1993;7:71.
Maurer HM: The intergroup rhabdomyosarcoma study-II. Cancer 1993;71:1904.

Raney RB et al: Rhabdomyosarcoma and the undifferentiated sarcomas. In: *Principles and Practice of Pediatric Oncology.* Pizzo PA, Poplack DG (editors). JB Lippincott, 1993.

RETINOBLASTOMA

Retinoblastoma is a neuroectodermal malignancy arising from embryonic retinal cells and accounts for 3% of malignant disease in children under 15 years of age. It is the most common intraocular tumor in pediatric patients and causes 5% of cases of childhood blindness. There are 200–300 new cases per year in the United States. This is a malignancy of early childhood, with 90% of tumors diagnosed before 5 years of age. Bilateral disease typically presents at a younger age (median age 14 months) than unilateral disease (median age 23 months).

Retinoblastoma is the prototype of hereditary cancers due to mutation in the retinoblastoma gene (RB1), which is located on the long arm of chromosome 13 (13q14). This gene is a tumor suppressor gene or anti-oncogene which normally controls cellular growth. When the gene is inactivated, cellular growth is uncontrolled. Uncontrolled cell growth leads to tumor formation. Inactivation of both RB1 alleles within the same cell are required for tumor formation.

Retinoblastoma is known to arise in heritable and nonheritable forms. Based on the different clinical characteristics of the two forms, Knudson proposed a two-mutation hypothesis for retinoblastoma tumor development. He postulated that two independent events were necessary for a cell to acquire tumor potential. Mutations at the RB1 locus can be inherited or arise spontaneously. In heritable cases, the first mutation arises during gametogenesis, either spontaneously (90%) or through transmission from a parent (10%). This mutation is present in every retinal cell as well as all other somatic and germ cells. Ninety percent of persons who carry this germline mutation will develop retinoblastoma. For tumor formation, the loss of the second RB1 allele within a cell must occur; loss of only one allele is insufficient for tumor formation. The second mutation occurs in a somatic (retinal) cell. In nonheritable cases (60%), both mutations arise in a somatic cell after gametogenesis has taken place.

Clinical Findings

A. Symptoms and Signs: Children with retinoblastoma generally come to medical attention while the tumor is still confined to the globe. Although congenital, retinoblastoma is not usually detected until it has grown to a considerable size. Leukocoria (white pupillary reflex) is the most common manifestation (60% of cases). Parents may note an unusual appearance of the eye or an asymmetry of the eyes in a photograph. The differential diagnosis of leukocoria includes *Toxocara canis* granuloma, astrocytic hamartoma, retinopathy of prematurity, Coats' disease, and persistent hyperplastic primary vitreous. Strabismus (20% of cases) is seen when tumor involves the macula and central vision is lost. Rarely (7% of cases), a painful red eye with glaucoma, a hyphema, or proptosis is the initial manifestation. A single focus or multiple foci of tumor may be seen in one or both eyes at diagnosis. Bilateral involvement occurs in 20–30% of children.

B. Evaluation: A child suspected of retinoblastoma must have a detailed ophthalmologic examination under anesthesia. An ophthalmologist makes the diagnosis of retinoblastoma by the appearance of the tumor within the eye without pathologic confirmation. A white to creamy pink mass protruding into the vitreous suggests the diagnosis; intraocular calcifications and vitreous seeding are virtually pathognomonic for retinoblastoma. A CT of the orbits detects intraocular calcification, evaluates the optic nerve for tumor infiltration, and detects extraocular extension of tumor. Metastatic disease of the marrow and meninges can be ruled out with a bone marrow aspirate and biopsy plus cerebrospinal fluid cytology. Under some circumstances, a bone scan or CT of the liver are indicated.

Treatment

Each eye is treated according to the potential for useful vision, and every attempt is made to preserve vision. The choice of therapy depends on the size, location, and number of intraocular lesions. Absolute indications for enucleation include no vision, neovascular glaucoma, inability to examine the treated eye, and inability to control tumor growth with conservative treatment. External beam irradiation is the mainstay of therapy. A total dose of 35–45 Gy is administered. Cryotherapy, photocoagulation, and radioactive plaques can be used for local tumor control. Patients with metastatic disease also receive chemotherapy.

Children with retinoblastoma confined to the retina (whether unilateral or bilateral) have an excellent prognosis, with 5-year survival rates greater than 90%. Mortality is directly correlated with extent of optic nerve involvement, orbital extension of tumor, and massive choroid invasion. Patients who have disease in the optic nerve beyond the lamina cribrosa have only a 40% 5-year survival rate. Patients with meningeal or metastatic spread rarely survive, though intensive chemotherapy and autologous bone marrow transplants have produced long-term survivors.

Patients with the germinal mutation (heritable form) have a significant risk for developing second malignant neoplasms. Second tumors develop within as well as outside the field of radiation. Tumors also develop in patients who have received no radiation therapy. Sarcomas are the most commonly occurring second malignant neoplasm, with osteosarcoma accounting for 40% of such tumors. The risk for a second neoplasm is 10% at 10 years from diagnosis in patients who did not receive radiation therapy and 20% in patients who received external-beam radiation therapy. The risk continues to increase over time. Although radiation contributes to the risk, it is the presence of the retinoblastoma gene itself that is primarily responsible for the development of nonocular tumors in these patients.

Donaldson SS et al: Retinoblastoma. In: *Principles and Practice of Pediatric Oncology.* Pizzo PA, Poplack DG (editors). JB Lippincott, 1993.

Doz F et al: The role of chemotherapy in orbital involvement of retinoblastoma. Cancer 1994;84:722.

Gallie BL: Retinoblastoma gene mutations in human cancer. N Engl J Med 1994;330:786.

HEPATIC TUMORS

The majority (57%) of liver tumors found in childhood are malignant. Ninety percent of hepatic malignancies are either hepatoblastoma or hepatocellular carcinoma. Hepatoblastomas are somewhat more frequent than hepatocellular carcinomas (51% versus 39%). A comparison of the features of these hepatic malignancies is found in Table 27–8. Of the benign tumors, 60% are hamartomas or vascular tumors such as hemangiomas.

Children with hepatic tumors usually come to medical attention because of an enlarging abdomen. Approximately 10% of hepatoblastomas are first discovered on a routine examination. Anorexia, weight loss, vomiting, and abdominal pain are seen more commonly in hepatocellular carcinoma. Serum alpha-fetoprotein is often elevated and is an excellent indicator for following response to treatment.

Imaging studies should include an abdominal ultrasound as well as an abdominal CT scan or MRI. Malignant tumors have a diffuse hyperechoic pattern on ultrasonography, whereas benign tumors are usually poorly echoic. Vascular lesions contain areas with varying degrees of echogenicity. Ultrasound is also useful for imaging the hepatic veins, portal veins, and inferior vena cava. CT scanning and in particular MRI are important for defining the extent of tumor within the liver. CT scanning of the chest and bone scan should be obtained to evaluate for metastatic spread.

The prognosis for children with hepatic malignancies depends on the tumor type and the resectability of the tumor. Complete resectability is essential for survival. Chemotherapy can decrease the size of most hepatic malignancies. Following biopsy of the lesion, neoadjuvant chemotherapy is administered prior to attempting a complete surgical resection. Chemotherapy can often convert an inoperable tumor to a completely resectable one as well as eradicate metastatic disease. Approximately 50–60% of hepatoblastomas are fully resectable, while only one third of hepatocellular carcinomas can be completely removed. Even with complete resection, only one-third of patients with hepatocellular carcinoma are long-term survivors. Continuous-infusion doxorubicin over 96 hours and cisplatin have been shown to be effective agents for hepatic malignancies. Other drugs that have demonstrated benefit include fluorouracil and cyclophosphamide. Etoposide, carboplatin, and ifosfamide are under investigation. Liver transplantation is being investigated for patients

Table 27–8. Comparison of hepatoblastoma and hepatocellular carcinoma in childhood.

	Hepatoblastoma	Hepatocellular Carcinoma
Median age at presentation	1 year (0–3 years)	12 years (5–18 years)
Male:female ratio	1.7:1	1.4:1
Associated conditions	Hemihypertrophy, Beckwith-Wiedemann syndrome	Hepatitis B virus infection, hereditary tyrosinemia, biliary cirrhosis, α_1-antitrypsin deficiency
Pathologic features	Fetal or embryonal cells; mesenchymal component (30%)	Large pleomorphic tumor cells and tumor giant cells
Solitary hepatic lesion	80%	20–50%
Unique features at diagnosis	Osteopenia (20–30%), isosexual precocity (3%)	Hemoperitoneum, polycythemia
Laboratory features Hyperbilirubinemia Elevated AFP Abnormal liver function tests	5% 60–70% 15–30%	25% 50% 30–50%

AFP = alpha-fetoprotein.

whose tumors cannot be completely resected following chemotherapy.

Greenberg M et al: Hepatic tumors. In: *Principles and Practice of Pediatric Oncology.* Pizzo PA, Poplack DG: (editors). JB Lippincott, 1993.

LANGERHANS CELL HISTIOCYTOSIS

Langerhans cell histiocytosis (formerly called histiocytosis X) is a rare and poorly understood spectrum of disorders. It can occur as an isolated lesion or as widespread systemic disease involving virtually any body site. Eosinophilic granuloma, Hand-Schuller-Christian disease, and Letterer-Siwe disease are all syndromes encompassed by this disorder. Langerhans cell histiocytosis is not a true malignancy but a reactive proliferation of normal histiocytic cells, perhaps resulting from an immunoregulatory defect.

The distinctive pathologic feature is proliferation of histiocytic cells beyond what would be seen in a normal inflammatory process. Langerhans histiocytes have typical features: On light microscopy, the nuclei are deeply indented ("coffee bean"–shaped) and elongate, and the cytoplasm is pale, distinct, and abundant. Additional diagnostic characteristics include Birbeck granules on electron microscopy, expression of CD1 on the cell surface, and positive immunostaining for S-100 protein.

Clinical Findings

Because Langerhans cell histiocytosis encompasses a broad spectrum of diseases, its presentation can be variable, from a single asymptomatic lesion to widely disseminated disease. Although it is clearly a continuum of disease, patients tend to present in distinct ways. Some present primarily with lesions limited to bone. Occasionally found incidentally on radiographs obtained for other reasons, these lesions are well-demarcated and frequently found in the skull, clavicles, ribs, and vertebrae. Lesions can be painful. Lesions are often solitary, but patients may develop other bone lesions and even visceral involvement.

Bony lesions, fever, weight loss, otitis media, exophthalmos, and diabetes insipidus are seen in a small number of children with the disease. Formerly called Hand-Schüller-Christian disease, this multifocal disease commonly presents with generalized symptoms and organ dysfunction.

Disseminated Langerhans cell histiocytosis (formerly referred to as Letterer-Siwe disease) typically presents in children under 2 years of age with a seborrheic skin rash, fever, weight loss, lymphadenopathy, hepatosplenomegaly, and hematologic abnormalities.

Treatment and Prognosis

The outcome of Langerhans cell histiocytosis is extremely variable, but the process usually resolves spontaneously.

Isolated lesions may need no therapy at all. However intralesional corticosteroids, curettage, or low-dose radiation therapy are useful local treatment measures for symptomatic lesions.

Multifocal disease is often treated with systemic chemotherapy. Prednisone, vinblastine. or etoposide, singly or in combination, can be given repeatedly or continuously until lesions heal and then is reduced and finally stopped. Single-agent therapy is as effective as multiagent therapy.

Patients with localized disease have an excellent prognosis. Multifocal disease is less predictable, but most cases resolve without sequelae. Age and degree of organ involvement are the most important prognostic factors. Infants with disseminated disease tend to do poorly, with mortality rates approaching 50%. New treatment approaches should be considered in this patient group. Cyclosporine is promising for this purpose.

Willman CL et al: Langerhans'-cell histiocytosis (histiocytosis X): A clonal proliferative disease. N Engl J Med 1994;331:154.

LATE EFFECTS OF PEDIATRIC CANCER THERAPY

Late effects of treatment by surgery, radiation, and chemotherapy have been identified in survivors of pediatric cancer. In some studies, up to 40% of survivors of pediatric cancer will have some disability secondary to treatment. Virtually any organ system can demonstrate sequelae related to previous cancer therapy. This has necessitated the creation of specialized oncology clinics whose function it is to identify and treat these patients.

Growth Complications

Growth complications of cancer therapy in the pediatric survivor are secondary to direct damage of endocrine tissue. Children with ALL, brain tumors, orbital tumors, and nasopharyngeal cancers who have received radiation are at highest risk.

Up to 90% of patients who receive greater than 30 Gy of radiation to the CNS will show evidence of growth hormone deficiency within 2 years. Approximately 50% of children receiving 24 Gy will have growth hormone problems. The effects of cranial radiation appear to be age-related, with children under 5 years at the time of therapy being particularly vulnerable. These patients may benefit from growth hormone therapy. There is currently no evidence that such therapy causes a recurrence of cancer.

Spinal radiation inhibits vertebral body growth. In 30% of such individuals, standing heights may be less than the fifth percentile. Asymmetric exposure of the spine to radiation may result in scoliosis. Chemotherapy alone may result in an attenuation of linear growth. This, however, is usually temporary, as a period of catch-up occurs when the drugs are discontinued.

Growth should be monitored closely. Follow-up studies should include height, weight, growth velocity, scoliosis examination, and, when indicated, growth hormone testing.

Endocrine Complications

In addition to growth hormone deficiency, prepubertal children given cranial radiation may experience early puberty secondary to premature activation of the hypothalamic-pituitary-gonadal axis. This results in premature closure of the epiphyses, with decreased growth and height. This sequela appears to be more common in girls. Luteinizing hormone analogue along with growth hormone is used to halt early puberty and facilitate continued growth.

Thyroid dysfunction is common in children receiving radiation therapy to the neck and those with brain tumors who receive greater than 30 Gy. Up to 65–90% of patients receiving more than 25–30 Gy to the neck region will develop hypothyroidism. The average time to develop thyroid dysfunction is 12 months after exposure, but dysfunction can occur as early as 6 months or as late as 7 years following radiation. Although signs and symptoms of hypothyroidism may be present, many patients will have a normal T_4 level with elevated TSH. These individuals should be considered for thyroid hormone replacement since persistent stimulation of the thyroid from an elevated TSH may predispose to thyroid nodules and carcinomas.

Gonadal dysfunction in males is usually the result of radiation to the testes, which can damage the germinal epithelium, producing azoospermia. Radiation to the testes can also produce Leydig cell damage with subsequent low testosterone levels and delayed sexual development. Patients who receive testicular radiation as part of their therapy for ALL, abdominal radiation for Hodgkin's disease, or total body irradiation in bone marrow transplantation are at highest risk. In boys, alkylating agents such as mechlorethamine and cyclophosphamide can also interfere with male gonadal function, resulting in oligospermia or azoospermia, low testosterone levels and abnormal FSH and LH levels. Determination of testicular size, semen analysis, and measurement of testosterone, FSH, and LH levels will help identify abnormalities in patients at risk.

Exposure of the ovaries during abdominal radiation may result in failure to undergo menarche, increased FSH and LH levels, and low estrogen levels. Girls given total body irradiation as preparation for bone marrow transplantation are at particularly high risk. Girls receiving craniospinal radiation for ALL (18–24 Gy) may also develop delayed menses and are at risk for early menopause. In patients at highest risk for development of gonadal complications, a detailed menstrual history should be obtained, and FSH and estrogen levels should be monitored if indicated.

There is no study to date that confirms an increased risk of miscarriage or spontaneous abortion, stillbirths or premature births, and major and minor congenital malformations in offspring of childhood cancer survivors. Women who have received abdominal radiation and who develop uterine vascular insufficiency or fibrosis of the abdominal and pelvic musculature or uterus may have an increased risk of perinatal death or low-birth-weight premature infants and should be considered high-risk pregnancies.

Cardiopulmonary Complications

Several chemotherapeutic agents are known to cause pulmonary dysfunction as a late effect: bleomycin, the nitrosoureas, cyclophosphamide, methotrexate, and busulfan. Bleomycin has been implicated most frequently in chemotherapy-related lung injury. Ten percent of patients who receive greater than 400 U (cumulative dose) of this drug will have pulmonary toxicity, which takes the form of pulmonary fibrosis. Pulmonary function tests in patients with chemotherapy-induced toxicity show restrictive lung disease, with decreased carbon monoxide diffusion and small lung volumes. Individuals exposed to this drug should be counseled to refrain from smoking and to give proper notification of the drug history if they should require general anesthesia.

Cardiac complications are usually due to anthracycline exposure (daunorubicin, doxorubicin), which destroys myocytes and leads to inadequate myocardial growth as the child ages. Inadequate left ventricular mass and decreased function can occur. Long-term survivors can present with arrhythmias or congestive heart failure. The latter is seen in at least 5% of patients who have received greater than 550 mg/m^2 of anthracyclines (cumulative dose). In a recent study, complications from these agents appeared 6–19 years following administration of the drugs. Pregnant women who have received anthracyclines should be followed up closely for signs and symptoms of congestive heart failure, since pregnancy is associated with an increase in intravascular volume.

Radiation therapy to the mediastinal region, which is common as part of therapy for Hodgkin's disease, has been linked to an increase risk of coronary artery disease and chronic restrictive pericarditis may also occur in these patients.

Current recommendations include an echocardiogram and electrocardiogram every 2–3 years in patients who have received anthracyclines. Closer follow-up may be indicated for those who have received more than 500 mg/m^2 of these drugs. Holter monitoring, exercise testing, or gated radionuclide angiography is indicated in patients who have received large cumulative doses, have a history of cardiac dysfunction, have had mediastinal radiation, or who were treated with anthracyclines under 4 years of age.

Renal Complications

Most of the renal long-term side effects stem from chemotherapy. Patients who have received cisplatin therapy may develop an abnormal glomerular filtration rate and persistent tubular dysfunction with hypomagnesemia. Alkylating agents such as cyclophosphamide and ifosfamide can cause hemorrhagic cystitis, which may continue after chemotherapy has been terminated. Patients with a history of hemorrhagic cystitis may also be at risk for bladder carcinoma. Ifosfamide can also cause Fanconi's syndrome (proteinuria, glycosuria, phosphaturia with hypophosphatemia, aminoaciduria, and hyposthenuria), which may result in clinical rickets if adequate phosphate replacement is not given.

Patients who are seen in long-term follow-up and who have received nephrotoxic agents should be monitored with urinalysis, appropriate electrolyte profiles, and blood pressure. Urine collection for creatinine clearance or renal ultrasound may be indicated in individuals with suspected renal toxicity. Cystoscopy and cytologic study of urine sediment are recommended in patients with suspected malignancy.

Neuropsychologic & Psychosocial Complications

Pediatric cancer survivors who have received cranial radiation for ALL or brain tumors appear to be at greatest risk for neuropsychologic problems. The severity of cranial radiation effects varies vary among individual patients and depends on the dose and dose schedule, the size and location of the radiation field, the amount of time elapsed after treatment, the age of the child when the radiation was administered, and the gender of the child. Girls may be more susceptible than boys to CNS toxicity, since they have more rapid brain growth and development during childhood.

The main effects of CNS radiation appear to be related to nonverbal tasks such as visual processing speed, visual motor integration, sequencing ability, and short-term memory.

Psychosocial dysfunction can be traced to absenteeism from school, which is seen frequently in pediatric cancer patients. One recent study found that leukemia survivors were perceived as having more behavior problems and as being less socially competent than the sibling control group. Adolescent survivors of cancer demonstrate an increased sense of physical fragility and vulnerability which manifests as hypochondriasis or phobic behaviors.

Pediatric cancer survivors may require ongoing counseling or other psychologic interventions once they have completed therapy. Children who have received CNS radiation may also require learning assistance in school, particularly in mathematics.

Second Malignancies

Approximately 3–12% of children treated for cancer will develop a new cancer within 20 years of their first diagnosis. This is a tenfold increased incidence when compared with age-matched controls. Exposure to alkylating agents and radiation therapy are risk factors in most of second malignancies. There are also genetic and familial conditions that are associated with an increased risk of second malignancies. These include Li-Fraumeni syndrome, retinoblastoma, neurofibromatosis, nevoid basal cell carcinoma, and having a sibling with cancer.

Recently, acute nonlymphocytic leukemia has been reported as a second malignancy in patients treated with mitotic inhibitors such as etoposide and teniposide for ALL. The frequency of administration of the drug and the total dose may be important factors in the development of this secondary leukemia.

Children receiving radiation therapy as part of treatment for ALL appear to be at an increased risk for developing brain tumors as a secondary malignancy. The population at highest risk appears to be those patients who were 5 years old or less at the time of diagnosis.

Blatt J, Copeland DR, Bleyer WA: Late effects of childhood cancer and its treatment. In: *Principles and Practice of Pediatric Oncology.* Pizzo PA, Poplack DG (editors). Lippincott, 1993.

Copeland DR: Neuropsychological and psychosocial effects of childhood leukemia and its treatment. CA Cancer J Clin 1992;42:283.

Delaat CA, Lampkin BC: Long-term survivors of childhood cancer: Evaluation and identification of treatment. CA Cancer J Clin 1992;42:263.

Monteleone PM, Rzejewski C, Kelleher JF: Prevalence of hepatitis C in transfused children with cancer. Am J Pediatr Hematol Oncol 1994;16:309.

Mustieles C et al: Male gonadal function after chemotherapy in survivors of childhood malignancy. Med Pediatr Oncol 1995;24:347.

Neglia JP et al: Second neoplasms after acute lymphoblastic leukemia in childhood. N Engl J Med 1991;325:1330.

Steinherz LJ, Steinherz PG, Tan C: Cardiac failure and dysrhythmias 6–19 years after anthracycline therapy: A series of 15 patients. Med Pediatr Oncol 1995;24:352.

Immunodeficiency

Erwin W. Gelfand, MD, & Anthony R. Hayward, MD, PhD

Recurrent or severe infection is the most common symptom of immunodeficiency, but most children with recurrent minor infections do not have an immunodeficiency that is definable by currently available tests. Host defenses against infection depend mainly on excluding pathogens at surfaces, together with mechanical means to decontaminate them. Specific and nonspecific immune mechanisms are needed only after an organism gains access to the body. Specific immunity in this context consists of antibody and cell-mediated immunity (CMI). Nonspecific immune mechanisms include mechanical barriers, complement, phagocytes, and natural killer cells. Nonspecific mechanisms may be guided by specific responses, such as the ability of antibody to direct killing by natural killer cells or to promote phagocytosis by opsonizing bacteria.

Before investigating a patient for a defined primary immunodeficiency (most of which are rare), one should exclude the more common conditions that increase local susceptibility to infection, such as cystic fibrosis and conditions that interfere with the integrity of the skin or the normal flora of mucous membranes (Table 28–1). Common causes of secondary immunodeficiency (HIV infection, drugs, protein loss) must also be excluded.

NONSPECIFIC FACTORS IN RESISTANCE TO INFECTION

DEFECTS OF COMPLEMENT

The complement series of proteins are activated by IgG or IgM antibody bound to surfaces. The split products of C3 and C5 activation attract neutrophils, and C3b bound to the surface of bacteria opsonizes them for phagocytosis by neutrophils. Deficiencies of individual classic pathway factors (C1–C9) occur as autosomal recessive traits and are rare. Deficiencies

of factors 1, 4, and 2 are associated with immune complex disorders, particularly systemic lupus erythematosus, chronic glomerulonephritis, dermatomyositis, and cutaneous vasculitis. Primary deficiency of C3 interferes with the opsonization of bacteria by the classic and alternative pathways of complement activation and results in recurrent bacterial infections similar to those seen in antibody deficiency. Treatment is mostly with antibiotics. Serum levels of C3 are occasionally low enough in membranoproliferative glomerulonephritis with nephritic factor to increase susceptibility to infection. Deficiency of two of the alternative pathway factors may also occasionally predispose to recurrent bacterial infection.

C5, C6, C7, C8, and C9 deficiencies are associated with dissemination of neisserial infections, resulting in an increase of gonococcal arthritis in those with gonorrhea and a recurrence of meningitis in the survivors of meningococcal meningitis. Complement function should be screened with a hemolytic assay in patients with recurrent meningitis.

The serum "opsonizing defect" associated with Leiner's disease and originally attributed to C5a deficiency is now known to result from low plasma levels of mannan-binding protein. About 7% of the population has the defective gene. Affected infants can have recurrent bacterial infections in infancy, which tend to get better with age.

Hereditary angioedema is a rare disorder, which causes recurrent angioedema without itching or wheals, usually beginning in late childhood or adolescence. It results from C1 esterase inhibitor deficiency in which susceptibility to infection is not increased. Transmission is autosomal dominant. Affected persons typically have recurrent episodes of edema lasting 48–72 hours affecting the face or a limb. Edema affecting the bowel can be very painful. Laryngeal edema is life-threatening. Diagnosis is by measurement of esterase inhibitor levels in serum; those who are symptomatic have levels below 30%. C4 levels are often low. Danazol, a synthetic androgen, prevents attacks by increasing C1 inhibitor levels. The diagnosis is suggested by decreased activity

Table 28–1. Host defense mechanisms and examples of nonspecific defects.

Protection by	Defect
Intact skin	Burns, eczema, sinus tracks, indwelling catheters
Drainage	Auditory tube obstruction, cystic fibrosis, foreign body, urinary obstruction
Normal flora	Antibiotic-induced diarrhea, postantibiotic candidiasis

of whole complement, C4, and C2 and confirmed by direct assay of the C1 inhibitor.

Derkx HH et al: Inherited complement deficiency in children surviving tulminant meningococcal septic shock. Eur J Peds 1996;154:735.

Lipscombe RJ et al: Identical point mutation leading to low levels of mannose binding protein and poor C3b mediated opsonisation in Chinese and Caucasian populations. Immunol Lett 1992;32:253.

Ruddy S: Rheumatic diseases and inherited complement deficiencies. Bull Rheum Diseases 1996;45:6.

DEFECTS OF PHAGOCYTE FUNCTION

Useful phagocyte function requires that the marrow makes adequate numbers of neutrophils, which migrate to sites of inflammation, where they ingest and kill bacteria. Defects may exist at one or more levels. Neutropenia is described in Chapter 26.

1. CHEMOTAXIS DEFECTS

Defects of chemotaxis can result in progressive local infections without much pus formation. Examples of primary cellular abnormalities are Chédiak-Higashi syndrome (see Chapter 26) and leukocyte functional antigen (LFA-1) deficiency. Most chemotaxis defects are probably secondary. Burns; infections such as HIV, rubella, and influenza; metabolic and nutritional disorders, including diabetes mellitus; the hypophosphatemia associated with hyperalimentation; uremia; and a wide variety of other conditions can be associated with depressed motility of phagocytic cells. The association of **impaired neutrophil chemotaxis with hyperimmunoglobulinemia E** (levels are usually more than 2000 units IgE/mL), recurrent staphylococcal abscesses of the skin, eczema, and otitis media is clinically recognizable and sometimes described as Job's syndrome. These patients can have impaired CMI, and the disorder also occurs in some patients with AIDS. Treatment is symptomatic.

Other infections that occur in patients with chemotactic defects include furunculosis, subcutaneous abscesses, oral ulcers, gingivitis, and pneumonia. The pathogenesis of these associations is obscure. Familial chemotactic defects are reported, but these are the exception.

Hall RA et al: Fungal pulmonary abscess in an adult secondary to hyperimmunoglobulin E (Job's) syndrome. Ann Thorac Surg 1995;59:759.

Jung LK: Association of aberrant F-actin formation with defective leukocyte chemotaxis and recurrent pyoderma. Clin Immunol Immunopathol 1991;61:41.

Van Eendenburg JP, Smitt JH, Weening RS: Hyperimmunoglobulin E recurrent infection (Job's) syndrome. Br J Dermatol 1991;125:397.

2. BACTERIAL KILLING DEFECTS

Chronic granulomatous disease patients have recurrent infections of lymph nodes, liver, or bone with catalase-positive organism (mostly staphylococci, sometimes *Serratia, Nocardia,* or other opportunists). The patient's neutrophils fail to reduce nitroblue tetrazolium in the NBT test and fail to kill staphylococci in a bacterial killing test. X-linked recessive chronic granulomatous disease results from coding abnormalities of the gp91 membrane cytochrome b. Most autosomal recessive chronic granulomatous disease is due to abnormalities of the p47 or p67 proteins, which are functionally part of the cytochrome redox system.

Patients usually have staphylococcal infections in the first months of life and develop groin, cervical, or axillary abscesses requiring incision and drainage. The infections cause high neutrophil counts and fever and sometimes spread to cause osteomyelitis or lung or liver abscesses. Colitis, leading to diarrhea and slow growth, is common. The abscesses require drainage and appropriate antibiotics for lengthy courses (3 weeks or more). All forms of the disease appear to benefit from interferon-γ in doses of 0.1 mg/m^2 on 2 or more days per week. This does not correct the underlying defect. Long-term antibiotic treatment—either with trimethoprim-sulfamethoxazole or dicloxacillin—may be required, and good dental care is necessary because of the increased risk of gingivitis and periodontitis. Bacterial infections can usually be controlled by antibiotics. It is invasive fungal infections of lung and bone, especially by *Aspergillus,* that are most often fatal. Bone marrow transplantation has not been very successful because of difficulty in obtaining long-term engraftment of donor neutrophils. Patients with chronic granulomatous disease seem to have fewer abscesses as they grow older, so that the outlook for a working life is good for those who pass puberty.

Defective bacterial killing by neutrophils also results from deficiency of leukocyte glucose-6-phosphate dehydrogenase (G6PD), glutathione dehydrogenase, and other metabolic defects. The severity is variable. A bacterial killing test should be used to screen for these abnormalities, since the NBT test is not always abnormal.

Forehand JR, Johnston RB Jr: Chronic granulomatous disease: Newly defined molecular abnormalities explain disease variability and normal phagocyte physiology. Curr Opin Pediatr 1994;6:668.

Weening RS, Leitz GJ, Seger RA: Recombinant human interferon-gamma in patients with chronic granulomatous disease: European follow up study. Eur J Pediatr 1995;154:295.

3. LEUKOCYTE ADHESION DEFICIENCY

Patients present with infections ranging from progressive, necrotic periumbilical infections with onset in infancy to recurrent surface infections starting in adult life. The severity of the clinical picture depends on the underlying defect. Leukocytes, monocytes, and some activated T cells normally express cell surface adhesion molecules that have a common beta subunit and cell-specific but related alpha subunits. Defects or deficiency of the beta subunit (called CD18) results in defective expression of this entire family of proteins: LFA-1 (CD11a), Mac-1 (CD11b), and p150,95 (CD11c).

The infections are caused by a range of organisms. The neutrophil count is normal or high, but there is relatively little pus formation. In childhood, the infections are often around body orifices, but they also involve the skin, esophagus, and respiratory tract. Death in childhood is common. Other patients with a milder phenotype have survived for 20 or more years. Diagnosis is by phenotyping blood mononuclear cells for LFA-1 or Mac-1; this approach can also be used for antenatal diagnosis.

Treatment of infections is with antibiotics, and prophylactic antibiotics may suffice for the more mildly affected patients. Mixed but stable chimerism, sufficient to reduce the risk of infections, has followed bone marrow transplantation.

Thomas C et al: Results of allogeneic bone marrow transplantation in patients with leukocyte adhesion deficiency. Blood 1995;86:1629.

DEFICIENCIES OF SPECIFIC IMMUNITY

Defects of specific immunity are broadly subdivided into those affecting predominantly antibody formation, those affecting cellular immunity, and those in which both mechanisms are impaired. The classification in Table 28–2 is based on combinations of clinical and laboratory results and includes only the more common conditions. Family studies in which a mode of inheritance can be shown are the most secure basis for classification, and in a few instances the underlying single gene defect is known, as in adenosine deaminase and purine nucleoside phosphorylase deficiencies. Occasionally, as in ataxia-telangiectasia, the phenotypic features are sufficiently characteristic to facilitate recognition. The fact that most cases of immunodeficiency are still reported as "varied immunodeficiency, largely unclassified" indicates that major advances remain to be made.

Primary immunodeficiency diseases: Report of a WHO scientific group. Immunodefic Rev 1992;3:195.

IMMUNOGLOBULIN & ANTIBODY DEFICIENCY SYNDROME

1. HYPOGAMMAGLOBULINEMIA SYNDROMES

Patients with hypogammaglobulinemia usually present with recurrent or severe bacterial infection of the respiratory tract (sinusitis, otitis, pneumonia) or skin (cellulitis, abscesses). Without antibiotic treatment, these infections tend to spread to cause septicemia and meningitis. Infections usually start after 4 months of age, when passively acquired maternal IgG levels have declined and in "acquired" forms of

Table 28–2. Classification of defects of specific immunity.

Deficiency of immunoglobulin	Deficiency of all Ig's = hypogamma-globulinemia Congenital (sometimes with high IgM) Acquired Unclassified (common variable hypogammaglobulinemia) Selective immunoglobulin deficiency IgA deficiency IgG subclass deficiencies IgM deficiency Antibody deficiency with immunoglobulins
Deficiency of cell-mediated immunity	Purine nucleoside phosphorylase DiGeorge syndrome Cartilage-hair hypoplasia Unclassified (common variable immunodeficiency affecting cell-mediated immunity)
Deficiency of both antibody and cell-mediated immunity	Severe combined immunodeficiency (various types) Ataxia-telangiectasia Wiskott-Aldrich syndrome

antibody deficiency may not start until adult life. The infections are mostly caused by encapsulated bacteria but following courses of antibiotics, *Mycoplasma* strains such as *Ureaplasma* become important. Several types of hypogammaglobulinemia are distinguished on biochemical or genetic grounds (see Table 28–2) but their treatment is similar. Congenital X-linked agammaglobulinemia (XLA) occurs in about $1:10^5$ live births, and some of these boys have an asymmetric arthritis, mostly of the knee or ankle, at the time of diagnosis, which may resolve after adequate IgG replacement. These patients typically have little or no tonsil and adenoid tissue. The severity of infections varies, so the diagnosis may not be made for many years. XLA results from mutations in the B-cell tyrosine kinase gene and patients have few if any B cells in their blood, although they have normal blood lymphocyte counts. Carrier detection is available. Some of these patients have impaired growth due to primary or secondary deficiency of growth hormone.

Other types of hypogammaglobulinemia are a little more common and may develop at any age. The diagnosis of hypogammaglobulinemia based on low serum immunoglobulin levels for age with absence of serum isohemagglutinins and of antibody response to immunization. Causes of secondary hypogammaglobulinemia (nephrotic syndrome, HIV infection, and protein-losing enteropathy) should be excluded by measuring serum albumin.

Buzi F et al: X-linked agammaglobulinemia, growth hormone deficiency and delay of growth and puberty. Acta Paediatr 1994;83:99.

Kinnon C et al: Physical and genetic approaches to the isolation of the gene for X-linked agammaglobulinemia. Immunodeficiency 1995;5:179.

Immunodeficiency With High IgM Levels

Boys with immunodeficiency with high levels of IgM have low IgG and IgA levels, often with lymphadenopathy and episodes of neutropenia. The disease results from mutation in the CD40 ligand gene so that the patients' T cells are unable to switch their B cells from making IgM to IgG and IgA. CMI is also impaired so these patients have *Pneumocystis* infections, cryptosporidiosis of the biliary tree and intestine, sclerosing cholangitis, and a high incidence of biliary tract carcinomas. Children with autosomal recessive forms of hyper-IgM immunodeficiency have normal expression of CD40L.

Kroczek RA et al: Defective expression of CD40 ligand on T cells causes "X linked Immunodeficiency with Hyper IgM (XHIM)." Immunol Rev 1994;138:39.

Common Variable Immunodeficiency Syndromes

Patients with congenital or acquired antibody defi-

ciency syndromes not classified elsewhere are often included in this group, and they outnumber patients with all other types of antibody deficiency except selective IgA deficiency. Onset of the immunodeficiency may be at any age. Susceptibility to common variable immunodeficiency is inherited, linked with the same class III histocompatibility gene deletions (for C4 and 21-hydroxylase, on chromosome 6) as selective IgA deficiency, but the factors that precipitate expression of common variable immunodeficiency in susceptible individuals are not known. The circulating B cells of these patients are immature and do not generally differentiate normally in tissue culture.

Infections follow the patterns described for other types of antibody deficiency. Some patients have remarkably few infections despite longstanding, very low immunoglobulin levels. The laboratory findings are variable. Low levels of one or more immunoglobulin classes are associated with varying degrees of impairment of T-cell proliferative responses. Autoantibody formation, raised IgE levels, and positive immediate hypersensitivity skin reactions occur, as do neutropenia and thrombocytopenia. Almost all these patients have B cells in their blood, although their number may be low. Patients with hypogammaglobulinemia and patients with facial anomalies may have the immunodeficiency-chromosome instability-facial anomaly (ICF) syndrome where a satellite DNA methylation anomaly is associated with instability of the pericentromeric heterochromatin of, in particular, chromosomes 1, 9, and 16. Inheritance of this variant is probably autosomal recessive.

Jaffe JS et al: T-cell abnormalities in common variable immunodeficiency. Pediatr Res 1993;33(1 Suppl):S24 (see discussion on p S27).

Puck JM: Molecular basis for three X-linked immune disorders. Hum Mol Gen 1994;3:1457.

Smeets DF et al: ICF syndrome: A new case and review of the literature. Hum Genet 1994;94:240.

Sneller MC et al: NIH conference: New insights into common variable immunodeficiency. Ann Intern Med 1993;118:720.

Complications of Hypogammaglobulinemia

Many patients have B-cell hyperplasia in the gut. About 10% of patients develop diarrhea and malabsorption that may be severe enough to resemble Crohn's disease. Infection is the likeliest cause of the diarrhea, and efforts should be made to exclude treatable agents such as *Giardia lamblia* or *Cryptosporidium*. In adult life, the patients often develop gastric atrophy with achlorhydria, sometimes followed by pernicious anemia. Affected boys occasionally develop optic atrophy or ataxia, evolving slowly or rapidly into fatal encephalitis. Echoviruses have sometimes been isolated from their cerebrospinal fluid or brains at biopsy or necropsy. A smaller proportion develop a dermatomyositis-like syndrome, with prominent peripheral cyanosis and myopathy but little heliotrope coloration. There is an impression that both of these complications are less commonly seen now that much higher immunoglobulin replacements are given. There are reports of an increased rate of cancer in patients with antibody deficiency. The association is predominantly with lymphoreticular proliferation and may sometimes result from EBV infection. Lymphoreticular proliferations in hypogammaglobulinemic patients are not always malignant.

Filipovich AH et al: Lymphoproliferative disorders and other tumors complicating immunodeficiencies. Immunodeficiency 1994;5:91.

Rudge P: Encephalomyelitis in primary hypogammaglobulinemia. Brain 1996;119:1.

Treatment

Patients with hypogammaglobulinemia should have serum IgG replaced to protect against infection. IgG is usually given by intravenous infusions of specially prepared deaggregated IgG (200–600 mg/kg every 4 weeks). If intravenous treatment is very difficult in young children, they may be temporarily managed on intramuscular injections of IgG concentrate (0.6 mL/kg every 2–3 weeks). Some adults are managed more cheaply with subcutaneous infusions of the intramuscular IgG preparation, given overnight on several nights per week. The aim of treatment must be to avoid—or minimize progression of—chronic lung disease (bronchitis, bronchiectasis). Productive cough and purulent sputum or conjunctivitis must be taken seriously and antibiotics given until there has been radiologic and clinical resolution. *Mycoplasma* infections of the respiratory or urinary tract should be sought for and treated with doxycycline or other appropriate antibiotics.

Reactions to immunoglobulin infusions or injections are not uncommon, especially with the initial infusion. They include headache, back and limb pain, anxiety, and tightness of the chest. Signs are tachycardia, shivering, fever, and, in severe cases, shock. Reactions are frequent in some patients and rare in others; their occurrence is sporadic and not generally due to hypersensitivity (anti-IgA reactions may be an exception but are rare). Skin tests are not helpful. When indicated, immunoglobulin replacement should be maintained for life and the severity of the reactions limited by premedication with acetaminophen, an antihistamine, or intravenous hydrocortisone immediately before the infusion. Alternative brands of IgG should be tried if reactions persist despite premedication.

Buckley RH: Breakthroughs in the understanding and therapy of primary immunodeficiency. Pediatr Clin North Am 1994;41:665.

2. OTHER TYPES OF HYPOGAMMAGLOBULINEMIA

Transient Hypogammaglobulinemia

Infants' IgG levels fall during the first 4–5 months of life, as maternal IgG is diluted and catabolized. The physiologic trough that occurs before the infant's IgG production maintains adult levels is accentuated in premature and dysmature infants. IgG levels of 250–300 mg/dL lie within 2 SD of the mean at 3–4 months of age, and the diagnosis of transient hypogammaglobulinemia is often made in infants with infections and IgG levels in this range. Immunoglobulin levels should return to normal by 30 months of age, and the diagnosis can only be made retrospectively. The only diagnostic laboratory findings are of low IgG, with or without low IgA and IgM, and subsequent return to normal levels. Salivary IgA is generally detectable, and, despite the low immunoglobulin levels, antibody activity (isohemagglutinin or antidiphtheria or tetanus antibody) is present in serum. IgG antibody is generally made following immunization, and tests for cellular immunity are normal. No treatment is usually required for infants who make antibody following immunization other than appropriate antibiotics for bacterial infections. Infants with severe infection and hypogammaglobulinemia could rationally be given IgG injections, since maternal antibody to the infecting organism will be rapidly depleted, but this is rarely necessary. The prognosis for affected infants is excellent, provided they do not succumb to infection before normal immunity is achieved.

Selective Immunoglobulin Deficiencies

A. IgA Deficiency: This disorder occurs in about 1:800 whites and is by far the most common defect of specific immunity. Susceptibility is linked to HLA histocompatibility genes, perhaps because an autoimmune mechanism interferes with the differentiation of IgA B lymphocytes. Fifty percent or more of IgA-deficient subjects have no symptoms arising from the deficiency, perhaps because they can protect their mucosa adequately with IgG and IgM antibodies. Failure of antibody responses in the IgG2 subclass is reported in many symptomatic patients. When symptoms are present, they are predominantly upper respiratory tract infections or diarrhea. There are also strong associations with inflammatory bowel disease, allergy (mainly respiratory and gut), and autoimmune disorders (thyroiditis, arthritis, vitiligo, thrombocytopenia, and diabetes).

The serum IgA is less than 5 mg/dL in selective IgA deficiency, and below −2 SD from the age-specific mean in "partial IgA deficiency." Serum IgM and IgG are normal, as is cellular immunity. The selective lack of IgA antibody responses and the presence of normal antibody responses in other immunoglobulin classes distinguish IgA deficiency from unclassified variable immunodeficiency. IgA has a short half-life in serum, and replacement is impractical. It is conceivable but unproved that colostrum feeding could modify severe gut symptoms. Symptomatic IgA-deficient subjects who are also IgG2-deficient have sometimes been treated with IgG replacement. This approach has been both advocated and condemned on theoretical grounds but without controlled data. A subset of IgA-deficient patients make antibodies to IgA, which are an important cause of transfusion reactions. Most IgA-deficient patients manage reasonably well with antibiotics only; atopic or autoimmune symptoms should be treated conventionally.

French MA, Denis KA, Dawkins R, Peter JB: Severity of infections in IgA deficiency: Correlation with decreased serum antibodies to pneumococcal polysaccharides and deceased serum IgG2 and/or IgG4. Clin Exp Immunol 1995;100:47.
Koskinen S, Tolo H, Hirvonen M, Koistenen J: Long-term follow-up of anti-IgA antibodies in healthy IgA-deficient adults. J Clin Immunol 1995;15:194.

B. Other Selective Subclass Deficiencies:

The possibility that deficiency of an IgG subclass might predispose to recurrent upper respiratory tract infections in patients who have normal serum immunoglobulin levels is still debated. Subclass levels are usually obtained on patients whose total IgG is in the normal or low normal range who have recurrent bacterial infections, particularly of the respiratory tract. It can be difficult to be confident of an immunoglobulin subclass deficiency because the levels are age dependent. The IgG heavy chain genes on chromosome 11 (grouped with IgG1 close to IgG3 and IgG2 close to IgG4) are usually normal in subclass deficiencies. Normally, IgG1 comprises over 60% of total IgG and IgG2 over 10%. IgG3 accounts for about 5%, and IgG4 may be undetectable in up to 20% of healthy persons. When IgG1 is deficient, IgG2 and IgG3 are generally low also, giving the clinical picture of hypogammaglobulinemia. IgG1 and IgG2 contain much of the antibody to capsular polysaccharides. IgG2 (and IgG4) deficiency is also associated with IgA deficiency. IgG3 deficiency is less common but has been incriminated in subjects with antibody deficiency syndromes with normal total IgG or IgG1 subclass levels. Even in adults it has been difficult to establish a link between IgG subclass deficiencies and any consistent pattern of infections. IgG replacement should be reserved for patients with defects of antibody production; many patients are managed with antibiotics alone.

Selective deficiencies of IgM, IgE, and kappa or lambda light chains due to gene deletions may be symptomless and are very rare. Selective IgM deficiency is reported in Bloom's syndrome and, in adults, predisposes to septicemia. Since IgM replacement is impractical on a long-term basis, reliance is placed mainly on antibiotics.

Avanzini MA et al: Qualitative and quantitative analyses of the antibody response elicited by *Haemophilus influenzae* type b capsular polysaccharide-tetanus toxoid conjugates in adults with IgG subclass deficiencies and frequent infections. Clin Exp Immunol 1994;96:54.
Herrod HG: Management of the patient with IgG subclass deficiency and/or selective antibody deficiency. Ann Allergy 1993;70:3.
Hoeger PH, Niggemann B, Haeuser G: Age related IgG subclass concentrations in asthma. Arch Dis Child 1994;70:179.
Mochizuki S et al: Systemic immunization against IgA in immunoglobulin deficiency. Clin Exp Immunol 1994;94:334.
Plebani A et al: Extensive deletion of immunoglobulin heavy chain constant region genes in the absence of recurrent infections: When is IgG subclass deficiency clinically relevant? Clin Immunol Immunopathol 1993; 68:46.
Smith LJ et al: Familial enteropathy with villous edema and immunoglobulin G2 subclass deficiency. J Pediatr 1996;128:722.

SELECTIVE DEFECTS OF CELL-MEDIATED IMMUNITY

Purine Nucleoside Phosphorylase Deficiency

Purine nucleoside phosphorylase deficiency causes a relatively selective CMI defect. It results in increased intracellular levels of deoxyguanosine triphosphate, which inhibit ribonucleotide reductase and interfere with DNA synthesis, especially in T cells. T-cell help to B cells is not prevented, probably because it is not dependent on cell division. The structural locus for purine nucleoside phosphorylase is on chromosome 14, and transmission is recessive. Presenting features may be neurologic (developmental retardation, behavior disorders, and spasticity), with immunodeficiency (severe varicella, anemia, and failure to thrive) developing later. The age at presentation has ranged from 6 months to 7 years. Investigations show low blood uric acid, lymphopenia, absent delayed hypersensitivity skin responses, and low or absent lymphocyte responses to mitogens. Serum immunoglobulins and antibody responses to injected antigens may be normal. Several patients developed an autoimmune hemolytic anemia. Diagnosis depends on enzyme measurement, and all patients with severely impaired cellular immunity who make immunoglobulin should probably be tested. Antenatal diagnosis is possible. It has been difficult to achieve stable engraftment following bone marrow transplantation.

Nelson DM et al: Correction of proliferative responses in purine nucleoside phosphorylase (PNP)-deficient T lymphocytes by retroviral-mediated PNP gene transfer and expression. J Immunol 1995;154:3006.

Tam DA Jr, Leshner RT: Stroke in purine nucleoside phosphorylase deficiency. Pediatr Neurol 1995;12:146.

Thymic hypoplasia (DiGeorge Syndrome)

DiGeorge syndrome is one of the "CATCH 22" (Cardiac defects, Abnormal facies, Thymic hypoplasia, Cleft palate, and Hypocalcaemia) range of disorders caused by microdeletions in the chromosome 22q11.2 region. Other associated syndromes are the velocardiofacial syndrome and isolated conotruncal cardiac disease. In most instances, the defective chromosome is inherited from the mother. The diagnostic criteria for thymic hypoplasia are a small or absent thymus, lack of parathyroid glands, and major vessel abnormalities such as truncus arteriosus, anomalous pulmonary venous drainage, or right-sided aortic arch. Other features include a small jaw, low-set ears, and a short philtrum. The term "partial DiGeorge syndrome" is commonly applied to infants who have impaired rather than absent parathyroid or thymus function. Clinical presentation usually results from cardiac failure or, after 24–48 hours, from hypocalcemia, and the diagnosis is sometimes made during the course of cardiac surgery, when no thymus is found in the mediastinum. Postoperative hypocalcemia can be severe and persistent, requiring both calcium and vitamin D supplements. Despite receiving fresh blood transfusions during cardiopulmonary bypass, patients do not usually develop graft-versus-host disease. Their susceptibility to infection is variable—a few have died with septicemia, and some have had chronic candidiasis, but many appear to respond normally. This may reflect the tendency for the number of T cells in the patient's blood to rise spontaneously over the course of several years. The differential diagnosis includes hypocalcemia and a small or absent thymus on chest x-ray secondary to infection.

A subset of DiGeorge patients has severe problems with production of autoantibodies to red cells, white cells, and platelets. These may respond to intravenous IgG or to corticosteroids. Treatment of other DiGeorge features may require surgery for the cardiac defects and vitamin D and calcium to correct hypocalcemia. Blood for these patients should be irradiated. Grafting thymic hypoplasia patients with fetal thymus or thymic epithelial cells is often followed by rapid improvement in the lymphocyte response to mitogens. The improvement is so rapid that thymic humoral factors are thought to be responsible, but factors currently available for treatment have not been useful. Infusions of HLA-matched sibling blood or marrow has been tried in a few patients who did not improve spontaneously and carries a risk for graft-versus-host disease.

Demczuk S et al: Excess of deletions of maternal origin in the DiGeorge/velo-cardio-facial syndromes: A study of 22 new patients and review of the literature. Hum Genet 1995;96:9.

Driscoll DA: Genetic basis of DiGeorge and velocardiofacial syndromes. Curr Opin Pediatr 1994;6:702.

Other Defects of Cell-Mediated Immunity

Many patients with the American (but not Finnish) type of **cartilage-hair hypoplasia** have a moderate degree of lymphopenia, low lymphocyte responses to mitogens, and higher than normal morbidity and mortality rates from herpesvirus and poxvirus infections. There is no established treatment. Short-limbed dwarfs who are immunodeficient should probably be tested for adenosine deaminase deficiency, since this is treatable. Other types of immunodeficiency affecting predominantly cellular immunity exist but are poorly classified. These are currently included in the "varied immunodeficiency" group. Their infections resemble those described above, with the frequent addition of chronic diarrhea and malabsorption and lung infections due to atypical mycobacteria, fungi, and *Pneumocystis carinii*. Treatment is experimental.

Brooks EG et al: Thymic hypoplasia and T-cell deficiency in ectodermal dysplasia: Case report and review of the literature. Clin Immunol Immunopathol 1994;71:44.

Fischer A et al: Bone marrow transplantation (BMT) in Europe for primary immunodeficiencies other than severe combined immunodeficiency: A report from the European Group for BMT and the European Group for Immunodeficiency. Blood 1994;83:1149.

COMBINED IMMUNODEFICIENCY DISORDERS

Severe combined immunodeficiency disease (SCID) comprises a heterogeneous group of conditions that have in common a primary severe impairment of both antibody- and cell-mediated immunity. The term SCID is usually restricted to infants with congenital immunodeficiency, but equally severe defects can be caused by AIDS or lymphocyte loss. The heterogeneity of the congenital forms reflects the range of underlying defects that may interfere with lymphocyte development at different stages and the varying degrees of engraftment with maternal lymphocytes that can occur during gestation or at birth. X-linked SCID results from mutations in the gamma chain shared by the cell surface receptors for the cytokines IL2, IL4, IL7, and IL9. These mutations vary in their interference with gamma-chain function, and this allows for a range of clinical severity in X-linked SCID syndromes.

Diarrhea, vomiting, and cough are common symptoms. The diarrhea causes failure to thrive, and although it may briefly remit after dietary changes, it recurs after a few days. The cough is usually persistent; it is often due to *P carinii* infection and can cause cyanosis. Skin rashes are common and frequently evanescent, except for rash following blood transfusion, which is due to graft-versus-host disease (qv). A *Candida* diaper rash is usual. Findings initially include absence of tonsils or palpable lymph nodes; later, there is emaciation.

All patients with SCID have some degree of hypogammaglobulinemia and failure of antibody production (although maternal IgG is present in infants). SCID infants with some immunoglobulin have been called "Nezelof's syndrome," but this separation is not very helpful in terms of pathogenesis or treatment. Lymphopenia is inconstant but, with rare exceptions, all have very low or absent T (CD3) cells from blood, with normal numbers of NK (CD16) cells. B lymphocytes (with surface IgM) are usually present in blood. In vitro lymphocyte responses to mitogens are generally absent. Antigen-specific responses (T cell or antibody) are difficult to test for in infancy because of uncertainty about prior experience and because they are generally too time-consuming for clinical purposes. Antenatal diagnosis of X-linked SCID is possible by molecular methods. All other SCID syndromes may be detected by fetal blood sampling at 15 weeks of gestation and phenotyping the lymphocytes obtained.

Arpaia E et al: Defective T cell receptor signaling and CD8+ thymic selection in humans lacking zap-70 kinase. Cell 1994;76:947.

Leonard WJ: The defective gene in X-linked severe combined immunodeficiency encodes a shared interleukin receptor subunit: Implications for cytokine pleiotropy and redundancy. Curr Opin Immunol 1994;6:631.

Stephan JL et al: Severe combined immunodeficiency: A retrospective single-center study of clinical presentation and outcome in 117 patients. J Pediatr 1993;123:564.

Differential Diagnosis & Treatment

The combination of diarrhea and hypogammaglobulinemia in infancy is suggestive of SCID. The main differential is between severe varied immunodeficiency and secondary immunodeficiency due to HIV infection or severe gastrointestinal disease with loss of protein and cells. Some T cells are usually present in these secondary immunodeficiencies, with a weak lymphocyte response to phytohemagglutinin, and the serum albumin concentration may be low. Infants in whom the diagnosis is suspected should receive antibiotics for infection and IgG replacement. They should not be transfused with blood unless it has first been irradiated. With confirmation of the diagnosis, they may be started on trimethoprim-sulfamethoxazole for *Pneumocystis* prophylaxis. Bone marrow grafting offers the best hope for cure. If an HLA-matched sibling is available, there is a high chance of success; the treatment can be given without depleting the marrow of T cells or immunosuppressing the recipient. Most SCID patients do not have HLA-matched donors and are treated with grafts of parental bone marrow from which the T cells are removed by lectins or monoclonal antibodies. Pregraft suppression, with the attendant hazards of thrombocytopenia and neutropenia, may be required; reconstitution can take 4 months; and the overall rate of T-cell engraftment is between 50% and 70%. Reconstitution for antibody responses may not occur even if B cells are produced.

Filipovich AH: Bone marrow transplantation from unrelated donors for congenital immunodeficiencies. Bone Marrow Transplant 1993;11(Suppl)1:78.

van Leeuwen JE et al: Relationship between patterns of engraftment in peripheral blood and immune reconstitution after allogeneic bone marrow transplantation for (severe) combined immunodeficiency. Blood 1994;84:3936.

VARIANTS OF SEVERE COMBINED IMMUNODEFICIENCY

1. ADENOSINE DEAMINASE DEFICIENCY

Adenosine deaminase converts adenosine and deoxyadenosine to inosine and deoxyinosine, respectively. Individuals homozygous for a null gene account for about 20% of cases of SCID. ADA deficiency impairs immunity through inhibition of ribonucleotide reductase by raised deoxy-ATP, so that T lymphocytes are prevented from dividing. There is also increased DNA fragmentation and interference with methylation reactions. Affected infants may be near-normal at birth (presumably because their mothers keep deoxyadenosine levels down in utero). Their cellular immunity fails first; they become lymphopenic and then become antibody-deficient, though they may continue to make immunoglobulin for months or years. Diagnosis is by assay of adenosine deaminase in red cell lysates. A bone marrow graft from a matched normal sibling is the ideal treatment (see below). Immune competence is also restored by weekly infusions of polyethylene glycol-stabilized ADA enzyme conjugate. Transfection of blood lymphocytes and stem cells are being evaluated for subjects who lack matched donors.

Hershfield MS. PEG-ADA: an alternative to haploidentical bone marrow transplantation and an adjunct to gene therapy for adenosine deaminase deficiency. Hum Mutat 1995;5:107.

Hoogerbrugge PM et al: Gene therapy for adenosine deaminase deficiency. Br Med Bull 1995;51:72.

2. SCID WITH LEUKOPENIA (Reticular Dysgenesis)

SCID with leukopenia occurs in infants with SCID who also have severe neutropenia, often with reduced numbers of granulocyte precursors in the marrow. Only about 20 cases have been reported. There is a familial trend, but the severity of the neutropenia varies between affected siblings, so this may be a secondary feature.

Gasparetto C et al: Dyshematopoiesis in combined immune deficiency with congenital neutropenia. Am J Hematol 1994;45:63.

3. SCID WITH DEFECTIVE EXPRESSION OF HLA ANTIGENS

This condition is difficult to diagnose because affected patients generally make immunoglobulins and have low to normal numbers of B and T cells in their blood, together with positive responses to phytohemagglutinin stimulation. Their clinical symptoms are nevertheless those of SCID. The defect is of class II (HLA-DR, DP, and DQ) histocompatibility antigen expression, and the T cells do not make antigen-specific responses, so the patients remain antibody-deficient. Diagnosis is by phenotyping blood lymphocytes for HLA-DR antigen expression. A number of affected families has been of North African descent. Patients with selective defects of class I histocompatibility antigen expression have milder degrees of immunodeficiency.

Casper JT et al: Successful treatment with an unrelated-donor bone marrow transplant in an HLA-deficient patient with severe combined immune deficiency (bare lymphocyte syndrome). J Pediatr 1990;116:262.

4. ZAP-70 DEFICIENCY

Affected infants have CD4 but no CD8 cells in blood. Their lymphocytes do not proliferate in response to antigen or mitogens because they lack an essential kinase in the T-cell activation pathway. Immunoglobulin production is variable.

Roifman CM: Selection transduction defect (STD) due to Zap-70 kinase deficiency. Immunodeficiency 1995; 5:193.

Other Combined Immunodeficiency Disorders

There is a poorly defined group of infants with more severe impairment of antibody and CMI than occurs in CVID but who have more T cells than are usually seen in SCID. These patients have severe and particularly protracted infections, mainly of the respiratory tract and gut. A subgroup with multiple intestinal atresias, hypogammaglobulinemia and impaired CMI has recently been recognized: the mechanism for this association is unknown. Many have severe herpes viruses infections. Autoimmune neutropenia, anemia, and thrombocytopenia are common, as are allergies. Immune deficiency in some of these patients has been corrected by bone marrow transplantation.

Rothenberg ME, White FV, Chilmonczyk B, Chatila T: A syndrome involving immunodeficiency and multiple intestinal atresias. Immunodeficiency. 1995;5:171.

5. SCID WITH RETICULO-ENDOTHELIOSIS (Omenn's Syndrome)

Omenn described a familial immunodeficiency with a severe eczematoid skin rash, lymphadenopathy, hepatosplenomegaly with diarrhea, and failure to thrive. Most of these patients have eosinophilia with high IgE with low IgG and IgM; blood B cells are low or absent. The blood T-cell numbers may be normal or low and a very restricted T-cell repertoire is reported. At autopsy the thymus has lacked Hassall's corpuscles. The absence of consistent laboratory abnormalities makes diagnosis difficult. Some cases have been successfully treated by marrow ablation followed by transplantation. The condition is probably different from maternal engraftment of an infant with SCID resulting in graft-versus-host disease.

Appleton AL, Curtis A, Wilkes J, Cant AJ: Differentiation of materno-fetal GVHD from Omenn's syndrome in pre-BMT patients with severe combined immunodeficiency. Bone Marrow Transpl 1994;14:157.
Berthet F et al: Clinical consequences and treatment of primary immunodeficiency syndromes characterized by functional T and B lymphocyte anomalies (combined immune deficiency). Pediatrics 1994;93:265–70.
Gomez L et al: Treatment of Omenn syndrome by bone marrow transplantation. J Pediatr 1995;127(1):76.

OTHER DISORDERS ASSOCIATED WITH IMMUNODEFICIENCY

WISKOTT-ALDRICH SYNDROME

Wiskott-Aldrich syndrome patients have thrombocytopenia, eczema, and recurrent infection (originally draining ears) and results from deletion of the WASP gene at X11p. Inheritance is X-linked recessive; the incidence is about 4 per million male births, and the gene has been localized to the p11 region of the X chromosome. The disorder is associated with deficient expression of a 115 kDa cell surface sialophorin identified as CD43. Common presenting symptoms are bloody diarrhea, cerebral hemorrhage, or septicemia followed by severe infections with polysaccharide-encapsulated bacteria. However, some patients have little if any eczema, while others have few infections. The main causes of death in infancy are bleeding and infections, but with increasing age lymphomas become increasingly common. Survival through the teens is rare in untreated patients, although partial syndromes are sometimes diagnosed in adults. A specific diagnosis should be easier now that the gene has been identified. Routine laboratories that suggest the diagnosis are a low platelet count, low or absent isohemagglutinins, and reduced antibody response to polysaccharides. IgM may be low, IgA and IgE are often high. Bone marrow transplantation with matched sibling marrow offers the best hope for long-term correction of the defect. The platelet count generally rises following splenectomy, but this operation must be followed by antibiotic prophylaxis because of the increased risk of septicemia and sudden death.

Rosen FS: The enigma of the Wiskolt-Aldrich syndrome. J Clin Invest 1996;97:2407.
Sullivan KE et al: A multiinstitutional survey of the Wiskott Aldrich syndrome. J Pediatr 1994;125:876.

ATAXIA-TELANGIECTASIA

Ataxia-telangiectasia (AT) is characterized by cerebellar ataxia (due to degeneration of Purkinje cells) usually developing between 2 and 5 years of age and followed by the appearance of telangiectases, particularly on the conjunctiva and over exposed areas: the nose, ears, and shoulders. The disorder has an autosomal recessive inheritance pattern, but there are six or more different complementation groups. The abnormal gene is on chromosome 11–11q22-23 in one study, but its mechanism of action is unknown. The Nijmegen breakage syndrome is probably a variant of AT with more severe clinical features, including microcephaly and "bird-like" facies. Abnormal findings in AT include raised serum α-fetoprotein levels (useful diagnostically), thymic hypoplasia, low or absent serum IgE, low IgA in 50%, abnormal carbohydrate tolerance, and defective ability to repair radiation-induced DNA fragmentation. Clinically, the most important symptom is the progressive loss of motor coordination, followed by weakness. Respiratory tract infections and many types of malignancy (including carcinomas) are the major causes of death. About 10% of patients develop lymphomas, the majority of which are T-cell–derived. Many of the lymphomas have translocations or inversions at sites where T-cell receptor genes are normally rearranged. Radiotherapy has been followed by skin breakdown, presumably the result of the DNA repair defect. The heterozygote frequency is 0.5–5%, depending on geographic and ethnic factors, and these individuals have an increased incidence of breast cancer.

Taylor AM et al: Genetic and cellular features of ataxia telangiectasia. Int J Radiat Biol 1994;65:65.
Telatar M et al: Ataxia telangiectasia. American J Hum Genet 1996;59:40.
Weemaes CM, Smeets DF, Van der Burgt CJ: Nijmegen breakage syndrome: A progress report. Int J Radiat Biol 1994;66(Suppl 6): S185.

CHRONIC MUCOCUTANEOUS CANDIDIASIS

Diagnosis requires chronic candidiasis affecting skin or nails and mucous membranes, which is not attributable to antibiotic treatment or another defined immunodeficiency. Involvement of scalp and flexures is common, usually as erythema and scaling but occasionally as granulomas with skin hypertrophy. The recurrent candidiasis points to an underlying immunodeficiency, but the faulty mechanism has not been identified. Affected patients make anti-*Candida* antibodies, and their in vitro lymphocyte responses may be positive even when *Candida* skin tests are negative. Evidence for the complexity of this form of immunodeficiency includes the frequent association with endocrinopathy, sometimes autoimmune (affecting parathyroid, thyroid, pituitary, or gonads), and, less commonly, susceptibility to staphylococcal infections with defective neutrophil mobility. There is usually some control of the candidiasis with continuous fluconazole treatment.

X-LINKED LYMPHOPROLIFERATIVE SYNDROME

This term is applied to boys who develop bone marrow aplasia, hypogammaglobulinemia, or a lymphoproliferative syndrome following Epstein-Barr virus (EBV) infection. The gene responsible has been mapped to Xq2s, and antenatal diagnosis is possible. Affected boys are immunologically normal prior to EBV infection, and during acute mononucleosis they make some antibody to the EBV. In most instances, the EBV infection results in a lethal lymphoproliferative syndrome characterized by liver failure, disseminated intravascular coagulation, and multiple monoclonal serum IgM bands. Acyclovir is sometimes beneficial, and α-interferon and monoclonal anti–B-cell antibodies are being investigated as treatments. Only 10–20% of affected boys who are infected with EBV survive to develop hypogammaglobulinemia.

Pracher E et al: Successful bone marrow transplantation in a boy with X-linked lymphoproliferative syndrome and acute severe infectious mononucleosis. Bone Marrow Transpl 1994;13:655.

Purtilo DT et al: The X-linked lymphoproliferative disease: From autopsy toward cloning the gene, 1975–1990. Pediatr Pathol 1991;11:685.

GRAFT-VERSUS-HOST DISEASE

Graft-versus-host disease (GvHD) follows the transfusion of immunocompetent but incompatible lymphocytes into a person incapable of rejecting them. It causes significant morbidity in about 30% of bone marrow transplant recipients and causes death in infants with SCID. It has been reported in infants receiving transfusions from HLA homozygous donors, so blood products for infants should be irradiated. An erythematous, macular and then bullous skin rash is variably followed by diarrhea, hepatitis, nephritis, pulmonary infiltrates, and fever, whereas marrow damage results in neutropenia and then thrombocytopenia. Many patients develop high IgE levels. Diagnosis is suspected on the basis of transplantation, an unirradiated blood or blood product transfusion, usually into an immunodeficient patient and is confirmed by skin or lip biopsy. Prophylaxis in transplant recipients is with corticosteroids and cyclosporine, and when the disease becomes severe it may be slowed by high-dose corticosteroids or at least temporarily halted by anti–T-cell antibodies (OKT3 or anti-lymphocyte serum). Chronic GvHD after allogeneic bone marrow transplantation causes scleroderma and bile duct destruction. The liver damage can be severe enough to require transplantation.

Henslee-Downey PJ: Mismatched bone marrow transplantation. Curr Opin Oncol 1995;7:115.

Takanashi M, Nishimura M, Tadokoro K, Juji T: Graft-versus-host disease associated with transfusions of HLA-matched, HLA-homozygous platelets. Transfusion 1995;35:535.

BIOCHEMICAL DEFECTS SOMETIMES ASSOCIATED WITH IMMUNODEFICIENCY

Several primary errors of metabolism affect immunity adversely. Transcobalamin 2 deficiency causes a megaloblastic anemia with impaired bacterial killing by neutrophils and reduced serum immunoglobulins of all classes. **Biotin-dependent decarboxylase deficiencies** may be associated with convulsions, alopecia, candidiasis, low serum IgA, and a reduced number of T cells. Lymphopenia and impaired CMI are reported in **hereditary orotic aciduria.** Chromosomal instability syndromes impair CMI, as in Bloom's syndrome, which may be severe enough to cause antibody deficiency (mostly of IgM) and malabsorption.

Prigent C et al: Aberrant DNA repair and DNA replication due to an inherited enzymatic defect in human DNA ligase I. Mol Cell Biol 1994;14:310.

SECONDARY IMMUNODEFICIENCY

Secondary immunodeficiency is a common cause of pediatric illness. The mechanisms that may be impaired are summarized in Table 28–3, and the symptoms are generally those that would be anticipated from the combination of the primary disorder and the complicating immunodeficiency. Whenever possible,

Table 28–3. Mechanisms of secondary immunodeficiency.

Mechanism	Example
Loss	
Immunoglobulin	Renal, in nephrotic syndrome
Immunoglobulin	Skin, from burns
Immunoglobulin and cells	Gut, in intestinal lymphangiectasia
Phagocytes	Following splenectomy
Malnutrition	Kwashiorkor
Zinc deficiency	Impaired cell-mediated immunity
Copper and iron deficiency	Impaired neutrophil function
Drugs	Steroids, cancer chemotherapy
	Specific immunosuppressants
	Phenytoin → IgA deficiency
Infections	HIV, EBV, CMV, measles, rubella, hepatitis, malaria

treatment should be directed at the primary disorder. Occasionally, immunologic methods may help; for example, varicella-zoster immune globulin may prevent varicella in patients with leukemia and intravenous IgG replacement might provide added protection where antibody production is diminished. IgG replacement is unlikely to help when loss (as in nephrotic syndrome) is responsible for hypogammaglobulinemia.

THERAPEUTIC IMMUNOSUPPRESSION

Therapeutic immunosuppression is increasingly used in pediatrics for transplant recipients and for autoimmune disease. Corticosteroids at 2 mg/kg of prednisolone interfere with cytokine production and cause lymphopenia by directing lymphocytes to the marrow: the duration of action is about 24 hours. Much higher doses, 20–30 mg/kg prednisolone/day are used for 3–5-day courses for treatment of life-threatening conditions, or to evaluate the potential for more powerful immunosuppressive agents. Corticosteroids are satisfactory anti-inflammatory and immunosuppressive agents when they can be given on alternate days as a single morning dose (as is sometimes the case for systemic lupus erythematosus or autoimmune anemias). Immunosuppression by corticosteroids is limited by the growth arrest and severe cushingoid changes, which result from daily doses with even 2 mg/kg of prednisolone per day. Transplant recipients require additional powerful immunosuppressives such as Cyclosporine A (CyA) or tacrolimus (FK 506). Both bind to immunophilins to form a complex that reversibly inhibits calcineurin dependent signalling in lymphocytes, blocking cytokine production and release. Immunosuppression achievable by both agents is limited by their nephrotoxicity, and trough blood levels need to be monitored carefully and drugs that affect their metabolism (erythromycin, theophylline) tracked. Preventing organ rejection usually requires two drugs, such as CyA and mycophenolate mofentil (MMF) or azathioprine. MMF is new and likely to be very useful. It inhibits purine synthesis and is relatively specific for lymphocytes: it may replace azathioprine, which causes much more general marrow suppression.

Severe organ rejection episodes, or graft-versus-host disease, can be controlled acutely with antibodies to T lymphocytes such as anti-thymocyte globulin and monoclonal CD3 antibody. Both deplete T cells and clear antigen receptors off the T-cell surface. Some T cells are activated too, causing a cytokine syndrome of fever, malaise, and pulmonary edema. This syndrome is minimized by giving corticosteroids or CyA.

Antimitotic agents (cyclophosphamide, chlorambucil) that block T-cell proliferation are effective but toxic immunosuppressants. The risks of immunosuppression include reactivation of latent herpesviruses (CMV, HSV, VZV), although antiviral treatments have made these less life-threatening. EBV reactivation is hazardous if it results in a lymphoproliferation with marrow phagocytosis of red and white cells. The appearance of serum oligoclonal immunoglobulin bands may give advance warning of this dangerous complication. Combined immunosuppression with agents having different modes of action tends to be much more potent, with a greater potential for opportunistic infections, than immunosuppression by single agents. The risk of infection is greatest when the neutrophil count is depressed by antimitotic agents at the same time as specific immunity is suppressed by corticosteroids and cyclosporine.

Lake KD, Canafax DM: 1995 Important interactions of drugs with immunosuppressive agents used in transplant recipients. J Antimicrob Chemother 1995 36SupplB:11.

INVESTIGATION OF IMMUNODEFICIENCY

Physical and anatomic defects are the most common causes of recurrent infections, and if a single site is affected it should be searched for a local abnormality. The age at onset of infections is important because defects of phagocytes, C3, or cellular immunity become symptomatic in the first months of life, whereas maternal antibody protects infants with hypogammaglobulinemia for 3–6 months. Antibody, complement, and phagocyte defects predispose mainly to bacterial infections; diarrhea, superficial candidiasis, and severe herpesvirus infections are typical of cellular immunodeficiency. A simple protocol for testing these mechanisms is presented in Table 28–4, and the level of investigation should reflect the frequency and severity of infections. A complete blood cell count and quantitative immunoglobulin measurement will identify more than 90% of *primary* immunodeficiency syndromes.

Kavanaugh A: Evaluation of patients with suspected immunodeficiency. Am Fam Phys 1994;49:1167.

Phagocyte Function

Tests of phagocytic cell function should first rule out neutropenia with white blood count and differential. A blood film is useful to exclude the Howell-Jolly bodies of asplenia and to look for normal lysosomal granules in neutrophils. Chemotaxis is generally measured in migration chambers in the laboratory and can also be assessed by migration of cells

Table 28–4. Hierarchy of tests for investigation of primary immunodeficiency.

Test Level	Complement	Phagocytes	Antibody	CMI
Screening	CH_{50}	Count, morphology	Ig measurement	Delayed hypersensitivity skin tests.
First level		NBT, LFA-1[1]	IHA,[2] TT	T-cell counts[3]
Second level	Factor assays	Killing and chemotaxis	Immunize	In vitro tests

[1]Only when chronic granulomatous disease or LFA-1 deficiency is suspected.
[2]IHA = isohemagglutinins, after age 1; TT = tetanus toxoid.
[3]Identify all T cells with CD3, subsets with CD4, CD8. CD45RO for memory cells.

from abraded skin onto a sterile coverslip. Results of chemotaxis tests must be interpreted cautiously, since secondary and transient defects in chemotaxis are common. Quantitation of ingestion and microbicidal activity requires special techniques available chiefly in research laboratories. However, the chemical reduction of nitroblue tetrazolium by phagocytes requires normal oxidation metabolism, so this test screens for chronic granulomatous disease (the most common bacterial killing defect) and for leukocyte G6PD deficiency. Myeloperoxidase deficiency is excluded by histochemical stain available in most oncology laboratories.

Complement

Deficiency of a classic pathway component can be excluded by a normal hemolytic complement titer, for which the patient's serum must be separated and frozen to –70 °C within 30 minutes of collection. Alternative pathway function is tested by lysis of rabbit red blood cells. There is little point in measuring individual complement component levels if the hemolytic titer is normal, unless it is to follow the activity of an immune complex–associated disease in which C4 and C3 may be low. The common form of opsonizing defect of yeast is now known to be due to deficiency of mannan-binding protein.

Antibodies & Immunoglobulins

In patients who are not blood group AB, isohemagglutinins are the most easily tested naturally occurring antibodies. They are of the IgM class, become detectable by 6 months of age, and reach adult levels about 1 year later. The importance of antibody tests is illustrated by the inverse correlation between isohemagglutinin titer and susceptibility to meningitis in patients with hypogammaglobulinemia, regardless of their serum IgM levels. Tetanus and diphtheria antibody tests are widely available, as are antibodies to pneumococcal polysaccharide, rubella, and mumps. In practice, it is often easier to measure serum immunoglobulins as a screening procedure than to test for antibodies, but it should be appreciated that some patients with varied immunodeficiency syndromes and some infants with severely im-

paired CMI make immunoglobulin that does not have useful antibody activity. Properly performed immunoglobulin estimations are reproducible to +10% for IgG and IgA and +20% for IgM, so small changes are of no significance. Measurement of serum IgD is not generally of diagnostic value in pediatrics. Immunoglobulin concentrations are lower in infants than in adults, and laboratories may erroneously report normal children's values as low. Comparisons of results from different laboratories may be difficult, because few commercial kit suppliers calibrate their control sera against the international standard. Simple protein electrophoresis is not sufficiently sensitive to make a confident diagnosis of hypogammaglobulinemia, although it is valuable for identifying the monoclonal excesses seen in macroglobulinemia, the oligoclonal gammopathy of EBV infections in X-linked lymphoproliferative syndrome, and in heavy chain diseases. Serum albumin should be measured at least once in patients with hypogammaglobulinemia to exclude secondary deficiencies due to loss. IgG or IgA subclass measurements may be abnormal in patients with varied immunodeficiency syndromes, but they are rarely helpful.

Cell-Mediated Immunity

Positive delayed hypersensitivity skin tests give good evidence for antigen-specific T-cell immunity. Only a positive response is interpretable—particularly in infancy, when prior immunization may not have been adequate to elicit good skin responses.

Phenotyping blood lymphocytes gives a good view of the number and maturity of lymphocytes that have come from the thymus. Only small volumes of blood are required, and results are rapidly available. Some of the more useful antibodies—and common deviations from normal—are summarized in Table 28–5. When abnormalities are suspected, it is important to check absolute numbers of lymphocytes and their subsets. Tests of T-cell proliferation and cytokine production are useful to characterize immunodeficiency detected by simpler tests, but they are not useful screening tests for children with recurrent infections.

Table 28–5. Blood lymphocyte phenotyping.

Antigen	Commercial Antibodies	Cells Stained	Normal Range and Changes Seen Clinically
CD2	OKT11	T, NK	70–90%. Falls to 10–20% when T cells absent.
CD3	OKT3, Leu4	All T	55–85%. Falls when T-cell number reduced. Increases to 90% when B cells absent.
CD4	OKT4, Leu3	HLA-D restricted T cells	35–60%. Selectively reduced in HIV infections. Reduced with other T cells by steroids, defect of cell-mediated immunity.
CD5		T cells, immature B cells	55–85%. Falls when T-cell number reduced. Increased with immature B cells.
CD8	OKT8, Leu2	HLA-A/B restricted T cells	25–50%. Selectively increased in response to some viral infections. Reduced with other T-cell defects.
CD11	OKM1, Mac-1	Monocytes	Lacking in LFA-1 deficiency.
CD16	Leu11	NK cells	Increased by viral infections.
CD19		B cells	Increased when T cells lacking.
CD20		B cells	Increased when T cells lacking.
CD25		IL-2 receptor	Activated T cells. Increased in graft-versus-host disease.
CD45RO	UCHL1	T cells	Memory T cells, low in newborns.
CD56	NKH-1	NK cells	Raised in active viral infections.

From Thompson RA (editor): Laboratory investigation of immunological disorders. Clin Immunol Allergy 1985;5:No. 3. See also Spickett GP, Matamoros N, Farrant J: Lymphocyte surface phenotype in common variable immunodeficiency. Dis Markers 1992;10:67.

Herrod HG, Blaiss MS, Valenski WR, Gross S: Cell-mediated immune status of children with recurrent infection. J Pediatr 1995;126:530.

Pacheco SE, Shearer WT: Laboratory aspects of immunology. Pediatr Clin North Am 1994;41:623.

Genetic Diagnosis

Molecular biology approaches are important for antenatal diagnosis, for carrier identification, and for characterizing an increasing number of primary immunodeficiencies. The X-linked defects have mostly been mapped, and others, such as adenosine deaminase deficiency, are well defined.

Di Santo JP et al: Prenatal diagnosis of X-linked hyper IgM syndrome. N Engl Med 1994;330:969.

Hirschhorn R: Overview of biochemical abnormalities and molecular genetics of adenosine deaminase deficiency. Pediatr Res 1993;33(1 Suppl):S35.

Nelson DL, Kurman CC: Molecular genetic analysis of the primary immunodeficiency disorders. Pediatr Clin North Am 1994;41:657.

Puck JM: Prenatal diagnosis and genetic analysis of X-linked immunodeficiency disorders. Pediatr Res 1993; 33(1 Suppl):S29 (see discussion on p S33).

29

Endocrine Disorders

Ronald W. Gotlin, MD, Michael S. Kappy, MD, PhD. & Robert H. Slover, MD

GENERAL CONCEPTS

One of the major functions of the endocrine system is to regulate the enzymatic and other metabolic processes (eg, molecular transport) responsible for maintaining the equilibrium (homeostasis) of the internal environment to ensure survival of the individual. Other critical roles for the endocrine system are regulation of growth (in utero and postnatal), pubertal development and reproduction, energy production, and, to a lesser extent, behavior.

The classic concept of endocrine effects representing the result of hormones secreted into the blood to reach a target cell has been updated to account for other ways in which hormonal effects are realized. Specifically, some hormone systems involve the stimulation or inhibition (or both) of metabolic processes in *neighboring* (as opposed to distant) cells (eg, within the pancreatic islets or cartilage). This phenomenon is termed, "paracrine."

Other hormone effects reflect the action of particular hormones *on the same cells that produced them.* This is termed, "autocrine." The discoveries of local production of insulin, glucagon, atrial natriuretic hormone, and many other hormones in the brain and gut support the concept of paracrine and autocrine processes in these tissues.

Another significant discovery in endocrine physiology was an appreciation of the role of specific hormone receptors in target tissues, without which the hormonal effects could not be manifested. In the complete androgen insensitivity (resistance) syndrome, androgen receptors are absent, and the individual develops normal female external genitalia despite the presence of testes (usually intra-abdominal) and adequate testosterone production. Similarly, in Albright's hereditary osteodystrophy (pseudohypoparathyroidism), affected persons have abnormal parathyroid hormone (PTH) receptor function and show the metabolic effects of hypoparathyroidism (low serum calcium and high phosphate), despite the secretion of more than adequate PTH.

HORMONE TYPES

There are three main structural types of hormones: peptides and proteins, steroids, and amines. The peptide hormones include the releasing factors secreted by the hypothalamus, the hormones of the anterior and posterior pituitary gland, the pancreatic islet cells, the parathyroid glands, insulin-like growth factor I (IGF-I) from the liver and other tissues, angiotensin II, atrial natriuretic hormone, and many local growth factors. The steroid hormones are secreted primarily by the adrenal cortex, the gonads, and the liver (active vitamin D), whereas the amine hormones are secreted by the adrenal medulla (epinephrine) and the thyroid gland (T_4 and T_3).

As a general rule, the peptide hormones and epinephrine are more rapid-acting than the others and bind to specific receptors on the target cell surface. The metabolic effects of these hormones are usually manifested by their stimulating or inhibiting the activity of preexisting enzymes or transport proteins (post-translational effects). The steroid hormones and active vitamin D, on the other hand, are more slow-acting and bind to their specific receptors within the target cell in the cytoplasm or directly to DNA in the nucleus. Their metabolic effects are generally caused by stimulating or inhibiting the synthesis of new enzymes or transport proteins (transcriptional effects), thereby increasing or decreasing the amount rather than the activity of these proteins in the target cell.

Metabolic processes that must be regulated rapidly (eg, blood glucose or calcium homeostasis) are usually under the control of the peptide hormones and epinephrine (Table 29–1), whereas those processes that may be regulated more slowly (eg, pubertal development, metabolic rate) are under the control of the steroid hormones (see Table 29–1). The control of electrolyte homeostasis is intermediate and is regulated by a combination of peptide and steroid hormones (see Table 29–1).

Table 29–1. Hormonal regulation of metabolic processes.

First Level (Most Direct)

Metabolite or Other Parameter	Abnormality	Endocrine Gland	Hormone
Glucose	Hyperglycemia	Pancreatic beta cell	Insulin
Glucose	Hypoglycemia	Pancreatic alpha cell	Glucagon
Glucose	Hypoglycemia	Adrenal medulla	Epinephrine
Calcium	Hypercalcemia	Thyroid C cell	Calcitonin (?)
Calcium	Hypocalcemia	Parathyroid	PTH
Sodium/plasma osmolality	Hypernatremia/hyperosmolality	Hypothalamus (posterior pituitary gland)	ADH
Plasma volume	Hypervolemia	Heart	ANH

Second Level: Sodium and Potassium Balance

Metabolite or Other Parameter	Abnormality	Endocrine Gland	Hormone
Sodium/potassium	Hyponatremia	Kidney	Renin (an enzyme)
	Hyperkalemia	Liver and others	Angiotensin I
	Hypovolemia	Lung	Angiotensin II
		Adrenal cortex	Aldosterone

Third Level (Most Complex)

Releasing Hormone	Tropic Hormone	Endocrine Gland	Endocrine Gland Hormone
CRH	ACTH	Adrenal cortex	Cortisol
GHRH	GH	Liver	IGF-I
GnRH	LH	Testis	Testosterone
GnRH	FSH/LH	Ovary	Estradiol/progesterone
TRH	TSH	Thyroid gland	T_4 (some T_3)

ADH = antidiuretic hormone; ACTH = corticotropin; CRH = corticotropin-releasing hormone; FSH = follicle-stimulating hormone; GH = growth hormone; GHRH = growth hormone releasing hormone; GnRH = gonadotropin-releasing hormone; IGF = insulin-like growth factor; LH = luteinizing hormone; PTH = parathyroid hormone; TRH = thyrotropin-releasing hormone; TSH = thyroid-stimulating hormone.

FEEDBACK CONTROL OF HORMONE SECRETION

Hormonal secretion is regulated, for the most part, by feedback in response to changes in the internal environment (see Table 29–1). When the metabolic imbalance is corrected, stimulation of the initial hormone's secretion ceases and may even be inhibited. Overcorrection of the imbalance stimulates a counterregulatory hormone secretion, so the circulating concentrations of metabolites are kept within relatively narrow limits.

Hypothalamopituitary control of hormonal secretion is also regulated by feedback, so that end-organ failure (endocrine gland insufficiency) leading to decreased circulating concentrations of endocrine gland hormones results in increased secretion of hypothalamic releasing and pituitary hormones (see Table 29–1; Figure 29–1). If restoration of normal circulating concentrations of endocrine gland hormones occurs, feedback inhibition at the pituitary and hypothalamus results in a cessation of the previously stimulated secretion of releasing and pituitary hormones, and a restoration of their circulating concentrations to normal.

Similarly, if there is autonomous endocrine gland hyperfunction (eg, in McCune-Albright syndrome, Graves' disease, and adrenal tumor), then the specific hypothalamic releasing and pituitary hormones are suppressed (see Figure 29–1). An understanding of the basic phenomenon of feedback control of hormonal secretion is fundamental to the understanding of endocrinologic disorders and their evaluation in children.

DISTURBANCES OF GROWTH

Disturbances of growth and development are the most common presenting complaints in the pediatric endocrine clinic. Knowledge of the endocrine system is essential to differentiate disturbances in hormonal secretion and action from normal variations in the timing and pattern of development (ie, "constitutional" deviations from the average). It has been estimated that over 1 million children in the United States have abnormal short stature.

Tall stature has become an increasingly unusual

Figure 29–1. General scheme of the hypothalamus-pituitary-endocrine gland axis. Releasing hormones synthesized in the hypothalamus are secreted into the hypothalamohypophyseal portal circulation. Tropic hormones are then secreted by the pituitary gland (hypophysis) in response, and they in turn act on specific endocrine glands to stimulate the secretion of their respective hormones. The endocrine gland hormones exert their respective effects on various target tissues (end organs), and, in addition, exert an indirect negative feedback (feedback inhibition) on their own secretion by acting at the level of the pituitary gland and the hypothalamus. This system is characteristic of those hormones listed in Table 29–1.

presenting complaint in our society. Because of the preference for tallness in both males and females, the number of young people evaluated and treated for tall stature has decreased.

SHORT STATURE

Most short stature is familial, racial, or genetic. Pathologic short stature follows malnutrition, intrauterine growth retardation, dysmorphism, psychosocial problems, and a wide range of systemic and chronic diseases (Table 29–2). The history, physical examination, growth curve, and radiograph bone age are most helpful in the differential diagnosis.

1. CONSTITUTIONAL SHORT STATURE

Familial or genetic short stature implies that a child is small because he or she is "programmed" to be so. In children with constitutional short stature, the growth pattern is normal, and bone age correlates with chronologic age. **Constitutional delay of growth,** on the other hand, implies a delayed growth pattern with delayed maturity and normal final height. Bone age in these children is delayed relative to chronologic age. Children with constitutional delay of growth (constitutional short stature) and skeletal maturation appear entirely normal in all other respects. In children with constitutional short stature, birth weight and length are not affected, but typically the rate of growth is decreased during infancy. There is often a history of a similar pattern of growth in one of the parents or in other members of the family. Puberty is delayed and these children characteristically reach normal height at a later than average age.

Treatment with low doses of testosterone over a 3- to 6-month period in boys may be useful in hastening the timing of puberty and accelerating growth, but final adult height is not enhanced. Whether growth hormone will have a place in treating these normal children is unknown; there are ethical, economic, and social concerns. Early studies have not shown that growth hormone increases final adult height.

2. GROWTH HORMONE & GROWTH HORMONE DEFICIENCY

The human growth hormone (hGH) gene on chromosome 17 codes for a 191 amino acid peptide, which is available as a pharmaceutical recombinant product.

hGH is released from the anterior pituitary in response to a delicate interplay of hypothalamic releasing and inhibitory factors. Moreover, a variety of stimuli, including adrenergic and serotonergic agents, arginine, glucagon, and insulin-induced hypoglycemia, have been used clinically as provocative tests of hGH secretion. Serum concentrations of hGH vary considerably; episodic surges occur in relation to nutrients, to activity, and particularly to natural sleep. The latter typically is associated with significant sustained elevation of hGH during the first 2 hours after the onset of sleep. Electroencephalographic monitoring during this interval reflects slow wave or deep sleep, suggesting a role for specific neurotransmitter influence.

Following secretion, hGH binds to specific receptors in a large variety of tissues and triggers direct and indirect actions. The latter category is used to designate the activity of the IGFs generated in response to hGH (Figure 29–2).

Growth hormone deficiency occurs in approximately 1 in 4000 children. About two thirds of cases are idiopathic (rarely familial): a deficiency or impairment in the hypothalamic secretion of hGH-releasing hormone is suspected. The remainder are secondary to pituitary or hypothalamic disease,

Table 29–2. Causes of short stature.

Familial, racial, or genetic
Constitutional short stature and delayed adolescence
Endocrine disturbances
  Growth hormone deficiency
    Hereditary—gene deletion
    Idiopathic—deficiency of growth hormone or growth hor-
      mone releasing hormone (or both) with and without
      associated abnormalities of midline structures of the
      central nervous system
    Acquired
      Transient—eg, psychosocial short stature
      Organic—tumor, irradiation of the central nervous
        system, infection, or trauma
  Hypothyroidism
  Adrenal insufficiency
  Cushing's disease and Cushing's syndrome (including
    iatrogenic causes)
  Sexual precocity (androgen or estrogen excess)
  Diabetes mellitus (poorly controlled)
  Diabetes insipidus
  Hyperaldosteronism
Primordial short stature
  Intrauterine growth retardation
    Placental insufficiency
    Intrauterine infection
  Primordial dwarfism with premature aging
    Progeria (Hutchinson-Gilford syndrome)
    Progeroid syndrome
      Werner's syndrome
      Cachectic (Cockayne's syndrome)
  Short stature without dysmorphism
  Short stature with dysmorphism (eg, Seckel's bird-headed
    dwarfism, leprechaunism, Silver's syndrome, Bloom's
    syndrome, Cornelia de Lange syndrome, Hallerman-
    Streiff syndrome)
Inborn errors of metabolism
  Altered metabolism of calcium or phosphorus (eg, hypo-
    phosphatemic rickets, hypophosphatasia, infantile hyper-
    calcemia, pseudohypoparathyroidism)
  Storage diseases
    Mucopolysaccharidoses (eg, Hurler's syndrome,
      Hunter's syndrome)
    Mucolipidoses (eg, generalized gangliosidosis,
      fucosidosis, mannosidosis)

Inborn errors of metabolism (cont'd)
    Sphingolipidoses (eg, Tay-Sachs disease, Niemann-Pick
      disease, Gaucher's disease)
    Miscellaneous (eg, cystinosis)
  Aminoacidemias and aminoacidurias
  Epithelial transport disorders (eg, renal tubular acidosis,
    cystic fibrosis, Bartter's syndrome, vasopressin-resistant
    diabetes insipidus, pseudohypoparathyroidism)
  Organic acidemias and acidurias (eg, methylmalonic acid-
    uria, orotic aciduria, maple syrup urine disease, isovaleric
    acidemia)
  Metabolic anemias (eg, sickle cell disease, thalassemia,
    pyruvate kinase deficiency)
  Disorders of mineral metabolism (eg, Wilson's disease,
    magnesium malabsorption syndrome)
  Body defense disorders (eg, Bruton's agammaglobulinemia,
    thymic aplasia, chronic granulomatous disease)
Constitutional (intrinsic) diseases of bone
  Defects of growth of tubular bones or spine (eg, achondro-
    plasia, metatropic dwarfism, diastrophic dwarfism, meta-
    physeal chondrodysplasia)
  Disorganized development of cartilage and fibrous compo-
    nents of the skeleton (eg, multiple cartilaginous exosto-
    ses, fibrous dysplasia with skin pigmentation, precocious
    puberty of McCune-Albright)
  Abnormalities of density of cortical diaphyseal structure or
    metaphyseal modeling (eg, osteogenesis imperfecta
    congenita, osteopetrosis, tubular stenosis)
Short stature associated with chromosomal defects
  Autosomal (eg, Down's syndrome, cri du chat syndrome,
    trisomy 18)
  Sex chromosomal (eg, Turner's syndrome-XO, penta X,
    XXXY)
Chronic systemic diseases, congenital defects, and can-
cers (eg, chronic infection and infestation, inflammatory
  bowel disease, hepatic disease, cardiovascular disease,
  hematologic disease, central nervous system disease, pul-
  monary disease, renal disease, malnutrition, cancers, colla-
  gen vascular disease)
Psychosocial short stature (deprivation dwarfism)
Miscellaneous syndromes (eg, arthrogryposis multiplex congenita, cerebrohepatorenal syndrome, Noonan's syndrome,
  Prader-Willi syndrome, Riley-Day syndrome)

infection, trauma, reticuloendotheliosis, and cranio-pharyngioma or other tumors (eg, gliomas). The deficiency of hGH may be an isolated defect, or it may occur in combination with other pituitary hormone deficiencies. Idiopathic hGH deficiency affects both sexes equally. There are also children who appear growth hormone-deficient, but defy traditional testing. This group includes children with hGH receptor defects. The most severely affected of these children have been called "Laron syndrome children," a group in whom the defective receptor for hGH leads to resistance to high growth hormone levels. These children benefit from treatment with IGF-I.

Other children who have defied traditional diagnostic criteria have been termed "idiopathic short children." These children seem to have normal growth hormone responses to testing, but very poor growth rates. Recently, some of these children have been found to have lower serum IGF-I concentrations, suggesting again a partial insensitivity to hGH

based on receptor gene defects. IGF-I may also help this group.

At birth, classic hGH-deficient children are of normal weight, but length may be reduced. The most characteristic clinical feature of the child with hGH deficiency is a linear growth rate as little as 50% of that of the normal child. Growth retardation may begin during infancy or may be delayed until later childhood. Other findings include infantile fat distribution, youthful facial feature, midfacial hypoplasia, and delayed sexual maturation. Skeletal maturation (bone age) is delayed. Headaches, visual field defects, polyuria, and polydipsia may precede or accompany the onset of growth failure in cases resulting from central nervous system disease. Abnormalities on skull radiography, computed tomography (CT), and magnetic resonance imaging (MRI) are common in organic hypopituitarism.

The diagnosis of growth hormone deficiency has remained problematic. Traditionally, provocative

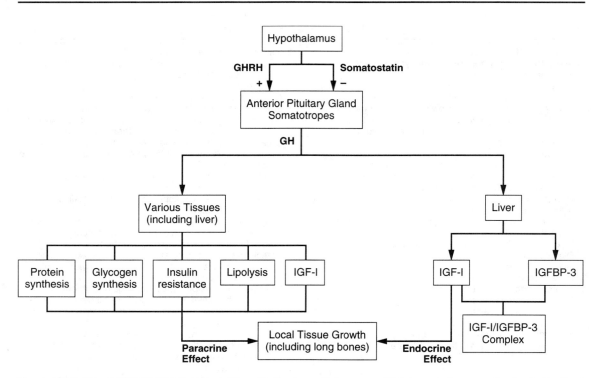

Figure 29–2. The GHRH/GH/IGF-I system. The effects of growth hormone (GH) on growth are partly due to its direct anabolic effects in muscle, liver, and bone. In addition, GH stimulates many tissues to produce IGF-I locally, which stimulates the growth of the tissue itself (**paracrine** effect of IGF-I). The action of GH on the liver results in the secretion of IGF-I (circulating IGF-I), which in turns stimulates growth in other tissues (**endocrine** effect of IGF-I). The action of growth hormone on the liver also enhances the secretion of IGF binding protein-3 (IGFBP-3), which forms a large molecular weight complex with IGF-I. The function of this complex is to transport IGF-I to its target tissues, but the complex also serves as a reservoir and possible inhibitor of IGF-I action. In various chronic illnesses, the direct metabolic effects of growth hormone are inhibited; the secretion of IGF-I in response to GH is blunted, and in some cases IGFBP-3 synthesis is enhanced, resulting in marked inhibition in the growth of the child. GHRH, growth hormone releasing hormone; IGF, insulinlike growth factor.

studies have been performed using a variety of agents including insulin-induced hypoglycemia, arginine, L-dopa, and clonidine. When results of growth hormone testing are equivocal, a trial of hGH treatment may be useful in determining whether an abnormally short child will benefit from growth hormone. Currently, the treatment of choice is synthetic hGH alone or in combination with other hormones. The dose of hGH is 0.15–0.3 mg/kg/wk administered subcutaneously; this dose is divided into six or seven equal daily doses.

Results of clinical trials with hGH-releasing hormone (somatotropin-releasing hormone) have been encouraging, and this agent may be used in the future in patients with hypothalamic hGH-releasing hormone deficiency. IGF-I, as previously described, has proved useful in growth hormone–resistant conditions. Physiologic doses of protein anabolic agents (eg, oxandrolone) may be effective in promoting linear growth but may accelerate epiphyseal closure, thus lessening adult height. Anabolic agents should

ideally be used at the time of puberty and in combination with hGH.

The efficacy of hGH treatment for conditions associated with severe short stature and normal hGH secretion (eg, intrauterine growth retardation, chronic renal disease, steroid-dependent asthma) is currently under clinical investigation. In Turner's syndrome (see Primary Amenorrhea), results over a 9-year study have demonstrated significant improvement in final adult height. The role of hGH as an anabolic agent in adults is under investigation. Early studies demonstrate significant benefit in bone metabolism and sense of well-being.

Growth hormone therapy is expensive and indications other than classic growth hormone deficiency remain controversial. Reported side effects of recombinant growth hormone therapy include benign intracranial hypertension, slipped capital femoral epiphysis, and leukemia, all subject to ongoing safety studies. Creutzfeld-Jakob disease has occurred in children previously treated with hGH.

3. HYPOTHYROIDISM

Hypothyroidism in childhood (discussed in a subsequent section) is invariably associated with poor growth and delayed skeletal maturation. In occasional cases, short stature may be the principal finding.

4. INTRAUTERINE GROWTH RETARDATION (Primordial Short Stature)

Intrauterine growth retardation may occur in craniofacial disproportion (eg, Seckel's dwarfism, Silver's syndrome, Noonan's syndrome), some cases of progeria (eg, Hutchinson-Gilford syndrome), and cachectic dwarfism, or in individuals with no accompanying significant dysmorphism. The birth weight and length of affected children are below normal for gestational age. They grow parallel with, but below, the fifth percentile. Most (85%) healthy full-term infants achieve catch-up in height during the first year of life, with half of those remaining short as adults. In most instances, skeletal maturation (bone age) corresponds to chronologic age or is only mildly delayed, in contrast to the striking delay often present in children with hGH and thyroid deficiency.

There is no satisfactory long-term treatment for primordial short stature, although growth hormone in large doses may be efficacious and is being evaluated in clinical trials.

5. SHORT STATURE DUE TO EMOTIONAL FACTORS (Psychosocial Short Stature, Deprivation Dwarfism)

Psychologic deprivation with disturbances in motor and personality development may be associated with short stature. Undernutrition contributes to the growth retardation of some but not all affected persons. Sometimes the child has an increased or even voracious appetite; polydipsia and polyuria are sometimes present. These children are of normal size at birth and grow normally for a variable period of time before growth slows. A history of feeding problems in early infancy is common. Sleep is often restless. Emotional disturbances in the family are the rule. Skeletal maturation is delayed, and serum hGH concentrations during sleep or in response to pharmacologic stimulation may be diminished.

Foster home placement or a change in the psychological and emotional environment at home usually results is significantly improved growth, normalization of personality, appetite, and dietary intake, and return of normal hGH secretion.

DIFFERENTIAL DIAGNOSIS OF SHORT STATURE

The following tests are useful when the history, physical examination, and growth chart do not point clearly to one of the conditions in Table 29–2.

1. Complete blood count (to detect chronic anemia, infection, leukemia).
2. Erythrocyte sedimentation rate (often elevated in collagen-vascular disease, cancer, chronic infection, inflammatory bowel disease).
3. Urinalysis and microscopic examination (eg, occult pyelonephritis, glomerulonephritis, renal tubular disease)
4. Stool examination for fat, occult blood, parasites, and parasite ova (inflammatory bowel disease, overwhelming parasitism).
5. Serum electrolytes and phosphorus (eg, mild adrenal insufficiency, renal tubular diseases, parathyroid disease, rickets); endomysial antibody (for celiac disease).
6. Blood urea nitrogen and serum creatinine (occult renal insufficiency).
7. Karyotyping (should be performed in all short girls with delayed sexual maturation with or without phenotypic features of Turner's syndrome).
8. Thyroid function assessment: total thyroxine (T_4), free thyroxine (FT_4), and thyroid-stimulating hormone (TSH) concentrations (short stature may be the only sign of hypothyroidism).
9. Controversy persists concerning the diagnosis of hGH deficiency. The authors prefer a combination of physiologic assessments: hGH levels obtained during natural sleep and following administration of the provocative agents clonidine and arginine. Measurement of IGF-I and IGF binding protein-3 has proved to be a useful adjunct to diagnosis. Both are typically lower in hGH deficiency.

Blizzard R, Johanson A: Disorders of growth. In: *Wilkins: The Diagnosis and Treatment of Endocrine Disorders in Childhood and Adolescence,* 4th ed. Kappy MS, Blizzard RM, Migeon CJ (editors). Charles C Thomas, 1994:383.

Goddard A, Covello R: Mutations of the growth hormone receptor in children with idiopathic short stature. J Pediatr 1995;127:244.

Hintz R: The prismatic case of Creutzfeld-Jakob disease associated with pituitary growth hormone treatment. J Clin Endocrinol Metab 1995;80:2298.

Inzucchi S, Robbins R: Effects of growth hormone on human bone biology. J Clin Endocrinol Metab 1994; 79:691.

Kallberg J, Albertsson-Wikland K: Growth in full-term small-for-gestational age infants: From birth to final height. Pediatr Res 1995;38:733.

Rappaport R, Oberfield S: Relationship of growth hormone deficiency and leukemia. J Pediatr 1995;126:759.

Rosenfeld R: Recommendations for diagnosis, treatment,

and management of individuals with Turner syndrome. The Endocrinologist 1994;4:351.

Rosenfeld R, Albertsson-Wikland K: Diagnostic controversy: The diagnosis of childhood growth hormone deficiency revisited. J Clin Endocrinol Metab 1995;80:1532.

Smith W, Nam T: Use of insulin-like growth factor-binding protein-2 (IGFBP-2), IGFBP-3, and IGF-I for assessing growth hormone status in short children. J Clin Endocrinol Metab 1993;77:1294.

Tanner J: Auxology. In: *Wilkins: The Diagnosis and Treatment of Endocrine Disorders in Childhood and Adolescence,* 4th ed. Kappy MS, Blizzard RM, Migeon CJ (editors). Charles C Thomas, 1994:137.

Zadik Z, Chalen S: Effect of long-term growth hormone therapy on bone age and pubertal maturation in boys with and without classic growth hormone deficiency. J Pediatr 1995;126:478.

TALL STATURE

Tall stature has been of concern primarily to adolescent and preadolescent girls. However, the upper limit of acceptable height in both sexes appears to be increasing, and concerns about excessive growth for girls are infrequent. When such concerns arise, the family history, growth curve, pubertal stage, and assessment of epiphyseal maturation (bone age) allow assessment of predicted final adult height. Although several conditions may produce tall stature, by far the most common cause is a constitutional or familial variation from the average (Table 29–3). Reassurance, counseling, and education may alleviate the subject's or family's concerns. In rare instances in which the predicted height appears to be excessive and unacceptable, hormonal therapy with estrogen (eg, ethinyl estradiol, 0.2–0.3 mg daily), cycled with a progestational agent for 7 out of 28 days, may be attempted to accelerate bone maturation and shorten the growth period. Estrogens are ineffective when the

physiologic age (as determined by stage of sexual maturity and epiphyseal development) has reached the 12-year-old level and may be of little value even when administered at earlier ages. Of greater concern, however, are pathologic conditions that cause acceleration of growth (see Table 29–3). Excessive growth in childhood warrants investigation to exclude early growth hormone excess, androgen excess, precocious puberty, and other genetic and syndromatic causes.

GIGANTISM & ACROMEGALY

Although growth hormone treatment is being introduced for an increasing number of indications, endogenous hGH excess is rare in childhood. As with adults, hGH excess is the result of a pituitary adenoma, which may appear in response to excessive growth hormone releasing hormone levels. The clinical presentation includes headaches and visual disturbance in most cases. Biochemical confirmation consists of elevations of serum concentrations of IGF-1 and IGF binding protein-3 (IGFBP-3), and failure of hGH to be suppressed below 2 mg/mL during an oral glucose tolerance test.

Treatment consists of transsphenoidal surgery after localization by CT scanning or MRI. Somatostatin analogue or bromocriptine may be useful when resection is incomplete or there is a recurrence. Monitoring the serum concentration of IGFBP-3 is useful in assessing efficacy of treatment.

Grinspoon S, Clemmons D: Serum insulin-like growth factor-binding protein-3 levels in the diagnosis of acromegaly. J Clin Endocrinol Metab 1995;80:927.

Wettenhall HNB, Cahill C, Roche AF: Tall girls: A survey of 15 years of management and treatment. J Pediatr 1975;86:602.

Zimmerman D, Young W: Congenital gigantism due to growth hormone-releasing hormone excess and pituitary hyperplasia with adenomatous transformation. J Clin Endocrinol Metab 1993;76:216.

Table 29–3. Causes of tall stature.

Constitutional (familial)
Endocrine causes
  Somatotropin excess (pituitary gigantism)
  Androgen excess (tall as children, short as adults)
    True sexual precocity
    Pseudosexual precocity
  Androgen deficiency (normal height as children, tall as adults)
    Klinefelter's syndrome
    Anorchia (infection, trauma, idiopathic)
  Hyperthyroidism
Genetic causes
  Klinefelter's syndrome
  Syndromes of XYY, XXYY (tall as adults)
Miscellaneous syndromes and entities
  Marfan's syndrome
  Cerebral gigantism (Soto's syndrome)
  Total lipodystrophy
  Diencephalic syndrome
  Homocystinuria

THE POSTERIOR PITUITARY GLAND

The posterior pituitary (neurohypophysis) is an extension of the ventral hypothalamus. The two principal neurohormones of the posterior pituitary, oxytocin and vasopressin, are synthesized in the supraoptic and paraventricular nuclei. After synthesis, these neurohormones are packaged in granules with specific neurophysins and transported via the axons to their storage site in the neurohypophysis.

Oxytocin is primarily important during parturition and breast-feeding and is not discussed further.

Antidiuretic Hormone (Vasopressin)

Osmoreceptors in the anterolateral hypothalamus and baroreceptors in the cardiac atria regulate antidiuretic hormone (ADH) release. Chemical mediators within the central nervous system, nausea, vomiting, and a variety of drugs and hormones influence the release of vasopressin. Disorders of vasopressin release and action include (1) central neurogenic diabetes insipidus (discussed in the following section), (2) nephrogenic diabetes insipidus (Chapter 22), and (3) the syndrome of inappropriate antidiuretic hormone (SIADH) (Chapter 40).

CENTRAL DIABETES INSIPIDUS

Essentials of Diagnosis

- Polydipsia and polyuria (>4 L/d).
- Urine specific gravity (<1.010; osmolality <280 mOsm/kg).
- Inability to concentrate urine after fluid restriction.
- Hyperosmolality of plasma (>300 mOsm/kg).
- Subnormal plasma ADH concentration.
- Responsiveness to ADH administration.

General Considerations

Hypofunction of the hypothalamus or posterior pituitary with deficiency of ADH (neurogenic, central diabetes insipidus) is usually due to loss of neurosecretory neurons in the neurohypophysis. The condition may be idiopathic, congenital, or acquired, or it may be associated with lesions of the posterior pituitary or hypothalamus (trauma, infections, suprasellar cysts, tumors, reticuloendotheliosis, or some development abnormality). Among the group previously considered to be idiopathic, improved imaging and biopsies have demonstrated frequent lymphocytic infiltrates and infundibular neurohypophysitis. Familial ADH deficiency may be transmitted as an autosomal dominant or X-linked recessive trait.

In nephrogenic diabetes insipidus, the renal tubules fail to respond to physiologic or pharmacologic doses of vasopressin, and no lesion of the pituitary or hypothalamus can be demonstrated. This disease is believed to be X-linked with variable degrees of penetrance, with a milder variant present in carrier females.

Clinical Findings

The onset of diabetes insipidus is often sudden, with polyuria, intense thirst, constipation, fever, and dehydration, particularly in infants. A desire for very cold beverages is common. The child awakens at night to urinate, is very thirsty, and drinks copiously.

It may be difficult to recognize polyuria and polydipsia in a young infant on an ordinary feeding regimen, and the infant may present with severe dehydration manifested by high fever, circulatory collapse, and convulsions. In longstanding cases, growth retardation, lack of sexual maturation, and central nervous system damage may occur. The serum osmolality exceeds 300 mOsm/kg. Familial diabetes insipidus may have a more insidious onset and a slowly progressive course.

Symptoms and signs of ADH deficiency may be absent in patients with panhypopituitarism. Treating these patients with glucocorticoids may unmask their polyuria and polydipsia.

Differential Diagnosis

Diabetes insipidus may be differentiated from psychogenic polydipsia (compulsive water drinking, potomania) and polyuria by limiting the usual excessive intake of fluid for 2–3 days and then withholding water for 7 hours. The test should be terminated if distress is clinically notable or if there is a weight loss exceeding 3% of body weight. The preliminary fluid limitation is necessary because patients with longstanding psychogenic polydipsia lose the ability to concentrate urine. Such a loss seems to correlate with the loss of the posterior pituitary signal (bright spot) on the MRI over time. Normal children and those with psychogenic polydipsia respond to dehydration with urinary osmolality above 450 mOsm/kg (specific gravity >1.020). With neurogenic and nephrogenic diabetes insipidus, the urine osmolality usually does not increase above 280 mOsm/kg (specific gravity >1.010) even after the period of dehydration. Measurement of serum ADH concentration at the time of dehydration and the administration of parenteral ADH help to distinguish between central neurogenic and nephrogenic forms of diabetes insipidus.

Decreased ability to concentrate urine may also occur with hypokalemia (eg, hyperaldosteronism) and with various forms of hypercalcemia (including hypervitaminosis D) and renal tubular abnormalities (eg, Fanconi's syndrome).

MRI may demonstrate anatomic abnormalities in central diabetes insipidus and may differentiate congenital from acquired (eg, post-traumatic) causes. The MRI in neurogenic diabetes insipidus demonstrates loss of the posterior pituitary bright spot. Gadolinium contrast is necessary to delineate small posterior pituitary tumors. Serial MRI is useful in following up post-traumatic diabetes insipidus.

Treatment

A. Medical Treatment: The treatment of choice for partial and total diabetes insipidus is desmopressin acetate administered intranasally. Typically, the dose rather than the dose interval must be adjusted, because the duration of action is generally at least 12 hours.

Chlorpropamide has been found to have an antidiuretic action through its potentiation of endogenous ADH effect; hypotension and hypoglycemia are, however, uncommon side effects limiting its use.

B. Other Therapy: Specific therapy is directed toward treatment of specific causative diseases when they are identified. Radiation therapy, surgery, and chemotherapy are used for such diseases as reticuloendotheliosis, histiocytosis, and craniopharyngioma.

Prognosis

In the absence of central nervous system damage in infancy resulting from severe dehydration and if there are no significant associated defects, life expectancy should be normal. Patients with infundibular neurohypophysitis may, in fact, have transient self-limited disease. Hydronephrosis and hydroureter are not uncommon sequelae of prolonged polyuria; patients should also be observed carefully for urinary tract infection.

Appignani B, Landy H: MR in idiopathic central diabetes insipidus of childhood. Am J Nucl Radiol 1993;14:1407.

Fujisawa I, Yamabe H: Lymphocytic infundibulohypophysitis as a cause of central diabetes insipidus. N Engl J Med 1993;329:683.

Kappy M, Ganong C: Cerebral salt wasting in children. Adv Pediatr 1996:43.

Perheentupa J, Czernichow P: Water regulation and its disorders. In: *Wilkins: The Diagnosis and Treatment of Endocrine Disorders in Childhood and Adolescence,* 4th ed. Kappy MS, Blizzard RM, Migeon CJ (editors). Charles C Thomas, 1994:1093.

THE PINEAL GLAND

The pineal gland in animals other than humans may have parenchymal cells (pinealocytes) and is often assigned an endocrine function (eg, regulation of somatic growth, sexual maturation, body pigmentation, blood glucose regulation, and day/night-sensitive neuroendocrine regulatory function). In humans, the pineal gland does not grow after the first year of life, resulting in a drop in serum melatonin concentration over childhood. About 25% of pineal glands are cystic. Pineal tumors are associated rarely with sexual precocity in the male. Cases of gonadotropin-secreting choriocarcinomas of the pineal gland with secondary Leydig cell activation and resultant sexual precocity have been reported.

Schmidt F, Penka B: Lack of pineal growth during childhood. J Clin Endocrinol Metab 1995;80:1221.

AUTOIMMUNE POLYGLANDULAR SYNDROMES (APS)

Two autoimmune syndromes causing multiple endocrine deficiencies are distinguished by their clinical, laboratory, and epidemiologic characteristics, as well as their associated nonendocrine pathology. APS type I is thought to have an autosomal recessive inheritance and usually presents in infancy. Males and females are equally affected and there is no relation to HLA type. The children (often sibling pairs) have hypoparathyroidism, Addison's disease, or mucocutaneous candidiasis singly or in combination. Other features include hypogonadism, alopecia, vitiligo, hepatitis, pernicious anemia and insulin-dependent diabetes mellitus. Autoimmune thyroid disease is rare in APS type I.

Persons with APS type II are generally adults with the HLA-DR3 and DR4 haplotypes; there is a 2–3:1 female preponderance. As seen in APS type I, Addison's disease is common, but in contrast to type I, autoimmune thyroid disease is often present, whereas diabetes is rare. Vitiligo, alopecia, hypogonadism, and pernicious anemia may be present (as in type I), and, in addition, rheumatoid arthritis and celiac disease can be seen.

Treatment is specific for each complication seen, and a recognition of the associations of disorders in these syndromes may help to detect them early in their course.

Smith BR, Furmaniak J: Adrenal and gonadal autoimmune diseases. J Clin Endocrinol Metab 1995;80:1502.

THE THYROID GLAND

FETAL DEVELOPMENT OF THE THYROID

The thyroid is capable of hormone synthesis in the 14th week of gestation, when thyroid-stimulating hormone (TSH) is detected in the fetal serum and pituitary gland. TSH does not normally cross the placenta, T_4 and T_3 cross in limited amounts, and the fetal pituitary-thyroid axis functions largely independent of the maternal pituitary-thyroid axis. Antithyroid drugs, including radioactive iodine, freely cross the placenta, and goitrous hypothyroid newborns may be born to hyperthyroid mothers who undergo treatment during pregnancy.

Mothers who have thyroid-stimulating immunoglobulins (TSI) can transmit these antibodies transplacentally, resulting in thyrotoxic newborns who may develop goiter and exophthalmos. Because

TSI may be present in the serum of controlled, previously hyperthyroid mothers, or even in women who have had surgical or radioiodine-induced removal of their thyroid glands, the possible transmission of TSI should be considered in all mothers who are or have been hyperthyroid. In addition, thyroid-binding inhibitory immunoglobulins (TBII) can cross the placenta, so that the newborn is also at risk for hypothyroidism. Both maternal TSI and TBII usually disappear from the infant's circulation by 6–8 weeks.

Physiology

Pituitary TSH stimulates the thyroid gland to take up iodine and synthesize mono-iodotyrosine and diiodotyrosine. Active hormone produced in excess of physiologic needs is stored within the thyroid follicles as colloid. The release of active thyroid hormones into the circulation is regulated by a negative feedback mechanism involving pituitary TSH and free thyroid hormone (see Figure 29–2).

Most T_4 and T_3 circulates bound to thyroid hormone-binding globulin (TBG), albumin, and prealbumin and 1% of T_3 and T_4 is free. T_4 is deiodinated in the tissues to either T_3 (active) or reverse T_3 (inactive), and the physiologic activity of thyroid hormone depends primarily on the amount of FT_4 presented to the cells. Receptors for T_3 are present on the cell surface, the nucleus, in the cytosol and on mitochondria.

At birth, the T_4 approximates that of the mother but levels increase rapidly during the first to fifth days of life in response to a TSH surge following birth. TSH levels subsequently decrease to childhood levels by 2–4 weeks of age. This physiologic neonatal TSH surge can cause falsely positive neonatal screens for hypothyroidism (ie, "high" TSH), since most of these are obtained on the first day of life.

The total T_4 is low in hypothyroidism and may be reduced in premature infants (particularly those with sepsis or respiratory distress), subacute and chronic thyroiditis, hypopituitarism, nephrosis, cirrhosis, hypoproteinemia, malnutrition, and following therapy with T_3. Prolonged administration of high doses of adrenocorticosteroids—as well as sulfonamides, testosterone, phenytoin, and salicylates—may also produce a decrease in total T_4. TSH and "free" T_4 levels remain in the normal range. The total T_3 and T_4 are high in hyperthyroidism and may be elevated in the acute forms of thyroiditis and acute hepatitis; in some types of inborn errors in thyroid hormone synthesis, release, or binding of thyroid hormone; following the administration of estrogens or clofibrate or during pregnancy; and following the administration of various iodine-containing globulins.

TBG is increased in pregnancy, after estrogen therapy (including oral contraceptives), occasionally as a genetic variation, in certain hepatic disorders, following administration of phenytoin, phenothiazines, and occasionally from an unknown cause. TBG is decreased in familial TBG deficiency; following the administration of glucocorticoids, androgens, or anabolic steroids; in nephrotic syndrome with marked hypoproteinemia; in some forms of hepatic disease; or as an idiopathic finding.

HYPOTHYROIDISM
(Congenital &
Acquired Hypothyroidism)

Essentials of Diagnosis

- Growth retardation, diminished physical activity, impaired tissue perfusion, constipation, thick tongue, poor muscle tone, hoarseness, anemia; intellectual retardation (these findings can arise in the first 2 months of life).
- Thyroid hormone concentrations low (TT_4, FT_4, and T_3 resin uptake [RU]); TSH levels elevated in primary hypothyroidism.
- *Note:* Most newborns with congenital hypothyroidism appear normal at birth and grow normally, even if untreated, for the first 3–4 months of life. Since congenital hypothyroidism must be treated as early as possible to avoid intellectual impairment, the diagnosis should be based on the newborn screening test and not on abnormal physical findings. Any suspected abnormality in the results of the newborn screen should be promptly investigated.

General Considerations

Thyroid hormone deficiency may be either congenital or acquired (juvenile hypothyroidism). Although there are many causes of hypothyroidism in the newborn (Table 29–4), most result from hypoplasia or aplasia of the thyroid gland, or failure of the gland to migrate into its normal anatomic location (ie, lingual or sublingual thyroid glands). Juvenile hypothyroidism, particularly in the presence of a history of goiter, usually results from chronic lymphocytic (Hashimoto's) thyroiditis (see below).

Of the genetically determined enzymatic defects that cause hypothyroidism (Table 29–5), only Pendred's syndrome (a defect in iodide organification with congenital nerve deafness) has distinguishing clinical features. In children who have enzymatic defects, thyroid enlargement is usually not present in the newborn period but occurs within the first two decades of life. Although thyroid function test (including radioactive iodide uptake studies) may be helpful in diagnosis, final clarification of the defect generally requires chromatographic fractionation of iodinated compounds in the serum, urine, and thyroid tissue.

Cabbage, soybeans, aminosalicylic acid, thiourea derivatives, resorcinol, phenylbutazone, cobalt, and iodides have been reported to cause goiter and hypothyroidism during pregnancy. Because many of these agents cross the placenta freely, they should be used with great caution during pregnancy.

Table 29–4. Causes of hypothyroidism.

A. Congenital (cretinism):
1. Aplasia, hypoplasia, or associated with maldescent of thyroid
   a. Embryonic defect of development
   b. Autoimmune disease (?)
2. Familial iodine-induced goiter secondary to metabolic inborn errors
   a. Iodide transport defect (defect 1)
   b. Organification defect (defect 2)
      (1) Lack of iodine peroxidase
      (2) Lack of iodine transferase: Pendred's syndrome, associated with congenital nerve deafness
   c. Coupling defect (defect 3)
   d. Iodotyrosine deiodinase defect (defect 4)
   e. Abnormal iodinated polypeptide (defects 5a and 5b)
      (1) Resulting from defect in intrathyroidal proteolysis of thyroglobulin
      (2) Abnormal plasma binding preventing use of T_4 by peripheral cells
   f. Inability of tissues to convert T_4 to T_3
3. Maternal ingestion of medications during pregnancy
   a. Maternal radioiodine
   b. Goitrogens (propylthiouracil, methimazole)
   c. Iodides
4. Iodide deficiency (endemic cretinism)
5. Idiopathic

B. Acquired (juvenile hypothyroidism):
1. Thyroidectomy or radioiodine therapy for
   a. Thyrotoxicosis
   b. Cancer
   c. Lingual thyroid
   d. Isolated midline thyroid
2. Destruction by x-ray
3. Thyrotropin deficiency
   a. Isolated
   b. Associated with other pituitary tropic hormone deficiencies
4. TRH deficiency due to hypothalamic injury or disease
5. Autoimmune disease (lymphocytic thyroiditis)
6. Chronic infections
7. Medications
   a. Iodides
      (1) Prolonged, excessive ingestion
      (2) Deficiency
   b. Cobalt
8. Idiopathic

Several hundred patients with clinical and laboratory features of resistance to thyroid hormone have been described. These syndromes are generally familial and are classified on the basis of the site of the resistance (eg, generalized; pituitary or peripheral tissue [see Refetoff et al, 1993]).

Clinical Findings

The severity of the findings in cases of thyroid deficiency depends on the age of onset and the degree of deficiency.

A. Symptoms and Signs: Even with congenital absence of the thyroid gland, the first finding may not appear for several days or weeks. Findings include physical and mental sluggishness; pale, gray, cool, or mottled skin; nonpitting myxedema; constipation; large tongue; poor muscle tone giving rise to a protuberant abdomen, umbilical hernia, and lumbar lordosis; hypothermia; bradycardia; diminished sweating (variable); decreased pulse pressure; hoarse voice or cry; delayed transient deafness; and a slow relaxation component of deep tendon reflexes (best appreciated in the ankles). Nasal obstruction and discharge and persistent jaundice may be present in the neonatal period.

The skin may be dry, thick, scaly, and coarse, with a yellowish tinge due to excessive deposition of carotene. The hair is dry, coarse, and brittle (variable) and may be excessive. Lateral thinning of the eyebrows may occur. The axillary and supraclavicular fat pads may be prominent in infants. Muscular hypertrophy (Kocher-Debré-Semelaigne syndrome)

is an unusual association with congenital hypothyroidism.

Growth changes include short stature; infantile skeletal proportions with relatively short extremities; infantile naso-orbital configuration (bridge of nose flat, broad, and underdeveloped; eyes seem to be widely spaced); delayed epiphyseal development; delayed closure of fontanelles; and retarded dental eruption. Treatment of acquired hypothyroidism may not result in the predicted final adult target height. Menometrorrhagia may be seen in older girls; galactorrhea has been reported.

In hypothyroidism resulting from enzymatic defects, ingestion of goitrogens, or chronic lymphocytic thyroiditis, the thyroid gland may be enlarged. Thyroid enlargement in children is usually symmetric, and the gland is moderately firm and without nodularity. In chronic lymphocytic thyroiditis, however, a cobblestone surface frequently is present; size and shape are readily apparent on inspection in children. Slowing of mental responsiveness and retardation of development of the brain may occur in neonates and infants, and in some cases a coincidental congenital malformation of the brain is present.

B. Laboratory Findings: Total TT_4 and FT_4 are decreased. Radioiodine uptake is below 10% (normal: 10–30%). The binding of T_3 by erythrocytes or resin in vitro (T_3RU test) is lowered. With primary hypothyroidism, the serum TSH concentration is elevated. A normocytic anemia is common, but microcytic or macrocytic anemia may occur as a result of decreased iron, folate, and cobalamin ab-

Table 29–5. Parathyroid deficiency states.

Disease or Condition	Synonym	Inheritance Pattern	Major Clinical Features	Serum Concentration Ca²⁺	P	Alk Ptase	PTH	Urinary Excretion Basal Conditions Ca²⁺	P	Response to Parathyroid Hormone[1] P	Cyclic AMP
"Idiopathic" (spontaneous), surgical, or "autoimmune" hypoparathyroidism	Autoimmune polyendocrinopathy. Thyroiditis and hypoparathyroidism (Schmidt's syndrome). Absence of parathyroid glands and thymic aplasia (DiGeorge's syndrome)	Familial in autoimmune type and associated with certain HLA types	Tetany, seizures, photophobia, diarrhea, positive Chvostek's and Trousseau's signs, candidiasis. In autoimmune type, other autoimmune diseases (eg, adrenal insufficiency, thyroiditis, pernicious anemia, diabetes mellitus).	↓(N)	↑	↓(N)	↓	N(↑,↓)	↓	N	N
Pseudohypoparathyroidism and pseudopseudohypoparathyroidism	Albright's syndrome	X-linked dominant	Brachymetacarpal and metatarsal short stature; mental subnormality; ectopic calcification of lenses, basal ganglia, and subcutaneous tissue.	↓(N)	↑(N)	↓↑(N)	↑	↓(N)	↓	↓	↓
Pseudohypoparathyroidism type II	PTH unresponsiveness	Unknown	Seizures. Phenotype normal.	↓	↑		↑	↓	↓	↓	N
Pseudohypohyperparathyroidism with osteitis fibrosa	Renal resistance to parathyroid hormone with osteitis fibrosa[2]	Probably familial	Clinical features of hypocalcemia. Phenotype normal.	↓	N	N	N(↓)	N(↑)	↓(N)	↓	↓
Pseudoidiopathic hypoparathyroidism[3]			Clinical features of hypoparathyroidism. Phenotype normal.	↓	↑		↑	↓	↑	N	N

[1]PTH is not commercially available for testing.
[2]The opposite (ie, skeletal unresponsiveness to parathyroid hormone [PTH] with normal renal responsiveness) has been described.
[3]Structural anomaly of PTH molecule has been proposed.

sorption. Serum cholesterol and carotene are usually elevated in childhood but may be low or normal in infants. Cessation of therapy in previously treated hypothyroid patients produces a marked rise in serum cholesterol levels in 6–8 weeks. Urinary creatine excretion is decreased, and urinary hydroxyproline is low. Circulating autoantibodies to thyroid constituents may be present. Erythrocyte glucose-6-phosphate dehydrogenase activity may be decreased. Serum growth hormone may be decreased, with subnormal hGH response to insulin-induced hypoglycemia and arginine stimulation.

C. Imaging: Skeletal maturation (bone age) is delayed. Centers of ossification, especially of the hip, may show multiple small centers or a single, stippled, porous, or fragmented center (epiphyseal dysgenesis). Vertebrae may show anterior beaking. Coxa vara and coxa plana may occur. Cardiomegaly is common.

Screening Programs for Neonatal Hypothyroidism

Congenital hypothyroidism should by diagnosed by neonatal screening within 60 days of birth. It may be clinically recognized during the first month of life or may be so mild that it remains unrecognized clinically for months. Adequate treatment started before the second month of life gives a good prognosis.

Differential Diagnosis

The various causes of primary hypothyroidism due to intrinsic defects of the thyroid gland must be differentiated from pituitary and hypothalamic failure with secondary thyroid insufficiency. TSH and FT_4 levels are the most useful tests and are usually sufficient in directing treatment or the need for further investigations.

Down's syndrome, chondrodystrophy, generalized gangliosidosis, I-cell disease, Hurler's and Hunter's syndromes, and certain other causes of short stature and coarse features can all be readily distinguished by the clinical manifestations and by laboratory studies.

Treatment

Levothyroxine is the drug of choice in a dose of 75–100 μg/m² once daily. In newborns and infants, the dose is 10–12 μg/kg. The hypothyroid patient may be very responsive to thyroid and may be sensitive to slight excesses of thyroid hormone. A dose of 0.025 mg (25 μg) of levothyroxine is often recommended initially with subsequent increases to full replacement in 1–2 weeks. Serum T_4 or FT_4 concentrations should be used to monitor the adequacy of therapy initially, since the elevated TSH may not fall into the normal range for several days to weeks. Later on, elevations of serum TSH are sensitive, early indicators of the need for increased medication (or increased compliance).

In the treatment of neonatal goiter with or without hypothyroidism resulting from drugs and goitrogens taken by the pregnant woman, temporary use of levothyroxine may be helpful in decreasing the size of the goiter.

Fisher DA: Management of congenital hypothyroidism. J Clin Endocrinol Metab 1991;72:523.

Glorieux J et al: Useful parameters to predict the eventual mental outcome of hypothyroid children. Pediatr Res 1988;24:6.

Refetoff S, Weiss RE, Usala SJ: The syndrome of resistance to thyroid hormones. Endocr Rev 1993;14:348.

Rivkees SA, Bode HH, Crawford JD: Long-term growth in juvenile acquired hypothyroidism: The failure to achieve normal adult stature. N Engl J Med 1988;318:599.

Sklar CA, Oazi R, David R: Juvenile autoimmune thyroiditis: Hormonal status at presentation after long-term follow-up. Am J Dis Child 1986;140:877.

THYROIDITIS

Chronic lymphocytic (Hashimoto's) thyroiditis, is perhaps the most common pediatric endocrinopathy, particularly in adolescent females. Acute and subacute thyroiditis are uncommon in all age groups.

1. ACUTE SUPPURATIVE THYROIDITIS

Acute thyroiditis is rare. Oropharyngeal organisms are thought to reach the thyroid via a patent foramen cecum and thyroglossal duct track. The most common pathogens are group A streptococci, pneumococci, *Staphylococcus aureus,* and anaerobes. The patient is invariably toxic, and the thyroid gland is exquisitely tender. There may be radiation of pain to adjacent areas of the neck or to the ear or chest. There is usually no consistently associated endocrine disturbance. Specific antibiotic therapy should be administered.

2. SUBACUTE NONSUPPURATIVE THYROIDITIS

Subacute thyroiditis (de Quervain's thyroiditis) is rare in the United States. In most cases, the cause is a virus (mumps, influenza, echovirus, coxsackievirus, Epstein-Barr virus, or adenovirus). Presenting features are similar to those of acute thyroiditis: fever, malaise, sore throat, dysphagia, pain in the thyroid gland that may radiate to the ears, and mild and transient manifestations of hyperthyroidism. In contrast to acute thyroiditis, the onset is generally insidious. The thyroid gland is firm, and the enlargement may be confined to one lobe. Radioiodine uptake is usually reduced, but thyroid hormone levels in the blood are normal or elevated. The differentiation from bacterial thyroiditis is difficult, and antibiotic therapy is consequently necessary.

3. CHRONIC LYMPHOCYTIC THYROIDITIS (Chronic Autoimmune Thyroiditis, Hashimoto's Thyroiditis, Lymphadenoid Goiter)

Essentials of Diagnosis

- Firm, freely movable, nontender, and diffusely enlarged goiter.
- Serum T_4 and TSH concentrations are generally normal but may be elevated or decreased, depending on the stage of the disease.

General Considerations

Chronic lymphocytic thyroiditis is being seen increasingly in all age groups and currently is the most common cause of goiter and hypothyroidism in childhood. In children and adolescents, the incidence peaks between the ages of 8 and 15 years and occurs most commonly in females (4:1). The disease is the result of an autoimmune attack on the thyroid. Susceptibility to thyroid autoimmunity (and other endocrine autoimmune disorders) is associated with inheritance of certain histocompatibility alleles in the APS type II (see above).

Clinical Findings

A. Symptoms and Signs: The goiter is characteristically firm, freely movable, nontender, and symmetric, with a pebbly consistency. Onset is usually insidious, and except for painless goiter; clinical manifestations are unusual. Occasionally, a sensation of tracheal compression or fullness, hoarseness, and dysphagia are described by the patient. There are no local signs of inflammation and no evidence of systemic infection.

B. Laboratory Findings: Laboratory findings are variable. Serum concentrations of T_4, FT_4, and T_3RU are usually normal but may be elevated or depressed. TSH levels may be slightly elevated during sleep. Thyroid antibodies (antithyroglobulin; antithyroid peroxidase) are usually present, although titers are frequently low. A variety of abnormalities in radioactive iodide uptake studies have been described; thyroid scans usually show a diffuse or patchy pattern, and cold (nonfunctioning) nodules have been reported. Thyroid scans and uptake studies add little to the diagnosis. Surgical or needle biopsy is diagnostic but seldom indicated.

Treatment

The treatment for chronic lymphocytic thyroiditis is controversial. Full therapeutic doses of thyroid hormone (levothyroxine, 100 μg/m²/d) may decrease the size of the goiter within 3 months, but in controlled trials the efficacy of thyroid hormone therapy is unsupported. Hypothyroidism is believed to be a common end-result of autoimmune thyroiditis in the second to third decades of life; consequently, patients with adolescent goiter require lifelong surveillance.

4. RIEDEL'S STRUMA (Chronic Fibrous Thyroiditis, Woody Thyroiditis, Invasive Thyroiditis)

Riedel's struma is extremely rare in the United States, particularly in children. It is characterized by marked and invasive fibrosis that extends beyond the thyroid gland to involve the trachea, esophagus, blood vessels, nerves, and muscles of the neck, so that the gland becomes fixed to these tissues. Surgery may be necessary to relieve fibrotic obstruction or constriction of neighboring structures and to eliminate thyroid carcinoma from the differential diagnosis.

Dayan CM, Daniels, GH: Chronic autoimmune thyroiditis. N Engl J Med 1996;335:99.

Rich EJ, Mendelman PM: Acute suppurative thyroiditis in pediatric patients. Pediatr Infect Dis J 1987;6:936.

Weetman AP, McGregor AM: Autoimmune thyroid disease: Developments in our understanding. Endocr Rev 1984;5:309.

HYPERTHYROIDISM

Essentials of Diagnosis

- Nervousness, irritability, emotional lability, tremor, excessive appetite, weight loss, smooth, moist, warm skin, increased perspiration, and heat intolerance.
- Goiter, exophthalmos, tachycardia, widened pulse pressure (systolic hypertension).
- Thyroid function studies elevated (eg, TT_4, FT_4, T_3RU). TSH concentration suppressed.

General Considerations

Most cases of hyperthyroidism in children are likely to have an autoimmune cause. Hyperthyroidism occurs with certain diseases that have an autoimmune basis, and a familial pattern with a predilection for females supports a role for a heritable and autoimmune basis. IgG antibody to thyroid receptors (TSI) stimulates thyroid hormone production. Transient congenital hyperthyroidism may occur in infants or thyrotoxic mothers. Hyperthyroidism may be associated with acute, subacute, or chronic thyroiditis, tumors of the thyroid, other tumors producing thyrotropin-like substances, and exogenous thyroid hormone excess.

Clinical Findings

A. Symptoms and Signs: Hyperthyroidism is four times more common in females than in males. The disease most frequently occurs in childhood between ages 12 and 14 years; only 2% of patients present before 10 years of age. The course of hyperthyroidism tends to be cyclic, with spontaneous remissions and exacerbations. A deterioration in school performance is a common feature in the history. Findings include weakness, dyspnea, dysphagia, amenorrhea, emotional instability, nervousness, marked variability in mood, personality disturbances, and (rarely) tremors and movements that may simulate chorea. The skin is warm and moist; the face is flushed. Palpitations, tachycardia, and systolic hypertension with increased pulse pressure are common. Proptosis and exophthalmos are common in hyperthyroid children. Goiter is present in more than 90% of cases and is characteristically diffuse and usually firm. A bruit and thrill may be present. Variable degrees of accelerated growth and development occur, and loss of weight is common despite polyphagia. In neonatal hyperthyroidism, hepatosplenomegaly and thrombocytopenia with antiplatelet antibodies are occasionally seen.

B. Laboratory Findings: TT_4, FT_4 and T_3RU are elevated, except in rare cases in which only the serum T_3 radioimmunoassay concentration is elevated (T_3 thyrotoxicosis). Radioiodine uptake is elevated and does not suppress with T_3 (cytomel), 25 µg three or four times daily for 7 days. The basal metabolic rate is elevated, and serum cholesterol is low. Antibodies to thyroglobulin are found in most patients. Circulating TSH concentrations measured by very sensitive assays are depressed, and TSI is often present in plasma.

C. Imaging: Skeletal maturation assessed radiographically is advanced in younger children. In newborns, accelerated bony maturation may be associated with subsequent premature closure of the cranial sutures. Longstanding hyperthyroidism is associated with osteoporosis.

Differential Diagnosis

Although the well-established case of hyperthyroidism seldom presents a problem in diagnosis, the findings in the early stages of the disease may be confused with chorea or, more commonly, with euthyroid goiter. Typically, the patient is an adolescent with a recent decline in school performance, nervousness, emotional lability, and increased perspiration. Repeated clinical and laboratory evaluations may be required to make the diagnosis. Disease states associated with hypermetabolism (severe anemia, leukemia, chronic infections, pheochromocytoma, as well as muscle-wasting disease) may resemble hyperthyroidism clinically but differ in the thyroid function studies.

Treatment

The symptoms of hyperthyroidism can fluctuate and in some mild cases may not require treatment.

A. General Measures: Bed rest is advisable only in severe cases, in preparation for surgery, or at the beginning of a medical regimen. The diet should be high in calories, carbohydrates, and vitamins (particularly vitamin B_1).

B. Medical Treatment: It takes 2–3 weeks to see a clinical response, and adequate control may take 2–3 months. The thyroid frequently increases in size as treatment is started, but then usually decreases within several months.

1. β-Adrenergic blocking agents (propranolol, atenolol)–These agents may be helpful in controlling symptoms of nervous instability and tachycardia and are indicated in severe disease with cardiovascular abnormalities (tachycardia, hypertension). In mild cases, β-blockade without other antithyroid treatment may be adequate. In large doses, propranolol decreases the peripheral conversion of T_4 to T_3.

2. Propylthiouracil–This drug interferes with thyroid hormone synthesis and, in large doses, with the peripheral conversion of T_4 to T_3. The correct dose must always be individually determined. Propylthiouracil is frequently used in the initial treatment of children with hyperthyroidism. Short-term therapy is occasionally successful, but treatment usually must be continued for at least 2–3 years with the smallest drug dosage that will produce a euthyroid state. If T_4 levels rise rapidly with reduction in drug dosage after 18–24 months of therapy, continued or alternative therapy will be necessary. Relapse occurs in 10–30% of cases, and severe cases may not respond.

a. Initial dosage–Give 75–300 mg/d in three or four divided doses 6–8 hours apart until tests of thyroid function are normal and all signs and symptoms have subsided. Larger doses are frequently necessary.

b. Maintenance–Give 50–100 mg/d in two or three divided doses. Some authors recommend continuing the drug at higher levels until the euthyroid state is approached or reached and, then, as the TSH level rises, adding thyroid hormone. The role of adjunctive thyroxine therapy in preventing recurrence of hyperthyroidism in Graves' disease is controversial. T_4 and TSH levels should be monitored during antithyroid treatment to determine whether the patient is becoming hypothyroid; thyroid hormone is added when indicated.

c. Toxicity–Granulocytopenia, fever, rash, and arthralgia may occur. The drug must be discontinued, and antibiotics and a short course of one of the adrenocorticosteroids should be prescribed if indicated.

3. Methimazole–This drug may be used in one-fifteenth to one-tenth the dosage of propylthiouracil and may be effective with a once-to-twice daily dosage schedule. Toxic reactions are similar to those seen with propylthiouracil.

4. Iodide–Medical treatment with continuous iodide administration alone usually produces a rapid but brief response. Because the efficacy of iodide is short-lived, it is generally recommended only for acute management. A progressive increase in dosage is often required for satisfactory control, and toxic reactions to iodide are not uncommon.

C. Radiation Therapy: Radioactive iodide (^{131}I) is currently being used as initial therapy for children and adolescents. Reports do not support the fear of an increased incidence of thyroid cancer, particularly when an ablative dose of ^{131}I is used. Therapy with thyroid hormone is necessary after thyroid ablation.

D. Surgical Measures: Subtotal thyroidectomy is considered by some to be the treatment of choice, especially when a close follow-up of the patient is difficult or impossible. In childhood, surgery should be used in patients when medical treatment is impossible or has been unsuccessful. The patient should be prepared first with bed rest, diet, and propranolol (as above) and with iodide and propylthiouracil as follows: Propylthiouracil should be given for 2–4 weeks. Iodide (as saturated solution of potassium iodide) is added 10–21 days before surgery is scheduled. Iodides act by blocking the effect of TSH on the thyroid, with a resultant decrease in iodine trapping and reduction of vascularity, and by inhibiting the release of hormone, thus reducing the possibility of thyroid storm. Give 1–10 drops daily for 10–21 days. Continue the drug for 1 week after surgery.

Management of Congenital (Transient) Hyperthyroidism

Congenital hyperthyroidism has a significant death rate in the neonatal period, but the eventual prognosis in surviving infants is excellent. Temporary treatment of congenital hyperthyroidism may be necessary, in which case iodides appear to be the drug of choice. Reserpine or propranolol may be necessary to control cardiac arrhythmias. Transection of an enlarged thyroid isthmus may be of value if respiratory distress due to tracheal compression is present.

Course & Prognosis

Improvement may occur without therapy in up to one third of cases, but partial remissions and exacerbations may continue for several years. With medical treatment alone, prolonged remissions may be expected in one half to two thirds of cases. Surgical therapy yields similar results. Postoperative hypothyroidism is not uncommon, and hypoparathyroidism and other complications may occur. Because of the comparatively high incidence of carcinoma in nodular goiters of childhood, such glands should be removed routinely once the thyrotoxicosis is in remission. Progressive exophthalmos following surgery is uncommon in childhood.

Becker DV: Choice of therapy during pregnancy. N Engl J Med 1984;311:464.

Burros GN: Hyperthyroidism during pregnancy. N Engl J Med 1978;298:150.

Collen RJ et al: Remission rates of children and adolescents with thyrotoxicosis treated with antithyroid drugs. Pediatrics 1980;65:550.

Heshizume K et al: Administration of thyroxine in treated Graves' disease. N Engl J Med 1991;324:947.

Levy WJ, Schumacher OP, Gupta M: Treatment of childhood Graves' disease. Cleve Clin J Med 1988;55:373.

CARCINOMA OF THE THYROID

Carcinoma of the thyroid is uncommon in childhood. The presentation is usually with asymptomatic asymmetric thyroid enlargement. Neck discomfort, dysphagia, voice changes, and respiratory difficulty are unusual but may occur. Fifty percent of children have metastatic disease at the time of presentation, usually to regional lymph nodes. Pulmonary metastasis occurs in 5% of cases.

Thyroid functions tests are usually normal. A technetium or iodine scan of the thyroid show a "cold" nodule and is the most definitive diagnostic test. Pulmonary metastases should be excluded by a CT scan of the chest.

Papillary carcinoma is the most common form in childhood, and the prognosis with treatment is relatively good (survival rate greater than 80% after 10–20 years). The treatment of choice is surgical excision of the entire gland and removal of all involved lymph nodes. Radical neck dissection is usually not indicated. If metastatic disease is not identified at surgery or by radioactive iodide scan postoperatively, replacement thyroid hormone is generally the only additional therapy required. Follow-up thyroid scans every 2–5 years are recommended.

Other, less common malignant tumors of the thyroid are follicular, medullary, and undifferentiated carcinomas, lymphomas, and sarcomas. Medullary carcinoma of the thyroid may be familial (autosomal dominant), usually occurring as a component of type 2 multiple endocrine neoplasia (MEN). This condition may be associated with excessive elaboration of gastrin and calcitonin, with pheochromocytoma, parathyroid hyperplasia, "marfanoid habitus," and mucosal neuromas (MEN type 2B). The treatment and prognosis depend on the cell type present, but the outcome is generally less favorable.

Gagel RF et al: Medullary thyroid carcinoma: Recent progress. J Clin Endocrinol Metab 1993;76:809.

Samuel AM, Sharma SH: Differentiated thyroid carcinomas in children and adolescents. Cancer 1991;67:2168.

DISORDERS OF CALCIUM HOMEOSTASIS

The integrated action of parathyroid hormone (PTH) and vitamin D on bone, small intestine, and kidney maintains the serum calcium level within a narrow normal range and contributes to normal bone mineralization. Deficiencies and excesses of these agents, as well as abnormalities in their receptors or of vitamin D metabolism, lead to the clinical disturbances described below and shown in Tables 29–5, 29–6, and 29–7. Less important factors contributing to calcium homeostasis include calcitonin, magnesium, pyrophosphate, and phosphorus.

HYPOPARATHYROIDISM

Essentials of Diagnosis

- Tetany with facial and extremity numbness, tingling, cramps, spontaneous muscle contractures, carpopedal spasm, positive Trousseau's and Chvostek's signs, loss of consciousness, convulsions.
- Diarrhea, photophobia, prolongation of electrical systole (QT interval) and laryngospasm.
- Defective nails and teeth, cataracts, and ectopic calcification in the subcutaneous tissues and basal ganglia.
- Serum and urine calcium normal or low; serum phosphorus high; urine phosphorus low; alkaline phosphatase normal or low; azotemia absent. Inappropriately low ratio of PTH to ionized calcium.

General Considerations

PTH deficiency results either from an absolute deficiency of PTH, an abnormality in the PTH molecule, or from "hormone resistant states" related to abnormalities of the PTH-receptor complex or its postreceptor action in the face of normal hormonal secretion (ie, pseudohypoparathyroid states; see Table 29–5). Hypoparathyroidism may be idiopathic or may result from autoimmune damage or from parathyroidectomy. Hypoparathyroidism may develop following thyroidectomy, with either an acute or an insidious onset, and may be transient or permanent. Parathyroid deficiency has been reported following irradiation of the neck or the administration of therapeutic doses of radioactive iodine for carcinoma of the thyroid.

Two types of transient hypoparathyroidism ("early" and "late") may be present in the newborn, both of which are due to a relative deficiency of PTH or hormone action. The early form occurs within the first 2 weeks of life in newborns with a history of birth asphyxia of those born to mothers with diabetes mellitus or hyperparathyroidism.

Hypomagnesemia may also be seen in the early form and augments the severity of hypocalcemia. The most common late form occurs almost exclusively in infants fed a milk formula with a high phosphate:calcium ratio.

Autoimmune hypoparathyroidism may be associated with candidal infection, Addison's disease, insulin-dependent mellitus, pernicious anemia, alopecia, vitiligo, thyroiditis, hypogonadism, steatorrhea, and hepatitis (see APS type I in previous text). This form of hypoparathyroidism is often familial (autosomal recessive). Infections resulting from lack of immune reaction to *Candida* may lead to severe intractable cutaneous and gastrointestinal candidiasis. Because of the frequent association of adrenocortical insufficiency with parathyroid insufficiency, adrenocortical function should be tested repeatedly.

Congenital absence of the parathyroids may occur in association with congenital absence of the thymus (with resultant thymic-dependent immunologic deficiency) and cardiovascular (DiGeorge syndrome), cerebral, and ocular defects.

Clinical Findings

A. Symptoms and Signs: Prolonged hypocalcemia causes tetany, photophobia, blepharospasm, and diarrhea.

Tetany is manifested by numbness, cramps, and twitchings of the extremities; carpopedal spasm and laryngospasm; positive Chvostek's sign (tapping of the face in front of the ear produces spasm of the facial muscles); positive Trousseau's sign (compression of the upper arm with a blood pressure cuff inflated to a pressure above systole for 2–4 minutes produces carpopedal spasm); unexplained bizarre behavior; irritability; loss of consciousness; convulsions; and retarded physical and mental development. Headache, vomiting, diarrhea, photophobia, increased intracranial pressure, papilledema, and pseudopapilledema may occur. In early infancy, respiratory distress may be the presenting finding.

B. Laboratory Findings (see Table 29–5): Serum calcium is decreased, serum phosphorus increased, and serum alkaline phosphatase is usually low-normal. Urinary excretion of calcium and phosphorus is usually decreased but is influenced by the dietary intake. Renal clearance of phosphorus is decreased, and the maximum tubular reabsorption of phosphate falls by 12–30% from a normal value of 85%. PTH levels are inappropriately reduced in relation to the ionized calcium concentration.

C. Imaging: Soft tissue and basal ganglia calcification may occur in idiopathic hypoparathyroidism or in pseudohypoparathyroidism.

Differential Diagnosis

The differential diagnosis of hypoparathyroid

Table 29–6. Rickets and disorders of calcium metabolism.[1]

Disease or Condition	Synonym	Inheritance Pattern	Clinical Features	Metabolic Features						Treatment
				Serum Concentrations				Urinary Excretion		
				Ca²⁺	P	Alk Ptase	PTH	Ca²⁺	P	
Hypoparathyroid states	See Table 29–5.									Vitamin D and calcium
Transient tetany of the newborn			Tetany, focal seizures; more common in prematures and infants of diabetic mothers; rarely described in association with maternal hyperparathyroidism	↓	↓ (N)	↓ (N)	↓ (N)	↓ (N)	↑ (N)	Diet high in calcium, low in phosphate; vitamin D may be necessary
Malabsorption syndrome	Disease entities associated with malabsorption include cystic fibrosis, celiac disease, sprue, Shwachman syndrome; hypoplasia of cartilage and hair.	Generally familial with mode of inheritance related to specific disease	Steatorrhea, failure to thrive. Some forms associated with neutropenia, skeletal anomalies, immunologic deficiencies, and abnormalities of cartilage and hair	↓ (N)	(N) ↓	↑ (N)	↑ (N)	↓	N (↑↓)	Vitamin D, calcium, and magnesium (hypomagnesemic states)
Chronic renal insufficiency			Growth failure, undernutrition, skeletal changes	↓ (N)	↑	↑ (N)	↑	↓ (N)	↓	Diet high in calcium, low in phosphorus; vitamin D
Vitamin D-deficient rickets	Infantile rickets		Rickets	↓ (N)	↓	↑	↑	↑	↑	Vitamin D and calcium
Familial hypophosphatemic vitamin D-resistant rickets[2]	(1) Hereditary vitamin D-resistant rickets (2) Phosphate diabetes (3) X-linked hypophosphatemia	X-linked dominant (occasionally autosomal dominant or sporadic)	Skeletal deformities, growth retardation	N (↓)	↓	N	N (↑)	N	↑	Oral phosphate and vitamin D
Hereditary vitamin D-refractory rickets[3] Type I Type II	(1) Hypophosphatemic vitamin D-refractory rickets (2) Pseudo-vitamin D-deficiency rickets	Autosomal recessive	Severe rachitic bone changes; generalized aminoaciduria	↓	↓ (N)	↑	↑	↓	↑	Vitamin D (calciferol) in large doses or approximately physiologic doses of 1,25-dihydroxycholecalciferol

[1] Normal tubular reabsorption of phosphate (TRP) is 83–98%; the lower values are associated with higher serum levels of phosphorus. In hypoparathyroidism, TRP varies from 40 to 70%. Low values for TRP are also found in some forms of inherited renal tubular disease, eg, vitamin D-resistant rickets.

[2] A variety of diseases (cystinosis, galactosemia, tyrosinosis, Wilson's disease, hereditary fructose intolerance) are associated with renal tubular defects and should be considered in the differential diagnosis.

[3] Type I has been shown to be the result of defective renal 1α-hydroxylation of 25-hydroxycholecalciferol; type II is due to tissue unresponsiveness to normal levels of 1,25-dihydroxycholecalciferol; in this type, the vitamin D receptor complex fails to bind to DNA.

Table 29–7. Hypercalcemic states.

I. **Primary hyperparathyroidism**
  A. Hyperplasia
  B. Adenoma
  C. Familial, including MEN I and II
  D. Ectopic PTH secretion
II. **Hypercalcemic states other than primary hyperpara-thyroidism associated with increased intestinal or re-nal absorption of calcium**
  A. Hypervitaminosis D (including idiopathic hypercalcemia of infancy)
  B. Familial hypocalciuric hypercalcemia
  C. Lithium therapy
  D. Sarcoidosis
  E. Phosphate depletion
  F. Aluminum intoxication
III. **Hypercalcemic states other than hyperparathyroid-ism associated with increased mobilization of bone minerals**
  A. Hyperthyroidism
  B. Immobilization
  C. Thiazides
  D. Vitamin A intoxication
  E. Malignant neoplasms
    1. Ectopic PTH secretion
    2. Prostaglandin-secreting tumor and perhaps prostaglandin release from subcutaneous fat necrosis
    3. Tumors metastatic to bone
    4. Myeloma

MEN = multiple endocrine neoplasia; PTH = parathyroid hormone.

states is outlined in Table 29–5. Convulsions may suggest epilepsy and other chronic disorders of the central nervous system. Central nervous system features (headache, vomiting, increased intracranial pressure, and convulsions) may require differentiation from other causes of increased intracranial pressure, such as brain tumor.

Treatment

A. Acute or Severe Tetany: The objective of treatment is to correct hypocalcemia immediately with calcium intravenously and orally.

B. Maintenance Management of Hypoparathyroidism and Chronic Hypocalcemia: The objective of treatment is to maintain the serum calcium and phosphate at an approximately normal level.

1. Drugs—Give ergocalciferol (vitamin D_2), cholicalciferol (vitamin D_3), dihydrotachysterol, or calcitriol (1,25-dihydroxyvitamin D_3). These preparations may not reach their peak effects for 3–7 days; since they are fat-soluble and are stored in the adipose tissue and the liver, their activity persists for weeks or months. Careful control of dosage with frequent determinations of serum and urine calcium and the ability to concentrate urine is essential to avoid hypercalcemia with resultant nephrocalcinosis and potential renal damage.

2. Diet—A low-phosphate, high-calcium diet, with added calcium lactate or carbonate (300–1200 mg three or four times daily with meals) is the treatment of choice for prolonged oral therapy both for raising serum calcium and lowering serum phosphate. Because calcium is efficiently absorbed, large doses of vitamin D are rarely necessary.

Course & Prognosis

Abnormal mineral concentrations in extracellular fluid are easily corrected. Central nervous system manifestations are usually reversible, and the prognosis for intellectual development is excellent. Hypercalcemia and consequent renal damage must be avoided: patients receiving high doses of long-acting vitamin D preparations must be carefully monitored.

Canalis E: The hormonal and local regulation of bone formation. Endocr Rev 1983;4:62.
Sanchez GJ et al: Hypercalcitonemia and hypocalcemia in acutely ill children: Studies in serum calcium, blood ionized calcium, and calcium, and calcium-regulating hormones. J Pediatr 1989;114:952.

PSEUDOHYPOPARATHYROIDISM (Albright's Syndrome, Albright's Hereditary Osteodystrophy, & Pseudopseudohypoparathyroidism)

Pseudohypoparathyroidism is an X-linked disease with a female:male ratio of approximately 2:1. PTH production is adequate, but there is a failure of response of the target organ (renal tubule, bone, or both) to the hormone. The failure of responses results from deficiency of the G unit of the trimolecular cyclase complex. This messenger pathway is used in other hormone target tissues. Therefore, resistance to other adenylyl cyclase–dependent hormones (eg, ADH, TSH) has been described in pseudohypoparathyroidism.

Patients with pseudohypoparathyroidism may have the same clinical features and chemical findings seen in idiopathic hypoparathyroidism (see Table 29–5). In addition, these patients have distinct phenotypes consisting of short stature; round, full faces; irregularly shortened hands and feet (with the index and third metacarpal bones often longer than the first, fourth, and fifth ones); a short, thick-set body; delayed and defective dentition; and mild mental retardation. The hair is dry and coarse, and nails and skin are thickened; candidiasis is not a feature. X-ray films may show thickness of the long bones with limitation of growth at the metaphyseal ends. There may be chondrodysplastic changes in the bones of the hands, demineralization of the bones, thickening of the cortices, and exostoses. Corneal and lenticular opacities and ectopic calcification of the basal ganglia and subcutaneous tissues may occur with or without abnormal serum calcium levels. Treatment is the same as that for hypoparathyroidism.

Similar phenotypic findings may be found in pseudopseudohypoparathyroidism, a variant of pseudohypoparathyroidism in which the blood chemistry findings are normal. No treatment is necessary.

In both pseudo- and pseudopseudohypoparathyroidism, the parathyroid glands are hyperplastic, serum levels of PTH are elevated, and the kidneys are relatively unresponsive to PTH.

Patten JL et al: Mutation in the gene encoding the stimulatory G protein of adenylate cyclase in Albright's hereditary osteodystrophy. N Engl J Med 1990;322:1412.

Spiegel AM, Shenker A, Weinstein LS: Receptor-effector coupling by G-proteins: Implications for abnormal signal transduction. Endocr Rev 1992;13:536.

HYPERPARATHYROIDISM & HYPERCALCEMIC STATES

Essentials of Diagnosis

- Abdominal pain, polyuria, polydipsia, hypertension, nephrocalcinosis, renal stones, intractable peptic ulcer, constipation, uremia, and pancreatitis.
- Bone pain and, rarely, pathologic fractures. X-ray film shows subperiosteal resorption, loss of the lamina dura of the teeth, renal parenchymal calcification or stones, and bone cysts or "brown tumors."
- Unusual (often bizarre) behavior and mood swings.
- Elevated serum concentrations of PTH.
- Serum (and urine) ionized calcium elevated; urine phosphate high, with low or normal serum phosphate; alkaline phosphatase normal or elevated.
- Short-term or mild hypercalcemia possibly entirely asymptomatic; hypercalcemia and mild hyperparathyroidism noted frequently as incidental findings in routine laboratory screening.

General Considerations

Over 80% of hypercalcemic children or adolescents have either hyperparathyroidism or a malignant tumor (see Table 29–7). The latter condition is invariably associated with additional significant clinical features, and the diagnosis is readily established. Hyperparathyroidism is rare in childhood and may be primary or secondary. The most common cause of primary hyperparathyroidism is a parathyroid adenoma. The most common causes of the secondary form are chronic renal disease (glomerulonephritis, pyelonephritis), congenital anomalies of the genitourinary tract, or rickets (see Table 29–6). Diffuse parathyroid hyperplasia or multiple adenomas has also been described in families. Familial hyperparathyroidism may be an isolated disease, or it may be associated with other endocrine neoplasias of the type 1 and, rarely, type 2 MEN syndromes.

Clinical Findings

A. Symptoms and Signs:

1. Due to hypercalcemia–Findings include hypotonicity and weakness of muscles; apathy, mood swings, and bizarre behavior; nausea, vomiting, abdominal pain, constipation, and loss of weight; hyperextensibility of joints; and hypertension, cardiac irregularities, bradycardia, and shortening of the QT interval. Coma occurs rarely. Calcium deposits may occur in the cornea or conjunctiva (band keratopathy). Detection of this important finding may require slit-lamp examination of the eye. Intractable peptic ulcer and pancreatitis occur in adults and rarely in children.

2. Due to increased calcium and phosphorus excretion–Findings include loss of renal concentrating ability with polyuria, polydipsia, precipitation of calcium phosphate in the renal parenchyma or as urinary calculi, and progressive renal damage.

3. Due to changes in the skeleton–Findings may include bone pain, osteitis fibrosa, subperiosteal absorption of phalanges, absence of lamina dura around the teeth, spontaneous fractures, and a "motheaten" appearance of the skull.

B. Imaging: Bone changes may be subtle in children even when radiography shows nephrocalcinosis. When bone changes occur, the distal clavicle and middle phalanges are initially affected. Later, there is a generalized demineralization with a predilection for subperiosteal cortical bone.

Treatment

Treatment consists of complete removal of the tumor or subtotal removal of hyperplastic parathyroid glands. Preoperatively, intake of dietary calcium should be restricted and hypercalcemia controlled with normal saline infusion and nonthiazide diuretics. Postoperatively, hypocalcemia tetany may occur. A diet high in calcium and vitamin D is recommended immediately postoperatively and is continued until serum calcium concentrations are normal and stable.

Treatment of secondary hyperparathyroidism is directed at the underlying disease. Diminution in the absorption of phosphate with aluminum hydroxide orally is helpful. The hypocalcemia of severe renal disease (creatinine clearance less than 15 mL/min) results from increased complexing with the elevated phosphate, metabolic acidosis, and impaired renal activation of vitamin D. Treatment with calcitriol is useful in this disorder.

Course & Prognosis

The prognosis following removal of a single adenoma is excellent. The prognosis following subtotal parathyroidectomy for diffuse hyperplasia or removal of multiple adenomas is usually good and depends on correction of the underlying defect. In patients with multiple sites of parathyroid adenoma or hyperplasia,

MEN is likely, and other family members may be at risk. Genetic counseling and DNA analysis to determine the specific gene defect are indicated.

A variety of drugs (excessive vitamin A or D, lithium, aluminum, thiazide diuretics) may result in hypercalcemia. Sarcoidosis, immobilization, hyperthyroidism, and hypothyroidism are additional disease conditions associated with hypercalcemia.

Ross AJ: Parathyroid surgery in children. Prog Pediatr Surg 1991;26:48.

IDIOPATHIC FAMILIAL HYPOCALCIURIC HYPERCALCEMIA

As the name implies, this interesting condition is distinguished by extremely high renal calcium reabsorption with consequent low to normal urinary calcium excretion. Since the renal response to PTH is calcium reabsorption, hypercalciuria is seen in hyperparathyroidism only when bone resorption exceeds renal calcium reabsorption. The condition appears explicable on the basis of mild hyperparathyroidism.

Idiopathic familial hypocalciuric hypercalcemia is usually familial (autosomal dominant). There appears to be an abnormality in the ion (eg, calcium)-sensing receptor site in the renal tubule resulting in an increased set point for the serum calcium excretion threshold. Patients are invariably asymptomatic, and treatment is unnecessary. Parathyroidectomy is contraindicated. The prognosis is excellent.

Page LA, Haddow JE: Self-limited neonatal hyperparathyroidism in familial hypocalciuric hypercalcemia. J Pediatr 1987;111:261.

HYPERVITAMINOSIS D

Exposure to sunlight and ingestion of vitamin D in a normal diet do not result in hypervitaminosis D and hypercalcemia, except possibly in Williams syndrome or sarcoidosis. Vitamin D intoxication is the result of ingestion of excessive amounts of vitamin D, some forms of which may be stored for months in adipose tissue.

Signs and symptoms of vitamin D-induced hypercalcemia are the same as those in other hypercalcemic states and include abdominal, renal, central nervous system, and bone findings. Renal insufficiency may be irreversible and is the result of renovascular effects of hypercalcemia and precipitation of calcium phosphate in renal interstitial tissue. Ectopic calcification can occur in many other tissues, including the cornea and the gastric mucosa.

Treatment depends on the stage of hypercalcemic toxicity. Because of adipose tissue storage of vitamin D, several months of treatment may be necessary. Dietary intake of foods fortified with vitamin D (eg, milk) and calcium should be reduced or eliminated, if possible. Hypercalcemia can be treated with intravenous fluids and nonthiazide diuretics. Adrenocorticosteroids, salmon calcitonin, and the antineoplastic agent plicamycin have also been used with success.

The central nervous system manifestations may be dramatic, and deaths have occurred during acute crises. Chronic brain damage in young infants has been reported. Asymptomatic renal damage may cause failure before the diagnosis is made.

IDIOPATHIC HYPERCALCEMIA OF INFANCY

Idiopathic hypercalcemia (Williams syndrome) is an uncommon disorder of infancy characterized in its severe form by peculiar ("elfin") facies (receding mandible, depressed bridge of nose, relatively large mouth, prominent eyes, occasional esotropia, and hypertelorism). Failure to thrive, mental and motor retardation, cardiovascular abnormalities, irritability, purposeless movements, constipation, hypotonia, polyuria, polydipsia, and hypertension are common. Cardiac defects include supravalvular aortic stenosis, peripheral pulmonary stenosis, and aortic valve calcifications. A gregarious and affectionate personality is the rule in older children with the syndrome. Generalized osteosclerosis is common, and there may be premature craniosynostosis and nephrocalcinosis with evidence of urinary tract disease.

Clinical manifestations may not appear for several months after birth. Serum concentrations of 1,25-dihydroxycholecalciferol (1,25-dihydroxyvitamin D_3) were frequently elevated in cases reported after World War II in England when excessive vitamin D was introduced into the diet. Currently, a defect in the metabolism of, or responsiveness to, vitamin D is postulated, rather than excessive dietary vitamin D intake and elevated serum 1,25-dihydroxycholecalciferol levels. Elastin deletions localized to chromosome 7 have been identified in over 90% of patients; thus, fluorescent in situ hybridization (FISH) analysis may be the best initial diagnostic tool.

Treatment consists of rigid restriction of dietary calcium and vitamin D and, in severe, unresponsive cases, moderate doses of glucocorticoids.

IMMOBILIZATION HYPERCALCEMIA

Abrupt immobilization of a rapidly growing adolescent following an injury may lead to a rapid decrease in bone deposition with continued bone resorption, calcium mobilization, and hypercalcemia. The condition is reversible when the patient becomes ambulatory.

HYPOPHOSPHATASIA

Hypophosphatasia is an uncommon inherited (autosomal recessive) condition characterized by a specific deficiency of alkaline phosphatase activity in serum, bone, and tissues. Radiographically, there is inadequate mineralization of epiphyseal cartilage and osteoid, with localized areas of radiolucency. The disease is radiographically and histologically similar to rickets. The earlier the age at onset, the more severe the condition. Failure to thrive, feeding problems, dwarfing, hyperpyrexia, delayed dentition or premature loss of teeth, widening of the sutures, bulging fontanelles, convulsions, bony deformities indistinguishable from rickets, hyperpigmentation, conjunctival calcification, bank keratopathy, and renal lesions have been reported. Premature closure of cranial sutures may occur. Calcium and phosphate concentrations in the extracellular fluid are usually normal; calcium levels, however, may be elevated. In the latter case, signs and symptoms may be similar to those of idiopathic hypercalcemia; late features include osteoporosis, osteopenia, and pseudofractures. The plasma and urine of patients and heterozygote carriers contain phosphoethanolamine in excessive amounts. In some cases, marked metaphyseal irregularities may occur. A condition known as **pseudohypophosphatasia** has been described in which the clinical features of hypophosphatasia are seen in association with normal levels of alkaline phosphatase.

No specific treatment is available, but glucocorticoids may be of value. The mortality rate is high in infancy. Adults are usually asymptomatic.

Russo AF et al: Characterization of the calcitonin/CGAP gene in Williams syndrome. Am J Med Genet 1991; 39:28.

THE GONADS
(Ovaries & Testes)

DEVELOPMENT & PHYSIOLOGY

The gonads develop from a bipotential anlage in the genital ridge of the celomic cavity. The primordial germ cells, which will become oocytes and spermatocytes, arise in the yolk sac and migrate to the genital ridge by the fourth week after conception, when the gonad is identifiable. Between the fourth and eighth weeks of gestation, differentiation into an ovary or testis occurs; by 7–9 weeks, the fetal testis begins to produce androgens, and granulosa cells can be identified in the ovary. Testicular androgen production at this time occurs in response to placental

human chorionic gonadotropin (hCG) and is necessary for male sexual differentiation. Between 9 and 12 weeks of gestational age, the fetal pituitary starts to produce luteinizing hormone (LH) and follicle-stimulating hormone (FSH); these fetal pituitary hormones are important for continued gonadal development. In response to fetal gonadotropins, ovarian development proceeds, and at the time of birth, ovarian maturation has reached the follicular stage. In the testis, Leydig cell production of testosterone continues until several months after birth.

Throughout childhood, pulsatile secretion of FSH and LH occurs at 60- to 90-minute intervals and stimulates the output of gonadal hormones (see Figure 29–1; Table 29–1). As puberty approaches, the amplitude and frequency of the peaks increase, initially at night during sleep. As puberty progresses, the basal serum LH concentrations rise, and estrogen production from the ovaries or testosterone production from the testes increases to adult levels.

SEXUAL DIFFERENTIATION

Normal Sexual Differentiation
Normal sexual differentiation requires a specific sequence of events. The bipotential gonad requires at least two X chromosomes to develop into an ovary; in the absence of a second X chromosome, a fibrous streak develops along the genital ridge (eg, in Turner's syndrome). Alternatively, in the presence of the testicular determining factor (TDF) gene located on the Y chromosome, a testis develops. Between the 7th and 14th weeks of gestation, testosterone produced locally by fetal Leydig's cells transforms wolffian ducts into the male genital tract. In target tissues, the enzyme 5α-reductase converts circulating testosterone to dihydrotestosterone (DHT), which virilizes the urogenital sinus and external genitalia. The tissue response to testosterone and DHT is dependent on functional androgen receptors. The gene coding for androgen receptors is located on the X chromosome, and various point mutations and deletions have been described that result in complete or partial androgen insensitivity (see below). Growth of the penis occurs mainly in the late second and third trimesters, requiring stimulation of the testis by fetal pituitary gonadotropins. Müllerian duct inhibiting factor (MIF), a glycoprotein produced by Sertoli's cells in the testes, causes regression of the internal female duct structures during the first 8 weeks of gestation. In the absence of this factor, the uterus and uterine (fallopian) tubes develop and mature. The homologous internal and external female and male genital structures are listed in Table 29–8.

Abnormal Sexual Differentiation
There are four major categories of abnormal sex-

Table 29–8. Sexual differentiation in the female and male.

Internal Duct Derivatives

Müllerian Duct Derivatives	Wollfian Duct Derivatives[1]
Fallopian tubes (oviducts) and fimbria	Epididymis
	Vas deferens
Uterus	Seminal vesicles
Cervix	Ejaculatory duct
Vagina (posterior two thirds)	Prostatic urethra

External Genitalia Homologues

Primitive Structure	Female Genitalia	Male Genitalia[2]
Undifferentiated gonad	Ovary	Testis
Genital tubercle	Clitoris	Glans penis
Genital swelling	Labia majora	Scrotum
Genital/urethral fold	Labia minora	Penile urethra/corpora

[1]Normal wollfian duct development is dependent on the *local* production of testosterone by Leydig's cells of the adjacent testis and on *testosterone's diffusion into the surrounding embryonic tissues.* Thus, females with congenital adrenal hyperplasia who are virilized as the result of *circulating* androgens do not have wolffian duct development. Normal male development is also dependent on regression of müllerian duct derivatives through the *local action of müllerian inhibiting factor* elaborated by the Sertoli cells of the adjacent testis.

[2]The normal development of male external genitalia is dependent on an adequate circulating concentration of testosterone, which is then further converted to dihydrotestosterone in the target tissues through the action of the enzyme, 5α-reductase. Significantly elevated circulating concentrations of other (adrenal) androgens, as in females with congenital adrenal hyperplasia, can virilize the genital tubercle, genital swelling, and genital/urethral folds along the lines of their male homologues, resulting in varying degrees of female pseudohermaphroditism (ambiguity) (see text).

ual differentiation resulting in ambiguous external genitalia.

A. Abnormalities in Normal Gonadal Differentiation: These usually result from an abnormality in the number of sex chromosomes. Klinefelter's syndrome (see Chapter 32), with a 47,XXY karyotype, is associated with a male phenotype, but with poorly functioning testes. Turner's syndrome with a 45,XO karyotype (see Chapter 32) is associated with a female phenotype, but with streak ovaries (gonadal dysgenesis). Mosaic forms of gonadal dysgenesis that contain a Y-bearing cell line have variable ambiguous internal and external phenotypes. Idiopathic testicular failure prior to completion of sexual differentiation results in ambiguous genitalia (incomplete virilization). True hermaphroditism, with the presence of both testicular and ovarian tissue, is rare and associated with external genitalia that range from fully masculine to almost completely feminine.

B. Abnormalities in Testosterone Synthesis or Action: These disorders cause male pseudohermaphroditism, in that only testicular tissue is present, but its decreased function results in incomplete viril-

ization with ambiguous genitalia. The enzyme defects in testosterone synthesis may affect only testosterone synthesis, or they may also affect the synthesis of cortisol, as in variants of congenital adrenal hyperplasia (CAH) (Figure 29–3). Defects in testosterone action result from either absent or defective androgen receptors or a defect in the peripheral conversion of testosterone metabolism to DHT due to 5α-reductase deficiency. The androgen receptor defect may be complete or incomplete, resulting in varying degrees of ambiguity.

C. Presence of Excessive Androgens in a Female Fetus: These disorders cause female pseudohermaphroditism (excessive virilization) and usually result in ambiguous genitalia. Excessive adrenal androgen production secondary to an enzyme defect in cortisol synthesis (ie, CAH, see below) is the cause of 95% of 46,XX patients with female pseudohermaphroditism and approximately 50% of all cases of patients with ambiguous genitalia. Occasionally, maternally derived androgens (eg, maternal CAH, luteoma of pregnancy) may cause virilization of the female fetus.

D. Miscellaneous Syndromes: These may be associated with multiple congenital anomalies, especially of the urinary tract and kidney. Occasionally, teratogenic agents (eg, drugs, radiation) may result in anomalous sexual development.

Migeon CJ, Berkovitz G, Brown T: Sexual differentiation and ambiguity. In: *Wilkins: The Diagnosis and Treatment of Endocrine Disorders in Childhood and Adolescence,* 4th ed. Kappy MS, Blizzard RM, Migeon CJ (editors). Charles C Thomas, 1994:573.

Quigley CA et al: Androgen receptor defects: Historical, clinical and molecular perspectives. Endocrine Rev 1995;16:271.

ABNORMALITIES IN OVARIAN FUNCTION

The ovary is composed of follicles (germ cells surrounded by granulosa cells), theca cells immediately surrounding the follicle, and stromal or supporting tissue. The ovary produces several hormones, primarily estrogens and progesterone, but androgens are also produced. At least three natural estrogens have been identified: estrone, 17β-estradiol (the most potent), and estriol. Production of the major ovarian estrogen, estradiol, is stimulated by pituitary LH secretion (see Figure 29–1; Table 29–1), but significant quantities of estrogen are not produced until the onset of puberty. Estrogens stimulate the growth of the uterus, vagina, and breasts. They also contribute to the normal adolescent growth spurt occurring in girls.

Patients with significant ovarian abnormalities in childhood may exhibit precocious puberty, delayed

Figure 29–3. The corticosteroid hormone synthetic pathway. The pathways illustrated are present in differing amounts in the "steroid-producing" tissues: adrenal glands, ovaries, and testes. In the adrenal glands, mineralocorticoids from the zona glomerulosa, glucocorticoids from the zona fasciculata, and androgens (and estrogens) from the zona reticularis are produced. The major adrenal androgen is androstenedione, since the activity of 17-ketoreductase is relatively low. The adrenal gland does secrete some testosterone and estrogen, however. The pathways leading to the synthesis of mineralocorticoids and glucocortcoids are not present in any significant degree in the gonads; however, the testes and ovaries each produce both androgens and estrogens. Further metabolism of testosterone to dihydrotestosterone occurs in target tissues as a result of the action of the enzyme, 5α-reductase. The current nomenclature for the adrenal steroidogenic enzymes is given as follows: [1], P450scc (side chain cleavage); [2], P450c17; [3], P450c21; [4], P450c11.

puberty (primary amenorrhea), or secondary amenorrhea.

1. PRECOCIOUS PUBERTY IN GIRLS

Puberty is considered precocious if the onset of secondary sexual characteristics occurs prior to 8 years of age, but recent studies in girls suggest that these criteria may need to be decreased to 6 years of age. Precocious puberty is thought to be more common in girls than in boys, but this may be due to the inclusion of a large group of 6- to 8-year-old girls in published studies who have a benign, slowly progressing form that is probably a normal variant.

True (complete; gonadotropin-releasing hormone [GnRH]–dependent) precocious puberty refers to early sexual maturation in response to hypothalamic-pituitary stimulation (GnRH/FSH/LH). In pseudoprecocity (ie, GnRH-independent precocity), the cause is elsewhere (eg, adrenal gland or ovary, or the result of exogenous hormones). GnRH-dependent precocious puberty is always isosexual and may progress to the production of mature ova. In pseudoprecocity, sexual characteristics may be isosexual or heterosexual; secondary sexual characteristics develop, but the hypothalamic-pituitary gonadal axis (see Figure 29–1) does not mature, and oocyte maturation does not occur.

Clinical Findings

A. Symptoms and Signs: Sexual development in girls usually starts with breast development, followed by pubic hair growth and menarche, but there are exceptions. The interval between breast development and menarche can range from 1 to 6 years but is usually about 2 years. Girls with ovarian or adrenal tumors may have a palpable abdominal mass also visualized by ultrasonography. A history of excessive mood changes and emotional lability is common. Children with precocious puberty usually have accelerated growth and may be tall during childhood, but because skeletal maturation (bone age) advances at a more rapid rate than linear growth (particularly in the female), adult short stature may occur.

B. Laboratory Findings: In true precocious puberty, the basal serum concentrations of FSH and LH may be in the pubertal range, but early in the course of the disorder, they may be within the prepubertal range. Thus, the documentation of the maturity of the hypothalamic-pituitary axis depends on finding a pubertal LH response (serum concentration greater than 10 IU/L) 30 minutes after stimulation with GnRH. In pseudoprecocity, the LH response to GnRH stimulation is suppressed as a result of feedback inhibition of the hypothalamic-pituitary axis by the autonomously secreted gonadal steroids (see Figure 29–1).

C. Imaging: Determination of skeletal maturation at onset and then every 6–12 months is helpful in predicting the effect of the precocity on adult height and may be used as one of the several criteria to determine if treatment of the precocity is warranted.

Abdominal and pelvic ultrasonography can usually identify an ovarian mass or follicular cysts or adrenal masses greater than 5 cm. Serial examinations are useful in demonstrating significant changes. A cranial CT scan or MRI of the hypothalamic and pituitary regions can identify mass lesions and other structural abnormalities of the central nervous system. Since some of these legions produce no clinical manifestations for prolonged periods, examinations should be performed periodically.

Differential Diagnosis

The causes of true and pseudoprecocious puberty are listed in Table 29–9. Of girls with precocious puberty, 90% have true precocious puberty, and most of these have no definable abnormality on CT or MRI. With newer scanning techniques, static (presumably congenital) mass lesions in the hypothalamus, including benign hypothalamic hamartomas, can be seen. The most common cause of pseudoprecocious puberty is McCune-Albright syndrome. Clinical manifestations of this disorder include polyostotic fibrous dysplasia, café au lait lesions with irregular borders, and autonomous hyperfunction of several endocrine glands, resulting in sexual precocity and other findings (eg, hyperthyroidism). Laboratory and x-ray findings helpful in differentiating true and pseudoprecocious puberty are discussed above.

Premature thelarche—benign early breast development—occurs most commonly between 12 and 36 months of age. It is most often bilateral but may begin or remain as unilateral breast enlargement. In the absence of other signs of pubertal development (eg, accelerated growth rate or skeletal maturation, pubic hair, or vaginal mucosal maturation), no laboratory evaluation is necessary. Treatment consists of reassurance regarding the self-limited nature of this condition, but observation of the child at regular (eg, 6-month) intervals may also be useful.

Premature adrenarche is benign early adrenal maturation, manifested by gradual increase in pubic hair and body odor, and, less commonly, axillary hair and acne. The average age at onset is 5–6 years. Again, no increase in growth rate or skeletal maturation occurs, and no abnormal virilization (eg, clitoromegaly) is present.

Premature adrenarche requires only reassurance and regular observation.

Treatment

In pseudoprecocious puberty, removal of the adrenal or ovarian tumor or correction of the adrenal enzyme disorder usually halts abnormal pubertal development. True precocious puberty can be treated with analogues of GnRH but some long-term outcomes (eg, fertility rate) have not been established. The analogues—given either by daily injection or as a depot sustained-release preparations—interrupt the physiologic pulsatile secretion. "Down-regulation" of the pituitary GnRH receptor also occurs, resulting in a block in pituitary LH secretion and release and the return of plasma estrogen concentrations to prepubertal values. If present initially, menses cease, secondary sexual development stabilizes or regresses, and linear growth and skeletal maturation slow to normal prepubertal rates.

Table 29–9. Causes of isosexual precocious pubertal development.

True (GnRH-dependent) precocious puberty
  Constitutional (idiopathic)
  Hypothalamic lesions (hamartomas, tumors, congenital malformations)
  Dysgerminomas
  Hydrocephalus
  CNS infections
  CNS trauma, irradiation
  Pineal tumors (rare)
  Neurofibromatosis with CNS involvement
  Tuberous sclerosis
  hCG-secreting tumors (eg, hepatoblastomas, choriocarcinomas)
Pseudo (GnRH-independent)-precocious puberty
  CAH in males
  Adrenal tumors
  McCune-Albright syndrome (polyostotic fibrous dysplasia)
  Familial Leydig cell hyperplasia (testotoxicosis)—males
  Gonadal tumors
  Exogenous estrogen—oral (contraceptive pills) or topical
Premature adrenarche—males
Premature thelarche—females

CAH = congenital adrenal hyperplasia.

In patients with McCune-Albright syndrome, analogues of GnRH are not initially helpful. Therapy with antiestrogens (eg, tamoxifen) or agents that block estrogen synthesis (eg, ketoconazole), or both, may be effective. Regardless of the cause of precocious puberty or the medical therapy selected, attention to the psychological needs of the patient and family is essential.

Clemons RD et al: Long-term effectiveness of depot gonadotropin releasing hormone analogue in the treatment of children with central sexual precocity. Am J Dis Child 1993;147:653.
Ganong CA, Kappy MS: Advances in the treatment of precocious puberty. Adv Pediatr 1994;41:223.

2. AMENORRHEA

Primary amenorrhea is the absence of menarche in a female 14 years of age or older or in a female of any age who is over 2½–3 years postpubertal maturation. Secondary amenorrhea is cessation of established menses after an interval of time equal to at least 6 months postmenarche or three menstrual cycles. A history and physical examination (including pelvic examination) often identify possible causes of amenorrhea (Table 29–10).

Table 29–10. Causes of amenorrhea.

I. With obstruction of outflow tract
  A. Fusion or stenosis of labia, hymen (imperforate), vagina, or cervix
  B. Müllerian agenesis (Mayer-Rokitansky-Küster-Hauser)
  C. Postabortion infection, cesarean section, hysterectomy
  D. Complete androgen resistance syndrome (46,XY female)
II. Estrogen deficiency
  A. Primary ovarian insufficiency
    1. Gonadal agenesis
    2. Gonadal dysgenesis (Turner's syndrome variants, true gonadal dysgenesis)
    3. Ovarian steroid biosynthesis deficiency (enzyme defects)
    4. Premature ovarian failure
      a. Autoimmune disease
      b. Infection, surgery, radiation, chemotherapy
  B. Secondary/tertiary ovarian insufficiency
    1. Hypothalamic or pituitary tumor, infection, irradiation
    2. Kallman's syndrome (GnRH/FSH/LH deficiency associated with anosmia)
    3. Eating disorders (eg, anorexia nervosa, bulimia)
    4. Excessive exercise (swimmers, runners, gymnasts)
    5. Chronic illness, malnutrition
III. Androgen excess
  A. Polycystic ovary syndrome
  B. Adrenal androgen excess (CAH, Cushing's disease or syndrome)
IV. Ovarian tumors—granulosa-theca cell, and others

CAH = congenital adrenal hyperplasia, FSH = follicle-stimulating hormone; GnRH = gonadotropin-releasing hormone; LH = luteinizing hormone.

Primary Amenorrhea

The most common cause of primary amenorrhea is physiologic or constitutional delay. Turner's syndrome, chronic illness, and severe undernutrition or strenuous exercise are also common causes.

The term "pseudoamenorrhea" is used when the patient is menstruating but has a genital tract obstruction that prevents release of menstrual blood. Sexual development is usually at Tanner stage III or IV (where stage I is prepubertal and stage V is fully mature), and cyclic abdominal pain without menstruation is noted. Pelvic examination may reveal an imperforate hymen, transverse vaginal ridge, or other obstruction. Treatment is surgical.

Turner's syndrome (45,XO syndrome and its variants) should be considered in patients with short stature and sexual infantilism or adrenarche without normal pubertal progression. This is a form of hypergonadotropic hypogonadism in which serum concentrations of FSH and LH are elevated but plasma estrogen concentration is low owing to a total or relative lack of ovarian tissue. Skeletal maturation is usually delayed. The phenotypic features of Turner's syndrome (described in Chapter 32) may be absent in 40–50% of girls with the syndrome. Current treatment for the short stature includes hGH with or without anabolic steroids. Low doses of estrogens are added to the treatment regimen when breast development is desired, but usually at a later age than the average girl, to ensure that maximal height will be achieved. After 2–3 years of estrogen therapy, a combination of estrogen and progesterone in physiologic doses is indicated, so that the patient does not have the increased risks associated with long-term unopposed estrogen treatment.

Mayer-Rokitansky-Küster-Hauser syndrome is characterized by congenital müllerian agenesis with normal ovaries, normal ovarian function, and normal breast development. Pelvic examination reveals an absent vagina and various uterine abnormalities with or without additional renal and skeletal anomalies. Full evaluation is necessary, including karyotyping, intravenous pyelography, and laparoscopy. Therapy for this syndrome is surgical vaginoplasty.

Secondary Amenorrhea

Common causes of secondary amenorrhea include stress, pregnancy, major weight loss, polycystic ovary syndrome, and hyperprolactinemia. Stress-induced amenorrhea is often noted in teenagers, but it should be diagnosed only after careful evaluation. Pregnancy is the most common cause of secondary amenorrhea in sexually active teenagers.

Irregular menses (oligomenorrhea) or amenorrhea may result from severe weight loss secondary to dieting, vigorous exercise (eg, in marathon runners, swimmers, ballet dancers, and gymnasts), depression, anorexia nervosa, or chronic illness. In the normally ovulating female, it is believed that a major source of estrogen is aromatization of androgens in peripheral adipose tissue. When the proportion of body weight represented by fat falls below a critical level (15–25%), estrogen production is decreased. This hypothesis has been advanced to explain amenorrhea in athletes and patients with anorexia nervosa.

In polycystic ovary syndrome (Stein-Leventhal syndrome), secondary amenorrhea is the result of chronic anovulation. Occasionally, dysfunctional uterine bleeding is the only finding; the full syndrome consists of obesity, hirsutism, secondary amenorrhea, bilaterally enlarged ovaries and, in some cases, clitoromegaly. Tests show normal circulating FSH concentrations, elevated LH, borderline-to-elevated adrenal or ovarian androgens, and increased plasma free testosterone concentrations. Polycystic ovary syndrome may be idiopathic or secondary to adrenocortical hyperplasia or an adrenocortical neoplasm. Laparoscopy, ovarian biopsy, endometrial biopsy, or a combination of these procedures may be necessary for diagnosis. Treatment consists of correction of the estrogen-androgen ratio by estrogen-progesterone combinations, with later induction of ovulation in adult patients who wish to become pregnant. Agents with antiandrogen activity (eg, spironolactone) may be helpful in controlling hirsutism.

Other causes of amenorrhea are shown in Table 29–10. Chronic illness and central nervous system disorders should always be considered. When galactorrhea and amenorrhea occur together, hyperprolactinemia due to adenoma or ingestion of antidepressants or marijuana, hypothyroidism, stress, and hypothalamic injury should be considered.

Apter D et al: Metabolic features of polycystic ovary syndrome are found in adolescent girls with hyperandrogenism. J Clin Endocrinol Metab 1995;80:2966.

Constantini NW, Warner MP: Menstrual dysfunction in swimmers: A distinct entity. J Clin Endocrinol Metab 1995;80:2740.

Franks S: Polycystic ovary syndrome. N Engl J Med 1995;333:853.

Spratt DI et al: Reproductive axis suppression in acute illness is related to disease severity. J Clin Endocrinol Metab 1993;76:1548.

OVARIAN TUMORS

Ovarian tumors are not rare in children. They may occur at any age and are usually large, benign, and unilateral. They may be estrogen-producing; ovarian tumors account for about 1% of cases of female sexual precocity. The most common estrogen-producing tumor is the granulosa cell tumor. Others that may cause sexual precocity include thecomas, luteomas, mixed types, theca-lutein and follicular cysts, and ovarian tumors (teratomas, choriocarcinomas, and dysterminomas). Ovarian tumors are usually palpated on rectal examination and readily seen by ovarian ul-

trasonography. Treatment is surgical removal. Recurrences are uncommon.

Mann JR et al: Results of United Kingdom Children's Cancer Study Group: Malignant germ cell tumor studies. Cancer 1989;63:1657.

ABNORMALITIES IN TESTICULAR FUNCTION

The major testicular hormone, testosterone, is produced by Leydig's (interstitial) cells. Production of testicular androgens is stimulated by LH secretion (see Figure 29–1; Table 29–1). Appreciable amounts of adrenal and testicular androgen usually begin to appear in boys at 12 years of age and are responsible, wholly or in part, for growth of the internal (wolffian) duct (see Table 29–8) and external genitalia and for development of secondary sexual characteristics, including pubic, axillary, and facial hair. Androgens induce nitrogen retention, accelerated growth rate (pubertal growth spurt), and skeletal maturation.

The seminiferous tubules are composed of germinal epithelium and Sertoli's cells. Testicular androgens in combination with pituitary FSH stimulate the development and maturation of the germinal epithelium and thus promote spermatogenesis. Sertoli's cells provide structural support for the germinal epithelium.

Patients with abnormalities in testicular function may present with delayed or precocious sexual development or cryptorchidism.

1. PRECOCIOUS PUBERTY IN BOYS

Puberty is considered precocious in boys if secondary sexual characteristics appear prior to 9 years of age. Precocious puberty appears to be much less common in boys than in girls, but this may be more apparent than real. In boys presenting with sexual precocity, pseudoprecocious puberty is as common as true, GnRH-dependent, precocious puberty. In addition, boys with true precocious puberty are more likely to have an identifiable pathologic process (eg, central nervous system tumor) rather than idiopathic precocious puberty.

Two main GnRH-independent forms of precocious puberty have been described in boys: McCune-Albright syndrome (described previously) and familial Leydig cell hyperplasia or *testotoxicosis*, a condition in which the LH receptor on the Leydig cell is hypersensitive to LH, resulting in testicular overproduction of testosterone in the face of prepubertal LH concentrations. As in McCune-Albright syndrome or other causes of autonomous gonadal or adrenal androgen secretion, the LH response to GnRH stimulation testing is suppressed.

Clinical Findings

A. Symptoms and Signs: In precocious development, increases in growth rate and growth of pubic hair are the common presenting signs. Testicular size may differentiate true precocity, in which the testes enlarge, from pseudoprecocity (most commonly due to CAH), in which the testes usually remain small. There are some exceptions: In advanced cases of pseudoprecocity, for example, some testicular enlargement may occur because seminiferous tubule elements may be stimulated by prolonged elevated androgen levels. In the very young child with early true precocity, minimal increases of testosterone may result in dramatic increases in penis size and pubic hair growth with very little testicular enlargement. Tumors of the testis present with asymmetric testicular enlargement.

B. Laboratory Findings: Basal serum LH and FSH concentrations may be elevated in boys with true sexual precocity, and the LH response to GnRH stimulation testing is pubertal (greater than 10 IU/L). Sexual precocity caused by CAH is usually associated with abnormal plasma concentrations of dehydroepiandrosterone (DHEA), androstenedione, 17-OH P (in CAH due to 21-hydroxylase deficiency), 11-deoxycortisol (in CAH due to 11-hydroxylase deficiency), or a combination of these steroids (see Adrenal Cortex section below). Determining serum hCG concentrations to confirm the presence of an hCG-producing tumor (eg, central nervous system dysgerminoma, hepatoma) may be necessary in boys who present with apparent true sexual precocity (accompanied by testicular enlargement).

C. Imaging: Diagnostic studies are similar to those used to evaluate sexual precocity in girls (see previous text). Ultrasonography may be useful in detection of hepatic, presacral, and testicular tumors.

Differential Diagnosis

The causes of isosexual precocity are outlined in Table 29–9. In boys, it is particularly important to differentiate pseudoprecocity from true sexual precocity. Seventy percent of boys with pseudoprecocious puberty have an adrenal enzyme abnormality (CAH). Of boys with true precocious puberty, 70% have benign central nervous system mass lesions. Premature adrenarche (described above) may occur in males as well as females.

Treatment

Specific therapy should be provided whenever possible. Treatment of idiopathic true precocious puberty in boys is similar to that in girls (see previous text). Treatment of McCune-Albright syndrome or familial Leydig cell hyperplasia with agents that block steroid synthesis (eg, ketoconazole), antiandrogen (eg, spironolactone), or with a combination of both has been successful.

Blizzard RM, Rogol AD: Variations and disorders of pubertal development. In: *Wilkins: The Diagnosis and Treatment of Endocrine Disorders in Childhood and Adolescence,* 4th ed. Kappy MS, Blizzard RM, Migeon CJ (editors). Charles C Thomas, 1994.

Ganong CA, Kappy MS: Advances in the treatment of precocious puberty. Adv Pediatr 1994;41:223.

Holland FJ: Gonadotropin-independent precocious puberty. Endocrinol Metab Clin North Am 1991;29:191.

Latronico AC et al: A novel mutation of the LH receptor gene causing male gonadotropin-independent precocious puberty. J Clin Endocrinol Metab 1995;80:2490.

2. SEXUAL INFANTILISM (Primary & Secondary Testicular Failure)

Lack of development of secondary sexual characteristics after the age of 17 years suggests abnormal testicular maturation. Although delay of puberty until 17 years of age may be physiologically normal, boys generally become concerned if pubertal changes do not occur by 14–15 years of age, and evaluation should be initiated at that time. Sexual infantilism may be difficult to differentiate from constitutionally delayed adolescence. Although the latter may be associated with a delay in testicular function, normal puberty occurs at a later date.

Testicular failure or insufficiency may be primary, resulting from the absence, malfunction, or destruction of testicular tissue, or secondary, due to pituitary (or hypothalamic) insufficiency. Primary testicular failure may be due to anorchia, surgical castration, Klinefelter's syndrome or other sex chromosome abnormalities, enzymatic defects in testosterone synthesis or action, or inflammation and destruction of the testes following infection (eg, mumps), autoimmune disorders, radiation, trauma, or tumor.

Secondary testicular failure may accompany panhypopituitarism, empty sella syndrome, Kallmann's syndrome (gonadotropin deficiency accompanied by anosmia), or isolated deficiencies of LH or FSH. Destructive lesions in or near the anterior pituitary, especially craniopharyngiomas, gliomas, or infection, may also result in hypothalamic or pituitary dysfunction. Prader-Willi syndrome and Laurence-Moon syndrome (Bardet-Biedl syndrome, Biemond syndrome II) are frequently associated with LH and FSH deficiency secondary to deficiency of GnRH. Miscellaneous causes of secondary testicular failure include chronic debilitating disease and hypothyroidism.

Clinical Findings

A. Symptoms and Signs: Physical examination may not be helpful in differentiating primary from secondary testicular insufficiency. Whereas cryptorchidism suggests primary testicular failure, hypothalamic or pituitary insufficiency as well as anatomic abnormalities may lead to failure of testicular descent.

B. Laboratory Findings: In primary testicular failure, the plasma testosterone concentration is low, whereas LH and FSH values are elevated into the castrate range. In secondary testicular failure, circulating concentrations of all three hormones are below the normal adult range. To establish the presence of the testes and their ability to respond to stimulation, two to three doses of hCG, 2000 U/m^2 are given intramuscularly. They can be given every other day. The plasma testosterone should rise to above 200 mg/dL 48 hours after the final dose. A karyotype should be determined in primary testicular failure of unknown cause.

C. Imaging: Skeletal (epiphyseal) maturation is usually delayed. A cranial CT scan or MRI should be performed in cases of secondary testicular failure.

Treatment

Specific therapy is indicated when the cause of testicular failure is known. Treatment with depot testosterone (eg, testosterone enanthate), beginning with 75–100 mg intramuscularly and increasing to 200 mg every 3–4 weeks, may be continued indefinitely. Specific therapy (pulsatile subcutaneous delivery of GnRH) may result in fertility in patients with hypothalamic-pituitary insufficiency.

Ghaik K, Cara JF, Rosenfield RL: GnRHa (Nafarelin) test to differentiate gonadotropin deficiency from constitutionally delayed puberty in teenage boys: A clinical research study. J Clin Endocrinol Metab 1995;80:2980.

3. CRYPTORCHIDISM

Cryptorchidism (undescended testis) is a common disorder in children. It may be unilateral or bilateral and may be classified as ectopic cryptorchidism or true cryptorchidism.

Approximately 3% of term male newborns and 3% of premature males have undescended testes at birth. In over 50% of these cases, the testes descend by the second month; by the age of 1 year, 80% of all undescended testes are in the scrotum. Further descent may occur through puberty, the latter perhaps stimulated by endogenous gonadotropins. If cryptorchidism persists into adult life, failure of spermatogenesis occurs, but testicular androgen production usually remains intact. The incidence of malignant neoplasm (usually seminoma) is appreciably greater in those testes that remain in the abdomen after puberty.

Ectopic testes are presumed to develop normally but are diverted as they descend through the inguinal canal. They are subclassified on the basis of their location; surgery is indicated once the diagnosis is established.

True cryptorchidism in most cases is thought to be the result of an abnormality in testicular development (dysgenesis). Cryptorchid testes frequently have a short spermatic artery, poor blood supply, or both. Although early scrotal positioning of these testes will obviate further damage related to intra-abdominal location, the testes generally remain abnormal, spermatogenesis is rare, and the risk of malignant neoplasm is increased. These testes should probably be removed if spermatogenesis does not occur after a reasonable period of observation.

Bilateral cryptorchidism is a common feature in prepubertal castrate syndrome (the vanishing testes syndrome), Noonan's syndrome, and disorders of androgen synthesis or action; it is seen less commonly with Klinefelter's syndrome, Sertoli-cell-only syndrome, and hypogonadotropin states.

Note: The diagnosis of bilateral cryptorchidism in an apparently male newborn should never be made until the possibility that the child is actually a fully virilized female with potentially fatal salt-losing CAH has been ruled out (see Adrenal Cortex below).

Clinical Findings

Plasma testosterone concentrations may be obtained after hCG stimulation to confirm the presence or absence of abdominal testes (see previous text). The child with bilaterally undescended testes should be evaluated for sex chromosome abnormalities; evaluation should include consideration of the possibility that the child is actually a virilized female.

Differential Diagnosis

In palpating for the testes, the cremasteric reflex may be elicited, with a resultant ascent of the testes into the inguinal canal or abdomen (pseudocryptorchidism). To prevent this, the fingers first should be placed across the abdominal ring and the upper portion of the inguinal canal, obstructing ascent. Examination while the child is in the squatting position or a warm bath is also helpful. No treatment of retractile testes is necessary, and the prognosis for testicular descent and competence is excellent.

Treatment

The best age for medical or surgical treatment has not been determined, but there is a trend toward operation in infancy or early childhood. Surgical repair is indicated for cryptorchidism persisting beyond puberty.

Gonadotropin therapy (hCG, 4000–5000 U intramuscularly three to five times per week for 2–3 weeks) is generally ineffective unless the child has retractile testes (pseudocryptorchidism) rather than true cryptorchidism.

Androgen treatment (eg, depot testosterone) is indicated as replacement therapy in the male beyond the normal age of puberty who has been shown to lack functional testes.

4. GYNECOMASTIA

Adolescent gynecomastia is a common, self-limited finding in boys. It may sometimes be seen as part of Klinefelter's syndrome, or it may be seen in boys who are on certain drugs, such as antidepressants or marijuana. This topic is discussed in more detail in Chapter 5.

TESTICULAR TUMORS

The major primary malignant tumors of the testis are seminomas and teratomas. Seminomas are rare in childhood; they may be hormone-producing. The major hormone-producing tumor of the testis is Leydig's cell tumor. It is frequently associated with sexual precocity. Other testicular tumors (choriocarcinomas and dysgerminomas) have been reported in association with sexual precocity.

Treatment of testicular tumors is surgical removal; chemotherapy and radiation therapy are not used in childhood unless there is a high-grade malignancy or metastasis. The prognosis in patients with Leydig's cell tumors is generally good.

Leonard MP et al: Pediatric testicular tumors: The Johns Hopkins experience. Urology 1991;37:253.

ADRENAL CORTEX

The adrenal cortex develops from the dorsal celomic mesothelium between the fourth and sixth weeks of fetal life. By 8–9 weeks of gestation, the fetal adrenal cortex contains the enzymes necessary to produce cortisol from progesterone. At 7–9 weeks of gestation, the fetal pituitary seems capable of producing and releasing ACTH to provide regulation of adrenal hormone production.

The zona glomerulosa, the outermost zone of the adult cortex, is the exclusive source of aldosterone, the major mineralocorticoid. The zona fasciculata makes cortisol, the major glucocorticoid, as well as small amounts of mineralocorticoids. The innermost zona reticularis appears to produce mainly adrenal androgens and estrogens.

During fetal life, a fetal zone, or provisional cortex, predominates. It produces glucocorticoids, mineralocorticoids, androgens, and estrogens but is relatively deficient in 3β-ol dehydrogenase (see Figure 29–3). Therefore, placentally produced progesterone serves as the major precursor for the fetal adrenal production of cortisol and aldosterone.

The adrenal cortex produces cortisol under the control of pituitary ACTH (see Figure 29–1; Table 29–1). This negative feedback control is superimposed on a diurnal pattern of ACTH release. ACTH concentrations are greatest during the early morning hours and least around midnight.

Glucocorticoids are catabolic and antianabolic; that is, they promote the release of amino acids from muscle and increase gluconeogenesis while decreasing incorporation of amino acids into muscle protein. They also antagonize insulin action and facilitate lipolysis. Glucocorticoids help maintain blood pressure through their "permissive" effect on peripheral vascular tone and by causing sodium and water retention.

Mineralocorticoids (primarily aldosterone in humans) promote sodium retention and stimulate potassium excretion. Although ACTH can stimulate aldosterone production, the predominant regulator of aldosterone secretion is the volume and sodium-sensitive renin-angiotensin-II-aldosterone system. Elevations in serum potassium concentrations also directly influence aldosterone release.

Androgen (DHEA and androstenedione) production by the zona reticularis is insignificant in normal children. At the onset of puberty, androgen production increases and may be an important factor in the dynamics of puberty in both sexes. The adrenal gland is the major source of androgen in the pubertal and adult female.

ADRENOCORTICAL INSUFFICIENCY
(Adrenal Crisis, Addison's Disease)

General Considerations

The leading causes of adrenal insufficiency today are hereditary enzymatic defects with CAH and loss of adrenal function due to autoimmune destruction of the glands. A rare form of familial Addison's disease may be seen in association with cerebral sclerosis and spastic paraplegia (adrenoleukodystrophy). Autoimmune Addison's disease may be familial and has been described in association with hypoparathyroidism, candidiasis, hypothyroidism, pernicious anemia, hypogonadism, and diabetes mellitus as one of the polyglandular autoimmune syndromes. The finding of circulating antibodies to adrenal tissue and other tissues involved in these conditions suggests that an autoimmune mechanism, probably related to a defect in immunoregulation involving suppressor T-cell function, is the cause. Occasionally, the gland is destroyed by tumor, calcification, or hemorrhage (Waterhouse-Friderichsen syndrome). In adults with AIDS, adrenal disease secondary to opportunistic infections (fungi, tuberculosis) is increased. A similar relationship is likely in children. Rarely, adrenal insufficiency is the result of ACTH or corticotropin releasing hormone deficiency due to anterior pituitary or hypothalamic disease. Any acute illness, surgery, trauma, or exposure to excessive heat may precipitate an adrenal crisis in susceptible individuals. A temporary salt-losing disorder due to partial mineralocorticoid deficiency or renal underresponsiveness may occur during infancy.

Clinical Findings

A. Symptoms and Signs:

1. Acute form (adrenal crisis)–Manifestations include nausea and vomiting, diarrhea, abdominal pain, dehydration, fever (which may be followed by hypothermia), weakness, hypotension, circulatory collapse, and confusion or coma. Increased pigmentation may be seen as the result of the intrinsic melanocyte stimulating hormone activity of the parent molecule of ACTH.

2. Chronic form (Addison's disease)–These include fatigue, hypotension, weakness, failure to gain or loss of weight, increased appetite for salt, vomiting (which may become forceful and sometimes projectile), and dehydration. Diffuse tanning with increased pigmentation over pressure points, scars, and mucous membranes may be present. A small heart may be seen on chest x-ray.

B. Laboratory Findings:

1. Suggestive of adrenocortical insufficiency–Serum sodium and bicarbonate, PCO_2, blood pH, and blood volume are decreased. Serum potassium and urea nitrogen are increased. Urinary sodium is elevated, and the urine sodium:potassium ratio is high despite low serum sodium. Eosinophilia and moderate lymphopenia may be present.

2. Confirmatory tests–The following tests measure the functional capacity of the adrenal cortex:

a. The ACTH (Cortrosyn) stimulation test is the most definitive test of adrenal gland function. In primary adrenal insufficiency (ie, originating in the gland itself), plasma cortisol concentrations fail to increase significantly over baseline 60 minutes after an intravenous dose of ACTH.

b. Baseline serum ACTH concentrations are elevated.

c. Urinary free cortisol and 17-hydroxycorticosteroid excretion are decreased.

d. The metyrapone (an inhibitor of 11-hydroxylase) test is helpful in diagnosing adrenal insufficiency due to pituitary or hypothalamic disease. After a dose of metyrapone is given at midnight, the next morning's plasma concentration of 11-deoxycortisol should be high, and the cortisol concentration low (because of the induced enzyme block) if the CRH-ACTH-adrenal axis is intact, since the transient inhibition of cortisol biosynthesis should lead to elevations of ACTH in normal individuals. In children with pituitary or hypothalamic disease, ACTH secretion is compromised, and the 11-deoxycortisol does not rise.

Caution: This test may provoke acute adrenal insufficiency in an individual with compromised hypo-thalamic, pituitary, or adrenal function, and the test is best done in the hospital with monitoring of the patient's vital signs.

Differential Diagnosis

Acute adrenal insufficiency must be differentiated from severe acute infections, diabetic coma, various disturbances of the central nervous system, and acute poisoning. In the neonatal period, adrenal insufficiency may be clinically indistinguishable from respiratory distress, intracranial hemorrhage, or sepsis.

Chronic adrenocortical insufficiency must be differentiated from anorexia nervosa, certain muscular disorders (eg, myasthenia grazvis, and other conditions), salt-losing nephritis, and chronic debilitating infections (eg, tuberculosis) and must be considered in cases of recurrent spontaneous hypoglycemia.

Treatment

A. Acute Form (Adrenal Crisis):

1. Replacement therapy–

a. Hydrocortisone sodium succinate (Solu-Cortef), 2 mg/kg diluted in 2–10 mL of water, is given intravenously over 2–5 minutes, followed by 5% dextrose/0.9% saline. Thereafter, it is given intravenously, 1.5 mg/kg in infants or 12.5 mg/m² in older children, every 4–6 hours until stabilization is achieved and oral therapy tolerated.

b. Fluids and electrolytes–Five to ten percent glucose in saline, 10–20 mL/kg intravenously, is given over the first hour and at 1½–2 times the maintenance fluid requirements thereafter. In addition, intravenous boluses of glucose (2 mL 10% glucose/kg) may be needed every 4–6 hours. **Caution:** Chronic overtreatment with fluids must be avoided. Total parenteral fluid in the first 8 hours should not exceed the maintenance fluid requirement of the normal child.

c. Fluorocortisone–When oral intake is tolerated, fludrocortisone (Florinef), 0.1 mg daily, is started and continued as necessary every 12–24 hours.

Rarely, inotropic agents such as dopamine or dobutamine are needed.

2. Waterhouse-Friderichsen syndrome with fulminant infections–The use of adrenocorticosteroids and norepinephrine in the treatment of prophylaxis of fulminant infections is still controversial; corticosteroids may augment the generalized Shwartzman reaction in fatal cases of meningococcemia. However, corticosteroids should always be considered in the presence of adrenal insufficiency, particularly with hypotension and circulatory collapse.

B. Maintenance Therapy of Chronic Form (Addison's Disease):

Following initial stabilization, the most effective substitution therapy is hydrocortisone given with fludrocortisone. Overtreatment should be avoided because it may result in obesity, growth retardation, and other cushingoid features. Additional hydrocortisone, fludrocortisone, or sodium chloride, singly or in combination, may be necessary with acute illness, surgery, trauma, or other stress reactions.

Supportive adrenocortical therapy should be given whenever surgical operations are performed in patients who have at some time received prolonged therapy with adrenocorticosteroids (see below).

1. Glucocorticoids (hydrocortisone or equivalent)–The dosage of all glucocorticoids is increased to two to four times the usual dosage during intercurrent illness or times or stress.

a. Hydrocortisone–A maintenance dosage of 10–15 mg/m^2/d is given orally in three divided doses. For adrenal enzyme defects, 25% of the dose is given in the morning and afternoon and 50% at night. For all other causes of adrenocortical insufficiency, 50% of the daily dose is given in the morning.

b. Prednisone–Two to three mg/m^2/d is given orally in two divided doses. Its potency may preclude necessary minor modulations in dosage.

2. Fludrocortisone–A dose of 0.05–0.2 mg is given orally once a day or in two divided doses. Periodic monitoring of blood pressure is recommended to avoid overdosing.

3. Salt–The child should be given ready access to table salt. Frequent blood pressure determinations in the recumbent position should be made to ensure that hypertension is avoided.

C. Corticosteroids in Patients With Adrenocortical Insufficiency Who Undergo Surgery:

1. Before operation–Hydrocortisone sodium succinate, 30 mg/m^2 intravenously, is given 1 hour before surgery.

2. During operation–Hydrocortisone sodium succinate, 25–100 mg intravenously, is administered with 5–10% glucose in saline throughout surgery.

3. During recovery–Hydrocortisone sodium succinate, 12.5 mg/m^2 intravenously, is given every 4–6 hours until oral doses are tolerated. The oral dose of three to five times the maintenance dose is gradually tapered to the maintenance dose as the patient recovers.

Course & Prognosis

A. Acute: The course of acute adrenal insufficiency is rapid, and death may occur within a few hours, particularly in infants, unless adequate treatment is given. Spontaneous recovery is unlikely. Patients who have received long-term treatment with adrenocorticosteroids may exhibit adrenal collapse if they undergo surgery or other acute stress. Pharmacologic doses of glucocorticoids during these episodes may be needed throughout life.

In all forms of acute adrenal insufficiency, the patient should be observed carefully once the crisis has passed and evaluated with laboratory tests to assess the degree of permanent adrenal insufficiency.

B. Chronic: Adequately treated chronic adrenocortical insufficiency is consistent with a relatively normal life. Patients on maintenance doses of glucocorticoids may require increases (two- to fourfold) during severe illnesses and operations.

Falorini A et al: High diagnostic accuracy for idiopathic Addison's disease with a sensitive radiobinding assay for autoantibodies against recombinant human 21-hydroxylase. J Clin Endocrinol Metab 1995;80:2752.

Migeon CJ, Donohoue P: Adrenal disorders. In: *Wilkins: The Diagnosis and Treatment of Endocrine Disorders in Childhood and Adolescence,* 4th ed. Kappy MS, Blizzard RM, Migeon CJ (editors). Charles C Thomas, 1994:717.

Smith BB, Furmaniak J: Adrenal and gonadal autoimmune disease. J Clin Endocrinol Metab 1995;80:1502.

Winter WE: Autoimmune endocrinopathies. In: *Wilkins: The Diagnosis and Treatment of Endocrine Disorders in Childhood and Adolescence,* 4th ed. Kappy MS, Blizzard RM, Migeon CJ (editors). Charles C Thomas, 1994:317.

CONGENITAL ADRENAL HYPERPLASIAS

Essentials of Diagnosis

- Pseudohermaphroditism in females, with urogenital sinus, enlargement of clitoris, and other evidence of virilization.
- Isosexual precocity in males with infantile testes.
- Increased linear growth in young children; advancement of skeletal maturation.
- Urinary and plasma androgen elevation; plasma 17-OH P and urinary pregnanetriol concentrations increased in the common form; may be associated with electrolyte and water disturbances (hyponatremia, hyperkalemia, and metabolic acidosis), particularly in the newborn period.

General Considerations

Congenital adrenal hyperplasia (CAH) is most commonly (>80%) the result of homozygous 21-hydroxylase (P450c21) deficiency (see Figure 29–3), an autosomal recessive disorder. In the severe form, excess adrenal androgen production beginning in the first trimester of fetal development results in virilization and life-threatening hypovolemic, hyponatremic shock (adrenal crisis). Other autosomal recessive enzyme defects involved in adrenal steroidogenesis will also result in CAH, since they have in common a defect in cortisol biosynthesis with resultant increased ACTH secretion during fetal life. These other enzymes are 20,22-desmolase, 3β-ol dehydrogenases, 18-hydroxylase/17,22-desmolase, and 11-hydroxylase. The clinical syndromes associated with each of these defects can be predicted from Figure 29–3 and Table 29–11. Recently, all of these enzymes except 3β-ol dehydrogenase have been shown to be associated with the cytochrome P450 complex. A new en-

Table 29–11. Clinical and laboratory findings in adrenal enzyme defects resulting in CAH.

Enzyme Deficiency[1]	Urinary 17-Ketosteroids	Elevated Plasma Metabolite	Plasma Androgens	Aldosterone	Hypertension/ Salt Loss	External Genitalia
20,22-Desmolase [1]	↓↓↓	—	↓↓↓	↓↓↓	−/+	Males: ambiguous Females: normal
3β-ol dehydroge-nase	↑↑ (DHEA)	17-OH pregnenol-one (DHEA)	↑ (DHEA)	↓↓↓	−/+	Males: ambiguous Females: virilized (?)
17-Hydroxylase [2]	↓↓↓	Progesterone	↓↓	Normal to ↑	+/−	Males: ambiguous Females: normal
21-Hydroxylase [3][2]	↑↑↑	17-OHP	↑↑	↓↓	−/+	Males: normal Females: virilized
11-Hydroxylase [4]	↑↑	11-Deoxycortisol	↑↑	↓↓ (↑ Deoxycor-ticosterone)	+/−	Males: normal Females: virilized
17,20-Desmolase [2]	↓↓↓	17-Hydroxysteroids (?)	↓↓	Normal	−/−	Males: ambiguous Females: normal

[1]Bracketed numbers correspond to those in Figure 29–3.
[2]Children with "simple virilizing (non–salt-wasting)" forms of 21-hydroxylase deficiency congenital adrenal hyperplasia (CAH) may have normal aldosterone production and serum electrolytes, but some children have normal aldosterone production and serum electrolytes at the expense of elevated plasma renin activity and are therefore *compensated salt-wasters* by definition. These children are usually treated with mineralocorticoid as well as glucocorticoid. Children with 21-hydroxylase deficiency CAH should therefore have documented normal plasma renin activity in addition to normal serum electrolytes before they are considered non–salt-wasters.

zyme nomenclature has been established, and it is given along with the older, more familiar nomenclature in shown in Figure 29–3 to avoid confusion.

Approximately 10% of CAH cases are caused by an 11-hydroxylase enzyme deficiency, and the remainder by deficiencies of the other enzymes (see Figure 29–3). In some forms, the infant may appear normal at birth, with symptoms occurring later. In all forms except isolated 17,20-desmolase deficiency, diminished secretion of cortisol results in excessive secretion of ACTH. ACTH excess results in adrenal hyperplasia with increased production of various adrenal hormone precursors, including androgens, and increased urinary excretion of their metabolites. Increased pigmentation, especially of the scrotum, labia majora, and nipples, frequently results from excessive ACTH secretion.

Studies in patients with 21-hydroxylase deficiency indicate that the clinical type (salt-wasting versus non–salt-wasting) is usually consistent within a family and that there is a close genetic linkage of the 21-hydroxylase gene to the HLA complex on chromosome 6. The latter finding has allowed more precise heterozygote detection and prenatal diagnosis. Population studies indicate that the defective gene is present in 1:100–1:250 people and that the incidence of the disorder is 1:15,000–1:5000. Hormonal evaluation of unaffected family members following ACTH stimulation allows detection of the heterozygote with a certainty of 80–90%, and a combination of hormonal and HLA studies can increase the number of cases detected. HLA typing in combination with the measurement of 17-OH P and androstenedione in amniotic

fluid has been used in the prenatal diagnosis of 21-hydroxylase deficiency. Mass screening for this enzyme defect, using a microfilter paper technique to measure 17-OH P is used in some centers.

Nonclassic presentations of 21-hydroxylase deficiency have been reported with increasing frequency. Affected persons have a normal phenotype at birth and develop evidence of virilization during later childhood, adolescence, or early adulthood. In these cases, previously referred to as late-onset or acquired enzyme deficiencies, results of hormonal studies are characteristic of 21-hydroxylase deficiency. An asymptomatic form has also been identified, in which individuals have none of the phenotypic features of the disorder but have hormonal study results identical with those in patients with nonclassic 21-hydroxylase deficiency. The nonclassic form appears to be less severe than the classic form. Because members of the same family may have classic, nonclassic, and asymptomatic forms, the disorders may be due to allelic variations of the same enzyme.

Female pseudohermaphroditism can be caused by factors other than enzyme deficiencies. In females, these include virilizing maternal conditions or related hormones taken by the mother during the first trimester of pregnancy. In such cases, the condition does not progress after birth, and cortisol deficiency with abnormal steroidogenesis is not present. Male pseudohermaphroditism may be seen in children with 17,20-desmolase deficiency, since that enzyme is necessary for normal androgen biosynthesis (see Table 29–11).

Virilization of female or male fetus may result

from tumors of the adrenal gland, ovary, or testis or from nonclassic CAH later in life. Symptoms begin after birth and progress until treated.

Clinical Findings

A. Symptoms and Signs:

1. CAH in females—In the female with potentially normal ovaries and uterus, virilization occurs, and sexual development is therefore along heterosexual lines. The abnormality of the external genitalia may vary from mild enlargement of the clitoris to complete fusion of the labioscrotal folds, forming a scrotum, a penile urethra, a penile shaft, and enlargement of the clitoris to form a normal-sized gland (see Table 29–8). When the enzyme defect is milder, signs of adrenal insufficiency may not occur, and evidence of virilization predominates (simple virilizing form). In the untreated complete form of 21-hydroxylase or 11-hydroxylase deficiency CAH, growth rate and skeletal maturation are accelerated, and patients may also become muscular. Pubic hair appears early (often before the second birthday); acne may be excessive; and the voice may deepen. Excessive pigmentation may develop. Signs of adrenal insufficiency may be present during the first days of life (typically in the first or second week). In rare cases, adrenal insufficiency does not occur for months or years.

2. CAH in males—In males, sexual development proceeds along isosexual lines, that is, virilization. The male infant usually appears normal at birth, but may present in an emergency department with an adrenal insufficiency crisis accompanying a relatively mild infection in the first 2–4 weeks of life. During the first few months of life, enlargement of the penis will be noted. There my be increased pigmentation resulting from excessive secretion of β-lipotropin and ACTH. Other symptoms and signs are similar to those of the congenital form in females. The testes are soft and not enlarged, except in the rare male in whom aberrant adrenal cells (adrenal rests) are present in the testes and produce unilateral or bilateral enlargement, often asymmetric. In the rare, isolated defect of 17,20-desmolase activity, ambiguous genitalia may be present because of the compromise in androgen production (see Figure 29–3).

3. Tumor—The findings may be identical with those of CAH, except that they appear at a later age. The tumor may be palpably enlarged. Rarely, an adrenal tumor in a male may also produce feminization with gynecomastia.

B. Laboratory Findings:

1. Blood and urine—Hormonal studies are essential for accurate diagnosis. Findings characteristic of the enzyme deficiencies are shown in Table 29–11. With adrenal tumor, secretion DHEA is greatly elevated, and determining plasma concentrations of DHEA sulfate may be useful in the diagnosis.

2. Genetic studies—When available, rapid chromosomal diagnosis should be obtained in any newborn with ambiguous genitalia.

3. Dexamethasone suppression test—If low-dose dexamethasone (2–4 mg/d in four divided doses for 7 days) reduces urinary 17-ketosteroids to normal, adrenal hyperplasia rather than adenoma is the probable diagnosis.

C. Imaging:

Adrenal ultrasonography, CT scanning, and MRI may be useful in defining pelvic anatomy or enlarged adrenals or in localizing an adrenal tumor. Vaginograms using contrast material and pelvic ultrasonography may be helpful in delineating the internal anatomy in a newborn with ambiguous genitalia.

Treatment

Treatment goals in CAH consist of normalizing growth velocity and skeletal maturation using the smallest dose of glucocorticoids that will suppress adrenal function by suppressing ACTH. Mineralocorticoid replacement helps to sustain normal electrolyte homeostasis. The use of excessive amounts of glucocorticoids results in the undesirable side effects of Cushing's syndrome, and excessive mineralocorticoid dosing results in hypertension (see Uses of Glucocorticoids & ACTH in Treatment of Nonendocrine Diseases for a more complete discussion of the effects of pharmacologic glucocorticoid therapy).

1. Initially, hydrocortisone given in a dosage of 25–30 $mg/m^2/d$ orally suppresses abnormal adrenal steroidogenesis within 2 weeks. The patients are then continued on maintenance doses of 10–15 $mg/m^2/d$ in three divided doses. Fifty percent of the daily dose should be given in the late evening to suppress the early morning ACTH rise. Dosage is regulated to maintain a normal growth rate and a normal rate of skeletal maturation. In adolescent females, normal menses are a sensitive index of the adequacy of therapy. Therapy should be continued throughout life in both males and females because of the possibility of malignant degeneration of the hyperplastic adrenal gland. In the pregnant female with CAH, adequate suppression of adrenal androgen secretion is critical to avoid virilization of the fetus, particularly a female fetus.

2. Other aspects of treatment are as for Addison's disease (ie, mineralocorticoid therapy leads to increased plasma renin activity and elevated 17-OH P production in the face of adequate or excessive glucocorticoid therapy, since 17-OH P is a salt-wasting hormone.

3. Clitororecession is often indicated in the first year of life. Vaginoplasty for labial fusion should be performed in early childhood, but it may be necessary during infancy if vaginal-urinary reflux and genitourinary tract infections occur. Partial clitoridec-

tomy is occasionally indicated if the clitoris is abnormally large or sensitive.

Course & Prognosis

When therapy is initiated in early infancy, abnormal metabolic effects are not observed, and masculinization does not progress. Unless adequately controlled, CAH results in sexual precocity and masculinization throughout childhood. Affected individuals will be tall as children but short as adults, because the rate of skeletal maturation is excessive and leads to premature closure of the epiphyses. Treatment with glucocorticoids permits normal growth, development, and sexual maturation. If treatment is delayed or inadequate until somatic development is over 12–14 years as determined by skeletal maturation (bone age), true sexual precocity may occur in males and females.

Patient education stressing lifelong therapy is important to ensure compliance in adolescence and later life.

Female pseudohermaphrodites mistakenly raised as males for more than 3 years may have serious psychological disturbances if their sex is changed after that time. Extensive psychological evaluation is mandatory in determining the optimal course of action.

When virilization of the patient (male or female) is caused by a tumor, the progression of signs and symptoms ceases after surgical removal; however, evidence of masculinization, particularly deepening of the voice, may persist.

Einaudi S et al: Auxological and biochemical parameters is assessing treatment of infants and toddlers with congenital adrenal hyperplasia due to 21-hydroxylase deficiency. J Pediatr Endocrinol 1993;6:173.

Mercado AB et al: Prenatal treatment and diagnosis of congenital adrenal hyperplasia owing to steroid 21-hydroxylase deficiency. J Clin Endocrinol Metab 1995;80:2014.

Migeon CJ, Donohoue P: Adrenal disorders. In: *Wilkins: The Diagnosis and Treatment of Endocrine Disorders in Childhood and Adolescence,* 4th ed. Kappy MS, Blizzard RM, Migeon CJ (editors). Charles C Thomas, 1994.

Wilson RC et al: Steroid 21-hydroxylase deficiency: Genotype may not predict phenotype. J Clin Endocrinol Metab 1995;80:2322.

ADRENOCORTICAL HYPERFUNCTION
(Cushing's Disease, Cushing's Syndrome)

Essentials of Diagnosis

- "Truncal type" adiposity with thin extremities, moon face, muscle wasting, weakness, plethora, easy bruisability, purplish striae, decreased growth rate, delayed skeletal maturation.
- Hypertension, osteoporosis, glycosuria.
- Elevated serum and urine adrenocorticosteroids; low serum potassium; eosinopenia, lymphopenia.

General Considerations

The syndrome is nonspecific; that is, it may result from excessive secretion of adrenal steroids autonomously (adenoma or carcinoma), as the result of excessive ACTH secretion from the pituitary (Cushing's disease) or ectopic sources, or from the chronic ingestion of pharmacologic doses of glucocorticoids (cortisol, cortisone, prednisone). Depletion of body protein is typical, owing to the catabolic (proteolytic) effects of the glucocorticoids. It has been suggested that Cushing's disease, with subsequent bilateral adrenal hyperplasia, is the result of a decreased responsiveness of the hypothalamopituitary feedback mechanism that regulates the release or production of ACTH. This would then result in a constant but only slightly excessive elevation in the secretion of ACTH and an elevation in its serum concentration. Alternatively, hypersecretion of ACTH could be caused by a micro- or macroadenoma of the pituitary gland.

Cushing's syndrome is more common in females. In children under 12 years, it is usually iatrogenic (secondary to pharmacologic doses of ACTH or one of the glucocortisoids). It may rarely be due to an adrenal tumor, adrenal hyperplasia, an adenoma of the pituitary gland or, even more rarely, an extrapituitary (ectopic) ACTH-producing tumor.

Clinical Findings

A. Symptoms and Signs:

1. Due to excessive glucocorticoid effect—Findings include "buffalo-type" adiposity, most marked on the face, neck, and trunk (a fat pad in the interscapular area is characteristic); easy fatiguability and weakness; plethoric facies; purplish striae; easy bruisability; ecchymoses; hirsutism; osteoporosis; hypertension; diabetes mellitus (usually latent); pain in the back; muscle wasting and weakness; and marked retardation of growth and skeletal maturation.

2. Due to excessive mineralocorticoid effect—Hypokalemia, mild hypernatremia with water retention, increased blood volume, edema, and hypertension may be found.

3. Due to excessive androgen effect—Manifestations include hirsutism, acne, and varying degrees of virilization. Menstrual irregularities occur during puberty in older girls.

B. Laboratory Findings:

1. Blood—

a. Plasma cortisol concentrations are elevated, and there may be a loss of the normal diurnal variation in cortisol secretion.

b. Serum chloride and potassium may be lowered. Serum sodium and bicarbonate concentrations may be elevated (metabolic alkalosis).

c. Serum ACTH concentrations are slightly elevated with adrenal hyperplasia (Cushing's disease), decreased in cases of adrenal tumor, and greatly increased with ACTH-producing pituitary or extrapituitary tumors.

d. The leukocyte count shows polymorphonuclear leukocytosis with lymphopenia, and the eosinophil count is low. The erythrocyte count may be elevated.

2. Urine–

a. Urinary free cortisol excretin is elevated. This is the most useful diagnostic test.

b. Urinary 17-hydroxycorticosteroid excretion (excretion products of the glucocorticoids) is elevated.

c. Urinary 17-ketosteroid excretion is usually elevated in association with adrenal tumors.

d. Glycosuria may be present.

3. Response to dexamethasone suppression testing–There is diminished suppression of adrenal function after a small dose (0.5 mg) of dexamethasone; larger doses of dexamethasone cause suppression of adrenal activity when the disease is due to adrenal hyperplasia. Adenomas and adrenal carcinomas may rarely be suppressed by large doses of dexamethasone (4–16 mg/d in four divided doses).

C. Imaging: Pituitary imaging may demonstrate a pituitary adenoma. Adrenal imaging (eg, CT scan) may demonstrate adenoma or bilateral hyperplasia. Radionuclide studies of the adrenals may be useful in complex cases. Osteoporosis (evident first in the spine and pelvis) with compression fractures may be seen in advanced cases, and skeletal maturation is usually delayed.

Differential Diagnosis

Children with exogenous obesity, particularly when accompanied by striae and hypertension, are frequently suspected of having Cushing's syndrome. The child's height, growth rate, and skeletal maturation are helpful in differentiating the two, since children with Cushing's syndrome have a poor growth rate, relatively short stature, and delayed skeletal maturation, whereas those with exogenous obesity usually have a normal or slightly increased growth rate, normal to tall stature, and advanced skeletal maturation. In addition, the color of the striae (purplish in Cushing's syndrome, pink in obesity) and the distribution of the obesity assist in the differentiation. The urinary free cortisol excretion (μg/g creatinine) is always normal in obesity.

Treatment

In all cases of primary adrenal hyperfunction due to tumor, surgical removal, if possible, is indicated. Corticotropin (ACTH) should be given preoperatively and postoperatively to stimulate the nontumorous, contralateral adrenal cortex, which is generally atrophied. Glucocorticoids should be administered parenterally in pharmacologic doses during and after surgery until the patient is stable. Supplemental oral glucocorticoids, potassium, salt, and mineralocorti-coids may be necessary until the suppressed contralateral adrenal gland has recovered, sometimes over a period of several months. (See above section on corticosteroid administration in surgical patients.)

The use of mitotane, a DDT derivative toxic to the adrenal cortex, and aminoglutethimide, an inhibitor of steroid synthesis, has been suggested, but the efficacy of these agents in children with adrenal tumors has not been determined.

Adrenal hyperplasia resulting from a pituitary microadenoma may respond to pituitary surgery or irradiation.

Prognosis

If the tumor is malignant, the prognosis is poor if it cannot be completely removed, because of the lack of effective chemotherapy. If it is benign, cure is to be expected following proper preparation and surgery.

Leinung MC et al: Long term follow-up of transsphenoidal surgery for the treatment of Cushing's disease in children. J Clin Endocrinol Metab 1995;80:2475.

Magiakou MA, Mastorakos G, Chrousos GP: Final stature in patients with endogenous Cushing's syndrome. J Clin Endocrinol Metab 1994;79:1082.

Migeon CJ, Donohoue P: Adrenal disorders. In: *Wilkins: The Diagnosis and Treatments of Endocrine Disorders in Childhood and Adolescence,* 4th ed. Kappy MS, Blizzard RM, Migeon CJ (editors). Charles C Thomas, 1994:717.

PRIMARY HYPERALDOSTERONISM

Primary hyperaldosteronism may be caused by a benign adrenal tumor or by adrenal hyperplasia. It is characterized by paresthesias, tetany, weakness, polyuria (nocturnal enuresis is common in young children), periodic paralysis, low serum potassium, elevated serum sodium, hypertension, metabolic alkalosis, and production of a large volume of alkaline urine with a low fixed specific gravity; the latter does not respond to vasopressin. Edema is rare. The glucose tolerance test is frequently abnormal. Plasma and urinary aldosterone are elevated, but other steroid levels are variable. Plasma renin activity is suppressed, in contrast to the secondary hyperaldosteronism due to renal vascular disease and Bartter's syndrome). In patients with adrenal tumor, the administration of ACTH may further increase the excretion of aldosterone. Marked decrease of aldosterone-induced hypokalemia, alkalosis, hypochloremia, or hypernatremia after the administration of an aldosterone antagonist such a spironolactone, may be of diagnostic value.

Treatment is with glucocorticoid or spironolactone administration, subtotal or total adrenalectomy for hyperplasia, and surgical removal if a tumor is present.

White PC: Disorders of aldosterone biosynthesis and action. N Engl J Med 1994;331:250.

USES OF GLUCOCORTICOIDS & ACTH IN TREATMENT OF NONENDOCRINE DISEASES

Glucocorticoids are commonly used for their anti-inflammatory and immunosuppressive properties in a variety of conditions in childhood. Pharmacologic doses are necessary to achieve these effects, and side effects are common. Numerous synthetic preparations possessing variable ratios of glucocorticoid to mineralocorticoid activity are available (Table 29–12).

Actions

Glucocorticoids exert a direct or permissive effect on virtually every tissue of the body; major known effects include the following:

1. Gluconeogenesis in the liver
2. Stimulation of fat breakdown (lipolysis) and redistribution of body fat
3. Catabolism of protein with an increase in nitrogen and phosphorus excretion
4. Decrease in lymphoid and thymic tissue and a decreased cellular response to inflammation and hypersensitivity
5. Alteration of central nervous system excitation
6. Retardation of connective tissue mitosis and migration, decreased wound healing
7. Improved capillary tone and increased vascular compartment volume and pressure

8. In the case of mineralocorticoids, control of cation flux across membranes, with sodium retention and potassium excretion

Uses

Glucocorticoids are commonly used in physiologic doses to treat adrenal insufficiency (eg, Addison's disease and CAH), but are used in pharmacologic doses to treat a wide variety of inflammatory and autoimmune malignant conditions in childhood. Corticosteroid use is contraindicated in active, questionably healed, or suspected tuberculosis. Corticosteroids should be used with extreme caution in the presence of herpes simplex of the eye, osteoporosis, peptic ulcer, active infections, emotional instability, and thrombophlebitis.

Side Effects of Therapy

When prolonged use of pharmacologic doses of glucocorticoids are necessary, clinical manifestations of Cushing's syndrome are common. Side effects may result either from the use of synthetic exogenous agents by any route, including inhalation and topical administration (inflamed skin), or from the use of ACTH, which stimulates excessive production of endogenous corticosteroids. Use of a larger dose of glucocorticoids given once every 48 hours (alternate-day therapy) lessens the incidence and severity of some of their side effects.

A. Endocrine/Metabolic Effects:

1. Hyperglycemia and glycosuria (chemical diabetes)
2. Cushing's syndrome
3. Persistent suppression of pituitary-adrenal responsiveness to stress with resultant hypoadrenocorticism

B. Effects on Electrolytes and Minerals:

Table 29–12. Potency equivalents for adrenocorticosteroids.

Adrenocorticosteroid	Trade Names	Potency/mg Compared With Cortisol (Glucocorticoid Effect)	Potency/mg Compared With Cortisol (Sodium-Retaining Effect)
Glucocorticoids Hydrocortisone (cortisol)	Cortef	1	1
Cortisone	Cortone Acetate	0.8	1
Prednisone	Meticorten, others	4–5	0.4
Methylprednisolone	Medrol, Meprolone	5–6	Minimal
Triamcinolone	Aristocort, Kenalog Kenacort, Atolone	5–6	Minimal
Dexamethasone	Decadron, others	25–40	Minimal
Betamethasone	Celestone	25	Minimal
Mineralocorticoid Fludrocortisone	Florinef	15–20	300–400

1. Marked retention of sodium and water, producing edema, increased blood volume, and hypertension (more common in endogenous hyperadrenal states)

2. Potassium loss with symptoms of hypokalemia

3. Hypocalcemia, tetany

C. Effects on Protein Metabolism and Skeletal Maturation:

1. Negative nitrogen balance, with loss of body protein and bone protein, resulting in osteoporosis, pathologic fractures, and aseptic bone necrosis

2. Suppression of growth, retarded skeletal maturation

3. Muscular weakness and wasting

D. Effects on the Gastrointestinal Tract:

1. Excessive appetite and intake of food

2. Activation or production of peptic ulcer

3. Gastrointestinal bleeding from ulceration or from unknown cause (particularly in children with hepatic disease)

4. Fatty liver with embolism, pancreatitis, nodular panniculitis

E. Lowering of Resistance to Infectious Agents; Silent Infection; Decreased Inflammatory Reaction:

1. Susceptibility to fungal infections; intestinal parasitic infections

2. Activation of tuberculosis; false-negative tuberculin reaction

3. Stimulation of activity of herpes simplex virus

F. Neuropsychiatric Effects:

1. Euphoria, excitability, psychotic behavior, and status epilepticus with electroencephalographic changes

2. Increased intracranial pressure with pseudotumor cerebri syndrome

G. Hematologic/Vascular Effects:

1. Bleeding into the skin as a result of increased capillary fragility

2. Thrombosis, thrombophlebitis, cerebral hemorrhage

H. Miscellaneous Effects:

1. Myocarditis, pleuritis, and arteritis following abrupt cessation of therapy

2. Cardiomegaly

3. Nephrosclerosis, proteinuria

4. Acne (in older children), hirsutism, amenorrhea, irregular menses

5. Posterior subcapsular cataracts; glaucoma

Tapering of Pharmacologic Doses of Steroids

Prolonged use of pharmacologic doses of glucocorticoids may result in suppression of ACTH secretion and consequent adrenal atrophy. Thus, the abrupt discontinuation of glucocorticoids may result in adrenal insufficiency. A gradual reduction in the steroid dose may allow resumption of ACTH secretion and stimulation of the adrenal glands, thereby lessening the risk of adrenal insufficiency. ACTH secretion generally does not occur until the administered steroid has been given in *subphysiologic* doses ($10 mg/m^2/d$ orally) for several weeks. If pharmacologic glucocorticoid therapy has been given for less than 2–3 weeks, the drug can be discontinued abruptly (if the condition for which it was prescribed allows) because adrenal suppression is unlikely. If tapering is necessary, a reduction of 25–50% every 2–7 days is sufficiently rapid to permit observation of clinical symptomatology. Moreover, withdrawal through use of an alternate-day schedule (ie, a single dose given every 48 hours) may allow for a 50% decrease in the total 2 days' dosage while providing the desired pharmacologic effect.

Once a physiologic equivalent is achieved, the dose may be reduced by 25% every 5–7 days until a subphysiologic dose is reached. At this point, assessment of endogenous adrenal activity is estimated by obtaining fasting plasma cortisol concentrations drawn prior to the morning steroid dose. When an alternate-day schedule is followed, a plasma cortisol is measured the morning prior to treatment. A plasma cortisol concentration within the physiologic range (8–15 µg/dL) demonstrates return of basal physiologic adrenal function; exogenous steroids may then be safely discontinued. After basal physiologic adrenal function returns, the adrenal reserve or capacity to respond to stress and infection is estimated by the ACTH stimulation test, in which 0.25 mg of synthetic ACTH (Cortrosyn) is administered intravenously. Plasma cortisol is measured prior to (zero time) and at 60 minutes after the infusion. A plasma cortisol concentration of greater than 20 µg/dL at 60 minutes, or a doubling of the zero time value, indicates a satisfactory adrenal reserve. The ACTH test should be performed in all patients who have received pharmacologic doses of corticosteroids for more than 2–3 weeks. Even if the results of the test are normal, patients who have received prolonged treatment with glucocorticoids may exhibit signs and symptoms of adrenal insufficiency during acute stress, infection, or surgery for months to years after they have been withdrawn. Careful monitoring and, when necessary, the use of pharmacologic doses of glutocorticoids should be considered during severe illnesses and surgery for life.

Allen DB: Growth suppression by glucocorticoid therapy. Pediatr Rounds 1995;4:1.

Crowley S et al: Growth and the growth hormone axis in prepubertal children with asthma. J Pediatr 1995; 126:297.

Louard RJ et al: Glucocorticoids antagonize insulin's antiproteolytic action on skeletal muscle in humans. J Clin Endocrinol Metab 1994;79:278.

Rivkees SA, Danon M, Herrin J: Prednisone dose limitation of growth hormone treatment of steroid-induced growth failure. J Pediatr 1994;125:322.

ADRENAL MEDULLA

PHEOCHROMOCYTOMA

Pheochromocytoma is an uncommon tumor. Only 10% of the total number of reported cases occur in childhood. The tumor may be located wherever there is any chromaffin tissue (eg, adrenal medulla, sympathetic ganglia, carotid body). It may be multiple, familial (autosomal dominant, in which case a high prevalence of MEN exists), recurrent, and sometimes malignant.

Although clinical manifestation of pheochromocytoma may result from physical expansion of lesions into surrounding tissue (eg, spinal cord), manifestations are generally due to excessive secretion of epinephrine or norepinephrine. Attacks of anxiety, unexplained perspiration, and headaches should arouse suspicion. Other findings are palpitation and tachycardia, dizziness, weakness, nausea and vomiting, diarrhea, dilated pupils with blurring of vision, abdominal and precordial pain, hypertension (usually persistent), heat intolerance, and vasomotor instability (flushing, postural hypotension). The symptoms may be sustained, producing all of the above findings plus papilledema, retinopathy, and enlargement of the heart. There is an increased incidence of pheochromocytomas in patients and families with neurofibromatosis, and MEN type 2 (see above). Neuroblastomas, neurogangliomas, and other neural tumors may cause increased secretion of pressor amines and occasionally simulate the findings of pheochromocytoma. Carcinoid tumors may produce cardiovascular changes similar to those associated with pheochromocytoma.

Laboratory diagnosis is possible in over 90% of cases. Serum catecholamines are elevated, particularly while the patient is symptomatic, and urinary excretion of catecholamines parallels this elevation. Elevated levels are characteristically high enough to be diagnostic but may be limited to the period of a paroxysm. The 24-hour urine excretion of metanephrines and vanillylmandelic acid is increased. Provocative tests employing histamine, tyramine, or glucagon and the phentolamine tests may be abnormal, but are dangerous, and these agents are rarely necessary for diagnosis. Displacement of the kidney may be shown by intravenous pyelogram, and the tumor may be identified by CT scans or MRI. Angiocatheterization with localized measurement of circulating concentrations of catecholamines may be helpful in localizing the tumor prior to surgery.

Surgical removal of the tumor is the treatment of choice; however, the procedure must be undertaken with great caution and with the patient properly stabilized because manipulation of the tumor may cause sudden and profound, potentially fatal changes in blood pressure. Oral phenoxybenzamine or intravenous phentolamine is used preoperatively. Profound hypotension may occur as the tumor is removed but may be controlled with an infusion of norepinephrine, which may have to be continued for 1–2 days.

Complete relief of symptoms is to be expected after recovery from removal of the tumor if it is benign, unless irreversible secondary vascular changes have occurred. If the disorder remains untreated, severe cardiac, renal, and cerebral damage may result.

Blizzard RM, Rogol AD: Variations and disorders of pubertal development. In: *Wilkins: The Diagnosis and Treatment of Endocrine Disorders in Childhood and Adolescence,* 4th ed. Kappy MS, Blizzard RM, Migeon CJ (editors). Charles C Thomas, 1994:857.

Bravo EB, Gifford RW Jr: Pheochromocytoma: Diagnosis, localization and management. N Engl J Med 1984; 311:1298.

Migeon CJ, Donohoue P: *Wilkins: The Diagnosis and Treatments of Endocrine Disorders in Childhood and Adolescence,* 4th ed. Kappy MS, Blizzard RM, Migeon CJ (editors). Charles C Thomas, 1994:717.

Diabetes Mellitus

30

H. Peter Chase, MD, & George S. Eisenbarth, MD, PhD

Essentials of Diagnosis

- Polyuria, polydipsia, and weight loss
- Hyperglycemia and glucosuria with or without ketonuria

General Considerations

Insulin-dependent (type I) diabetes mellitus (previously called juvenile diabetes) is the most common type of diabetes in people under age 40 years. It is associated with diminished insulin production and being ketosis-prone, although about 85% of persons affected still make some insulin 1 year after diagnosis and 42% still make small amounts of insulin 3 years after diagnosis. Type I diabetes differs from non–insulin-dependent (type II) diabetes mellitus, which is the most common type of diabetes occurring in a person over age 40 years; it is associated with being overweight, not prone to ketosis, and insensitive to insulin. Non–insulin-dependent diabetes is rarely seen in persons younger than 18 years of age, but it does occur in overweight teenagers and is referred to as *maturity-onset diabetes of youth* (MODY). Diet, exercise, and oral hypoglycemic agents constitute the main therapy for patients with MODY, as for adults with type II diabetes. The remainder of this discussion deals with type I diabetes.

Etiology

Type I diabetes results from immunologic damage to the insulin-producing beta cells of the pancreatic islets. This damage occurs gradually, over months or years in most people, and symptoms do not appear until about 90% of the pancreatic islets have been destroyed. The immunologic damage requires a genetic predisposition and is probably affected by environmental factors.

The importance of genetics is shown by the fact that 35–50% of second identical twins develop diabetes after the first twin develops the disease. About 6% of siblings or offspring of persons with type I diabetes also develop diabetes (compared with the usual incidence of 2–3 out of 1000). The condition is more common in white children but occurs in all racial groups. There is an association with HLA groups DR3 and DR4, and about 95% of white diabetic children have at least one of these HLA types. Fifty-three percent have both one DR3 and one DR4 (one from each parent) compared with only 6% of the general population having this combination. The presence of the amino acid, aspartic acid, on position 57 of the DQ beta chain of the HLA complex is considered protective of type I diabetes; conversely, its absence provides a marker for susceptibility.

The importance of environmental factors in the etiology is suggested because less than 50% of second identical twins develop diabetes. If the condition were purely genetic, the second twin would always develop the disease. Important environmental factors may be viral disease or chemicals in the diet. For example, 40% of infants with congenital rubella develop diabetes or an abnormal glucose tolerance test by 20 years of age, and the incidence of diabetes was high after eating foods accidentally preserved with excessive nitrates. The early introduction of cow's milk also has been suggested as a possible environmental factor.

The immunologic basis of diabetes is demonstrated by the ability of a potent immunosuppressive agent, cyclosporine, to preserve islet tissue for 1–2 years when given to newly diagnosed patients. However, renal damage from cyclosporine precludes its long-term use. White blood cells are found in the islets of newly diagnosed patients and may release toxic products (free radicals, interleukin-1, tumor necrosis factor) that injure the islets. Antibodies to islet cells (ICA), insulin, "64 K" or glutamic acid decarboxylase (GAD), ICA512, and other antibodies are present in the serum of over 90% of patients for months to years prior to diagnosis. These antibodies are likely the effect, not the cause of islet destruction.

Many centers now screen for prediabetes using an ICA test or other antibody test. An intravenous (IV) glucose tolerance test helps to define those at highest risk so that they may enter prevention trials. Initial pilot data suggest a preventive role for nicotinamide, azathioprine, and early insulin administration.

Intervention trials on antibody-positive first-degree relatives based on data from the pilot trials have begun. European investigators are doing a double-blind study of nicotinamide, whereas US centers are doing a randomized study of IV and subcutaneous insulin compared with no therapy (see Keller et al, 1993).

Diagnosis

The classic symptoms of polyuria and polydipsia are now so well recognized that friends or family members usually suspect the diagnosis of type I diabetes. Other cases may be detected by finding glucosuria on routine office urinalysis. Up to 50% of patients with new cases of diabetes used to present in coma, but most are now diagnosed before developing severe ketonuria, ketonemia, and secondary acidosis. An oral glucose tolerance test is rarely necessary in children. A random blood glucose level above 300 mg/dL (16.6 mmol/L) or a fasting blood glucose above 200 mg/dL (11 mmol/L) is all that is needed to make the diagnosis of type I diabetes. If the presentation is mild, hospitalization is usually not necessary.

Good education for all family members is paramount to the family's handling the condition in the home. All parent figures need to learn about diabetes and know how to give insulin injections and perform home blood glucose monitoring. There is also much stress for the family around the time of the initial diagnosis, and feelings of shock, denial, sadness, anger, fear, and guilt may be present. Meeting with a counselor to express these feelings at the time of diagnosis helps with long-term adaptation.

Treatment

The five major variables in the treatment of type I diabetes are (1) insulin dosage, (2) diet, (3) exercise, (4) stress management, and (5) blood glucose and urine ketone monitoring. All must be taken into account to obtain safe, effective metabolic control for each patient-family unit. Although teenagers can be taught to do much of their own diabetes management, they do better when supportive, not overbearing, parents remain involved. Children younger than 10 or 11 years of age cannot reliably administer insulin without adult supervision, because they lack fine motor control and may not understand the importance of accurate dosage.

A. Insulin: Insulin functions (1) to allow glucose to pass into the cell, (2) to decrease the body's (particularly the liver's and muscle's) own production of glucose, and (3) to turn off ketone production.

1. Treatment of new-onset diabetes—If ketonuria is large, the pH low (<7.30), and the patient dehydrated, then IV insulin and fluid therapy should be given (as described in Ketoacidosis in the following text). If moderate or large ketonuria is present at first diagnosis and the child is adequately hydrated and has a normal venous pH, one or two intramuscular injections of 0.1–0.2 U of regular (short-acting) insulin per kilogram body weight about 1 hour apart

will help shut off the ketone production. If ketonuria is small or absent, this regimen is not necessary and subcutaneous shots can be started.

When ketonuria is not present, the child is usually more sensitive to insulin and a total daily dose of 0.25–0.50 U/kg/24 h (by subcutaneous injection) can be used. If ketonuria is or was present, the child usually does not produce as much insulin and will require 0.5–1.0 U per kg body weight of total insulin per 24 hours.

These doses are adjusted with each injection during the first week. Most physicians begin newly diagnosed children on synthetic human insulin. About two thirds of the total dose is usually given 30–60 minutes before breakfast and the other one third 30–60 minutes before dinner. Children under age 4 years usually need 1 or 2 U of regular insulin to cover meals, and the remainder of the dosage is neutral protamine Hagedorn (NPH) insulin. Children 4–10 years of age may require up to 4 U of regular insulin to cover breakfast and dinner (Table 30–1), whereas proportionately higher dosages (usually 4–10 U) of regular insulin are used for older children.

A new more rapid-acting form of regular insulin called Humalog will soon be available. Humalog's onset of activity is 10–15 minutes rather than 30–60 minutes, as with regular insulin (see Table 30–2). It is thus not necessary to wait 30–60 minutes to eat after the injection of Humalog is taken. Humalog also peaks sooner than regular insulin and is gone within 4 hours. The shorter duration reduces the risk of later hypoglycemia. It is likely that most people will be changed form regular to Humalog insulin.

2. Continuing insulin dosage—The total daily insulin dosage may need to be increased gradually to 1 U/kg (especially if ketonuria is present at onset). When gluconeogenesis and glycolysis are suppressed by insulin, the "honeymoon" or "grace" period is often seen. This may occur 1–8 weeks after diagnosis in more than 50% of children. Continuing small doses of insulin at levels that do not cause frequent hypoglycemia may be important at this time to help preserve later beta-cell function.

In helping families with day-to-day dosing of regular insulin, some physicians use sliding scales, more recently referred to as "thinking scales," to emphasize that the family must always be thinking about food recently eaten or to be eaten and recent or forthcoming exercise, in addition to the blood glucose level. Table 30–1 is an example of a thinking scale for a 4- to 10-year-old.

After the initial correct dosage of NPH (long-acting) insulin is attained, daily adjustments usually are not needed. However, small decreases may be made for heavy activity (eg, afternoon sports or overnight events). Many families gradually learn to make small (0.5–1.0 U) weekly adjustments in their child's insulin dosage, based on home blood glucose testing

Table 30–1. Example of a thinking scale to adjust regular insulin dose for a 4- to 10-year-old child.[1]

	Active			Not Active		
Blood Sugar mg/dL	Blood Sugar mmol/L	Regular Insulin		Blood Sugar mg/dL	Blood Sugar mmol/L	Regular Insulin
<100	<5.5	0		<70	<3.9	0
100–200	5.5–11.1	1		70–150	3.9–8.3	1
201–300	11.2–16.6	2		151–200	8.4–11.1	2
>300	>16.6	3		201–250	11.2–13.9	3
				>250	>13.9	4

[1]Blood sugar should be measured 30 minutes before breakfast and dinner and at least 2 hours after eating. The regular insulin dose shown should then be added to the long-acting insulin.

results. Understanding the times of insulin activity is essential (Table 30–2).

Most children receive two injections of insulin daily. The most common combinations are mixtures of regular and NPH insulins twice daily (see Table 30–2), or regular and NPH insulin in the morning and regular and ultralente insulin at dinner. Ultralente insulin is sometimes preferred at dinner, because it does not peak as much as NPH insulin during the night and it is also more apt to last through the night. Ultralente insulin delays the action of regular insulin slightly, but does not delay the action of Humalog insulin.

When children and families are willing to use three insulin injections per day, the evening shot is often split, with regular insulin given before dinner and NPH insulin at bedtime (to help maintain coverage through the night). Some physicians use injections of regular and ultralente insulin before breakfast and dinner and an injection of regular insulin before lunch. Continuous subcutaneous insulin injection therapy by insulin pump is sometimes used in emotionally mature, older teens who are willing to invest more time in blood glucose monitoring and dietary therapy. This is particularly true when glucose control (monitored by HbA_{1c} levels; see following text) remains suboptimal in spite of receiving three or more injections per day. The following constitutes "intensive diabetes management":

- Three or more insulin injections per day or insulin pump therapy
- Four or more blood sugar determinations per day
- Careful attention to dietary intake
- Frequent contact with the health care provider

This was shown in the Diabetes Control and Complications Trial (DCCT; see text that follows and References) to result in improved glucose control and to reduce the risk for the eye, kidney, and neurologic complications of diabetes. All teenagers who have suboptimal glucose control and who are willing should be considered for intensive diabetes management.

B. Diet: The following are the mainstays of dietary treatment:

1. Eat a well-balanced diet.
2. Keep the day-to-day intake consistent.
3. Eat meals and snacks at the same time each day.
4. Use snacks to prevent insulin reactions (encourage solid protein at bedtime every night).
5. Manage carbohydrate intake carefully.
6. Avoid overtreating low blood sugars.
7. Reduce cholesterol, total fat, and saturated fat intake.
8. Maintain appropriate weight for height; avoid becoming overweight.
9. Increase fiber intake.
10. Avoid foods high in salt.
11. Avoid excessive protein intake.

Table 30–2. Times of insulin activities.

Type of Insulin	Begins Working	Main Effect	All Gone
Short-acting			
Regular	½ h	2–4 h	4–8 h
Humalog	10–15 min	30–60 min	4 h
Semilente	1–2 h	2–5 h	8–12 h
Longer-acting			
NPH	2–4 h	6–8 h	12–15 h
Ultralente	4–6 h	8–15 h	15–18 h
Premixed			
Lente (3 parts Semilente and 7 parts Ultralente)	1–2 h	6–12 h	15–18 h
NPH/Regular	½ h	Variable[1]	12–15 h

[1]Available in various combinations to fit individual needs.

These recommendations are discussed in detail in *Understanding Insulin Dependent Diabetes* (see References). Of these recommendations, number 2 (consistency) and number 5 (careful management of carbohydrate intake) are essential to any form of dietary treatment.

The American Diabetes Association (ADA) no longer recommends any one "diabetic" or "ADA" diet. Instead, medical nutrition therapy for diabetics should be individualized, with consideration given to usual eating habits and other lifestyle changes. Some families and children (particularly those with weight problems) find exchange diets helpful initially while they are learning categories of foods. An exchange diet is a food plan in which foods are grouped into one of six food lists having similar nutritional composition. Caloric intake and numbers of exchanges are set, but foods within a group can be exchanged with one another. Working with a knowledgeable dietitian is important in diabetes management.

The DCCT found that four nutrition factors contributed to better sugar control (lower hemoglobin A_{1C} levels). These factors are (1) adherence to a meal plan, (2) avoidance of extra snacks, (3) avoidance of overtreatment of low blood sugars (hypoglycemia), and (4) prompt treatment of high blood sugars. Two other nutrition factors include adjusting insulin levels for meals and maintaining a consistent schedule of night snacks. The DCCT did popularize a "carbohydrate-counting" dietary plan in which the dosage of regular insulin is altered with each injection to adjust for the amount of carbohydrate to be eaten and exercise.

C. Exercise: Regular aerobic exercise is important for children with diabetes because exercise fosters a sense of well-being, helps increase insulin sensitivity, and helps maintain proper weight, blood pressure, and blood fat levels. Exercise may also help maintain normal peripheral circulation in later years.

The prevention of hypoglycemia during exercise or in the 2–8 hours after exercise (delayed hypoglycemia) is obviously important. This is done with careful monitoring of blood sugar levels (before, during, and after exercise), sometimes reducing the dosage of the insulin having activity at the time of the exercise, and by providing extra snacks. In general, the longer and more vigorous the activity, the more food that should be eaten before exercising. One "carbohydrate count" is 15 g of glucose in the United States (10 g in Canada and the United Kingdom); 15 g of glucose usually covers about 30 minutes of exercise. The use of drinks containing 5–10% dextrose, such as Gatorade, during the period of exercise, is often beneficial.

D. Stress Management: The management of stress is important on a short-term basis because stress hormones increase blood glucose levels. Chronic emotional upsets may lead to missed injections or other compliance problems. When this hap-

pens, counseling for the family and child becomes an important part of diabetes management.

E. Blood Glucose Measurements: All families must be able to monitor blood glucose levels at least three to four times daily, and more frequently in small infants or patients who have glucose control problems or have illness. Blood glucose levels can be done using visual strips or by meter with an accuracy of 10% or more. Blood glucose levels to aim for when no food has been eaten for 2 or more hours vary according to the age of the child (Table 30–3).

Blood glucose results must be recorded even if the meter has a memory feature. This allows the family to look for patterns and make changes in the insulin dosage. If more than 50% of the values are above the desired range for age or more than 12% below the desired range, the insulin dosage usually needs to be adjusted. Some families are able to make these changes on their own (particularly after the first year), whereas other families need help from their physician. The recommendation of the ADA in the 1994 Standards of Care is that children with diabetes have clinic visits every 3 months (see References). This provides the opportunity to adjust insulin dosages according to changes in growth and blood glucose levels, as well as to check for changes on the physical examination (eg, eyes, thyroid).

Laboratory Evaluations

In addition to the home measurements of blood glucose and urine ketone levels, glycosylated hemoglobin should be measured every 3 months. This test reflects the frequency of elevated blood glucose levels over the previous 3 months. Normal values vary among laboratories, but are usually below 6.2% (hemoglobin A_{1C}) or below 8.0% (total glycosylated hemoglobin). The desired ranges vary according to the ages of the children. For the hemoglobin A_{1C} method, these ranges are 12 years old or older, less than 7.8%; 5–11 years old, less than 8.5%; and under 5 years of age, 7.5–9.0%. Higher levels are allowed in younger children to reduce their risk for hypoglycemia, because their brains are still developing and they may not relate hypoglycemia symptoms to a need for treatment. Low hemoglobin A_{1C} values are generally associated with a greater risk for low blood sugars (see Hypoglycemia). Using either method, longitudinal averages more than 33% above the upper limit of normal are associated with a higher risk

Table 30–3. Ideal glucose levels after 2 or more hours of fast.

Age	Glucose Level
≤4 years	100–200 mg/dL (5.5–11 mmol/L)
5–12 years	80–180 mg/dL (4.6–10 mmol/L)
≥13 years	70–150 mg/dL (3.9–8.3 mmol/L)

for the later renal and retinal complications of diabetes. In the intensive treatment group of the DCCT, the lower hemoglobin A_{1C} values resulted in greater than 50% reductions in the eye, kidney, and nerve complications of diabetes.

It is also important to measure serum cholesterol levels once yearly, although elevations may be secondary to poor glucose control.

When puberty is reached and the person has had diabetes for 5 years or longer, the 24-hour urinary excretion of albumin should be measured (as "microalbumin") in two separate urines once yearly (see Chronic Complications). This can be done using timed overnight urine collections, since teens tend to hate collecting 24-hour specimens. Normal values vary with the methodology of the laboratory, but are generally below 20 μg/min.

If the thyroid is enlarged (about 20% of youths with type I diabetes), the thyroid-stimulating hormone (TSH) level should be measured once or twice yearly. This is the first test to become abnormal in the autoimmune thyroiditis that is commonly associated with type I diabetes.

A checklist of physician's contributions to good diabetes care is shown in Table 30–4.

Acute Complications

A. Hypoglycemia: Hypoglycemia (or insulin reaction) is defined as a blood glucose level below 60 mg/dL (or 3.2 mmol/L). For preschool children, values below 70 mg/dL (3.9 mmol/L) should be cause for concern. The common symptoms of hypoglycemia are hunger, weakness, shakiness, sweating, drowsiness (at an unusual time), headache, and behavior changes. Children learn to recognize hypoglycemia at different ages, but can often report "feeling funny" as young as 4–5 years of age. If low blood sugar is not treated immediately with simple

Table 30–4. Physician's checklist of good diabetes management.

Variable	Frequency of Measurement	Tests and Values
Blood sugars	3–4 times daily	See age-appropriate values.
Hemoglobin A_{1c}	Every 3 months	See age-appropriate values.
Urine microalbumin	Annually after 5 years of diabetes (pubertal patients)	<20 μg/min
Ophthalmology referral	Annually after 5 years of diabetes (pubertal patients)	Retinal photographs
Signs of other endocrinopathy	Evaluate annually (eg, thyroid enlargement)	(eg, TSH: 0.5–5.0 IU/dL)

TSH = thyroid-stimulating hormone.

sugar, the hypoglycemia may result in loss of consciousness or convulsions. If not treated for several hours, brain damage or death can occur.

Consistency in daily routine, correct insulin dosage, regular blood glucose monitoring, controlled snacking, compliance of patients and parents, and good education all are important in preventing severe hypoglycemia.

The treatment of mild hypoglycemia involves giving 4 ounces of juice, sugared soda pop, or milk, and waiting 10 minutes. If the blood glucose level is still below 60 mg/dL (3.2 mmol/L), the liquids are repeated. If the glucose level is above this, solid foods are given. Moderate hypoglycemia, in which the person is conscious but incoherent, is treated by squeezing one-half tube of concentrated glucose (eg, Insta-Glucose) or of cake frosting between the gums and lips and stroking the throat to encourage swallowing.

In the DCCT study, 10% of patients with standard management and 25% of patients with intensive insulin management (insulin pumps or three or more insulin shots per day) had one or more severe hypoglycemic reactions each year. All families are advised to have glucagon in their homes and to give 0.3 mL (0.3 mg) to children less than 5 years old and 0.5 mL (0.5 mg) to children over 5 years old for hypoglycemia by either subcutaneous or intramuscular injection. Some people (usually those who have had diabetes for more than 10 years) fail to recognize the symptoms of low blood sugar (hypoglycemic unawareness). For these people, glucose control must be liberalized to prevent severe hypoglycemic reactions. School personnel, sports coaches, and babysitters must be trained to recognize and treat hypoglycemia.

B. Ketonuria and Ketoacidosis: Families must be educated to check urine ketones during any illness (including vomiting even once) or any time a blood glucose level is above 240 mg/dL (13.3 mmol/L). If moderate or large ketonuria is detected, the physician must be called and 10–20% of the total daily insulin dose given subcutaneously as regular insulin every 3 hours until the urine ketones are small or negative. This prevents ketonuria from progressing to ketoacidosis and allows most patients to be treated at home by telephone management. Juices and other fluids are encouraged, and suppositories to prevent vomiting may be indicated. If deep breathing (Kussmaul's respirations) or excessive weakness occurs, the patient should be evaluated promptly by a physician.

Acidosis (pH <7.30) is now present in less than 25% of newly diagnosed children. Acidosis may also occur in those with known diabetes who do not check for ketonuria and call the physician when moderate or large urine ketones are present. Repeated episodes of ketoacidosis usually result from missed insulin injections and require that a responsible adult take over the diabetes management. If this adult participation is not possible, a change in the child's living situation may be necessary.

Treatment of diabetic ketoacidosis (DKA) is based on four physiologic principles: (1) restoration of fluid volume, (2) inhibition of lipolysis and return to glucose utilization, (3) replacement of body salts, and (4) correction of acidosis. Laboratory tests at the start of treatment should include a venous pH, a blood glucose, and an electrolyte panel. Mild DKA is defined as a venous pH of 7.2–7.3, moderate DKA as a pH of 7.10–7.19, and severe DKA as a pH below 7.10. **Patients with severe DKA should be hospitalized and not treated in a clinic or emergency room.** More severe cases may benefit from determination of osmolarity, calcium and phosphorus, and blood urea nitrogen levels. Severe and moderate episodes of DKA generally require hourly determinations of serum glucose, electrolyte, and venous pH levels, whereas these parameters can be measured every 2 hours if the pH level is between 7.2 and 7.30.

1. Restoration of fluid volume–Dehydration is judged by (a) acute loss in body weight (if a recent weight is known), (b) dryness of oral mucous membranes, (c) low blood pressure, and (d) high heart rate. Initial treatment is physiologic saline (0.9%), 10–20 mL/kg during the first hour. If indicated, this is repeated during the second hour. The total volume of initial reexpansion fluid should not exceed 40 mL per kg body weight because of the danger of cerebral edema (see Management of Cerebral Edema). Albumin, 10 mL/kg of 5% solution, can be given for 30 minutes if the patient is in shock. After initial reexpansion, half-physiologic (0.45%) saline usually is given at 1.5 times maintenance.

2. Inhibition of lipolysis and return to glucose utilization–Insulin turns off fat breakdown and ketone formation. IV regular insulin is usually given at 0.1 U/kg/h. The insulin solution should be administered by pump and can be made by diluting 30 U of regular insulin in 150 mL of 0.9% saline (1 U/5 mL). If the glucose level falls below 250 mg/dL, (13.9 mmol/L) 5% dextrose is added to the IV fluids. If the glucose level continues to decrease below 120 mg/dL (6.6 mmol/L), 10% dextrose can be added. If necessary, the insulin dose can be reduced to 0.05 U/kg/h, but it should not be discontinued before the venous pH reaches 7.30. The half-life of IV insulin when discontinued is 6 minutes, whereas subcutaneous insulin takes 30–60 minutes to act. Thus, often it is better to continue the IV insulin until the subcutaneous insulin can begin acting.

3. Replacement of body salts–In patients with DKA, both sodium and potassium pass into the urine with the ketones and are depleted. Serum sodium concentrations may be falsely lowered by hyperglycemia, causing water to be drawn into the IV space, and by hyperlipemia if fat replaces some of the water in the serum used for electrolyte analysis. Sodium is usually replaced adequately by the use of physiologic and half-physiologic saline in the rehydration fluids as previously discussed.

Serum potassium levels initially may be elevated because of the inability of potassium to stay in the cell in the presence of acidosis (although the total body potassium is low). Potassium should not be given until the serum potassium level is known to be low or normal and the pH is above 7.10. It is then usually given at a concentration of 40 mEq/L with 50% of the potassium (20 mEq/L) as either potassium acetate or potassium chloride and the other half as potassium phosphate (s0 mEq/L). Hypocalcemia can occur if all of the potassium is given as the phosphate salt; hypophosphatemia occurs if none of the potassium is of the phosphate salt.

4. Correction of acidosis–Acidosis is corrected as the fluid volume and aerobic glycolysis are restored and as insulin is administered to inhibit ketogenesis. As noted earlier, measuring the venous pH (identical with the arterial pH) reveals the severity of acidosis. Bicarbonate is usually reserved for patients with a pH lower than 7.0 and is given as 1–2 mEq/kg body weight over 1 or 2 hours. The pH is monitored every hour and the bicarbonate discontinued when the pH reaches 7.10.

5. Management of cerebral edema–Some degree of cerebral edema has been shown by computed tomography (CT) scan to be common in DKA (see References). Associated clinical symptoms are rare, unpredictable, and often associated with mortality. Cerebral edema may be related to overhydration with hypotonic fluids, although the cause is not well understood. Early neurologic signs may include headache, excessive drowsiness, and dilated pupils. Prompt initiation of therapy should include elevation of the head of the bed, hyperventilation, mannitol (1.0 g/kg by IV bolus), and fluid restriction. If the cerebral edema is not recognized early, over 50% of patients will die or have permanent brain damage.

Chronic Complications

About 30–40% of persons with type I diabetes eventually develop renal failure or loss of vision. Factors that greatly reduce this likelihood are longitudinal hemoglobin A_1 levels in a good range, maintenance of blood pressure below the 90th percentile level for age, and abstinence from smoking or chewing tobacco. Annual retinal examinations and urine microalbumin measurements are important for pubertal children who have had diabetes for 5 years or longer (see Laboratory Evaluations). Preliminary data now show that the use of angiotensin-converting enzyme (ACE) inhibitors may reverse or delay kidney damage when it is detected in the microalbuminuria stage (20–300 µg/min). Similarly, laser treatment to coagulate proliferating capillaries prevents bleeding and leakage of blood into the vitreous fluid or behind the retina. This treatment thus prevents retinal detachment and saves the vision for many diabetics with proliferative diabetic retinopathy.

REFERENCES

American Diabetes Association: Standards of medical care for patients with diabetes mellitus. Diabetes Care 1994;17:616.

Chase HP: *Understanding Insulin Dependent Diabetes,* 8th ed. Denver: Hirschfeld Press, 1995. [Available for $10.00 from The Children's Diabetes Foundation, 777 Grant St. Suite 302, Denver, CO 80203.]

Chase HP, Garg SK, Jelley DH: Diabetic ketoacidosis in children and the role of outpatient management. Pediatr Rev 1990;11:297.

Davies JL, Kawaguchi Y, Bennett ST, et al: A genome-wide search for human type I diabetes susceptibility genes. Nature 1994;371:130.

Delahanty LM, Halford BN: The role of diet behaviors in achieving improved glycemic control in intensively treated patients in the Diabetes Control and Complications Trial. Diabetes Care 1994;16:1453.

The Diabetes Control and Complications Trial Research Group: The effect of intensive treatment of diabetes on the development and progression of long-term complications in insulin-dependent diabetes mellitus. N Engl J Med 1993;329:977.

Keller RJ, Eisenbarth GS, Jackson RA: Insulin prophylaxis in individuals at high risk of type I diabetes. Lancet 1993;341:927.

Krane EJ, Rockoff MA, Wallman JK, Wolfsdorf JI: Subclinical brain swelling in children during treatment of diabetic ketoacidosis. N Engl J Med 1985;312:1147.

Leslie RDG, Elliott RB: Early environmental events as a cause of IDDM: Evidence and implications. Diabetes 1994;43:843.

Position Statement. Nutrition recommendations and principles for people with diabetes mellitus. Diabetes Care 1994;17:519.

31

Inborn Errors of Metabolism

Carol L. Greene, MD, & Stephen I. Goodman, MD

Disorders in which defects of single genes cause clinically significant blocks in metabolic pathways are called **inborn errors of metabolism.** For many years after Garrod first described them in 1908, these conditions were considered esoteric and rare. The number of known inborn errors has increased rapidly in recent years, however, and they are now recognized as important causes of disease in the pediatric age group. Many of them can now be treated effectively. Even when treatment is not available, correct diagnosis permits couples to make informed decisions about future offspring.

Pathogenesis is almost always due to accumulation of enzyme substrate behind the metabolic block or to deficiency of the reaction product. In some cases, the accumulated enzyme substrate is diffusible and has an adverse effect on distant organs; in others, as in lysosomal storage diseases, the substrate accumulates only locally.

The clinical manifestations of inborn errors vary significantly; there are mild and severe forms of virtually every disorder, and many patients do not match the classic phenotype. In many cases, this is because the mutations in different patients, even though they are in the same gene, are not identical.

Strategies used to treat inborn errors include avoiding enzyme substrate in the diet (eg, low-phenylalanine diet for phenylketonuria), removing accumulated substrate by pharmacologic means (eg, glycine therapy for isovaleric acidemia), supplementing an inadequately produced metabolite (eg, arginine administration for urea cycle disorders), providing additional coenzyme (eg, vitamin B_{12} therapy for methylmalonic acidemia), and providing normal enzyme (eg, enzyme infusion in Gaucher's disease or liver transplantation for Wilson's disease). Gene replacement is a long-term goal, and trials of treatment of adenine deaminase deficiency began in 1990. However, problems of delivery to target organs and control of gene action make this an unrealistic option at present for most of these disorders.

Inborn errors can present at any time, affect virtually any organ system, and cause all but the most common pediatric problems. This chapter focuses

first on when these conditions should be considered in the differential diagnosis of common pediatric problems. A few of the more important disorders are then discussed in detail.

DIAGNOSIS

SUSPECTING INBORN ERRORS

Some important clinical situations are considered later in this section. In general, inborn errors must be considered in the differential diagnosis of the critically ill newborn and of the child with seizures, Reye-like syndromes, parenchymal liver disease, mental retardation or developmental delay, recurrent vomiting, unusual odor, unexplained acidosis, hyperammonemia, and hypoglycemia.

Inborn errors should be strongly suspected when (1) symptoms accompany changes in diet, (2) there is developmental slowing or regression, (3) there is a history of food preferences or aversions, or (4) there is a history of parental consanguinity or a history of problems that could be due to an inborn error, such as retardation or unexplained death in sibs, cousins, or other relatives.

Physical findings that should always raise the suspicion of an inborn error include alopecia or abnormal hair, retinal cherry-red spot or retinitis pigmentosa, cataracts or corneal opacity, hepatomegaly or splenomegaly, coarse features, skeletal changes (including gibbus), and ataxia. Features that may be important, in combination with a suspicious history, include failure to thrive, microcephaly, rash, jaundice, hypotonia, and hypertonia.

Finding an immediate cause of symptoms does not rule out an underlying inborn error. For example, renal tubular acidosis and cirrhosis are often due to an underlying inborn error. Some inborn errors predispose to infection, eg, gram-negative septicemia in patients with galactosemia. In other inborn errors, acute crises may be brought on by intercurrent infections. Presentation of some inborn errors has been mistaken for non-accidental trauma (eg, Glutaric Acidemia Type I) or poisoning (eg, methylmalonic acidemia); in addition, children with inborn errors of metabolism may be at higher risk of child abuse or neglect because of the much greater irritability that some of these infants often demonstrate.

LABORATORY STUDIES

Table 31–1 lists common clinical and laboratory features of different groups of inborn errors. Table 31–2 lists laboratory tests used to diagnose these diseases and gives some comments about their use.

Laboratory studies are almost always needed for the diagnosis of inborn errors. Serum electrolytes and pH can be determined in any hospital laboratory and should be used to estimate anion gap as well as acid-base status. Analysis of serum lactate, pyruvate, and ammonia may be available in laboratories of large hospitals. Amino acid and organic acid studies must be performed at specialized facilities to ensure adequate analysis and interpretation. It is becoming possible to diagnose an increasing number of inborn errors with DNA probes. For most disorders, this requires an extensive genealogic chart or a knowledge of the precise mutation carried in the family.

The physician should know what conditions a test will detect and when it will detect them. For example, urine organic acids may be normal in patients with medium-chain acyl-CoA dehydrogenase deficiency or biotinidase deficiency, glycine may be elevated only in cerebrospinal fluid in patients with glycine encephalopathy, and a result that is normal in one physiologic state may be abnormal in another. For instance, the urine of a hypoglycemic child should be positive for ketones; in such children, a ketone-negative urine test may suggest the presence of a defect in fatty acid oxidation.

Samples used to diagnose metabolic disease may be obtained at autopsy. They may be analyzed directly or stored frozen until a particular analysis is justified by the results of postmortem examination, new clinical information, or new developments in the field. Studies of other family members may also help to establish the diagnosis in a deceased patient; these include demonstrating that the parents are heterozygous carriers of a particular disorder or showing that another sibling has the condition.

COMMON CLINICAL SITUATIONS

Mental Retardation

Many inborn errors can cause mental retardation without other distinguishing characteristics. Labora-

tory studies of serum and urine amino acids should be obtained for every patient with nonspecific mental retardation. Because physical stigmas of certain mucopolysaccharidoses are subtle, urine screens for mucopolysacchariduria are also useful. Electrolytes should be examined because the presence of a high anion gap or renal tubular acidosis significantly increases the chance of finding an underlying inborn error. If developmental regression or specific neurologic findings are present, the evaluation should be expanded accordingly.

Acute Presentation in Neonate

Acute metabolic disease in the newborn may be clinically indistinguishable from sepsis and is most often caused by disorders of protein or carbohydrate metabolism. Initial symptoms may be poor feeding or vomiting, altered mental status or tone, jitteriness or seizures, and jaundice. Acidosis or altered mental status out of proportion to systemic symptoms should increase suspicion of metabolic disorder. Laboratory studies should include determination of electrolytes, ammonia, glucose, urine pH, and urine ketones. Glycine in cerebrospinal fluid should be measured if glycine encephalopathy is suspected. Serum and urine to be used for amino and organic acid analysis should be collected before oral intake is stopped and sent for analysis if indicated by the results of initial studies.

Vomiting & Encephalopathy in the Infant or Older Child

Even though vomiting and altered consciousness in the infant or child are more often due to infection and trauma than to an inborn error, the physician should order laboratory studies of electrolytes, ammonia, glucose, urine pH, urine-reducing substances, and urine ketones in all patients before the results are altered by treatment. Samples for amino and organic acid analysis should be obtained early and frozen pending the results of initial studies. An inborn error is even more likely when the presentation is judged "typical" of Reye's syndrome (vomiting, encephalopathy, and hepatomegaly), and amino and organic acids should be studied immediately. If there is hypoglycemia with inappropriately low urine or serum ketones, disorders of fatty acid oxidation should be considered.

Hypoglycemia

Studies of electrolytes, ammonia, uric acid, urine-reducing substances, and urine ketones should be performed, and urine should be obtained to measure levels of organic acids. Ketone body production is usually not efficient in the neonate, and ketonuria in a hypoglycemic neonate suggests an inborn error. In the older child, however, the absence of ketonuria suggests inborn error, particularly of fatty acid oxidation.

Table 31–1. Presenting clinical and laboratory features of inborn errors.[1]

	Defects of Carbohydrate Metabolism	Defects of Amino Acid Metabolism[2]	Organic Acid Disorders[3]	Defects of Fatty Acid Oxidation	Defects of Purine Metabolism	Lysosomal Storage Diseases	Disorders of Peroxisomes
Neurodevelopmental							
Mental/developmental retardation	+++	+++	+++	+	++	+++	+++
Developmental regression	–	–	+	–	–	+++	+++
Acute encephalopathy	+++	+++	+++	+++	–	–	–
Seizures	++	+++	+++	+	–	+++	++
Ataxia/movement disorder	–	+	++	–	+++	–	–
Hypotonia	++	++	++	+++	–	+	+++
Hypertonia	–	++	+++	–	++	+	–
Abnormal behavior	–	++	++	–	++	+++	–
Growth							
Failure to thrive	+++	+++	+++	+	–	+	–
Short stature	++	–	+	–	–	++	–
Macrocephaly	–	–	+	–	–	+++	++
Microcephaly	+	++	+++	–	–	+	–
General							
Vomiting/anorexia	++	+++	+++	+++	–	–	++
Food aversion or craving	++	+++	+++	+++	–	–	–
Odor	–	++	++	–	–	–	–
Dysmorphic features	–	+	+	–	–	++	++
Congenital malformations	–	++	++	–	–	–	++

Organ specific

	1	2	3	4	5	6	7
Hepatomegaly	+++	–	++	+++	–	+++	+++
Liver disease/cirrhosis	++	+	–	+	–	–	+
Splenomegaly	–	–	–	–	–	++	+
Skeletal dysplasia	–	–	–	–	–	++	++
Cardiomyopathy	++	–	+	+++	–	++	–
Tachypnea/hyperpnea	++	++	++	++	–	–	–
Rash	–	++	++	–	–	–	–
Alopecia or abnormal hair	–	+	++	–	–	–	+
Cataracts or corneal opacity	++	–	–	–	–	++	–
Retinal abnormality	–	+	+	+	–	++	++
Frequent infections	++	–	++	–	++	–	–
Deafness	–	–	+	–	–	++	–

Laboratory-general

	1	2	3	4	5	6	7
Hypoglycemia	+++	+	++	++	–	–	–
Hyperammonemia	–	++	++	++	–	–	–
Metabolic acidosis	++	++	+++	+++	–	–	–
Respiratory alkalosis	–	++	–	–	–	–	–
Elevated lactate/pyruvate	++	–	+++	++	–	–	–
Elevated liver enzymes	++	++	++	+++	–	+	+
Neutropenia or thrombocytopenia	+	–	+	–	++	+	–
Ketosis	+++	++	+++	–	–	–	–
Hypoketosis	–	–	+	+++	–	–	–

[1] +++, most conditions in group; ++, some; +, one or few; –, not found.
[2] Includes disorders of urea cycle but not maple syrup urine disease.
[3] Includes maple syrup urine disease and disorders of pyruvate oxidation.

Table 31–2. Obtaining and handling samples to diagnose inborn errors.

Test	Comments
Acid-base status	Accurate estimation of anion gap must be possible. Samples for blood gases should be kept on ice and analyzed immediately.
Blood ammonia	Sample should be collected without a tourniquet, kept on ice, and analyzed immediately.
Blood lactic acid and pyruvic acid	Sample should be collected without a tourniquet, kept on ice, and analyzed immediately. Reduction of pyruvic acid to lactic acid must be prevented. Normal literature values are for the fasting, rested state.
Amino acids	Blood and urine should be examined. CSF glycine should be measured if nonketotic hyperglycinemia is to be ruled out. Normal literature values are for the fasting state. Growth of bacteria in urine should be prevented. At autopsy: liver, kidney, or vitreous may be analyzed if urine is not available.
Organic acids	Urine preferred for analysis. At autopsy: liver, kidney, or vitreous may be analyzed if urine is not available.
Carnitine and acylcarnitine profile	Blood (plasma) may be analyzed for total, free, and esterified carnitine; normal values are for the healthy, nonfasted state. Acylcarnitine profile in blood may identify compounds esterified to carnitine, and urine and tissue studies may be needed for certain conditions.
Urine mucopolysaccharides	Variations in urine concentration may cause errors in screening tests. Diagnosis requires knowing which mucopolysaccharides are increased. Some patients with Morquio's disease do not have abnormal mucopolysacchariduria.
Enzyme assays	Specific assays must be requested. Exposure to heat may cause loss of enzyme activity. Enzyme activity in whole blood may become normal after transfusion or vitamin therapy. Leukocyte or fibroblast pellets should be kept frozen prior to assays. Fibroblasts may be grown from skin biopsies taken up to 72 hours after death. Tissues such as liver and kidney should be taken as soon as possible after death, frozen immediately, and kept at −70 °C until assayed.

Hyperammonemia

Symptoms of hyperammonemia may appear and progress rapidly or insidiously. Decreased appetite and irritability usually appear first, with vomiting, lethargy, seizures, and coma appearing as ammonia levels increase. Tachypnea is caused by a direct effect on respiratory drive. Physical examination cannot exclude the presence of hyperammonemia, and serum ammonia should be measured whenever hyperammonemia is possible.

Severe hyperammonemia may be due to urea cycle disorders, to organic acidemias, or, in the neonate, to transient hyperammonemia of the newborn. The cause can usually be ascertained by measuring citrulline and electrolytes in serum and measuring amino acids, organic acids, and orotic acid in urine. Respiratory alkalosis is usually present in transient hyperammonemia of the newborn and hyperammonemia due to a urea cycle defect, whereas metabolic acidosis is usually associated with hyperammonemia due to organic acidemia. Urine organic acid analysis will demonstrate the cause if the condition is due to organic acidemia. Serum citrulline is usually low or undetectable in early urea cycle defects; normal or slightly high in transient hyperammonemia of the newborn; and very high in citrullinemia and argininosuccinic acidemia, and argininosuccinic acid is found in urine only in the latter. Of infants with early urea cycle defects, only those with hyperammonemia due to ornithine transcarbamoylase deficiency have increased urine orotic acid levels and (often) a family history of male newborn deaths due to defects that appear to be transmitted as an X-linked trait.

Acidosis

Inborn errors may cause chronic or acute acidosis at any age, and with or without an increased anion gap. Inborn errors should be considered when acidosis occurs with recurrent emesis or hyperammonemia, and when acidosis is out of proportion to the clinical state of the patient. Acidosis due to an inborn error is usually, but not always, difficult to correct. The presence of renal tubular acidosis does not exclude an underlying inborn error.

Serum glucose and ammonia, and urine pH and ketones should always be examined. Samples for amino and organic acids should be obtained at once and sent to the laboratory or saved in the freezer, depending on how strongly an inborn error is suspected. It is useful to test blood lactate and pyruvate levels in the chronically acidotic patient even if urine organic acid levels are normal. Lactate and pyruvate levels are difficult to interpret in the acutely ill patient, but in the absence of shock very high levels of lactic acid suggest primary lactic acidosis.

MANAGEMENT OF METABOLIC EMERGENCIES

Patients with severe acidosis, hypoglycemia, and hyperammonemia may be very ill; initially mild symptoms may worsen quickly, and coma and death may ensue within hours. With prompt and vigorous treatment, however, patients can recover completely, even from deep coma. All oral intake should be stopped. Glucose should be given intravenously in amounts sufficient to stop catabolic processes or to prevent development of catabolism in a patient with a known inborn error at risk for crisis. Most conditions respond favorably to glucose administration, and few (eg, primary lactic acidosis due to pyruvate dehydrogenase deficiency) do not. Severe or increasing hyperammonemia should be treated pharmacologically or with dialysis, and severe acidosis should be treated with bicarbonate administration. More specific measures can be instituted when a diagnosis is established.

NEWBORN SCREENING

Criteria used to decide whether or not to screen newborns for a disorder include its frequency, the significance of consequences if it is not treated, the availability and cost of screening and diagnostic tests, and the availability and cost of treatment. All states in the United States screen newborns for phenylketonuria and hypothyroidism, and most states also screen for galactosemia. Other metabolic disorders for which newborns are frequently screened include maple syrup urine disease, homocystinuria due to cystathionine synthase deficiency, and biotinidase deficiency.

Some screening tests measure a metabolite (eg, phenylalanine) that becomes abnormal only with time and exposure to diet, and in such instances the disease cannot be detected reliably until intake of the enzyme substrate has become established. Other tests (eg, for biotinidase deficiency) assay an enzyme and can be performed at any time; however, transfusions may cause false-negative results, and exposure of the sample to heat may cause false-positive results. Screening tests are not diagnostic, and diagnostic tests must be undertaken when an abnormal screening result is obtained. Also, because false-negative results are not unknown, a normal newborn screening test does not rule out a condition if symptoms develop.

The time of newborn screening recommended by the American Academy of Pediatrics is appropriate for the detection of phenylketonuria; hypothyroidism, for instance, can be missed when screening is carried out at this time. Early discharge of neonates causes significant problems with newborn screening, both with false-negative and false-positive results. Nevertheless, all babies should be screened before discharge from hospital. Physicians should combine current AAP recommendations and law and regulations in each state to arrive at appropriate strategies for each hospital and practice.

American Academy of Pediatrics, Committee on Genetics: Newborn screening fact sheet. Pediatrics 1989;83:449.

Buist NRM, Tuerck JM: The practitioner's role in newborn screening. Pediatr Clin North Am 1992;39:199.

Chaves-Carballo E: Detection of inherited neurometabolic disorders: A practical clinical approach. Pediatr Clin North Am 1992;39:801.

Childs B: Sir Archibald Garrod's conception of chemical individuality: A modern appreciation. N Engl J Med 1970;282:71.

Emery JL et al: Investigation of inborn errors of metabolism in unexpected infant deaths. Lancet 1988;2:29.

Fernandez J et al (editors): *Inborn Metabolic Diseases: Diagnosis and Treatment,* 2nd ed. Springer-Verlag, 1995.

Goodman SI, Greene CL: Metabolic disorders of the newborn. Pediatr Rev 1994;15:359.

Greene CL, Blitzer MG, Shapira E: Inborn errors of metabolism and Reye syndrome: Differential diagnosis. J Pediatr 1988;113:156.

Ozand PT, Gascon GG: Organic acidurias: A review. Part 1. J Child Neurol 1991;6:196.

Phillip M et al: An algorithmic approach to diagnosis of hypoglycemia. J Pediatr 1987;110:387.

Roth KS: Inborn errors of metabolism: The essentials of clinical diagnosis. Clin Pediatr 1991;30:183.

Rowe PC, Valle D, Brusilow SW: Inborn errors of metabolism in children referred with Reye's syndrome: A changing pattern. JAMA 1988;260:3167.

Scriver CR et al (editor): *The Metabolic Basis of Inherited Diseases,* 7th ed. McGraw-Hill, 1995.

Shih VE: Detection of hereditary metabolic disorders involving amino acids and organic acids. Clin Biochem 1991;24:301.

Surtees R, Leonard JV: Acute metabolic encephalopathy: A review of causes, mechanism and treatment. J Inherit Metab Dis 1989;12:42.

Valle D: Treatment of genetic disease: Current status and prospects for the future. Semin Perinatol 1991;15:52.

Ward JC: Inborn errors of metabolism of acute onset in infancy. Pediatr Rev 1990;11:205.

DISORDERS OF CARBOHYDRATE METABOLISM

GLYCOGEN STORAGE DISEASES

Glycogen is a highly branched polymer of glucose that is stored in liver and muscle. Many different disorders of its biosynthesis and degradation have been described, and the enzyme defects responsible have been identified. The most common forms of glycogenosis are characterized by growth failure, hepatomegaly, and fasting hypoglycemia. Defects that cause these so-called hepatic forms of the disease include glucose-6-phosphatase (type I; von Gierke disease), debrancher enzyme (type III), hepatic phosphorylase (type VI), and phosphorylase kinase (type IX), which normally regulates hepatic phosphorylase activity. Further, there are two forms of glucose-6-phosphatase deficiency; in one, the enzyme defect can be demonstrated in fresh or frozen liver; in the other, the defect can be demonstrated only in fresh tissue.

Forms of the disease affecting primarily muscle include acid maltase deficiency (type II; Pompe disease), which may be seen in infancy with cardiomegaly and macroglossia, and muscle phosphorylase (type V) and phosphofructokinase (type VII) deficiencies, in which the most striking features are easy fatigability and muscle weakness and stiffness.

Diagnosis

Precise diagnosis is by appropriate biochemical tests, such as responsiveness of blood glucose to fasting and glucagon, and enzyme assays on leukocytes, liver, or muscle. Disorders that can be diagnosed using red or white blood cells include deficiencies of debrancher enzyme (type III) and phosphorylase kinase (IX). Pompe's disease can usually be diagnosed by assaying acid maltase in fibroblasts or peripheral leukocytes.

Treatment

In general, treatment is designed to prevent hypoglycemia while avoiding storage of even more glycogen in liver. In the most severe hepatic forms, this requires careful monitoring of specific diets, using restriction of free sugars and measured amounts of cornstarch, and some good results have been reported following continuous nighttime carbohydrate feeding.

Fernandes J, Chen Y-T: Glycogen storage diseases: In: *Inborn Metabolic Diseases: Diagnosis and Treatment,* 2nd ed. Fernandez J et al (editors). Springer-Verlag, 1995.

Greene HL et al: Type I glycogen storage disease: A metabolic basis for advances in treatment. Adv Pediatr 1979;26:63.

Hers HG et al: Glycogen storage diseases. In: *The Metabolic Basis of Inherited Disease,* 7th ed. Scriver CR et al (editors). McGraw-Hill, 1995.

GALACTOSEMIA

Classic galactosemia is caused by almost total deficiency of galactose-1-phosphate uridyltransferase. Accumulation of galactose-1-phosphate in liver, brain, and renal tubules causes hepatic parenchymal disease, mental retardation, and renal Fanconi syndrome. Accumulation of galactitol (dulcitol) in the lens produces cataracts. With prompt institution of a galactose-free diet, the prognosis for life is excellent.

In the severe form of the disease, onset is marked by vomiting, jaundice, and hepatomegaly in the newborn period after milk feeding. Without treatment, death frequently occurs in the first month of life, often from *Escherichia coli* sepsis. Cataracts usually develop within 2 months in untreated cases, and hepatic cirrhosis is progressive. In less severe cases, survival is possible, but mental retardation is irreversible. Even when dietary restrictions are instituted early, patients with galactosemia are at increased risk for speech and language deficits and ovarian failure, and some patients develop progressive delay, tremor, and ataxia. Clinical and laboratory evidence of the disease abates gradually with effective treatment.

The disorder is inherited as an autosomal recessive trait with an incidence of approximately one in 40,000 live births. Because disease in infancy may be severe and diagnosed late, newborn screening is becoming increasingly common. Screening is accomplished by demonstrating enzyme deficiency in red cells with the Beutler test and/or by demonstrating increased serum galactose. Prenatal diagnosis of fetal is possible.

Diagnosis

In infants receiving foods containing galactose, laboratory findings include galactosuria and hypergalactosemia together with proteinuria and aminoaciduria. It is important not to exclude the diagnosis simply because the urine does not contain reducing substances. When the diagnosis is suspected, galactose-1-phosphate uridyltransferase should be assayed in erythrocytes; only blood transfusions will cause this test to be falsely negative, and only sample deterioration will cause it to be falsely positive.

Treatment

A galactose-free diet should be instituted as soon as the diagnosis is made, and compliance with the diet monitored. The diet is not a simple exclusion of milk and requires extensive knowledge of the galactose content of foods. Avoidance of galactose should be lifelong in severe cases, with appropriate calcium replacement. Additional therapies, such as supplementations with uridine, are under investigation. Heterozygous mothers are advised to follow a galactose-free diet during pregnancies.

Donnel G (editor): Galactosemia: New frontiers in research. NIH Publication No. 93-3438, 1993.

Gross KC, Acosta PB: Fruits and vegetables are a source of galactose: Implications in planning the diets of patients with galactosemia. J Inherit Metab Dis 1991:253.

Kaufman FR et al: Correlation of ovarian function with galactose-1-phosphate uridyl transferase levels in galactosemia. J Pediatr 1988;112:755.

Levy HL et al: Sepsis due to *Escherichia coli* in neonates with galactosemia. N Engl J Med 1977;297:823.

Lo W et al: Neurologic sequelae in galactosemia. Pediatrics 1984;73:309.

Sardharwalla IB, Wraith JE: Galactosemia. Nutr Health 1987;5:175.

HEREDITARY FRUCTOSE INTOLERANCE

Hereditary fructose intolerance is an autosomal recessive disorder in which deficient activity of fructose-1-phosphate aldolase causes hypoglycemia and tissue accumulation of fructose-1-phosphate on fructose ingestion. Other abnormalities include failure to thrive, vomiting, jaundice, hepatomegaly, proteinuria, and generalized aminoaciduria. The untreated condition can progress to death as a result of liver failure.

Diagnosis

The diagnosis is supported by the demonstration of fructosuria following an inpatient, closely monitored fructose load. The appearance of hypoglycemia and hypophosphatemia after fructose loading (200 mg/kg) is diagnostic, as is reduced activity of fructose-1-phosphate aldolase in liver. Some patients may be diagnosed by identification of one of the common mutations on DNA analysis.

Treatment

Treatment consists of eliminating fructose from the diet and is complicated by the fact that many proprietary drugs and vitamins are in a sucrose base. If the diet is relaxed, there may be retardation of physical growth, but growth will resume when more stringent dietary restrictions are instituted. If the disorder is recognized early, the prospects for normal development are good. As affected individuals grow up, they may recognize the association of nausea and vomiting with fructose-containing foods and selectively avoid them.

Brooks CC, Tolan DR: Association of the widespread A149P hereditary fructose intolerance mutation with newly identified sequence polymorphisms in the aldolase B gene. Am J Hum Genet 1993;52:835.

Odierre M et al: Hereditary fructose intolerance in childhood: Diagnosis, management and course in 55 patients. Am J Dis Child 1978;132:605.

Steinmann B, Gitzelmann R: The diagnosis of hereditary fructose intolerance. Helv Paediatr Acta 1981;36:297.

PRIMARY LACTIC ACIDEMIAS & OTHER DISORDERS OF ENERGY METABOLISM

Primary lactic acidemia is a diagnosis made with increasing frequency and may be one of the more common causes of static, progressive, or self-limited neurodevelopmental problems in children. The range of severity and prognosis in these disorders is illustrated by extremes. For example, defects in the mitochondrial respiratory chain including Complex IV deficiency may cause Leigh disease, a fatal neurodegenerative disease, whereas another presentation of Complex IV deficiency is benign, resolving congenital hypotonia. Lactic acidemia is said to be primary when it is due to a defect in the metabolism of pyruvic acid and secondary when a change in cellular redox potential favors the reduction of pyruvate to lactate (as in shock). Some causes of primary lactic acidosis are shown in Table 31–3. In general, such disorders may present at any age with neurologic findings and, when the defect is in gluconeogenesis, with hypoglycemia. Patients with a defect in the E_1 component of the pyruvate dehydrogenase complex often show central nervous system malformations or mild facial dysmorphism. Recurrent altered mental status, recurrent ataxia, and recurrent acidosis are typical of many disturbances of pyruvate metabolism.

Table 31–3. Causes of primary lactic acidosis in childhood.

Defects of the pyruvate dehydrogenase complex
1. E_1 (pyruvate decarboxylase) deficiency
2. E_2 (dihydrolipoyl transacetylase) deficiency
3. E_3 (lipoamide dehydrogenase) deficiency
4. Pyruvate decarboxylase phosphate phosphatase deficiency

Abnormalities of gluconeogenesis
1. Pyruvate carboxylase deficiency
   a) Isolated
   b) Biotinidase deficiency
   c) Holocarboxylase synthetase deficiency
2. Fructose-1,6-diphosphatase deficiency
3. Glucose-6-phosphatase deficiency (von Gierke disease)

Defects in mitochondrial respiratory chain
1. Complex I deficiency
2. Complex IV deficiency (cytochrome C oxidase deficiency; frequent cause of Leigh disease)
3. ATPase deficiency (frequent cause of Leigh disease)
4. Other respiratory chain disorders

Defects in the mitochondrial respiratory chain are also may present with nonspecific findings such as hypotonia or renal tubular acidosis or with more specific features such as ophthalmoplegia. Ragged red fibers and mitochondrial abnormalities may be noted on histologic examination of muscle. Thirteen of the more than 100 genes that control activity of the respiratory chain are part of the mitochondrial genome. Therefore, inheritance of defects in the respiratory chain may be mendelian or maternal.

Diagnosis

Diagnosis of primary lactic acidemia may be based on (1) demonstrating significant elevations of blood lactic acid concentration (more than 2 mmol/L venous/fasting/resting/free flowing sample) or pyruvic acid in blood or spinal fluid and excluding secondary lactic acidemia; or (2) demonstration of classic features of mitochondrial disorder such as ragged red fibers. Primary lactic acidemia may be present even if blood lactic acid concentration is normal, since lactate levels may vary according to the state of the patient (eg, resting versus active; fasting versus fed). Carefully controlled and monitored provocative testing such as fasting, challenge with carbohydrates, or exercise may identify clinical categories leading to suggestions for diagnosis and treatment. If a specific diagnosis is suggested by clinical symptoms, diagnostic tests of blood samples for enzyme assays (eg, biotinidase, pyruvate carboxylase) may lead to diagnosis, but enzyme analysis of fibroblasts or skeletal muscle is often required. For some clinical presentations, mitochondrial DNA analysis of blood or tissue may identify a diagnostic mutation. In many patients, the cause of the disorder cannot be defined. For some diagnoses, the genetics and prognosis may be clear, but, in many cases, neither recurrence risk nor prognosis can be predicted.

Treatment

In some patients, defects in gluconeogenesis can be treated with glucose administration, fructose avoidance, or administration of pharmacologic amounts of biotin. Modified ketogenic diet has been reported to be useful in some cases of proved or presumed pyruvate dehydrogenase deficiency. Other treatments are of theoretic or empiric value, with little data on efficacy. Thiamine or lipoic acid can be tried in patients with pyruvate dehydrogenase complex deficiencies, and coenzyme Q and riboflavin have been reported to be helpful in some patients with respiratory chain defects. Dichloroacetic acid has been tried in pyruvate dehydrogenase complex deficiencies and in respiratory chain disorders, with variation in both clinical response and adverse effects.

Brown GK et al: "Cerebral" lactic acidosis: Defects in pyruvate metabolism with profound brain damage and minimal systemic acidosis. Eur J Pediatr 1988;147:10.

Clarke LA: Mitochondrial disorders in pediatrics: Clinical, biochemical and genetic implications. Pediatr Clin North Am 1992;39:319.

DeVivo DC, DiMauro S: Mitochondrial defects of brain and muscle. Biol Neonate 1990;581(Suppl 1):54.

Eymard B, Hauw J-J: Mitochondrial encephalomyopathies. Curr Opin Neurol Neurosurg 1992;5:909.

Hart Z, Chang C: A newborn infant with respiratory distress and persistent stridulous breathing. J Pediatr 1988;113:150.

Kerr DS: Lactic acidosis and mitochondrial disorders. Clin Biochem 1991;24:33.

Robinson BH et al: Variable clinical presentation in patients with defective E_1 component of pyruvate dehydrogenase complex. J Pediatr 1987;111:525.

Shoffner JM, Wallace DC: Mitochondrial genetics: Principles and practice. Am J Hum Genet 1992;51:1179.

Tulinius MH et al: Mitochondrial encephalomyopathies in childhood: I. Biochemical and morphologic investigations. J Pediatr 1991;119:242.

Tulinius MH et al: Mitochondrial encephalomyopathies in childhood: II. Clinical manifestations and syndromes. J Pediatr 1991;119:251.

DISORDERS OF AMINO ACID METABOLISM

DISORDERS OF THE UREA CYCLE

Ammonia is converted to an amino group in urea by enzymes of the urea cycle. Defects in early urea cycle enzymes, such as carbamoyl phosphate synthetase or ornithine transcarbamoylase, usually present in infancy with severe and rapidly fatal hyperammonemia, vomiting, and encephalopathy, but the course may also be milder, with vomiting and encephalopathy following protein ingestion or infections. Although defects in argininosuccinic acid synthetase (citrullinemia) and argininosuccinic acid lyase (argininosuccinic acidemia) may also present with severe hyperammonemia in infancy, a chronic course with mental retardation is more usual in these conditions.

Except for ornithine transcarbamoylase deficiency, which is X-linked, urea cycle disorders are inherited as autosomal recessive traits. Citrullinemia and argininosuccinic acidemia can be diagnosed in utero by appropriate enzyme assays, but carbamoyl phosphate synthetase and ornithine transcarbamoylase deficiency states can be diagnosed in utero only by using specific gene probes, and then only in certain families.

Diagnosis

Blood ammonia levels should be measured in any newborn who is acutely ill without obvious cause. A urea cycle defect should be suspected when severe hyperammonemia is associated with respiratory alkalosis. Serum citrulline is low or undetectable in carbamoyl phosphate synthetase and ornithine transcarbamoylase deficiency, high in argininosuccinic acidemia, and very high in citrullinemia. Large amounts of argininosuccinic acid are found in the urine of patients with argininosuccinic acidemia. Urine orotic acid is increased in infants with ornithine transcarbamoylase deficiency, and there may also be a family history of male newborn deaths that appear to be transmitted as an X-linked trait.

Age of onset of symptoms varies with protein intake, growth, and stress such as infection. Individual families with ornithine transcarbamoylase deficiency illustrate variable age of onset, with age of onset of symptoms in related males extending over decades. Many female carriers of ornithine transcarbamoylase deficiency show protein intolerance; some develop migraine-like symptoms after protein loads and others develop potentially fatal episodes of vomiting and encephalopathy after protein ingestion, certain infections, or labor and delivery. Trichorrhexis nodosa is common in patients with the chronic form of argininosuccinic acidemia.

Treatment

In the newborn, measures to reduce serum ammonia by hemodialysis, peritoneal dialysis, or double-volume exchange transfusion should be instituted as soon as hyperammonemia is documented. Protein intake should be stopped, and glucose should be given to reduce endogenous protein breakdown. Arginine should be given intravenously, both because it is an essential amino acid for patients with urea cycle defects and because it increases the excretion of waste nitrogen in patients with citrullinemia and argininosuccinic acidemia. Sodium benzoate, sodium phenylacetate, and sodium phenylbutyrate can also be given intravenously, and one or more of these drugs is needed intravenously for treatment of hyperammonemic coma.

Long-term treatment includes oral administration of arginine (or citrulline), adherence to a low-protein diet, and administration of sodium benzoate and sodium phenylacetate or sodium phenylbutyrate to increase excretion of nitrogen as hippuric acid and phenylacetylglutamine. Female ornithine transcarbamoylase-deficient heterozygotes who develop hyperammonemia should also receive such treatment.

The outcome of argininosuccinic acidemia and citrullinemia is better than that of ornithine transcarbamoylase and carbamoyl phosphate synthetase deficiency. Most patients with urea cycle defects, no matter what the enzyme defect, develop permanent neurologic and intellectual impairments, with cortical atrophy and ventricular dilatation seen on CT scan. The prognosis may be improved if the initial hyperammonemic episode is rapidly identified and treated.

Batshaw ML et al: Risk of serious illness in heterozygotes for ornithine transcarbamylase deficiency. J Pediatr 1986;108:236.

Brusilow SW et al: Treatment of episodic hyperammonemia in children with inborn errors of urea synthesis. N Engl J Med 1984;310:1630.

Cederbaum SD: The treatment of urea cycle disorders. Int Pediatr 1992;7:61.

Hudak ML, Jones MD, Brusilow SW: Differentiation of transient hyperammonemia of the newborn and urea cycle enzyme defects by clinical presentation. J Pediatr 1985;107:712.

Leonard JV: Urea cycle disorders. In: *Inborn Metabolic Disorders: Diagnosis and Treatment,* 2nd ed. Fernandez et al (editors). Springer-Verlag, 1995.

Nagata N et al: Retrospective survey of urea cycle disorders: Part 2. Neurological outcome in forty-nine Japanese patients with urea cycle enzymopathies. Am J Med Genet 1991;40:477.

PHENYLKETONURIA & THE HYPERPHENYLALANINEMIAS

Probably the best-known disorder of amino acid metabolism is the classic form of phenylketonuria. It was first recognized in 1934 by Fölling in several retarded children who excreted phenylpyruvic acid in the urine. The disorder is due to decreased activity of phenylalanine hydroxylase, the enzyme that converts phenylalanine to tyrosine. Phenylketonuria is inherited as an autosomal recessive trait, with an incidence in whites of approximately 1 in 10,000 live births. On normal phenylalanine intake, affected patients develop hyperphenylalaninemia and produce and excrete phenylpyruvic, phenyllactic, phenylacetic, and 2-hydroxyphenylacetic acid. The untreated patient shows severe mental retardation, hyperactivity, seizures, a light complexion, and eczema. The patient's urine has a "mouse-like" odor.

Clinicians had early success preventing severe mental retardation in phenylketonuric children by restricting phenylalanine from the diet starting in early infancy. This success led to the development of screening programs to detect the disease early. Since the outcome is best when treatment is begun in the first month of life, infants should be screened during the first few days of life. A second test is necessary when newborn screening is done before 24 hours of age, and in such cases the second test should be completed by the third week of life. Infants receiving hyperalimentation and premature infants should be screened at or near 7 days, and re-screened if they were transfused or not fed at the time of the initial test.

Enzymes involved with the interconversion of phenylalanine and tyrosine, and whose deficiencies can produce hyperphenylalaninemia, are shown in Figure 31–1. In classic phenylketonuria, there is little or no phenylalanine hydroxylase activity, but in the

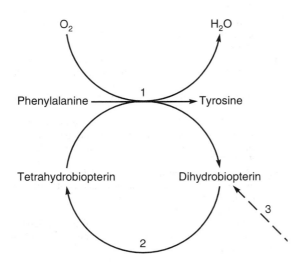

Figure 31–1. Oxidation of phenylalanine to tyrosine. **1.** Phenylalanine hydroxylase. **2.** Dihydropteridine reductase. **3.** Enzymes of biopterin biosynthesis.

less severe hyperphenylalaninemias there is significant residual activity. Rare variants can be due to deficiency of dihydrobiopterin reductase or to defects in biopterin synthesis. All are inherited as autosomal recessive traits.

Prenatal diagnosis of phenylketonuria is often possible using DNA probes. Molecular approaches are replacing serum measurements of phenylalanine and tyrosine to determine carrier status. Prenatal diagnosis of defects in pterin metabolism can often be made.

Diagnosis & Treatment

The diagnosis of phenylketonuria in a severely retarded older child with typical biochemical and physical characteristics is straightforward, but in the newborn period, especially when there is no family history, the condition must be differentiated from other forms of hyperphenylalaninemia. This is usually done by determining serum phenylalanine and tyrosine levels on a normal diet, and by examining pterins and metabolites of phenylalanine in urine.

A. Classic Phenylketonuria: Findings include persistently elevated serum levels of phenylalanine (> 20 mg/dL on a regular diet), normal or low serum levels of tyrosine, urinary excretion of phenylpyruvic and 2-hydroxyphenylacetic acids, and normal pterins. Poor phenylalanine tolerance persists throughout life. Restriction of dietary phenylalanine intake (see below) is indicated, and a favorable outcome is the rule.

B. Persistent Hyperphenylalaninemia: In infants receiving a normal protein intake, serum phenylalanine levels are usually 4–20 mg/dL, and pterins are normal. Phenylalanine restriction may or may not be indicated, depending on the phenylalanine tolerance.

C. Transient Hyperphenylalaninemia: Serum phenylalanine levels are elevated early but progressively decline toward normal. If required at all, dietary restriction is only temporary.

D. Dihydropteridine Reductase Deficiency: Serum phenylalanine levels vary. The pattern of pterin metabolites is abnormal. Seizures and psychomotor regression occur even with diet therapy, probably because the enzyme defect also causes neuronal deficiency of serotonin and dopamine. These deficiencies require treatment with levodopa, carbidopa, and 5-hydroxytryptophan, and possibly also with tetrahydrobiopterin.

E. Defects in Biopterin Biosynthesis: Serum phenylalanine levels vary. Total pterins are low, and their pattern may suggest the specific defect, which can be at one of several steps in the biosynthetic pathway. Clinical findings include myoclonus, tetraplegia, and other movement disorders. Treatment is the same as for dihydropteridine reductase deficiency, but in general is not as effective.

F. Tyrosinemia of the Newborn: Serum phenylalanine levels are lower than those seen in phenylketonuria and are accompanied by marked hypertyrosinemia. This usually occurs in premature infants and is due to immaturity of 4-hydroxyphenylpyruvic acid oxidase. The condition resolves spontaneously within 3 months, almost always without sequelae. If necessary, intramuscular injection of 100 mg ascorbic acid will normalize serum tyrosine (and phenylalanine) within 48 hours.

G. Maternal Phenylketonuria: Offspring of phenylketonuric mothers may have transient hyperphenylalaninemia at birth. Elevated maternal phenylalanine causes mental retardation, microcephaly, growth retardation, and often congenital heart disease or other malformations. The risk to the fetus is considerably lessened if phenylalanine restriction is begun before conception and maintained throughout pregnancy.

Treatment of Classic Phenylketonuria

Treatment of classic phenylketonuria is to limit dietary phenylalanine intake to amounts that permit normal growth and development. Products deficient in phenylalanine but otherwise similar to milk are commercially available but must be supplemented with normal milk and other foods to supply enough phenylalanine to permit normal growth and development. Serum phenylalanine concentrations must be monitored frequently, while ensuring that growth, development, and nutrition are adequate. This monitoring is best done in clinics experienced in dealing with such problems. Although dietary treatment is most effective when initiated during the first months of life, it may also be of benefit in reversing behaviors such as hyperactivity, irritability, and distractibility when started later in life.

Phenylalanine restriction should continue throughout life, because of subtle changes in IQ and behavior in persons treated early who go off diet and because of the risk of late development of potentially irreversible neurologic damage after stopping diet. Females with phenylketonuria merit special attention during the childbearing years. Counseling should be given during adolescence, and the woman's diet should be closely monitored prior to conception and throughout pregnancy.

Children with classic phenylketonuria who are treated promptly after birth and achieve phenylalanine and tyrosine homeostasis will develop well physically and can be expected to have normal or nearly normal intellectual development.

Blau N et al: Tetrahydrobiopterin deficiency: From phenotype to genotype. Pteridines 1993;4:1.

Cleary MA et al: Magnetic resonance imaging in phenylketonuria: Reversal of cerebral white matter change. J Pediatr 1995;127:251.

Hanly WB et al: Malnutrition with early treatment of phenylketonurea. Pediatr Res 1970;4:318.

Koch R et al: The effects of diet discontinuation in children with phenylketonurea. Eur J Pediatr 1987;146(Suppl):A12.

Matalon R, Michals K: Phenylketonuria: Screening, treatment and maternal PKU. Clin Biochem 1991;24:337.

O'Flynn ME: Newborn screening for phenylketonuria: Thirty years of progress. Curr Probl Pediatr 1992:159.

Potocnik U, Widhalm K: Long-term follow-up of children with classical PKU after diet discontinuation: A review. J Am Coll Nutr 1994;13:232.

Thompson AJ et al: Neurologic deterioration in young adults with phenylketonuria. Lancet 1990;336:602.

Villasana D et al: Neurological deterioration in adult phenylketonuria. J Inherited Metab Dis 1989;12:451.

HEREDITARY TYROSINEMIA

Hereditary tyrosinemia is caused by deficiency of fumarylacetoacetase and is characterized by progressive hepatic parenchymal damage, renal tubular dystrophy with generalized aminoaciduria and hypophosphatemic rickets, hypermethioninemia, and tyrosine metabolites, succinylacetone, and δ-aminolevulinic acid in the urine. The course may be rapidly fatal in infancy or somewhat more chronic, with liver cell carcinoma almost invariable.

The condition is inherited as an autosomal recessive trait and is especially common in Scandinavia and in the Chicoutimi-Lac St Jean region of Quebec. Prenatal diagnosis can be established.

Diagnosis

Similar clinical and biochemical findings may occur in galactosemia and hereditary fructose intolerance, but increased succinylacetone occurs only in fumarylacetoacetase deficiency, and diagnosis is based on demonstrating this compound in urine.

Treatment

A diet low in phenylalanine and tyrosine (50 mg each/kg/d) is indicated but not usually successful in preventing or reversing liver disease, and liver transplantation appears to be the only effective therapy for these children. Pharmacologic therapy to inhibit 4-hydroxyphenylpyruvate dehydrogenase improves biochemistry and acute clinical status, and studies are in progress to determine to what extent risk of hepatocellular carcinoma is altered.

Kvittingen EA et al: Tyrosine. In: *Metabolic Diseases: Diagnosis and Treatment.* Fernandez J et al (editors). Springer-Verlag, 1995.

Lindstedt S et al: Treatment of hereditary tyrosinaemia type I by inhibition of 4-hydroxyphenylpyruvate dioxygenase. Lancet 1992;340:813.

MAPLE SYRUP URINE DISEASE (Branched-Chain Ketoaciduria)

Maple syrup urine disease is due to deficiency of the enzyme that catalyzes oxidative decarboxylation of the branched-chain keto acid derivatives of leucine, isoleucine, and valine. The accumulated keto acids of leucine and isoleucine cause the characteristic odor, while only the keto acid of leucine has been implicated in causing central nervous system dysfunction. Many variants of this disorder have been described, including mild, intermittent, and thiamine-dependent forms, and all are inherited as autosomal recessive traits.

Patients with classic maple syrup urine disease are normal at birth but soon develop the characteristic odor, lethargy, feeding difficulties, coma, and seizures. Unless diagnosis is made and dietary restriction of branched-chain amino acids is begun, most will die in the first month of life, but nearly normal growth and development may be achieved if treatment is begun before about 10 days of age.

Diagnosis

Marked elevations of branched-chain amino acids, including alloisoleucine, in serum and urine are characteristic. Alloisoleucine, a transamination product of the keto acid of isoleucine, is almost pathognomonic. The magnitude and consistency of amino and organic acid changes are altered in mild and intermittent forms of the disease. Prenatal diagnosis is possible.

Treatment

Products deficient in branched-chain amino acids but in other respects similar to milk are commercially available but must be supplemented with normal milk and other foods to supply enough branched-chain amino acids to permit normal growth and development. Serum levels of branched-chain amino acids must be monitored frequently, even at intervals of 1 or 2 days in the first months of life, to cope with changing protein requirements. Acute episodes must be aggressively treated to *prevent* catabolism and negative nitrogen balance.

Biggeman B, Zass R, Wendel U: Postoperative metabolic decompensation in maple syrup urine disease is completely prevented by insulin. J Inherited Metab Dis 1993;16:912.

Giacoia GP, Berry GT: Acrodermatitis enteropathic-like syndrome secondary to isoleucine deficiency during treatment of maple syrup urine disease. Am J Dis Child 1993;147:954.

Nord A et al: Developmental profile of patients with maple syrup urine disease. J Inherit Metab Dis 1991;14:881.

Ogier deBaulny H et al: Branched chain organic acidurias. In: *Inborn Metabolic Disease: Diagnosis and Treatment,* 2nd ed. Fernandez J et al (editors). Springer-Verlag, 1995.

Treacy E et al: Maple syrup urine disease: Interrelation between branched-chain amino, oxo, and hydroxy acids; implications for treatment; associations with CNS dysmyelination. J Inherit Metab Dis 1992;15:121.

HOMOCYSTINURIA

Homocystinuria is most often due to deficiency of cystathionine synthase, but it may also be due to deficiency of methylenetetrahydrofolate reductase or to defects in the biosynthesis of methyl-B_{12}, which is the coenzyme for N^5-methyltetrahydrofolate methyltransferase. All known inherited forms of homocystinuria are transmitted as autosomal recessive traits and can be diagnosed in the fetus.

About half of untreated patients with cystathionine synthase deficiency are retarded, and most have arachnodactyly, osteoporosis, and a tendency to develop dislocated lenses and thromboembolic phenomena. A relationship between risk of arteriosclerotic heart disease and mild hyperhomocystinemia due to carrier status for cystathionine synthase deficiency or other conditions is increasingly evident. Patients with remethylation defects usually show failure to thrive and a variety of neurologic symptoms, including microcephaly and seizures in infancy and early childhood.

Diagnosis

Diagnosis is made by demonstrating homocystinuria in a patient who is not severely deficient in vitamin B_{12}. Serum methionine levels are usually high in patients with cystathionine synthase deficiency and often low in patients with remethylation defects. When the remethylation defect is due to deficiency of methyl-B_{12}, megaloblastic anemia may be present, and an associated deficiency of adenosyl-B_{12} may cause methylmalonic aciduria. Studies of cultured fibroblasts may be necessary to make a specific diagnosis.

Treatment

About 50% of patients with cystathionine synthase deficiency respond to large oral doses of pyridoxine. Early treatment of pyridoxine nonresponders by dietary methionine restriction may prevent mental retardation and delay lens dislocations, perhaps justifying screening of newborn infants for the condition. Oral administration of betaine (250 mg/kg/d) will increase methylation of homocystine to methionine in patients with remethylation defects and may also improve neurologic function. Large doses of cobalamin (eg, 1 mg hydroxy-B_{12} administered intramuscularly every other day) are indicated in some patients.

Andrea G, Sebastio G: Homocystinuria due to cystathionine β-synthase deficiency and related disorders. In: *Inborn Metabolic Diseases: Diagnosis and Treatment,* 2nd ed. Fernandez J et al (editors). Springer-Verlag, 1995.

Malinow MR: Hyperhomocyst(e)inemia: A common and easily reversible risk factor for occlusive atherosclerosis. Circulation 1990;81:2004.

Mudd SH et al: The natural history of homocystinuria due to cystathionine β-synthase deficiency. Am J Hum Genet 1985;37:1.

Rosenblatt DS, Shevell MI: Inherited disorders of cobalamin and folate absorption and metabolism. In: *Inborn Diseases: Diagnosis and Treatment,* 2nd ed. Fernandez J et al (editors). Springer-Verlag, 1995.

NONKETOTIC HYPERGLYCINEMIA

Inherited deficiency of various subunits of the glycine cleavage enzyme causes nonketotic hyperglycinemia. In its most severe form, also termed **glycine encephalopathy,** the condition presents in the newborn period with unremitting seizures, hypotonia, hiccups, a burst suppression pattern on EEG, and (usually) death in infancy. Forms that present with seizures later in infancy or with developmental delay in childhood are observed. All forms of the condition are inherited as autosomal recessive traits.

Diagnosis

This deficiency should be suspected in any infant with intractable seizures, especially when hiccupping, and is confirmed by demonstrating a large increase in glycine in cerebrospinal fluid, with the CSF:serum glycine ratio being abnormally high. Demonstrating the specific enzyme defect by liver biopsy is necessary only if the couple is contemplating having more children, as prenatal diagnosis is possible only by assaying the enzyme in chorionic villus.

Treatment

Treatment is generally unsuccessful. Early efforts to use sodium benzoate therapy were thought to be without effect on long-term outcome, but recent studies suggest that this drug may be useful in seizure control.

Eyskens FJM et al: Neurologic sequelae in transient nonketotic hyperglycinemia of the neonate. J Pediatr 1992; 121:620.

Hamosh et al: Dextromethorphan and high dose benzoate therapy for nonketotic hyperglycinemia in an infant. J Pediatr 1992;121:131.

Hayasaka K et al: Nonketotic hyperglycinemia: Analyses of glycine cleavage system in typical and atypical cases. J Pediatr 1987;110:873.

Tada K, Hayasaka K: Non-ketotic hyperglycinaemia: Clinical and biochemical aspects. Eur J Pediatr 1987; 146:221.

Toone JR, Applegate DA, Levy HL: Prenatal diagnosis of non-ketotic hyperglycemia: Experiences in 50 at risk pregnancies. J Inherited Metab Dis 1994;17:342.

ORGANIC ACIDEMIAS

Organic acidemias are disorders of amino (and fatty) acid metabolism in which nonamino organic acids accumulate in serum and urine. These conditions are usually diagnosed by examining organic acids in urine, a complex procedure that requires considerable interpretive expertise and is usually performed only in specialized laboratories. Clinical features of organic acidemias are given in Table 31–4, together with the urine organic acid patterns typical of each. Additional details about some of the more important organic acidemias are provided below.

KETOTIC HYPERGLYCINEMIAS
(Propionic and Methylmalonic Acidemia)

Idiopathic hyperglycinemia was first reported in 1961 as a syndrome of mental retardation and episodic ketoacidosis, neutropenia, thrombocytopenia, osteoporosis, and hyperglycinemia induced by protein intake or infection. It was then renamed ketotic hyperglycinemia to distinguish it from nonketotic hyperglycinemia, described above. It is now known that the syndrome is almost always due to propionic or methylmalonic acidemia.

The oxidation of threonine, valine, isoleucine, and methionine through propionyl- and L-methylmalonyl-CoA is shown in Figure 31–2. Propionic acidemia is due to a defect in the biotin-containing enzyme propionyl-CoA carboxylase, and methylmalonic acidemia is due to a defect in methylmalonyl-CoA mutase. In most cases the latter is due to a defect in the mutase apoenzyme, but in others it is due to a defect in the biosynthesis of its adenosyl-B_{12} coenzyme. In some of these defects only the synthesis of adenosyl-B_{12} is blocked; in others, the synthesis of methyl-B_{12} is also blocked.

Clinical symptoms in propionic and methylmalonic acidemia vary according to the location and severity of the enzyme block. Those with severe blocks present with acute, life-threatening metabolic acidemia and hyperammonemia early in infancy or with metabolic acidemia, vomiting, and failure to thrive during the first few months of life. Children with less severe blocks may show only mild or moderate mental retardation.

All known forms of propionic and methylmalonic acidemia are transmitted as autosomal recessive traits and can be diagnosed in utero.

Diagnosis

Laboratory findings include hyperglycinemia and hyperglycinuria, a positive methylmalonic aciduria screening test, the presence of diagnostic changes on urine organic acid chromatography (Table 31–4) and, in certain blocks of B_{12} metabolism, hypomethioninemic homocystinuria.

Treatment

Patients with enzyme blocks in B_{12} metabolism usually respond to massive (1 mg/d) doses of vitamin B_{12}, given orally or intramuscularly, whereas nonresponders require amino acid restriction and correction of their rather constant metabolic acidemia. Secondary carnitine deficiency has been reported, and blood carnitine should be measured and supplemented if required.

Ogier deBaulny H et al: Branched chain organic acidurias. In: *Inborn Metabolic Disease: Diagnosis and Treatment,* 2nd ed. Fernandez J et al (editors). Springer-Verlag, 1995.

Shevell MI et al: Varying neurological phenotypes among mut^E and mut$^-$ patients with methylmalonyl-CoA mutase deficiency. Am J Med Genet 1993;45:619.

Shinnar S, Singer HS: Cobalamin C mutation (methylmalonic aciduria and homocystinuria) in adolescence: A treatable cause of dementia and myelopathy. N Engl J Med 1984;311:451.

Werlin SL: E. coli sepsis as a presenting sign in neonatal propionic acidemia. Am J Med Genet 1993;46:455.

ISOVALERIC ACIDEMIA

This condition, due to deficiency of isovaleryl-CoA dehydrogenase in the leucine oxidative pathway, was the first organic acidemia to be described in humans. It usually presents with poor feeding, metabolic acidosis, seizures, and an odor of "sweaty feet" during the first few days of life, with coma and death occurring if the condition is not recognized and appropriate therapy quickly begun. Other patients show a more chronic course, with episodes of vomit-

Table 31–4. Clinical and laboratory features of organic acidemias.

Disorder	Enzyme Defect	Clinical and Laboratory Features
Isovaleric acidemia	Isovaleryl-CoA dehydrogenase	Acidosis and "odor of sweaty feet" in infancy, or growth retardation and episodes of vomiting, lethargy, acidosis, and odor. Isovalerylglycine always present in urine, with 3-hydroxy-isovaleric acid during acute episodes.
3-Methylcrotonyl-CoA carboxylase deficiency	3-Methylcrotonyl-CoA carboxylase	Acidosis and feeding problems in infancy, or Reye-like episodes in older child. 3-Methylcrotonylglycine in urine, usually with 3-hydroxyisovaleric acid.
Combined carboxylase deficiency	Holocarboxylase synthetase	Hypotonia and lactic acidosis in infancy. 3-Hydroxyisovaleric acid in urine, often with small amounts of 3-hydroxypropionic and methylcitric acids. Often biotin responsive.
	Biotinidase	Alopecia, seborrheic rash, and ataxia in infancy or childhood. Urine organic acids as above. Usually biotin responsive.
3-Hydroxy-3-methylglutaric acidemia	Hydroxymethylglutaryl-CoA lyase	Hypoglycemia and acidosis in infancy; Reye-like episodes with nonketotic hypoglycemia in older children. 3-Hydroxy-3-methyl-glutaric, 3-methylglutaconic, and 3-hydroxyisovaleric acids in urine.
3-Ketothiolase deficiency	3-Ketothiolase	Ketotic hyperglycinemia syndrome in infancy, or developmental and growth retardation with episodes of vomiting, acidosis, and encephalopathy. 2-Methyl-3-hydroxybutyric and 2-methylacetoacetic acids and tiglyglycine in urine, especially after isoleucine load.
Propionic acidemia	Propionyl-CoA carboxylase	Hyperammonemia and metabolic acidosis in infancy; ketotic hyperglycinemia syndrome later. 3-Hydroxypropionic and methylcitric acids in urine, with 3-hydroxy- and 3-ketovaleric during ketotic episodes.
Methylmalonic acidemia	Methylmalonyl-CoA mutase	Clinical features same as propionic acidemia. Methylmalonic acid in urine, often with 3-hydroxypropionic and methylcitric acids.
	Defects in B_{12} biosynthesis	Clinical features same as above when only adenosyl-B_{12} synthesis is decreased: early neurologic features prominent when accompanied by decreased synthesis of methyl-B_{12}. In latter instance, hypomethioninemia and homocystinuria accompany methylmalonic aciduria.
Pyroglutamic acidemia	Glutathione synthetase	Acidosis and hemolytic anemia in infancy; chronic acidosis later. Pyroglutamic acid in urine.
Glutaric acidemia type I	Glutaryl-CoA dehydrogenase	Progressive extrapyramidal movement disorder in childhood, with episodes of acidosis, vomiting, and encephalopathy. Glutaric acid in urine, usually with 3-hydroxyglutaric acid.
Glutaric acidemia type II	Electron transfer flavoprotein (ETF) ETF: ubiquinone oxidoreductase (ETF dehydrogenase)	Hypoglycemia, acidosis, hyperammonemia, and "smell of sweaty feet" in infancy, often with polycystic and dysplastic kidneys. Later onset may be with episodes of hypoketotic hypoglycemia, or slowly progressive skeletal myopathy. Glutaric, ethylmalonic, 3-hydroxy-isovaleric, isovalerylglycine, and 2-hydroxyglutaric acids in urine, often with sarcosine in serum and urine.
4-Hydroxybutyric acidemia	Succinic semialdehyde dehydrogenase	Seizures and developmental retardation. 4-Hydroxybutyric acid in urine.

Threonine
Valine
Methionine
Isoleucine

↓

Propionyl–CoA $\xrightarrow{1}$ D–methylmalonyl–CoA → L–methylmalonyl–CoA $\xrightarrow{2}$ Succinyl–CoA

Adenosyl–B_{12}

Vitamin B_{12} ——•—— <

Methyl–B_{12}

Figure 31–2. Oxidation of propionyl-CoA to succinyl-CoA. *1.* Propionyl-CoA carboxylase. *2.* Methylmalonyl-CoA mutase.

ing, lethargy, and urine (and body) odor precipitated by intercurrent infections or increased protein intake. The condition is inherited as an autosomal recessive trait, and disease can be diagnosed in utero.

Diagnosis

Isovaleric acidemia and glutaric acidemia type II are the only conditions in which the characteristic odor of "sweaty feet" occurs. Isovalerylglycine is consistently detected in the urine by organic acid chromatography.

Treatment

Providing a low-protein diet or diets low in leucine or all three branched-chain amino acids is effective. Oral administration of glycine appears to prevent complications during acute infections, but poses the risk of neurotoxicity due to severe hyperglycinemia. Oral administration of L-carnitine may also be indicated.

Cohn RM et al: Isovaleric acidemia: Use of glycine therapy in neonates. N Engl J Med 1978;299:996.

de Sousa C et al: The response to L-carnitine and glycine therapy in isovaleric acidaemia. Eur J Pediatr 1986; 144:451.

Ogier deBaulny H et al: Branched chain organic acidurias. In: *Inborn Metabolic Disease: Diagnosis and Treatment*, 2nd ed. Fernandez J et al (editors). Springer-Verlag, 1995.

COMBINED CARBOXYLASE DEFICIENCY

Holocarboxylase synthetase and biotinidase are two enzymes of biotin metabolism in mammals. Holocarboxylase synthetase covalently binds biotin to the apocarboxylases for pyruvate, 3-methylcrotonyl-CoA and propionyl-CoA; and biotinidase releases biotin from these proteins and from proteins in the diet. Recessively inherited deficiency of either enzyme causes deficiency of all three carboxylases, that is, multiple carboxylase deficiency. Holocarboxylase synthetase deficiency usually presents in the neonatal period with hypotonia, and biotinidase deficiency more often presents somewhat later with a syndrome of ataxia, seborrhea, and alopecia. Because many patients with biotinidase deficiency do not show typical symptoms but do develop neurologic sequelae, newborn screening for the condition may be justified.

Diagnosis

This diagnosis should be considered in patients with typical symptoms or in those with primary lactic acidosis. Urine organic acids are usually, but not always, abnormal (Table 31–4). Diagnosis is usually by enzyme assay. Biotinidase can be assayed in serum; holocarboxylase synthetase, in leukocytes or fibroblasts.

Treatment

Oral administration of biotin in large doses, 10–20 mg/d, often reverses the organic aciduria within days and the clinical symptoms within days to weeks. Incidence of hearing loss is high, even in treated patients.

Burri BJ, Sweetman L, Nyhan WL: Heterogeneity of holocarboxylase synthetase in patients with biotin-responsive multiple carboxylase deficiency. Am J Hum Genet 1985;37:326.

Kalayci O et al: Infantile spasms as the initial symptom of biotinidase deficiency. J Pediatr 1994;124:103.

McVoy JRS et al: Partial biotinidase deficiency: Clinical and biochemical features. J Pediatr 1990;116:78.

Wolf B, Heard GS: Screening for biotinidase deficiency in newborns: Worldwide experience. Pediatrics 1990;85:512.

GLUTARIC ACIDEMIA TYPE I

Glutaric acidemia type I is due to deficiency of glutaryl-CoA dehydrogenase and causes a progressive extrapyramidal movement disorder in childhood, with dystonia and athetosis and neuronal degeneration in the caudate and putamen. Macrocephaly at birth is common. Death often occurs during the first decade of life, but the clinical course is highly variable, and several patients have only mild neurologic abnormalities. Children with Glutaric acidemia type I may present with retinal hemorrhages and intracranial bleeding, strongly resembling shaken baby syndrome. The condition is inherited as an autosomal recessive trait.

Diagnosis

Glutaric acidemia type I should be suspected in any patient with progressive dystonia or athetosis. The diagnosis is confirmed by demonstration of glutaric and 3-hydroxyglutaric acids in urine by organic acid analysis. Deficiency of glutaryl-CoA dehydrogenase can be demonstrated in fibroblasts, leukocytes, and, for prenatal diagnosis, amniotic cells.

Treatment

Restriction of dietary lysine and tryptophan are indicated, but neurologic symptoms, once present, do not resolve. A variety of drugs that alter neurotransmitter levels, especially GABA, may be used to control dystonia. Studies suggest that early dietary treatment and aggressive management of intercurrent illness may prevent neurologic deterioration in some patients.

Goodman SI, Frerman FE: Organic acidemias due to defects in lysine oxidation: 2-ketoadipic acidemia and glutaric acidemia. In: *The Metabolic Basis of Inherited Disease*, 6th ed. Scriver CR et al (editors). McGraw-Hill, 1989.

Haworth JC et al: Phenotypic variability in glutaric aciduria type I: Report of fourteen cases in five Canadian Indian kindreds. J Pediatr 1991;118:52.

Hoffman GF et al: Glutaryl-coenzyme A dehydrogenase deficiency: A distinct encephalopathy. Pediatrics 1991;88:1194.

Iafolla AK, Kahler SG: Megalencephaly in the neonatal period as the initial manifestation of glutaric aciduria type I. J Pediatr 1989;115:1004.

DISORDERS OF FATTY ACID OXIDATION & CARNITINE

LONG-CHAIN AND MEDIUM-CHAIN ACYL-COA DEHYDROGENASE DEFICIENCIES

Deficiencies of long-chain and medium-chain acyl-CoA dehydrogenase (LCAD, MCAD), and long-chain hydroxyacyl-CoA dehydrogenase (LCHAD), three enzymes of fatty acid β-oxidation, usually cause Reye-like episodes of hypoketotic hypoglycemia, mild hyperammonemia, hepatomegaly and encephalopathy, or less often, sudden death in infancy. The long- and medium-chain defects can usually be distinguished clinically, with the long-chain defects more often causing early severe hypotonia and cardiomyopathy. MCAD deficiency is common, occurring in perhaps 1:5000 live births, and recent studies suggest that LCHAD may also be common. Although Reye-like episodes may be fatal, they tend to become less frequent and severe with time, and prolonged survival is typical of MCAD, with few deaths after diagnosis is made and treatment instituted. In LCAD and LCHAD deficiency, cardiomyopathy is the direct result of the defect in the oxidation of long chain fatty acids, and progressive liver disease and renal tubular acidosis may also be present. These conditions are inherited as autosomal recessive traits.

Diagnosis

Suspicion should be aroused by the lack of an appropriate ketone response to fasting. Patients with MCAD deficiency excrete phenylpropionylglycine and hexanoylglycine in the urine and acylcarnitine profile is abnormal in blood; urine and blood findings may be highly variable in LCAD and LCHAD. A common mutation has been found in MCAD, which may be useful to prove the diagnosis. Reports suggest a common mutation in LCHAD may be similarly used. Assays of MCAD activity in fibroblasts are necessary only when typical biochemistry is not found. However, fibroblast studies may be required for diagnosis of LCAD or LCHAD. The finding of normal urine organic acids does not exclude these conditions, since excretion of dicarboxylic acids and other products of microsomal and peroxisomal oxidation of fatty acids can be intermittent.

Treatment

Acute management is directed toward preventing or reversing catabolism and hypoglycemia. Long-term measures include providing carbohydrate snacks before bedtime and vigorous treatment of intercurrent infections. Because cardiomyopathy and muscle weakness in MCAD deficiency may be due to secondary carnitine deficiency, oral administration of carnitine is typically prescribed. Medium-chain triglycerides are contraindicated in MCAD deficiency, because they may raise serum octanoic acid to rise to neurotoxic concentrations, but they appear to be a useful energy source for patients with LCAD and LCHAD deficiency.

Duran M et al: Sudden child death and "healthy" affected family members with medium-chain acyl-coenzyme A dehydrogenase deficiency. Pediatrics 1986;78:1052.

Hale DE, Bennett MJ: Fatty acid oxidation disorders: A new class of metabolic diseases. J Pediatr 1992;121:1.

Pollitt RJ: Disorders of mitochondrial β-oxidation: Prenatal and early postnatal diagnosis and their relevance to Reye's syndrome and sudden infant death. J Inherited Metab Dis 1989;12:215.

Rhead WJ: Inborn errors of fatty acid oxidation in man. Clin Biochem 1991;24:319.

Stanley CA: Disorders of fatty oxidation. In: *Inborn Metabolic Disease: Diagnosis and Treatment,* 2nd ed. Fernandez J et al (editors). Springer-Verlag, 1995.

Taubman B, Hale DE, Kelley RI: Familial Reye-like syndrome: A presentation of medium-chain acyl-coenzyme A dehydrogenase deficiency. Pediatrics 1987;79:382.

Vockley J: The changing face of disorders of fatty acid oxidation. Mayo Clin Proc 1994;69:249.

Wanders RJ et al: Long chain 3-hydroxyacyl-CoA dehydrogenase deficiency: Different clinical expression in three unrelated patients. J Inherited Metab Dis 1991; 14:325.

GLUTARIC ACIDEMIA TYPE II

Glutaric acidemia type II (multiple acyl-CoA dehydrogenation deficiency) was first described in 1976 in a baby who died at 3 days of age with profound hypoglycemia, metabolic acidosis, and the "smell of sweaty feet." Since that time, many others have been diagnosed. Some have renal cysts and die in early infancy, and others have Reye-like episodes or skeletal muscle weakness (or both) beginning in childhood or adolescence. Some patients are deficient in electron transfer flavoprotein and others in ETF:ubiquinone oxidoreductase, proteins that transfer electrons from many flavin-containing enzymes of fatty- and amino acid oxidation into the respiratory chain. Both enzyme deficiencies are inherited as autosomal recessive traits, and the infantile form of the disease can be diagnosed in utero.

Diagnosis

Diagnosis can be made by demonstrating derivatives of the substrates of mitochondrial flavin-containing dehydrogenases on organic acid analysis of urine (Table 31–4). Tissue assays of electron transfer flavoprotein and ETF:ubiquinone oxidoreductase are not usually necessary.

Treatment

Dietary measures (carbohydrate feedings before bedtime, provision of bicarbonate, and restriction of fat) are variably effective, and administration of riboflavin and carnitine has shown promise, usually in older patients.

Frerman FE, Goodman SI. Glutaric acidemia type II and defects of the mitochondrial respiratory chain. In: *The Metabolic Basis of Inherited Disease,* 6th ed. Scriver CR et al (editors). McGraw-Hill, 1989.

Goodman SI, Loehr JP, Frerman FE: Clinical and biochemical aspects of glutaric acidemia Type II. In: *Fatty Acid Oxidation: Clinical Biochemical and Molecular Aspects.* Liss, 1990.

CARNITINE

Carnitine is an essential nutrient that is found in highest concentrations in red meats. Its primary function is to transport long-chain fatty acids into mitochondria for oxidation. Primary defects of carnitine biosynthesis and transport exist and may present with Reye's syndrome, myoglobinuria, hypotonia, or cardiomyopathy. These disorders are exceedingly rare compared with secondary carnitine deficiency or insufficiency, which may be due to diet (especially hyperalimentation), renal losses, drug therapy (especially valproic acid), and other metabolic disorders (especially disorders of fatty acid oxidation and organic acidemias). The prognosis depends on the cause of the carnitine abnormality.

Carnitine can be measured in blood. Unless the purpose is solely to monitor dietary deficiency, amounts of free and esterified carnitine should be determined. In some situations, muscle carnitine may be low despite normal blood levels. Free and esterified carnitine also can be measured in urine, and specialized laboratories can identify the specific ester present. If carnitine insufficiency is suspected, the patient should be evaluated to rule out disorders that might cause secondary carnitine deficiency.

Oral carnitine is used in carnitine deficiency or insufficiency in doses of 25–100 mg/kg/d or higher. Intravenous carnitine may be added to hyperalimentation, and high dose intravenous carnitine is available. Treatment is aimed at maintaining normal free carnitine levels. Carnitine supplementation in patients with disorders of fatty acid oxidation and organic acidosis may also augment excretion of accumulated metabolites, in addition to ameliorating carnitine insufficiency. Supplementation may not prevent metabolic crises in such patients, however, even when serum carnitine has been returned to normal.

DeVivo DC, Tein I: Primary and secondary disorders of carnitine metabolism. Int Pediatr 1990;5:134.

Kelly KJ et al: Fatal rhabdomyolysis following influenza infection in a girl with familial carnitine palmityl transferase deficiency. Pediatrics 1988;84:312.

Matsuda I et al: Carnitine deficiency and hyperammonemia with valproate therapy. J Pediatr 1986;109:131.

Moukarzel AA et al: Carnitine status of children receiving long-term total parenteral nutrition: A longitudinal prospective study. J Pediatr 1992;120:759.

Schmidt-Sommerfeld E, Werner D, Penn D: Carnitine plasma concentrations in 353 metabolically healthy children. Eur J Pediatr 1988;147:356.

Shapira Y, Glick B, Gutman A: Carnitine deficiency. Int Pediatr 1993;8:219.

Stanley CA: Disorders of fatty acid oxidation. In: *Inborn Metabolic Disorders: Diagnosis and Treatment,* 2nd ed. Fernandez J et al (editors). Springer-Verlag, 1995.

DISORDERS OF PURINE METABOLISM

HYPOXANTHINE-GUANINE PHOSPHORIBOSYLTRANSFERASE DEFICIENCY (Lesch-Nyhan Syndrome)

Hypoxanthine-guanine phosphoribosyltransferase (HPRT) is the enzyme that converts the purine bases hypoxanthine and guanine to inosine monophosphate (IMP) and guanosine monophosphate (GMP), respectively. The X-linked recessive disorder with complete deficiency is characterized by central nervous system dysfunction and purine overproduction with hyperuricemia and hyperuricuria. Depending on the residual activity of the mutant enzyme, male hemizygotes may be severely retarded and show choreoathetosis, spasticity, and compulsive, mutilating lip and finger biting, or they may present with only gouty arthritis and urate ureterolithiasis. The enzyme deficiency can be demonstrated in erythrocytes, fibroblasts, and cultured amniotic cells; this disorder can thus be diagnosed in utero.

Although the cause of the central nervous system dysfunction in Lesch-Nyhan syndrome remains obscure, the absent or less severe central nervous system manifestations of purine nucleoside phosphorylase deficiency suggest that the problem relates to accumulation of substrate behind the block.

Diagnosis

Diagnosis is made by demonstrating elevated uric acid:creatinine ratio in urine, followed by demonstration of enzyme deficiency in red blood cells.

Treatment

Allopurinol and probenecid may be given to reduce hyperuricemia but do not affect neurologic status. Insertions of the HPRT gene into cultured cells from affected patients and into experimental animals have been effective and offer promise as models for human gene therapy in the future.

Van den Berghe G, Vincent MF: Disorders of purine and pyrimidine metabolism. In: *Inborn Metabolic Disorders: Diagnosis and Treatment,* 2nd ed. Fernandez J et al (editors). Springer-Verlag, 1995.

LYSOSOMAL DISEASES

Lysosomes are cellular organelles in which complex macromolecules are degraded by specific acid hydrolases. Deficiency of a lysosomal enzyme causes its substrate to accumulate in lysosomes of tissues that degrade it, creating a characteristic clinical picture. These so-called storage disorders are classified as mucopolysaccharidoses, lipidoses, or mucolipidoses, depending on the nature of the stored material. Two additional disorders, cystinosis and Salla disease, are caused by defects in lysosomal proteins that normally transport material from the lysosome to the cytoplasm.

Clinical and laboratory features of these conditions are shown in Table 31–5. Most are autosomal recessive traits, and all can be diagnosed in utero.

The diagnosis of mucopolysaccharidosis is suggested by certain clinical and radiologic findings and urine screening tests. Further tests are needed to determine which particular mucopolysaccharides are present. Diagnosis should be confirmed by enzyme assays of cultured fibroblasts or leukocytes; this is especially important when the parents are contemplating having more children.

When a lipidosis or mucolipidosis is suspected, diagnosis is made by appropriate enzyme assays of biopsy specimens, cultured skin fibroblasts, and peripheral leukocytes.

Most of these conditions cannot be treated effectively, although there is increasing evidence that bone marrow transplantation may affect the course of some lysosomal diseases. Gaucher's disease is treated effectively with infusions of natural enzyme modified to allow uptake of the enzyme by lysosomes.

Barth PG: Springolipids. In: *Inborn Metabolic Disorders: Diagnosis and Treatment,* 2nd ed. Fernandez J et al (editors). Springer-Verlag, 1995.

Beck M, Spranger J: Mucopolysaccharides and oligosaccharides. In: *Inborn Metabolic Disorders: Diagnosis and Treatment,* 2nd ed. Fernandez J et al (editors). Springer-Verlag, 1995.

Grabowski G: Clinical and therapeutic perspectives on Gaucher disease. Int Pediatr 1993;8:22.

Muenzer J: Mucopolysaccharidoses. Acta Pediatr 1986; 33:269.

Sidransky E, Ginns EI: Clinical heterogeneity among patients with Gaucher's disease. JAMA 1993;269:1154.

Whitley CB et al: Long-term outcome of Hurler syndrome following bone marrow transplantation. Am J Med Genet 1993;46:209.

PEROXISOMAL DISEASES

Peroxisomes are intracellular organelles that contain a large number of enzymes, many of which are oxidases linked to catalase or peroxidase. Among the enzyme systems in peroxisomes is one for β-oxidation of very long chain fatty acids (which is analogous in many ways to the system for fatty acid oxidation in mitochondria) and another for plasmalogen biosynthesis. In addition, peroxisomes contain oxidases for D- and L-amino acids, pipecolic acid and phytanic acid, and an enzyme (alanine-glyoxylate aminotransferase) that effects transamination of glyoxylate to glycine.

In some peroxisomal diseases, many enzymes are deficient. Zellweger (cerebrohepatorenal) syndrome, the best known among these, is probably due to a defect in organelle assembly. Patients present in infancy with seizures, hypotonia, characteristic facies with a large forehead, and hepatomegaly, and at autopsy show renal cysts and absent peroxisomes. Neonatal adrenoleukodystrophy and hyperpipecolic acidemia are similar conditions, with similar clinical and laboratory findings and multiple enzyme deficiencies in cultured fibroblasts, but peroxisomes are usually detected in tissues.

In other peroxisomal diseases, only a single enzyme is deficient. Primary hyperoxaluria (alanine-glyoxalate aminotransferase deficiency), X-linked adrenoleukodystrophy and adrenomyeloneuropathy (very long chain acyl-CoA ligase deficiency), and adult Refsum's disease (phytanic acid oxidase deficiency) are disorders due to deficiency of single peroxisomal enzymes.

Except for childhood adrenoleukodystrophy, which is X-linked, all peroxisomal diseases are transmitted as autosomal recessive traits and can be diagnosed in utero. Bone marrow transplantation may be

Table 31–5. Clinical and laboratory features of lysosomal storage diseases.

Disorder	Enzyme Defect	Clinical and Laboratory Features
I. Mucopolysaccharidoses		
Hurler syndrome	α-Iduronidase	Autosomal recessive. Mental retardation, hepatosplenomegaly, umbilical hernia, coarse facies, corneal clouding, dorsolumbar gibbus, severe heart disease. Heparan sulfate and dermatan sulfate in urine.
Scheie syndrome	α-Iduronidase (incomplete)	Autosomal recessive. Corneal clouding, stiff joints, normal intellect. Clinical types intermediate between Hurler and Scheie common. Heparan sulfate and dermatan sulfate in urine.
Hunter syndrome	Sulfoiduronate sulfatase	X-linked recessive. Coarse facies, hepatosplenomegaly, mental retardation variable. Corneal clouding and gibbus not present. Heparan sulfate and dermatan sulfate in urine.

Sanfilippo syndrome:
  Type A
  Type B
 	
  Type C
 	
  Type D
	
	Sulfamidase
	α-N-Acetylglucos-
	  aminidase
	Acetyl-CoA: α-
	  glucosaminide-N-
	  acetyltransferase
	α-N-acetylglucosamine-
	  6-sulfatase
		Autosomal recessive. Severe mental retardation with comparatively mild skeletal changes, visceromegaly, and facial coarseness. Types cannot be differentiated clinically. Heparan sulfate in urine.

Morquio syndrome	N-Acetylgalactosamine- 6-sulfatase	Autosomal recessive. Severe skeletal changes, platyspondylisis, corneal clouding. Keratan sulfate in urine.
Maroteaux-Lamy syndrome	N-Acetylgalactosamine- 4-sulfatase	Autosomal recessive. Coarse facies, growth retardation, dorsolumbar gibbus, corneal clouding, hepatosplenomegaly, normal intellect. Dermatan sulfate in urine.
β-Glucuronidase deficiency	β-Glucuronidase	Autosomal recessive. Varies from mental retardation, dorsolumbar gibbus, corneal clouding, and hepatosplenomegaly to mild facial coarseness, retardation, and loose joints. Hearing loss common. Dermatan sulfate or heparan sulfate in urine.
II. Mucolipidoses		
Mannosidosis	α-Mannosidase	Autosomal recessive. Varies from severe mental retardation, coarse facies, short stature, skeletal changes, and hepatosplenomegaly to mild facial coarseness and loose joints. Hearing loss common. Abnormal oligosaccharides in urine.
Fucosidosis	α-Fucosidase	Autosomal recessive. Variable: coarse facies, skeletal changes, hepatosplenomegaly, occasional angiokeratoma corporis diffusum. Abnormal oligosaccharides in urine.
I-cell disease (mucolipidosis II)	N-Acetylglucosaminyl- phosphotransferase	Autosomal recessive; severe and mild forms known. Very short stature, mental retardation, early facial coarsening, clear cornea, stiffness of joints. Increased lysosomal enzymes in serum. Abnormal sialyl oligosaccharides in urine.
Sialidosis	N-Acetylineuraminidase (sialidase)	Autosomal recessive. Mental retardation, coarse facies, skeletal dysplasia, myoclonic seizures, cherry-red macular spot. Abnormal sialyl oligosaccharides in urine.
III. Lipidoses		
Niemann-Pick disease	Sphingomyelinase	Autosomal recessive. Acute and chronic forms known. Acute neuronopathic form common in eastern European Jews. Accumulation of sphingomyelin in lysosomes of RE system and CNS. Hepatosplenomegaly, developmental retardation, macular cherry-red spot. Death by 1–4 years.
Metachromatic leuko-dystrophy	Arylsulfatase A	Autosomal recessive. Late infantile form, with onset at 1–4 years, most common. Accumulation of sulfatide in white matter. Gait disturbances (ataxia), motor incoordination, and dementia. Death usually in first decade.
Krabbe disease (globoid cell leukodystrophy)	Galactocerebroside β-galactosidase	Autosomal recessive. Globoid cells in white matter. Onset at 3–6 months with seizures, irritability, and retardation. Death by 1–2 years. Juvenile and adult forms are rare.

(continued)

Table 31–5. Clinical and laboratory features of lysosomal storage diseases. (continued)

Disorder	Enzyme Defect	Clinical and Laboratory Features
Fabry disease	α-Galactosidase A	X-linked recessive. Storage of trihexosylceramide in endothelial cells. Pain in extremities, angiokeratoma corporis diffusum and (later) poor vision, hypertension, and renal failure.
Farber disease	Ceramidase	Autosomal recessive. Storage of ceramide in tissues. Subcutaneous nodules, arthropathy with deformed and painful joints, and poor growth and development. Death within first year.
Gaucher disease	Glucocerebroside β-glucosidase	Autosomal recessive. Acute neuronopathic form: Accumulation of glucocerebroside in lysosomes of RE system and CNS. Retardation, hepatosplenomegaly, macular cherry-red spot, and Gaucher cells in bone marrow. Death by 1–2 years. Chronic form common in eastern European Jews. Accumulation of spingomyelin in lysosomes of RE system. Hepatosplenomegaly and flask-shaped osteolytic bone lesions. Consistent with normal life expectancy.
G_{M1} gangliosidosis	GM_1 ganglioside β-galactosidase	Autosomal recessive. Accumulation of G_{M1} ganglioside in lysosomes of RE system and CNS. Infantile form: Abnormalities at birth with dysostosis multiplex, hepatosplenomegaly, macular cherry-red spot, and death by 2 years. Juvenile form: Normal development to 1 year of age, then ataxia, weakness, dementia, and death by 4–5 years. Occasional inferior beaking of vertebral bodies of L1 and L2.
G_{M2} gangliosidoses Tay-Sachs disease Sandhoff disease	β-N-Acetylhexos-aminidase A β-N-Acetylhexos-aminidase A & B	Autosomal recessive. Tay-Sachs disease common in eastern European Jews; Sandhoff disease is panethnic. Clinical phenotypes are identical, with accumulation of G_{M2} ganglioside in lysosomes of CNS. Onset at age 3–6 months, with hypotonia, hyperacusis, retardation, and macular cherry-red spot. Death by 2–3 years. Juvenile and adult onset forms of Tay-Sachs disease are rare.
Wolman disease	Acid lipase	Autosomal recessive. Accumulation of cholesterol esters and triglycerides in lysosomes of reticuloendothelial system. Onset in infancy with gastrointestinal symptoms and hepatosplenomegaly, and death by 3–6 months. Adrenals commonly enlarged and calcified.

effective treatment for males with adrenoleukodystrophy. Dietary treatment may have some promise for female carriers of X-linked adrenomyeloneuropathy, and diet therapy is being attempted in other peroxisomal disorders.

Diagnosis

The best screening test for Zellweger syndrome, hyperpipecolic acidemia, X-linked adrenoleukodystrophy, neonatal adrenoleukodystrophy, and infantile Refsum's disease is determination of very long chain fatty acids in serum or plasma; these acids are increased in all these conditions. Urine bile acids are abnormal in other peroxisomal disorders; together, these studies identify most peroxisomal diseases. Tissue biopsy and appropriate enzyme assays are needed for confirmation, especially when a family plans further pregnancies.

Aubourg P et al: A two-year trial of oleic and erucic acids ("Lorenzo's oil") as treatment for adrenomyeloneuropathy. N Engl J Med 1993;329:745.

Moser HW: Peroxisomal disorders. Clin Biochem 1991;24:343.

Moser HW et al: Adrenoleukodystrophy: Phenotypic variability and implications for therapy. J Inherit Metab Dis 1992;15:645.

Sadeghi-Nejad A, Senior B: Adreno-myeloneuropathy presenting as Addison's disease in childhood. N Engl J Med 1990;322:13.

REFERENCES

Cohn RM, Roth KS: *Metabolic Disease: A Guide to Early Recognition.* Saunders, 1983.

Fernandez J, Saudubray J-M, Tada K (editors): *Inborn Metabolic Diseases: Diagnosis and Treatment,* 2nd ed. Springer-Verlag, 1995.

Goodman SI, Markey SP: *Diagnosis of Organic Acidemias by Gas Chromatography-Mass Spectrometry.* AR Liss, 1981.

Scriver CR et al (editors): The Metabolic Basis of Inherited Diseases, 7th ed. McGraw-Hill, 1995.

Genetics & Dysmorphology

32

Eva Sujansky, MD, Janet M. Stewart, MD, & David K. Manchester, MD

New techniques in molecular biology and biochemistry have changed the way clinicians think about and approach birth defects. Scientific reports that advance the understanding of human genetics and development appear almost daily. Molecular approaches to clinical problems now support "reverse genetics," the characterization of human disorders at the level of the gene before their clinical biochemistry and pathophysiology are described. Worldwide, scientists have united to map the human genome.

The clinical implications of these advances are too numerous to discuss completely in this text. This chapter reviews human chromosomes and chromosome abnormalities, briefly describes diagnostic and therapeutic applications of recombinant DNA technology, and then outlines clinically important aspects of mendelian genetics, dysmorphology, and teratology. The chapter concludes with a review of the scope and approach of genetic counseling and some comments about fetal surgery. The reader is directed to the referenced publications for more comprehensive treatments of the rapidly expanding field of clinical genetics.

I. CHROMOSOMES & CELL DIVISIONS

Human chromosomes consist of deoxyribonucleic acid (DNA) and specific proteins. In a nondividing cell, chromosomes are tightly packaged in the nucleus. Chromosomes contain most of the genetic information necessary for growth and differentiation. Chromosome aberrations lead to physical and mental abnormalities. Documentation of chromosome abnormality is important for appropriate management of the affected child and for assessment of the risk of recurrence; sometimes this risk affects many family members.

Although the correct number of chromosomes was established in 1956, it was not until the early 1970s that newly developed cytogenetic techniques allowed recognition of the more detailed characteristics of chromosomes and identification of a whole array of chromosome abnormalities.

The nuclei of all normal human cells, with the exception of gametes, contain 46 chromosomes, consisting of 23 pairs (Figure 32–1). Of these, 22 pairs are called **autosomes.** They are numbered according to their size; chromosome 1 is the largest, and chromosome 22 is the smallest. In addition, there are two **sex chromosomes:** two X chromosomes in females and one X and one Y chromosome in males. The two members of a chromosome pair are called **homologous chromosomes.** One homolog of each chromosome pair is maternal in origin (from the egg); the second is paternal (from the sperm). The egg and sperm each contain 23 chromosomes (**haploid cells**). During the formation of the zygote, they fuse into a cell with 46 chromosomes (**diploid cell**). The subsequent prenatal and postnatal growth of the human organism is through somatic cell divisions, called mitoses.

Mitosis (Figure 32–2) is a cell division of somatic cells. The process has different stages, during which the DNA replication takes place and two daughter cells, genetically identical to the original parent cells, are formed. During **metaphase,** the phase following DNA replication but preceding cell division, individual chromosomes can be visualized. They consist of two arms, a short arm and a long arm separated by a centromere. Each arm consists of two identical parts, called **chromatids.** Chromatids of the same chromosome are called **sister chromatids.**

Meiosis (Figure 32–3), during which eggs and sperm are formed, is cell division limited to gametes. During meiosis, three unique processes take place:

(1) Crossing over of genetic material between two homologous chromosomes; this is preceded by the pairing of both members of each chromosome pair, thus facilitating the physical exchange of homologous genetic material between them.

(2) Random assortment of maternally and paternally derived homologous chromosomes into the

Figure 32–1. Normal male human karyotype.

daughter cells. The distribution of maternal or paternal chromosomes to a particular daughter cell is independent for each such cell.

(3) Two cell divisions, the first of which is a **reduction division,** that is, a parental cell with 46 chromosomes divides into two daughter cells with 23 chromosomes each.

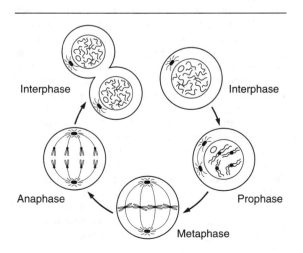

Figure 32–2. Diagram demonstrating the various stages of the mitotic cycle.

CHROMOSOME PREPARATION & ANALYSIS

Because the structure of chromosomes can be visualized only during mitosis, the tissue obtained for chromosome analysis must contain many cells in a dividing state. This condition exists naturally only in bone marrow. Because bone marrow is not readily accessible, it is used for chromosome analysis only when immediate identification of a patient's chromosome constitution is necessary for appropriate management (eg, to rule out trisomy 13 in a newborn with a complex congenital heart disease requiring immediate intervention).

The peripheral blood lymphocytes are easy to obtain and are therefore most frequently used for chromosome analysis. Other tissues used for this purpose include skin or internal organs, such as thymus or gonads. Chorionic villi or amniocytes are used for prenatal diagnosis. If tissue other than bone marrow is used, the cells must be exposed to a mitogenic agent to increase the rate of mitosis.

Lymphocytes require 3 days' growth in a culture medium, and other tissues require 1–2 weeks' growth before enough mitoses are present to allow complete analysis. The chromosome preparation protocol calls

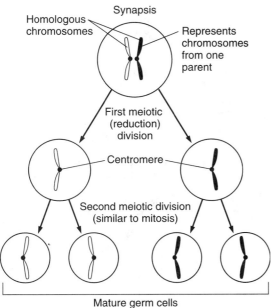

Figure 32–3. Diagram of meiosis, demonstrating the conversion from the diploid somatic cell to the haploid gamete.

for the processed cells to be placed on a glass slide and stained using new techniques that produce a light-and-dark band pattern across the arms of the chromosomes (Figure 32–1). This band pattern is characteristic and reproducible for each chromosome, allowing the chromosomes to be arranged in homologous pairs and numeric and structural abnormalities to be identified. The layout of chromosomes on a sheet of paper in a predetermined order is called a **karyotype.**

In addition to the previously described **routine chromosome analysis,** the following specific studies can be requested:

(1) **High-resolution chromosome analysis** of more elongated chromosomes, allowing visualization of more detailed chromosome bands and detection of abnormalities in a smaller segment of chromosome.

(2) **Fluorescent in situ hybridization (FISH).** This technique involves the use of specific fluorescent-labeled DNA probes that hybridize to the corresponding regions of chromosomes, thus allowing their visualization under a fluorescent microscope. If a cocktail of probes from the same chromosome is used, the whole chromosome may be stained (**chromosome painting**). FISH can be used for the detection of submicroscopic structural rearrangements, undetectable by classic cytogenetic techniques, or the identification of marker chromosomes in metaphase cells (Figure 32–10). In addition, it allows interphase cells (lymphocytes, amniocytes) to be screened for

numerical abnormalities, such as trisomy 21. However, the study of interphase nuclei is not 100% accurate, and any abnormality must be confirmed by a conventional chromosome analysis.

(3) **Fragile X study** (see the section on fragile X syndrome, later).

(4) **Assessment of chromosome breaks and sister chromatid exchanges** requires special techniques that may lead to enhancement of the breaks or special staining that allows visualization of the exchanged chromatids.

CHROMOSOME NOMENCLATURE

A uniform nomenclature consisting of a simple system of symbols has been developed to describe normal and abnormal chromosome findings.

The symbols for normal male and female constitution are 46,XY and 46,XX, respectively. The sign (+) or (−) in front of the chromosome number indicate trisomy or monosomy, respectively, for that particular whole chromosome. For example, 47,XY,+21 designates a male with trisomy 21. The sign (+) or (−) after the chromosome number describes extra material or missing material, respectively, on one of the arms of the chromosome. The symbol for the short arm is p; for the long arm, q. Thus, 46,XX,8q− denotes a deletion on the long arm of chromosome 8. More detailed description of structural abnormalities includes break points in the rearrangement. For example, 46,XY,t(4:8)(q22;p21) means a reciprocal translocation (letter *t*) between the long arm of chromosome 4, at band 22, and the short arm of chromosome 8, at band 21. Other common symbols include *del* (deletion), *dup* (duplication), and *inv* (inversion).

CHROMOSOME ABNORMALITIES

Errors during cell division may result in numerical or structural abnormalities of chromosomes.

Numerical abnormalities are the result of unequal division, called **nondisjunction,** of chromosomes into the daughter cells. Any deviation from the normal diploid number of chromosomes is called **aneuploidy.** This most frequently involves the presence of an additional chromosome, called **trisomy** (eg, trisomy 21, Down syndrome) (Figure 32–4), or the presence of only a single copy of a chromosome, called **monosomy** (eg, monosomy X, Turner syn-

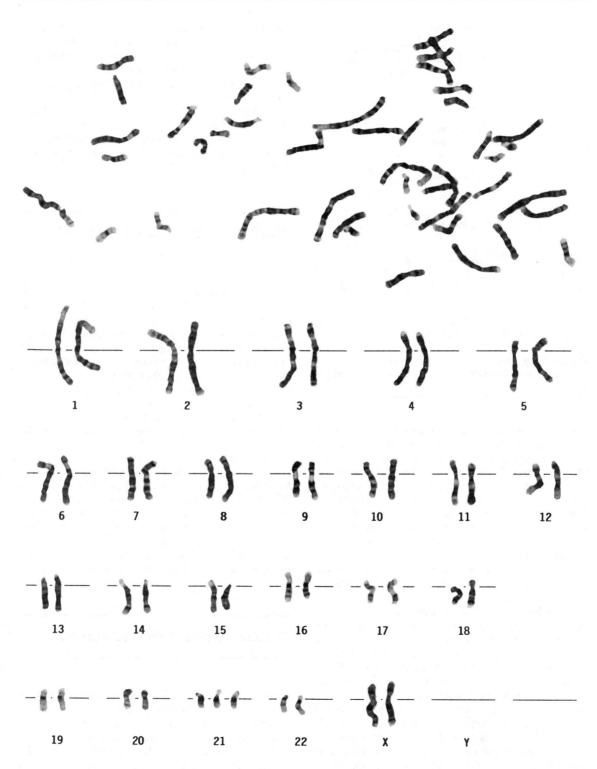

Figure 32–4. Karyotype of trisomy 21.

drome). Rarely, three copies (**triploidy**) of the whole set of 23 chromosomes are found. Four sets of chromosomes (**tetraploidy**) are not found in liveborns.

Structural abnormalities are the result of breaks in chromosomes, which join randomly to form new combinations. In contrast to the numerical abnormalities, which result in trisomy or monosomy of a whole chromosome, structural chromosome abnormalities result in trisomy or monosomy (or both) of only part of a chromosome. The number of possible chromosome abnormalities is infinite. The following types of chromosome rearrangements, according to the mechanism leading to the abnormality, are recognized (Figure 32–5):

(1) **Deletion** is the absence of a part of a chromosome. The deletion is called **terminal** if the distal end of a chromosome arm is included and **interstitial** if it is not included in the deletion. A terminal deletion of both arms of a chromosome may result in reattachment of the remaining arms, leading to formation of a **ring chromosome.**

(2) **Translocation** is detachment of a chromosome segment from its normal location and its attachment to another chromosome. The translocation is **balanced** if the cell contains two complete copies of all the chromosome material, although in a different order. In an **unbalanced** translocation, the rearrangement results in partial trisomy or monosomy.

Translocations can be reciprocal or robertsonian. A **reciprocal** translocation involves exchange of segments between two chromosomes; for example, part of the short arm of chromosome 4 trades places with part of the long arm of chromosome 10. In **robertsonian** translocations, two acrocentric chromosomes fuse at their centromeres. The most frequent robertsonian translocation is formed between chromosomes 14 and 21.

(3) **Inversion** is the result of a double break in the same chromosome. The detached middle section turns upside down before reattaching. If both breaks are on the same side of the centromere, the inversion is **paracentric**; if the breaks are on the opposite arms of a chromosome, the inversion is **pericentric.**

MOSAICISM

Mosaicism is the presence of two or more different chromosome constitutions in different cells of the same individual. For example, a patient may have some cells with 47 chromosomes and others with 46 chromosomes; 46,XX/47,XX,+21 indicates mosaicism for trisomy 21; 45,X/46,XX/47,XXX indicates mosaicism for a monosomy and a trisomy X. Mosaicism should be suspected if clinical symptoms are milder than expected in a nonmosaic patient with

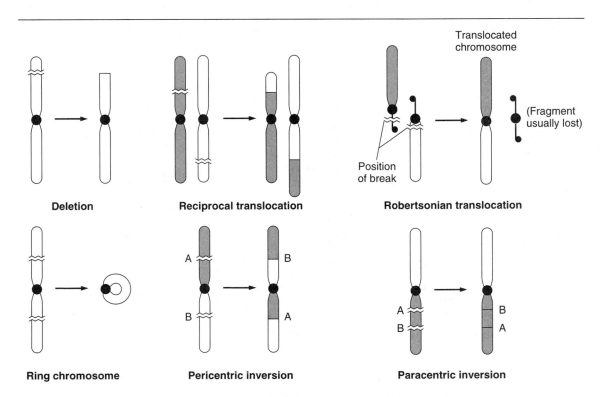

Figure 32–5. Schematic examples of structural chromosome abnormalities.

the same chromosome abnormality. The prognosis is frequently better for a patient with mosaicism than for one with a corresponding chromosome abnormality without mosaicism. In general, the smaller the proportion of the abnormal cell line, the better the prognosis. In the same patient, however, the proportion of normal and abnormal cells in various tissues, such as in skin and peripheral blood, may be significantly different. A prognosis frequently cannot be reliably assessed and should be made with caution or deferred. Mosaicism for structural abnormalities is very rare.

UNIPARENTAL DISOMY

Under normal circumstances, one member of each homologous pair of chromosomes is of maternal origin from the egg and the other is of paternal origin from the sperm (Figure 32–6A). In uniparental disomy, **both copies of a particular chromosome pair originate from the same parent.** If the uniparental disomy is caused by chromosome error in the first meiotic division, both homologous chromosomes of that parent will be present in the gamete. This is called **heterodisomy** (Figure 32–6B). If the disomy is caused by an error in the second meiotic division, two copies of the same chromosome will be present. This is called **isodisomy** (Figure 32–6C). The union of a disomic gamete with a nullisomic gamete from the other parent will result in a zygote with a normal karyotype. Therefore, a uniparental disomy would not

be detected by chromosome analysis. However, DNA analysis would reveal that the child inherited two copies of DNA of a particular chromosome from one parent without the contribution from the other parent. Uniparental disomy has been documented for human chromosomes 7, 11, 15, and X. It has been found in patients with Prader-Willi, Angelman, and Beckwith-Wiedemann syndromes. In addition, cystic fibrosis with only one carrier parent (caused by maternal isodisomy) has been reported. Hemophilia A has been passed from father to son as a result of paternal heterodisomy of X and Y.

Uniparental disomy causes severe prenatal and postnatal growth retardation. Furthermore, it is suspected that uniparental disomy of some chromosomes is lethal. The possible mechanisms for the adverse effects of uniparental disomy include possible homozygosity for deleterious recessive genes and the consequences of imprinting. (See principles of imprinting in the section on dysmorphology, later.)

CLINICAL SIGNIFICANCE OF CHROMOSOME ABNORMALITIES

Chromosome abnormalities result in dysmorphic features, major malformations, developmental delays, or mental retardation. As a rule, abnormalities of autosomes have more severe consequences than abnormalities of sex chromosomes, some of which result only in behavioral problems. Numerical abnormalities resulting in complete trisomy or monosomy

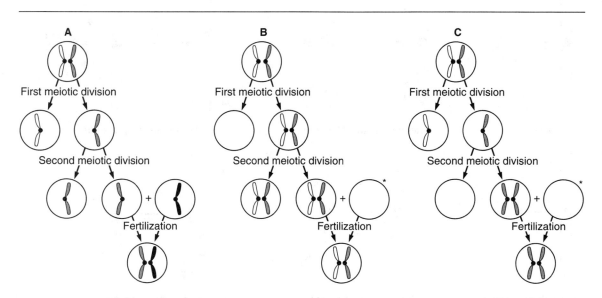

Figure 32–6. Diagram demonstrating the assortment of homologous chromosomes during normal gametogenesis and uniparental disomy. **A:** Fertilization of normal gametes. **B:** Heterodisomy. **C:** Isodisomy. The asterisks (∗) in **B** and **C** indicate the nullisomic gametes from the other parent.

are more deleterious than structural chromosome abnormalities resulting in duplication or deletion of a chromosome segment. Frequently, the smaller the duplicated or deleted segment, the milder the clinical symptoms. However, comparison of patients with duplications or deletions of different sizes in a particular chromosome indicates that involvement of a small specific segment sometimes has a disproportionately great effect on mortality and morbidity.

ABNORMALITIES OF AUTOSOMES

DOWN SYNDROME

The term *Down syndrome* is preferred to the previously used term *mongolism.* The most constant characteristic of the disease is mental retardation. IQs vary between 20 and 80, with the great majority between 45 and 55. Down syndrome occurs in about 1:600 newborns; however, the incidence is greater among children of mothers over 35 years of age. The mother's age at the time of conception and the nature of the chromosome abnormality are important in genetic counseling.

Clinical Findings

A. Symptoms & Signs: The principal findings are a small, brachycephalic head, a characteristic face, and other dysmorphic features. (For details, see Jones's *Smith's Recognizable Patterns of Human Malformation.*) About one-third of children with Down syndrome have congenital heart disease, most often an endocardial cushion defect or other septal defect. Generalized hypotonia is often present. Sexual development is retarded, especially in males, who are usually sterile. The affected newborn is prone to have prolonged physiologic jaundice, polycythemia, and a transient leukemoid reaction. Later, there is an increased tendency for thyroid dysfunction, hearing loss, and atlanto-occipital instability. Leukemia is 20 times more common than in unaffected children. Susceptibility to intercurrent infections is increased. Patients with Down syndrome display an increased sensitivity to the mydriatic effects of atropine instilled into the conjunctiva.

B. Laboratory Findings: The chromosome abnormalities are pathognomonic. The great majority of cases (95%) have 47 chromosomes with trisomy of 21. However, about 4% of sporadic cases and about one-third of the familial cases have 46 chromosomes, including an abnormal translocated chromosome formed as the result of a centric fusion between two acrocentric chromosomes (robertsonian translocation), one of which is chromosome 21. The transloca-

tion is found in 10% of patients whose mothers are younger but in only 3% of those with older mothers. In structural chromosome rearrangements, only band q22 on the long arm of chromosome 21 need be trisomic for Down syndrome to occur.

Mosaicism of the 46/47 type can also occur in persons with Down syndrome. These patients may have milder symptoms, especially higher than expected IQs. Occasionally, normal parents of affected children have inapparent mosaicism.

Prevention

Down syndrome is sporadic in most families; however, the recurrence risk may be increased under certain circumstances. The risk of having a child affected with trisomy 21 varies with **maternal age** (1:2000 for mothers under 25 years of age; 1:50 for mothers 35–39 years of age; 1:20 for mothers over 40 years of age).

In counseling parents who have one child with Down syndrome about the risk of having a second affected child, the geneticist must study the karyotype of the affected child and sometimes the parents to achieve diagnostic accuracy. Several situations may occur.

A. Child With Trisomy 21, Parents With Normal Karyotypes: The risk is only slightly greater than for parents in the general population (1–2%).

B. Trisomic Child, One Parent With Mosaicism: The risk depends on the degree of gonadal mosaicism of the affected parent.

C. Child With 14/21 or 21/21 Translocation, Parents With Normal Karyotypes: The risks are unknown but should be considered only slightly increased.

D. Child With 14/21 Translocation, One Parent Is a Balanced Translocation Carrier:

1. When the mother is the carrier, there is a 10–15% chance that the child will be affected, a 33% chance that the child will be a balanced translocation carrier, and a 43–48% chance that the child will have a normal karyotype.

2. When the father is the carrier, there is a 3–5% chance of having another affected child, and 50% of the apparently unaffected children may be carriers.

E. Child With 21/21 Translocation and One Parent With the Translocation: The recurrence risk is 100%.

Treatment

There is no convincing documentation of the merit of any of the forms of specific therapy that have been attempted, ranging from megadoses of vitamins to exercise programs proposed to overcome the physical and developmental abnormalities of the syndrome. Therapy is thus directed toward specific problems, for example, cardiac surgery or digitalis administration for heart problems, antibiotic administration for infections, tests of thyroid function, infant stimulation programs, special education, and occupational training. The goal of treatment is to help affected children develop to their full potential. Parents' participation in support groups should be encouraged.

TRISOMY 18 SYNDROME

The incidence of trisomy 18 syndrome is about 1:4000 live births, and the ratio of affected males to females is approximately 1:3. The mean maternal age is advanced. Affected babies frequently die in early infancy, although patients occasionally survive into childhood.

Clinical Findings

A. Symptoms & Signs: Trisomy 18 is characterized by prenatal and postnatal growth retardation; hypertonicity; dysmorphic features, including a characteristic face (Figure 32–7) and extremities (see Jones's *Smith's Recognizable Patterns of Human Malformation*); and congenital heart disease (often ventricular septal defect or patent ductus arteriosus). Surviving children show significant developmental delay and mental retardation.

B. Laboratory Findings: In place of uniform trisomy 18, chromosome analysis occasionally reveals mosaicism for trisomy 18 or an unbalanced translocation involving a third number 18 and another chromosome. Rarely, double trisomies have been found in which trisomy X or trisomy 21 is present in addition to trisomy 18.

Complications

Complications are related to associated lesions. Death is often caused by heart failure or pneumonia.

Treatment & Prognosis

There is no treatment other than general supportive care. Death usually occurs in infancy or early childhood, although some patients have reached adulthood.

TRISOMY 13 SYNDROME

The incidence of trisomy 13 is about 1:12,000 live births, and 60% of the patients are female. The mean maternal age is increased. Death usually (but not always) occurs in infancy or by the second year of life, commonly as a result of heart failure or infection.

The symptoms and signs include prenatal and postnatal growth deficiency, arrhinencephaly, eye malformations (anophthalmia, colobomas), cleft lip and palate, polydactyly or syndactyly, and congenital heart disease (usually ventricular septal defect). The facies of an infant with trisomy 13 is shown in Figure 32–8. For other abnormal findings, see Jones's *Smith's Recognizable Patterns of Human Malformation.* Surviving children demonstrate failure to thrive, developmental retardation, apneic spells, seizures, and deafness.

Treatment is supportive. Because it is sometimes necessary to decide immediately after birth how extensive therapy should be for a severely malformed infant, this diagnosis (as well as one of trisomy 18) can be immediately confirmed by direct examination of mitotic figures obtained from bone marrow. Prevention in the form of genetic counseling is indicated. Prenatal diagnosis is available. The recurrence risks are analogous to those of similar chromosome situations in Down syndrome.

Figure 32–7. Child with trisomy 18.

Figure 32–8. Child with trisomy 13.

ABNORMALITIES OF SEX CHROMOSOMES

TURNER SYNDROME

The incidence of Turner syndrome is 1:10,000 among females. However, it is estimated that 95% of conceptuses with monosomy X are miscarried and only 5% are liveborn. Turner syndrome must be ruled out in all females with shortness of stature, webbing of the neck, coarctation of the aorta, or amenorrhea. The diagnosis is made by chromosome analysis. Patients with pseudohypoparathyroidism and Noonan syndrome have a similar phenotype with normal chromosomes.

Clinical Findings

A. Symptoms & Signs: In a newborn, Turner syndrome may be manifested by webbing of the neck, edema of the hands and feet, coarctation of the aorta, and a characteristic triangular face. Later symptoms include short stature, a shield chest with wide-set nipples, streak ovaries, amenorrhea, absence of secondary sex characteristics, and infertility. However, only short stature and amenorrhea and none of the other characteristics may be seen in some affected girls.

Complications relate primarily to the dangers of coarctation of the aorta, when present. Rarely, the dysgenetic gonads may become neoplastic (go-

nadoblastoma). The incidence of malformations of the urinary tract is increased. Sexual infantilism and the perceptual motor difficulties to which these patients are prone may pose psychologic hazards.

B. Laboratory Findings: Monosomy X (45,X) is found in a majority of patients with Turner syndrome. Mosaicism 45,X/46,XX or 45,X/46,XX/47,XXX may be present. Occasionally, the patient has two X chromosomes, one of which has a structural abnormality, for example, a deletion or a translocation of part of one X to one of the autosomal chromosomes. Rarely, mosaicism 45,X/46,XY is found. The presence of a Y chromosome significantly increases the risk for gonadoblastoma.

Treatment & Prognosis

Treatment consists of identifying and treating perceptual problems before they become established. Estrogen replacement therapy will cause development of secondary sex characteristics, permit normal menstruation, and prevent development of osteoporosis. Teenage patients need counseling to cope with the stigma of their condition and to understand the need for hormone therapy. In recent years, growth hormone therapy has been used successfully to increase the height of affected girls. Females with 45,X or 45,X mosaicism have a low fertility rate, and those who become pregnant have been reported to have a high risk of fetal wastage (spontaneous miscarriage, approximately 30%; stillbirth, 6–10%). Furthermore, their liveborn offspring have an increased frequency of chromosome abnormalities involving either sex chromosomes or autosomes (14/102), and congenital malformations (19/102). Thus, prenatal ultrasonography and chromosome analysis are indicated for females with sex chromosome abnormalities.

KLINEFELTER SYNDROME

The incidence of Klinefelter syndrome in the newborn population is roughly 1:500, but it is about 1% among mentally retarded males and about 3% among males seen at infertility clinics. The maternal age at birth is often advanced. The diagnosis is rarely made before puberty, except as a result of prenatal diagnosis. Unlike gonadal dysgenesis, Klinefelter syndrome is rarely the cause of spontaneous abortions.

Clinical Findings

A. Symptoms & Signs: The characteristic findings do not usually appear until after puberty. Micro-orchidism associated with otherwise normal external genitals, azoospermia, and sterility are almost invariable in diagnosed cases. Gynecomastia, normal to borderline IQ, diminished facial hair, lack of libido and potency, and a tall, eunuchoid build are frequent features. In chromosome variants with three and four X chromosomes (XXXY and XXXXY), mental retardation may be severe, and radioulnar synostosis may be present as well as anomalies of the external genitalia and cryptorchidism. In the XXXXY cases, these findings are especially prominent, as well as microcephaly, short stature, and dysmorphic features.

The adult XXYY patient tends to be taller and more retarded than the average XXY patient.

In general, the physical and mental abnormalities associated with Klinefelter syndrome increase as the number of sex chromosomes increases.

B. Laboratory Findings: The majority of cases have a 47,XXY constitution. Rare variants are 48,XXXY, 49,XXXXY, and 48,XXYY. A variety of mosaicisms containing combinations of the above, as well as 46,XY/47,XXY mosaicism, have been reported. Some patients with 46,XY/47,XXY mosaicism are fertile.

Urinary excretion of gonadotropins is high in adults. Levels are comparable to those found in postmenopausal women.

XYY SYNDROME

The incidence of the 47,XYY karyotype in the newborn population is as yet unknown, although current estimates are that it occurs in about 1:1000 male births. Affected newborns in general are perfectly normal. This syndrome may be present in 10% of men over 6 ft tall who come into conflict with the law because of their aggressive personalities.

Affected individuals may on occasion exhibit an abnormal behavior pattern from early childhood and may be slightly retarded. Fertility may be normal.

There is no treatment. Many males with an XYY karyotype are normal. Long-term problems may relate to low IQ and environmental stress.

RECURRENCE RISKS

Most numerical chromosome abnormalities occur sporadically. However, occurrences in siblings or other relatives have been reported, suggesting a hereditary predisposition to nondisjunction in some kindreds. Attempts to identify a single cause have been unsuccessful. It is reasonable to assign parents of a child with aneuploidy an empirical recurrence risk of 1–2% and offer prenatal diagnosis for subsequent pregnancies. Determination of the recurrence risk in structural chromosome abnormalities requires chromosome analysis of the patient's parents to assess whether the abnormality was a de novo event in the patient or if a parental balanced rearrangement of chromosomes exists in one of the parents. If a balanced rearrangement is found, chromosome analysis of other family members must be attempted until all family members with the rearrangement are identified. This analysis is important because, although members of kindreds with normal chromosomes are not at increased risk of recurrence (except in a rare case of gonadal mosaicism), those with balanced structural rearrangements are. The specific risk varies according to the type of rearrangement and the chromosomes involved.

OTHER CHROMOSOME ABNORMALITIES

FRAGILE X SYNDROME

Fragile X syndrome, present in approximately 1:1000 males, accounts for 30–50% of cases of X-linked mental retardation. It is associated in a high proportion of gene carriers with a fragile site (a chromatin gap) on the long arm of the X chromosome (Xq27.3) (Figure 32–9). This fragile site is visible only when the tissue culture medium used for chromosome analysis is deficient in folate or thymidine. Thus, the laboratory performing chromosome analysis must be informed in advance that a fragile X study is desired. Even under optimal circumstances, the fragile site is not expressed in all cells. In affected males, 1–50% of cells are positive. In female carriers of the gene, the fragile site is usually expressed in a low percentage of cells. Furthermore, approximately 40% of carrier females and 20% of males who carry the gene do not express the fragile site at all.

Recently, direct DNA testing became available.

Figure 32–9. Partial karyotype showing fragile X and normal Y chromosomes. The arrows point to the fragile sites.

The fragile X mental retardation 1 gene has been identified and named FMR-1. The gene was found to have unstable CGG repeats at the 5′ end. Normal individuals have up to a 200-bp (base pair) fragment of cytidine phosphate guanosine dinucleotides. In asymptomatic carriers, this fragment is increased up to 500 bp (**premutation**) and in persons expressing the fragile X phenotype to over 600 bp (**full mutation**). Abnormal methylation of this region, found in persons with the full mutation, shuts off the expression of the adjacent genes. DNA analysis is more reliable in detecting fragile X than the cytogenetic study and should be used when fragile X is highly suspicious, especially in known fragile X families. However, in the case of isolated developmental delay or behavior problems, cytogenetic analysis is preferable as it may detect another chromosome abnormality.

Typically, the majority of males with fragile X syndrome present with mental retardation, oblong face with large ears, and large testicles, especially after puberty. Other physical signs include evidence of connective tissue disorder, for example, hyperextensible joints and mitral valve prolapse. The majority are hyperactive and exhibit infantile autism or autistic-like behavior. However, some males with the abnormal gene are of normal phenotype.

In contrast, only about one-third of females with the fragile X show some degree of mental retardation. Typical physical features and behavioral problems are also less common. There is a difference in the clinical expression of fragile X in male and female offspring, depending on which parent is transmitting the gene. The premutation can change into the full mutation only when passed through a female. Persons with the premutation have minimal or no risk of retardation.

Genetic counseling in families with this disorder used to be difficult because the incomplete penetrance of cytogenetic and clinical symptoms in both sexes precluded identification of all carriers of the gene. Identification of the abnormal DNA amplification by direct DNA analysis can detect nearly all asymptomatic gene carriers of both sexes. Therefore, it is a reliable test for prenatal and postnatal diagnosis of fragile X and facilitates genetic counseling.

SYNDROMES ASSOCIATED WITH CHROMOSOME FRAGILITY

It is well known that such environmental factors as exposure to radiation, certain chemicals, and viruses contribute to chromosome breaks and rearrangements. However, some well-defined autosomal recessive syndromes are associated with a greatly increased risk of chromosome aberrations. These include **Bloom syndrome,** characterized by small stature and development of telangiectasia upon exposure to sunlight; **Fanconi anemia,** frequently associated with a radial ray defect, pigmentary changes, hypogonadism, mild mental retardation, and development of pancytopenia; **ataxia telangiectasia** (Louis-Bar syndrome), characterized by telangiectasia of the skin and eyes, immunodeficiency, and progressive ataxia; **xeroderma pigmentosum,** resulting in the formation of skin lesions secondary to sun exposure; and **Werner syndrome,** which is associated with premature senility.

The knowledge that specific chromosome aberrations are associated with these syndromes is frequently the basis for cytogenetic confirmation of their diagnosis. For example, Bloom syndrome is associated with an increased tendency to exchange segments between homologous chromosomes during mitosis; this tendency is called sister chromatid exchange. In Fanconi anemia, translocations between nonhomologous chromosomes take place, resulting in the formation of so-called quadriradii.

CONTIGUOUS GENE SYNDROMES

Syndromes are disorders with recognizable patterns of malformations. Some syndromes are caused by chromosome abnormalities; others, by single-gene defects. In many syndromes, the cause is unknown. In some of these syndromes, which usually occur sporadically but in uncommon instances are familial, high-resolution chromosome analysis can lead to the identification of small interstitial deletions. The deletion is visible under the microscope in the chromosomes of some but not all affected individuals. It is postulated that the syndrome is caused by the absence of a cluster of genes located in the deleted segment. In some cases with normal karyotypes, the deletion is submicroscopic, subject to detection by FISH (Figure 32–10) or DNA analysis. In other cases, other mechanisms interfere with the normal activity of the genes believed to be responsible for the syndrome. Uniparental disomy has been documented in some patients with Prader-Willi syndrome (short stature, obesity, hypogonadism, mental retardation), Angelman syndrome (happy puppet syndrome with mental retardation, inappropriate laughter and hand flapping), Beckwith-Wiedemann syndrome (overgrowth, macroglossia, omphalocele, mental retardation) with normal high-resolution chromosomes. Abnormal imprinting, caused by the uniparental origin of the responsible chromosome segment, is implicated in the etiology. (See the discussion on imprinting in the section on dysmorphology, later.) The group of genes causing the syndrome are related only through their linear placement on the same chromosome segments and do not influence each other's functions directly (thus the term *contiguous gene syndrome*). Table 32–1 lists examples of the currently known contiguous gene syndromes and their associated chromosome abnormalities.

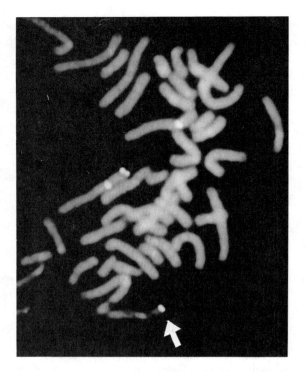

Figure 32–10. Fluorescent in situ hybridization (FISH) showing the brightly fluorescent probes of Wolf-Hirschhorn syndrome (4p deletion syndrome). One probe is hybridized to the normal location on chromosome 4; the other (arrow) documents 4/11 translocation, which was not detectable by a classic cytogenetic analysis.

Table 32–1. Currently recognized contiguous gene syndromes.

Syndrome	Abnormal Chromosome Segment
Prader-Willi syndrome	del 15q11
Shprintzen/DiGeorge spectrum	del 22q11
Langer-Gideon syndrome	del 8q24
Miller-Dieker syndrome	del 17p13
Retinoblastoma/mental retardation	del 13q14
Beckwith-Wiedemann syndrome	11p15
Wilms' tumor with aniridia, genitourinary malformations, and mental retardation	del 11p13

Clarke A: Genetic imprinting in clinical genetics. Development 1990(Suppl 131).

Emanuel BS: Molecular cytogenetics: Toward dissection of the contiguous gene syndrome. (Invited editorial.) Am J Hum Genet 1988;43:575.

Hagerman RJ, Cronister-Silverman A (editors): *Fragile X Syndrome.* Johns Hopkins Univ Press, 1991.

Hall JG: How imprinting is relevant to human disease. Development 1990(Suppl 141).

Jones KL: *Smith's Recognizable Patterns of Human Malformation,* 5th ed. Saunders, 1996, in press.

Kaneko N, Kawagoe S, Hiroi M: Turner's syndrome: Review of the literature with reference to a successful pregnancy outcome. Gynecol Obstet Invest 1990;29:81.

Mittleman F, Heim S: Chromosome abnormalities in cancer. Cancer Detect Prev 1990;14:527.

Rooney DE, Czepulkowski BH (editors): *Human Cytogenetics: A Practical Approach.* Oxford Univ Press, 1986.

Rousseau F et al: Direct diagnosis by DNA analysis of the fragile X syndrome of mental retardation. N Engl J Med 1991;325:1673.

Smith AN, Scott JA (editors): *Genetic Applications: A Health Perspective.* Learner Managed Designs, 1988.

Spence JE et al: Uniparental disomy as a mechanism for human genetic disease. Am J Hum Genet 1988;42:217.

Tkachuk DC et al: Clinical applications of fluorescence in situ hybridization. Genet Anal Tech Appl 1991;8:67.

Trask BJ: Fluorescence in situ hybridization: Applications in cytogenetics and gene mapping. Trends Genet 1991; 7:149.

CHROMOSOME ABNORMALITIES IN CANCER

Numerical and structural chromosome abnormalities have been identified in numerous hematopoietic and solid tumor malignancies of individuals with otherwise normal chromosomes. The cytogenetic abnormalities have been categorized as follows: In **primary abnormalities,** their presence is necessary for initiation of the malignancy. (*Example:* 13q– in retinoblastoma.) **Secondary abnormalities** appear only after the malignancy has developed. (*Example:* Philadelphia chromosome, t[9;22][q34;q11], in acute and chronic myeloid leukemia.) **Cytogenetic noise** is the term used to denote a variety of random chromosome abnormalities.

The primary and secondary chromosome abnormalities are specific for particular malignancies and can be utilized for diagnosis or prognosis. For example, the presence of Philadelphia chromosome is a good prognostic sign in CML and indicates a poor prognosis in ALL. The sites of chromosome breaks coincide with the known loci of oncogenes and antioncogenes.

II. PRINCIPLES OF RECOMBINANT DNA

The revolutionary progress made in molecular biology during the past 2 decades has led to the development of recombinant DNA methods, which have greatly advanced our understanding of the structure and function of human genes. The recombinant DNA technology has major implications for all medical disciplines and especially for human genetics, since it allows location of genes on chromosomes, isolation and characterization of genes, and determination of DNA sequences and encoded protein sequences.

The development of recombinant DNA technology was based on the discovery of bacterial enzymes (restriction enzymes). These endonucleases cleave DNA at sites specific for each enzyme. Each restriction endonuclease recognizes a specific nucleotide sequence consisting of 4, 6, 8, or 10 nucleotides and cleaves DNA within that sequence, thus producing DNA fragments. A difference in DNA sequence caused by a normal variation of DNA or by a gene mutation either produces or eliminates an endonuclease recognition site, resulting in a DNA fragment of a different size. Thus, the number and arrangement of restriction sites (called a "restriction map") are characteristic of a given DNA sequence. Before a DNA fragment of interest can be analyzed, multiple copies of it must be produced. This can be achieved by incorporating the human DNA fragment into a **vector,** that is, a DNA segment containing the means of replication and selection in bacteria. The vector-containing human DNA insert is replicated, thus producing multiple copies of the segment of interest. The source of inserts can be **genomic DNA,** obtained directly from the cleaving of the target organism, or **complementary DNA** (cDNA), obtained by copying messenger RNA (mRNA) into DNA by reverse transcription.

A **genomic library** can be constructed by randomly fragmenting human genomic DNA with restriction enzymes and then inserting the fragments into a vector. Such a library contains large numbers of different DNA sequences. Some of these specific DNA fragments are used to manufacture human proteins (eg, insulin, growth hormone, interferon, and blood clotting factors) for pharmacologic applications; others are used as **probes,** which may be thought of as DNA segment-specific, radioactively labeled reagents for mapping and diagnosis.

Molecular genetics is most commonly used to look for changes in genomic DNA detected by Southern blot analysis, but a similar technique of Northern blot analysis is being used increasingly to look for mRNA abnormalities. **Southern blot analysis** relies on the use of restriction endonucleases to cleave human genomic DNA at specific nucleotide sequences and to produce DNA fragments of different lengths. These DNA fragments are then separated by agarose gel electrophoresis, transferred to a membrane, and overlaid with a radioactive probe, which hybridizes only with a fragment having cDNA. This fragment is identified by autoradiography, and its size is determined.

In recent years, a gene amplification technique called **polymerase chain reaction** (PCR) has been developed. This technique is having a tremendous effect on the use of DNA probes in diagnosis, because it is simpler and less time-consuming than older methods. PCR substantially increases the amount of DNA sequence to be analyzed by easy enzymatic synthesis of 100,000 to 1 million copies of the original DNA segment in a short time. Oligonucleotides, which usually consist of 120 bases and are complementary to the DNA flanking the target segment, are synthesized and used to prime DNA synthesis by DNA polymerase. Each cycle, consisting of denaturation of genomic DNA, primer annealing, and polymerase extension, produces new DNA strands complementary to the target DNA. During each cycle, the amount of amplified DNA doubles, accumulating rapidly in an exponential fashion. After 20 cycles, the DNA is amplified 1 million–fold.

The amplified DNA can be labeled with **synthetic oligonucleotide probes.** DNA sequence variation can be analyzed in a crude cell lysate of fewer than 100 cells in a dot blot format. This method, therefore, eliminates the need for DNA purification, gel electrophoresis, and the use of radioactive probes. It can be performed on a small DNA sample in a short time. The disadvantage is that a small contamination with a foreign DNA can result in an incorrect diagnosis.

APPLICATION OF RECOMBINANT DNA TECHNOLOGIES IN CLINICAL GENETICS

GENETIC DIAGNOSIS

Genetic diagnosis can be performed by direct detection of a mutant gene or by indirect methods.

Direct detection of an abnormal gene is possible only when the nature of the mutation is known. If the abnormal gene has a partial deletion, insertion, or rearrangement, restriction endonuclease analysis with the Southern blot technique is used. Cloned DNA fragments of the gene are used as molecular probes to label the gene, demonstrating the altered size of the gene in comparison with a normal control. Gene deletions have been found in α- and β-thalassemias, antithrombin III deficiency, congenital adrenal hyperplasia secondary to 21-hydroxylase deficiency, Duchenne muscular dystrophy, hemophilias A and B, Lesch-Nyhan syndrome, ornithine transcarbamoylase deficiency, neurofibromatosis, and other disorders.

An abnormal gene with a point mutation can be diagnosed by restriction analysis if the mutation either created or abolished a restriction recognition site, but a restriction recognition site is created or abolished in only 5–10% of point mutations. In the remainder,

PCR can be used for DNA amplification, and the mutation can be documented by a mutant-specific oligonucleotide probe, which recognizes the mutant but not the normal alleles. In addition to point mutations, deletions, and insertions, a new phenomenon called **unstable expansion of trinucleotide repeats** was found to be responsible for human gene mutations. These repeats were found to be CGG in fragile X syndrome, CTG in myotonic dystrophy (autosomal dominant), and CAG in both Huntington disease (autosomal dominant) and spinobulbar muscular atrophy (Kennedy disease, X-linked). The repeats are found in the 3′ or 5′ region of the genes, and their size varies within the normal population. Mutations result in the increase in the number of repeats; the number of repeats frequently corresponds with the severity of the disorder. The tendency of the repeats to increase in number in each successive generation is the molecular basis for so-called anticipation, that is, increased severity of the disorder in successive generations.

The advantage of a diagnostic study using the direct detection of the mutant gene is that it requires the affected individual only, and it need not involve other family members.

Indirect detection of abnormal genes is used (1) when the gene is known but there is extensive heterogeneity of the molecular defect between families, and (2) when the gene responsible for a disease is unknown but its chromosome location is known. In the former situation—when the gene is known—it is not always necessary to know the exact molecular defect to determine the presence of the gene. It is, however, necessary to mark and trace the inheritance of the abnormal gene. This can be done on the basis of intragenic DNA polymorphism, which is characterized by the addition or removal of a restriction site and is thus identifiable by restriction fragment length polymorphism (RFLP) analysis. This DNA polymorphism, although it is intragenic, is not the mutation that causes the disorder—it simply marks and helps to differentiate the abnormal gene from the normal one. RFLP cannot be used, however, unless both parents of the tested individual are heterozygous. Thus, a family study is necessary to determine the haplotypes of the chromosomes with and without the mutant gene. However, crossover and recombination are not a problem, because the polymorphism is intragenic or in very close proximity to the gene. Examples of disorders that can be screened by this method are phenylketonuria, hemophilia, β-thalassemia, and Fabry disease.

The latter situation—when the abnormal gene is unknown—exists in the majority of single-gene disorders. In this case, linkage analysis using a large number of DNA polymorphic markers may reveal a close link between one or more such markers and the presence of the clinical disorder. Such a linkage study localizes the gene of interest to a specific chromosome or to a specific region of a chromosome. Once the location of the gene is known, the same technique (using probes known to be linked to the gene locus of interest) can be used to trace the presence or absence of the gene through the family. This method assumes that the two loci—the locus of the gene and the locus of the DNA polymorphism used to mark the gene—are so close that they will not segregate independently but will be transmitted together. The presence of the marker, therefore, is a reliable indication of the presence of the gene of interest. Thus, the distance between the two loci is of utmost importance in determining the reliability of any linkage analysis, because crossing over and recombination between the gene and the marker during meiosis will result in an error in the diagnosis. To minimize the errors, multiple linked markers should be used in linkage analysis of any gene.

DETECTION OF GENETIC HETEROGENEITY

Genetic heterogeneity is occasionally suspected on the basis of clinical variability. In other instances, there is no clinical clue. For example, enzyme deficiencies may be caused by a number of different mutations, such as an abnormal active site in one case and an abnormal coenzyme in another. Alternatively, the phenotype may be caused in different families by different enzyme defects. Such heterogeneity cannot be suspected on a clinical basis; however, it can be detected using DNA technology.

PREVENTION

Recombinant DNA technology has the potential to prevent genetic disease by facilitating the detection of carriers of defective genes and permitting prenatal diagnosis. Family studies can also clarify the mode of inheritance, thus allowing more accurate determination of recurrence risks and appropriate options. For example, differentiation of a gonadal mosaicism from decreased penetrance of a dominant gene has important implications for genetic counseling.

In the past, the diagnosis of a genetic disease characterized by a late onset of symptoms, for example, Huntington disease, could not be made prior to the appearance of clinical symptoms. In some inborn errors of metabolism, diagnostic tests (eg, measurement of enzyme activities) could be conducted only on inaccessible tissues. Gene identification techniques can enormously enhance our ability to diagnose symptomatic and presymptomatic individuals, conduct prenatal diagnosis, and detect heterozygous carriers.

TREATMENT

Recombinant DNA technology could facilitate treatment in the following ways:

(1) By production of large amounts of therapeutic agents, for example, growth hormone and interferon, which are present naturally in small quantities and are therefore very expensive. This is already being done.

(2) By gene therapy—the introduction of a normal gene into an individual affected with a serious inherited disorder. In principle, genes could be introduced either during embryonic life (germ line therapy), in which case the gene could be transmitted to future generations; or the gene could be introduced only into somatic cells (somatic therapy), in which case it would be present only during the life of the recipient. Gene therapy through bone marrow transplantation has been done experimentally on patients with severe combined immunodeficiency and with the non-neurologic form of Gaucher disease.

Korf B: Molecular medicine: Molecular diagnosis. N Engl J Med 1995;332:1218, 1499.

Mandel JL: Questions of expansion. Nature Genet 1993;4:8.

Nelson DL: Fragile X syndrome: Review and current status. Growth Genet Horm 1993;9:1.

III. MENDELIAN GENETICS

SINGLE-GENE DEFECTS

A **gene** is the unit of inheritance that determines the genetic makeup of an individual. Genes occur in pairs at a single locus or site on specific chromosomes. These paired genes, called **alleles,** determine the genotype of an individual at that locus. If the genes at a specific locus are identical, the individual is **homozygous;** if they are different, **heterozygous.** During normal meiosis, these alleles separate, one going to each of the two gametes. An understanding of this process is necessary for an understanding of single-gene inheritance.

Disorders caused by an abnormality in a single gene are either autosomal or X-linked, depending on the location of the gene on an autosome in the former and on the X chromosome in the latter. If the abnormality is present when the defective gene is in either the heterozygous or the homozygous state, it is dominantly inherited. If, however, it is present only when the gene involved is in the homozygous state, the disorder is recessively inherited.

AUTOSOMAL DOMINANT INHERITANCE

Autosomal dominant inheritance has the following characteristics:

(1) Individuals in the same family may show very different manifestations of the same disorder. This phenomenon is called **variable expressivity.** Typically, at least some persons who carry the gene are mildly affected, because an individual must be healthy enough and fertile enough to reproduce and pass on the trait. In some disorders, such as Huntington disease, manifestations do not appear until after the childbearing years. In others, which tend to be more severe (eg, achondroplasia), there is a high mutation rate.

(2) Some persons who are obligatory carriers of the gene (ie, both their parent and their child are affected) may have no apparent manifestations. This phenomenon is called **nonpenetrance,** and the penetrance rate varies for each dominantly inherited condition.

(3) Males and females are equally affected, although the manifestations may vary according to sex. For example, baldness is a dominant trait but affects only males. In this case, the trait is said to be **sex-limited.** Both males and females can pass on the abnormality to children of either sex.

(4) Dominant inheritance is typically said to be "vertical," that is, the condition passes from one generation to the next in a vertical fashion (Figure 32–11).

(5) In some cases, the family history seems to be completely negative, and the affected individual appears to be the first abnormal case. This spontaneous appearance may be caused by a point mutation or a change in the structure of a specific gene. Such a change may be a deletion, a duplication, or an amino acid substitution. The mutation rate varies with each dominant condition, and in some cases the mutation rate increases with advancing paternal age. There are, however, several other possible explanations for a negative family history:

(a) Nonpaternity.

(b) Decreased penetrance or mild manifestations in one of the parents. For this reason, both parents must be carefully examined and a thorough family history taken.

(c) Germ cell mosaicism. In rare cases, there may be mosaicism in the germ cell line of either parent, in which case the risk of recurrence increases. This is a

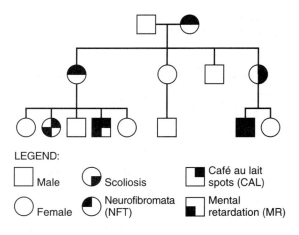

LEGEND:

☐ Male ◖ Scoliosis ◳ Café au lait spots (CAL)

○ Female ◐ Neurofibromata (NFT) ◲ Mental retardation (MR)

Figure 32–11. Autosomal dominant inheritance: Neurofibromatosis, showing variable expressivity.

proposed explanation for cases in which two children of completely normal parents are affected with a dominant condition. The best example of this is osteogenesis imperfecta. Earlier it was thought that there were two forms of the disorder—one autosomal dominant, milder and later in onset; and one autosomal recessive, perinatal in onset and severe (often lethal). The latter was felt to be recessive because of affected siblings born to clinically normal parents. However, newer studies have shown that only one of the paired collagen genes is abnormal in the severe form instead of two, as would be expected in a recessive disease. Recurrent cases, therefore, must be the result of germ cell mosaicism, and indeed, prenatal diagnosis has shown that the actual recurrence risk in this form of osteogenesis imperfecta is 7%.

It is not known how common germ cell mosaicism is, but it has been described in two X-linked disorders as well (Duchenne muscular dystrophy and hemophilia A). The incidence of germ cell mosaicism may depend on many factors which are just beginning to be understood.

(d) The possibility that the abnormality is not truly an autosomal dominant condition. It may be a phenocopy, that is, a nongenetic condition that mimics a certain genotype, or it may be a similar but genetically different abnormality with a different mode of inheritance.

(6) As a general rule, dominant conditions are not caused by enzyme defects, since most biochemical defects are substrate-limited rather than enzyme-limited. Therefore, enzyme levels at 50% of the normal value are sufficient for normal function. There are exceptions, such as acute intermittent porphyria. Dominant traits are more often related to structural abnormalities of protein, for example, as in the Marfan syndrome.

(7) The risk of any offspring carrying an abnormal

dominant gene is 50%, or 1:2 for each pregnancy. This is true whether the gene is penetrant or not, and the severity in the offspring is not related to the severity in the affected parent but may be related to the sex of the parent transmitting the gene. For example, if the gene for myotonic dystrophy is passed through the mother, there is a 10–20% chance that the child (regardless of sex) may have a severe congenital form of the disease. Conversely, if the gene for Huntington disease is passed through the father, there is a 5–10% possibility that the offspring may have the severe, rigid juvenile form. This is independent of the severity of the condition in the transmitting parent. It has been attributed to imprinting, although we know in these two conditions that it is associated with an expansion of the repeat segment that causes the disease in question. There are certainly other mechanisms of imprinting in other conditions. If an abnormality represents a new mutation of a dominant trait, the parents of the affected individual run a low risk during subsequent pregnancies, but the risk for the offspring of the affected individual is 50%.

(8) Options available for future pregnancies include prenatal diagnosis in an increasing number of cases and artificial insemination or egg donation, depending on which parent carries the abnormal gene.

NEUROFIBROMATOSIS

Essentials of Diagnosis (Neurofibromatosis 1)

Two or more of the following:

- Six or more café au lait macules, at least 15 mm in diameter in postpubertal and at least 5 mm in prepubertal individuals.
- Two or more neurofibromas of any type or one plexiform neurofibroma.
- Axillary or inguinal freckling.
- Two or more Lisch nodules (iris hamartomas).
- Distinctive bony lesions such as sphenoid dysplasia or pseudarthrosis.
- An affected first-degree relative.

General Considerations

Neurofibromatosis is one of the most common autosomal dominant disorders, occurring in 1:4000 to 1:3000 births and seen in all races and ethnic groups. It has a wide range of variability and can present in many ways. In general, however, the disorder is progressive, and new manifestations appear over time. There are at least two types of neurofibromatosis: Neurofibromatosis 1 is characterized by multiple skin findings, and neurofibromatosis 2 is characterized by bilateral acoustic neuromas, with minimal or no skin manifestations. A third category includes all of the atypical forms. Because neurofibromatosis 2 is less common and rarely presents before late adolescence, this discussion is limited to type 1.

Clinical Findings

Café au lait macules may be present at birth, and in about 80% of individuals with neurofibromatosis 1, they are apparent by 1 year of age. The typical skin lesion is 10–30 mm, ovoid, and smooth-bordered, but there is great variation. Neurofibromas are benign tumors consisting of Schwann cells, nerve fibers, and fibroblasts; they may be discrete or plexiform. Discrete tumors are more common and can occur at any age. They are well demarcated and can present in cutaneous, subcutaneous, or internal tissues. Plexiform neurofibromas are more diffuse and can invade normal tissue. They are congenital and are frequently detected during periods of rapid growth. If the face or a limb is involved, there may be associated hypertrophy or overgrowth. The incidence of Lisch nodules, which can be seen with a slit lamp, also increases with age. Common features of affected individuals include a large head (although only a small percentage have true hydrocephalus), bony abnormalities on x-ray studies, scoliosis, and a wide spectrum of developmental problems ranging from learning disabilities to true mental retardation. The most common problems in childhood are secondary to plexiform neurofibromas and learning disabilities. Although the average IQ is within the normal range, it is lower than in unaffected family members. The learning problem seems to be specific and involves a visual-perceptual disability that could lead to difficulties in reading and writing or to behavioral impulsivity.

Differential Diagnosis

Areas of hyperpigmentation can be seen in other conditions (eg, the Albright, Noonan, and LEOPARD syndromes), but the lesions are either single or different in character. Isolated neurofibromas and familial café au lait spots (fewer than six and with no other manifestations of neurofibromatosis) have been described. The relationship of such cases to classic neurofibromatosis 1 is uncertain.

Complications

It is difficult to differentiate a complication from a rare manifestation of the underlying disorder. Seen in less than 25% of persons with neurofibromatosis are seizures, optic glioma, deafness, constipation, short stature, early puberty, and hypertension. Optic glioma seems to occur in about 15% of individuals with neurofibromatosis 1. Although the tumor may be apparent at an early age, it rarely causes functional problems and is usually nonprogressive. There is an increased risk for a variety of malignancies. Other tumors may be benign but may cause significant morbidity and mortality because of their location in a vital and closed space.

Treatment

Appropriate therapy should be initiated as each new manifestation arises. Neurofibromas can be removed, but removal is of limited help if they are multiple or in a vital area. The most important part of therapy is close, ongoing follow-up. Because this disorder is progressive, affected individuals should be seen at regular intervals and have regular eye examinations, hearing tests, and developmental screening, as well as other evaluations (eg, computed tomography [CT] scans) as indicated. This is best done in a multidisciplinary neurocutaneous clinic.

Prognosis

Because there is such variability in neurofibromatosis, it is difficult to assess the prognosis. However, most affected persons have only skin lesions and few other problems. Severely affected individuals are rare in the pediatric age range, and close follow-up and early intervention may ameliorate some complications.

Genetic Counseling

The gene for neurofibromatosis 1 was localized to the long arm of chromosome 17 in 1987 and partially cloned in 1990. It is very long and seems to code for a protein similar to a tumor suppressor factor. There are a variety of mutations in the gene for neurofibromatosis, including substitutions, deletions, and additions. Only a small percentage of the mutations can be identified, but the majority seem to code for a truncated protein. It is possible to screen for this truncated protein and identify an abnormality in about 70% of individuals with neurofibromatosis. In those cases, other affected family members can be identified and prenatal diagnosis is possible. If no abnormality is identified, there are numerous informative, flanking DNA probes that can be used in a high percentage of families for linkage analysis to identify those carrying the gene, including affected fetuses through prenatal diagnosis.

Approximately 50% of all cases of neurofibromatosis are felt to be caused by new mutations. Before attributing an individual case to a new mutation, however, both parents must be carefully evaluated, including a thorough examination of the skin and a slit-lamp examination to look for Lisch nodules. Recent evidence suggests that penetrance is close to 100% if individuals are carefully examined.

AUTOSOMAL RECESSIVE INHERITANCE

Autosomal recessive inheritance also has some distinctive characteristics:

(1) There is less variability among affected persons. Parents are carriers and are clinically normal. (There are exceptions to this rule, however. For example, sickle cell disease is considered recessive. Under normal circumstances, carriers—those with the sickle cell trait—are normal but may become symptomatic if they become hypoxic.)

(2) Both males and females are affected equally.

(3) Inheritance is horizontal; siblings may be affected, but both parents are normal (Figure 32–12).

(4) Recessive conditions are frequently rare; the rarer the condition, the more likely there is to be consanguinity. Conversely, if a child whose parents are related presents with an unrecognized abnormality, a recessive condition is likely.

(5) A negative family history is not unusual. In common conditions such as cystic fibrosis, there may be an affected second- or third-degree relative, but usually not. Because parents are clinically normal even though they are carriers, one must not be lulled into a false sense of security by the negative family history.

(6) Recessive conditions are frequently associated with enzyme defects. (See Chapter 26.)

(7) The recurrence risk is 25%, or 1:4 for each pregnancy. With a new partner, however, the risk drops and can be recalculated on the basis of the gene frequency in the population.

(8) In rare instances, a child with a recessive disorder and a normal karyotype may have inherited both copies of the abnormal gene from one parent and none from the other. This **uniparental disomy** was first described in a girl with cystic fibrosis and growth retardation. This phenomenon is of unknown frequency, but it is more likely to be present in a child with several autosomal recessive conditions or one who has some unexpected and seemingly unrelated abnormalities or severe growth retardation. Molecular testing can confirm the presence of uniparental disomy. The recurrence risk is obviously lower in such a situation, although it is not known what factors predispose an individual to uniparental disomy.

(9) Options available for future pregnancies include prenatal diagnosis in many cases and artificial insemination.

CYSTIC FIBROSIS

The gene for cystic fibrosis is one of the most common abnormal genes in the white population. Approximately 1:22 persons is a carrier. In 1985, the cystic fibrosis gene was located on the long arm of chromosome 7. In 1989, the gene for cystic fibrosis was cloned, and it was discovered that a three-base deletion coding for phenylalanine was present in the majority of cases. Subsequent studies have shown that the incidence of this delta F508 mutation varies with ethnic background and is present in about 75% of patients in North America and the United Kingdom, 50% in Spain, 43% in Italy, and 30% of individuals with Ashkenazic ethnic backgrounds. This gene is called the cystic fibrosis transmembrane conductance regulator (CFTR), which codes for a protein that functions as a chloride channel important in secreting chloride from the cell. It has been shown that the introduction of normal CFTR into cells with the cystic fibrosis gene will correct the biologic abnormality, raising the possibility of gene therapy. Trials have begun in which the gene is attached to a vector and delivered to the respiratory epithelium via an aerosol. This therapy is directed at somatic cells and will in no way affect the cystic fibrosis gene in germ cells. Although many unanswered questions remain, gene therapy for cystic fibrosis has exciting promise.

Cloning of the gene for cystic fibrosis and identification of the mutation in the majority of cases have completely changed genetic counseling and prenatal diagnosis for this disorder. Today, the affected child

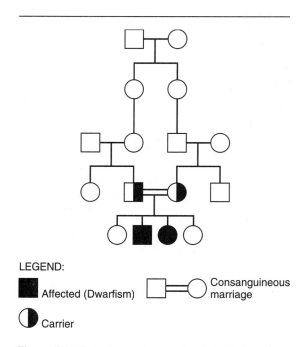

LEGEND:

■ Affected (Dwarfism)

◗ Carrier

□—○ Consanguineous marriage

Figure 32–12. Autosomal recessive inheritance: Rare form of dwarfism.

is studied using polymerase chain reaction (PCR) techniques to search for an identifiable mutation. If this is found, carriers can be identified and specific prenatal diagnosis can be performed, identifying both carriers and affected fetuses. If a mutation cannot be identified, then linkage analysis, DNA haplotyping, and amniotic fluid enzyme studies can be done. With continuing research, more mutations are being identified, but linkage analysis available today can achieve 90–99% accuracy.

The identification of the mutation in the cystic fibrosis gene has also raised the issue of mass screening because of the high frequency of this gene in the white population. While screening is definitely indicated in families with an affected member, mass population screening has not been recommended. Because all of the mutations have not yet been identified, a significant number of "negative" individuals will still carry a gene for cystic fibrosis. Although a specific risk could be calculated for each couple, the high false-negative rate and the counseling required for each couple tested make the value and cost-effectiveness of mass screening questionable at this time.

X-LINKED INHERITANCE

When a gene for a specific disorder is on the X chromosome, the condition is said to be X-linked, or sex-linked. Females may be either homozygous or heterozygous, because they have two X chromosomes. Males, by contrast, have only one, and an affected male is said to be hemizygous. The severity of any disorder is more consistent in males than in females (within a specific family). According to the Lyon hypothesis, because one of the two X chromosomes is inactivated and because this inactivation is random, the clinical picture in females depends on the percentage of mutant versus normal alleles inactivated. The X chromosome is not inactivated until about 14 days of gestation, and parts of the short arm remain active throughout life.

X-LINKED RECESSIVE INHERITANCE

The following features are characteristic of X-linked recessive inheritance:

(1) Males are affected, and heterozygous females are either normal or have mild manifestations.

(2) Inheritance is "diagonal" through the maternal side of the family (Figure 32–13).

(3) A female carrier has a 50% chance of having

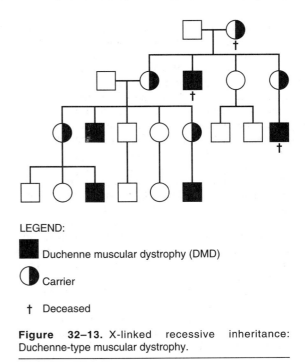

LEGEND:

■ Duchenne muscular dystrophy (DMD)

◑ Carrier

† Deceased

Figure 32–13. X-linked recessive inheritance: Duchenne-type muscular dystrophy.

carrier daughters and a 50% chance of having affected sons.

(4) All of the daughters of an affected male are carriers, and none of his sons are affected. Because a father can give only his Y chromosome to his sons, male-to-male transmission excludes X-linked inheritance except in the rare case of uniparental disomy, where a son receives both the X and the Y from his father.

(5) The mutation rate is high in some X-linked disorders, particularly when the affected male is infertile. In such instances, the mutation is felt to occur in the propositus in one-third of cases, in the mother in one-third of cases, and in earlier generations in one-third of cases. For this reason, genetic counseling may be difficult in families with an isolated case.

(6) On rare occasions, a female may be fully affected. Several possible mechanisms may account for a fully affected female: (a) unfavorable lyonization, (b) 45,X karyotype, (c) homozygosity in the female, (d) an X-autosome translocation in which the X chromosome of normal structure is preferentially inactivated, (e) uniparental disomy, and (f) nonrandom inactivation.

DUCHENNE-TYPE MUSCULAR DYSTROPHY

Duchenne-type muscular dystrophy has been recognized as an X-linked recessive condition for many years. There is also a milder type, Becker muscular dystrophy, which is allelic. The gene, now known to be in band Xp21, is one of the largest genes in the human genome, which may explain its high mutation rate. About 60–65% of families have a deletion in the gene. In rare cases, this may be visible on cytogenetic analysis, but molecular studies are usually required. Because of the length of the gene, there are many available informative restriction fragment length polymorphisms (RFLPs) both flanking and within the gene itself. This gene has been shown to encode mRNA for a protein called dystrophin, which is localized to the muscle surface membrane, the sarcolemma. Males with low or undetectable levels of dystrophin have Duchenne-type muscular dystrophy, whereas those with nearly normal levels but dystrophin of an abnormal size have Becker muscular dystrophy. New treatments, such as corticosteroids and even gene therapy, are being tried, but should be done only on a research protocol in a center for muscle disease.

If a deletion is present, it is usually apparent in the female carrier as well, using gene dosage studies. If there is no deletion, linkage studies, combined with creatinine kinase levels, help to predict female carriers in informative families with a high degree of probability. Negative studies in the mother, however, do not guarantee a negligible risk because of germ cell mosaicism. This may be present in 20–25% of the women, giving an actual recurrence risk of about 5–7% even with negative studies. Both deletion testing and linkage studies can be used to identify an affected fetus.

X-LINKED DOMINANT INHERITANCE

The X-linked dominant inheritance pattern is much less common than the X-linked recessive type. Examples include incontinentia pigmenti and hypophosphatemic or vitamin D–resistant rickets.

(1) The heterozygous female is symptomatic, and the disease is twice as common in females because they have two X chromosomes that can be affected.

(2) Clinical manifestations are more variable in females than in males.

(3) The risk for the offspring of heterozygous females is 50% regardless of sex.

(4) All of the daughters but none of the sons of affected males will have the disorder.

(5) Although a homozygous female is possible (particularly in an inbred population), she would be severely involved. All of her children would also be affected, but more mildly.

(6) Some disorders (eg, incontinentia pigmenti) are lethal in males (and in homozygous females). Affected women have twice as many daughters as sons and an increased incidence of miscarriages, because all affected males will be spontaneously aborted.

For more complete information about specific single-gene defects, see the McKusick reference cited at the end of this chapter.

MITOCHONDRIAL INHERITANCE

Some unusual disorders seem to be transmitted only by female members of a family and affect a high proportion of offspring, both male and female. Examples include Leber hereditary optic neuropathy, Leigh disease, MELAS (mitochondrial encephalomyopathy, lactic acidosis, and stroke-like episodes), and MERRF (myoclonic epilepsy and ragged red fibers). It is now known that these diseases are caused by mutations in mitochondrial DNA (mtDNA). Mitochondrial DNA is double-stranded, circular, and smaller than nuclear DNA and is found in the cytoplasm. It codes for enzymes involved in oxidative phosphorylation, which generates ATP.

There are several characteristics of mitochondrial disorders:

(1) All mitochondrial disorders show remarkable phenotypic variability.

(2) They are maternally inherited, because only the egg has any cytoplasmic material.

(3) All cells are heteroplasmic—that is, all cells contain both normal and mutated or abnormal mtDNA. The proportion of normal to abnormal mtDNA seems to determine the severity of the disease and the age at onset in most cases.

(4) Those tissues with the highest ATP requirements—specifically, central nervous system and skeletal muscle—seem to be most susceptible to mutations in mtDNA.

(5) There is an increase in somatic cell mtDNA mutations and a decline in oxidative phosphorylation function with age. This explains the later onset of some of these disorders and may indeed be a clue to the whole aging process.

POLYGENIC DISEASE
(Multifactorial Inheritance)

The inheritance of many common traits and abnormalities does not seem to be caused by a single gene. In the past, multiple genes, each with a small effect, as well as a variety of environmental factors were felt to be important, and the terms *polygenic* and *multifactorial inheritance* have been used. It is now felt that there may be a smaller number of genes involved, with one or more major genes important in each condition. The terms *oligogenic* and *multilocus* have been used to denote this more limited concept. Inherited in this way are a variety of normal traits, for example, height and intelligence, as well as a variety of common abnormalities, such as hypertension and allergies. It is important to realize that many of these conditions do not have a single cause and represent genetic heterogeneity or a group of diseases with common manifestations and different causes. In some conditions, there is an association with certain HLA types. For example, there is a high correlation between ankylosing spondylitis and HLA-B27. It is important to understand the difference between an association such as this and linkage of a certain disease with the HLA locus. In the latter instance, the gene for the disease is on chromosome 6, close to the HLA locus, but there is no association with a specific HLA type. Although the concept of polygenic inheritance has been questioned, many of the principles still hold true. The actual recurrence risks remain the same unless a broad category (eg, coronary artery disease, diabetes) can be subdivided and the consultand can be identified as being in a higher- or lower-risk group. For these reasons, the earlier terminology will be used in this section.

Many common congenital abnormalities, such as cleft lip and palate, neural tube defects, and some kinds of congenital heart disease, are inherited in a polygenic manner. If the combination of predisposing genes from both parents and certain environmental factors (mostly unknown) exceeds the "threshold," the abnormality then becomes manifest. Twin studies have been helpful in determining the relative importance of genetic versus environmental factors. If genetic factors are of little or no importance, then the concordance between monozygotic and dizygotic twins should be the same. (Dizygotic twins are no more genetically similar to each other than to other siblings.) If an abnormality is completely genetic, the concordance between identical twins should be lower than 100%. In polygenic conditions, the concordance rate for identical twins is higher than that seen in dizygotic twins, but lower than 100%, indicating both genetic and environmental factors.

Polygenic or multifactorial inheritance has some distinctive characteristics:

(1) The risk for relatives of affected persons is increased, and the risk is higher for first-degree relatives (those who have 50% of their genes in common) and lower for more distant relations, although the risk for the latter is higher than for the general population (Table 32–2).

(2) The recurrence risk varies with the number of affected family members. For example, after one child is born with a neural tube defect, the recurrence risk is 2–3%. If a second affected child is born, the risk increases to 10–12%. This is in contrast to single-gene disorders, in which the risk is the same no matter how many family members are affected.

Table 32–2. Empiric risks for some congenital disorders.

Mental deficiency of unknown cause: Incidence 3:1000
  Risks for siblings
    Both parents normal: 5–13% retarded
    One parent retarded: 20% retarded
    Both parents retarded: 42% retarded
Anencephaly and spina bifida: Incidence (average) 1:1000
  One affected child: 2–3%
  Two affected children: 10–12%
  One affected parent: 2–3%
Hydrocephalus: Incidence 1:2000 newborns
  Occasional X-linked recessive
  Often associated with neural tube defect
  Some environmental etiologies (eg, toxoplasmosis)
  Recurrence risk, one affected child
    Hydrocephalus: 1%
    Some central nervous system abnormality: 3%
Cleft lip and/or palate: Incidence (average) 1:1000
  One affected child: 2–4%
  One affected parent: 2–4%
  Two affected children: 10%
  One affected parent, one affected child: 10–20%
Cleft palate: Incidence 1:2000
  One affected child: 2%
  Two affected children: 6–8%
  One affected parent: 4–6%
  One affected parent, one affected child: 15–20%
Congenital heart disease: Incidence 8:1000
  One affected child: 2–3%
  One affected parent, one affected child: 10%
Clubfoot: Incidence 1:1000 (male:female = 2:1)
  One affected child: 2–3%
Congenital dislocated hip: Incidence 1:1000
  (female > male) with marked regional variation
  One child affected: 2–14%
Pyloric stenosis: Incidence, males: 1:200; females: 1:1000

Male index parent	
Brothers	3.2%
Sons	6.8%
Sisters	3.0%
Daughters	1.2%
Female index patient	
Brothers	13.2%
Sons	20.5%
Sisters	2.5%
Daughters	11.1%

(3) The risk is higher if the defect is more severe. In Hirschsprung disease, another polygenic condition, the longer the aganglionic segment, the higher the recurrence risk.

(4) Sex ratios may not be equal. If there is a marked discrepancy, the recurrence risk is higher if a child of the less commonly affected sex has the disorder. This assumes that more genetic factors are required to raise the more resistant sex above the threshold. For example, pyloric stenosis is more common in males. If the first affected child is a female, the recurrence risk is higher than if the child is a male.

(5) The risk for the offspring of an affected person is approximately the same as the risk for siblings, assuming that the spouse of the affected person has a negative family history.

CLEFT LIP & CLEFT PALATE

From a genetic standpoint, cleft lip with or without cleft palate is distinct from isolated cleft palate. The former is more common in males; the latter, in females. Although both can occur in a single family, particularly in association with certain syndromes, this pattern is unusual. There is racial variation in the incidence of facial clefting. Among Asians, whites, and blacks, the incidence is 1.61, 0.9, and 0.31, respectively, per 1000 live births.

Clinical Findings

A cleft lip may be unilateral or bilateral and complete or incomplete. It may occur with a cleft of the entire palate or just the primary (anterior and gingival ridge) or secondary (posterior) palate. An isolated cleft palate can involve only the soft palate or both the soft and hard palates. It can be a V-shaped or wide horseshoe cleft. A cleft associated with micrognathia and glossoptosis (a tongue that falls back and causes respiratory or feeding problems) is called Pierre Robin syndrome. Among individuals with facial clefts—more commonly those with isolated cleft palate—there is an increased incidence of other congenital abnormalities. The incidence of congenital heart disease, for example, is between 1% and 2%, but among those with Pierre Robin syndrome, it can be as high as 15%. Associated abnormalities should be identified in the period immediately after birth and before surgery.

Differential Diagnosis

It is important to remember that a facial cleft may occur in many different circumstances. It may be an isolated abnormality or part of a more generalized syndrome. Prognosis, management, and accurate determination of recurrence risks all depend on an accurate diagnosis. The following causes must be considered in individuals with cleft lip and cleft palate or isolated cleft palate:

(1) Environmental factors, for example, a history of use of anticonvulsants (especially phenytoin) by the mother, fetal alcohol syndrome, and amniotic band syndrome.

(2) Chromosome abnormalities, particularly trisomies 13 and 18 and 4p–.

(3) Single-gene disorders, including Van der Woude syndrome (an autosomal dominant condition characterized by lip pits and either cleft lip and palate or cleft palate). Treacher Collins syndrome (cleft palate), or Stickler syndrome (Pierre Robin syndrome with severe myopia, hearing loss, and arthropathies).

(4) Syndromes of unknown cause, such as Möbius syndrome (cleft palate) or Cornelia de Lange syndrome (cleft palate).

(5) Nonsyndromic. In the past, nonsyndromic cleft lip or cleft palate has been considered a classic example of polygenic or multifactorial inheritance. More recently, however, this mode of inheritance has been questioned, and several studies have suggested one or more major autosomal loci, both recessive and dominant or codominant. Empirically, however, the recurrence risk is still in the range of 2–3% because of nonpenetrance or the presence of other contributing genes.

Complications & Treatment

There are many problems associated with facial clefts, such as early feeding difficulties, which may be severe; recurrent serous otitis media associated with fluctuating hearing and language delays; speech problems, including hypernasality and articulation errors; and dental/orthodontic complications. Long-term management should ideally be through a multidisciplinary cleft palate clinic.

Genetic Counseling

Accurate counseling depends on accurate diagnosis. A complete family history must be taken, and both parents must be examined. The choice of laboratory studies is guided by the presence of other abnormalities and clinical suspicions. They may include chromosome analysis, eye examination, and x-ray studies. Clefts of both the lip and the palate have been detected on ultrasound prenatally, but intrauterine diagnosis is most likely in syndromes in which other, more serious abnormalities can be identified.

NEURAL TUBE DEFECTS

The term *neural tube defect* encompasses a variety of malformations, including anencephaly, spina bifida or myelomeningocele, sacral agenesis, sacral lipomas, and other spinal dysraphisms. Hydrocephalus associated with the Arnold-Chiari malformation is commonly seen with spina bifida at all levels. Sacral agenesis, also called the caudal regression syndrome, is seen more frequently in infants of diabetic mothers than in other infants.

Clinical Findings

At birth, neural tube defects can present as rachischisis at any level, as a fluid-filled sac that may or may not be leaking, or as a variety of skin-covered lesions associated with a fatty mass, a hemangioma, a tuft of hair, or asymmetric buttock creases. In the latter cases, CT or magnetic resonance imaging (MRI) studies should be conducted to look for bony and neural involvement. The extent of associated abnormalities depends on the level of the lesion and may include a variety of foot deformities, flexion contractures, dislocated hips, or total flaccid paralysis below the level of the lesion. Hydrocephalus may be apparent at birth, but more often there is an increase in head circumference, irritability, and poor feeding, with vomiting beginning shortly after the back has been closed. Neurogenic bladder and bowel may present as constant urinary dribbling, frequent stooling, and occasionally rectal or even vaginal prolapse. Urinary retention may also occur, particularly in the immediate postoperative period. There is also a higher incidence of unassociated abnormalities, particularly with higher lesions and anencephaly.

Differential Diagnosis

It is important to look for syndromes that may present as neural tube defects. Some chromosome abnormalities, congenital rubella, and the fetal valproic acid syndrome have been associated with neural tube defects.

Complications & Management

If the spinal defect is leaking or open at birth, the major concerns are infection and drying of the nerve roots, leading to further loss of function. For this reason, surgical closure is recommended as soon as possible. The infant should be closely monitored, and a shunt, usually ventriculoperitoneal, should be inserted as soon as signs of hydrocephalus become apparent. The shunt may need to be replaced if it becomes obstructed, infected, or separated, or it may need to be lengthened as the child grows. There has been much discussion about whether true shunt independence ever develops. The signs and symptoms of chronic shunt malfunction may be very insidious and consist only of slow deterioration of school performance or staring spells. Hydromyelia may develop and lead to progressive scoliosis; sudden death has also been ascribed to shunt malfunction in adults with spina bifida.

The child's ability to walk varies according to the level of the lesion. Children with low lumbar and sacral lesions walk with minimal support, those with high lumbar and thoracic lesions are rarely functional walkers, and those with midlumbar lesions vary. In any case, the child should receive physical therapy and assume the upright position at the appropriate developmental age. Orthopedic surgery may be necessary to get the child upright and ambulatory.

Concerns about the bladder begin at birth. The bladder may be small and spastic or large and hypotonic; the sphincter may be flaccid or tight. The child may therefore be constantly wet because the bladder holds little urine, or there may be incomplete emptying of the bladder and ureteral reflux. In the latter case, there is a high risk for urinary tract infections. In addition, there may be a problem called "bladder dyssynergy." Normally, when the bladder contracts, the sphincter relaxes, allowing for an unimpeded flow of urine. In a dyssynergic state, the sphincter also contracts, predisposing the patient to urethral reflux. Management is guided by the results of early studies to determine the type of bladder present. Continence can be achieved in a variety of ways. In most cases, medications are necessary, such as anticholinergic agents to relax the smooth muscle of the bladder or alpha-sympathomimetic drugs to increase bladder outlet resistance. The mother and ultimately the child are taught the technique for clean intermittent catheterization. If the child still cannot achieve continence, a surgical procedure may be required. If the bladder is small, with increased tone, augmentation using a portion of bowel may be necessary to prevent reflux and upper tract deterioration. These procedures improve urinary retention and decrease leakage, but they usually require intermittent catheterization as well to ensure complete emptying. Renal function should be monitored regularly and an ultrasound examination should be performed annually. Symptomatic infections should be treated.

Bowel control can be more of a problem, because a lax sphincter and poor peristalsis predispose to constipation and poor emptying. The principles of management include increasing the bulk of the stool to facilitate spontaneous and more complete evacuation and at the same time keep the child as free from accidents as possible. This is done with a combination of a high-fiber diet, fluids, and suppositories. Enemas, digital stimulation or evacuation, and surgical procedures have been used as well.

Areas of skin anesthesia or hypesthesia roughly correlate to motor level. Skin breakdown is always a threat, and skin care must be meticulous. If skin breakdown does occur, all pressure must be relieved, the wound kept clean, and an artificial skin dressing used to promote healing. Surgical closure is sometimes required. The advantages of prevention over treatment cannot be emphasized too strongly.

Recently, it has become apparent that children with spina bifida and urinary tract anomalies have a significant risk for type I (IgE-mediated) allergic reactions to latex. Symptoms may vary from urticaria to anaphylaxis during surgery. Some but not all children will have a history of allergic reactions to rubber. It is difficult to predict who has this sensitivity. Skin tests are poorly standardized and carry some risk. The IgE radioallergosorbent test (RAST) is helpful if positive, but it is not 100% sensitive. It has been predicted that up to 40% of children with spina bifida are latex-sensitive, with the incidence increasing with age. Recognition of this problem and the avoidance of latex products is essential.

There is a wide range of intellectual capacity in children with neural tube defects, but most function at the low normal to borderline levels. Most children are now mainstreamed, but they have a higher incidence of fine motor and visual-perceptual problems. Because of early aggressive care, most children with neural tube defects now survive into adolescence, when different problems become apparent. The introduction of MRI has demonstrated that most individuals with spina bifida have tethered cords. Many are asymptomatic, but others develop back or leg pain, change in bladder function, change in motor or sensory level, spasticity, or scoliosis. These symptoms may develop at any age, and prompt surgical intervention is necessary, as lost function may not be regained. Scoliosis may also become apparent in adolescence and may be associated with syringomyelia or a tethered cord. Neurologic evaluation is indicated before scoliosis surgery. Respiratory compromise and even sleep apnea may occur. A small percentage of patients have progressive loss of renal function secondary to chronic infection and stones despite aggressive treatment, and some develop renal failure. Problems with bowel management and skin breakdown increase as individuals become obese and less ambulatory. The major problems, however, are psychosocial. The transition into independent adulthood is very difficult because of poor social skills, limited social contacts, inferior education, and poor preparation for the competitive work world.

Individuals with closed spinal cord abnormalities (eg, sacral lipomas) have similar problems, although hydrocephalus is rarely seen and intelligence is usually normal. Early surgical treatment is important to preserve function and prevent further disability secondary to cord tethering. Because needs are ongoing and management approaches change with time, all children with spinal defects of any type should be followed up in a multidisciplinary clinic.

Genetic Counseling

Recurrence risks vary according to etiology, but most neural tube defects are polygenic, with a recurrence risk of 2–3%. The risk for the offspring of an affected person is essentially the same. There would be a considerably higher risk if the anencephaly or encephalocele were associated with renal abnormalities or polydactyly, as seen in Meckel-Gruber syndrome. Prenatal diagnosis is available, and pregnancies can be monitored in a variety of ways. In fetuses with open neural tube defects, serum alpha-fetoprotein levels, measured at 16–18 weeks of gestation, are elevated. Routine screening has also been recommended by the American Academy of Obstetrics and Gynecology. Alpha-fetoprotein levels in amniotic fluid are also elevated, and amniocentesis combined with experienced ultrasound studies will detect more than 90% of neural tube defects. Recent studies have shown that folic acid can significantly lower the incidence of neural tube defects, but the folic acid must be taken *prior* to conception. It is now recommended that all women of childbearing age take 0.4 mg of folic acid daily. This can be achieved by dietary modification (see Table 11–8) or by taking a multivitamin capsule once daily that contains 0.4 mg of folic acid. For the woman at increased risk because of a previous child with a neural tube defect, the current recommendation is to increase folic acid intake to 4 mg when a pregnancy is planned. There is no evidence that the use of folic acid will prevent other midline defects or other types of anomalies.

American Academy of Pediatrics Committee on Genetics: Health supervision for children with neurofibromatosis. Pediatrics 1995;96:368.

Austin KD, Hall JG: Nontraditional inheritance. Pediatr Clin North Am 1992;39:335.

Carey JC: Health supervision and anticipatory guidance for children with genetic disorders (including specific recommendations for trisomy 21, trisomy 18, and neurofibromatosis 1). Pediatr Clin North Am 1992;39:25.

Coutelle C et al: Gene therapy for cystic fibrosis. Arch Dis Child 1993;68:437.

Hardesty RA (editor): Advances in management of cleft lip and palate. Clin Plastic Surg 1993;20(4).

Heim RA et al: Screening for truncated NF1 proteins. Nature Genet 1994;8:218.

Huson SM, Hughes RCA (editors): *The Neurofibromatoses: A Pathologic and Clinical Overview.* Chapman & Hall, 1994.

Korf B: Molecular medicine: Molecular diagnosis. N Engl J Med 1995;332:1218, 1499.

Miller RG, Hoffman EP: Molecular diagnosis and modern management of Duchenne muscular dystrophy. Neurol Clin 1994;12:699.

Recommendations for use of folic acid to reduce number of spina bifida cases and other neural tube defects. JAMA 1993;269:1233.

Rekate HL (editor): *Comprehensive Management of Spina Bifida.* CRC Press, 1991.

Shoffner JM, Wallace DC: Mitochondrial genetics: Principles and practice. Am J Hum Genet 1992;51:1179.

Shprintzen RJ, Bardach J: *Cleft Palate Speech Management: A Multidisciplinary Approach.* Mosby, 1995.

IV. DYSMORPHOLOGY

Morphogenesis is the complex process that forms the structures necessary for survival; dysmorphology tries to understand how this process is altered to produce birth defects. Birth defects affect 2–3% of infants and can be found in up to 7% of adults. They are now the leading cause of death in the first year of life.

MECHANISMS OF DYSMORPHOGENESIS

Most birth defects occur because normal development has been altered by abnormal interactions between genetic and environmental factors. Specific causes, however, are recognized in only about 30% of cases.

GENETIC FACTORS

Single-gene defects and chromosome abnormalities account for about 25% of birth defects. Several recognizable phenotypes have now been associated with specific chromosomal lesions, and the mapping of individual genes that contribute to morphogenesis is gaining momentum.

Two recent advances that have revolutionized the field of teratology, the study of mechanisms of birth defects, are (1) the recognition that the genetic control of development is homologous across species and (2) development of transgenic animals.

The major themes of embryology and the genes that regulate them have been conserved throughout evolution. The picture of development that is emerging from experimental data attributes the regulation of axis formation, segmentation, and position to transcription factors, proteins that bind DNA to regulate gene expression. Three families of genes encoding transcription factors—Hox (also called homeobox or homeotic genes), Pax, and Sox—initiate cellular differentiation and organogenesis in *Drosophila,* rodent, and human embryos. Structures then take shape under the guidance of growth factors, peptides, and sterols that communicate the messages of organogenesis to groups of cells expressing specific receptors. Fibroblast growth factor 4 (FGF4), for example, plays a critical role in limb formation. Cellular adhesion molecules accomplish the same kinds of communication through cell-cell interactions.

Much of the spatial information needed to assemble and complete an organism is contained in the extracellular matrix. Matrix proteins interact to form polymers that bring growth factor–like motifs into fixed positions. They provide frameworks for differentiation and paths for cell migration.

Human birth defects are now becoming understood in light of these embryologic insights. Among these are achondroplasia, now known to result from mutations in the gene for FGF4 receptor protein; aniridia and other eye defects, caused by mutations in PAX 6; X-linked hydrocephalus, resulting from mutations in the gene for the cellular adhesion molecule L1CAM; and craniosynostosis syndromes, resulting both from FGF receptor mutations and from mutations in homeotic genes.

Perhaps the most powerful tool in the field of developmental biology is now the transgenic mouse. Briefly, mice are made chimeric at the blastocyst stage of development by addition of multipotential stem cells into which various exogenous genes (transgenes) have been incorporated. These chimeric animals are then bred, and their offspring that carry the experimental gene are referred to as "transgenic."

Transgenic mice provide a powerful experimental model because, depending on how the addition of the transgene has been accomplished, its function during development can be studied by causing its overexpression or by knocking it out and then observing the effects.

Genes that contribute to multifactorial disorders, including birth defects, are also being isolated through linkage studies. Mapping and sequencing the human genome is making it possible to track the segregation of multiple loci through families in which genetic predisposition to multifactorial processes is evidenced in affected members. This strategy is now beginning to localize candidate genes whose altered expression is involved in such common abnormalities as cleft lip and palate.

ENVIRONMENTAL FACTORS

Epidemiologic studies consistently indicate that certain environmental factors (eg, season, residence, occupation, socioeconomic status, and exposures to drugs, chemicals, and environmental contaminants) contribute to risks for congenital malformations, but few specific human teratogens have been identified. Among these are congenital infections (see Chapter 34), a dozen or so prescribed drugs, a growing list of abused substances, and a few well-documented environmental agents, including ionizing radiation in doses exceeding 10–50 cGy, methyl mercury, lead, and industrial products contaminated with dioxins.

Although animal studies have traditionally been used to assess reproductive risks, more recent applications attest to their greater value as models for investigation of teratogenic mechanisms. The following principles of reproductive toxicology were formulated in animal models but are directly relevant to human birth defects:

(1) Most chemicals and drugs capable of being absorbed into the maternal circulation will also equilibrate across the placenta.

(2) Drugs, toxins, and hazardous physical agents are teratogenic through dose-dependent mechanisms. Hence, the level of exposure is an important consideration in risk assessment. For prescribed and abused substances, transplacental levels are expected to be high enough to be pharmacologically active. For environmental contaminants, transplacental levels will reflect the level of exposure. Most exposures that do not produce maternal signs and symptoms will not achieve toxic concentrations in the conceptus. Exceptions such as lead and other heavy metals that are concentrated by placental mechanisms, however, demonstrate the need for caution and continued surveillance.

(3) Extensive preclinical testing of pharmaceuticals and selection of agents with low reproductive toxicities are useful and provide some measure of re-

assurance, particularly for over-the-counter agents. However, idiosyncratic reactions, that is, toxicities or hypersensitivities that occur in predisposed individuals, probably do occur during development. Most idiosyncratic reactions will reflect genetically determined sensitivities.

(4) Genetic polymorphisms for drug receptor-effector systems and for drug metabolism contribute significantly to risks for reproductive toxicity. Excellent examples of these effects are provided by animal models of facial clefting and spina bifida. Associations between birth defects and polymorphisms in drug-metabolizing enzymes indicate the role that drug distribution may play in dysmorphogenesis.

DEVELOPMENTAL FACTORS

Embryonic and fetal development are classically presented in morphogenetic stages during which individual organs pass through their critical periods (Figure 32–14). Some familiarity with both developmental biology and descriptive human embryology is essential for a clinical approach to birth defects.

Development begins through the ordered expression of genes; first, maternal transcripts present in the ovum, then products expressed from the newly conceived genome.

Research into the regulation of gene expression during development has intensified following the discovery that epigenetic modification of DNA, called imprinting, is active during mammalian development. **Parental imprinting** is the term geneticists use to describe the process whereby the expression of a gene is determined by the sex of the parent from which it is inherited. The phenomenon is readily demonstrated in transgenic mice. Its molecular basis is not entirely understood, but involves at least sex-dependent modification of DNA by addition of methyl groups (DNA methylation).

Parental imprinting is becoming an important clinical consideration. Examples include the central role of imprinting in the expression of the Angelman and Prader-Willi phenotypes, as discussed above, where the syndrome produced depends on the respective loss of maternally or paternally inherited portions of chromosome 15. Imprinting also affects expression of the gene for insulin-like growth factor 2 (IGF-2), a developmentally important protein. The gene for IGF-2 is located on chromosome 11, and it is the paternally derived allele that is expressed. Partial duplication of this region of paternally derived chromosome 11 results in Beckwith-Wiedemann syndrome (a syndrome of multiple congenital anomalies, including omphalocele, macroglossia, hemihypertrophy, and neonatal hypoglycemia that is associated with increased risk for development of Wilms tumor), which can also be produced by loss ("relax-

ation") of maternal imprinting leading to overexpression of IGF-2 during fetal development.

Although the contributions of developmental biology to clinical dysmorphology are rapidly expanding, it remains practical to consider maldevelopment within a descriptive division of gestation into five phases.

The **first phase**—preconception—includes gametogenesis and fertilization, during which new mutations frequently occur. The **second phase**—implantation—begins with fertilization and is complete by 13–14 days. During this period, the blastocyst invades endometrium, and the placenta differentiates and begins to function. In humans, placentation precedes organogenesis. Although the trophoblastic tissues that separate maternal and embryonic circulation are readily permeable by most xenobiotics (compounds foreign to the biologic system), environmental exposures during this stage of development are not often associated with birth defects. The reason for this is unclear, but the phenomenon could be explained by spontaneous abortion during implantation. A final common pathway for pregnancy loss during this period may be trophoblast failure.

The **third phase** of prenatal development is organogenesis, extending from the second to the eighth weeks following conception. Most critical periods of organ formation occur during this stage; thus, most structural abnormalities can be traced to these or preceding weeks. Although considerations of teratogenic mechanisms necessarily concentrate on this stage of development, it should not be assumed that adverse effects of environmental agents or genetic disorders are limited to this period.

The **fourth phase**—fetal development (weeks 9–38 postconception)—is the longest phase of human gestation. During this stage, cytotoxicity is less likely to be expressed as a structural defect but is not necessarily less likely to occur. Although organs are formed by this time, functional differentiation and growth occur during these weeks. This is an especially important period for the brain. Investigators in the field of behavioral teratology are just beginning to study relationships between events in fetal life and later brain function.

The **fifth** and **final phase** of intrauterine development is the intrapartum period. Fetal presentation at the time of delivery as well as the route of delivery and any trauma sustained can affect morphologic features in the neonate. Many apparently abnormal findings are related to molding of the head or the position of the extremities and are transient in nature.

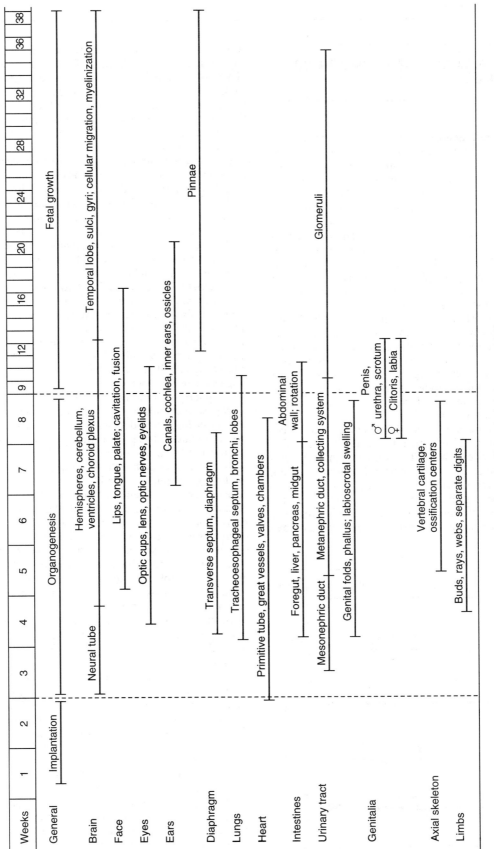

Figure 32–14. Critical periods in human gestation.

CLASSIFICATION OF DYSMORPHIC FEATURES

Accurate diagnosis is the key to prognosis and management of birth defects. Recognition of specific syndromes and patterns of maldevelopment can be extremely valuable but is often difficult in the neonatal period. A dysmorphologist should be consulted, if possible, but classification of defects by etiology can also be useful and requires less expertise than does recognition of specific syndromes. The approach to classification taken here begins with an attempt to distinguish intrinsic from extrinsic causes on the basis of the history and physical examination. The goal is to assign anomalies found to one of the etiologic categories listed in Figure 32–15.

Malformations are the result of intrinsically abnormal processes of development. The conceptus is abnormal from the outset of gestation, and malformations are generally attributed to genetic processes. The characteristic morphologic features of Down syndrome and the hypoplastic thumbs and pancytopenia associated with Fanconi syndrome are classified as malformations.

Disruptions are the result of extrinsic processes. Development is perceived as proceeding normally when factors external to the conceptus interfere at a cellular level. Note that "external factors" also include maternal factors. Drug-related embryopathies such as those attributed to the use of thalidomide are prototypical disruptions, but multifactorial processes also include neural tube defects. The distinction between a disruption and a malformation may be difficult to discern on the basis of form alone. Careful histories—especially family histories and cytogenic studies—are imperative. It is easier to establish the classification of malformation on the basis of a positive family history or abnormal karyotype than it is to rule out a disruption. Disruptions, however, may be far more common.

Deformations are the result of extrinsic mechanical forces. Deformations rarely involve internal organs but may range from minor malpositioning of limbs to major disturbances of the head and trunk. Intrauterine problems resulting in deformations include multiple pregnancies, abnormal uterine shape, fetal positioning, rupture of the amnion, and oligohydramnios caused by loss of or failure to produce fluid or by failure of the fetus to urinate. Deformations are characteristically asymmetric. Deforming processes may bend, amputate, or fuse structures.

Dysplasias occur as a result of abnormal tissue differentiation. In theory, extrinsic processes may be involved, but intrinsic, genetically determined factors are most often responsible. Dysplasias emphasize the link between cell function and morphogenesis. Examples include osteogenesis imperfecta (a disorder in which poorly ossified bone is easily fractured) and mucopolysaccharidoses (inborn errors of metabolism that result in growth deficiency, skeletal abnormalities, and unusual facies). Most dysplasias are the result of single-gene mutations.

Recognition of pathogenesis influences prognosis. Finding a deformation, for instance, means that the development and function of unaffected organs will be normal. However, deformation that arises from neurologic abnormality carries a poorer prognosis. Many dysplasias are not recognizable in the neonatal period. Those presenting at birth (eg, thanatophoric dwarfism) frequently have poor prognoses. Disruptions are probably the most common cause of birth defects and demonstrate the vulnerability of the developing human to extrinsic factors. Isolated disruptions, such as congenital heart defects, have excellent prognoses if repair is possible. Malformations are often multiple and, like dysplasias, often have poor prognoses.

Pathogenetic categorization may also help estimate risks for recurrence. The highest risks are associated with single gene disorders, producing dysplasias and malformations. Most chromosomally mediated malformations occur sporadically, but careful cytogenetic analyses of family members may be required. Risks for recurrence are higher if parents carry balanced translocations. Disruptions also tend to occur sporadically, but many are the result of multifactorial processes with substantial genetic input, as evidenced by higher risks for recurrence in relatives of affected infants. Isolated deformations that do not occur as a result of uterine abnormalities have a low risk for recurrence.

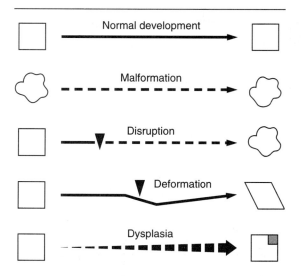

Figure 32–15. Etiologic classification of congenital anomalies.

MULTIPLE MALFORMATIONS

Many dysmorphic infants have more than one abnormality. Recognition of relationships between multiple malformations also provides important clues to etiology and prognosis.

A **developmental field** is a region or a group of cells in an embryo that responds as a coordinated unit to intrinsic or extrinsic stimuli. The pathogenesis of developmental field defects may involve functional disturbances in primordial cells, interactions among tissues, or processes common to multiple tissues. Disturbances of rostral mesoderm, for instance, may lead to multiple anomalies of the head and face. Genital and cardiac abnormalities may be related through disturbances in other organs, such as the hypothalamus or vascular structures.

A **sequence** is a pattern of anomalies caused by a single event. Renal agenesis, for instance, results in decreased amniotic fluid, fetal compression, pulmonary hypoplasia, and limb deformation. This same sequence may occur as a result of loss of amniotic fluid or urethral obstruction. The sequence of micrognathia, glossoptosis, and cleft soft palate (Pierre Robin syndrome) may begin with mandibular hypoplasia, which pushes the developing tongue posteriorly so that it interferes with movements of the posterior palatal shelves.

The term **association,** when used to describe multiple anomalies, refers to their nonrandom occurrence outside any known developmental field. It denotes statistical but not necessarily causal relationships. The pathogenesis may involve both developmental field defects and sequences. Knowledge of associations is useful because it alerts the clinician to investigate other specific organs further if a defect is recognized in one.

The term **syndrome** is applied to patterns of multiple anomalies that recur with such regularity that they are considered to be pathogenetically related. Down syndrome and Williams syndrome are disorders with morphologic features found in individuals with specific chromosome abnormalities: trisomy 21 and deletion chromosome 7q11.2, respectively.

DYSMORPHIC PATTERNS IN NEONATES

The following are examples of patterns of maldevelopment recognizable in the neonate. Numerous other patterns have been described in older children. Photographs of these entities are available in Jones's *Smith's Recognizable Patterns of Human Malformation.*

It should be emphasized that many syndromes and conditions presenting in childhood are not recognizable in the neonate. Clinicians may frequently be forced to wait for infants to "grow into" recognizable syndromes.

Chromosome Abnormalities

Several chromosome abnormalities are recognizable in neonates. These include trisomies 21, 13, and 18 and monosomy X (Turner syndrome). Chromosome abnormalities should be considered in the evaluation of all infants with multiple anomalies.

The triad of intrauterine growth retardation, major or multiple minor malformations, and poor adaptation to extrauterine life should always be investigated cytogenetically. Note that breech presentation at term, polyhydramnios, and unexplained low Apgar scores may be important symptoms of central nervous system maldevelopment.

Of the numerous other conditions presenting in newborns, the following recognizable patterns are emphasized because they have important prognostic implications.

Cornelia de Lange Syndrome

Cornelia de Lange syndrome, a sporadically occurring constellation of congenital anomalies, has typical features that can be recognized in the newborn. Intrauterine growth retardation and characteristic facial features, including prominent eyebrows with central fusion (synophrys) and thin, downturned lips, are invariable. These infants are hirsute, and limb abnormalities occur in over 50%. Hypoplasia of the hands and feet is common, but major limb reductions occur in 30% and frequently involve the ulnar—rather than the radial—ray. One affected infant in four has congenital heart disease. No specific chromosome abnormalities have been found. The immediate prognosis depends largely on the presence of congenital heart disease or respiratory failure. Subsequent failure to thrive and severe mental deficiency are the rule.

Shprintzen-DiGeorge Spectrum

DiGeorge syndrome was originally reported as a constellation of congenital heart disease (abnormalities of the great vessels), thymic aplasia, and hypoparathyroidism. It was often clinically recognized by unusual facial features and hypocalcemia in newborns with heart disease. Shprintzen syndrome (velocardiofacial syndrome) was associated with cleft palate with congenital heart disease of various types, nasal prominence, and elongated fingers. Both disorders are now recognized as members of a dysmorphologic sequence resulting from deficient input and migration of rostral neural crest cells. An exciting development is the association of both phenotypes with deletions at chromosome 22q11. These can be detected by FISH probes. Such deletions may account for as many as 5% of congenital heart defects.

Smith-Lemli-Opitz Syndrome

Smith-Lemli-Opitz syndrome is a recessive condition characterized by intrauterine and postnatal growth failure, microcephaly, large ears, and unusual facies typified by a short, upturned nose and palatal ridging. Hypogenitalism and at least partial syndactyly of the toes are invariable. Polydactyly may also be present. The disorder has recently been shown to be the result of deficient synthesis of cholesterol and can be diagnosed by detecting elevated levels of cholesterol precursors.

VATER (VACTERL) Association

Vertebral anomalies and abnormalities of the heart, trachea, esophagus, kidneys, and limbs are found in association with each other and in association with anal atresia more often than would be expected by chance alone. The acronym VATER (*ver*tebral defects, imperforate *a*nus, *t*racheo*e*sophageal fistula, and *r*adial and *r*enal dysplasia) is sometimes written as VACTERL to include *c*ardiac and *l*imb anomalies. The limb defects seen are usually preaxial (radial or fibular). The association occurs sporadically. Although the anomalies themselves may be immediately or ultimately life-threatening, neurologic abnormalities are absent, and the prognosis for intellectual development is good if the VATER association is recognized early enough for proper treatment to be instituted.

CHARGE Association

The CHARGE association—*c*oloboma, *h*eart disease, choanal *a*tresia, *r*etarded growth, *g*enital anomalies, and *e*ar anomalies—was recognized through nonrandom association of facial anomalies. More recently, maldevelopment within a developmental field involving neural crest cells has been suggested. The importance of recognizing this condition is that the central nervous system is involved and that hypothalamic maldevelopment may affect secretion of pituitary trophic hormones.

Arthrogryposis Multiplex

Lack of movement in utero produces joint contractures. These may affect a single extremity, as in clubfoot, but are potentially much more ominous when they involve multiple joints. This phenotype is etiologically extremely heterogeneous. The differential diagnosis of multiple joint contractures in the neonate must carefully consider external causes (deformation); abnormalities of bones, joints, and connective tissue; maldevelopment or injury of the central nervous system; and myopathic processes. The prognosis in this condition is also extremely variable and usually cannot be determined without evaluation by multiple disciplines (neurology, clinical genetics, orthopedics, etc). Imaging and cytogenetic, biochemical, and electrophysiologic studies are frequently indicated. Muscle biopsy may also need to be considered.

Amnion Rupture Sequence

Rupture of the amniotic membrane in early gestation may lead to loss of fluid and entrapment of the developing conceptus. Early rupture is often associated with major structural abnormalities that are incompatible with life. Later rupture may lead to complex deformations of the head and limbs or to amputation of structures by constricting amniotic bands. It may be difficult to distinguish these deformations from malformations unless the placenta is carefully examined for the presence of amniotic bands. If the head has escaped significant deformation, neurologic development proceeds normally. The amniotic rupture sequence occurs sporadically, and its recognition allows counseling for low recurrence risks.

Twins

Multiple pregnancies are at high risk for abnormal development. Crowding may result in deformations in both identical and nonidentical twins. In one sense, monozygosity itself is a "birth defect," because it occurs after conception. Depending on the timing of division, placental circulations and amniotic sacs may or may not be shared. Division after day 13 of gestation results in conjoined twins. Despite genetic concordance, congenital abnormalities in monozygotes are frequently discordant. This observation demonstrates the role of environmental factors in multifactorial birth defects. Monochorionic twins are particularly at risk for abnormalities resulting from vascular accidents, because emboli are more likely to form in shared circulations.

Skeletal Dysplasias

Several distinct dysplasias of bone and cartilage produce a phenotype with short, curved, or malformed limbs. The head and trunk may appear normal in a few of these disorders, but more frequently there is a protuberant abdomen with or without ascites. Many of these dysplasias result in death from pulmonary hypoplasia associated with small or poorly compliant chest walls. The differential diagnosis of skeletal dysplasias presenting with respiratory compromise includes achondrogenesis, osteogenesis imperfecta, camptomelic syndrome, asphyxiating thoracic dystrophy, thanatophoric dwarfism, and several other rare syndromes. Achondroplasia, the most common short-limbed skeletal dysplasia, does not compromise development of the chest. Many of these disorders are the result of new dominant mutations, but recessive inheritance must always be considered. Accurate diagnosis is extremely important and is best made radiographically. Films should include all extremities. A lateral view of the spine, which may be critical to the diagnosis, should be obtained as well. The immediate prognosis depends largely on the extent of pulmonary hypoplasia. Long-term prognoses are variable.

DYSMORPHIC PATTERNS IN CHILDREN

The reader is referred to the general references at the end of this chapter for detailed information about the large number of recurrent patterns of maldevelopment now recognized in older children. Recognition of these phenotypes (ie, physical, developmental, and behavioral characteristics) often requires direct experience with rare syndromes. Diagnosis usually requires consultation with experienced clinical geneticists. The four examples that follow are phenotypic diagnoses commonly suspected by general pediatric practitioners. They are presented to illustrate the approach taken by clinical geneticists to confirm diagnoses in referred cases.

Noonan syndrome is recognized in children who have short stature, low-set ears, characteristic facies with downslanting palpebral fissures, webbed neck, and congenital heart disease, typically atrial septal defects or abnormalities of the pulmonary outflow tract. Arrhythmias and abnormal conduction are frequent. The syndrome can be inherited as an autosomal dominant trait, but because its features change with age, affected parents or other older relatives may be difficult to recognize. Affected children are large for gestational age at birth and may have had mild subcutaneous edema recognized prenatally by ultrasonography. The classic phenotype is usually present by school age, but by adulthood it may have further evolved in less predictable fashion, with variability in stature and associated findings such as hearing loss. The diagnosis may require follow-up of suspected cases over years with careful attention paid to ruling out other conditions.

Williams syndrome is also recognized by a phenotype that evolves over years. The classic pattern of findings includes supravalvular aortic or pulmonary stenosis, growth and developmental delays, blue eyes with stellate irides, and characteristic facies often described as elfin in young children but which tend to coarsen with age. An overly friendly, outgoing personality characteristically develops. The disorder is not typically familial. Disturbances of calcium metabolism with increased absorption and urinary excretion can sometimes be documented, but these findings appear to be transient in many cases. Because the phenotype evolves over time, it may not be suspected until after urinary calcium excretion has normalized. The diagnosis was formerly made on the basis of accumulating clinical findings after other disorders affecting growth and development had been ruled out. The diagnosis can now be confirmed in more than 90% of cases by cytogenetic studies utilizing fluorescent in situ hybridization (FISH) with a chromosome 7q probe specific for the region of the elastin gene. Follow-up of this diagnosis is particularly important because significant medical problems such as hypertension, renal complications, and degenerative spinal problems may develop in adults.

Disorders of connective tissue are frequently suspected in children with hyperextensible joints. Important diagnoses included in the differential for this finding are **Ehlers-Danlos syndrome** (for which 10 clinical subtypes have been described) and **Marfan syndrome,** an autosomal dominant disorder in which abnormal elastic tissue can lead to dislocation of lenses and development of aortic aneurysms. Many connective tissue disorders are dominantly inherited, in which case positive family histories and findings become important diagnostic criteria. However, both disorders also are encountered as new mutations, in which case the diagnosis may again depend on evolution of the phenotype over years. Minimal criteria for Ehlers-Danlos syndrome include clinically apparent involvement of skin and, for subtype classification, changes in other structures, such as joints and teeth. Care must be taken in distinguishing between connective tissue disorders, in which low muscle tone is the rule, and myopathies, in which muscle weakness leads to hyperextension of joints in young children. Careful neurologic examination with attention to reflexes is imperative. In Marfan syndrome, hyperextensibility of joints is accompanied by alterations in growth, especially of extremities. Lens dislocation, which can be pathognomonic, is inconsistently present and may not develop until late childhood or adulthood. Widening of the aortic root, another hallmark of the disorder, also may not develop for years. Marfan syndrome results from mutations in genes for fibrillin, an elastin-associated protein. Mutation analysis is not yet a clinically practical approach to diagnosis in isolated cases, but, in the presence of a positive family history, linkage studies can confirm clinical impressions.

DRUG-RELATED DISORDERS

Thalidomide is the classic example of a human teratogen producing a specific syndrome. The compounds discussed below are also associated with specific abnormalities. Regional teratogen information services can provide additional information.

Anticonvulsants

There is now general agreement that exposure to anticonvulsant drugs increases risks for maldevelopment. Significant abnormalities may occur as frequently as once in every 10 pregnancies in this population. Growth of the brain and mid face are consistently affected. A recognizable "fetal anticonvulsant syndrome," initially described in association with phenytoin use, has now also been reported in children exposed in utero to carbamazepine and valproic acid. Additional structural anomalies are also associated with exposures to individual agents. Maternal use of phenytoin has been associated with cleft lip and palate, hypoplasia of distal phalanges and nails, and sacral teratomas. Maternal use of trimethadione has also been associated with growth retardation, decreased mentation, and unusual facies (fetal trimethadione syndrome). An increased risk for neural tube defects has recently been linked to maternal use of valproic acid.

Isotretinoin

Excessive doses of vitamin A have long been recognized as teratogenic in animals. The potent vitamin A analogue isotretinoin (Accutane) was therefore considered a potential teratogen when it was introduced as treatment for acne. Despite warnings, some women have taken this drug during pregnancy, and several infants with multiple anomalies have been born. A specific syndrome that includes abnormalities of the central nervous system, ears, and great vessels along with hypoplasia of the thymus and parathyroid gland has been described. This condition is a partial phenocopy of the **DiGeorge sequence** that occurs as a contiguous gene syndrome related to microdeletions of chromosome 22. It is now clear that both isotretinoin and the deletion produce the same developmental field defect. The mechanism involves failure of cells to migrate normally from the neural crest to form structures in the head and neck.

Ethyl Alcohol

Admonitions against heavy use of alcohol during pregnancy have been given since ancient times. More recently, a specific syndrome has been recognized in the offspring of heavy drinkers. The fetal alcohol syndrome consists of intrauterine and postnatal growth retardation, microcephaly, significant mental dysfunction, and craniofacial changes including short palpebral fissures, short nose, and a long, smooth philtrum. A variety of other structural abnormalities has also been reported.

Although it is clear that high concentrations of alcohol are cytotoxic, the mechanisms of alcohol toxicity are poorly understood. The dose-response relationship is not entirely clear, but maternal alcohol intake exceeding 2–3 oz daily is considered toxic. The timing of fetal exposure to alcohol is important. Structural abnormalities occur with increased frequency in the offspring of chronic alcohol abusers, but neurologic abnormalities can be decreased if women stop drinking by 16–20 weeks of gestation. Approximately two-thirds of pregnancies in active alcoholics will have significant complications, including prematurity, growth retardation, and perinatal asphyxia. Fetal alcohol syndrome is seen in about one-third of offspring of active alcoholics. Previous attempts to associate a specific phenotype with fetal alcohol effects (FAEs) have proven unreliable, and this terminology is now being dropped from the lexicon of dysmorphology.

Cocaine

As use of cocaine has increased, its effects on pregnancy have become more evident. Stimulation of the central and peripheral sympathetic nervous systems by cocaine can produce intense uterine vasoconstriction, leading to placental ischemia and abruption. Cocaine readily crosses the placenta and is active in the fetal circulation. Ischemic injury occurs in fetal limbs, intestines, and kidneys, and the central nervous system appears to be particularly vulnerable. Intracranial hemorrhage and porencephalic cysts have been reported in as many as one-third of infants born to women abusing crack cocaine in combination with alcohol and other substances.

Inhalants

Abuse of inhalants is widespread and includes sniffing glue, gasoline, spray paints, and other hydrocarbons. Toxic effects in users lead to a chronic organic brain syndrome and hepatotoxicity. These agents are absorbed into the maternal central circulation through pulmonary veins and delivered as highly concentrated boluses to the placenta and fetal circulation. It is now recognized that inhalant neurotoxicity in fetuses results in microcephaly and a syndrome of growth retardation similar to fetal alcohol syndrome.

CLINICAL APPROACH TO THE DYSMORPHIC INFANT

Physicians caring for neonates with birth defects must frequently provide care and make accurate diagnoses under conditions of great stress. The extent of an infant's abnormalities may not be immediately apparent, and parents who feel grief and guilt are often desperate for information. As with any medical problem, however, the history and physical examination provide most of the clues to diagnosis. Special aspects of these procedures are outlined below.

HISTORY

Environmental, family, and pregnancy histories may contain important clues to the diagnosis. Parental recall after delivery of an infant with an anomaly is better than recall after a normal birth. An obstetric wheel can help document gestational age and events of the first trimester: the last menstrual period, the onset of symptoms of pregnancy, the date of diagnosis of the pregnancy, the date of the first prenatal visit, and the physician's impressions of fetal growth at that time.

To investigate fetal growth and development, prenatal visits should be noted and, with the aid of the obstetric wheel, a record should be made of the patterns of fetal growth, the onset of fetal movement (usually at 16 weeks), and the mother's perceptions of fetal movements. Normal fetal movement is usually strong enough to hurt the mother and be visible to the father. Abnormal fetal movement may indicate neuromuscular dysfunction or fetal constraint. A history of decreased fetal movement will often distinguish neuromuscular abnormalities (which result in a low Apgar score) from intrapartum events (which depress the infant).

Abnormal patterns of uterine growth may also provide clues to fetal function. Increased uterine size may indicate accumulation of amniotic fluid (hydramnios). Fluid may accumulate if the fetus fails to swallow as a result of a neuromuscular disorder, obstruction of the fetal esophagus or proximal small bowel, or fetal heart failure. Hydramnios is also associated with diabetes and high-output renal failure in the fetus. Lack or delay of uterine growth may reflect fetal growth directly or may indicate too little amniotic fluid (oligohydramnios). Amniotic fluid may be lost through premature rupture of membranes with or without formation of amniotic bands, or it may be the result of compromised function of fetal kidneys. The mother should be questioned about loss or leakage of amniotic fluid, which may have been mistaken for a vaginal discharge.

The history should also include details about the onset and progression of labor. Breech presentation at term may indicate a uterine anomaly or abnormality of the fetal central nervous system.

Family histories should always be included but may seem threatening to parents or relatives attempting to cope with strong feelings about birth defects. The interviewer should be prepared to respond to specific questions from family members.

Finally, an environmental history that includes descriptions of parental habits, their work, and the home should be obtained.

PHYSICAL EXAMINATION

Meticulous physical examination is crucial to accurate diagnosis in dysmorphic infants. Delivery of an affected infant may necessitate immediate attention to potentially life-threatening problems, but it is precisely because intensive support may be required that a complete examination becomes urgent. The examination should be performed as soon as possible.

In addition to the routine procedures described in Chapter 4, special attention should be paid to the neonate's physical measurements (Figure 32–16). Photographs are very helpful and should include a scale of measurements for reference. The placenta should also be examined.

Measurement	Range (cm)	
	Term (38–40 weeks)	Preterm (32–33 weeks)
1 Head circumference	32–37	27–32
2 Anterior fontanelle $\left(\frac{L-W}{2}\right)$	0.7–3.7	. . .
3 Interpupillary distance	3.3–4.5	3.1–3.9
4 Palpebral fissure	1.5–2.1	1.3–1.6
5 Inner canthal distance	1.5–2.5	1.4–2.1
6 Outer canthal distance	5.3–7.3	3.9–5.1
7 Philtrum	0.6–1.2	0.5–0.9
8 Ear length	3–4.3	2.4–3.5
9 Chest circumference	28–38	23–29
10 Internipple distance*	6.5–10	5–6.5
11 Height	47–55	39–47
12 13 Ratio $\dfrac{\text{Upper body segment}}{\text{Lower body segment}}$	1.7	. . .
14 Hand (palm to middle finger)	5.3–7.8	4.1–5.5
15 Ratio of middle finger to hand	0.38–0.48	0.38–0.5
16 Penis (pubic bone to tip of glans)	2.7–4.3	1.8–3.2

*Internipple distance should not exceed 25% of chest circumference.

Figure 32–16. Neonatal measurements.

LABORATORY STUDIES

Radiologic and ultrasonographic examinations can be extremely helpful in the evaluation of dysmorphic infants. In general, films of infants with apparent limb or skeletal anomalies should include views of the skull and all of the long bones in addition to frontal and lateral views of the axial skeleton. Chest and abdominal films should be obtained when indicated. The pediatrician should consult a radiologist for further workup. Nuclear scans and imaging by CT, MRI, and ultrasonography are all useful diagnostic tools, but their interpretation in the presence of birth defects may require considerable experience.

Cytogenetic analysis provides specific diagnoses in approximately 5% of dysmorphic infants who survive the newborn period. Chromosome abnormalities are recognized in 10–15% of infants who die. Karyotypes can be determined rapidly through analysis of cells in bone marrow. These allow limited interpretation and should always be accompanied by complete analysis of cultured cells. Any case requiring rapid diagnosis should be discussed with an experienced dysmorphologist. A normal karyotype does not rule out the presence of significant genetic disease.

PERINATAL AUTOPSY

When a dysmorphic infant dies, postmortem examination can provide important diagnostic information and should include sampling of tissue for cytogenetic analysis. The pediatrician and the pathologist should consider whether samples of blood, urine, or tissue should be obtained for metabolic analyses. X-ray studies should be done whenever limb anomalies or disproportionate growth is present. Placental as well as fetal tissue can be used for viral culture. The pediatrician should discuss the case thoroughly with the pathologist, and photographs should always be taken.

Hall JG, Fnoster-Iskenium UG, Allanson JE: *Handbook of Normal Physical Measurements.* Oxford Univ Press, 1989.

Spranger J et al: Errors of morphogenesis: Concepts and terms. Recommendations of an international working group. J Pediatr 1982;100:160.

Stevenson RE, Hall JG, Goodman RM (editors): *Human Malformations and Related Anomalies,* Vols 1 and 2. Oxford Univ Press, 1993.

Wynne-Davies R, Hall C, Apley A: *Atlas of Skeletal Dysplasias.* Churchill Livingstone, 1987.

V. GENETIC COUNSELING

ISSUES

Genetic counseling is more than just a communication process about the risk for recurrence of genetic disorders in a family. When families come for counseling, specific questions need to be addressed:

(1) What is the problem? An accurate *diagnosis* is the sine qua non of genetic counseling.

(2) What does it mean? For a family to make informed decisions concerning future pregnancies, they must understand the *prognosis* of the disorder. The

birth of an infant with anencephaly is undoubtedly a traumatic experience, but caring for a child with a high myelomeningocele poses greater long-term stresses.

(3) What caused the abnormality? Determination of *etiology* is essential for correct counseling. The risk for recurrence of cleft lip and palate caused by amniotic bands is minimal, whereas the risk for recurrence of Van der Woude syndrome could be 50%.

(4) Is it curable or treatable? Possible *therapy*—its success, burden, and expense—needs to be discussed.

(5) Will the problem recur in future pregnancies? Only after the first four questions have been addressed can meaningful *recurrence risk figures* be given. At this time, it is often necessary to review with the family some basic genetic information, showing pictures of chromosomes, explaining the difference between chromosomes and genes, and diagramming the more common mechanisms of inheritance.

(6) Can the abnormality be prevented or anticipated in future pregnancies? This question brings up the issue of *prenatal diagnosis* and other options available to the couple.

This may appear to be a formidable list of questions for the counselor to address, and answers may come from other members of the genetic counseling team and appropriate consultants. In addition, ongoing psychologic support is essential throughout the counseling process.

PROCESS

History

The cornerstone of a genetic evaluation is a thorough history, both of any pregnancy that resulted in an abnormal infant and of the family in general. Issues to be addressed in the pregnancy history include problems conceiving, bleeding, maternal illnesses or exposures, medications, smoking, the use of alcohol or other recreational drugs, possible exposures to teratogens, and lifetime histories of both parents' exposure to x-rays. Information such as onset, intensity, and distribution of fetal activity may help to differentiate a prenatal from a postnatal problem. It is often helpful to ask whether this pregnancy was "different" from others in any way. Information about the delivery should be obtained from birth records whenever possible. A family history should always be taken in a pedigree form. Parental ages, recurrent miscarriages, stillbirths, and infant deaths are all important. The possibility of consanguinity should be explored by asking for common family names and family origins. The general health and development of all first- and second-degree relatives should be ascertained. Information about ethnic background may be valuable. It is sometimes hard to know how extensive the family history should be. This depends to some extent on what may be suspected, but the major limiting factor is availability of information. Often, couples need to explore their family history in more depth, and objective documentation should be assembled if that is possible.

Physical Examination

The type of examination done as part of a genetic evaluation differs from others in that minor abnormalities are stressed as well as more obvious defects. It may also be necessary to examine parents, siblings, and even more distant relatives to make or confirm a diagnosis. Photographs should be obtained when relatives cannot be examined.

Laboratory Tests

The need for specific laboratory tests varies with the situation. Because these tests are expensive, they should be ordered with care, but they should certainly be done when important information can be gained. Chromosome analysis is indicated in any child with multiple major or minor anomalies, particularly if associated with mental retardation or developmental delay. High-resolution analysis or parental chromosomes may also be appropriate. Fragile X testing should be done in instances of mental retardation of unknown cause. Molecular testing is not routine but may be of value in particular families.

COUNSELING

Much has been written about directive versus nondirective genetic counseling, but in the United States at least, the latter is recommended and more widely practiced. Although it is difficult to be totally objective, particularly if the geneticist is familiar with the long-term burden of a disorder, it is important to remember that the ultimate choice belongs to the parents. A geneticist may have concerns about society at large, but a counselor should be the advocate for the family, not for society. The timing of genetic counseling is also important. There is a fine line between counseling that is too early (because the family, still concerned about the welfare of the affected person, is emotionally unprepared) and counseling that is too late (because another at-risk fetus has already been conceived). The possibility of a genetic basis for the mishap should be mentioned early, but continuing contact is needed to refine the diagnosis and help the family understand the implications.

There are many ways to communicate information to the parents, but all explanations should be given in language that the family can understand and in a relaxed and unhurried atmosphere. The baseline risk for congenital abnormalities should be discussed and put into the perspective of the risk being quoted. The actual risk should be compared with the burden (or

the parents' perception of the burden) of the abnormality in question. Examples can be helpful. The issues of guilt and blame must be addressed. This part of counseling can be difficult if one of the parents carries an abnormal gene or used a teratogenic substance, such as cocaine or alcohol. Ongoing psychologic counseling may be needed. It may be difficult for parents to understand how an isolated abnormality in a family can still be genetic and be associated with a significant recurrence risk; it may be necessary to review with them such concepts as phenocopy, new mutations, decreased penetrance, and variable expressivity.

All too often, no specific diagnosis can be made and no cause can be determined. In these cases, recurrence risks can only be estimated. It may be helpful for families to explore possible mechanisms and for the geneticist to discuss the implications for subsequent pregnancies. In any case, parents should consider their own emotional response to the birth of a second affected child.

Genetic counseling is not a static process. Families often continue to have questions. A letter explaining clearly and concisely the information covered in the counseling session is helpful. Although a geneticist cannot assume responsibility for all problems a family may have, appropriate referrals can be made. Continued contact is advisable to ensure adequate understanding and reopen counseling as new information and testing become available. A social worker, genetic nurse, or genetic associate who is a member of the counseling team is an ideal person to maintain contact.

A word should be said about responsibility to the extended family. As more genetic disorders become diagnosable by new molecular techniques, counseling needs to be expanded to the family at large. This requires both the cooperation of the consultand and collaboration between genetic units throughout the country. During counseling, it is necessary to educate families concerning this need and at the same time respect confidentiality.

OPTIONS

In situations of increased risk, families have a variety of options. They can have no further children or they can take the risk, but in many cases there are more and better choices. Some families for whom prenatal diagnosis is unacceptable or unavailable may prefer adoption. Artificial insemination is genetically appropriate if a disease is recessive or if the father is the carrier, and in vitro fertilization with donor ova if the mother is the carrier. Preimplantation diagnosis of an embryo obtained after in vitro fertilization with maternal eggs and paternal sperm is theoretically possible in many single-gene conditions. A successful pregnancy has followed this procedure done to rule out cystic fibrosis in the embryo. However, this is still experimental and is of limited availability. Even if it were more available, cost might be a determining factor in its application. Some families may consider sterilization, but they should realize that the risk for each of the parents may drop markedly if in the future the couple should separate and remarry. For most families, however, some type of prenatal diagnosis is requested and often available. All of these options are expensive. Prevention of an abnormality is, of course, the ideal. To date, the use of periconceptional folic acid is the only known effective preventive agent other than the avoidance of teratogenic substances such as alcohol and cocaine. Technology has outstripped society's responsiveness to the needs of these families. This problem must be addressed in the future.

PRENATAL DIAGNOSIS

It has been estimated that prenatal diagnosis is indicated in 7–8% of all pregnancies. As technology improves, the indications for and the accuracy of prenatal diagnosis can only increase. Today, a large proportion of pregnant women undergo at least one ultrasound study during pregnancy, and more congenital abnormalities are being detected prior to birth even in low-risk women. Prenatal diagnosis introduces options for management that range from interruption of abnormal pregnancies to preparation for specialized perinatal care.

METHODS

Prenatal diagnosis techniques analyze maternal blood, image the conceptus, and sample fetal and placental tissues.

Maternal Blood

The use of maternal serum alpha-fetoprotein as a screening test was originally introduced because elevated values were found in association with neural tube defects. It was also noted that women who carried a fetus with Down syndrome had a 25% lower value compared to those in whom the fetus was normal. Combining this test with maternal age enabled about 20% of fetuses with trisomy 21 to be detected in women under 35 years of age. Subsequent studies have shown that adding measurements of human chorionic gonadotropin and unconjugated estradiol can increase rates of detection.

Fetal cells, including lymphocytes, trophoblasts, and nucleated red blood cells, are present in maternal circulation. Research is being directed toward isolating these cells for prenatal diagnosis using culture, hybridization, and PCR-based techniques.

Testing of Fetal Tissue

Amniocentesis has been available for many years. Its accuracy and safety are well established. Fluid surrounding the fetus is sampled and cells are cultured for cytogenetic or metabolic analysis. Alpha-fetoprotein and other molecules can also be measured. This is a safe procedure with a complication rate (primarily for miscarriage) of less than 1% in experienced hands.

Chorionic villus sampling (placental) is now available in most centers and can be performed late in the first trimester. Tissue obtained by chorionic villus sampling provides DNA for molecular analysis and contains dividing cells (cytotrophoblast) that can be rapidly karyotyped. However, direct cytogenetic preparations may be of poor quality. In addition, chromosomal abnormalities detected by this technique may be confined to the placenta (confined placental mosaicism). Cultured preparations may be more accurate. Certainly, if an unusual cytogenetic picture is found on chorionic villus sampling, further studies should be considered before management decisions are made. Numerous studies have been done comparing the safety of first-trimester chorionic villus sampling with amniocentesis. Of some concern is the possible association of chorionic villus sampling prior to 11 weeks with terminal transverse limb defects, perhaps secondary to vascular disruption.

Fetal blood can be directly sampled in late gestation through ultrasound-guided percutaneous umbilical blood sampling (PUBS).

It is occasionally necessary to biopsy fetal tissues such as liver (eg, in ornithine transcarbamylase deficiency) or muscle (eg, in cases of Duchenne muscular dystrophy in which mutation analyses and linkage studies are uninformative) for accurate prenatal diagnosis. These procedures are available in only a few perinatal centers.

Fetal Visualization

Transabdominal real-time **ultrasonography** can view all major fetal organs, including the kidneys, heart, brain, spinal cord, bladder, and limbs beginning as early as 16–18 weeks' gestation. Transvaginal ultrasonography is now providing even earlier imaging. It is therefore possible to look for almost any genetic syndrome that includes a specific defect. Routine ultrasound screening has demonstrated many unexpected abnormalities. Most of these are major defects, however, and minor anomalies are easily missed, especially if unexpected.

X-ray studies of the fetus are rarely necessary because ultrasonography has improved so greatly. If a skeletal abnormality or bone dysplasia is suspected, however, x-ray films may be helpful.

INDICATIONS

Amniocentesis or chorionic villous sampling is indicated in the following instances:

(1) Maternal age over 35 years.

(2) Previous child with a chromosome abnormality.

(3) Either parent a translocation carrier. In this case, the risk for a fetus with an unbalanced chromosome abnormality depends on the type of translocation.

(4) A history of any genetic disorder diagnosable by biochemical techniques or by DNA analysis. The list of such conditions changes daily, and a genetic center should be contacted for the most recent information.

(5) A request by the parents for fetal sexing because of a history of an X-linked disorder that is not otherwise diagnosable.

(6) Maternal blood testing (eg, triple test) indicating increased risks for chromosomal abnormalities.

(7) As part of the workup of fetal anomalies found by ultrasonography.

Fetal ultrasonography is indicated whenever an abnormality characterized by a structural defect is suspected. The defect may be suspected because of the family history, potential teratogenic exposure during pregnancy, or questionable abnormalities noted on a routine ultrasound examination done in the obstetrician's office. In any case, the patient should be referred to a medical center experienced in fetal ultrasonography for further evaluation.

D'Alton ME, DeCherney AH: Prenatal diagnosis. N Engl J Med 1993;328:114.

Simpson JL, Elias S (editors): *Essentials of Prenatal Diagnosis.* Churchill Livingstone, 1993.

REFERENCES

Buyse ML: *Birth Defects Encyclopedia.* Blackwell, 1990.

Emery AEH, Rimoin DL: *Principles and Practice of Medical Genetics,* 2nd ed. Churchill Livingstone, 1990.

Gorlin RJ, Cohen MM, Levin LS: *Syndromes of the Head and Neck,* 3rd ed. Oxford Univ Press, 1990.

Jones KL: *Smith's Recognizable Patterns of Human Malformation,* 5th ed. Saunders, 1996.

King RA, Rotter JI, Motulsky AG: *The Genetic Basis of Common Diseases.* Oxford Univ Press, 1993.

McKusick VA: *Mendelian Inheritance in Man,* 11th ed. Johns Hopkins Univ Press, 1994.

Stevenson RE, Hall JG, Goodman RM (editors): *Human Malformations and Related Anomalies,* Vols 1 and 2. Oxford Univ Press, 1993.

33

Allergic Disorders

David S. Pearlman, MD, Leon S. Greos, MD,
& Joanne M. Vitanza, MD

Allergic disorders include a variety of local and systemic manifestations of the union between antigen (allergen) and antibody. Although this union triggers the chain of events that culminates in the clinical allergic reaction, nonimmune factors are important in modifying this chain of events and, in some instances, can be completely responsible for clinical reactions which are indistinguishable from immune-induced reactions.

Allergic reactivity involves a variety of immune mechanisms and is one way the body deals with foreign substances. Some forms of allergic reactivity, however, occur only in certain members of the population. These disorders (allergic rhinitis, asthma, atopic dermatitis) are called **atopic disorders,** a term signifying a form of reactivity for which there is a familial and genetic association. An individual with such a disorder commonly responds to substances usually considered innocuous to other people. These include animal danders, spores from molds, house dust mites, pollens, and foods. Responses are caused by IgE antibody produced to these substances. However, atopic disorders can occur even in the apparent absence of sensitization.

It is a misconception that allergic disorders are commonly outgrown. Rather, they frequently are lifelong and can take an enormous toll in morbidity, on physical and emotional development, on family economics, and, in a small but significant number, in mortality. The pediatrician alone and with the allergist and other specialists has an opportunity to make an important impact in controlling disease activity and in preventing the chronicity of allergic disease which begins in childhood.

PRINCIPLES OF DIAGNOSIS

The diagnosis of allergic disease is based primarily on clinical findings. Diagnosis requires a detailed history and physical examination. Laboratory procedures, including allergy testing, can be very helpful, but results should be interpreted in light of the history.

History

Obtain the chief complaint.

History of the Present Illness: Inquire about the nature of symptoms, their severity, date of onset, occurrence in relation to location, and seasons in which symptoms occur. Note daily activities with which the symptoms interfere (school, work, sleep, recreation). Ask which environmental factors and exposures trigger symptoms. (However, in the case of chronic symptoms, patients may not be aware of specific triggers.) Obtain details of and responses to treatments utilized.

History of Other Allergic Diseases: Inquire about associated atopic disease (past or present), including allergic rhinitis/hay fever, asthma, atopic dermatitis, and other allergic problems, such as food allergy, hives, insect allergy, and drug allergy.

History of Complicating Illnesses: Ask the patient about a history of and frequency of infections, including pneumonia, bronchitis, croup, otitis media, and sinusitis.

Family History: Inquire whether immediate family members (parents, siblings) have a history of allergic rhinitis, asthma, or atopic dermatitis. There is approximately a 30–60% chance of a child's having atopic disease when one parent is allergic, and a 60% or greater chance when both parents are affected.

Environmental History: A thorough history is important, including the age of the home, length of time in the home, any relationship between moving into the home and the onset of or change in symptoms, and exposures to animals and cigarette smoke. Inquire about the type of heating (including wood-burning stoves) and air conditioning, use of humidifiers, presence of mold or mildew in the home, details of the patient's bedroom (mattress, bedding, pillow types, types of floor and window coverings, amount of toys and stuffed animals, location of the bedroom within the home). Information regarding the patient's school, day care center, or baby-sitter's home (amount of time spent there, number of children, presence of pets and cigarette smoke) is important.

Other: The history should include immunization

history, hospitalizations, surgeries (including tonsillectomy, adenoidectomy, ear ventilation tubes), all other medical problems, and systems review. In addition, a complete list of current medications should be obtained (prescription and over-the-counter).

Physical Examination

The following signs deserve special emphasis:

General Appearance of the Patient: State of health, nourishment and physical development, presence of cough and its character, coloration, presence of respiratory distress, adenoidal facies, mouth breathing.

Vital Signs: Height and weight.

Skin: Presence, location, and type of rash; degree of dryness of the skin; cyanosis.

Eyes: "Allergic shiners" (lower lid edema, eye shadowing), conjunctival injection, eye discharge and watering, cataract formation, blepharitis.

Nose: Degree of nasal mucosal edema, mucosal color, presence and type of nasal secretions (clear, mucoid, or purulent), polyps, septal position and integrity, nasal crease (horizontal skin fold across the nose), allergic salute.

Ears: Appearance and movement of the tympanic membrane, movement, evidence of fluid in the middle ear.

Mouth: Palatal malformations.

Throat: Appearance of the tonsils, presence of posterior pharyngeal lymphoid tissue, presence and character of secretions, stridor.

Chest: Configuration of the chest, evidence of hyperinflation, pattern of breathing, use of accessory muscles of respiration, presence of retractions.

Lungs: Presence of wheezing and its relationship to the inspiratory and expiratory cycles, whether wheezing can be heard after exertion or with forced exhalation or chest compression; presence of rhonchi or rales; degree and equality of air exchange.

Heart: Murmurs, arrhythmias, accentuation of the pulmonic (second) heart sound (as would be found with pulmonary hypertension in severe asthma).

Abdomen: Hepatic or splenic enlargement.

Lymphatic: Lymph node enlargement in the cervical, axillary, and inguinal regions.

Diagnostic Procedures

Allergy Testing: In all atopic disorders, testing for the presence of IgE antibodies to allergens is potentially useful in identifying or excluding allergens that may play a role in the disease.

Skin Tests: There are two methods of skin testing: the prick-puncture method, wherein an allergen extract is introduced into the epidermis; and intradermal testing, wherein the extract is injected into the dermis. Generally, prick-puncture testing should be done before intradermal testing because it is less likely to cause severe reactions in highly sensitive individuals. Intradermal testing is more sensitive than prick-puncture testing, but more false-positive reactions occur. Intradermal testing to foods is not recommended because of the potential for severe adverse reactions and because of frequent false-positive or irritant responses. Allergy skin tests make use of the biologic amplification of the allergen–IgE antibody reaction on mast cells, which release chemical mediators responsible for the manifestations of allergic reactions. IgE antibody is formed elsewhere in response to allergen exposure, circulates, and adheres to receptors in mast cells, which are abundant in skin and other tissues; the skin serves as a sensitive and readily accessible site to test for allergic sensitivity. A positive test is indicated by erythema and wheal formation at the test site and by itself only indicated the presence of specific antibody in the skin. Whether a positive test is of clinical importance can be determined only in the context of the patient's history. Skin testing should be performed with allergens that are likely to be relevant to the patient's exposure. Negative and positive control tests are important to ensure the validity of test results. Skin testing is potentially dangerous in highly sensitive individuals.

Serologic Tests: Immunoassays that detect the presence of circulating IgE can be used. There are many different types of assays; the prototype for these is the radioallergosorbent test (RAST). Results of RAST generally correlate well with those of skin tests, although they are somewhat less sensitive than skin tests. Thus, they are not as reliable when high sensitivity is of the utmost importance (eg, when detecting specific IgE to a potentially life-threatening allergen, such as venom or penicillin in a patient with a history of anaphylaxis). RAST is useful for testing individuals in whom skin testing is difficult (eg, patients with extensive eczema or dermatographia). False-positive immunoassays may occur if the total IgE level is extremely elevated. As with skin tests, the clinical significance of RAST results must be interpreted in light of the patient's history; a laboratory or a physician who does not have information from evaluating the patient directly is not in a position to make the best judgment for the patient.

Measurement of Total IgE Level: Elevated IgE levels suggest an atopic disorder, but the correlation is so imperfect that this is not a generally useful procedure. Greatly elevated IgE levels in infancy (>2 SD above the mean) are highly predictive of an atopic diathesis, and elevated IgE levels in bronchiolitis suggest the diagnosis of asthma. However, a normal or low level of IgE does not rule out an atopic disorder or allergic sensitization.

Provocative Testing: This procedure involves challenging a patient with a suspected allergen and observing the response. Provocative tests are most valuable in determining clinical sensitivity to foods, especially since false-positive skin and serologic tests to foods are common. Elimination and subsequent challenge may be revealing if done properly, but also can be misleading if an objective protocol for assessing the response is not followed. Provocative testing to a food should not be performed with a substance suspected of causing a life-threatening reaction. Provocative inhalant testing is potentially hazardous and generally is not used in clinical practice. Provocative testing (eg, to exercise, for bronchial hyper-responsiveness to methacholine) can be helpful in establishing or supporting a diagnosis of asthma when diagnosis in uncertain.

Eosinophilia: Increased numbers of eosinophils in the blood or bodily secretions (nasal, bronchial, gastrointestinal) are frequently present in a variety of allergic conditions; the presence of eosinophilia may strengthen a suspicion of allergic diathesis. Nasal eosinophilia (>15%) is highly suggestive of allergic rhinitis, but eosinophilia can occur in the absence of clinical allergy. Conversely, the absence of eosinophilia does not rule out allergy, particularly because of a variety of factors (eg, concurrent infection, use of corticosteroid) that may suppress eosinophilia. Nasal eosinophilia in infants up to 3 months of age may be normal.

Controversial Techniques for Diagnosis & Treatment: Intracutaneous end-point titration, measurement of food-specific antibody, measurement of food immune complexes, sublingual and intracutaneous provocation-neutralization tests, and cytotoxic tests all have been claimed to be of value in diagnosing and treating allergic disorders. Their merit has yet to be validated scientifically, however, and they remain techniques of unproved value that are not recommended.

Nelson HS: Variable in allergy skin testing. Allergy Proc 1994;15:265.
O'Connell EJ et al: Selecting the right test for presumed allergy. J Respir Dis 1995;16:476.
Ownby DR, Adinoff AD: The appropriate use of skin testing and allergen immunotherapy in young children. J Allergy Clin Immunol 1994;94:662.
Terr AI: Unconventional theories and unproven methods in allergy. In: *Allergy: Principles and Practice,* 4th ed. Middleton E Jr et al (editors). Mosby, 1993.

GENERAL PRINCIPLES OF TREATMENT

Environmental Control of Exposure

Avoidance of offending agents, both allergic and nonallergic, is the most effective means of therapy for all atopic disorders. As continued exposure to an allergen can heighten sensitivity to other, unrelated allergens and to nonallergic irritant by a "priming" phenomenon, avoidance measures are essential to therapy, particularly in chronic allergic disorders. In many instances, complete avoidance of significant al-

lergens is impossible, but it is frequently feasible to reduce the incidence and severity of reactions by minimizing exposure. Many nonimmune factors can precipitate or aggravate atopic disorders (eg, cigarette smoke, fumes, odor, cold air in asthma), and avoidance of such known or suspected irritants is also important to effective management.

Environmental control measures to reduce exposure to common indoor allergens are important to implement in the patient's bedroom, but the principles should be kept in mind throughout the rest of the home as well.

The ingredients of house dust (mites, cockroaches, indoor mold spores, dander from cats, dogs, and other mammalian house pets) are common offenders. The accumulation of dust may be minimized by the avoidance of dust collectors and dust producers, including wool (rugs, blankets), flannel (bedding, pajamas), cotton stuffing (upholstered furniture, stuffed toys, quilts), chenille (bedspreads, drapes, rugs), kapok (rug pads), venetian blinds, and carpets. For maximal elimination of dust mite exposure in particular, carpet should be removed from the child's bedroom and replaced with linoleum, tile, or a wooden floor. A washable throw rug may be a satisfactory alternative to carpeting.

Mattresses, box springs, and polyester pillows in the bedroom should be completely enclosed in impermeable casings. Inexpensive plastic casings may be obtained from department stores; better-quality casings may be obtained from medical suppliers. All bedding above this encasing should be washed weekly in hot water. Furniture and bedding stuffed solely with synthetic or "hypoallergenic" materials are preferred; foam rubber may harbor molds. Toys may be restuffed with old nylon stockings and should also be washed regularly. Even products stuffed solely with synthetic material will accumulate dust and its component allergens in time; these products should be covered or periodically replaced. The bedroom should be dusted and vacuumed at least weekly. This cleaning should not be done with the allergic child present.

Forced air ducts act as a reservoir for dust and mold and thus should be commercially cleaned periodically or should be sealed off. An electric radiator may be substituted as a source of heat, if necessary. If pollinosis is a problem, windows should be kept closed during the pollen seasons; air conditioners are useful to keep homes closed up in warm weather months. Air cleaners (central or room) are helpful to reduce both irritant and allergen exposure: electrostatic or high-efficiency particulate air (HEPA) filters are most effective. Automatic humidifiers with provision for humidity not to exceed 50% can be helpful in dry climates. Humidifiers should be cleaned frequently to be kept as free of mold as possible. In humid climates where dust mite and mold sensitivity is more of a problem, dehumidification to relative humidity less than 50% is appropriate.

Sensitization to animals develops so frequently in atopic individuals that close contact with furry animals of any kind is best avoided—pelt danders, saliva, and urine (rodents) are the important sources of animal allergen. Despite many myths, length of animal hair has not been demonstrated to be relevant to allergenicity. However, different animals excrete differing quantities of allergenic proteins, which may explain patients' observations of differing responses to individual animals of the same species. Depending on the degree of sensitivity, it may be important to rid the environment of animals altogether. If this is not possible, keeping the animal out of the bedroom at all times and the use of a HEPA filter in the bedroom may help.

Immunotherapy (Hyposensitization)

If avoidance of offensive allergens is not possible, allergen-specific immunotherapy may be indicated. There are a variety of immunotherapy procedures, but the same general principle applies to all: extremely small amounts of allergen are injected subcutaneously at frequent intervals and in increasing amounts until a maximal dose is reached; this is usually the highest tolerated dose of a given allergen extract or that amount which has been demonstrated to reduce clinical reactivity to the allergen as observed after natural contact. The effectiveness of immunotherapy is dose-related. Most commonly, perennial therapy is utilized, and the maximally tolerated dose is continued as a "maintenance" dose at gradually lengthened intervals, generally up to 4 weeks. The majority of well-selected patients with allergic asthma or allergic rhinitis ("hay fever") are significantly improved after 1–2 years of immunotherapy; therapy is given for at least 3 years to achieve lasting benefit.

The beneficial effects of immunotherapy in perennial and seasonal allergic rhinitis and in allergic asthma have been demonstrated in double-blind, placebo-controlled trials. Although immunotherapy against house dust mites and cats has been substantiated, it should not replace appropriate environmental control. Venom immunotherapy for sensitivity to stinging insects (Hymenoptera) is efficacious and essential for those patients who have experienced a life-threatening systemic reaction following a sting. The use of bacterial extracts is not considered effective. Immunotherapy to foods in general has not been proved efficacious and can be dangerous in highly sensitive individuals.

Drug Therapy

Many drugs are effective in the treatment of allergic disorders (Table 33–1). The principal groups include adrenergic agents, antihistamines, corticosteroids, noncorticosteroid anti-inflammatory agents, methylxanthines, anticholinergic agents, and expectorants. The selection of drugs depends on the pathologic processes involved.

Adrenergic Agents: As a group, adrenergic agents exhibit many different pharmacologic effects. Their usefulness in allergic disorders depends mainly on their ability to constrict blood vessels (α_1-adrenergic activity) and relax other smooth muscle (β_2-adrenergic activity). Allergic reactions are mediated by chemical mediators such as histamine and leukotrienes that produce varying degrees of vasodilatation, angioedema, and smooth muscle spasm. The pharmacologic actions of adrenergic agents antagonize the actions of these chemical mediators and at times may even reverse their effects completely. The drugs in this group have been developed for their selective activity at the α-adrenergic and β-adrenergic receptors, and thus have markedly differing effects. For example, phenylephrine, a relatively potent α_1-agonist agent, is especially useful in rhinitis. On the other hand, albuterol is devoid of α_1-adrenergic activity but is a potent β_2-agonist and an effective bronchodilator, which makes it useful in the treatment of asthma. Vasodilatation, angioedema, and asthma may all be present in anaphylaxis, and thus epinephrine, a potent α_1-agonist and β_2-agonist, is the drug of choice.

Adrenergic drugs are not always completely effective when given alone and are not without undesirable effects. For example, epinephrine "resistance" may occur in severe asthma because of the presence of significant inflammation. Repeated use of this drug may increase the patient's anxiety and, in the presence of severe hypoxemia and acidosis, may produce cardiac dysrhythmia leading to cardiac arrest. β_2-Agonist aerosols can be effective in acute asthma, but rare paradoxic bronchospasm has been reported with several of these agents. Also, there is an unsettled issue as to whether chronic routine use of β_2-agonist aerosols is detrimental in some patients.

Antihistamines: Antihistamines act through competitive inhibition of histamine at receptor sites, thereby preventing histamine from exerting its activity. Three classes of antihistamines have been recognized: H_1-receptor inhibitors, the classic (first-generation) antihistamines, have been used for many years in allergic disorders; H_2-receptor inhibitors, which are useful in inhibiting gastric acid secretion, also have mild antipruritic effects; and finally, agents that affect a newly identified H_3 receptor. H_1 antihistamines have antipruritic properties and are particularly useful in urticaria and allergic rhinitis, in which histamine plays a major role. It must be noted that their effectiveness is limited in many allergic disorders because various mediators besides histamine are also operative. In the treatment of chronic urticaria and anaphylaxis, the combination of H_1 and H_2 antihistamines has therapeutic benefit when neither alone is sufficiently effective.

Although antihistamines are useful in milder aller-

Table 33–1. Preparations and dosages of drugs commonly used in allergic disorders.

Agent	Route	Dosage
Adrenergic agents		
Albuterol	PO	Short-acting syrup[1]: 0.1 mg/kg per dose every 8 h Short-acting tablet[2]: 2–4 mg every 6–8 h Extended-release[3]: 4–8 mg every 12 h
	Inhaled	1 or 2 inhalations from pressurized aerosol or inhale contents of one Rotacap.[4] May use as often as every 4 h, but *avoid excessive use.* **or** 0.1–0.15 mg/kg (up to 0.5 mL) of 0.5% inhalant solution[3] diluted with 2 mL of water or saline administered by compressor-driven nebulizer. May use every 4 h. May use 0.15 mg/kg up to 1.0 mL every 20 min for three doses, then decrease frequency.
Bitolterol[3]	Inhaled	1 or 2 inhalations from pressurized aerosol. May use as often as every 4 h, but *avoid excessive use.*
Epinephrine Aqueous 1:1000	SC, IM	0.01 mL/kg up to 0.3 mL. May repeat at intervals of 15–20 min for a total of three doses.
Suspension 1:200	SC	0.005 mL/kg up to 0.15 mL. May repeat in 8–12 h. (Shake well before administering.)
Metaproterenol	PO[2]	10–20 mg every 6–8 h
	Inhaled[3]	1 or 2 inhalations from pressurized aerosol. May be used as often as every 4 h, but *avoid excessive use.* **or** 0.1–0.3 mL of 5% inhalant solution 2 diluted with 2 mL of water or saline and administered by compressor-driven nebulizer. May use every 4 h.
Pirbuterol[3]	Inhaled	1 or 2 inhalations from pressurized or breath activated aerosol. May use as often as every 4 h, but *avoid excessive use.*
Salmeterol[3]	Inhaled	1 or 2 inhalations every 12 h for maintenance therapy or to prevent nocturnal symptoms
Terbutaline[3]	PO	2.5 mg every 8 h
	SC	0.01 mL/kg up to 0.25 mL. May repeat once after 20 min.
	Inhaled	1 or 2 inhalations from pressurized aerosol. May use as often as every 4 h, but *avoid excessive use.*
Antihistamines		
Astemizole[3]	PO	10 mg once daily
Chlorpheniramine	PO	Short-acting: 2–4 mg three or four times a day Long-acting: 2–3 mg twice a day
Clemastine fumarate	PO	6–12 y: Up to 3 mg/d in two divided doses Over 12 y: Up to 6 mg/d in two divided doses
Cyproheptadine[1]	PO	0.25 mg/kg/d in two or three divided doses, not to exceed 16 mg daily
Diphenhydramine hydrochloride	PO	1 mg/kg per dose (up to 50 mg) four times daily
	IM, IV	25–50 mg (if IV, give slowly)
Hydroxyzine hydrochloride	PO	0.2–0.5 mg/kg per dose (up to 50 mg) three times daily
Loratadine[3]	PO	10 mg once daily
Terfenadine[3]	PO	60 mg twice daily
Systemic corticosteroids		
Hydrocortisone, dexamethasone, prednisolone/prednisone, methylprednisolone	IV, PO	Most rapid therapeutic effect follows IV or PO administration, but there may be no perceptible effect for hours. In acute situations, high doses of corticosteroids (eg, 1 mg/kg per dose of methylprednisolone every 4–6 h) are generally used the first day and the dose is tapered as rapidly as possible or withdrawn completely. **Approximate equivalents of activity:** 100 mg of hydrocortisone = 4 mg of dexamethasone = 25 mg of prednisolone/prednisone = 20 mg of methylprednisolone

(continued)

Table 33–1. Preparations and dosages of drugs commonly used in allergic disorders. (continued)

Agent	Route	Dosage
Topical corticosteroids for asthma and rhinitis		
Beclomethasone[2]	Inhaled	6–12 y: Up to 10 inhalations per day in 2–4 divided doses Over 12 y: Up to 16 inhalations per day
	Intranasal	1 spray in each nostril up to three times a day, or 2 sprays in each nostril twice a day[5]
Budesonide[2]	Intranasal	2 sprays in each nostril twice a day or 4 sprays in each nostril in the morning[5]
Dexamethasone sodium phosphate	Intranasal	1 or 2 sprays in each nostril twice a day (should be used for short periods only)[5]
Flunisolide[2]	Inhaled	1 or 2 inhalations twice a day
	Intranasal	1 spray in each nostril 3 times a day, or 2 sprays in each nostril twice a day[5]
Fluticasone[3]	Intranasal	1 spray in each nostril once a day[5]
Triamcinolone	Inhaled[2]	6–12 y: Up to 12 inhalations per day in 2–4 divided doses Over 12 y: Up to 16 inhalations per day
	Intranasal[3]	1 or 2 sprays in each nostril once daily; up to 2 sprays in each nostril twice daily[5]
Other drugs used in allergic disorders		
Cromolyn sodium	Inhaled[1]	2 inhalations from pressurized aerosol or 1 ampule (20 mg/2 mL) by compressor-driven nebulizer three or four times a day. May also be used just prior to exercise or contact with an asthma-precipitating agent (eg, animals).
	Intranasal[2]	1 or 2 sprays in each nostril three or four times a day
Nedocromil sodium[3]	Inhaled	2 inhalations from pressurized aerosol four times a day initially. This may be reduced to three or four times a day maintenance dosage.
Aminophylline, theophylline	IV	3–5 mg/kg[6] every 4–6 h (infuse over 20 min) or 0.6–1 mg/kg/h[6] as constant infusion
	PO	16–24 mg/kg/d[6] (use with extreme caution in children under 1 y of age) Short-acting: Every 6 h Long-acting: Every 8–12 h

[1]Safety and efficacy for children under 2 y of age has not been established.
[2]Safety and efficacy for children under 6 y of age has not been established.
[3]Safety and efficacy for children under 12 y of age has not been established.
[4]Safety and efficacy for children under 4 y of age has not been established.
[5]Discontinue if nasal bleeding occurs.
[6]Refers to theophylline dose.

gic disorders, they are not the drug of first choice in a severe allergic reaction. In this clinical setting, epinephrine must be given first, and antihistamines should be administered as adjunctive therapy.

Sedation is the most common side effect of most first-generation H_1 antihistamines. This central nervous system (CNS) depressant property may interfere with normal functions, overtly or subtly. On the other hand, this sedation effect may be useful in helping an itching child sleep. H_1 antihistamines also possess anticholinergic drying activity. Nonsedating second-generation antihistamines are now available which avoid the CNS depression and anticholinergic effects of the first-generation H_1 antihistamines. Although previously considered to be potentially harmful in asthma, it is now generally agreed that antihist-

amines are not contraindicated for other allergic disorders when asthma is present.

Corticosteroids: Corticosteroids have been helpful in the treatment of all of the allergic disorders. Their effectiveness results from their multiple anti-inflammatory actions. The potential untoward side effects of prolonged systemic corticosteroid administration (eg, growth suppression, hypertension, peptic ulcer, diabetes, cataracts, osteoporosis, myopathy, other features of Cushing's syndrome) limit their use. The main indications for their use are in anaphylaxis, acute severe asthma, and chronic severe disorders such as asthma that are refractory to other appropriate therapy. Their slow onset of action (several hours) precludes administration of these drugs as first choice in acute allergic emergencies. For chronic asthma therapy, topical therapy by the inhaled oral route is preferred. When chronic systemic therapy is necessary for any disorder, alterative-day early morning therapy with a short-acting preparation (eg, prednisone) should be attempted.

Most atopic syndromes are amenable to other forms of therapy, and the chronic use of systemic corticosteroids is rarely necessary and may be confined to several days of therapy. The development of corticosteroids with high topical potency but limited systemic activity makes the topical route of administration a more attractive option in respiratory syndromes and atopic dermatitis. However, topical use retains the potential for inducing steroid side effects depending on dosage, duration of therapy, and individual patient sensitivity.

Noncorticosteroid Anti-inflammatory Agents: Cromolyn sodium is used in the management of asthma and allergic rhinitis and conjunctivitis; in the United States at this time, nedocromil sodium is approved only for the treatment of asthma. Both are considered to have anti-inflammatory activity, although the exact mechanisms of action are unclear. Since asthma is a disease of inflammation and because of their impressive safety profile, cromolyn sodium and nedocromil sodium are among the first-line agents for chronic asthma therapy, especially in children. However, these agents do not reverse inflammatory tissue changes already present and are of no value in the treatment of acute asthmatic paroxysms. In addition, they are not as potent as corticosteroids. These agents are useful in blocking allergen-, irritant-, and exercise-induced asthma if used prior to anticipated exposure.

Methylxanthines: Theophylline and its ethylenediamine derivative, aminophylline, are effective bronchodilators that appear to act at a different point in the same pathway in which β_2 agonists exert their dilating effect on smooth muscle. When used properly, these drugs are useful in the management of chronic asthma, but because they do not appear to have potent anti-inflammatory activity, they are not considered principal first-line agents in chronic asthma therapy. There is great patient variation in the metabolism of methylxanthines, and dosage must be highly individualized. The optimal therapeutic blood level may vary with the severity of the asthma, but the therapeutic index is relatively narrow. Levels over 20 μg/mL are considered most likely to be associated with toxicity, although side effects may occur at lower levels. Because infections, medications, and other factors can significantly change theophylline metabolism, therapeutic levels between 5 and 15 μg/mL are recommended. *In early to mid infancy, metabolism is markedly diminished, and methylxanthines should be used with particular caution.*

For chronic administration of methylxanthines, long-acting preparations given orally (once or twice daily) are preferred. These drugs can also be given at bedtime in order to control nocturnal asthma. Theophylline levels should be monitored periodically in patients on chronic therapy. Factors known to accelerate theophylline clearance include young age (postinfancy to 16 years), high-protein diet, smoking (tobacco, marijuana), and anticonvulsant drugs (phenobarbital, phenytoin). Theophylline clearance is inhibited by extremes in age (infancy and over 50 years), high-carbohydrate diet, ciprofloxacin, erythromycin, cimetidine, viremia, and congestive heart failure.

The use of these agents has been associated with severe toxic reaction, in some cases resulting in death. Overdosage frequently occurs as a result of failure to appreciate the variability of rate and extent of absorption with different preparations. Side effects include headache, palpitations, dizziness, stomachache, nausea, vomiting, and convulsions. Nausea and stomachache may be related to local irritation or to a CNS-mediated toxic effect observed when these drugs are administered by any route. In recent years, subtle effects on behavior, attention span, and learning have been observed by some investigators, but not by others.

Anticholinergic Agents: Anticholinergic agents (atropine sulfate, ipratropium bromide) have mild bronchodilatory effects that add little to the effects of selective β_2 agonists in the treatment of asthma. However, some potentiation of the duration of bronchodilatory effect from β_2-agonist agents has been demonstrated. Newer quaternary ammonium products (eg, ipratropium bromide) have markedly reduced systemic absorption, thereby giving these drugs a large therapeutic margin. These agents may be useful for patients with a strong cough, irritant, or psychologic component.

Expectorants: *Adequate hydration is essential to effective expectoration.* Expectorants such as guaifenesin (glyceryl guaiacolate) may be used in asthma to liquefy thick, tenacious mucus, but it is not clear whether any therapeutic benefit is derived from these agents. Iodides seem to be more effective than guaifenesin, but with prolonged use, goiter, salivary gland inflammation, gastric irritation, and skin eruptions, including acne, may occur.

Antibiotics: Antibiotics do not provide specific therapy for any of the allergic disorders. Antibiotics should be used when specific evidence of bacterial infection exists (eg, impetiginous superinfection of atopic dermatitis). Their excessive use in children with allergic disorders should be avoided to reduce the risk of developing either allergic sensitization or bacterial resistance to these drugs.

Sedatives: Sedatives have been misused in asthma and have been responsible for some deaths. The anxiety associated with an extreme asthma episode is likely a reflection of the severity of the respiratory distress and hypoxemia rather than the cause of it. Sedatives that suppress the respiratory center (eg, barbiturates) should not be used in the therapy of severe asthma.

Other Prospective Drugs: Major pharmacologic advances in the control of allergic diseases have occurred in recent years. Currently, various drugs—many with novel pharmacologic properties—are under investigation. Some are already available in other countries. Among the more interesting drugs on the nearer horizon in the United States are newer topical corticosteroids, other second-generation antihistamines, and leukotriene inhibitors.

Prophylaxis of Atopic Disorders

There are suggestions that the avoidance of cow's milk products, eggs, and wheat during the first 12 months of life significantly lessens the likelihood of developing allergy in early childhood. There is also some evidence that a diet excluding cow products, fish, and eggs for the first 6 months of life coupled with general environmental precautions to minimize contact with house dust and animal dander is associated with a diminished likelihood of developing atopic dermatitis, at least in the first year. It seems prudent, therefore, to institute these dietary and environmental restrictions for the first few months of life in children with a strong family history of atopy.

Abramson MJ, Puy RM, Weiner JM: Is allergen immunotherapy effective in asthma? A meta-analysis of randomized controlled trials. Am J Respir Crit Care Med 1995;151:969.

Ledford DK, Lockey RF: Immunotherapy for allergic disease. In: *Allergy, Asthma, and Immunology From Infancy to Adulthood,* 3rd ed. Bierman CW et al (editors). Saunders, 1996.

Luskin AT: Environmental control: Key to asthma management. J Respir Dis 1995;16:253.

Meltzer EO: Prevalence, economic and medical impact of tobacco smoking. Ann Allergy 1994;73:381.

Rakes GP, Platts-Mills TA: Principles of avoidance. In: *Allergy, Asthma, and Immunology From Infancy to Adulthood,* 3rd ed. Bierman CW et al (editors). Saunders, 1996.

Simons FER, Simons KJ: The pharmacology and use of H_1-receptor–antagonist drugs. N Engl J Med 1994; 330:1663.

Szefler SJ: Anti-inflammatory drugs in the treatment of allergic disease. Med Clin North Am 1992;76:953.

ANAPHYLAXIS

Anaphylaxis is an acute, life-threatening clinical syndrome resulting from the release of inflammatory mediators and characterized by cutaneous (urticaria, angioedema), respiratory (bronchospasm, upper airway edema), cardiovascular (hypotension), and gastrointestinal (nausea, pain, vomiting, diarrhea) signs and symptoms, which may occur alone or in combination. Anaphylactic shock, upper airway angioedema, and bronchial obstruction are the principal life-threatening manifestations of severe allergic reactions. The reaction usually starts rapidly after contact with the offending substance and can be short-lived, protracted, or biphasic (acute with recurrence several hours later), despite treatment. Anaphylaxis may be IgE-mediated (eg, anaphylaxis secondary to foods, certain drugs, insect stings, skin testing, immunotherapy, latex, possibly exercise-induced anaphylaxis) or non–IgE-mediated (eg, through immune complex formation) or mediated through nonimmune mast cell degranulating agents. Clinical reactions that stem from nonimmune mechanisms are often called "anaphylactoid." Idiopathic anaphylaxis has been described as an entity.

Treatment

Emergency Measures: *Anaphylaxis is a medical emergency.* Immediate recognition and treatment are essential. Maintain a patent airway. Monitor blood pressure and pulse. Place the patient in the supine position with the legs elevated. Begin oxygen therapy.

1. Epinephrine: Epinephrine 1:1000, 0.01 mL/kg to a maximum of 0.3 mL, should be injected subcutaneously or intramuscularly without delay. This may be repeated at intervals of 15–20 minutes two or three times as necessary. If the reaction is caused by a recent sting or injection into an extremity, a tourniquet nay be applied proximal to the site for 15–20 minutes, briefly releasing it every 3–5 minutes. If the offending substance has been injected intradermally or subcutaneously, absorption may be delayed by injecting 0.1 mL of epinephrine subcutaneously at the injection site. Subsequent therapy depends on the clinical manifestations and the response to treatment.

2. Antihistamines: Antihistamines (see Table 33–1), given intramuscularly or intravenously, may be especially useful for cutaneous symptoms, and possibly for hypotension. Intravenous infusion of antihistamines should be given slowly, over a period of 5–10 minutes, to avoid inducing hypotension. A combination of an H_1 and an H_2 antihistamine may be superior to an H_1 alone.

3. Corticosteroids: Corticosteroids do not provide immediate benefit but, when given early, may be helpful in preventing biphasic or protracted anaphylaxis.

4. Bronchodilators: These medications, including aerosolized β_2 agonists and aminophylline, may be useful when bronchospasm occurs.

5. Fluids: Anaphylactic shock is, in part, produced by hypovolemia secondary to massive loss of intravascular fluids; treatment of persistent hypotension requires restoration of intravascular volume by fluid replacement.

6. Vasopressors: Hypotension that is refractory to the above medications and fluid replacement may require an intravenously administered vasopressor such as epinephrine or dopamine.

Follow-up Measures: The patient should be observed for an adequate time after the initial symptoms have subsided. If anaphylaxis is severe, the patient should be observed in the hospital for 24 hours, especially since biphasic or protracted anaphylaxis may occur despite initial and continued therapy.

Prevention

When the causative agent is known, it should be avoided. If it is not known, an effort to determine the cause should be made, starting with a detailed, careful history. In selected cases, testing may be indicated, such as in Hymenoptera sting or food anaphylaxis. With exercise-induced anaphylaxis, patients should be instructed to exercise with another person and to stop exercising at the first sign of symptoms. In this disorder, symptoms may not occur each time the patient exercises. The prior ingestion of food or nonsteroidal anti-inflammatory drug has been implicated in some cases; therefore, eating within 4 hours of exercise or taking aspirin or related compounds before exercise should be avoided. Patients with a history of anaphylaxis should carry epinephrine for self-administration (eg, EpiPen, EpiPen Jr, Ana-Kit), and they and all caretakers should be instructed thoroughly on its use.

Children who have experienced respiratory or cardiovascular compromise following an insect sting and who have venom-specific IgE should receive venom immunotherapy. Children with a large local reaction or cutaneous symptoms have only a low likelihood of having a life-threatening reaction to a future sting, and immunotherapy generally is not recommended. The main allergens responsible for severe allergic reactions are found in venom of Hymenoptera (bees, wasps, yellow jackets, hornets, fire ants). Immunotherapy with venom extracts is highly efficacious. It is unknown for how long venom immunotherapy should be continued, but there is evidence that 3–5 years may be sufficient.

Laboratory Findings

The diagnosis of anaphylaxis generally is based on signs and symptoms. An elevated serum tryptase level obtained during or shortly after the reaction may be helpful to support the diagnosis when it is in question. Electrocardiographic changes, including those indicative of ischemia, may occur. The chest x-ray may show hyperinflation. Hemoconcentration and increased creatine kinase and aspartate aminotransferase (SGOT) may be seen.

Differential Diagnosis

Classic signs and symptoms may make the diagnosis of anaphylaxis obvious. However, if symptoms are mild or subtle or if the history is only suggestive, other diagnoses to consider include vasovagal reactions, other forms of shock, primary cardiac events, asthma, vocal cord dysfunction, mastocytosis, hereditary angioedema, and anxiety attacks.

Prognosis

The prognosis is good when signs and symptoms are promptly recognized and treated and the offending agent is strictly avoided. Accidental exposure to the causative substance may occur, so patients must be prepared to recognize and treat anaphylaxis themselves. Anaphylaxis can be fatal. Idiopathic and exercise-induced anaphylaxis tends to be recurrent, which can be frightening for patients and parents.

Lieberman P: Distinguishing anaphylaxis from other serious disorders. J Respir Dis 1995;16:411.

Lieberman P: Anaphylaxis: Guidelines for prevention and management. J Respir Dis 1995;16:456.

Reisman RE: Venom hypersensitivity. J Allergy Clin Immunol 1994;94:651.

Sampson H, Mendelson L, Rosen JP: Fatal and near fatal anaphylactic reactions to food in children and adolescents. N Engl J Med 1992;327:380.

BRONCHIAL ASTHMA
("Reactive Airways Disease")

Bronchial asthma is a largely reversible chronic inflammatory process of the lower respiratory tract manifest by recurrent obstruction of airflow throughout the tracheobronchial tree. The inflammation results in epithelial denudation, mucosal edema, increased and unusually viscid secretions, and smooth muscle contraction. This inflammation and bronchoconstriction result in paroxysmal exacerbations or chronic symptoms, including dyspnea, cough, and wheezing.

The incidence of asthma is reportedly less than 5% of the general population, with suggestions of a much greater prevalence in school-age children (perhaps 12–15%). Before adolescence, boys are affected twice as frequently as girls. Onset in early childhood is common, but may occur at any age.

Numerous factors trigger or aggravate asthma and may vary with age. In infancy and early childhood, viral upper and lower respiratory tract infections are principal triggers of asthma. As the child gets older, allergic reactivity becomes increasingly important; evidence of sensitization to inhalant allergens is found eventually in the majority of children with asthma. Allergic sensitization probably plays a major role in the pathogenesis of asthma in many, if not most, children. The most common allergens are aeroallergens (animal danders, dust mites, cockroaches, molds, pollens). Foods occasionally provoke asthma, mainly in infants. However, allergy does not appear to be a requisite for asthma and, in some patients, offensive allergens cannot be identified by history or by allergy testing. Furthermore, allergens are rarely the sole significant triggering factor involved. Asthma "triggers" vary with the individual, but common triggers include parental cigarette smoke (a risk factor for the development, worsening, or persistence of asthma), air pollutants, odors, paint fumes, cold air, exercise, and rapid changes in temperature or barometric pressure. Bacterial sinus infections can exacerbate asthma symptoms, but evidence is lacking for a role of other bacterial infections (pharyngitis, even pneumonia). Psychologic factors appear to be important in some cases but are seldom the sole cause of asthma. Aspirin idiosyncrasy can be problematic in asthma in children as in adults.

An important pathogenetic feature of asthma is "nonspecific" hyper-reactivity of the airways to various chemical mediators (eg, acetylcholine, histamine, leukotrienes). Exposure to asthma triggers also increases this hyper-reactivity, and because of this feature, asthma is sometimes called "reactive airways disease." Although a common feature of asthma, airways hyper-reactivity is not always present, and its correlation with airway inflammation is imperfect.

Clinical Findings

History: Wheezing is a common symptom in the first 3 years of life, occurring probably in at least one-third of children. In about two-thirds of those children, there is a single or minimal number of episodes and there is no recurrence later in childhood. Parental asthma, allergic sensitization, other atopic disorders, and exposure to maternal smoking are risk factors for persistence, that is, asthma. Onset of symptoms may occur as early as the first few weeks of life. Particularly in early childhood, the first episode usually is associated with a lower respiratory tract infection or bronchiolitis. As age increases, there is a progressively greater tendency for initial and subsequent episodes to be associated with inhalant allergens or irritants. The initial inciting event appears to render the tracheobronchial tree more hyperactive to both similar and unrelated precipitants.

Episodes of asthma associated with infections are usually slow in onset and prolonged; those caused by specific, identifiable allergens tend to be acute in onset and relatively brief if the causative agent is removed. However, *chronic allergen exposure to house dust mites, cockroaches, and animal allergens, for instance, may produce chronic inflammatory changes predisposing the patient to later symptoms without an obvious cause-and-effect association.*

Bronchial asthma in infants (under 2 years of age) deserves special comment. The first episode usually follows the onset of a viral respiratory infection by a few days; some degree of cough or wheezing may persist for prolonged periods and becomes worse with subsequent "colds." In infants, the predominant symptoms may be dyspnea, excessive secretions, noisy and rattly breathing, cough, and, in many cases, some intercostal and suprasternal retractions—rather than the typical pronounced expiratory wheezes that occur in older children. These episodes are often mistaken for croup, bronchiolitis, or pneumonia.

Asthma can occur in the absence of overt wheezing. Complaints may include "chest congestion," prolonged cough, exercise intolerance, dyspnea, and recurrent bronchitis or pneumonia. *Prolonged or recurrent cough in childhood should raise the suspicion of asthma.* In **cough-variant asthma,** wheezing and signs of lower respiratory tract obstruction are absent initially. However, more typical symptoms and signs of asthma may develop as the child gets older. Bronchodilator drugs are usually effective in this condition.

Physical Examination: Chest auscultation during a forced expiratory maneuver rather than on simple tidal volume can be revealing, especially when the patient's symptoms are absent or mild. With increasing severity of an episode, prolongation of the expiratory phase and wheezes and rhonchi occur. As the obstruction becomes more severe, however, wheezes become more high-pitched, breath sounds may diminish in intensity, and with severe obstruction, the chest may be "silent" because of very poor air exchange. Dyspnea with marked labor of breathing, retractions, and use of accessory muscles of respiration may be observed. Cough, restlessness, apprehension, and fatigue may be present. Flushed, moist skin may be noted with dry mucous membranes. Cyanosis of lips, gums, and nail beds may be noted with progression of severity of the episode. Increasing tachycardia and later pulsus paradoxus are also observed. Tachycardia may *improve* after effective treatment with β_2 agonists (including epinephrine!) because of improved oxygenation and reduced work of breathing.

Laboratory Findings: Eosinophil accumulations (eg, clumps of eosinophils on sputum smear) and blood eosinophilia are commonly found. Their presence tends to reflect disease activity and does not necessarily mean that allergic factors are involved. Leukocytosis is common in acute severe asthma without any evidence of bacterial infection; also, high counts can be seen immediately after epinephrine administration. Hematocrit can be elevated with dehydration as in prolonged attacks or in severe chronic disease.

During severe acute asthma, hypoxemia, in part because of ventilation/perfusion mismatch, is commonly present early with a normal or low PCO_2 level secondary to hyperventilation. Respiratory acidosis and increasing CO_2 tension may ensue, with further obstruction of airflow, and signals impending respiratory failure.

Radiographic Imaging: Bilateral hyperinflation, bronchial thickening, peribronchial infiltration, and areas of density from patchy atelectasis or bronchopneumonia may be present. Patchy atelectasis is common and often misinterpreted as pneumonia. The pulmonary arteries may appear prominent. Flattening of the diaphragms frequently is present.

Pulmonary Function Studies: (See Chapter

18.) Increased airway resistance results in a decrease in flow rates (peak expiratory flow rate [PEFR], forced expiratory volume in 1 second [FEV_1]), decreased vital capacity (VC), and increased functional residual capacity (FRC) and residual volume (RV). Residual hyperinflation frequently is chronic. Reversal or significant improvement of these abnormalities in response to inhaled bronchodilator therapy alone or with anti-inflammatory therapy is observed.

Allergy and Provocative Tests: Exercise challenges or methacholine or histamine challenge may be helpful in establishing the diagnosis of suspected asthma when history, examination, and pulmonary function tests are not definitive. Allergy testing is discussed elsewhere in this chapter.

Differential Diagnosis

Bronchial asthma may be confused with croup, acute bronchiolitis, bronchopneumonia, and pertussis, especially in the very young. Immunodeficiency (primarily defects in immunoglobulin production or function) may have associated coughing and wheezing because of chronic lower respiratory tract infection. Nasal and pharyngeal "wheezes" (mainly inspiratory) may be transmitted to the chest, especially in infants, from upper airway edema, secretions, or other obstructing factors, such as allergic rhinitis, upper respiratory tract infections, and adenoidal hypertrophy. Gastroesophageal reflux may cause wheezing and coughing. Laryngeal stridor is usually a history of intubation (eg, for prematurity) or is congenital and associated with other anomalies. In cases of tracheal or bronchial foreign body, dyspnea or wheezing is usually of sudden onset; on auscultation, the wheezes are usually unilateral. Characteristic x-ray findings are not always present. Paradoxic inspiratory closure of the vocal cords (vocal cord dysfunction) or a paralyzed cord can masquerade as or occur with asthma and must be considered in refractory disease.

The differentiation between bronchial asthma and cystic fibrosis is usually made on the basis of history. Patients with cystic fibrosis have recurrent or serious pulmonary infections and (usually) profuse, bulky stools, and high sweat chloride; often they have clubbing of the nails; more recently, genetic markers have become available. Chronic inflammatory changes seen on chest x-ray in cystic fibrosis also can be a helpful differential point. There is evidence for a significant reactive airway (asthmatic) component with or without allergic precipitants in many children with cystic fibrosis, and cystic fibrosis and asthma can coexist.

Tracheal or bronchial compression by extramural forces may resemble asthma and may be caused by a foreign body in the esophagus, aortic ring, anomalous vessels, or inflammatory or neoplastic lymphadenopathy.

Wheezing may be present in immotile cilia syndrome, but chronic upper and lower respiratory tract infections (sinusitis, otitis media, pneumonia) are recurrent because of the lack of mucociliary clearance.

TREATMENT OF CHRONIC ASTHMA

Goals of therapy include minimal or no chronic symptoms, no sleep interference, minimal acute exacerbations, no need for emergency visits, minimal need for PRN bronchodilators, no limitation of activity (including exercise), optimization of lung function, and minimal or no adverse effects from treatment. These are accomplished by (1) controlling the environment; (2) using appropriate medications; (3) utilizing immunotherapy when appropriate; (4) educating the patient, family, and other caregivers; and (5) closely monitoring the child with periodic follow-up visits and pulmonary function tests.

General Measures: *Avoidance of aggravating factors* is the mainstay of therapy. (See Environmental Control of Exposure, earlier.) Avoidance of allergens and irritants that drive the patient's asthma is potentially the most effective form of anti-inflammatory therapy. *Immunotherapy* is used for allergens that cannot be avoided (eg, pollens, molds, house dust mites, possibly animal danders).

Patient and family education is also fundamental to effective asthma management. The patient and his or her family must understand the role of asthma triggers, the importance of chronicity of disease activity even without obvious symptoms, how to use objective (eg, peak flow) measurements as indicators of disease activity, the importance of airway inflammation, and identification of the patient's early warning signs of worsening asthma, which allows for early intervention. A *step-care plan* should be developed for all patients with asthma. This educational process extends to school personnel, baby-sitters, and all those who care for the child with asthma.

Peak flow meters (PFMs) are useful in monitoring acute and chronic asthma. Since perception of the degree of airflow limitation is poorly perceived by many patients, PFMs can assist assessment of airflow and disease activity on a day-to-day basis and with acute symptoms, as well as in the physician's office and the emergency room. Monitoring peak flow rates may forewarn worsening asthma and signal the need for increased asthma medications. They are also helpful in monitoring the effects of changes in asthma medications, and their use enhances patient-physician communication.

Spacer devices optimize delivery of medication to the lungs and, with inhaled steroids, also minimize side effects. These devices are especially useful in younger children when metered-dose inhalers are used. Several effective devices are currently available. However, with acute exacerbations, nebulization treatments are more effective in young children.

Exercise should be encouraged rather than restricted. Exercise-induced bronchospasm can be ameliorated, if necessary, by cromolyn sodium, nedocromil sodium, or β_2-agonist aerosols prior to exercise. It may be necessary to use a combination of these medications before exercise. Optimizing lung functions and long-term asthma control is also important in minimizing bronchospasm from exercise. In children with chronic or recurrent asthma, breathing and fitness exercises under the guidance of a properly trained physical therapist may help improve the patient's cardiopulmonary status, including muscular function of the thoracic cage.

Specific Measures: See General Principles of Treatment (earlier).

PHARMACOTHERAPY OF CHRONIC ASTHMA

Stepwise Therapy

Inhalant short-acting β_2-agonists are used PRN as rescue medication and for symptom relief for all levels of asthma. They are **symptom relievers.** Even in very young children, the inhaled route is preferred over oral medication. For very mild asthma, other medications may not be needed. β_2 Agonists do not control inflammation.

Control of Inflammation: Evidence for chronic inflammation even in mild asthma dictates that anti-inflammatory agents be considered first-line therapy of all chronic symptomatic disease. Anti-inflammatory agents are considered **disease controllers.** These agents should be implemented when the patient has symptoms greater than three times weekly that require bronchodilator therapy or interfere with routine daily activities, including sleep. Anti-inflammatory drugs include cromolyn sodium, nedocromil sodium, and inhaled corticosteroids. With inhaled corticosteroids, once disease control is established using the dosage necessary, dosage should be decreased gradually to the lowest amount necessary to maintain symptom control and optimal lung function. Dosage can be increased during exacerbations. Cromolyn sodium often is tried first, especially in young children, or nedocromil sodium in older children; inhaled corticosteroids are the most potent agents of the group and can be used initially or when other agents are not effective. Maximum efficacy may not be obtained for weeks to months.

For asthma that not controlled with recommended dosages of anti-inflammatory drugs, or for steroid-sparing effect, methylxanthines, long-acting inhaled β_2 agonists (salmeterol, approved for age 12 and older), anticholinergic agents (ipratropium bromide), or long-acting oral β_2 agonists may be added. (Steroid sparing does not equal inflammation sparing, however.) Nedocromil sodium may have an effect additive to inhaled corticosteroids.

"Continuity" symptoms of night cough, breathlessness, and wheezing provoked by exercise or exposure to allergens or irritants usually indicate more severe disease than do occasional, spontaneous, and brief episodes caused by recognizable allergens with symptom-free periods in between. Interference with sleep generally connotes serious obstruction.

Referral to an Asthma Specialist: Asthma is a chronic disorder with significant variation in course and therapeutic requirements and in which the degree of obstruction and underlying etiologic and aggravating factors often are not appreciated. Early involvement of the asthma specialist to help in assessing disease severity and lability, in identification of causative allergens and other factors, and in construction of an individual treatment plan is recommended and plays an effective role in decreasing morbidity and costs associated with inadequately controlled disease. Specialist assessment should be considered for patients who require daily maintenance therapy, who have potentially life-threatening disease, or whose asthma is otherwise difficult to manage.

TREATMENT OF ACUTE EXACERBATIONS OF ASTHMA

It is important that the child, parents, and other caregivers, including physicians and their staffs, be able to assess asthma severity accurately. Respiratory rate, respiratory effort, movement of air in the chest, color, alertness, and objective measures of airflow (eg, using a peak flow meter to measure the peak expiratory flow rate [PEFR]) are important aspects of that assessment. Note that peak flow rates may be falsely high in severe obstruction.

Home Care

Older Children: Begin with inhaled β_2-agonist therapy metered-dose inhaler, preferably through a spacer device. Two to four sprays or an aerosolized bronchodilator (eg, 0.50 mL of 0.5% solution of albuterol) can be used every 20 minutes, three times, initially. If the response is good (symptom relief, improvement in PEFR to >70% of the patient's best), give the β_2 agonist every 3–4 hours.

Young Children: Give 0.25 (<1 year of age) or 0.5 (>1 year of age) mL of albuterol 0.5% solution in 2 mL of saline or water, at 20- minute intervals up to three times.

If there is no improvement with these measures, if there is marked distress, or if PEFR persists at less than 50% (older children), the patient should be seen in the physician's office or sent to the emergency room.

Office or Emergency Room

Inhaled β_2 agonists are the drugs of first choice in the treatment of acute asthma; they are as effective as subcutaneously administered epinephrine and have minimal systemic side effects. However, in severe asthma unresponsive to initial aerosolized therapy, or in patients who cannot cooperate with or who resist inhalation therapy, epinephrine or terbutaline may be administrated subcutaneously. Relative or apparent complete lack of responsiveness to these drugs may be the result of bronchial obstruction from mucosal edema and thick mucus plugs or complicating problems such as pneumothorax. Sensitivity to adrenergic drugs may improve after initiation of corticosteroids.

For the treatment of acute asthma, give 0.25 (<1 year old) up to 1.00 mL of albuterol 0.5% solution by nebulizer at 20-minute intervals up to three times. Administer oxygen and measure oxygen saturation (SaO_2) by oximetry. With good response (at least moderate symptom relief, PEFR >70% of the patient's personal best or predicted normal), space albuterol treatments to every 1–2 hours and observe. Consider a short course (5–7 days) of an oral corticosteroid (prednisone, 1–2 mg/kg/d). If the response is poor (poor symptom relief, PEFR <70%), add prednisone, 1–2 mg/kg orally, or methylprednisolone intravenously; continue albuterol treatments every hour and observe for at least 2 hours after adequate response is obtained. If the PEFR continues below 50%, consider hospital admission. If SaO_2 by oximetry is above 90%, the PEFR exceeds 70%, the child is not showing signs of distress (eg, retraction, use of accessory muscles of respiration), and there is reasonable confidence of reliable care at home, the patient can be discharged with written instructions and scheduled follow-up.

Hospital Care

When outpatient therapy fails, admission to the hospital becomes necessary for more aggressive care and support. Hospitalization should be seriously considered in any patient with a prior history of ventilation for asthma, as risk of respiratory failure is substantially increased.

1. Adequate hydration is important. If fluid intake is poor or vomiting is present, fluids may be administered intravenously. Fluids should be given at maintenance requirements. Care should be taken not to overhydrate. Overhydration may contribute to pulmonary edema related to high intrapleural pressures generated in severe asthma. Potassium requirements should be kept in mind; corticosteroid and β_2-agonist use can be associated with hypokalemia.

2. Administer moisturized oxygen; titrate by oximetry to maintain SaO_2 above 90%. All children with acute severe asthma are hypoxemic, largely as a result of ventilation/perfusion mismatch, and will benefit from supplemental oxygen.

3. Arterial blood determination for pH, PCO_2, and PO_2, may be critical in severe asthma, at least to establish baseline status. Further monitoring depends on the clinical status and the degree of obstruction assessed by PEFR or spirometry. Determination of blood gases or pH on capillary blood generally is unreliable. SaO_2 may be monitored by pulse oximetry.

4. Continue albuterol, 0.5–1.0 mL of 0.5% solution, by inhalation every 1–4 hours. In an intensive care unit setting, albuterol may be given by continuous nebulization.

5. Patients who require hospitalization should receive corticosteroids promptly, even though patients may not realize benefit from the medication for several hours. The use of corticosteroids in status asthmaticus reduces morbidity and mortality and accelerates recovery by reducing inflammation and potentiating the effectiveness of β_2 agonists. (For dosage schedule, see Table 33–1.)

6. The effectiveness of aminophylline when given in addition to aggressive therapy with β_2 agonists is controversial. If aminophylline is used, a loading does of 5 mg/kg intravenously over 20 minutes can be given if the patient is not already receiving theophylline; if the patient is already receiving theophylline and the blood level is unknown, give 2–3 mg/kg. The aminophylline dose should be repeated every 4–6 hours (3–5 mg/kg) or given as a continuous infusion; assess theophylline blood levels and adjust the dosage to maintain levels in the 8- to 14-µg/mL range. Conservative therapeutic levels are suggested, since the risk for toxicity may be increased with concomitant β_2-agonist therapy.

7. Give antibiotics as indicated.

8. Severe airflow limitation that does not respond to the above therapy may require assisted ventilation by a mechanical respirator. Intubation and assisted ventilation should be performed only by medical personnel trained in such techniques.

Precautions in Therapy

Do not use narcotics or barbiturates. They depress the respiratory center; tranquilizers may do the same in the presence of severe hypoxemia. Severe cough caused by irritation may necessitate use of nondepressant doses of antitussives, however.

Do not use epinephrine excessively, as it may thicken secretions, deplete glycogen stores, and increase apprehension.

Discharge and Follow-up Therapy: General criteria for discharge include over 90% SaO_2 on room air, PEFR above 70% of the patient's personal best or predicted normal, and reasonable confidence for adequate continued care at home. Close follow-up after discharge from the emergency room or hospital is essential. Bronchodilators and systemic corticosteroids should be continued at home. If the patient has not been on prolonged corticosteroid therapy within the past year, corticosteroids can be discontinued abruptly when the patient's response is adequate and asthma is stable rather than tapered. Many clinicians use a course of 5–10 days, depending on the severity of the episode and the patient's prior history of corticosteroid use. Maintenance medications should be resumed, and inhaled corticosteroids should be considered. A follow-up outpatient visit must be arranged. Instructions should be clear and in writing. Relapses at home signal the need for prompt re-examination at the office or hospital.

Prognosis

In the past 25–30 years, morbidity and mortality rates for asthma have increased. Mortality statistics indicate that a high percentage of deaths have resulted from *under-recognition of asthma severity and undertreatment,* particularly in labile asthmatics and asthmatics whose perception (and/or parental and physician perception) of pulmonary obstruction is poor.

There is no proof that bronchial asthma can be "cured," and there is evidence for ongoing inflammation even in asthmatics who are asymptomatic for prolonged periods. There is also evidence that the rate of decline of lung function in adulthood is abnormally high in many asthmatics and that there may be decreased growth of lung function in children with moderate to severe asthma. On the other hand, the prognosis for symptom-free control in childhood asthma is fairly good. The majority of asthmatic children have fewer symptoms in their teens, and some appear to achieve freedom from any asthmatic symptoms, perhaps for life. Unfortunately, however, only a minority (probably <30%) fall into this category, and it is usually the pediatrician rather than the asthma that the child outgrows. Many asthmatics have persistent, significant (though often unrecognized) chronic pulmonary obstruction, and others later redevelop symptomatic obstruction. Mild asthma is more likely to be outgrown than is moderate or severe asthma.

In some cases of occupational asthma in adults, early elimination of environmental exposure to causative agents is associated with complete remission of the disease. It is conceivable, therefore, that early intervention in childhood asthma may be able to at least prevent the chronicity and perhaps even facilitate complete recession of this disease. Since important risk factors for the development and severity of asthma are environmental factors over which there is possible control, the pediatrician and the allergist have a critical opportunity to markedly alter the course of this disorder.

Clark NM, Evans D, Mellins RB: Patient use of peak flow monitoring. Am Rev Respir Dis 1992;145:722.

Global Initiative for Asthma: Global Strategy for Asthma Management and Prevention, National Heart, Lung, and Blood Institute/World Health Organization workshop report (publication No. 95-3659). National Institutes of Health, 1995.

Lapin CD, Cloutier MM: Outpatient management of acute exacerbations of asthma in children. J Asthma 1995; 32:5.

McFadden ER Jr, Gilbert IA: Exercise-induced asthma. N Engl J Med 1995;330:1362.

National Heart, Lung, and Blood Institute National Asthma Education Program Expert Panel Report: Guidelines for the Diagnosis and Management of Asthma (publication No. 91-3042). Department of Health & Human Services, 1991.

Nelson HS: Drug therapy: Beta-adrenergic bronchodilators. N Engl J Med 1995;333:499.

Toogood JH: Making better—and safer—use of inhaled steroids. J Respir Dis 1993;14:221.

ALLERGIC RHINITIS

Allergic rhinitis is the most common atopic disease, perhaps because the nose is anatomically vulnerable to inhalant allergens. The pathologic changes are chiefly hyperemia, edema, and increased serous and mucoid secretions caused by mediator release, all of which lead to variable degrees of nasal obstruction, pruritus, and rhinorrhea. This process may involve the eyes and other structures, including the sinuses and possibly the middle ear. Inhalant allergens are principally responsible for symptoms, but food allergens can cause symptoms on rare occasion. Children with allergic rhinitis seem to be more susceptible to upper respiratory infections, which, in turn, intensify symptoms of existing allergic rhinitis.

Classification

Allergic rhinitis may be perennial, seasonal ("hay fever"), or episodic, but these entities frequently occur together.

Perennial Allergic Rhinitis: Rhinitis occurs to some degree all year long but may be more severe in winter. Nasal congestion-obstruction tends to be the prominent symptom. Greater exposure to allergens in house dust during the winter months is the result of closed-up homes, an increase in the amount of time spent indoors, and heating systems that raise, disperse, and circulate dust. The increased dryness of heated air and greater exposure to pets housed indoors may also add to the problem.

This disease can begin before the second year of life. It often accompanies bronchial asthma and may be provoked by the same allergens. Dental abnormalities, including disturbances in dental arch growth and malocclusion, have been attributed to longstanding rhinitis with nasal obstruction.

Seasonal Allergic Rhinitis ("Hay Fever"): This disease occurs seasonally as a result of exposure to specific wind-borne pollens. The major pollen groups in the temperate zones are trees (late winter to early spring), grasses (late spring to early summer), and weeds (late summer to early fall), but seasons can vary significantly in different parts of the country. Mold spores also cause seasonal allergic rhinitis, principally in the summer and fall. Seasonal allergy symptoms may be aggravated by coincident exposure to perennial allergens.

The age at onset is generally later than that of perennial allergic rhinitis, usually after 3 years of age. Worsening or extension of sensitivities over a period of several years after onset can be expected.

Clinical Findings

Symptoms & Signs: Nasal obstruction is manifested by mouth breathing, difficulty in eating, nasal speech, inability to clear the nose with blowing, "allergic salute," and snoring. Nasal seromucoid secretions are increased, with anterior rhinorrhea, sniffling, postnasal drip, and loose cough. Nasopharyngeal mucus frequently causes poor appetite, fatigue, and pharyngeal irritation. Nasal itching leads to nose rubbing, paroxysmal sneezing, and epistaxis. In perennial rhinitis, nasal obstruction tends to be a predominant symptom; sneezing is often most pronounced in the morning shortly after waking. In seasonal rhinitis, there tend to be more intense itching, coryza, and sneezing. Eye symptoms are more common in seasonal rhinitis and include itching, tearing, and, in extreme cases, photophobia. The intense itching of the nose and eyes, violent sneezing, and florid conjunctival injection and coryza experienced by older children and adults are not so commonly seen in young children.

Examination shows decreased patency of nasal airways and increased seromucoid discharge (usually more serious in seasonal rhinitis). The mucous membranes range from pale blue and swollen ("boggy") with dimpling in the turbinates to reddened with little edema. Conjunctival injection, periorbital edema, and circumorbital cyanosis ("allergic shiners") are frequently observed. Increased pharyngeal lymphoid tissue ("cobblestoning") from chronic pharyngeal drainage and enlarged tonsillar and adenoid tissue may be present. Bleeding or ulceration may be seen on the anterior nasal septum. A horizontal crease extending across the lower third of the nose ("allergic crease") as a result of frequent upward rubbing of the nose ("allergic salute") is frequently observed.

Laboratory Findings: Eosinophilia often can be demonstrated on smears of nasal secretions (>15%) or blood. This is a frequent but not universal finding in allergic rhinitis. Skin or serologic tests may reveal IgE antibody to offending allergens.

Associated Conditions: Sinusitis may accompany allergic rhinitis. Allergic mucosal swelling of the sinus ostia is believed to obstruct sinus drainage, predisposing the patient to and/or interfering with the normal resolution of sinus disease. Vigorous treatment is indicated until there is resolution of clinical findings.

Auditory tube dysfunction and chronic or recurrent otitis media can also be a complication of allergic rhinitis. The atopic child seems particularly prone to the development of serous otitis media. The middle ear is rarely a "shock organ" for allergy per se; rather, otitis media probably is related to auditory tube dysfunction that can be associated with allergic rhinitis. There is little evidence that allergy is a major cause of serous otitis media in the first 2–3 years of life, however.

Nasal polyps are unusual in children and generally are not caused by allergy. When polyps are present, cystic fibrosis should be considered.

Differential Diagnosis

The most common disorder that must be differentiated from allergic rhinitis is vasomotor (nonallergic, noninfectious) rhinitis. This form of perennial rhinitis masquerades as allergic rhinitis. Symptoms include variable degrees of serous or mucoid rhinorrhea and nasal stuffiness, often with pharyngeal drainage. Nasal itching may or may not be present. Occasionally, nasal eosinophilia is observed ("nonallergic rhinitis with eosinophilia" [NARES]). Diagnosis depends on ruling out sinusitis or an allergic cause.

Other disorders to consider include frequent common colds, infectious rhinitis and sinusitis, adenoidal hypertrophy, foreign bodies (usually unilateral symptoms), nasal polyposis associated with cystic fibrosis or aspirin idiosyncrasy, choanal stenosis or atresia, nasopharyngeal neoplasms, and palatal malformations.

Treatment

Avoidance: The value of identification and avoidance of causative allergens cannot be overstated (see General Principles of Treatment).

Medications: Medications are most effective when used regularly.

Antihistamines help to control symptoms of itching and sneezing and rhinorrhea (see Table 33–1). Oral decongestants help to relieve nasal stuffiness. Topical decongestants (eg, phenylephrine) can be used for no more than 5 days for severe episodes; beware of a "rebound" effect (rhinitis medicamentosa) with prolonged use.

Intranasal cromolyn may be used alone or in conjunction with antihistamines and decongestants. Intranasal corticosteroid sprays can be used for nasal symptoms and are extremely effective in controlling allergic rhinitis. Care must be taken to prevent complications, including nasal bleeding and, rarely, nasal septal perforation. They may be effective alone or with antihistamines.

Immunotherapy: Immunotherapy should be considered when symptoms are severe and other symptomatic measures have failed.

Surgery: Surgical procedures (removal of nasal polyps, sinus surgery, insertion of ventilating tubes for chronic otitis media, adenoidectomy) should be considered only when medical therapy fails.

Prognosis

Unless specific allergens can be identified and

eliminated from the environment, perennial allergic rhinitis tends to be protracted. However, nasal obstruction may become less troublesome as the child grows and the nasal airway increases in caliber. In seasonal allergic rhinitis, patients tend to suffer repeatedly from their seasonal symptoms. Symptoms are usually most severe from adolescence through midadult life. On moving to a region devoid of problem allergens, patients may be free of seasonal allergic rhinitis for 1–3 years but may acquire sensitivity to airborne allergens prominent in the area to which they move.

Bielory L, Frohman LP: Allergic and immunologic disorders of the eye. J Allergy Clin Immunol 1992;89:1.

Druce HM: Allergic and nonallergic rhinitis. In: *Allergy: Principles and Practice,* 4th ed. Middleton E Jr et al (editors). Mosby, 1993.

International Rhinitis Management Working Group: International consensus report on the diagnosis and management of rhinitis. Allergy 1994;49S:1.

Virant FS (editor): Chronic sinus disease. Immunol Allergy Clin North Am 1994;14:1.

Wright AL et al: Epidemiology of physician-diagnosed allergic rhinitis in childhood. Pediatrics 1994;94:895.

ATOPIC DERMATITIS
(Eczema)

Atopic dermatitis is a chronic or chronically relapsing, pruritic dermatitis. It commonly occurs in patients with a personal or family history of atopy. A common denominator of atopic dermatitis is a lowered threshold for itching; this disorder has been called "an itch that rashes." Much of the skin damage is secondary to scratching, excoriation, and chronic rubbing. Scratching also predisposes the patient to skin infection. Factors that aggravate itching include dryness, sweating, contact with rough materials and detergents, and psychologic factors.

There is a high incidence of elevated IgE total and specific IgE antibodies in children with this disorder. In some infants and children, specific IgE to food or inhalant allergens plays a role in atopic dermatitis. A young child with severe atopic dermatitis that is poorly responsive to therapy appears particularly likely to have food hypersensitivity. A careful history with supporting tests for specific IgE can be helpful to identify allergens that may be aggravating or precipitating the disease. Foods most frequently implicated include milk, eggs, and legumes (including peanuts). Aeroallergens may play an important role in the pathogenesis of atopic dermatitis; cutaneous contact may be an important route of exposure. Many patients have specific IgE of no apparent clinical relevance to the disease.

The origin of atopic dermatitis is unknown; evidence suggests a role for IgE-mediated immediate-phase and late-phase reactions. Dry skin, which appears to be present in all patients with atopic dermatitis, may allow increased penetration of potentially allergenic proteins. Patients with atopic dermatitis have increased histamine releasability from basophils and mast cells. Histologic findings vary with the stage of the dermatitis; biopsy of acute lesions reveals a mononuclear cell infiltrate (lymphocytes, macrophages); increased mast cell numbers; a few neutrophils, basophils, and eosinophils; and eosinophil major basic protein deposition. The presence of the latter suggests that eosinophils participate in causing the disorder.

Clinical Findings

Symptoms & Signs: Atopic dermatitis usually begins in infancy, but can begin at almost any time in childhood. In infants, lesions typically appear after 2 months of age, beginning on the cheeks and the forehead and spreading in a patchy or generalized distribution over the trunk and the extensor surfaces of extremities. After infancy, involvement of flexural creases (antecubital, popliteal, neck) predominates; frequently, the wrists, hands, feet, face, and eyelids also are involved. The appearance of the rash varies depending on the stage of the dermatitis (acute, subacute, chronic). As the child grows older, the eczema tends to wax and wane, sometimes disappearing completely for months. Although it may abate altogether by age 3–5 years, it is not uncommon for the dermatitis to persist through childhood and adulthood; that is, frequently it is not outgrown. Although scarring is unusual, hyperpigmentation and hypopigmentation may occur. As noted, excessive skin dryness is a frequent concomitant finding, and a form of congenital ichthyosis often accompanies atopic dermatitis.

Laboratory Findings: No laboratory tests are diagnostic of atopic dermatitis, but they may help to substantiate the diagnosis. The IgE level is frequently elevated, with a higher level corresponding to more severe disease, but the level may be normal. Specific IgE antibodies to various inhalant and food allergens are found on skin testing or RAST in approximately 80% of children. Eosinophilia may occur. Routine skin biopsy does not differentiate atopic dermatitis from other eczematous processes and is not ordinarily indicated.

Differential Diagnosis

Seborrheic dermatitis may be distinguished by a lack of significant pruritus, its predilection for the scalp ("cradle cap"), and its coarse, yellowish scales. Lack of dermatitis in the axillae favors the diagnosis of atopic dermatitis. Seborrheic dermatitis may occur in association with atopic dermatitis. Contact dermatitis is distinguished chiefly by the distribution of lesions (usually on extensor and exposed areas), generally with a greater demarcation of dermatitis than in atopic dermatitis. Nummular eczema is characterized by coin-shaped plaques. Scabies is more papulovesicular and relatively nonerythematous, occurring chiefly in the interdigital and waistline areas; itching may be intense, particularly at night. Because of scratching, an eczematous dermatitis may develop. If erythema and scaling without itching are present, the diagnosis of ichthyosis vulgaris should be considered. Various other disorders have associated skin eruptions that may resemble atopic dermatitis, including Wiskott-Aldrich syndrome, agammaglobulinemia, ataxia-telangiectasia, phenylketonuria, Hurler syndrome, Job syndrome (hyper-IgE), histiocytosis X, and cutaneous lymphoma.

Complications & Sequelae

Bacterial skin infection, particularly with *Staphylococcus aureus,* occurs with some frequency. Honey-colored crusting, folliculitis, pyoderma, and furunculosis indicate bacterial infection. Viral infections with herpes and molluscum contagiosum can occur. Generalized herpesvirus infection of the skin is known as eczema herpeticum or Kaposi's varicelliform eruption. Varicella occasionally is unusually severe in children with atopic dermatitis. Fungal skin infections (eg, with a dermatophyte fungus) also may occur.

Nutritional disturbances may result from unwarranted and unnecessarily vigorous dietary restrictions imposed by physicians and parents. Chronic, severe, generalized atopic dermatitis may lead to a catabolic state, with resultant growth retardation. This process reverses with adequate control of the dermatitis. Cataracts in late childhood or adulthood occur in a small percentage of cases, even when corticosteroids are not used in treatment. Temporary or chronic emotional disturbances may occur as a result of feelings of disfigurement, imposed restrictions, and unhealthy attitudes of parents and others toward a child with this disease. Poor academic performance and behavioral disturbances may be a result of uncontrolled intense or frequent itching, sleep loss, and poor self-image.

Treatment
(See Chapter 14.)

Allergen Avoidance: Known causative allergens should be avoided. If an ingested allergen is suspected as aggravating the atopic dermatitis based on history and tests for specific IgE, it should be removed from the diet for approximately 1 week while maximizing therapy to keep the dermatitis under control. If the skin improves without this food in the diet, a relationship between the food and the dermatitis is suggested. The food is then added back to the diet and the patient is observed for worsening of dermatitis. However, it may be difficult to determine in this type of unblinded "elimination-challenge" diet the impact of a food on the dermatitis because many other factors may also contribute to dermatitis and

because of potential observer bias by parents. In these cases, a single-blind or double-blind challenge with the suspected food in an office setting may be indicated. If one or more food allergens are found to be causative, one must be sure that the patient's diet remains nutritionally adequate. Maternal avoidance of important food allergens during breast-feeding, delayed addition of solid foods to the infant's diet until after 6 months of age, and avoidance of highly allergenic foods during infancy may prevent or delay the development of atopic dermatitis. Avoidance of relevant aeroallergens (especially animal dander and dust mites) may be beneficial.

Immunotherapy: This therapy is of unclear general value but may be helpful in cases in which aggravation by unavoidable allergens occurs. Immunotherapy also can aggravate atopic dermatitis.

Other: Treatment with immunomodulating agents and phototherapy may prove useful in treating patients with severe, refractory disease, but their use thus far generally has been experimental.

Prognosis

Many cases of atopic dermatitis resolve spontaneously in early childhood, but the disease may persist even into adult life. There is a high likelihood that a child with atopic dermatitis will develop allergic rhinitis, asthma, or both. Consequently, it seems wise to institute simple environmental control measures in the homes of children with atopic dermatitis and to follow up these children closely for the development of these disorders. In patients in whom controlled, blinded food challenges result in a flare of dermatitis, avoidance of the specific food has been shown to be beneficial. Breast-feeding may delay but will not eliminate the onset of atopic dermatitis.

Adinoff AD, Clark RAF: Atopic dermatitis. In: *Allergy, Asthma, and Immunology From Infancy to Adulthood,* 3rd ed. Bierman CW et al (editors). Saunders, 1996.

Burks AW et al: Atopic dermatitis and food hypersensitivity in children. Allergy Proc 1992;13:285.

Charlesworth EN: Practical approaches to the treatment of atopic dermatitis. Allergy Proc 1994;15:269.

Sampson HA: Atopic dermatitis. Allergy 1992;69:469.

ADVERSE REACTIONS TO FOODS

Foods are frequently suspected of causing a myriad of symptoms. Adverse reactions to foods can be classified on the basis of the mechanism of the reaction. Although these reactions are often diagnosed by patients or physicians as "allergic," the majority, in fact, are nonimmune in origin. Examples of the latter include pharmacologic or metabolic mechanisms and reactions to food toxins (see Table 33–2). The term *allergic reaction* to food is used only to describe re-

Table 33–2. Adverse reactions to foods: mechanisms of hypersensitivity.

Food allergy (IgE-mediated reactions): Classic "allergic" reactions caused by IgE antibody and release of mediators from mast cells and basophils
Immune non–IgE-mediated food hypersensitivity
    Milk or soy protein gastroenteritis
    Gluten sensitivity (celiac sprue)
Metabolic mechanisms
    Carbohydrate enzyme deficiencies (eg, lactase deficiency)
    Glucose-6-phosphate dehydrogenase deficiency
    Phenylketonuria
    Ceruloplasmin deficiency (Wilson's disease)
Pharmacologic mechanisms
    Histamine intoxication (scombroid poisoning as from tuna or mackerel)
    Vasoactive amines occurring naturally in foods (eg, strawberries, melons, cheese, chocolate, some wines and beers)
    Methylxanthines (caffeine)
Food intolerance (idiosyncratic or unknown mechanism)
    Anaphylactoid (unable to demonstrate IgE-mediated process yet syndrome resembles anaphylaxis)
    Food-associated, exercise-induced anaphylaxis (IgE may play a role in some cases)
    Dyes
    Preservatives

actions in which an immune mechanism is responsible, the most common of which is IgE-mediated.

Several factors influence a patient's potential to react to food, including a predisposition to develop IgE antibody. Early introduction of cow's milk or solid foods may increase a risk of food allergy. In general, allergy to foods in early childhood is likely to be a problem as the child grows. For example, most children (60–90%) who develop a milk allergy in infancy are able to tolerate milk in the diet by the age of 4 years (but skin tests and RAST to milk may remain positive). On the other hand, severe and potentially life-threatening sensitivity to such allergens as peanuts, nuts, and seeds may be lifelong.

IgE-Mediated Syndromes of Food Hypersensitivity

Reactions can occur in all body tissues. A wide variety of signs and symptoms can be encountered, many of which may appear extremely vague. *Skin or gastrointestinal involvement is characteristic of IgE-mediated reactions but may be absent even in life-threatening allergic reactions to foods.* Less commonly, the airway and the cardiovascular system are involved. Such reactions usually occur from minutes to 2 hours, rarely beyond 4 hours after allergen ingestion. The most common food allergens in young children are cow's milk, eggs, peanuts, soy, and wheat. In older children and adults, fish, shellfish, and nuts are most often involved in allergic reactions. However, severe reactions can occur to almost any food. The presence of IgE can be demonstrated by prick skin testing or RAST.

Gastrointestinal Signs & Symptoms: In mild cases, symptoms may include mouth itching or paresthesias, abdominal discomfort, bloating, nausea, vomiting, and diarrhea. In severe cases, there may be forceful vomiting, severe abdominal pain, bloody and mucoid diarrhea, and dehydration.

Urticaria & Angioedema: In mild cases, findings may include periorbital and lip angioedema, hives, flushing, or any combination of these. In severe cases, there may be tongue, pharyngeal, and laryngotracheal edema. *Angioedema of the uvula is always a reason for concern and warrants management;* death may occur from asphyxia.

Anaphylaxis: Life-threatening reactions result from massive mediator release and generally involve several organ systems. However, food anaphylaxis may present only as shock! (See Anaphylaxis, earlier.) Anaphylactoid reactions also occur which are anaphylaxis-like in clinical appearance but result from nonimmune release of chemical mediators.

Atopic Dermatitis: Food allergy often plays an important role in atopic dermatitis. (See Atopic Dermatitis, earlier.)

Respiratory Tract Symptoms: Rarely, food hypersensitivity can cause isolated rhinitis or asthma. More commonly, respiratory tract involvement occurs as part of a generalized and life-threatening reaction.

Non–IgE-Mediated Syndromes of Food Hypersensitivity

Tension-Fatigue Syndrome: A combination of the following symptoms has been reported: fatigue, lassitude, irritability, sleeplessness, disturbed behavior, apathy, pallor, "shadowy" eyes with "allergic pleats," and sometimes a generalized headache with vague abdominal complaints. This syndrome is claimed to be associated in particular with foods commonly and abundantly eaten, such as cow's milk, cereal grains, chocolate, eggs, and pork. Similar symptoms have also been attributed to yeast "allergy" (the "yeast connection"), but neither a relationship to colonization with or ingestion of yeast nor an IgE-mediated process has been established.

Hyperactivity: Claims that dyes, sugar, and other food additives may contribute to hyperactivity in children with attention- deficit disorder (ADD) are controversial. In the occasional case in which a child appears to benefit from restricted diets (eg, the "Feingold diet"), there is no evidence of an IgE-mediated reaction. On the other hand, allergic disorders in children with ADD may be poorly tolerated and complicate ADD.

Migraine: In addition to other causes, foods may precipitate a migrainous episode on an allergic or nonallergic basis. Foods containing significant amounts of vasoactive amines (eg, chocolate, cheese, liver, and some wines and beers) may precipitate migraine headaches in some patients.

Clinical Findings

A history of the temporal association of ingestion of suspected food to reaction and the nature and duration of symptoms observed are often helpful in establishing the diagnosis of food allergy. Alternatively, acute symptoms suggestive of food allergy may occur, but the cause may not be obvious from the history. With chronic symptoms such as atopic dermatitis or urticaria, the association with food may be less obvious.

A symptom diary kept for 7–14 days is helpful in establishing a temporal association of ingestion of foods to symptoms and also serves to provide a baseline observation for symptom pattern. It is important to note both the form in which the food was ingested (eg, raw versus cooked) and other foods ingested at the same time.

Skin testing is useful to confirm a suspected food allergy or to identify a previously unrecognized allergen (use prick test only). Large positive reactions in skin tests are often clinically relevant; mild (<3 mm) reactions correlate poorly with clinical sensitivity. Negative reactions to skin tests do not rule out a nonimmune clinical reaction or even an allergic reaction to some elements of food (eg, partially hydrolyzed product). RAST scores of less than 3 usually are not associated with clinical sensitivity. Measurement of IgG to foods is not clinically useful. Eosinophilia of stool mucus may be present in cases of gastrointestinal allergy; blood eosinophilia may occur.

Provocative food tests are helpful in evaluating less serious reactions. Elimination (at least 1 week) and rechallenge may be useful to confirm suspected diagnosis. In very serious reactions such as angioedema, anaphylaxis, and bronchial asthma, the causative food is usually known by the patient or his or her parents or can identified by the physician with the aid of a history and skin testing. Food challenges are potentially hazardous in these situations.

Differential Diagnosis

With chronic gastrointestinal symptoms, consider carbohydrate enzyme deficiencies (eg, lactase), cystic fibrosis, celiac disease, chronic intestinal infections, gastrointestinal malformations, and irritable bowel syndrome as other possible causes. With repeated vomiting in infancy, consider pyloric stenosis or gastroesophageal reflux (in infants <8 weeks of age). With acute involvement of the laryngeal or tracheal airway, consider acute epiglottis and foreign body.

Treatment & Prognosis

Treatment consists of eliminating the offending food, but the physician must be careful to provide specific advice for ensuring the nutritional adequacy of the diet. If milk products are withdrawn from the diet for over 1 month, the daily requirement of calcium should be administered. *Especially in the grow-ing child, the unnecessary and unjustified restriction of many foods over an indefinite period merely because they might be involved or because they happened to give a positive skin reaction is condemned.* The majority of proved offending foods in young children can be tolerated as time passes and, unless the symptoms have been life-threatening, should be rechallenged at 6- to 12-month intervals until the food can be reintroduced without symptoms.

The prognosis is good if the offending food can be identified and avoided. In some of the vague chronic syndromes, identification may not be possible and the patient may remain symptomatic. With severe sensitivity, the offending food is usually known.

Anderson JA (editor): Food allergy. Immunol Allergy Clin North Am 1991;11:701.

Anderson JA: Milestones marking the knowledge of adverse reactions to food in the decade of the 1980s. Ann Allergy 1994;72:143.

Burks W: A step-by-step approach to food allergy. Contemp Pediatr 1993;10:32.

Hoffman KM, Sampson HA: Evaluation and management of patients with adverse food reactions. In: *Allergy, Asthma, and Immunology From Infancy to Adulthood*, 3rd ed. Bierman CW et al (editors). Saunders, 1996.

Metcalfe DD, Sampson HA, Simon RA (editors): *Food Allergy: Adverse Reactions to Foods and Food Additives.* Blackwell, 1991.

DRUG HYPERSENSITIVITY

Drugs are so widely used that drug reactions of one type or another are common. It is helpful to categorize drug reactions according to the mechanism of the reaction. **Toxic drug reactions** are caused by the inherent pharmacologic properties of the drug and are most frequently encountered after drug overdosage. However, some individuals exhibit inordinate sensitivity to the recognized pharmacologic effects of a drug and develop toxicity after administration of amounts that are usually nontoxic. **Drug idiosyncrasy** is an unusual response to the pharmacologic action of the drug (eg, hyperactivity rather than sedation following the administration of phenobarbital). **Allergic reactions** to drugs are independent of the drug's pharmacologic action and are the result of immune processes. These reactions can be classified as (1) IgE-mediated hypersensitivity reactions, (2) cytotoxic antibody-mediated reactions, (3) antigen-antibody immune complex–mediated reactions, and (4) cell-mediated hypersensitivity reactions. **Pseudoallergic ("anaphylactoid") reactions** mimic IgE-mediated reactions but are caused by non-immune release of histamine and other mediators from mast cells (eg, reactions to radiocontrast media, opiates, and vancomycin). Drug reactions that are suspected to involve immune processes in which the specific mechanisms have not been identified include erythema multiforme, Stevens-Johnson syndrome, toxic epidermal necrolysis, fixed drug eruptions, drug fever, interstitial nephritis, and eosinophilic pneumonitis.

Clinical Manifestations

Manifestations of drug allergy are extremely varied and depend on the type of immune process responsible for the reaction. Urticaria is a common cutaneous manifestation of IgE-mediated hypersensitivity reactions, resulting from mast cell mediator release. Systemic anaphylaxis is a manifestation of this type of reaction as well. Serum sickness, which is caused by immune complex formation, at least when foreign proteins are involved, is characterized by fever, rash, lymphadenopathy, myalgias, and arthralgias occurring 7–21 days after the first encounter with a substance. Re-exposure to the antigen in an already sensitized individual may result in symptoms in as early as 12–36 hours. A cytotoxic drug reaction occurs when a drug binds to the surface of a cell such as a red blood cell or a platelet. IgG antibodies directed against the cell-bound drug or the altered cell surface membrane bind to the cell surface, with resultant cell destruction. An example of this type of immune drug reaction is penicillin-induced hemolytic anemia. Finally, delayed-type hypersensitivity may occur to a topically applied drug, such as neomycin, with resultant contact dermatitis.

Various adverse reactions to aspirin and related medications have been recognized in children. One example is the syndrome of nasal polyposis, severe aspirin-induced bronchospasm, and rhinosinusitis. The mechanism of aspirin-induced bronchospasm is unknown but is thought to relate to abnormal arachidonic acid pathway metabolism. In these cases, most nonsteroidal anti-inflammatory drugs (NSAIDs) are likely to cause the same response. Urticaria or angioedema may also occur with a specific NSAID, in some cases because of the presence of IgE antibodies to the specific drug. In addition, NSAIDs commonly aggravate chronic idiopathic urticaria by an apparently nonimmune mechanism.

The parenteral route of drug administration is generally more sensitizing than the oral route. Topical administration of drugs, especially over inflamed skin, is particularly sensitizing. Exposure to sunlight may lead to skin reactions to photosensitizing drugs such as sulfonamides and tetracyclines. Although an immune reaction is highly specific, cross-reactions with chemically related drugs are not infrequent, for example, among β-lactam antibiotics (ie, penicillins, cephalosporins).

Tests for drug allergy have been limited to patch testing in contact dermatitis and to skin testing for the presence of IgE to certain drugs, including penicillin, insulin, heterologous antiserum, chymopapain, vaccines, local anesthetics, and muscle relaxants. Serologic tests, when available, tend to be less sensitive than skin tests. In some cases, the allergic reaction is caused by a metabolite of the drug or the mechanism of the reaction is unknown, making it difficult to develop tests to identify drug allergy. The principal metabolites responsible for allergic reactions to penicillin have been identified; although some are available commercially for use in skin testing, reagents which are most predictive of severe reactivity are not. Finally, certain compounds, such as radiocontrast media, cause nonimmune mediator release; therefore, skin tests cannot be used to identify or predict a reaction to these materials. Thus, a clear history of a previous reaction to a drug often must be relied on for diagnosing drug sensitivity.

Treatment & Prognosis

Regardless of the manifestation, the treatment of drug allergy includes discontinuation of the offending drug at the first sign of an adverse reaction and avoidance of that drug. An alternative drug should be used, if possible, when a reaction to a drug is known or suspected. Individuals with extreme hypersensitivity to a given drug should be warned of hidden sources of the drug, such as vaccines and other substances. In selected cases, if there is no acceptable alternative to a given drug and the drug is required, desensitization may be indicated (eg, penicillin desensitization). The use of a small "test dose" of radiocontrast medium in patients with a history of reaction is not a valid test for predicting reactivity to the agent.

Symptomatic treatment of drug reactions is usually effective. Antihistamines may be used to treat pruritus. Corticosteroids are used for severe or prolonged drug reactions, such as in anaphylaxis and serum sickness. (See also Anaphylaxis, earlier.) Guidelines to prevent reactions to radiocontrast media include the use of newer, low-osmolality agents and pretreatment with an antihistamine and a corticosteroid. Protocols have been developed.

The prognosis is good, especially when drug allergens are identified early and avoided.

Anderson JA: Allergic reactions to drugs and biological agents. JAMA 1992;268:2845.

Patterson R et al: Drug allergy and protocols for management of drug allergies. Allergy Proc 1994;15:239.

Roujeau JC, Stern RS: Severe adverse cutaneous reactions to drugs. N Engl J Med 1994;331:1272.

URTICARIA & ANGIOEDEMA

Urticaria is a relatively common vascular reaction of the upper dermis consisting mainly of vasodilation and perivascular transudation, resulting in the classic "hive" or wheal and flare. Lesions are characteristically pruritic. Ordinarily, this vascular reaction is largely caused by to the liberation of histamine, but various other mediators may be major participants. Angioedema is essentially a similar vascular reaction of the deep dermis and subcutaneous tissue, resulting in the production of a more diffuse edema.

Traditionally, urticaria has been classified as acute or chronic if the hives have been recurrent for less or more than 6 weeks, respectively. Urticaria and angioedema also may be classified based on the pathophysiology of the lesions. Urticaria and angioedema may be caused by the interaction of an antigen (eg, food, drug, inhalant, venom) with IgE that is bound to skin mast cells and/or circulating basophils. Complement activation resulting from non-IgE immune complex formation may lead to mediator release, with resultant urticaria and angioedema (eg, serum sickness, transfusion reactions, collagen-vascular diseases). Urticaria may be caused by agents which directly release mast cell mediators, such as opiates, radiocontrast media, and mannitol. Various types of physical urticarias occur wherein hives develop upon exposure to cold, heat, vibration, sunlight, pressure, or water.

In *cold urticaria,* exposure to cold induces localized urticaria or angioedema. Death from massive mast cell mediatory release can occur after swimming in cold water. *Cholinergic urticaria* results from elevation of the core body temperature; it is characterized by small wheals with large surrounding erythema associated with overheating (eg, during exercise). *Dermatographism* is the appearance of a wheal and erythema on the skin when "written on" (eg, stroked with a fingernail). Dermatographism, which can occur in allergic and nonallergic individuals, generally is of no pathologic significance but may accompany chronic urticaria or urticaria pigmentosa (mastocytosis). Other forms of physical urticarias are *pressure urticaria/angioedema, solar urticaria,* and *aquagenic urticaria. Papular urticaria* is a term used to characterize multiple papules from insect bites, found especially on the extremities. It is not true urticaria. Urticarial reactions to aspirin, other nonsteroidal anti-inflammatory drugs, and, rarely, azo dyes and benzoates, may occur, possibly as a result of abnormal arachidonic acid metabolism. *Chronic idiopathic urticaria/angioedema* occurs in both atopic and nonatopic patients and is characterized by distinct pathologic features on skin biopsy. As the name implies, a causative agent cannot be found. Some patients with this disorder have IgG autoantibodies against mast cell surface IgE or IgE receptors. Urticaria may occur in association with other disorders, such as hepatitis, thyroid disease, and cancer. Urticaria can occur as a component of vasculitis and may be present as an early component of Schönlein-Henoch purpura.

Hereditary angioedema is a rare, autosomal dominant disorder caused by a quantitative or functional deficiency of C1-esterase inhibitor and characterized by episodic, frequently severe, nonpruritic angioedema of the skin, gastrointestinal, and/or upper respiratory tract mucosa. It is not associated with urticaria. Life-threatening laryngeal angioedema may occur.

Clinical Evaluation

History: The history is of prime importance in ascertaining the possible cause. Specific areas of inquiry should include a history of exposure to drugs, vaccines, foods, inhalants (pollens, animal dander, molds), physical factors (cold, heat, vibration, sunlight, pressure, exercise, water), stress (probably overrated as a cause of hives), and infections (viral, fungal, parasitic). It is important to note when the urticaria and angioedema began and how long individual lesions persist. Characteristically, lesions rarely persist for more than a couple of hours in the same place; persistence suggests another diagnosis. Rare familial urticarial disorders are suggested by family history. Approximately 50% of acute-onset urticaria cannot be linked to a specific cause.

Symptoms & Signs: Urticarial lesions appear as erythematous areas, classically with a raised pale center, but may be only erythematous; they usually occur in large numbers and may be located anywhere on the body. Pruritus is the rule and is frequently intense; it may precede the appearance of the lesions. Angioedema often involves the face, tongue, extremities, or genitalia. Typically, there is little or no pruritus associated with angioedema. Angioedema without urticaria frequently occurs as a solitary lesion. Angioedema and urticaria also often occur together in the same patient. Mild purpura may be observed secondary to vascular trauma from scratching. Extensive petechiae or purpura suggests other vascular or systemic disorders.

Laboratory Findings: Laboratory tests are done based on the history and physical findings. Extensive laboratory evaluation, without focus on the suggested causes of the disorder based on the patient's history or examination, is not recommended. In chronic urticaria, selected "screening" laboratory studies to look for an important underlying disease may be indicated, such as a complete blood count, erythrocyte sedimentation rate, urinalysis, and chemistry profile. Other specific tests should be done according to the suspected presence of specific underlying disease. Testing for IgE antibody to food and inhalant allergens may be helpful to verify the patient's history of a causative agent or to implicate a potential cause of the urticaria and angioedema. Specific tests for physical urticarias, such as an ice cube test or a pressure test, may be indicated based on history. If the history or appearance of the urticarial lesions suggests vasculitis, a skin biopsy is indicated. Hereditary angioedema is diagnosed by finding a low C4 level and a low level of or functionally abnormal C1-esterase inhibitor.

Patient diaries occasionally may be helpful to determine the cause of recurrent hives. A trial of food or drug elimination may be considered.

Differential Diagnosis

Urticarial lesions generally are typical in appearance and easily recognized. The major diagnostic dilemma relates to determining the underlying cause. Angioedema usually can be distinguished from other forms of edema because it is transient, asymmetric, and nonpitting and does not occur predominantly in dependent areas of the body.

Treatment & Prognosis

Treatment consists mainly of the detection and elimination of the causative agents, when possible. Aspirin and related compounds, alcohol, and heat should be avoided because they may aggravate urticaria and angioedema. Antihistamines (especially hydroxyzine) are usually the most useful therapeutic agents for treating urticaria. In resistant cases, combining an H_1 antihistamine with an H_2 antihistamine may be helpful. Corticosteroids may be indicated for severe or refractory urticaria and angioedema. Cyproheptadine is especially helpful for cold urticaria. Epinephrine is usually effective for acute urticaria and angioedema. Intubation may be indicated for life-threatening laryngeal edema. Hereditary angioedema can be treated with the prophylactic use of anabolic agents.

The prognosis is generally good for patients with urticaria and angioedema. Symptomatic treatment is generally effective, although some patients have refractory symptoms. Spontaneous remission of urticaria and angioedema is frequent, but some patients have a prolonged course. Reassurance of patients is important, as this disorder can cause significant frustration. Periodic follow-up is important to continue to monitor patients for a possible serious underlying cause. Follow-up is particularly important in patients with laryngeal edema.

Greaves MW: Chronic urticaria. N Engl J Med 1995; 332:1767.

Hanifin JM: Management strategies for atopic dermatitis and urticaria. J Respir Dis 1992;13:S14.

Kaplan AP: Urticaria and angioedema. In: *Allergy: Principles and Practice,* 4th ed. Middleton E Jr et al (editors). Mosby, 1993.

SUGGESTED ADDITIONAL READING

References for Physicians

Bierman CW et al (editors): *Allergy, Asthma, and Immunology From Infancy to Adulthood,* 3rd ed. Saunders, 1996.

deShazo RD, Smith DL (editors): Primer on allergic and immunologic diseases, 3rd ed. JAMA 1992;268:2785.

Middleton E Jr et al (editors): *Allergy: Principles and Practice,* 4th ed. Mosby, 1993.

Patterson RC et al (editors): *Allergic Diseases: Diagnosis and Management,* 4th ed. Lippincott, 1993.

References for Parents and Patients

Boggs PB: *Sneezing Your Head Off.* Patient Education, 1994.

Sander N: *Consumer Update on Asthma.* Asthma and Allergy Network/Mothers of Asthmatics, 1993.

Sander N: *A Parent's Guide to Asthma.* Doubleday, 1989.

Wood RA: *Taming Asthma and Allergy by Controlling Your Environment: A Guide for Patients.* Asthma and Allergy Foundation of America, 1995.

Young SH, Dobozin BS, Miner M: *Allergies: The Complete Guide to Diagnosis, Treatment and Daily Management.* Consumer Reports Books, 1992.

Organizations for Parents & Patients

Asthma and Allergy Foundation of America: 1125 15th St NW, Suite 502, Washington, DC 20005; (800) 7-ASTHMA.

Asthma and Allergy Network/Mothers of Asthmatics: 3554 Chain Bridge Rd, Suite 200, Fairfax, VA 22030-2709; (800) 878-4403.

Eczema Association for Science and Education: 1221 SW Yamhill, Suite 303, Portland, OR 97205; (503) 728-4430.

34

Antimicrobial Therapy of Pediatric Infections

John W. Ogle, MD

PRINCIPLES OF ANTIMICROBIAL THERAPY

Antimicrobial therapy of bacterial infection is arguably the most important scientific development of 20th century medicine. Antimicrobial therapy contributes significantly to the quality of life of many people and reduces the morbidity and mortality due to infectious diseases. The remarkable success of antimicrobial therapy has been achieved with comparatively little toxicity and expense. The relative ease of administration and the availability of these drugs have led many to adopt a philosophy of broad-spectrum empiric antimicrobial therapy for many common infections.

Unfortunately, this era of cheap, safe, and reliable therapy may be coming to a close owing to the increasing antimicrobial resistance that is encountered in previously susceptible microorganisms. The problem of antimicrobial resistance is certainly not new; resistance was recognized in sulfonamides and penicillins shortly after their introduction into practice. Rather, what is new and of concern is the worldwide dissemination of resistant clones of microorganisms, such as *Streptococcus pneumoniae* and *Staphylococcus aureus,* which are inherently virulent and common causes of serious infection, not only among hospitalized patients, but also among outpatients.

Until recently, the recognition of new resistance clones was balanced by the promise of newer and more potent antimicrobial agents. Now, since relatively fewer new agents are under development, clinicians are beginning to encounter limitations in their ability to treat some serious bacterial infections. Many factors contribute to the selection of antimicrobial-resistant clones. Our success in treating patients with chronic diseases and immune-compromising conditions has resulted in additional years of life for such patients, but has facilitated selection of resistant strains in inpatient units and chronic care facilities.

Overuse of antimicrobial agents by well-intentioned clinicians also significantly contributes to the selection of resistant strains. Examples of overuse include medications for mildly ill patients with self-limited conditions, such as viral infections, and broad-spectrum antimicrobials for patients whose condition can be treated with narrow-spectrum agents. Similarly, the failure to document infection with appropriate cultures, obtained prior to therapy, limits our willingness to stop or narrow the spectrum of antimicrobials. In addition, little research has been conducted to determine the necessary duration of therapy and, as a result, we probably often treat longer than is necessary. Similarly, prophylactic strategies, as used for prevention of recurrent otitis media, contribute a selection pressure for antibiotic resistance.

The decision-making process for choosing an appropriate antimicrobial agent is summarized in Table 34–1. Accurate clinical diagnosis is based on history, physical examination, and initial laboratory tests. The clinical diagnosis then leads to a consideration of the organisms that are most commonly associated with the clinical condition, of the usual pattern of antimicrobial susceptibility for the most likely organism or organisms, and of the past experience with successful treatment regimens.

Appropriate cultures should be obtained in potentially serious infections. Empiric antimicrobial therapy may be initiated, then modified according to the patient's response and the culture results. Often there are several equally safe and efficacious antimicrobials. In this circumstance, the relative cost of the different choices should be considered.

Other important considerations include the age, immune status, and exposure history of the patient. Neonates and young infants may present with nonspecific signs of infection, making the differentiation of serious disease from mild illness difficult. In older children, clinical diagnosis is more precise, which may allow no therapy or use of a more narrow spectrum antibiotic. The presence of an immune deficiency may increase the number and types of potential infecting organisms that need to be considered, including organisms that are usually avirulent, but that may be serious and difficult to treat once infection is established. An abnormal immune response may also diminish the severity of the clinical signs

Table 34–1. Steps in decision making for use of antimicrobial agents.

Step	Action	Example
1	Determine diagnosis.	Septic arthritis
2	Consider age and preexisting condition.	Normal 2-year-old child
3	Consider common organisms.	*Staphylococcus aureus, Haemophilus influenzae*
4	Consider organism susceptibility.	Penicillin- or ampicillin-resistant
5	Obtain proper cultures.[1]	Blood, joint fluid
6	Initiate empiric therapy based on above considerations and past experience (eg, personal, literature).	Nafcillin and cefotaxime
7	Modify therapy based on culture results and patient response.	*S aureus* isolated. Discontinue cefotaxime.
8	Follow clinical response.	

[1]Indicated for serious or unusual infections or those with unpredictable clinical response to empiric therapy.

and symptoms of infection and thereby lead to underestimation of the severity of the illness. The exposure history of the patient is another important factor that may influence the likelihood of certain types of infecting organisms. This history includes exposures from family members, classmates, or day-care environments or exposure to unusual organisms by virtue of travel, diet, or animal contact. Final important considerations are the pace and seriousness of the illness. A rapidly progressive, serious illness should be treated initially with broad-spectrum antimicrobials until the nature of the illness and infecting organism or organisms are identified. In contrast, a mildly ill outpatient should be treated preferentially with narrow-spectrum antimicrobials.

Antimicrobial susceptibility, antimicrobial families, and dosing recommendations are listed in Tables 34–2 through 34–6.

ANTIMICROBIAL SUSCEPTIBILITY TESTING

It is critically important to obtain cultures and other diagnostic material from patients prior to initiating antimicrobial therapy. This is especially important when the patient has a serious infection, when initial attempts at therapy have failed, or when the use of multiple antimicrobial agents is anticipated. Whenever cultures identify the causative agent, therapy can be narrowed or optimized according to susceptibility results. Antimicrobial susceptibility testing should be done in a laboratory using carefully defined procedures (National Committee for Clinical Laboratory Standards). The use of nonstandard media, inoculum size, or growth conditions may give markedly different and undependable results.

There are several different ways to test antimicrobial susceptibility. The identification of an antibiotic-destroying enzyme (eg, β-lactamase) implies resistance to that group of antimicrobial agents. Tube or microtiter broth dilution techniques can be used to determine the minimum inhibitory concentration (MIC) of antibiotic, which is the amount of antibiotic (μg/mL) necessary to inhibit the organism under specific laboratory conditions. The physician, who also has a knowledge of the clinical pharmacology of the antimicrobial agent, can infer antibiotic susceptibility if the MIC is less than the antibiotic concentration achievable in the patient using appropriate antibiotic dosages. Disk susceptibility testing (again, only under carefully controlled conditions) yields similar results. The E-test is standardized for some organisms and correlates well with MICs. Clinical laboratories usually define antimicrobial susceptibility (susceptible, intermediate, resistant) in relation to levels of the test antibiotic achievable in the blood (or serum).

In general, organisms are considered susceptible to an antibiotic if the MIC of the antibiotic for an organism is lower than levels of that antimicrobial agent achievable in the blood using appropriate parenteral dosages. This assumption of susceptibility should be reconsidered whenever the patient has a focus of infection (eg, meningitis, osteomyelitis, abscess) in which poor antibiotic penetration might occur, since the levels of antibiotic might be lower than the MIC in such areas. Conversely, although certain organisms may be reported resistant to an antibiotic because sufficiently high blood concentrations cannot be achieved, urine concentrations may be much higher. If so, a urinary tract infection would respond to that antibiotic, whereas septicemia would not.

Thus, antimicrobial susceptibility testing, although a very important part of therapeutic decision making,

Table 34–2. Susceptibility of some common pathogenic microorganisms to various antimicrobial drugs.

Organism	Potentially Useful Antibiotics[1]
BACTERIA	
Anaerobic bacteria[2]	Cefoxitin,[3] cefotetan,[3] chloramphenicol, clindamycin, imipenem[3] metronidazole, penicillins with or without β-lactamase inhibitor
Bordetella pertussis	Erythromycin, clarithromycin, amoxicillin, trimethoprim-sulfamethoxazole
Campylobacter spp	Erythromycin, tetracyclines
Clostridium spp	Clindamycin, penicillins, tetracyclines, metronidazole
Clostridium difficile	Bacitracin (PO), metronidazole, vancomycin (PO)
Corynebacterium diphtheriae	Erythromycin, penicillins
Enterobacteriaceae[4]	Aminoglycosides,[5] ampicillins, cephalosporins, imipenem, monobactams, trimethoprim-sulfamethoxazole, [quinolones][3]
Enterococcus	Ampicillin (with aminoglycoside), vancomycin
Haemophilus influenzae	Amoxicillin/clavulanate, ampicillins (if β-lactamase negative),[6] cephalosporins (II and III),[7] chloramphenicol, rifampin, trimethoprim-sulfamethoxazole
Listeria monocytogenes	Ampicillin with aminoglycoside, trimethoprim-sulfamethoxazole
Moraxella catarrhalis	Amoxicillin/clavulanate, ampicillins (if β-lactamase-negative),[6] cephalosporins (III),[7] erythromycin, trimethoprim-sulfamethoxazole
Neisseria gonorrhoeae	Ampicillins (if β-lactamase-negative),[6] cephalosporins (II and III),[7] penicillins, spectinomycin, tetracyclines, trimethoprim-sulfamethoxazole [quinolones][5]
Neisseria meningitidis	Ampicillins, cephalosporins (II and III),[7] chloramphenicol, penicillins, rifampin
Pasteurella multocida	Amoxicillin/clavulanate, ampicillins, penicillins, tetracyclines
Pseudomonas aeruginosa	Aminoglycosides,[5] antipseudomonas penicillins,[8] aztreonam, ceftazidime, imipenem, [quinolones][3]
Salmonella spp	Ampicillin, cephalosporins (III),[7] chloramphenicol, trimethoprim-sulfamethoxazole
Shigella spp	Ampicillin, cephalosporins (III), chloramphenicol, tetracyclines, trimethoprim-sulfamethoxazole
Staphylococcus aureus	Antistaphylococcal penicillins,[9] cephalosporins (I and II), clindamycin, erythromycin, rifampin, trimethoprim-sulfamethoxazole, vancomycin
Staphylococci (coagulase-negative)	Cephalosporins (I and II),[10] clindamycin, rifampin, vancomycin
Streptococci (most species)	Ampicillins, cephalosporins, clindamycin, erythromycin, penicillins, vancomycin
Streptococcus pneumoniae[11]	Ampicillins, cephalosporins, erythromycin, penicillin, vancomycin[11]
INTERMEDIATE ORGANISMS	
Chlamydia spp	Clarithromycin, erythromycin, tetracyclines (quinolones)[3]
Mycoplasma spp	Erythromycin, tetracyclines
Rickettsia spp	Chloramphenicol, tetracyclines
FUNGI	
Candida spp	Amphotericin B, fluconazole, flucytosine, ketoconazole
Fungi, systemic[2]	Amphotericin B, fluconazole, itraconazole,[3] ketoconazole, miconazole
Dermatophytes	Griseofulvin, topical antifungals, itraconazole[3]
VIRUSES	
Herpes simplex	Acyclovir
Human immunodeficiency virus	Dideoxyinosine (ddI), dideoxycytodine (ddC), zidovudine (AZT), stavudine (d4T)
Influenza A virus	Amantadine, rimantidine
Respiratory syncytial virus	Ribavirin
Varicella-zolster virus	Acyclovir, famciclovir,[5] valacyclovir[3]
Cytomegalovirus	Foscarnet, ganciclovir

[1]In alphabetical order. Selection depends on patient's age, diagnosis, site of infection, severity of illness, antimicrobial susceptibility of suspected organism, and drug risk.
[2]Species-dependent.
[3]Not FDA-approved for use in children.
[4]Includes *E coli, Klebsiella* spp, *Enterobacter* spp, and others; antimicrobial susceptibilities should always be measured.
[5]Amikacin, gentamicin, kanamycin, tobramycin.
[6]Also applies to amoxicillin and related compounds.
[7]Refer to second- (II) or third- (III) generation cephalosporins.
[8]Carbenicillin, mezlocillin, piperacillin, ticarcillin.
[9]Cloxacillin, dicloxacillin, methicillin, nafcillin, oxacillin.
[10]Only if the coagulase-negative *Staphylococcus* is also methicillin- or oxacillin-sensitive.
[11]Because of increasing frequency of *S pneumoniae* strains resistant to penicillin and cephalosporins, therapy for presumed severe infections (eg, meningitis) should include vancomycin until susceptibility studies are available.

Table 34–3. Groups of common antibacterial agents.

Group	Examples	Some Common Susceptible Organisms (Genus)[1]	Common Resistant Organisms (Genus)	Common or Unique Adverse Reactions
PENICILLIN GROUP				
Penicillins	Penicillin G, V	*Streptococcus, Neisseria*	*Staphylococcus, Haemophilus,* enterobacteriaceae	Rash, anaphylaxis, drug fever, bone marrow suppression
Ampicillins	Ampicillin, amoxicillin	(Same as penicillins), plus *Haemophilus* (β-lactamase negative), *Escherichia coli, Enterococcus*	*Staphylococcus,* many enterobacteriaceae	Diarrhea
Antistaphylococcal penicillins	Cloxacillin, dicloxacillin, methicillin, nafcillin, ox-acillin	*Streptococcus, Staphylococcus aureus*	Gram-negative, *Staphylococcus* (coagulase-negative), enterococci	Renal (interstitial nephritis)
Antipseudomonas penicillins	Azlocillin, carbenicillin, piperacillin, ticarcillin	(Same as ampicillins), plus *Pseudomonas*	(Same as ampicillins)	Decreased platelet adhesiveness, hypokalemia, hypernatremia
Penicillin/β-lactamase inhibitor combination	Amoxicillin-clavulanate, ampicillin-sulbactam, ticarcillin-clavulanate	Broad-spectrum	Some enterobacteriaceae, *Pseudomonas*	Diarrhea
Carbapenems	Imipenem/cilastatin	Broad-spectrum, gram-negative rods, anaerobes, *Pseudomonas*	MRSA,[2] many enterococci	CNS, seizures
CEPHALOSPORIN GROUP				
First generation (I)	Cefazolin, cephalexin, cephalothin, cephapirin, cephradine	Gram-positive	Gram-negative, enterococci, some staphylococci (coagulase-negative)	Rash; anaphylax, drug fever
Second generation (II)	Cefaclor, cefamandole, cefonicid, cefuroxime loracarbef	Gram-positive, some *Haemophilus,* some enterobacteriaceae	*Enterococcus, Pseudomonas,* some staphylococci (coagulase-negative)	Serum sickness (cefaclor)
	Cefoxitin, cefotetan	Same as second-generation plus anaerobes		
Third generation (III)	Cefotaxime, ceftizoxime, ceftriaxone, cefixime, cefpodoxine	*Streptococcus, Haemophilus,* Enterobacteriaceae, *Neisseria*	*Pseudomonas,* staphylococci	Biliary sludging (ceftriaxone)
	Ceftazidime	(Same as other third-generation cephalosporisn), plus *Pseudomonas*	Staphylococci	
OTHER DRUGS				
Clindamycin	Clindamycin	Gram-positive, anaerobes	Gram-negative, *Enterococcus*	Nausea, vomiting, hepatotoxicity
Vamcomycins	Vancomycin	Gram-positive	Gram-negative	"Redman" Syndrome, shock, ototoxicity, renal
Macrolide agents	Erythromycin, clarithromycin, azithromycin	Gram-positive *Bordetella, mycoplasma, chlamydia*	Gram-negative	Nausea and vomiting
Quinolones[3]	Ciprofloxacin, norfloxacin, ofloxacin	Gram-negative	*Enterococcus, Streptococcus S pneumoniae,* anaerobes	GI, rash, CNS

(*continued*)

Table 34–3. Groups of common antibacterial agents. (continued)

Group	Examples	Some Common Susceptible Organisms (Genus)[1]	Common Resistant Organisms (Genus)	Common or Unique Adverse Reactions
Tetracyclines	Chlortetracycline, tetracycline, doxycycline, minocycline	Anaerobes, *Mycoplasma, Chlamydia*	Many enterobacteriaceae, *Staphylococcus*	Teeth staining, rash, flora overgrowth, hepatotoxicity, pseudotumor cerebri
Chloramphenicol	Chloramphenicol	*S pneumoniae, H influenzae, Salmonella*	*Staphylococcus,* many enterobacteriaceae	Bone marrow suppression, gray syndrome, neuritis
Sulfonamides	Many	Gram-negative (urine)	Gram-positive	Rash, renal, bone marrow suppression, Stevens-Johnson syndrome
Trimethoprim-sulfamethoxazole	Trimethoprim-sulfamethoxazole	*S aureus,* gram-negative *S pneumoniae H influenzae*	*Streptococcus, Pseudomonas* anaerobes	Rash, renal, bone marrow suppression, Stevens-Johnson syndrome
Rifampin	Rifampin	*Neisseria, Haemophilus, Staphylococcus Streptococcus*	Resistance develops rapidly if used as sole agent	Rash, GI, hepatotoxicity, CNS, bone marrow suppression
Aminoglycosides	Amikacin, gentamicin, kanamycin, streptomycin, tobramycin	Gram-negative, including *P aeruginosa*	Gram-positive, anaerobes, some pseudomonads	Renal, ototoxicity, potentiates neuromuscular blocking agents

[1]Not all strains susceptible; always obtain antimicrobial susceptibility tests on significant isolates.
[2]Methicillin-resistant S aureus
[3]Not recommended for children.

reflects assumptions that the clinician must understand, especially for management of patients with serious infections. Ultimately, the true test of the efficacy of therapy is patient response. Patients who do not respond to seemingly appropriate therapy may require assessment, including reculturing and repeat susceptibility testing, to determine whether resistant strains have evolved or superinfection with a resistant organism is present. In addition, antimicrobial therapy cannot be expected to cure some infections unless additional supportive treatment (usually surgical) is undertaken.

ALTERATION OF DOSE & MEASUREMENT OF BLOOD LEVELS

Certain antimicrobial agents have not been approved (and often not tested) for use in newborns. For those that have been approved, it is important to recognize that both dose and frequency of administration may need to be altered (see Tables 34–4 and 34–5), especially in young (7 days or less) or low birth weight (2000 g or less) neonates.

Antimicrobial agents are excreted or metabolized through various physiologic mechanisms (eg, renal, hepatic). It is important to consider these routes of excretion and alter the antimicrobial dosage appropriately in any patient with some degree of organ dysfunction (see Chapter 40). As indicated in Table 34–4, an assessment of renal or hepatic function may be routinely necessary for patients receiving certain drugs (eg, renal function for aminoglycosides, hepatic function for chloramphenicol); otherwise, harmful drug levels may accumulate. If significant organ dysfunction is present, dosage modification may be necessary (see detailed description in individual drug information packet), and the measurement of drug levels may be indicated.

Serum levels of drugs posing a high risk of toxicity (eg, aminoglycosides, vancomycin, chloramphenicol) are ordinarily measured. For certain other serious bacterial infections (eg, bacterial endocarditis), measurement of the serum concentration of an antimicrobial may be important to deliver optimal therapy.

THE USE OF NEW ANTIMICROBIAL AGENTS

New antibiotics are introduced frequently, often with claims to unique features that distinguish these usually more expensive products from their predecessors. The role that any new antimicrobial will play can only be determined over time, during which new or previously unrecognized side effects might be described and the clinical efficacy is established in

Table 34–4. Guidelines for use of common parenteral antibacterial agents[1] in children ≥ 1 month of age.

Agent	Route	Dose[2] (mg/kg/d)	Maximum Daily Dose	Interval (hours)	Adjustment[3]	Blood Levels[4] (µg/mL) Peak	Trough
Amikacin	IM, IV	15–22.5	1.5 g	8	R	15–25	5–10
Ampicillin	IM, IV	100–400	12 g	4–6	R		
Aztreonam	IM, IV	90–120	6 g	6–8	R		
Cefazolin	IM, IV	50–100	6 g	8	R		
Cefotaxime	IM, IV	100–200	12 g	6–8	R		
Cefoxitin	IM, IV	80–160	12 g	4–6	R		
Ceftazidime	IM, IV	100–150	6 g	8	R		
Ceftizoxime	IM, IV	150–200	12 g	6–8	R		
Ceftriaxone	IM, IV	50–100	4 g	12–24	R		
Cefuroxime	IM, IV	100–150	6 g	6–8	R		
Cephalothin	IM, IV	75–125	12 g	4–6	R		
Cephradine	IM, IV	50–100	8 g	6	R		
Chloramphenicol	IV	50–100	4 g	6	R, H	15–25	5–10
Clindamycin	IM, IV	25–40	4 g	6–8	R, H		
Gentamicin	IM, IV	3–7.5	300 mg	8	R	5–10	< 2.0
Methicillin	IM, IV	150–200	12 g	6	R		
Metronidazole	IV	30	4 g	6	H		
Nafcillin	IM, IV	150	12 g	6	None		
Penicillin G	IV	100,000–250,000 units/kg	20 million units	4–6	H, R		
Pencillin G (benzathine)	IM	50,000 units/kg	2.4 million units	Single dose	None		
Penicillin G (procaine)	IM	25,000–50,000 units/kg	4.8 million units	12–24	R		
Tetracycline[5]	(IV)[5]	20–30	2 g	12	R		
Ticarcillin	IV	200–300	24 g	4–6	R		
Tobramycin	IM, IV	3–6	300 mg	8	R	5–10	< 2
Vancomycin	IV	40–60	2 g	6	R	20–40	

[1]Not including some newly released drugs, ones not recommended for use in children, or ones not widely used.
[2]Always consult package insert for complete prescribing information. Dosage may differ for alternative routes, newborns (see Table 34–6), or patients with liver or renal failure (see Adjustment column) and may not be recommended for use in pregnant women or newborns. Maximum dosage may be indicated only in severe infections or by parenteral routes.
[3]Mode of excretion (R = renal, H = hepatic) of antimicrobial agent should be assessed at the onset of therapy and dosage modified or levels determined as indicated in package insert.
[4]Suggested levels to reduce toxicity.
[5]Not recommended in children 8 years of age and under.

large numbers of patients. Because this may take many years, a conservative approach to using new antibiotics seems fitting, especially since the costs are often higher and appropriate antimicrobial choices for most common infections already exist. It is appropriate to ask if a new antimicrobial therapy has been proved to be as effective as (or more effective than) the current drug of choice and, if so, whether its side effects are comparable or less common and its cost reasonable.

The development of new antibiotics is important as a response to the emergence of resistant organism and for treatment of infections that are clinically difficult to treat (eg, viruses, fungi, and some resistant bacteria). Fortunately, these infections are either rare or (usually) self-limited in normal hosts.

Table 34–5. Guidelines for use of common oral antibacterial agents in children ≥ 1 month of age.

Agent[1]	Dose[2] (mg/kg/d)	Interval (hours)	Other Considerations
Amoxicillin	40	8	GI side effects
Amoxicillin/clavulanate	40	8	GI side effects
Ampicillin	50	6	GI side effects
Cefaclor	40	8	Serum sickness-like illness
Cefadroxil	30	12	
Cefixime	8	12–24	
Cefpodoxime	10	12	Taste (suspension)
Cefprozil	30	12	GI side effects
Cefuroxime	30–40	12	GI side effects
Cephalexin	25–50	6	
Cephradine	25–50	6	
Chloramphenicol	50–75	6	Aplastic anemia
Clarithromycin	15	12	GI side effects
Clindamycin	20–30	6	GI side effects
Cloxacillin	50–100	6	GI side effects
Dicloxacillin	12–25	6	GI side effects
Doxycycline[3]	2–4[3]	12–24	Teeth staining ≤ 8 years
Erythromycin	20–50[4]	6–12[4]	GI side effects
Erythromycin/sulfisoxazole	40 (erythromycin)	6–8	
Furazolidone	5–8	6	
Loracarbef	19, 30 for otitis	12	
Metronidazole	15–35	8	
Nitrofurantoin	5–7	6	
Oxacillin	50–100	6	
Penicillin V	25–50	6	Taste (suspension)
Rifampin	10–20	12–24	
Sulfisoxazole	120–150	6	
Tetracycline[3]	25–50[3]	6	Teeth staining ≤ 8 years
Trimethoprim-sulfamethoxazole	8–12 (TMP)	12	Stevens-Johnson syndrome

[1]Not including some newly released drugs, ones not recommended for use in children, or ones not widely used.
[2]Always consult package insert for complete prescribing information. Dosage may differ for alternative routes, newborns (see Table 34–6), or patients with liver or renal failure (see Adjustment column) and may not be recommended for use in pregnant women or newborns. Maximum dosage may be indicated only in severe infections or by parenteral routes.
[3]Not recommended in children 8 years of age and under.
[4]Preparation-dependent.

PROPHYLACTIC ANTIMICROBIAL AGENTS

Antimicrobials can be used to decrease the incidence of postoperative infections (Table 34–7). A dose of an antimicrobial is given 30 minutes to 2 hours prior to surgery. The goal is to achieve high levels of antimicrobial agents in the serum at the time of the surgical incision and by this means, combined with good surgical technique, to reduce the bacterial contamination of the wound. During a lengthy procedure, a second dose may be given. No evidence ex-

Table 34–6. Guidelines for use of selected antimicrobial agents in newborns.[1]

Antibiotic Drug	Route	Body Wt (g)	Maximum Dosage (mg/kg/d) [Frequency] < 7 Days	Maximum Dosage (mg/kg/d) [Frequency] 8–30 Days	Blood Levels (µg/mL) Peak	Blood Levels (µg/mL) Trough
Amikacin[2]	IV, IM	< 2000 > 2000	15 [q12h] 20 [q12h]	22.5 [q8h] 30 [q8h]	15–25	5–10
Ampicillin	IV, IM	< 2000 > 2000	100 [q12h] 150 [q8h]	150 [q8h] 200 [q6h]		
Cefotaxime	IV, IM		100 [q12h]	150 [q8h]		
Ceftazidime	IV, IM	< 2000 > 2000	100 [q12h] 150 [q8h]	150 [q8h] 150 [q8h]		
Chloramphenicol[3]	IV, PO	< 2000 > 2000	25 [q24h] 25 [q24h]	25 [q24h] 50 [q12h]	15–25	5–10
Clindamycin	IV, IM, PO	< 2000 > 2000	10 [q12h] 15 [q8h]	15 [q8h] 20 [q6h]		
Erythromycin	PO		20 [q12h]	30 [q8h]		
Gentamicin[2]	IV, IM		5 [q12–18h]	7.5 [q8h]	5–10	< 2
Methicillin	IV, IM	< 2000 > 2000	100 [q12h] 150 [q8h]	150 [q8h] 200 [q6h]		
Nafcillin	IV	< 2000 > 2000	50 [q12h] 60 [q8h]	75 [q8h] 150 [q6h]		
Oxacillin	IV, IM	< 2000 > 2000	50 [q12h] 75 [q8h]	75 [q8h] 150 [q6h]		
Penicillin G[4]	IV	< 2000 > 2000	100,000[4] [q12h] 150,000[4] [q8h]	150,000[4] [q8h] 200,000[4] [q6h]		
Ticarcillin	IV, IM	< 2000 > 2000	150 [q12h] 225 [q8h]	225 [q8h] 300 [q6h]		
Tobramycin[2]	IV, IM		4 [q12–18h]	6 [q8h]	5–10	< 2
Vancomycin	IV		20 [q12h]	30 [q8h]	20–40	

[1]Adapted from Nelson JD: *Pocketbook of Pediatric Antimicrobial Therapy,* 11th ed. Williams & Wilkins, 1995.
[2]Neonates weighting < 1200 g may require even smaller doses. Antibiotic levels should be closely monitored.
[3]Chloramphenicol must be used with extreme caution. Levels should be measured in all patients to ensure proper dosing.
[4]Penicillin dosages are in units/kg/d. Other preparations (eg, benzathine penicillin) may be given IM. See specific diseases for dosage.

ists that subsequent multiple doses of antimicrobials add additional benefit. The antimicrobial used for prophylaxis is directed toward the flora that most commonly cause postoperative infection. Usually gram-positive cocci such as *S aureus* are targeted and a first-generation cephalosporin (such as cefazolin) is a cost-effective choice. Third-generation cephalosporins and other broad-spectrum agents are more expensive and offer less benefit because they are less active against *S aureus* than cefazolin. Cefoxitin or cefotetan is useful for surgical procedures such as colorectal surgery, although cefazolin is appropriate for most gynecologic patients.

In hospitals where the predominant *S aureus* strains are methicillin-resistant or in cases where the patient is allergic to penicillin and cephalosporins, vancomycin can be considered. However, prophylactic vancomycin has caused hypotension at the time of induction of general anesthesia. In addition, frequent use of vancomycin as a prophylactic antimicrobial will undoubtedly contribute to the development of vancomycin-resistant strains such as *Enterococcus faecalis*. For these reasons, vancomycin should generally not be used for prophylaxis, although it might prove useful for individual patients at extremely high risk.

Prophylactic antimicrobials are given in several other circumstances. Endocarditis prophylaxis is indicated during dental and colorectal or genitourinary procedures on patients with high-risk heart lesions. Prophylaxis against infection with group A streptococcal infection reduces the recurrence rate for acute rheumatic fever. Postexposure prophylaxis is given after exposure to pertussis, *Haemophilus influenzae* type b infection (depending on age), meningococcus, household exposure to tuberculosis, plague,

Table 34–7. Antimicrobial prophylaxis and preferred prophylactic agents: Selected conditions and pathogens.[1,2]

Pathogen/Condition	Agent
Bacterial endocarditis[3]	Ampicillin, ampicillin and gentamicin, amoxicillin, or other approved regimens
Group A streptococci–rheumatic fever[4]	Benzathine penicillin G, penicillin, sulfadiazine
Bordetella pertussis (exposure to respiratory secretions)	Erythromycin
Haemophilus influenzae type b[5] (household exposure)	Rifampin
Neisseria meningiditis (household exposure)	Rifampin, sulfadiazine[6]
Mycobacterium tuberculosis (household exposure)	Isoniazid
N gonorrhoeae—ophthalmia neonatorum	Erythromycin, silver nitrate ophthalmic
N gonorrhoeae (sexual contact)	Ceftriaxone, cefixime
Treponema pallidum (sexual contact)	Penicillin
Streptococcus pneumoniae—sickle cell disease, asplenia	Penicillin
Postoperative wound infection[7]	Cefazolin, other regimens
Group B streptococcal sepsis	Ampicillin to mother prior to delivery
Pneumonic *Yersinia pestis*[8] (exposure)	Tetracycline,[9] chloramphenicol
Francisella tularensis[8] (aerosolized exposure)	Tetracycline,[9] chloramphenicol
Vibrio cholera	Tetracycline,[9] trimethoprim-sulfamethoxazole (TMP-SMX)
Recurrent otitis media	Amoxicillin, sulfadiazine
Recurrent urinary tract infection	Nitrofurantoin, TMP-SMX
Pseudomonas carinii—HIV, some immunocompromised)	TMP-SMX, pentamidine

[1]Modified, with permission, from the report of the Committee on Infectious Diseases, 23rd ed. American Academy of Pediatrics, 1994:522.
[2]Decisions for prophylaxis must take a number of factors into account, including the evidence for efficacy of therapy, the degree of the exposure to an infecting agent, the risk and consequences of infection, the susceptibility of the infecting agent to antimicrobials, and the patient's ability to tolerate and comply with the antimicrobial agent. See individual chapters of the text for discussion.
[3]See discussion in chapter.
[4]Oral prophylaxis may be indicated in some patients. Alternative regimens indicated for penicillin-allergic patients. See discussion in chapter.
[5]Prophylaxis provided to family if contacts include children < 4 years old. Some experts provide prophylaxis in day care settings after one case and some after two cases of HiB.
[6]Only for known sulfadiazine-susceptible strains.
[7]Alternative regimens may be used, depending on the site of surgery and the degree of contamination.
[8]Prophylaxis not well established. Carefully assess risk on a case-by-case basis.
[9]Indicated for children > 8 years old.

aerosolized tularemia, and other high-risk infections. Silver nitrate, erythromycin, or tetracycline can be used in ophthalmic preparations for prevention of gonococcal ophthalmia neonatorum. Children with asplenia and sickle cell disease receive prophylactic penicillin to protect against overwhelming *S pneumoniae* sepsis.

Prophylactic antimicrobials are also useful during the viral respiratory season in children at high risk for recurrent otitis media and for some children with recurrent urinary tract infection. However, because

of the emergence of resistant *S pneumoniae,* as well as its frequency, decisions for antimicrobial prophylaxis should be carefully considered for each child.

INITIAL EMPIRIC ANTIMICROBIAL CHOICES FOR SELECTED CONDITIONS

General recommendations for specific conditions are included in the sections that follow. A specific selection depends on the patient's age, diagnosis, site of infection, severity of illness, antimicrobial susceptibility of bacterial isolates, and history of drug allergy. Always consult the package insert for detailed prescribing information. Tables 34–2 through 34–6 include further information.

Neonatal Sepsis & Meningitis

The newborn with sepsis may have signs of focal infection such as pneumonia or respiratory distress syndrome or may have subtle nonfocal signs. Group B streptococcus, *E coli,* other gram-negative rods, and *Listeria monocytogenes* are commonly encountered. Ampicillin and gentamicin (or another aminoglycoside) are preferred. If meningitis is present, many substitute a third-generation cephalosporin for the aminoglycoside. In the newborn with cellulitis, *S aureus* and group A streptococci are additional considerations. Usually, nafcillin, oxacillin, or a first-generation cephalosporin are added. Omphalitis is often polymicrobial and *Enterococcus* spp, gram-negative aerobes, and anaerobes may be causative. Clindamycin, ampicillin, and an aminoglycoside or third-generation cephalosporin cover the most likely organisms; early surgical intervention is indicated.

Sepsis in an Infant

S pneumoniae, Neisseria meningiditis and *H influenzae* type b are most commonly encountered in infants. A third-generation cephalosporin is appropriate. Intermediate-level penicillin and cephalosporin resistance in *S pneumoniae* usually do not cause therapy to fail unless meningitis or another difficult-to-treat infection such as endocarditis or osteomyelitis is present.

Nosocomial Sepsis

Many bacterial pathogens are possible. Usually, recent local experience is the best guide to the infecting species. For example, some neonatal units experience frequent infections due to *Enterobacter cloacae,* whereas in other units *Klebsiella pneumoniae* is the most common nosocomial isolate. Initial therapy should be effective for methicillin-resistant *S aureus* (MRSA) and resistant *Pseudomonas aeruginosa* if these are frequent isolates. *E faecalis* is a common cause of nosocomial bacteremia in patients with central catheters, particularly in units where cephalosporins are heavily used. Coagulase-negative staphylococci are commonly isolated from patients with indwelling central catheters. In seriously ill patients where the local experience suggests that *Enterococcus* spp or coagulase-negative staphylococci are common, the initial regimen should include vancomycin. Regimens containing ampicillin are effective for *Enterococcus* spp unless the local isolates have a high rate of resistance.

Meningitis

Bacterial meningitis in neonates is usually caused by infection with group B streptococci, *E coli,* or *L monocytogenes.* A combination of ampicillin and gentamicin or another aminoglycoside, or ampicillin and a third-generation cephalosporin are started initially. In an infant or older child, *S pneumoniae* is the most common isolate, and *N meningiditis* or *H influenzae* type b also occur. Initial therapy should include vancomycin, a third-generation cephalosporin, and rifampin.

Meningitis in a child with a ventriculoperitoneal shunt is most commonly caused by coagulase-negative staphylococci, many of which are methicillin-resistant. Many of these patients are not seriously ill, and therapy should await obtaining the appropriate shunt fluid for Gram's stain and culture. Seriously ill patients should be treated initially with vancomycin and a third-generation cephalosporin, because *S aureus* and gram-negative rods are also possible and more serious causes of infection.

Urinary Tract Infection

E coli is the most common isolate in the urinary tract. Outpatients with symptoms of lower urinary tract disease or with mild illness can be treated with ampicillin, cephalexin, or a sulfonamide. For hospitalized patients with suspected bacteremia, ampicillin and gentamicin or a cephalosporin are appropriate. Gram's stain may be used to guide the initial choice. For patients with known or suspected resistant organisms, such as *P aeruginosa,* or for patients with urosepsis, an aminoglycoside or ceftazidime and ticarcillin may be started. Unit-specific data on typical bacterial species and their patterns of susceptibility should guide the antimicrobial choice for nosocomial urinary tract infections.

Bacterial Pneumonia

Newborns with bacterial pneumonia generally should be treated the same as for sepsis. Infants and older children are frequently infected with *S pneumoniae.* Ampicillin, a second- or third-generation cephalosporin, erythromycin-sulfisoxazole, or trimethoprim-sulfamethoxazole may be used, depending on the local rates of resistant organisms and the seriousness of the illness. A rapidly progressive pneumonia, with pneumatoceles or large pleural effusions, may be due to *S aureus* or group A streptococci, *H influenzae* type b, or another gram-negative rod. Oxacillin, nafcillin, or another effective antistaphylococcal agent should be used in addition to a third-generation cephalosporin.

Children 6 years and older frequently have infection with *Mycoplasma pneumoniae, Chlamydia pneumoniae,* or *S pneumoniae.* Erythromycin, or other macrolide antibiotic, is usually indicated for initial empiric therapy.

SPECIFIC ANTIMICROBIAL AGENTS

Penicillins/Aminopenicillins

Penicillin remains the drug of choice for streptococcal infections, prophylaxis of acute rheumatic fever, syphilis, oral anaerobic infections, dental infections, *N meningitidis* and *N gonorrhoeae* (where susceptibility is known), Lyme disease, leptospirosis, rat-bite fever, actinomycetes, and infections due to *Clostridium* and *Bacillus* spp. For oral therapy of minor infections, amoxicillin or ampicillin is usually equivalent. For systemic therapy, aqueous penicillin G is preferable. For dog or cat bites, where *Pasteurella multocida* is commonly encountered, amoxicillin-clavulanate provides good coverage of *Pasteurella,* as well as *Staphylococcus.* An alternate is separate prescriptions for penicillin and an antistaphylococcal drug such as cephalexin (Keflex). As for human bites, amoxicillin-clavulanate provides adequate therapy for *Eikenella corrodens* and other mixed oral aerobes and anaerobes.

Penicillinase-Resistant Penicillins (PRPs)

S aureus is usually resistant to penicillin and amoxicillin owing to the penicillinase production by these organisms. Nafcillin, oxacillin, methicillin, and first- and second-generation cephalosporins are stable to penicillinase and are usually equivalent for intravenous therapy. Methicillin is associated with more frequent interstitial nephritis. Oxacillin and methicillin are renally excreted, whereas nafcillin is excreted through the biliary tract. These properties occasionally are advantageous in children with renal or liver failure. Cost should usually be the deciding factor for choosing one agent over another. Often both *S aureus* and *S pyogenes* are suspected initially, for example, in cellulitis or postoperative wound infections. The PRPs and first- and second-generation cephalosporins are efficacious for most streptococcal infections.

Methicillin-resistant *S aureus* (MRSA) is an uncommon community-acquired infection in children, but may cause nosocomial infection in some hospitals. MRSA infections are also resistant to other PRPs, and first- and second-generation cephalosporins. Vancomycin is effective against MRSA and coagulase-negative staphylococci.

For outpatient therapy, cloxacillin, dicloxacillin, and first- or second-generation cephalosporins are usually equally effective for infections due to *S aureus.* Cost may be used to determine the choice between drugs.

Antipseudomonas Penicillins

Carbenicillin and ticarcillin are active drugs against streptococci, ampicillin-susceptible enterococci, *H influenzae,* gram-negative rods, including more resistant gram-negative rods such as *Enterobacter, Proteus,* and *P aeruginosa,* and gram-negative anaerobes such as *Bacteroides fragilis. P aeruginosa* is inherently resistant to most antimicrobials, and high levels of these drugs are usually required. The combination of carbenicillin or ticarcillin and an aminoglycoside is synergistic against *P aeruginosa* and many other enteric gram-negative rods. Ticarcillin in a fixed combination with clavulanic acid has activity against β-lactamase-producing strains of *Klebsiella, S aureus,* and *Bacteroides.* Piperacillin is more active in vitro against many gram-negative enteric infections and may be advantageous in some circumstances, but is not approved in children. Piperacillin-tazobactam is another combination antimicrobial/β-lactamase inhibitor that has enhanced activity against many β-lactamase producers.

Antipseudomonal penicillins cause the same toxicities as penicillin, and therefore are usually very safe. Carbenicillin, ticarcillin, and piperacillin contain large amounts of sodium, which may cause problems for some patients with cardiac or renal disease.

Glycopeptide Agents

Vancomycin and teicoplanin are glycopeptide antimicrobial agents active against the cell wall of gram-positive organisms. Only vancomycin is licensed in the United States. Vancomycin is useful for parenteral therapy of resistant gram-positive cocci such as MRSA, methicillin-resistant coagulase-negative staphylococci, and ampicillin-resistant enterococci. Vancomycin is also used orally for therapy of colitis due to *Clostridium difficile,* although it should not be used as the first drug of choice. The empiric use of vancomycin has increased tremendously over the last several years. As a result, vancomycin-resistant enterococci and coagulase-negative staphylococci have become problems, particularly in inpatient units, intensive care units, and oncology wards. Vancomycin usage should be carefully monitored in hospitals and in high-use units within hospitals. Vancomycin should not be used empirically when an infection is mild or when other antimicrobial agents are likely to be effective. Vancomycin should be stopped promptly if infection is due to organisms susceptible to other antimicrobials.

Infection control guidelines for prevention of spread of vancomycin-resistant enterococcus were recently published by the Centers for Disease Control and Prevention. The potential of spread of the vancomycin resistance gene to *S aureus* is so worrisome that a recent publication listed recommendations for laboratory-based monitoring to detect this event in addition to infection control steps to take if it is encountered.

Rapid infusion of vancomycin is associated with the "red man" syndrome, which is characterized by diffuse red flushing, at times pruritus, and occasionally tachycardia and hypotension. As a result, vancomycin is infused slowly over 1 hour or longer in some cases. Diphenhydramine or hydrocortisone or both may also be used as premedication.

Vancomycin peak-and-trough serum concentrations are commonly measured despite the lack of data associating these levels with either toxicity or a positive therapeutic outcome. Vancomycin accumulation may occur in patients with abnormal or unpredictable renal function. Similarly, vancomycin dosing may be unpredictable in patients with an altered volume of distribution such as nephrotic syndrome or in patients in shock. Measuring vancomycin peak serum concentrations is helpful in these patients.

Cephalosporins

Cephalosporin agents make up a large and often confusing group of antimicrobials. Many of these drugs are similar in antibacterial spectrum and side effects and may have similar names. Clinicians should learn well the properties of one or two drugs in each class. Cephalosporins are often grouped as "generations" to signify their similar antimicrobial activity. First-generation cephalosporins such as cephapirin intravenously and cephalexin orally are primarily useful for *S aureus* infection and urinary tract infection due to susceptible *E coli*. Second-generation cephalosporins, such as cefuroxime intravenously and cefaclor orally, have somewhat reduced but acceptable activity against gram-positive cocci, but greater activity against gram-negative rods. They are active against *H influenzae, Moraxella (Branhamella) catarrhalis,* and *N gonorrhoeae,* including strains that produce β-lactamase capable of inactivating ampicillin. Third-generation cephalosporins have substantially less activity against gram-positive cocci such as *S aureus,* but greatly augmented activity against aerobic gram-negative rods. Cefotaxime and ceftriaxone are examples of intravenous drugs, whereas cefixime, cefpodoxime, and cefprozil are representative oral drugs.

No cephalosporin agent has substantial activity against *L monocytogenes,* enterococci, or MRSA. The cephalosporins have little value for treating anaerobic infections except for cefoxitin and cefotetan, two second-generation cephalosporins with excellent activity against *B fragilis.* Ceftazidime is a third-generation cephalosporin with appreciable activity against *P aeruginosa.*

Cephalosporin is seldom the drug of choice for a given infection, and despite popularity, it is often more expensive than other antimicrobials with similar side effects. Resistance to cephalosporin is common among aerobic gram-negative rods. The presence of inducible cephalosporinases in the chromosome of some gram-negative rod organisms such as *P aeruginosa, Serratia marcescens,* and *Enterobacter* spp has led to some clinical failures because of the emergence of resistance while on therapy. Similarly, extended-spectrum cephalosporinases that hydrolyze third-generation cephalosporins have become widespread in some hospitals. Active laboratory-based surveillance is necessary to predict the usual susceptibility encountered in gram-negative infections.

Aztreonam

Aztreonam is the only monobactam antimicrobial agent that is approved in the United States. Although it is not approved for use in children, there is considerable pediatric experience with its use, including in neonates and premature infants. Aztreonam is active against streptococcal species and aerobic gram-negative rods, including *P aeruginosa.* Aztreonam has activity against *H influenzae* and *M catarrhalis* including those that are β-lactamase producers. Most patients with allergy to penicillin or cephalosporin are not sensitized to aztreonam, except that children with prior reactions to ceftazidime may have reactions to aztreonam because aztreonam and ceftazidime have a common side chain.

Imipenem

Imipenem-cilastatin is a combination of an active antibiotic and cilastatin, which inhibits the metabolism of imipenem in the kidney and thereby results in high urinary levels of imipenem. Although imipenem-cilastatin is not approved for children younger than 12 years, there is considerable experience with its use. Imipenem-cilastatin is a broadly active antimicrobial agent with good activity against streptococci, some staphylococci, and enterococci, gram-negative rods such as *P aeruginosa,* β-lactamase-producing *H influenzae,* and gram-negative anaerobes. Because imipenem-cilastatin is active against so many species of bacteria, there is a strong temptation to use it as single-drug empiric therapy. Units that have used imipenem-cilastatin heavily have encountered resistance in many different species of gram-negative rods. A more appropriate use is to reserve imipenem for patients who have infections that are unresponsive or have proved resistant to other antimicrobial agents.

Macrolide Agents

Erythromycin is the most commonly used of the macrolide antimicrobial agents. It is active against many bacteria that are resistant to cell wall–active antimicrobials and is the drug of choice for *Bordetella pertussis, C pneumoniae, M pneumoniae,* and *C trachomatis* infections (in children for whom tetracycline is not an option). Erythromycin is used for outpatient therapy of mild infections and streptococcal and staphylococcal infections and is used instead of penicillin in patients with penicillin allergy. More serious infections are usually treated with penicillins, PRPs, or cephalosporins because of significant incidence of erythromycin resistance in both species. The combination erythromycin-sulfisoxazole is very useful for otitis media, but erythromycin alone does not have sufficient activity against *H influenzae* to be recommended. Gastrointestinal side effects are common.

Erythromycin is available in many formulations including the base, estolate, ethyl succinate, and stearate. Transient hepatic toxicity is seen in adults, but is much less common in children. Erythromycin base and stearate should be taken with meals for best absorption.

Clarithromycin and azithromycin are new macrolide antimicrobials that are much less likely to cause nausea, vomiting, and diarrhea than erythromycin. Therefore, these agents are useful in children who cannot tolerate erythromycin. Clarithromycin is more active than erythromycin against *H influenzae, M catarrhalis,* and *N gonorrhoeae* and is the drug of choice, sometimes in combination, for nontuberculous mycobacterial infections. Azithromycin can be used for single-dose therapy of *C trachomatis* infections, although it is not approved in children younger than 16 years. It is beneficial in adolescents when compliance with erythromycin is a concern. Clarithromycin and azithromycin are considerably more expensive than most erythromycin formulations, which are usually therefore preferred.

Clindamycin

Clindamycin is active against *S aureus, S pyogenes,* other streptococcal species except enterococci, and both gram-positive and gram-negative anaerobes. Clindamycin or metronidazole are frequently combined with other antimicrobials for empiric therapy of suspected anaerobic or mixed anaerobic and aerobic infection. Examples are pelvic inflammatory disease, necrotizing enterocolitis, other infections in which the integrity of the gastrointestinal or genitourinary tracts is compromised, and sinusitis. Clindamycin may be superior for treatment of serious streptococcal infections that appear to be toxin-mediated. For the usual oral anaerobes, penicillin is more active than clindamycin. Empiric use of clindamycin is justified in suspected anaerobic infection, because cultures frequently cannot be obtained and, if obtained, may be slow in confirming anaerobic infection. Clindamycin has been associated with the occurrence of pseudomembranous colitis. Although diarrhea is a frequent side effect, pseudomembranous colitis is uncommonly due to clindamycin in children.

Sulfonamides

Sulfonamides, which make up the oldest class of antimicrobials, remain useful for many infections. Sulfonamide agents are often used to treat urinary tract infections and otitis media in combination with erythromycin or trimethoprim. They are also used for other infections due to *E coli* and for *Nocardia.* Although useful for rheumatic fever prophylaxis in penicillin-allergic patients, sulfonamides fail to eradicate group A streptococci and cannot be used for treatment of acute infections.

Trimethoprim-sulfamethoxazole (TMP-SMX) is a fixed combination, which is more active than either drug alone. Gram-positive cocci including *S pneumoniae,* some staphylococci, *Haemophilus,* and many gram-negative rods are susceptible. Unfortunately, resistance to TMP-SMX has developed in recent years, which limits its usefulness. Most *Shigella* and *Salmonella enteriditis* strains remain susceptible, as do most *E coli.* TMP-SMX is therefore very useful for treatment of urinary tract infections, respiratory infections such as otitis media, sinusitis, and pneumonia, and bacterial dysentery. TMP-SMX is also the drug of choice for treatment of and prophylaxis against *Pneumocystis carinii* infection. Dermatologic and myelosuppressive side effects limit the use of TMP-SMX in some children infected with HIV.

Sulfonamide is associated with several cutaneous reactions including urticaria, photosensitivity, Stevens-Johnson syndrome, purpura, and macular-papular rashes. Hematologic side effects such as leukopenia, thrombocytopenia, and hemolytic anemia are uncommon. Common gastrointestinal side effects are nausea and vomiting. The dermatologic and hematologic side effects are thought to be more common with TMP-SMX than with sulfonamide alone.

Tetracyclines

Tetracycline agents are effective against a broad range of bacteria, but are not commonly used in children because alternative effective drugs are available. Many different tetracycline formulations are available. Tetracycline agents are effective against many *E coli,* rickettsiae, *Chlamydia* spp, *Mycoplasma* spp, and *B pertussis.* Doxycycline or minocycline is the drug of choice for eradication of *C trachomatis* in pelvic inflammatory disease and nongonococcal urethritis.

Staining of the permanent teeth was noted in young children treated with repeated courses of tetracyclines. As a result, tetracyclines are generally not given to children younger than 9 years of age unless alternative drugs are unavailable. A single course of tetracycline does not pose a significant risk of tooth staining. Mucous membrane candidiasis, photosensitivity, nausea, and vomiting are other common side effects.

Tetracycline is used for therapy of rickettsial infections such as Rocky Mountain spotted fever, rickettsial pox, typhus, and Q fever, as an alternative to erythromycin for *M pneumoniae, C pneumoniae,* and for treatment of psittacosis, chancroid, melioidosis, brucellosis, *P multocida,* infection, and relapsing fever.

Aminoglycosides

The aminoglycoside antimicrobial agents are protein synthesis inhibitors and are active against aerobic gram-negative rods including *P aeruginosa*. Streptomycin was the first drug in this class, but today is used only for tuberculosis and the occasional cases of plague and tularemia. Kanamycin was subsequently introduced and was used extensively in newborn nurseries, but when resistance developed, gentamicin, tobramycin, and then amikacin supplanted kanamycin.

Aminoglycoside agents are used for serious gram-negative infections and are given intravenously or intramuscularly. Aminoglycoside is used for urinary tract infections, pyelonephritis, suspected gram-negative sepsis, *P aeruginosa* infections in patients with cystic fibrosis or burns, and other gram-negative pneumonias. Aminoglycoside also has activity against gram-positive organisms and, combined with penicillin or ampicillin, may give synergistic killing of *L monocytogenes* and group B streptococci. Penicillin or ampicillin combined with an aminoglycoside is indicated for therapy of serious enterococcal infections, such as sepsis or endocarditis. Aminoglycosides have activity against *S aureus* but are not used for therapy except in combination with other antistaphylococcal antibiotics.

Aminoglycosides are not active in an acidic environment and may not be effective against loculated abscesses. Aminoglycosides diffuse poorly into the cerebrospinal fluid and achieve about 10% of serum concentrations. As a result, a third-generation cephalosporin is preferred for bacillary meningitis.

Aminoglycoside is associated with both renal and eighth-nerve injury. Therapeutic serum concentrations are not very different from the range associated with toxicity. Careful monitoring is necessary, particularly in children with abnormal or changing renal function, premature infants, and infants with rapidly changing volumes of distribution. Aminoglycoside is usually infused over 30–45 minutes, and the peak serum concentration is measured 30–45 minutes after the end of the infusion. A trough serum concentration is measured prior to the next dose. The efficacious and nontoxic serum concentrations are gentamicin and tobramycin trough less than 2 μg/mL, peak serum concentrations 5–10 μg/mL, amikacin trough concentrations less than 10 μg/mL, and peak serum concentrations 15–25 μg/mL.

Aminoglycoside has a prolonged effect on the regrowth of susceptible organisms (the "postantibiotic effect"). Some investigators have used this principle to establish guidelines for once-daily dosing of aminoglycosides, using larger initial doses given each 24 hours. The published studies in adult patients suggest that this dosing method is as efficacious as traditional dosing and associated with less renal toxicity. There is little pediatric experience with this approach, and because toxicity in children is less common than in adults, the traditional dosing regimens are still appropriate. However, daily or less frequent dosing has been carried out in small premature infants for many years. It is likely that once-daily dosing regimens will be investigated and may also be advantageous for the general pediatric population.

Quinolones

Nalidixic acid, the prototype quinolone antimicrobial is over 20 years old and is useful only for urinary tract infections. Modification of the quinolone structure has resulted in many new compounds called fluoroquinolones, which are well absorbed after oral administration and possess excellent antibacterial activity against resistant gram-negative pathogens. The many different fluoroquinolones vary in their activity against specific organisms. Fluoroquinolones are active against most of the Enterobacteriaceae, including *E coli, Enterobacter, Klebsiella,* in some cases *P aeruginosa,* and many other gram-negative bacteria such as *H influenzae, M catarrhalis, N gonorrhoeae,* and *N meningitidis.* The fluoroquinolones are active against some enterococci, *S aureus* and coagulase-negative staphylococci, but not against methicillin-resistant *S aureus.* The activity of fluoroquinolones against streptococci and anaerobic organisms is too limited for clinical usefulness.

Quinolone antibiotics are currently contraindicated in children, although they are potentially very attractive alternatives to current therapy. The contraindication is based on the recognition that nalidixic acid and other quinolones cause arthropathy when used experimentally in newborn animals of many species. The fear that children would also be susceptible to cartilage injury has not been realized in clinical experience. Both retrospective long-term follow-up studies of children treated with nalidixic acid and prospective studies of children treated under protocol with fluoroquinolones have not shown toxicity. As such, despite the contraindications listed, quinolone is considered for use in children when the benefit clearly outweighs the risk, when no alternative drug is available, and after informed discussion with the parents.

Quinolone is useful for oral therapy of resistant gram-negative urinary tract infections such as *P aeruginosa,* single-dose therapy of gonorrhea, therapy of resistant cases of shigellosis, therapy of patients with cystic fibrosis infected with *P aeruginosa,* and therapy for patients with chronic suppurative otitis media and in some cases nontuberculous mycobacterial infection.

Metronidazole

Metronidazole has excellent activity against most anaerobes, particularly gram-negative anaerobes such as bacteroides and fusobacterium, and gram-positive anaerobes such as clostridium, prevotella and porphyromonas. Gram-positive anaerobic cocci such as peptococcus and peptostreptococcus are often more susceptible to penicillin or to clindamycin. Because metronidazole lacks activity against aerobic organisms, it is usually given with one or more other antibiotics.

Metronidazole is well absorbed after oral administration and has excellent penetration into the central nervous system.

Chloramphenicol

Chloramphenicol has been used for many years to treat infections due to a broad spectrum of bacteria. Streptococci, many enterococci, gram-negative rods such as *E coli, H influenzae,* gram-negative cocci such as *Neisseria* spp, and anaerobic organisms are usually susceptible. Chloramphenicol is very well absorbed after oral administration, and cerebrospinal fluid levels are about 70% of serum levels.

Chloramphenicol causes a reversible suppression of bone marrow with prolonged use. Aplastic anemic is a rare idiosyncratic (non–dose-related) complication, which occurs in about 1 in 20,000 to 1 in 100,000 patients. Chloramphenicol given by any route may cause aplastic anemia, but most cases of aplastic anemia follow oral therapy. Because of this toxicity and because other antimicrobials choices are usually equally efficacious, chloramphenicol is not often used in general practice. However, Rocky Mountain spotted fever and resistant *S typhi* infections are treated with chloramphenicol.

Chloramphenicol was historically associated with the gray baby syndrome, a syndrome of cardiovascular collapse associated with high serum levels of chloramphenicol. Accordingly, chloramphenicol serum concentrations should be obtained whenever the drug is used. Peak serum concentrations between 15 and 30 µg/mL are safe and efficacious.

REFERENCES

Antimicrobial prophylaxis in surgery. The Medical Letter 1992;34(862):5.

Classen DC et al: The timing of prophylactic administration of antibiotics and the risk of surgical-wound infection. N Engl J Med 1992;326(5):281.

Committee on Infectious Diseases: Report of the Committee on Infectious Diseases, 23rd ed. American Academy of Pediatrics, 1994.

Edmond MB, Wenzel RP, Pasculle AW: Vancomycin-resistant *Staphylococcus aureus*: Perspectives on measures needed for control. Ann Intern Med 1996;124(3):329.

Jacobson KL et al: The relationship between antecedent antibiotic use and resistance to extended-spectrum cephalosporins in Group I β-lactamase-producing organisms. Clin Infect Dis 1995;21:1107.

Moellering RCJ: Monitoring serum vancomycin levels: Climbing the mountain because it is there? (Editorial). Clin Infect Dis 1994;18:544.

Nelson JD: *Pocketbook of Pediatric Antimicrobial Therapy,* 11th ed. Williams & Wilkins, 1995.

Nicolau D: Once-daily aminoglycosides. Connecticut Med 1992;56(10):561.

Physicians' Desk Reference, 49th ed. Medical Economics, 1995.

Prins JM et al: Once versus thrice daily gentamicin in patients with serious infections. The Lancet 1993;341:335.

Recommendations for preventing the spread of vancomycin resistance: Recommendations of the Hospital Infection Control Practices Advisory Committee. Am J Infect Control 1995;23:87.

Sanders CC, Sanders WEJ: β-Lactam resistance in gram-negative bacteria: Global trends and clinical impact. Clin Infect Dis 1992;15:824.

Sanford JP, Gilbert DN, Sande MA: *Sanford Guide to Antimicrobial Therapy.* Antimicrobial therapy, Inc, 1995.

Schaad JB et al: Use of fluoroquinolones in pediatrics: Consensus report of an International Society of Chemotherapy Commission. Pediatr Infect Dis J 1995;14:1.

Skopnik H, Heimann G: Once daily aminoglycoside dosing in full term neonates. Pediatr Infect Dis J 1995;14:71.

Todd JK: Antimicrobial susceptibility testing in the office laboratory. Pediatr Infect Dis 1983;2:481.

Tomasz A: Multiple-antibiotic-resistant pathogenic bacteria: A report on the Rockefeller University Workshop. N Engl J Med 1994;330(17):1247.

Infections: Viral & Rickettsial

35

Myron J. Levin, MD, & Jose R. Romero, MD

I. VIRAL INFECTIONS

Viruses cause most pediatric infections. Although immunizations have decreased the incidence of some viral infections, new viruses have been discovered. Mixed viral or viral-bacterial infections of the respiratory and intestinal tracts are rather common, as is prolonged, asymptomatic shedding of some viruses in childhood. Thus, the detection of a virus is not always proof that it is the cause of a given illness. Viruses are often a predisposing factor for bacterial respiratory infections (eg, otitis, sinusitis, and pneumonia).

Diagnosis of many viral illnesses is now possible through antigen or nucleic detection techniques. These are more rapid than isolation of viruses in tissue culture and in many cases almost as sensitive. Polymerase chain reaction (PCR) amplification of the viral genome permits recognition of previously undetectable infections. New diagnostic tests are changing many basic concepts about viral diseases and make diagnosis of viral infections increasingly complex. Only laboratories with excellent quality control procedures should be used, and the results of new tests must be interpreted cautiously. The availability of specific antiviral agents increases the value of early diagnosis for some serious viral infections. Table 35–1 lists viral agents associated with common clinical signs, and Table 35–2 lists diagnostic tests. The local viral diagnostic laboratory should be contacted for details regarding specimen collection, handling, and shipping.

RESPIRATORY INFECTIONS

Many virus infections cause upper or lower respiratory tract signs and symptoms. Those that produce a predominance of these signs and symptoms are described in this section. However, many "respiratory" viruses can also produce distinct nonrespiratory disease (eg, enteritis or cystitis caused by adenoviruses; parotitis caused by parainfluenza viruses). It is also important to realize that respiratory viruses can cause disease in any area of the respiratory tree. Thus, they can cause coryza, pharyngitis, bronchitis, tracheitis, bronchiolitis, and pneumonia, although certain viruses tend to be closely associated with one anatomic area (eg, parainfluenza with croup; respiratory syncytial virus (RSV) with bronchiolitis) or discrete epidemics (eg, influenza, RSV, parainfluenza). Nevertheless, it is not possible to be certain of the viral cause of an infection in a given child. This information is provided by the virology laboratory and is often important for epidemiologic, therapeutic, and preventive reasons.

INFECTIONS DUE TO ADENOVIRUSES

There are over 40 types of adenoviruses, which account for 2–10% of all respiratory illnesses. In addition, enteric adenoviruses are an important cause of childhood diarrhea. Adenoviral infections are common early in life. Epidemic disease occurs in the winter and spring, especially in closed environments, such as day care and institutions. Because of latent infection in lymphoid tissue, asymptomatic shedding from the respiratory or intestinal tract is common.

Diagnosis is by culture of conjunctival, respira-

Table 35–1. Common viral causes of clinical syndromes.

Rash
  Enterovirus
  Adenovirus
  Measles
  Rubella
  Human herpes virus type 6 or 7
  Varicella
  Parvovirus B19[1]
  Epstein-Barr virus
  Dengue
Fever
  Enterovirus
  Adenovirus
  Epstein-Barr virus
  Human herpes virus type 6[2]
  Cytomegalovirus
  Influenza
  Rhinovirus
  Many others
Conjunctivitis
  Adenovirus
  Enterovirus 70
  Influenza
  Measles
  Herpes simplex[3]
Parotitis
  Mumps
  Parainfluenza
  Enterovirus
  Influenza
  Cytomegalovirus
  Epstein-Barr virus
  Human immunodeficiency virus
Pharyngitis
  Adenovirus
  Enterovirus
  Epstein-Barr virus
  Herpes simplex virus[4]
  Influenza
Adenopathy
  Epstein-Barr virus
  Cytomegalovirus
  Rubella[5]
  Human immunodeficiency virus
Croup
  Parainfluenza
  Influenza
  Adenovirus
  Measles

Bronchiolitis
  Respiratory syncytial virus[6]
  Adenovirus
  Parainfluenza
  Influenza
Pneumonia
  Respiratory syncytial virus[7]
  Adenovirus
  Parainfluenza
  Measles
  Varicella[8]
  Rhinovirus[7]
  Cytomegalovirus[7,9]
Enteritis
  Rotavirus
  Enteric adenovirus
  Hepatitis A[10]
  Enterovirus
  Norwalk agent
  Calicivirus
Hepatitis
  Hepatitis[10] A, B, C, D, E
  Epstein-Barr virus
  Adenovirus
  Cytomegalovirus
Arthritis
  Parvovirus B19
  Rubella
  Hepatitis B
Congenital infection
  Cytomegalovirus
  Hepatitis B
  Hepatitis C[11]
  Rubella
  Human immunodeficiency virus
  Parvovirus B19
  Enterovirus
  Varicella
  Herpes simplex virus
Meningoencephalitis
  Enterovirus
  Mumps
  Arthropod-borne encephalitis
  Herpes simplex virus
  Cytomegalovirus
  Lymphocytic choriomeningitis virus
  Measles
  Varicella
  Adenovirus
  Human immunodeficiency virus
  Epstein-Barr virus

[1]Erythema infectiosum agent.
[2]Roseola agents.
[3]Conjunctivitis rare, only in primary infections; keratitis in older patients.
[4]May cause isolated pharyngeal vesicles at any age.
[5]May cause adenopathy without rash.
[6]Over 70% of cases.
[7]Usually only in young infants.
[8]Immunosuppressed, pregnant, rarely other adults.
[9]Severely immunosuppressed at risk.
[10]Anicteric cases more common in children; these may resemble viral gastroenteritis.
[11]Especially when the mother is HIV-positive.

Table 35–2. Diagnostic tests for viral infections.

Agent	Rapid Antigen Detection (Specimen)	Tissue Culture Days to Positive (Mean, Range)	Serology		Poly-merase Chain Reaction[1]	Comments
			Acute	Paired		
Adenovirus	+ (respiratory secretions)	+ 10 (1–21)	–	+	RL	"Enteric" strains detected by culture on special cell line, electron microscopy, or antigen detection.
Arboviruses	–	–	+	+		Acute serum may diagnose many forms.
Astrovirus	–	–	–	–		Diagnosis by electron microscopy.
Calicivirus	–	–	–	–		Diagnosis by electron microscopy.
Colorado tick fever	–	–	–	RL, CDC		
Cytomegalovirus	+ (tissue biopsy, blood, respiratory secretions)	+ 2	+	+	+	EIA may be done on tissue culture.
Enterovirus	–	+ 4 (2–15)	–	+	+	Serology for coxackie B viruses.
Epstein-Barr virus	–	–	+	+	+	Single serologic panel defines infection status; heterophil titer less sensitive.
Hantavirus	–	–	+	ND	+	Diagnosis by presence of IgM antibody.
Hepatitis A virus	–	–	+	ND		Diagnosis by presence of IgM antibody.
Hepatitis B virus	+ (blood)	–	+	ND		Diagnosis by presence of surface antigen or anti-core IgM antibody.
Hepatitis C	–	–	+	NA	+	Postitive acute result suggests that hepatits C is causative agent.
Herpes simplex virus	+ (skin, tissue biopsy)	+ 1 to + 2	+	+	+	Serology rarely used for herpes simplex. IgM antibody used in selected cases. Tzanck preparation of vesicle easy, 70% sensitive.
Human herpes-virus-6	–	–	RL, CDC	RL, CDC	+	Roseola agent.
Human immuno-deficiency virus	+ (blood) (acid dissociation of immune complexes)	+ 15 (5–28)	+		+	Antibody proves infection unless passively acquired (< age 15 months); culture not widely available.
Influenza virus	+ (respiratory secretions)	+ 3 (2–7)	–	+	RL	Antigen detection 70–90% sensitive.
Lymphocytic choriomeningitis virus	–	Blood, CSF 7 (5–20)	–	+		Can be isolated in suckling mice.
Measles virus	+ (respiratory secretions)	+ (5–14)	+	+	RL	Difficult to grow; IgM serology diagnostic.
Mumps virus	–	+ (>5)	+	+		Complement fixation titers may allow single-specimen diagnosis.
Parvovirus B19	–	–	+	+	+	Erythema infectiosum agent; antigen detection not yet commercially available.
Parainfluenza virus	+ (respiratory secretions)	+ 5 (2–10)	–	+		
Rabies virus	+ (skin, conjunctiva, tissue biopsy	–	–	+		Usually diagnosed by antigen detection.
Respiratory syncytial virus	+ (respiratory secretions)	+ 5 (3–14)	–	+		Rapid antigen detection; 85–90% sensitive.
Rhinovirus	–	+ 4 (2–7)	–	–		Too many types to diagnose serologically.
Rotavirus	+ (feces)	–	–	–		Electron microscopy useful for many enteric viruses.
Rubella virus	–	+ (> 10)	+	+		Recommended that paired sera be tested simultaneously.
Varicella-zoster virus	+ (skin scraping, tissue biopsy)	+ 3	RL	+	+	Tzanck preparation 70% sensitive.

[1]Useful only when performed on selected specimens by qualified laboratories

Key: + = Commercially or widely available. ***Note:*** Results from some commercial laboratories are unreliable.
  – = Not available commercially.
  RL, CDC = Specific antibody titers or PCR available by arrangement with individual research laboratories or the Centers for Disease Control and Prevention.
  ND = Not done.

tory, or stool specimens. Several days to weeks are required for growth in conventional cultures. Rapid culture using the shell vial technique detects virus in 48 hours. Adenovirus infection can also be diagnosed by direct fluorescent antibody stains of respiratory secretions. This is quicker, but is less sensitive than the culture methods. Special cells are needed to isolate enteric adenoviruses. Respiratory adenovirus infections can be detected by serology using acute and convalescent serum. Detection of enteric adenoviruses in diarrheal specimens can now be done rapidly with EIA.

Specific Adenoviral Syndromes

A. Pharyngitis: The most common adenoviral disease in children. Fever and adenopathy are common. Tonsillitis may be exudative. An influenza-like systemic illness may be present. Laryngotracheitis or bronchitis may accompany pharyngitis.

B. Follicular Conjunctivitis: This form of conjunctivitis may be prolonged and associated with preauricular adenopathy and corneal damage. Association with fever and pharyngitis is called "pharyngoconjunctival fever."

C. Epidemic Keratoconjunctivitis: Severe conjunctivitis with punctate keratitis and occasionally visual impairment. Preauricular adenopathy is common.

D. Pneumonia: Severe pneumonia may occur at all ages. It is especially common in young children (< 3 years). Chest radiographs show bilateral peribronchial and interstitial infiltrates. Symptoms persist for 2–4 weeks. This adenoviral pneumonia can be necrotizing and can cause permanent lung damage.

E. Rash: A diffuse morbilliform (rarely petechial) rash resembling measles, rubella, or roseola. Koplik's spots are absent.

F. Diarrhea: Enteric adenoviruses (types 40 and 41) are the second most common cause of short-lived diarrhea in an afebrile child.

G. Mesenteric Lymphadenitis: Fever and abdominal pain may mimic appendicitis. Pharyngitis is often associated. Adenovirus-induced adenopathy may be a factor in appendicitis and intussusception.

H. Other: Immunosuppressed patients, including neonates, may develop severe or fatal pulmonary or gastrointestinal infections or multisystem disease. Other rare complications include encephalitis, hepatitis, and myocarditis. Hemorrhagic cystitis can be a serious problem in immunocompromised children.

Treatment

There is no specific treatment. Intravenous immune globulin may be tried in immunocompromised patients with severe pneumonia.

Abzug MJ, Levin MJ: Neonatal adenovirus infection: Four patients and a review of the literature. Pediatrics 1991;87:890.

Krajden M et al: Clinical features of adenoviral enteritis: A review of 127 proven cases. Pediatr Infect Dis J 1990; 9:636.

Krilov LR et al: Disseminated adenovirus infection with hepatic necrosis in patients with human immunodeficiency virus infection and other immunodeficiency states. Rev Infect Dis 1990;12:303.

Murtagh P et al: Adenovirus type 7H respiratory infections: A report of 29 cases of acute lower respiratory disease. Acta Paediatr 1993;82:557.

INFLUENZA

Because young children have little prior experience with influenza, clinical infection with influenza is common. Although only three main types (A/H1N1, A/H3N2, B) have been prevalent recently, antigenic shift and drift ensure a supply of susceptible hosts of all ages. Outbreaks occur in fall and winter. Each year's strain tends to first occur in the Far East.

Clinical Findings

Spread of influenza occurs by way of respiratory secretions. The incubation period is 2–7 days. An influenza epidemic is often present in the community.

A. Symptoms and Signs: Influenza infection in older children and adults produces a characteristic syndrome of sudden onset of high fever, severe myalgia, headache, and chills. These overshadow the associated coryza, pharyngitis, and cough. Usually absent are rash, marked conjunctivitis, adenopathy, exudative pharyngitis, and dehydrating enteritis. Fever, diarrhea, vomiting, and abdominal pain are common in young children. Chest examination is usually unremarkable. Unusual clinical findings or variants include croup (most severe with type A influenza), exacerbation of asthma, myositis (especially calf muscles), myocarditis, parotitis, encephalopathy (distinct from Reye's syndrome), nephritis, and a transient maculopapular rash.

Acute illness lasts 2–5 days. Cough and fatigue may last several weeks.

B. Laboratory Findings: The leukocyte count is normal to low, with variable shift. The virus may be found in respiratory secretions by fluorescent antibody staining or enzyme immunoassay (EIA; for influenza A only). It can also be cultured within 3–5 days from pharyngeal swabs or throat washings. Many laboratories obtain positive cultures within 48 hours by centrifuging specimens onto cell layers and using antigen detection. Other body fluids or tissues (except lung) rarely yield the virus. A late diagnosis may be made with paired serology, using hemagglutination inhibition assays.

C. Imaging: The chest radiograph is nonspecific; it may show hyperaeration, peribronchial thickening, diffuse interstitial infiltrates, or bronchopneumonia in severe cases. Pneumothorax may occur. Hilar nodes are not enlarged. Pleural effusion is rare in uncomplicated influenza.

Differential Diagnosis

The following may be considered: all other respiratory viruses, *M pneumoniae* or *C pneumoniae* (longer incubation period, prolonged illness), streptococcal pharyngitis (pharyngeal exudate or petechiae, adenitis, no cough), bacterial sepsis (petechial or purpuric rash may occur), meningitis, toxic shock syndrome (rash, hypotension), mosquito-borne encephalitis virus (formerly called arbovirus) infections (fewer respiratory symptoms, summer onset), and rickettsial infections (rash, different season, insect exposure).

Complications & Sequelae

Lower respiratory tract symptoms are most common in children younger than 5 years. Secondary bacterial infections (classically staphylococcal) of the middle ear, sinuses, or lungs are most common. Of the viral infections that precede Reye's syndrome, varicella and influenza (usually type B) are most notable. During an influenza outbreak, ill children who develop protracted vomiting or irrational behavior should be evaluated for Reye's syndrome (see Chapter 21). Influenza can also cause a viral or postviral encephalitis, with cerebral symptoms much more prominent than those of the accompanying respiratory infection. Although the myositis is usually mild and resolves promptly, severe rhabdomyolysis and renal failure have been reported.

Children with underlying cardiopulmonary, metabolic, neuromuscular, or immunosuppressive disease may develop severe viral pneumonia.

Prevention

Influenza vaccine is moderately protective in older children (see Chapter 10). Medical staff and family members should also be immunized to protect high-risk patients. Type A infections may be prevented by amantadine or rimantadine (5 mg/kg; maximum 150 mg/d under age 10; 200 mg/d if older). Amantadine is divided into two daily doses; rimantadine can be given in a single dose. The physician should consider administering chemoprophylaxis during an epidemic to high-risk children who cannot be immunized or who have not yet developed immunity (about 6 weeks after primary vaccination or 2 weeks after a booster dose). These agents are inactive against influenza B.

Treatment & Prognosis

Treatment consists of general support and management of pulmonary complications, especially bacterial superinfections. Amantadine and rimantadine are of some benefit against influenza A (but not influenza B) if begun within 48 hours of onset. Their value in compromised hosts or others with severe disease is uncertain. Ribavirin is active in vitro against influenza A and B. The efficacy of aerosolized ribavirin in humans is controversial, but it may be tried in severe infections, especially in compromised hosts.

Recovery is usually complete unless severe cardiopulmonary or neurologic damage has occurred.

Brady MT: Amantadine and rimantadine. Rep Pediatr Infect Dis 1994;4:29.

Christenson JC, San Joaquin VH: Influenza-associated rhabdomyolysis in a child. Pediatr Infect Dis J 1990; 9:60.

Glezen WP: Indication for amantadine in otherwise healthy children. Pediatr Infect Dis J 1993;12:106.

Kondos AK: The effects of influenza virus infection on FEV_1 in asthmatic children. Chest 1991;100:1235.

Rimantadine for prevention and treatment of influenza. Med Lett Drugs Ther 1993;35:109.

Rodriguez WJ et al: Efficacy and safety of aerosolized ribavirin in young children hospitalized with influenza: A double-blind, multicenter, placebo-controlled trial. J Pediatr 1994;125:129.

Serwint JR, Hiller RM, Korsch BM: Influenza type A and B infections in hospitalized pediatric patients who should be immunized. Am J Dis Child 1991;145:623.

Sugaya N et al: Impact of influenza virus infection as a cause of pediatric hospitalization. J Infect Dis 1992;165: 373.

PARAINFLUENZA

Parainfluenza viruses (types 1–4) are the most important cause of croup. Most infants are infected with type 3 in the first 3 years of life; all types may cause outbreaks. Infection with types 1 and 2 are experienced gradually over the first 5 years of life. Type 1 occurs in the fall of odd-numbered years; type 3 appears annually, with a peak in the spring or summer. Most primary infections are symptomatic and frequently involve the lower respiratory tract.

Clinical Findings

A. Symptoms and Signs: Clinical diseases include febrile upper respiratory infection (especially in older children with re-exposure), laryngitis, tracheobronchitis, croup, and bronchiolitis (second most common cause after respiratory syncytial virus). The relative incidence of these manifestations is type-specific. Croup is the most prominent manifestation in young children in whom a virus is identified. Parainfluenza viruses cause 65% of cases of croup in young children, 25% of tracheobronchitis, and 50% of laryngitis. Pneumonia occurs in infants and immunodeficient children. Onset is acute. Most children are febrile. Symptoms of upper respiratory tract infection often accompany croup.

B. Laboratory Findings: Diagnosis is often

based on clinical findings. These viruses can be identified by rapid culture techniques (48 hours).

Differential Diagnosis

Parainfluenza-induced respiratory syndromes are difficult to distinguish from those caused by other respiratory viruses. Croup must be distinguished from epiglottitis caused by *H influenzae* (abrupt onset, toxicity, drooling, dyspnea, little cough, left shift of blood smear, and a history of inadequate immunization).

Therapy

There is no specific therapy or vaccine. Croup management is discussed in Chapter 20. Ribavirin is active in vitro and has been used in immunocompromised children, but its efficacy is unproved.

Heidemann SM: Clinical characteristics of parainfluenza virus infection in hospitalized children. Pediatr Pulmonol 1992;13:86.

Husby et al: Treatment of croup with nebulized steroid (budesonide): A double blind, placebo controlled study. Arch Dis Child 1993;68:352.

Knott AM, Long CE, Hall CB: Parainfluenza viral infections in pediatric outpatients: Seasonal patterns and clinical characteristics. Pediatr Infect Dis J 1994;13:269.

Welliver RC et al: Parainfluenza virus bronchiolitis. Am J Dis Child 1986;140:34.

RESPIRATORY SYNCYTIAL VIRUS (RSV) DISEASE

Essentials of Diagnosis

- Diffuse wheezing and tachypnea following upper respiratory symptoms in an infant (bronchiolitis).
- Epidemics in late fall to early spring.
- Hyperinflation on chest radiograph.
- RSV antigen detected in nasal secretions.

General Considerations

Respiratory syncytial virus is the most important cause of lower respiratory tract illness in young children, accounting for more than 70% of cases of bronchiolitis and 40% of cases of pneumonia. Outbreaks occur annually, and attack rates are high; 60% of children are infected in the first year of life. During peak season, the clinical diagnosis of RSV infection in infants with bronchiolitis is as accurate as most laboratory tests. Despite the presence of serum antibody, reinfection is common. No vaccine is available. Immunosuppressed patients may develop progressive severe pneumonia. Children with congenital heart disease with increased pulmonary blood flow, children with chronic lung disease, and premature infants under 6 months of age are also at higher risk for severe illness.

Clinical Findings

A. Symptoms and Signs: Initial symptoms are those of upper respiratory infection. Fever may be present. The classic disease is bronchiolitis, characterized by diffuse wheezing, variable fever, cough, tachypnea, difficulty feeding, and cyanosis in severe cases. Hyperinflation, crackles, prolonged expiration, wheezing, and retractions are present. The liver and spleen may be palpable because of lung hyperinflation but are not enlarged. The disease usually lasts 3–7 days in previously healthy children.

Apnea may be the presenting manifestation, especially in premature infants in the first few months of life; it usually resolves in the first few days of illness, often being replaced by obvious signs of bronchiolitis. No explanation for apnea has been found.

RSV infections in subsequent years are more likely to cause tracheobronchitis or upper respiratory tract infection except in compromised hosts or children with severe chronic lung or heart disease, who may have additional attacks of severe pneumonitis.

B. Laboratory Findings: Routine tests are nonspecific. Rapid detection of RSV antigen in nasal or pulmonary secretions by fluorescent antibody staining or EIA is more than 90% sensitive and specific. Rapid tissue culture methods take 48 hours and have comparable sensitivity.

C. Imaging: Diffuse hyperinflation and peribronchiolar thickening are most common; atelectasis and patchy infiltrates also occur in uncomplicated infection, but pleural effusions are rare. Consolidation occurs in 25% of children with lower tract disease.

Differential Diagnosis

Although almost all cases of bronchiolitis are due to RSV during an epidemic, other viruses cannot be excluded. Mixed infections with other viruses, chlamydia, or bacteria are not uncommon. Wheezing may be due to asthma, a foreign body, or other airway obstruction. Respiratory syncytial virus may closely resemble *Chlamydia* pneumonitis when fine crackles are present and fever and wheezing are not prominent. The two may also coexist. Cystic fibrosis may resemble RSV infection; a positive family history or failure to thrive associated with hyponatremia or hypoalbuminemia should prompt a sweat chloride test. Pertussis should also be considered in this age group, especially if cough is prominent and if the infant is under 6 months of age. A markedly elevated leukocyte count should suggest bacterial superinfection (neutrophilia) or pertussis (lymphocytosis).

Complications

Secondary bacterial infection of the middle ear (usually due to pneumococci or *H influenzae*) is the most common complication. However, bacterial pneumonia occurs in only 0.5–1% of hospitalized cases. Sudden exacerbations of fever and leukocytosis should suggest bacterial infection. Respiratory failure or apnea may require mechanical ventilation. Cardiac failure may occur as a complication of pulmonary disease or myocarditis. Respiratory syncytial virus—as well as parainfluenza and influenza viruses—commonly causes acute exacerbations of asthma. Nosocomial infection is so common during outbreaks that elective hospitalization or surgery, especially for those with underlying illness, should be postponed. Well-designed hospital programs to prevent nosocomial spread are imperative (see below).

Treatment

Children who are very hypoxic or cannot feed because of respiratory distress must be hospitalized and given humidified oxygen and tube or intravenous feedings. Antibiotics, decongestants, expectorants, and steroids are of no value in routine infections. The child should be kept in respiratory isolation. Cohorting ill infants in respiratory isolation during peak season (with or without rapid diagnostic attempts) and emphasizing good hand-washing may greatly decrease nosocomial transmission.

Often a trial of bronchodilator therapy is given to determine if bronchospasm coexists. Patients appear to respond differently to bronchodilator therapy. Discontinue these if there is no improvement. If they do help, nebulized salbutamol (0.10 mg/kg) treatments (every 2–6 hours as needed) may be tried (see Chapter 20).

Ribavirin is the only licensed antiviral therapy used for RSV infection. It is given by continuous aerosolization (6 g in a 300 mL vial of water) by a special nebulizer (Small Particle Aerosol Generator, ICN Pharmaceuticals) for 12–18 hours of every day for 3–5 days. This agent has minimal effect on viral shedding. There is some controversy about its efficacy. At best, there is a very modest effect on disease severity in normal infants. Even in high-risk infants, the clinical response varies among studies. Nevertheless, ribavirin is often used in severely ill children who are immunologically or anatomically compromised. It is very expensive. It is teratogenic in animals, but the significance of that observation in humans is unknown. It should be used in a negative-pressure room, preferably fitted with additional respiratory care equipment capable of preventing contamination of room air. Caregivers should wear masks, and pregnant women should not be in a room when ribavirin is being administered.

Bronchospasm may be exacerbated by this drug. It should be used with extreme caution in ventilated patients and only by therapists expert in pediatric ventilator management. In general, it should be considered for use only for very young infants (≤ 8 weeks), former premature infants (< 35 weeks) who are under 6 months old, children with underlying cardiopulmonary or immunologic diseases, and normal infants with evidence of severe RSV infection (ventilated or with $PO_2 < 65$ mm Hg; PCO_2 rising).

Monthly administration of gamma-globulin containing high titers of anti-RSV antibody is now available to prevent severe disease in high-risk preterm patients during epidemic periods.

Prognosis

Although mild bronchiolitis does not produce long-term problems, 30–40% of patients hospitalized with this infection will wheeze later in childhood. Chronic restrictive lung disease and bronchiolitis obliterans are rare sequelae.

Groothuis JR et al: Prophylactic administration of respiratory syncytial virus immune globular to high risk infants and young children. N Engl J Med 1993;329:1524.

Groothuis JR, Salbenblatt CK, Lauer BA: Severe respiratory syncytial virus infection in older children. Am J Dis Child 1990;144:346.

Hall CB et al: Risk of secondary bacterial infection in infants hospitalized with respiratory syncytial viral infection. J Pediatr 1988;113:266.

Hammer J, Numa A, Newth CJL: Albuterol responsiveness in infants with respiratory failure caused by respiratory syncytial virus infection. J Pediatr Med 1995;127:485.

La Via WV, Marks MI, Stutman HR: Respiratory syncytial virus puzzle: Clinical features, pathophysiology, treatment, and prevention. J Pediatr 1992;121:503.

MacDonald NE et al: Respiratory syncytial viral infection in infants with congenital heart disease. N Engl J Med 1982;307:397.

Madge P et al: Prospective controlled study of four infection-control procedures to prevent nosocomial infection with respiratory syncytial virus. Lancet 1992;340:1079.

Meart KL et al: Aerosolized ribavirin in mechanically ventilated children with respiratory syncytial virus lower respiratory tract disease: A prospective, double-blind, randomized trial. Intensive Care Med 1994;22:566.

Smith DW et al: A controlled trial of aerosolized ribavirin in infants receiving mechanical ventilation for severe respiratory syncytial virus infection. N Engl J Med 1991;325:24.

Wildin SR, Chonmaitree T, Swischuk LE: Roentgenographic features of common pediatric viral respiratory infections. Am J Dis Child 1988;142:43.

MEASLES
(Rubeola)

Essentials of Diagnosis

- Exposure to measles 9–14 days previously.
- Prodrome of fever, cough, conjunctivitis, and coryza.
- Koplik's spots (few to countless small white papules on a diffusely red base on the buccal mucosa) 1–2 days prior to and after onset of rash.
- Maculopapular rash spreading down from the face and hairline over 3 days and later becoming confluent.
- Leukopenia.

General Considerations

This classic childhood exanthem had greatly decreased in incidence in the United States because of vaccination. The recent increase in cases is more the result of improper immunization than of vaccine failures. It is now recommended that all children be revaccinated upon entrance into primary or secondary school (Chapter 10). The attack rate in susceptibles is extremely high; spread is respiratory. Morbidity and mortality rates in the developing world are substantial because of underlying malnutrition and secondary infections.

Clinical Findings

A history of contact with a suspected case is often obtainable during an epidemic, but since airborne spread is efficient and patients are contagious during the prodrome, no contact history may be obtained. In temperate climates, measles is a winter-spring disease. Many suspected cases are misdiagnoses of other viral infections.

A. Symptoms and Signs: High fever and lethargy are prominent. Sneezing, eyelid edema, tearing, copious coryza, photophobia, and harsh cough ensue and worsen. Koplik's spots are almost pathognomonic for rubeola, though they may be absent.

The discrete maculopapular rash spreads quickly over the face and trunk, coalescing to a bright red. As it involves the extremities, it fades from the face and is completely gone within 6 days; fine desquamation may occur. Fever usually falls 2–3 days after the onset of the rash.

The use of killed-virus vaccine until 1967 resulted in partial immunity; upon exposure to wild virus, some vaccinees develop a severe atypical measles characterized by peripheral rash, pneumonia, headache, high fever, and abdominal pain. Koplik's spots are absent. Many adults who were not reimmunized with live-virus vaccines are still at risk for this atypical disease. Partial immunity may be seen in infants with residual maternal antibody, those given immune globulin in any form, and some who have been "appropriately" immunized. These individuals may develop mild cases of measles that can be easily missed because of a nonspecific rash or the absence of fever.

B. Laboratory Findings: Lymphopenia is characteristic. Total leukocyte counts may fall to 1500/μL. An experienced cytologist may see multinucleated giant cells in oral mucosal scrapings and in nasal secretions, but diagnosis is usually made by detection of measles IgM antibody in serum drawn at least 2 days after the onset of rash or by detection of a significant rise in antibody. Tissue culture may also be used, but it takes longer and is less sensitive. Direct detection of measles antigen by fluorescent antibody staining of nasopharyngeal cells is a useful rapid method.

C. Imaging: Chest radiographs often show hyperinflation, perihilar infiltrates, or parenchymal patchy, fluffy densities. Secondary bacterial infection produces consolidation or effusion.

Differential Diagnosis

Table 35–3 lists other illnesses that may resemble measles.

Complications & Sequelae

A. Respiratory Complications: These occur in up to 15% of cases. Bacterial superinfections of lung, middle ear, sinus, and cervical nodes are most common. Fever that persists after the third or fourth day of rash suggests such a complication, as does leukocytosis. Bronchospasm, severe croup, and progressive viral pneumonia or bronchiolitis (in infants) also occur. Immunosuppressed patients are at much greater risk for fatal pneumonia.

B. Cerebral Complications: Encephalitis occurs in 1:2000 cases. Onset is usually within a week after appearance of rash. Symptoms include combativeness, ataxia, vomiting, seizures, and coma. Lymphocytic pleocytosis and a mildly elevated protein are usual cerebrospinal fluid findings, but the fluid may be normal. Fifty percent of patients so affected die or are severely damaged.

Subacute sclerosing panencephalitis is a slow measles virus infection of the brain that becomes symptomatic years later in about 1:100,000 previously infected children. This progressive cerebral deterioration is associated with myoclonic jerks and a typical electroencephalographic pattern. It is fatal in 6–12 months. It may occur following administration of vaccine, with an estimated incidence of 1:1,000,000. High titers of measles antibody are present in serum and spinal fluid.

C. Other Complications: These include hemorrhagic or "black" measles (severe disease with multiorgan bleeding, fever, cerebral symptoms), thrombocytopenia, appendicitis, keratitis, myocarditis, optic neuritis, reactivation or progression of tuberculosis in untreated children (including transient cutaneous anergy), and premature delivery or stillbirth.

Mild liver function test elevation has been detected in up to 50% of cases in young adults; frank jaundice may also occur.

Treatment, Prognosis, & Prevention

Recovery generally occurs 7–10 days after onset of symptoms. Therapy is supportive: eye care, cough relief (avoid narcotic suppressants in infants), and fever reduction (acetaminophen, lukewarm baths; avoid salicylates). Secondary bacterial infections should be treated promptly; antimicrobial prophylaxis is not indicated. Ribavirin is active in vitro and may be useful in infected immunocompromised children. In malnourished children, acute vitamin A supplementation should be given to attenuate the illness.

The current two-dose active vaccination strategy is successful. Vaccine should not be withheld for concurrent mild acute illness, tuberculosis or positive PPD, breast feeding, or exposure to an immunodeficient contact.

Table 35–3. Red rashes in children.

Condition	Incubation Period (Days)	Prodrome	Rash	Laboratory Tests	Comments, Other Diagnostic Features
Measles	9–14	Cough, rhinitis, conjunctivitis	Maculopapular; face to extremities; lasts 7–10 d; Koplik's spots in mouth	Leukopenia	Toxic. Bright red rash becomes confluent, may desquamate.
Rubella	14–21	Usually none	Mild maculopapular; rapid spread face to extremities; gone by day 4	Normal or leukopenia	Postauricular, occipital adenopathy common. Polyarthralgia in some older girls. Mild clinical illness.
Roseola (exanthem subitum)	10–14	Fever (3–4 d)	Pink, macular rash occurs at end of illness; transient	Normal	Fever often high, and disappears when rash develops; child appears well. Usually occurs in children 6 m–2 y of age.
Erythema infectiosum	13–18	None	Erythematous "slapped" cheeks; then reticular rash on extremities, trunk	Normal (reticulocytopenia)	Rash may reappear over weeks, especially with exposure to heat, sunlight. May cause arthralgia/arthritis, usually in older children or adults. Red cell maturation arrest in children with chronic hemolysis can cause aplastic crisis.
Enterovirus	2–7	Variable fever, chills, myalgia, sore throat	Usually macular, maculopapular on trunk or palms, soles; vesicles, petechiae also seen	Variable	Varied rashes may resemble those of many other infections. Pharyngeal or hand-foot-mouth vesicles may occur.
Streptococcal scarlet fever	1–7	Fever, abdominal pain, headache, sore throat	Diffuse erythema, "sandpaper" texture; neck, axillae, inguinal areas; spreads to rest of body; desquamates 7–14 d	Leukocytosis; positive group A streptococcus culture of throat or wound	Strawberry tongue, red pharynx with or without exudate. Eyes, perioral and periorbital area, palms, and soles spared. Pastia's lines. Brief prodrome. Cervical adenopathy, mild variant, scarlatina. Usually occurs in children 2–10 y of age.
Staphylococcal scarlet fever	1–7	Variable fever	Diffuse erythroderma; resembles streptococcal scarlet fever except eyes may be hyperemic, no "strawberry" tongue, pharynx spared	Variable leukocytosis if infected	Focal *Staphylococcus aureus* infection usually present.

(continued)

Table 35–3. Red rashes in children. (continued)

Condition	Incubation Period (Days)	Prodrome	Rash	Laboratory Tests	Comments, Other Diagnostic Features
Staphylococcal scalded skin	Variable	Irritability, absent to low fever	Painful erythroderma, followed in 1–2 d by dry cracking around eyes, mouth; bullae form with friction (Nikolsky's sign)	Normal if only colonized by staph; leukocytosis and sometimes bacteremia if infected	Normal pharynx. Look for focal staph infection. Usually occurs in infants.
Toxic shock syndrome	Variable	Fever, myalgia, headache, diarrhea, vomiting	Nontender erythroderma: red eyes, palms, soles, pharynx, lips	Leukocytosis; abnormal liver enzymes, coagulation tests; proteinuria	*S aureus* infection, multiorgan involvement. Swollen hands, feet. Hypotension or shock.
Erythema multiforme	—	Usually none or related to underlying cause	Discrete, red maculopapular lesions; symmetric, distal, palms and soles; target lesions classic	Normal or eosinophilia	Reaction to drugs (especially sulfas), or infectious agents. Urticaria, arthralgia also seen.
Stevens-Johnson syndrome	—	Pharyngitis, conjunctivitis, fever, malaise	Bullous erythema multiforme; may slough in large areas; hemorrhagic lips; purulent conjunctivitis	Leukocytosis	Classic precipitants are drugs (especially sulfas), *Mycoplasma pneumoniae* and herpes simplex infections. Pneumonitis and urethritis also seen.
Drug allergy	—	None, fever alone, or fever, myalgia, pruritus	Macular, maculopapular, urticarial, or erythroderma	Leukopenia, eosinophilia	Rash variable. Severe reactions may resemble measles, scarlet fever; adenopathy, hepatosplenomegaly, marked toxicity possible.
Kawasaki disease	Unknown	Fever, cervical adenopathy, irritability	Polymorphous (may be erythroderma) on trunk and extremities; red palms and soles, lips, tongue, pharynx	Leukocytosis, thrombocytosis, elevated ESR; pyuria; negative cultures and streptococcal serology	Swollen hands, feet; prolonged illness; bulbar hyperemia; uveitis; aseptic meningitis; no response to antibiotics. Vasculitis and aneurysms of coronary and other arteries occur.
Leptospirosis	4–19	Fever, myalgia, chills	Variable erythroderma	Leukocytosis; hematuria, proteinuria; hyperbilirubinema	Conjunctivitis; toxic. Hepatitis, aseptic meningitis may be seen. Rodent, dog contact.

Vaccination prevents the disease in susceptible exposed individuals if given within 72 hours (see Chapter 10). Immune globulin (0.25 mL/kg intramuscularly) will prevent or modify measles if given within 6 days. Suspected cases should be diagnosed promptly and reported to the local health department.

Fortenberry JD et al: Severe laryngotracheobronchitis complicating measles. Am J Dis Child 1992;146:1040.

Gellin BG, Katz SL: Measles: State of the art and future directions. J Infect Dis 1994;170(Suppl):53.

Hussey GD, Klein M: Randomized, controlled trial of vitamin A in children with severe measles. N Engl J Med 1990;323:160.

Kaplan LJ et al: Severe measles in immunocompromised patients. JAMA 1992;267:1237.

Kipps A, Dick G, Moodie JW: Measles and the central nervous system. Lancet 1983;2:1406.

Mason WH et al: Epidemic measles in the postvaccine era: Evaluation of epidemiology, clinical presentation and complications during an urban outbreak. Pediatr Infect Dis J 1993;12:42.

INFECTIONS DUE TO ENTEROVIRUSES

Enteroviruses are a major cause of illness in children. They are physically and biochemically similar and may produce identical syndromes. The multiple types make vaccine development impractical and have hindered development of antigen-detection and serologic tests. However, common RNA sequences and group antigens have led to diagnostic tests for viral nucleic acid and proteins. A rapid polymerase chain reaction assay will soon be commercially available, but tissue culture is the commonly used diagnostic method for echoviruses, polioviruses, and coxsackie B viruses. Since cultures may turn positive in 2–4 days, they should be inoculated promptly and may be clinically useful, particularly in cases of meningoencephalitis. Many coxsackie A viruses fail to grow.

Transmission is fecal-oral. Multiple enteroviruses circulate in the community at any one time; summer-fall outbreaks are common in temperate climates, but illness is seen year-round. After poliovirus, coxsackie B virus is most virulent, followed by echovirus. Neurologic, cardiac, and overwhelming neonatal infections are the severest forms of illness.

ACUTE FEBRILE ILLNESS

Accompanied by nonspecific upper respiratory or enteric symptoms, sudden onset of fever and irritability in infants or young children is often enteroviral in origin, especially in late summer and fall. Occasionally, a petechial rash is seen; more often, a diffuse maculopapular eruption (often prominent on palms and soles) occurs on the second to fourth days of fever. Purpura is rare and should suggest bacterial sepsis. Rapid recovery is the rule. More than one febrile enteroviral illness can occur in the same patient in one season. Leukocyte counts are usually normal. Many types of coxsackievirus and echovirus infections present in this manner. Infants, especially, often undergo an evaluation for bacteremia or meningitis and may be hospitalized to rule out sepsis.

RESPIRATORY TRACT ILLNESSES

1. FEBRILE UPPER RESPIRATORY INFECTION WITH PHARYNGITIS

This syndrome is most common in older children, who complain of headache, sore throat, myalgia, and abdominal discomfort. The usual duration is 3–4 days. Vesicles or papules may be seen in the pharynx. There is no exudate. Occasionally, enteroviruses are the cause of croup, bronchitis, or pneumonia. They may also exacerbate asthma.

2. HERPANGINA

Herpangina is characterized by an acute onset of fever and posterior pharyngeal ulcers, often linearly arranged on the anterior fauces. Bilateral faucial ulcers may also be seen. Dysphagia, vomiting, and anorexia also occur and, rarely, parotitis or vaginal ulcers. Symptoms disappear in 1 week. The epidemic form is due to a variety of coxsackie A viruses; coxsackie B viruses and echoviruses cause sporadic cases.

The differential diagnosis includes primary herpes simplex gingivostomatitis (ulcers are more prominent anteriorly, and gingivitis is present), aphthous stomatitis (fever absent, recurrent episodes, anterior lesions), trauma, hand-foot-and-mouth disease (see below), and Vincent's angina (spreading painful gingivitis from the gum line, underlying dental disease).

3. ACUTE LYMPHONODULAR PHARYNGITIS

Coxsackievirus A10 has been associated with a febrile pharyngitis characterized by nonulcerating yellow-white posterior pharyngeal papules. The duration is 1–2 weeks; therapy is supportive.

4. PLEURODYNIA
(Bornholm Disease, Epidemic Myalgia)

Caused by coxsackie B virus (epidemic form) or many nonpolio enteroviruses (sporadic form), pleurodynia presents with an abrupt onset of unilateral pleuritic pain of variable intensity. Symptoms are episodic, and relapses occur. Associated symptoms include headache, fever, vomiting, myalgias, and abdominal and neck pain. Physical findings include fever, chest muscle tenderness, decreased thoracic excursion, and occasionally a friction rub. The chest radiograph is normal. Hematologic tests are nondiagnostic.

The differential diagnosis includes bacterial pneumonia, empyema, tuberculosis, and coccidioidomycosis (all excluded radiographically), costochondritis (no fever or other symptoms), and a variety of abdominal problems, especially those causing diaphragmatic irritation.

There is no specific therapy. Potent analgesic agents and chest splinting alleviate the pain.

RASHES
(Including Hand-Foot-and-Mouth Disease)

The rash may be macular, maculopapular, urticarial, scarlatiniform, petechial, or vesicular. One of the most characteristic is that of hand-foot-and-mouth disease (caused by coxsackievirus, especially types A5, A10, and A16), in which vesicles or red papules are found on the tongue, oral mucosa, hands, and feet. Associated fever and malaise are mild. The rash may appear when fever abates, simulating roseola.

CARDIAC INVOLVEMENT

Myocarditis and pericarditis may be caused by a number of nonpolio enteroviruses, particularly type B coxsackieviruses; disease may be mild or fatal. In infants, other organs may be involved at the same time; in older patients, cardiac disease is usually isolated (see Chapter 19 for therapy). Enteroviral genomes are present in cardiac tissue in some cases of dilated cardiomyopathy or myocarditis; the significance of this finding is not known.

SEVERE NEONATAL INFECTION

Sporadic and nosocomial nursery cases of severe systemic enteroviral disease occur. Clinical manifestations include combinations of fever, rash, pneumonitis, encephalitis, hepatitis, gastroenteritis, myocarditis, pancreatitis, and myositis. The infants may appear septic, with cyanosis and dyspnea. The differential diagnosis includes bacterial and herpes infections, necrotizing enterocolitis, other causes of heart or liver failure, and metabolic diseases. Diagnosis is suggested by the finding of cerebrospinal fluid mononuclear pleocytosis and confirmed by the isolation of virus from urine, stool, cerebrospinal fluid, or pharynx. Strict isolation is needed; therapy is supportive. Intravenous immunoglobulin is often administered, but its value is uncertain. Passively acquired maternal antibody may protect newborns from severe disease. For this reason, labor should not be induced in pregnant women near term with suspected enteroviral disease.

Abzug M, Levin MJ, Rotbart HA: Profile of enterovirus disease in the first two weeks of life. Pediatr Infect Dis J 1993;12:820.

Modlin JF: Perinatal echovirus and group B coxsackie infections. Clin Perinatol 1988;15:233.

CENTRAL NERVOUS SYSTEM ILLNESSES

1. POLIOMYELITIS

Essentials of Diagnosis
- No prior immunization or underlying immune deficiency.
- Headache, fever, muscle weakness.
- Asymmetric, flaccid paralysis; muscle tenderness and hyperesthesia; intact sensation; late atrophy.
- Aseptic meningitis.

General Considerations
Poliovirus infection is subclinical in 90–95% of cases; causes nonspecific febrile illness in about 5%; and causes aseptic meningitis or paralytic disease in 1–3%. In endemic areas, most older children and adults are immune because of prior inapparent infections. Occasional cases in the United States occur in patients who have traveled to foreign countries; most cases are in immunodeficient patients who receive the poliovirus vaccine or are exposed to recent vaccines. Severe poliovirus infections rarely follow oral poliovirus vaccination as a result of reversion of the vaccine virus. The incidence varies from 1:1,000,000 to 1:10,000,000, depending on virus type and the age of the vaccinee. The risk of this complication is about 2600 times greater in immunodeficient children.

Clinical Findings
A. Symptoms and Signs: The initial symptoms are fever, myalgia, sore throat, and headache for 2–6 days. Several symptom-free days are followed by recurrent fever and signs of aseptic meningitis—headache, stiff neck, spinal rigidity, and nau-

sea. Mild cases resolve completely. High fever, severe myalgia, and anxiety usually portend progression to loss of reflexes and subsequent flaccid paralysis. Sensation remains intact, although hyperesthesia of skin overlying paralyzed muscles is common and pathognomonic. The disease progression is variable, especially in infants.

Paralysis is usually asymmetric. Bulbar involvement affects swallowing, speech, and cardiorespiratory function and accounts for most deaths. Bladder distention and marked bowel constipation characteristically accompany lower limb paralysis. Paralysis is usually complete by the time the temperature normalizes. Weakness often resolves completely. Atrophy is usually apparent by 4–8 weeks. Most improvement of muscle paralysis will take place within 6 months.

B. Laboratory Findings: In patients with meningeal symptoms, the cerebrospinal fluid shows up to several hundred leukocytes (mostly lymphocytes); glucose level is normal, and protein concentration is mildly elevated. Poliovirus is easy to grow in cell culture and can be readily differentiated from other enteroviruses. It is rarely isolated from spinal fluid but usually from throat and stool for several weeks following infection. Paired serology is also diagnostic. Differentiation of wild from live attenuated vaccine strains requires expertise.

Differential Diagnosis

Aseptic meningitis due to poliovirus is indistinguishable from that due to other viruses. Paralytic disease in the United States is usually due to nonpolio enteroviruses. Polio may resemble Guillain-Barré syndrome (variable sensory loss, symmetric loss of function; minimal pleocytosis, high protein concentration in spinal fluid), polyneuritis (sensory loss), pseudoparalysis due to bone or joint problems (eg, trauma, infection), botulism, or tick paralysis.

Complications & Sequelae

Complications are the result of the acute and permanent effects of paralysis. Respiratory, pharyngeal, bladder, and bowel malfunction are most critical. Deaths are usually due to complications arising from respiratory dysfunction. Limbs with provocation paralysis (such as intramuscular injections, excessive prior use, or trauma) tend to be most severely involved and have the worst prognosis for recovery of functions. Postpolio muscular atrophy occurs in 30–40% of paralyzed limbs 20–30 years later, characterized by increasing paralysis and fasciculations in previously affected, partially recovered limbs.

Treatment & Prognosis

Therapy is supportive. Bed rest, fever and pain control (heat therapy is helpful), and careful attention to progression of weakness (particularly of respiratory muscles) are important. No intramuscular injections should be given during the acute phase. Intuba-

tion or tracheostomy for secretion control and catheter drainage of the bladder may be needed. Assisted ventilation and enteral feeding may also be needed. Paralysis is mild in about 30%, permanent in 15%, and results in death in 5–10%. Disease is worse in adults and pregnant women than in children.

Agre JC, Rodriguez AA: Neuromuscular function in polio survivors at one-year follow-up. Arch Phys Med Rehabil 1991;72:7.

Nikowane BM et al: Vaccine associated paralytic poliomyelitis. JAMA 1987;257:1335.

Strebel PM et al: Epidemiology of poliomyelitis in the United States one decade after the last reported case of indigenous wild virus-associated disease. Clin Infect Dis 1992;14:568.

Strebel PM et al: Intramuscular injections within 30 days of immunization with oral poliovirus vaccine: A risk factor for vaccine-associated paralytic poliomyelitis. N Engl J Med 1995;332:500.

Wright PF et al: Strategies for the global eradication of poliomyelitis by the year 2000. N Engl J Med 1991; 325:1774.

2. ASEPTIC MENINGITIS

Nonpolio enteroviruses cause over 80% of cases of aseptic meningitis at all ages. In the summer and fall, multiple cases may be seen associated with circulation of neurotropic strains. Nosocomial outbreaks also occur; severe disease and death may occur in neonates. Spread is fecal-oral.

Clinical Findings

The usual enteroviral incubation period is 4–6 days. Since enteroviral infections are often subclinical, a history of contact with a patient with meningitis is unusual. Neonates may acquire infection from maternal blood, vaginal secretions, or feces at birth; occasionally, the mother has had a febrile illness just prior to delivery.

A. Symptoms and Signs: Onset is usually acute with variable fever, marked irritability, and lethargy in infants. Incidence is much greater in children less than 1 year of age. Older children also describe frontal headache, photophobia, and myalgia. Abdominal pain, diarrhea, and vomiting may occur. The incidence of rash varies with the infecting strain. If rash occurs, it is usually seen after several days of illness and is diffuse, macular or maculopapular, occasionally petechial, but not purpuric. Oropharyngeal vesicles and rash on the palms and soles suggest an enteroviral cause. The anterior fontanelle may be full. In older children, it is easier to demonstrate meningeal signs. Seizures are unusual, and focal neurologic findings are so rare that they suggest another agent or diagnosis. Frank encephalitis is rare at all ages, though more common in neonates.

B. Laboratory Findings: Blood leukocyte

counts are nonspecific and often within the normal range. The spinal fluid leukocyte count is 100–1000/μL. Early in the illness, polymorphonuclear cells predominate; a shift to mononuclear cells occurs within 8–36 hours. In about 95% of cases, spinal fluid parameters include a total leukocyte count less than 3000/μL, protein less than 80 mg/dL, and glucose more than 40% of serum values. Marked deviation from any of these findings should prompt consideration of another diagnosis (see below). The syndrome of inappropriate secretion of antidiuretic hormone may occur but is rarely clinically significant.

Culture of cerebrospinal fluid may yield an enterovirus within a few days; virus may be found in acellular spinal fluids. Polymerase chain reaction for enteroviruses will soon be available in the United States. This can give an answer within 24–48 hours. Isolation of an enterovirus from throat or stool suggests but does not prove enteroviral meningitis. Vaccine poliovirus present in feces in infants being evaluated for aseptic meningitis may confuse the diagnosis. It can usually be distinguished by growth characteristics from other enteroviruses. Rarely, vaccine poliovirus causes ventriculoperitoneal shunt infections.

C. Imaging: Cerebral imaging is not often indicated; if done, it is usually normal; subdural effusions, infarcts, edema, or focal abnormalities seen in bacterial meningitis are absent, except for the very rare case of focal encephalitis.

Differential Diagnosis

In the prevaccine era, mumps and polio were leading causes of aseptic meningitis. Other viruses include mosquito-borne viruses and herpes simplex. In adolescents, herpesvirus type 2 may cause aseptic meningitis with initial genital infection. In neonates, early herpesvirus meningoencephalitis may mimic enteroviral disease (see the section on herpesviruses, below). This is an important alternate diagnosis to exclude because of complications for urgent specific therapy.

Other causes of aseptic meningitis that may resemble enteroviral infection include partially treated bacterial meningitis (recent antibiotic treatment; spinal fluid parameters resembling those seen in bacterial disease and bacterial antigen sometimes present); parameningeal foci of bacterial infection such as brain abscess, subdural empyema, mastoiditis (predisposing factors, glucose level in cerebrospinal fluid possibly lower, focal neurologic signs, and imaging); tumors or cysts (malignant cells detected by cytologic examination, a history of neurologic symptoms, higher protein concentration or lower glucose level in cerebrospinal fluid); trauma (presence, without exception, of red blood cells, which are often assumed to be due to traumatic lumbar puncture but are crenated and fail to clear); vasculitis (other systemic or neurologic signs; older children); tuberculous or fungal meningitis (see Chapters 37 and 38); cysticercosis; parainfectious encephalopathies (*Mycoplasma pneumoniae*, respiratory viruses); Lyme disease; leptospirosis; and rickettsial diseases.

Treatment & Prevention

There is no specific therapy. Infants are usually hospitalized, isolated, and treated with fluids and antipyretics. If they are moderately to severely ill, infants are given appropriate antibiotics for bacterial pathogens until cultures are negative for 48–72 hours. This practice will change somewhat when the polymerase chain reaction assay for enteroviruses is available. If patients—especially older children—are mildly ill, antibiotics may be withheld and the child observed. A repeat lumbar puncture in 8–12 hours may be helpful; with viral infection, the Gram stain is again negative, the cell count does not rise substantially, and there is a further shift to mononuclear cells. In these cases, children who are clinically stable may be closely observed in the hospital or at home. The illness usually lasts less than 1 week. Adequate analgesia, including codeine compounds or other strong pain relievers, may be needed. C-reactive protein and lactate levels are usually low in the cerebrospinal fluid of children with viral meningitis; both may be elevated with bacterial infection. With clinical deterioration, repeat lumbar puncture, cerebral imaging, neurologic consultation, and more aggressive diagnostic tests (eg, viral cultures, brain biopsy) should be considered. Herpesvirus encephalitis is of graver concern in such cases, particularly in infants under 1 month of age. Newborns may receive empiric acyclovir therapy until an etiologic diagnosis is made.

Measures to prevent enteroviral infection include good hygiene, scrupulous hand washing, and proper isolation in the hospital.

Prognosis

In general, enteroviral meningitis has no significant short-term neurologic or developmental sequelae. Frank encephalitis may cause diffuse brain damage. Developmental delay may follow infection in the first few months of life. Unlike mumps, enterovirus infections rarely cause hearing loss.

Dalton M, Newton RW: Aseptic meningitis. Dev Med Child Neurol 1991;33:446.

Modlin JF et al: Focal encephalitis with enterovirus infections. Pediatrics 1991;88:841.

Rotbart HA: Meningitis and encephalitis. In: *Human Enterovirus Infections.* ASM Press, 1995.

Schlesinger Y, Sawyer MM, Storck GA: Enteroviral meningitis in infancy: Potential role for polymerase chain reaction in patient management. Pediatrics 1994;94:157.

Sumaya CV, Corman LI: Enteroviral meningitis in early infancy: Significance in community outbreaks. Pediatr Infect Dis J 1982;1:151.

Wilfert CM, Lehrman SN, Katz SL: Enteroviruses and meningitis. Pediatr Infect Dis J 1983;2:333.

INFECTIONS DUE TO HERPESVIRUSES

HERPES SIMPLEX

Essentials of Diagnosis

- Grouped vesicles on an erythematous base.
- Tender regional adenopathy, especially with primary infection.
- Fever and malaise with primary infection.
- Recurrent episodes in many patients.

General Considerations

There are two types of herpes simplex viruses. Type 1 causes most oral, skin, and cerebral disease. Type 2 causes most (80–85%) genital and congenital infections. Latent infection in sensory ganglia routinely follows primary infection. Recurrences may be spontaneous, induced by external events (eg, fever, menstruation, or sunlight) or immunosuppression. Transmission is by direct contact with infected secretions. Herpes simplex viruses are very susceptible to antiviral drugs.

Primary infection usually occurs early in childhood, though many adults (20–50%) have never been infected. Primary infection with HSV-1 is subclinical in 80% of cases and causes gingivostomatitis in the remainder. Type 2 HSV, which is transmitted sexually, is also usually (80%) subclinical or produces mild, nonspecific symptoms. Infection with one type usually precludes infection with other strains of the same type, but individuals can be infected with both type 1 and type 2 HSV. Recurrent episodes are due to reactivation of latent virus.

Clinical Findings

The source of primary infection is often an asymptomatic excreter; at any one time, 1–3% of normal seropositive adults excrete HSV-1 in the saliva or HSV-2 in genital secretions. A history of contact with an active HSV infection is rarely obtained.

A. Symptoms and Signs:

1. Gingivostomatitis–High fever, irritability, and drooling are seen in infants. Multiple oral ulcers are seen on the tongue and on the buccal and gingival mucosa, occasionally extending to the pharynx. Pharyngeal ulcers may predominate in older children and adolescents. Diffusely swollen red gums that are friable and bleed easily are typical. Cervical nodes are swollen and tender. Duration is 7–14 days. Herpangina, aphthous stomatitis, thrush, and Vincent's angina should be excluded.

2. Vulvovaginitis or urethritis–Genital herpes (especially type 2) in a prepubertal child should suggest sexual abuse. Vesicles or ulcers on the vulva, vagina, or penis and tender adenopathy are seen. Systemic symptoms (fever, flu-like illness, myalgia) are common with the initial episode. Painful urination may cause retention. Primary infections last 10–21 days. Lesions may resemble trauma, syphilis, or chancroid in the adolescent and bullous impetigo, trauma, and severe chemical irritation in younger children.

3. Cutaneous infections–Direct inoculation onto cuts (eg, herpetic whitlow on a thumb) or abrasions may produce localized or extensive vesicles or ulcers. A deeper HSV infection on the fingers may be mistaken for a bacterial felon or paronychia; surgical drainage is of no value and is contraindicated. HSV infection of eczematous skin may result in extensive areas of vesicles and shallow ulcers (eczema herpeticum), which may be mistaken for impetigo or varicella.

4. Recurrent cutaneous infection–Recurrent oral shedding is usually asymptomatic. Perioral recurrences often begin with a prodrome of tingling or burning limited to the vermilion border, followed by vesiculation, scabbing, and crusting around the lips over the next few days. Rarely, intraoral lesions recur. Fever, adenopathy, and other symptoms are absent. Recurrent cutaneous herpes most closely resembles impetigo; the latter is often outside the perinasal and perioral region, responds to antibiotics, and yields *Streptococcus pyogenes* or *Staphylococcus aureus* on culture. Recurrent genital disease is common after episodes of type 2 genital herpes. The disease is shorter (65–67 days) and milder (mean, four lesions) and is not associated with systemic symptoms.

5. Keratoconjunctivitis–Keratoconjunctivitis may be part of a primary infection due to spread from infected saliva. Most cases are caused by reactivation of virus latent in the ciliary ganglion. Keratoconjunctivitis produces photophobia, pain, and conjunctival irritation. With recurrences, dendritic corneal ulcers may be demonstrable with fluorescein staining. Stromal invasion may occur. Steroids should never be used without ophthalmologic consultation. Other causes of these symptoms include trauma and bacterial and viral infection (especially adenovirus if pharyngitis is present).

6. Encephalitis–Although unusual in infants outside the neonatal period, encephalitis may occur at any age, usually without cutaneous herpes lesions. In older children, HSV encephalitis often represents a reactivation of latent virus. HSV is probably the most common cause of sporadic severe encephalitis. It is the most important because it can be treated with specific antiviral therapy. Fever, headache, behavioral changes, and neurologic deficits and/or focal seizures occur (the latter as a result of the typical temporal lobe involvement). Early in infection, all studies may be normal. Later, mild mononuclear pleocytosis (often with erythrocytes) is present along with elevated protein concentration, which continues to rise on repeat lumbar punctures. Hypodense areas with a temporal lobe predilection are seen on CT scan, especially after 3–5 days. MRI is more sensitive and is positive sooner. Periodic focal epileptiform discharges are seen on EEGs but are not diagnostic of HSV infection. Viral cultures of spinal fluid are usually negative. The polymerase chain reaction to detect HSV DNA in spinal fluid is a sensitive rapid test. Without early antiviral therapy, the prognosis is very poor. The differential diagnosis includes mumps and mosquito-borne encephalitis, rabies, parainfectious encephalopathy, brain abscess, acute demyelinating syndromes, and bacterial meningoencephalitis.

7. Neonatal infections–The infection is acquired by ascending spread (5–10% of cases) prior to delivery or at the time of vaginal delivery from a mother with genital infection. Occasionally, the infection is acquired in the postpartum period from oral secretions of family members or hospital personnel. A history of genital herpes in the mother is usually absent. Within a few days to weeks, skin vesicles (especially at sites of trauma, such as where scalp monitors were placed) appear in about 50% of infected infants. Some infants are acutely ill, presenting with jaundice, shock, bleeding, or respiratory distress. Others appear well initially, but dissemination to brain or other organs becomes evident over the next week if the infection is untreated. Some infants present with only neurologic symptoms at 2–3 weeks after delivery: apnea, lethargy, fever, poor feeding, or persistent overt seizures. The brain infection in these children is often diffuse and is best appreciated by MRI. The skin lesions may resemble impetigo, bacterial scalp abscesses, or miliaria. These lesions may occur over weeks or occasionally months. The systemic signs are nonspecific.

B. Laboratory Findings: Routine test results are nonspecific. With multisystem disease, abnormalities in platelets, clotting factors, and liver function test results are often present. A finding of lymphocytic pleocytosis is the rule in aseptic meningitis or encephalitis. Virus may be cultured from infected epithelial sites (vesicles, ulcers, or corneal scrapings) and from infected tissue (skin, brain) obtained by biopsy. Cultures of spinal fluid are positive in about 50% of cases. Isolation from throat, eye, urine, or stool of a newborn is diagnostic. Vaginal culture of the mother may offer circumstantial evidence for the diagnosis.

Herpes simplex virus will be detected within 2 days in tissue culture. Rapid diagnostic tests include cytology of scrapings from the base of vesicles or ulcers using chemical stains (Tzanck test) to look for characteristic multinucleated giant cells, immunofluorescent stains to detect viral antigen, or EIA. The positive polymerase chain reaction for HSV DNA is in the cerebrospinal fluid when there is brain involvement. Serum is often positive in the presence of multisystem disease.

Complications, Sequelae, & Prognosis

Gingivostomatitis may result in dehydration due to dysphagia; severe chronic oral disease and esophageal involvement may occur in immunosuppressed patients.

Primary vulvovaginitis may be associated with aseptic meningitis, paresthesias, autonomic dysfunction due to neuritis (urinary retention, constipation), and secondary candidal infection.

Extensive cutaneous disease (as in eczema) may be associated with dissemination, bacterial superinfection, and death.

Keratitis may result in corneal opacification or perforation.

Untreated encephalitis is fatal in 70% of patients and causes severe damage in most of the remainder. When acyclovir treatment is instituted early, 20% die and 40% are neurologically impaired.

Disseminated neonatal infection is often fatal in spite of therapy.

Treatment

A. Specific Measures: Herpes simplex virus is very sensitive to antiviral therapy. Topical antivirals are most effective for corneal disease and include 1% trifluridine, 3% acyclovir, and 3% vidarabine. Trifluridine appears superior; cure rates over 95% are reported. The dose is 1 drop every 2 hours while the patient is awake until the ulcer heals, then 1 drop every 4 hours for 7 more days. Vidarabine ointment requires fewer treatments and may be more practical for young children.

Mucocutaneous HSV infections respond to oral administration of acyclovir. The main indication is severe genital HSV infection in adolescents; acyclovir (400 mg three times daily for 7 days) is beneficial for primary disease when therapy is begun early. Recurrent disease rarely requires therapy. Frequent recurrences may be suppressed by oral administration of acyclovir (400 mg twice a day), but this regimen should be used sparingly. Other forms of severe cutaneous disease, such as eczema herpeticum and HSV infections in immunocompromised children, also respond to therapy with acyclovir. Intravenous therapy is often used in this setting (250 mg/m^2 every 8 hours). Oral acyclovir is also used for severe gingivostomatitis in infants (5–10 mg/kg per dose four times a day for 5–7 days).

Severe HSV infections are treated with acyclovir

at 500 mg/m^2 every 8 hours intravenously for 14 days for encephalitis and 14–21 days for neonates.

Antiviral therapy does not alter the incidence or severity of recurrences of genital infection. Development of resistance to acyclovir is rare after standard courses but is increasingly reported in immunocompromised patients after prolonged therapy.

B. General Measures:

1. Gingivostomatitis–Gingivostomatitis is treated with pain relief and temperature control. Maintaining hydration is important because of the long duration of illness (7–14 days). Nonacidic, cool fluids are best. Topical anesthetic agents (such as viscous lidocaine or an equal mixture of Kaopectate, diphenhydramine, and viscous lidocaine) may be used as a mouthwash for older children who will not swallow it; ingested lidocaine may be toxic to infants or may lead to aspiration. Antiviral therapy is not generally indicated in normal hosts, though it could be considered for those with severe disease. Antibiotics are not helpful.

2. Genital infections–Genital infections require pain relief, assistance with voiding (warm baths, topical anesthetics, rarely catheterization), and psychologic support. Lesions should be kept clean; drying decreases the potential for spread and may shorten the duration of infection. Sexual contact should be avoided during the interval from prodrome to crusting stages.

3. Cutaneous lesions–Skin lesions should be kept clean, dry, and covered if possible to prevent spread. Systemic analgesics may be helpful. Secondary bacterial infection is uncommon in patients with lesions on the mucosa or involving small areas. Secondary infection should be considered and treated if necessary (usually with an antistaphylococcal agent) in patients with more extensive lesions. *Candida* superinfection occurs in 10% of women with primary genital infections.

4. Recurrent cutaneous disease–Recurrent disease is usually milder than primary infection. Sun block lip balm helps prevent labial recurrences after intense sun exposure. There is no evidence that the many popular topical or vitamin therapies are efficacious.

5. Keratoconjunctivitis–An ophthalmologist should be consulted regarding the use of cycloplegics, anti-inflammatory agents, local debridement, and other therapies.

6. Encephalitis–See Chapter 23.

7. Neonatal infection–The affected infant should be isolated and treated with acyclovir for 14–21 days. Cesarean section is indicated if there are obvious maternal cervical or vaginal lesions, especially if these represent primary infection. In women with a history of genital herpes infection, vaginal delivery with peripartum cultures of maternal cervix is the standard. Clinical follow-up is recommended when maternal cultures are positive. Repeated cervical cultures during pregnancy are not useful.

Arvin AM: Oral therapy with acyclovir in infants and children. Pediatr Infect Dis J 1987;6:56.

Brown ZA et al: Neonatal herpes simplex virus infection in relation to asymptomatic maternal infection at the time of labor. N Engl J Med 1991;324:1247.

Corey L, Spear PG: Infections with herpes simplex viruses. (Two parts.) N Engl J Med 1986;314:686, 749.

Gasecki AP, Steg RE: Correlation of early MRI with CT scan, EEG, and CSF: Analyses in a case of biopsy-proven herpes simplex encephalitis. Eur Neurol 1991;31:372.

Kimura H et al: Relapse of herpes simplex encephalitis in children. Pediatrics 1992;89:891.

Koskiniemi M et al: Neonatal herpes simplex virus infection: A report of 43 patients. Pediatr Infect Dis 1989;8:30.

Kuzushima K et al: Clinical manifestations of primary herpes simplex type 1 infection in a closed community. Pediatrics 1991;87:152.

Monney MA, Janniger CK, Schwartz RA: Kaposi's varicelliform eruption. Cutis 1994;53:243.

Toltzis P: Current issues in neonatal herpes simplex virus infections. Clin Perinatol 1991;18:193.

Troendle-Atkins J, Demmler GJ, Buffone GJ: Rapid diagnosis of herpes simplex virus encephalitis by using the polymerase chain reaction. J Pediatr 1993;123:376.

VARICELLA (Chickenpox) & HERPES ZOSTER (Shingles)

Essentials of Diagnosis

Varicella:

- Exposure to varicella or herpes zoster 10–20 days previously; no prior history of varicella.
- Widely scattered macules and papules concentrated on the face and trunk, rapidly progressing to clear vesicles, pustules, and then crusting, over 5–6 days. Variable fever and nonspecific systemic symptoms.

Herpes zoster:

- History of varicella.
- Local paresthesias and pain prior to eruption (more common in older children).
- Dermatomal distribution of grouped vesicles on an erythematous base.

General Considerations

Primary infection with varicella zoster virus results in varicella, which almost always confers lifelong immunity; the virus remains latent in sensory ganglia and reappears as herpes zoster in 10–15% of individuals. The incidence of herpes zoster is increased in immunosuppressed patients. Spread from a contact with varicella during primary infection is by respiratory secretions or fomites from vesicles or pustules, with a greater than 95% infection rate in susceptibles. Herpes zoster is about one-third as infectious. Over 95% of young adults with a history of varicella are immune, as are 90% of native-born Americans who are unaware of having had varicella.

Many individuals from tropical or subtropical areas never have childhood exposure. Humans are the only reservoir.

Clinical Findings

Exposure to varicella or herpes zoster has usually occurred 14–16 days previously (range, 10–21 days). Contact may not have been recognized. Although varicella is the most distinctive childhood exanthem, inexperienced observers may mistake other diseases for varicella. A 1- to 3-day prodrome of fever and respiratory symptoms may occur, especially in older children. The preeruptive pain of herpes zoster may last several days and be mistaken for other illnesses.

A. Symptoms and Signs:

1. Varicella–The usual case consists of mild systemic symptoms followed by crops of red macules that rapidly become tiny vesicles with surrounding erythema ("dew drop on a rose petal"), form pustules, become crusted and then scab over, and leave no scar. The rash appears predominantly on the trunk and face. Lesions occur in the scalp, nose, mouth (where they are nonspecific ulcers), conjunctivae, and vagina. The magnitude of systemic symptoms usually parallels skin involvement. Up to five crops of lesions may be seen. New crops usually stop forming after 5–7 days. Pruritus is often intense. If varicella occurs in the first few months of life, it is often mild as a result of persisting maternal antibody. Once crusting begins, the patient is no longer contagious.

2. Herpes zoster–The eruption of shingles involves a single dermatome, usually truncal or cranial. The rash does not cross the midline. Ophthalmic zoster may be associated with corneal involvement. The closely grouped vesicles, which resemble a localized version of varicella or herpes simplex, often coalesce. The duration is 7–10 days before crusting. Postherpetic neuralgia is rare in children. A few vesicles are occasionally seen outside the involved dermatome. This disease is a common problem in HIV-infected children. Herpes zoster is also common in children who had varicella in early infancy or whose mothers had varicella during their pregnancy.

B. Laboratory Findings: Leukocyte counts are normal or low. Leukocytosis suggests secondary bacterial infection. Multinucleated giant cells in a stained cytologic scraping from a vesicle base (Tzanck test) will indicate the presence of either a varicella-zoster virus or herpes simplex infection. Further distinction is usually made on clinical grounds. The virus may also be identified by fluorescent antibody staining of a lesion smear. Rapid culture methods take 48 hours. Diagnosis may also be made with paired serology. Serum transaminase levels may be modestly elevated during normal varicella.

C. Imaging: Varicella pneumonia classically produces numerous bilateral nodular densities and hyperinflation. This is very rare in normal children.

Abnormal chest radiographs are seen more frequently in adults.

Differential Diagnosis

Varicella is usually distinctive. Similar rashes include those of coxsackievirus infection (fewer lesions, lack of crusting), impetigo (fewer lesions, no classic vesicles, Gram stain response to antimicrobial agents, perioral or peripheral lesions), papular urticaria (insect bite history, nonvesicular rash), scabies (burrows, no typical vesicles), parapsoriasis (rare in children under 10 years of age; chronic or recurrent; often a history of prior varicella), rickettsialpox (eschar where the mite bites, smaller lesions, no crusting), dermatitis herpetiformis (chronic, urticaria, residual pigmentation), and folliculitis.

Complications & Sequelae

Secondary bacterial infection with staphylococci or group A streptococci is most common, presenting as impetigo, cellulitis, abscesses, scarlet fever, or sepsis.

Protracted vomiting or a change in sensorium suggests Reye's syndrome or encephalitis. Since Reye's syndrome usually occurs in patients who are also using salicylates, this drug should be especially avoided in patients with varicella. Encephalitis occurs in less than 0.1% of cases, usually in the first week of illness. It is often limited to cerebellitis with ataxia and resolves completely. Diffuse encephalitis can be severe.

Varicella pneumonia usually afflicts immunocompromised, pregnant, or older patients and may be fatal. Cough, dyspnea, tachypnea, rales, and cyanosis occur several days after onset of rash.

Hemorrhagic varicella lesions may be seen without other complications. Usually owing to autoimmune thrombocytopenia, hemorrhagic lesions can occasionally represent idiopathic disseminated intravascular coagulation (purpura fulminans).

Varicella may be life-threatening in immunosuppressed patients (especially those with leukemia or lymphoma or those receiving high doses of steroids). Their disease is complicated by severe pneumonitis, hepatitis, and encephalitis. Varicella exposure in such patients must be evaluated immediately (see Chapter 10).

Neonates born to mothers who develop varicella from 5 days before to 2 days after delivery are at high risk for severe or fatal (5%) disease and must be given varicella-zoster immune globulin and followed closely (see Chapter 10).

Unusual complications of varicella include optic neuritis, myocarditis, transverse myelitis, orchitis, and arthritis.

Complications of herpes zoster include secondary bacterial infection, motor or cranial nerve paralysis, encephalitis, keratitis, and dissemination in immunosuppressed patients. Prolonged pain does not occur in normal children.

Treatment

A. General Measures: Supportive measures include maintenance of hydration, administration of acetaminophen for discomfort, cool soaks or antipruritics for itching (diphenhydramine, 1.25 mg/kg every 6 hours; or hydroxyzine, 0.5 mg/kg every 6 hours), and observance of general hygiene measures (keep nails trimmed and skin clean). Care must be taken to avoid overdosage with antihistaminic agents. Topical or systemic antistaphylococcal antibiotics may be needed.

B. Specific Measures: Although acyclovir is more active against herpes simplex, it is the preferred drug for varicella and herpes zoster infections. Recommended parenteral acyclovir dosage for severe disease is 30 mg/kg/d intravenously in three divided doses, each infused over 1 hour. Parenteral therapy should be started early in immunosuppressed patients or high-risk infected neonates. Varicella-zoster immune globulin is of no value. The effect of oral acyclovir (80 mg/kg/d in four doses) on varicella in normal children was modestly beneficial and nontoxic, but only when administered within 24 hour after the onset of varicella. This should be used selectively in normal children (intercurrent illness; possibly second attacks in the household or adolescent age—both of which are associated with more severe disease) and in children with underlying chronic illnesses. Valacyclovir and famciclovir are new antiviral agents that are superior because of better absorption. These will be studied in children in the near future.

Prevention

Varicella-zoster immune globulin (VZIG) is available for postexposure prevention of varicella in high-risk persons (see Chapter 10). The live attenuated vaccine is recommended for all susceptible children and adults.

Prognosis

Except for secondary bacterial infections, serious complications are rare and recovery complete in normal hosts.

Abzug MJ, Cotton MF: Severe chickenpox after intranasal use of corticosteroids. J Pediatr 1993;123:577.

American Academy of Pediatrics Committee on Infectious Diseases: The use of oral acyclovir in otherwise healthy children with varicella. Pediatrics 1993;91:674.

American Academy of Pediatrics Committee on Infectious Diseases: Pediatrics 1995;95:791.

Fleischer G et al: Life-threatening complications of varicella. Am J Dis Child 1981;135:896.

Gerhon AA: Varicella zoster virus: Prospects for control. Adv Pediatr Infect Dis 1995;10:93.

Jackson MA, Burry VF, Olson LC: Complications of vari-

cella requiring hospitalization in previously healthy children. Pediatr Infect Dis J 1992;11:441.

Srugo I et al: Clinical manifestations of varicella-zoster virus infections in human immunodeficiency virus-infected children. Am J Dis Child 1993;147:742.

Wurzel CL et al: Prognosis of herpes zoster in healthy children. Am J Dis Child 1986;140:477.

ROSEOLA INFANTUM
(Exanthema Subitum)

Roseola infantum is a benign illness caused by human herpesvirus 6 (HHV-6). HHV-6 is a major cause of acute febrile illness in young children. Its significance is its ability to mimic more serious causes of high fever and its role in inciting febrile seizures. This disease may also result from infection with the recently discovered human herpesvirus 7 (HHV-7).

Clinical Findings

The most prominent historical feature is the abrupt onset of fever, often reaching 40.6 °C, which lasts up to 8 days (mean, 4 days) in an otherwise mildly ill child. The fever then ceases abruptly, and a characteristic rash may appear. Roseola occurs predominantly in children 6 months to 4 years old, with 90% of cases occurring before the second year. It is the most common recognized cause of exanthematous rash in this age group.

A. Symptoms and Signs: Mild lethargy and irritability may be present, but generally there is a dissociation between systemic symptoms and the febrile course. The pharynx, tonsils, and tympanic membranes may be injected. Conjunctivitis, coryza, cough, and pharyngeal exudate are notably absent. Adenopathy of the head and neck often occurs. If rash appears (10–20% incidence), it begins on the trunk and spreads to the face, neck, and extremities. Rose-pink macules or maculopapules, 2–3 mm in diameter, are nonpruritic, tend to coalesce, and disappear in 1–2 days without pigmentation or desquamation. Rash may occur without fever.

B. Laboratory Findings: Early leukocytosis gives way to leukopenia and a relative lymphocytosis with atypical lymphocytes. Laboratory evidence of hepatitis occurs in some patients, especially adults.

Differential Diagnosis

The initial high fever may require exclusion of serious bacterial infection. However, the relative well-being of most children and the typical course and rash soon clarify the diagnosis. The erythrocyte sedimentation rate is normal. If the child has a febrile seizure, it is important to exclude bacterial meningitis. The cerebrospinal fluid is normal in children with roseola. In children who receive antibiotics or other medication at the beginning of the fever, the rash may be incorrectly attributed to a drug allergy.

Complications & Sequelae

Febrile seizures occur. There is some evidence that HHV-6 can directly infect the central nervous system, causing meningoencephalitis or aseptic meningitis. Multiorgan disease (pneumonia, hepatitis, encephalitis) may occur in immunocompromised patients.

Treatment & Prognosis

Fever is readily managed with acetaminophen and sponge baths. Fever control should be a major consideration in children with a history of febrile seizures. Roseola infantum is otherwise entirely benign.

Barone SR, Kaplon MH, Krilov LR: Human herpesvirus 6 infection in children with first febrile seizures. J Pediatr 1995;127:95.

Caserta MT and Hall CB: Human herpesvirus-6. Annu Rev Med 1993;44:377.

Hall CB et al: Human herpesvirus 6 infection in children: A prospective study of complications and reactivation. N Engl J Med 1994;331:432.

Okada K et al: Exanthema subitum and human herpesvirus 6 infection: clinical observations in fifty-seven cases. Pediatr Infect Dis J 1993;12:204.

Pruksananonda P et al: Primary human herpesvirus 6 infection in young children. N Engl J Med 1992;326:1445.

Suga S et al: Clinical and virological analyses of 21 infants with exanthem subitum (roseola infantum) and central nervous system complications. Ann Neurol 1993;33:597.

CYTOMEGALOVIRUS (CMV) INFECTIONS

Cytomegalovirus is a ubiquitous human herpesvirus transmitted by many routes. It can be acquired following maternal viremia or from birth canal secretions and maternal milk. Young children are infected by the saliva of playmates; older individuals are infected by sexual partners (saliva, vaginal secretions, and semen). Transfused blood products and transplanted organs can be a source of CMV infection. Clinical illness is largely determined by the immune competence of the patient. Normal individuals usually develop a mild, self-limited illness, whereas immunocompromised children can develop severe, progressive, often multiorgan disease. In addition, in utero infection can be teratogenic.

1. IN UTERO CYTOMEGALOVIRUS INFECTION

Clinical Findings

Approximately 0.5–1.5% of children are born with CMV infections acquired during maternal viremia. Over 90% of them are asymptomatic and are usually born to mothers who had experienced reactivation of latent CMV infection during the pregnancy. Symptomatic infants are born to mothers with primary CMV infection. Even after primary maternal infection, less than 50% of fetuses are infected, and only 10% of those infected are symptomatic at birth. Primary infection in the first half of pregnancy poses the greatest risk for severe fetal damage.

A. Symptoms and Signs: Severely affected infants are born ill; they are often small for gestational age, floppy, and lethargic. They feed poorly and have poor temperature control. Hepatosplenomegaly, jaundice, petechiae, seizures, and microcephaly are often present. Characteristic signs are a distinctive chorioretinitis and periventricular calcification. A purpuric ("blueberry muffin") rash similar to that seen with congenital rubella may be present. The mortality rate is 20–30%. Survivors usually have significant sequelae. Less severely ill children are born with one or more of the above findings. Isolated hepatosplenomegaly or thrombocytopenia may occur. Even mildly affected children may subsequently manifest mental retardation and psychomotor delay. Most infected infants (90%) are born to mothers with preexisting immunity and have no clinical manifestations at birth. Of these, 10–15% develop sensorineural hearing loss, which is often bilateral.

B. Laboratory Findings: Anemia, thrombocytopenia, hyperbilirubinemia, and elevated aminotransferase levels are common. Lymphocytosis is occasionally seen. Pleocytosis and an elevated protein content are seen in cerebrospinal fluid. The diagnosis is readily confirmed by isolation of CMV from urine or saliva within 48 hours, using rapid culture methods combined with immunoassay. The presence in the infant of IgM-specific CMV antibodies suggests the diagnosis. Some commercial EIA kits are 90% sensitive and specific.

C. Imaging: Skull radiographs show microcephaly and periventricular calcification. CT scan shows calcification and ventricular dilatation. Long bone films show the "celery stalk" pattern characteristic of congenital viral infections. Interstitial pneumonia may be present.

Differential Diagnosis

Cytomegalovirus infection should be considered in any newborn who is seriously ill shortly after birth, especially once bacterial sepsis, metabolic disease, intracranial bleeding, and cardiac disease have been excluded. Other congenital infections to be considered in the differential diagnosis include toxoplasmosis (serology, more diffuse calcification of the central nervous system, specific type of retinitis, macrocephaly), rubella (serology, specific type of retinitis, cardiac lesions, eye abnormalities), enteroviral infections (time of year, maternal illness, severe hepatitis), herpes simplex (skin lesions, cultures, severe hepatitis), and syphilis (serology for both infant and mother, skin lesions, bone involvement).

Treatment & Prevention

Support is rarely required for anemia and thrombocytopenia. The antiviral drug ganciclovir is under study in severely ill children. Most children with symptoms at birth have significant neurologic, intellectual, visual, or auditory impairment. Children who are asymptomatic at birth have a 5–15% incidence of hearing loss but few other sequelae. It is possible that the late sequelae of CMV infection—including abnormalities occurring in initially asymptomatic infants—may be ameliorated by ganciclovir use. Delayed development and hearing loss should be discovered and treated as soon as possible.

2. PERINATAL CYTOMEGALOVIRUS INFECTION

Cytomegalovirus infection can be acquired from birth canal secretions or shortly after birth from maternal milk. In some socioeconomic groups, 10–20% of infants are infected at birth and excrete CMV for many months. Infection can also be acquired in the postnatal period from unscreened transfused blood products.

Clinical Findings

A. Symptoms and Signs: Ninety percent of normal infants infected by their mothers at birth develop subclinical illness (ie, virus excretion only) or a minor illness within 1–3 months. The remainder develop an illness lasting several weeks which is characterized by hepatosplenomegaly, lymphadenopathy, and interstitial pneumonitis in various combinations. The severity of the pneumonitis may be increased by the simultaneous presence of *Chlamydia trachomatis*. Infants who receive blood products are often premature and immunologically impaired. If they are born to CMV-negative mothers and subsequently receive CMV-containing blood, they frequently develop severe infection and pneumonia after a 2- to 6-week incubation period.

B. Laboratory Findings: Lymphocytosis, atypical lymphocytes, anemia, and thrombocytopenia may be present, especially in premature infants. Liver function is abnormal. CMV can be isolated from urine and saliva. Secretions obtained at bronchoscopy contain CMV and epithelial cells bearing CMV antigens. Serum levels of CMV antibody rise significantly.

C. Imaging: Chest films show a diffuse interstitial pneumonitis.

Differential Diagnosis

Cytomegalovirus infection should be considered as a cause of any prolonged illness in early infancy, especially if hepatosplenomegaly, lymphadenopathy, or atypical lymphocytosis is present. This must be distinguished from granulomatous or malignant diseases and from congenital infections (syphilis, toxoplasmosis, hepatitis B) not previously appreciated. Other viruses (Epstein-Barr virus, HIV, adenovirus) can cause this syndrome. CMV is a recognized cause of viral pneumonia in this age group. However, since asymptomatic CMV excretion is common in early infancy, care must be taken to establish the diagnosis and to rule out concomitant pathogens such as *Chlamydia* and RSV.

Treatment & Prevention

The self-limited disease of normal infants requires no therapy. Severe pneumonitis in premature infants requires oxygen administration and often intubation. Very ill infants should receive ganciclovir (5 mg/kg every 12 hours). CMV infection acquired by transfusion can be prevented by excluding CMV-seropositive blood donors. Milk donors should also be screened for prior CMV infection. It is likely that high-risk infants receiving large doses of intravenous immune globulin for other reasons will be protected against severe CMV disease.

3. CYTOMEGALOVIRUS INFECTION ACQUIRED IN CHILDHOOD & ADOLESCENCE

Young children are readily infected by playmates, especially since CMV continues to be excreted in saliva and urine for many months after infection. The annual incidence of CMV excretion by children in day care centers exceeds 75%. In fact, young children in a family are often the source of primary CMV infection of the mother during subsequent pregnancies. An additional peak of CMV infection occurs in sexually active individuals.

Clinical Findings

A. Symptoms and Signs: Most young children who acquire CMV are asymptomatic or have a minor febrile illness, occasionally with adenopathy. They provide the reservoir of virus shedders that facilitate spread of CMV. Occasionally, a child may have a prolonged fever with hepatosplenomegaly and adenopathy. Older children and adults are more likely to be symptomatic in this fashion and can present with a syndrome that mimics the infectious mononucleosis syndrome which follows infection by Epstein-Barr virus (1–2 weeks of fever, malaise, anorexia, splenomegaly, and some adenopathy). This syndrome can also occur 2–4 weeks after transfusion of CMV-infected blood.

B. Laboratory Findings: In the CMV mononucleosis syndrome, lymphocytosis and atypical lymphocytes are common, as is a mild rise in aminotransferase levels. CMV is present in saliva and urine, and diagnosis is made as above.

Differential Diagnosis

In older children, CMV infection should be included as a possible cause of fever of unknown origin, especially when lymphocytosis and atypical lymphocytes are present. CMV infection is distinguished from Epstein-Barr virus infection by the absence of pharyngitis, the relatively minor adenopathy, and the absence of serologic evidence of acute Epstein-Barr virus infection. Mononucleosis syndromes are also caused by *Toxoplasma gondii,* rubella virus, adenovirus, hepatitis A virus, and HIV.

Prevention

Screening of transfused blood would prevent cases related to this source.

4. CYTOMEGALOVIRUS INFECTION IN IMMUNOCOMPROMISED CHILDREN

Cytomegalovirus infection in this setting can be acquired from infused blood products or transplanted tissue as well as from playmates. In addition, reactivation of latent CMV can cause symptomatic disease. This is clearly seen in children with AIDS or congenital immunodeficiencies. However, in most other immunocompromised patients, primary infection is much more likely to cause severe symptoms than is reactivation disease. The severity of the resulting disease is generally proportionate to the degree of immunosuppression.

Clinical Findings

A. Symptoms and Signs: A mild febrile illness with myalgia, malaise, and arthralgia may occur, especially with reactivation disease. Severe disease often includes subacute onset of dyspnea and cyanosis as manifestations of an interstitial pneumonitis. Auscultation reveals only coarse breath sounds and scattered rales. A rapid respiratory rate may precede clinical or x-ray evidence of pneumonia. Hepatitis without jaundice or hepatomegaly is common. Diarrhea, which can be severe, occurs with CMV colitis, and CMV can cause esophagitis with symptoms of odynophagia or dysphagia. These enteropathies are most common in AIDS, as is the presence of a retinitis that often progresses to blindness. Encephalitis and polyradiculitis also occur in AIDS.

B. Laboratory Findings: Neutropenia and thrombocytopenia are common. Atypical lymphocytosis is not frequent. Serum aminotransferase levels are often elevated. The stools may contain occult blood if enteropathy is present. CMV is readily isolated from saliva, urine, buffy coat, and bronchial secretions. Results are available in 48 hours.

C. Imaging: Bilateral interstitial pneumonitis is present on chest radiographs.

Differential Diagnosis

The initial febrile illness must be distinguished from treatable bacterial and fungal infection. Similarly, the pulmonary disease must be distinguished from intrapulmonary hemorrhage, drug-induced or radiation pneumonitis, pulmonary edema, and bacterial, fungal, and parasitic infection in this population. In this regard, it is noteworthy that CMV infection is bilateral and interstitial on x-ray films of the chest, cough is nonproductive, chest pain is absent, and the patient is not usually toxic. *Pneumocystis carinii* infection may present in a similar manner. Polymicrobial disease may be present in these patients. It is suspected that bacterial and fungal infections are enhanced by the neutropenia that can accompany CMV infection. Infection of the gastrointestinal tract is diagnosed by endoscopy, mainly to exclude candidal and herpes simplex infections.

Treatment & Prognosis

Blood donors should be screened to exclude those with prior CMV infection. Ideally, seronegative transplant recipients should receive organs from seronegative donors. Severe symptoms, most commonly pneumonitis, often respond to early therapy with intravenous ganciclovir (5 mg/kg every 12 hours for 14–21 days). Foscarnet is an alternate antiviral therapy. Neutropenia is a frequent side effect of this therapy. Prophylactic use of oral acyclovir or intravenous ganciclovir may prevent this problem in organ transplant recipients.

Boppana SB et al: Symptomatic congenital cytomegalovirus infection: Neonatal morbidity and mortality. Pediatr Infect Dis J 1992;11:93.

Jordan CJ et al: Spontaneous cytomegalovirus mononucleosis. Ann Intern Med 1973;79:153.

Kumar ML et al: Postnatally acquired cytomegalovirus infections in infants of CMV-excreting mothers. J Pediatr 1984;104:669.

Lynch L et al: Prenatal diagnosis of fetal cytomegalovirus infection. Am J Obstet Gynecol 1991;165:714.

Stagno S, Whitley RJ: Herpesvirus infections of pregnancy: Part 1. Cytomegalovirus and Epstein-Barr virus infections. N Engl J Med 1985;313:1270.

INFECTIOUS MONONUCLEOSIS

Mononucleosis is the most characteristic syndrome produced by infection with the Epstein-Barr virus (EBV). Its elements are fever, pharyngitis, lymphadenopathy, splenomegaly, atypical lymphocytosis, and the production of heterophil antibodies. Young children infected with EBV have either no symptoms or a mild nonspecific febrile illness. As the age of the host increases, EBV infection is more likely to produce the mononucleosis syndrome, occurring in 20–25% of infected adolescents. Epstein-Barr virus is readily acquired from asymptomatic carriers (15–20% of whom excrete the virus on any given day) and from recently ill patients, who excrete virus for many months. Young children are infected from the saliva of playmates and family members. Adolescents may be infected through sexual activity. Epstein-Barr virus can also be transmitted by blood transfusion and organ transplantation.

Clinical Findings

A. Symptoms and Signs: After an incubation period of 1–2 months, a 2- to 3-day prodrome of malaise and anorexia yields, abruptly or insidiously, to a febrile illness with temperatures exceeding 39 °C. The major complaint is pharyngitis, which is often (50%) exudative. Lymph nodes are enlarged, firm, and mildly tender. Any area may be affected, but posterior and anterior cervical nodes are almost always enlarged. Splenomegaly is present in 50–75% of patients. Hepatomegaly is common (30%), and the liver is frequently tender. Five percent of patients have a rash, which can be macular, scarlatiniform, or urticarial. Rash is almost universal in patients taking penicillin or ampicillin. Soft palate petechiae and eyelid edema are also observed.

B. Laboratory Findings:

1. Peripheral blood–Leukopenia may occur early, but an atypical lymphocytosis (comprising over 10% of the total leukocytes at some time in the illness) is most notable. Hematologic changes may not be seen until the third week of illness and may be entirely absent in some EBV syndromes, eg, neurologic ones.

2. Heterophil antibodies–These nonspecific antibodies appear in over 90% of older patients with mononucleosis but in fewer than 50% of children under age 5. They may not be detectable until the second week of illness and may persist for up to 12 months after recovery. Rapid screening tests (slide agglutination) are usually positive if the titer is significant; a positive result strongly suggests but does not prove EBV infection.

3. Anti-EBV antibodies–It may be necessary to measure specific antibody titers when heterophil antibodies fail to appear, as in young children. Epstein-Barr virus infection is established by detecting IgM antibody to the viral capsid antigen (VCA); or by detecting a fall over several weeks of IgG antibody to the VCA antigen (IgG antibody peaks by the time symptoms appear). Seroconversion of antibody to EBNA confirms the above indicators.

4. Aminotransferase, γ-glutamyl transferase, and bilirubin levels–Aminotransferase and γ-glutamyl transferase levels are mildly elevated in 80% of patients; bilirubin is mildly elevated in 25%.

Differential Diagnosis

Severe pharyngitis may suggest group A streptococcal infection. Enlargement of only anterior cervical lymph nodes, a neutrophilic leukocytosis, and the absence of splenomegaly suggest bacterial infection. Although a child with a positive throat culture usually requires therapy, up to 10% of children with mononucleosis are asymptomatic carriers. In this group, penicillin therapy is unnecessary and often causes a rash. Severe primary herpes simplex pharyngitis, occurring in adolescence, may also mimic infectious mononucleosis. In this type of pharyngitis, some anterior mouth ulcerations should suggest the correct diagnosis. Epstein-Barr virus infection should be considered in the differential diagnosis of any perplexing prolonged febrile illness. Some similar illnesses that produce atypical lymphocytosis include rubella (pharyngitis not prominent, shorter illness, less adenopathy and splenomegaly), adenovirus (upper respiratory symptoms and cough, conjunctivitis, less adenopathy, fewer atypical lymphocytes), hepatitis (more severe liver function abnormalities, no pharyngitis or splenomegaly), and toxoplasmosis (negative heterophil test and less pharyngitis). Serum sickness-like drug reactions and leukemia (smear morphology is important) may be confused with infectious mononucleosis. Cytomegalovirus mononucleosis is a close mimic except for minimal pharyngitis and less adenopathy; it is much less common. Serologic tests for EBV and cytomegalovirus should clarify the correct diagnosis. The acute, initial manifestation of HIV infection is a mononucleosis-like syndrome in some children.

Complications

Splenic rupture is a very rare complication, which usually follows significant trauma. Hematologic complications, including hemolytic anemia, thrombocytopenia, or neutropenia, are more common. Neurologic involvement can include aseptic meningitis, encephalitis, isolated neuropathy such as Bell's palsy, and Guillain-Barré syndrome. Any of these may appear prior to or in the absence of the more typical signs and symptoms of infectious mononucleosis. Rare complications include myocarditis, pericarditis, and atypical pneumonia. Very rarely, EBV infection becomes a progressive lymphoproliferative disorder characterized by persistent fever, multiple organ involvement, neutropenia or pancytopenia, and agammaglobulinemia. Hemocytophagia is often present in the bone marrow. An X-linked genetic defect in immune response has been inferred for some patients (Duncan's syndrome, X-linked lymphoproliferative disorder). Children with other congenital immunodeficiencies or chemotherapy-induced immunosuppression can also develop progressive EBV infection or EBV-induced lymphomas.

Treatment & Prognosis

Bed rest may be necessary in severe cases. Acetaminophen controls high fever. Potential airway obstruction due to swollen pharyngeal lymphoid tissue responds rapidly to systemic corticosteroids. Corticosteroids may also be given for hematologic and neurologic complications, though no controlled trials have proved their efficacy in these conditions. Fever and pharyngitis disappear by 10–14 days. Adenopathy and splenomegaly can persist several weeks longer. Some patients complain of fatigue, malaise, or lack of well being for several months. Although steroids may shorten the duration of fatigue and malaise, their long-term effects on this potentially oncogenic viral infection are unknown, and indiscriminate use is discouraged. Patients with splenic enlargement should avoid contact sports for 6–8 weeks.

Chetham MM, Roberts KB: Infectious mononucleosis in adolescents. Pediatr Ann 1991;20:206.

Connelly KP, DeWitt LD: Neurologic complications of infectious mononucleosis. Pediatr Neurol 1994;10:181.

Schaller RJ, Counselman FL: Infectious mononucleosis in young children. Am J Emerg Med 1995;13:438.

Schuster V, Kreth HW: Epstein-Barr virus infection and associated diseases in children: II. Diagnostic and therapeutic strategies. Eur J Pediatr 1992;151:794.

Sumaya CV: Epstein-Barr virus serologic testing: Diagnostic indications and interpretations. Pediatr Infect Dis J 1986;5:337.

VIRAL INFECTIONS SPREAD BY INSECT VECTOR (Table 35–4)

In the United States, mosquitoes are the most common insect vectors that spread viral infections. As a consequence, these infections often occur as summer-fall epidemics. Encephalitis is the common severe manifestation. Subclinical infection is common, as is milder central nervous system disease, such as meningitis.

Goodpasture HC et al: Colorado tick fever: Clinical, epidemiologic, and laboratory aspects of 228 cases in Colorado in 1973-74. Ann Intern Med 1978;88:303.

Hayes EB, Gubler DJ: Dengue and dengue hemorrhagic fever. Pediatr Infect Dis J 1992;11:311.

INFECTIONS DUE TO MISCELLANEOUS VIRUSES

ERYTHEMA INFECTIOSUM

This benign exanthematous illness of school-age children is caused by a human parvovirus designated B19. It is not related to the canine parvoviruses. Spread is respiratory, occurring in winter-spring epidemics. A nonspecific mild flu-like illness may occur during the initial viremia at 7–10 days; the characteristic rash occurring at 10–17 days actually represents an immune response. The patient is viremic and contagious prior to—but not after—the onset of rash. The disease is mildly contagious; only about half of susceptible household contacts are infected.

Approximately one-half of infected individuals have a subclinical illness. Most cases (70%) occur in children between the ages of 5 and 15, with an additional 20% occurring later in life. Forty percent of adults are seronegative. The secondary attack rate in a school or household setting is 50% among susceptible children and 20–30% among susceptible adults. Rare complications of parvovirus infection include aplastic crises in children with chronic hemolytic anemia, occasionally hydrops fetalis when susceptible pregnant women are infected, and persistent anemia or pancytopenia in immunocompromised patients.

Clinical Findings

Owing to the nonspecific nature of the exanthem and the many subclinical cases, a history of contact with an infected individual is often absent or unreliable. Recognition of the illness is easier during outbreaks.

A. Symptoms and Signs: Typically, the first sign of illness is the rash, which begins as raised maculopapular lesions on the cheeks that coalesce to give a "slapped cheek" appearance. The lesions are warm, nontender, and sometimes pruritic. They may be scattered on the forehead, chin, and postauricular areas, but the circumoral region is spared. Within 1–2 days, similar lesions appear on the proximal extensor surfaces of the extremities and spread distally in a symmetric fashion. Palms and soles are usually spared. The trunk, neck, and buttocks are also commonly involved. Central clearing of confluent lesions produces a characteristic lace-like pattern. The rash fades in several days to several weeks but frequently reappears in response to local irritation, heat (bathing), sunlight, and stress. Almost one-half of infected children have some rash remaining (or recurring) for 10 days. Fine desquamation may be present.

Mild systemic symptoms occur in up to 50% of

Table 35–4. Some virus diseases spread by insects in the United States.

Disease	Natural Reservoir (Vector)	Geographic Distribution	Incubation Period	Clinical Presentation	Laboratory Findings	Complications, Sequelae	Diagnosis, Therapy, Comments[1]
St. Louis encephalitis (SLE)	Birds (*Culex* mosquitoes)	Southern Canada, Central USA, South America	2–5 days (up to 3 weeks)	Abrupt onset of fever, chills, headache, nausea, vomiting; may develop generalized weakness, seizures, coma, paralysis; aseptic meningitis is common in children.	Modest leukocytosis, neutrophilia. CSF: 100–200 wbc/μL (PMNs predominate early).	Mortality rate 2–5% in children (especially <age 5). Neurologic sequelae in 1–20%.	Most important mosquito-borne encephalitis in USA: 20–500 cases a year, < 20% symptomatic. (Worse in elderly.) Therapy: supportive. Diagnosis: serology. Specific antibody often present within 5 days.
California encephalitis (LaCrosse, Jamestown Canyon, 3 others)	Chipmunks and other small mammals (*Aedes* mosquitoes)	Northern and mid Central USA, southern Canada	2–5 days	Similar to SLE; focal neurologic signs in up to 25%.	Variable white counts. CSF: 30–200 (up to 600) wbc/μL; variable PMNs; protein often normal.	Mortality rate < 1%. Seizure disorder if this appeared during acute illness.	About 50–150 cases a year in USA, 5% symptomatic. Therapy: supportive. Diagnosis: serology. Up to 90% have specific IgM antibody in first week; 25% of population has IgG antibody.
Western equine encephalitis	Birds (*Culex* mosquitoes)	Canada, USA, and Mexico west of Mississippi River longitude; South America	2–5 days	Similar to that of SLE. Most infections are subclinical.	Variable white counts. CSF: 10–300 wbc/μL.	Permanent brain damage, 10% overall; 30% in infants < 1 year of age.	About 10–150 cases a year in USA. Worse in infants. Equine illness precedes human outbreaks. Therapy: supportive. Diagnosis: serology. Often IgM antibody in first week.
Eastern equine encephalitis	Birds (*Culex Aedes* mosquitoes)	Eastern seaboard USA; Caribbean, South America	2–5 days	Similar to that of SLE but more severe. Progresses rapidly in one-third to coma and death.	Leukocytosis with neutrophilia. CSF: 500–2000 wbc/μL; PMNs predominate early.	Mortality rate 20–70%; neurologic sequelae in over 50% of children.	Most severe mosquito-borne encephalitis in USA. Fewer than 20 cases a year. Only 3–10% of cases are symptomatic. Therapy: supportive. Diagnosis: serology. Background seropositivity very low. Titers often positive in first week.
Colorado tick fever	Small mammals (*Dermacentor andersoni*, or wood tick)	Rocky Mountain region of USA and Canada	3–34 days (range, 1–14 days)	Fever, myalgia, conjunctivitis, headache, retro-orbital pain; rash in < 10%. No respiratory symptoms. Biphasic in 50%.	Leukopenia (maximum at 4–6 days), mild thrombocytopenia.	Rare encephalitis, coagulopathy.	Patient may have no known tick bite. Acute illness lasts 7 days; prolonged fatigue in adults. Therapy: supportive. Diagnosis: serology.
Dengue (4 types)	Humans (*Aedes* mosquitoes)	Asia, Africa, Central and South America, Caribbean; rarely in southern USA	2–7 days	Fever, headache, myalgia, retro-ocular pain, pharyngitis, cough; maculopapular or petechial rash in 20%; adenopathy.	Leukopenia, thrombocytopenia.	Hemorrhagic fever, shock syndrome, prolonged weakness.	High infection rate. Biphasic course may occur. Therapy: supportive. Ribavirin is experimental. Diagnosis: serology.

children. These include low-grade fever (38–38.5 °C), mild malaise, sore throat, and coryza. They appear for 2–3 days and are followed by a week-long asymptomatic phase before the rash appears.

B. Laboratory Findings: A mild leukopenia occurs early in some patients, followed by leukocytosis and lymphocytosis. Specific IgM and IgG serum antibody tests are available and preferred. Antigen and nucleic acid detection tests are available. The disease is not diagnosed by routine viral culture.

Differential Diagnosis

The characteristic rash and the mild nature of the illness distinguish erythema infectiosum from other childhood exanthems. It lacks the prodromal symptoms of measles and the lymphadenopathy of rubella. Systemic symptoms and pharyngitis are more prominent with enteroviral infections and scarlet fever.

Complications & Sequelae

A. Arthritis: This is more common in older patients, beginning with late adolescence. Approximately 10% of children have severe joint symptoms. Girls are affected more than boys. Pain and stiffness occur symmetrically in the peripheral joints. Arthritis usually follows the rash and may persist for 2–6 weeks but resolves without permanent damage in most patients.

B. Aplastic Crisis: Parvovirus B19 replicates primarily in erythroid progenitor cells. Consequently, reticulocytopenia occurs for approximately 1 week during the illness. This goes unnoticed in normal individuals but results in severe anemia in patients with chronic hemolytic anemia. The rash of erythema infectiosum follows the hemolysis in these patients.

Pure red cell aplasia, chronic pancytopenia, idiopathic thrombocytopenic purpura, and a hemophagocytic syndrome have also been described. Patients with AIDS and other immunosuppressive illnesses may develop prolonged anemia or pancytopenia. Patients with hemolytic anemia and aplastic crisis or immunosuppressed patients may still be contagious and should be isolated while in the hospital. Parvovirus is under study as a cause of a variety of collagen-vascular diseases.

C. In Utero Infections: Infection of susceptible pregnant women may produce fetal infection with hydrops fetalis; fetal death occurs in about 6%, with most fatalities occurring in the first 20 weeks—compared with a fetal loss of 3.5% in controls. The risk of fetal infection is not known. Congenital anomalies have not been associated with parvovirus B19 infection during pregnancy.

Treatment & Prognosis

Erythema infectiosum is a benign illness for normal individuals. Patients with aplastic crisis may require blood transfusions. It is unlikely that this complication can be prevented by quarantine measures,

since acute parvovirus infection in contacts is often unrecognized and is most contagious prior to the rash. Pregnant women who are exposed to erythema infectiosum or who work in a setting where an epidemic occurs should be tested for evidence of prior infection. Susceptible pregnant women should then be followed for evidence of parvovirus infection. If maternal infection occurs, the fetus should be followed by ultrasonography for evidence of hydrops and distress. In utero transfusion or early delivery may salvage some fetuses. Pregnancies should not be terminated because of parvovirus infection. The risk of fetal death among exposed pregnant women of unknown serologic status is less than 2.5% for homemakers and less than 1.5% for school teachers.

Standard immune globulin is not protective. High-dose intravenous immune globulin has stopped viremia and led to marrow recovery in some cases of prolonged aplasia. Its role in normal patients and pregnant women is unknown.

Bell LM: Parvovirus B19 infection: A decade of discovery. Rep Pediatr Infect Dis 1992;2:6.

Heegaard ED, Hornsleth A: Parvovirus: The expanding spectrum of disease. Acta Paediatr 1995;84:109.

Koch WC et al: Manifestations and treatment of human parvovirus B19 infections in immunocompromised patients. J Pediatr 1990;116:355.

Rodis J et al: Management and outcome of pregnancies complicated by human B19 parvovirus infection: A prospective study. Am J Obstet Gynecol 1990;163:1168.

HANTAVIRUS INFECTION

Essentials of Diagnosis

- Influenza-like prodrome (fever, myalgia, headache, cough).
- Rapid onset of unexplained pulmonary edema.
- Residence or travel in epidemic area; exposure to aerosols from deer mouse droppings or secretions.
- Confirmation by serology.

General Considerations

A new severe viral disease appeared in an epidemic cluster in the Southwestern United States in 1993. This unique viral illness is the first native bunyavirus epidemic in this country. *Hantavirus* disease is distinctly different in mode of spread (no arthropod vector) and clinical picture from other bunyavirus diseases.

Clinical Findings

The initial cases of hantavirus infection involved travel to or residence in an area where New Mexico, Colorado, Utah, and Arizona are contiguous and involved potential exposure to the habitat of the reservoir, ie, the deer mouse. This rodent and other, selected rodents that harbor the virus live in many other locales. Thus, many cases have been confirmed in 20 other states west of the Mississippi River.

A. Symptoms and Signs: Onset is sudden, with a nonspecific virus-like prodrome: fever; back, hip, and leg pain; chills; headache, dry cough, and nausea and vomiting. Abdominal pain may be present. Sore throat, conjunctivitis, rash, and adenopathy are absent. After 1–10 days (usually 4–5), dyspnea, tachypnea, and evidence of a pulmonary capillary leak syndrome appear. This often progresses rapidly over a period of hours. Hypotension is common not only from hypoxemia but also from decreased cardiac output. This distinguishes the disease from early bacterial sepsis.

B. Laboratory Findings: The hemogram is significant for leukocytosis with a prominent left shift and hemoconcentration. LDH is elevated, as are liver function tests; serum albumin is low. Urinalysis is normal. A serum IgM ELISA test is positive early in the illness. Otherwise the diagnosis is made by specific staining of tissue or PCR, usually at autopsy.

C. Imaging: Initial chest x-rays are normal. This is followed by bilateral interstitial infiltrates with the typical butterfly pattern of acute pulmonary edema, bibasilar airspace disease, or both. Significant pleural effusions are often present.

Differential Diagnosis

In the same geographic areas, plague and tularemia are possibilities. Viral respiratory pathogens and *Mycoplasma* have a slower tempo, do not elevate the LDH, and do not cause the hematologic changes. Q fever, psittacosis, toxin exposure, *Legionella,* and fungi are possibilities, but the history and tempo of the illness should be distinguishing features. Hantavirus pulmonary syndrome is a consideration in previously healthy persons with a febrile illness that results in unexplained pulmonary edema.

Treatment & Prognosis

When given early for other bunyavirus infections, intravenous ribavirin has been effective. A trial of this therapy for is under way. Management should concentrate on oxygen therapy and mechanical ventilation as required. Because of capillary leakage, Swan-Ganz catheter to monitor cardiac output and inotropic agents, rather than fluid therapy, should be used to maintain perfusion. The virus is not spread by person-to-person contact. No isolation is required. Thus far, the case-fatality rate is approximately 50%.

Butler JC, Peters CJ: Hantavirus, and hantavirus pulmonary syndrome. Clin Infect Dis 1994;19:387.

Khan AS et al: Fatal hantavirus pulmonary syndrome in an adolescent. Pediatrics 1995;95:276.

Outbreak of hantavirus infection—southwestern United States, 1993. MMWR Morb Mortal Wkly Rep 1993; 42:495.

MUMPS

Essentials of Diagnosis

- No prior mumps vaccine; exposure 14–21 days previously.
- Parotid gland swelling.
- Aseptic meningitis with or without parotitis.
- Orchitis, pancreatitis, or oophoritis.

General Considerations

Mumps was one of the classic childhood infections; the virus spread by the respiratory route, attacked almost all unimmunized children (asymptomatically in 30–40% of cases), and produced lifelong immunity. The vaccine is so efficacious that clinical disease is rare in immunized children. As a result of subclinical infections, 95% of adults—regardless of the history—are immune. The epidemiology of this illness is changing, however. The vaccine was not in broad use until 1977. Geographic differences in vaccine requirements for school also existed. Thus, there is a large group of adolescents and young adults who are not immune. Since 1986, mumps has been reported with increasing frequency. College outbreaks are notable.

Clinical Findings

A history of exposure to a child with parotitis is not proof of mumps exposure. In an adequately immunized individual, parotitis is usually due to another cause.

A. Symptoms and Signs:

1. Salivary gland disease—Tender swelling of one or more glands, variable fever, and facial lymphedema are typical. Parotid involvement is most common. The ear is displaced upward and outward; the mandibular angle is obliterated. Systemic toxicity is usually absent. Parotid stimulation with sour foods may be quite painful. The orifice of Stensen's duct may be red and swollen; yellow secretions may be expressed, but pus is absent.

2. Meningoencephalitis—Prior to widespread immunization, mumps was the most common cause of aseptic meningitis, which occurs in up to 50% of cases, usually manifested by mild headache or asymptomatic mononuclear pleocytosis. Cerebral symptoms do not correlate with parotid symptoms. Although neck stiffness, nausea, and vomiting can occur, encephalitic symptoms are rare (1:1000 cases of mumps); recovery in 3–10 days is the rule. Vaccine-related meningoencephalitis, which occurs with a similar frequency, is usually mild and self-limited.

3. Pancreatitis—Abdominal pain may represent transient pancreatitis. Because salivary disease may elevate serum amylase, specific markers of pancreatic function (lipase, amylase isoenzymes) are required for assessing pancreatic involvement.

4. Orchitis, oophoritis—Involvement of the gonads is associated with fever, local tenderness, and swelling. Orchitis is unusual in children but occurs in up to one-third of affected postpubertal males. Usually it is unilateral and resolves in 1–2 weeks. Although one-third of infected testes atrophy, bilateral involvement and sterility are rare. Atrophic testes have rarely been reported to develop malignant tumors.

5. Other–Thyroiditis, mastitis (especially adolescent females), arthritis, and presternal edema (occasionally with dysphagia or hoarseness) may be seen.

B. Laboratory Findings: Peripheral blood leukocyte count is usually normal. Up to 1000/μL (predominantly lymphocytes) may be present in the spinal fluid, with mildly elevated protein and normal to slightly decreased glucose. Viral culture of saliva, throat, urine, or spinal fluid may be positive. Spinal fluid often yields the vaccine strain in cases of meningitis following the Urabe vaccine. It is not easily distinguishable from the wild strain. Paired sera assayed by EIA are currently used for diagnosis. Complement-fixing antibody to the soluble antigen disappears in several months; its presence in a single specimen thus indicates recent infection.

Differential Diagnosis

Mumps parotitis may resemble the following: cervical adenitis (the jaw angle may be obliterated, but the ear does not usually protrude; Stensen's duct orifice is normal; leukocytosis and neutrophilia are observed), bacterial parotitis (pus in Stensen's duct, toxicity, exquisite tenderness); recurrent parotitis (idiopathic or associated with calculi), tumors or leukemia, and tooth infections. Many viruses, including parainfluenza, enteroviruses, Epstein-Barr virus, CMV, and influenza, can cause parotitis. Parotid swelling in HIV infection is less painful and tends to be chronic.

Unless parotitis is present, mumps meningitis resembles that caused by enteroviruses or early bacterial infection. An elevated amylase is a useful clue in this situation. Isolated pancreatitis is not distinguishable from many other causes of epigastric pain and vomiting. Mumps is a classic cause of orchitis, but torsion, epididymitis, *Mycoplasma,* other viruses, hematomas, hernias, and tumors must also be considered.

Complications

The major neurologic complication is nerve deafness (usually unilateral), which may be transient but usually results in inability to hear high tones. It may occur without meningitis. Permanent damage is rare, occurring in less than 0.1% of cases of mumps. Aqueductal stenosis and hydrocephalus (especially following congenital infection), myocarditis, transverse myelitis, and facial paralysis are other rare complications.

Treatment & Prognosis

Treatment is supportive and includes provision of fluids, analgesics, and scrotal support for orchitis. Systemic steroids have been used for orchitis, but their value is anecdotal. Surgery is not recommended.

Harel L et al: Mumps arthritis in children. Pediatr Infect Dis J 1990;9:928.

Hersh BS et al: Mumps outbreak in a highly vaccinated population. J Pediatr 1991;119:187.

Koskiniemi M et al: Clinical appearance and outcome in mumps encephalitis in children. Acta Paediatr Scand 1983;72:603.

Manson AL: Mumps orchitis. Urology 1990;36:355.

McDonald JC, Moore DL, Quennec P: Clinical and epidemiologic features of mumps meningoencephalitis and possible vaccine-related disease. Pediatr Infect Dis J 1989;8:751.

Sugiura A, Yamada A: Aseptic meningitis as a complication of mumps vaccination. Pediatr Infect Dis J 1991; 10:209.

RABIES

Essentials of Diagnosis

- History of animal bite 10 days to 1 year (usually 20–90 days) previously.
- Paresthesias or hyperesthesia in bite area.
- Irritability followed by fever, confusion, combativeness, muscle spasms (especially pharyngeal with swallowing).
- Progressive symptoms, death.
- Rabies antigen detected in corneal scrapings or tissue obtained by brain or skin biopsy; Negri bodies seen in brain tissue.

General Considerations

Rabies remains a serious public health problem wherever animal immunization is not widely practiced. Although infection does not always follow a bite by a rabid animal (about 40% infection rate following rabid dog bites), infection is usually fatal. Any warm-blooded animal may be infected, but susceptibility and transmissibility vary with different species. Bats may be well yet carry and excrete the virus in saliva or feces for prolonged periods; they are the major cause of rabies in the United States. Dogs and cats are usually clinically ill within 10 days after becoming contagious (the standard quarantine period for suspect animals). Valid quarantine periods or signs of illness are not fully known for many species. Rodents rarely transmit infection. Animal vaccines are only partially immunogenic; a single inoculation may fail to produce immunity in up to 20% of dogs.

Clinical Findings

The risk is assessed according to the type of animal (bats always considered rabid); the animal's behavior (unprovoked bite or unusual behavior); wound extent and location (infection more common after head or arm bites, or if wounds have extensive salivary contamination or are not quickly and thoroughly cleaned); geographic area (urban rabies rare to nonexistent in many US cities; rural rabies always possible, especially outside the United States); and animal vaccination history (risk low if documented). Owing partially to the long incubation period, a bite history is not always obtained. Aerosolized virus in caves inhabited by bats has caused infection.

A. Symptoms and Signs: Paresthesias at the bite site are usually the first symptom. Nonspecific anxiety excitability or depression follows, then muscle spasms, drooling, hydrophobia, delirium, and lethargy. Swallowing or even the sensation of air blown on the face may cause pharyngeal spasms. Seizures, fever, cranial nerve palsies, coma, and death follow within 7–14 days of onset. In a minority of patients, the disease lacks the spastic components and is characterized primarily by flaccid paralysis and cranial nerve defects.

B. Laboratory Findings: Leukocytosis is common. The spinal fluid is usually normal or may show elevation of protein and mononuclear cell levels. Cerebral imaging and electroencephalography are not diagnostic.

Infection in an animal may be determined by use of the fluorescent antibody test to examine brain tissue for antigen.

Rabies virus is excreted in the saliva of infected humans, but the diagnosis is usually made by antigen detection in scrapings or tissue samples of richly innervated epithelium, such as the cornea or hairline of the neck. Classic Negri cytoplasmic inclusion bodies in brain tissue are not always present.

Seroconversion occurs after 7–10 days.

Differential Diagnosis

Failure to elicit the bite history in areas where rabies is rare may delay diagnosis. Other disorders to be considered include pseudorabies (hysterical belief that one has the disease); parainfectious encephalopathy; encephalitis due to herpes simplex, mosquito-borne viruses, other viruses, and Guillain-Barré syndrome.

Prevention

See Chapter 10 for information regarding vaccination and postexposure prophylaxis. The development of human immune globulin and diploid cell vaccine has made prophylaxis more effective and minimally toxic. Since rabies is almost always fatal, presumed exposures must be managed carefully.

Treatment & Prognosis

Survival is rare but has been reported in three patients receiving meticulous intensive care. No antivi-

ral preparations are of proven benefit. Early diagnosis is important for the protection and prophylaxis of individuals exposed to the patient.

Alvaraz L et al: Partial recovery from rabies in a nine-year-old boy. Pediatr Infect Dis J 1994;13:1154.

Baevsky RH, Bartfield JM: Human rabies: A review. Am J Emerg Med 1993;11:279.

Fishbein DB, Robinson LE: Rabies. N Engl J Med 1993; 329:1632.

Shah U, Jaswal GS: Victims of a rabid wolf in India: Effect of severity and location of bites on development of rabies. J Infect Dis 1976;134:25.

RUBELLA

Essentials of Diagnosis

- History of rubella vaccination usually absent.
- Prodromal nonspecific respiratory symptoms and adenopathy (postauricular and occipital).
- Maculopapular rash beginning on face, rapidly spreading to entire body, and disappearing by fourth day.
- Few systemic symptoms.

Congenital infection:

- Retarded growth, development.
- Cataracts, retinopathy.
- Purpuric "blueberry muffin" rash at birth, jaundice, thrombocytopenia.
- Deafness.
- Congenital heart defect.

General Considerations

If it were not teratogenic, rubella would be of little clinical importance. Clinical diagnosis is difficult in some cases because of its variable expression. In one study, over 80% of infections were subclinical. Because of inadequate vaccination, many outbreaks now occur in adolescents or adults.

The number of reported rubella cases in the United States decreased until 1989, when a resurgence was noted. Congenital rubella, both in infants of unimmunized women and in some who have apparently been reinfected in pregnancy, is also increasing.

Clinical Findings

The incubation period is 14–21 days. The nondistinctive signs may make exposure history unreliable. A history of immunization makes rubella unlikely but still possible.

Congenital rubella usually follows maternal infection in the first trimester.

A. Symptoms and Signs:

1. Infection in children—Young children may only have rash. Older patients often have a nonspecific prodrome of low-grade fever, ocular pain, sore throat, and myalgia. Postauricular and suboccipital adenopathy (sometimes generalized) is characteristic. This often precedes the rash or may occur without rash. The rash consists of discrete maculopapules beginning on the face. A "slapped cheek" appearance or pruritus may occur. The rash quickly spreads to the trunk and extremities after it fades from the face; it is gone by the fourth day. Enanthem is usually absent.

2. Congenital infection—More than 80% of women infected in the first 4 months of gestation are delivered of affected infants; less than 10% of those infected later in pregnancy are delivered of affected infants. Later infections can result in isolated defects, such as deafness. The main manifestations are as follows:

a. Growth retardation—Fifty to 85 percent are small at birth and remain so.

b. Cardiac anomalies—Pulmonary artery stenosis, patent ductus arteriosus, ventricular septal defect.

c. Ocular anomalies—Cataracts, microphthalmia, glaucoma, retinitis.

d. Deafness.

e. Cerebral disorders—Chronic encephalitis.

f. Hematologic disorders—Thrombocytopenia, dermal nests of extramedullary hematopoiesis or purpura ("blueberry muffin" spots), lymphopenia.

g. Others—Hepatitis, osteomyelitis, immune disorders, malabsorption, diabetes.

B. Laboratory Findings: Leukopenia is common, and platelet counts may be low. Congenital infection is associated with low platelet counts, abnormal liver function tests, hemolytic anemia, pleocytosis, and very high rubella IgM antibody titers. Total serum IgM is elevated, and IgA and IgG levels may be depressed.

C. Imaging: Pneumonitis and bone metaphysial longitudinal lucencies may be present in films of children with congenital infection.

Diagnosis

Virus may be isolated from throat or urine from 1 week before to 2 weeks after onset of rash. Children with congenital infection are infectious for months. The virus laboratory must be notified that rubella is suspected. Serologic diagnosis is best made by demonstrating a fourfold rise in antibody titer between specimens drawn 1–2 weeks apart. The first should be drawn promptly, since titers increase rapidly after onset of rash. Both specimens must be tested simultaneously by a single laboratory. Specific IgM titers are used, but specificity and sensitivity vary with the testing site diagnosing disease. Because the decision to terminate a pregnancy is usually based on serologic results, testing must be done carefully.

Differential Diagnosis

Rubella may resemble infections due to enterovirus, adenovirus, measles, Epstein-Barr virus, roseola, parvovirus (erythema infectiosum), and *Toxoplasma gondii*. Because public health implications are great, sporadic suspected cases should be serologically or virologically confirmed.

Congenital rubella must be differentiated from congenital CMV infection, toxoplasmosis, and syphilis.

Complications & Sequelae

A. Arthralgia and Arthritis: Both occur more often in adult women. Polyarticular involvement (fingers, knees, wrists), lasting a few days to weeks, is typical. Frank arthritis occurs in a small percentage. It may resemble acute rheumatoid arthritis.

B. Encephalitis: With an incidence of about 1:6000, this is a nonspecific parainfectious encephalitis associated with a low mortality rate. A syndrome resembling subacute sclerosing panencephalitis (see rubeola) has also been described in congenital rubella.

C. Rubella in Pregnancy: Infection in the mother is self-limited and not severe (see previous text for sequelae).

Prevention

See Chapter 10 for the indications for and efficacy of rubella vaccine. Standard prenatal care should include rubella antibody testing. Seropositive mothers are at no risk; seronegative mothers are vaccinated after delivery.

A pregnant woman possibly exposed to rubella should be tested immediately; if seropositive, she is immune and need not worry. If she is seronegative, a second specimen should be drawn in 4–6 weeks, and both specimens should be tested simultaneously. Seroconversion in the first trimester suggests high fetal risk; such women require counseling regarding therapeutic abortion.

When pregnancy termination is not an option, some experts recommend intramuscular administration of 20 mL of standard immune globulin within 72 hours after exposure in an attempt to prevent infection. (This negates the value of subsequent antibody testing.) The efficacy of this practice is unknown.

Treatment & Prognosis

Symptomatic therapy is sufficient. Arthritis may improve with administration of anti-inflammatory agents. The prognosis is excellent in those with acquired disease but poor in congenitally infected infants, in whom most defects are irreversible or progressive. The severe cognitive defects seem to correlate closely in these infants with the degree of growth failure.

Chantler JK et al: Persistent rubella virus infection associated with chronic arthritis in children. N Engl J Med 1985;313:1117.

Freij BJ, South MA, Sever JL: Maternal rubella and the

congenital rubella syndrome. Clin Perinatol 1988; 15:247.

Kaplan KM et al: A profile of mothers giving birth to infants with congenital rubella syndrome: An assessment of risk factors. Am J Dis Child 1990;144:118.

Weber B et al: Congenital rubella syndrome after maternal reinfection. Infection 1993;21:118.

II. RICKETTSIAL INFECTIONS

The rickettsiae are pleomorphic, gram-negative coccobacilli which are obligate intracellular parasites. Rickettsial diseases are often included in the differential diagnosis of febrile rashes, although some (notably Q fever) are not characterized by rash. Severe headache is a prominent symptom. The endothelium is the primary target tissue, and the ensuing vasculitis is responsible for severe illness.

All rickettsioses except Q fever are transmitted by cutaneous arthropod contact, either by bite or fecal contamination of skin breaks. Evidence of such contact by history or physical examination may be completely lacking, especially in young children. The geographic distribution of the vector is often the primary determinant for suspicion of these infections. Therapy often must be empirical. Most new broad-spectrum antimicrobials are inactive against these cell wall–deficient organisms; chloramphenicol and tetracycline are usually effective.

HUMAN EHRLICHIOSIS

Ehrlichia species are responsible for febrile pancytopenia in animals. In humans, *Ehrlichia sennetsu* is responsible for a mononucleosis-like syndrome seen in Japan and Malaysia. One agent of North American human ehrlichiosis has been identified as a new species, *Ehrlichia chaffeensis*. The reservoir is currently unknown; ticks are the presumed vectors. Most cases caused by this agent are reported in the south central and mid to southern Atlantic states. Almost all cases occur between March and October, when ticks are active. A second ehrlichiosis syndrome, which was recently described in the upper Midwest, is caused by *E phagocytophila* or *E cqui*, which are known large animal pathogens. *E chaffeensis* presumably has a predilection for mononuclear cells, whereas intracytoplasmic inclusion in granulocytes are common with the *E phagocytopila* and *E cqui* infections. Hence, diseases caused by these agents are referred to as human monocytic ehrlichiosis or human granulocytic ehrlichiosis, respectively. Recent evidence suggests that human ehrlichiosis is underrecognized; 10% of adults suspected of having Rocky Mountain spotted fever or Lyme disease had serologic evidence of human ehrlichiosis.

Clinical Findings

In approximately 75% of cases, a history of tick bite can be elicited. The majority of the remaining patients report having been in a tick-infested area. The usual incubation period ranges from 5 to 21 days.

A. Symptoms and Signs: Fever is universally present. Gastrointestinal symptoms (anorexia, nausea and vomiting) are reported in 70% of pediatric cases. Headache, myalgia, and rash are seen in over 50%. The rash may be erythematous, macular, papular, petechial, scarlatiniform, or vasculitic. Meningitis occurs. Interstitial pneumonitis occurs in severe cases. The physical examination, except for rash, is usually normal. Conjunctival injection, mild cervical adenopathy, and organomegaly have been described but are usually absent.

B. Laboratory Findings: Laboratory abnormalities include leukopenia, lymphopenia with eye shift, thrombocytopenia, and elevated aminotransferase levels. Anemia is seen in one-third of cases.

The definitive diagnosis is made serologically. CDC uses appropriate antigens in an immunofluorescent antibody test in order to distinguish between the etiologic agents. Intracytoplasmic inclusions (morulae) may occasionally be observed in mononuclear cells in monocytic ehrlichiosis and are usually observed in polymorphonuclear cells from the peripheral blood or bone marrow in granulocytic ehrlichiosis.

Differential Diagnosis

The differential diagnosis includes other rickettsial infections (especially Rocky Mountain spotted fever), Colorado tick fever, leptospirosis, Epstein-Barr virus infection, CMV infection, other viral infections, Kawasaki disease, systemic lupus erythematosus, and leukemia.

Treatment & Prognosis

Children have an excellent prognosis. Although the disease may last several weeks, it is usually self-limited. In vitro and in vivo evidence suggest that tetracycline is effective.

Anderson BE et al: *Ehrlichia chaffeensis,* a new species associated with human ehrlichiosis. J Clin Microbiol 1991;29:2838.

Bakken JS et al: Human granulocytic ehrlichiosis in the upper Midwest United States. JAMA 1994;272:212.

Barton LL et al: Infection with *Ehrlichia* in childhood. J Pediatr 1992;120:998.

Harkness JR: Ehrlichiosis. Infect Dis Clin North Am 1991;5:37.

Roland WE et al: Ehrlichiosis: A cause of prolonged fever. Clin Infect Dis 1995;20:212.

RICKETTSIALPOX

Rickettsia akari is transmitted by mites from infected house mice. Infection is rarely diagnosed; most cases in the United States have occurred in northeastern cities, particularly New York. The bite site becomes a papule, then a pustule; it ulcerates and then forms a characteristic black eschar at about the time fever develops at 9–14 days. Local adenopathy is the rule. Headache, myalgia, and photophobia are followed in 2–4 days by a generalized, maculopapular rash. Palms and soles may be involved. Vesicles develop on the papules and form crusts. The fever lasts about a week.

The differential diagnosis includes varicella, enteroviral infections, the other rickettsial spotted fevers, meningococcemia, and gonococcemia. Mild cases require no therapy. Tetracyclines or chloramphenicol is effective.

Kass EM et al: Rickettsialpox in a New York City hospital, 1980 to 1989. N Engl J Med 1994;331:1612.

ROCKY MOUNTAIN SPOTTED FEVER

Rickettsia rickettsii infection causes one of many similar tick-borne illnesses characterized by fever and a rash. Most are named for their geographic area. In all except Rocky Mountain spotted fever, there is a characteristic eschar at the bite site, the "tache noire." Dogs and rodents are reservoirs of *R rickettsii*.

Rocky Mountain spotted fever is the most severe of these infections and the most important in the United States. It occurs predominantly in the eastern seaboard, in the southeastern states, and in Arkansas, Texas, Missouri, Kansas, and Oklahoma—rarely in the West. Most cases occur in children exposed in rural areas from April to September. Since tick attachment lasting 4 hours or longer is needed, frequent tick removal is a preventive measure.

Clinical Findings

A. Symptoms and Signs: After the incubation period of 3–12 days (mean, 7 days), there is high fever (over 40 °C, often hectic) of abrupt onset, myalgia, severe and persistent headache (less obvious in infants), general toxicity, myalgia, vomiting, and diarrhea. The characteristic rash occurs in 90–95% of patients and appears 2–6 days after fever onset as macules and maculopapular rash on the palms, soles, and extremities, becoming petechial and spreading centrally. Conjunctivitis, splenomegaly, edema, meningismus, irritability, and confusion may be seen.

B. Laboratory Findings: Laboratory findings are nonspecific and reflect diffuse vasculitis: thrombocytopenia, hyponatremia, early mild leukopenia, proteinuria, abnormal liver function tests, hypoalbuminemia, and hematuria. Cerebrospinal fluid pleocytosis is common. Serologic diagnosis is achieved with indirect fluorescent or latex agglutination antibody methods, but generally only 7–10 days after onset of the illness. Skin biopsy with specific fluorescent staining may give the diagnosis within the first week of the illness.

Differential Diagnosis

The differential diagnosis includes meningococcemia, measles, meningitis, staphylococcal sepsis, enteroviral infection, leptospirosis, Colorado tick fever, scarlet fever, murine typhus, Kawasaki disease, and ehrlichiosis.

Treatment & Prognosis

To be effective, therapy for Rocky Mountain spotted fever must be started early and is often based on a presumptive diagnosis in endemic areas prior to rash onset. It is important to remember that atypical presentations, such as the absence of pathognomonic rash, often lead to delay in appropriate therapy. Chloramphenicol is the agent of choice for children under 8 years of age; a doxycycline is preferable for older children. Treatment should be continued for 2 or 3 days after the temperature has returned to normal for a full day. A minimum of 10 days of therapy is recommended.

Complications and death result from severe vasculitis, especially in the brain, heart, and lung. The mortality rate is 5–7%. Delay in therapy is an important determinant of mortality.

Kirk JL et al: Rocky Mountain spotted fever: A clinical review based on 48 confirmed cases. Medicine 1990; 69:35.

Sexton DJ, Corey CR: Rocky Mountain "spotless" and "almost spotless" fever: A wolf in sheep's clothing. Clin Infect Dis 1992;15:439.

Walker DH: Rocky Mountain spotted fever: A second alert. Clin Infect Dis 1995;20:1111.

ENDEMIC TYPHUS
(Murine Typhus)

Endemic typhus is present in the United States mainly in southern Texas. The disease is transmitted by fleas from infected rodents, either by bite, from rodent feces in scratches, or by inhalation. Domestic cats and opossums may play a role in the transmission of suburban cases. There is no eschar at the bite, which may go unnoticed. The incubation period is 6–14 days. Headache, myalgia, and chills slowly worsen. Fever may last 10–14 days. After 3–8 days, a rash appears. Truncal macules and papules spread to the extremities; the rash may become petechial.

The centrifugal nature of the rash in typhus, with sparing of the palms and soles, is a distinction from Rocky Mountain spotted fever. Rash may be absent in 20–40% of patients. Intestinal and respiratory symptoms may occur. The illness is usually self-limited and milder than epidemic typhus. More prolonged neurologic symptoms have been described. Therapy is usually not needed. Doxycycline is the drug of choice. Therapy for 3 days is usually sufficient. The OX-19 tube of the Weil-Felix panel is positive. Specific serologic tests are available.

Esperanza L et al: Murine typhus: Forgotten but not gone. Southern Med J 1992;85:754.

Samra Y, Shaked Y, Maier MK: Delayed neurologic toxicity in murine typhus: Report of two cases. Arch Intern Med 1989;149:949.

Q FEVER

Coxiella burnetii is transmitted by inhalation, rather than by an arthropod bite. The birth tissues and excreta of domestic animals and of some rodents are the infectious source. Unpasteurized milk from infected animals may also transmit disease. Q fever is also distinguished from other rickettsial diseases by the absence of cutaneous manifestations and by the prominence of pulmonary disease.

Clinical Findings

A. Symptoms and Signs: Chills, fever, severe headache, and myalgia occur 10–20 days after exposure. Abdominal pain, vomiting, chest pain, and cough are prominent in children. Examination of the lung may produce few findings, as in other atypical pneumonias. Hepatosplenomegaly is common.

B. Laboratory Findings: Leukopenia with left shift is characteristic. Thrombocytopenia is unusual and another distinction from other symptomatic rickettsial diseases. Transaminase levels are elevated. Diagnosis is made by finding a complement-fixing antibody response (fourfold rise or single high titer) to the phase II organism. IgM ELISA is also available.

C. Imaging: Pneumonitis occurs in 50% of patients. Multiple segmental infiltrates are common. Consolidation and pleural effusion are exceptional.

Differential Diagnosis

In the appropriate epidemiologic setting, Q fever should be considered in evaluating causes of atypical pneumonias (mycoplasma, viruses, *Chlamydia pneumoniae*). It should also be included among the causes of mild hepatitis without rash or adenopathy.

Treatment & Prognosis

Typically the illness lasts 1–2 weeks without therapy. One complication is chronic disease, which often implies myocarditis or granulomatous hepatitis. *C burnetii* is also one of the causes of "culture-negative" endocarditis. Both types of complication are rare. The endocarditis is difficult to treat; mortality approaches 50%. The course of the uncomplicated illness is shortened with tetracycline or chloramphenicol; tetracycline is preferred.

Ruiz-Contreras J et al: Q fever in children. Am J Dis Child 1993;147:300.

Pinsky RK et al: An outbreak of cat-associated Q fever in the United States. J Infect Dis 1991;164:202.

REFERENCES

Feigin RD, Cherry JD (editors): *Textbook of Pediatric Infectious Diseases,* 3rd ed. Saunders, 1992.

Galasso GH, Merigan TC, Buchanan RA (editors): *Antiviral Agents and Viral Diseases of Man,* 32nd ed. Raven Press, 1990.

Myers SA, Sexton DJ: Dermatologic manifestations of arthropod-borne disease. Infect Dis Clin North Am 1994;8:689.

Remington JS, Klein JO: *Infectious Disease of the Fetus and Newborn Infant.* Saunders, 1990.

36 Human Immunodeficiency Virus (HIV) Infections: Acquired Immunodeficiency Syndrome (AIDS)

Elizabeth J. McFarland, MD

Essentials of Diagnosis

Children less than 18 months
- A child known to be HIV-seropositive or born to an HIV-infected mother.

And
- Has positive results on two separate determinations on blood or tissue (excluding cord blood) for one or more of the following HIV detection tests: HIV culture, HIV polymerase chain reaction, HIV antigen (p24).

Or
- Meets criteria for acquired immunodeficiency syndrome (AIDS) diagnosis based on the 1987 CDC AIDS surveillance case (specific opportunistic infections, lymphoid interstitial pneumonitis, Kaposi's sarcoma, primary brain lymphoma, others; see CDC case definition, MMWR, 1994).

Or
- Has HIV antibody and evidence of cellular and humoral immunodeficiency (without an obvious cause) and symptoms compatible with HIV infections (multiple serious bacterial infections, encephalopathy, recurrent *Salmonella* septicemia, HIV wasting syndrome, certain non-Hodgkin's lymphomas, disseminated fungal infections, or mycobacterial infections).

Children older than 18 months
- HIV-seropositive by repeatedly reactive enzyme immunoassay (EIA) and confirmatory test.

Or
- Meets any of the criteria listed for children less than 18 months.

General Considerations

Human immunodeficiency virus (HIV) is the most common cause of AIDS in children. It is a retrovirus that infects helper T lymphocytes (CD4 lymphocytes), monocytes, macrophages, and other cell types. Helper T lymphocytes—the primary target cells—are infected following binding of the virus's glycosylated envelope protein, gp120, to the CD4 surface protein found on these cells. Both the function and the number of helper T lymphocytes are diminished by infection. The destruction of helper T cells profoundly affects both humoral and cell-mediated immunity and results in generalized immune incompetence and progression to AIDS. AIDS is a clinical syndrome, which was originally defined before HIV was identified as the etiologic agent. The diagnosis of AIDS is made after an HIV-infected child suffers any of the opportunistic infections or malignant conditions listed for category C symptoms (see Table 36–3). In adults, the criteria for a diagnosis of AIDS also includes absolute helper T-lymphocyte (CD4+ lymphocytes) counts of 200/μL or less.

HIV infection begins with a high viral burden in the bloodstream during primary infection, which declines without therapy concurrent with the appearance of an HIV-specific host immune response. In most cases, this is followed by a period of "clinical latency" of variable duration. During this time, the infected person is generally asymptomatic, but high levels of virus can be detected primarily in lymph node tissue. The virus and anti-HIV immune responses are in a steady state with high levels of virus production and destruction balanced with production and destruction of CD4 lymphocytes. Eventually, the balance favors the virus, viral burden increasing as CD4 lymphocyte counts decline.

Perinatal transmission accounts for over 90% of prepubertal AIDS cases and almost all new pediatric HIV infections. Perinatal transmission may occur transplacentally, at the time of delivery, and via breast feeding. Indirect evidence suggests that about 30–70% of the perinatal infections occur in utero; however, the timing of transmission remains an area of active investigation. Formerly, most nonperinatal cases were acquired via transfusion or hemophilia therapy. Of hemophiliacs who received blood products prior to 1985 (when screening began), 65–90% are infected. Sexual activity (both heterosexual and homosexual) and sharing of contaminated needles account for most infections after puberty.

About 84% of HIV-infected women are of childbearing age: 41% are intravenous drug abusers, and most of the remainder are sexual partners of infected men. Women exposed by heterosexual contact make up the the most rapidly increasing transmission group in the United States. About 15–30% of infants born to untreated HIV-infected pregnant women will be infected. Risk factors associated with mother-to-infant transmission include advanced disease stage, high viral burden, low CD4 lymphocyte count, and factors related to increased exposure to maternal blood or cervical secretions at the time of delivery (ie, duration of rupture of membranes, presence of blood in infants gastric secretions, twin A delivery). Recently, clinical trials have demonstrated that transmission can be reduced by 65% with antiretroviral treatment of the mother and infant during pregnancy and delivery and during the first 6 weeks after birth.

AIDS ranks among the top 10 causes of mortality in children aged 1–4 years. In the United States during recent years, about 7000 HIV-infected women deliver live infants each year, resulting in 1000–2000 newly infected infants. The number of infected children in other parts of the world, particularly Africa, India, Thailand, and parts of South America is even greater.

In the United States, risk factors for HIV infection among adults include exposure to blood products from 1978 to the spring of 1985, parenteral illicit drug use, multiple heterosexual or homosexual contacts, and a heterosexual partner with one of the above risk factors. Casual, classroom, or household contact with an HIV-infected person poses no risk. Many individuals, particularly women, are unaware of their risk factors. Adolescents are also likely to be unaware or unwilling to admit risk factors. A high level of suspicion is required for making the diagnosis in these cases.

About 20–30% of HIV-infected infants develop an AIDS-defining illness by 1 year of age, have a rapidly progressive course, and die before age 2–3 years. In the remainder, the disease progresses more slowly with a mortality rate of 3.5% per year up to age 7 years. Median survival is over 7 years. It is not uncommon for an HIV-infected child to survive into early adolescence. Children who acquire HIV at older ages by transfusion or other means are likely to progress at the slower rate. Although little has been reported regarding the natural history of HIV infection acquired in adolescence, it is generally assumed that disease progression will be similar to that observed in adults. There are rare HIV-infected children and adults who have been infected over 8–10 years with no evidence of immune suppression. It is not yet clear whether these patients will escape disease progression.

Clinical Findings

A. Symptoms and Signs:

1. Primary, acute infection–The incubation period for primary infection is 2–4 weeks. Symptoms associated with primary infection are nonspecific ("flu" or mild mononucleosis-like illness) and often subclinical. Adolescents may present with fever, fatigue, malaise, pharyngitis, enlarged lymph nodes, hepatosplenomegaly. Signs seen more frequently with HIV than with other similar viral syndromes are mild oral ulcerations, a diffuse macular, erythematous rash, and mild encephalopathy. Occasionally, thrush or *Candida* esophagitis is observed. These early symptoms associated with primary infection resolve spontaneously within 1–2 weeks, although some persons have fatigue and depression for weeks or months.

Following perinatal acquisition, a primary infection syndrome is rarely recognized. Likewise, newborns with perinatal HIV infection are rarely symptomatic (less than 7%) at birth. Size and physical features are not different from uninfected infants. However, 75–95% will demonstrate some sign (most nonspecific signs) by age 1 year. The median time to appearance of any sign is 5 months.

2. Nonspecific symptoms–Frequent illness is a typical historical feature (especially recurrent otitis media or sinusitis or both), in addition to poor weight gain (sometimes progressing to wasting syndrome), chronic cough, chronic diarrhea, *Candida* infection, developmental delay, unexplained fevers, night sweats, generalized lymphadenopathy, or hepatosplenomegaly. Delayed growth may be observed as early as 4 months in some infants. These common, early findings may be present for years in an otherwise well child.

3. Infections related to immunodeficiency–Progressive immune dysfunction in both humoral and cell-mediated responses results in susceptibility to infections. Children lack prior experience with many bacterial pathogens; hence, recurrent bacterial infections are more common than in HIV-infected adults. The most common types of serious bacterial infections in order of frequency are bacteremia, pneumonia, urinary tract infections, cellulitis, abscesses, bone and joint infections, and meningitis. Common organisms include *Streptococcus pneumoniae, Salmonella* spp, *Enterococcus* spp, *Staphylococcus aureus, Haemophilus influenzae,* other gram-negative rods, and *Streptococcus viridans.* Infections with *Mycobacterium* tuberculosis (usually acquired from adults in the household) may be severe. Persistent candidal mucocutaneous infections (oral, skin, and vaginal) are extremely common. *Candida* esophagitis is reported in about 15% of pediatric cases. Cryptococcal infections and histoplasmosis have been described, although much less frequently than among HIV-infected adults.

Abnormal responses to viral infections, particularly herpesviruses are common. Primary varicella infections may be prolonged or severe. Recurrent varicella-zoster infections occur with progressive immune dysfunction. Cytomegalovirus (CMV) infections may result in disseminated disease, hepatitis, gastroenteritis, retinitis, and encephalitis. Epstein-Barr virus (EBV) is associated with oral hairy leukoplakia and perhaps other conditions such as cardiomyopathy and lymphoid interstitial pneumonitis. Herpes simplex lesions may be large, painful, and persistent.

The onset of late-stage immunodeficiency is accompanied by susceptibility to a variety of opportunistic pathogens. Pneumonia caused by *Pneumocystis carinii* is the most common, accounting for 30% of the AIDS-defining diagnoses among children. The incidence is highest between age 2 months and 6 months, and *Pneumocystis carinii* pneumonia (PCP) is often fatal during this time period. Symptoms are difficult to distinguish from a viral or atypical pneumonia. Usually, patients have fever, tachypnea, retractions, progressive hypoxemia, and an elevated lactate dehydrogenase (LDH). Disseminated infection with *Mycobacterium avium* complex (MAC) occurs in approximately 11% of HIV-infected children. The rate increases to about 25% in infected children who have CD4 lymphocyte counts under 50–100. Symptoms and signs associated with this opportunistic pathogen include fever, night sweats, weight loss, diarrhea, fatigue, lymphadenopathy, hepatomegaly, anemia, and granulocytopenia. A variety of diarrheal pathogens that cause mild, resolving symptoms in healthy persons may result in severe, chronic diarrhea in HIV-infected persons. These include *Rotavirus, Cryptosporidium, Isospora belli, Giardia,* and bacterial pathogens (*Campylobacter, Salmonella, Shigella, Clostridium difficile*). Reactivation of toxoplasmosis is uncommon in pediatric HIV, but causes encephalitis in up to 28% of HIV-infected adults. It may present as an encephalitis, a central nervous system mass lesion, or disseminated disease during early infancy.

4. Organ system disease—HIV infection may cause a variety of organ system symptoms. In most cases, the pathogenesis is not fully understood; however, symptoms may occur in the absence of other obvious pathogens and are thought to result from HIV infection itself.

Encephalopathy is a particularly common problem, afflicting 20% or more HIV-infected children. Following perinatal transmission, affected patients may present with acquired microcephaly, progressive motor deficit, ataxia, pseudobulbar palsy, and failure to attain (or surrender previously attained) developmental milestones. The child may demonstrate a static course, associated with steady but below-normal developmental progress; may reach a plateau; or may lose developmental skills. Children who are older when they acquire HIV infection may have symptoms similar to those observed in infected adults, that is, characterized by gradual mental status changes, initially affecting attention and memory. Other treatable causes of central nervous system disease should be sought especially when an acute change in symptoms occurs.

Lymphoid interstitial pneumonitis, which is uncommon among adults, affects almost 50% of children with AIDS. Histologically, it is characterized by a diffuse peribronchial and interstitial infiltrate composed of lymphocytes and plasma cells. It may be asymptomatic or associated with dry cough, hypoxemia, dyspnea or wheezing on exertion, and clubbing of the digits. Auscultatory findings may be few. Children with this disorder frequently have enlargement of the parotid glands and generalized lymphadenopathy.

Hematologic signs are common. Immune thrombocytopenia associated with antiplatelet antibodies occurs, but does not correlate with the degree of immune suppression. Many cases are low grade with no clinical symptoms or therapy required. However, some cases result in serious bleeding complications. Anemia is frequently present in late-stage disease. Likewise, granulocytopenia may occur as the disease progresses. Often patients are also on drugs, which may result in bone marrow suppression; distinguishing between the effects of HIV or the drug therapy may be difficult.

Subclinical cardiac abnormalities detected only by echocardiogram are common. Symptomatic cardiomyopathy is also observed in some cases, primarily infants with rapid disease progression. Symptoms are those of congestive heart failure and may respond to diuretics and digitalis.

Mild to moderate elevation of liver enzymes is frequently observed and, more rarely, overt clinical hepatitis due to HIV infection itself. However, patients are often taking drugs with potential hepatotoxicity, and superinfection with other infectious pathogens (CMV, EBV, hepatitis C) that affect the liver may occur. Thus, causes other than HIV should be sought in the face of significant liver pathology. Chronic diarrhea may occur with HIV infection. However, as with hepatitis, it is commonly associated with other gastrointestinal infections, which may respond to treatment. Severe diarrhea warrants an aggressive evaluation including cultures, microscopic examinations, and possible colonoscopy with biopsy. Lactose intolerance exacerbated by diarrhea is not infrequent among HIV-infected children. Nephropathy, myopathy, and neuropathy all are recognized in pediatric HIV but are relatively uncommon.

5. Malignancy—Malignancy is AIDS-defining in 2% of HIV-infected children. The malignancies most commonly associated with pediatric HIV infection are non-Hodgkin's lymphomas (NHL). Unlike NHL in immunocompetent persons, NHL in HIV-infected children commonly manifests at extranodal sites (bone, gastrointestinal tract, liver, or lungs) and is usually high grade and of B-cell origin. Presenting symptoms include fever, night sweats, and weight loss. Central nervous system primary lesions are common. Symptoms are those of a central nervous system mass lesion or increased intracranial pressure or both. Kaposi's sarcoma, a common malignancy among HIV-infected homosexual males, rarely occurs among children. There is an increased frequency of leiomyosarcomas, a rare soft tissue tumor not otherwise associated with immunodeficiency, among HIV-infected children. Cervical neoplasia associated with human papillomavirus (HPV) is more common and aggressive in adolescent females with HIV infection.

B. Laboratory Findings: In children older than 18 months (after loss of maternal antibody), HIV antibody is positive by enzyme immunoassay (EIA). A confirmatory test, usually a Western blot, must be performed since occasionally individuals have nonviral cross-reacting antibodies, which result in a false-positive EIA. Rarely (less than 1%) an infected child may fail to make antibody. However, they are usually obviously ill, and tests for virus or viral antigen are positive. During primary infection of adolescents, HIV antibody may be absent; tests for the presence of virus (p24 antigen, HIV culture, or DNA detection) are positive.

Children born to HIV-infected mothers will have positive tests for HIV antibody, regardless of infection status, owing to transplacental passage of maternal antibody for many months. The median time to loss of maternal HIV antibody is 10 months; all children lose maternal antibody by 18 months. No reliable IgM antibody test is available. In these infants, a diagnosis of HIV infection can be made in over 95% by age 2–5 months using tests for virus in blood or tissue (HIV culture or nucleic acid detection). Detection of viral antigen (p24 antigen), using an immune complex dissociation step in the assay, is an alternative, less expensive test, requiring only frozen serum and less technical expertise; however, it is 10–20% less sensitive.

A proportion of infected infants will have negative results by these sensitive assays during the first 0–12 weeks of life, presumably because of low viral burden, perhaps indicating that the infection was acquired at the time of birth. Hence, negative tests during the early period do not reliably rule out infection. However, in an infant who is otherwise well and has had at least two negative HIV cultures or nucleic acid detection tests, performed at when over 1 month of age—at least one of which was performed at over 4 months of age—is unlikely to be infected. These infants can be followed up for clinical symptoms and tested at age 15–18 months for reversion to seronegative status to confirm the absence of infection. Most experts recommend a final antibody test performed at 24 months.

There are rare reports of children who had blood tests that were repeatedly positive for HIV by culture or nucleic acid detection and who demonstrated no symptoms of HIV infection and have subsequently reverted to negative serology. In a few cases, evidence suggests that these test results were the result of transient viremia rather than laboratory error. This phenomenon has only recently been recognized and appears to be extremely uncommon.

Lymphocyte numbers and lymphocyte subclasses are altered as the disease progresses. The absolute number and percentage of helper T (CD4) lymphocytes declines; suppressor/killer T (CD8) lymphocytes may be increased and the ratio of helper/suppressor lymphocytes, normally more than 1, is reversed. Helper T-lymphocyte numbers and percentages in infants are normally much higher than in adults and decline to adult levels by age 6 years. Hence, age-adjusted values must be used in evaluating these tests.

In the absence of a secondary infection or organ system disease, routine laboratory tests (complete cell count [CBC], blood chemistry profiles) are often normal. Some children will have thrombocytopenia due to autoimmune antibodies at a relatively early stage of disease. As disease progresses, anemia becomes common and granulocytopenia unrelated to drug therapy may occur. Mild elevation of liver enzymes is common. Serum LDH levels are high in children with *P carinii* infection. Hypergammaglobulinemia is characteristic and may be observed as early as 9 months of age. Some children fail to make specific antibody to antigens (eg, tetanus, *Haemophilus influenzae* type b, *Pneumococcus*). This failure contributes to subsequent infections. With brain involvement, the cerebrospinal fluid (CSF) may be normal or the protein elevated and a mononuclear pleocytosis present.

C. Imaging: Cerebral images demonstrate atrophy and calcification in the basal ganglia and frontal lobes in patients with encephalopathy. Chest radiographs of children with lymphoid interstitial pneumonitis show diffuse interstitial reticulonodular infiltrates, occasionally with hilar adenopathy. The chest radiograph in *P carinii* pneumonia typically demonstrates early perihilar infiltrates progressing to bilateral diffuse alveolar disease. Infection with other opportunistic pathogens usually results in x-ray findings typical of each agent. The more severe the immunodeficiency, however, the more atypical these presentations can be.

Differential Diagnosis

Differential diagnosis of HIV will correlate with the presenting sign or symptom. Infants with evidence of immunodeficiency may resemble infants with other types of congenital immunodeficiencies such as hypogammaglobulinemia or severe combined immunodeficiency syndrome. In the case of poor growth, other causes of failure to thrive should be considered. Children or adolescents presenting with generalized lymphadenopathy or hepatosplenomegaly may resemble those infected with other viruses such as EBV or CMV. The symptoms of acute primary infection in the adolescent may be similar to EBV, CMV, toxoplasmosis, rubella, syphilis, viral hepatitis and other viral infections, or disseminated gonococcal infection.

The diagnosis can be made or excluded with HIV antibody testing in a child greater than 18 months of age. In younger children, a negative result usually excludes HIV infection but a positive result must be followed by careful confirmatory testing for the presence of virus. In these children, other congenital immunodeficiencies, congenital infections (CMV, toxoplasmosis, syphilis) and many other illnesses may cause similar presenting clinical signs.

Prevention

Awareness of modes of transmission is crucial for prevention of HIV. As a result of careful donor screening and testing of the donated blood, HIV transmission resulting from transfusion of blood products is now an extremely rare event. An aggressive educational campaign promoted by the gay community resulted in a marked decrease in the annual incidence of HIV infections in that population. However, ongoing and expanded educational efforts are necessary to maintain the decreased rates and to reach other populations at risk. Caregivers should encourage developmentally appropriate AIDS education for children beginning at early ages and continuing into adolescence.

The only 100% effective method of avoiding sexual transmission of HIV infection is abstinence or limiting sexual contact to a mutually monogamous partner who is not HIV-infected. However, condoms, when used consistently and correctly have been highly effective at preventing transmission between sexually active discordant couples. In two studies, seroconversions occurred in 0–2% among discordant couples using condoms consistently compared with 10–15% among couples with inconsistent condom use. A third study reported 1.1 seroconversions per 100 person-years of observation among consistent condom users compared with 9.7 among inconsistent users. The Centers for Disease Control and Prevention (CDC) provides detailed instructions on correct condom use.

All medical equipment that can penetrate the skin should be sterile. Infected blood and secretions should be handled according to the recommendations made by the CDC. Injecting drug users without access to sterile needles or needle exchange programs can reduce the risk of transmission by cleaning the needles with bleach.

Vertical transmission can be substantially prevented by antiretroviral therapy of the mother and early prophylaxis of the newborn. A multicenter clinical trial, ACTG 076, compared placebo with zidovudine (ZDV) treatment of the mother and infant during the second or third trimester, at the time of delivery, and during the first 6 weeks of life (Table 36–1). Among HIV-infected asymptomatic women with no prior antiretroviral treatment, a 65% lower transmission rate was observed with ZDV therapy. Short-term adverse events were minor and reversible. With the availability of this potentially preventive therapy, the CDC and the American College of Obstetrics and Gynecology now recommend offering routine HIV testing with informed consent to all pregnant women. Women found to be infected should be counseled regarding all HIV-related pregnancy care issues, including the risks and benefits of ZDV therapy. Trials are ongoing to study the long-term effects on women and infants receiving ZDV during pregnancy as well as to investigate other dosing regimens and treatment agents.

Since breast milk can carry the virus, breast-feeding by HIV-infected mothers is contraindicated when access to safe formula can be ensured, as is the case in the United States.

Therapy

The rate of disease progression in HIV-infected infants and children may vary greatly. Susceptibility to opportunistic pathogens increases as CD4 lymphocyte numbers decline. Thus, the risk/benefit ratio for many prophylactic treatments increases or the disease progresses. Appropriate specific and general treatment measures depend on the child's disease stage and CD4 lymphocyte count. The CDC has recently revised the disease staging criteria for HIV-infected children (Tables 36–2 and 36–3). The criteria incorporate both age-adjusted CD4 lymphocyte counts associated with none, moderate, or severe immune suppression (categories 1, 2, and 3, respectively) and clinical symptoms ranging from none, nonspecific, moderate, and severe symptoms (categories N, A, B, and C, respectively). Each child is classified by both CD4 count and clinical category. In general, category C diagnoses correlate with diseases indicating an AIDS diagnosis, with the exclusion of lymphoid interstitial pneumonitis, which was included as an AIDS-defining illness but is not a sign

Table 36–1. Treatment regimen used in ACTG 076 trial of zidovudine (ZDV) for the reduction of mother-to-infant HIV transmission.

Maternal treatment	
During pregnancy, starting 14–34 weeks' gestation	ZDV 100 mg/PO 5 times daily
During labor and delivery	ZDV 2 mg/kg intravenous loading dose, then continuous infusion 1 mg/kg/h
Infant treatment	
Begun within 12 hours of delivery and continued for 6 weeks	ZDV 2 mg/kg PO 4 times daily

Adapted from Centers for Disease Control. MMWR 1994;43 (No. RR-11):3.

Table 36–2. Immunologic categories based on age-specific CD4 T-lymphocyte counts and percent of total lymphocytes.

	Age of Child					
	<12 mo		1–5 y		6–12 y	
Immunologic Category	μL	(%)	μL	(%)	μL	(%)
1. No evidence of suppression	≥1500	(≥ 25)	≥1000	(≥ 25)	≥500	(≥ 25)
2. Evidence of moderate suppression	750–1499	(15–24)	500–999	(15–24)	200–499	(15–24)
3. Severe suppression	<750	(<15)	<500	(<15)	<200	(<15)

Adapted from Centers for Disease Control. MMWR 1994;43(No. RR-12):4.

Table 36–3. Clinical categories of children with HIV infection.

Category N: Not symptomatic
No signs or symptoms or only one of the conditions listed in category A
Category A: Mildly symptomatic
Having two or more of the following conditions:
  Lymphadenopathy
  Hepatomegaly
  Splenomegaly
  Dermatitis
  Parotitis
  Recurrent or persistent upper respiratory infection, sinusitis or otitis media
Category B: Moderately symptomatic
Having symptoms attributed to HIV infection other than those in category A or C
Examples:
  Anemia, neutropenia, thrombocytopenia
  Bacterial meningitis, pneumonia, sepsis (single episode)
  Candidiasis, oropharyngeal, persisting >2 mo
  Cardiomyopathy
  Cytomegalovirus infection with onset <1 mo of age
  Diarrhea, recurrent or chronic
  Hepatitis
  Herpes simplex virus recurrent stomatitis, bronchitis, pneumonitis, esophagitis at <1 mo of age
  Herpes zoster, two or more episodes or more than one dermatome
  Leiomyosarcoma
  Lymphoid interstitial pneumonia
  Nephropathy
  Nocardiosis
  Persistent fever
  Toxoplasmosis with onset <1 mo of age
  Varicella, complicated
Category C: Severely symptomatic
  Serious bacterial infections, multiple or recurrent
  Candidiasis, esophageal or pulmonary
  Coccidiomycosis, disseminated
  Cryptosporidiosis or isosporiasis with diarrhea > 1 month
  Cytomegalovirus with onset > 1 month of age
  Encephalopathy
  Herpes simplex virus: persistent oral lesions, or bronchitis, pneumonitis, esophagitis at > 1 month of age
  Histoplasmosis
  Kaposi's sarcoma
  Lymphoma
  Mycobacterium tuberculosis, extrapulmonary
  Mycobacterium, other species, disseminated
  Pneumocystis carinii pneumonia
  Progressive multifocal leukoencephalopathy
  Salmonella septicemia, recurrent
  Toxoplasmosis of the brain with onset > 1 month of age
  Wasting syndrome

Adapted from Centers for Disease Control. MMWR 1994;43(No. RR-12):6, 8.

of late-stage disease. Initial studies suggest that these criteria are useful in predicting prognosis.

Technologic advances in the measurement of virus in the blood have recently made possible accurate estimates of viral burden. Declines in viral burden following initiation of antiretroviral therapy have correlated with improved clinical outcome. Although these measurements are still being validated, it is likely that they will serve as surrogate markers for the expected clinical responses to treatment. Sensitive viral burden measurements will speed drug development and may soon provide an additional surrogate marker to use with CD4 lymphocyte counts and clinical symptoms in guiding therapeutic choices.

A. Specific Measures: Determining when to begin therapy and which antiretroviral drugs to use is a complicated decision. Most children need an individualized treatment plan. Current recommendations are to initiate antiretroviral therapy when the child demonstrates significant immune suppression or HIV-associated symptoms. Trials of earlier therapy during infancy, the time of primary infection, are underway. Whenever possible, children should be enrolled in collaborative treatment studies. Current information on clinical trials may be obtained by calling the AIDS Clinical Trials Information Line (800-TRIALS-A) or the Pediatric Branch, National Cancer Institute (301-402-0696).

The FDA has approved five antiretroviral drugs that are nucleoside analogues that prevent viral DNA synthesis and secondarily inhibit viral replication. These drugs differ in toxicities, pharmacokinetics, and efficacy. Zidovudine (azidothymidine [AZT, ZDV]) was the first drug approved and has been the most thoroughly studied. Toxicities include anemia, neutropenia, headache, myalgia, and insomnia. Didanosine (dideoxyinosine [ddI]) was approved as alternative drug for patients who cannot tolerate or no longer respond to ZDV. Side effects include pancreatitis, peripheral neuropathy, and retinal depigmentation. The drug is poorly absorbed in the presence of gastric acid and must be taken in conjunction with antacid preparations 1–2 hours before and after food. For adolescents and adults, zalcitabine (dideoxycytidine [ddC]) was approved for use in combination with ZDV. In adults, peripheral neuropathy is seen in up to one third of patients receiving this agent. Clinical trials in children have been completed. It appears that this toxicity is less common in children.

Stavudine (didehydrodideoxythymidine [d4T]) has a better safety profile than ddI and ddC and is more easily administered than ddI; however, there are less efficacy data available at this time.

The fifth nucleoside analogue, lamivudine (3TC) is generally well tolerated. Although viral isolates resistant to 3TC develop rapidly on treatment, the drug remains useful in combination with ZDV because the mmutation conferring lamivudine resistance results in phenotypic ZDV sensitivity, even in ZDV-resistant mutants.

Three new drugs, saquinavir, ritonavir, and indinavir, have been recently approved by the FDA. These drugs inhibit the HIV protease, an enzyme required for the production of infectious virions. These drugs result in major decreases in viral titer in plasma especially when used in combination with one of the nucleoside analogue drugs. Experience with the protease inhibitors for the treatment of children is limited.

Although ZDV has been demonstrated to be more effective than placebo in preventing disease progression among symptomatic HIV-infected adults and children, subsequent trials have demonstrated that long-term ZDV monotherapy is not optimal in preventing disease progression. ZDV delays disease progression in asymptomatic adults with CD4 counts under 500 compared with placebo. However, in longer trials of asymptomatic adults with CD4 counts both under and over 500 cells/μL treated with ZDV monotherapy, no difference in morbidity or mortality was observed when compared with what was observed when initiation of ZDV was delayed until HIV-related symptoms developed. A trial that compared the outcomes for individuals with at least 16 weeks of ZDV monotherapy, who were then maintained longer on ZDV or changed to ddI, demonstrated a benefit to changing the medication. A recent trial in children demonstrated greater disease progression among antiretroviral naive children treated with ZDV monotherapy than among those treated with either of the two other regimens, ddI alone, or ZDV plus ddI. The other two regimens were not significantly different. A similar trial for HIV-infected adults also demonstrated that initial therapy with ZDV combined with either ddI or ddC, or ddI alone, was superior to initial ZDV monotherapy in naive patients. On the basis of these data, generally ZDV in combination with either ddI or ddC, or ddI alone, would be standard choices for initial treatment of an infected child. Additional clinical trials are ongoing, which may lead to revised recommendations; antiretroviral choices should be made only after expert consultation.

HIV has a high spontaneous mutation rate, and emergence of drug resistance during treatment is now well documented. This observation and the failure of monotherapy to prevent disease progression in clinical trials have led to increased interest in the use of combinations of antiretroviral drugs begun at an earlier disease stage as a potentially more effective treatment strategy. Trials testing these concepts are under way. Likewise, several potent antiretroviral drugs that interrupt other aspects of viral function are now in clinical trials. The use of viral burden measurements as a surrogate marker for clinical efficacy is likely to speed results in both development of new agents and to make trials in early disease stage feasible.

B. General Measures:

1. Immunizations–Combined diphtheria-tetanus-pertussis (DPT), conjugated *Haemophilus influenzae* type b (HIB), hepatitis B, pneumococcal and influenza vaccines should be given at the recommended times. Because of the possibility of development of vaccine-associated polio in the patient or in the patient's immunodeficient contacts (eg, mother) after administration of oral polio vaccine, the inactivated polio vaccine is recommended both for the patient and for healthy children in their households. The risk of measles is considered greater than the potential risk of the vaccine in asymptomatic children; thus, measles-mumps-rubella vaccine should be given at the usual time. The varicella vaccine, also a live virus, has not been approved for use in immunocompromised patients; studies of its safety and immunogenicity in HIV-infected children are underway. Varicella and measles may be fatal in HIV-infected children. Since antibody titers to vaccines decline with time and progressive immunodeficiency, prophylaxis with immune globulin for measles exposure should be given, regardless of immunization status. Varicella-zoster immune globulin should be given after each exposure to HIV-infected children without prior varicella-zoster infection. Infected children with a tetanus-prone wounds should receive tetanus immune globulin, regardless of immunization status.

2. Prophylactic treatments for infections–A number of effective prophylactic therapies for the prevention of opportunistic infections are available. Since patients taking all potential prophylactic therapies require extremely complicated medication regimens, which may result in a reduced quality of life, harmful drug interactions, or synergistic toxicities, caregivers need to prioritize the choice of prophylactic therapies for each child on the basis of specific risk factors or patient desires.

Antibiotic prophylaxis for *P carinii* has been extremely effective. Since this infection has its highest incidence during the first year of life, at a time when the infection status of the infant may still be unknown and during which rapid decline of CD4 lymphocyte count may occur within weeks, current recommendations are to treat all infants born to HIV-infected mothers from 4–6 weeks of age until a reasonably certain determination of HIV infection status can be made, usually by age 6 months. At that point, uninfected infants may have discontinued prophylaxis. Infected infants should continue on prophylactic drugs until 12 months, when further treatment will be based on assessment of age-adjusted CD4 lymphocyte counts during the first year of life and every 3 months thereafter. Published guidelines from the CDC are summarized in Table 36–4. The first choice for prophylaxis is trimethoprim-sulfamethoxazole (TMP/SMX) which is clearly more effective than other alternatives. For patients intolerant to TMP/SMX, dapsone or pentamidine (aerosolized for older children, intravenous for younger children) are secondary options (Table 36–5).

Monthly intravenous immune globulin (IVIG) is effective in reducing the number of bacterial infections and hospitalizations in HIV-infected children who are not receiving PCP prophylaxis with TMP/SMX. No criteria for the routine use of IVIG have been defined. Appropriate candidates for IVIG might be children with hypogammaglobulinemia, poor functional antibody development, or a history of serious or multiple bacterial infection.

Rifabutin has been approved for use as prophylaxis for MAC in adults and is recommended by the CDC for use in adults with CD4 counts less than 100. The frequency of disseminated MAC was reduced by 50% in HIV-infected adults with CD4 counts of less

Table 36–4. PCP prophylaxis for HIV-exposed and infected infants by age and HIV infection status.

Age/HIV Infection Status	PCP Prophylaxis
Birth to 4–6 wk	No prophylaxis
4–6 wk to 4 mo	Prophylaxis
4–12 mo	
HIV-infected or indeterminate	Prophylaxis
HIV infection reasonably excluded[1]	No prophylaxis
1–5 y, HIV-infected	Prophylaxis if: CD4 count <500 cells/μL or CD4 <15%[2,3]
6–12 y, HIV-infected	Prophylaxis if: CD4 count <200 cells/μL or CD4 15%[3]

Adapted from Centers for Disease Control. MMWR 1995; 44(No. RR-4):6.
[1]Among children who have had two or more negative HIV cultures or polymerase chain-reaction tests, both of which are performed at ≥ 1 months of age and one of which is performed at ≥4 months of age, or two or more negative HIV IgG antibody tests performed at >6 months of age among children who have no clinical evidence of HIV disease.
[2]Children 1–2 years of age who were receiving PCP prophylaxis and had a CD4 count <750 cells/μL or percentage of < 15% at <12 months of age should continue prophylaxis.
[3]Prophylaxis should be considered on a case-by-case basis for children who might otherwise be at risk for PCP, such as those with rapidly declining CD4 counts or percentages or children with category C conditions; children who have had PCP should receive lifelong PCP prophylaxis.
PCP = *Pneumocystis carinii* pneumonia.

Table 36–5. Drug regimens for PCP prophylaxis for children > 4 weeks of age.

Recommended regimen
Trimethoprim-sulfamethoxazole (TMP-SMX) 150 mg TMP/M[2]/d with 750 mg SMX/M[2]/d administered orally, divided into two doses per day 3 times weekly on consecutive days.
Acceptable alternative TMP-SMX dosage schedule (using same total daily dosage)
  Single daily dose 3 times per week on consecutive days
  Divided bid dose 7 days per week
  Divided bid dose 3 times per week on alternate days
Alternative regimens if TMP-SMX is not tolerated
Dapsone 2 mg/kg (not to exceed 100 mg) administered orally once daily
Aerosolized pentamidine (children > 5 y) 300 mg administered via Respirgard II inhaler monthly
Intravenous pentamidine 4 mg/kg administered every 2–4 weeks

Adapted from Centers for Disease Control. MMWR 1995: 44(No. RR-4);6.

than 200. Survival rates were not different in two large placebo-controlled trials. There are no data on the efficacy of rifabutin prophylaxis in children and no specific recommendations have been made for its use in children. The major adverse events have been elevated liver enzymes and uveitis, especially when used concurrently with fluconazole. Azithromycin and clarithromycin also have activity against MAC and are currently under study for MAC prophylaxis.

CMV-seropositive children with very low CD4 lymphocyte counts (less than 50–100) may benefit from ophthalmologic examinations every 3–6 months for early detection of retinitis, although this has not been studied rigorously. After CMV retinitis has been diagnosed, patients require induction treatment with intravenous ganciclovir and subsequent lifelong prophylaxis with ganciclovir. A clinical trial has recently demonstrated that prophylactic oral ganciclovir was nearly as effective in reducing the recurrence of CMV retinitis in infected adults as intravenous ganciclovir. Initial pharmacokinetic studies of this agent are ongoing in children.

Recurrent mucocutaneous and esophageal candidiasis can sometimes be prevented with topical treatments such as nystatin or clotrimazole. Some patients require chronic fluconazole treatment for effective control. Unfortunately, chronic treatment with this drug often result in emergence of fluconazole-resistant *Candida* isolates, subsequently requiring amphotericin B treatment for symptomatic disease. Some patients suffer recurrent severe herpes simplex or varicella-zoster infections. These may respond to or be prevented with oral acyclovir treatment.

HIV-infected children have a higher risk of progression of infections due to *Mycobacterium* tuberculosis. These children should have yearly Mantoux skin tests with several concurrent control skin tests (tetanus, candida, mumps). If the control skin tests are not reactive, the child may be anergic and results of the tuberculosis skin test are not reliable. Since the child's infection is usually acquired from adult household contacts, other household members should be also skin-tested for tuberculosis yearly, regardless of the anergy status of the HIV-infected child. Adults and children found to have positive tuberculosis skin tests should be further evaluated for disease and treated according to guidelines for HIV-infected persons.

3. Infections and other conditions–Unusual infections may require invasive diagnostic techniques such as biopsy or bronchoscopy. Bacterial infections should be diagnosed and treated aggressively. Varicella-zoster and herpes simplex virus infections should be treated with acyclovir. Mucocutaneous *Candida* infections that fail to resolve with topical antifungal medications may be treated with fluconazole. Symptomatic CMV infection should be treated with ganciclovir or foscarnet. MAC requires treatment with a multidrug regimen to delay the emergence of resistance. Lymphoid interstitial pneumonitis may respond to corticosteroid therapy. The long-term toxicity of corticosteroids in patients with HIV infection is unknown. Organ system disease (eg, encephalopathy, cardiomyopathy, and nephropathy) and chronic infections may improve with the initiation of or change in antiretroviral therapy. ZDV treatment has been associated with marked improvement in encephalopathic symptoms. Autoimmune thrombocytopenia may improve with IVIG or corticosteroid treatments. Anemia and granulocytopenia, whether drug-induced or HIV-induced, may respond to erythropoietin and granulocyte colony-stimulating factor (G-CSF), respectively. Transfusions may be needed; CMV-seronegative blood should be used. Most of these conditions are likely to be recurrent or chronic and most, following acquisition, will require either repeated or lifelong treatment.

4. General support–Growth failure (weight and height) is one of the earliest and most sensitive markers of disease progression. The cause is likely to be a complex combination of increased metabolic needs related to chronic infection and decreased caloric intake. Although controlled trials of the effects of nutritional intervention have been difficult to carry out, malnutrition is known to contribute to immunodeficiency and well-nourished HIV-infected children appear to have fewer infections, less fatigue, and a better quality of life. Nutritional evaluation and counseling should be a part of early care before problems arise. When a child's routine diet fails to provide adequate nutrition, supplemental nutrition in the form of oral supplements and nutritious snacks is often required. Supplemental feeding by gastrointestinal tubes may be required for children who are unable to consume adequate calories by the oral route.

Evaluation and support for psychosocial needs of HIV-affected families is imperative. As with other chronic illnesses, HIV infection has an impact on all family members and an additional social stigma. Emotional concerns and financial needs are often more prominent than medical needs at many stages of the disease and make an impact on the family's ability to carry out a medical treatment regimen. Ideally, care should be coordinated by a team of caregivers familiar with this disease, the newest therapies, and community resources.

Prognosis

Recent prospective natural history studies have demonstrated a median survival of more than 7 years. This is distinctly different from results of initial natural history studies, which suggested that over 80% of infants with vertically acquired HIV infection would be symptomatic during infancy and 80% would die by age 3 years. Poor prognosis in perinatal infection is associated with encephalopathy, infections with *P carinii,* early development of AIDS, and rapidly declining helper T-lymphocyte counts. Detection of HIV in the blood within 48 hours of birth (implying in utero infection) and viral burdens, which remain high during the first months of life may be associated with more rapid disease progression. The presence of lymphoid interstitial pneumonitis or parotitis is a sign of relatively good prognosis. Some perinatally infected children and many of those infected at older ages by blood products survive into adolescence. Because of the great variability in individual responses to infection and treatment, definite statements regarding the life expectancy or quality of life should not be made.

Public Health Issues

In general, the infant or child who is well enough to attend day care or school should be treated no differently from other children. The exception may be a toddler with uncontrollable biting behavior or bleeding lesions that cannot be adequately covered; in these situations, the child may be excluded from group day care. Routine good hygiene used for the prevention of transmission of other infectious diseases is appropriate for the prevention of common infections, which may be severe in the HIV-infected child. Optimally, the school health care provider and teacher will be aware of the diagnosis, but there is no legal requirement that any individual at the school or care center be informed. Parents and child may prefer to keep the diagnosis confidential, since the social consequences of HIV infection often overshadow the medical problems.

Horizontal transmission (ie, in the absence of sexual contact or injecting drug use) of HIV is exceedingly rare and is associated with exposure of broken skin or mucous membranes to HIV-infected blood or bloody secretions. Since undiagnosed, HIV-infected infants and children might be enrolled, all schools and care centers should have policies with simple guidelines for blood precautions to prevent transmission of HIV infection in these settings. Saliva, tears, urine, and stool are not contagious if there is no gross blood in these fluids. A barrier protection (eg, latex or rubber gloves, thick pads of fabric, or paper) should be used when possible contact with blood or bloody body fluids may occur. Sharp objects that might be contaminated with blood, such as razors or toothbrushes, should not be shared. No special care is required for dishes, towels, toys, or bedclothes. Blood-soiled clothing may be washed routinely with hot water and detergent. Contaminated surfaces may be easily disinfected with a variety of agents, including household bleach (1:10 dilution), some commercial disinfectants (eg, Lysol), and 70% isopropyl alcohol.

Conclusion

Pediatric HIV infection is a complex and multifaceted disease. Many aspects of care are under intense investigation, and recommendations for clinical care change frequently. Updated information should be sought whenever a child is diagnosed with HIV infection. With the recognition of the longer survival time in most infected children, this disease is now approached as a chronic illness. Primary care physicians are encouraged to participate in the care of HIV-infected children in collaboration with centers with expertise in pediatric HIV issues.

REFERENCES

American Academy of Pediatrics: HIV infection and AIDS. In: Peter G (editor). *1994 Red Book: Report of the Committee on Infectious Diseases,* 23rd ed. American Academy of Pediatrics, 1994:254.

Bryson Y et al: Clearance of HIV infection in a perinatally infected infant. N Engl J Med 1995;332:833.

Bryson Y, Luzuriaga K, Sullivan J, Wara D: Proposed definitions for in utero versus intrapartum transmission of HIV-1 [letter]. N Engl J Med 1992;327:1246.

Cao Y et al: Virologic and immunologic characterization of long-term survivors of human immunodeficiency virus type 1 infection. N Engl J Med 1995;332:201.

Centers for Disease Control and Prevention: Recommendations and Reports: 1993 Sexually Transmitted Diseases Treatment Guidelines. MMWR 1993;42(No. RR-14):1.

Centers for Disease Control and Prevention: Recommendations of the U.S. Public Health Service Task Force on the use of zidovudine to reduce perinatal transmission of human immunodeficiency virus. MMWR 1994;43:1.

Centers for Disease Control and Prevention: Recommendations on prophylaxis and therapy for disseminated *Mycobacterium avium* complex for adults and adolescents infected with human immunodeficiency virus. MMWR 1993;42:17.

Centers for Disease Control and Prevention: Update—barrier protection against HIV infection and other sexually transmitted diseases. MMWR 1993;43:589.

Centers for Disease Control and Prevention: 1994 revised classification system for human immunodeficiency virus infection in children less than 13 years of age. MMWR 1994;43:1.

Centers for Disease Control and Prevention: Human immunodeficiency virus transmission in household settings—United States. MMWR 1994;43:347, 353.

Centers for Disease Control and Prevention: USPHS/IDSA Guidelines for the prevention of opportunistic infections in persons infected with human immunodeficiency virus: A summary. MMWR 1995;44(No. RR-8):1.

Centers for Disease Control and Prevention: 1995 Revised guidelines for prophylaxis against *Pneumocystis carinii* pneumonia for children infected with or perinatally exposed to human immunodeficiency virus. MMWR 1995;44(No. RR-4):1.

Centers for Disease Control and Prevention: US Public Health Service recommendations for human immunodeficiency virus counseling and voluntary testing for pregnant women. MMWR 1995;44(No. RR-7):1.

Centers for Disease Control and Prevention: Update: AIDS among women—United States, 1994. MMWR 1995; 44:81.

Working Group on Antiretroviral Therapy: National Pediatric HIV Resource Center: Antiretroviral therapy and medical management of the human immunodeficiency virus-infected child. Pediatr Infect Dis J 1993;12:5132.

Church J: The diagnostic challenge of the child born "at risk" for HIV infection. Pediatr Clin North Am 1994;41:715.

Connor E et al: Reduction of maternal-infant transmission of human immunodeficiency virus type 1 with zidovudine treatment: Pediatric AIDS Clinical Trials Group Protocol 076 Study Group. N Engl J Med 1994; 331:1173.

Daar E, Moudgil T, Meyer R, Ho D: Transient high levels of viremia in patients with primary human immunodeficiency virus type 1 infection. N Engl J Med 1991; 324:961.

Denny T et al: Lymphocyte subsets in healthy children during the first 5 years of life. JAMA 1992;267:1484.

Drew W et al: Group for the Syntex Cooperative Oral Ganciclovir Study Group: Oral ganciclovir as maintenance treatment for cytomegalovirus retinitis in patients with AIDS. N Engl J Med 1995;333:615.

Ho D et al: Rapid turnover of plasma virions and CD4 lymphocytes in HIV-1 infection. Nature 1995;373:123.

Horsburgh C, Caldwell M, Simonds R: Epidemiology of disseminated nontuberculous mycobacterial disease in children with acquired immunodeficiency syndrome. Pediatr Infect Dis J 1993;12:219.

McKinney RJ, Wilfert C: Growth as a prognostic indicator in children with human immunodeficiency virus infection treated with zidovudine: AIDS Clinical Trials Group Protocol 043 Study Group. J Pediatr 1994; 125:728.

Pantaleo G, Graziosi C, Fauci A: New concepts in the immunopathogenesis of human immunodeficiency virus infection. N Engl J Med 1993;328:327.

Pantaleo G et al: HIV infection is active and progressive in lymphoid tissue during the clinically latent stage of disease. Nature 1993;362:355.

Peckham C, Gibb D: Mother-to-child transmission of the human immunodeficiency virus. N Engl J Med 1995; 333:298.

Pizzo P, Wilfert C: Antiretroviral therapy for infection due to human immunodeficiency virus in children. Clin Infect Dis 1994;19:177.

Simonds R, Chanock S: Medical issues related to caring for human immunodeficiency virus-infected children in and out of the home. Pediatr Infect Dis J 1993;12:845.

Spector S et al: Group, Pediatric AIDS Clinical Trials Group: A controlled trial of intravenous immune globulin for the prevention of serious bacterial infections in children receiving zidovudine for advanced human immunodeficiency virus infection. N Engl J Med 1994; 331:1181.

Task Force on Pediatric AIDS: Pediatric guidelines for infection control of human immunodeficiency virus (acquired immunodeficiency virus) in hospitals, medical offices, schools and other settings. Pediatrics 1988;82:801.

Tindall B, Cooper D: Primary HIV infection: Host responses and intervention strategies. AIDS 1991;5:1.

Tovo P et al: Prognostic factors and survival in children with perinatal HIV-1 infection: The Italian Register for HIV infections in children. Lancet 1992;339:1249.

Wilfert C, Wilson C, Luzuriaga K, Epstein L: Pathogenesis of pediatric human immunodeficiency virus type 1 infection. J Infect Dis 1994;170:286.

Infections: Bacterial & Spirochetal

37

John W. Ogle, MD

BACTERIAL INFECTIONS

GROUP A STREPTOCOCCAL INFECTIONS

Essentials of Diagnosis

Streptococcal pharyngitis:
- Clinical diagnosis based entirely on symptoms; signs and physical examination unreliable.
- Throat culture or rapid antigen detection test positive for group A streptococci.

Impetigo:
- Rapidly spreading, highly infectious skin rash.
- Erythematous denuded areas and honey–colored crusts.
- On culture, group A streptococci are grown in most (not all) cases.

General Considerations

Group A streptococci are common gram–positive bacteria capable of producing a wide variety of clinical illnesses. Prominent among these are acute pharyngitis; impetigo; cellulitis; and scarlet fever, the generalized illness caused by strains that elaborate erythrogenic toxin. Group A streptococci can also cause pneumonia, septic arthritis, osteomyelitis, meningitis, and numerous other less common infections. Group A streptococcal infections may also produce nonsuppurative sequelae (rheumatic fever or acute glomerulonephritis).

The cell walls of streptococci contain both carbohydrate and protein antigens. The C-carbohydrate antigen determines the *group*, and the M- or T-protein antigens determine the specific *type*. In most strains, the M protein appears to confer virulence, and antibodies developed against the M protein are protective against reinfection with that type.

Group A streptococci are almost all β-hemolytic. These organisms may be carried asymptomatically on the skin and in the pharynx, rectum, and vagina. Ten to 15 percent of school children in some studies are asymptomatic pharyngeal carriers of group A streptococci. Streptococcal carriers are asymptomatic individuals who do not mount an immune response to the organism and are therefore believed to be at low risk for nonsuppurative sequelae. Unfortunately, there are no accepted criteria for identification of streptococcal carriers.

All group A streptococci are sensitive to penicillin. Resistance to erythromycin is common in some countries and has increased in the United States.

Clinical Findings
A. Symptoms and Signs:
1. Respiratory infections–
a. Infancy and early childhood (under 3 years of age)–The onset of infection is insidious, with mild symptoms, eg, low-grade fever, serous nasal discharge, and pallor. Otitis media is common. Pharyngitis with exudate and cervical adenitis are uncommon in this age group.

b. Childhood type–Onset is sudden, with fever and marked malaise and often with repeated vomiting. The pharynx is sore and edematous, and the tonsillar area generally shows exudate. Anterior cervical lymph nodes are tender and enlarged. Small petechiae are frequently seen on the soft palate. Fine discrete petechiae occasionally appear also on the upper abdomen and trunk. In scarlet fever, the skin is diffusely erythematous and appears sunburned and roughened (sandpaper rash). The rash is most intense in the axillas and groin and on the abdomen and trunk. It blanches on pressure except in the skin folds, which do not blanch and are pigmented (Pastia's sign). The rash usually appears 24 hours after the onset of fever and rapidly spreads over the next 1–2 days. Desquamation begins on the face at the end of the first week and becomes generalized by the third week. Early, the surface of the tongue is coated white, with the papillae enlarged and bright red ("white strawberry tongue"). Subsequently, desquamation occurs, and the tongue appears beefy red ("red strawberry tongue"). The face generally shows circumoral pallor. Petechiae may be seen on all mucosal surfaces.

c. Adult type–The adult type is characterized by exudative or nonexudative tonsillitis with fewer systemic manifestations, lower fever, and no vomiting. Scarlet fever is uncommon in this age group.

2. Impetigo–Streptococcal impetigo begins as a papule that vesiculates and then breaks, leaving a denuded area covered by a honey-colored crust. Both *Staphylococcus aureus* and group A streptococci are isolated in some cases. The lesions spread readily and diffusely. Local lymph nodes may become swollen and inflamed. Although the affected child often lacks systemic symptoms, occasionally a high fever and toxicity are present. If flaccid bullae are present, the disease is called bullous impetigo and is caused by an epidermolytic toxin-producing strain of *S aureus*.

3. Cellulitis–The portal of entry is often an insect bite or superficial abrasion on an extremity. There is a diffuse and rapidly spreading cellulitis that involves the subcutaneous tissues and extends along the lymphatic pathways with only minimal local suppuration. Local acute lymphadenitis occurs. The child is usually acutely ill, with fever and malaise. In classic erysipelas, the involved area is bright red, swollen, warm, and very tender. The infection may extend rapidly from the lymphatics to the bloodstream.

Streptococcal perianal cellulitis is an entity peculiar to young children. Pain with defecation often leads to constipation, which may be the presenting complaint. The child is afebrile and otherwise well. Perianal erythema and tenderness and painful rectal examination are the only abnormal physical findings. Culture of a perianal swab specimen usually yields a heavy growth of group A streptococcus. A variant of this syndrome is streptococcal vaginitis in prepubertal girls. Symptoms are dysuria and pain; marked erythema and tenderness of the introitus and blood-tinged discharge are seen.

4. Necrotizing fasciitis–This dangerous disease is being more frequently reported, particularly complicating varicella. Only 20–40% of cases are due to group A streptococci. About 30–40% are due to *S aureus* and the rest to mixed bacterial infections. The disease is characterized by extensive necrosis of superficial fasciae, with undermining of surrounding tissue and extreme systemic toxicity. Initially, the skin overlying the infection is pale red without distinct borders, resembling subcutaneous cellulitis. Blisters or bullae may appear. The color deepens to a distinct purple. The involved area may develop mild to massive edema. Early recognition and aggressive debridement of necrotic tissue are essential.

5. Group A streptococcal infections in newborn nurseries–Group A streptococcal epidemics still occasionally occur in nurseries. The organism may be introduced into the nursery from the vaginal tract of a mother or from the throat or nose of a mother or member of the staff. The organism then spreads from infant to infant. The umbilical stump is colonized while the infant is in the nursery. As is true also in staphylococcal infections, there may be no or few clinical manifestations while infants are still in the nursery; most often, a colonized infant develops a chronic, oozing omphalitis days later at home. The organism may spread from the infant to other family members. More serious and even fatal infections may develop, including sepsis, meningitis, empyema, septic arthritis, and peritonitis.

6. Streptococcal sepsis–Serious illness from group A streptococcal sepsis is now more common both in children and in adults. Rash and scarlet fever may be present; prostration and shock result in high mortality rates. Pharyngitis is uncommon as an antecedent illness. Underlying disease is a predisposing factor. Some authors hypothesize that a more virulent clone of group A streptococci is responsible for the increase in cases of streptococcal sepsis.

B. Laboratory Findings: Leukocytosis with a marked shift to the left is seen early. Eosinophilia regularly appears during convalescence. β-Hemolytic streptococci are cultured from the throat. The organism may be cultured from the skin and by needle aspiration from subcutaneous tissues and other involved sites, such as infected nodes. Occasionally, blood cultures are positive. Group A streptococci may be identified most easily by demonstrable sensitivity to bacitracin. Grouping by immunofluorescence or coagglutination studies correlates best with the original precipitin reactions described by Lancefield. M and T typing is not routinely done.

Rapid antigen detection tests are 60–95% sensitive and over 95% specific for detecting group A streptococci in throat swabs. The predictive value of negative tests is about 80%, meaning that one in five patients with a positive throat culture will have a negative rapid antigen test. Rapid tests may be useful when early antibiotic therapy is considered, but because the currently available tests lack sensitivity, a standard culture should be done on specimens testing negative.

Antistreptolysin O (ASO) titers rise about 150 units within 2 weeks after an acute infection. Elevated ASO and anti-DNase B titers are useful in documenting prior throat infections in cases of acute rheumatic fever. However, elevated anti-DNase B and antihyaluronidase titers are most useful in associating pyoderma and acute glomerulonephritis. The streptozyme test is a 2-minute slide test that detects antibodies to streptolysin O, hyaluronidase, streptokinase, DNase B, and NADase. It is somewhat more sensitive than the measurement of ASO titers.

Proteinuria, cylindruria, and minimal hematuria may be seen early in children with streptococcal infection. True poststreptococcal glomerulonephritis is seen 1–4 weeks after the respiratory or skin infection.

Differential Diagnosis

Streptococcal infection in early childhood must be differentiated from adenovirus and other respiratory virus infections.

Adenoviruses, coxsackieviruses (both A and B), echoviruses, Epstein-Barr virus (infectious mononucleosis), and many respiratory viruses can produce pharyngitis. The pharyngitis in herpangina (coxsackie A viruses) is vesicular or ulcerative. Herpes simplex also causes ulcerative lesions, which most commonly involve the anterior pharynx, tongue, and gums. With other viruses (coxsackieviruses and echoviruses), rashes are common. In infectious mononucleosis, the pharyngitis is often exudative. Splenomegaly and generalized adenopathy are typical, and laboratory findings are often diagnostic (atypical lymphocytes, elevated liver enzymes, and a positive heterophil or other serologic test for mononucleosis). Uncomplicated streptococcal pharyngitis improves within 24–48 hours if penicillin is given and by 72–96 hours without antimicrobials.

Group G and group C streptococci are uncommon causes of pharyngitis but have been implicated in epidemics of sore throat in college students. Acute rheumatic fever does not occur following group G or C infection, though acute glomerulonephritis is a complication.

Arcanobacterium hemolyticum is also a cause of pharyngitis. Scarlatinal or maculopapular truncal rashes may be been seen.

In diphtheria, systemic symptoms, vomiting, and fever are less marked; pharyngeal pseudomembrane is confluent and adherent; the throat is less red; and cervical adenopathy is prominent.

Pharyngeal tularemia causes white rather than yellow exudate. There is little erythema, and cultures for β-hemolytic streptococci are negative. A history of exposure to rabbits and a failure to respond to antimicrobials may suggest the diagnosis Response to specific antibiotic therapy is prompt.

Leukemia and agranulocytosis may present with pharyngitis and are diagnosed by bone marrow examination.

Scarlet fever must be differentiated from other exanthematous diseases, principally rubella, erythema due to sunburn, drug reactions, Kawasaki disease, toxic shock syndrome, and staphylococcal scalded skin syndrome. (See also Table 38–3.)

Complications

Suppurative complications of group A streptococcal infections include sinusitis, otitis, mastoiditis, cervical lymphadenitis, pneumonia, empyema, septic arthritis, and meningitis. Spread of streptococcal infection from the throat to other sites—principally the skin (impetigo) and vagina—is common and should be considered in every instance of chronic vaginal discharge or chronic skin infection, such as that complicating childhood eczema.

Both acute rheumatic fever and acute glomerulonephritis are nonsuppurative complications of group A streptococcal infections.

A. Acute Rheumatic Fever: See Chapter 19.

B. Acute Glomerulonephritis: Acute nephritis can follow streptococcal infections of either the pharynx or the skin—in contrast to rheumatic fever, which follows pharyngeal infection only. Glomerulonephritis may occur at any age, including infancy. In most reported series of acute glomerulonephritis, males predominate by a ratio of 2:1, whereas acute rheumatic fever occurs with equal frequency in both sexes.

Certain M types are strongly associated with poststreptococcal glomerulonephritis ("nephritogenic types"). Moreover, the serotypes resident on or producing disease on the skin often differ from those found in the pharynx.

The incidence of acute glomerulonephritis after streptococcal infection is variable and has ranged from nil to 28%. Several outbreaks of acute glomerulonephritis in families have involved 50–75% of siblings of affected patients in 1- to 7-week periods. Second attacks of glomerulonephritis are rare. The median latent period between infection and the development of glomerulonephritis is 10 days. This contrasts with acute rheumatic fever, which occurs after a median latent period of 18 days.

Treatment

A. Specific Measures: Treatment is directed not only toward eradication of acute infection but also toward the prevention of rheumatic fever. In patients with pharyngitis, antibiotics should be started early to relieve symptoms and should be continued for 10 days to prevent rheumatic fever. Although early therapy has not been shown to prevent glomerulonephritis, it seems advisable to promptly treat impetigo in sibling contacts of patients with poststreptococcal nephritis. Neither sulfonamides nor trimethoprim-sulfamethoxazole is effective in the treatment of streptococcal infections.

Although topical therapy for impetigo with antimicrobial ointments (eg, bacitracin, mupirocin) is as effective as systemic therapy, it does not eradicate pharyngeal carriage and is less practical for extensive disease.

1. Penicillin–A single dose of benzathine penicillin G given intramuscularly (0.6 million units for children weighing < 60 lb and 1.2 million units for children weighing > 60 lb) is preferred for treatment of pharyngitis and impetigo. Phenoxymethyl penicillin (penicillin V) (250 mg for children weighing < 40 lb and 500 mg for children weighing > 40 lb) administered orally three or four times daily between meals for 10 days is successful in about 90% of cases. Giving penicillin V (250 mg) twice daily is as effective as more frequent oral administration or intramuscular therapy and may achieve better compliance, but a single daily dose results in a higher failure rate. Parenteral therapy is indicated if there is vomiting or sepsis. Mild cellulitis may be similarly treated. Cellulitis requiring hospitalization should be treated with aqueous penicillin G (150,000 units/kg/d intravenously in four to six divided doses) or procaine penicillin (50,000 units/kg intramuscularly once or twice a day) until there is marked improvement. Penicillin V, 125–250 mg every 6 hours, may then be given orally to complete a 10-day course. Acute cervical lymphadenitis may require incision and drainage. Treatment of necrotizing fasciitis requires emergency surgical debridement followed by high-dose parenteral antibiotics appropriate to the organisms cultured.

2. Other antibiotics–For pharyngitis or impetigo, erythromycin estolate (20–40 mg/kg/d in two to four divided doses) should be given for 10 days. Erythromycin ethyl succinate (40–50 mg/kg/d) is best tolerated if given in four divided doses. Both erythromycin preparations are best absorbed and tolerated when taken with food. Clindamycin, cephalexin, cefuroxime, cefaclor, loracarbef, cefprozil, cefpodoxime, cefixime, and cefadroxil are also effective oral antimicrobials. Cefixime and cefadroxil may be given once daily, whereas cefuroxime, loracarbef, cefprozil, and cefaclor may be used twice daily. In most studies, bacteriologic failures after cephalosporin therapy are less frequent than failures following penicillin. However, cephalosporins are far more expensive than penicillin, and penicillin currently remains the agent of choice. The dosage of clindamycin is 10–20 mg/kg/d in four divided doses. Each of these drugs should be given for 10 days. Many strains are resistant to tetracycline. For serious infections in patients with known penicillin allergy, cefazolin (100–150 mg/kg/d intravenously or intramuscularly in three divided doses), clindamycin (25–40 mg/kg/d intravenously in four divided doses), or vancomycin (40 mg/kg/d intravenously in four divided doses) should be given. Clindamycin is preferred by many and may be superior to penicillin for necrotizing fasciitis.

3. Treatment failure–Even when compliance is perfect, organisms will be found in 5–15% of children cultured after cessation of therapy. Reculture is indicated only in the patient with pharyngitis who has a personal or family history of rheumatic fever. Re-treatment at least once with an oral cephalosporin or clindamycin is indicated in patients with recurrent culture positive pharyngitis.

4. Prevention of recurrences in rheumatic individuals–The preferred prophylaxis for rheumatic individuals is benzathine penicillin G, 1.2 million units intramuscularly every 3 weeks. One of the following alternative oral prophylactic regimens may be used: sulfadiazine, 0.5–1 g daily; penicillin G, 200,000 units twice daily; or erythromycin, 250 mg twice daily. Most authorities feel that lifelong prophylaxis is indicated, particularly in the presence of rheumatic heart disease. A similar approach to the prevention of recurrences of glomerulonephritis is debatable but may be indicated during childhood when there is a suspicion that repeated streptococcal infections coincide with flare-ups of acute glomerulonephritis.

B. General Measures: Analgesic lozenges or gargles with 30% glucose or warm saline solution may be used for relief of sore throat. A soft, bland diet that includes noncarbonated high-glucose drinks (such as apple, grape, and pear juice) and iced milk or sherbet is helpful. Acetaminophen is useful for pain or fever.

With impetigo, local treatment may promote earlier healing. Crusts should first be soaked off; areas beneath the crusts should then be washed with soap daily.

C. Treatment of Complications: Acute complications are best treated with penicillin. Rheumatic fever is best prevented by early and adequate penicillin treatment of the streptococcal infection (see above).

D. Treatment of Carriers: Identification and management of group A streptococcal carriers is difficult. There are no established clinical or serologic criteria for differentiating carriers from the truly infected. Some children receive multiple courses of antimicrobials, with persistence of group A streptococci in the throat, leading to a "streptococcal neurosis" on the part of families.

Clindamycin (20 mg/kg/d in four divided doses) given orally or a combination of rifampin (20 mg/kg/d for 4 days) given orally and penicillin in standard dosage given orally has been used to improve bacteriologic cure rates after streptococcal pharyngitis and may be useful in selected streptococcal carriers.

Prognosis

Death is rare except in infants or young children with sepsis or pneumonia. The febrile course is shortened and complications eliminated by early and adequate treatment with penicillin.

Bisno AL: Group A streptococcal infections and acute rheumatic fever. N Engl J Med 1991;325:783.

Bisno AL, Stevens DL: Streptococcal infections of skin and soft tissues. N Engl J Med 1996;334:240.

Chaudhary S et al: Penicillin V and rifampin for the treatment of group A streptococcal pharyngitis: A randomized trial of 10 days penicillin vs 10 days penicillin with rifampin during the final 4 days of therapy. J Pediatr 1985;106:481.

Dajani A et al: Treatment of acute streptococcal pharyngitis and prevention of rheumatic fever: A statement for health professionals. Pediatrics 1995;96:758.

Gerber MA, Randolph MF, Mayo DR: The group A streptococcal carrier state. Am J Dis Child 1988;142:562.

Moses AE et al: Increased incidence and severity of *Streptococcus pyogenes* bacteremia in young children. Pediatr Infect Dis J 1995;14:767.

Shulman ST et al: Streptococcal pharyngitis: The case for penicillin. Pediatr Infect Dis J 1994;13:1.

GROUP B STREPTOCOCCAL INFECTIONS

Essentials of Diagnosis

Early-onset neonatal infection:
- Newborn infant, age birth to 7 days, with rapidly progressing overwhelming sepsis, with or without meningitis.
- Pneumonia with respiratory failure frequently present; chest x-ray resembles that seen in hyaline membrane disease.
- Leukopenia with a shift to the left.
- Blood or spinal fluid cultures growing group B streptococci.

Late-onset infection:
- Meningitis, sepsis, or other focal infection in a child 1–16 weeks old with spinal fluid or blood cultures growing group B streptococci.

General Considerations

Although most patients with group B streptococcal disease are infants under 3 months of age, cases are seen in infants 4–5 months of age. Serious infection also occurs in women with puerperal sepsis, in immunocompromised patients, in patients with cirrhosis and spontaneous peritonitis, and in diabetics with cellulitis. Group B streptococcal infections occur as frequently as gram-negative infections in the newborn period. Two distinct clinical syndromes distinguished by differing perinatal events, age at onset, and serotype of the infecting strain have been described in these infants.

Clinical Findings

Early-onset illness is observed in newborns less than 7 days old. The onset of symptoms in the majority of these infants occurs in the first 48 hours of life, and most are ill within 6 hours. Apnea is often the first sign. There is a high incidence of associated maternal obstetric complications, especially premature labor and prolonged rupture of the membranes. Newborns with early-onset disease are severely ill at the time of diagnosis, and the mortality rate is more than 50%. Although most infants with early-onset infections are full term, premature infants are at increased risk for the disease. Newborns with early-onset infection acquire group B streptococci from the maternal genital tract in utero or during passage through the birth canal. When early-onset infection is complicated by meningitis, as occurs in approximately 30% of cases, more than 80% of the bacterial isolates belong to serotype III. Postmortem examination of infants with early-onset disease almost always reveals pulmonary inflammatory infiltrates and hyaline membranes containing large numbers of group B streptococci.

Late-onset infection occurs in infants between 7 days and 4 months of age; the median age at onset is about 4 weeks. Maternal obstetric complications are infrequently associated with late-onset infection. These infants are usually not as severely ill at the time of diagnosis as those with early-onset disease, and the mortality rate is significantly lower. In recent series, about 37% of patients have meningitis and 46% have sepsis. Other clinical manifestations, such as septic arthritis and osteomyelitis, "occult" bacteremia, otitis media, ethmoiditis, conjunctivitis, cellulitis (particularly of the face or submandibular area), lymphadenitis, breast abscess, empyema, and impetigo, have been described. Strains of group B streptococci possessing the capsular type III polysaccharide antigen are isolated from more than 95% of infants with late-onset disease, regardless of clinical manifestations. The exact mode of transmission of the organisms is not well defined.

Type III group B streptococci that cause neonatal disease are genetically closely related. Dissemination of a clone of high virulence in neonates is responsible for the increase in cases of disease reported from many nurseries in the 1970s and 1980s.

Prevention

Many women of childbearing age possess circulating antibody to the polysaccharide antigen of type III group B streptococci. This antibody is transferred to the newborn via the placental circulation. Carriers delivering healthy infants have significant serum levels of IgG antibody to this antigen. In contrast, women delivering infants who develop type III group B streptococcal disease of either the early- or late-onset type rarely have detectable antibody in their sera. Similar findings have recently been described for type Ia infections.

A vaccine prepared with type III polysaccharide has been evaluated in pregnant women. Although the vaccine is not optimally immunogenic, 63% of mothers produced IgG antibody.

The American Academy of Pediatrics recommends screening all pregnant women for group B streptococcus at 26–28 weeks of gestation by cultures obtained from both the rectum and the lower vagina using a selective broth medium. Women with positive cultures or rapid antigen tests who also have one or more risk factors should receive ampicillin intravenously intrapartum. The risk factors are (1) preterm labor at less than 37 weeks of gestation, (2) premature rupture of membranes at less than 37 weeks of gestation, (3) fever during labor, (4) multiple births, and (5) rupture of membranes beyond 18 hours at any gestation. Mothers who deliver an infant infected with group B streptococci should receive intrapartum antibiotic chemoprophylaxis with each subsequent delivery. Application of these guidelines would significantly reduce early-onset disease, but the practice is controversial because they are difficult and expensive to implement.

Diagnosis

Culture of group B streptococci from a normally sterile site such as blood or cerebrospinal fluid provides proof of diagnosis. Frequent false-positive results limit the usefulness of testing for group B streptococcal antigen.

Treatment

Penicillin G is the drug of choice. Group B streptococci are less susceptible than other streptococci to penicillin, and high doses are recommended, especially for meningitis (at least 250,000 units/kg/d, given in three doses per day to infants less than 1 week old and in four doses per day to older infants). Aminoglycosides act synergistically with penicillin in vitro; for this reason, both penicillin and gentamicin should be used for meningitis and other serious infections. Penicillin dosage for nonmeningeal infections is 50,000 units/kg/d (in divided doses every 12 hours) for infants less than 1 week old and 75,000–100,000 units/kg/d (in divided doses every 8 hours) for older infants. Duration of therapy is 3 weeks for meningitis, at least 4 weeks for osteomyelitis or endocarditis, and 10–14 days for other infections. Therapy does not eradicate carriage of the organism. Ceftriaxone is active in vitro against group B streptococci, and because of its long serum half-life it may be given once or twice daily intramuscularly or intravenously. Ceftriaxone is sometimes used to complete a course of therapy when intravenous access has become difficult.

Adams WG et al: Outbreak of group B streptococcal sepsis, Pediatr Infect Dis J 1993;12:565.

American Academy of Pediatrics Committee on Infectious Diseases: Guidelines for prevention of group B streptococcal (GBS) infection by chemoprophylaxis. Pediatrics 1992;90:775.

Baker CJ et al: Immunization of pregnant women with a polysaccharide vaccine of group B streptococcus. N Engl J Med 1988;319:1180.

Edwards MS et al: Long-term sequelae of group B streptococcal meningitis in infants. J Pediatr 1985;106:717.

Fischer GW: Immunoglobulin therapy of neonatal group B streptococcal infections: An overview. Pediatr Infect Dis J 1988;7(Suppl):13.

Gibbs RS et al: Consensus: Perinatal prophylaxis for group B streptococcal infection. Pediatr Infect Dis J 1992; 11:179.

Hussain SM et al: Invasive group B streptococcal disease in children beyond infancy. Pediatr Infect Dis J 1995; 14:278.

Katz V et al: Group B streptococci: Results of a protocol of antepartum screening and intrapartum treatment. Am J Obstet Gynecol 1994;170:521.

Larsen JW, Dooley SL: Group B *Streptococcus* infections: An obstetrical viewpoint. Pediatrics 1993;91:148.

Noya FJ, Baker CJ: Prevention of group B streptococcal infection. Infect Dis Clin North Am 1992;6:41.

Perkins MD, Mirrett S, Reller LB: Rapid bacterial antigen detection is not clinically useful. J Clin Microbiol 1995;33:1486.

STREPTOCOCCAL INFECTIONS WITH ORGANISMS OTHER THAN GROUP A OR B

Streptococci of groups other than A and B are part of the normal flora of humans and can cause disease. Group C or G organisms occasionally produce pharyngitis (with an ASO rise) but without risk of subsequent rheumatic fever, though acute glomerulonephritis may occasionally occur. Group D streptococci and *Enterococcus* are normal inhabitants of the gastrointestinal tract and may produce urinary tract infections, meningitis and sepsis in the newborn, and endocarditis. Nosocomial infections caused by *Enterococcus* are frequent in neonatal and oncology units. Nonhemolytic aerobic streptococci and α-hemolytic streptococci are normal flora of the mouth. They are involved in the production of dental plaque and probably dental caries and are the most common cause of subacute infective endocarditis. Finally, there are numerous anaerobic and microaerophilic streptococci, normal flora of the mouth, skin, and gastrointestinal tract, which alone or in combination with other bacteria may cause sinusitis, dental abscesses, brain abscesses, and intra-abdominal or lung abscesses.

Treatment

A. Enterococcal Infections: Urinary tract infections can be treated with oral amoxicillin alone. Sepsis or meningitis in the newborn should be treated intravenously with a combination of ampicillin (100–200 mg/kg/d in three divided doses) and gentamicin (6–7.5 mg/kg/d in three divided doses). Endocarditis requires at least 30 days of intravenous treatment. Penicillin G (250,000 units/kg/d in six to eight divided doses) plus streptomycin (30 mg/kg/d) or gentamicin (6–7.5 mg/kg/d in three divided doses) is most often used. Third-generation cephalosporins are not effective. Ampicillin-resistant enterococci are usually susceptible to vancomycin (40–60 mg/kg/d in four divided doses). Careful monitoring of aminoglycoside levels is required, both to avoid toxicity and to ensure therapeutic levels.

Whenever endocarditis is being treated, peak and trough serum killing powers should be obtained. A bactericidal level of 1:8 or greater immediately before the next penicillin dose should be maintained.

High-level resistance to aminoglycosides (MIC > 1000 µg/mL) is an increasing problem in many hospitals. Vancomycin resistance has also increased. Patients with serious enterococcal infections require consultation with infectious disease experts and with the clinical microbiology laboratory to determine the optimal combination of antimicrobials.

B. Viridans Streptococcal Infections (Subacute Infective Endocarditis): It is important to determine the penicillin sensitivity of the infecting strain as early as possible in the treatment of viridans streptococcal endocarditis. Resistant organisms are most commonly seen in patients receiving chronic penicillin prophylaxis for rheumatic heart disease. Strains sensitive to penicillin G (MIC < 0.1 µg/mL) may be treated for 4 weeks with penicillin, 150,000–200,000 units/kg/d intravenously, with gentamicin added during the first 2 weeks. If the MIC is 0.5 µg/mL or higher, longer therapy and higher doses of penicillin G must be used (200,000–300,000 units/kg/d intravenously in combination with streptomycin or gentamicin for 4–6 weeks). If the MIC is 0.1–0.5 µg/mL, penicillin G at the higher dose for a minimum of 4 weeks is recommended, with gentamicin added for the first 2 weeks. Vancomycin, 40 mg/kg/d, is usually preferred for resistant strains and patients allergic to penicillin.

Boulanger JM, Ford-Jones EL, Matlow AG: Enterococcal bacteremia in a pediatric institution: A four-year review. Rev Infect Dis 1991;13:847.

Chia JKS et al: Use of bacitracin therapy for infection due to vancomycin-resistant *Enterococcus faecium* Clin Infect Dis 1995;21,1520.

Moellering RC: Emergency *Enterococcus* as a significant pathogen. Clin Infect Dis 1992;14:1173.

Norris AN et al: Chloramphenicol for vancomycin-resistant enterococcal infections. Clin Infect Dis 1995;20:1137.

Rice LB, Shales DM: Vancomycin resistance in the *Enterococcus*: Relevance in Pediatrics. Pediatr Clin North Am 1995;42:601.

Simon RM, Dobson MB, Baker CJ: Enterococcal sepsis in neonates: Features by age at onset and occurrence of focal infection. Pediatrics 1990;85:165.

PNEUMOCOCCAL INFECTIONS

Essentials of Diagnosis

Bacteremia:
- High fever (≥ 39.4 °C).
- Leukocytosis (≥ 15,000/µL).
- Age 6–24 months.

Pneumonia:
- Fever, leukocytosis, and tachypnea.
- Localized chest pain.
- Localized or diffuse rales. Chest x-ray may show lobar infiltrate (with effusion).

Meningitis:
- Fever, leukocytosis.
- Bulging fontanelle, neck stiffness.
- Irritability and lethargy.

All types:
- Diagnosis confirmed by cultures of blood, spinal fluid, pleural fluid, or other body fluid.

General Considerations

Pneumococcal sepsis, sinusitis, otitis media, pneumonitis, meningitis, osteomyelitis, cellulitis, arthritis, vaginitis, and peritonitis are all part of a spectrum of pneumococcal infection. Clinical findings that correlate with occult bacteremia in ambulatory patients include age (6–24 months), degree of temperature elevation (≥ 39.4 °C), and leukocytosis (≥ 15,000/µL). Although each of these findings is in itself nonspecific, a combination of them should arouse suspicion. This constellation of findings in a child who has no focus of infection may be an indication for blood cultures and antibiotic therapy. The cause of two thirds of such bacteremic episodes is pneumococci.

Streptococcus pneumoniae is the most common cause of acute purulent otitis media.

Pneumococci are the organisms responsible for most cases of acute bacterial pneumonia in children. The disease is indistinguishable on clinical grounds from other bacterial pneumonias. Effusions are common, though frank empyema is less common. Abscesses also occasionally occur.

Pneumococcal meningitis is now more common than *H influenzae* type b meningitis because of widespread vaccination. Pneumococcal meningitis, sometimes recurrent, may complicate serious head trauma, particularly if there is persistent leakage of cerebrospinal fluid. This has led some physicians to recommend the prophylactic administration of penicillin or other antimicrobials in such cases.

Children with sickle cell disease, other hemoglobinopathies, congenital or acquired asplenia, and some immunoglobulin and complement deficiencies are unusually susceptible to overwhelming pneumococcal sepsis and meningitis. These children often have a catastrophic illness with shock and disseminated intravascular coagulation. Even with excellent supportive care, the mortality rate is 20–50%. The spleen is important in the control of pneumococcal infection by clearing organisms from the blood and producing an opsonin that enhances phagocytosis. Autosplenectomy may explain why children with sickle cell disease are at increased risk for developing serious pneumococcal infections.

S pneumoniae rarely causes serious disease in the neonate. Although *S pneumoniae* does not normally colonize the vagina, transient colonization does occur. Serious neonatal disease—including pneumonia, sepsis, and meningitis—may occur and clinically is similar to group B streptococcal infection.

For more than 30 years, penicillin has been the agent of choice for pneumococcal infections. Most strains are still highly susceptible to penicillin; however, there have been increasing reports of pneumococci with moderately increased resistance to penicillin and reports of treatment failure, particularly in meningitis. The prevalence of these relatively penicillin-resistant strains in North America varies from 3% to 35%. Pneumococci with high-level resistance to penicillin and multiple other drugs are increasingly encountered throughout the United States. Pneumococci from normally sterile body fluids should be screened routinely for susceptibility to penicillin as well as other drugs.

Pneumococci have been classified into 83 serotypes based on capsular polysaccharide antigens. Serotypes 6, 14, 18, 19, and 23 cause most pneumococcal infections in children. The frequency distribution of serotypes varies at different times, in different geographic areas, and with different sites of infection. The most recently developed polyvalent pneumococcal vaccine contains capsular polysaccharides of 23 serotypes and is discussed in Chapter 10. Specific antibody induced by the vaccine protects only against the serotypes included in the vaccine. Children under age 18–24 months generally do not have a good antibody response to this vaccine, and the protective efficacy of the vaccine in older children is controversial. Despite these limitations, the vaccine is recommended for high-risk children over 2 years of age. The successful development of conjugate vaccines that protect against *H influenzae* type b has spurred the development of protein-polysaccharide conjugates to protect against pneumococci.

Clinical Findings

A. Symptoms and Signs: In pneumococcal sepsis, fever usually appears abruptly, often accompanied by chills. There may be no respiratory symptoms. In pneumococcal sinusitis, mucopurulent nasal discharge may occur. In infants and young children with pneumonia, fever, and tachypnea without auscultatory changes are the usual presenting signs. Respiratory distress is manifested by flaring of the alae nasi, chest retractions, and tachypnea. Abdominal pain is common. In older children, the adult form of pneumococcal pneumonia with signs of lobar consolidation may occur, but sputum is rarely bloody. Thoracic pain resulting from pleural involvement is sometimes present, but less often in children than in adults. With involvement of the right hemidiaphragm, pain may be referred to the right lower quadrant, suggesting appendicitis. Vomiting is common at onset but seldom persists. Convulsions are relatively common at onset in infants.

Meningitis is characterized by fever, irritability, convulsions, and neck stiffness. The most important sign in very young infants is a tense, bulging anterior fontanelle. In older children, fever, chills, headache, and vomiting are common symptoms. Classic signs are nuchal rigidity associated with positive Brudzinski and Kernig signs. With progression of untreated disease, the child may develop opisthotonos, stupor, and coma.

B. Laboratory Findings: Leukocytosis is often pronounced (20,000–45,000/μL), with 80–90% polymorphonuclear neutrophils. Neutropenia may be seen early in very serious infections. The presence of pneumococci in the nasopharynx is not a helpful finding, because up to 40% of normal children carry pneumococci in the upper respiratory tract. Large numbers of organisms seen on gram-stained smears of endotracheal aspirates are seen with pneumonia. In meningitis, cerebrospinal fluid usually shows an elevated white cell count of several thousand, chiefly polymorphonuclear neutrophils, with decreased glucose and elevated protein levels. Gram-positive diplococci are seen on stained smears of cerebrospinal fluid sediment in 70–90% of cases. Antigen detection tests are not useful.

Differential Diagnosis

There are many causes of high fever and leukocytosis in young infants; 80–90% of children presenting with these signs have a disease other than pneumococcal bacteremia, such as herpesvirus 6, enterovirus, or other viral infection, urinary tract infection, unrecognized focal infection elsewhere in the body, or early acute shigellosis (diarrhea will appear later).

Infants with upper respiratory tract infection who subsequently develop signs of lower respiratory disease are most likely to be infected with a respiratory virus. Hoarseness or wheezing is often present. X-ray of the chest typically shows perihilar infiltrates and increased bronchovascular markings. It must be remembered, however, that viral respiratory infection often precedes pneumococcal pneumonia and that the clinical picture may be mixed.

Staphylococcal pneumonia frequently causes cavities and empyema, but it may be indistinguishable early in its course from pneumococcal pneumonia. It is most common in infants.

In primary pulmonary tuberculosis, children are not toxic, and x-rays show a primary focus associated with hilar adenopathy and often with pleural involvement. Miliary tuberculosis presents a classic x-ray appearance.

Pneumonia caused by *Mycoplasma pneumoniae* is most common in children 5 years of age and older. Onset is insidious, with infrequent chills, low-grade fever, prominent headache and malaise, cough, and, often, striking x-ray changes. Marked leukocytosis (eg, > 18,000/μL) is unusual.

Pneumococcal meningitis is diagnosed by lumbar puncture. Without a gram-stained smear and culture of spinal fluid, it is not distinguishable from other types of acute bacterial meningitis.

Complications

Complications of sepsis include meningitis and osteomyelitis; complications of pneumonia include empyema, parapneumonic effusion, and, rarely, lung abscess. Mastoiditis, subdural empyema, and brain abscess may follow untreated pneumococcal otitis media. Both pneumococcal meningitis and peritonitis are more likely to occur independently without coexisting pneumonia. Shock, disseminated intravascular coagulation, and Waterhouse-Friderichsen syndrome resembling meningococcemia are occasionally seen in pneumococcal sepsis, particularly in asplenic patients. Hemolytic uremic syndrome may be seen as a complication of pneumococcal pneumonia or sepsis.

Treatment

A. Specific Measures: Penicillin is the drug of choice, but erythromycin and cephalosporins are also effective. All significant *S pneumoniae* isolates should be confirmed as susceptible to penicillin. Both relatively resistant and absolutely penicillin-resistant *S pneumoniae* are reported. Multiply resistant strains may be difficult management problems that require infectious disease consultation.

1. Sepsis—All children with blood cultures that grow pneumococci must be reexamined as soon as possible. The child who has a focal infection such as meningitis or who appears septic should be admitted to the hospital and should receive parenteral antimicrobials. Only if the child is afebrile and appears well should management on an ambulatory basis be considered. If the physician is assured of close follow-up, lumbar puncture is not mandatory; penicillin V (50–100 mg/kg/d orally for 10 days) is prescribed, and the initial dose is given at once. Ceftriaxone (50 mg/kg intramuscularly) is preferred by some and may be associated with a lower need for hospitalization. Some children may be intermittently afebrile yet still progress to meningitis.

2. Pneumonia—For infants, severely ill patients, and immunocompromised hosts, aqueous penicillin G (150,000–200,000 units/kg/d intravenously in four to six divided doses) is given. Mild pneumonia may be treated with phenoxymethyl penicillin (50 mg/kg/d orally in four divided doses for 7–10 days). Erythromycin (40–50 mg/kg/d orally in two to four divided doses) is given to patients allergic to penicillin. Oral cephalosporins may be used.

3. Otitis media—Treat with oral ampicillin, amoxicillin, trimethoprim-sulfamethoxazole, or erythromycin for 10 days.

4. Meningitis—Until bacteriologic confirmation and susceptibility testing are completed, vancomycin (60 mg/kg/d intravenously in four divided doses) should be given. Failures are reported with lower-dose therapy. Corticosteroids are recommended by many as adjunctive therapy for pneumococcal meningitis, but they are controversial because they may reduce the entry of vancomycin into the cerebrospinal fluid. Vancomycin, ceftriaxone, and rifampin are given by many initially when corticosteroids are also administered. After bacteriologic

confirmation of susceptibility, aqueous penicillin G (300,000 units/kg/d intravenously in six divided doses for 10–14 days) should be given. Third-generation cephalosporins are acceptable if in vitro testing shows the isolate is susceptible, but uncommon resistant strains are associated with clinical failures.

B. General Measures: Supportive and symptomatic care is required.

Prognosis

In children, case fatality rates of less than 1% should be achieved except in meningitis, in which rates of 5–20% still prevail. The presence of large numbers of organisms without a prominent cerebrospinal fluid inflammatory response or of meningitis due to a penicillin-resistant strain indicates a poor prognosis. Serious neurologic sequelae, particularly hearing loss, are more frequent following pneumococcal meningitis than following meningococcal or *H influenzae* type b meningitis.

Adcock PM, Paul RI, Marshall GS: Effect of urine latex agglutination tests on the treatment of children at risk for invasive bacterial infection. Pediatrics 1995;96:951.

Baraff LJ et al: Practice guideline for management of infants and children 0 to 36 months of age with fever without source. Pediatrics 1993;92:1.

Barnett E, Klein J: The problem of resistant bacteria for the management of acute otitis media. Pediatr Clin North Am 1995;42;509.

Bradley JS, Kaplan SL, Klugman, KP, Leggiadro RJ: Consensus: Management of infections in children caused by *Streptococcus pneumoniae* with decreased susceptibility to penicillin. Pediatr Infect Dis 1005;14:1037.

Burman LA, Norrby R, Trollfors B: Invasive pneumococcal infections: Incidence, predisposing factors, and prognosis. Rev Infect Dis 1985;7:133.

Friedland IR et al: Dilemmas in diagnosis and management of cephalosporin-resistant *Streptococcus pneumoniae* meningitis. Pediatr Infect Dis J 1993;12:196.

Jacobs NM: Pneumococcal osteomyelitis and arthritis in children: A hospital series and literature review. Am J Dis Child 1991;145:70.

Kornelisse RF et al: Pneumococcal meningitis in children: Prognostic indicators and outcome. Clin Infect Dis 1995;21:1390.

Murdoch IA, Dos Anjos R: Continued need for pneumococcal prophylaxis after splenectomy. Arch Dis Child 1991;65:1268.

Tuomanen EI, Austrian R, Masure HR: Pathogenesis of pneumococcal infections. N Engl J Med 1995;332:1280.

Wald EER et al: Dexamethasone therapy for children with abacterial meningitis. Pediatrics 1995;95:21.

Zenni MK et al: *Streptococcus pneumoniae* colonization in the young child: Association with otitis media and resistance to penicillin. J Pediatr 1995;127:535.

STAPHYLOCOCCAL INFECTIONS

Staphylococcal infections are common and important in childhood. Staphylococcal skin infections range from minor furuncles to the varied syndromes now collected under the encompassing term "scalded skin syndrome." Staphylococci are the major cause of osteomyelitis and of septic arthritis. They are an uncommon but important cause of bacterial pneumonia. A toxin produced by certain strains causes staphylococcal food poisoning. Staphylococci are now responsible for most infections of artificial heart valves. They cause toxic shock syndrome (see below). Finally, they are found in infections at all ages and in multiple sites, particularly when infection is introduced from the skin or upper respiratory tract or when closed compartments become infected (pericarditis, sinusitis, cervical adenitis, surgical wounds, abscesses in the liver or brain, and abscesses elsewhere in the body).

Staphylococci, which do not produce the enzyme coagulase, are termed coagulase-negative but are seldom speciated in the clinical microbiology laboratory. Most *Staphylococcus aureus* strains produce coagulase. *S aureus* and coagulase-negative staphylococci are normal flora of the skin and respiratory tract. The latter rarely causes disease except in compromised hosts, the newborn, or patients with plastic-negative staphylococci infection occurs frequently.

Most strains of *S aureus* elaborate a β-lactamase that confers penicillin resistance. This can be overcome in clinical practice by the use of a nonpenicillin antibiotic, a cephalosporin, or a penicillinase-resistant penicillin such as methicillin, oxacillin, nafcillin, cloxacillin, or dicloxacillin. Methicillin-resistant strains are found worldwide and are now common in certain hospitals and areas in the United States. Most of these strains retain β-lactamase production, and many are resistant to other antibiotics as well. Methicillin-resistant strains are also resistant in vivo to all of the penicillinase-resistant penicillins and cephalosporins.

S aureus produces a variety of exotoxins, most of which are of uncertain importance. Two toxins are recognized as playing a central role in specific diseases: exfoliatin and staphylococcal enterotoxin. The former is largely responsible for the various clinical presentations of the scalded skin syndrome. Most strains that elaborate exfoliatin are of phage group II. Enterotoxin causes staphylococcal food poisoning. The exoprotein toxin most commonly associated with toxic shock syndrome has been termed TSST-1. However, *S aureus* strains isolated from patients with toxic shock syndrome who have focal infections do not produce detectable TSST-1. Their organisms have been found to produce enterotoxins B or C, suggesting that the syndrome may be caused by more than one *S aureus* exoprotein.

Clinical Findings

A. Symptoms and Signs:

1. Staphylococcal skin diseases–Dermal infection with *S aureus* causes furuncles or cellulitis.

S aureus are often found along with streptococci in impetigo. If the strains produce exfoliatin, localized lesions become bullous (bullous impetigo).

Generalized exfoliative disease (scalded skin syndrome) is thought to result from systemic spread of exfoliatin. The infection may begin at any site but appears to be introduced through the respiratory tract in most cases. There is a prodromal phase of erythema, often beginning around the mouth, accompanied by fever and irritability. The involved skin becomes tender, and a sick infant will cry when picked up or touched. A day or so later, exfoliation begins, usually around the mouth. The inside of the mouth is red, and a peeling rash is present around the lips, often in a radial pattern resembling rhagades. Generalized, painful peeling may follow, involving the limbs and trunk but often sparing the feet. More commonly, peeling is confined to areas around body orifices. If erythematous but unpeeled skin is rubbed sideways, superficial epidermal layers separate from deeper ones and sloughs (Nikolsky's sign). In the newborn, the disease is termed Ritter's disease and may be fulminant. If there is tender erythema but not exfoliation, the disease is termed nonstreptococcal scarlet fever. The scarlatiniform rash is sandpaper-like, but strawberry tongue is not seen, and cultures grow *S aureus* rather than streptococci.

2. Osteomyelitis and septic arthritis–See Chapter 24.

3. Staphylococcal pneumonia–Staphylococcal pneumonia in infancy is characterized by abdominal distention, high fever, respiratory distress, and toxemia. It often occurs without predisposing factors or after minor skin infections. The organism is necrotizing, producing bronchoalveolar destruction. Pneumatoceles, pyopneumothorax, and empyema are frequently encountered. Rapid progression of disease is characteristic. Frequent chest x-rays to monitor the progress of disease are indicated. Presenting symptoms may be typical of paralytic ileus, suggestive of an abdominal catastrophe.

Staphylococcal pneumonia usually is peribronchial and diffuse and begins with a focal infiltrative lesion progressing to patchy consolidation. Most often only one lung is involved (80%), more often the right. Purulent pericarditis occurs by direct extension in about 10% of cases, with or without empyema.

4. Staphylococcal food poisoning–Staphylococcal food poisoning is produced by enterotoxin. The most common source is poorly refrigerated and contaminated food. The disease is characterized by vomiting, prostration, and diarrhea occurring 2–6 hours after ingestion of contaminated foods.

5. Staphylococcal endocarditis–*S aureus* may produce infection of normal heart valves, of valves or endocardium in children with congenital or rheumatic heart disease, or of artificial valves. About 25% of all cases of endocarditis are due to *S aureus*.

The great majority of artificial heart valve infections involve either *S aureus* or coagulase-negative staphylococci. Infection usually begins in an extracardiac focus, often the skin. Involvement of the endocardium must be suspected in every case of *S aureus* bacteremia, regardless of the presence of signs. Suspicion must be highest in the presence of congenital heart disease, particularly ventricular septal defects with aortic insufficiency, but also simple ventricular septal defect, patent ductus arteriosus, and tetralogy of Fallot.

The presenting symptoms in staphylococcal endocarditis are fever, weight loss, weakness, muscle pain or diffuse skeletal pain, poor feeding, pallor, and cardiac decompensation. Signs include splenomegaly, cardiomegaly, petechiae, hematuria, and a new or changing murmur. The course of *S aureus* endocarditis is rapid, though subacute disease is occasionally seen. Peripheral septic embolization and uncontrollable cardiac failure are common, even when optimal antibiotic therapy is administered, and may be indications for surgical intervention (see below).

6. Toxic shock syndrome—Toxic shock syndrome is characterized by fever, blanching erythroderma, diarrhea, vomiting, myalgia, prostration, hypotension, and multiple organ dysfunction involvement associated with cultures of *S aureus*. Bacteremia does not occur.

Large numbers of cases have been described in menstruating adolescents and young women using vaginal tampons. Toxic shock syndrome has also been seen in both boys and girls with focal staphylococcal infections as well as in individuals with postoperative wound infections due to *S aureus*. Additional clinical features include sudden onset; conjunctival suffusion; mucosal hyperemia; desquamation of skin on the palms, soles, fingers, and toes during convalescence; disseminated intravascular coagulation in severe cases; renal and hepatic functional abnormalities; and evidence of myolysis. The mortality rate with early treatment is now about 2%. Recurrences were seen during subsequent menstrual periods in as many as 60% of untreated women who continued to use tampons. Recurrences were reported in up to 15% of those who were treated with antistaphylococcal antibiotics and stopped using tampons. The disease is caused by strains of *S aureus* that produce TSST-1 or one of the related enterotoxins.

7. Coagulase-negative staphylococcal infections—Localized and systemic coagulase-negative staphylococcal infections occur primarily in immunocompromised patients, high-risk newborns, and patients with plastic prostheses or catheters. In low-birth-weight infants, coagulase-negative staphylococci are the commonest nosocomial pathogen in nurseries in the United States. Intravenous administration of lipid emulsions and indwelling central venous catheters are risk factors contributing to coagu-

lase-negative staphylococcal bacteremia in newborn infants. In patients with an artificial heart valve, Dacron patch, ventriculoperitoneal shunt for hydrocephalus, or a Hickman or Broviac vascular catheter, coagulase-negative staphylococci are one of the common causes of sepsis or catheter infection, often necessitating removal of the foreign material and prolonged antibiotic therapy. Because blood cultures are frequently contaminated by this organism, diagnosis of genuine localized or systemic infection is often difficult or uncertain.

B. Laboratory Findings: Moderate leukocytosis (15,000–20,000/μL) with a shift to the left is occasionally found, although normal counts are common, particularly in infants. The sedimentation rate is elevated. Blood cultures are frequently positive in systemic staphylococcal disease and should always be obtained when it is suspected. Similarly, pus from sites of infection should always be aspirated or obtained surgically, examined with Gram's stain, and cultured both aerobically and anaerobically.

There are no useful serologic tests for staphylococcal disease.

Differential Diagnosis

Staphylococcal skin disease has many morphologic forms and therefore many differential diagnoses. Bullous impetigo must be differentiated from chemical or thermal burns, from drug reactions, and, in the very young, from the various congenital epidermolytic syndromes or even herpes simplex infections. Staphylococcal scalded skin syndrome resembles scarlet fever in some instances and in others appears similar to Kawasaki disease, Stevens-Johnson syndrome, erythema multiforme, and other drug reactions. A skin biopsy may be critical in establishing the correct diagnosis. The skin lesions of varicella may become superinfected with exfoliatin-producing staphylococci and produce a combination of the two diseases (bullous varicella).

Osteomyelitis of the long bones and septic arthritis must often be differentiated (see Chapter 24).

Severe, rapidly progressing pneumonia is typical of *S aureus* infection and group A streptococci but may occasionally be produced by pneumococci. Abscesses and pneumatoceles may be seen in pneumonia due to pneumococci, *Haemophilus influenzae*, and group A streptococci. Empyema formation occurs with all bacterial pneumonias.

Staphylococcal food poisoning is often epidemic. It is differentiated from other common-source gastroenteritis syndromes (*Salmonella, Clostridium perfringens, Vibrio parahaemolyticus*) by the short incubation period (2–6 hours), the prominence of vomiting (as opposed to diarrhea), and the absence of fever.

Endocarditis must be suspected in any instance of *S aureus* bacteremia, particularly when there is a significant heart murmur or preexisting cardiac disease (see Chapter 19).

Newborn infections with *S aureus* can resemble infections with streptococci and a variety of gram-negative organisms. Umbilical and respiratory tract colonization occurs with many pathogenic organisms (group B streptococci, *Escherichia coli, Klebsiella*), and both skin and systemic infections occur with virtually all of these.

Toxic shock syndrome must be differentiated from Rocky Mountain spotted fever, leptospirosis, Kawasaki disease, drug reactions, adenovirus, and measles. (See also Table 38–3.)

Treatment

A. Specific Measures: Since 85% of *S aureus* strains are penicillin-resistant, it is important to use a β-lactamase-resistant penicillin as the first drug in treatment. In serious systemic disease, in osteomyelitis, and in the treatment of large abscesses, intravenous therapy is indicated initially (oxacillin or nafcillin, 100–200 mg/kg/d in four divided doses, or methicillin, 200–300 mg/kg/d in four divided doses). When high doses over a long period are required, it is preferable not to use methicillin, because of the frequency with which interstitial nephritis is seen. In life-threatening illness, an aminoglycoside antibiotic (gentamicin or tobramycin) or nifompin may be used in addition for its possible synergistic action. *S aureus* is penicillin-sensitive, penicillin G may be used for treatment.

When children with established penicillin sensitivity are treated, cephalosporins may be used (cefazolin, 100–150 mg/kg/d intravenously in three divided doses; or cephalexin, 50–100 mg/kg/d orally in four divided doses). The third-generation cephalosporins should not generally be used for staphylococcal infections.

For methicillin-resistant infections, vancomycin (40 mg/kg/d intravenously in three or four divided doses) should be used. Infections due to methicillin-resistant staphylococci frequently do not respond to cephalosporins despite in vitro testing that suggests susceptibility. For treatment of meningitis, vancomycin must be given in higher doses (60 mg/kg/d divided into four doses). Combinations including rifampin may be either synergistic or antagonistic.

1. Skin infections–See Chapter 14.

2. Osteomyelitis and septic arthritis–Treatment should be begun intravenously, with antibiotics selected to cover the most likely organisms (staphylococci in hematogenous osteomyelitis; *H influenzae,* meningococci, pneumococci, staphylococci in children with septic arthritis under the age of 3 years; staphylococci and gonococci in arthritis in older children). Antibiotic levels should be kept high at all times.

In osteomyelitis, clinical studies support the use of intravenous treatment until fever and local symptoms

and signs have subsided—usually after at least 1 week—followed by oral therapy (dicloxacillin, 100–150 mg/kg/d in four divided doses; or cephalexin, 100–50 mg/kg/d in four divided doses) for at least 3 additional weeks. Longer treatment may be required, particularly when x-rays show extensive involvement. In arthritis, where drug diffusion into synovial fluid is good, intravenous therapy need be given only for a few days, followed by adequate oral therapy for at least 3 weeks. In all instances, oral therapy should be administered under careful supervision, either in the hospital or, in some instances, at home with frequent support and reinforcement from physicians or visiting nurses. Monitoring serum bacteriocidal concentrations is recommended by some experts, but has not been proved necessary in all cases. The erythrocyte sedimentation rate is a good indicator of response to therapy.

Surgical drainage of osteomyelitis or septic arthritis is often required (see Chapter 24).

3. Staphylococcal pneumonia–Antibiotic therapy should consist of a parenteral penicillinase-resistant penicillin with or without an aminoglycoside. Empyema or pyopneumothorax require chest tube drainage. The tube should be removed as soon as drainage has become clinically insignificant.

If staphylococcal pneumonia is promptly treated and empyema promptly drained, resolution in children is almost always complete—despite evidence of widespread parenchymal destruction and the persistence of bullae, blebs, and even pockets of empyema or abscess fluid well into convalescence. Surgical decortication or segmental resection is usually not required.

4. Staphylococcal food poisoning–Therapy is supportive and usually not required except in severe cases or for small infants with marked dehydration.

5. Staphylococcal endocarditis–As outlined above, high-dose, prolonged, parenteral treatment with oxacillin, nafcillin, or methicillin plus gentamicin or tobramycin is indicated. In penicillin-allergic patients, vancomycin should be used. With penicillin-sensitive organisms, penicillin G is the drug of choice. Therapy lasts in all instances for at least 6 weeks.

In some patients, medical treatment may fail. Signs of this are (1) recurrent fever without apparent treatable other cause (eg, thrombophlebitis, incidental respiratory or urinary tract infection, drug fever), (2) persistently positive blood cultures, (3) intractable and progressive congestive heart failure, and (4) recurrent (septic) embolization. In such circumstances—particularly (2), (3), and (4)—valve replacement becomes necessary. Antibiotics are continued for at least another 4 weeks. Persistent or recurrent infection may require a second surgical procedure.

6. Toxic shock syndrome–Treatment is first

with volume expansion and inotropic agents and later with oxacillin, nafcillin, or cephalosporins. If a tampon is in place, it should be removed. All focal staphylococcal infections should be drained without delay. Some experts feel that corticosteroid therapy may be effective if given to patients with severe illness early in the course of their disease. Antibiotic treatment reduces risk of recurrence.

7. Coagulase-negative staphylococcal infections–Bacteremia and other serious coagulase-negative staphylococcal infections are treated initially with vancomycin. Coagulase-negative staphylococci are uncommonly resistant to vancomycin (see Chapter 34 for dosing). Strains susceptible to penicillin or oxacillin are treated with those agents.

B. General Measures: Localized pus should be drained. Oxygen, intravenous fluids, and other supportive care are indicated in staphylococcal pneumonia and other systemic infections. Blood transfusion may be indicated if the patient is severely anemic.

Prognosis

Septicemia, endocarditis, and widespread pneumonitis in infancy all have a serious prognosis. Infants and children who recover from serious staphylococcal pneumonia have a good long-term prognosis without development of chronic respiratory disease. Osteomyelitis is never fatal if promptly treated.

Baltimore RS: Infective endocarditis in children. Pediatr Infect Dis J 1992;11:907.

Choux M et al: Shunt implantation: Reducing the incidence of shunt infection. J Neurosurg 1992;77:875.

Dagan R: Management of acute hematogenous osteomyelitis and septic arthritis in the pediatric patient. Pediatr Infect Dis J 1993;12:88.

Ferguson MA, Todd JK: Toxic shock syndrome associated with *Staphylococcus aureus* sinusitis in children. J Infect Dis 1990;161:953.

Freeman J et al: Association of intravenous lipid emulsion and coagulase negative staphylococcal bacteremia in neonatal intensive care units. N Engl J Med 1990;2:30.

Freeman J et al: Extra hospital stay and antibiotic United Statesge with nosocomial coagulase-negative staphylococcal bacteremia in two neonatal intensive care unit populations. Am J Dis Child 1990;144:324.

Friedland IR, du Plessis J, Cilliers A: Cardiac complications in children with *Staphylococcus aureus* bacteremia. J Pediatr 1995;127:746.

Givner LB, Kaplan SL: Meningitis due to *Staphylococcus aureus* in children. Clin Infect Dis 1993;16:766.

Hieber JP, Nelson AJ, McCracken GH: Acute disseminated staphylococcal disease in childhood. Am J Dis Child 1977;131:181.

Huebner J et al: Endemic nosocomial transmission of *Staphylococcus epidermidis* bacteria isolates in a neonatal intensive care unit over 10 years. J infect Dis 1994;169:526.

Moreira BM, Daum RS: Antimicrobial resistance in staphylococcus. Pediatr Clin North Am 1995;42:619.

Raad II, Sabbagh MF: Optimal duration of therapy for catheter-related Staphylococcus aureus bacteremia: A study of 35 cases and review. Clin Infect Dis 1992;14:75.

Schwalbe RS, Stapleton JT, Gilligan PH: Emergence of vancomycin resistance in coagulase-negative staphylococci. N Engl J Med 1987;316:927.

Shulman ST, Ayoub EM: Severe staphylococcal sepsis in adolescents. Pediatrics 1976;58:59.

Todd JKT: Toxic shock syndrome. Clin Microbiol Rev 1988;1:432.

Tolan RW Jr et al: Operative intervention in active endocarditis in children: Report of a series of cases and review. Clin Infect Dis 1992;14:852.

MENINGOCOCCAL INFECTIONS

Essentials of Diagnosis

- Fever, headache, vomiting, convulsions, shock (meningitis).
- Fever, shock, petechial or purpuric skin rash (meningococcemia).
- Diagnosis confirmed by culture of normally sterile body fluids.

General Considerations

Meningococci may be carried asymptomatically for many months in the upper respiratory tract. Fewer than 1% of carriers develop disease. Meningitis and sepsis are the two commonest forms of illness, but septic arthritis, pericarditis, pneumonia, chronic meningococcemia, otitis media, conjunctivitis, and vaginitis also occur. The highest attack rate for meningococcal meningitis is in the first year of life. The incidence in the United States is about 1.2 cases per 100,000 people. There were nearly 3000 reported cases in 1994.

Meningococci are classified serologically into groups A, B, C, D, X, Y, Z, 29-E, and W-135. The serologic groups serve as specific markers for studying outbreaks and transmission of disease. Major epidemics of meningococcal disease in the United States prior to 1950 were caused by group A strains. In recent years, however, group A organisms have accounted for only about 2% of meningococcal isolates. Group B accounts for about 40%; group C, for 30%; and group Y, for 20%. Sulfonamide resistance is common in non-group A strains. *N meningitidis* resistant to penicillin G are reported from South Africa and Spain but not in the United States. Resistant isolates are susceptible to third-generation cephalosporins. Few isolates are resistant to rifampin. Pathogenic strains differ in their virulence and in their potential for epidemic spread. Serogroup A meningococci have the greatest propensity to cause widespread outbreaks.

Children develop immunity from asymptomatic carriage of meningococci (usually nontypable, nonpathogenic strains) or other cross-reacting bacteria.

Patients deficient in one of the late components of complement (C6, C7, or C8) are uniquely susceptible to meningococcal infection, particularly group A meningococci. Deficiencies of early and alternate pathway complement components are also reported.

Meningococci are gram-negative organisms containing endotoxin in their cell walls. Endotoxins may cause capillary vascular injury and leak and may also cause disseminated intravascular coagulation. The development of irreversible shock with multiple organ failure is a significant factor in the fatal outcome of acute meningococcal infections.

Vaccines prepared from purified meningococcal polysaccharides (A, C, Y, and W-135) are available for controlling outbreaks and preventing spread in special high-risk groups such as household contacts and military recruits. Unfortunately, the vaccines, except for the A component, are ineffective in children under 2 years of age (see Chapter 10).

Clinical Findings

A. Symptoms and Signs: Many children with clinical meningococcemia also have meningitis, and some may have other foci of infection. All children with suspected meningococcemia should have a lumbar puncture.

1. Meningococcemia–A prodrome of upper respiratory infection is followed by high fever, headache, nausea, marked toxicity, and hypotension. Purpura, petechiae, and occasionally bright pink, tender macules or papules over the extremities and trunk are seen. The rash usually progresses rapidly.

Fulminant meningococcemia (Waterhouse-Friderichsen syndrome) progresses rapidly and is characterized by disseminated intravascular coagulation, massive skin and mucosal hemorrhages, and shock. This syndrome also may be due to *H influenzae, S pneumoniae,* or other bacteria.

Chronic meningococcemia is characterized by periodic bouts of fever, arthralgia or arthritis, and recurrent petechiae. Splenomegaly is often present. The patient may be free of symptoms between bouts. Chronic meningococcemia occurs primarily in adults and mimics Henoch-Schönlein purpura.

2. Meningitis–In many children, meningococcemia is followed within a few hours by symptoms and signs of acute purulent meningitis, with severe headache, stiff neck, nausea, vomiting, and stupor. Children with meningitis and meningococcemia generally fare better than children with meningococcemia alone.

B. Laboratory Findings: The peripheral white blood cell count may be either low or elevated. Thrombocytopenia may be present with or without disseminated intravascular coagulation (see Chapter 26). If petechial or hemorrhagic lesions are present, meningococci can sometimes be demonstrated on smear by puncturing the lesions and expressing a drop of tissue fluid. Organisms may be demonstrated by Gram's stain of buffy coat preparations of blood. The spinal fluid is generally cloudy and contains more than 1000 white cells/μL, with many polymorphonuclear cells and gram-negative intracellular diplococci.

A total hemolytic complement assay may reveal absence of late components as an underlying cause.

Differential Diagnosis

The lesions of *H influenzae* or pneumococci, enterovirus infection, endocarditis, leptospirosis, Rocky Mountain spotted fever, other rickettsial diseases, Henoch-Schönlein purpura, and blood dyscrasias. Other causes of sepsis and meningitis are distinguished by appropriate Gram's stain and cultures.

Complications

Meningitis may lead to permanent central nervous system damage, with deafness, convulsions, paralysis, or impairment of intellectual function. Hydrocephalus may develop and requires ventriculo-peritoneal shunt. Subdural collections of fluid are common but usually resolve spontaneously. Extensive skin necrosis, loss of digits or extremities, intestinal hemorrhage, and late adrenal insufficiency may complicate fulminant meningococcemia.

Prevention

Household contacts, day-care center contacts, and hospital personnel directly exposed to the respiratory secretions of patients are at increased risk of developing meningococcal infection and should be given chemoprophylaxis with rifampin. The secondary attack rate among household members is 1–5% during epidemics and less than 1% in nonepidemic situations. Children 3 months to 2 years of age are at the greatest risk, presumably because they lack protective antibodies. Secondary cases are reported in day-care centers, but school classroom outbreaks are rare. Hospital personnel are not at increased risk unless they have had contact with a patient's oral secretions, eg, during mouth-to-mouth resuscitation, intubation, or suctioning procedures. Approximately 50% of secondary cases in households have their onset within 24 hours of identification of the index case. Exposed children should be examined promptly. If they are febrile, they should be fully evaluated and treated with high doses of penicillin or another effective antimicrobial pending the results of blood cultures.

All intimate contacts should receive chemoprophylaxis with rifampin given orally in the following dosages twice daily for 2 days: 600 mg for adults, 10 mg/kg for children 1 month to 12 years of age, and 5 mg/kg for infants under 1 month of age. An alternate dosing schedule for rifampin is 20 mg/kg/d (maximum adult dose, 600 mg/d) once daily for 4 days. If the organism is sensitive to sulfonamides, sulfadiazine may be used. Penicillin and most other antibiotics (even with parenteral administration) are not effective chemoprophylactic agents, since they do not eradicate upper respiratory tract carriage of meningococci. Cephalosporins, such as ceftriaxone intramuscularly or cefixime orally, are effective for prophylaxis. Ciprofloxacin has been used to eradicate nasopharyngeal carriage in adults but is not approved for use in children. In some situations, meningococcal polysaccharide vaccine should be given to contacts in addition to chemoprophylaxis. Throat cultures to identify carriers are not useful.

Treatment

Blood cultures should be obtained for all children with fever and purpura or other signs of meningococcemia, and antibiotics should be administered immediately as an emergency procedure. There is a good correlation between survival rates and initiation of prompt antibiotic therapy. Purpura and fever should be considered a medical emergency.

Children with meningococcemia or meningococcal meningitis should be managed as though shock were imminent even if their vital signs are stable when they are first seen. If hypotension already is present, supportive measures should be aggressive, because the prognosis is grave in such situations. It is optimal to initiate treatment in an intensive care setting. Treatment should not be delayed for the sake of transporting the patient. Shock may worsen following antimicrobial therapy due to endotoxin release. To minimize the risk of nosocomial transmission, patients should be treated in respiratory isolation for the first 24 hours of antibiotic treatment.

A. Specific Measures: Antibiotics should be begun promptly. Since other bacteria, such as *S pneumoniae, S aureus,* or other gram-negative organisms, can cause identical syndromes, initial therapy should be broadly effective. Cefotaxime or ceftriaxone are preferred (see Chapter 34 for dosages). When the diagnosis is confirmed, penicillin G (250,000 units/kg/d in six doses) intravenously for seven days is the drug of choice. Relative penicillin resistance is uncommon.

B. General Measures:

1. Cardiovascular–See Chapter 12 for management of septic shock. Corticosteroids are not beneficial. Sympathetic blockade has been used to improve limb perfusion. Topically applied nitroglycerin has been used locally to improve perfusion.

2. Hematologic–Since hypercoagulability is frequently present in patients with meningococcemia, administration of heparin should be considered for patients with disseminated intravascular coagulation. A loading dose of 100 units/kg is followed by 15 units/kg/h as a continuous drip. The patient is monitored by following the partial thromboplastin time. Recombinant tissue plasminogen activator and concentrated antithrombin III have been tried experimentally to reserve coagulopathy. See Chapter 26 for the management of disseminated intravascular coagulation.

Prognosis

Unfavorable prognostic features include shock, disseminated intravascular coagulation, and extensive skin lesions. The case fatality rate in fulminant meningococcemia is very high—over 50%. In uncomplicated meningococcal meningitis, the fatality rate is much lower—generally 10–20%.

Algren JT et al: Predictors of outcome in acute meningococcal infection in children. Crit Care Med 1993;21:447.

Boyer D, Gordon RC, Baker T: Lack of clinical usefulness of a positive latex agglutination test for *Neisseria meningitidis/Escherichia coli* antigens in the urine. Pediatr Infect Dis J 1993;12:779.

Dashefsky B, Teele DW, Klein JO: Unsuspected meningococcemia. J Pediatr 1983;102:69.

Edwards MS, Baker CJ: Complications and sequelae of meningococcal infections in children. J Pediatr 1981; 99:540.

Leggiadro RJ, Winkelstein JA: Prevalence of complement deficiencies in children with systemic meningococcal infections. Pediatr Infect Dis J 1987;6:75.

Lennon D et al: Successful intervention in a group A meningococcal outbreak in Auckland, New Zealand. Pediatr Infect Dis J 1992;11:617.

Mayatepek E et al: Deafness, complement deficiencies and immunoglobulin status in patients with meningococcal diseases due to uncommon serogroups. Pediatr Infect Dis J 1993;12:808.

Nguyen QV, Nguyen EA, Weiner LB: Incidence of invasive bacterial disease in children with fever and petechiae. Pediatrics 1984;74:77.

Perez-Trallero E et al: Meningococci with increased resistance to penicillin. Lancet 1990;335:1096.

Reido FX, Plikaytis BD, Broome CV: Epidemiology and prevention of meningococcal disease. Pediatr Infect Dis J 1995;14:643.

Shay DK, Goldman DA, Jarvis WR: Reducing the spread of meningococcemia. Pediatrics 1995;96:144.

Wong VK et al: Meningococcal infections in children: A review of 100 cases. Pediatr Infect Dis J 1989;8:224.

Woods CR et al: Invasive disease caused by *Neisseria meningitidis* relatively resistant to penicillin in North Carolina. J Infect Dis 1994;170:453.

Zens W et al: Recombinant tissue plasminogen activator treatment in two infants with fulminant meningococcemia. Pediatrics 1995;96:144.

GONOCOCCAL INFECTIONS

Essentials of Diagnosis

- Purulent urethral discharge showing intracellular gram-negative diplococci on smear in male patient (usually adolescent).
- Purulent, edematous, sometimes hemorrhagic conjunctivitis showing intracellular gram-negative diplococci on smear in infant 2–4 days of age.
- Fever, arthritis (often polyarticular) or tenosynovi-

tis, and maculopapular peripheral rash that may be vesiculopustular or hemorrhagic.
- Positive culture of blood or pharyngeal or genital secretions.

General Considerations

Neisseria gonorrhoeae is a gram-negative diplococcus. Although morphologically similar to other neisseriae, it differs in its ability to grow on selective media and to ferment carbohydrates. The cell wall of *N gonorrhoeae* contains endotoxin, which is liberated when the organism dies and is responsible for the production of a cellular exudate. The incubation period is short, usually 2–5 days.

Antimicrobial-resistant gonococci are now a serious problem. Nationally, 2% of *N gonorrhoeae* are highly resistant as a result of plasmid-encoded penicillinase; 1% are highly resistant as a result of plasmid-encoded resistance to tetracycline; and 16% have chromosomal resistance to penicillin, tetracycline, or cefoxitin.

Gonococcal disease in children may be transmitted sexually or nonsexually. Prepubertal girls usually manifest gonococcal vulvovaginitis because of the neutral-alkaline pH of the vagina and thin vaginal mucosa.

Prepubertal gonococcal infection outside the neonatal period should be considered presumptive evidence of sexual contact or child abuse. In the adolescent or adult, the workup of every case of gonorrhea should include a careful and accurate inquiry into sexual practices, since pharyngeal infection must be detected if present and may be difficult to eradicate. In addition, efforts should be made to identify and treat all sexual contacts. When prepubertal children are infected, all family members should be cultured, and epidemiologic investigation should be thorough.

Clinical Findings

A. Symptoms and Signs:

1. Asymptomatic gonorrhea–The ratio of asymptomatic to symptomatic gonorrheal infections in adolescents and adults is probably 3–4:1 in women and 0.5–1:1 in men. Asymptomatic infections are considered as infectious as symptomatic ones.

2. Uncomplicated genital gonorrhea–

a. Male with urethritis–Urethral discharge is sometimes painful and bloody and may be white, yellow, or green. There may be associated dysuria. The patient is usually afebrile.

b. Prepubertal female with vaginitis–The only clinical findings initially may be dysuria and polymorphonuclear neutrophils in the urine. Vulvitis characterized by erythema, edema, and excoriation accompanied by a purulent discharge may follow.

c. Postpubertal female with cervicitis–Symptomatic disease is characterized by a purulent discharge, dysuria, and, occasionally, dyspareunia.

Lower abdominal pain is absent. Physical examination reveals an afebrile patient with a yellow, foul-smelling discharge. The cervix is frequently hyperemic and tender when touched by the examining finger. This tenderness is not worsened by moving the cervix, nor are the adnexa tender to palpation.

d. Rectal gonorrhea–Rectal gonorrhea is often asymptomatic. There may be purulent discharge, edema, and pain during evacuation.

3. Pharyngeal gonorrhea–Pharyngeal involvement is usually asymptomatic. There may be some sore throat and, rarely, acute exudative tonsillitis with bilateral cervical lymphadenopathy and fever.

4. Conjunctivitis and iridocyclitis–Copious exudate is characteristic of gonococcal conjunctivitis. Newborns are symptomatic on days 2–4. In the adolescent or adult eye, infection probably is spread from infected genital secretions by the fingers.

5. Pelvic inflammatory disease (salpingitis)–The interval between initiation of genital infection and its ascent to the uterine tubes is variable and may range from days to months, with menses frequently the initiating factor. With the onset of a menstrual period, gonococci invade the endometrium, causing transient endometritis. Subsequently, salpingitis may occur, resulting in pyosalpinx or hydrosalpinx; rarely, it leads to peritonitis or perihepatitis. Gonococcal salpingitis occurs in an acute, subacute, or chronic form. All three forms have in common tenderness on gentle movement of the cervix and bilateral tubal tenderness during pelvic examination.

Gonococci or *Chlamydia trachomatis* are the cause of about 50% of pelvic inflammatory disease. A mixed infection caused by enteric bacilli, *Bacteroides fragilis* or other anaerobes occurs in the other 50%.

6. Gonococcal perihepatitis (Fitz-Hugh and Curtis syndrome)–In the typical clinical pattern, there is right upper quadrant tenderness in association with signs of acute or subacute salpingitis. Pain may be pleuritic and referred to the shoulder. Hepatic friction rub is a valuable but inconstant sign.

7. Disseminated gonorrhea–Dissemination follows asymptomatic more often than symptomatic genital infection and often results from gonococcal pharyngitis or anorectal gonorrhea. The most common form of disseminated gonorrhea is polyarthritis or polytenosynovitis, with or without dermatitis. Monarticular arthritis is less common, and gonococcal endocarditis and meningitis are fortunately rare.

a. Polyarthritis–Disease usually begins with the simultaneous onset of low-grade fever, polyarthralgia, and general malaise. After a day or so, the joint symptoms become acute, and swelling, redness, and tenderness occur, frequently over the wrists, ankles, and knees but also in the fingers, feet, and other peripheral joints. Skin lesions may be noted at the same time: individual, tender, evolving 5- to 8-mm maculopapular lesions that may become vesicular, pustular, and then hemorrhagic. They are few in number and noted on the fingers, palms, feet, and other distal surfaces and may be single or multiple. In patients with this form of the disease, blood cultures are often positive, but joint fluid rarely yields organisms. Skin lesions often are positive by Gram's stain but rarely by culture. Genital, rectal, and pharyngeal cultures must always be performed.

b. Monoarticular arthritis–In this somewhat less common form of disseminated gonorrhea, fever is often absent. Arthritis evolves in a single joint. Dermatitis usually does not occur. Systemic symptoms are minimal. Blood cultures are negative, but joint aspirates may yield gonococci on smear and culture. Genital, rectal, and pharyngeal cultures must always be performed.

B. Laboratory Findings: Demonstration of gram-negative, kidney bean–shaped diplococci on smears of urethral exudate in males is presumptive evidence of gonorrhea. Positive culture confirms the diagnosis. Negative smears do not rule out gonorrhea. Gram-stained smears of cervical or vaginal discharge in girls are more difficult to interpret because of normal gram-negative flora, but they may be useful when technical personnel are experienced. In girls with suspected gonorrhea, both the cervical os and the anus should be cultured. Gonococcal pharyngitis requires culture for diagnosis.

Cultures for *N gonorrhoeae* are plated on a selective chocolate agar containing antibiotics (eg, Thayer-Martin agar) to suppress normal flora. If bacteriologic diagnosis is critical, suspected material should be cultured on chocolate agar as well. Since gonococci are labile, agar plates should be inoculated immediately and placed without delay in an atmosphere containing CO_2 (candle jar). When transportation is necessary, material should be directly inoculated into Transgrow medium prior to shipment to an appropriate laboratory. In cases of possible sexual molestation, notify the laboratory that definite speciation is needed, since nongonococcal *Neisseria* spp can grow on the selective media.

All children or adolescents with a suspected or established diagnosis of gonorrhea should have serologic tests for syphilis and HIV.

Differential Diagnosis

Urethritis in the male may be gonococcal or "nonspecific." The latter is a syndrome characterized by discharge (rarely painful), mild dysuria, and a subacute course. The discharge is usually scant or moderate in amount but may be profuse. The responsible microorganisms cannot all be identified, but about half of cases are due to *C trachomatis*. The remainder are probably due to *Ureaplasma,* trichomonads, or other as yet unknown agents. Most cases respond to tetracycline therapy (500 mg orally four times a day for 7 days in adolescents). *C trachomatis* has

been shown to cause epididymitis in males and salpingitis in females.

Vulvovaginitis in a prepubertal female may be due to infection caused by miscellaneous bacteria, including *Shigella* sp and group A streptococci, *Candida,* and herpes simplex; discharges may be caused by trichomonads, *Enterobius vermicularis* (pinworm), or foreign bodies. Symptom-free discharge (leukorrhea) normally accompanies rising estrogen levels.

Cervicitis in a postpubertal female, alone or in association with urethritis and involvement of Skene's and Bartholin's glands, may be due to infection caused by *Candida,* herpes simplex, *Trichomonas,* or discharge resulting from inflammation caused by foreign bodies (usually some form of contraceptive device). Leukorrhea may be associated with birth control pills.

Salpingitis may be due to infection with other organisms. The symptoms must be differentiated from those of appendicitis, urinary tract infection, ectopic pregnancy, endometriosis, or ovarian cysts or torsion.

Disseminated gonorrhea presents a wide differential diagnosis that must include meningococcemia, acute rheumatic fever, Henoch-Schönlein purpura, juvenile rheumatoid arthritis, lupus erythematosus, leptospirosis, secondary syphilis, certain viral infections (particularly rubella, but also enteroviruses and parvovirus), serum sickness, type B hepatitis (in the prodromal phase), infective endocarditis, and even acute leukemia and other types of cancer. The fully evolved skin lesions of disseminated gonorrhea are remarkably specific, and genital, rectal, or pharyngeal cultures, plus cultures of blood and joint fluid, usually yield gonococci from at least one source.

Prevention

Prevention of gonorrhea is principally a problem of sex education and treatment of contacts.

Treatment

A. Uncomplicated Urethral, Endocervical, or Rectal Gonococcal Infections in Adolescents: Due to increasing penicillin resistance, current recommended therapy is ceftriaxone (125 mg or 250 mg intramuscularly once) plus, for potential concurrent *Chlamydia trachomatis* infection, doxycycline (100 mg orally twice daily for 7 days). Erythromycin base (500 mg orally four times daily for 7 days) should be substituted for the doxycycline in pregnant patients. Alternatives to ceftriaxone include cefixime 400 mg orally, ciprofloxacin 500 mg orally, or ofloxacin 400 mg orally, each given in one dose. Spectinomycin (2 g intramuscular once) is used for resistant strains. Quinolone antibiotics should not be used in pregnant women or children. Quinolone resistance has been recognized in several cities If the contact's infecting strain was proved susceptible to penicillin, the patient may be treated orally with amoxicillin, 50 mg/kg to a maximum of 3 g, and probenecid, 25 mg/kg to a maximum of 1 g, taken together as a single dose. A "test of cure" culture is not necessary after the ceftriaxone/doxycycline regimen; repeat screening in 1–2 months is preferable.

B. Pharyngeal Gonococcal Infection: Ceftriaxone (125 mg or 250 mg intramuscularly once) should be used; ciprofloxacin (0.5 g orally once) is an alternative. Neither spectinomycin nor amoxicillin is recommended. A repeat culture is recommended 4–7 days after therapy.

C. Disseminated Gonorrhea: Recommended regimens include ceftriaxone (1 g intramuscularly or intravenously once daily) or cefotaxime (1 g intravenously every 8 hours). Proved penicillin-sensitive organisms may be treated with ampicillin (1 g intravenously every 6 hours) or an equivalent penicillin regimen. Oral therapy may follow parenteral therapy after clinical resolution. Recommended regimens include cefixime (400 mg orally twice daily) or ciprofloxacin (0.5 g twice daily; not used for pregnant patients) to complete 7 days of therapy. If concurrent infection with *Chlamydia* is present or has not been excluded, a course of doxycycline or erythromycin should also be prescribed.

Total duration of therapy is 7 days for disseminated infections.

D. Pelvic Inflammatory Disease: Therapy is given with cefoxitin (2 g intramuscularly or intravenously every 6 hours) and doxycycline (100 mg twice daily orally.) until the patient is clinically improved, then continuing doxycycline to complete 7 days. Clindamycin and gentamicin given intravenously until the patient is clinically unproved may be used rather than cefoxitin.

E. Prepubertal Gonococcal Infections:

1. Uncomplicated genitourinary, rectal, or pharyngeal infections–These infections may be treated with ceftriaxone (25–50 mg/kg/d to a maximum of 125 mg intramuscularly once). Children over 8 years of age should also receive doxycycline (100 mg orally twice daily for 7 days). The physician should evaluate all children for evidence of sexual abuse and coinfection with syphilis, *Chlamydia,* and HIV.

2. Disseminated gonorrhea–This should be treated with ceftriaxone (50 mg/kg once daily parenterally).

Alexander ER: Misidentification of sexually transmitted organisms in children: Medicolegal implications. Pediatr Infect Dis J 1988;7:1.

Fluoroquinolone resistance in *Neisseria gonorrhoeae*: Colorado and Washington, 1995. MMWR 1995;44:761.

Gorwitz RJ et al: Sentinel surveillance for antimicrobial resistance in *Neisseria gonorrhoeae*—United States, 1988–1991. The Gonococcal Isolate Surveillance Project Study Group. MMWR Morb Mortal Wkly Rep 1993;42:29.

Hammerschlag MR et al: Efficacy of neonatal ocular prophylaxis for the prevention of chlamydial and gonococcal conjunctivitis. N Engl J Med 1989;320:769.

Handsfield HH et al: A comparison of single-dose cefixime with ceftriaxone as treatment for uncomplicated gonorrhea. N Engl J Med 1991;325:1337.

McCormack W: Pelvic inflammatory disease. N Engl J Med 1994;320:115.

Schwarcz SK et al: National surveillance of antimicrobial resistance in *Neisseria gonorrhoeae.* JAMA 1990;264:1413.

Sexually transmitted diseases: Treatment guidelines MMWR Morb Mortal Wkly Rep 1993;42(RR-14):75.

Siegel RM et al: The prevalence of sexually transmitted diseases in children and adolescents evaluated for sexual abuse in Cincinnati: Rationale for limited STD testing in prepubertal girls. Pediatrics 1995;96:1090.

BOTULISM

Essentials of Diagnosis

- Dry mucous membranes.
- Nausea and vomiting.
- Diplopia; dilated, unreactive pupils.
- Descending paralysis.
- Difficulty in swallowing and speech occurring within 12–36 hours after ingestion of toxin contaminated home-canned food.
- Multiple cases in a family or group.
- Hypotonia and constipation in infants.
- Diagnosis by clinical findings and identification of toxin in blood, stool, or implicated food.

General Considerations

Botulism is a paralytic disease caused by *Clostridium botulinum,* an anaerobic, gram-positive, spore-forming bacillus normally found in soil. The organism produces an extremely potent neurotoxin. Of the seven types of toxin (A–G), types A, B, and E cause most human diseases. The toxin, a polypeptide, is so potent that 0.1 μg is lethal for humans.

Food-borne botulism usually results from ingestion of toxin-containing food. Preformed toxin is absorbed from the gut and produces paralysis by preventing acetylcholine release from cholinergic fibers at myoneural junctions.

In the United States, home-canned vegetables are usually the cause. Commercially canned foods rarely are responsible. Virtually any food will support the growth of *C botulinum* spores into vegetative toxin-producing bacilli if an anaerobic, nonacid environment is provided. The food may not appear or taste spoiled. The toxin is heat-labile, but the spores are heat-resistant. Inadequate heating during processing (temperature < 115 °C) allows the spores to survive and later resume toxin production. Boiling of foods for 10 minutes or heating at 80 °C for 30 minutes before eating will destroy the toxin.

Infant botulism is seen in infants less than 6 months of age. About 80 cases were reported in

1994. It usually presents as constipation and severe hypotonia at a median age of 10 weeks. Uncommonly, infants less than 2 weeks of age develop botulism. The toxin appears to be produced by *C botulinum* organisms residing in the gastrointestinal tract. In some instances, honey has been the source of spores. Clinical findings include constipation, weak suck and cry, pooled oral secretions, cranial nerve deficits, generalized weakness, and, on occasion, sudden apnea. A characteristic electromyographic pattern termed "brief, small, abundant motor-unit action potentials" (BSAP) is observed.

Wound botulism was recognized in 11 (21%) of 53 adult botulism cases reported in 1994. All occurred in drug users at the injection site.

Clinical Findings

A. Symptoms and Signs: The incubation period for food-borne botulism is 8–36 hours. Initially, there is lassitude or fatigue, generally with headache. This is followed by double vision, dilated pupils, ptosis, and, within a few hours, difficulty in swallowing and in speech. Pharyngeal paralysis occurs in some cases, and food may be regurgitated. The mucous membranes often are very dry. Descending skeletal muscle paralysis may be seen. The sensorium is clear, and the temperature normal. Death usually results from respiratory failure.

B. Laboratory Findings: Feces, vomitus, serum, and suspect food should be examined for the presence of toxin by injection into mice. The organism also may be cultured from feces or the suspect food. Laboratory findings, including cerebrospinal fluid examination, are usually normal. Electromyography (EMG) suggests the diagnosis if the characteristic abnormalities—small amplitude, brief polyphasic potentials with an incremental response to repeated stimuli—are seen.

A nondiagnostic EMG does not exclude the diagnosis and should be repeated.

Differential Diagnosis

Carbon monoxide poisoning causes unconsciousness without cranial nerve paralysis, and carboxyhemoglobin can be detected in blood. Guillain-Barré syndrome is characterized by ascending paralysis, sensory deficits, and elevated cerebrospinal fluid protein without pleocytosis.

Other illnesses that should be considered include poliomyelitis, postdiphtheritic polyneuritis, certain chemical intoxications, tick paralysis, and myasthenia gravis. The history and elevated cerebrospinal fluid protein characterize postdiphtheritic polyneuritis.

Poisoning with methyl alcohol, organic phosphorus compounds, methyl chloride, sodium fluoride, or atropine may have to be ruled out.

Tick paralysis is characterized by a flaccid ascending motor paralysis that begins in the legs. An attached tick should be sought.

Myasthenia gravis usually occurs in adolescent girls. It is characterized by ocular and bulbar symptoms, with normal pupils, fluctuating weakness, the absence of other neurologic signs, and clinical response to cholinesterase inhibitors.

Complications

Difficulty in swallowing leads to aspiration pneumonia. Serious respiratory paralysis may be fatal despite assisted ventilation and modern intensive supportive measures.

Treatment

A. Specific Measures: Equine botulism antitoxin is of probable value in the treatment of botulism. Trivalent antitoxin (types A, B, and E) should be given intramuscularly as soon as the diagnosis is made after skin testing for horse serum sensitivity. The antitoxin, 24-hour diagnostic consultation, epidemic assistance, and laboratory testing services are available from the Centers for Disease Control. Botulism immune globulin is available from the Infant Botulism Prevention Program (510-540-2646). A clinical trial is under way to evaluate this product. Guanidine hydrochloride, 15–35 mg/kg/d orally in three doses, may reverse the neuromuscular block, but its efficacy is questionable.

B. General Measures: General and supportive therapy consists of bed rest, ventilatory support (if necessary), fluid therapy, and administration of purgatives and high enemas. In cases of infant botulism, some authorities recommend penicillin to eliminate organisms continuing to produce toxin within the gastrointestinal tract. Aminoglycoside antimicrobials may exacerbate neuromuscular blockage and should be avoided.

Prognosis

The mortality rate (about 25%) is lower in children than adults. In nonfatal cases, symptoms subside over 2–3 months and recovery is complete.

Dowell VR Jr: Botulism and tetanus: Selected epidemiologic and microbiologic aspects. Rev Infect Dis 1984; 6(Suppl 1):S202.

Graf WD et al: Electrodiagnosis reliability in the diagnosis of infant botulism. J Pediatr 1992;120:747.

Infant Botulism Prevention Program. Wound botulism—California, 1995. MMWR 1995;44:889.

Mills DC, Arnon SS: The large intestine as the site of *Clostridium botulinum* colonization in human infant botulism. J Infect Dis 1987;156:997.

Schreiner MS et al: Infant botulism: A review of 12 years experience at the Children's Hospital of Philadelphia. Pediatrics 1991;87:159.

Schwartz PJ, Arnon SS: Botulism immune globulin for infant botulism arrives: One year and a Gulf war later. West J Med 1992;156:197.

Thilo EH, Townsend SF: Infant botulism at 1 week of age: Report of two cases. Pediatrics 1993;92:151.

Wilcox P et al: Long-term follow-up of symptoms, pulmonary function, respiratory muscle strength, and exercise performance after botulism. Am Rev Respir Dis 1989; 139:157.

TETANUS

Essentials of Diagnosis

- Unimmunized or partially immunized patient.
- History of skin wound.
- Spasms of jaw muscles (trismus).
- Stiffness of neck, back, and abdominal muscles, with hyperirritability and hyperreflexia.
- Episodic, generalized muscle contractions.
- Diagnosis is based on clinical findings and the immunization history.

General Considerations

Tetanus is caused by *Clostridium tetani,* an anaerobic, gram-positive bacillus that produces a potent neurotoxin. In unimmunized or incompletely immunized individuals, infection follows contamination of a wound by soil containing clostridial spores from animal manure. The toxin reaches the central nervous system by retrograde axon transport, is bound to cerebral gangliosides, and is thought to increase reflex excitability in neurons of the spinal cord by blocking function of inhibitory synapses. Intense muscle spasms result. Two-thirds of cases in the United States follow minor puncture wounds of the hands or feet. In many cases, no history of a wound can be obtained. In the newborn, usually in underdeveloped countries, infection generally results from contamination of the umbilical cord. The incubation period typically is 4–14 days but may be longer.

Although 36 cases of tetanus were reported in the U.S. in 1994, an estimated 1 million cases occur globally.

Clinical Findings

A. Symptoms and Signs: In children and adults, the first symptom is often minimal pain at the site of inoculation, followed by hypertonicity and spasm of the regional muscles. Characteristically, difficulty in opening the mouth (trismus) is evident within 48 hours. In newborns, the first signs are irritability and inability to suck at the breast. The disease may then progress to stiffness of the jaw and neck, increasing dysphagia, and generalized hyperreflexia with extreme rigidity and spasms of all muscles of the abdomen and back (opisthotonos). The facial distortion resembles a grimace (risus sardonicus). Difficulty in swallowing and convulsions triggered by minimal stimuli such as sound, light, or movement may occur. Individual spasms may last seconds or minutes. Recurrent spasms are seen several times each hour, or they may be almost continuous. In most cases, the temperature is normal or only mildly elevated. A high or subnormal temperature is a bad prognostic sign. Patients are fully conscious and lucid. A profound circulatory disturbance associated with sympathetic overactivity may occur on the second to fourth day, which may contribute to the mortality rate. This is characterized by elevated blood pressure, increased cardiac output, tachycardia (> 20 beats/min), and arrhythmia.

B. Laboratory Findings: The diagnosis is made on clinical grounds. There may be a mild polymorphonuclear leukocytosis. The cerebrospinal fluid is normal with the exception of some elevation of pressure. Serum muscle enzymes may be elevated. Transient electrocardiographic and electroencephalographic abnormalities may occur. Anaerobic culture and microscopic examination of pus from the wound can be helpful, but *C tetani* is difficult to grow, and the drumstick-shaped gram-positive bacilli often cannot be found.

Differential Diagnosis

In areas where tetanus is rarely seen, physicians may not recognize the infection until classic findings are present. Poliomyelitis is characterized by asymmetric paralysis in an incompletely immunized child. The history of an animal bite, absence of trismus, and pleocytosis suggest rabies. Local infections of the throat and jaw should be easily recognized. Bacterial meningitis, phenothiazine reactions, decerebrate posturing, narcotic withdrawal, spondylitis, and hypocalcemic tetany may be confused with tetanus.

Complications

Complications include sepsis, malnutrition, pneumonia, atelectasis, asphyxial spasms, decubitus ulcers, and fractures of the spine due to intense contractions. They can be prevented in part by skilled supportive care.

Prevention

A. Tetanus Toxoid: Active immunization with tetanus toxoid is the cornerstone of prevention of tetanus (see Chapter 10) and almost always is achieved after the third dose of vaccine. A booster at the time of injury is needed if none has been given in the past 10 years—or within 5 years in case of a heavily contaminated wound. Nearly all cases of tetanus (99%) in the United States are in unimmunized or incompletely immunized individuals. Many adolescents and adults lack protective antibody.

B. Tetanus Antitoxin: Human tetanus immune globulin (TIG) should be used in nonimmunized individuals with soil-contaminated wounds. For children who have had no or one tetanus toxoid immunization, 250–500 units should be given intramuscularly.

Tetanus toxoid and TIG should be administered concurrently at different sites using different syringes.

C. Treatment of Wounds: Proper surgical cleansing and debridement of contaminated wounds will decrease the risk of tetanus.

D. Prophylactic Antimicrobials: Prophylactic antimicrobials are useful if the child is unimmunized and TIG is not available.

Treatment

A. Specific Measures: Serotherapy lowers the mortality rate from tetanus, but not dramatically. TIG, 500 units intramuscularly is recommended by most experts. Surgical debridement of wounds is indicated, but more extensive surgery or amputation to eliminate the site of infection is not necessary. Penicillin G and tetanus toxin are both GABA antagonists; therefore, some experts prefer metronidazole.

B. General Measures: The patient is kept in a quiet room with minimal stimulation. Control of spasms and prevention of hypoxic episodes are crucial. Diazepam is useful (0.6–1.2 mg/kg/d intravenously in six divided doses). In the newborn, two or three divided doses should be given. Large doses (up to 25 mg/kg/d) may be required for older children. Diazepam is given intravenously until muscular spasms become infrequent and the generalized muscular rigidity much less prominent. The drug may then be given orally and the dose reduced as the child improves. Barbiturates, chlorpromazine, and paraldehyde may also be useful.

Mechanical ventilation and muscle paralysis are necessary in severe cases.

Prognosis

The fatality rate in newborns and heroin addicts is high (70–90%). The overall mortality rate in the United States is 65%. In a recent series of 44 neonates treated in Mexico City, the mortality rate was 25%. The fatality rate depends primarily on the quality of supportive care. Many deaths are due to pneumonia or respiratory failure. If the patient survives 1 week, recovery is likely.

Bleck TP: Tetanus: Pathophysiology, management and prophylaxis. Dis Mon (Sept) 1991;37:545.

Bowen V et al: Tetanus: A continuing problem in minor injuries. Can J Surg 1988;31:7.

Gergen PJ et al: A population based serologic survey of immunity to tetanus in the United States. N Engl J Med 1995;332:761.

Sanford JP: Tetanus: Forgotten but not gone. N Engl J Med 1995;322:812.

Simental PS et al: Neonatal tetanus experience at the National Institute of Pediatrics in Mexico City. Pediatr Infect Dis J 1993;12:722.

Sutton DN: Management of autonomic dysfunction in severe tetanus: The use of magnesium sulphate and clonidine. Intensive Care Med 1990;16:75.

GAS GANGRENE

Essentials of Diagnosis

- Contamination of a wound with soil or feces.
- Massive edema, skin discoloration, bleb formation, and pain in an area of trauma.
- Serosanguineous exudate from wound.
- Crepitation of subcutaneous tissue.
- Rapid progression of signs and symptoms.
- Clostridia cultured or seen on stained smears.

General Considerations

Gas gangrene (clostridial myonecrosis) is a necrotizing infection that follows trauma or surgery and is caused by several anaerobic, gram-positive, spore-forming bacilli of the genus *Clostridium*. These are soil, genital tract (female), and fecal organisms. In devitalized tissue, the spores germinate into vegetative bacilli that proliferate and produce toxins causing thrombosis, hemolysis, and tissue necrosis. *Clostridium perfringens,* the species causing approximately 80% of cases of gas gangrene, produces at least 8 such toxins. The areas involved most often are the extremities, abdomen, and uterus. *Clostridium septicum* may also cause myonecrosis and causes septicemia in patients with neutropenia. Nonclostridial infections with gas formation can mimic clostridial infections and are more common.

Clinical Findings

A. Symptoms and Signs: The onset of gas gangrene is sudden, usually 1–20 days (mean, 3–4 days) after trauma or surgery. The skin around the wound becomes discolored, with hemorrhagic bullae, serosanguineous exudate, and crepitation in the subcutaneous tissues. Pain and swelling are usually intense. Systemic illness appears early and progresses rapidly to intravascular hemolysis, jaundice, shock, toxic delirium, and renal failure.

B. Laboratory Findings: Isolation of the organism requires anaerobic culture. Gram-stained smears may demonstrate many gram-positive rods and few inflammatory cells.

C. Imaging: X-ray films may demonstrate gas in tissues, but this is a late finding and is also seen in infections with other gas-forming organisms or may be due to air introduced into tissues during trauma or surgery.

D. Surgical Findings: Direct visualization of the muscle at surgery may be necessary to diagnose gas gangrene. Early, the muscle is pale and edematous and does not contract normally; later, the muscle may be frankly gangrenous.

Differential Diagnosis

Gangrene and cellulitis caused by other organisms and clostridial cellulitis (not myonecrosis) must be distinguished. Necrotizing fasciitis may resemble gas gangrene.

Prevention

Gas gangrene can be prevented by the adequate cleansing and debridement of all wounds. It is essential that foreign bodies and dead tissue be removed. A clean wound does not provide a suitable anaerobic environment for the growth of clostridial species.

Treatment

A. Specific Measures: Penicillin G (300,000–400,000 units/kg/d intravenously in six divided doses) should be given.

B. Surgical Measures: Surgery should be prompt and extensive, with removal of all necrotic tissue.

C. Hyperbaric Oxygen: Hyperbaric oxygen therapy has been shown to be effective, but it is not a substitute for surgery. A patient may be exposed to 2–3 atm in pure oxygen for 1- to 2-hour periods for as many sessions as necessary until there is clinical remission.

Prognosis

Clostridial myonecrosis is fatal if untreated. With early diagnosis, antibiotics, and surgery, the mortality rate is about 20–60%. Involvement of the abdominal wall, leukopenia, intravascular hemolysis, renal failure, and shock are ominous prognostic findings.

Bessman AN, Wagner W: Nonclostridial gas gangrene: Report of 48 cases and review of the literature. *Clostridium septicum* JAMA 1975;233:958.

Bratton SL et al: Clostridium septicum infections in children. Pediatr Infect Dis J 1992;11:569.

Hart GB et al: Gas gangrene. J Trauma 1983;23:991.

Rudge FW: The role of hyperbaric oxygen in the treatment of clostridial myonecrosis. Mil Med 1993;158:80.

Stevens DL et al: Comparison of clindamycin, rifampin, tetracycline, metronidazole, and penicillin for efficacy in prevention of experimental gas gangrene due to *Clostridium perfringens*. J Infect Dis 1987;155:220.

DIPHTHERIA

Essentials of Diagnosis

- A gray, adherent pseudomembrane, most often in the pharynx but also in the nasopharynx or trachea.
- Sore throat, serosanguineous nasal discharge, hoarseness, and fever in a nonimmunized child.
- Peripheral neuritis or myocarditis.
- Positive culture.
- Treatment should *not* be withheld pending culture results.

General Considerations

Diphtheria is an acute infection of the upper respiratory tract or skin caused by toxin-producing *Corynebacterium diphtheriae*. Five or fewer cases per year are reported in the United States, but significant numbers of elderly adults and unimmunized children are susceptible to infection. Travelers to foreign countries such as the former Soviet Union, where an epidemic of diphtheria occurred in May 1994, may also acquire disease. Corynebacteria are gram-positive club-shaped rods with a beaded appearance on Gram's stain.

The capacity to produce exotoxin is conferred by a lysogenic bacteriophage and is not present in all strains of *C diphtheriae*. In immunized communities, infection probably occurs through spread of the phage among carriers of susceptible bacteria rather than through spread of phage-containing bacteria themselves. Diphtheria toxin kills susceptible cells by irreversible inhibition of protein synthesis.

The toxin is absorbed into the mucous membranes and causes destruction of epithelium and a superficial inflammatory response. The necrotic epithelium becomes embedded in exuding fibrin and red and white cells, forming a grayish "pseudomembrane" commonly present over the tonsils, pharynx, or larynx. Any attempt to remove the membrane exposes and tears the capillaries, resulting in bleeding. The diphtheria bacilli within the membrane continue to produce toxin, which is absorbed and may result in toxic injury to heart muscle, liver, kidneys, and adrenals, and is sometimes accompanied by hemorrhage. The toxin also produces neuritis, resulting in paralysis of the soft palate, eye muscles, or extremities. Death may occur as a result of respiratory obstruction or acute toxemia and circulatory collapse. The patient may succumb after a somewhat longer time as a result of cardiac damage. The incubation period is 1–6 days.

Clinical Findings

A. Symptoms and Signs:

1. Pharyngeal diphtheria–Early manifestations of diphtheritic pharyngitis are mild sore throat, moderate fever, and malaise, followed fairly rapidly by severe prostration and circulatory collapse. The pulse is more rapid than the fever would seem to justify. A pharyngeal membrane forms and may spread into the nasopharynx or the trachea, producing respiratory obstruction. The membrane is tenacious and gray and is surrounded by a narrow zone of erythema and a broader zone of edema. The cervical lymph nodes become swollen, and swelling is associated with brawny edema of the neck ("bull neck"). Laryngeal diphtheria presents with stridor, which can lead to obstruction of the airway.

2. Other forms–Cutaneous, vaginal diphtheria and wound diphtheria currently account for as many as 33% of cases and are characterized by ulcerative lesions with membrane formation.

B. Laboratory Findings: Diagnosis is clinical. Direct smears are unreliable. Material is first obtained from the nose, throat, or skin lesions, if present, for culture on Loeffler's and tellurite agar. Sixteen to 48 hours are required before identification of the organism is possible. A toxigenicity test is then performed. Cultures may be negative in individuals who have received antibiotics. The white blood cell count is usually normal, but hemolytic anemia and thrombocytopenia are frequent. The red blood cell count may show evidence of rapid destruction of erythrocytes. Thrombocytopenia due to peripheral destruction is frequent.

Differential Diagnosis

Pharyngeal diphtheria resembles acute streptococcal pharyngitis, mononucleosis, and occasionally, other viral pharyngitis. Nasal diphtheria may be mimicked by a foreign body or purulent sinusitis. Other causes of laryngeal obstruction are epiglottitis and viral croup. Neuropathy may be a manifestation of Guillain-Barré syndrome, poliomyelitis, or acute poisoning.

Complications

A. Myocarditis: Diphtheritic myocarditis is characterized by a rapid, thready pulse; indistinct heart sounds, ST-T wave changes, conduction abnormalities, dysrhythmias, or cardiac failure; hepatomegaly; and fluid retention. Myocardial dysfunction may occur from 2 to 40 days after the onset of pharyngitis.

B. Polyneuritis: Neuritis of the nerves innervating the palate and pharyngeal muscles occurs during the first or second week. Nasal speech and regurgitation of food through the nose are seen. Diplopia and strabismus occur during the third week or later. Neuritis may also involve peripheral motor nerves supplying the intercostal muscles and diaphragm and other muscle groups. Generalized paresis usually occurs after the fourth week.

C. Bronchopneumonia: Secondary pneumonia is common in fatal cases.

Prevention

A. Immunization: Immunization with diphtheria toxoid combined with pertussis and tetanus toxoids (DTP) should be used routinely for infants and children (see Chapter 10).

B. Care of Exposed Susceptibles: Children exposed to diphtheria should be examined, and nose and throat cultures obtained. If signs and symptoms of early diphtheria are found, treatment should be as for diphtheria. Immunized asymptomatic individuals should receive diphtheria toxoid if a booster has not been received within 5 years. Unimmunized close contacts should receive either erythromycin orally (40 mg/kg/d in four divided doses) for 7 days or benzathine penicillin G intramuscularly (25,000 units/kg), active immunization with diphtheria toxoid and be observed daily.

Treatment

A. Specific Measures:

1. Antitoxin–Diphtheria antitoxin should be ad-

ministered within 48 hours to be effective (see Chapter 10).

2. Antibiotics–Penicillin G (150,000 units/kg/d intravenously) should be given for 10 days. For the patient allergic to penicillin, erythromycin, 40 mg/kg/d, is given orally for 10 days.

B. General Measures: Bed rest in the hospital for 10–14 days is usually required. All patients must be strictly isolated for 1–7 days until respiratory secretions are noncontagious. Isolation may be discontinued when three successive nose and throat cultures at 24-hour intervals are negative. These cultures should not be taken until at least 24 hours have elapsed since the cessation of antibiotic treatment.

C. Treatment of Carriers: All carriers should be treated. Erythromycin (40 mg/kg/d orally in three or four divided doses), penicillin V potassium (50 mg/kg/d for 10 days), or benzathine penicillin G (600,000–1,200,000 units intramuscularly) should be given. All carriers must be confined at home. Before they can be released, carriers must have three negative cultures of both the nose and the throat taken 24 hours apart and obtained at least 24 hours after the cessation of antibiotic therapy.

Prognosis

Mortality rates vary from 3% to 25% and are particularly high in the presence of early myocarditis. Neuritis is reversible; it is fatal only if an intact airway and adequate respiration cannot be maintained. Permanent damage due to myocarditis occurs rarely.

Bethell DB et al: Prognostic value of electrocardiographic monitoring of patients with severe diphtheria. Clin Infect Dis 1995;20:1259.

Diphtheria acquired by US citizens in the Russian Federation and Ukraine—1994. MMWR 1995;44:237.

English PC: Diphtheria and theories of infectious disease: Centennial appreciation of the critical role of diphtheria in the history of medicine. Pediatrics 1985;76:1.

Pappenheimer AM Jr, Murphy JR: Studies on the molecular epidemiology of diphtheria. Lancet 1983;2:923.

Thisyakorn United States, Wongvanich J, Kumpeng V: Failure of corticosteroid therapy to prevent diphtheritic myocarditis or neuritis. Pediatr Infect Dis J 1984;3:126.

INFECTIONS DUE TO ENTEROBACTERIACEAE

Essentials of Diagnosis

- Diarrhea by several different mechanisms due to *Escherichia coli.*
- Neonatal sepsis or meningitis.
- Urinary tract infection.
- Opportunistic infections.
- Diagnosis confirmed by culture.

General Considerations

Enterobacteriaceae are a family of gram-negative

bacilli that are part of the normal flora of the gastrointestinal tract and are also found in water and soil. They cause gastroenteritis, urinary tract infections, neonatal sepsis and meningitis, opportunistic infections, and, occasionally, other infections. *Escherichia coli* is the organism in this family that most commonly causes infection in children, but *Klebsiella, Morganella, Enterobacter, Serratia, Proteus,* and other genera are also important, particularly in the compromised host. *Shigella* and *Salmonella* are discussed in separate sections.

E coli strains capable of causing diarrhea were originally termed enteropathogenic (EPEC) and were recognized by serotype. It is now known that *E coli* may cause diarrhea by several distinct mechanisms. The mechanisms responsible for diarrhea in the originally described EPEC strains are not known. Enterotoxigenic *E coli* (ETEC) cause a secretory, watery diarrhea. ETEC adhere to enterocytes and secrete one or more plasmid-encoded enterotoxins. One of these toxins resembles cholera toxin in structure, function, and mechanism of action. Enteroinvasive *E coli* are very similar to *Shigella* in pathogenetic mechanism. Enterohemorrhagic *E coli* (EHEC) are the cause of hemorrhagic colitis and the hemolytic uremic syndrome. The most common EHEC serotype is O157:H7, though several other serotypes cause the same syndrome. These strains elaborate a toxin, closely related to Shiga toxin produced by *S dysenteriae,* and termed verotoxin or Shiga-like toxin. Several outbreaks of hemolytic uremic syndrome associated with EHEC have followed consumption of inadequately cooked ground beef. Thorough heating to 68–71 °C is necessary.

Eighty percent of *E coli* strains causing neonatal meningitis possess specific capsular polysaccharide (K1 antigen), which, alone or in association with specific somatic antigens, confers virulence. K1 antigen is also present on approximately 40% of strains causing neonatal septicemia. The *E coli* K1 organisms do not appear to cause gastrointestinal disease.

Approximately 90% of urinary tract infections in children are caused by *E coli*. *E coli* bind to the uroepithelium by P-fimbria, which are present in greater than 90% of E coli that cause pyelonephritis. Other bacterial cell-surface structures, such as O and K antigens, and host factors are also important in the pathogenesis of urinary tract infections.

Klebsiella, Enterobacter, Serratia, and *Morganella* are normally found in the gastrointestinal tract and in soil and water. *Klebsiella* may cause a bronchopneumonia with cavity formation. *Klebsiella, Enterobacter,* and *Serratia* are often opportunists associated with antibiotic United Statesge, debilitating states, and chronic respiratory conditions. They frequently cause urinary tract infection or sepsis. In many newborn nurseries, nosocomial outbreaks caused by aminoglycoside-resistant *Klebsiella pneumoniae* are a major problem.

Many of these infections are difficult to treat because of antibiotic resistance. Antibiotic susceptibility tests are necessary. Parenteral third-generation cephalosporins are usually more active than ampicillin, but resistance due to high level production of chromosomal cephalosporinase may occur. *Enterobacter* and *Serratia* strains broadly resistant to cephalosporins also cause infections in hospitalized newborns and children. Aminoglycoside antibiotics (gentamicin, tobramycin, amikacin) are usually effective but require monitoring of serum levels to assure therapeutic, non-toxic levels.

Clinical Findings
A. Symptoms and Signs:
1. *E coli* gastroenteritis–*E coli* may cause diarrhea of varying type and severity. Enterotoxigenic *E coli* usually produce mild, self-limiting illness without significant fever or systemic toxicity, often known as traveler's diarrhea. However, diarrhea may be severe in newborns and infants, and occasionally an older child or adult will have a cholera-like syndrome. Enteroinvasive strains cause a shigellosis-like illness characterized by fever, systemic symptoms, blood and mucus in the stool, and leukocytosis, but currently are uncommon in the United States. Enterohemorrhagic strains cause hemorrhagic colitis. Diarrhea is initially watery, and fever is usually absent. Abdominal pain and cramping occur, and diarrhea progresses to blood streaking or grossly bloody stools. Hemolytic uremic syndrome occurs within a few days of diarrhea in 2–5% of children and is characterized by microangiopathic hemolytic anemia, thrombocytopenia, and renal failure (see Chapter 22).

E coli are transmitted from person to person and in food and water. Spread of *E coli* in day-care centers is probably common. Undercooked ground beef may transmit enterohemorrhagic *E coli*.

2. Neonatal sepsis–Findings include jaundice, hepatosplenomegaly, fever, temperature lability, apneic spells, irritability, and failure to suck vigorously. Meningitis is associated with sepsis in 25–40% of cases. Other metastatic foci of infection may be present, including pneumonia and pyelonephritis. Sepsis may lead to severe metabolic acidosis, shock, disseminated intravascular coagulation, and death.

3. Neonatal meningitis–Findings include high fever, full fontanelles, vomiting, coma, convulsions, pareses or paralyses, poor or absent Moro reflex, opisthotonos, and, occasionally, hypertonia or hypotonia. Sepsis coexists or precedes meningitis in most cases. Thus, signs of sepsis often accompany those of meningitis. Cerebrospinal fluid usually shows a cell count of over 1000/μL, mostly polymorphonuclear neutrophils, and bacteria on Gram's stain. Cerebrospinal fluid glucose concentration is low (usually less than half that of blood), and the protein is elevated above the levels normally seen in newborns and premature infants (> 150 mg/dL).

4. Acute urinary tract infection–Symptoms include dysuria, increased urinary frequency, and fever in the older child. Nonspecific symptoms such as anorexia, vomiting, irritability, failure to thrive, and unexplained fever are seen in children under 2 years of age. Young infants may present with jaundice. As many as 1% of girls of school age and 0.05% of boys have asymptomatic bacteriuria. Screening for and treatment of asymptomatic bacteriuria is not recommended.

B. Laboratory Findings: Because *E coli* are normal flora in the stool, a positive stool culture alone does not prove that the *E coli* in the stool are causing disease. Serotyping, tests for enterotoxin production or invasiveness, and tests for P-fimbria are performed in research laboratories. MacConkey's agar with sorbitol substituted for lactose (SMAC agar) is useful to screen stool for enterohemorrhagic *E coli*. Serotyping and testing for enterotoxin are available at many state health departments. Blood cultures are positive in neonatal sepsis. Cultures of cerebrospinal fluid and urine should also be obtained. The diagnosis of urinary tract infections is discussed in Chapter 22.

Differential Diagnosis

The clinical picture of enteropathogenic *E coli* infection may resemble that of salmonellosis, shigellosis, or viral gastroenteritis.

Neonatal sepsis and meningitis caused by *E coli* can be differentiated from other causes of neonatal infection only by blood and cerebrospinal fluid culture.

Treatment

A. Specific Measures:

1. *E coli* gastroenteritis–Gastroenteritis due to enteropathogenic *E coli* seldom requires antimicrobial treatment. Fluid and electrolyte therapy, preferably given orally, may be required to avoid dehydration. Bismuth subsalicylate reduces stool volume by about one third in infants with watery diarrhea, probably including toxigenic *E coli*. In nursery outbreaks, infants have been treated with neomycin (100/mg/kg/d orally in three divided doses for 5 days) or colistin (10–15 mg/kg/d orally in three divided doses for 5 days). Clinical efficacy is not established. Traveler's diarrhea may be treated with trimethoprim-sulfamethoxazole in children and with fluoroquinolones in adults. It is not clear whether the risk of hemolytic uremic syndrome increases or decreases following treatment of enterohemorrhagic colitis, but many experts withhold antimicrobials in this setting.

2. *E coli* sepsis, pneumonia, or pyelonephritis–The drugs of choice are ampicillin (150–200 mg/kg/d intravenously or intramuscularly in divided doses every 4–6 hours), cefotaxime (150–200 mg/kg/d intravenously or intramuscularly in divided doses every 6–8 hours), ceftriaxone (50–100 mg/kg/d intramuscularly as single dose or in two divided doses), and gentamicin (5–7.5 mg/kg/d intramuscularly or intravenously in divided doses every 8 hours). Treatment is for 10–14 days. Amikacin or tobramycin may be used instead of gentamicin if the strain is susceptible. Third-generation cephalosporins are often an attractive alternative as single-drug therapy and do not require monitoring for toxicity.

3. *E coli* meningitis–Third-generation cephalosporins such as cefotaxime (200 mg/kg/d intravenously in four divided doses) are given for a minimum of 3 weeks. Ampicillin (200–300 mg/kg/d intravenously in four to six divided doses) and gentamicin (5–7.5 mg/kg/d intramuscularly or intravenously in three divided doses) are also effective. Treatment with intrathecal and intraventricular aminoglycosides does not improve outcome. Newborns treated with aminoglycosides must have serum levels monitored.

4. Acute urinary tract infection–See Chapter 22.

Prognosis

Death due to gastroenteritis leading to dehydration can be prevented by early fluid and electrolyte therapy. Neonatal sepsis with meningitis is still associated with a mortality rate of over 50%. Most children with recurrent urinary tract infections do well if they have no serious underlying anatomic defects. The mortality rate in opportunistic infections usually depends on the severity of infection and the underlying condition.

Belongia EA et al: Transmission of *Escherichia coli* 0157:H7 infection in Minnesota day care facilities. JAMA 1993;269:883.

Bonadio WA et al: Escherichia coli bacteremia in children: A review of 91 cases in 10 years. Am J Dis Child 1991; 145:671.

Boyce TG, Swerdlow DL, Griffin PM: *Escherichia coli* 0157:H7 and the hemolytic uremic syndrome. N Engl J Med 1995;333:364.

Ericsson CD, DuPont HL: Travelers' diarrhea: Approaches to prevention and treatment. Clin Infect Dis 1993; 16:616.

Figueroa-Quintanilla D et al: A controlled trial of bismuth subsalicylate in infants with acute watery diarrheal disease. N Engl J Med 1993;328:1654.

Gallagher PG: Enterobacter bacteremia in pediatric patients. Rev Infect Dis 1990;12:808.

Keene WE et al: A swimming-associated outbreak of hemorrhagic colitis caused by *Escherichia coli* 0157:H7 and *Shigella sonnei*. N Engl J Med 1994;331:579.

Levine MM: *Escherichia coli* that cause diarrhea: Enterotoxigenic, enteropathogenic, enteroinvasive, enterohemorrhagic, and enteroadherent. J Infect Dis 1987;155:377.

MacDonald KL et al: *Escherichia coli* O157:H7, an emerging gastrointestinal pathogen. JAMA 1988;259:3567.

Murry BE: Can antibiotic resistance be controlled? N Engl J Med 1994:330:1229.

Pickering LK, Obrig, TG, Stapleton FB: Hemoytic-uremic syndrome and enterohemorrhagic *Escherichia coli* Pediatr Infect Dis J 1994;13:459.

Siitonen A et al: Invasive *Escherichia coli* infections in children: bacterial characteristics in different age groups and clinical entities. Pediatr Infect Dis J 1993;12:606.

Stull TL: Epidemiology and natural history of urinary tract infections in children. Med Clin North Am 1991;75:287.

PSEUDOMONAS INFECTIONS

Essentials of Diagnosis

- Opportunistic infection.
- Confirmed by cultures.

General Considerations

Pseudomonas aeruginosa is an important cause of infection in children with cystic fibrosis, neoplastic disease, neutropenia, or extensive burns and in those receiving antibiotic therapy. Infections of the urinary and respiratory tracts, ears, mastoids, paranasal sinuses, eyes, skin, meninges, and bones are seen. *Pseudomonas* pneumonia is a common nosocomial infection in patients receiving assisted ventilation. *P aeruginosa* sepsis may be accompanied by characteristic peripheral lesions called ecthyma gangrenosum. Ecthyma gangrenosum also may occur by direct invasion through intact skin in the groin, axilla, or other skinfolds. *P aeruginosa* is an infrequent cause of sepsis in previously healthy infants, and may be the initial sign of underlying medical problems. *P aeruginosa* osteomyelitis often complicates puncture wounds of the feet. *P aeruginosa* is a frequent cause of malignant external otitis media and of chronic suppurative otitis media. Outbreaks of vesiculopustular skin rash have been associated with exposure to contaminated water in whirlpool baths and hot tubs.

P aeruginosa is an aerobic gram-negative rod with versatile metabolic requirements. *P aeruginosa* may grow in distilled water and in commonly used disinfectants, complicating the problem of infection control. *P aeruginosa* is both invasive and destructive to tissue, and toxigenic due to secreted exotoxins, which contribute to virulence. Other *Pseudomonas* species occasionally cause nosocomial infections. *Xanthomas maltophilia* (previously *P maltophilia*) and *Butkholderia cepacia* (previously *P cepacia*) are the most frequent.

P aeruginosa infects the tracheobronchial tree of nearly all patients with cystic fibrosis. Mucoid exopolysaccharide, an exuberant capsule, is characteristically overproduced by isolates from patients with cystic fibrosis. Although bacteremia seldom occurs, patients with cystic fibrosis ultimately succumb to chronic lung infection with *P aeruginosa*. Infection due to *B cepacia* has caused a rapidly progressive pulmonary disease in some colonized patients and may be spread by close personal contact.

Clinical Findings

The clinical findings depend on the site of infection and the patient's underlying disease. Sepsis with these organisms resembles gram-negative sepsis with other organisms, though the presence of ecthyma gangrenosa suggests the diagnosis. The diagnosis is made by culture. *Pseudomonas* infection should be suspected in neonates and neutropenic patients with clinical sepsis.

A severe necrotizing pneumonia occurs in patients on ventilators.

Patients with cystic fibrosis have a persistent bronchitis which progresses to bronchiectasis and ultimately to respiratory failure. During exacerbations of illness, cough and sputum production increase with low grade fever, malaise, and diminished energy.

The purulent aural drainage without fever in patients with chronic suppurative otitis media is not distinguishable from that due to other cause.

Prevention

A. Infections in Debilitated Patients: Colonization of extensive second- and third-degree burns by *P aeruginosa* can lead to fatal septicemia. Aggressive debridement and topical treatment with 0.5% silver nitrate solution, 10% mafenide cream, or gentamicin ointment will greatly inhibit *P aeruginosa* contamination of burns. (See Chapter 12 for a discussion of burn wound infections and prevention.)

B. Nosocomial Infections: Faucet aerators, communal soap dispensers, disinfectants, improperly cleaned inhalation therapy equipment, infant incubators, and back rub lotions have all been associated with *Pseudomonas* epidemics. Infant-to-infant transmission by nursery personnel carrying *Pseudomonas* on the hands is frequent in neonatal units. Careful maintenance of equipment and enforcement of infection control procedures are essential to minimize nosocomial transmission.

C. Patients With Cystic Fibrosis: Chronic infection of the lower respiratory tract occurs in nearly all patients with cystic fibrosis. The infecting organism is seldom cleared from the respiratory tract, even with intensive antimicrobial therapy, and the resultant injury to the lung eventually leads to pulmonary insufficiency. Treatment is aimed at controlling signs and symptoms of the infection.

Treatment

P aeruginosa is inherently resistant to many antimicrobials and may develop resistance during therapy. Mortality rates in hospitalized patients exceed 50%, due both to the severity of underlying illnesses in patients predisposed to *Pseudomonas* infection and to the limitations of therapy. Aminoglycoside antimicrobials; ureidopenicillins such as ticarcillin or piperacillin; the combination of β-lactamase inhibitor with a ureidopenicillin such as ticarcillin/clavulanate piperacillin/tazobactam; expanded-spectrum cephalosporins, such as ceftazidime; imipenem; and the fluoroquinolones are active against most *P aeruginosa* strains, as well as other enteric gram-negative rods. However, antimicrobial susceptibility patterns vary from area to area, and resistance tends to appear as new drugs become popular. Treatment of infections is best guided by clinical response and susceptibility tests.

Use of gentamicin or tobramycin (5–7.5 mg/kg/d intramuscularly or intravenously in three divided doses) or amikacin (15–22 mg/kg/d in two or three divided doses) in combination with ticarcillin (200–300 mg/kg/d intravenously in six divided doses) or with another anti-*Pseudomonas* β-lactam antibiotic is recommended for treatment of serious *Pseudomonas* infections. Ceftazidime (150–200 mg/kg/d in four divided doses) is a third-generation cephalosporin with excellent activity against *P aeruginosa*. Treatment should be continued for 10–14 days. Treatment with two active drugs is recommended for all serious infections.

Pseudomonas osteomyelitis requires surgical debridement and antimicrobial therapy for 2 weeks. *Pseudomonas* folliculitis does not require antibiotic therapy.

Chronic suppurative otitis media responds to intravenous ceftazidime (150–200 mg/kg/d in three or four divided doses) given until the drainage has ceased for 3 days. Twice-daily ceftazidime with aural debridement and cleaning given on an outpatient basis has also been successful. Oral ciprofloxacin is also effective but is not FDA-approved in children because of concerns about skeletal toxicity.

Swimmer's ear may be caused by *P aeruginosa* and responds well to topical drying agents (alcohol, vinegar mix) and cleansing.

Prognosis

Because debilitated patients are most frequently affected, the mortality rate is high. These infections may have a protracted course, and eradication of the organisms may be difficult.

Agger WA, Mardan A: *Pseudomonas aeruginosa* infections of intact skin. Clin Infect Dis 1995;20:302.

Bodey GP et al: Infections caused by Pseudomonas aeruginosa. Rev Infect Dis 1983;5:279.

Boisseau AM et al: Perineal ecthyma gangrenosum in infancy and early childhood: Septicemic and non septicemic forms. J Am Acad Dermatol 1992;27:415.

Dagan R et al: Outpatient management of chronic suppurative otitis media without cholesteatoma in children. Pediatr Infect Dis J 1992;11:542.

Fergie JE, Patrick CC, Lott L: *Pseudomonas aeruginosa* cellulitis and ecthyma gangrenosum in immunocompromised children. Pediatr Infect Dis J 1991;10:469.

Fiel SB: Clinical management of pulmonary disease in cystic fibrosis. Lancet 1993;341:1070.

Fisher MC et al: Sneakers as a source of *Pseudomonas aeruginosa* in children with osteomyelitis following puncture wounds. J Pediatr 1985;106:607.

Flores G, Stavola JJ, Noel GJ: Bacteremia due to *Pseudomonas aeruginosa* in children with AIDS. Clin Infect Dis 1993;16:706.

Grundmann H et al: *Pseudomonas aeruginosa* in a neonatal intensive care unit: Reservoirs and ecology of the nosocomial pathogen. J Infect Dis 1993;168:943.

Jackson MA, Wong KY, Lampkin B: Pseudomonas aeruginosa septicemia in childhood cancer patients. Pediatr Infect Dis J 1982;1:239.

Jacobs RF, McCarthy RE, Elser JM: *Pseudomonas* osteochondritis complicating wound punctures of the foot in children: A ten year evaluation. J Infect Dis 1989; 160:657.

Leigh I et al: *Pseudomonas aeruginosa* infection in very low birth weight infants: A case-control study. Pediatr Infect Dis J 1995;12:367.

Martin-Ancel A, Borque C, del Castillo F: *Pseudomonas sepsis* in children without previous medical problems. Pediatr Infect Dis J 1993;12:258.

SALMONELLA GASTROENTERITIS

Essentials of Diagnosis

- Nausea, vomiting, headache, meningismus.
- Fever, diarrhea, abdominal pain.
- Culture or organism from stool, blood, or other specimens.

General Considerations

Salmonellae are gram-negative rods that frequently cause food-borne gastroenteritis and occasionally bacteremic infection of bone, meninges, and other foci. Three species—*Salmonella typhi, Salmonella choleraesuis,* and *Salmonella enteritidis*—and approximately 2000 serotypes are recognized. *S typhimurium* is the most frequently isolated serotype in most parts of the world. Approximately 50,000 cases of salmonellosis are reported annually in the United States, but many cases are either not reported or not recognized.

Salmonellae are able to penetrate the mucin layer of the small bowel and attach to epithelial cells. Organisms penetrate the epithelial cells and multiply in the submucosa. Infection results in fever, vomiting, watery diarrhea, and occasionally, mucus with some polymorphonuclear leukocytes in the stool. Although the small intestine is generally regarded as the principal site of infection, colitis also occurs. *S typhimurium* frequently involves the large bowel.

Salmonella infections in childhood occur in two major forms: (1) gastroenteritis (including food poisoning), which may be complicated by sepsis and focal suppurative complications; and (2) enteric fever (typhoid fever and paratyphoid fever). (See next section.) Although the incidence of typhoid fever has decreased in the United States, the incidence of *Salmonella* gastroenteritis has greatly increased in the past 15–20 years. The highest attack rates occur in children under 6 years of age, with a peak in the age group from 6 months to 2 years old.

Salmonellae are widespread in nature, infecting domestic and wild animals. Fowl and reptiles have a particularly high carriage rate. Transmission results primarily from ingestion of contaminated food. Transmission from human to human occurs by the fecal-oral route via contaminated food, water, and fomites. Numerous foods are associated with outbreaks including meats, milk, cheese, ice cream, chocolate and other foods. Contaminated egg powder and frozen whole egg preparations used to make ice cream, custards, and mayonnaise are responsible for outbreaks. Eggs with contaminated shells that are consumed raw or undercooked have been incriminated in outbreaks and sporadic cases.

Salmonellae are susceptible to gastric acidity and, therefore, the elderly, infants, and patients treated with antacids or H_2 blocking drugs are at increased risk of infection. Most cases of Salmonella meningitis (80%) and bacteremia occur in infancy. Newborns may acquire the infection from their mothers during delivery and may precipitate outbreaks in nurseries. Newborns are at special risk of developing meningitis.

Clinical Findings

A. Symptoms and Signs: Infants usually develop fever, vomiting, and diarrhea. The older child may also complain of headache, nausea, and abdominal pain. Stools are often watery or may contain mucus and, in some instances, blood, suggesting shigellosis. Drowsiness and disorientation may be associated with meningismus. Convulsions occur less frequently than with shigellosis. Splenomegaly is occasionally noted. In the usual case, diarrhea is moderate and subsides after 4–5 days, but it may be protracted.

B. Laboratory Findings: Diagnosis is made by isolation of the organism from stool, blood, or, in some cases, from urine, cerebrospinal fluid, or pus from a suppurative lesion. The white blood cell count usually shows a polymorphonuclear leukocytosis but may show leukopenia. Typing of isolates is done with specific antisera. *Salmonella* isolates should be reported to public health authorities for epidemiologic purposes.

Differential Diagnosis

In staphylococcal food poisoning, the incubation period is shorter (2–4 hours) than in *Salmonella* food poisoning (12–24 hours). Fever is absent, and vomiting rather than diarrhea is the main symptom. In shigellosis, many pus cells are likely to be seen on a stained smear of stool, and there is more likely to be a marked shift to the left in the peripheral white count, although some cases of salmonellosis are indistinguishable from shigellosis. *Campylobacter* gastroenteritis commonly resembles salmonellosis clinically. (Organisms previously classified as *Arizona* are considered *Salmonella* and cause a similar illness.) Culture of the stools is necessary to distinguish the causes of bacterial gastroenteritis.

Complications

Unlike most types of infectious diarrhea, salmonellosis is frequently accompanied by bacteremia, especially in newborns and infants. Septicemia with extraintestinal infection is seen, most commonly with *S choleraesuis* but also with *S enteritidis, S typhimurium,* and *S paratyphi* B and C. The organism may localize in any tissue and may cause arthritis, osteomyelitis, cholecystitis, endocarditis, meningitis, pericarditis, pneumonia, or pyelonephritis. In patients with sickle cell anemia or other hemoglobinopathies, there is a predilection for osteomyelitis to develop. Severe dehydration and shock are more likely to occur with shigellosis but may occur with *Salmonella* gastroenteritis.

Prevention

Measures for the prevention of *Salmonella* infections include thorough cooking of foodstuffs derived from potentially infected sources; proper refrigeration during storage; and recognition and control of infection among domestic animals, combined with proper meat and poultry inspections. Raw and undercooked fresh eggs should be avoided. Adults with salmonellosis who are food handlers or who have occupations involving care of young children should have three negative stool cultures before resuming work.

Treatment

A. Specific Measures: In uncomplicated *Salmonella* gastroenteritis antibiotic treatment does not shorten the course of the clinical illness and may prolong convalescent carriage of the organism. Colitis or secretory diarrhea due to *Salmonella* may improve with antibiotic therapy.

However, to prevent sepsis and focal disease, antibiotic treatment is recommended for newborns and infants less than 3 months of age, for severely ill children, and for children with sickle cell disease, liver disease, recent gastrointestinal surgery, cancer, depressed immunity, and chronic renal or cardiac disease. Infants with positive stool cultures or suspected salmonellosis sepsis at less than 3 months of age should be admitted to hospital, evaluated for focal infection including blood culture and cerebrospinal fluid examination, and treated intravenously. Ampicillin (150–200 mg/kg/d intravenously in four divided doses for 5–10 days), or trimethoprim-sulfamethoxazole is recommended. Older patients developing bacteremia during the course of gastroenteritis should receive parenteral treatment initially, and a careful search should be made for additional foci of infection. After signs and symptoms subside, these patients should receive oral medication. Parenteral and oral treatment should last a total of 7–10 days. Longer treatment is indicated for specific complications. If susceptibility tests indicate resistance to ampicillin, chloramphenicol, third-generation cephalosporins or trimethoprim-sulfamethoxazole should be given. Fluoroquinolones also are efficacious but are not FDA-approved for administration to children.

Salmonella meningitis is best treated with a combination of chloramphenicol (100 mg/kg/d intravenously in four divided doses) and ampicillin (200–300 mg/kg/d intravenously in four to six divided doses) for 3 weeks or a third-generation cephalosporin (cefotaxime, ceftriaxone) for 3 weeks. If the child improves rapidly and the cerebrospinal fluid is sterile, treatment may be completed with a single drug, the choice guided by results of susceptibility tests.

Outbreaks on pediatric wards are difficult to control. Strict hand washing, cohorting of patients and personnel, and ultimate closure of the unit may be necessary.

B. Treatment of the Carrier States: About half of patients are still infectious after 4 weeks. Infants tend to remain convalescent carriers for up to a year. Antibiotic treatment of carriers is not effective.

C. General Measures: Careful attention must be given to maintaining fluid and electrolyte balance, especially in infants.

Prognosis

In gastroenteritis, the prognosis is good. In sepsis with focal suppurative complications, the prognosis is more guarded.

The case fatality rate of *Salmonella* meningitis is high in infants. There is a strong tendency to relapse if treatment is not prolonged.

Ackman DM, Drabkin P, Birkhead G, Cieslak P: Reptile-associated salmonellosis in New York State. Pediatr Infect Dis J 1995;14:955.

Chalker RB, Blaser MJ: A review of human salmonellosis: III. Magnitude of Salmonella infection in the United States. Rev Infect Dis 1988;10:111.

Rennels MB, Leving MM: Classical bacterial diarrhea: Perspectives and update—*Salmonella, Shigella, Escherichia coli, Aeromonas,* and *Plesiomonas.* Pediatr Infect Dis J 1986;5(Suppl):21.

Sanchez C et al: Ciprofloxacin and trimethoprim-sulfamethoxazole versus placebo in acute uncomplicated *Salmonella* enteritis: A double blind trial. J Infect Dis 1993;168:1304.

St Geme JW III et al: Consensus: management of *Salmonella* infection in the first year of life. Pediatr Infect Dis J 1988;7:615.

Telzak EE et al: A nosocomial outbreak of *Salmonella enteriditis* infection due to the consumption of raw eggs. N Engl J Med 1990;323:394.

TYPHOID FEVER & PARATYPHOID FEVER

Essentials of Diagnosis

- Insidious or acute onset of headache, anorexia, vomiting, constipation or diarrhea, ileus, and high fever.
- Meningismus, splenomegaly, and rose spots.
- Leukopenia; positive blood, stool, bone marrow, and urine cultures.

General Considerations

Typhoid fever is caused by the gram-negative bacillus *Salmonella typhi;* paratyphoid fevers, which are usually milder but may be clinically indistinguishable, are caused by *Salmonella paratyphi* A, *Salmonella schottmülleri,* or *Salmonella hirschfeldii* (formerly *Salmonella paratyphi* A, B, and C). Children have a shorter incubation period than do adults (usually 5–8 days instead of 8–14 days). The organism enters the body through the walls of the intestinal tract and, following a transient bacteremia, multiplies in the reticuloendothelial cells of the liver and spleen.

Persistent bacteremia and symptoms then follow. Reinfection of the intestine occurs as organisms are excreted in the bile. Bacterial emboli produce the characteristic skin lesions (rose spots). Symptoms in children may be mild or severe, but children younger than age 5 uncommonly have clinically severe typhoid fever.

Typhoid fever is transmitted by the fecal-oral route and by contamination of food or water. Unlike other *Salmonella* species, there are no animal reservoirs of *S typhi*; each case is the result of direct or indirect contact with the organism or with an individual who is actively infected or a chronic carrier.

About 500 cases per year are reported in the United States, 60% of which are acquired during foreign travel.

Clinical Findings

A. Symptoms and Signs: In children, the onset of typhoid fever is apt to be sudden rather than insidious, with malaise, headache, crampy abdominal pains and distention, and sometimes constipation followed within 48 hours by diarrhea, high fever, and toxemia. An encephalopathy may be seen with irritability, confusion, delirium, and stupor. Vomiting and meningismus may be prominent in the young. The classic prolonged three-stage disease seen in adult patients is often shortened in children. The prodrome may be only 2–4 days; the toxic stage may last only 2–3 days; and the defervescence stage may last 1–2 weeks.

During the prodromal stage, physical findings may

be absent, or there may merely be some abdominal distention and tenderness, meningismus, mild hepatomegaly, and minimal splenomegaly. The typical typhoidal rash (rose spots) is present in 10–15% of children. It appears during the second week of the disease and may erupt in crops for the succeeding 10–14 days. Rose spots are erythematous maculopapular lesions 2–3 mm in diameter that fade on pressure. They are found principally on the trunk and chest, and they generally disappear within 3–4 days. The lesions usually number less than 20.

B. Laboratory Findings: Typhoid bacilli can be isolated from many sites, including blood, stool, urine, and bone marrow. Blood cultures are positive in 50–80% of cases during the first week and less often later in the illness. Stool cultures are positive in about 50% of cases after the first week. Urine and bone marrow cultures are also valuable. Most patients will have negative cultures (including stool) by the end of a 6-week period. Serologic tests (Widal reaction) are not as useful as cultures because both false-positive and false-negative results occur. A fourfold rise in titer of O (somatic) agglutinins is suggestive but not diagnostic of infection.

Leukopenia is common in the second week of the disease, but in the first week, leukocytosis may be seen. Proteinuria, mild elevation of liver enzymes, thrombocytopenia, and disseminated intravascular coagulation are common.

Differential Diagnosis

Typhoid and paratyphoid fevers must be distinguished from other serious prolonged fevers. These include typhus, brucellosis, tularemia, miliary tuberculosis, psittacosis, vasculitis, lymphoma, mononucleosis, and Kawasaki disease.

The diagnosis of typhoid fever if often made clinically in developing countries. In developed countries, where typhoid fever is uncommon and physicians are unfamiliar with the clinical picture, the diagnosis is often not suspected until late. Positive cultures confirm the diagnosis.

Complications

The most important complications of typhoid fever are gastrointestinal hemorrhage (2–10%) and perforation (1–3%). They occur toward the end of the second week or during the third week of the disease.

Intestinal perforation is one of the principal causes of death. The site of perforation generally is the terminal ileum or cecum. The clinical manifestations are indistinguishable from those of acute appendicitis, with pain, tenderness, and rigidity in the right lower quadrant. The x-ray finding of free air in the peritoneal cavity is diagnostic.

Bacterial pneumonia, meningitis, septic arthritis, abscesses, and osteomyelitis are uncommon complications, particularly if specific treatment is given promptly. Shock and electrolyte disturbances may lead to death.

About 1–3% of patients become chronic carriers of *S typhi*. Chronic carriage is defined as excretion of typhoid bacilli for more than a year, but carriage is often lifelong. Adults with underlying biliary or urinary tract disease are much more likely than children to become chronic carriers.

Prevention

Routine typhoid vaccine is not recommended in the United States but should be considered for some foreign travel to endemic areas. An attenuated oral typhoid vaccine produced from strain Ty21a has better efficacy and causes minimal side effects but is not approved for children under 6 years. A newly licensed capsular polysaccharide vaccine (ViCPS) requires one intramuscular injection and may be given to children 2 years and older (see Chapter 10).

Treatment

A. Specific Measures: Equally effective regimens for susceptible strains include the following: trimethoprim-sulfamethoxazole (10 mg/kg trimethoprim and 50 mg/kg sulfamethoxazole per day orally in two or three divided doses), amoxicillin (100 mg/kg/d orally in four divided doses), and ampicillin (100–200 mg/kg/d intravenously in four divided doses). Aminoglycosides and first- and second-generation cephalosporins are clinically ineffective regardless of in vitro susceptibility results. Third-generation cephalosporins are used for resistant strains. Ceftriaxone and cefotaxime may be used parenterally. Cefixime is efficacious orally. Occasionally, the presence of multiple resistant strains requires the use of chloramphenicol (50–100 mg/kg/d orally or intravenously in four doses).

Treatment duration is 14–21 days. Patients remain febrile for 3–5 days even with appropriate therapy.

B. General Measures: General support of the patient is exceedingly important and includes rest, good nutrition, and careful observation, with particular regard to evidence of intestinal bleeding or perforation. Blood transfusions may be needed even in the absence of frank hemorrhage.

Prognosis

A prolonged convalescent carrier stage in children often continues 3–6 months. This does not require retreatment with antibiotics or exclusion from school or other activities.

With early antibiotic therapy, the prognosis is excellent. With early treatment, the mortality rate is less than 1%. Relapse occurs 1–3 weeks later in 10–20% of cases despite appropriate antibiotic treatment.

Bitar R, Tarpley J: Intestinal perforation in typhoid fever: A historical and state-of-the-art review. Rev Infect Dis 1985;7:257.

Butler T et al: Patterns of morbidity and mortality in typhoid fever dependent on age and gender: Review of 552 hospitalized patients with diarrhea. Rev Infect Dis 1991;13:85.

Girgis NI et al: Comparison of the efficacy, safety, and cost of cefixime, ceftriaxone, and aztreonam in the treatment of multi-drug-resistant *Salmonella typhi* septicemia in children. Pediatr Infect Dis J 1995;14:603.

Hall CB: A single shot of *Salmonella typhi:* A new typhoid vaccine with pediatric advantages. Pediatrics 1995; 96:348.

Hoffman SL et al: Reduction of mortality in chloramphenicol-treated severe typhoid fever by high-dose dexamethasone. N Engl J Med 1984;310:82.

Mahle WT, Levine MM: *Salmonella typhi* infection in children younger than five years of age. Pediatr Infect Dis J 1993;12:627.

Meloni T et al: Ceftriaxone treatment of *Salmonella* enteric fever. Pediatr Infect Dis J 1988;7:734.

Thisyakorn U, Mansuwan P, Taylor DN: Typhoid and paratyphoid fever in 192 hospitalized children in Thailand. Am J Dis Child 1987;141:862.

SHIGELLOSIS
(Bacillary Dysentery)

Essentials of Diagnosis

- Cramps and bloody diarrhea.
- High fever, malaise, convulsions.
- Pus and blood in diarrheal stools examined microscopically.
- Diagnosis confirmed by stool culture.

General Considerations

Shigellae are nonmotile gram-negative rods of the family Enterobacteriaceae and are closely related to *Escherichia coli*. The genus *Shigella* is divided into four major groups, A–D: *Shigella dysenteriae, Shigella flexneri, Shigella boydii,* and *Shigella sonnei*. Approximately 20,000 cases of shigellosis are reported each year in the United States. *S sonnei* followed by *S flexneri* are the most common isolates. *S dysenteriae*, which causes the most severe diarrhea of all species and the greatest number of extraintestinal complications, accounts for fewer than 1% of all Shigella infections in the United States.

Shigellosis is often a serious disease, particularly in children under 2 years of age, and without supportive treatment there is an appreciable mortality rate. In older children and adults, the disease tends to be self-limited and milder. Shigellosis is unusual in infants under 3 months of age, although in rare cases shigellae may be transmitted from the mother to the newborn during delivery. Diarrhea and refusal to take feedings are the most common symptoms in neonatal shigellosis, and bloody diarrhea and fever occur less frequently. Vomiting, convulsions, or high fever is almost never encountered.

Shigella is usually transmitted by the fecal-oral route. Food- and water-borne outbreaks occur but are less important overall than person-to-person transmission. The disease is very communicable; as few as 200 bacteria can produce illness in an adult. The secondary attack rate in families is high, and shigellosis is a serious problem in day-care centers and custodial institutions. *Shigella* organisms produce disease by invading the colonic mucosa, causing mucosal ulcerations and microabscesses. A plasmid-encoded gene is required for enterotoxin production, chromosomal genes are required for invasiveness, and smooth lipopolysaccharide are required for virulence.

Clinical Findings

A. Symptoms and Signs: The incubation period of shigellosis usually is 2–4 days. Onset is abrupt, with abdominal cramps, urgency, tenesmus, chills, fever, malaise, and diarrhea. In severe forms, blood and mucus are seen in small volume in the watery stool (dysentery), and meningismus and convulsions may occur. In older children, the disease may be mild and may be characterized by watery diarrhea without blood. In young children, a fever of 39.4–40 °C is common. Rarely, there is rectal prolapse. Symptoms generally last 3–7 days.

B. Laboratory Findings: The total white blood cell count varies, but often there is a marked shift to the left. The stool may contain gross blood and mucus, and many neutrophils are seen if mucus from the stool is examined microscopically. Stool cultures usually are positive; however, they may be negative because the organism is somewhat fragile and present in small numbers late in the disease, and because laboratory techniques are suboptimal for the recovery of shigellae.

Differential Diagnosis

Diarrhea due to rotavirus infection is a winter rather than a summer disease, usually children are not as febrile or toxic, and stool does not contain gross blood or neutrophils. Intestinal infections caused by *Salmonella* or *Campylobacter* are differentiated by culture. Amebic dysentery is diagnosed by microscopic examination of fresh stools or sigmoidoscopy specimens; intussusception is characterized by an abdominal mass, "currant jelly" stools without leukocytes, and absence of fever. Mild shigellosis is not distinguishable clinically from other forms of infectious diarrhea.

Complications

Dehydration, acidosis, shock, and renal failure are the major complications. In some cases, a chronic form of dysentery occurs, characterized by mucoid stools and poor nutrition. Bacteremia and metastatic infections are rare but serious complications. Febrile seizures are common. Fulminating fatal dysentery and hemolytic uremic syndrome occur rarely.

Treatment

A. Specific Measures: Trimethoprim-sulfamethoxazole (10 mg/kg/d trimethoprim and 50 mg/kg/d sulfamethoxazole, in two divided doses orally for 5 days) is the treatment of choice. Amoxicillin is not effective. Ampicillin (100 mg/kg/d in four divided doses) is also efficacious if the strain is sensitive. Ceftriaxone parenterally or cefixime orally is effective and should be used for resistant strains. Ciprofloxacin, 500 mg twice daily for 5 days, is efficacious in adults but is not approved in children. Successful treatment results in reduced duration of fever, cramping, and diarrhea and in termination of fecal excretion of *Shigella*. Strains resistant to ampicillin and trimethoprim-sulfamethoxazole are common in Mexico and underdeveloped countries. In the United States, 7% of isolates are resistant to trimethoprim-sulfamethoxazole and one-third are resistant to ampicillin. Tetracycline and chloramphenicol are also effective, but resistance is common. Presumptive therapy should be based on the susceptibility pattern of recent local isolates.

B. General Measures: In severe cases, immediate rehydration is critical. A mild form of chronic malabsorption syndrome may supervene and require prolonged dietary control.

Prognosis

The prognosis is excellent if vascular collapse is treated promptly by adequate fluid therapy. The mortality rate is high in very young, malnourished infants who do not receive fluid and electrolyte therapy. Convalescent fecal excretion of *Shigella* lasts 1–4 weeks in patients not receiving antimicrobial therapy. Long-term carriers are rare.

Ashkenazi S et al: Convulsions in shigellosis: Evaluation of possible risk factors. Am J Dis Child 1983;137:985.

Ashkenazi S et al: A randomized, double-blind study comparing cefixime and trimethoprim-sulfamethoxazole in the treatment of childhood shigellosis. J Pediatr 1993; 123:817.

Bennish ML: Potentially lethal complications of shigellosis. Rev Infect Dis 1991;13:5319.

DeWitt TG, Humphrey KF, McParthy P: Clinical predictors of acute bacterial diarrhea in young children. Pediatrics 1985;76:551.

Dupont HL, Nornick RB: Adverse effects of Lomotil therapy in shigellosis. JAMA 1973;226:1525.

Eidlitz-Marcus T et al: Comparative efficacy of two- and five-day courses of ceftriaxone for treatment of severe shigellosis in children. J Pediatr 1993;123:822.

Huskins WC et al: Shigellosis in neonates and young infants. J Pediatr 1994;125:14.

Tacket CO, Cohen ML: Shigellosis in day-care centers: Use of plasmid analysis to assess control measures. Pediatr Infect Dis 1983;2:127.

Tauxe RV et al: Antimicrobial resistance of Shigella isolates in the United States: The importance of international travelers. J Infect Dis 1990;162:1107.

CHOLERA

Essentials of Diagnosis

- Sudden onset of severe watery diarrhea.
- Persistent vomiting without nausea or fever.
- Extreme and rapid dehydration and electrolyte loss, with rapid development of vascular collapse.
- Contact with a case of cholera, with shellfish, or the presence of cholera in the community.
- Diagnosis confirmed by stool culture.

General Considerations

Cholera is an acute diarrheal disease caused by the gram-negative organism *Vibrio cholerae*. It is transmitted by contaminated water or food, especially contaminated shellfish. The disease is generally so dramatic that in endemic areas the diagnosis is obvious. Individuals with mild illness and young children may play an important role in transmission of the infection.

Asymptomatic infection is far more common than clinical disease. In endemic areas, rising titers of vibriocidal antibody are seen with increasing age; infection occurs in individuals with low titers. The age-specific attack rate is highest in children under 5 years and declines with age. Cholera is unusual in infancy.

Cholera toxin is a protein enterotoxin that is primarily responsible for symptoms. Cholera toxin binds to a regulatory subunit of adenyl cyclase in enterocytes, causing increased cyclic adenosine monophosphate and an outpouring of NaCl and water into the lumen of the small bowel.

Nutritional status is an important factor determining the severity of the diarrhea. Duration of diarrhea is prolonged in adults and children suffering from severe malnutrition.

Cholera is endemic in India and southern and Southeast Asia and in parts of Africa. Seven major pandemics have occurred since 1817. The most recent pandemic, caused by the El Tor biotype of *cholerae* 01, began in 1961 in Indonesia. In 1982, 37 countries were affected and 54,000 cases reported. Epidemic cholera spread in Central and South America, with a total of 1 million cases and 9500 deaths reported through 1994. Cases in the United States occurred in the course of foreign travel or as a result of consumption of contaminated imported food. Cholera is increasingly associated with consumption of shellfish. Interstate shipments of oysters have resulted in cholera in several inland states.

Several recent studies provide evidence that *V cholerae* is a natural inhabitant of shellfish and copepods in estuarine environments. Seasonal multiplication of *V cholerae* may provide a source for outbreaks in endemic areas. Chronic cholera carriers are rare. The incubation period is short, usually 1–3 days.

Clinical Findings

A. Symptoms and Signs: Many patients infected with *V cholerae* have mild disease, with 1–2% developing severe diarrhea. During severe cholera, there is a sudden onset of massive, frequent, watery stools, generally light gray in color ("rice water") and containing some mucus but no pus. Vomiting may be projectile and is not accompanied by nausea. Within 2–3 hours, the tremendous loss of fluids results in severe and life-threatening dehydration, hypochloremia, and hypokalemia, with marked weakness and collapse. Renal failure with uremia and irreversible peripheral vascular collapse will occur if fluid therapy is not administered. The illness lasts 1–7 days and is shortened by appropriate antibiotic therapy.

B. Laboratory Findings: Markedly elevated hemoglobin (20 g/dL) and marked acidosis, hypochloremia, and hyponatremia are seen, and marked acidosis may complicate isotonic dehydration.

Cultural confirmation using thiosulfate-citrate-bile-salt-sucrose (TCBS) agar takes 16–18 hours for a presumptive diagnosis and 36–48 hours for a definitive bacteriologic diagnosis.

Prevention

Cholera vaccine is available in the United States and provides 50% efficacy. Protection lasts 3–6 months. Cholera vaccine is not generally recommended for travelers. In endemic areas, all water and milk must be boiled, food protected from flies, and sanitary precautions observed. Thorough cooking of shellfish prevents transmission. All patients with cholera should be isolated.

Chemoprophylaxis is indicated for household and other close contacts of cholera patients. It should be initiated as soon as possible after the onset of the disease in the index patient. Tetracycline (500 mg daily for 5 days) is effective in preventing infection. Trimethoprim-sulfamethoxazole may be substituted in children.

Tourists visiting endemic areas are at little risk if they exercise common sense in what they eat and drink and maintain good personal hygiene.

Treatment

Physiologic saline or lactated Ringer's solution should be administered intravenously in large amounts to restore blood volume and urine output and to prevent irreversible shock. Potassium supplements are required. Sodium bicarbonate, given intravenously, may also be needed initially to overcome profound acidosis. Moderate dehydration and acidosis can be corrected in 3–6 hours by oral therapy alone, because the active glucose transport system of the small bowel is normally functional. The optimal composition of the oral solution (in meq/L) is as follows: Na$^+$ 90, Cl$^-$ 80, and K$^+$ 20—with glucose, 110 mmol/L.

Treatment of children with tetracycline (50 mg/kg/d orally in four divided doses for 2–5 days) shortens the duration of the disease and prevents clinical relapse but is not as important as fluid and electrolyte therapy. Tetracycline resistance occurs in some regions, and ciprofloxacin may be used. Trimethoprim-sulfamethoxazole should be used in children under 9 years of age.

Prognosis

With early and rapid replacement of fluids and electrolytes, the case fatality rate is 1–2% in children. If significant symptoms appear and no treatment is given, the mortality rate is over 50%.

Carpenter CC: The treatment of cholera: Clinical science at the bedside. J Infect Dis 1992;166:2.

Finkelstein RA et al: Epitopes of the cholera family of enterotoxins. Rev Infect Dis 1987;9:544.

Fukuda JM et al: Clinical characteristics and risk factors for *Vibrio cholerae* infection in children. J Pediatr 1995; 126:882.

Gotuzzo E et al: Ciprofloxacin for the treatment of cholera: A randomized, double-blind, controlled clinical trial of a single daily dose in Peruvian adults. Clin Infect Dis 1995;20:1485.

Johnston JM et al: Cholera on a Gulf Coast oil rig. N Engl J Med 1983;309:523.

Lacey SW: cholera: Calamitous past, ominous future. Clin Infect Dis 1995;20:1409.

MMWR Update: *Vibrio cholerae* 01—western hemisphere, 1991–1994, and *V. cholerae* 0139—Asia, 1994. MMWR 1995;44:215.

CAMPYLOBACTER INFECTION

Essentials of Diagnosis

- Fever, vomiting, abdominal pain, diarrhea.
- Blood, mucus, pus in stools (dysentery).
- Presumptive diagnosis by darkfield or phase contrast microscopy of stool wet mount or modified Gram's stain.
- Definitive diagnosis by stool culture.

General Considerations

Campylobacter species (formerly grouped with vibrios and known as *Vibrio fetus*) are small, gram-negative, curved or spiral bacilli that are commensals or pathogens in many animals. *Campylobacter jejuni* frequently causes acute enteritis in humans, and *Campylobacter fetus* causes bacteremia and meningitis in immunocompromised patients. *Campylobacter fetus* may cause maternal fever, abortion, stillbirth, and severe neonatal infection. *Helicobacter pylori* (previously called *Campylobacter pylori*) has been associated with gastritis and peptic ulcer disease in both adults and children (see Chapter 20).

In the past decade, *C jejuni* has been responsible for 3–11% of cases of acute gastroenteritis in North

America and Europe; in many areas, enteritis due to *C jejuni* is more common than that due to *Salmonella* or *Shigella.*

Campylobacter colonizes domestic and wild animals, especially poultry. Numerous cases have been associated with sick puppies or other animal contacts. Contaminated food and water, improperly cooked poultry, and person-to-person spread by the fecal-oral route are important in transmission. Outbreaks associated with day-care centers, contaminated water supplies, and raw milk have been reported. Raw milk consumption, often during visits to dairy farms, was responsible for 20 outbreaks involving nearly 500 children from 1981 to 1990. Newborns may acquire the organism from their mothers at delivery.

Clinical Findings

A. Symptoms and Signs: *C jejuni* enteritis can be mild or severe. In tropical countries, asymptomatic stool carriage is common. The incubation period is usually 1–7 days. The disease usually begins with sudden onset of high fever, malaise, headache, abdominal cramps, nausea, and vomiting. Diarrhea follows and may be watery or bile-stained, mucoid, and bloody. Passage of up to 20 stools per day is not uncommon. The illness is self-limiting, lasting 2–7 days, but relapses occur in 15–25% of cases. Without antimicrobial treatment, the organism remains in the stool for 1–6 weeks.

B. Laboratory Findings: The peripheral white blood cell count generally is elevated, with many band forms. Microscopic examination of stool reveals erythrocytes and pus cells, and darkfield or phase contrast microscopic examination of wet mounts may reveal darting bacilli characteristic of *Campylobacter.* Other bacteria, particularly *Vibrio* species, may exhibit similar motility, but in areas where cholera and *Vibrio parahaemolyticus* diarrhea are rare, a positive darkfield examination has a predictive value of about 90%. Isolation of *C jejuni* from stool is not difficult but requires selective agar, incubation at 42 °C, rather than 35 °C, and incubation in an atmosphere of about 5% oxygen and 5% CO_2 (candle jar is satisfactory).

Differential Diagnosis

Campylobacter enteritis may resemble viral gastroenteritis, salmonellosis, shigellosis, amebiasis, or other infectious diarrheas. Because it also mimics ulcerative colitis, Crohn's disease, intussusception, and appendicitis, mistaken diagnosis can lead to unnecessary surgery.

Complications

The most important complications are dehydration and inappropriate treatment due to misdiagnosis as inflammatory bowel disease. Other complications are uncommon but include erythema nodosum, convul-

sions, reactive arthritis, bacteremia, urinary tract infection, and cholecystitis. Guillain-Barré syndrome is associated with *Campylobacter jejuni* infection in the preceding 1–3 weeks.

Prevention

No vaccine is yet available. Hand washing and adherence to basic food sanitation practices help prevent disease. Handwashing and cleaning kitchen utensils after contact with raw poultry are important.

Treatment

Treatment of fluid and electrolyte disturbances is most important. Antimicrobial treatment with erythromycin in children (30–50 mg/kg/d orally in four divided doses for 5 days) or with tetracycline or clindamycin in adults terminates fecal excretion and may prevent relapses, but antimicrobial treatment does not shorten or modify the illness unless given early in the disease. Antimicrobials used for shigellosis, such as trimethoprim-sulfamethoxazole and ampicillin, are inactive against *Campylobacter.* Supportive therapy is sufficient in most cases.

Prognosis

The outlook is excellent if dehydration is corrected and misdiagnosis does not lead to inappropriate diagnostic or surgical procedures.

Allos BM, Blaser MJ: *Campylobacter jejuni* and the expanding spectrum of related infections. Clin Infect Dis 1995;20:1092.

Paisley JW et al: Dark-field microscopy of human feces for presumptive diagnosis of *Campylobacter fetus* subsp jejuni enteritis. J Clin Microbiol 1982;15:61.

Rees JH et al: *Campylobacter jejuni* infection and Guillain-Barré syndrome. N Engl J Med 1995;333:1374.

Wong S-N et al: *Campylobacter* infection in the neonate: Case report and review of the literature. Pediatr Inf Dis J 1990;9:665.

Wood RC et al: Campylobacter enteritis outbreaks associated with drinking raw milk during youth activities. JAMA 1992;268:3228.

TULAREMIA

Essentials of Diagnosis

- A cutaneous or mucous membrane lesion at the site of inoculation and regional lymph node enlargement.
- Sudden onset of fever, chills, and prostration.
- History of contact with infected animals, principally wild rabbits, or history of tick exposure.
- Positive culture or immunofluorescence of mucocutaneous ulcer or regional lymph nodes.
- High serum antibody titer.

General Considerations

Tularemia is caused by *Francisella tularensis,* a

gram-negative organism usually acquired from infected animals, principally wild rabbits; occasionally from infected domestic dogs or cats; by contamination of the skin or mucous membranes with infected blood or tissues; by inhalation of infected material; by bites of ticks, fleas, or deer flies that have been in contact with infected animals; or by ingestion of contaminated meat or water. Strains of high virulence for humans and rabbits (Jellison type A) and strains with lowered virulence (Jellison type B) for humans, which are avirulent in rabbits, are present throughout the United States. The incubation period is short, usually 3–7 days, but may vary from 2 to 25 days.

Ticks are the most important vector. Rabbits are the classic vectors of tularemia. It is important to seek a history of rabbit hunting, skinning, or food preparation in any patient who has a febrile illness with tender lymphadenopathy, often in the region of a draining skin ulcer.

Clinical Findings

A. Symptoms and Signs: Several clinical types of tularemia are seen in children. Sixty percent of infections are of the ulceroglandular form and start as a reddened papule that may be pruritic, quickly ulcerates, and is not very painful. Shortly thereafter, the regional lymph nodes become large and tender. Fluctuance quickly follows. At the same time, there may be marked systemic manifestations, including high fever, chills, weakness, and vomiting. Pneumonitis occasionally accompanies the ulceroglandular form or may be seen as the sole manifestation of infection (pneumonic form). A detectable skin lesion is occasionally absent, and localized lymphoid enlargement exists alone (glandular form). Oculoglandular and oropharyngeal forms also occur in children. The latter is characterized by tonsillitis, often with membrane formation, cervical adenopathy, and high fever. In the absence of any primary ulcer or localized lymphadenitis, a prolonged febrile disease reminiscent of typhoid fever can be seen (typhoidal form). Splenomegaly is common in all forms.

B. Laboratory Findings: *F tularensis* can be recovered from ulcers, regional lymph nodes, and sputum of patients with the pneumonic form. However, the organism grows only on an enriched medium (blood-cystine-glucose agar), and laboratory handling is dangerous owing to the risk of airborne transmission to laboratory personnel. Immunofluorescent staining of biopsy material or aspirates of involved lymph nodes is diagnostic, although it is not widely available.

The white blood cell count is not remarkable. Agglutinins are present after the second week of illness, and in the absence of a positive culture their development confirms the diagnosis. An agglutination titer of 1:160 or higher is considered positive.

Differential Diagnosis

The typhoidal form of tularemia may mimic typhoid, brucellosis, miliary tuberculosis, Rocky Mountain spotted fever, and infectious mononucleosis. Pneumonic tularemia resembles atypical and mycotic pneumonitis. The ulceroglandular type of tularemia resembles pyoderma caused by staphylococci or streptococci, rat-bite fever, plague, anthrax, and cat-scratch fever. The oropharyngeal type must be distinguished from streptococcal or diphtheritic pharyngitis, infectious mononucleosis, herpangina, or other viral pharyngitides.

Prevention

Reasonable attempts should be made to protect children from bites of insects, principally ticks, fleas, and deer flies, by the use of proper clothing and repellents. Since rabbits are the source of most human infections, the dressing and handling of such game should be performed with great care. If contact occurs, thorough washing with soap and water is indicated.

Treatment

A. Specific Measures: Streptomycin (30 mg/kg/d intramuscularly in two divided doses for 8–10 days, maximum dose 1 g) with drug of choice, although gentamycin is probably equally efficacious. Tetracycline is effective, but relapse rates are higher. Chloramphenicol is less effective. Failures are also higher with ceftriaxone.

B. General Measures: Antipyretics and analgesics may be given as necessary. Skin lesions are best left open. Glandular lesions occasionally require incision and drainage.

Prognosis

The prognosis is excellent with appropriate therapy in patients recognized early.

Cross JT, Jacobs RF: Tularemia: Treatment failures with outpatient use of ceftriaxone. Clin Infect Dis 1993; 17:976.

Enderlin G et al: Streptomycin and alternative agents for the treatment of tularemia: Review of the literature. Clin Infect Dis 1994;19:42.

Jacobs RF, Condrey YM, Yamauchi T: Tularemia in adults and children: A changing presentation. Pediatrics 1985;76:818.

Liles WC, Burger RJ: Tularemia from domestic cats. West J Med 1993;158:619.

Rohrbach BW et al: Epidemiological and clinical characteristics of tularemia in Oklahoma, 1979 to 1985. South Med J 1991;84:1091.

Spach DH et al: Tick-borne diseases in the United States. N Engl J Med 1993;329:936.

Uhari M, Syrjala H, Salminen A: Tularemia in children caused by Francisella tularensis biovar palaearctica. Pediatr Infect Dis J 1990;9:80.

PLAGUE

Essentials of Diagnosis
- Sudden onset of fever, chills, and prostration.
- Regional lymphadenitis with suppuration of nodes (bubonic form).
- Hemorrhage into skin and mucous membranes and shock (septicemia).
- Cough, dyspnea, cyanosis, and hemoptysis (pneumonia).
- History of exposure to infected animals.

General Considerations
Plague is an extremely serious, acute infection caused by a gram-negative bacillus, *Yersinia pestis.* It is a disease of rodents that is transmitted to humans by the bites of fleas. Plague bacilli have been isolated from rodents in 15 of the western states in the United States. Direct contact with rodents, rabbits, or domestic cats may transmit fleas infected with plague bacilli. During the 1980s, a mean of 18 cases per year was reported in the United States, primarily from the southwestern region. Most cases occur from June through September.

Human plague in the United States appears to occur in cycles that reflect cycles in wild animal reservoirs.

Clinical Findings
A. Symptoms and Signs: Plague assumes several clinical forms, the two most common being bubonic and septicemic. Pneumonic plague, the form that occurs when organisms enter the body through the respiratory tract, is now very uncommon.

1. Bubonic plague—Bubonic plague begins after an incubation period of 6 days with a sudden onset of high fever, chills, headache, vomiting, and marked delirium or clouding of consciousness. A less severe form also exists, with a less precipitous onset, but with progression over several days to severe symptoms. Although the flea bite is rarely seen, the regional lymph node, usually inguinal and unilateral, is painful and tender, 1–5 cm in diameter. The node usually suppurates and drains spontaneously after 1 week. The plague bacillus is known to produce an endotoxin that causes vascular necrosis. Bacilli may overwhelm regional lymph nodes and enter the circulation to produce septicemia. Severe vascular necrosis results in widely disseminated hemorrhage in skin, mucous membranes, liver, and spleen. Myocarditis and circulatory collapse may result from damage by the endotoxin.

Plague meningitis or pneumonia may occur following bacteremic spread from an infected lymph node.

2. Septicemic plague—The septicemic form is defined as any case of plague without evidence of lymphadenopathy. Regional lymphadenopathy and bubo formation occur after 3–5 days. This form is less common than bubonic plague but carries a worse prognosis, largely because it is less likely to be recognized and treated early. Patients may present initially with a nonspecific febrile illness characterized by fever, myalgia, chills, and anorexia. It is frequently complicated by pneumonia.

B. Laboratory Findings: Aspiration of a bubo leads to visualization of bipolar staining gram-negative bacilli on a stained smear. Pus, sputum, and blood all yield the organism, although laboratory infections are common enough to make isolation dangerous. A buffy coat Gram's stain may reveal the organism, and blood-agar cultures yield positive results in 48 hours. The white blood cell count is markedly elevated, with a shift to the left.

Sera obtained during disease and convalescence should be collected and stored for use in confirming the diagnosis in cases where the organism may not be recovered.

Differential Diagnosis
The septic phase of the disease may be confused with such illnesses as meningococcemia, sepsis, and rickettsioses. The bubonic form resembles tularemia, anthrax, cat-scratch fever, streptococcal adenitis, and cellulitis. Primary gastroenteritis and appendicitis may have to be distinguished.

Prevention
Proper disposal of household and commercial wastes and chemical control of rats are basic for control of plague. Flea control is instituted and maintained with the liberal use of insecticides. Children vacationing in remote camping areas should be warned not to handle dead or dying animals. Domestic cats that roam freely in suburban areas may contact infected wild animals and acquire infected fleas. Travelers to wild areas in the enzootic western states are at low risk of infection, and immunization of visitors to these areas is not recommended.

Vaccination is recommended for those traveling or living in areas of high incidence (see Chapter 10).

Treatment
A. Specific Measures: Streptomycin is the drug of choice in a dosage of 20–40 mg/kg intramuscularly in three divided doses for 5–7 days. For patients not requiring parenteral therapy, tetracycline, 20–30 mg/kg/d in four divided doses, or chloramphenicol (75–100 mg/kg/d intravenously or orally in four divided doses) may be given for 10–14 days. Tetracycline is not recommended for children under 9 years of age.

In septicemia and pneumonic plague, specific antibiotic treatment must be started in the first 15–24 hours of the disease if survival is to be expected. Treatment with streptomycin started 36–48 hours after onset of the disease may result in death due to liberation of plague toxin.

Bubonic plague is not highly contagious. Every effort is made to effect resolution of buboes without resorting to surgery. Pus from draining lymph nodes should be handled with gloves.

B. General Measures: Pneumonic plague is highly infectious, and strict isolation is required. All contacts should receive prophylaxis with sulfadiazine (100–200 mg/kg/d orally in four divided doses for 7 days) or tetracycline (30 mg/kg/d in four divided doses for 7 days).

Prognosis

The mortality rate in untreated bubonic plague is about 50%; it is 90% in the septicemic form and nearly 100% in the pneumonic form. Recent mortality rates in New Mexico were 3% for bubonic plague and 71% for the septicemic form.

Craven BB, Barnes AM: Plague and tularemia. Infect Dis Clin North Am 1991;5:165.
Crook LD: Plague: A clinical review of 27 cases. Arch Intern Med 1992;152:1253.
Hull HF, Montes JM, Mann JM: Septicemic plague in New Mexico. J Infect Dis 1987;155:113.
Human plague—United States, 1993–1994. MMWR Morb Mortal Wkly Rep 1994;43:243.
Mann JM, Shandler L, Cushing AH: Pediatric plague. Pediatrics 1982;69:762.

HAEMOPHILUS INFLUENZAE TYPE b INFECTIONS

Essentials of Diagnosis

- Purulent meningitis in children under age 4 years with direct smears of cerebrospinal fluid showing gram-negative pleomorphic rods.
- Acute epiglottitis: High fever, drooling, dysphagia, aphonia, and stridor.
- Septic arthritis: Fever, local redness, swelling, heat, and pain with active or passive motion of the involved joint in a child 4 months to 4 years of age.
- Cellulitis: Sudden onset of fever and distinctive cellulitis in an infant, often involving the cheek or periorbital area.
- In all cases, a positive culture from the blood, cerebrospinal fluid, or aspirated pus confirm the diagnosis.

General Considerations

H influenzae type b (HIB) has become uncommon because of widespread immunization in early infancy. The 95% reduction in disease seen in many parts of the United States is due to high rates of vaccine coverage and reduced nasopharyngeal carriage after vaccination. Although the incidence is reduced, HIB remains important because of its potential for serious invasive disease. It causes meningitis, bacteremia, epiglottitis (supraglottic croup), septic

arthritis, periorbital and facial cellulitis, pneumonia, and pericarditis. HIB infections occur most frequently in the age group from 4 months to 4 years (epiglottitis: 2–5 years), although 340 cases of HIB were reported in the United States in 1994. Recognition and prompt therapy of the many serious manifestations of HIB infection will become more challenging as physicians encounter fewer infections.

Antibody to the HIB capsular polysaccharide, polyribose-phosphate (PRP) is protective against invasive disease. PRP is a poor immunogen, particularly in infants less than 2 years old. Vaccines consisting of PRP chemically conjugated to protein are far more immunogenic and raise protective levels of antibody in infants beginning at age 2 months. Four separate interchangeable PRP protein conjugate vaccines are available (see Chapter 10).

Disease due to *H influenzae* types A, C, D, E, F, or unencapsulated strains is uncommonly seen but now comprises a larger proportion of positive cultures. Ampicillin-resistant HIB were first reported in 1974. Resistance is due to the production of plasmid-encoded β-lactamase in most cases. Currently, 25–40% of HIB strains in the United States are ampicillin-resistant. HIB resistant to chloramphenicol—or to both ampicillin and chloramphenicol—are uncommon in the United States. Third-generation cephalosporins are preferred for initial therapy of suspected HIB infections. Resistance of HIB to the third-generation cephalosporins has not been reported, and the cephalosporins lack the hematologic toxicity of chloramphenicol. Ampicillin is adequate for culture-proved HIB where susceptibility to ampicillin has been proved by the microbiology laboratory.

Unencapsulated, nontypable *H influenzae* frequently colonize the mucous membranes and cause otitis media, sinusitis, bronchitis, and pneumonia in both children and adults. Bacteremia is uncommon but does occur. Neonatal sepsis similar to early onset group B streptococci is recognized. Obstetric complications of chorioamnionitis and bacteremia are associated with these neonatal cases.

Ampicillin resistance occurs in 25–40% of nontypable *H influenzae*.

Clinical Findings
A. Symptoms and Signs:
1. Meningitis–In the United States, HIB is an uncommon cause of bacterial meningitis except in unimmunized children. Infants usually present with fever, irritability, lethargy, poor feeding with or without vomiting, and a high-pitched cry. Signs of localized disease elsewhere should be looked for carefully, including otitis, cellulitis, arthritis, and pneumonia.

2. Acute epiglottitis–The most useful clinical finding in the early diagnosis of HIB epiglottitis is evidence of dysphagia characterized by a refusal to eat or swallow saliva and by drooling. This finding, plus the presence of a high fever in a "toxic" child—even in the absence of cherry-red epiglottis on direct examination of the epiglottis—should strongly suggest the diagnosis and lead to prompt intubation. Stridor is a late sign. (See Chapter 17 for details.)

3. Septic arthritis–HIB is a common cause of septic arthritis in unimmunized children under 4 years of age in the United States. Disease may involve multiple joints and is complicated by osteomyelitis in about 20% of cases. The child is febrile and refuses to move the involved joint and limb because of pain. Examination reveals swelling, warmth, redness, tenderness on palpation, and severe pain on attempted movement of the joint.

4. Cellulitis–Cellulitis due to HIB occurs almost exclusively in the 3-month to 4-year age group. Fever is usually noted at the same time as the cellulitis, and many infants appear toxic. The cheek or periorbital (preseptal) area is usually involved. There is mild swelling with central erythema, rapidly progressing to a lesion without a distinct border that exhibits central reddish discoloration surrounded by a purplish area. Superficial trauma is characteristically absent. Bacteremia is frequent.

Periorbital cellulitis due to HIB must be distinguished from two other similar entities. The first is periorbital cellulitis caused by local infection of the skin due to trauma. Staphylococci, streptococci, or a combination of the two are usually isolated. The second is periorbital or occasionally orbital cellulitis, which is an extension of ethmoid or splenic sinusitis. Typical nasopharyngeal flora, *S pneumoniae,* nontypable *H influenzae,* and *M catarrhalis* are commonly involved. Bacteremia is uncommon in these two types of periorbital cellulitis.

5. Pneumonia–Pneumonia due to HIB usually presents clinically in much the same fashion as pneumonia due to the pneumococcus. Disease is most common in the age group from 3 months to 4 years, just as it is with *H influenzae* meningitis. Most cases are segmental or lobar in distribution, but diffuse bronchopneumonia or interstitial involvement is occasionally seen. Both empyema and lung abscesses occur. HIB involvement of other organs (meningitis, epiglottitis, otitis media) may be present.

The true incidence of HIB pneumonia is not known. Pneumonia due to unencapsulated *H influenzae* is difficult to diagnose because a small percentage have positive blood cultures.

6. Bacteremia–Acutely ill children 4–36 months of age, with temperatures higher than 39 °C and nonspecific symptoms associated with an elevated white blood cell count, may have HIB bacteremia. This syndrome is associated most frequently with pneumococcal bacteremia.

B. Laboratory Findings: The white blood cell count in HIB infections may be high or normal with a shift to the left. Blood culture is frequently positive.

Positive culture of aspirated pus or fluid from the involved site proves the diagnosis.

In meningitis (before treatment), spinal fluid smear may show the characteristic pleomorphic gram-negative rods.

The diagnosis of HIB pneumonia depends on isolation of the organism from blood, lung tissue, or empyema fluid. A positive culture from the upper respiratory tract is not diagnostic. Antigen detection tests are generally not helpful.

C. Imaging: A lateral view of the neck in suspected acute epiglottitis may suggest the diagnosis, but misinterpretation is common. Intubation should not be delayed to obtain films. Haziness of maxillary and ethmoid sinuses occurs with orbital cellulitis.

Differential Diagnosis

A. Meningitis: Meningitis must be differentiated from head injury, brain abscess, tumor, lead encephalopathy, and other forms of meningoencephalitis, including mycobacterial, viral, fungal, and bacterial agents.

B. Acute Epiglottitis: In croup caused by viral agents (parainfluenza 1, 2, and 3, respiratory syncytial virus, influenza A, adenovirus), the child has more definite upper respiratory symptoms, cough, hoarseness, slower progression of obstructive signs, and fever. Spasmodic croup occurs typically at night in a child with a history of previous attacks; these attacks may be of allergic origin. A history of sudden onset of choking and paroxysmal coughing suggests aspiration of a foreign body. Occasionally, retropharyngeal abscess or rarely laryngeal diphtheria may have to be differentiated from epiglottitis.

C. Septic Arthritis: Differential diagnosis includes acute osteomyelitis, prepatellar bursitis, cellulitis, rheumatic fever, and fractures and sprains.

D. Cellulitis: Erysipelas, streptococcal cellulitis, insect bites, and trauma (including Popsicle panniculitis or other types of freezing injury) may occur. Periorbital cellulitis must be differentiated from paranasal sinus disease without cellulitis, allergic inflammatory disease of the lids, conjunctivitis, and herpes zoster infection.

E. Pneumonia: See Chapter 18.

F. Bacteremia: Sepsis due to other bacteria, including *S pneumoniae* and *N meningitidis,* must be differentiated by blood culture.

Complications

A. Meningitis: See Chapter 23.

B. Acute Epiglottitis: The disease may rapidly progress to complete airway obstruction with complications owing to hypoxia. Mediastinal emphysema and pneumothorax may occur.

C. Septic Arthritis: Septic arthritis may result in rapid destruction of cartilage and ankylosis if diagnosis and treatment are delayed. Even with early treatment, the incidence of residual damage and disability after septic arthritis in weight-bearing joints may be as high as 25%.

D. Cellulitis: Bacteremia may lead to meningitis or pyarthrosis.

E. Pneumonia: Complications include empyema and, rarely, pneumatocele and pneumothorax.

F. Bacteremia: Meningitis, pneumonia, or other infected foci may develop. Children with HIB bacteremia should be evaluated thoroughly (including lumbar puncture) for infected foci. Inpatient management with intravenous antimicrobials is indicated until the child is afebrile and appears well.

Prevention

Epidemiologic studies have demonstrated that families and close contacts of patients with HIB infections are at increased risk of acquiring infection. The index case and all household contacts should be given rifampin, 20 mg/kg/d (maximum adult dose 600 mg/d), orally for 4 successive days. There is controversy regarding a recommendation for chemoprophylaxis for day-care-center contacts. Some authorities recommend rifampin chemoprophylaxis for young contacts (especially children age 2 or less) of a case who regularly attended a day-care center. Other authorities believe that the risk to day-care-center contacts is low and do not recommend prophylaxis unless two cases of systemic HIB disease have occurred in children in the day-care center within a 60-day period. Rifampin, if used, should be given to children in the same classroom as the index case and to adults working in that classroom.

Treatment

All bacteremic or potentially bacteremic HIB diseases require hospitalization for treatment. The drugs of choice in hospitalized cases are a third-generation cephalosporin (cefotaxime or ceftriaxone) until the sensitivity of the organism is known.

Second-generation cephalosporins (cefuroxime, cefamandole, cefoxitin, and cefaclor) should not be used for any HIB infection in which meningitis is a possibility, since these drugs do not reach cerebrospinal fluid in concentrations adequate to treat or prevent infection. Ceftriaxone or cefotaxime is preferred for meningitis because of more rapid and reliable sterilization of cerebrospinal fluid. Meningitis is treated intravenously. Other patients may be switched to oral therapy after initial therapy. Oral therapy with amoxicillin is preferred for susceptible strains. Several agents may be used for ampicillin-resistant strains or for those of unknown susceptibility. These include trimethoprim-sulfamethoxazole, erythromycin-sulfonamide combinations, cefaclor, amoxicillin-clavulanic acid, cefixime, loracarbef, cefpodoxime, and cefprozil. Penicillin, erythromycin alone, and first-generation cephalosporins are not reliable. Oral chloramphenicol is very effective but is

not preferred because it is associated with hematologic toxicity.

A. Meningitis: Therapy is begun as soon as bacterial meningitis has been identified and cerebrospinal fluid, blood, and other appropriate cultures have been obtained. Therapy is begun with cefotaxime (50 mg/kg intravenously every 6 hours) or ceftriaxone (50 mg/kg intravenously every 12 hours). If the organism is sensitive to ampicillin, it is the drug of choice. Therapy should preferably be given intravenously for the entire course; chloramphenicol may be given orally when tolerated (if it is used levels must be monitored), and ceftriaxone may be given intramuscularly if venous access becomes difficult.

Duration of therapy is 10 days. Although a 7-day regimen appears effective in most uncomplicated cases, it has not been studied in children who have also been treated with steroids to prevent hearing loss (see below). Longer treatment is reserved for those children who respond slowly or in whom septic complications have occurred. Antibiotics can be discontinued after 10 days in a febrile child if the clinical response was rapid and satisfactory, but the source of prolonged or recurrent fevers must always be sought with great care. The most common causes for recurrence of fever or persistence of fever beyond 6 days are the following: phlebitis, hospital-acquired viral or bacterial superinfection, metastatic disease requiring drainage (eg, subdural empyema, septic pericarditis, arthritis), drug fever, and subdural effusions. Fever commonly recurs after steroids are discontinued.

Repeated lumbar taps are usually not necessary in HIB meningitis. They should be obtained in the following circumstances: unsatisfactory or questionable clinical response, seizure occurring after several days of therapy, and prolonged (7 days) or recurrent fever if the neurologic examination is abnormal or difficult to evaluate. Routine lumbar tap at the end of therapy is not recommended. (See Chapter 23 for additional information.)

Supportive therapy with intravenous fluids and oxygen, should be given as required. Patients should be observed carefully for development of the syndrome of inappropriate ADH secretion (SIADH). Dexamethasone given immediately after diagnosis and continued for a period of 4 days may reduce the incidence of hearing loss in children with HIB meningitis. The use of dexamethasone is controversial, but when it is used, the dose is 0.6 mg/kg/d in four divided doses for 4 days. Therapy for longer than 4 days, for neonates, or for viral meningitis is not recommended. In animal models, it is important to give the dexamethasone prior to beginning antimicrobials; this maximally blocks formation of inflammatory mediators (interleukin-1β and tumor necrosis factor) thought responsible for eighth nerve damage.

B. Acute Epiglottitis: See Chapter 17.

C. Septic Arthritis: Initial therapy should include nafcillin (or another effective antistaphylococcal antibiotic), 150 mg/kg/d in four divided doses, and cefotaxime or ceftriaxone (dosage as for meningitis). If the isolate is sensitive to ampicillin, it is given in a dosage 200–300 mg/kg/d intravenously in four divided doses. If a child is improved following initial intravenous therapy, then oral amoxicillin (75–100 mg/kg/d in four divided doses every 6 hours) may be administered under careful supervision to complete a 2-week course. Alternative oral agents for ampicillin-resistant organisms include chloramphenicol, cefaclor, trimethoprim-sulfamethoxazole, amoxicillin-clavulanic acid, and cefixime. Ideally, susceptibility to these agents should be proved prior to use. Drainage of infected joint fluid is an essential part of treatment. In joints other than the hip, this can often be accomplished by one or more needle aspirations. In hip infections—and in arthritis of other joints where treatment is delayed or clinical response is slow—surgical drainage is advised. Local instillation of antibiotics is not necessary and may be injurious.

The joint should be immobilized. Antipyretics and analgesics are given as required, and adequate hydration is maintained.

D. Cellulitis and Orbital Cellulitis: Initial therapy should include an agent effective against staphylococci in combination with cefotaxime or ceftriaxone. Ampicillin may be used if the isolate is shown to be susceptible. Therapy is given parenterally for 3–7 days, followed by oral treatment as for septic arthritis, and supportive and symptomatic treatment as required. There is usually marked improvement after 72 hours of treatment. Antibiotics should be given for 10–14 days.

E. Pneumonia: Initial therapy is with cefotaxime, ceftriaxone, or cefuroxime. In seriously ill children with pneumatocele or empyema, initial therapy should include nafcillin, 150–200 mg/kg/d in four divided doses, until *Staphylococcus* is proved not to be the cause. Ampicillin may be used if the HIB isolate is shown to be susceptible. Oxygen, intravenous fluids, and supportive care are given as needed. Treatment lasts 3 weeks. Empyema should be treated by placement of one or more chest tubes into the pleural space. When possible, a chest tube should be removed after 4 or 5 days.

Prognosis

The case fatality rate for HIB meningitis is less than 5%. Young infants have the highest mortality rate. One of the most common neurologic sequelae, which develops in approximately 5–10% of patients with HIB meningitis, is significant sensory neural hearing loss. All patients with HIB meningitis should have their hearing checked at some time during the course of the illness or shortly after recovery.

Children in whom invasive HIB develops despite appropriate immunization should have tests to investigate immune function and to rule out HIV.

The case fatality rate in acute epiglottitis is 2–5%; deaths are associated with bacteremia and the rapid development of airway obstruction.

The prognosis for the other diseases requiring hospitalization is good with the institution of early and adequate antibiotic therapy.

Falla TJ et al: Population-based study of non-typable Haemophilus influenzae invasive disease in children and neonates. Lancet 1993;341:851.

Farley MM et al: Invasive *Haemophilus influenzae* disease in adults. Ann Int Med 1992;116:806.

Ginsburg CM et al: Report of 65 cases of *Haemophilus influenzae* b pneumonia. Pediatrics 1979;64:283.

Gorelick MH, Baker MD: Epiglottis in children, 1979 through 1992. Arch Pediatr Adolesc Med 1994;148:47.

Kinney JS et al: Early onset *Haemophilus influenzae* sepsis in the newborn infant. Pediatr Infect Dis J 1993;12:739.

Korones DN, Marshall GS, Shapiro ED: Outcome of children with occult bacteremia caused by *Haemophilus influenzae* type b. Pediatr Infect Dis J 1992;11:516.

Makintubee S, Istre GR, Ward JI: Transmission of invasive *Haemophilus influenzae* type b disease in day care settings. J Pediatr 1987;111:180.

Progress toward elimination of *Haemophilus influenzae* type b disease among infants and children—United States, 1993–1994. MMWR 1995;44:545.

Rittenhouse SF et al: A survey of β-lactamase-producing *Haemophilus influenzae*. Diagn Microbiol Infect Dis 1995;21:223.

Rotbart HA, Glode MP: *Haemophilus influenzae* type b septic arthritis in children: Report of 23 cases. Pediatrics 1985;75:254.

Takala AK et al: Vaccination with *Haemophilus influenzae* type b meningococcal protein conjugate vaccine reduces oropharyngeal carriage of *Haemophilus influenzae* type b among American Indian children. Pediatr Infect Dis J 1993;12:593.

Taylor HG et al: The sequelae of *Haemophilus influenzae* meningitis in school-age children. N Engl J Med 1990; 323:1657.

Vadheim CM et al: Eradication of *Haemophilus influenzae* type b disease in southern California. Arch Pediatr Adolesc Med 1994;148:51.

Valdepena HG et al: Epiglottitis and *Haemophilus influenzae* immunization: The Pittsburgh experience—a five-year review. Pediatrics 1995;96:424.

PERTUSSIS
(Whooping Cough)

Essentials of Diagnosis

- Prodromal catarrhal stage (1–3 weeks) characterized by mild cough, coryza, and fever.
- Persistent staccato, paroxysmal cough ending with a high-pitched inspiratory "whoop."
- Leukocytosis with absolute lymphocytosis.
- Diagnosis confirmed by fluorescent stain or culture of nasopharyngeal secretions.

General Considerations

Pertussis is an acute, highly communicable infection of the respiratory tract caused by *Bordetella pertussis* and characterized by severe bronchitis. Children usually acquire the disease from symptomatic family contacts. Adults who have mild respiratory illness, not recognized as pertussis, frequently are the source of infection. Asymptomatic carriage of *B pertussis* is not documented. Infectivity is greatest during the catarrhal and early paroxysmal cough stage (for about 4 weeks after onset).

The disease is most common and most severe in early infancy. From 1992 to 1994, 13,615 cases were reported in the United States. Forty-one percent of the case patients were less than 1 year of age. Seventy-four percent of infants aged 6 months or less were hospitalized. Fifteen percent had pneumonia, 1.9% had seizures, 0.2% had encephalopathy, and 0.6% died.

Active immunity follows natural pertussis. Reinfections occur years to decades later but are usually mild. Immunity following immunization wanes in 5–10 years. The majority of young adults in the United States are susceptible to pertussis infection and disease is probably common but unrecognized.

Bordetella parapertussis causes a similar but milder syndrome and is reported frequently in central Europe.

B pertussis organisms attach to the ciliated respiratory epithelium and multiply there; deeper invasion does not occur. Disease is due to several bacterial toxins; the most potent is pertussis toxin, which is responsible for lymphocytosis and many of the symptoms of pertussis.

Clinical Findings

A. Symptoms and Signs: The onset of pertussis is insidious, with catarrhal upper respiratory tract symptoms (rhinitis, sneezing, and an irritating cough). Slight fever may be present; temperature greater than 38.3 °C suggests bacterial superinfection or another cause of respiratory tract infection. After about 2 weeks, cough becomes paroxysmal, characterized by 10–30 forceful coughs ending with a loud inspiration (the "whoop"). Infants and adults with otherwise typical, severe pertussis often lack characteristic whooping. Vomiting commonly follows a paroxysm. Coughing is accompanied by cyanosis, sweating, prostration, and exhaustion. This stage lasts for 2–4 weeks, with gradual improvement. Cough suggestive of chronic bronchitis lasts for another 2–3 weeks. Paroxysmal coughing may continue for some months and may worsen with intercurrent viral respiratory infection. In adults, older children, and partially immunized individuals, symptoms may consist only of irritating cough lasting 1–2 weeks. In the younger unimmunized child, symptoms of pertussis last about 8 weeks or longer. Clinical pertussis is milder in immunized children.

B. Laboratory Findings: White blood cell counts of 20,000–30,000/μL with 70–80% lympho-

cytes typically appear near the end of the catarrhal stage. Many older children and adults with mild infections never demonstrate lymphocytosis. The blood picture may resemble lymphocytic leukemia or leukemoid reactions. Identification of *B pertussis* by culture from nasopharyngeal swabs or nasal wash specimens proves the diagnosis. The organism may be found in the respiratory tract in diminishing numbers beginning in the catarrhal stage and ending about 2 weeks after the beginning of the paroxysmal stage. After 4–5 weeks of symptoms, cultures and fluorescent antibody tests are almost always negative. Fresh Bordet-Gengou agar or charcoal agar containing an antimicrobial should be inoculated as soon as possible; *B pertussis* does not tolerate drying or prolonged transport. Enzyme-linked immunosorbent assays for detection of antibody to pertussis toxin or filamentous hemagglutinin may be useful for diagnosis but are currently not widely available. The chest x-ray reveals thickened bronchi and sometimes shows a "shaggy" heart border, indicating bronchopneumonia and patchy atelectasis.

Differential Diagnosis

The differential diagnosis of pertussis includes bacterial, tuberculous, chlamydial, and viral pneumonia. Cystic fibrosis and foreign body aspiration may be considerations.

Adenoviruses and respiratory syncytial virus may cause paroxysmal coughing with an associated elevation of lymphocytes in the peripheral blood, mimicking pertussis.

Complications

Bronchopneumonia due to superinfection is the most common serious complication. It is characterized by abrupt clinical deterioration during the paroxysmal stage, accompanied by high fever and sometimes a striking leukemoid reaction with a shift to predominantly polymorphonuclear leukocytes. Atelectasis is a second common pulmonary complication. Atelectasis may be patchy or extensive and may shift rapidly to involve different areas of lung. Intercurrent viral respiratory infection is also a common complication and may provoke worsening or recurrence of paroxysmal coughing. Otitis media is common. Residual chronic bronchiectasis is infrequent despite the severity of the illness. Apnea and sudden death may occur during a particularly severe paroxysm. A diffuse encephalopathy of uncertain cause may complicate severe cases and frequently is fatal. It is unclear whether anoxic brain damage, cerebral hemorrhage, or pertussis neurotoxins are to blame, but anoxia is most likely the cause. Epistaxis and subconjunctival hemorrhages are common.

Prevention

Active immunization (see Chapter 10) with pertussis vaccine in combination with diphtheria and tetanus toxoids (DTP) should be given in early infancy. Acellular pertussis vaccines cause less fever and fewer local and febrile systemic reactions, but they are recommended only for the fourth and fifth doses. Pertussis cases have greatly increased recently, probably due in part to the large number of children who are not adequately immunized and in part due to an increased incidence of the disease in adults.

Chemoprophylaxis with erythromycin should be given to exposed family and hospital contacts, particularly those under age 2 years, for 14 days. Hospitalized children with pertussis should be isolated because of the great risk of transmission to patients and staff. Several large hospital outbreaks have been reported in the last decade.

Treatment

A. Specific Measures: Antibiotics may ameliorate early infections but not those in the paroxysmal stage. Erythromycin is the drug of choice since it promptly terminates respiratory tract carriage of *B pertussis*. A single resistant strain has been reported. Patients should be treated with erythromycin estolate (40–50 mg/kg/24 h in four divided doses for 14 days). Erythromycin ethylsuccinate is efficacious, but the higher dose recommended causes considerable gastrointestinal intolerance. There is no clinical experience with clarithromycin or azithromycin. Ampicillin 100 mg/kg/d divided in four doses may be used for erythromycin-intolerant patients. Household or other close contacts such as in day-care centers should be treated with erythromycin to reduce secondary transmission. This prophylaxis should be used regardless of age or immunization status.

Corticosteroids reduce the severity of disease but may mask signs of bacterial superinfection. Albuterol, 0.3–0.5 mg/kg/d in 4 doses, has reduced the severity of illness, but tachycardia is common when the drug is given orally, and aerosol administration may precipitate paroxysms.

B. General Measures: Nutritional support during the paroxysmal phase is very important. Frequent small feedings, tube feeding, or parenteral fluid supplementation may be needed. Minimizing stimuli that trigger paroxysms is probably the best way of controlling cough. In general, cough suppressants are of little benefit.

C. Treatment of Complications: Respiratory insufficiency due to pneumonia or other pulmonary complications should be treated with oxygen and assisted ventilation if necessary. Convulsions are treated with oxygen and anticonvulsants. Bacterial pneumonia or otitis media requires additional antibiotics.

Prognosis

The prognosis for patients with pertussis has improved in recent years because of adequate nursing care, treatment of complications, nutrition, and modern intensive care. However, the disease is still very serious in infants under 1 year of age; most deaths occur in this age group. Children with encephalopathy have a poor prognosis.

Bortolussi R et al: Clinical course of pertussis in immunized children. Pediatr Infect Dis J 1995;14:870.

Christie CDC et al: The 1993 epidemic of pertussis in Cincinnati. N Engl J Med 1994;331:16.

Etkind P et al: Pertussis outbreaks in groups claiming religious exemptions to vaccinations. Am J Dis Child 1992;146:173.

Gan VN, Murphy TV: Pertussis in hospitalized children. Am J Dis Child 1990;144:1130.

Hoppe JE: Comparison of erythromycin estolate and erythromycin ethylsuccinate for treatment of pertussis. Pediatr Infect Dis J 1992;11:189.

Lewis K et al: Pertussis caused by an erythromycin-resistant strain of *Bordetella pertussis*. Pediatr Infect Dis J 1995;14:388.

Long SS et al: Widespread silent transmission of pertussis in families: Antibody correlates of infection and symptomatology. J Infect Dis 1990;161:480.

Pertussis—United States, January 1992–June 1995. MMWR 1995;44:525.

Rabinovich R, Robbins A: Pertussis vaccines: A progress report. JAMA 1994;271:68.

Roberts I, Gavin R, Lennon D: Randomized controlled trial of steroids in pertussis. Pediatr Infect Dis J 1992;11:982.

Schmitt-Grohe S et al: Pertussis in German adults. Clin Infect Dis 1994;21:860.

Trollfors B et al: A placebo-controlled trial of a pertussis-toxoid vaccine. N Engl J Med 1995;333:1045.

LISTERIOSIS

Essentials of Diagnosis

Early-onset neonatal disease:
- Signs of sepsis a few hours after birth in an infant born with fetal distress; hepatosplenomegaly. Maternal fever.

Late-onset neonatal disease:
- Meningitis, sometimes with monocytes in the cerebrospinal fluid and peripheral blood. Onset at 9–30 days of age.

General Considerations

Listeria monocytogenes is a gram-positive, non-spore-forming aerobic rod distributed widely in the animal kingdom and in food, dust, and soil. It causes systemic infections in newborn infants and immunosuppressed older children. In pregnant women, infection is relatively mild, with fever, aches, and chills, but it is accompanied by bacteremia and sometimes results in intrauterine or perinatal infection with grave consequences for the fetus or newborn. One-fourth of the cases occurred in pregnant women, and 20% of these perinatal cases resulted in stillbirth or neonatal death. *Listeria* is present in the stool of approximately 10% of the normal population. Persons in contact with animals seem to be at particular risk. Recent large food-borne outbreaks have been traced to contaminated cabbage in coleslaw, contaminated soft cheese, and milk. The role of contaminated food in sporadic listeriosis is now recognized.

Like group B streptococcal infections, *Listeria* infections in the newborn can be divided into early and late forms. Early infections are more common, leading to a severe congenital form of infection. Later infections are often characterized by meningitis.

Clinical Findings

A. Symptoms and Signs: In the early neonatal form, symptoms of listeriosis usually appear on the first day of life and always by the third day. Infants are frequently premature and have signs of fetal distress. Respiratory distress, diarrhea, and fever occur. On examination, hepatosplenomegaly and a papular rash are found. A history of maternal fever is common. Meningitis may accompany the septic course.

The late neonatal form usually occurs after 9 days of age and can occur as late as 5 weeks. Meningitis is common, characterized by irritability, fever, and poor feeding.

Listeria infections occur rarely in older children, usually in those with animal contact or those who are immunosuppressed. Signs and symptoms are those of meningitis, usually with insidious onset.

B. Laboratory Findings: In all patients except those receiving white cell depressant drugs, the white blood cell count is elevated, with 10–20% monocytes. When meningitis is found, the characteristic cerebrospinal fluid cell count is high (> 500/μL) with a predominance of polymorphonuclear leukocytes in 70% of cases; monocytes predominate in up to 30%. Gram-stained smears of cerebrospinal fluid are usually negative, but the short gram-positive rods may be seen. The chief pathologic feature in severe neonatal sepsis is miliary granulomatosis with microabscesses in liver, spleen, central nervous system, lung, and bowel.

Cultures are frequently positive from multiple sites, including blood in the infant and the mother. The organisms form small, weakly hemolytic colonies on blood agar and may be mistaken for streptococci.

Differential Diagnosis

Early-onset neonatal disease resembles hemolytic disease of the newborn, group B streptococcal sepsis or severe cytomegalovirus infection, rubella, or toxoplasmosis. Late-onset disease must be differentiated from meningitis due to echovirus and coxsackievirus, group B streptococci, and gram-negative enteric bacteria.

Prevention

Immunosuppressed, pregnant, and elderly patients can decrease the risk of *Listeria* infection by avoiding soft cheeses and by thoroughly reheating or avoiding ready-to-eat foods. These recommendations include avoiding raw meat and milk and thorough washing of vegetables.

Treatment

Ampicillin (150–300 mg/kg/d every 6 hours intravenously) is the drug of choice in most cases of listeriosis. Gentamicin (2.5 mg/kg every 8 hours intravenously) should also be given, since it has a synergistic effect with ampicillin in vitro. If ampicillin cannot be used, trimethoprim-sulfamethoxazole is also effective. Cephalosporins are not effective. Treatment of severe disease should continue for at least 2 weeks.

Prognosis

In a recent outbreak of early-onset neonatal disease, the mortality rate was 27% despite aggressive and appropriate management. Meningitis in older infants has a good prognosis. In immunosuppressed children, prognosis depends to a great extent on that of the underlying illness.

Cherubin CE et al: Epidemiological spectrum and current treatment of listeriosis. Rev Infect Dis 1991;13:1108.

Foodborne listeriosis, United States 1988–1990: Update. MMWR Morb Mortal Wkly Rep 1992:41:251.

Gellin BG et al: The epidemiology of listeriosis in the United States—1986. Listeriosis Study Group. Am J Epidemiol 1991;133:392.

Lennon D et al: Epidemic perinatal listeriosis. Pediatr Infect Dis J 1984;3:30.

Linnan MJ et al: Epidemic listeriosis associated with Mexican-style cheese. N Engl J Med 1988;319:823.

Schuchat A et al: Role of foods in sporadic listeriosis. I. Case-control study of dietary risk factors. JAMA 1992; 267:2041.

Visintine AM, Oleske JM, Nahmias AJ: *Listeria monocytogenes*. Infection in infants and children. Am J Dis Child 1977;131:393.

TUBERCULOSIS

Essentials of Diagnosis

- All types: Positive tuberculin test in patient or members of household, suspicious chest x-ray, history of contact, and demonstration of organism by stain and culture.
- Pulmonary: Fatigue, irritability, and undernutrition, with or without fever and cough.
- Glandular: Chronic cervical adenitis.
- Miliary: Classic "snowstorm" appearance of chest x-ray; choroidal tubercles.
- Meningitis: Fever and manifestations of meningeal irritation and increased intracranial pressure. Characteristic cerebrospinal fluid.

General Considerations

Tuberculosis is a granulomatous disease caused by *Mycobacterium tuberculosis*. It remains a leading cause of death throughout the world. Children under 3 years of age are most susceptible. Lympho-hematogenous dissemination through the lungs to extrapulmonary sites, including the brain and meninges, eyes, bones and joints, lymph nodes, kidneys, intestines, larynx, and skin, is more likely to occur in infants. Increased susceptibility occurs again in adolescence, particularly in girls within 2 years of menarche. Tuberculosis in the United States has increased substantially since 1986 following three decades of decline. In 1994, 24,361 cases were reported. Certain high-risk groups are identified, including ethnic minorities, foreign-born persons, prisoners, residents of nursing homes, indigents, migrant workers, and health care providers. HIV infection is an important risk factor both for development and spread of disease. Pediatric tuberculosis is also increasing, with 1695 cases in children under age 15 reported in 1994. Exposure to an adult at risk for tuberculosis is the most common risk factor in children. The primary complex in infancy and childhood consists of a small parenchymal lesion in any area of the lung with caseation of regional nodes and calcification. Postprimary tuberculosis in adolescents and adults occurs in the apexes of the lungs and is likely to cause chronic, progressive cavitary pulmonary disease with less tendency for hematogenous dissemination.

Clinical Findings

A. Symptoms and Signs:

1. Pulmonary–See Chapter 18.

2. Miliary–Diagnosis is made on the basis of a classic snowstorm or millet seed appearance of lung fields on x-ray, though early in the course of disseminated tuberculosis the chest x-ray may show no or only subtle abnormalities. The majority also have a fresh primary complex and pleural effusion. Choroidal tubercles are sometimes seen on funduscopic examination. Other lesions may be present and produce osteomyelitis, arthritis, meningitis, tuberculomas of the brain, enteritis, or infection of the kidneys and liver.

3. Meningitis–Symptoms include fever, vomiting, headache, lethargy, and irritability, with signs of meningeal irritation and increased intracranial pressure, including cranial nerve palsies, convulsions, and coma. Choroidal tubercles are pathognomonic when associated with these signs and symptoms. Otorrhea or acute otitis media may be seen.

4. Glandular–The primary complex may be associated with a skin lesion drained by regional nodes or chronic cervical node enlargement and infection of the tonsils. Involved nodes may become fixed to the overlying skin, suppurate, and drain.

B. Laboratory Findings: The Mantoux test

(0.1 mL of intermediate strength PPD [5 TU] inoculated intradermally) is read as positive at 48–72 hours if there is significant induration (Table 37–1). False-negative results are seen in malnourished patients, those with overwhelming disease, and in a few percent of children with isolated pulmonary disease. Temporary suppression of tuberculin reactivity may be seen with viral infections (eg, measles, influenza, varicella, mumps), after live virus immunization, and when corticosteroids or other immunosuppressive drugs are present. The two commercially available reagents for Mantoux testing give discrepant results in some cases. For this reason, every Mantoux test should be accompanied by intradermal injection of control antigens such as *Candida*, or diphtheria-tetanus toxoids. Unfortunately, some normal children have no reaction to control antigens. When tuberculosis is suspected and the child is anergic, household members and adult contacts (eg, teachers) should also be tested immediately. Multiple puncture tests (tine tests) are associated with false-negative and false-positive reactions. Furthermore, a positive tine test is not sufficient for diagnosis, necessitating a Mantoux test. The subsequent Mantoux test may lead to "boosting" and a false-positive reaction. Because of these problems, tine tests should not be used.

The erythrocyte sedimentation rate is usually elevated. Cultures of pooled early morning gastric aspirates from three successive days will yield *M tuberculosis* in about 40% of cases. Biopsy may be necessary to establish the diagnosis in some cases. Therapy should not be delayed in suspected cases. The cerebrospinal fluid in tuberculous meningitis shows slight to moderate pleocytosis (50–300 white blood cells, predominantly lymphocytes), decreased glucose, and increased protein.

Table 37–1. Interpretation of tuberculin skin test reactions.

Degree of Risk	Risk Factors	Positive Reaction
High	Recent close contact with a case of active tuberculosis; chest radiograph compatible with tuberculosis; immunocompromise; HIV infection	≥ 5-mm induration
Medium	Current or previous residence in high-prevalence area (Asia, Africa, Latin America); recent skin test converters within 2 years; intravenous drug use; homelessness, or residence in a correctional institution; recent weight loss or malnutrition; leukemia, Hodgkin's disease, diabetes mellitus; age < 4 years	≥ 10-mm induration
Low	Children ≥ 4 years without any risk factor	≥ 15-mm induration

Standard intradermal Mantoux test, 5 test units.

The direct detection of mycobacteria in body fluids or discharges is best done by staining specimens with auramine O and examining them with blue-light fluorescence microscopy; this is superior to the Ziehl-Neelsen method.

C. Imaging: Chest x-ray should be obtained in all children with suspicion of tuberculosis at any site or with a positive skin test. Segmental consolidation with some volume loss and hilar adenopathy are common findings in children. Pleural effusion also occurs with primary infection. Cavities and apical disease are unusual.

Differential Diagnosis

Pulmonary tuberculosis must be differentiated from fungal, parasitic, mycoplasmal, and bacterial pneumonias; lung abscess; foreign body aspiration; lipoid pneumonia; sarcoidosis; and mediastinal cancer. Cervical lymphadenitis is most apt to be due to streptococcal or staphylococcal infections. Cat-scratch fever and infection with atypical mycobacteria may need to be distinguished from tuberculous lymphadenitis also. Viral meningoencephalitis, head trauma (battered child), lead poisoning, brain abscess, acute bacterial meningitis, brain tumor, and disseminated fungal infections must be excluded in tuberculous meningitis. The skin test in the patient or family contacts is frequently valuable in differentiating these conditions from tuberculosis.

Prevention

A. BCG Vaccine: BCG vaccines are live attenuated strains of *M bovis*. Although this BCG is often routinely given to infants and children in countries with a high prevalence of tuberculosis, protective efficacy varies greatly with vaccine potency and method of delivery. In the United States, BCG vaccination is considered only for tuberculin-negative children and neonates in high-risk situations who are unlikely to receive isoniazid (INH) prophylaxis or close follow-up , or who are at high risk of exposure to persons infected with *M tuberculosis* resistant to isoniazid and rifampin (see Chapter 10).

B. Isoniazid (INH) Chemoprophylaxis: Daily administration of isoniazid (10 mg/kg/d orally; maximum 300 mg) is advised for children who cannot avoid intimate household contact with adolescents or adults with active disease. Isoniazid is given until 3 months after last contact. At the end of this time, a Mantoux test should be done, and therapy should be continued for 9 months if it is positive. BCG is not recommended during the period of isoniazid chemoprophylaxis.

C. Other Measures: Tuberculosis in infants and young children is evidence of recent exposure to active infection in an adult. The source contact (index case) should be identified, isolated, and treated to prevent other secondary cases. Reporting cases to local health departments is essential for contact tracing. Exposed tuberculin-negative children should be skin-tested every 2 months for 6 months after contact has been terminated. Routine tuberculin skin testing is advised at 12–15 months of age, prior to school entry, and again in adolescence. Yearly testing of school children is recommended in high-risk populations, including children from socioeconomically deprived neighborhoods and those from high-risk foreign countries.

Treatment

A. Specific Measures: Most children in the United States are hospitalized initially. If the infecting organism has not been isolated for susceptibility testing from the presumed contact, reasonable attempts should be made to obtain it from the child using gastric aspirates, sputum induction, bronchoscopy, thoracentesis, and so on. Cooperation with outpatient therapy must be assured. Direct observed therapy given twice weekly by a trained professional is carried out when compliance cannot be ensured.

All children with positive skin tests (see Table 37–1) without overt disease should receive 9 months of isoniazid (10 mg/kg/d orally, maximum 300 mg) therapy. In children with overt pulmonary disease, therapy for 6–9 months using isoniazid (10 mg/kg/d), rifampin (15 mg/kg/d), and pyrazinamide (25–30 mg/kg/d) in a single daily oral dose for 2 months, followed by isoniazid plus rifampin (either in a daily or twice-weekly regimen) for 4 months appears effective for isoniazid-susceptible organisms. For more severe disease, such as miliary or central nervous system infection, duration is increased to 12 months or more, and a fourth drug (streptomycin or ethambutol) is added for the first 2 months.

1. Isoniazid–The hepatotoxicity seen in adults and some adolescents is rare in children. Transient elevation of transaminases (up to three times normal) may be seen at 6–12 weeks, but therapy is continued unless clinical illness occurs. Routine monitoring of liver function tests is unnecessary. Peripheral neuropathy associated with pyridoxine deficiency is rare in children, and it is not necessary to add pyridoxine unless significant malnutrition coexists.

2. Rifampin–Although an excellent bactericidal agent, rifampin is never used alone due to rapid development of resistance. Hepatotoxicity may be seen but rarely with recommended doses. The orange discoloration of secretions is benign.

3. Pyrazinamide–This excellent sterilizing agent has most effect during the first 2 months of therapy; with the recommended duration and dosing, it is well tolerated. Although it elevates the uric acid level, it rarely causes symptoms of hyperuricemia in children. Use of this drug is now common for tuberculous disease in children; resistance is almost unknown. Oral acceptance and central nervous system penetration are good.

4. Ethambutol–Since color blindness and optic

neuritis are the major side effects, ethambutol is usually given only to children who can be reliably vision tested every 2 months. This complication occurs in a few percent of patients, usually those receiving more than the recommended dosage of 15 mg/kg/d.

5. Streptomycin–Streptomycin (20–30 mg/kg/d intramuscularly in one or two doses) should be given for 1 or 2 months in severe disease. Hearing should be tested periodically during use.

B. Chemotherapy for Drug-Resistant Tuberculosis: The incidence of drug resistance is increasing and nationally averages 5–10%. Transmission of multiply resistant strains to contacts have resulted in some epidemics. In areas with high rates of resistance, it may be necessary to begin therapy with four drugs pending susceptibility testing. Consultation of local laboratories or experts in treating tuberculosis is important. Therapy should continue for 12 months or longer.

C. General Measures:

1. Corticosteroids–These drugs may be used for suppressing inflammatory reactions in meningeal, pleural, and pericardial tuberculosis and for the relief of bronchial obstruction due to hilar adenopathy. Prednisone is given orally, 1 mg/kg/d for 6–8 weeks, with gradual withdrawal at the end of that time. The use of corticosteroids may mask progression of disease. Accordingly, the clinician needs to be sure that an effective regimen is being used.

2. Bed rest–Rest in bed is indicated only while the child feels ill. Isolation is necessary only for children with draining lesions or renal disease and those with chronic pulmonary tuberculosis. Most children with tuberculosis are noninfectious and can attend school while being treated.

Prognosis

If bacteria are sensitive and treatment is completed, most patients make lasting recovery. Re-treatment is more difficult and less successful. With antituberculosis chemotherapy (especially isoniazid), there should now be nearly 100% recovery in miliary tuberculosis. Without treatment, the mortality rate in both miliary tuberculosis and tuberculous meningitis is almost 100%. In the latter form, about two-thirds of treated patients survive. There may be a high incidence of neurologic abnormalities among survivors if treatment is started late.

Cieslak TJ et al: A pseudoepidemic of tuberculin skin test conversions caused by a particular lot of purified protein derivative of tuberculin test solution. Pediatr Infect Dis J 1995;14:392.

Essential components of a tuberculosis prevention and control program: Screening for tuberculosis and tuberculosis infection in high-risk populations. MMWR 1995; 44(RR-11):1.

Iseman MD: Treatment of multidrug-resistant tuberculosis. N Engl J Med 1993;329:784.

Jacobs RF et al: Intensive short course chemotherapy for tuberculous meningitis. Pediatr Infect Dis J 1992; 11:194.

Kent SJ et al: Tuberculous meningitis: A 30-year review. Clin Infect Dis 1993;17:987.

Nemir RL, Krasinski K: Tuberculosis in children and adolescents in the 1980's. Pediatr Infect Dis J 1988;7:375.

Schaaf HS et al: Respiratory tuberculosis in childhood: The diagnostic value of clinical features and special investigations. Pediatr Infect Dis J 1995;14:189.

Starke JR, Correa AG: Management of mycobacterial infection and disease in children. Pediatr Infect Dis J 1994;14:455.

Swanson DS, Starke JR: Drug-resistant tuberculosis in pediatrics. Pediatr Clin North Am 1995;42:553.

INFECTIONS WITH NONTUBERCULOUS MYCOBACTERIA

Essentials of Diagnosis

- Chronic unilateral cervical lymphadenitis.
- Granulomas of the skin.
- Chronic bone lesion with draining sinus (chronic osteomyelitis).
- Reaction to PPD-S (standard) of 5–8 mm, negative chest x-ray, and negative history of contact with tuberculosis.
- Positive skin reaction to a specific atypical antigen.
- Diagnosis by positive acid-fast stain or culture.
- Disseminated infection in patients with AIDS.

General Considerations

Various species of acid-fast mycobacteria other than *Mycobacterium tuberculosis* may cause subclinical infections and, occasionally, clinical disease closely simulating tuberculosis. Strains of nontuberculous mycobacteria are common in soil, food and water. Organisms enter the host by small abrasions in skin, oral mucosa, or gastrointestinal mucosa. Strain cross-reactivity with *M tuberculosis* can be demonstrated by simultaneous skin testing (Mantoux) with PPD-S (standard) and PPD prepared from one of the atypical antigens. The larger skin reaction suggests infection with the homologous strain.

The Runyon classification of mycobacteria includes the following:

Group I: Photochromogens (PPD-Y): Yellow color develops upon exposure to light in previously white colony grown 2–4 weeks in the dark. Group 1 includes *Mycobacterium kansasii* and *Mycobacterium marinum*.

Group II: Scotochromogens (PPD-G): Colonies are definitely yellow-orange after incubation in the dark. Organisms may be found in small numbers in the normal flora of some human saliva and gastric contents. Subclinical infection is widespread in the United States, but clinical disease appears rarely. Group II includes *Mycobacterium scrofulaceum*.

Group III: Nonphotochromogens (PPD-B):

"Battey avian-swine group" grows as small white colonies after incubation in the dark, with no significant development of pigment upon exposure to light. Infection with *Mycobacterium avium* complex is prevalent on the East Coast of the United States, particularly the Southeast. Patients with acquired immunodeficiency syndrome (AIDS).

Group IV: "Rapid growers": *Mycobacterium fortuitum* and *Mycobacterium chelonei* are the recognized pathogens. Within 1 week after inoculation, they form colonies closely resembling *M tuberculosis* morphologically.

Clinical Findings

A. Symptoms and Signs:

1. Lymphadenitis–In children, the commonest form of infection due to mycobacteria other than tuberculosis is cervical lymphadenitis. *M scrofulaceum* or *M avium* complex is almost always the cause. A submandibular node swells slowly and is firm and usually nontender. Over time, the node suppurates and may drain chronically. Nodes in other areas of the head and neck and elsewhere are sometimes involved. There is no fever or toxicity.

2. Pulmonary disease–In the western United States, this is usually due to *M kansasii;* in the eastern United States, it may be due to *M avium* complex. In other countries, disease is usually caused by *M avium* complex. In adults, there is usually underlying chronic pulmonary disease, but in children, this is often not the case. Immunologic deficiency may be present. Presentation is clinically indistinguishable from that of tuberculosis. Patients with cystic fibrosis may be infected with nontuberculous mycobacteria. It may be difficult to differentiate infection from colonization in these patients with chronic symptoms.

3. Swimming pool granuloma–This is due to *M marinum.* A solitary chronic granulomatous lesion, frequently on the elbow, develops after minor trauma in infected swimming pools. Minor trauma in home aquariums or other aquatic environments also may lead to infection.

4. Chronic osteomyelitis–Osteomyelitis is caused by *M kansasii, M scrofulaceum,* or "rapid growers." Findings include swelling and pain over a distal extremity, radiolucent defects in bone, fever, and clinical and x-ray evidence of bronchopneumonia. Such cases are rare.

5. Meningitis–Disease is due to *M kansasii* and may be indistinguishable from tuberculous meningitis.

6. Disseminated infection–Rarely apparently immunologically normal children develop disseminated infection due to nontuberculous mycobacteria. Children are ill, with fever and hepatosplenomegaly, and organisms are demonstrated in bone lesions, lymph nodes, or liver. Chest x-rays are usually normal. Sixty to 80 percent of patients with AIDS will acquire *M avium* complex infection characterized by fever, night sweats, weight loss, and diarrhea. Infection usually indicates severe immune dysfunction and is associated with low CD4 lymphocyte counts.

B. Laboratory Findings: In most cases, there is a small reaction (< 10 mm) when Mantoux testing is done with PPD-S. Larger reactions may be seen. The chest x-ray is negative, and there is no history of contact with tuberculosis. Needle aspiration of the node excludes bacterial infection and may yield acid-fast bacilli on stain or culture. Fistulization should not be a problem because total excision follows if the infection is due to atypical mycobacteria. If other organisms are found, formal excision may be avoided. Excision is usually required if aspiration is nondiagnostic and the clinical findings support the diagnosis.

Cultures of any normally sterile body site will yield *M avium* complex in immunocompromised patients with disseminated disease. Blood cultures are positive, with a large density of bacteria.

Differential Diagnosis

See section on differential diagnosis in the previous discussion of tuberculosis and in Chapter 20.

Treatment

A. Specific Measures: The usual treatment of lymphadenitis is complete surgical excision. Chemotherapy is neither necessary nor sufficient for cure. Occasionally, excision is impossible because of proximity to branches of the facial nerve. Chemotherapy may then be necessary. Occasionally, resolution of the adenopathy is under way when the diagnosis is made. In these cases, careful follow-up is adequate.

Response of extensive adenopathy or other forms of infection varies according to the infecting species and susceptibility. Recent data suggest that isoniazid, rifampin, and streptomycin with or without ethambutol (depending on sensitivity to isoniazid) will result in a favorable response in almost all patients with *M kansasii* infection. Chemotherapeutic treatment of *M avium* complex is much less satisfactory as resistance to isoniazid, rifampin, and pyrazinamide is usual. Susceptibility testing is necessary to optimize therapy. Most clinicians favor surgical excision of involved tissue if possible and treatment with at least three drugs to which the organism has been shown to be sensitive. Disseminated disease in patients with AIDS calls for a combination of three or more active drugs. Clarithromycin, in addition to two or more of the following drugs, is started immediately: ethionamide, capreomycin, amikacin, clofazimine, rifabutin, ciprofloxacin, and cycloserine. *M fortuitum* and *M chelonei* are usually susceptible to amikacin plus erythromycin or doxycycline and may be successfully treated with such combinations. Swimming pool granuloma due to *M marinum* is usually self-limited but may be treated either with drugs or by surgical excision with good results.

B. General Measures: Isolation of the patient is usually not necessary. General supportive care is indicated for the child with disseminated disease.

Prognosis

The prognosis is good for localized disease, though fatalities occur in immunocompromised children with disseminated disease.

Contreras MA et al: Pulmonary infection with nontuberculous mycobacteria. Am Rev Respir Dis 1988;137:149.

Hofer M et al: Disseminated osteomyelitis from *Mycobacterium ulcerans* after a snakebite. N Engl J Med 1993; 328:1007.

Horsburgh CR Jr: Mycobacterium avium complex infection in the acquired immunodeficiency syndrome. N Engl J Med 1991;324:1332.

Lowry PW et al: Mycobacterium chelonei causing otitis media in an ear-nose-and-throat practice. N Engl J Med 1988;319:978.

Starke JR, Correa AB: Management of mycobacterial infection and disease in children. Pediatr Infect Dis J 1995;14:455.

Street ML et al: Nontuberculous mycobacterial infections of the skin. Report of 14 cases and a review of the literature. J Am Acad Dermatol 1991;24:208.

Woods GL, Washington JA: Mycobacteria other than Mycobacterium tuberculosis: Review of microbiologic and clinical aspects. Rev Infect Dis J 1987;9:275.

LEGIONELLA INFECTION

Essentials of Diagnosis

- Severe progressive pneumonia in a child with compromised immunity.
- Diarrhea and neurologic signs are common.
- Positive culture requires buffered charcoal yeast extract media and proves infection.
- Direct fluorescent antibody staining of respiratory secretions proves infection.

General Considerations

Legionella pneumophila is an ubiquitous gram-negative bacillus that causes two distinct clinical syndromes: Legionnaires' disease and Pontiac fever. Legionnaires' disease is an acute, severe pneumonia that is frequently fatal in immunocompromised patients. Pontiac fever is a mild, nonpneumonic, flu-like illness characterized by fever, headache, myalgia, and arthralgia. The disease is self-limited and is described in outbreaks in otherwise healthy adults.

Twenty-two species of *Legionella* have been discovered. *Legionella* is present in many natural water sources as well as domestic water supplies (faucets, showers). Contaminated cooling towers and heat exchangers have been implicated in several large institutional outbreaks. Sporadic, community-acquired cases also occur, and the source of infection is not usually clear. Person-to-person transmission has not been documented.

Few cases of Legionnaires' disease have been reported in children. Most have been children with compromised cellular immunity or children receiving steroids. In adults, risk factors include smoking, underlying cardiopulmonary or renal disease, alcoholism, and diabetes.

L pneumophila is thought to be acquired by inhalation of a contaminated aerosol. The bacteria are phagocytosed but proliferate within macrophages. Cell-mediated immunity is necessary to activate macrophages to kill intracellular bacteria.

Clinical Findings

A. Signs and Symptoms: Onset of fever, chills, anorexia, and headache is abrupt. Pulmonary symptoms occur within 2–3 days but progress rapidly. The cough is nonproductive early on. Purulent sputum occurs late. Hemoptysis, diarrhea, and neurologic signs (including lethargy, irritability, tremors, and delirium) are seen.

B. Laboratory Findings: White blood count is usually elevated. Chest radiographs show rapidly progressive, patchy consolidation. Cavitation and large pleural effusions are uncommon. Cultures from sputum, tracheal aspirates, or bronchoscopic specimens, when grown on buffered yeast charcoal extract media, are positive in 50–70% of patients at 3–7 days. Direct fluorescent antibody staining of sputum or other respiratory specimens is only 70–75% sensitive but 95% specific. As such, a negative culture or direct fluorescent antibody staining of sputum or tracheal secretions does not rule out Legionnaires' disease. Serologic tests are available and aid in diagnosis, but a maximum rise in titer may require 6–8 weeks.

Differential diagnosis

Legionnaires' disease is usually a rapidly progressive pneumonia in a patient who appears very ill with unremitting fevers. Other bacterial pneumonias, viral pneumonias, *Mycoplasma* pneumonia, and fungal disease are all possibilities and may be difficult to differentiate on clinical grounds in an immunocompromised patient.

Complications

In sporadic untreated cases, mortality rates are 5–25%. In untreated immunocompromised patients, mortality approaches 80%. Hematogenous dissemination may result in extrapulmonary foci of infection, including pericardium, myocardium, and renal involvement. *Legionella* may present as "culture-negative" endocarditis.

Prevention

No vaccine is available. Hyperchlorination and periodic superheating of water supplies in hospitals have been shown to reduce the number of organisms and the frequency of cases.

Treatment

Erythromycin (40–50 mg/kg/d in four divided doses, orally or intravenously) results in clinical improvement in 48–72 hours. Rifampin (20 mg/kg/d divided in two doses) is very active in vitro and is also given to gravely ill patients. Therapy is continued for 21 days to reduce the likelihood of relapse.

Prognosis

Mortality rate is high if Legionnaires' disease is not recognized and appropriately treated. Malaise, problems with memory, and fatigue are common problems in patients after recovery.

Carlson NC et al: Legionellosis in children: An expanding spectrum. Pediatr Infect Dis J 1990;9:133.

Esposito AL, Gantz NM: Legionnaires' disease: The distance travelled since Philadelphia. Pediatr Infect Dis J 1986;5:163.

Greene KA et al: Fatal postoperative *Legionella* pneumonia in a newborn. J Perinatol 1990;10:183.

Helms CM et al: Legionnaires' disease associated with a hospital water system. JAMA 1988;259:2423.

Lowry PW et al: A cluster of *Legionella* sternal wound infection due to postoperative topical exposure to contaminated tap water. N Engl J Med 1991;324:109.

Meyer RD: Legionella infections: A review of five years of research. Rev Infect Dis 1983;5:258.

Tompkins LS: *Legionella* prosthetic-valve endocarditis. N Engl J Med 1988;318:530.

PSITTACOSIS (ORNITHOSIS) & *CHLAMYDIA PNEUMONIAE* INFECTION

Essentials of Diagnosis

- Fever, cough, malaise, chills, headache.
- Diffuse rales; no consolidation.
- Long-lasting x-ray findings of bronchopneumonia.
- Isolation of the organism or rising titer of complement-fixing antibodies.
- Exposure to infected birds.

General Considerations

Psittacosis is caused by *Chlamydia psittaci*. When the agent is transmitted to humans from psittacine birds (parrots, parakeets, cockatoos, and budgerigars), the disease is often called **psittacosis** or **parrot fever.** However, other avian genera (pigeons, turkeys) are common sources of infection in the United States, and the general term **ornithosis** is often used. Thirty-eight cases were reported in 1994. The agent is an obligatory intracellular parasite. Human-to-human spread occurs rarely. The incubation period is 5–21 days with a mean of 15 days. The bird from whom the disease was transmitted may not be clinically ill.

Recently, a new strain of *Chlamydia,* designated the TWAR agent or *C pneumoniae,* has been found to cause an atypical pneumonia. Transmission is by respiratory spread. Infection appears to become prevalent during the second decade; half of surveyed adults are seropositive. Only a small percentage of infections result in clinical pneumonia. The disease may be more common than atypical pneumonia due to *M pneumoniae.* Lower respiratory tract infection due to *C pneumoniae* is uncommon in infants and young children.

Clinical Findings

A. Symptoms and Signs:

1. *C psittaci*–The disease is extremely variable but tends to be mild in children. The onset is rapid or insidious, with fever, chills, headache, backache, malaise, myalgia, and dry cough. Signs include those of pneumonitis, alteration of percussion note and breath sounds, and rales. Pulmonary findings may be absent early. Splenomegaly, epistaxis, prostration, and meningismus are occasionally seen. Delirium, constipation or diarrhea, and abdominal distress may occur. Dyspnea and cyanosis may occur later.

2. *C pneumoniae*–Clinically, *C pneumoniae* infection is very similar to *M pneumoniae* infection. Most are mild upper respiratory infections. Lower tract infection is characterized by fever, sore throat (perhaps more severe with *C pneumoniae*), cough, and bilateral pulmonary findings and infiltrates. Prolonged symptoms in some patients suggest that therapy with erythromycin or tetracycline may have to be more prolonged than that usually given for *Mycoplasma.*

B. Laboratory Findings:
In psittacosis, the white blood cell count is normal or decreased, often with a shift to the left. Proteinuria is frequently present. *C psittaci* is present in the blood and sputum during the first 2 weeks of illness and can be isolated by inoculation of clinical specimens into mice or embryonated hens' eggs, but culture is available only in research laboratories. Complement-fixing antibodies appear during or after the second week, and a fourfold rise or a single titer of 1:32 or higher suggests the diagnosis. The rise in titer may be minimized or delayed by early chemotherapy. Infection with *C pneumoniae* may lead to diagnostic confusion because cross-reactive antibody may cause falsely positive *C psittaci* titers. Serologic tests for *C pneumoniae* are now available in reference laboratories. A fourfold rise in MIF or CF antibody, or IgM titers of 1:16 or more support the diagnosis.

C. Imaging:
The x-ray findings in psittacosis are those of central pneumonia, which later becomes widespread or migratory. Psittacosis is indistinguishable from viral pneumonias by x-ray. Signs of pneumonitis may appear by x-ray in the absence of clinical suspicion of pulmonary involvement.

Differential Diagnosis

Psittacosis can be differentiated from acute viral or

mycoplasmal pneumonias only by the history of contact with potentially infected birds. In severe or prolonged cases with extrapulmonary involvement, the differential diagnosis includes a wide spectrum of diseases such as typhoid fever, brucellosis, rheumatic fever, etc.

Complications

Complications of psittacosis include myocarditis, endocarditis, hepatitis, pancreatitis, and secondary bacterial pneumonia. *C pneumoniae* infection may be prolonged or recur.

Treatment

For psittacosis, tetracyclines in full doses should be given for 14 days. Erythromycin is an alternative for children under 9 years of age. Supportive oxygen may be needed. The patient should be kept in isolation. The role of the expanded-spectrum macrolides is not yet clear. *C pneumoniae* responds to either erythromycin or tetracycline.

Block S et al: *Mycoplasma pneumoniae* and *Chlamydia pneumonia* in pediatric community acquired pneumonia: Comparative efficacy and safety of clarithromycin vs erythromycin ethylsuccinate. Pediatr Infect Dis J 1995; 14:471.

Byrom NP, Wells J, Mair HJ: Fulminant psittacosis. Lancet 1979;1:353.

Crosse BA: Psittacosis: A clinical review. J Infect 1990; 21:251.

Grayston JT: *Chlamydia pneumoniae* (TWAR) infections in children. Pediatr Infect Dis J 1994;13:675.

Hammerschlag MR et al: Persistent infection with Chlamydia pneumoniae following acute respiratory illness. Clin Infect Dis 1992;14:178.

Jantos CA et al: Infection with *Chlamydia pneumonia* in infants and children with acute lower respiratory tract disease. Pediatr Infect Dis J 1995;14:117.

CAT-SCRATCH DISEASE

Essentials of Diagnosis

- History of a cat scratch or cat contact.
- Primary lesion (papule, pustule, conjunctivitis) at site of inoculation.
- Acute or subacute regional lymphadenopathy.
- Aspiration of sterile pus from a node.
- Laboratory studies excluding other causes.
- Biopsy of node or papule showing histopathologic findings consistent with cat-scratch disease and occasionally characteristic bacilli on Warthin-Starry stain.
- Positive cat-scratch serology (antibody to *Bartonella henselae*).

General Considerations

Cat-scratch disease is a benign, self-limited form of lymphadenitis. Patients often report a cat scratch

(67%) or contact with a cat or kitten (90%). The cat almost invariably is healthy. The clinical picture is that of a regional lymphadenitis associated with an erythematous papular skin lesion without intervening lymphangitis. The disease occurs worldwide and is more common in the fall and winter. It is estimated that more than 20,000 cases per year occur in the United States. The most common systemic complication is encephalitis.

After some years of controversy and vacillation, the etiologic agent of cat-scratch disease has now been identified as *Bartonella henselae,* a gram-negative bacillus that also causes bacillary angiomatosis.

Clinical Findings

A. Symptoms and Signs: About 50% of patients with cat-scratch disease develop a primary lesion at the site of inoculation, though some authors report a much higher percentage. The lesion usually is a papule or pustule and is located most often on the arm or hand (50%), head or leg (30%), or trunk or neck (10%). The lesion may be conjunctival (10%). Regional lymphadenopathy appears 10–30 days later and may be accompanied by mild malaise, lassitude, headache, and fever. Multiple sites are seen in about 10% of cases. Involved nodes may be hard or soft and 1–6 cm in diameter. They are usually tender, and about 25% of them suppurate. The overlying skin may or may not be inflamed. Lymphadenopathy usually resolves in about 2 months, but it may persist for up to 8 months.

Unusual manifestations include nonpruritic maculopapular rash, erythema multiforme or nodosum, purpura, conjunctivitis (Parinaud's oculoglandular fever), parotid swelling, pneumonia, chronic sinus drainage, osteolytic lesions, mesenteric and mediastinal adenitis, peripheral neuritis, hepatosplenomegaly, and encephalitis.

B. Laboratory Findings: Antigens prepared from pus aspirated from nodes of infected individuals have been used for skin testing. Because they are poorly standardized and are not available commercially, their use is discouraged. The skin test is positive in more than 90% of patients thought to have cat-scratch disease and 5% of normal controls.

Histopathologic examination of involved nodes shows characteristic changes that are nondiagnostic unless the organism is demonstrated. The lymph node architecture is distorted by multiple areas of central necrosis with acidophilic staining. These areas are surrounded by foci of epithelioid cells and scattered giant cells of the Langhans type. There is usually some elevation in the sedimentation rate. In cases with central nervous system involvement, the cerebrospinal fluid is usually normal but may show a slight pleocytosis and modest elevation of protein.

A serologic test for *B henselae* is now available and appears to be diagnostically useful.

Differential Diagnosis

Cat-scratch disease must be distinguished from pyogenic adenitis, tuberculosis (typical and atypical), tularemia, plague, brucellosis, Hodgkin's disease, lymphoma, rat-bite fever, primary toxoplasmosis, infectious mononucleosis, lymphogranuloma venereum, and fungal infections.

Treatment

The best therapy is reassurance that the adenopathy is benign and will subside spontaneously within 4–8 weeks in most cases. In cases of suppuration, node aspiration under local anesthesia with an 18- to 19-gauge needle relieves the pain. Excision of the involved node is indicated in cases of chronic adenitis. Antimicrobial therapy has not been proved to alter the course of illness; gentamicin and ciprofloxacin have been useful anecdotally in a few severe infections, and trimethoprim-sulfamethoxazole and erythromycin have also been useful in some cases.

Prognosis

The prognosis is good if complications do not occur.

Adal KA, Cockerell CJ, Petri WAJ: Cat scratch disease, bacillary angiomatosis, and other infections due to *Rochalimaea.* N Engl J Med 1994;330:1509.

Bogue CW et al: Antibiotic therapy for cat scratch disease. JAMA 1989;262:813.

Carithers HA: Cat-scratch disease: An overview based on a study of 1200 patients. Am J Dis Child 1985;139:1124.

Collipp PJ: Cat-scratch disease: therapy with trimethoprim-sulfamethoxazole. Am J Dis Child 1992;146:397.

Demers DM et al: Cat-scratch disease in Hawaii: Etiology and seroepidemiology. J Pediatr 1995;127:23.

Holley HP Jr: Successful treatment of cat-scratch disease with ciprofloxacin. JAMA 1991;265:1563.

Koehler JE, Glaser CA, Tappero JW: *Rochalimaea henselae* infection. JAMA 1994;271:531.

Malatack JJ, Jaffe R: Granulomatous hepatitis in three children due to cat-scratch disease without peripheral adenopathy: An unrecognized cause of fever of unknown origin. Am J Dis Child 1993;147:949.

Margileth AM, Hayden GF: Cat scratch disease. N Engl J Med 1993;329:53.

Zangwill KM et al: Cat scratch disease in Connecticut. N Engl J Med 1993;329:8.

SPIROCHETAL INFECTIONS

SYPHILIS

Essentials of Diagnosis

Congenital:
- All types: History of untreated maternal syphilis, a positive serologic test, and a positive darkfield examination.
- Newborn: Hepatosplenomegaly, characteristic x-ray bone changes, anemia, increased nucleated red cells, thrombocytopenia, abnormal spinal fluid, jaundice, edema.
- Young infant (3–12 weeks): Snuffles, maculopapular skin rash, mucocutaneous lesions, pseudoparalysis (in addition to x-ray bone changes).
- Children: Stigmas of early congenital syphilis (saddle nose, Hutchinson's teeth, etc), interstitial keratitis, saber shins, gummas of nose and palate.

Acquired:
- Chancre of genitals, lip, or anus in child or adolescent. History of sexual contact.

General Considerations

Syphilis is a chronic, generalized infectious disease caused by a slender spirochete, *Treponema pallidum.* In the acquired form, the disease is transmitted by sexual contact. Primary syphilis is characterized by the presence of an indurated painless chancre, which heals in 7–10 days. A secondary eruption involving the skin and mucous membranes appears in 4–6 weeks. After a long latency period, late lesions of tertiary syphilis involve the eyes, skin, bones, viscera, central nervous system, and cardiovascular system.

Congenital syphilis results from transplacental infection. Characteristic disease occurs after the fourth month of gestation and may result in stillbirth or manifest illness in the newborn, in early infancy, or later in childhood. First-trimester fetal infection has been found in the products of conception in therapeutic abortions. Syphilis occurring in the newborn and young infant is comparable to secondary disease in the adult but is more severe and life-threatening. Late congenital syphilis (developing in childhood) is comparable to tertiary disease.

Congenital syphilis is increasing in the United States due to increasing primary and secondary syphilis in women of childbearing age, and perhaps due to inadequate diagnosis and treatment of syphilis in prenatal care programs. Over 2200 cases of congenital syphilis and 20,600 cases of primary and secondary syphilis were reported in 1994. Prostitution in women addicted to crack cocaine has been associated with a more than 500% increase in congenital syphilis in New York City.

Clinical Findings

A. Symptoms and Signs:

1. Congenital syphilis–

a. Newborns–Most newborns with congenital syphilis are asymptomatic. If not detected and treated, symptoms develop within several weeks to months. When clinical signs are present, they usually consist of jaundice, anemia with or without thrombocytopenia, increase in nucleated red blood cells, hepatosplenomegaly, and edema. There may be overt signs of meningitis (bulging fontanelle, opisthotonos), but subclinical infection with cerebrospinal fluid abnormalities is more likely.

b. Young infants (3–12 weeks)–The infant may appear normal for the first few weeks of life only to develop "snuffles," a syphilitic skin eruption, mucocutaneous lesions, and pseudoparalysis of the arms or legs. Shotty lymphadenopathy may sometimes be felt. Hepatomegaly is universal, with splenomegaly in 50%. Other signs of disease seen in the newborn may be present. Anemia has been reported as the only presenting manifestation of congenital syphilis in this age group. "Snuffles" (rhinitis) is characterized by a profuse mucopurulent discharge that excoriates the upper lip and is present in 25%. A syphilitic rash is common on the palms and soles but may occur anywhere on the body; it consists of bright red, raised maculopapular lesions that gradually fade. Moist lesions occur at the mucocutaneous junctions (nose, mouth, anus, genitals) and lead to fissuring and bleeding.

Syphilis in the young infant may lead to stigmas recognizable in later childhood, such as rhagades (scars) around the mouth or nose, a "saddle" nose, and a high forehead (secondary to mild hydrocephalus associated with low-grade meningitis and frontal periostitis). The permanent upper central incisors may be peg-shaped with a central notch (Hutchinson's teeth), and the cusps of the sixth-year molars may have a lobulated mulberry appearance.

c. Children–Bilateral interstitial keratitis (at 6–12 years) is characterized by photophobia, increased lacrimation, and vascularization of the cornea associated with exudation. Chorioretinitis and optic atrophy may also be seen. Meningovascular syphilis (at 2–10 years) is usually slowly progressive, with mental retardation, spasticity, abnormal pupil response, speech defects, and abnormal spinal fluid. Deafness sometimes occurs. Thickening of the periosteum of the anterior tibias produces saber shins. A bilateral effusion into the knee joints (Clutton's joints) may occur but is not associated with sequelae. Gummas may develop in the nasal septum, palate, long bones, and subcutaneous tissues.

2. Acquired syphilis–The primary chancre of the genitals, mouth, or anus may occur as a result of intimate sexual contact. If the chancre is missed, signs of secondary syphilis, such as rash, fever, headache and malaise, may be the first manifestation of the disease.

B. Laboratory Findings:

1. Darkfield microscopy–Treponemes can be seen in scrapings from a chancre and from moist lesions.

2. Serologic tests for syphilis (STS)–There are two general types of serologic tests for syphilis: treponemal and nontreponemal. The latter (Venereal Disease Research Laboratory, or VDRL) is useful for screening and follow-up of known cases. A rapid test (the rapid plasma reagin, or RPR) is useful for screening, but positive sera should be further examined by quantitative nontreponemal and treponemal tests. Positive nontreponemal tests are confirmed with more specific fluorescent treponemal antibody absorption, or FTA-ABS test. False-positive FTA-ABS tests are uncommon except with other spirochetal disease.

One or 2 weeks after the onset of primary syphilis (chancre), the FTA-ABS test becomes positive. The VDRL or a similar nontreponemal test usually turns positive a few days later. By the time the secondary stage has arrived, virtually all patients show both positive FTA-ABS and positive nontreponemal tests. During latent and tertiary syphilis, the VDRL may become negative, but the FTA-ABS test usually remains positive. The quantitative VDRL or a similar nontreponemal test should be used to follow treated cases (see below).

Positive serologic tests in cord sera may represent passively transferred antibody rather than congenital infection and therefore must be supplemented by a combination of clinical and laboratory data. Elevated total cord IgM is a helpful but nonspecific finding. A specific IgM-FTA-ABS is available, but negative results are not conclusive and should not be relied upon. Demonstration of characteristic treponemes by darkfield examination of material from a moist lesion (skin, nasal or other mucous membranes) is definitive. Serial measurement of quantitative VDRL is also very useful, since passively transferred antibody in the absence of active infection should decay with a normal half-life of about 18 days.

In one study, 15% of infants with congenital syphilis had negative cord blood serology, presumably due to maternal infection late in pregnancy.

C. Imaging:
Radiographic abnormalities are present in 90% of infants with symptoms of congenital syphilis and 20% of asymptomatic infants. Metaphysial lucent bands, periostitis, and a widened zone of provisional calcification may be present. Bilateral symmetric osteomyelitis with pathologic fractures of the medial tibial metaphyses (Wimberger's sign) is almost pathognomonic.

Differential Diagnosis

A. Congenital Syphilis:

1. Newborns–Sepsis, congestive heart failure, congenital rubella, toxoplasmosis, disseminated herpes simplex, cytomegalovirus infection, and hemolytic disease of the newborn have to be differentiated. Positive Coombs' test and blood group incompatibility distinguish hemolytic disease.

2. Young infants–Pseudoparalysis (a flaccid paralysis) occurs in poliomyelitis. Signs of scurvy do not appear until the latter half of the first year of life. Injury to the brachial plexus, acute osteomyelitis, and septic arthritis must be differentiated from pseudoparalysis. Coryza due to viral infection often responds to symptomatic treatment. Rash (ammoniacal diaper rash) and scabies may be confused with a syphilitic eruption.

3. Children–Interstitial keratitis and bone lesions of tuberculosis are distinguished by positive tuberculin reaction and chest x-ray. Arthritis associated with syphilis is unaccompanied by systemic signs, and joints are not tender. Mental retardation, spasticity, and hyperactivity are shown to be of syphilitic origin by strongly positive serologic tests.

B. Acquired Syphilis:

Herpes genitalis, traumatic lesions, and other venereal diseases must be differentiated.

Prevention

A serologic test for syphilis should be performed at the initiation of prenatal care and repeated at delivery. In mothers at high risk of syphilis, repeated tests may be necessary. Serologic tests for syphilis may be negative on both the mother and the baby at the time of birth if the mother acquired syphilis near term. Adequate treatment of mothers with secondary syphilis before the last month of pregnancy reduces the incidence of congenital syphilis from 90% to less than 2%. Examination and serology of sexual partners and siblings should also be done.

Treatment

A. Specific Measures:

Penicillin is the drug of choice for *T pallidum*. If the patient is allergic to penicillin, erythromycin or one of the tetracyclines may be used.

1. Congenital syphilis–Infants with positive serology should be fully evaluated: history of maternal disease and therapy, CBC, liver function tests, long bone radiographs, cerebrospinal fluid examination, and quantitative serologic tests.

Treatment is indicated for infants with physical signs, abnormal radiographs, elevated cerebrospinal fluid protein or cell counts, or reactive cerebrospinal fluid VDRL. In addition, infants born to inadequately treated mothers or mothers treated with nonpenicillin drugs should be treated. If there are no clinical or laboratory signs of syphilis, the infant may be followed at monthly intervals with quantitative serologic tests and physical examinations if follow-up is ensured. Rising titers or clinical signs usually occur within 4 months in infants with infection. Infants with suspected congenital syphilis should have roentgenography of the long bones and a cerebrospinal fluid examination.

Infants with proved or suspected congenital syphilis should receive either of the following: (1) aqueous crystalline penicillin G, 50,000 units/kg/dose intramuscularly or intravenously every 12 hours (if < 1 week old) or every 8 hours (if between 1 and 4 weeks of age) for 10–14 days; or (2) aqueous procaine penicillin G, 50,000 units/kg/d intramuscularly for a minimum of 10 days. All infants diagnosed after 4 weeks of age should receive 50,000 units/kg/dose intramuscularly or intravenously every 6 hours for 10–14 days. Because treatment failures in early congenital syphilis may be due to low levels of benzathine penicillin in the cerebrospinal fluid and the eye—and because cerebrospinal fluid serology may fail to detect central nervous system infection—benzathine penicillin is no longer recommended for proved or strongly suspected congenital syphilis. Asymptomatic seropositive infants with normal cerebrospinal fluid born to adequately treated mothers may be given benzathine penicillin G (50,000 units/kg intramuscularly in a single dose) with follow-up serologic examinations at 1, 2, 3, 6, and 12 months. For larger children, the total dose of penicillin need not exceed the dosage used in adult syphilis of more than 1 year's duration.

Follow-up quantitative VDRL or RPR tests should be performed at 2, 4, 6, and 12 months after the end of therapy or should be repeated until they become nonreactive. Repeat cerebrospinal fluid examination every 6 months for 3 years is indicated for infants with a positive cerebrospinal fluid VDRL reaction. Titers decline with treatment and are usually negative by 12 months. Retreatment is indicated for rising titers or stable titers that do not decline.

2. Acquired syphilis–Benzathine penicillin G, 50,000 units/kg up to a maximum of 2.4 million units to adolescents with primary, secondary, or latent disease less than 1 year's duration. Late latent disease and neurosyphilis require weekly therapy for 3 weeks.

B. General Measures:

Care should be given to the maintenance of adequate nutrition.

Penicillin treatment of early congenital or secondary syphilis may result in a febrile Jarisch-Herxheimer reaction. Treatment is symptomatic, with careful follow-up and aspirin or acetaminophen, although transfusion may be necessary in infants with severe hemolytic anemia.

Prognosis

Severe disease, if unexpected, may be fatal in the newborn. Complete cure can be expected if the young infant is treated with penicillin. Serologic reversal usually occurs within 1 year. Treatment of primary syphilis with penicillin is curative. Permanent neurologic sequelae may be seen with meningovascular syphilis.

Azimi PH et al: Concentrations of procaine and aqueous penicillin in the cerebrospinal fluid of infants treated for congenital syphilis. J Pediatr 1994;24:649.

Beerman MR et al: Lumbar puncture in the evaluation of possible asymptomatic congenital syphilis in neonates. J Pediatr 1996;128:125.

Dorfman DH, Glaser JH: Congenital syphilis presenting in infants after the newborn period. N Engl J Med 1990; 323:1299.

Dunn RA, Zenker PN: Why radiographs are useful in evaluation of neonates suspected of having congenital syphilis. Radiology 1992;182:639.

Hook EW III, Marra CM: Acquired syphilis in adults. (Medical Progress.) N Engl J Med 1992;326:1060.

Paryani SG et al: Treatment of asymptomatic congenital syphilis: Benzathine versus procaine penicillin G therapy. J Pediatr 1994;125:471.

Rawstron SA et al: Maternal and congenital syphilis in Brooklyn, NY. Am J Dis Child 1993;147:727.

Sanchez PJ: Congenital syphilis. Adv Pediatr Infect Dis 1992;7:161.

Tramont EC: Syphilis in adults: From Christopher Columbus to Sir Alexander Fleming to AIDS. Clin Infect Dis 1995;21:1361.

Wright MS, Tecklenburg FW: Critical illness in congenital syphilis after the newborn period. Clin Pediatr 1992; 31:247.

Zenker PN, Berman FM: Congenital syphilis: Trends and recommendations for valuation and management. Pediatr Infect Dis J 1991;10:516.

RELAPSING FEVER

Essentials of Diagnosis

- Episodes of fever, chills, malaise.
- Occasional rash, arthritis, cough, hepatosplenomegaly, conjunctivitis.
- Diagnosis confirmed by direct microscopic identification of spirochetes in smears of peripheral blood.

General Considerations

Relapsing fever is a vector-borne disease caused by spirochetes of the genus *Borrelia*. Epidemic relapsing fever is transmitted to humans by body lice (*Pediculus humanus*) and endemic relapsing fever by soft-bodied ticks (genus *Ornithodoros*).

Tick-borne relapsing fever is endemic in the western United States. Transmission usually takes place during the warm months, when ticks are active and recreation or work brings people into contact with *Ornithodoros* ticks. Mountain camping areas and cabins are sites where infection often is acquired. The ticks are nocturnal feeders and remain attached for only 5–20 minutes. Consequently, the patient seldom remembers a tick bite.

Rarely, neonatal relapsing fever results from transplacental transmission of *Borrelia*. Both louseborne and tick-borne relapsing fever may be acquired during foreign travel.

Clinical Findings

A. Symptoms and Signs: The incubation period is 4–18 days. The attack is sudden, with high fever, chills, tachycardia, nausea and vomiting, headache, myalgia, arthralgia, bronchitis, and a dry, nonproductive cough. Hepatomegaly and splenomegaly appear later. Meningeal irritation may be present. An erythematous rash may be seen over the trunk and extremities, and petechiae may be present. After 3–10 days, the fever falls by crisis. Jaundice, iritis, conjunctivitis, cranial nerve palsies, and hemorrhage are more common during relapses.

The disease is characterized by relapses lasting 3–5 days, occurring at intervals of 1–2 weeks, with interim asymptomatic periods. The relapses duplicate the initial attack but become progressively less severe. In louse-borne relapsing fever, there is usually a single relapse; in tick-borne infection, there are two to six relapses.

B. Laboratory Findings: During febrile episodes, the urine contains protein, casts, and, occasionally, erythrocytes; there is a marked polymorphonuclear leukocytosis and, in about 25% of cases, a false-positive serologic test for syphilis. Spirochetes can be found in the peripheral blood by direct microscopy in approximately 70% of cases by darkfield examination or by Wright, Giemsa, or acridine orange staining of thick and thin smears. They are not found during afebrile periods. The blood may be injected into young mice and the spirochetes found 1–14 days later in the tail blood. OXK agglutinin titers in serum may be positive.

Differential Diagnosis

Relapsing fever may be confused with malaria, leptospirosis, dengue, typhus, rat-bite fever, Colorado tick fever, Rocky Mountain spotted fever, collagen vascular disease, or any fever of unknown origin.

Complications

Complications include facial paralysis, iridocyclitis, optic atrophy, hypochromic anemia, pneumonia, nephritis, myocarditis, endocarditis, and seizures. Central nervous system involvement is seen in 10–30% of cases.

Treatment

For children under 7 years of age with tick-borne relapsing fever, erythromycin (40–50 mg/kg/d orally in divided doses every 6 hours for 10 days) should be given. Older children may be given tetracycline. Penicillin and chloramphenicol are also efficacious.

In louse-borne relapsing fever, a single dose of tetracycline or erythromycin has been effective.

Severely ill patients should be hospitalized. Antibiotic treatment should be started after the fever has dropped; this will lessen the risk of severe or even fatal Jarisch-Herxheimer reaction. Isolation precautions are not necessary.

Prognosis

The mortality rate in treated cases of relapsing fever is very low, except in debilitated or very young children. With treatment, the initial attack is shortened and relapses prevented. The response to antimicrobial therapy is dramatic.

Le CT: Tick-borne relapsing fever in children. Pediatrics 1980;66:963.

Outbreak of relapsing fever—Grand Canyon National Park, Arizona, 1990. MMWR Morb Mortal Wkly Rep 1991; 40:296.

Sciotto CG et al: Detection of *Borrelia* in acridine orange-stained blood smears by fluorescence microscopy. Arch Pathol Lab Med 1983;107:384.

Spach DH et al: Tick-borne diseases in the United States. N Engl J Med 1993;329:936.

LEPTOSPIROSIS

Essentials of Diagnosis

- Biphasic course lasting 2 or 3 weeks.
- Initial phase: high fever, headache, myalgia, and conjunctivitis.
- Apparent recovery for 2–3 days.
- Return of fever associated with meningitis.
- Jaundice, hemorrhages, and renal insufficiency (severe cases).
- Culture of organism from blood and cerebrospinal fluid (early) and from urine (later), or direct microscopy of urine or cerebrospinal fluid.
- Positive leptospiral agglutination test.

General Considerations

Leptospirosis is a zoonosis caused by many antigenically distinct but morphologically similar spirochetes. The organism enters through the skin or respiratory tract. Classically, the severe form—Weil's disease, with jaundice and a high mortality rate—was associated with infection with *Leptospira icterohaemorrhagiae* following immersion in water contaminated with rat urine. It is now known that a variety of animals (dogs, rats, cattle, etc) may serve as reservoirs for pathogenic *Leptospira;* that a given serogroup may have multiple animal species as hosts; and that severe disease may be caused by many different serogroups other than *L icterohaemorrhagiae.*

In the United States, leptospirosis occurs in children, students, and housewives due to contact with dogs. Cattle, swine, or rodents may transmit the organism. Sewer workers, farmers, abattoir workers, animal handlers, and soldiers are at risk of occupational exposure. Outbreaks have resulted from swimming in contaminated streams and harvesting field crops.

In the United States, about 100 cases are reported yearly, and about one third are in children.

Clinical Findings

A. Symptoms and Signs:

1. Initial phase—The incubation period is 4–19 days, with a mean of 10 days. Chills, fever, headache, myalgia, conjunctivitis (episcleral injection), photophobia, cervical lymphadenopathy, and pharyngitis occur commonly. This leptospiremic phase lasts for 3–7 days.

2. Phase of apparent recovery—Symptoms typically (but not always) subside for 2–3 days.

3. Systemic phase—Fever reappears and is associated with headache, muscular pain and tenderness in the abdomen and back, and nausea and vomiting. Lung, heart, and joint involvement occasionally occurs. These manifestations are due to extensive vasculitis.

a. Central nervous system involvement—The central nervous system is involved in 50–90% of cases. Severe headache and mild nuchal rigidity are usual, but delirium, coma, and focal neurologic signs may be seen.

b. Renal and hepatic involvement—In about 50% of cases, the kidney or liver or both are affected. Gross hematuria and oliguria or anuria are sometimes seen. Jaundice may be associated with an enlarged and tender liver.

c. Gallbladder involvement—Leptospirosis may cause acalculous cholecystitis in children. An abdominal ultrasound study may reveal a dilated, nonfunctioning gallbladder. Pancreatitis is unusual.

d. Hemorrhage—Petechiae, ecchymoses, and gastrointestinal bleeding may be severe.

e. Rash—A rash is seen in 10–30% of cases. It may be maculopapular and generalized or may be petechial or purpuric. Occasionally, erythema nodosum is seen. Peripheral desquamation of the rash may occur. Gangrenous areas are sometimes noted over the distal extremities. In such cases, skin biopsy demonstrates the presence of severe vasculitis involving both the arterial and the venous circulations.

B. Laboratory Findings: Leptospires are present in the blood and cerebrospinal fluid only during the first 10 days of illness. They appear in the urine during the second week, where they may persist for 30 days or longer. The organism can be isolated from blood inoculated into Fletcher's semisolid medium or EMJH semisolid medium, but culture techniques are slow (7–10 days), difficult, and not generally available.

The white blood cell count often is elevated, especially when there is liver involvement. Serum bilirubin levels usually remain below 20 mg/dL. Other liver function tests may be abnormal, although the AST usually shows only slight elevation. An elevated serum creatinine phosphokinase is frequently found. Cerebrospinal fluid shows moderate pleocytosis (< 500/µL) predominantly mononuclear cells, increased protein (50–100 mg/dL), and normal glucose. Urine often shows microscopic pyuria, hematuria, and, less often, proteinuria (++ or greater). The erythrocyte sedimentation rate is markedly elevated. Chest x-ray may show pneumonitis.

The serologic test of choice is a microscopic agglutination test using live organisms (performed at the Centers for Disease Control and Prevention, Atlanta, GA 30333, or at research centers). Leptospiral agglutinins generally reach peak levels by the third to fourth week. A 1:100 titer is considered suspicious; a fourfold or greater rise is diagnostic.

Differential Diagnosis

Fever and myalgia associated with the characteristic conjunctival (episcleral) injection should suggest leptospirosis. During the prodrome, malaria, typhoid fever, typhus, rheumatoid arthritis, brucellosis, and influenza may be suspected. Later, depending on the organ systems involved, a variety of other diseases need to be distinguished, including encephalitis, viral or tuberculous meningitis, viral hepatitis, glomerulonephritis, viral or bacterial pneumonia, rheumatic fever, subacute infective endocarditis, acute surgical abdomen, and Kawasaki disease (see Table 35–3).

Prevention

Preventive measures include the avoidance of contaminated water and soil, the use of rodent control, immunization of dogs and other domestic animals, and good sanitation. Immunization or antimicrobial prophylaxis with doxycycline may be of value to certain high-risk occupational groups.

Treatment

A. Specific Measures: Aqueous penicillin G (150,000 units/kg/d in four to six divided doses intravenously for 7–10 days) should be given when the diagnosis is suspected. Recent studies in severely ill patients indicate a benefit even if started 4 days into the illness. A Jarisch-Herxheimer reaction may be seen. Tetracycline (40–50 mg/kg/d) may be used for mildly ill patients.

B. General Measures: Symptomatic and supportive care is indicated, particularly for renal and hepatic failure and hemorrhage.

Prognosis

Leptospirosis generally is anicteric and self-limiting. The disease usually lasts 1–3 weeks but may be more prolonged. Relapse may occur.

There are usually no permanent sequelae associated with central nervous system infection, though

headache may persist. The mortality rate in reported cases in the United States is 5%, usually from renal failure. The mortality rate may reach 20% or more in elderly patients who have severe kidney and hepatic involvement.

Farr RW: Leptospirosis. Clin Infect Dis 1995;21:1.
Van Crevel R et al: Leptospirosis in travelers. Clin Infect Dis 1994;19:132.
Watt G et al: Placebo-controlled trial of intravenous penicillin for severe and late leptospirosis. Lancet 1988; 1:433.
Watt G et al: Limulus lysate positivity and Herxheimer-like reactions in leptospirosis: A placebo controlled study. J Infect Dis 1990;162:564.

LYME DISEASE

Essentials of Diagnosis

- Presence of skin lesion (erythema migrans) 3–30 days after tick bite.
- Arthritis, usually pauciarticular, occurring about 4 weeks after appearance of skin lesion. Headache, chills, and fever.
- Residence or travel in an endemic area during the late spring, summer, or early fall.

General Considerations

Lyme disease is a subacute or chronic spirochetal infection caused by *Borrelia burgdorferi* and transmitted by the bite of an infected deer tick (*Ixodes* spp). The disease was known in Europe for many years as tick-borne encephalomyelitis, often associated with a characteristic rash (erythema migrans). Discovery of the agent and vector followed investigation of an outbreak of pauciarticular arthritis in Lyme, Connecticut, in 1977.

Although cases are reported from many countries and states, endemic areas include the Northeast, upper Midwest, and West Coast in the United States and the northern European countries. The disease appears to be spreading due to increased infection in and distribution of the tick vector. Most cases with rash are recognized in spring and summer, when most tick bites occur. Since the incubation period for joint and neurologic disease may be months, however, cases may present at any time. Ixodes ticks are very small, and the infecting bite is often unrecognized.

Clinical Findings

A. Symptoms and Signs: Erythema migrans is the most characteristic feature of Lyme disease and develops in 60–80% of patients. Three to 30 days after the bite, a ring of erythema develops at the site and spreads over days. It may attain a diameter of 20 cm. The center of the lesion may clear (resembling tinea corporis), remain red, or become raised (suggesting a chemical or infectious cellulitis). Many patients are otherwise asymptomatic; some have fever (usually low-grade), headache, and myalgias. Multiple satellite skin lesions, urticaria or diffuse erythema may occur. Untreated, the rash lasts days to 3 weeks and eventually disappears.

In up to 50% of patients, arthritis develops several weeks to months after the bite. Recurrent attacks of migratory, monoarticular or pauciarticular arthritis involving the knees and other large joints are seen. Each attack lasts for days to a few weeks. Fever is common and may be high. Complete resolution between attacks is typical. Chronic arthritis develops in less than 10%, more often in those with the DR4 haplotype.

Neurologic manifestations develop in up to 20% of cases and usually consist of Bell's palsy, aseptic meningitis (which may be indistinguishable from viral meningitis), or polyradiculitis. Peripheral neuritis, Guillain-Barré syndrome, encephalitis, ataxia, chorea and other cranial neuropathies are less common. Seizures suggest another diagnosis. Untreated, the neurologic symptoms are usually self-limited but may be chronic or permanent. Although the fatigue and nonspecific neurologic symptoms may be prolonged in a few patients, Lyme disease is not usually proved as a cause of the chronic fatigue syndrome.

Self-limited heart-block or myocardial dysfunction occur in about 5% of patients.

B. Laboratory Findings: Most patients with only rash have no abnormal laboratory tests. Children with arthritis may have moderately elevated sedimentation rates and white blood cell counts; the ANA and rheumatoid factor are negative or non-specific; streptococcal antibodies are not elevated. Circulating IgM cryoglobulins may be present. Joint fluid may show up to 100,000 cells with a polymorphonuclear predominance, normal glucose, elevated protein and immune complexes; Gram's stain and culture are negative. In patients with central nervous system involvement, the spinal fluid may show lymphocytic pleocytosis and elevated protein; the glucose and all cultures and stains are normal or negative. Abnormal nerve conduction may be present with peripheral neuropathy.

Diagnosis

Lyme disease is a clinical diagnosis. History, physical examination, and laboratory features are important to consider. The causative organism is difficult to culture. Serologic testing may support the clinical diagnosis. Antibody testing should be performed in experienced laboratories: The enzyme immunoassay is currently the most accurate test, and confirmation of positives by Western blot should be considered, especially with unusual clinical syndromes. Serologic tests are positive in only 30–60% of patients with early disease. Therapy early in disease may blunt antibody titers. Recent studies have shown considerable intralaboratory and interlaboratory variability in titers reported. Overdiagnosis of

Lyme disease based on atypical symptoms and "positive" serology appears to be common. Sera from patients with syphilis, HIV, and leptospirosis may give false-positive results for Lyme disease. Diagnosis of central nervous system disease requires both objective abnormalities of the neurologic examination, laboratory or radiographic studies, and consistent positive serology.

Differential Diagnosis

Aside from the disorders already mentioned, the rash may resemble pityriasis, erythema multiforme, a drug eruption, or erythema nodosum. Erythema migrans is nonscaly, minimally or nontender, and persists longer in the same place than many of the more common childhood erythematous rashes. The arthritis may resemble juvenile rheumatoid arthritis, reactive arthritis, septic arthritis, reactive effusion from a contiguous osteomyelitis, rheumatic fever, leukemic arthritis, lupus, and Henoch-Schönlein purpura. Spontaneous resolution in a few days to weeks helps differentiate it from juvenile rheumatoid arthritis, in which arthritis lasting a minimum of 6 weeks is required for diagnosis. The neurologic signs may suggest idiopathic Bell's palsy, viral or parainfectious meningitis or meningoencephalitis, lead poisoning, psychosomatic illness, and many other conditions.

Treatment

Although antimicrobial therapy is beneficial in most cases of Lyme disease, it is most effective if started early; prolonged treatment is important for all forms. Relapses are seen with all regimens in some patients.

A. Rash, Other Early Infections: Amoxicillin (40 mg/kg/d) orally in three divided doses, or penicillin V potassium, 25–50 mg/kg/d in three divided doses—some experts add probenecid, 10 mg/kg/dose—for 2–3 weeks. Use erythromycin (30 mg/kg/d) in penicillin-allergic children, although it may be less effective. Doxycycline (100 mg orally twice a day) or tetracycline (250 mg four times daily) may be used in children over age 9.

B. Arthritis: Use the amoxicillin or doxycycline regimen (same dosage as above), but treat for 4 weeks. Parenteral ceftriaxone, 75–100 mg/kg once daily, or penicillin G, 300,000 units/kg/d in four divided doses for 2–3 weeks, is used for persistent arthritis.

C. Bell's Palsy: The same oral drug regimens may be used for 4 weeks.

D. Other Neurologic Disease or Cardiac Disease: Parenteral therapy for 2 weeks is recommended with either ceftriaxone, 75–100 kg/d in one daily dose; or penicillin G, 300,000 units/kg/d in four divided doses.

Prevention

Prevention consists of avoidance of endemic areas,

wearing long sleeves and pants, frequent "tick checks," and applications of tick repellents. Permethrin sprayed on clothing decreases tick attachment. Repellents containing high concentrations of DEET may be neurotoxic and should be used cautiously and washed off when tick exposure ends. Prophylactic antibiotics should not be used.

Adams WV et al: Cognitive effects of Lyme disease in children. Pediatrics 1994;94:185.

Bingham PM et al: Neurologic manifestations in children with Lyme disease. Pediatrics 1995;96:1053.

Dattwyler RJ et al: Treatment of late Lyme borreliosis: Randomized comparison of ceftriaxone and penicillin. Lancet 1988;1:1191.

Luft EJ et al: Invasion of the central nervous system by *Borrelia burgdorferi* in acute disseminated infection. JAMA 1992;267:1364.

Malane MS et al: Diagnosis of Lyme disease based on dermatologic manifestations. Ann Intern Med 1991; 144:490.

Pfister HW et al: Randomized comparison of ceftriaxone and cefotaxime in Lyme neuroborreliosis. J Infect Dis 1991;163:311.

Rahn DW et al: Lyme disease: Recommendations for diagnosis and treatment. Ann Intern Med 1991;114:472.

Shapiro ED et al: A controlled trial of antimicrobial prophylaxis for Lyme disease after deer-tick bites. N Engl J Med 1992;327:1769.

Steere AC et al: The overdiagnosis of Lyme disease. JAMA 1993;269:1812.

Szer IL et al: The long term course of Lyme arthritis in children. N Engl J Med 1991;325:159.

Williams CL et al: Lyme disease in childhood: Clinical and epidemiologic features of 90 cases. Pediatr Infect Dis J 1990;9:10.

REFERENCES

Committee on Infectious Diseases: Report, 23rd ed. American Academy of Pediatrics, 1994.

Feigin RD, Cherry JD (editors): *Textbook of Pediatric Infectious Disease,* 3rd ed. Saunders, 1993.

Infections: Parasitic & Mycotic

38

Adriana Weinberg, MD, & Myron J. Levin, MD

I. INFECTIONS: PARASITIC

Parasitic diseases are common and may present clinically in a variety of ways (Table 38–1). Although travel to endemic areas suggests particular infections, many are acquired from contact with human carriers and can occur anywhere. The most common infections acquired abroad are giardiasis and malaria—at home, giardiasis, toxoplasmosis, and cryptosporidiosis. A list of antiparasitic agents is presented in Table 38–2.

Some of the less common parasitic infections and those seen primarily in the developing world are presented in abbreviated form in Table 38–3.

Selection of Patients for Evaluation

The incidence of parasitic infection varies greatly with geographic area. Children who have traveled or lived in endemic areas are at risk of infection with a variety of intestinal and tissue parasites. Children who have resided only in developed countries are usually free of tissue parasites (except perhaps *Toxoplasma*). Searching for intestinal parasites is expensive for the patient and time-consuming for the laboratory. More than 90% of ovum and parasite examinations performed in most hospital laboratories in the United States are negative; many have been ordered inappropriately. An approach to determining which children with diarrhea need such examinations is presented in Figure 38–1.

Children with underlying immunodeficiency, in both developed and developing countries, are uniquely susceptible to parasites, particularly protozoan intestinal infections. In these patients, normally commensal infestations may become debilitating infections, and multiple pathogens are frequently identified. The yield for diagnostic testing in compromised hosts is higher and the threshold for ordering tests must be lower.

Specimen Processing

For tissue parasites, contact the laboratory for proper collection procedure. Diarrheal stools may contain trophozoites that rapidly die during transport. The specimen should be either examined immediately or placed in a stool fixative such as polyvinyl alcohol. Several types of commercial vials containing fixatives are available and may be sent home with the child for outpatient specimen collection. Since they may contain toxic compounds, the vials should be safely stored. Fixed specimens are stable at room temperature. Formed stools usually contain cysts that are more stable. It is best to fix these also after collection, but they may be reliably examined after room temperature transport.

Eosinophilia & Parasitic Infections

Although parasites commonly cause eosinophilia, in developed countries other causes are much more common and include allergies, drugs, and other infections. Heavy intestinal nematode infections cause eosinophilia; they are easily detected on a single ovum and parasite examination. Light nematode infections and common protozoan infections—giardiasis, cryptosporidiosis, and amebiasis—rarely cause eosinophilia. Eosinophilia is also unusual or minimal in more serious infections such as amebic liver abscess, cysticercosis, toxoplasmosis, and malaria.

The most common parasitic infection in the United States that causes significant eosinophilia with negative stool examination is toxocariasis. In a young child with unexplained eosinophilia and a negative stool examination, a serologic test for *Toxocara* may be the next appropriate test. Trichinosis may rarely cause marked eosinophilia; strongyloidiasis may also be difficult to diagnose with stool examinations. Patients with eosinophilia who have lived in or traveled to developing regions of the world have a much broader differential diagnosis.

Table 38–1. Symptoms of parasitic infection.

Sign	Agent	Comments[1]
Abdominal pain	Anisakis	Shortly after raw fish ingestion.
	Ascaris	Heavy infection; may obstruct bowel, biliary tract.
	Clonorchis	Heavy, early infection. Hepatomegaly later.
	Entamoebal histolytica	Hematochezia, variable fever, diarrhea.
	Fasciola hepatica	Diarrhea, vomiting.
	Hookworm	Heavy infection. Iron deficiency anemia.
	Strongyloides	Eosinophilia, pruritus. May resemble peptic disease.
	Trichinella	Myalgia, periorbital edema, eosinophilia.
	Trichuris	Diarrhea, dysentery with heavy infection.
Cough	Ascaris	Wheezing, eosinophilia. During migration phase.
	Paragonimus westermani	Hemoptysis; chronic. May mimic tuberculosis.
	Strongyloides	Wheezing, pruritus, eosinophilia during migration or dissemination.
	Toxocara	Affects ages 1–5; hepatosplenomegaly; eosinophilia.
	Tropical eosinophilia	Pulmonary infiltrates, eosinophilia.
Diarrhea	Blastocystis	Possibly with heavy infection in immunosuppressed or normal individuals.
	Cryptosporidium	Watery; prolonged in normals, chronic in immunosuppressed.
	Dientamoeba fragilis	Only with heavy infection.
	Entamoeba histolytica	Hematochezia, variable fever; no eosinophilia.
	Giardia	Afebrile, chronic; anorexia; no hematochezia or eosinophilia.
	Schistosoma	Chronic; hepatosplenomegaly.
	Strongyloides	Abdominal pain; eosinophilia.
	Trichinella	Myalgia, periorbital edema, eosinophilia.
	Trichuris	With heavy infection.
Dysentery	Balantidium coli	Swine contact.
	Entamoeba histolytica	Few to no leukocytes in stool; fever; hematochezia
	Schistosoma	During acute infections.
	Trichuris	With heavy infection.
Dysuria	Enterobius	Usually girls with worms in urethra, bladder; nocturnal, perianal pruritus.
	Schistosoma	Hematuria. Exclude bacteriuria, stones.
Headache (and other cerebral symptoms)	Angiostrongylus	Eosinophilic meningitis.
	Naegleria	Fresh-water swimming; rapidly progressive meningoencephalitis.
	Plasmodium	Fever, chills, jaundice, splenomegaly. Cerebral ischemia (with P falciparum).
	Taenia solium	Cysticercosis. Focal seizures, deficits; hydrocephalus, aseptic meningitis.
	Toxoplasma	Meningoencephalitis (especially in the immunosuppressed); hydrocephalus in infants.
	Trypanosoma	African forms. Chronic lethargy (sleeping sickness).
Pruritus	Ancylostoma braziliense	Creeping eruption; dermal serpiginous burrow.
	Enterobius	Perianal, nocturnal.
	Filaria	Variable; seen in many filarial disease.
	Hookworm	Local at penetration site in heavy exposure.
	Strongyloides	Diffuse with migration; may be recurrent.
	Trypanosoma	African forms; one of many nonspecific symptoms.

(continued)

Table 38–1. Symptoms of parasitic infection. (continued)

Sign	Agent	Comments[1]
Fever	*Entamoeba histolytica*	With acute dysentery or liver abscess.
	Leishmania donovani	Hepatosplenomegaly, anemia, leukopenia.
	Plasmodium	Chills, headache, jaundice; periodic.
	Toxocara	Cough, hepatosplenomegaly, eosinophilia.
	Toxoplasma	Generalized adenopathy; splenomegaly.
	Trichinella	Myalgia, periorbital edema, eosinophilia.
	Trypanosoma	Early stage, African forms; lymphadenopathy.
Anemia	*Diphyllobothrium*	Megaloblastic due to B_{12} deficiency; rare.
	Hookworm	Iron deficiency.
	Leishmania donovani	Fever, hepatosplenomegaly, leukopenia (kala-azar).
	Plasmodium	Hemolysis.
	Trichuris	Heavy infection, due to iron loss.
Eosinophilia	*Angiostrongylus*	Eosinophilic meningitis.
	Fasciola	Abdominal pain.
	Filaria	Microfilariae in blood. Lymphadenopathy.
	Onchocerca	Nodules, keratitis.
	Schistosoma	Chronic; intestinal or genitourinary symptoms.
	Strongyloides	Abdominal pain, diarrhea.
	Toxocara	Hepatosplenomegaly, cough; affects ages 1–5.
	Trichinella	Myalgia, periorbital edema.
	Tropical eosinophilia	Unknown filarial agent. Cough.
Hematuria	*Schistosoma*	*S haematobium.* Bladder, urethral granulomas. Exclude stones, bacteriuria.
Hemoptysis	*Paragonimus westermani*	Lung fluke. Variable chest pain; chronic.
Hepatomegaly	*Clonorchis*	Heavy infection. Tenderness early; cirrhosis late.
	Echinococcus	Chronic; cysts.
	Entamoeba histolytica	Toxic hepatitis or abscess. No eosinophilia.
	Leishmania donovani	Splenomegaly, fever, pancytopenia.
	Schistosoma	Chronic; hepatic fibrosis, splenomegaly.
	Toxocara	Splenomegaly, eosinophilia, cough; no adenopathy.
Splenomegaly	*Leishmania donovani*	Hepatomegaly, fever, anemia.
	Plasmodium	Fever, chills, jaundice, headache.
	Schistosoma	Hepatomegaly.
	Toxocara	Eosinophilia, hepatomegaly.
	Toxoplasma	Lymphadenopathy, other symptoms.
Lymphadenopathy	Filaria	Inguinal typical; chronic.
	Leishmania donovani	Hepatosplenomegaly, pancytopenia fever
	Schistosoma	Acute infection; fever, rash, arthralgia, leptosplenomegaly.
	Toxoplasma	Cervical common; may involve single site; splenomegaly.
	Trypanosoma	Localized near bite or generalized hepatosplenomegaly (Chagas' disease); generalized (especially posterior cervical) in African forms.

[1]Symptoms usually related to degree of infestation. Infestation with small numbers of organisms is often asymptomatic.

Table 38–2. Manufacturers of commonly used antiparasitic drugs.

[1]Albendazole—*Zentel* (SmithKline Beecham)
[2]Aminosidine (paromomycin)
[2]Benznidazole—*Rochagan* (Roche, Brazil)
[3]Bithionol—*Bitin* (Tanabe, Japan)
Chloroquine—*Aralen* (Sanofi Winthrop), others
[1]Diethylcarbamazine—*Hetrazan* (Wyeth-Ayerst)
[3]Diloxanide furoate—*Furamide* (Boots, England)
[1]Eflornithine (difluoromethylornithine, DFMO)—*Ornidyl* (Merrell Dow)
Furazolidone—*Furoxone* (Roberts)
[2]Halofantrine—*Halfan* (SmithKline Beecham)
Hydroxychloroquine—*Plaquenil* (Sanofi Winthrop)
Iodoquinol (diiodohydroxyquin)—*Yodoxin* (Glenwood), others
[3]Ivermectin—*Mectizan* (Merck)
Mebendazole—*Vermox* (Janssen)
Mefloquine—*Lariam* (Roche)
[2]Meglumine antimonate—*Glucantime* (Rhône-Poulenc Rorer, France)
[3]Melarsoprol—*Arsobal* (Rhône-Poulenc Rorer, France)
Metronidazole—*Flagyl* (Searle), others
[3]Nifurtimox—*Lampit* (Bayer, Germany)
Oxamniquine—*Vansil* (Pfizer)
Paromomycin—*Humatin* (Parke-Davis)
Pentamidine isethionate—*Pentam* 300 (Fujisawa), *NebuPent* (Fujisawa)
Praziquantel—*Biltricide* (Miles)
Primaquine phosphate—(Sanofi Winthrop)
[2]Proguanil—*Paludrine* (Ayerst, Canada, ICI, England)
Pyantel pamoate—*Antiminth* (Pfizer)
Pyrimethamine—*Daraprim* (Glaxo-Wellcome)
Pyrimethamine-sulfadoxine—*Fansidar* (Roche)
Quinidine gluconate—(Lilly)
[2]Quinine dihydrochloride
Quinine sulfate—many manufacturers
[3]Sodium stibogluconate (antimony sodium gluconate)— *Pentostam* (Glaxo-Wellcome, England)
[1]Spiramycin—*Rovamycine* (Rhône-Poulenc Rorer)
Sulfadiazine—(Eon Labs, and others)
[3]Suramin—(Bayer, Germany)
Thiabendazole—*Mintezol* (Merck)
[2]Tinidazole—*Fasigyn* (Pfizer)
[2]Tryparsamide

Adapted from The Medical Letter 1995;37(961):107.
[1]Available in the United States only from the manufacturer.
[2]Not available in the United States.
[3]Available from the CDC Drug Service, Centers for Disease Control and Prevention, Atlanta, Georgia 30333; (404)639-3670 (evenings, weekends, or holidays: (404)639-2888).

PROTOZOAL INFECTIONS

MALARIA

Essentials of Diagnosis

- Residence in or travel to an endemic area.
- Cyclic paroxysms of chills, fever, and intense diaphoresis.
- Headache, backache, cough, abdominal pain, nausea, vomiting, diarrhea.
- Coma, seizures.
- Splenomegaly, anemia.
- Malaria parasites in peripheral blood smear.

General Considerations

Malaria kills a million children worldwide each year and is undergoing resurgence in areas where it was previously controlled. Imported cases diagnosed in the United States each year number approximately 1000. The female anopheline mosquito transmits the parasites—*Plasmodium vivax* (most common), *Plasmodium falciparum* (most virulent), *Plasmodium ovale* (similar to *P vivax*), and *Plasmodium malariae*. The gametocytes ingested from an infected human form sporozoites in the mosquito; when inoculated into a susceptible host, these sporozoites infect hepatocytes. Antibody—but not drug therapy—decreases sporozoite infectivity. The preerythrocytic phase (hepatic) is about 1–2 weeks for all but *P malariae* infection (3–5 weeks), but the initial symptoms may be delayed for up to a year in *P falciparum,* 4 years in *P vivax,* and decades in *P malariae* infections. Merozoites released into the circulation from hepatocytes infect red cells (young cells by *P vivax* and *P ovale,* old cells by *P malariae,* and all cells by *P falciparum*) and begin the synchronous erythrocytic cycles—rupturing the infected cells at intervals of 48 hours for all but *P malariae,* which has a 72-hour cycle. Asynchronous cycles causing daily fevers are most common in early stages of infection. Survival is associated with a progressive decrease in intensity of cycles; relapses years later may occur as a result of hepatic infection, which persists in all but *P falciparum* infections. Infection acquired congenitally or from transfusions or needle sticks does not result in a hepatic phase.

Susceptibility varies genetically; certain red cell phenotypes are partially resistant to *P falciparum* infection (hemoglobin S, hemoglobin F, thalassemia, and possibly G6PD deficiency). The worldwide distribution of the four species is determined, to some extent, by host genetic factors. The absence of *P vivax* from Africa reflects the lack of specific Duffy blood group substances among most native Africans. Recurrent infections result in some natural species-specific immunity; this does not prevent sporozoite infection but does decrease parasitemia and symptoms. Normal splenic function is an important factor because of the immunologic and filter function of the spleen. Asplenic persons develop rapidly progressive

Table 38–3. Some parasitic infections seen less commonly in developed regions.

Agent (Disease)	Geographic Region	Vector	Symptoms and Signs	Laboratory Findings	Diagnosis	Therapy and Comments
Trypanosoma cruzi (Chagas' disease)	South and Central America, Mexico	Reduviid bug	Acute: Painful red nodule at bite site, conjunctivitis, periorbital edema (Romaña's sign), fever, local ± generalized adenitis. Late: Myocarditis, megaesophagus, megacolon.	Mononuclear leukocytosis	Organisms in peripheral blood. Positive serology.	Nifurtimox may help early. No therapy for late disease. May be transmitted by blood transfusion or congenitally.
Trypanosomal brucei (sleeping sickness)	Africa	Tsetse fly	Hepatosplenomegaly, adenopathy. Nodule at bite site (resolves). Recurrent fever, headache, myalgia, progressive encephalitis.	Elevated ESR, anemia, CSF pleocytosis	Organisms in blood, CSF, marrow, nodes. Positive serology.	Suramin for non-CNS disease. Eflornithine promising.
Leishmania donovani (kala-azar)	Mideast, India, Mediterranean, South and Central America	Sandfly	Fever, generalized adenopathy, hepatosplenomegaly weeks to months after infection.	Pancytopenia, hypergamma-globulinemia	Organisms in marrow, nodes, spleen. Positive serology.	Sodium stibogluconate, meglumine antimonate, pentamidine, amphotericin
Leishmania tropica (Oriental sore)	Asia, India, North Africa	Sandfly	Papule at bite site (usually on face, limbs) develops after weeks to months, then ulcerates and scars.	...	Organisms in skin biopsy. Positive skin test, serology.	Same as for *L donovani*.
Leishmania braziliensis, L mexicana (chiclero ulcer)	South America	Sandfly	Painful mucocutaneous ulcers or granulomas. Nasolabial lesions common.	...	Skin biopsy. Positive skin test, serology.	Same as for *L donovani*.
Wuchereria, Brugia (filariasis)	Tropics, subtropics	Mosquito	Chronic adenopathy, often inguinal. Obstructive lymphedema.	Eosinophilia	Concentrated blood smears for larvae. Positive serology.	Ivermectin, diethylcarbamazine kill larvae. Surgery for lymphatic obstruction.
Angiostrongylus cantonensis (eosinophilic meningitis)	Hawaii, Asia, Pacific Islands	Snails, slugs	Ingestion (usually inadvertent) followed in 1–4 weeks by meningitis of variable severity. Paresthesias.	Eosinophils in CSF and blood	Positive serology. Larvae may be present in CSF.	Fever absent or low. No focal lesions on CNS imaging. No specific therapy. Steroids may be beneficial. Mebendazole may help.
Naegleria fowleri (amebic meningoencephalitis)	Worldwide	Fresh water (ponds, lakes)	Swimming (usually in warm, fresh water) followed in 7 days by rhinitis, altered sense of taste or smell, fever, headache, meningismus, coma.	CSF pleocytosis. Negative Gram stain.	Amebas in CSF by direct examination or cytologic stain. Cultures are positive.	Free-living amebas; may resemble leukocytes in CSF. Amphotericin B may be helpful. Usually fatal.
Paragonimus westermani (lung fluke infection)	Asia, South America, Africa	Raw crabs, crustaceans	Cough, hemoptysis. Rarely seizures, other CNS signs if migration to brain occurs.	...	Large ova in concentrated specimens, feces. Cystic nodular lesions on chest x-ray or CNS imaging.	Resembles pulmonary tuberculosis. Praziquantel, very effective.
Clonorchis sinensis (liver fluke infection)	Asia	Raw fish	Adult flukes obstruct biliary tree. Acute: Hepatomegaly, fever, jaundice, urticaria. Late: cirrhosis, carcinoma.	Variable liver function test abnormalities	Ova in feces.	Praziquantel. Advanced disease not treatable. Liver transplant.

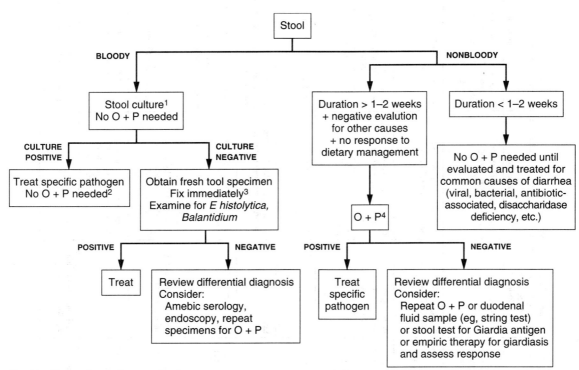

Figure 38–1. Parasitologic evaluation of acute diarrhea.

O + P = Ova and parasite examination.
[1]*Shigella, Salmonella, Campylobacter, E coli (Escheria coli)* 0157, *Yersinia*; assay for *Clostridium difficile* toxin
  if recent antimicrobial use.
[2]Unless critically ill, from endemic area for amebiasis, or unresponsive to standard therapy.
[3]In stool fixative, eg, polyvinyl alcohol.
[4]Include examination for *Cryptosporidium*; immediate stool fixation needed if stool is diarrheal.

malaria with many circulating infected erythrocytes (including mature forms of *P falciparum*). Maternal immunity protects the neonate despite the placental infection seen in active malarial infection in pregnancy.

Clinical Findings

A. Symptoms and Signs: Clinical manifestations vary according to species, strain, and host immunity. The infant presents with recurrent bouts of fever, irritability, poor feeding, vomiting, jaundice, and splenomegaly. Exanthem, rash, and significant dehydration are usually absent and help distinguish malaria from viral infections presenting with similar symptoms. Symptoms are similar in older children, with headache, backache, chills, myalgia, and fatigue more easily elicited. Fever may be cyclic (every 48 hours for all but *P malariae* infection, in which it occurs every 72 hours) or irregularly (most commonly observed with *P falciparum*. Between attacks, patients may look quite well. If the disease is untreated, relapses cease within a year in *P falciparum* and within several years in *P vivax* infections, but may recur decades later in *P malariae* infection. Infection during pregnancy often causes intrauterine growth retardation or premature delivery but rarely true fetal infection.

Physical examination in uncomplicated cases may show only mild splenomegaly an anemia.

B. Laboratory Findings: The diagnosis of malaria relies on detecting one or more of the four human plasmodia in blood smears. Most acute infections are caused by either *P vivax/P ovale,* although 5–7% are due to multiple species. Giemsa-stained thick smears offer the highest diagnostic accuracy for malaria parasites. Identification of the plasmodia species relies on morphologic criteria (Table 38–4) and requires an experienced observer.

Alternative techniques of similar or higher diagnostic accuracy for *P falciparum* include ELISA, DNA hybridization, and polymerase chain reactors. A unique feature of the microscopic examination is the semiquantitative estimate of the parasitemia, which is best done on thin smears. This information is particularly useful in the management of infections caused by *P falciparum,* in which high parasitemia

Table 38–4. Differentiation of malaria parasites on blood smears.

	P falciparum	*P vivax/P ovale*
Multiple infected erythrocytes	Common	Rare
Mature trophozoites or schizonts	Absent[1]	Common
Schüffner's dots	Absent	Common
Enlarged erythrocytes	Absent	Common
Banana-shaped gametocytes	Common	Absent

[1]Usually sequestered in the microcirculation. Rare cases with circulating forms have extremely high parasitemia and a poor prognosis.

(more than 10% infected erythrocytes or more than 500,000 infected erythrocytes/μL) is associated with high morbidity and mortality and requires hospitalization. Treatment response of *P falciparum* and chloroquine-resistant *P vivax* infections is best monitored by daily parasitemia assays: constant or increased number of infected erythrocytes after 48 hours of treatment or after the second hemolytic crisis suggest an inadequate therapeutic response. Other laboratory findings that reflect the severity of hemolysis include decreased hematocrit, hemoglobin, and haptoglobin; increased reticulocyte count; and hyperbilirubinemia and increased lactate dehydrogenase (LDH). Thrombocytopenia is common, but the incidence of leukocytosis is variable.

Differential Diagnosis

Relapsing fever may be seen with borreliosis, brucellosis, sequential common infections, Hodgkin's disease, juvenile rheumatoid arthritis, rat-bite fever, or one of the idiopathic periodic fevers. Other common causes of high fever and headache include influenza, *Mycoplasma pneumoniae* or enteroviral infection, sinusitis, meningitis, enteric fever, tuberculosis, occult pneumonia, or bacteremia. Fever, headache, and jaundice in a patient returning from tropical areas should include leptospirosis and yellow fever in the differential diagnosis. Malaria may also coexist with other diseases.

Complications & Sequelae

Severe complications are limited to *P falciparum* infection and result from microvascular obstruction and tissue ischemia. *P falciparum*-infected erythrocytes lose deformability and become more adherent to endothelial cells; this results in an accumulation in the microcirculation, thus hindering blood flow. Tissue ischemia, high-glucose consumption of malaria parasites, tumor necrosis factor release, and quinine therapy contribute to hypoglycemia and lactic acidosis observed in this disease. Impaired consciousness and seizures are the most common complications of malaria in children. Both impaired consciousness and

respiratory distress caused by cerebral and pulmonary edema, respectively, suggest life-threatening disease.

Additional complications of *P falciparum* infection include renal failure, gastroenteritis, and severe anemia. Hemolysis that occurs during the parasite life cycle, other factors such as tumor necrosis factor and induced suppression of hematopoiesis and quinine/quinidine-associated, immune-mediated anemia may contribute to anemia.

Prevention

Malaria chemoprophylaxis should be instituted 2 weeks before traveling to an endemic area to permit changes if the drug is not tolerated. Since the antimalarial drugs recommended for prophylaxis do not kill sporozoites, therapy should be continued for 4 weeks after returning from an endemic area to cover infection acquired at departure.

Chloroquine is the drug of choice for prophylaxis of *P vivax, P ovale, P malariae,* and chloroquine-sensitive *P falciparum* (Table 38–5). Chloroquine is safe for all ages and during pregnancy. Side effects (dizziness, blurred vision, headache) can be reduced by administering 50% of the weekly dose twice per week. Effects of chloroquine on heart rhythm are in-

Table 38–5. Chemoprophylaxis of malaria.

Drug	Dosage
Chloroquine-sensitive areas[1]	
Chloroquine	5 mg base/kg/wk up to 300 mg (adult dose)
Chloroquine-resistant areas	
Mefloquine	0.25 tablet (62.5 mg) once a week (15–19 kg)
	0.5 tablet (125 mg) (20–30 kg)
	0.75 tablet (187.5 mg) (31–45 kg)
	1 tablet (250 mg) (> 45 kg)
Doxycycline	2 mg/kg/d (age > 8 y) up to 100 mg (adult dose)
Chloroquine	5 mg base/kg/wk up to 300 mg (adult dose)
plus	
proguanil	50 mg daily (age < 2 y)
	100 mg (age 2–6 y)
	150 mg (age 7–10 y)
	200 mg (age > 10 y)
Relapse of *P vivax* or *P ovale*[2]	
Primaquine	0.3 mg base/kg/d up to 15 mg (adult dose) during the last 2 weeks of prophylaxis

Updated malaria chemoprophylaxis information may be obtained by calling the Centers for Disease Control and Prevention Hot Line at (404)332-4555.
[1]Chloroquine-resistant *Plasmodium falciparum* has not yet been identified in Central America west of the Panama Canal zone, Haiti, Dominican Republic, Mexico, and most of the Middle East.
[2]Optional. Observation and prompt initiation of treatment when relapse occurs are sufficient.

frequent and are typically associated with rapid intravenous infusion or overdosage. Chloroquine has immunosuppressive properties and has been reported to impair immunization against rabies, but not against yellow fever.

For chloroquine-resistant *P falciparum,* the drug of choice is mefloquine. The side effects of mefloquine are headache, dizziness, and blurred vision. Daily doxycycline is recommended for patients older than 8 years of age who are unable to tolerate mefloquine. Women on prolonged doxycycline therapy tend to develop yeast vaginitis, and it is advisable to supply them with nystatin suppositories. Mefloquine is not recommended for children under 15 kg or during pregnancy. Chloroquine plus chloroguanide (Proguanil) is the alternative regimen under these circumstances, although it is less effective than mefloquine. Daily primaquine also effectively prevents chloroquine-resistant *P falciparum,* and is used to prevent relapse of *P vivax* or *P ovale.*

No drug regimen guarantees protection against malaria. If fever develops within 1 year (particular within 2 months) after travel to an endemic area, patients should be advised to seek medical attention. Insect repellents, insecticide-impregnated bed nets and proper clothing are important adjuncts for malaria prophylaxis.

Treatment

Treatment for malaria includes a variety of supportive strategies in addition to the antimalarial drugs. It is advisable to hospitalize nonimmune patients with *P falciparum* until a response to treatment defined as a "decrease in daily parasitemias" is documented. At this time, severe complications are unlikely to occur.

Partially immune patients with uncomplicated *P falciparum* infection and nonimmune persons infected with *P vivax, P ovale,* or *P malariae* can be treated as outpatients if there is reliable follow-up. For children, hydration and treatment of hypoglycemia are of utmost importance. Anemia, seizures, pulmonary edema, and renal failure require conventional management. Corticosteroids are contraindicated for cerebral malaria. In face of severe malaria, exchange transfusion can be a life-saving procedure, particularly in nonimmune persons with parasitemia greater than 15%.

Chloroquine is the drug of choice for treatment of chloroquine-sensitive plasmodia (Table 38–6). In patients unable to take oral medication, treatment can be initiated with chloroquine or quinidine administered as a carefully controlled intravenous infusion (for potential arrhythmogenic effect) and later converted to oral chloroquine. For chloroquine-resistant *P falciparum,* oral therapy includes quinine in association with pyrimethamine-sulfadoxine, tetracycline, or clindamycin, or mefloquine or halofantrine. If the patient failed chemoprophylaxis, the same drug

Table 37–6. Treatment of malaria.

Drug	Dosage
Chloroquine-susceptible plasmodia	
Chloroquine	10 mg base/kg PO initially, followed by 5 mg base/kg 6 h later and on day 2 and 3 (total dose of 25 mg base/kg over 3 days)
Chloroquine-resistant *P falciparum*	
Oral regimens	
Quinine sulfate	25 mg/kg/d up to 2g/kg/d in 3 doses for 3–7 d
plus	
pyrimethamine-sulfadoxine	0.25 tablet on the last day of quinine (age < 1 y) 0.5 tablet (age 1–3 y) 1 tablet (age 4–8 y) 2 tablets (age 9–14 y) 3 tablets (age >15 y)
or	
tetracycline	20 mg/kg/d up to 1 g/d in 4 doses for 7 d
or	
clindamycin	20–40 mg/kg/d up to 2700 mg in 3 doses for 3 d
Mefloquine	25 mg/kg up to 1250 mg in a single dose
Halofantrine	8 mg/kg up to 500 mg/6 h for 3 doses; repeat in 1 wk
Parenteral regimens	
Quinidine gluconate	10 mg/kg up to 600 mg loading dose in normal saline slowly over 1–2 h followed by continuous infusion of 0.02 mg/kg/min until oral therapy can be started
Chloroquine-resistant *P vivax*	
Mefloquine	25 mg/kg up to 1250 mg in a single dose
Halofantrine	8 mg/kg up to 500 mg/6 h for 3 doses; repeat in 1 wk
Prevention of Relapse With *P vivax* or *P orale*	
Primaquine phosphate[1]	0.3 mg base/kg/d up to 15.3 mg base for 14 d

[1]Screen for G6PD deficiency.

should not be used for treatment. Halofantrine is not recommended for persons who failed mefloquine chemoprophylaxis because of cross-resistance. Patients infected with chloroquine-resistant *P falciparum* who cannot take oral medication should be treated with intravenous quinidine. This is two or three times more active than quinine, and serum levels can be measured in most North American hospitals. Chloroquine-resistant *P vivax,* which has been identified in Papua, New Guinea, Iran, Java, Indonesia, and Columbia, can be treated with mefloquine or halofantrine. Persons with *P vivax* or *P ovale* infection living in nonendemic areas are usually treated with primaquine to prevent late relapse.

Baird KJ et al: Treatment of chloroquine-resistant *Plasmodium vivax* with chloroquine and primaquine and halofantrine. J Infect Dis 1995;171:1678.

Marsh K et al: Indicators of life-threatening malaria in African children. N Engl J Med 1995;332:1399.

AMEBIASIS

Essentials of Diagnosis

- Acute dysentery: diarrhea with blood and mucus, pain, tenderness.
- Chronic nondysenteric diarrhea.
- Hepatic abscess.
- Lung abscess.
- Amebas or cysts in stools or abscesses; serologic evidence of amebic infection.

General Considerations

Amebiasis, because of *Entamoeba histolytica,* is a common problem in endemic areas with poor hygiene. An estimated 10% of the world's population is infected with *E histolytica* or *E dispar* amebiasis. Amebiasis should be suspected in patients with a history of travel to or in contact with individuals from endemic areas who may be asymptomatic carriers. In the United States, amebiasis may be seen in homes for the retarded or handicapped, where poor hygiene fosters the spread of enteric pathogens. *E histolytica* has been found in the stools of as many as 30% of gay men, in whom nonpathogenic variants of the organism may predominate. Individuals of any age may be infected. Transmission is usually fecal-oral, often from asymptomatic carriers who pass cysts. Trophozoites are killed by stomach acid and are not infectious. Infection with *E dispar,* which is morphologically identical with *E histolytica* but only results in asymptomatic carriage, is 10 times more common than infection with *E histolytica.* Furthermore, only 10% of *E histolytica* infections result in gastrointestinal or other symptoms. However, an estimated 100,000 people die of amebic infection each year.

Clinical Findings

Intestinal amebiasis can present as asymptomatic cyst passage, acute amebic proctocolitis, chronic nondysenteric colitis, or ameboma. Since all *E dispar* infections and up to 90% of *E histolytica* infections are asymptomatic, carriage is the most common presentation of the disease. Patients with acute amebic colitis present with a 1- to 2-week history of watery stools containing blood and mucus and abdominal pain and tenesmus. A minority of patients are febrile or dehydrated. Abdominal examination may reveal pain over the lower abdominal quadrants. Fulminant colitis is an unusual complication of amebic dysentery and is associated with a grave prognosis (more than 50% mortality). Patients with fulminant colitis present with severe bloody diarrhea, fever and diffuse abdominal pain. Children under the age of 2 years appear to be at increased risk for this condition. Chronic amebic colitis is clinically indistinguishable from idiopathic inflammatory bowel disease; patients present with recurrent episodes of bloody diarrhea over a period of years. Ameboma is a localized amebic infection, usually located in the cecum or ascending colon, which presents as a painful abdominal mass.

The most common complication of intestinal amebiasis is intestinal perforation and peritonitis, which can occur in association with both acute dysenteric or fulminant colitis. Perianal ulcers is a less common complication. The ulcers typically present as painful, punched-out lesions, which usually respond to medical therapy. Infrequently, colonic strictures may develop following colitis.

Extraintestinal amebiasis includes liver and lung, abscess and, less rarely, cerebral or genitourinary disease. Most patients with amebic liver abscess, the most common form of extraintestinal amebiasis, present with fever and right upper quadrant tenderness of less than 10 days' duration. The pain may be dull, pleuritic, and referred to the right shoulder. Physical examination reveals liver enlargement in less than 50% of affected patients. A subset of patients has a subacute presentation of 2 weeks to 6 months' duration. In these patients, hepatomegaly, anemia and weight loss are common findings, and fever is less common. Jaundice and diarrhea are rarely associated with an amebic liver abscess.

The most common complication of amebic liver abscess is pleuropulmonary amebiasis due to rupture of a right liver lobe, hepatic abscess with erosion of the diaphragm or invasion of the pleural space, and pulmonary parenchyma. In addition, lung abscesses may occur from hematogenous spread. Cough, dyspnea, and pleuritic pain can also be caused by the serous pleural effusions and atelectasis that frequently accompany amebic liver abscesses. Rupture of hepatic abscesses can lead to peritonitis and more rarely to pericarditis. Cerebral amebiasis is an infrequent manifestation. Genitourinary amebiasis is also uncommon and results from rupture of a liver abscess, hematogenous dissemination, or lymphatic spread.

Diagnosis

Intestinal amebiasis is diagnosed by observing the parasite on stool examination or mucosal biopsy. The differential diagnosis of acute amebic colitis includes bacillary diarrhea, *Balantidium coli,* and *B fragilis* infection. Chronic amebic colitis has to be distinguished from inflammatory bowel disease, *Cyclospora,* and *B coli.* Occult blood is present in virtually all cases of amebic colitis and can be used as an inexpensive screening test. Fecal leukocytes area noncontributory to the diagnosis of amebic dysentery. The presence of hematophagous trophozoites in feces indicates pathogenic *E histolytica* infection.

Ideally, a wet mount of the stool should be examined no longer than 20 minutes after collection to detect motile trophozoites. Otherwise, specimens should be fixed with polyvinyl alcohol or refrigerated to avoid disintegration of the trophozoites. Three separate stool examinations have 90% sensitivity for the diagnosis of amebic dysentery. However, infection of the ascending colon, amebomas, and extraintestinal infections frequently yield negative stool examination results. An antigen detection test, currently under clinical evaluation, may be sensitive and more specific, because it detects *E histolytica*-specific antigens that do not cross-react with *E dispar*. Colonoscopy and biopsy are most helpful in stool-negative amebic colitis. Barium studies are contraindicated for patients with acute amebic colitis because of the risk of perforation.

Treatment and Prevention

Treatment of amebic infection is complex because different agents are required for eradicating the parasite from the bowel or from tissue (Table 38–7). Whether treatment of asymptomatic cyst passers is indicated at all is a controversial issue. Currently, the prevalent opinion among experts is that asymptomatic infection with *E histolytica,* as evidenced by the presence of amebic cysts in the stool and a positive serologic test, should be treated in nonendemic areas. If serology is negative, the cysts are more likely to represent infection with the nonpathogenic *E dispar*, which does not require treatment. Among the drugs active against intraluminal cysts, iodoquinol is the most readily available, but also the most toxic (causes prominent gastrointestinal side effects, interferes with thyroid function, causes dose-dependent optic neuritis). Paromomycin, a nonabsorbable aminoglycoside, can be safely used during pregnancy and has only mild intestinal side effects including flatulence and increased number of stools. Dilox-

anide furoate is relatively nontoxic and widely used outside of the United States. The treatment of invasive amebiasis requires metronidazole. Metronidazole has a disulfiram-like effect and should be avoided in patients receiving ethanol-containing medications. Tinidazole, a more potent nitro-imidazole against amebic infection can be used for shorter treatment courses and is well tolerated in children.

In patients who cannot tolerate metronidazole or tinidazole, erythromycin and tetracycline are active against intestinal trophozoites, but are inactive against trophozoites in liver abscesses. Conversely, chloroquine is active only against hepatic amebiasis. Treatment of invasive amebiasis should always be followed with an intraluminal cysticidal agent, even if the stool examination is negative. Patients with large, thin-walled hepatic abscesses may need therapeutic aspiration to avoid abscess rupture. Patients with amebiases should be placed under enteric precautions. Travelers to endemic areas need to follow the same precautions that apply to prevention of enteric infections—drink bottled or boiled water, eat cooked vegetable and fruits, and eat only uncontrolled fruits with peels.

The presence of antibodies against *E histolytica* in the serum can differentiate *E histolytica* from *E dispar* infections. The antibody response follows both intestinal and extraintestinal invasive amebiasis. The presence of antibodies 7–10 days after initiation of symptoms constitutes strong evidence of invasive amebiasis. ELISA and indirect hemagglutination assays are positive in 85% to 95% of invasive *E histolytica* colitis or amebic abscess. However, these antibodies persist for years, and a positive result does not distinguish between acute or past infection. Asymptomatic cyst passers with negative serology are more likely to be infected with *E dispar*.

Noninvasive imaging studies have greatly improved the diagnosis of hepatic abscesses. Ultrasonographic examination is preferred because it is less expensive and rapid, and it distinguishes parenchymal from biliary tract disease. Computed tomography (CT) and magnetic resonance imaging (MRI) are slightly more sensitive and permit better resolution of the lesion. Because an amebic abscess may take up to 2 years to completely resolve on CT scans, imaging techniques are not recommended for therapeutic evaluation. Although the epidemiologic information, serology, and therapeutic response all can be used to support an amebic etiology, fine-needle aspiration under ultrasonography or CT guidance provides specimens for the definitive diagnosis.

Table 38–7. Treatment of amebiasis.

Type of Infection	Drug of Choice	Dosage
Asymptomatic	Iodoquinol	30–40 mg/kg/d up to 2 g/d in 3 doses for 20 d
	or	
	Paromomycin	25–35 mg/kg/d in 3 doses for 7 d
	or	
	Diloxanide furoate[1]	20 mg/kg/d up to 1.5 g/d in 3 doses for 10 d
Intestinal disease and hepatic abscess[2]	Metronidazole	35–50 mg/kg/d up to 2.25 g/d in 3 doses for 10 d
	or	
	Tinidazole[3]	50 or 60 mg/kg up to 2 g/d for 3 d

[1]Drug available from the CDC Drug Service, telephone: (404) 639-3670.
[2]Treatment should be followed by iodoquinol or other intraluminal cysticidal agent.
[3]Not marketed in the United States; higher dosage is for hepatic abscess.

Bruckner DA: Amebiasis. Clin Microbiol Rev 1992;5:356.
Merritt RJ et al: Spectrum of amebiasis in children. Am J Dis Child 1982;136:785.
Ravdin JI: Amebiasis. Clin Infect Dis 1995;20:1453.
Reed SL: Amebiasis: An update. Clin Infect Dis 1992; 14:385.

Rustgi AK, Richter JM: Pyogenic and amebic liver abscess. Med Clin North Am 1989;73:847.

FREE-LIVING AMEBAE

Essentials of Diagnosis

- Acute meningoencephalitis: fever, headache, meningismus, acute mental deterioration.
- Swimming in warm, fresh water in endemic areas.
- Chronic granulomatous encephalitis: insidious onset of focal neurologic deficits.
- Keratitis: pain, photophobia, conjunctivitis, blurred vision.

Clinical Findings

Infection with free-living amebae is uncommon. *Naegleria* spp, *Acanthamoeba* spp, and *Leptomixida* ameba have been associated with human disease.

Acute meningoencephalitis, caused by *N fowleri,* has been observed, especially in children and young adults. Patients present with abrupt fever, headache, nausea and vomiting, meningismus, and decreased mental status usually 3–5 (but not always) after swimming in fresh, warm-water lakes. Central nervous system invasion occurs after nasal inoculation of *N fowleri.* This disease is rapidly progressive, and death ensues within 1 week of onset of symptoms. Chronic granulomatous encephalitis, caused by *Acanthamoeba* or *Leptomixida* ameba, occurs most commonly in patient who are immunocompromised from corticosteroids, chemotherapy, or AIDS. There is no association with fresh water swimming. This disease has an insidious onset of focal neurologic deficits, and approximately 50% of patients present with headache. Skin, sinus, or lung infections with *Acanthamoeba* precede many of the central nervous system infections and may still be present at the onset of neurologic disease. The granulomatous encephalitis progresses to fatal outcome over a period of weeks to months (average 6 weeks). *Acanthamoeba* keratitis is a corneal infection associated with minor trauma or use of soft contact lenses in otherwise healthy persons. Frequently misdiagnosed as herpes simplex or bacterial keratitis, *Acanthamoeba* keratitis has a characteristic dendriform epithelial pattern, which suggests the diagnosis.

Diagnosis

Amebic encephalitis should be included in the differential diagnosis of acute meningoencehalitis in children with a history of recent fresh water swimming. The cerebrospinal fluid is usually hemorrhagic, with leukocyte counts that may be normal early in the disease but later range from 400 to 2600 with neutrophil predominance, low to normal glucose, and elevated protein. The etiologic diagnosis relies on finding trophozoites on a wet mount of the cerebrospinal fluid. Granulomatous encephalitis is diagnosed by brain biopsy of CT-identified nonenhancing lucent areas. The cerebrospinal fluid of these patients is usually nondiagnostic with intermediate blood cell counts, elevated protein, and decreased glucose. *Acanthamoeba* or *Leptomysida* amebae have not been found in the cerebrospinal fluid; however, they can be visualized in biopsies or grown from brain or other infected tissues. *Acanthamoeba* keratitis is diagnosed by finding the trophozoites in corneal scrapings or isolating the parasite from corneal specimens or contact lens cultures.

Treatment & Prevention

The few patients who have survived acute amebic meningoencephalitis received high-dose intravenous and intrathecal amphotericin B, accompanied by miconazole, rifampin, and sulfisoxazole in some cases. Little is known about the therapeutic response of granulomatous encephalitis because most cases have been diagnosed at autopsy. In vitro, *Acanthamoeba* is most sensitive to diamidine derivatives (pentamidine) followed by the azoles (miconazole, ketoconazole), paromomycin, neomycin, 5-fluorocytosine, and amphotericin B. *Leptomyxida* amebae are particularly sensitive to ketoconazole. Whenever an isolate is obtained, it is advisable to test for antimicrobial susceptibility. *Acanthamoeba* keratitis responds well to surgical debridement followed by 3–4 weeks of topical 1% miconazole, 0.1% propamidine isethionate, and Neosporin.

Because primary amebic meningitis occurs infrequently, active surveillance of lakes for *N fowleri* is not warranted. However, in the presence of a documented case, it is advisable to close the implicated lake to swimming. *Acanthamoeba* keratitis can be prevented by heat disinfection of contact lenses, by storage of lenses in sterile solutions, and by not wearing lenses when swimming in fresh water.

Sotelo-Avila C: *Naegleria* and *Acanthamoeba.* Free living amebas pathogenic for man. Perspect Pediatr Pathol 1987;10:51.

Visversvara GS et al: *Leptomyxida* ameba, a new agent of amebic meningoencephalitis in humans and animals. J Clin Microbiol 1990;28:2750.

BALANTIDIUM COLI

Balantidium coli rarely produces human disease. Patients with achlorhydria, poor nutritional status, or poor hygiene are at increased risk of developing invasion of the colonic mucosa with this organism. Patients typically present with chronic intermittent watery diarrhea or with acute colitis with blood and mucus. Complications include intestinal perforation and more rarely extraintestinal spread of *B coli* to mesenteric lymph nodes, liver, or pleura. The diagnosis is made by the finding of large, motile trophozoites in fresh stool or in scrapings taken from the periphery of ulcers on endoscopic examination. Cysts in stool is a less common finding. Tetracycline is the treatment of choice: 40 mg/kg/d up to g/d in four divided doses for 10 days. For children less than 8 years of age, iodoquinol for 20 days of metronidazole for 10 days are acceptable alternatives.

Ladas SD et al: Invasive balantidiasis presented as chronic colitis and lung involvement. Dig Dis Sci 1989;34:1621.

BLASTOCYSTIS HOMINIS

The pathogenic role of *Blastocystis hominis* in human disease has been debated for many years. The most recent information indicates that *B hominis* does not cause diarrhea and does not require specific treatment. In vitro, metronidazole, emetine, furazolidone, and TMP-SMX inhibit growth of this parasite.

Markell EK: Is there any reason to continue treating blastocystis infections? Clin Infect Dis 1995;21:104.

DIENTAMOEBA FRAGILIS

The pathogenicity of Dientamoeba fragilis is controversial. Purported symptoms include abdominal pain, diarrhea, nausea, anorexia, vomiting, and fatigue. Iodoquinol for 20 days has been used with success. Paromomycin or tetracycline for 10 days each are alternative drugs.

Spencer MJ, Garcia LS, Chapin MR: *Dientamoeba fragilis:* An intestinal pathogen in children? Am J Dis Child 1979;133:390.
Turner JA: Giardiasis and infections with *Dientamoeba fragilis.* Pediatr Clin North Am 1985;32:865.

GIARDIASIS

Essentials of Diagnosis

- Chronic, relapsing diarrhea, flatulence, bloating, anorexia, poor weight gain.
- Night-time vomiting.
- Absence of fever and hematochezia.
- Detection of trophozoites, cysts on *Giardia* antigens in stool.

General Considerations

Giardiasis is the most common intestinal protozoal infection in children in the United States and in most areas around the world. It is caused by *Giardia lamblia.* Endemic worldwide, it is classically associated with drinking contaminated water, either in rural areas or in areas with faulty purification systems. Acquisition in swimming pools has occurred. Because even ostensibly clean urban water supplies can be in-

termittently contaminated, giardiasis can be acquired by almost any traveler. Fecal-oral contamination allows person-to-person spread. Recently, day care centers have been recognized as major sources, with an incidence of up to 50% reported in some centers. Asymptomatic infections occur in 25% of infected persons and facilitate spread to household contacts. Food-borne outbreaks have also occurred. Although infection is rare in neonates, it may occur at any age.

Clinical Findings

A. Signs and Symptoms: Infection *Giardia* includes asymptomatic cyst passage, acute self-limited diarrhea, and a chronic syndrome of diarrhea, malabsorption, and weight loss. Acute diarrhea occurs 1–2 weeks after infection and is characterized by abrupt onset of diarrhea with greasy, malodorous stools; malaise; flatulence; bloating; and nausea. Fever and vomiting occur in a minority of patients. Vomiting often occurs at night during sleep. Urticaria, reactive arthritis, biliary tract disease, gastric infection, and constipation have occasionally been reported. The disease has a protracted course (more than 1 week) and frequently leads to weight loss. Patients who develop chronic diarrhea complain of profound malaise, lassitude, headache, and diffuse abdominal pain in association with bouts of diarrhea—most typically foul-smelling, greasy stools—intercalated with periods of constipation or normal bowel habits. This syndrome can persist for months until specific therapy is administered or until it spontaneously subsides. Chronic diarrhea frequently leads to malabsorption, steatorrhea, vitamin A and B_{12} deficiencies, and disaccharidase depletion. Lactose intolerance, which develops in 20–40% of patients, can persist for several weeks after treatment and needs to be differentiated from relapsing giardiasis or reinfection.

B. Laboratory Findings: The diagnosis of giardiasis relies on finding the parasite in stool or duodenal aspirates or detecting *Giardia* antigen in feces. For ova and parasite examination, a fresh stool provides the best examination results. Liquid stools have the highest yield of trophozoites. These are more readily found on wet mounts of fresh specimens. With semiformed stools, the examiner should look for cysts in fresh or fixed specimens, preferably using a concentration technique. When these techniques are carefully applied, one ova and parasite examination has a 50–70% sensitivity; three examinations increase the sensitivity to 90%. Antigen assays detect *Giardia* by means of immunofluorescence or enzyme-linked immunoassay. They are comparable in cost to a stool ova and parasite examination and are 85–90% sensitive and 95–100% specific. The antigen detection assays are limited to ruling in or ruling out giardiasis and are best applied for mass screening or testing patients after completion of therapy. With a careful stool ova and parasite examination or with the use of a new antigen test, direct sampling of the duodenal contents should be restricted to particularly difficult cases. Three methods are currently available: the string test (Entero-Test), duodenal aspiration, and duodenal biopsy.

Treatment & Prevention

The drug of choice for giardiasis in metronidazole. When given at 5 mg/kg (up to 250 mg) three times daily for 5 days, metronidazole has an efficacy of 80–95%. The drug is well tolerated in children. It has a disulfiram-like effect and should be avoided in patients receiving ethanol-containing medications.

Furazolidone is frequently used in children as an alternative drug because it is available in suspension. Administered at 1.5 mg/kg (up to 100 mg) four times daily for 7–10 days, it has only an 80% efficacy rate. Furazolidone may cause gastrointestinal side effects, turn urine red, and cause mild hemolysis in patients with G6PD deficiency. For pregnant women with giardiasis, paromomycin, a nonabsorbable aminoglycoside, constitutes a safe but only marginally effective alternative (efficacy 60–70%). For patients who fail one drug or suffer relapse, a second course with the same drug or switching to another drug is equally effective.

The prevention of giardiasis requires proper treatment of the water supply and interruption of person-to-person transmission. For travelers to developing countries or in wilderness areas, it is recommended to halogenate or boil (for over 10 minutes) the drinking water and avoid uncooked foods that might have been washed with contaminated water. Sexual transmission is prevented by avoiding oral-anal and oral-genital sex. Interrupting fecal-oral transmission requires strict hand-washing. However, outbreaks of diarrhea in day care centers might be particularly difficult to eradicate, and reinforcing hand-washing and treating both symptomatic and asymptomatic carriers may be necessary.

Addiss DG, Juranek DD, Spencer HC: Treatment of children with asymptomatic and non-diarrheal Giardia infection. Pediatr Infect Dis J 1991;10:843.

Bobb RR: Giardiasis: Taming the pervasive parasite infection. Postgrad Med 1995;98:155.

Thompson SC: *Giardia lamblia* in children and the child care setting: A review of the literature. J Paediatr Child Health 1994;30:202.

Wolf MS: Giardiasis. Clin Microbiol Rev 1992;5:93.

CRYPTOSPORIDIOSIS

Cryptosporidium parvum is an intracellular protozoan that has gained importance because it causes severe diarrhea in patients with AIDS and in other immunodeficient persons. The parasite is ubiquitous and infects and reproduces itself in the epithelial cell lining of the digestive and respiratory tracts of humans and most other vertebrate animals. Humans acquire the infection from contaminated water supplies or from close contact with infected humans or animals. Immunocompetent persons infected with *Cryptosporidium* usually develop self-limited diarrhea (2–26 days' duration) with or without abdominal cramps. Diarrhea is intermittent and scant, or continuous, watery, and voluminous. Low-grade fever, nausea, vomiting loss of appetite, and malaise may accompany the diarrhea. Other clinical manifestations associated with cryptosporidiosis include cholecystitis, pancreatitis, hepatitis, and respiratory symptoms. Young children (younger than 2 years of age) appear more susceptible to infection. Immunocompromised patients (either cellular or humoral deficiency) tend to develop prolonged disease, which usually subsides only after correcting the immunodeficiency. There are no characteristic laboratory features of cryptosporidiosis other than identification of the microorganism in feces or on biopsy. Examination of multiple stool specimens by at least two techniques (concentration and staining) may be necessary.

There is currently no reliable treatment for cryptosporidiosis. Immunocompetent patients and those with temporary immunodeficiencies do not require specific therapy but may benefit from antidiarrheal agents and hydration. Immunocompromised patients usually require more intense supportive care with parenteral nutrition in addition to hydration and nonspecific antidiarrheal agents. Octreotide acetate, a synthetic analogue of somatostatin that inhibits secretory diarrhea has been associated with symptomatic improvement, but not with parasitologic cure. Among the antiparasitic agents, paromomycin, azithromycin, nitazoxanide (a new antiparasitic drug available from Unimed on compassionate use), and hyperimmune bovine colostrum have been successfully used in some patients. In patients with AIDS, institution of effective antiretroviral therapy seems to have a positive impact on the outcome of cryptosporidiosis. Prevention of *Cryptosporidium* infection is limited by oocyst resistance to some of the standard water purification procedures and to common disinfectants. Enteric precautions are recommended for infected persons. Boiled or bottled drinking water may be considered for those at high risk for developing chronic infection (eg, patients with AIDS whose CD4 cells are less than 200).

Current WL, Garcia LS: Cryptosporidiosis. Clin Microbiol Rev 1991;4:325.

Fraser D: Epidemiology of xigiardia lamblia and *Cryptosporidium* infection in childhood. Isr J Med Sci 1994;30:356.

TRICHOMONIASIS

Trichomonas vaginalis resides in the genitourinary tract as an extracellular protozoan. It can damage the underlying epithelial cells through direct contact leading to ulcerations. Because it is sexually transmitted, *Trichomonas* is commonly associated with other venereal diseases. Thus, patients found to harbor *Trichomonas* should be screened for syphilis (in areas of high endemicity), *N gonorrhoeae, C trachomatis,* hepatitis B virus, and HIV, which may be clinically silent. Newborn females can acquire trichomoniasis at birth. Thereafter, trichomoniasis is rare until menarche. Although finding *Trichomonas* in a prepubertal child suggests sexual abuse, it cannot be used as definite proof because nonsexual transmission of the protozoan has been documented. The clinical features of *T vaginitis* and its management are discussed in Chapter 39.

Graves A, Gardner WA Jr: Pathogenicity of *Trichomonas vaginalis.* Clin Obstet Gynecol 1003;36:145.
Lossick JG: Treatment of sexually transmitted vaginosis/vaginitis. Rev Infect Dis 1990;12:S665.

TOXOPLASMOSIS

Essentials of Diagnosis

- Congenital toxoplasmosis: chorioretinitis, icterus, hepatosplenomegaly, abnormal blood count, microcephaly, hydrocephaly, convulsions, psychomotor retardation, abnormal cerebrospinal fluid, intracranial calcifications, microphthalmia, strabismus.
- Acquired toxoplasmosis in an immunocompetent host: lymphadenopathy sometimes accompanied by fever, hepatosplenomegaly, rash, and myalgias.
- Acquired or reactivated toxoplasmosis in an immunocompromised host: encephalitis, chorioretinitis, myocarditis, and pneumonitis.
- Ocular toxoplasmosis: chorioretinitis.
- Serologic evidence of infection with *Toxoplasma gondii* or demonstration of the agent in tissue or body fluids.

General Considerations

Toxoplasma gondii is a worldwide parasite of animals and birds. Felines, the definitive hosts, excrete oocysts in their feces. Ingested mature oocysts or tissue cysts lead to tachyzoite invasion of the intestinal cells. Intracellular replication of the tachyzoites determine cell lysis and spread of the infection to adjacent cells or to other tissues via the bloodstream. Extracellular tachyzoites are lysed by complement fixing antibodies and interferon-γ-activated macrophages. In chronic infection, *T gondii* appears as bradyzoite-containing tissue cysts that do not trigger an inflammatory reaction. Under special circumstances such as immunodepression, tachyzoites are released from the cysts and begin a new cycle of infection. Interferon-γ and other cytokines seem to be important in keeping the chronic infection quiescent.

The two major routes of *Toxoplasma* transmission to humans are oral (including pica) and congenital. Oocysts survive for up to 18 months in moist soil. Oral infection occurs after ingestion of cyst-containing undercooked meat or other food products. Oocyst survival is limited in dry, very cold, or very hot conditions, and at high altitude, which probably accounts for the lower incidence of toxoplasmosis in these climatic regions. In the United States, less than 1% of cattle and 25% of sheep and pigs are infected with toxoplasmosis. In humans of different geographic areas, seropositivity increases with age from 0% to 10% in children under 10 years of age to 3–70% in adults. Congenital transmission occurs during acute infection of the pregnant woman; this occurs in 0.2–1% of all pregnancies in the United States. Rarely, fetal infection has been documented in immunocompromised mothers with chronic toxoplasmosis. The rate of vertical transmission in untreated patients increases from 10% in the first trimester to 60% in the third. Symptomatic disease is more likely to follow infection in early gestation (20–25%) compared with late gestation (less than 11%). Treatment during pregnancy decreases transmission by about 60%.

Clinical Findings

A. Congenital Toxoplasmosis: Congenital toxoplasmosis has a wide variety of manifestations, including miscarriage, prematurity, and stillbirth. Most frequently, symptomatic infants present with a combination of fever, microcephaly or hydrocephaly, hepatosplenomegaly, jaundice, chorioretinitis, convulsions, abnormal cerebrospinal fluid (xanthochromia and mononuclear pleocytosis), and cerebral calcification. Other findings include strabismus, palsy, maculopapular rash, pneumonitis, myocarditis thrombocytopenia, lymphocytosis, monocytosis, and a erythroblastosis-like syndrome. The overall mortality rate for congenital toxoplasmosis is approximately 10% and is higher in neonates who are symptomatic at birth. Sequelae such as chorioretinitis, mental retardation, seizures, and palsies are common; these may also develop in children who are symptomatic at birth. Sequelae such as chorioretinitis, mental retardation, seizures, and palsies are common; these may also develop in children who are asymptomatic in the neonatal period. Congenital toxoplasmosis must be differentiated from cytomegalovirus (CMV) infection, rubella, herpes simplex, syphilis, Lyme disease, listeriosis, erythroblastosis, and the encephalopathies that accompany degenerative diseases.

B. Acquired *Toxoplasma* Infection in the Immunocompetent Host: Only 10–20% of acute *Toxoplasma* infections produce symptoms, and patients usually present with lymphadenopathy without fever. The nodes are discrete, may or may not be tender, and do no suppurate. Cervical lymph nodes are most frequently involved, but any nodes may be enlarged. Less common findings include fever, malaise, myalgias, fatigue, hepatosplenomegaly, atypical lymphocytes (usually less than 10%), and liver enzyme elevations. Unilateral chorioretinitis may occur. The disease is self-limited, although lymph node enlargement may persist or may wax and wane for a few months to 1 year or even longer. Rarely, an apparently healthy child may develop severe disseminated disease with myocarditis, pneumonitis, or encephalitis.

Toxoplasmic lymphadenitis must be distinguished from other causes of infectious mononucleosis-like syndromes (less than 1% are caused by toxoplasma), particularly Epstein-Barr virus and CMV, cat-scratch disease, tuberculosis, tularemia, and lymphoma.

C. Acute Toxoplasmosis in the Immunodeficient Host: Immunocompromised hosts tend to develop severe disease following acute infection or reactivation. Children born to HIV- and *Toxoplasma*-infected mothers may acquire both pathogens in utero. Most of these patients who acquire toxoplasmosis after birth frequently develop encephalitis, chorioretinitis, and pneumonia. Patients with lymphoma, leukemia, or transplantation are at high risk for acquiring *Toxoplasma* encephalitis, myocarditis, and pneumonitis.

D. Ocular Toxoplasmosis: In active congenital toxoplasmosis, chorioretinitis is usually bilateral and shows acute inflammatory foci on funduscopic examination. This generally resolves, leaving depigmented scars of the retina surrounded by areas of hyperpigmentation. Chorioretinitis may reactivate in a single eye later in life. The appearance of the ocular lesion is not specific and mimics other granulomatous ocular diseases.

Diagnosis

Active infection is diagnosed by isolation of *T gondii* from blood or body fluids; demonstration of tachyzoites in histologic sections or cytology preparations; demonstration of cysts in placenta or fetal tissues; characteristic lymph node histology; and demonstration of characteristic serologic test results. Serologic tests are most commonly used. IgG antibodies are reliably measured by the Sabin-Feldman dye test, immunofluorescence, ELISA, and particle agglutination. With use of these tests, IgG anti-*Toxoplasma* is first detected 1–2 weeks after infection, peaks at 1–2 months, and, after detecting at variable speeds, persists for life.

IgM antibodies are reliably measured by ELISA or particle agglutination. These antibodies appear earlier and decline faster than IgG antibodies. Absence of both serum IgG and IgM virtually rules out the diagnosis of toxoplasmosis. Acute toxoplasmosis in an immunocompetent host is best documented by analyzing IgG and IgM in paired blood samples drawn 3 weeks apart. Since high antibody titers (IgM or IgG)

can persist for several months after acute infection, a single high-titer determination is nonspecific. However, seroconversion or a fourfold increase in titer confirms the diagnosis.

In the immunocompromised host, serology is not sensitive, and active infection should be documented by polymerase chain reaction (PCR) or local antibody production in body fluids or by demonstration of tachyzoites. Patients with *Toxoplasma* chorioretinitis typically have low levels of specific IgG and absent IgM. The diagnosis can be confirmed by demonstrating high antibody titers in aqueous fluid. Congenital neonatal infection is documented by detecting anti-*Toxoplasma* IgM or IgA in the blood. Prenatal diagnosis of congenital infection requires a combination of ultrasonography (to detect ventricle enlargement), PCR in amniotic fluid, and serology in cord blood. Recent studies indicate that sampling the cord blood might be unnecessary by virtue of the high PCR sensitivity.

Differential Diagnosis

Congenital infection may resemble that due to cytomegalovirus, syphilis, rubella, or other agents. Acquired infection mimics a number of viral or lymphoproliferative diseases.

Prevention

Pregnant women and immunocompromised patients should wash hands thoroughly after handling raw meat. Cook meat to 66 °C or greater, wash fruits and vegetables before consumption, and avoid contact with cat feces. Serologic screening of pregnant women is warranted in areas of high prevalence. A first test should be performed by 10–12 weeks of pregnancy. Seronegative patients should be retested at 20–22 weeks and near term. Seroconverters require specific therapy.

Treatment

Although therapy does not alter established central nervous system damage, it does markedly decrease late sequelae. A year of treatment is recommended for all congenitally infected infants; symptomatic patients receive 6 months of pyrimethamine and sulfadiazine, followed by alternating spiramycin and pyrimethamine-sulfadiazine monthly for the next 6 months. Subclinical infection is treated with pyrimethamine and sulfadiazine for 6 weeks, followed by alternating spiramycin for 6 weeks with pyrimethamine-sulfadiazine for 4 weeks.

Pyrimethamine is given orally at a dosage of 1 mg/kg/d (maximum, 25 mg); gastrointestinal upset, leukopenia, thrombocytopenia, and, rarely, agranulocytosis are side effects. Frequent blood counts should be performed and the drug stopped if the counts fall very low. Leucovorin calcium (folinic acid), 5 mg intramuscularly every 3 days, decreases the myelotoxicity. The dosage of sulfadiazine or trisulfapyrimidines is 40-45 mg/kg twice a day orally (maximum, 8 g/d). Clindamycin can be substituted for sulfadiazine in patients who cannot tolerate sulfonamides. Spiramycin and trimethoprim-sulfamethoxazole are less active.

In acquired infection, usually self-limited, the potentially toxic therapy should be prescribed with discretion, usually only if the illness is complicated.

In chorioretinitis, antimicrobial therapy is used for 4 weeks. A course of corticosteroids (prednisone, 1.5 mg/kg up to 75 mg) is recommended when lesions involve the macula or the optic nerve. Lesions tend to improve after 10 days of therapy.

In pregnancy, spiramycin should be started immediately. Pyrimethamine plus sulfadiazine alternating every 3 weeks with spiramycin are used when fetal infection has been documented, because, although toxic, only the first two drugs ameliorate severity of the disease in the infected fetus.

Freij BG, Sever HL: Toxoplasmosis. Pediatr Rev 1991; 12:227.

McAuley J et al: Early and longitudinal evaluations of treated infants and children and untreated historical patients with congenital toxoplasmosis: the Chicago collaborative treatment trial. Clin Infect Dis 1994;18:38.

McCabe RE et al: Clinical spectrum in 107 cases of toxoplasmic lymphadenopathy. Rev Infect Dis 1987;9:754.

Wong SY, Remington JS: Toxoplasmosis in pregnancy. Clin Infect Dis 1994;18:853.

METAZOAL INFECTIONS

NEMATODE INFECTIONS

1. ENTEROBIASIS
(Pinworms)

Essentials of Diagnosis
- Nocturnal anal pruritus.
- Worms in the stool or eggs on perianal skin.

General Considerations
This worldwide infection is caused by *Enterobius vermicularis.* The adult worms are about 5–10 mm long and live in the colon; females deposit eggs on the perianal area, primarily at night, causing intense pruritus. Scratching contaminates the fingers and allows transmission back to the host (autoinfection) or to contacts.

Clinical Findings
A. Symptoms and Signs: Although blamed for a myriad of symptoms, pinworms are definitely associated only with localized pruritus. Adult worms may migrate within the colon or up the urethra or vagina in girls. They can be found within the bowel wall, in the lumen of the appendix (usually an incidental finding by the pathologist), in the bladder, and even the peritoneal cavity of girls. The granulomatous reaction that may be present around these ectopic worms is usually asymptomatic. Worm eradication may correspond with the cure of recurrent urinary tract infections in some young girls.

B. Laboratory Findings: The usual diagnostic test consists of pressing a piece of transparent tape on the child's anus in the morning prior to bathing, then placing it on a drop of xylene on a slide. Microscopic examination under low power usually demonstrates the ova. Occasionally, eggs or adult worms are seen in fecal specimens. Parents may also notice adult worms.

Differential Diagnosis
Nonspecific irritation or vaginitis, streptococcal perianal cellulitis (usually painful), and vaginal or urinary bacterial infections may at times resemble pinworm infection, although the symptoms of pinworms are often so suggestive that a therapeutic trial is justified without a confirmed diagnosis.

Treatment
A. Specific Measures: Treat all household members at the same time to prevent reinfections. Since the drugs are not active against the eggs, therapy should be repeated after 2 weeks to kill the recently hatched adults.

1. Pyrantel pamoate–This drug is given as a single dose (11 mg/kg [maximum, 1 g]); it is safe and very effective.

2. Mebendazole–and albendazole are also highly effective for this infection as well as for other helminthiases. A single oral dose of 100 mg mebendazole or 400 mg albendazole is used for all ages.

B. General Measures: Personal hygiene must be emphasized. Nails should be kept short and clean. Children should wear undergarments to bed to diminish contamination of fingers; bedclothes should be laundered frequently. Although eggs may be widely dispersed in the house and multiple family members infected, the disease is mild and treatable. Avoid creating "pinworm psychosis" in the parents.

Tornieporth NG et al: Ectopic enterobiasis: A case report and review. J Infect 1992;24:87.

2. ASCARIASIS

Essentials of Diagnosis
- Abdominal cramps and discomfort.
- Large, white or reddish, round worms or ova in the feces.

General Considerations

Ascaris lumbricoides is a worldwide human parasite. Ova passed by carriers may remain viable for months under the proper soil conditions. The ova contaminate food or fingers and are subsequently ingested by a new host. The larvae hatch, penetrate the intestinal wall, enter the venous system, reach the alveoli, are coughed up, and return to the small intestine, where they mature. The female lays thousands of eggs daily.

Clinical Findings

A. Symptoms and Signs: Infections usually remain asymptomatic; severe cases, however, can be associated with pain, weight loss, anorexia, diarrhea, or vomiting. Adult worms may be seen in feces or vomitus. Rarely, they perforate or obstruct the small bowel, biliary system, or appendix.

Large numbers of larvae migrating through the lungs may cause an acute, transient eosinophilic pneumonia (Löffler's syndrome). Otitis media has been occasionally reported.

B. Laboratory Findings: The diagnosis is made by observing the large, round worms in the stool or by microscopic detection of the ova.

Treatment

Because the adult worms live less than a year, asymptomatic infection need not be treated. Mebendazole (100 mg twice daily for 3 days), pyrantel pamoate (a single dose of 11 mg/kg [maximum, 1 g]), and albendazole (400 mg in a single dose) are highly and equally effective. In cases of intestinal or biliary obstruction, piperazine (150 mg/kg initially, followed by six doses of 65 mg/kg every 12 hours by nasogastric tube) is recommended because it narcotizes the worms and helps relieve obstruction. However, surgical removal is occasionally required.

Bratton RL, Nesse RE: Ascariasis: An infection to watch in immigrants. Postgrad Med 1993;1:171.

3. TRICHURIASIS (Whipworm)

Trichuris trichiura is a widespread human and animal parasite common in poor children living in warm, humid areas conducive to survival of the ova. The adult worms live in the cecum and colon; the ova are passed and become infectious after several weeks in the soil. Ingested infective eggs hatch in the upper small intestine. Unlike *Ascaris, Trichuris* does not have a migratory tissue phase. No symptoms are usually present unless the infection is severe, in which case it can cause pain, diarrhea, and mild abdominal distention. Massive infections may also cause rectal prolapse and dysentery. Detecting the characteristic barrel-shaped ova in the feces makes

the diagnosis. Adult worms may be seen in the prolapsed rectum or at proctoscopy; their thin heads are buried in the mucosa, and the thicker posterior portions extrude. Mild to moderate eosinophilia may be present.

Mebendazole (100 mg orally twice daily for 3 days) or albendazole (400 mg in a single dose) improve gastrointestinal symptoms as well as constitutional effects.

Nokes C et al: Parasitic helminth infection and cognitive function in school children. Proc R Soc Lond [Biol] 1992;247:77.
Robertson LJ et al: Trichuris trichiura and the growth of primary school children in Panama. Trans R Soc Trop Med Hyg 1992;86:656.

4. HOOKWORM

Essentials of Diagnosis

- Iron deficiency anemia.
- Hematochezia.
- Abdominal discomfort, weight loss.
- Ova in the feces.

General Considerations

The common human hookworms are *Ancylostoma duodenale* and *Necator americanus.* Both are widespread in the tropics and subtropics. The larger *Ancylostoma* is more pathogenic because it consumes more blood, up to 0.5 mL per worm per day.

The adults live in the jejunum. Eggs are passed in the feces and develop and hatch into infective larvae in warm, damp soil within 2 weeks. The larvae penetrate human skin on contact, enter the blood, reach the alveoli, are coughed up and swallowed, and develop into adults in the intestine. The adult worms attach with their mouth parts to the mucosa from which they suck blood. Blood loss is the major sequel of infection. Infection rates reach 90% in areas without sanitation.

A separate species, *Ancylostoma braziliense* (the dog or cat hookworm), causes creeping eruption (cutaneous larva migrans). This disease is seen mainly on the warm-water American coasts.

Clinical Findings

A. Symptoms and Signs: The larvae usually penetrate the skin of the feet and cause intense local itching ("ground itch"). This subsides as the larvae continue their migration. In creeping eruption, the nonhuman larvae migrate blindly in the skin before dying, creating serpiginous burrows. Löffler syndrome may supervene during every migration.

Mild intestinal infections produce no symptoms. Severe infections cause pain, iron deficiency anemia, and malnutrition. Occasionally, abdominal pain and diarrhea may be observed.

B. Laboratory Findings: The large ova of both species of hookworm are found in feces and are indistinguishable. Microcytic anemia, hypoalbuminemia, eosinophilia, and hematochezia are seen in severe cases.

Prevention

Fecal contamination of soil should be prevented; skin contact with potentially contaminated soil should also be avoided.

Treatment

A. Specific Measures: Mebendazole (100 mg orally twice daily for 3 days) or pyrantel pamoate (11 mg/kg [maximum, 1 g], daily for 3 days) are the drugs of choice. Topical thiabendazole and albendazole and oral thiabendazole are useful for creeping eruption.

B. General Measures: Iron therapy may be more important than worm eradication. Parenteral iron or transfusions may be needed in severe cases.

Prognosis

The outcome is usually excellent.

Hotez PJ: Hookworm disease in children. Pediatr Infect Dis J 1989;8:516.

5. STRONGYLOIDIASIS

Essentials of Diagnosis

- Abdominal pain, diarrhea.
- Eosinophilia.
- Larvae in stools and duodenal aspirates.
- Serum antibodies.

General Considerations

The responsible parasite, *Strongyloides stercoralis,* is unique in having both parasitic and free-living forms; the latter can survive in the soil for several generations. The parasite is found in most tropical and subtropical regions of the world. The adults live in the submucosal tissue of the duodenum and occasionally in the whole intestine. Eggs deposited in the mucosa hatch rapidly; the first-stage (rhabditiform) larvae, therefore, are the predominant form found in duodenal aspirates and feces. The larvae rapidly mature to the tissue-penetrating filariform stage and initiate internal autoinfection. The filariform larvae also inhabit the soil and can penetrate the skin of another host, subsequently migrating into veins and alveoli and reaching the intestine when coughed up and swallowed.

Older children and adults are more often infected than young children. Even low worm burden can result in significant clinical symptoms. Infestations due to poor sanitation and hygiene in homes for the retarded are noteworthy. Immunosuppressed patients may develop fatal disseminated strongyloidiasis, known as the hyperinfective cycle.

Clinical Findings

A. Symptoms and Signs: At the site of the skin penetration, there may be a pruritic rash. Large numbers of migrating larvae can cause wheezing, cough, and hemoptysis. Although one third of intestinal infections are asymptomatic, the most prominent features of strongyloidiasis include abdominal pain, distention, diarrhea, vomiting, and occasionally malabsorption.

Patients with cellular immunodeficiencies may develop disseminated infection involving the intestine, the lungs, and the meninges. Gram-negative sepsis may complicate disseminated strongyloidiasis.

B. Laboratory Findings: Finding larvae in the feces, in duodenal aspirates, or on a string test (Entero-Test) is diagnostic. IgG antibodies measured by ELISA or immunoblot are sensitive and specific for *Strongyloides* infection, but persist after successful therapy. Marked eosinophilia is common.

Differential Diagnosis

Strongyloidiasis should be differentiated from peptic disease, celiac disease, regional or tuberculous enteritis, hookworm infection, and other causes of intestinal symptoms or malabsorption. The pulmonary phase may mimic asthma or bronchopneumonia. Severe infection can present as an acute abdomen.

Treatment

Thiabendazole (25 mg/kg orally twice daily for 2 days [maximum, 3 g/d]) and ivermectin (200 mg/kg/d for 1 or 2 days) are the drugs of choice. In the hyperinfection syndrome, 2–3 weeks of therapy may be necessary. Patients from endemic areas should be tested for specific antibodies and treated before undergoing immunosuppression. Relapses are common.

Gann PH, Weva FH, Gani AA: A randomized trial of single- and two-dose ivermectin versus thiabendazole for treatment of strongyloidiasis. J Infect Dis 1994; 163:1076.

Lindo JF et al: Prospective evaluation of enzyme linked immunosorbent assay and immunoblot methods for the diagnosis of endemic *Strongyloides stercoralis* infection. Am J Trop Med Hyg 1994;51:175.

Wehner JH et al: The prevalence and response to therapy of *Strongyloides stercoralis* in patients with asthma from endemic areas. Chest 1994;106:762.

6. VISCERAL LARVA MIGRANS (Toxocariasis)

Essentials of Diagnosis

- Visceral involvement including hepatomegaly, marked eosinophilia, and anemia.

- Posterior or peripheral ocular inflammatory mass.
- Elevated antibody titers in serum or aqueous fluid; demonstration of *Toxocara* larvae on biopsy.

General Considerations

Visceral larva migrans is a worldwide disease. The agent is the cosmopolitan intestinal ascarid of dogs and cats, *Toxocara canis* or *Toxocara cati.* The eggs passed by infected animals contaminate parks and other areas that young children frequent. Children with pica are more at risk. In the United States, seropositivity ranges from 2.8% in unselected populations to 23% in southern United States to 54% in rural areas. Ingested eggs hatch and penetrate the intestinal wall, then migrate to the liver, lungs, eyes, and other organs, where they die and incite a granulomatous inflammatory reaction.

Clinical Findings & Diagnosis

A. Visceral Larva Migrans (VLM): Toxocariasis is usually asymptomatic, but young children (1–5 years of age) sometimes present with anorexia, fever, fatigue, pallor, abdominal distention, abdominal pain, nausea, vomiting, and cough. Hepatomegaly is common, splenomegaly is unusual, and adenopathy is absent. Lung involvement, usually asymptomatic, can be readily demonstrated by radiologic examination. Seizures are common, but more severe neurologic abnormalities are infrequent. Eosinophilia with leukocytosis and anemia are atypical laboratory findings. Most patients recover spontaneously, but disease may last up to 6 months.

B. Ocular Larva Migrans (OLM): This condition occurs in older children and adults who present with a unilateral posterior or peripheral inflammatory mass. Present or past history of VLM and eosinophilia are typically absent. Anti-*Toxocara* antibody titers are low in the serum and high in vitreous and aqueous fluids.

Hypergammaglobulinemia and elevated isohemagglutinins sometimes occur in consequence to cross-reactivity between *Toxocara* antigens and human group A and B blood antigens. The diagnosis is confirmed by finding larvae in granulomatous lesions. Positive serology in high titers (optical density > 0.5) and the exclusion of other causes of hypereosinophilia allow a presumptive diagnosis to be made in typical cases.

Differential Diagnosis

Diseases with hypereosinophilia must be considered. These include trichinosis (large liver and spleen not usually seen, muscle tenderness), eosinophilic leukemia (rare in children; eosinophils are abnormal in appearance), collagen vascular disease (those associated with eosinophilia are rare in young children), (strongyloidiasis (no organomegaly; enteric symptoms are common), early ascariasis, and tropical eosinophilia (seen mainly in India), allergies, and hypersensitivity syndromes.

Treatment & Prevention

A. Specific Measures: The clinical benefit of specific anthelminthic therapy is not defined. Treatment with thiabendazole (25 mg/kg [maximum, 3 g/d] orally twice a day for 5–7 days), diethylcarbamazine (2 mg/kg three times a day orally for 7–10 days), albendazole (400 mg twice a day for 3–5 days), or mebendazole (100–200 mg twice a day for 5 days) is indicated for severe complications of brain, lung, or heart VLM.

B. General Measures: Treating any cause of pica, such as iron deficiency, is important. Corticosteroids are used for marked inflammation of lung, eye, or other organs. Pets should be dewormed routinely. Other children in the household may be infected. Mild eosinophilia and positive serologic tests may be the only clue to their infection. Therapy is not necessary for these patients.

Blatia V, Sarin SK: Hepatic visceral larva migrans: Evolution of the lesion, diagnosis and role of high-dose albendazole. Am J Gastroenterol 1994;89:624.

Magnaval YF: Comparative efficacy of diethylcarbamazine and mebendazole for the treatment of human toxocariasis. Parasitology 1995;110:529.

Marmor M et al: Toxocara canis infection of children: Epidemiologic and neuropsychologic findings. Am J Pub Health 1987;77:554.

Taylor MR et al: The expanded spectrum of toxocaral disease. Lancet 1988;1:692.

7. TRICHINOSIS

Essentials of Diagnosis

- Vomiting, diarrhea, and pain within 1 week of eating infected meat.
- Fever, periorbital edema, myalgia, and marked eosinophilia.

General Considerations

Trichinella spiralis is a small roundworm. The adults inhabit the intestines of hogs and several other meat-eating animals. The cycle begins when the larvae in the muscle of hogs, bear, walrus, and other animals are ingested; they then enter the bowel mucosa, develop into adults, reemerge into the intestine, mate, and reenter the mucosa. The hundreds of larvae produced by each female over the next weeks enter the bloodstream and encyst in the striated muscle. Their migration causes marked inflammation. Humans are usually infected by eating undercooked pork. Smoking, salting, or drying the meat does not kill the larvae. Machines used to grind infected pork may contaminate other meat, such as beef.

Clinical Findings

A. Symptoms and Signs: Most infections are asymptomatic. The initial bowel penetration may cause nausea, vomiting, diarrhea, and cramps within

1 week after ingestion of contaminated meat. This may progress to the classic myopathic form, which consists of fever, periorbital edema (primarily of the face and eyelids), myalgia, and weakness. Many organs may be infected by the migrating larvae—diaphragm, heart, lungs, kidneys, spleen, skin, and brain. Severe cerebral involvement may be fatal. Myocarditis may also be severe or fatal. Symptoms usually peak after 2–3 weeks, but may last months. Another syndrome of chronic diarrhea has been described in the Inuit population in Canada.

B. Laboratory Findings: Marked eosinophilia is the rule. Serology confirms the diagnosis. Muscle biopsy is rarely necessary.

Differential Diagnosis

The classic symptoms are pathognomonic if one is aware of this disease. It has to be distinguished from influenza, dermatomyositic, typhoid fever, the L-tryptophan-associated eosinophilia-myalgia syndrome, sinusitis, and angioneurotic edema.

Prevention

Because a microscopic examination must be performed, meat in the United States is not inspected for trichinosis. Although all states require the cooking of hog swill, hog-to-hog or hog-to-rat cycles may continue. All pork and sylvatic meat (such as bear or walrus) should be heated to at least 65 °C. Freezing meat to at least −15 °C for 3 weeks may also prevent transmission. Animals used for food should not be fed or allowed access to raw meat.

Treatment

Mebendazole has activity against the intestinal, circulating, and tissue stages of infection. The adult dose is 200–400 mg three times daily for 3 days followed by 400–500 mg three times daily for 10 days. Pediatric dosing has not been standardized. Concurrent corticosteroids are used in attempt to prevent the Herxheimer reaction associated with treatment.

Prognosis

Death may occur within the first weeks, but most infections are self-limited.

MacLean JD et al: Trichinosis in the Canadian Arctic: Report of five outbreaks and a new clinical syndrome. J Infect Dis 1989;160:513.

Santos Duran-Ortiz J et al: Trichinosis with severe myopathic involvement mimicking polymyositis. Report of a family outbreak. J Rheumatol 1992;19:310.

CESTODE INFECTIONS
(Flukes)

1. TAENIASIS & CYSTICERCOSIS

Essentials of Diagnosis

- Mild abdominal pain; passage of worm segments (taeniasis).
- Focal seizures, headaches (neurocysticercosis).
- Cysticerci present in biopsy specimens, on plain films (as calcified masses), or on CT or MRI.
- Proglottids and eggs in feces; specific antibodies in serum or CSF.

General Considerations

Both the beef tapeworm (*Taenia saginata*) and the pork (*Taenia solium*) tapeworm cause taeniasis. The adults live in the intestines of humans; the egg-laden distal segments, or proglottids, break off and are passed in feces, disintegrating and releasing the ova in the soil. After ingestion in food or water by cattle or pigs, the eggs hatch and the larvae migrate to and encyst in skeletal muscle. When ingested by humans, these larvae mature into adults.

Humans can be an intermediate host for *T solium* (but not *T saginata*), and the larvae released from ingested eggs encyst in a variety of tissues, especially muscle and brain. Full larval maturation occurs in 2 months, but the cysts cause little inflammation until they die months to years later. Inflammatory edema ensues with calcification or disappearance of the cyst. A slowly expanding mass of sterile cysts at the base of the brain may cause obstructive hydrocephalus (racemose cysticercosis).

Both parasites are distributed worldwide. Contamination of foods by eggs in human feces allows infection without exposure to meat or travel to endemic areas. Asymptomatic cases are common, but neurocysticercosis is a leading cause of seizures in endemic areas.

Person–person spread may occur, resulting in infection of individuals with no exposure to infected meat.

Clinical Findings

A. Symptoms and Signs:

1. Taeniasis–In most tapeworm infections, the only clinical manifestation is the passage of fecal proglottids—white, motile bodies 1 × 2 cm in size. They occasionally crawl out onto the skin and down the leg, especially the larger *T saginata*.

Children may harbor the adult worm for years and complain of abdominal pain, anorexia, and diarrhea.

2. Cysticercosis–Most cases are asymptomatic. Subcutaneous nodules of 1–2 cm may be the only sign. After several years, the cysticerci calcify and appear as radiographic opacities. Brain cysts may remain silent or cause seizures, headache, hydrocephalus, and basilar meningitis. Rarely, the spinal cord is involved. Neurocysticercosis becomes manifest an average of 5 years after exposure but may cause symptoms in the first year of life. In the eye, cysts cause bleeding, retinal detachment, and uveitis. Definitive diagnosis requires histologic demonstration of larvae or cyst membrane. Presumptive diagnosis is often made by the characteristics of the cysts seen on CT or MRI studies; the differential diagnosis may include tuberculoma, brain abscess, arachnoid cyst, and tumor. The presence of *T solium* eggs in feces is uncommon but supports the diagnosis.

B. Laboratory Findings: Eggs or proglottids may be found in feces or on the perianal skin (using the tape method employed for pinworms). Eggs of both *Taenia* species are identical. The species are identified by examination of proglottids; more than 18 lateral uterine branches are present in *T saginata,* less than 12 branches in *T solium.*

Peripheral eosinophilia is minimal or absent. Spinal fluid eosinophilia is seen in 10–75% of cases of neurocysticercosis; its presence supports an otherwise presumptive diagnosis.

Enzyme immunoassay (EIA) antibody titers are eventually positive in up to 98% of serum specimens and over 75% of cerebrospinal fluid specimens from patients with neurocysticercosis. Solitary cysts are less often associated with seropositivity than are multiple cysts. High titers tend to correlate with more severe disease. Cerebrospinal fluid titers are higher if cysts are near the meninges.

Treatment

A. Taeniasis: Praziquantel (5–10 mg/kg once) is the drug of choice. Feces free of segments or ova for 3 months suggest cure.

B. Cysticercosis: Specific treatment is reserved for patients with meningitis or parenchymal cysts. In contrast, those with inactive disease require only symptomatic treatment (anticonvulsants). Praziquantel and albendazole cause disappearance of noninflamed cysts and possibly more rapid resolution of inflamed ring-enhancing cysts. The recommended dose of praziquantel is 50 mg/kg/d in three divided doses for 2 weeks; that for albendazole is 15 mg/kg divided into three doses daily for 8 days. Albendazole is more effective than praziquantel. Larval death may result in clinical worsening due to inflammatory edema. A short course of dexamethasone may decrease these symptoms. The racemose cysts contain no viable larvae and do not respond to medical therapy. Follow-up scans every several months help assess the response to therapy.

Prevention

The incidence in the United States is low, because beef and pork are inspected for taeniasis. Prevention requires proper cooking of meat, careful washing of raw vegetables and fruits, treatment of intestinal carriers, avoiding the use of human excrement for fertilizer, and providing proper sanitary facilities.

Prognosis

The prognosis is good in intestinal taeniasis. Symptoms associated with a few cerebral cysts may disappear in a few months; heavy infections may cause death or chronic neurologic impairment.

Del Brutto OH et al: Therapy for neurocysticercosis: A reappraisal. Clin Infect Dis 1993;17:730.

Sorvillo FJ et al: Cysticercosis surveillance: locally acquired and travel-related infections and detection of intestinal tapeworm carriers in Los Angeles County. Am J Trop Med Hyg 1992;47:365.

Sotelo J et al: Comparison of therapeutic regimens of anticysticercal drugs for parenchymal brain cysticercosis. J Neurol 1990;237:69.

St. Geme III JW et al: Consensus: Diagnosis and management of neurocysticercosis in children. Pediatr Infect Dis J 1993;12:455.

Takayanagui OM, Jardim E: Therapy for neurocysticercosis. Comparison between albendazole and praziquantel. Arch Neurol 1992;49:290.

2. HYMENOLEPIASIS

Hymenolepis nana, the cosmopolitan human tapeworm, is a common parasite of children; *Hymenolepis diminuta,* the rat tapeworm, is rare. The former is capable of causing autoinfection, because the entire life cycle may take place in the human intestine. The larvae hatched from the ingested eggs penetrate the intestinal wall and then reenter the lumen to mature into adults. Their eggs are immediately infectious for the same or a new host. The adult is only a few centimeters long. Finding the characteristic eggs in feces is diagnostic.

H diminuta has an intermediate stage in rat fleas and other insects; children are infected when they ingest these insects.

Light infections with either tapeworm are usually asymptomatic; heavy infection can cause diarrhea and abdominal pain. Therapy is with praziquantel (25 mg/kg once).

Drugs for parasitic infections. Med Lett Drugs Ther 1995;37:117.

Tanowitz HB et al: Diagnosis and treatment of intestinal helminths. I. Common intestinal cestodes. Gastroenterologist 1993;1:265.

3. ECHINOCOCCOSIS

Essentials of Diagnosis

- Cystic tumors of liver, lung, kidney, bone, brain, and other organs.
- Eosinophilia.
- Urticaria and pruritus if cysts rupture.

- Protoscoleces or daughter cysts in the primary cyst.
- Positive serology.

General Considerations

Dogs, cats, and other carnivores are the hosts for *Echinococcus granulosus*. Endemic areas include Australia, New Zealand, and southwestern USA, including Native American reservations where shepherding is practiced. The adult tapeworm lives in the intestine, and eggs are passed in the animals' feces. When ingested, the eggs hatch, and the larvae penetrate the intestinal mucosa and disseminate in the bloodstream. The larvae produce cysts; the primary sites of involvement are the liver (60–70%) and the lungs (20–25%). A unilocular cyst is most common. Over years, it may reach 25 cm in diameter, although most are much smaller. The cysts of *Echinococcus multilocularis* are multilocular and demonstrate more rapid growth.

Clinical Findings

A. Symptoms and Signs: Clinical disease is due to pressure from the enlarging cysts, vessel erosion, and sensitization to cyst or worm antigens. Liver cysts present as slowly expanding tumors that may cause biliary obstruction. Most are in the right lobe and extend inferiorly; 25% are on the upper surface and may be asymptomatic for years. Omental torsion or hemorrhage from vessel erosion may occur.

Rupture of a pulmonary cyst causes coughing, dyspnea, wheezing, urticaria, chest pain, and hemoptysis; cyst and worm remnants are found in sputum. Brain cysts may cause focal neurologic signs and convulsions; renal cysts cause pain and hematuria; bone cysts cause pain.

B. Laboratory Findings: Presumptive diagnosis is made by a combination of radiographic, cytologic, and serologic findings. The appropriate body fluid (tracheal aspirate, ascitic or pleural fluid, spinal fluid, or urine, depending on the site of the cyst) should be examined for protoscoleces. Passing a large amount of fluid through a 5 μm filter and then looking for protoscoleces with an acid-fast stain or other stain has been found to be a sensitive method.

Eosinophilia is variable and may be absent. Serologic tests are useful for diagnosis and follow-up of therapy.

Diagnostic titers vary among laboratories. The bentonite flocculation test is positive at a titer of 1:5, and the indirect hemagglutination test is positive at 1:128. Titers are much higher in secondary echinococcosis (due to cyst rupture). Titers remain high at least a year after surgery. They are usually negative by 10 years. Persistently elevated titers suggest persistent infection.

The skin test for echinococcosis (Casoni test) should not be used. It has never been standardized, and many false-positive results are seen.

C. Imaging: Pulmonary or bone cysts may be visible on plain films. Other imaging techniques are preferred for cysts in other organs. Visualization of daughter cysts is highly suggestive of echinococcosis.

Differential Diagnosis

Tumors, bacterial or amebic abscess, and tuberculosis (pulmonary) must be considered.

Complications

Sudden cyst rupture with anaphylaxis and death is the worst complication. If the patient survives, secondary infections from seeding of daughter cysts may occur. Segmental lung collapse, secondary bacterial infections, effects of increased intracranial pressure, and severe renal damage due to renal cysts are other potential complications.

Treatment

Definitive therapy of *E multilocularis* requires meticulous surgical removal of the cysts, preceded by careful injection of the cyst with formalin, iodine, or 95% alcohol solution to sterilize infectious protoscoleces. Freezing the cyst wall and injecting silver nitrate prior to removal is another technique. A surgeon familiar with this disease should be consulted. Medical therapy (see below) may be of some benefit. If the cyst leaks or ruptures, the allergic symptoms must be managed immediately.

Albendazole (15 mg/kg/d for 28 days with repeat courses as necessary following a 14-day "rest period") is effective in many, but not all, cases of *E granulosus* infection (hydatid disease).

Prognosis

Large liver cysts may be asymptomatic for years. Surgery is often curative for lung and liver cysts but not always for cysts in other locations. Secondary disease has a much worse prognosis; about 15% of patients with this disease die.

Ersahin Y, Mutluer S, Guzelbag E: Intracranial hydatid cysts in children. Neurosurgery 1993;33:219.

Force L et al: Evaluation of eight serological tests in the diagnosis of human echinococcosis and follow-up. Clin Infect Dis 1992;15:473.

Morris DL et al: Albendazole: Objective evidence of response in human hydatid disease. JAMA 1985;253:2053.

TREMATODE INFECTIONS

1. SCHISTOSOMIASIS

Essentials of Diagnosis

- Transient pruritic rash after exposure to fresh water.
- Fever, urticaria, arthralgias, cough, lymphadenitis, and eosinophilia.

- Weight loss, anorexia, hepatosplenomegaly.
- Hematuria, dysuria.
- Eggs in stool, urine, or rectal biopsy specimens.

General Considerations

One of the most common serious parasitic diseases, schistosomiasis is caused by several species of *Schistosoma* flukes; *Schistosoma japonicum, Schistosoma mekongi,* and *Schistosoma mansoni* involve the intestines, and *Schistosoma haematobium* the urinary tract. The first two are found in East and Southeast Asia; *S mansoni* in tropical Africa, the Caribbean, and parts of South America; and *S haematobium* in northern Africa.

Infection is caused by free-swimming larvae (cercariae), which emerge from the intermediate hosts, certain species of fresh-water snails. The cercariae penetrate human skin, migrate to the liver, and mature into adults, which then migrate through the portal vein to lodge in the bladder veins (*S haematobium*), superior mesenteric veins (*S mekongi, S japonicum*), or inferior mesenteric veins (*S mansoni*). Clinical disease results primarily from the inflammation caused by the many eggs that are laid in the perivascular tissues or embolize to the liver. Escape of ova into bowel or bladder lumen allows microscopic visualization and diagnosis from stool or urine specimens, as well as contamination of fresh water and infection of the snail hosts that ingest them.

Clinical Findings

Much of the population in endemic areas is infected but asymptomatic. Only heavy infections produce symptoms.

A. Symptoms and Signs: The cercarial penetration may cause a pruritic rash; larval migration may cause fever, urticaria, and cough; the maturation phase may cause tender hepatosplenomegaly followed by days to weeks of fever and malaise as the worms migrate to their final destination. Bladder infection results in dysuria, hematuria, reflux, stones, and incontinence. Secondary pyelonephritis and ureteral obstruction may occur. Intestinal infection is usually asymptomatic. The final stages of disease are characterized by hepatic fibrosis, portal hypertension, splenomegaly, ascites, and bleeding from esophageal varices. The chronic inflammation in the urinary tract associated with *S haematobium* infections may result in obstructive uropathy, stones, infection, bladder cancer, fistulas, and anemia due to chronic hematuria. Spinal cord granulomas and paraplegia due to egg embolization into Batson's plexus have been reported.

B. Laboratory Findings: The diagnosis is made by finding the species-specific eggs in feces (*S japonicum, S mekongi, S mansoni,* and occasionally *S haematobium*) or urine (*S haematobium,* occasionally *S mansoni*). A rectal biopsy may reveal *S man-* soni and should be done if other specimens are negative. Peripheral eosinophilia is common, and eosinophils may be seen in urine.

Prevention

The best prevention is to avoid contact with contaminated fresh water in endemic areas. Efforts to destroy the snail hosts have been successful in areas of accelerated economic development.

Treatment

A. Specific Measures: Praziquantel is the drug of choice for schistosomiasis. A dose of 40 mg/kg/d divided in two divided doses (*S mansoni* or *S haematobium*) or 20 mg/kg three times in 1 day (*S japonicum* or *S mekongi*) is very effective and nontoxic. Oxamniquine (20 mg/kg/d in two doses once per day is our alternative regimen for *S mansonii*.

B. General Measures: Medical therapy of nutritional deficiency or secondary bacterial infections may be needed. The urinary tract should be carefully evaluated in *S haematobium* infections; reconstructive surgery may be needed. Hepatic fibrosis requires careful evaluation of the portal venous system and surgical management of the portal hypertension when appropriate.

Prognosis

Medical therapy decreases the worm infection and liver size, despite continued exposure in endemic areas. Early disease responds well to therapy, but once significant scarring or severe inflammation has occurred, eradication of the parasites is of little benefit.

Dunn DW et al: Prospects for immunological control of schistosomiasis. Lancet 995;345:1488.

Mahmoud AAF: Schistosomiasis: An overview. Immunol Invest 1992;21:383.

McGarvey ST et al: Child growth and schistosomiasis japonica in northeastern Leyte, the Philippines: Cross-sectional results. Am J Trop Med Hyg 1992;46:571.

II. INFECTIONS: MYCOTIC

The three major categories of fungal infections are shown in Table 38–8. In the United States, systemic disease in normal hosts is commonly caused by three organisms—*Coccidioides, Histoplasma,* and *Blastomyces*—which are restricted to certain geographic areas. Prior residence in or travel to these areas, even for a brief time, is a prerequisite for inclusion in a differential diagnosis. Of these three, *Histoplasma* most often relapses years later in patients who are immunosuppressed.

Table 38–8. Pediatric fungal infections.

Type	Agents	Incidence	Diagnosis	Diagnostic Tests	Therapy	Prognosis
Superficial	Candida Dermatophytes Sporothrix Malassezia	Very common	Simple accurate[1]	KOH prep	Topical[2]	Good
Systemic: Normal host	Coccidioides Histoplasma Blastomyces	Common: regional	Often presumptive	Chest x-ray Serology Histology Culture examination of body fluids or tissue	None[3] or systemic	Good
Systemic: Opportunistic infection	Candida Pneumocystis[4] Aspergillus Malassezia Pseudallescheria Zygomycetes Cryptococcus	Uncommon	Difficult[5]	Tissue biopsy, culture	Systemic, prolonged	Poor if therapy delayed

[1]Sporotrichosis may require biopsy for diagnosis and is treated with systemic therapy.
[2]These fungi in immunocompromised patients may cause severe, rapidly progressive disease.
[3]Often self-limited in normal host.
[4]Now considered a yeast. May infect many normal individuals.
[5]Except Cryptococcus, which is often diagnosed by antigen detection.

Immunosuppression, foreign bodies (eg, central catheters), ulceration of gastrointestinal and respiratory mucosae, broad-spectrum antimicrobial therapy, and HIV infection are major risk factors for opportunistic fungal disease.

Laboratory diagnosis may be difficult because of the small number of fungi present in some lesions, slow growth of some of the organisms, and difficulty in distinguishing colonization of mucosal surfaces from infection. A tissue biopsy with fungal stains and culture is the best method for diagnosing systemic disease. Repeat blood cultures may be negative even in the presence of intravascular infections. Tests for antibody and antigen are currently too insensitive to diagnose most systemic infections, but serology is useful for coccidioidomycosis and histoplasmosis and antigen detection is useful in histoplasmosis.

The risk of empiric treatment is greater for fungal than for bacterial infections because of the toxicity of some antifungals (especially amphotericin B), the frequent need for prolonged parenteral administration, and the limited data available for choosing the best dose or regimen. Delay in treating systemic disease, however, may prove fatal.

Susceptibility testing of fungi is not well standardized, and the correlation of in vitro susceptibility to clinical response is not well defined.

Several less common fungal infections, are presented in Table 38–9. The common superficial fungal infection of the hair and skin are discussed in Chapter 14.

BLASTOMYCOSIS

The causative fungus, *Blastomyces dermatitidis,* is found in soil primarily in the Mississippi and Ohio River Valleys and the states bordering the Great Lakes. Transmission is by inhalation of spores. Outbreaks associated with construction have occurred. Severe disease is much more common in adults and males.

Primary infection is unrecognized or produces pneumonia. Acute symptoms include cough, chest pain, headache, weight loss, and fever occurring several weeks to months after inoculation. Infection is usually self-limited in normal patients. Progressive pulmonary disease may occur. Radiographic consolidation is typical; effusions, nodules, hilar nodes, and cavities are less common. Lower lobe disease is more common with acute infection. Chronic disease can develop in the upper lobes, with cavities and fibronodular infiltrations similar to that seen in tuberculosis, but, unlike tuberculosis or histoplasmosis, these lesions rarely caseate or calcify.

Cutaneous lesions usually represent disseminated disease; local primary inoculation is rare. Slowly progressive ulcerating nodules are typical. Verrucous lesions may be seen. Bone disease resembles other forms of chronic osteomyelitis. Skull lesions in children and spinal involvement in adults are typical. A total body radiographic examination is advisable when blastomycosis is diagnosed.

The genitourinary tract involvement characteristic of dissemination in adults is rare in prepubertal children. Lymph nodes, brain, and kidneys may be involved.

Table 38–9. Unusual fungal infections in children.

Organism	Predisposing Factors	Route of Infection	Clinical Disease	Diagnostic Tests	Therapy and Comments
Aspergillus species	None	Inhalation of spores	Allergic bronchopulmonary aspergillosis; wheezing, cough migratory infiltrates, eosinophilia.	Organisms in sputum; positive skin test; specific IgE antibody; elevated IgE levels.	Hypersensitivity to fungal antigens. Use steroids. No antifungals needed.
	Immuno-suppression	Inhalation of spores	Progressive pulmonary disease: Consolidation, nodules, abscesses. Sinusitis. Disseminated disease: Usually lung, brain; occasionally intestine, kidney, heart, bone.	Demonstrate organs in tissues by stain or culture; septate hyphae branching at 45° angle.	Amphotericin B for 4–6 weeks. Concomitant itraconazole may improve outcome.
Malassezia furfur; M pachydermatis	Central venous catheter, usually lipid infusion (can occur in the absence of lipid)	Line infection from skin colonization	Sepsis; pneumonitis, thrombocytopenia.	Culture of catheter blood specimen on lipid-enriched media (for *M furfur; M pachydermatis* does not need lipid). Fungus may be seen in buffy coat.	Discontinuation of lipid may be sufficient. Remove catheter. Short-term amphotericin B may be added. Organism ubiquitous on normal skin; requires long-chain fatty acids for growth.
Pseudallescheria boydii	Immuno-suppression	Inhalation	Disseminated abscesses (lung, brain, liver, spleen, other).	Culture of pus or tissue.	Surgical drainage; itraconazole.
	Minor trauma	Cutaneous	Mycetoma (most common).	Yellow-white granules in pus. Culture.	Aggressive surgery. Amputation may be needed.
Sporothrix schenkii	Minor trauma (thorns, splinters)	Cutaneous	Chronic skin ulcers, subcutaneous nodules along lymphatics. Pneumonia, osteomyelitis, or arthritis.	Gram or fungal stain of pus or tissue may show "hockey stick" organisms. Culture of pus, tissue.	Itraconazole, drainage, debridement.
Zygomycetes (*Mucor, Rhizopus*)	Immunosuppression, diabetic acidosis	Inhalation, mucosal colonization, invasion of vessels or tissue	Rhinocerebral: sinus, nose, necrotizing vasculitis; central nervous system spread. Pulmonary. Disseminated: Any organ.	Broad aseptate hyphae on tissue stains. Culture: rapidly growing, fluffy fungus.	Amphotericin B, surgical debridement; itraconazole may be a second agent for combined therapy. Poor prognosis.

Diagnosis requires isolation or visualization of the fungus. Pulmonary specimens (sputum, tracheal aspirates, lung biopsy) may be positive with conventional stains or fungal cell wall stains. Microscopically, the budding yeasts are thick-walled, have refractile walls, and are large and very distinctive. Sputum specimens are positive in 50–80% of cases; skin lesions are positive in 80–100%. The fungus can be grown readily in most laboratories. The blastomycin skin test is neither sensitive nor specific. Antibody measured by several immunoassays is sensitive for detecting infection.

Recommended therapy for life-threatening or central nervous system infections is amphotericin B. Itraconazole is suggested therapy for other forms of blastomycosis. Surgical debridement of devitalized bone or drainage of large abscesses is also important.

Alkrinawi S, Reed MH, Pastarkamp H: Pulmonary blastomycosis in children: Findings on chest radiographs. Am J Roentgenol 1995;165:651.

Bosso JA: Fungal infections in pediatric patients. Pharmacotherapy 1990;10:1505.

Brown LR et al: Roentgenographic features of pulmonary blastomycosis. Mayo Clin Proc 1991;66:29.

Dismukes ED et al: Itraconazole therapy for blastomycosis and histoplasmosis. Am J Med 1992;93:489.

Schutze GE et al: Blastomycosis in children. Clin Infect Dis 1996;22:496.

Steele RW, Abernathy RS: Systemic blastomycosis in children. Pediatr Infect Dis J 1983;2:304.

CANDIDIASIS

Essentials of Diagnosis

- Superficial infections in normal or immunosuppressed individuals: Oral thrush or ulcerations; vulvovaginitis; erythematous intertriginous rash with satellite lesions.
- Systemic infection in the immunosuppressed: Renal, hepatic, splenic, pulmonary, or cerebral abscesses; "cotton-wool" retinal lesions; cutaneous nodules.
- Budding yeast and pseudohyphae seen in biopsy specimens, fluid, or scrapings of lesions; positive culture.

General Considerations

Disease due to *Candida* is usually caused by *Candida albicans;* similar systemic infection may be due to *Candida tropicalis, C parapsilosis, C glabrata* formerly called *Torulopsis glabrata*, and other *Candida* species. Speciation is important because of differences in pathogenicity and sensitivity for azole therapy. In tissue, pseudohyphae are seen as well as the budding yeast phase. *Candida* grows on routine media more slowly than bacteria; growth is usually evident on agar after 2–3 days and in blood culture media in 2–7 days.

C albicans is ubiquitous and often present in small numbers on skin, mucous membranes, or in the intestinal tract. Normal bacterial flora, intact epithelial barriers, neutrophils and macrophages in conjunction with antibody, and normal lymphocyte function (manifested by skin test reactivity) are all factors in preventing invasion. Disseminated infection is almost always preceded by prolonged broad-spectrum antibiotic therapy, instrumentation, or immunosuppression. Patients with diabetes mellitus are especially prone to superficial *Candida* infection; thrush and vaginitis are most common. *Candida* is the third most common blood isolate in hospitals in the United States.

Clinical Findings

A. Symptoms and Signs:

1. Oral candidiasis (thrush)–Adherent creamy white plaques with mucosal ulceration are seen. Lesions may be few and asymptomatic, or they may be extensive, extending into the esophagus. Thrush is very common in otherwise normal infants in the first weeks of life; it may last weeks despite topical therapy. Spontaneous thrush in older children is unusual unless they have recently received antimicrobials. Steroid inhalation for asthma predisposes patients to thrush. Infection with HIV should be considered if there is no other reason for oral thrush, or if it is persistent or recurrent.

2. Skin infection–

a. Diaper dermatitis is often due entirely or partly to *Candida*. Pronounced erythema with a sharply defined margin, and satellite lesions is typical. Pustules, vesicles, papules, or scales may be seen. Eroded lesions with a scalloped border are common. Any moist area, such as axillae or neck folds, may be involved.

b. Congenital skin lesions may be seen in infants born to women with *Candida* amnionitis. A red maculopapular or pustular rash is seen. Dissemination may occur.

c. Vulvovaginitis is seen in sexually active girls or diabetics, and occurs at any age in girls receiving antibiotics. Thick, cheesy discharge with intense pruritus is typical. The vagina and labia are usually erythematous.

d. Scattered red papules or nodules may represent cutaneous dissemination.

e. Chronic mucocutaneous candidiasis may be associated with a specific lack of T-cell response to *Candida*.

f. Paronychia and onychomycosis occur in normal children, but are often associated with immunosuppression, hypoparathyroidism, and adrenal insufficiency.

3. Enteric infection–Esophageal involvement in immunosuppressed patients is the most common enteric manifestation. It is manifested by substernal pain, dysphagia, painful swallowing, and anorexia. Nausea and vomiting are common in young children. Only 50% of the patients have thrush. Stomach or intestinal ulcers also occur. A syndrome of mild diarrhea in normal individuals who have predominant *Candida* on stool culture has also been described, though *Candida* is not considered a true enteric pathogen. Its presence more often reflects recent antimicrobial therapy.

4. Pulmonary infection–Since the organism frequently colonizes the respiratory tract, it is commonly isolated from respiratory secretions. Thus, demonstration of tissue invasion is needed to diagnose *Candida* pneumonia or tracheitis. The infection may cause fever, cough, abscesses, nodular infiltrates, and effusion. It is rare, being seen in immunosuppressed patients and patients intubated for long periods.

5. Renal infection–Candiduria may be the only manifestation of disseminated disease. More often, candiduria is associated with instrumentation or anatomic abnormality of the urinary tract. Symptoms of cystitis may be present. Masses of *Candida* may obstruct ureters and cause obstructive nephropathy. Casts in the urine suggest renal tissue infection.

6. Other infections–Endocarditis, myocarditis, meningitis, and osteomyelitis are usually only seen in compromised patients or neonates.

7. Disseminated candidiasis–Mucosal colonization precedes but does not predict dissemination. Too often, dissemination mimics bacterial sepsis which fails to respond to antimicrobials. It is common in neonates, especially premature infants, in an

ICU setting. A careful search should be carried out for lesions highly suggestive of disseminated *Candida* (retinal "cotton-wool" spots or nodular dermal abscesses). If these findings are absent, diagnosis is often presumptively based on the presence of a compatible disease in a compromised patient, a burn patient, or a patient with prolonged postsurgical or ICU course, who has no other cause for the symptoms; who fails to respond to antimicrobials; and who usually has *Candida* colonization of mucosal surfaces. This approach is necessary because candidemia is not appreciated antemortem in many such patients.

Hepatosplenic candidiasis is increasingly recognized in immunosuppressed patients. The typical case consists of a severely neutropenic patient who develops chronic fever and variable abdominal pain. No bacteria are isolated, and there is no response to antimicrobials. Symptoms persist even when neutrophils return. Ultrasound or CT scan of the liver and spleen demonstrates multiple round lesions. Biopsy is needed to confirm the diagnosis.

B. Laboratory Findings: Budding yeast cells are easily seen in scrapings or other samples. The presence of pseudohyphae is suggestive of tissue invasion. Culture is definitive. Blood cultures may take 3 or more days to yield positive results, or they may remain negative, even with disseminated disease or endocarditis. *Candida* should never be considered a contaminant in cultures from normally sterile sites. *Candida* in any number in the urine may represent true infection.

Candida antigen tests are not sensitive or specific enough for clinical use. Antibody tests are not useful.

Differential Diagnosis

Thrush may resemble formula (which can be easily wiped away with a tongue blade or swab, revealing normal mucosa), other types of ulcers, (including herpes), or burns. Skin lesions may resemble contact, allergic, chemical, or bacterial dermatitis, miliaria, folliculitis, or eczema. Systemic infection may resemble that due to bacteria, herpes simplex, cytomegalovirus, toxoplasmosis, and other fungi.

Complications

Failure to recognize disseminated disease while it is still treatable is the greatest complication. Osteoarthritis and meningitis occur more often in neonates than older children. Blindness from retinitis, massive emboli from large vegetations of endocarditis, intestinal perforation, and abscesses in any organ are other complications; the greater the length or degree of immunosuppression, and the longer the delay before therapy, more complications are seen.

Treatment

A. Oral Candidiasis: In infants, oral nystatin suspension (100,000 units four to six times a day until resolution) usually suffices. It must come in contact with the lesions because it is not systemically absorbed. Older children may use it as a mouthwash (200,000–500,000 units four times a day), though it is poorly tolerated due to taste. Clotrimazole troches (10 mg) are an alternative in older children. Prolonged therapy with either agent and more frequent dosing may be needed. Painting the lesions with a cotton swab dipped in gentian violet (0.5–1%) is visually dramatic and messy but may help refractory cases. Eradication of *Candida* from pacifiers, bottle nipples, toys, or the mother's breasts (if the infant is breast-feeding and there is candidal infection of the nipples) may be helpful.

Oral azoles—ketoconazole (100–200 mg for 5–7 days) or fluconazole (100–200 mg)—are effective in older children with candidal infection refractory to nystatin. These drugs have not been evaluated in infants.

Discontinuation of antibiotics or corticosteroids is advised when possible.

B. Skin Infection: Cutaneous infection usually responds to a cream or lotion containing nystatin, amphotericin B, or an imidazole. Associated inflammation, such as severe diaper dermatitis, is also helped by concurrent use of a topical mild corticosteroid cream, such as 1% hydrocortisone. Covering the medicated areas with a thick coat of an occlusive ointment such as zinc oxide seems to promote healing and allows normal diapering.

Another approach is to keep the involved area dry; a heat lamp and nystatin powder may be used. Cornstarch is a yeast nutrient and should not be used as a drying agent.

Suppression of intestinal *Candida* with nystatin and eradicating thrush may help prevent recurrence of the diaper dermatitis.

Vaginal infection is treated with clotrimazole, miconazole, or nystatin (cheapest if generic is used) suppositories or creams, usually applied once nightly for 7–14 days. One clotrimazole formulation need be given only one night. *Candida* balanitis in sexual partners should be treated. Oral azole therapy is equally effective. A single dose of fluconazole is effective for vaginitis. It is more expensive, but very convenient.

C. Renal Infection: Candiduria limited to the bladder may be treated with amphotericin B bladder irrigation (if a catheter is already in place), or a short course of oral flucytosine or fluconazole. Removal of an indwelling catheter is imperative. Renal abscesses or ureteral fungus balls require amphotericin B therapy and surgical debridement in many cases. Amphotericin B may improve poor renal function due to renal candidiasis, even though the drug is nephrotoxic. Fluconazole, which is excreted in urine, is an acceptable alternative.

D. Systemic Infection: Systemic infection is dangerous and resistant to therapy. Surgical drainage of abscesses and removal of all infected tissue (such as a heart valve) are required for cure. Hepatosplenic candidiasis is never considered cured, and fungi may remain viable for life. Systemic infection is optimally treated with amphotericin B at 0.5–1 mg/kg/d, infused over 2–4 hours. It is continued for at least 4 weeks, depending on disease response. Correcting predisposing factors is important (eg, discontinuing antibiotics and immunosuppressives, and improving control of diabetes). Addition of flucytosine (50–75 mg/kg/d orally in four doses; keep serum levels below 75 µg/mL) may help. This is frequently done for neonatal infections, but clinical outcome seems to be similar when amphotericin is used alone. Unlike amphotericin B, it penetrates tissue well; it is also synergistic with amphotericin B against many organisms. It should not be used as a single agent in serious infections because resistance develops rapidly. Fluconazole is emerging as an acceptable alternative for serious candidal infections in nonneutropenic patients and is used more frequently in immunocompromised patients. The latter use must be considered in light of a significant incidence of fluconazole-resistant *Candida* in some clinical settings. Infected central venous lines must be removed immediately; this alone often is curative. However, persistent fever and candidemia suggest infected thrombus, endocarditis, or tissue infection. If the infection is considered limited to the line and environs, 10–14 days of an antifungal such as amphotericin B or fluconazole following line removal is recommended in compromised patients. Fluconazole should also be considered for immunocompetent patients because of the late occurrence of focal *Candida* infection in some cases.

Fluconazole is well absorbed (oral and intravenous therapy are equivalent), reasonably nontoxic, and effective for a variety of *Candida* infections. It is the drug of choice if amphotericin B is not tolerated. The dosage is 8–12 mg/kg/d in a single daily dose for initial therapy of severely ill children. The rile of severe cytokines that enhance anti-*Candida* defenses is under evaluation.

Prognosis

Superficial disease in normal hosts has a good prognosis; in abnormal hosts, it may be quite refractory to therapy. Early therapy of systemic disease is often curative if the underlying immune response is adequate. The outcome is poor when therapy is delayed or when host response is inadequate.

Chun CS, Turner, RB: The outcome of candiduria in pediatric patients. Diagn Microbiol Infect Dis 1991;14:119.

Faix RG: Invasive neonatal candidiasis: comparison of albicans and parapsilosis infection. Pediatr Infect Dis J 1992;11:88.

Hughes WT: Systemic candidiasis: A study of 109 fatal cases. Pediatr Infect Dis J 1982;1:11.

Rex JH et al: A randomized trial comparing fluconazole with amphotericin B for the treatment of candidemia in patients without neutropenia. N Engl J Med 1994; 331:1325.

Stamos JK: Candidemia in a pediatric population. Clin Infect Dis 1995;20:571.

Swerdloff JN, Filler SG, Edwards JE Jr: Severe candidal infections in neutropenic patients. Clin Infect Dis 1993;17:S457.

Thaler M et al: Hepatic candidiasis in cancer patients: The evolving picture of the syndrome. Ann Intern Med 1988;108:88.

COCCIDIOIDOMYCOSIS

Essentials of Diagnosis

- Travel to an endemic area.
- Primary pulmonary form: Fever, chest pain, cough, anorexia, weight loss, and often a macular rash or erythema nodosum or multiforme.
- Primary cutaneous form: Trauma followed in 1–3 weeks by an ulcer and regional adenopathy.
- Spherules seen in pus, sputum, cerebrospinal fluid, joint fluid; positive culture.
- Positive coccidioidin skin test.
- Appearance of precipitating and complement-fixing antibodies.

General Considerations

This disease is caused by the dimorphic fungus *Coccidioides immitis,* which is endemic in the southwestern United States (Sonoran Desert areas of western Texas, New Mexico, Arizona, and California), northern Mexico, and South America. Infection results from inhalation or inoculation of arthrospores (highly contagious and readily airborne in the dry climate). Even brief travel in or through an endemic area, especially during windy seasons, may allow infection. Human-to-human transmission does not occur. More than half of all infections are asymptomatic. Dissemination occurs in less than 1% of cases; the risk is much higher in Filipinos, Hispanics, and blacks, especially in older males.

Clinical Findings

A. Symptoms and Signs:

1. Primary disease–The incubation period is 10–16 days (range, 7–28 days). Symptoms vary from those of a mild fever and arthralgia to severe influenza-like illness with high fever, nonproductive cough, pleurisy, myalgias, arthralgias, headache, and anorexia. True upper respiratory tract signs are not common. Severe pleuritic chest pain suggests this diagnosis. Signs vary from none to rash, rales, pleural rubs, hilar adenopathy and signs of pulmonary consolidation. Weight loss may occur.

2. Skin disease–Up to 10% of children develop erythema nodosum or multiforme. Less specific maculopapular eruptions occur in a larger number of children. These imply a favorable host response to the organism. Primary skin inoculation sites develop indurated ulcers with local adenopathy. Contiguous involvement of skin from deep infection in nodes or bone also occurs.

3. Chronic pulmonary disease—This may be asymptomatic or associated with chronic cough (occasionally with hemoptysis), weight loss, pulmonary consolidation, effusion, cavitation, or pneumothorax.

4. Disseminated disease—This is less common in children than adults. It is more common in infants, neonates, pregnant women (especially during the third trimester), blacks, and Filipinos—or with HIV or any other type of immunosuppression. One or more organs may be involved. The most common sites involved are bone or joint (subacute or chronic swelling, pain, redness), node, meninges (slowly progressive meningeal signs, ataxia, vomiting, headache, cranial neuropathies), and kidney (dysuria, urinary frequency). As with most fungal diseases, the evolution of the illness is usually slow.

B. Laboratory Findings: Direct examination of respiratory secretions, pus, spinal fluid, or tissue may reveal the large spherules (30–60 μm). Phase-contrast microscopy is useful for demonstrating these refractile bodies; Gram or methylene blue stains are not helpful, but PAS, methenamine silver, and calcofluor stains are.

The fluffy, gray-white colonies grow within 2–5 days on routine fungal or other media. They are highly infectious. Spinal fluid cultures are often negative.

Routine laboratory tests are nonspecific. The sedimentation rate is usually elevated. Eosinophilia may occur, particularly prior to dissemination and is more common in coccidioidomycosis than in many other conditions with similar symptoms. Meningitis causes a mononuclear pleocytosis with elevated protein and mild hypoglycorrhachia.

Within 2–21 days, most patients develop a delayed hypersensitivity reaction to skin test antigen (coccidioidin 1:100 strength, or Spherulin 0.1 mL, intradermally, should produce 5 mm induration at 48 hours). Erythema nodosum predicts strong reactivity; when this is present the antigen should be diluted 10–100 times before use. The skin test may be negative in compromised patients or those with disseminated disease. Positive reactions may remain for years and do not prove active infection.

Antibodies consist of precipitins (usually measurable by 2–3 weeks in 90% of cases and gone by 12 weeks) and complement-fixing antibodies (elevated by several weeks and gone by 8 months, unless dissemination occurs). The extent of the complement-fixing antibody response reflects the severity of infection. Persistent high levels suggest dissemination. Serum precipitins usually indicate acute infection. Excellent ELISA assays are now available to detect IgM and IgG antibodies against the precipitin and complement-fixing antigens. The presence of anti-body in spinal fluid indicates central nervous system infection.

C. Imaging: Pulmonary consolidation, hilar adenopathy, effusion, thin-walled cavities, or solitary granulomas (coin lesions) may be seen. About 5% of infected people have asymptomatic nodules or cysts after recovery. Unlike reactivation tuberculosis, apical disease is not prominent. Bone infection causes osteolysis that enhances with technetium. Cerebral imaging may show hydrocephalus and meningitis; intracranial abscesses and calcifications are unusual. Radiographic evolution of all lesions is slow.

Differential Diagnosis

Primary pulmonary infection resembles acute viral, bacterial, or mycoplasmal infections; subacute presentation mimics tuberculosis, histoplasmosis and blastomycosis. Chronic pulmonary or disseminated disease must be differentiated from cancer, tuberculosis, or other fungal infections.

Complications

Dissemination of primary pulmonary disease is associated with ethnic background, prolonged fever (> 1 month), a negative skin test, high complement fixation antibody titer, and marked hilar adenopathy. Local pulmonary complications include effusion, empyema, and pneumothorax. Cerebral infection can cause noncommunicating hydrocephalus due to basilar meningitis.

Treatment

A. Specific Measures: Mild pulmonary infections require no therapy. Antifungal therapy is used for prolonged fever, severe pneumonitis > 4–6 weeks, and mediastinal adenopathy), or any form of disseminated disease. Neonates, those with genetic risk factors, and those with high antibody titer are also treated.

Amphotericin is used for severe disease (1 mg/kg/d until better; then reduce dose; total duration, 2–3 months). For less severe disease and for meningeal disease, fluconazole or itraconazole is preferred (duration of therapy is more than 6 months). Long-term suppression therapy is likely to be required after treating coccidioidal meningitis. Refractory meningitis may require prolonged intrathecal or intraventricular amphotericin B therapy.

B. General Measures: Most pulmonary infections require only symptomatic therapy, self-limited activity, and good nutrition. They are not contagious. Secondary bacterial infection is unusual.

C. Surgical Measures: Excision of pulmonary cavities or abscesses may be needed. Infected nodes, sinus tracts, and bone are other operable lesions. Azole therapy should be given prior to surgery to prevent dissemination; it is continued for 4 weeks arbitrarily or until other criteria for cure are met.

Prognosis

Most patients recover. Even with amphotericin B, however, disseminated disease may be fatal, especially in those racially predisposed to severe disease. Reversion of the skin test to negative or a rising complement-fixing antibody titer is an ominous sign. Meningitis may require lifetime therapy to prevent progression or relapse.

Catanzaro A et al: Fluconazole in the treatment of chronic pulmonary and nonmeningeal disseminated coccidioidomycosis. Am J Med 1995;98:249.

Child DC et al: Radiologic findings of pulmonary coccidioidomycosis in neonates and infants. Am J Radiol 1989;145:261.

Galgiani JN et al: Fluconazole therapy for coccidioidal meningitis. Ann Int Med 1993;119:28.

Kafka JA, Catanzaro A: Disseminated coccidioidomycosis in children. J Pediatr 1981;98:355.

Stevens DA: Coccidioidomycosis. N Engl J Med 1995; 332:1077.

CRYPTOCOCCOSIS

Essentials of Diagnosis

- Mainly a problem for immunosuppressed individuals.
- Meningitis: headache, vomiting, cranial nerve palsies, meningeal signs; mononuclear cell pleocytosis.
- Cryptococcal antigen detected in cerebrospinal fluid; also in serum and urine in some patients.
- Readily isolated on routine media.

General Considerations

Cryptococcus neoformans is a ubiquitous soil yeast. It appears to survive better in soil contaminated with bird excrement, especially that of pigeons. However, most human cases are not associated with a history of significant contact with birds. Inhalation is the presumed route of inoculation. Infections in children are quite rare, even in heavily immunocompromised patients such as those with HIV infection. It is much more common in compromised adults. Normal individuals can also be infected. Asymptomatic carriage is not seen.

Clinical Findings

A. Symptoms and Signs:

1. Meningitis—The most common clinical disease is meningitis, following hematogenous spread from a pulmonary focus. Symptoms of headache, vomiting, and fever occur over days to months. Meningeal signs and papilledema are common. Cranial nerve dysfunction and seizures may occur.

2. Pulmonary disease—Pulmonary infection is the next most common infection and may coexist with cerebral involvement. Symptoms are nonspecific and subacute—cough, weight loss, and fatigue.

Radiographic findings are usually lower lobe infiltrates or nodular densities, less often effusions, and rarely cavitation, hilar adenopathy, or calcification.

3. Other forms—Cutaneous forms are usually secondary to dissemination. Papules, pustules, and ulcerating nodules are typical. Bones (rarely joints) may be infected; osteolytic areas are seen, and the process may resemble osteosarcoma. Many other organs can be involved with dissemination.

B. Laboratory Findings: The spinal fluid usually has a lymphocytic pleocytosis; it may be completely normal in immunosuppressed patients with cryptococcal meningitis. Direct microscopy may reveal organisms in sputum, spinal fluid, or other specimens. The India ink stain demonstrates the capsules nicely, but it is insensitive; artifacts may give false-positive results. The capsular antigen can be detected by latex agglutination or enzyme immunoassay tests, which are both sensitive (> 90%) and specific. Serum, spinal fluid, and urine may be tested. False-negative cerebrospinal fluid tests have occurred. The organism grows well after several days on many routine media; for optimal culture, collecting and concentrating a large amount of spinal fluid (up to 10 mL) is recommended, because the number of organisms may be low.

Differential Diagnosis

Cryptococcal meningitis may mimic tuberculosis, viral meningoencephalitis, or a space-occupying central nervous system lesion.

Complications

Hydrocephalus may occur from chronic basilar meningitis. Significant pulmonary or osseous disease may accompany the primary infection or dissemination.

Treatment

Amphotericin B (0.7 mg/kg) and flucytosine (100 mg/kg/d) are used for most systemic infections, including meningitis. The combination is synergistic and allows lower doses of amphotericin B to be used. Therapy is usually 6 weeks for cerebral infections (or for 1 month after sterilization) and 8 weeks for osteomyelitis. Fluconazole (400 mg/d) is an alternative therapy, which may be as efficacious in patients with AIDS. Combinations of fluconazole with flucytosine or amphotericin B are under investigation. Fluconazole (200 mg/d) is the preferred maintenance therapy to prevent relapses in high-risk patients. Relapses occur in up to 25–50% of meningitis cases, especially with continued immunosuppression. Antigen levels should be followed every few weeks to assess the response.

Prognosis

Treatment failure, including death, is common in immunosuppressed patients, especially those with

AIDS. Lifelong maintenance therapy is required in these patients. Poor prognostic signs are the presence of extrameningeal disease; fewer than 20 cells/µL of initial cerebrospinal fluid; initial cerebrospinal fluid antigen titer greater than 1:32.

Dismukes WE: Management of cryptococcoses. Clin Infect Dis 1993;17(Suppl 2):5507.

Leggiadro RJ, Barrett FF, Hughes WT: Extrapulmonary cryptococcosis in immunocompromised infants and children. Pediatr Infect Dis J 1992;11:43.

Nelson MR, Fisher M: The role of azoles in the treatment and prophylaxis of cryptococcal disease in HIV infection. AIDS 1994;8:651.

Nightingale SD: Initial therapy for acquired immunodeficiency syndrome-associated cryptococcoses with fluconazole. Ann Intern Med 1995;155:538.

Ting SF, Glader BE, Prober CG: Cryptococcal infection in a nine year old child with hemophilia and the acquired immunodeficiency syndrome. Pediatr Infect Dis J 1991; 10:76.

HISTOPLASMOSIS

Essentials of Diagnosis

- Residence in or travel to endemic areas.
- Pneumonia with flu-like illness.
- Hepatosplenomegaly, anemia, leukopenia.
- Positive skin test.
- Detection of the organism in smears or tissue or by culture.

General Considerations

The dimorphic fungus, *Histoplasma capsulatum,* is found in the central and eastern United States (Ohio and Mississippi River Valleys). The small yeast form (2–4 µm) is seen in tissue, especially within macrophages; the mycelial form is a slowly growing, fluffy, gray-white fungus. Endemic infections are very common at all ages and are usually asymptomatic. Over two-thirds of children are infected in endemic areas. Reactivation is very rare in children; it may occur years later, usually due to significant immunosuppression. Infection is acquired by inhaling spores that transform into the pathogenic yeast phase. Soil contamination is enhanced by the presence of bat or bird feces.

Clinical Findings

Because human-to-human transmission does not occur, infection requires exposure to the endemic area—usually within the past weeks or months. Congenital infection is not seen.

A. Symptoms and Signs:

1. Asymptomatic infection (50% of infections)–This is usually diagnosed by the presence of scattered calcifications in lungs or spleen and a positive skin test. The calcification may resemble that due to tuberculosis but may be more extensive than the usual Ghon complex.

2. Pneumonia–Approximately 45% of patients have mild to moderate disease. Most of these are not recognized as a histoplasmal infection. Acute pulmonary disease may resemble influenza, with fever, myalgia, arthralgia, and cough occurring 1–3 weeks after exposure; the subacute form resembles infections such as tuberculosis, with weight loss, night sweats, and pleurisy. Chronic disease is unusual in children. Physical examination may be normal, or rales may be heard. Mediastinal nodes may be greatly enlarged. Effusion is uncommon. A small number of patients may have immune-mediated signs such as arthritis, pericarditis, and erythema nodosum. The usual duration of the disease is less than 2 weeks, followed by complete resolution. Symptoms may last several months and still resolve without antifungal therapy.

3. Disseminated infection (5% of infections)–Fungemia during primary infection is probably common; transient hepatosplenomegaly may occur, but resolution is the rule in normal individuals. Heavy infection, severe pulmonary disease, and immunosuppression may be followed by progressive reticuloendothelial cell infection, with anemia, fever, weight loss, organomegaly, bone marrow involvement, and death. Dissemination may occur in otherwise normal children; usually they are less than 2 years of age.

4. Other–Ocular involvement consists of multifocal choroiditis. This is usually seen in normal adults with other evidence of disseminated disease. Brain, heart valve, pericardium, intestine, and skin (oral ulcers, nodules) are other involved sites. Adrenal gland involvement is common with systemic disease.

B. Laboratory Findings: Routine tests are normal or nonspecific in the benign forms. Pancytopenia is present in many cases of dissemination. The diagnosis can be made by demonstrating the organism by histology or culture. Tissue yeast forms are small and may be mistaken for artifact. They are usually found in macrophages, occasionally in peripheral blood leukocytes in severe disease, but rarely in sputum, urine, or spinal fluid. Cultures of infected fluids or tissues may yield the organism after 1–6 weeks of incubation on fungal media, but even cultures of bronchoalveolar lavage or transbronchial biopsy specimens in immunocompromised patients are often negative. Thus, bone marrow and tissue specimens are needed. Detection of histoplasmal antigen in blood, urine, cerebrospinal fluid, and bronchoalveolar lavage is probably the most sensitive diagnostic test. The level of antigen correlates with the extent of the infection, and antigen levels can be used to follow the response to therapy and to indicate low-grade infection, which becomes apparent after completion of therapy (eg, in a child with HIV infection).

Antibodies may be detected by immunodiffusion, complement fixation, and precipitation; the latter two rise in the first few weeks of illness and fall unless dissemination occurs. A single high titer or rising titer indicates highly likely disease. Antigen detection has replaced serology as a rapid diagnostic test. Skin test reactivity to the yeast phase is a sensitive test of infection, but it is not useful in endemic disease, and patients with disseminated disease often have a negative test. Some antigens may induce a serologic response that may invalidate the use of serology for diagnosis. Thus, skin tests play no role in the management of individual cases.

C. Imaging: Scattered pulmonary calcifications in a well child is typical of past infection. Bronchopneumonia (focal midlung infiltrates) occurs with acute disease, often with hilar adenopathy, occasionally with nodules, but seldom with effusion or cavity formation.

Differential Diagnosis

Pulmonary disease resembles viral infection, tuberculosis, coccidioidomycosis, and blastomycosis. Systemic disease resembles disseminated fungal or mycobacterial infection or leukemia, histiocytosis, or cancer.

Treatment

Mild infections do not require therapy. Disseminated disease in infants may respond to as little as 10 days of amphotericin B, although 4–6 weeks (or 30 mg/kg total dose) is usually recommended. Amphotericin B is the preferred therapy for moderately severe forms of the disease. Surgical excision of local pulmonary disease may be useful. Itraconazole appears to be equivalent to amphotericin B therapy for mild disease and can be substituted for amphotericin B in severe disease after a favorable initial response has occurred. With chronic pulmonary or disseminated disease therapy may be required for prolonged periods.

Tests for fungal antigen are useful here. Chronically immunosuppressed patients (eg, those with HIV) may require lifelong maintenance therapy with an azole.

Prognosis

Mild infections do well. With early diagnosis and treatment, infants with disseminated disease usually recover; the prognosis worsens if immune response is poor.

Fojtasek MF et al: The *Histoplasma* capsulation antigen assay in disseminated histoplasmosis in children. Pediatr Infect Dis J 1994;19(Suppl 1):519.

Leggiadro RJ, Barrett FF, Hughes WT: Disseminated histoplasmosis of infancy. Pediatr Infect Dis J 1988;7:799.

Weinberg GA et al: Unusual manifestations of histoplasmosis in childhood. Pediatrics 1983;72:99.

Wheat J: Histoplasmosis: Recognition and treatment. Clin Infect Dis 1994;19(Suppl 1):519.

Wheat J: Itraconazole: Treatment for disseminated histoplasmosis in patients with the acquired immuno-deficiency syndrome. Am J Med 1995;98:336.

PNEUMOCYSTIS CARINII INFECTION

Essentials of Diagnosis

- Significant immunosuppression.
- Fever, tachypnea, cough, dyspnea.
- Hypoxemia; diffuse interstitial infiltrates.

General Considerations

Although classified as a fungus on the basis of structural and nucleic acid characteristics, *Pneumocystis* responds readily to antiprotozoal drugs. It is a ubiquitous pathogen. Infection is presumed to occur via inhalation. With normal immune function, there is usually no recognized clinical disease. A syndrome of afebrile pneumonia similar to that caused by *Chlamydia trachomatis* in normal infants has been described but is rarely diagnosed. Organisms dormant in the lung may be reactivated in heavily immunosuppressed children, chiefly those with abnormal T cell function such as occurs with HIV infection and hematologic malignancies. Prolonged, high-dose corticosteroid therapy is also a risk factor; onset of illness as steroids are tapered is a typical presentation. Severely malnourished infants with no underlying illness may also develop this infection, as can those with congenital humoral or cellular immune deficiency. The incubation period is usually at least a month after onset of immunosuppression.

Pneumocystis pneumonia is a common complication of advanced HIV infection and is one of the diseases that defines AIDS. Careful prophylaxis may prevent this infection (see Chapter 36).

Infection is generally limited to the lower respiratory tract. In advanced disease, spread to other organs occurs.

Clinical Findings:

A. Symptoms and Signs: A gradual onset of fever, tachypnea, dyspnea, and mild cough occurs over 1–4 weeks. Initially, the chest is clear, although retractions and nasal flaring are present. At this stage, the illness is nonspecific. Hypoxemia out of proportion to the clinical and radiographic signs is an early finding, however, and even minimally decreased arterial PO_2 values should suggest this diagnosis in immunosuppressed children. Tachypnea, nonproductive cough, and dyspnea progress. Respiratory failure and death are common if not treated. In very immunosuppressed children the onset may be abrupt and progression more rapid.

The general examination is unremarkable. There

are no upper respiratory signs, conjunctivitis, organomegaly, enanthem, or rash.

B. Laboratory Findings: These reflect the individual child's underlying illness and are not specific. Serum lactate dehydrogenase may be markedly elevated from pulmonary damage.

C. Imaging: Early chest radiographs are normal. The classic pattern in later films is that of bilateral, interstitial, lower lobe infiltrates without effusion, consolidation, or hilar adenopathy. Older HIV-infected patients may present with other patterns, including nodular infiltrates, lobar pneumonia, cavities, and upper lobe infiltrates—especially those receiving aerosolized pentamidine for prophylaxis.

Diagnosis

Diagnosis requires finding the round (6–8 μm) cysts in a lung biopsy specimen, bronchial brushings or alveolar washings, induced sputum, or tracheal aspirates. The latter specimens are less sensitive but are more rapidly and easily obtained. They are more often negative in children with leukemia compared to those with HIV infection; presumably, greater immunosuppression results in larger numbers of organisms. Since immunosuppressed patients may have many causes of pneumonia, negative results from tracheal secretions should prompt more aggressive diagnostic attempts. Bronchial washing using fiberoptic bronchoscopy is usually well tolerated and rapidly performed.

Several rapid stains—as well as the standard methenamine silver stain—are useful. The indirect fluorescent antibody method is most sensitive. All require competent laboratory evaluation, because few organisms may be present and there are many artifacts.

There are no commercially available clinically useful tests for antigen or antibody detection.

Differential Diagnosis

In normal infants, *Chlamydia* and cytomegalovirus pneumonia are the most common causes of the afebrile pneumonia syndrome described for *Pneumocystis.* In older immunocompromised children, the differential diagnosis includes influenza, respiratory syncytial virus, adenovirus, and other viral infections; bacterial and fungal pneumonia; pulmonary emboli or hemorrhage; congestive heart failure; and *Chlamydia pneumoniae* and *Mycoplasma* pneumonia. Lymphoid interstitial pneumonitis, which is seen in older infants with HIV infection, is more indolent and the lactase dehydrogenase is normal (see Chapter 36). *Pneumocystis* pneumonia is uncommon in children who are complying with prophylactic regimens.

Prevention

Children at high risk of developing *Pneumocystis* infection should receive prophylactic therapy immediately. This includes all those with hematologic malignancies or other reasons for receiving intensive chemotherapy and many children with organ transplants or advanced HIV infection. All children born to HIV-infected mothers should receive prophylaxis against *Pneumocystis* starting at 6 weeks of age. This should be maintained until the HIV infection status and immunologic status are clarified (see Chapter 36).

The drug of choice is trimethoprim-sulfamethoxazole (5 mg/kg/d of trimethoprim and 25 mg/kg/d of sulfamethoxazole) for 3 days of each week.

Many patients with HIV infection have rashes and other adverse reactions that preclude use of sulfonamides. Intravenous pentamidine every 2–4 weeks is a substitute. Aerosolized pentamidine (300 mg per dose via a jet nebulizer) every 4 weeks is a less toxic alternative in older children. It is a lung irritant in some children. Breakthrough infections, particularly in the upper lobes, are seen much more commonly than with trimethoprim-sulfamethoxazole prophylaxis. Dapsone and atovaquone are under study as alternative prophylaxis.

Treatment

A. General Measures: Supplemental oxygen and nutritional support may be needed. Bronchodilators may be tried but are usually not helpful. The patient should be in respiratory isolation.

B. Specific Measures: Trimethoprim-sulfamethoxazole (20 mg/kg/d of trimethoprim and 100 mg/kg of sulfamethoxazole in four divided doses intravenously or orally if well tolerated) is the drug of choice. It should be started immediately, since improvement may not be seen for 3–5 days. Duration of treatment is 3 weeks in HIV-infected children. Monitoring serum levels ensures delivery and may allow decreased dosage with less toxicity. Methylprednisolone (2–4 mg/kg/d in four divided doses intravenously) should also be given to HIV-infected patients with moderate-to-severe infection. If trimethoprim-sulfamethoxazole is not tolerated or there is no clinical response in 5 days, pentamidine isethionate (4 mg/kg once daily by slow intravenous infusion) should be given. Clinical efficacy is similar with pentamidine, but adverse reactions are more common. These include dysglycemias, pancreatitis, nephrotoxicity, and leukopenia. Other effective alternatives that were studied in adults include atovaquone, trimetrexate plus leucovorin, trimethoprim-dapsone, and primaquine plus clindamycin.

Prognosis

The mortality rate is high in immunosuppressed patients who are treated late in the illness.

Bartlett MS, Smith JW: *Pneumocystis carinii:* An opportunist in immunocompromised patients. Clin Microbiol Rev 1991;4:137.

Hughes WT: *Pneumocystis carinii* pneumonia. Rep Pediatr Infect Dis 1995;5:19.

Masur H: Prevention and treatment of pneumocystis pneumonia. N Engl J Med 1992;327:1853.

Sattler FR et al: Trimethoprim-sulfamethoxazole compared with pentamidine for treatment of *Pneumocystis carinii* pneumonia in the acquired immunodeficiency syndrome: A prospective, noncrossover study. Ann Intern Med 1988;109:280.

Simonds RJ: *Pneumocystis carinii* pneumonia among US children with perinatally acquired HIV infection. JAMA 1993;270:470.

Simonds RJ et al: Prophylaxis against *Pneumocystis carinii* pneumonia among children with perinatally acquired human immunodeficiency virus infection in the United States. N Engl J Med 1995;332:786.

Sleasman JW et al: Corticosteroids improve survival of children with AIDS and *Pneumocystis carinii* pneumonia. Am J Dis Child 1993;147(1):30–34.

REFERENCES

PARASITIC INFECTIONS

Drugs for parasitic infections. Med Lett Drugs Ther 1995;37:99.

MYCOTIC INFECTIONS

Barber GR et al: Catheter-related *Malassezia furfur* fungemia in immunocompromised patients. Am J Med 1993;95:365.

Cross JT Jr: Antifungal drugs. Pediatr Rev 1995;16:123.

Gallis HA et al: Amphotericin B: 30 years of clinical experience. Rev Infect Dis 1990;12:329.

Gupta AK et al: Antifungal agents: An overview. J Am Acad Dermatol 1994;30(pt I):677,30(pt II):911.

Kauffman CA: Newer developments in therapy for endemic mycoses. Clin Infect Dis 1994;19(Suppl):528.

Liu LY, Weller PF: Antiparasitic drugs. N Engl J Med 1996;334:1178.

Marcon MJ, Powell DA: Human infections due to Malassezia spp. Clin Microbiol Rev 1992;5:101.

Systemic antifungal drugs. Med Lett Drugs Ther 1994;36:11.

Sexually Transmitted Diseases

39

Eric J. Sigel, MD

The rate of sexually transmitted diseases (STDs) during adolescence continues to rise despite recent public health initiatives that encourage safer sex practices. By age 18, 56% of females and 76% of males have initiated sexual activity: 25% will develop an STD—an estimated 3 million teenagers per year. Adolescents contract STDs at a higher rate than adults because of both sexual risk taking and biologic factors. Practitioners need to carefully screen sexually active adolescents for STDs and use this opportunity to discuss risk reduction.

ADOLESCENT SEXUALITY

Adolescents continue to experiment sexually despite the threat of the human immunodeficiency virus (HIV). The average age of sexual debut has steadily declined, with about one third of all teenagers having initiated sex by age 15. A small but significant number of preteens have also begun having intercourse, often imitating older siblings and modeling behavior suggested by the media. Condom use is sporadic. Forty-three percent of teens overall used a condom during their last intercourse, whereas almost 50% used condoms during their first sexual encounter. Anal intercourse occurs in both heterosexual and homosexual populations: 20% of Hispanic girls may practice anal intercourse, often with the intent to preserve virginity.

Anywhere from 10% to 30% of males experiment with same-sex partners in some fashion, with 4–10% practicing anal sex. Frequently teenage males have their first homosexual experience with partners who are significantly older, which puts them at higher risk for STDs.

Unsafe sexual experimentation sometimes is related to alcohol and drug inebriation: 82% of high school students have experimented with alcohol, whereas 50% of high school senior boys have been drunk in the last 30 days. Sexual risk taking may follow alcohol intake; the incidence of date rape is strongly associated with intoxication.

RISK FACTORS

Certain behaviors and experiences put the adolescent at higher risk for developing STDs. Early age at sexual debut, lack of condom use, multiple partners, prior STD, history of STD in a partner, and having sex with a partner who is 3 or more years older are risk factors that predispose a teenager to an STD. Other risk-taking behaviors associated with STDs in adolescents are smoking, alcohol use, drug use, dropping out of school, and pregnancy. A thorough history will help elicit these risk factors.

The cervix of the adolescent female is predisposed to certain STDs, such as chlamydia, gonorrhea, and human papillomavirus. The columnar cells, which divide rapidly at the exposed squamocolumnar junction, are susceptible to contracting an infection. During early to mid puberty this junction slowly invaginates as the uterus and cervix mature, and by the late teens to early 20s, the columnar cells are inside the cervix, making it more difficult for organisms to attach.

PREVENTION OF STDS

Primary prevention focuses largely on education and risk reduction techniques. Primary care providers need to discuss these as part of well adolescent check-ups. Although adolescents are aware of HIV, they may not have much information about other more common STDs. Discussing prevalence, symptoms, and sequelae of STDs can raise awareness and help teenagers make informed decisions about whether to initiate sexual activity and about what kind of safer sex techniques they should use. Making condoms available reiterates the message that safe sex is vital to health, and this also facilitates safer sex practices.

Secondary prevention requires identifying patients with an STD (see Screening) and treating them before they infect others. Risk reduction and safer sex practices need to be discussed. Identifying partners is also essential in order to limit the continued spread of STDs. Working with the state or county health department proves valuable, since these agencies assume the responsibility for locating the contacts of infected persons and ensure appropriate treatment. Gonorrhea, syphilis, HIV, hepatitis B, and chancroid are reportable to government agencies.

Tertiary prevention is prevention of complications of a specific illness, such as treating pelvic inflammatory disease before infertility develops; following the serologic response to syphilis to ensure that secondary or neurosyphilis does not develop; treating cervicitis to prevent pelvic inflammatory disease; or treating a chlamydial infection before orchitis ensues.

SCREENING

Many STDs are asymptomatic; thus, a comprehensive approach to screening adolescents is essential. This begins during the interview; asking open-ended questions about sexual experience is essential. One must be explicit and make sure that the teen understands what is being asked. If the adolescent has ever engaged in sexual activity, the practitioner needs to determine what kind of sexual activity (mutual masturbation, oral, anal, or vaginal sex) and whether it has been heterosexual, homosexual, or both and whether it has been consensual or forced.

During the interview, while trying to assess degree of risk, an opportunity should be taken to discuss risk reduction techniques. After the practitioner has determined that a patient has engaged in sex; or if the patient denies it but is presenting with STD symptoms; or if a patient reports that a partner has an STD, a thorough clinical screening process is warranted.

For males, the first 10 mL of voided urine should be collected. If results are positive for leukocyte esterase, urethritis is likely. Testing for gonorrhea (culture) and chlamydia (culture, ELISA, or polymerase chain reaction [PCR]) is necessary and can be done from spun urine or from a urethral swab. In addition, a patient with urethritis needs evaluation for *Trichomonas*: a wet preparation for *trichomonas* can be made from the spun urine or from urethral discharge. If high-risk behavior is present (three or more partners in the last 6 months or more than two partners per year for several years), then screening for hepatitis B surface antigen is warranted.

In communities with a high prevalence of hepatitis B, screening with hepatitis B core antibody should be undertaken to determine previous infection. If the core antibody is present, a test for hepatitis B surface antigen is needed to determine whether the patient is a carrier. Patients who are negative for hepatitis B core antibody are candidates for immunization against hepatitis B.

In areas with a relatively high rate of syphilis (urban areas on the east and west coasts), an RPR/VDRL (rapid plasma reagin/Venereal Disease Research Laboratory) should be drawn yearly RPR should be done in all cases in which any STD is present. HIV antibody should be evaluated in all high-risk patients and those requesting an HIV test.

For females, screening criteria for syphilis, hepatitis B, and HIV are the same as for males. Cervical culture for gonorrhea and culture, ELISA, or PCR for chlamydia should be performed. The Papanicolaou (Pap) smear serves to evaluate the cervix for the presence of human papillomavirus. This should be done yearly for teenagers who are asymptomatic and in a monogamous relationship and for all females who are 18 years old. If a patient demonstrates high-risk sexual behavior or has frequent STDs, cervical cytology should be done every 6 months.

SIGNS & SYMPTOMS

For males, the most common symptom of an STD is urethritis, with dysuria and penile discharge. Less common symptoms are scrotal pain, hematuria, proctitis, and pruritus in the pubic region. Signs include epididymitis, orchitis, and urethral discharge. Rarely do males develop systemic symptoms.

For females, the most common symptoms include vaginal discharge and dysuria. Vaginal itching and irregular menses or spotting are also common. Abdominal pain, fever, and vomiting, though less common, are signs of pelvic inflammatory disease. Pain in the genital region and dyspareunia may also be present.

Signs that can be found in both males and females with an STD include ulcerations, adenopathy, and genital warts.

THE SPECTRUM OF STDs

Treatment of each STD is included in Table 39–1.

CHLAMYDIA TRACHOMATIS INFECTION

Chlamydia is the most common bacterial cause of STD, with 4 million cases annually. In females, it presents most commonly as cervicitis, but also causes proctitis, or salpingitis/pelvic inflammatory disease. It is an obligate intracellular organism that is often asymptomatic (50%). The presence of mucopus at the cervical os (mucopurulent cervicitis, or MPC)

Table 39–1. Treatment regimens. (Note: Alternative regimens are not as effective but are clinically useful if the recommended regimens cannot be used due to allergy or pregnancy.)

Disease	Recommended Regimens	Pregnancy
Gonorrhea, uncomplicated	Cefixime, 400 mg PO in a single dose	Safe
	or	
	Ofloxacin, 400 mg PO in a single dose	Contraindicated
	or	
Cervicitis/ Urethritis	Ciprofloxacin, 500 mg PO in a single dose	Safe
	or	
	Ceftriaxone, 125 mg IM in a single dose	Safe
	plus	
	Azithromycin, 1 g orally	Safe
	or	
	Doxycycline, 100 mg PO BID for 7 d	Contraindicated
Epididymitis, disseminated	Ofloxacin, 400 mg/d PO for 10 d	
	Ceftriaxone, 1 gm IM/IV/24 h	Safe
	or	
	Cefotaxime, 1 g IV/8 h	Safe
	Cefixime, 400 mg PO BID	Safe
	or	
	Ciprofloxacin, 500 mg PO BID	Contraindicated
Chlamydia trachomatis Cervicitis/urethritis	Azithromycin, 1 g PO in a single dose	Safe
	or	
	Doxycycline, 100 mg PO BID for 7 d	Contraindicated
Alternative Regimen	Erythromycin, 500 mg PO QID for 7 d	Safe
	or	
	Ofloxacin, 300 mg PO BID for 7 d	Contraindicated
Epididymitis	Doxycycline, 100 mg PO BID for 10 d	
	or	
	Ofloxacin, 300 mg PO BID for 10 d	
Nongonococcal, non-chlamydial urethritis	Doxycycline, 100 mg PO BID for 7 d	
	or	
	if no response to doxycycline, then Erythromycin, 500 mg PO QID for 7 d	
	or	
	Ofloxacin, 300 mg PO BID for 7 d	
Trichomonas vaginalis Vaginitis/urethritis	Metronidazole, 2 g in a single dose	Contraindicated in the first trimester
	or	
	Metronidazole, 500 mg PO BID for 7d	Contraindicated
Bacterial vaginosis	Metronidazole, 2 g PO in a single dose	Contraindicated in the first trimester
	or	
	Clindamycin cream, 2%, one full applicator intravaginally at night for 7 d	Safe
	or	
	Metronidazole, .75% gel, 5 g intravaginally BID for 5 d	Contraindicated
Alternative Regimen	Metronidazole, 500 mg PO BID for 7 d	Contraindicated
Syphilis Early (primary, secondary, or latent less than 1 y)	Benzathine penicillin G, 2.4 million units IM (for patients > 40 kg)	Safe
	Benzathine penicillin G, 50,000 units/kg IM (for patients < 40 kg)	Safe
Alternative Regimen	Doxycycline, 100 mg PO BID for 14 d	Contraindicated
Late (more than 1-year duration)	Benzathine penicillin G, 2.4 million units IM once/week for 3 consecutive weeks (for patients > 40 kg)	Safe
	Benzathine penicillin G, 50,000 units/kg IM once/week for 3 consecutive weeks (for patients < 40 kg)	Safe

(continued)

Table 39–1. Treatment regimens. (Note: Alternative regimens are not as effective but are clinically useful if the recommended regimens cannot be used due to allergy or pregnancy.) (continued)

Disease	Recommended Regimens	Pregnancy
Herpes Simplex		
First episode genital	Acyclovir, 400 mg PO 3 times/d for 7 d	Safe
First episode proctitis	Acyclovir, 400 mg PO 5 times/d for 7–10 d	Safe
Recurrent	Acyclovir, 400 mg PO 3 times/d for 5 d	Safe
	or	
	Acyclovir 800 mg PO 2 times/d for 5 d	Safe
Suppression	Acyclovir 400 mg PO 2 times/d	Safe
Note: valacyclovir and famciclovir are approved for use in herpes zoster; they are effective for HSV, but are more expensive.		
Chancroid	Azithromycin, 1 g PO once	Safe
	or	
	Ceftriaxone 250 mg IM once	Safe
	or	
	Erythromycin 500 mg PO QID for 7 d	Safe
Human papilloma virus		
External lesions penile, vulvar, and intravaginal lesions, uncomplicated	Podophyllin, 25% in benzoin tincture apply directly to warts; wash off in 1–4 h	Contraindicated
	or	
	Trichloroacetic acid (85%); apply directly to warts; wash off in 6–8 h	Safe
	or	
	Podofilox, 0.5% solution; apply BID for 3 d; used by the patient at home; practitioner needs to demonstrate how compound is applied (To be used **only** on external lesions)	Contraindicated
	or	
	Cryotherapy: liquid nitrogen, cryoprobe	Safe
	NOTE: Topical therapies usually require weekly treatments for 4 consecutive weeks	
	If patients fail to respond, alternative therapies by experienced clinicians include:	
	Electrocautery	Safe
	Electrodesiccation	Safe
	Intralesional α-interferon	Contraindicated
Cervical lesions	Laser therapy	Safe
	Cryosurgery	Safe
	Trichloroacetic acid, 85%	Safe
	Podophyllin, 25% in benzoin tincture; to be performed only by experienced practitioners	Contraindicated
Arthropod infections		
Pediculosis pubis	Lindane 1% shampoo: apply for 4 minutes, then wash off	Contraindicated
	Permethrin 1% cream rinse: wash off after 10 minutes	Safe
	NOTE: Bedding and clothing need to be decontaminated by washing in hot water or by getting dry-cleaned.	
	Regimen may be repeated in 1 week if complete response is not achieved.	
Scabies	Permethrin cream 5%: apply to entire body from the neck down; wash off in 8–12 h	Safe
	Lindane 1%: 1 ounce lotion or 30 g cream; apply thinly to all areas of the body from the neck down and wash off in 8 h.	Contraindicated
	NOTE: Bedding and clothing need to decontaminated as outlined.	
	Retreatment may be necessary in 1 week.	
Pelvic inflammatory disease		
Inpatient therapy	*Regimen A*	
	Cefoxitin, 2 g IV q 6 h	Safe
	or	
	Cefotetan, 2 g IV q 12 h	Safe
	plus	
	Doxycycline, 100 mg PO/IV 12 h	Contraindicated
	Once clinically improved for 48 h, patients can be discharged and continue Doxycycline 100 mg BID PO for 14 days total	
	Regimen B	
	Clindamycin, 900 mg IV/8 h	Safe
	and	
	Gentamicin, 2 mg/kg IV loading dose, then 1.5 mg/kg IV/8 h	Safe

Table 39–1. Treatment regimens. (Note: Alternative regimens are not as effective but are clinically useful if the recommended regimens cannot be used due to allergy or pregnancy.) (continued)

Disease	Recommended Regimens	Pregnancy
Outpatients	NOTE: Once clinically improved for 48 h, patients can be discharged and continue doxycycline 100 mg PO BID for 14 days total	
	Note: Pregnant patients with PID should be hospitalized and treated with parenteral antibiotics.	
	Regimen A	
	Ceftriaxone, 250 mg IM once	Safe
	or	
	Cefoxitin, 2 g IM plus	Safe
	Probenecid, 1 g PO	
	plus	
	Doxycycline, 100 mg, PO BID for 14 d	Contraindicated
	Regimen B	
	Ofloxacin, 400 mg PO BID for 14 d	
	plus, either	
	Clindamycin, 450 mg PO QID for 14 d	Safe
	or	
	Metronidazole, 500 mg PO BID for 14 d	Contraindicated

Therapy should be continued for 24–48 h after the patient has improved; therapy can then be switched to either oral regimen to complete a 7-day course.
Adapted from Centers for Disease Control and Prevention, 1993 Sexually Transmitted Diseases Treatment Guidelines. *MMWR* 1993; 42(No. RR-14):1–99; Drugs for sexually transmitted diseases. The Medical Letter, 1995;37:117.

is a sign of chlamydia or gonorrhea. Chlamydia can be detected by culture (90–95% sensitive) or PCR of the cervix. Culture has been recognized as the gold standard, but PCR is more sensitive and easier to process. PCR is also more sensitive than ELISA techniques.

A cervical sample should be obtained, after the gonorrhea culture and the Pap test, using the manufacturer's swab provided with the specific test being run. If symptomatic, a rectal specimen should be obtained. To optimize detection, columnar cells need to be collected by inserting the swab in the os and rotating it 360 degrees. The presence of MPC indicates either gonorrhea or chlamydia or both; since 30% of patients have both infections, treatment for both is necessary.

In males, chlamydia may be asymptomatic or may manifest as dysuria, urethritis, or epididymitis. Fifty percent may complain of urethral discharge, although an additional 30% have evidence of a discharge after milking the penis. The discharge is usually clear white. All males with a discharge, pyuria or urethritis, or complaints of dysuria (and when a urinary tract infection has been ruled out) should be evaluated and treated for both gonorrhea and chlamydia. A thorough genital examination will disclose any evidence of epididymitis or orchitis. Reiter's syndrome is a complication of chlamydia urethritis, which should be suspected in males who are sexually active and present with low back pain (sacroiliitis), arthritis (polyarticular), and conjunctivitis.

The first-void urine for leukocyte esterase is appropriate screening for asymptomatic, sexually active males. This test has a high false-positive rate, but is

the easiest way of screening large numbers of patients. Examination of the urine sediment for white blood cells (WBCs) is similar in sensitivity, but more labor-intensive. If either test is positive, then a test for chlamydia should be performed. Because of the false-positive rate of the screening test, patients should be told that there is a chance they have an STD and will need further evaluation.

Patients who are symptomatic and asymptomatic contacts, regardless of physical signs need to be treated. Evaluation of the symptomatic patient or the asymptomatic contact includes either a urethral swab inserted 2–4 cm and rotated 360 degrees or a swab of a spun sample of the first-void urine sent for culture or PCR.

Biro FM et al: A comparison of diagnostic methods in adolescent girls with and without symptoms of *Chlamydia* urogenital infection. Pediatrics 1994;93(3):476.

Centers for Disease Control and Prevention: Recommendations for Prevention and Management of *Chlamydia trachomatis* Infections. MMWR 1993;42(RR-12):1.

Shafer MA et al: Evaluation of urine-based screening strategies to detect *Chlamydia trachomatis* among sexually active asymptomatic young males. JAMA 1993; 270:2065.

NEISSERIA GONORRHOEAE INFECTION

Gonorrhea is the second most prevalent bacterial STD: 117 of 100,000 adolescent females and 954 of 100,000 males report having had gonorrhea. Sites of infection include the cervix, urethra, rectum, and pharynx. In addition, gonorrhea is a cause of pelvic inflammatory disease. In uncomplicated gonococcal cervicitis, females are symptomatic 57% of the time, presenting with vaginal discharge and dysuria. Urethritis and pyuria may be present. MPC with a yellowish discharge may be found on examination. The cervical swab should be cultured on Thayer-Martin agar. Gram's stain of the cervical discharge is not used as a diagnostic tool because nongonococcal *Neisseria* spp reside in the vagina, confounding the interpretation of the Gram's stain. If MPC is present, the patient should be treated presumptively for gonorrhea and chlamydia.

Ninty-five percent of males with gonorrhea are symptomatic, with a yellowish-green urethral discharge and burning on urination. Culture confirmation of gonorrhea can be achieved with a swab of the urethra or urine sediment, plated on Thayer-Martin agar. Gram's stain of the discharge showing gram-negative intracellular diplococci indicates gonorrhea. Rarely does gonorrhea cause systemic symptoms in males.

Both males and females can develop proctitis and pharyngitis. If proctitis is present, appropriate cultures should be obtained and treatment for both gonorrhea and chlamydia given. In the case of pharyngitis, streptococcal infection should be ruled out. If the history is strongly suggestive of oral sex exposure, the patient should be cultured and empirically treated for gonorrhea. Otherwise, it is appropriate to await culture results (24–48 hours).

Disseminated gonococcal infection occurs in a minority (0.5–3%) of patients with untreated gonorrhea. Hematogenous spread can lead directly to systemic symptoms, most commonly arthritis and dermatitis. Joints most frequently involved are the wrist, metacarpophalangeal, knee, and ankle. Skin lesions are typically tender, necrotic pustules on an erythematous base occurring on the distal extremities. Disseminated disease occurs more frequently in women, and risk factors include pregnancy and gonococcal pharyngitis. Treatment requires hospitalization.

Test of cure is considered only for patients who remain symptomatic. (See also Chapter 38.)

NONGONOCOCCAL NONCHLAMYDIAL URETHRITIS

About 15% of males with urethritis have cultures negative for *N. gonorrhoeae* and *C. trachomatis,* but continue to have symptoms despite empiric treatment for these organisms. *Ureaplasma urealyticum* has been identified as a causative organism in urethritis. Routine culture is not done but studies have shown an increased detection of *U. urealyticum* in a first-void urine specimen. Other organisms that have been implicated, but not definitively proved, are *Mycoplasma* spp and *Bacteroides ureolyticus.* Coliforms

may cause urethritis in men practicing anal intercourse.

A patient with urethritis needs to be evaluated for gonorrhea, chlamydia, and *Trichomonas* infection. If negative for *Trichomonas,* empiric therapy is given for gonorrhea and chlamydia. If symptoms persist after adequate therapy and cultures are negative, then nongonococcal, nonchlamydial urethritis (NGU) should be assumed and treated presumptively.

Stamm WE et al: Azithromycin for empirical treatment of the nongonococcal urethritis syndrome in men: A randomized double blind study. JAMA 1995;274(7):545.

TRICHOMONAS VAGINALIS INFECTION

Fifty percent of females with *Trichomonas* infection develop a symptomatic vaginitis with vaginal itching, a green-gray, malodorous frothy discharge, and dysuria. Occasionally, postcoital bleeding and dyspareunia may be present. On examination, the vulva may be erythematous with evidence of a discharge. The cervix may be friable. Vaginitis is the most common manifestation of trichomoniasis; rarely does pelvic inflammatory disease result from *Trichomonas* infection. Wet preparation—mixing the discharge with normal saline—permits the flagellated protozoan to be seen on microscopic examination. Seventy-five percent of symptomatic persons and 64% of asymptomatic patients will have a positive wet preparation. This infection also may be detected by the pathologist when reviewing the Pap smear. Culture and antigen detection are more sensitive (more than 95% and 80–90%, respectively), but are expensive and not readily available.

Males with urethral discharge should be evaluated for trichomoniasis, since 6% of males with a discharge have been found to have trichomoniasis. Almost 50% of males with a *Trichomonas* infection have a discharge, typically clear white, without being coinfected with other organisms. *Trichomonas* urethritis frequently has a positive urine leukocyte esterase test or WBCs on urethral smear. A wet preparation permits detection of the trichomonad. Male partners of females diagnosed with trichomoniasis have a 22% chance of having *Trichomonas* infection. Treatment is necessary for the symptomatic person as well as an asymptomatic contact.

Krieger JN et al: Clinical manifestations of trichomoniasis in men. Ann Intern Med 1993;118:844.
Wolner-Hanssen P et al: Clinical manifestations of vaginal trichomoniasis. JAMA 1989;261:571.

BACTERIAL VAGINOSIS

Women typically develop bacterial vaginosis after an alteration in normal vaginal flora has occurred. A decrease in the number of lactobacilli, the predominant bacteria that reside in the vagina normally, is observed, as well as an overgrowth of *Gardnerella vaginalis, Bacteroides* spp, *Mobiluncus* spp, or genital mycoplasmas. It is unclear whether bacterial vaginosis is sexually transmitted. The presenting symptom is a malodorous vaginal discharge, although 50% of patients are asymptomatic. Patients may report vaginal itching or dysuria. Risk factors for developing bacterial vaginosis include frequent sexual activity, multiple partners, uncircumcised partner, prior STD, low socioeconomic status, use of an intrauterine device, and smoking. Diagnosis can be made by finding three out of the four following features: presence of a fishy, malodorous vaginal discharge; vaginal pH higher than 4.5; a positive "whiff" test (mixing the discharge with potassium hydroxide releases an amine/fishy odor); and 20% of squamous cells positive for clue cells on wet preparation. Clue cells are squamous epithelial cells that have multiple bacteria adhering to them, making their borders irregular and giving them a speckled appearance.

Treating patients who do not complain of vaginal discharge or itching, but demonstrate bacterial vaginosis on routine pelvic examination has been debated. Some studies associate bacterial vaginosis and pelvic inflammatory disease. Because of this relationship, the recommendation is to have a low threshold for treating bacterial vaginosis in the asymptomatic patient.

Joesoef MR, Schmic GP: Bacterial vaginosis: Review of treatment options and potential clinical indications for therapy. Clin Infect Dis 1995;20(Suppl 1):S72.

Thomason JL: Bacterial vaginosis: Current review with indications for asymptomatic therapy. Am J Obstet Gynecol 1991;165:1210.

GENITAL LESIONS

A variety of microorganisms, both bacterial and viral, cause sexually transmitted genital lesions. A careful history, physical examination, and appropriate laboratory tests contribute to making the correct diagnosis. Associated pain, adenopathy (nature and duration), history of recurrence, number of lesions, and presence of systemic symptoms are differential points, as is the exposure history.

HERPES SIMPLEX

Herpes simplex virus (HSV) is the most common cause of visible genital lesions. An estimated 30 million people are infected in the United States. As with most oral HSV infections, many primary genital infections are asymptomatic or not recognizable as herpetic in origin. Symptomatic initial HSV infection causes vesicles of the external genitalia, quickly followed by shallow, painful ulcerations of the vulva, vagina, penis, rectum, and urethra. Atypical presentation of herpes infection includes vulvar erythema and fissures. Urethritis may occur. Initial infection can be severe, lasting up to 3 weeks and may be associated with fever and malaise, as well as localized tender adenopathy. The pain and dysuria can be extremely uncomfortable, requiring sitz baths, topical anesthetics, and occasionally catheterization for urinary retention.

HSV type II is the most common cause of genital herpes (80–90%). Symptoms tend to be more severe in females. Viral meningitis occurs in 10–20% of females with primary genital herpes. Recurrence in the genital area with HSV type II is likely (65–80%). Recurrent genital herpes is of shorter duration (7–10 days), with a smaller number of lesions and usually no systemic symptoms. Prodromal pain in the genital, buttock, or pelvic region is common prior to recurrences.

Diagnosis of genital herpes is often made presumptively. Culture of the vesicles confirms the diagnosis; recurrent attacks are suggestive. Acyclovir administered within the first 5 days of primary infection decreases the duration and severity of HSV infection. The effect of acyclovir on recurrent disease is minimal. For best results, therapy should be started with the prodrome or during the first day of the attack (patient has medicine at home). If recurrences are frequent and cause significant physical or emotional discomfort, patients can take acyclovir on a daily basis for suppression to reduce the number and duration of recurrences.

HSV type I, which accounts for 10–20% of genital herpes infections, is usually the consequence of oral-genital sex. Primary infection is as severe as with HSV type II, and treatment is the same. However, this virus is much less often associated with recurrent disease. Thus, determining the type of virus can be useful for prognosis.

Any genital ulcer should be cultured for HSV and differentiated from syphilis and chancroid ulcers. All patients with active lesions should be counseled to abstain from sexual contact. In addition, most patients have periodic asymptomatic shedding of HSV. This asymptomatic shedding is an important source of the current epidemic. Thus, herpes-infected individuals should be encouraged to use condoms at all times.

Koutsky LA et al: Underdiagnosis of genital herpes by current clinical and viral isolation procedures. N Engl J Med 1992;326:1533.

Lavoie SR, Kaplowitz L: Management of genital herpes infection. Semin Dermatol 1994;13(4):248.

Mertz G: Epidemiology of genital herpes infections. Infect Dis Clin North Am 1993;7:825.

CHANCROID

Chancroid is a relatively rare ulceration caused by *Haemophilus ducreyi*. It is endemic in many urban areas and has been associated with HIV infection, drug use, and prostitution. Ten percent of patients with *H ducreyi* are coinfected with HSV or syphilis. Typically, the lesion begins as a papule and after 24–48 hours erodes into an ulcer, which has ragged, sharply demarcated edges and a purulent base. The lesion is painful, solitary, and somewhat deeper than HSV infection. Tender, fluctuant inguinal adenopathy is usually present. Diagnosis of chancroid is made by ruling out the aforementioned infections and by Gram's stain showing gram-positive cocci arranged in a boxcar formation. Culture can be performed, but the test is not usually available.

After treatment, symptoms improve within 3 days. Most ulcers resolve in 7 days, although large ulcers may take 2 weeks to heal. All sexual contacts need to be examined and treated, even if asymptomatic.

Joseph AK, Rosen T: Laboratory techniques used in the diagnosis of chancroid, granuloma inguinale, and lymphogranuloma venereum. Dermatol Clin 1994;12(1):1.

Morse SA: Chancroid and *Haemophilus ducreyi*. Clin Microbiol Rev 1989;2:137.

SYPHILIS

The incidence of syphilis had risen steadily up to 1991, when it reached its highest level since the 1940s. The rate of syphilis has steadily declined through 1994, returning to 1986 levels. Although the absolute number of patients with syphilis has leveled off, incidence in the teen population is still rising; it more than doubled from 1986 to 1990 in women aged 15–19 and is especially prevalent in poor urban populations.

Primary syphilis presents as a chancre—a painless ulcer with an indurated base—usually solitary, with associated nontender, firm adenopathy. The chancre appears 10–90 days after exposure and spontaneously resolves 4–8 weeks later. Since it is painless, it may go undetected, especially if the lesion is within the vagina. Chancres may occur on the genitalia, lips, or anus. Secondary syphilis occurs 4–10 weeks after the chancre appears, presenting with generalized malaise, adenopathy, and a nonpruritic maculopapular rash that may include the palms and soles. Secondary syphilis resolves in 1–3 months, but can recur. Verrucous lesions known as condyloma lata

may develop on the genitalia. These must be distinguished from genital warts.

If the patient has a lesion, is high risk, or is a contact, or if secondary syphilis is suspected, a nontreponemal serum screen—either RPR or VDRL—should be drawn. If the nontreponemal test is positive, then a specific treponemal test, an FTA-ABS or MHA-TP is done to confirm the diagnosis. Titers from the RPR/VDRL are used to evaluate the degree of infection and are repeated at 3, 6, and 12 months to ensure that they fall at least fourfold as a measure of therapeutic response. If not, retreatment is necessary. An additional diagnostic tool is darkfield microscopy, which can be used to detect spirochetes in scrapings of the base of the chancre.

If a patient is engaging in high-risk sexual behavior or is living in an urban area in which syphilis is endemic, yearly RPRs should be drawn to screen for asymptomatic infections.

Syphilis is reportable to all state health departments, and all contacts need to be evaluated. Patients also need to be evaluated for other STDs, including HIV.

Untreated syphilis can lead to serious complications such as tertiary syphilis, which can in turn lead to serious multiorgan involvement including aortitis and neurosyphilis. Transmission to the fetus can occur from an untreated pregnant woman with syphilis. (See also Chapter 38.)

Martin DH, DiCarlo RP: Recent changes in the epidemiology of genital ulcer disease in the United States: The crack cocaine connection. Sex Transm Dis 1994;21(2 Suppl):S76.

GENITAL WARTS

Condyloma acuminata, or genital warts, is caused by the human papillomavirus (HPV). Genital warts are the most common STD: 12–40 million people are estimated to be infected. There are multiple serotypes of HPV. Types 6 and 11 are detected most frequently, whereas 16 and 18 are most commonly implicated in the etiology of cervical dysplasia. The infection is more common in persons with multiple sex partners and in women who have previously had an abnormal Pap smear. HPV is relatively more common in the adolescent population—the exposed and actively dividing cells of the cervical transition zone make teenagers more susceptible. The infection is usually asymptomatic in women and is often detected by cytology or by physical examination. Females may develop verrucous lesions on any genital mucosal surface. Lesions typically are fleshy, soft, and vascular. They can be flat or papular or solitary or clustered, and may range in size from microscopic to several centimeters. Visible, external lesions and internal vaginal lesions can be treated topically. Internal and cervical lesions should be treated by an experienced practitioner.

If a Pap smear shows signs of inflammation only and there is concomitant infection such as vaginitis or cervicitis, then the smear should be repeated after the infection has cleared. If the smear shows any degree of cervical intraepithelial neoplasia, then referral to a practitioner who performs colposcopy is essential in order to biopsy and treat the lesion and prevent progression to cervical cancer.

HPV is transmitted sexually: 30–60% of males whose partners have HPV have some evidence of condyloma on examination. Verrucous lesions may be found on the shaft or corona of the penis. Lesions also may develop in the urethra or rectum. Condyloma acuminata can be distinguished from condyloma lata (syphilis), skin tags, and molluscum contagiosum by application of 5% acetic acid solution. HPV lesions turn white. Microscopic lesions can be detected by wrapping the penis in gauze soaked with acetic acid. After 5 minutes, one may be able to detect small white papules, which represent HPV. All penile lesions need to be treated topically, and both males and females need weekly treatment for 4 consecutive weeks to clear the infection. If the lesions do not resolve, referral to a dermatologist or gynecologist is necessary. Insistence on condom use is essential to prevent the continued spread of HPV.

Baken L et al: Genital human papillomavirus infection among male and female sex partners: Prevalence and type-specific concordance. J Infect Dis 1995;171:429.

Eltabakh GH: Value of wet mount and cervical cultures at the time of cervical cytology in asymptomatic women. Obstet Gynecol 1995;85(4):499.

Fairly C et al: Human papillomavirus infection and its relationship to recent and distant sexual partners. Obstet Gynecol 1994;84:755.

VIRAL INFECTIONS

HEPATITIS B & C

Hepatitis B and hepatitis C are often STDs. Hepatitis B is at least 10 times more common than HIV in the adolescent population. It was the first STD to be prevented by immunization, and also, since sequelae of HBV includes hepatocellular carcinoma, the first neoplasm that can be prevented by immunization. Symptoms, diagnosis, and treatment are described in Chapter 21. Since HBV is an important STD in adolescents, high-risk teenagers need to be screened for HBV. If core antibody-positive, then a test for surface antigen should be sent to determine active infection. If this is positive, they should be followed up to detect carrier status and counseled about prevention. If they have not been exposed to the virus or are low risk, immunization should be initiated.

Hepatitis C generally is transmitted through blood products and sharing intravenous needles, although about 10% of hepatitis C infection has been linked to sexual transmission. Hepatitis C needs to be considered in teenagers who are symptomatic and have demonstrated high-risk sexual behavior or intravenous drug use.

Nowicki MJ, Baliestreri WF: Viral hepatitis. Principles Pract Pediatr Updates 1993;1-4:1.

Thomas D et al: Hepatitis C, hepatitis B and human immunodeficiency virus infections among non-intravenous drug using patients attending clinics for sexually transmitted diseases. J Infect Dis 1994;169:990.

HUMAN IMMUNODEFICIENCY VIRUS

HIV/AIDS is the sixth leading cause of death among 15–24-year-olds. Although the incidence of AIDS in the teen population is relatively small (less than 1% of the overall AIDS rate), the numbers of people in their 20s with HIV infection is substantial (20% of AIDS cases). Because of the long latency period between infection with HIV and progression to AIDS, it is felt that many HIV-positive young adults contracted HIV during adolescence. Blinded seroprevalence studies in certain urban areas show that anywhere from 1% of teens and 2.7% of young adults are HIV-positive.

Risk factors for contracting HIV include a prior STD, infrequent condom use, practicing active and receptive anal sex (both males and females), practicing survival sex (trading sex for money or drugs), intravenous drug use or using crack cocaine, homelessness, and being the victim of sexual abuse (males). The number of females who are becoming HIV-positive has increased dramatically in each of the last several years. HIV infection should be considered in any sexual risk-taking youth, whether they are practicing heterosexual or homosexual sex.

Screening for HIV should include risk-taking youths and those with an STD. Adolescents may also present to the office requesting an HIV test. In either case, a careful history of sexual behavior should be obtained to assess risk and intervene with risk reduction counseling. It is also necessary to determine how teens may respond to being told they are HIV-positive and what support systems they have in place. If the adolescent is homeless; does not have emotional support from family, friends, or a counselor; or threatens suicide or homicide in response to the idea of being be HIV-positive, then testing should be deferred until the practitioner is confident that the youth will be safe if the test is positive.

Hein K et al: Comparison of HIV+ and HIV– adolescents: Risk factors and psychosocial determinants. Pediatrics 1995;95:96.

ARTHROPOD INFESTATIONS

See Chapter 14 for discussion of skin diseases.

Pediculosis pubis, or pubic lice, live in the pubic hair. Either the louse itself or the nits can be transmitted by close contact from person to person. Patients complain of itching, and they may report having seen the insect. Examination of the pubic hair may reveal the louse crawling around or attached to the hair. Closer inspection may reveal the nit or sack of eggs, which is a gelatinous material (1–2 mm) stuck to the hair shaft.

Sarcoptes scabei or **scabies** is an organism smaller than the louse. It can be identified by the classic burrow, created by the organism laying eggs and traveling just below the skin surface. Scabies can be sexually transmitted by close contact and can be found in the pubic region, groin, lower abdomen, or upper thighs. The rash is intensely pruritic, erythematous, and scaly.

Both infestations can be treated with either premethrin or lindane. The entire area needs to be covered with the lotion or shampoo for the time specified by the manufacturer. One treatment usually clears the infestation, although a second treatment may be necessary. Partners should be treated also. In the case of pubic lice, bedsheets and clothes must be washed in hot water.

PELVIC INFLAMMATORY DISEASE

Pelvic inflammatory disease (PID) is a potential complication of STDs, caused by infection ascending from the vagina or cervix to the uterus, fallopian tubes, or ovaries. Causative agents include gonorrhea, chlamydia, and anaerobic bacteria that reside in the vagina. Over 1 million women develop PID annually, and 275,000 are hospitalized. The incidence is highest in the teen population. Teenage girls have a 1:8 chance of developing PID, whereas women in their 20s have a 1:80 chance. Predisposing risk factors include number of partners, younger age of initiating sexual intercourse, and lack of condom use. Low levels of protective antibody from lack of previous exposure to sexually transmitted organisms, and cervical ectopy, contribute to developing PID.

Vaginal douching may increase the risk of PID by promoting the access of lower genital tract organisms to internal pelvic organs. There is also an association between recent menses and development of PID.

Clinical Findings

A. Symptoms and Signs: Diagnosis of PID is usually made clinically. Typical patients have lower abdominal pain, nausea, vomiting, and fever. Vaginal discharge may or may not be present. Recent genital infection and menses may be associated. On physical examination, affected patients have lower abdominal, cervical motion, and adnexal tenderness. A pelvic/ovarian mass may be palpated. Signs of peritonitis may be present. Mucopurulent cervicitis is present in 50% of patients. Laparoscopy is the gold standard for detecting salpingitis; it can be used if the diagnosis is in question or to help differentiate between an ectopic pregnancy and ovarian cysts or torsion. Pelvic ultrasonography also is helpful in detecting tubo-ovarian abscesses. These are found in almost 20% of teens with PID.

B. Laboratory Findings: Laboratory findings include elevated WBCs with a left shift, and an elevated erythrocyte sedimentation rate (ESR). A positive cervical culture for *N gonorrhoeae* or *C trachomatis* are supportive. It is important to note that 25% of the time neither of these STDs are detected. Aerobic and anaerobic organisms that normally reside in the vagina are found to be causative or contributory agents in many cases of PID. Pregnancy needs to be ruled out, since an ectopic pregnancy can present with abdominal pain.

Table 39–2. Diagnostic criteria for PID.

Minimum criteria
Empiric treatment of PID should be instituted on the basis of the presence of all of the following three minimum clinical criteria for pelvic inflammation and in the absence of an established cause other than PID:
  Lower abdominal tenderness
  Adnexal tenderness
  Cervical motion tenderness
Additional criteria
For women with severe clinical signs, more elaborate diagnostic evaluation is warranted because incorrect diagnosis and management may cause unnecessary morbidity. These additional criteria may be used to increase the specificity of the diagnosis.
The following are the **routine** criteria for diagnosing PID:
  Oral temperature > 38.3 °C
  Abnormal cervical or vaginal discharge
  Elevated erythrocyte sedimentation rate
  Elevated C-reactive protein
  Laboratory documentation of cervical infection with *Neisseria gonorrhoeae* or *Chlamydia trachomatis*
The following are the **elaborate** criteria for diagnosing PID:
  Histopathologic evidence of endometritis on endometrial biopsy
  Tubo-ovarian abscess on sonography or other radiologic tests
  Laparoscopic abnormalities consistent with PID
Although initial treatment decisions can be made before bacteriologic diagnosis of *C trachomatis* or *N gonorrhoeae* infection, such a diagnosis emphasizes the need to treat sex partners.

Adapted from Centers for Disease Control and Prevention, 1993 Sexually Transmitted Diseases Treatment Guidelines. MMWR 1993;42(RR-14):1.

Treatment

With increasing frequency PID is being managed at the outpatient level. Some argue that all adolescents should be hospitalized because of the significant rate of complications. Severe systemic symptoms and toxicity, signs of peritonitis, inability to take fluids, pregnancy, and elevated WBCs and ESR support hospitalization. In addition, if the practitioner believes that the patient will not comply with medication, then hospitalization is warranted. Treatment regimens for hospitalized patients can be found in Table 39–1.

Outpatient management should be reserved for compliant patients who have classic signs of PID without systemic symptoms. Close follow-up is mandatory to evaluate possibility of persistent disease or treatment failure.

Sequelae

Scarring of the fallopian tubes is one of the major sequelae of PID. With one episode of PID, 17% of patients become infertile, 17% develop chronic pelvic pain, and 10% will have an ectopic pregnancy. Infertility rates increase with each episode of PID: three episodes of PID result in a 73% infertility rate. Fitz-Hugh–Curtis syndrome is inflammation of the liver capsule (perihepatitis) from either hematogenous or lymphatic spread of the precipitating organism from the uterine tubes. This causes right upper quadrant pain; liver function tests may be elevated. Symptoms resolve with therapy, but subsequent adhesions from the liver capsule to surrounding tissue can develop.

Tubo-ovarian abscesses, another sequalae of PID, can be detected by careful physical examination (feeling a mass or fullness in the adnexa) and confirmed by pelvic ultrasonography. Surgical drainage is often required to ensure adequate treatment.

McCormack WM: Pelvic inflammatory disease. N Engl J Med 1994;330:115.

Rome E: Pelvic inflammatory disease in the adolescent. Curr Opin Pediatr 1994;6:383.

REFERENCES

Centers for Disease Control and Prevention: 1993 Sexually Transmitted Diseases Treatment Guidelines. MMWR 1993;42(RR-14):1.

Centers for Disease Control and Prevention: Health Risk Behaviors Among Persons Aged 12–21 Years: US, 1992. MMWR 1994;43:233.

Centers for Disease Control and Prevention: Premarital Sexual Experience Among Adolescent Women—US 1970–1988. MMWR 1991;39:51.

Drugs for sexually transmitted diseases. Med Lett 1995; 37:117.

Gittes EB, Irwin C: Sexually transmitted diseases in adolescents. Pediatr Rev 1993;14:180.

Sexually Transmitted Diseases in the United States. *Facts in Brief.* Alan Guttmacher Institute, 1993.

40

Fluid & Electrolyte Therapy

James V. Lustig, MD

BODY FLUIDS

In term infants, the total body water (TBW) accounts for approximately 70–75% of the body weight. Following the normal postnatal fluid adjustment with its attendant weight loss, the TBW represents about 65% of the total body weight. This fraction remains constant until puberty, when the TBW decreases to 55–60% of the body weight. Approximately two-thirds of the TBW is intracellular water (ICW), and one-third is extracellular water (ECW). The ECW is further divided into plasma volume and interstitial fluid (ISF) (Figure 40–1).

The intracellular and extracellular fluids are separated by the cell membranes of the body. For the purposes of discussing clinical disorders of hydration, these membranes may be conceptualized as one aggregate cell membrane that is water-permeable. Furthermore, the cell membrane facilitates the passage into and the maintenance of sodium (Na^+) concentration in the ECW, whereas potassium (K^+) is moved into and maintained in the intracellular environment via a membrane-associated "pump" (Figure 40–2).

Because the cell membrane is water-permeable and particles are dissolved in the water on each side of the cell membrane, shifts of water would occur if the number of particles dissolved on each side of the cell membrane were not the same. Normally, the volumes of the ECW and ICW do not change, because the concentration of dissolved particles is identical on each side of the membrane. If this relationship were not maintained, there would be fluid shifts from one compartment to the other because of the permeable nature of the membrane. The actual number of dissolved particles per unit of water is seldom computed. In clinical situations, the concept of osmolality is used. Osmolality is expressed as mosm/kg of water, which is equivalent to mmol/g of water times the number of particles formed when a molecule dissociates; for example, two particles for NaCl and one particle for glucose. Osmolarity is equal to mosm/L of plasma. Technically, therefore, osmolality and osmolarity are slightly different, but for clinical purposes they are very similar and often used interchangably.

Osmolality is the same throughout the body water. Conceptualizing osmotic shifts between the ECW and ICW is fundamental to understanding disorders of hydration. Shifts occur only if there is an inequality on each side in the concentration of solutes that cannot permeate the membrane. Normally, Na^+, Cl^-, and HCO_3^- are primarily excluded from most cellular environments, whereas K^+ is maintained within cells. In addition to the isosmolality maintained between fluid compartments, electroneutrality is maintained within body fluids.

The extracellular fluid (ECF) is the only fluid compartment that can be readily monitored, and its composition reflects interactions between the ECF and intracellular fluid (ICF). Figure 40–2 is a depiction of the composition and distribution of the body fluids.

CONTROL OF THE ECF

The more important mechanisms controlling the ECF volume are thirst, aldosterone, and antidiuretic hormone (ADH).

Aldosterone from the adrenal cortex enhances the tubular reabsorption of Na^+ in the kidney. As a constant osmolality is maintained, retention of Na^+ leads to increased ECF volume.

Thirst controls the need to drink and reflects changes in the volume of ECF. Thirst provides precise control over a wide range of fluid volumes and can even be a response to an inhibition or absence of ADH with its attendant copious, dilute urine. However, thirst acts to maintain volume even at the expense of osmolality. An individual who cannot perceive thirst rapidly develops a significant problem with fluid balance. Neurologically impaired children or children who cannot respond to thirst pose serious management problems.

Under normal physiologic conditions, plasma osmolality, as opposed to plasma volume, is the variable primarily regulated. Plasma osmolality and volume are maintained through the interaction of thirst and ADH. Thirst controls fluid intake, whereas ADH controls the volume of urine output.

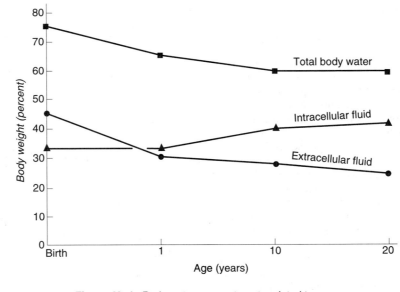

Figure 40–1. Body water compartments related to age.

Atrial natriuretic factor (ANF) has been a topic of recent interest, as ANF plays an important role in the control of blood volume and blood pressure. In the brain, ANF inhibits drinking and desire for salt while acting to decrease blood pressure rise and inhibiting the release of vasopressin. Diuresis and sodium loss are mediated both by a direct effect on the renal tubules and by increasing the glomerular filtration rate. Low-dose infusions of ANF in animals appear to decrease the pressor effects of norepinephrine. Thus, it appears that in the normal state, ANF plays a significant role in diuresis, sodium excretion, and renin secretion.

Figure 40–2. Composition of body fluids. ICF = intracellular fluid, ISF = interstitial fluid.

ACID-BASE EQUILIBRIUM

The pH of arterial blood is maintained between 7.38 and 7.42, except in infants, in whom it ranges from 7.35 to 7.45. Over 50% of the blood's buffering capacity is in the bicarbonate system. The action of buffers is strengthened by the lung's effect on carbonic acid and the alkalinization or acidification of urine, which alters the concentration and amount of bicarbonate in the blood.

The bicarbonate system can interact with the non-bicarbonate system, and the lung and the kidney can act to alter or stabilize pH. In respiratory alkalosis, there is effective alveolar hyperventilation.

In metabolic acidosis, which results from an increase of a strong acid or loss of bicarbonate, the respiratory center increases respiratory drive, CO_2 is exhaled, and P_{CO_2} decreases.

Renal regulation of acid-base status primarily alters HCO_3^- concentration. Unwanted acid or base can be excreted in the urine, and subsequently the HCO_3^- concentration can be altered throughout the entire ECF. Bicarbonate can be altered in two ways via the kidneys, since the urine may be either alkalinized or acidified. When the urine is alkalinized, HCO_3^- enters the kidney and is ultimately lost in the urine. This alkalinization of the urine can occur at any time that there is a relative or absolute excess of bicarbonate. This mechanism does not function if there is a deficiency of Na^+ or K^+, because the body could not maintain electroneutrality in this situation. A chloride deficiency also inhibits this mechanism.

If there is a relative or absolute decrease in HCO_3^-, the urine can be acidified. In this situation, water and CO_2 combine in the tubular cell to form carbonic acid, which then dissociates. H^+ is exchanged for Na^+, and the sodium bicarbonate gains access to the peritubular plasma and the ECF. This reaction facilitates the excretion of significant amounts of H^+. The reaction is limited by salt depletion or dehydration. Some of the processes controlling pH are illustrated schematically in Figure 40–3.

PRINCIPLES OF FLUID & ELECTROLYTE MANAGEMENT

The therapy for any disorder of fluids and electrolytes is predicated on providing the patient with maintenance requirements of fluids and electrolytes, replacing any previous losses, and replenishing ongoing abnormal losses. In planning therapy, these three components should be addressed individually so that no basic needs are overlooked. Therapy should be phased in order to (1) maintain adequate perfusion, (2) restore fluid and electrolyte deficits while correcting acid-base defects, (3) meet nutritional needs, and (4) replace ongoing losses.

The cornerstone of therapy is understanding main-

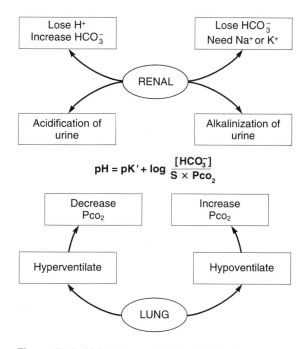

$$pH = pK' + \log \frac{[HCO_3^-]}{S \times P_{CO_2}}$$

Figure 40–3. Maintaining metabolic stability via compensatory mechanisms.

tenance requirements. The phrase *maintenance requirements* means enough water and electrolytes to prevent deterioration of body stores. When short-term (2–3 days') parenteral therapy is given, enough calories are given to blunt hunger and inhibit protein breakdown and ketosis. However, the amount given is usually little more than 20% of the patient's true caloric needs.

Different models have been devised to calculate maintenance fluid needs based on body weight, surface area, or caloric expenditures. A system based on caloric expenditures is helpful since we know that 1 mL of water is needed every 24 hours for each calorie expended and that metabolic needs, not size, determine the use of body stores (see Figure 40–4).

Calories consumed per unit of body weight (metabolic rate) decrease as size and age increase. The schema presented, which is based on caloric needs, is applicable to youngsters weighing over 3 kg (see Table 40–1).

As Table 40–1 shows, a child weighing 25 kg would need 1600 kcal daily and 1600 mL of water. If the child were admitted to the hospital for an elective procedure and received fluids intravenously for 2 days, the fluid would probably contain 5% glucose, which would provide 320 kcal/d, or about 20% of the maintenance needs. Maintenance fluid requirements take into account insensible water loss and water lost in sweat, urine, and stool. Patients are assumed to be relatively inactive and afebrile.

Figure 40–4. Estimate of caloric needs per day. For each calorie expended, 1 mL of water is needed. (Adapted, with permission, from Holliday MA, Segar WE: The maintenance need for water in parenteral fluid therapy. Pediatrics 1957;19:823.)

Table 40–2. Alterations of maintenance fluid requirements.

Factor	Altered Requirement
Fever	12% per °C[1]
Hyperventilation	10–60 mL/100 kcal
Sweating	10–25 mL/100 kcal
Hyperthyroidism	Variable: 25–50%
Gastrointestinal loss and renal disease	Monitor and analyze output. Adjust therapy accordingly.

[1]Do not correct for 38 °C; correct 24% for 39 °C.

Electrolyte needs can be similarly approximated, although maintenance estimates vary considerably. Reasonable initial approximations for maintenance needs are 3 meq Na^+/100 kcal and 2.5 meq K^+/100 kcal.

Altered metabolic states alter maintenance needs. Allowances must be made for such occurrences. Fever and hyperventilation are among the most commonly encountered of these conditions. For every degree (centigrade) of body temperature, fluid needs increase by 12.5%. Corrections are made for temperatures above 38 °C. A fever of 39 °C would require maintenance fluid to be increased by 25%. Table 40–2 lists factors commonly altering fluid requirements.

Normally, one need not measure individual components of output to ensure appropriate fluid balance. It is useful to monitor the patient's weight, urinary output, fluid input, and urine specific gravity. If there is an alteration of fluid or electrolyte balance, determination of electrolyte concentrations, urine osmolality, and pH may be necessary. These measurements help the physician monitor the efficacy of therapy. In patients with significant burns, anuria, oliguria, or abnormal ongoing losses (eg, from a stoma), it is important to measure output and its frac-

tions so that appropriate replacement can be instituted.

DEHYDRATION

Depletion of body fluids—dehydration—is one of the most commonly encountered problems in pediatrics. The problems associated with dehydration remain common not only because of the frequency of gastroenteritis in young children but also because infants and young children often decrease their intake when ill. Furthermore, renal function in the first year of life does not maximally conserve water, the infant's high ratio of surface area to volume promotes evaporative fluid losses, and fever significantly increases fluid needs. Caregivers who treat both children and adults should remember that young children and adults have significant differences among compartments of body water as well as differences in TBW. As a result, perfusion is compromised at a lower percentage of dehydration in adults than in children, but children require a greater proportionate deficit replacement when they are dehydrated.

The clinical effects of dehydration are proportionate both to the degree of dehydration and to the relative ratio of salt to water lost. Briefly, dehydration decreases the extracellular volume, leading to decreased tissue perfusion. The decreased volume results in compensatory increases in pulse rate as the heart attempts to increase output in the face of decreased stroke volume. The decreased tissue perfusion also impairs renal function, leading to acidosis and uremia. Decreased oxygen delivery caused by dehydration may lead to lactic acidosis. These changes are illustrated in Figure 40–5.

The clinical sequelae of dehydration reflect the amount of fluid depletion. A number of clinical profiles have been suggested as a way to correlate the appearance of symptoms and physical signs with the degree of dehydration. Such a system is illustrated in Table 40–3. Such schema are imprecise at best. The primary utility of such systems is to remind the physician to estimate the degree of dehydration (be-

Table 40–1. Caloric and water needs per unit of body weight.

| Body Weight (kg) | Maintenance Needs | |
	kcal/kg	mL of Water/kg
3–10	100	100
11–20	50	50
>20	20	20

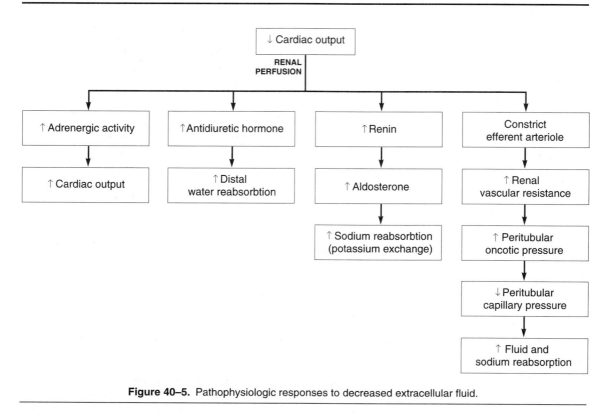

Figure 40–5. Pathophysiologic responses to decreased extracellular fluid.

cause treatment varies with the degree of dehydration) and, more importantly, to assess the adequacy of perfusion. Simple measures—for example, checking the patient's last recorded weight and comparing it to the present weight; carefully assessing blood pressure, capillary refill, and orthostatic blood pressure changes; and meticulously reviewing the history of fluids ingested and frequency of output—are often most helpful. Physicians dealing with growing children must remember the fluid shift that occurs around the time of puberty. Young children may not suffer shock until the degree of dehydration is approximately 15%. However, after the fluid shift at puberty, shock may occur when the degree of dehydration is 9–10%. The significance of this shift underscores the need to constantly assess the adequacy of perfusion and the patient's response to treatment.

Dehydration is further characterized by the elec-

Table 40–3. Clinical manifestations of dehydration.[1]

Clinical Signs	Degree of Dehydration		
	Mild	**Moderate**	**Severe**
Decrease in body weight	3–5%	8–10%	12–15%

Skin
  Turgor
  Color
  Mucous membranes
	Normal (+/−)
	Normal
	Dry ⟶
		Decreased
		Pale
		
			Markedly decreased
			Markedly decreased
			Mottled or gray; parched

Hemodynamic
  Pulse
  Blood pressure
  Perfusion
	Normal ⟶
	Normal ⟶
	Normal ⟶
			Tachycardia
			Low
			Circulatory collapse

Fluid loss
  Urinary output
  Tears
	Mild oliguria ⟶
	Decreased ⟶
			Anuria
			Absent

[1]The manifestations of dehydration reflect the extracellular fluid in general and the plasma in particular. Therefore, hypotonic dehydration is clinically more apparent, and hypertonic dehydration is less apparent.

Table 40–4. Estimated water and electrolyte deficits in dehydration (moderate to severe).[1]

Type of Dehydration	H_2O (mL/kg)	Na^+ (meq/kg)	K^+ (meq/kg)	Cl^- and HCO_3^- (meq/kg)
Isotonic	100–150	8–10	8–10	16–20
Hypotonic	50–100	10–14	10–14	20–28
Hypertonic	120–180	2–5	2–5	4–10

[1]Adapted, with permission, from Winters RW: *Principles of Pediatric Fluid Therapy.* Little, Brown, 1982.

trolyte composition of the plasma. If relatively more solute than water is lost, the sodium concentration falls, and hyponatremic dehydration ($[Na^+]$ <130 meq/L) results. This finding is important because the hypotonicity of the plasma results in further volume loss from the ECF, and perfusion is therefore more significantly impaired for a given degree of hyponatremic dehydration than for the same degree of isotonic or hypertonic dehydration. It is important to remember that significant solute losses do occur in hypernatremic dehydration. Because plasma volume is protected, this might appear to be the least dangerous form of dehydration, but it poses the risk of an underestimation of the severity of dehydration. Further, if the hypertonicity is corrected too rapidly (a drop in $[Na^+]$ of >0.5–1 meq/L in 1 hour), cerebral edema, seizures, and severe central nervous system injury may occur. Typical electrolyte losses associated with each form of dehydration are listed in Table 40–4.

METABOLIC DERANGEMENTS

1. METABOLIC ACIDOSIS

Metabolic acidosis results from either abnormally increased abnormal production of a strong acid or loss of a buffer base, such as bicarbonate. Ketone body production is increased in starvation, diabetic ketoacidosis, and salicylism. Lactic acidosis usually reflects poor tissue perfusion or hypoxia, although primary lactic acidosis may rarely occur. Loss of bicarbonate is most often associated with loss of alkaline fluid from the small intestine. Such losses often accompany diarrheal disease or the use of suction to remove fluid from the intestine. Diarrheal stool is often acidic. The acidic pH reflects the bacterial fermentation of the intestinal fluid, which results in the production of organic acids. Loss of bicarbonate is also seen in renal tubular acidosis.

Metabolic acidosis is associated with a significant negative base excess and compensatory hyperventilation. Effective treatment depends on treating the underlying disorder. Bicarbonate may be used to ameliorate severe acidosis. Normalization which is too

rapid or too aggressive may have serious deleterious sequelae. Therefore, only severe acidosis should be treated. In general, one need not attempt to correct the pH if it is greater than 7.10, and one need not correct to values greater than 7.25 with bicarbonate. The dose of sodium bicarbonate used to correct pH is given by the following formula:

$$\textbf{Dose (meq)} = 0.3 \times \textbf{body weight (kg)} \times \textbf{base excess}$$

If sodium bicarbonate is given, the amount of sodium administered in maintenance fluids should be adjusted.

The use of $NaHCO_3$ remains controversial. When administered to a patient with normal renal function with normal metabolic balance, an increase in $[HCO_3]$ ensues. Subsequently, renal excretion should result in elimination of any excess. However, in the setting of severe metabolic acidosis, this may not occur, and in fact, deleterious effects may ensue. This is a result of the production of CO_2 which comes from titrating acid with HCO_3. Under normal conditions, the lungs would rapidly excrete the CO_2. However, in the face of poor tissue perfusion and/or decreased pulmonary function, the CO_2 may diffuse across cell membranes, precipitating an exacerbation of intracellular acidosis. This would result in decreased cardiac function and hemodynamic instability. Further problems with the administration of $NaHCO_3$ may result from hyperosmolarity, excess expansion of the ECF, and increased lactate production. Proponents of HCO_3 administration believe that failure to administer HCO_3 in the face of severe acidosis may result in loss of extracellular buffering capacity.

The problems articulated here have resulted in the development of new buffering agents such as Carbicarb, which is a mixture of disodium carbonate and sodium bicarbonate. This mixture increases the extracellular $[HCO_3]$ while consuming the CO_2 which is produced. This buffer also appears to improve cardiac function. Although it is not yet available in the clinical setting, preliminary studies are promising.

Other considerations must be taken into account when correcting an acidosis. Mild to moderate acidosis is associated with increased use of lactate for metabolic use, yielding increased energy production in the heart and the liver as well as an increase in gluconeogenesis. In ischemic states and during reperfusion, such considerations appear to be important and protective of compromised tissue. This is balanced by decreased response to catecholamines, decreased cardiac output, and dilation of vascular beds, contributing to hypotension in the acidotic patient. The clinician, in dealing with an acidotic compromised patient, thus has multiple mechanisms of protection and injury to consider in establishing a therapeutic plan for a patient with altered acid-base balance.

Many physicians rely on determination of the anion gap to detect cases of metabolic acidosis caused by the production of strong acid. The anion gap may be calculated as:

$$\text{Anion gap} = ([Na^+] + [K^+]) - ([Cl^-] + [HCO_3^-])$$

Small variations are not significant, and the anion gap determinations should not be overinterpreted. The anion gap tends to be normal in diarrhea with its attendant hyperchloremic acidosis and bicarbonate loss. However, if azotemia ensues because of dehydration, the increase in phosphate and sulfate may increase the anion gap. Clinical situations in which an exaggerated anion gap is encountered include diabetic ketoacidosis, uremia, salicylate intoxication, lactic acidosis, hypokalemia, hypocalcemia, methanol intoxication, ethylene glycol, or other causes of metabolic acidosis. Therapy with various antibiotics, including carbenicillin and large doses of sodium penicillin, can also elevate the anion gap. A low anion gap is associated with hypoalbuminemia, dilution, hyperkalemia, hypercalcemia, and lithium intoxication.

2. METABOLIC ALKALOSIS

Metabolic alkalosis is the result of gaining buffer base or losing strong acid, most commonly because of the loss of gastric juice from vomiting or nasogastric suctioning. Pyloric stenosis is the prototypical situation leading to the development of metabolic alkalosis. Other situations that may lead to metabolic alkalosis include chronic diarrhea, the administration of diuretics, and the use of silver nitrate in the treatment of burns. Metabolic anomalies in which sodium is conserved without chloride, such as 11β-hydroxylase deficiency, predispose patients to the development of metabolic alkalosis.

The laboratory profile of metabolic alkalosis includes, in addition to an elevated pH, a positive base excess and a normal or mildly elevated PCO_2.

The volume of ECF is an important determinant in maintaining a metabolic alkalotic state. Volume depletion increases the reabsorption of sodium and HCO_3 in the proximal tubule, while in the distal tubule a mineralocorticoid-dependent process results in further sodium reabsorption and HCO_3 generation. In states in which there is associated NaCl deficiency, the NaCl deficiency contributes to the maintenance of the metabolic alkalosis, as does the depleted ECF. The decrease in readily reabsorbable chloride results in enhanced bicarbonate reabsorption. These processes indicate that ECF volume is preferentially maintained before the alkalosis is corrected.

Parallel to the contraction alkalosis described above, situations that result in a rapid expansion of ECF volume with fluids not containing bicarbonate result in a transient dilutional acidosis as a result of a drop in $[HCO_3]$. This transient acidosis is corrected easily and rapidly unless renal function is impaired.

The treatment of metabolic alkalosis includes, in addition to the treatment of the underlying disorder, the administration of chloride. Chloride may be supplied by a number of salts.

3. RESPIRATORY ACIDOSIS

Respiratory acidosis denotes a decrease in alveolar ventilation with an attendant increase in PO_2 (both in the alveoli and in plasma). In acute respiratory acidosis, CO_2 is retained. In addition to a drop in pH and an increase in PO_2, patients are likely to demonstrate an increased level of bicarbonate and a decreased level of chloride, which is lost as the urine is acidified. Clinically, these patients are air-hungry, and their respiration is characterized by retractions and the use of accessory muscles. Cyanosis may be present. This scenario may be seen in upper or lower airway obstruction, ventilation/perfusion disturbances, inadequate perfusion, or respiratory failure. The goal of treatment is to provide adequate ventilation. HCO_3^- therapy is not efficacious because the elevated PCO_2 inhibits the shifting of the equation $H^+ + HCO_3^- \leftrightarrow H_2CO_3$ to the right.

4. RESPIRATORY ALKALOSIS

Respiratory alkalosis occurs when hyperventilation results in a decrease in PO_2. Patients describe tingling in the extremities, paresthesia, dizziness, and palpitations. Syncope may occur, and very occasionally tetany associated with hypocalcemia or even seizures may be seen. The hyperventilation is the result of central nervous system stimulation. Causes of respiratory alkalosis include hysteria, central nervous system irritation from meningitis or encephalitis, and salicylism. Treatment varies from providing a paper bag to facilitate rebreathing by the hysterical patient to increasing the dead space in a patient with a central nervous system anomaly who requires ventilation.

POTASSIUM DISORDERS

Maintenance of the appropriate potassium distribution and size of the body pool is maintained by the Na^+-K^+ pump at the cell membrane and by the kidney. Potassium is filtered by the glomerulus, reabsorbed in the proximal tubule, and excreted in the distal tubule. The kidney can either excrete or conserve K^+ readily, but secretion of potassium occurs via the mechanism that results in acidification of the urine. Therefore, potassium secretion depends on the body's Na^+ level and pH. The kidney cannot conserve K^+ on short notice. Adrenal corticosteroids promote Na^+ retention, whereas Addison's disease results in Na^+ loss and K^+ retention. The concentration of K^+ in the ECF is increased by acidemia, whereas alkalosis, hypochloremia, and glycogen deposition result in decreased levels of K^+ in the ECF. Alkalosis promotes the entry of K^+ into cells, whereas acidemia results in K^+ leaving cells and entering the ECF. Treatment of a diabetic in ketoacidosis results in a decrease in the serum potassium concentration ($[K^+]_s$) as the pH rises, and insulin administration results in glycogen deposition.

Potassium excretion continues for a significant period even if the intake of K^+ is decreased. By the time that a lowered urinary $[K^+]$ occurs, the body's K^+ pool has already been significantly depleted.

Diuretics, especially thiazides, acetazolamide, and mercurials, enhance the secretion of K^+. Aberrations in the concentration of potassium in the ECF alter myocardial contractility and can cause death from arrhythmia or cardiac standstill. When hypokalemia occurs with a loss of 10–20% of the body's potassium stores, apathy and muscle weakness occur. Occasionally, paresthesias are reported, and tetany may be seen. Further losses may result in flaccid paralysis and decreased respiration. Electrocardiographic changes associated with hypokalemia include T-wave depression, the appearance of U waves, ST-segment depression, and arrhythmia (see Figure 40–6). Arrhythmias associated with hypokalemia include premature ventricular contractions, atrial or nodal tachycardia, and ventricular tachycardia or fibrillation. Hypokalemia also heightens responsiveness to digitalis and may precipitate digitalis toxicity.

The first priority in the treatment of hypokalemia is maintaining an adequate concentration of K^+ in the serum. The magnitude of the total K^+ loss cannot be readily calculated because the vast majority of the body's K^+ is located intracellularly. Providing maintenance amounts of K^+ is usually sufficient to prevent problems. In those situations in which $[K^+]_s$ in the serum is dangerously low and K^+ must be administered intravenously, it is imperative that the patient have a cardiac monitor, and the physician must be prepared to treat any arrhythmias. Potassium should not be administered at a rate exceeding 0.5 meq/kg/h outside an intensive care unit.

Hyperkalemia is characterized by muscle weakness, occasional paresthesias and tetany, and ascending paralysis. Electrocardiographic changes associated with hyperkalemia include heightened T waves, widening of the QRS complex, and arrhythmias (see Figure 40–6). The arrhythmias seen with hyperkalemia include sinus bradycardia or sinus arrest, atrioventricular block, nodal or idioventricular rhythms, and ventricular tachycardia or fibrillation. The clinical severity of hyperkalemia depends on the electrocardiographic changes, the status of the other electrolytes, and the progression of the underlying disorder. If the $[K^+]_s$ is less than 6.5 meq/L, the physician seldom needs to do anything more than discontinue the administration of potassium. If potentiating factors (eg, hyponatremia, a brisk rise in $[K^+]_s$, alkalemia, digitalis toxicity, or renal failure) are present, one needs to be more aggressive. Any suggestions of a dysrhythmia must be evaluated and treated aggressively. A rhythm strip should be obtained immediately whenever significant hyperkalemia is suspected. If electrocardiographic changes or arrhythmias are present, treatment must be promptly initiated. Intravenous Ca^{2+}, usually administered as 10% calcium gluconate (0.2–0.5 mL/kg over 2–10 minutes), will briefly ameliorate depolarization. The calcium should be administered with a

Hypokalemia	Hyperkalemia
Apathy, muscle weakness, paresthesias, tetany	Ascending paralysis; occasional tetany and paresthesias, muscle weakness
Depressed T wave, U wave; ST-segment depression	Peaked T wave, prolonged PR interval, ST-segment depression, wide QRS complex
Arrhythmias	Arrhythmias
Premature beats	Sinus bradycardia
Atrial or nodal tachycardia	Atrioventricular block
Ventricular tachycardia or fibrillation	Idioventricular tachycardia or fibrillation
	Cardiac arrest

Figure 40–6. Clinical sequelae of hypokalemia and hyperkalemia.

cardiac monitor in place and should be discontinued immediately if bradycardia occurs. Administering Na^+ and increasing the pH with bicarbonate therapy will cause K^+ to move from the extracellular to the intracellular environment. The administration of insulin will result in glycogen deposition and a shift of K^+ to the intracellular environment. Insulin (0.1 U/kg/h) must be accompanied by glucose (approximately 3.5 g/U of insulin) to prevent hypoglycemia. Potassium may be removed by ion exchange resins, such as sodium polystyrene sulfonate (Kayexalate), which may be given orally or as a retention enema (0.2 g/kg orally or 1 g/kg as an enema). Because ion exchange is not rapid, other measures must be used simultaneously. Dialysis is efficacious, although it is costly and poses its own risks.

HYPERNATREMIA & HYPONATREMIA

Extreme care is required to treat hypernatremic dehydration successfully. The cellular space of the brain cannot equilibrate as rapidly as the ECF. If the $[Na^+]_s$ decreases too rapidly, the osmolality of the ECF drops more rapidly than that of the brain. As a result, water leaves the ECF and enters the brain to maintain osmotic neutrality. This shift can lead to cerebral edema, seizures, and death. To prevent this, the $[Na^+]_s$ should not drop more than about 15 meq/L in 24 hours. A drop in $[Na^+]_s$ of more than 1 meq/L/h should be avoided. To effect this gradual decrease in $[Na^+]_s$, the physician should order isotonic solutions to restore deficits in ECW. Electrolyte concentrations and serum osmolality must be monitored frequently. If metabolic acidosis is present, it must be corrected gradually to avoid central nervous system irritability. If hypernatremia has developed gradually and the ECF and blood urea nitrogen (BUN) are not significantly compromised, hypotonic solutions may be used for rehydration. However, the rate of fall of the serum sodium must not be greater than indicated above. This method involves very gradual administration of fluid and may not be of use if the degree of dehydration is significant and perfusion is altered. Alterations of blood glucose levels and BUN may contribute to the hyperosmolar state. Hyperglycemia is often seen in hypernatremic dehydration. Hyperglycemia should be monitored closely, since it may contribute significantly to the osmolal disequilibrium.

The typical symptoms and signs of dehydration are present in patients with hyponatremic dehydration. This form of dehydration brings the patient to medical attention rapidly because, in contrast to hypernatremic dehydration, the vascular space is selectively compromised as water leaves the vascular space to maintain osmotic neutrality.

The treatment of hyponatremic dehydration is straightforward. The magnitude of the sodium loss may be calculated by the following formula:

$$Na^+_{deficit} = [Na^+]_{desired} - [Na^+]_{observed} \times BW \times V_d$$

where BW = body weight (in kilograms) and V_d = volume of distribution. Similar formulas exist for calculating chloride and bicarbonate deficits.

The presence of hyponatremia without a deficit in the ECF is troublesome because it implies a change in osmotic regulation. In these situations, water restriction and treatment of the underlying defect are the primary keys to therapy.

Whenever there is a rapid decrease in serum osmolality, the central nervous system is at risk. Fluid shifts out of the vascular space and into the central nervous system may occur with intravenous water overload, with overly rapid dialysis, or in the treatment of diabetic ketoacidosis if glucose levels are allowed to drop precipitously. Nausea, vomiting, headaches, irritability, twitchiness, or neurologic changes should alert the physician to the possible presence of this disequilibrium syndrome, and steps should be taken to prevent central nervous system injury.

Although most patients tolerate a water load easily, patients with compromised renal function or an obstructive uropathy cannot. Such patients require fluid restriction in addition to treatment of the primary problem.

The syndrome of inappropriate secretion of ADH (SIADH) is also characterized by hyponatremia. SIADH may be seen in a wide variety of clinical settings, including meningitis, head injury, pneumonia, cystic fibrosis, intracranial tumors, stress, drugs (barbiturates and opiates), severe pain, and surgery. Patients with this syndrome pass small volumes of concentrated urine and experience thirst. For this reason, water is retained and $[Na^+]_s$ is decreased. Aldosterone secretion is eventually inhibited by the expansion of the ECF. The clinical manifestations of SIADH depend not only on the magnitude of the hyponatremia but also on the rapidity with which the syndrome evolved. The effective treatment of SIADH depends on fluid restriction.

In cases of severe water intoxication, a solution of 3% NaCl may be administered intravenously in the face of frank neurologic disturbances. This should be done to elevate the sodium only to a level at which seizures will not occur.

REHYDRATION

Because of the high worldwide incidence of dehydration caused by infantile diarrhea, the development of effective, inexpensive, technologically independent rehydration fluid has been a major priority. The demonstration of effective oral rehydration in developing countries has led to the introduction of easily administered oral rehydration solutions in developed nations.

The first solutions endorsed by the World Health Organization contained 90 meq/L of Na^+. This concentration was reasonable in areas with a high incidence of cholera, but such solutions may cause hypernatremia in patients who lose less Na^+ or who live in cooler areas, where insensible losses are not as great. In the United States today, a typical effective solution for oral rehydration of patients with mild to moderate dehydration contains 50–60 meq/L of Na^+, 20–30 meq/L of K^+, 30 meq/L of HCO_3^-, and enough chloride to provide electroneutrality. Glucose in a concentration of 2–3% provides adequate calories for the short term and facilitates absorption of electrolytes. Some manufacturers offer another oral rehydration formula with greater concentrations of sodium and chloride for more severe cases of dehydration.

Compromised perfusion (as evidenced by inadequate capillary refill, poor color, increased pulse, decreased urine output, or low blood pressure) constitutes an emergency that must be addressed at once. A 20-mL/kg bolus of fluid should be given intravenously as rapidly as possible. Either colloid or crystalloid may be used. The fluid may be administered intraosseously (the marrow space of the tibia is accessible) if no intravenous site is available. If there is no response to the first bolus, a second may be given. It is important to document urine formation and output.

The magnitude of electrolyte deficit may be estimated from tables such as those presented previously or in the case of hypotonic dehydration may be estimated from:

Deficit (meq) = [Desired concentration – observed concentration] $\times$ BW $\times$ V_d

where BW = body weight (in kilograms) and V_d = volume of distribution. Potassium defects must be estimated because potassium is primarily an intracellular ion, so the serum concentration does not reflect the balance of the ion in the body.

Typically, one-half the previous deficits are administered in the first 8 hours of therapy, and the remainder are given over the next 16 hours. Maintenance needs are provided at a steady rate. Ongoing losses are analyzed as needed and replaced at a steady rate as well. If the patient is unable to eat for a prolonged period, nutritional needs must be anticipated and met through either enteral nutrition or hyperalimentation.

The treatment of hypertonic dehydration presents special problems, as previously discussed. It is currently popular to use hypotonic solutions to treat patients with hypertonic/hypernatremic dehydration. A number of formulas have been developed to estimate the free water loss in such cases. These are similar to the formula shown for the calculation of electrolyte deficits in hypotonic dehydration, with an additional factor such as $[Na^+]_{observed}/[Na^+]_{desired}$ added to account for the effect of the increased concentration of sodium on the ECF. A popular guideline is the estimate that 4 mL/kg of free water will lower the serum sodium concentration by 1 meq/L in cases of hypertonic dehydration. The real key to successfully treating patients with these disorders is meticulous monitoring and attention to the patient's clinical response.

It is, unfortunately, fashionable simply to provide twice the maintenance fluids needed and to assume that time will cure the problem that precipitated the dehydration. This prevents early detection of secondary problems, such as fluid shifts or deficits caused by ongoing losses. By calculating deficits and needs, the physician can monitor the efficacy of therapy as the patient is being treated.

REFERENCES

Holliday MA, Segar WE: The maintenance need for water in parenteral fluid therapy. Pediatrics 1957;19:823.

Ichikawa I (editor): *Pediatric Textbook of Fluids & Electrolytes.* Williams & Wilkins, 1990.

Schrier RW (editor): *Renal and Electrolyte Disorders,* 4th ed. Little, Brown, 1992.

Winters RW (editor): *The Body Fluids in Pediatrics.* Little, Brown, 1973.

41

Drug Therapy

Christopher M. Paap, PharmD, BCPS

INTRODUCTION

Drug therapy in pediatric patients can be a rational and safe process when the concepts of developmental physiology, physical assessment, and pharmacology are understood and taken into consideration. Treatment must be carefully based on the patient's acuity and physical examination, the pharmacology of the therapies being considered, and the desired outcome. This chapter provides a systematic approach to the optimal use of drugs in pediatric patients.

DEVELOPING A PEDIATRIC DRUG REGIMEN

Drug Selection

A. Patient-Specific Factors: Patient age is one of the most important parameters to consider when developing a drug therapy regimen. Both the physiologic and the psychological age should significantly influence the drug selection, route of administration, dosing regimen, and monitoring parameters. Physiologic factors such as the inability of newborns and infants to reliably absorb oral medications limit this route of administration. Psychological issues are more important when considering treatment in older children and adolescents or when the parents of a young child have limited cognitive functioning. The ability of the patient or parent to accurately use a drug therapy can affect its efficacy and safety. Examples of physiologic and psychological factors to keep in mind when selecting drug therapy are given in Table 41–1.

Since nearly all drugs are eliminated from the body by the liver and kidneys, organ function should be assessed both before selecting drug therapy and during the treatment course. Renal function can be easily assessed by monitoring serum creatinine concentrations to estimate glomerular filtration rate (GFR), also known as creatinine clearance (CLcr) (equation 1).

$$\text{Clcr} = \frac{0.48 \times \text{Ht(cm)}}{\text{Serum creatinine}} = \text{mL/min/1.73m}^2 \quad (1)$$

Since there is a lack of data regarding drug dosage adjustment in children with renal dysfunction, generalization from the adult literature is commonly done. Since the GFR calculated from equation 1 is based on body surface area (BSA), extrapolation from the adult literature can be more reliably assumed. It is also important to recognize that many of the metabolites of drugs that are primarily degraded by liver enzyme systems are ultimately excreted by the kidneys and can accumulate in patients with renal dysfunction. Assessment of liver function is difficult clinically. Decreased drug metabolism via the liver has not been correlated with elevated transaminases (AST/ALT) or decreased albumin. In late stages of liver dysfunction, changes in bleeding times (prothrombin time/partial thromboplastin time [PT/PTT]) are strong indicators that hepatic drug metabolism may be impaired. However, this cannot be reliably quantified. Therefore, close monitoring for drug toxicity is necessary when decreased hepatic metabolism is suspected in patients being treated with hepatically metabolized drugs. Table 41–2 lists some commonly used drugs and their primary route of elimination.

The acuity of the patient should always be taken into consideration when determining appropriate drug therapy regimens. Children who appear toxic warrant more aggressive therapy, which may include multiple drug therapies, invasive administration procedures (eg, intravenous [IV]), and close monitoring (hospitalization). Likewise, children with conditions characterized by a limited physiologic reserve can deteriorate more rapidly, and a more aggressive drug therapy regimen should be considered. Alternatively, drug therapy may not be appropriate when the child has mild symptoms, such that the side effects of treatment may be worse than the disease (eg, decongestant use in infants with a cold).

As the child's acuity changes, so should the drug therapy regimen. After a child has responded to an initial treatment regimen, the drug therapy plan should be reevaluated and adjusted to meet the changing needs of the patient. Table 41–3 provides several examples of acuity changes that may indicate the need for a change in drug therapy.

Table 41–1. Physiologic and psychological factors that can affect drug therapy.

Factors	Drug and Interactions
Physiologic	
Hyperbilirubinemia	Drugs such as ceftriaxone or sulfisoxazole can displace bilirubin and induce kernicterus in newborns.
Newborn immaturity	
GI malabsorption	Oral antibiotics are unreliably absorbed during the first month of life, but may otherwise be useful in older infants and children.
Renal insufficiency	Renally eliminated drugs such as the penicillins and aminoglycosides in newborns require extended dosing intervals.
Hepatic insufficiency	Hepatically eliminated drugs such as phenobarbital, morphine, and diazepam require lower doses and extended intervals.
Malnutrition (decreased albumin)	Drugs such a phenytoin, warfarin, and ibuprofen can have enhanced pharmacologic action due to decreased protein binding and increased "free" drug concentrations.
Short bowel syndrome	Oral medications of all types can have erratic absorption when the amount of bowel available to absorb the drug is reduced.
Cerebral palsy or mental retardation	Drugs such as narcotics, anticonvulsants, and anticholinergics can produce central nervous system side effects which are difficult to recognize.
Psychological	
Addictive personality	Older children or parents given narcotics, stimulants, or tranquillizers such as codeine, methylphenidate, or diazepam may abuse or misuse these drugs at home.
Limited cognitive functioning	Decreased understanding of directions, indications, or monitoring of drug therapy can lead to noncompliance or delayed recognition of side effects.

B. Drug-Specific Factors:

Therapeutic index (ratio of maximum tolerated dose to minimum curative dose)–Individualization of drug therapy requires specific knowledge about the patient and the potential drug treatment alternatives. The therapeutic index of a particular drug therapy identifies the relative benefits and risks of a selected drug regimen. Drugs with a wide therapeutic index have a greater margin of safety than drugs with a narrow therapeutic index. The therapeutic index can be visualized by examining the relation between a drug's therapeutic effect and its toxic effect in terms of blood concentration (Figure 41–1). If a choice exists between a drug with a wide therapeutic index and one with a narrow therapeutic index, the wide therapeutic index is preferred. Examples of drugs with wide and narrow therapeutic indices are given in Table 41–4.

Compliance

Drug therapy can be successful only if the patient is amenable to it. Factors that affect compliance with drug regimens deserve careful consideration. Since many patients (about 50% of children) do not have comprehensive medical insurance, if the prescribed medication is expensive, the prescription may never be filled. Also, in the managed-care setting, formulary restrictions (which are largely cost-driven) may limit drug therapy selection. In pediatric dosing, the palatability and frequency of administration affect compliance. Finally, drugs that have undesirable side effects have lower compliance rates (eg, erythromycin and stomach upset). Although efficacy of the drug therapy is of major importance, the drug regimen is effective only if the patient takes it as prescribed.

Drug Dosing

A. Methods Based on Weight: Nearly every drug that has been safely used in pediatric patients has an established milligram per kilogram (mg/kg) dosing range. Drug dosing based on a child's weight in kilograms is simple, convenient, and widely accepted. Depending on the therapeutic index of the drug, dosing may fall within a range or require a specific initial dose (see Figure 41–1; Table 41–5). In

Table 41–2. Primary route of elimination for drugs commonly used in pediatrics.

Renal Elimination	Hepatic Elimination
Penicillins	Anticonvulsants (phenytoin, carbamazepine)
Cephalosporins	
Aminoglycosides	Acetaminophen
Digoxin	Theophylline
Ranitidine and cimetidine	Antidepressants (imipramine, fluoxetine)
	Steroids (anti-inflammatory and hormonal)
Furosemide	Opiate narcotics (morphine, codeine)
Fluconazole	Benzodiazepines (diazepam, lorazepam)
Acyclovir	Erythromycin
	Clindamycin

Table 41–3. Effect of changing clinical acuity on drug selection.

Initial Acuity Level	Subsequent Acuity Level	Impact on Drug Selection
Serious bacterial infection with lethargy, decreased oral intake, and fever	Resolving fever, increased oral intake, normal playful activities	Initial therapy with intravenous medication(s) may be switched to oral.
Mild bacterial infection with low-grade fever, cough, and sore throat	Persistant fever, decreased activity, focal signs of infection, worsened cough and tachypnea	Initial oral therapy may be switched to intravenous therapy and hospitalization.
Wheezing patient with asthma, with tachypnea, dyspnea, and retractions requiring supplemental oxygen	Asthma, wheezing with normal respiratory rate, breathing room air	Initial aggressive nebulization and intravenous corticosteroids may be switched to metered-dose inhaler and oral/inhaled corticosteroids.
Active generalized seizure	No seizure activity for 24–48 h	Change from intravenous to oral therapy with same or different anticonvulsant.

general, drugs with a wide therapeutic index have wider dosing ranges, and dose rounding to a standard dose (eg, amoxicillin, 250 mg rather than 236 mg) is recommended.

Drugs with a narrow therapeutic index should be dosed based on the specific mg/kg dosing guidelines and adjusted during therapy with careful therapeutic drug monitoring. Frequent recalculation of dosages should be incorporated into the care of children who are on long-term drug therapy, since their growth will eventually necessitate increased dosages.

There are specific dosing recommendations for the most commonly prescribed drugs in children throughout the various chapters of this book. Other resources for mg/kg dosing guidelines are provided here in the section on Pediatric Drug Information. In older children over 40–50 kg, in whom pediatric doses based on body weight might exceed the normal adult dose, it is recommended that the normal adult dosage be used as the upper limit to prevent toxicity and still maintain desired efficacy.

B. Methods Based on BSA: Drug dosing based on BSA may be more accurate, but it is more difficult and has not been shown to have clear advantages over mg/kg dosing. Many drugs with a narrow therapeutic index have dosing guidelines based on patient BSA. There are several different methods for estimating BSA. The nomogram in Figure 41–2 is simple to use. An equation can be easily programmed into a calculator or a computerized database spreadsheet to produce a rapid estimate of BSA for a medical record (equation 2).

$$\text{BSA (m}^2\text{)} = \text{wt (kg)}^{0.51436} \times \text{ht (cm)}^{0.42246} \times 0.0235 \quad (2)$$

Some drugs have both mg/kg- and BSA-based dosing recommendations (eg, acyclovir), and the calculated dosages by the two methods can be discrepant. There are limited data evaluating the differences in efficacy and safety of drugs dosed by each method; however, many clinicians believe that dosing based on the BSA is a more accurate method.

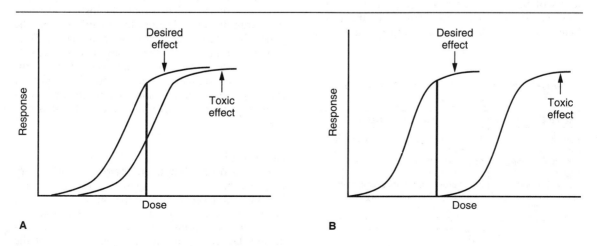

Figure 41–1. Graphs of therapeutic index defined as the difference between desired (therapeutic) effect and toxic effect of a drug at a given dose. **A:** Narrow therapeutic index. **B:** Wide therapeutic index.

Table 41–4. Therapeutic indices of selected drugs.

Wide[1]	Narrow[2]
Penicillins	Aminoglycosides
Cephalosporins	Anticonvulsants
Acetaminophen	Cancer chemotherapy agents
Ibuprofen	Catecholamines (dopamine, epi-
Decongestants and	nephrine)
antihistamines	Amphotericin B
Sucralfate	Opiate narcotics (morphine, codeine)
Benzodiazepines	Heparin and warfarin
Ranitidine and	Lidocaine
cimetidine	Digoxin
	Theophylline

[1]Relatively safe; can round doses.
[2]Increased toxicity; requires specific dosing.

Although extrapolation of adult doses to pediatric patients is not recommended, this is best done by dosage adjustment on the basis of BSA (equation 3).

$$\text{Approximate dose for child} \atop (\text{mg/dose or mg/d}) =$$

$$\frac{\text{BSA of child (m}^2)}{1.73 \text{ m}^2 \text{ (normal BSA for adult)}} \times \frac{\text{Average adult dose}}{(\text{mg/dose or mg/d})} \quad (3)$$

C. Individualization: Many factors can affect a patient's response to a medication, and individualized dosage adjustments may be necessary to achieve the desired response or outcome. Drugs that require

Table 41–5. Therapeutic blood levels.[1]

Drug	Expressed as Fraction of g/mL	Expressed as Fraction of mol/L (SI Units)
Acetaminophen	10–20 µg/mL[2]	65–130 µmol/L
Amikacin	15–30 µg/mL (peak) < 5 µg/mL (trough)	
Aspirin	150–300 µg/mL	1–2.2 mmol/L
Carbamazepine	4–12 µg/mL	16–48 µmol/L
Chloramphenicol	15–25 µg/mL	40–75 µmol/L
Digoxin	0.9–2.4 ng/mL	1–2 nmol/L
Ethanol	1000 µg/mL	20 mmol/L
Ethosuximide	40–100 µg/mL	280–700 µmol/L
5-Flucytosine	<100 µg/mL <80 µg/mL in newborns and infants	
Gentamicin	6–10 µg/mL (peak) <2 µg/mL (trough)	
Lidocaine	<100 ng/mL (newborn) 1.5–2.5 µg/mL (adult)	<0.4 µmol/L (newborn) 6–9 µmol/L (adult)
Methsuximide as the metabolite of N-des-methsuximide	10–40 µg/mL	50–200 µmol/L
Phenobarbital	15–40 µg/mL	60–160 µmol/L
Phenytoin	10–20 µg/mL	40–80 µmol/L
Primidone	4–12 µg/mL	20–55 µmol/L
Procainamide	4–6 µg/mL	15–20 nmol/L
Quinidine	3–5 µg/mL	10–15 µmol/L
Theophylline	5–20 µg/mL	25–110 µmol/L
Tobramycin	6–10 µg/mL (peak) <2 µg/mL (trough)	17–21 µmol/L (peak)
Valproic acid	50–120 µg/mL	350–800 µmol/L
Vancomycin	20–40 µg/mL (peak) 4–12 µg/mL (trough)	

[1]Therapeutic level or range for drugs that can be routinely analyzed.

Figure 41–2. Body surface area: Children. To determine the body surface area in a child, use a straight edge to connect the height and mass. The point of intersection on the body surface line gives the area in m². (Reproduced with permission from *Geigy Scientific Tables,* 8th ed, vol. 1. Lentner C ed: CIBA-Geigy;1981.)

routine blood concentration monitoring should have doses adjusted to achieve therapeutic and nontoxic concentrations (see Table 41–5). Three important pharmacokinetic principles govern appropriate individualization of drug doses based on blood concentration determinations.

First is the concept of **steady state,** which is the time it takes for the drug concentration to reach its equilibrium in the body and is directly related to the elimination half-life of the drug. In general, a drug is considered to be at steady state after it has been continuously administered at the same dosage and interval (eg, gentamicin, 25 mg/8 h) for at least five half-lives. For some drugs, the half-life may be short (eg, gentamicin half-life—2–4 h), and steady state is achieved in 1 day. Some drugs have a long half-life (eg, phenobarbital half-life—24–36 h) and require

days to weeks to achieve steady state. Interpreting drug levels and making dosage adjustments on the basis of blood concentrations that are not at steady state can lead to overdosing and toxicity. Likewise, after a dosage adjustment has been made, a new steady state must be achieved and an additional five half-lives are needed before rechecking the blood concentration.

A second principle is the "linear" relation between blood concentration of the drug and dosing rate and body clearance (equation 4).

$$\begin{array}{l} \text{Drug} \\ \text{Concentration} \\ \text{(mg/L, μg/mL)} \end{array} = \dfrac{\begin{array}{c}\text{Dosing rate}\\ \text{(mg/d, mg/kg/d, etc)}\end{array}}{\begin{array}{c}\text{Total body clearance}\\ \text{(renal and hepatic)}\\ \text{(mL/d, mL/kg/d, etc)}\end{array}} \quad (4)$$

The blood concentration of a given drug is directly related to the dosing rate at steady state. Therefore, if a steady-state blood concentration is 50% of that desired, doubling the dosage will achieve the desired concentration after it achieves its new steady state.

A third concept is the "nonlinear" relation between clearance, dosing rate, and blood concentration, which exists for a select group of drugs (salicylates, ethanol, phenytoin, and theophylline). These drugs do not have predictable correlation between dosing rate and steady-state blood concentration and require close drug monitoring by clinicians experienced with their pharmacokinetics (Figure 41–3).

Dosage individualization and close monitoring of drug concentrations can also be useful in evaluating suspected malabsorption of oral medications. This is encountered during long-term therapy in which oral drugs are preferred, such as in the treatment of HIV, osteomyelitis, and seizure disorders. Assessment of oral drug absorption by means of blood concentration monitoring allows for safe dose escalation to overcome decreased absorption.

D. Routes of Administration:

1. Oral route–Oral administration is the easiest, least expensive, and most convenient route of drug administration in children. Oral therapy is not appropriate in very young infants less than 1–2 months of age or in children with short bowel syndrome because of unpredictable bioavailability (absorption). Oral therapy is also inappropriate in a severely ill child. When oral therapy is indicated and desired, the appropriate dosage form for the age of the child should be selected. Oral suspensions and liquids are available for many medications and are preferred for infants and young children, although most adolescents prefer tablets and capsules. A number of drugs are not available in a liquid from the manufacturer but can be compounded by pharmacies (Table 41–6).

Table 41–6. Common drugs that can be compounded into suspensions or liquids for oral administration.

Azathioprine	Metolazone
Baclofen	Metronidazole
Caffeine	Midazolam
Captopril	Ondansetron
Cisapride	Rifampin
Clonazepam	Spironolactone
Lorazepam	Verapamil

There are several "sprinkle" formulations, which can be sprinkled onto food and used for infants on baby foods or for older children. Chewable tablets can be given to young children when they have molar teeth to crush the tablets in their mouth (generally 12–18 months).

Oral medication absorption can be affected by dietary factors and should be considered when selecting and monitoring oral drug therapy. Recommendations for the administration of oral drugs with or without food are specific for each drug and should be followed. Drugs that require administration on an empty stomach generally have significantly decreased absorption when given with food, and these recommendations should be closely adhered to. The recommendation that a drug be administered with food is generally made to decrease gastrointestinal upset associated with the drug and not to improve absorption. Thus, most drugs can be taken on an empty stomach to achieve therapeutic response, but some are best administered with food to decrease gastrointestinal complaints.

2. Rectal route–Rectal administration of medications should be reserved for children who cannot take oral medications. It is important to stress to the parent or child the need to remove the wrapping from suppositories prior to insertion. Incomplete dose administration can occur if the suppository does not remain in the rectum for sufficient time. Drug distribution within a suppository may not be uniform and therefore administering half of a suppository may not provide half the dose, leading to either a subtherapeutic or a toxic response in the child.

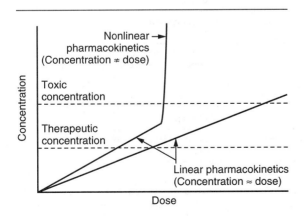

Figure 41–3. Differences between linear and nonlinear concentration-dose profiles. Drugs with nonlinear pharmacokinetics can produce unexpected toxic concentrations with only small incremental changes in dose.

Table 41–7. Duration of an adequate therapeutic trial for commonly prescribed drugs in pediatrics.

Drug	Length of Trial
Albuterol (inhaled)	Response generally occurs within the first 12 hours of starting therapy.
Antibacterial antibiotics	Response generally occurs within 48–72 hours after starting therapy.
Corticosteroids (inhaled)	Maximal response takes 1–2 weeks of continuous therapy.
Antidepressants	Maximal response takes 3–6 weeks of continuous therapy.

Table 41–8. Monitoring parameters for organ toxicities from drug therapy.

Organ-Specific Toxicity	Parameters
Gastrointestinal	Frequency of nausea, vomiting, diarrhea, cramping, abdominal pain, and decrease in oral intake
Renal	Blood urea nitrogen (BUN), creatinine, urinalysis (casts, enzymes, electrolytes), urine output
Hepatic	Liver function tests (AST/ALT/bilirubin/alk phos); sclera coloring, bleeding times (PT/PTT), nausea, vomiting, pruritis, mental status, jaundice, liver size
Neurologic	Lethargy, anxiety, irritability, orientation, hallucinations, confusion, mental status
Dermatologic	Type of rash (eg, macular, papular, vesicular), location and extent, itching, temporal onset
Hematologic	Complete blood count with differential, bleeding time (PT/PTT), platelet count, bruising, infection

3. Parenteral route–Intravenous administration of drugs is the most reliable method of delivery and is preferred in severely ill children. Many physical incompatibilities have been identified with the coadministration of IV medications and maintenance fluids. If an incompatibility is suspected, a pharmacist should be contacted for documentation and management of the incompatibility. The site of drug administration into an IV line should be as proximal to the patient as possible, particularly in infants who have maintenance fluid flow rates of less than 40 mL/h, because significant delay in drug delivery can occur from more distal sites in the IV system.

Monitoring Drug Therapy

A. Efficacy: The efficacy of a particular drug regimen should be continuously evaluated throughout the treatment. Resolution of patient-specific signs and symptoms are excellent indicators of effective therapy. The drug therapy must be given an adequate trial before it is considered ineffective and a change in treatment considered. The time course of response to therapy defines an adequate therapeutic trial. Several examples are given in Table 41–7.

B. Safety: Monitoring the safety of a drug regimen requires knowledge of the specific toxicities of the prescribed medication and continuous evaluation of the patient for signs and symptoms of these toxicities. Toxicities are generally categorized by organ

Table 41–9. Common pediatric drugs associated with drug interactions.

Drug	Potential Interaction	Comments
Carbamazepine	Increases hepatic metabolism of other drugs causing decreased levels	Can increase its own metabolism. Has an active epoxide metabolite.
Phenobarbital	Increases hepatic metabolism of other drugs causing decreased levels	No effect on phenytoin. Primidone is metabolized to phenobarbital and can cause similar interactions.
Phenytoin	Increases hepatic metabolism of other drugs causing decreased levels	Has nonlinear pharmacokinetics.
Rifampin	Increases hepatic metabolism of other drugs causing decreased levels	Rapid onset. Can occur with 4 day prophylaxis regimens. Decreases efficacy of oral contraceptives.
Erythromycin Clarithromycin	Decreases hepatic metabolism of other drugs causing increased levels	Erythromycin is a component of Pediazole suspension; can use azithromycin as alternative without interactions
Cimetidine	Decreases hepatic metabolism of other drugs causing increased levels	Can use ranitidine or famotidine as alternatives without interactions
Valproate	Decreases hepatic metabolism of other drugs causing increased levels	
Antacids	Increases gastric pH and decreases oral absorption of some drugs	All H_2 blockers can cause the same interaction. Decreases ketoconazole and itraconazole absorption.
Mg^{2+}, Ca^{2+}, and Fe^{2+} salts	Bind to some drugs and inactivate or decrease oral absorption	Tetracyclines and fluoroquinolones should not be given within 2 hours of these salts.

Table 41–10. Important drug information resources for pediatric practitioners.

Resource	Information Content
Harriet Lane Handbook (Johns Hopkins Hospital and Year Book Medical Publishers)	Drug dosing for standard indications; some side effects information. Available dosage forms; plenty of other useful clinical information not related to drug therapy. Pocket size.
Pediatric Dosing Handbook (American Pharmaceutical Association and Lexicomp Publishing)	Comprehensive dosing and side effect information. Available dosage forms, drug interactions, and pharmacokinetics; useful appendices. Pocket size.
American Hospital Formulary Service (American Society of Health-System Pharmacists)	Most pediatric dosing, comprehensive side effects, dosage forms, drug interactions, and pharmacokinetics. Large book.
Physicians' Desk Reference (Medical Economics)	Incomplete or no pediatric dosing for many drugs. Little or no pediatric pharmacokinetics or side effects. Contains available dosage forms. Large book.
Drugs During Pregnancy and Lactation (Williams & Wilkins)	"The book" on drug use during pregnancy and lactation. No dosing, but well referenced with primary literature. Large book.

system effects. Monitoring parameters for specific organ system dysfunction is summarized in Table 41–8. It is important for clinicians to have appropriate drug information resources available to identify drug-specific toxicities (see Table 41–10).

C. Drug Interactions: When a patient is receiving multiple drug therapies, it is important to evaluate these regimens for clinically important drug interactions. Drug interactions can occur among several drugs or between drugs and food. Table 41–9 lists several common drug interactions that occur in pediatric patients (see also Table 41–10). Drug interactions are not a contraindication for the use of interacting drugs. With appropriate identification and drug therapy adjustment, interacting drug regimens can be safely used.

D. Endpoints: When drug therapy is initiated, a desired therapeutic endpoint should be identified. After the desired endpoint has been reached, drug therapy should be reevaluated for discontinuation or for establishment of a new endpoint. The benefits of treatment must always be weighed against the relative risks of the drug therapy to optimize outcome and reduce drug-related complications.

PEDIATRIC DRUG INFORMATION

The Pharmacist

Pharmacists, particularly pharmacists who practice in a pediatric care environment, are extremely useful sources of drug information. They often know drug doses and side effects as well as practical issues regarding the appropriate therapeutic uses of pharmaceuticals. Their services are usually at no cost and are available 24 hours per day 7 days per week. Also, pharmacists usually have current drug information resources.

Reference Books

Table 41–10 summarizes several useful drug references. Clinicians who care for pediatric patients should be familiar with these resources.

Computer Sources

There is a trend toward computerized drug information databases in institutional and managed-care settings, which allow for the rapid retrieval of current drug information. Several of these databases also provide specific citations from the primary literature from which the information is derived. Access to these powerful drug information resources will facilitate rapid development of drug therapy decisions. Several examples of such databases are Drugdex from Micromedex, Inc, and Clinical Pharmacology from Gold Standard.

REFERENCES

Gelman CR, Rumack BH (editors): *DRUGDEX Information Systems.* Micromedex, 1995.

Radde IC, MacLeod SM: *Pediatric Pharmacology & Therapeutics,* 2nd ed. CV Mosby, 1993.

Yaffe SJ, Aranda JV: *Pediatric Pharmacology,*. WB Saunders, 1992.

42

Normal Biochemical & Hematologic Values

Keith B. Hammond, MS, FIMLS

Pediatricians and other health professionals caring for children have the responsibility to insist on accurate, rapid, and comprehensive laboratory testing. Collecting large blood samples for biochemical assay is not suitable for the proper care of children—especially for premature infants or older children in intensive care, where repetitive sampling may be essential. Technology for performing biochemical assays on blood samples of 100 μL or less has been available for 30 years or more. Most of the earlier automated systems for assay were better adapted to larger samples. However, the newest automated systems have the capacity to work with small volumes.

In infants and young children, blood samples taken by heel-prick are better collected by laboratory personnel than by physicians or nurses.

INTERPRETATION OF LABORATORY VALUES

Accreditation by the College of American Pathologists and by state or federal agencies has done much to ensure standardized laboratory performance. Methods used in various laboratories differ, as do normal values for the methods. Normal range is, of course, a combination of biologic variation and intrinsic laboratory variation; thus, an acceptable range of normal values should ideally be composed of data developed within the laboratory for the population it serves. Any laboratory should be able to provide information on the coefficient of variation and standard deviation applicable to each test performed in that laboratory. Each laboratory should maintain a rigorous procedure of checks with daily standards and control specimens. Errors may still occur but can usually be detected by retesting before a questionable result is reported. Fortunately, errors occur much less commonly today than in the past.

The clinical value of a test is related to its sensitivity and specificity. Sensitivity is an expression of the incidence of positive test results in those who have the disease. Specificity is an expression of the incidence of negative test results in those free of the disease. Sensitivity and specificity are calculated as follows:

$$\text{Sensitivity (\%)} = \frac{TP}{TP + FN} \times 100$$

(ie, how many TP are missed)

$$\text{Specificity (\%)} = \frac{TN}{TN + FP} \times 100$$

(ie, how many TN are missed)

where TP = a true-positive result, FP = a false-positive result, TN = a true-negative result, and FN = a false-negative result.

Screening tests must be interpreted with appreciation of sensitivity and specificity. These expressions are illustrated in Figure 42–1 in terms of a screening test for phenylketonuria in newborns. The values are not strictly correct but serve the purpose of illustration. According to Figure 42–1, a blood phenylalanine level of 4 mg/dL is the discriminating point above which all infants are presumed to have the disease and below which they are presumed to be normal. However, no test is ever quite that exact. Some normal infants will have levels above 4 mg/dL; the test results in these will be false-positive. Some abnormal infants will have levels below 4 mg/dL; the test results in these will be false-negative. The discriminating point is a compromise between sensitivity and specificity. Moving the point to 2 mg/dL would effect 100% sensitivity, but there would be a large increase in the number of false-positive results. Moving it to 6 mg/dL would make it very specific, but this would increase the number of false-negative responses, which would result in failure to detect phenylketonuria in a much larger proportion of affected children.

These concepts can be viewed in yet another way. Suppose that this test were set at a specificity of 99.9%. This would mean that in a sample of 10,000 tests, there would be 10 false-positive results. In a rare condition such as phenylketonuria, however, the true incidence of the disease may be only 1 in

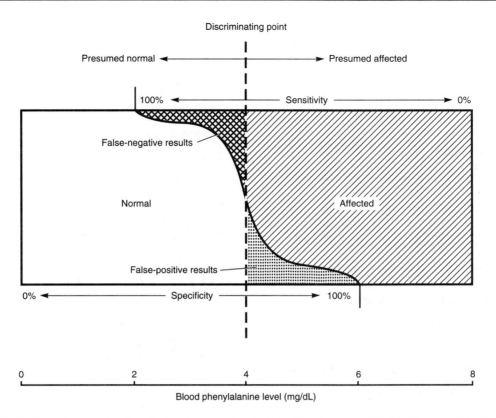

Figure 42–1. Screening test for phenylketonuria in newborns. Data have been simplified to illustrate the concepts of sensitivity and specificity (see text).

12,000. The ratio of true-positive to false-positive results is thus 1:12; this is a reflection of the low incidence of the disease and the relatively high incidence of false-positive results because of the nature of the assay. These considerations, of course, apply to the interpretation of all laboratory tests.

LABORATORY VALUES

Normal blood chemistry values and miscellaneous other laboratory values are shown in Tables 42–1 to 42–3.

Table 42–1. Normal blood chemistry values and miscellaneous other hematologic values.[1]
(Values may vary with the procedure used.)

Determinations for	
(S) = Serum	(P) = Plasma
(B) = Whole blood	(RBC) = Red blood cells

Acid-Base Measurements (B)
pH: 7.38–7.42 from 14 min of age and older
PaO_2: 65–76 mm Hg (8.66–10.13 kPa)
$PaCO_2$: 36–38 mm Hg (4.8–5.07 kPa)
Base excess: –2 to +2 meq/L, except in newborns (range, –4 to –0)

Acid Phosphatase (S, P)
Values using *p*-nitrophenyl phosphate buffered with citrate (end-point determination)
Newborns: 7.4–19.4 IU/L at 37 °C
2–13 y: 6.4–15.2 IU/L at 37 °C
Adult males: 0.5–11 IU/L at 37 °C
Adult females: 0.2–9.5 IU/L at 37 °C

Alanine Aminotransferase (ALT, SGPT) (S)
Newborns (1–3 d): 1–25 IU/L at 37 °C
Adult males: 7–46 IU/L at 37 °C
Adult females: 4–35 IU/L at 37 °C

Alkaline Phosphatase (S)
Values in IU/L at 37 °C using *p*-nitrophenyl phosphate buffered with AMP (kinetic)

Group	Males	Females
Newborns (1–3 d)	95–368	95–368
2–24 mo	115–460	115–460
2–5 y	115–391	115–391
6–7 y	115–460	115–460
8–9 y	115–345	115–345
10–11 y	115–336	115–437
12–13 y	127–403	92–336
14–15 y	79–446	78–212
16–18 y	58–331	35–124
Adults	41–137	39–118

Ammonia (P)
Newborns: 90–150 µg/dL (53–88 µmol/L); higher in premature and jaundiced infants
Thereafter: 0–60 µg/dL (0–35 µmol/L) when blood is drawn with proper precautions

Amylase (S)
Values using maltotetrose substrate (kinetic)
Neonates: Undetectable
2–12 mo: Levels increase slowly to adult levels
Adults: 28–108 IU/L at 37 °C

Anticoagulation Factors (P)
Values in U/mL. Shown are mean values and –2 SD or lower range (in parentheses)

Factor	Preterm (25–32 wk)	Term Infant	Infant (6 mo)	Adult
AT III	0.35 (0.20)	0.56 (0.32)	1.04 (0.84)	1.0 (0.8)
PC	0.29 (0.20)	0.50 (0.30)	0.59 (0.37)	1.0 (0.6)
PS, total	. . .	0.24 (0.10)	0.87 (0.55)	1.0 (0.6)
PS, free	0.48	0.42	. . .	1.0 (0.5)
HcF II	0.25 (0.10)	0.49 (0.36)	0.97 (0.59)	1.0 (0.7)

AT III = antithrombin III, PC = protein C, PS = protein S, Hcf II = heparin cofactor II.

α_1-Antitrypsin (antiprotease) (S)
1–3 mo: 127–404 mg/dL
3–12 mo: 145–362 mg/dL
1–2 y: 160–382 mg/dL
2–15 y: 148–394 mg/dL

Ascorbic Acid: See Vitamin C.

Aspartate Aminotransferase (AST, SGOT) (S)
Newborns (1–3 d): 16–74 IU/L at 37 °C
Adult males: 8–46 IU/L at 37 °C
Adult females: 7–34 IU/L at 37 °C

Base Excess: See Acid-Base Measurements.

Bicarbonate, Actual (P)
Calculated from pH and $PaCO_2$
Newborns: 17.2–23.6 mmol/L
2 mo–2 y: 19–24 mmol/L
Children: 18–25 mmol/L
Adult males: 20.1–28.9 mmol/L
Adult females: 18.4–28.8 mmol/L

Bilirubin (S)
Values in mg/dL (µmol/L)
Levels after 1 mo are as follows:
Conjugated: 0–0.3 mg/dL (0–5 µmol/L)
Unconjugated: 0.1–0.7 mg/dL (2–12 µmol/L)

Peak Newborn Level	Percentage of Newborns (Birth Weight) Exceeding Peak Level		
	<2001 g	2001–2500 g	>2500 g
20 (342)	8.2%	2.6%	0.8%
18 (308)	13.5%	4.6%	1.5%
16 (274)	20.3%	7.6%	2.6%
14 (239)	33.0%	12.0%	4.4%
11(188)	53.8%	23.0%	9.3%
8 (137)	77.0%	45.4%	26.1%

Bleeding Time (Simplate)
2–9 min

Blood Volume
Premature infants: 98 mL/kg
At 1 y: 86 mL/kg (range, 69–112 mL/kg)
Older children: 70 mL/kg (range, 51–86 mL/kg)

BUN: See Urea Nitrogen.

C Peptide (S)
5–15 y (8:00 AM fasting): 1–4 ng/mL
Adults (8:00 AM fasting): <4 ng/mL
Adults (nonfasting): <8 ng/mL

C-Reactive Protein (S)
3–16 y: 0.1–1.5 mg/dL

(*continued*)

Table 42–1. Normal blood chemistry values and miscellaneous other hematologic values.[1]
(Values may vary with the procedure used.) (continued)

Calcium, Ionized (P)
  0–2 d: 1.1–1.4 mmol/L
  3–4 d: 1.1–1.5 mmol/L
  5–8 d: 1.2–1.5 mmol/L
  9–14 d: 1.3–1.6 mmol/L
  2 mo–18 y: 1.2–1.4 mmol/L

Calcium, Total (S)
  Premature infants (first week): 3.5–4.5 meq/L (1.7–2.3 mmol/L)
  Full-term infants (first week): 4–5 meq/L (2–2.5 mmol/L)
  Thereafter: 4.4–5.3 meq/L (2.2–2.7 mmol/L)

Carbon Dioxide, Total (S, P)
  Cord blood: 15–20.2 mmol/L
  Children: 18–27 mmol/L
  Adults: 24–35 mmol/L

Cation-Anion Gap (S, P)
  5–15 mmol/L

Ceruloplasmin (Copper Oxidase) (S, P)
  21–43 mg/dL (1.3–2.7 µmol/L)

Chloride (S, P)
  Premature infants: 95–110 mmol/L
  Full-term infants: 96–116 mmol/L
  Children: 98–105 mmol/L
  Adults: 98–108 mmol/L

Cholesterol, Total (S, P)
  Values in mg/dL (mmol/L)

Group	Males	Females
6–7 y	115–197 (2.97–5.09)	126–199 (3.25–5.14)
8–9 y	112–199 (2.89–5.14)	124–208 (3.20–5.37)
10–11 y	108–220 (2.79–5.68)	115–208 (2.97–5.37)
12–13 y	117–202 (3.02–5.21)	114–207 (2.94–5.34)
14–15 y	103–207 (2.66–5.34)	102–208 (2.63–5.37)
16–17 y	107–198 (2.76–5.11)	106–213 (2.73–5.50)

Coagulation Factors (P)
  Values in U/mL. Shown are mean values and –2 SD or lower range (in parentheses).

Factor	Preterm (25–32 wk)	Term Infant	Infant (6 mo)	Adult
II	0.32 (0.18)	0.52 (0.25)	0.88 (0.60)	1.0 (0.7)
V	0.80 (0.43)	1.00 (0.54)	0.91 (0.55)	1.0 (0.6)
VII	0.37 (0.24)	0.57 (0.35)	0.87 (0.50)	1.0 (0.6)
VIII	0.75 (0.40)	1.50 (0.55)	0.90 (0.50)	1.0 (0.6)
vWF	1.50 (0.90)	1.60 (0.84)	1.07 (0.60)	1.0 (0.6)
IX	0.22 (0.17)	0.35 (0.15)	0.86 (0.36)	1.0 (0.5)
X	0.38 (0.20)	0.45 (0.30)	0.78 (0.38)	1.0 (0.6)
XI	0.20 (0.12)	0.42 (0.20)	0.86 (0.38)	1.0 (0.6)
XII	0.22 (0.09)	0.44 (0.16)	0.77 (0.39)	1.0 (0.6)
XIII	. . .	0.61 (0.36)	1.04 (0.50)	1.0 (0.6)
PreK	0.26 (0.14)	0.35 (0.16)	0.86 (0.56)	1.1 (0.6)

vWF = von Willebrand factor, PreK = prekallikrein.

Complement (S)
  C3: 96–195 mg/dL
  C4: 15–20 mg/dL
Copper (S)
  Cord blood: 26–32 µg/dL (4.1–5.2 µmol/L)
  Newborns: 26–32 µg/dL (4.1–5.2 µmol/L)
  1 mo: 73–93 µg/dL (11.5–14.6 µmol/L)

  2 mo: 59–69 µg/dL (9.3–10.9 µmol/L)
  6 mo–5 y: 27–153 µg/dL (4.2–24.1 µmol/L)
  5–17 y: 94–234 µg/dL (14.8–36.8 µmol/L)
  Adults: 70–118 µg/dL (11–18.6 µmol/L)

Copper Oxidase: See Ceruloplasmin.

Cortisol (S, P)
  Morning (8:00 AM): 5–25 µg/dL (0.14–0.68 µmol/L)
  Evening: 5–15 µg/dL (0.14–0.41 µmol/L)

Creatine (S, P)
  0.2–0.8 mg/dL (15.2–61 mmol/L)

Creatine Kinase (S, P)
  Newborns (1–3 d): 40–474 IU/L at 37 °C
  Adult males: 30–210 IU/L at 37 °C
  Adult females: 20–128 IU/L at 37 °C

Creatinine (S,P)
  Values in mg/dL (µmol/L)

Group	Males	Females
Newborns (1–3 d)[1]	0.2–1.0 (17.7–88.4)	0.2–1.0 (17.7–88.4)
1 y	0.2–0.6 (17.7–53.0)	0.2–0.5 (17.7–44.2)
2–3 y	0.2–0.7 (17.7–61.9)	0.3–0.6 (26.5–53.0)
4–7 y	0.2–0.8 (17.7–70.7)	0.2–0.7 (17.7–61.9)
8–10 y	0.3–0.9 (26.5–79.6)	0.3–0.8 (26.5–70.7)
11–12 y	0.3–1.0 (26.5–88.4)	0.3–0.9 (26.5–79.6)
13–17 y	0.3–1.2 (26.5–106.1)	0.3–1.1 (26.5–97.2)
18–20 y	0.5–1.3 (44.2–115.0)	0.3–1.1 (26.5–97.2)

[1]Values may be higher in premature newborns.

Creatinine Clearance
  Values show great variability and depend on the specificity of the analytical methods used.
  Newborns (1 d): 5–50 mL/min/1.73 m (mean, 18 mL/min/1.73 m)
  Newborns (6 d): 15–90 mL/min/1.73 m² (mean, 36 mL/min/1.73 m²)
  Adult males: 85–125 mL/min/1.73 m²
  Adult females: 75–115 mL/min/1.73 m²

2,3-Diphosphoglycerate (B)
  Values vary with the method used and with altitude.
  4.5–6 mmol/L

Factor: See Anticoagulation Factors and Coagulation Factors.

Fatty Acids, "Free" (P)
  Newborns: 435–1375 µeq/L
  4 mo–10 y (14-h fast): 500–900 µeq/L
  4 mo–10 y (19-h fast): 730–1200 µeq/L
  Adults (14-h fast): 310–590 µeq/L
  Adults (19-h fast): 405–720 µeq/L

Ferritin (S)
  Newborns: 20–200 ng/mL (mean, 117 ng/mL)
  1 mo: 60–550 ng/mL (mean, 350 ng/mL)
  1–15 y: 7–140 ng/mL (mean, 31 ng/mL)
  Adult males: 50–225 ng/mL (mean, 140 ng/mL)
  Adult females: 10–150 ng/mL (mean, 40 ng/mL)

Fibrinogen (P)
  200–500 mg/dL (5.9–14.7 µmol/L)

(continued)

Table 42–1. Normal blood chemistry values and miscellaneous other hematologic values.[1]
(Values may vary with the procedure used.) (continued)

Galactose (S, P)
1.1–2.1 mg/dL (0.06–0.12 mmol/L)

Galactose 1-Phosphate (RBC)
Normal: 1 mg/dL of packed erythrocyte lysate; slightly higher in cord blood
Infants with congenital galactosemia on a milk-free diet: <2 mg/dL
Infants with congenital galactosemia taking milk: 9–20 mg/dL

Galactose-1-Phosphate Uridyl Transferase (RBC)
Normal: 308–475 mIU/g of hemoglobin
Heterozygous for Duarte variant: 225–308 mIU/g of hemoglobin
Homozygous for Duarte variant: 142–225 mIU/g of hemoglobin
Heterozygous for congenital galactosemia: 142–225 mIU/g of hemoglobin
Homozygous for congenital galactosemia: <8 mIU/g of hemoglobin

Glomerular Filtration Rate
Newborns: About 50% of values for older children and adults
Older children and adults: 75–165 mL/min/1.73 m^2 (levels reached by about 6 mo)

Glucose (S, P)
Premature infants: 20–80 mg/dL (1.11–4.44 mmol/L)
Full-term infants: 30–100 mg/dL (1.67–5.56 mmol/L)
Children and adults (fasting): 60–105 mg/dL (3.33–5.88 mmol/L)

Glucose-6-Phosphate Dehydrogenase (RBC)
150–215 U/dL

Glucose Tolerance Test (S): See Table (p. 1128).

γ-Glutamyl Transpeptidase (S)
0–1 mo: 12–271 IU/L at 37 °C (kinetic)
1–2 mo: 9–159 IU/L at 37 °C (kinetic)
2–4 mo: 7–98 IU/L at 37 °C (kinetic)
4–7 mo: 5–45 IU/L at 37 °C (kinetic)
7–12 mo: 4–27 IU/L at 37 °C (kinetic)
1–15 y: 3–30 IU/L at 37 °C (kinetic)
Adult males: 9–69 IU/L at 37 °C (kinetic)
Adult females: 3–33 IU/L at 37 °C (kinetic)

Glycohemoglobin (Hemoglobin A$_{1c}$) (B)
Normal: 6.3–8.2% of total hemoglobin
Diabetic patients in good control of their condition ordinarily have levels <10%
Values tend to be lower during pregnancy; they also vary with technique

Growth Hormone (GH) (S)
After infancy (fasting specimen): 0–5 ng/mL
In response to natural and artificial provocation (eg, sleep, arginine, insulin, hypoglycemia): >8 ng/mL
During the newborn period (fasting specimen), GH levels are high (15–40 ng/mL) and responses to provocation are variable

Haptoglobin (S)
50–150 mg/dL has hemoglobin-binding capacity.

Hematocrit (B)
At birth: 44–64%
14–90 d: 35–49%
6 mo–1 y: 30–40%
4–10 y: 31–43%

Hemoglobin A$_{1c}$: See Glycohemoglobin

Hemoglobin Electrophoresis (B)
A$_1$ hemoglobin: 96–98.5% of total hemoglobin
A$_2$ hemoglobin: 1.5–4% of total hemoglobin

Hemoglobin, Fetal (B)
At birth: 50–85% of total hemoglobin
At 1 y: <15% of total hemoglobin
Up to 2 y: Up to 5% of total hemoglobin
Thereafter: <2% of total hemoglobin

Immunoglobulins (S)
Values in mg/dL

Group	IgG	IgA	IgM
Cord blood	766–1693	0.04–9	4–26
2 wk–3 mo	299–852	3–66	15–149
3–6 mo	142–988	4–90	18–118
6–12 mo	418–1142	14–95	43–223
1–2 y	356–1204	13–118	37–239
2–3 y	492–1269	23–137	49–204
3–6 y	564–1381	35–209	51–214
6–9 y	658–1535	29–384	50–228
9–12 y	625–1598	60–294	64–278
12–16 y	660–1548	81–252	45–256

Glucose tolerance test results in serum.

Normal levels based on results in 13 normal children given glucose.
1.75 g/kg orally in one dose, after 2 wk on a high-carbohydrate diet.

Time	Glucose		Insulin		Phosphorus	
	mg/dL	mmol/L	μU/mL	pmol/L	mg/dL	mmol/L
Fasting	59–96	3.11–5.33	5–40	36–287	3.2–4.9	1.03–1.58
30 min	91–185	5.05–10.27	36–110	258–789	2.0–4.4	0.64–1.42
60 min	66–164	3.66–9.10	22–124	158–890	1.8–3.6	0.58–1.16
90 min	68–148	3.77–8.22	17–105	122–753	1.8–3.6	0.58–1.16
2 h	66–122	3.66–6.77	6–84	43–603	1.8–4.2	0.58–1.36
3 h	47–99	2.61–5.49	2–46	14–330	2.0–4.6	0.64–1.48
4 h	61–93	3.39–5.16	3–32	21–230	2.7–4.3	0.87–1.39
5 h	63–86	3.50–4.77	5–37	36–265	2.9–4.4	0.94–1.42

(continued)

Table 42–1. Normal blood chemistry values and miscellaneous other hematologic values.[1]
(Values may vary with the procedure used.) (continued)

Insulin: See Glucose Tolerance Test and Table (top of page).

Inulin Clearance
<1 mo: 29–88 mL/min/1.73 m²
1–6 mo: 40–112 mL/min/1.73 m²
6–12 mo: 62–121 mL/min/1.73 m²
<1 y: 78–164 mL/min/1.73 m²

Iron (S, P)
Newborns: 20–157 µg/dL (3.6–28.1 µmol/L)
6 wk–3 y: 20–115 µg/dL (3.6–20.6 µmol/L)
3–9 y: 20–141 µg/dL (3.6–25.2 µmol/L)
9–14 y: 21–151 µg/dL (3.8–27 µmol/L)
14–16 y: 20–181 µg/dL (3.6–32.4 µmol/L)
Adults: 44–196 µg/dL (7.2–31.3 µmol/L)

Iron-Binding Capacity (S, P)
Newborns: 59–175 µg/dL (10.6–31.3 µmol/L)
Children and adults: 275–458 µg/dL (45–72 µmol/L)

Lactate (B)
Venous blood: 5–18 mg/dL (0.5–2 mmol/L)
Arterial blood: 3–7 mg/dL (0.3–0.8 mmol/L)

Lactate Dehydrogenase (LDH) (S, P)
Values using lactate substrate (kinetic)
Newborns (1–3 d): 40–348 IU/L at 37 °C
1 mo–5 y: 150–360 IU/L at 37 °C
5–8 y: 150–300 IU/L at 37 °C
8–12 y: 130–300 IU/L at 37 °C
12–14 y: 130–280 IU/L at 37 °C
14–16 y: 130–230 IU/L at 37 °C
Adult males: 70–178 IU/L at 37 °C
Adult females: 42–166 IU/L at 37 °C

LDH: See Lactate Dehydrogenase.

Lead (B)
<10 µg/dL (<0.48 µmol/L)
When a large proportion of a population of children have blood lead levels in the range of 10–19 µg/dL (0.48–0.92 µmol/L), communitywide childhood lead poisoning activities are warranted.
Levels >20 µg/dL (>0.97 µmol/L) indicate the need for medical and environmental evaluation and possible pharmalogic intervention.
Levels >70 µg/dL (>3.38 µmol/L) indicate the immediate need for medical and environmental management.

Lipase (S, P)
20–136 IU/L based on 4-h incubation

Lipoprotein Cholesterol, High-Density (HDL) (S)
Values in mg/dL (mmol/L)

Group	Males	Females
6–7 y	35–77 (0.90–1.98)	24–76 (0.62–1.96)
8–9 y	31–80 (0.80–2.06)	34–77 (0.87–1.98)
10–11 y	34–81 (0.87–1.09)	30–74 (0.77–1.91)
12–13 y	30–82 (0.77–2.11)	33–73 (0.85–1.88)
14–15 y	26–72 (0.67–1.86)	29–73 (0.74–1.88)
16–17 y	25–66 (0.72–1.70)	27–78 (0.69–2.01)

Lipoprotein Cholesterol, Low-Density (LDL) (S)
Values in mg/dL (mmol/L)

Group	Males	Females
6–7 y	56–134 (1.44–3.46)	52–149 (1.34–3.85)
8–9 y	52–129 (1.34–3.33)	57–143 (1.47–3.69)
10–11 y	45–149 (1.16–3.85)	56–140 (1.44–3.61)
12–13 y	55–135 (1.42–3.48)	58–138 (1.49–3.56)
14–15 y	48–143 (1.24–3.69)	47–140 (1.21–3.61)
16–17 y	53–134 (1.36–3.36)	44–147 (1.13–3.79)

Magnesium (S, P)
Newborns: 1.5–2.3 meq/L (0.75–1.15 mmol/L)
Adults: 1.4–2 meq/L (0.7–1 mmol/L)

Methemoglobin (B)
0–0.3 g/dL (0–186 µmol/L)

Osmolality (S, P)
270–290 mosm/kg

Oxygen Capacity (B)
1.34 mL/g of hemoglobin

Oxygen Saturation (B)
Newborns: 30–80% (0.3–0.8 mol/mol of venous blood)
Thereafter: 65–85% (0.65–0.85 mol/mol of venous blood)

Paco₂: See Acid-Base Measurements.

Pao₂: See Acid-Base Measurements.

Partial Thromboplastin Time (P)
Children: 42–54 s

pH: See Acid-Base Measurements.

Phenylalanine (S, P)
0.7–3.5 mg/dL (0.04–0.21 mmol/L)

Phosphatase: See Acid Phosphatase and Alkaline Phosphatase.

Phosphorus, Inorganic (S, P)
Premature infants:
At birth: 5.6–8 mg/dL (1.81–2.58 mmol/L)
6–10 d: 6.1–11.7 mg/dL (1.97–3.78 mmol/L)
20–25 d: 6.6–9.4 mg/dL (2.13–3.04 mmol/L)
Full-term infants:
At birth: 5–7.8 mg/dL (1.61–2.52 mmol/L)
3 d: 5.8–9 mg/dL (1.87–2.91 mmol/L)
6–12 d: 4.9–8.9 mg/dL (1.58–2.87 mmol/L)
Children:
1 y: 3.8–6.2 mg/dL (1.23–2 mmol/L)
10 y: 3.6–5.6 mg/dL (1.16–1.81 mmol/L)
Adults: 3.1–5.1 mg/dL (1–1.65 mmol/L)
(See also Glucose Tolerance Test.)

Potassium (S, P)
Premature infants: 4.5–7.2 mmol/L
Full-term infants: 3.7–5.2 mmol/L
Children: 3.5–5.8 mmol/L
Adults: 3.5–5.5 mmol/L

Prealbumin: See Transthyretin.

Proteins (S): SeeTable (top of page 1129).

Prothrombin Time (P)
Children: 11–15 s

(continued)

Table 42–1. Normal blood chemistry values and miscellaneous other hematologic values.[1]
(Values may vary with the procedure used.) (continued)

Proteins in serum.

Values are for cellulose acetate electrophoresis and are
in g/dL. SI conversion factor: g/dL × 10 = g/L.

Group	Total Protein	Albumin	α_1-Globulin	α_2-Globulin	β-Globulin	λ-Globulin
At birth	4.6–7.0	3.2–4.8	0.1–0.3	0.2–0.3	0.3–0.6	0.6–1.2
3 mo	4.5–6.5	3.2–4.8	0.1–0.3	0.3–0.7	0.3–0.7	0.2–0.7
1 y	5.4–7.5	3.7–5.7	0.1–0.3	0.5–1.1	0.4–1.0	0.2–0.9
>4 y	5.9–8.0	3.8–5.4	0.1–0.3	0.4–0.8	0.5–1.0	0.4–1.3

Protoporphyrin, "Free" (FEP, ZPP) (B)
Values for free erythrocyte protoporphyrin (FEP) and zinc
protoporphyrin (ZPP) are 1.2–2.7 µg/g of hemoglobin.

Pyruvate (B)
Resting adult males (arterial blood): 50.5–60.1 µmol/L
Adults (venous blood): 34–102 µmol/L

Retinol-Binding Protein (S)

3–5 y	1.0–5.0 mg/dL
6–8 y	1.5–5.9 mg/dL
9–11 y	1.5–6.5 mg/dL
12–16 y	1.5–7.0 mg/dL

Sedimentation Rate (Micro) (B)
<2 y: 1–5 mm/h
>2 y: 1–8 mm/h

SGOT: See Aspartate Aminotransferase.

SGPT: See Alanine Aminotransferase.

Sodium (S, P)
Children and adults: 135–148 mmol/L

Sugar: See Glucose.

T_3: See Triiodothyronine.

T_4: See Thyroxine.

TBG: See Thyroxine-Binding Globulin.

Thrombin Time (P)
Children: 12–16 s

Thyroid-Stimulating Hormone (TSH) (S)
Values in µIU/mL

	Males	Females
1–30 d	0.52–16.0	0.72–13.1
1 mo–5 y	0.55–7.1	0.46–8.1
6–18 y	0.37–6.0	0.36–5.8

Thyroxine (T_4) (S)
1–2 d: 11.4–25.5 µg/dL (147–328 nmol/L)
3–4 d: 9.8–25.2 µg/dL (126–324 nmol/L)
1–6 y: 5–15.2 µg/dL (64–196 nmol/L)
11–13 y: 4–13 µg/dL (51–167 nmol/L)
>18 y: 4.7–11 µg/dL (60–142 nmol/L)

Thyroxine, "Free" (Free T_4) (S)
1–2.3 ng/dL

Thyroxine-Binding Globulin (TBG) (S)
1–7 mo: 2.9–6 mg/dL

7–12 mo: 2.1–5.9 mg/dL
Prepubertal children: 2–5.3 mg/dL
Pubertal children and adults: 1.8–4.2 mg/dL

α-Tocopherol: See Vitamin E.

Transaminase: See Alanine Aminotransferase and
Aspartate Aminotransferase.

Transthyretin (S, P)
2–5 mo: 14–33 mg/dL
6–11 mo: 12–27 mg/dL
12–17 mo: 11–26 mg/dL
18–23 mo: 14–24 mg/dL
24–36 mo: 11–26 mg/dL
3–5 y: 9.1–33.0 mg/dL
6–8 y: 15.3–45.5 mg/dL
9–11 y: 16.0–47.6 mg/dL
12–16 y: 19.0–50.0 mg/dL

Triglyceride (S, P)
Fasting (>12 h) values in mg/mL (mmol/L)

Group	Males	Females
6–7 y	32–79 (0.36–0.89)	24–128 (0.27–1.44)
8–9 y	28–105 (0.31–1.18)	34–115 (0.38–1.29)
10–11 y	30–115 (0.33–1.29)	39–131 (0.44–1.48)
12–13 y	33–112 (0.37–1.26)	36–125 (0.40–1.41)
14–15 y	35–136 (0.39–1.53)	36–122 (0.40–1.37)
16–17 y	38–167 (0.42–1.88)	34–136 (0.38–1.53)

Note: Lower values represent the 5th percentile, whereas
upper values are calculated from the mean + 2 SD.

Triiodothyronine (T_3) (S)
1–3 d: 89–405 ng/dL
1 wk: 91–300 ng/dL
1–12 mo: 85–250 ng/dL
Prepubertal children: 119–218 ng/dL
Pubertal children and adults: 55–170 ng/dL

TSH: See Thyroid-Stimulating Hormone.

Tyrosine (S, P)
Premature infants: 3–30.2 mg/dL (0.17–1.67 mmol/L)
Full-term infants: 1.7–4.7 mg/dL (0.09–0.26 mmol/L)
1–12 y: 1.4–3.4 mg/dL (0.08–0.19 mmol/L)
Adults: 0.6–1.6 mg/dL (0.03–0.09 mmol/L)

Urea Clearance
Premature infants: 3.5–17.3 mL/min/1.73 m²
Newborns: 8.7–33 mL/min/1.73 m²
2–12 mo: 40–95 mL/min/1.73 m²
≥2 y: >52 mL/min/1.73 m²

Urea Nitrogen (S, P)
1–2 y: 5–15 mg/dL (1.8–5.4 mmol/L)
Thereafter: 10–20 mg/dL (3.5–7.1 mmol/L)

(continued)

Table 42–1. Normal blood chemistry values and miscellaneous other hematologic values.[1]
(Values may vary with the procedure used.) (continued)

Uric Acid (S, P)
Males:
  0–14 y: 2–7 mg/dL (119–416 µmol/L)
  >14 y: 3–8 mg/dL (178–476 µmol/L)
Females:
  0–14 y: 2–7 mg/dL (119–416 µmol/L)
  >14 y: 2–7 mg/dL (119–416 µmol/L)

Vitamin A (S, P)
Total vitamin A: 19–81 µg/dL (0.66–2.82 µmol/L)
Retinol: 19–77 µg/dL (0.66–2.68 µmol/L)
Retinyl esters: 0.1–4.7 µg/dL (0.01–0.16 µmol/L)

Vitamin C (Ascorbic Acid) (S, P)
0.2–2 mg/dL (11–114 µmol/L)

Vitamin D (S)
1,25-Dihydroxycholecalciferol:
  Normal: 37 ± 12 pg/mL
  X-linked vitamin D–resistant disease: 16 ± 8 pg/mL
  Vitamin D dependency: 9.5 ± 3 pg/mL in type I. Normal
    in type II.
  Hypophosphatemic bone disease: 30 ± 6 pg/mL
  Lead poisoning: 20 ± 1 pg/mL
25-Hydroxycholecalciferol:
  Normal: 26–31 ng/mL

Vitamin E (Tocopherol) (S, P)
α-Tocopherol:
  <12 y: 3.8–15.5 µg/mL (9.1–37.2 µmol/L)
  >12 y: 4.7–203 µg/mL (11.3–48.7 µmol/L)
γ-Tocopherol:
  The γ isomer contributes 10–20% of the total
    tocopherols in plasma but is only 10% as active as the
    α form in vivo.
Vitamin E status is best assessed by performing chromatographic separation of the isomers and determining both
  α- and γ-tocopherol levels. Levels should be expressed
  in terms of vitamin E/total lipid ratio:
  <12 y: >0.6 mg/g (>1.4 µmol/g)
  >12 y: >0.8 mg/g (>1.9 µmol/g)

Volume (B)
Premature infants: 98 mL/kg (mean)
Full-term infants: 75–100 mL/kg
1 y: 69–112 mL/kg (mean, 86 mL/kg)
Older children: 51–86 mL/kg (mean, 70 mL/kg)

Volume (P)
Full-term neonates: 39–77 mL/kg
Infants: 40–50 mL/kg
Older children: 30–54 mL/kg

Water (B, S, RBC)
Whole blood: 79–81 g/dL
Serum: 91–92 g/dL
Red blood cells: 64–65 g/dL

Xylose Absorption Test (B)
Following a 5-g loading dose, the laboratory will report the
  D-xylose concentration of the baseline and 60-min
  samples in mg/dL. The difference between these 2
  values should be corrected to a constant surface area of
  1.73 m[2] according to the formula shown below.
The actual surface area can be derived from a number of
  available nomograms using the patient's weight and
  height.
Normal corrected blood values[2]: 9.8–20 mg/dL
Effect of age and sex: No significant differences between
  males and females. No significant differences in ages
  14–92 y.

Zinc (S)
Males: 83–88 µg/dL (12.7–13.5 µmol/L)
Females: 85–91 µg/dL (13–13.9 µmol/L)
Females taking oral contraceptives: 86–93 µg/dL
  (13.2–14.2 µmol/L)
At 16 wk of gestation: 66–70 µg/dL (10.1–10.7 µmol/L)
At 38 wk of gestation: 54–58 µg/dL (8.3–8.9 µmol/L)

---

[1]Adapted from Meites S (editor): *Pediatric Clinical Chemistry,* 2nd ed. American Association for Clinical Chemistry, 1982, and
many other sources.

[2]

$$\text{Corrected blood value} = \frac{(\text{Value}_{60\,\text{min}} - \text{Value}_{\text{baseline}}) \times \text{Actual surface area}}{1.73}$$

Table 42–2. Normal values: urine, duodenal fluid, feces, sweat, and miscellaneous.[1]

URINE

Acidity, Titratable
20–50 meq/d

Addis Count
Red blood cells (12-h specimen): <1 million
White blood cells (12-h specimen): <2 million
Casts (12-h specimen): <10,000
Protein (12-h specimen): <55 mg

Albumin
First mo: 1–100 mg/L
Second month: 0.2–34 mg/L
2–12 mo: 0.5–19 mg/L

δ-**Aminolevulinic Acid:** See Porphyrins.

Ammonia
2–12 mo: 4–20 μeq/min/m^2
1–16 y: 6–16 μeq/min/m^2

Calcium
4–12 y: 4–8 meq/L (2–4 mmol/L)

Catecholamines (Norepinephrine, Epinephrine)
Values in μg/24 h (nmol/24 h)
(See Table, bottom of page.)

Chloride
Infants: 1.7–8.5 mmol/24 h
Children: 17–34 mmol/24 h
Adults: 140–240 mmol/24 h

Copper
0–30 μg/24 h

Coproporphyrin: See Porphyrins.

Creatine
18–58 mg/L (1.37–4.42 mmol/L)

Creatinine
Newborns: 7–10 mg/kg/24 h
Children: 20–30 mg/kg/24 h
Adult males: 21–26 mg/kg/24 h
Adult females: 16–22 mg/kg/24 h

Epinephrine: See Catecholamines.

Homovanillic Acid
Children: 3–16 μg/mg of creatinine
Adults: 2–4 μg/mg of creatinine

5-Hydroxyindoleacetic Acid
0.11–0.61 μmol/kg/7 h, based on results in 15 well-nourished, apparently healthy, mentally defective children on a tryptophan load

Hydroxyproline, Total
5–14 y: 38–126 mg/24 h (290–961 μmol/24 h)

Mercury
<50 μg/24 h (249 nmol/24 h)

Metanephrine and Normetanephrine
<2 y: <4.6 μg/mg of creatinine (23.3 nmol)
2–10 y: <3 μg/mg of creatinine (15.2 nmol)
10–15 y: <2 μg/mg of creatinine (10.3 nmol)
>15 y: <1 μg/mg of creatinine (5.1 nmol)

Mucopolysaccharides
Acid mucopolysaccharide screen should yield negative results. Positive results after dialysis of the urine should be followed up with a thin-layer chromatogram for evaluation of the acid mucopolysaccharide excretion pattern.

Norepinephrine: See Catecholamines.

Normetanephrine: See Metanephrine and Normetanephrine.

Osmolality
Infants: 50–600 mosm/L
Older children: 50–1400 mosm/L

Phosphorus, Tubular Reabsorption
78–97%

Porphobilinogen: See Porphyrins.

Porphyrins
δ-Aminolevulinic acid: 0–7 mg/24 h (0–53.4 μmol/24 h)
Porphobilinogen: 0–2 mg/24 h (0–8.8 μmol/24 h)
Coproporphyrin: 0–160 μg/24 h (0–244 nmol/24 h)
Uroporphyrin: 0–26 μg/24 h (0–31 nmol/24 h)

Potassium
26–123 mmol/L

Sodium
Infants: 0.3–3.5 mmol/24 h (6–10 mmol/m^2)
Children and adults: 5.6–17 mmol/24 h

Urobilinogen
<3 mg/24 h (<5.1 μmol/24 h)

Uroporphyrin: See Porphyrins.

Vanilmandelic Acid (VMA)
Because of the difficulty in obtaining an accurately timed 24-h collection, values based on micrograms per milligram of creatinine are the most reliable indications of VMA excretion in young children.
1–12 mo: 1–35 μg/mg of creatinine
(31–135 μg/kg/24 h)

Catecholamines in urine.

Group	Total Catecholamines	Norepinephrine	Epinephrine
<1 y	20	5.4–15.9 (32–94)	0.1–4.3 (0.5–23.5)
1–5 y	40	8.1–30.8 (48–182)	0.8–9.1 (4.4–49.7)
6–15 y	80	19.0–71.1 (112–421)	1.3–10.5 (7.1–57.3)
>15 y	100	34.4–87.0 (203–514)	3.5–13.2 (19.1–72.1)

(continued)

Table 42–2. Normal values: urine, duodenal fluid, feces, sweat, and miscellaneous.[1] (continued)

1–2 y: 1–30 µg/mg of creatinine
2–5 y: 1–15 µg/mg of creatinine
5–10 y: 1–14 µg/mg of creatinine
10–15 y: 1–10 µg/mg of creatinine (1–7 mg/24 h;
    5–35 µmol/24 h)
Adults: 1–7 µg/mg of creatinine (1–7 mg/24 h;
    5–35 µmol/24 h)

VMA: See Vanilmandelic Acid.

Xylose Absorption Test
Mean 5-h excretion expressed as a percentage
   of the ingested load
<6 mo: 11–30%
6–12 mo: 20–32%
1–3 y: 20–42%
3–10 y: 25–45%
>10 y: 25–50%
Or: % excretion > (0.2 × age [mo]) + 12

DUODENAL FLUID VALUE

Enzymes
Amylase: (Anderson)
   0–2 mo: 0–10 U/mL
   2–6 mo: 10–20 U/mL
   6–12 mo: 40–150 U/mL
   1–2 y: 100–225 U/mL
   2–5 y: 125–275 U/mL
Carboxypeptidase:
   0.4–1 U (Ravin)
Chymotrypsin:
   11–65 U (Ravin)
Protease:
   18–70 U (Free-Meyers)
Trypsin: (Anderson or as noted)
   0–2 mo: 110–160 U/mL
   2–6 mo: 115–160 U/mL
   6–12 mo: 120–290 U/mL; 3–10 U
    (Nothman et al)
   1–2 y: 200–300 U/mL
   2–5 y: 200–275 U/mL

pH
6–8.4

Viscosity
<3 min (Shwachman)

FECES

Chymotrypsin
3–14 mg/kg 72 h

Fat, Percentage of Dry Weight
2–6 mo: 5–43%
6 mo–6 y: 6–26%

Fat, Total
2–6 mo: 0.3–1.3 g/d
6 mo–1 y: <4 g/d
Children: <3 g/d
Adolescents: <5 g/d
Adults: <7 g/d

Lipids, Split Fat
Adults: >40% of total lipids

Lipids, Total
Adults: Up to 7 g/d on normal diet, 10–27% of dry weight

Nitrogen
Infants: <1 g/d
Children: <1.2 g/d
Adults: <3 g/d

Urobilinogen
2–12 mo: 0.03–14 mg/d
5–10 y: 2.7–39 mg/d
10–14 y: 7.3–99 mg/d

SWEAT

Electrolytes
Values for chloride. Elevated values in the presence of a
   family history or clinical findings of cystic fibrosis are
   diagnostic of cystic fibrosis.
Normal: <40 mmol/L
Borderline: 40–60 mmol/L
Elevated: >60 mmol/L

MISCELLANEOUS

Amylo-1,6-Glucosidase Debrancher (Liver)
>1 µmol/min/g of wet tissue

Chloride
Breast milk: 2.5–30 mmol/L
Cow's milk: 20–80 mmol/L
Muscle: 20–26 mmol/kg of wet fat-free tissue
Spinal fluid: 120–128 mmol/L

Copper (Liver)
<20 µg/g of wet tissue

Glucose-6-Phosphatase (Liver)
>5 µmol/min/g of wet tissue

Lactate Dehydrogenase (LDH) (Cerebrospinal Fluid)
17–59 IU/L at 37 °C

Potassium
Breast milk: 12–17 mmol/L
Cow's milk: 20–45 mmol/L
Muscle: 160–180 mmol/kg of wet fat-free tissue

Proteins (Cerebrospinal Fluid)
Total proteins:
   Newborn: 40–120 mg/dL (0.4–1.2 g/L)
   1 mo: 20–70 mg/dL (0.2–0.7 g/L)
   Thereafter: 15–40 mg/dL (0.15–0.4 g/L)
Gamma globulin:
   Children: Up to 9% of total
   Adults: Up to 14% of total

Sodium
Breast milk: 4.7–8.3 mmol/L
Cow's milk: 22–26 mmol/L
Muscle: 33–43 mmol/kg of wet fat-free tissue

[1]Adapted from Meites S (editor): *Pediatric Clinical Chemistry,* 2nd ed. American Association for Clinical Chemistry, 1982, and many other sources.

Table 42–3. Normal values: common hematologic measurements and indices.

RED BLOOD CELL VALUES AT VARIOUS AGES: MEAN AND LOWER LIMIT OF NORMAL (–2 SD)[1]

Age	Hemoglobin (g/dL)		Hematocrit (%)		Red Cell Count (10^{12}/L)		MCV (fl)		MCH (pg)		MCHC (g/dL)	
	Mean	–2 SD	Mean	–2 SD	Mean	–2 SD	Mean	–2 SD	Mean	–2 SD	Mean	–2 SD
Birth (cord blood)	16.5	13.5	51	42	4.7	3.9	108	98	34	31	33	30
1 to 3 d (capillary)	18.5	14.5	56	45	5.3	4.0	108	95	34	31	33	29
1 wk	17.5	13.5	54	42	5.1	3.9	107	88	34	28	33	28
2 wk	16.5	12.5	51	39	4.9	3.6	105	86	34	28	33	28
1 mo	14.0	10.0	43	31	4.2	3.0	104	85	34	28	33	29
2 mo	11.5	9.0	35	28	3.8	2.7	96	77	30	26	33	29
3–6 mo	11.5	9.5	35	29	3.8	3.1	91	74	30	25	33	30
0.5–2 y	12.0	10.5	36	33	4.5	3.7	78	70	27	23	33	30
2–6 y	12.5	11.5	37	34	4.6	3.9	81	75	27	24	34	31
6–12 y	13.5	11.5	40	35	4.6	4.0	86	77	29	25	34	31
12–18 y												
Female	14.0	12.0	41	36	4.6	4.1	90	78	30	25	34	31
Male	14.5	13.0	43	37	4.9	4.5	88	78	30	25	34	31
18–49 y												
Female	14.0	12.0	41	36	4.6	4.0	90	80	30	26	34	31
Male	15.5	13.5	47	41	5.2	4.5	90	80	30	26	34	31

NORMAL LEUKOCYTE COUNTS[2]

Age	Total Leukocytes		Neutrophils			Lymphocytes			Monocytes		Eosinophils	
	Mean	(Range)	Mean	(Range)	%	Mean	(Range)	%	Mean	%	Mean	%
Birth	18.1	(9.0–30.0)	11.0	(6.0–26.0)	61	5.5	(2.0–11.0)	31	1.1	6	0.4	2
12 h	22.8	(13.0–38.0)	15.5	(6.0–28.0)	68	5.5	(2.0–11.0)	24	1.2	5	0.5	2
24 h	18.9	(9.4–34.0)	11.5	(5.0–21.0)	61	5.8	(2.0–11.5)	31	1.1	6	0.5	2
1 wk	12.2	(5.0–21.0)	5.5	(1.5–10.0)	45	5.0	(2.0–17.0)	41	1.1	9	0.5	4
2 wk	11.4	(5.0–20.0)	4.5	(1.0–9.5)	40	5.5	(2.0–17.0)	48	1.0	9	0.4	3
1 mo	10.8	(5.0–19.5)	3.8	(1.0–9.0)	35	6.0	(2.5–16.5)	56	0.7	7	0.3	3
6 mo	11.9	(6.0–17.5)	3.8	(1.0–8.5)	32	7.3	(4.0–13.5)	61	0.6	5	0.3	3
1 y	11.4	(6.0–17.5)	3.5	(1.5–8.5)	31	7.0	(4.0–10.5)	61	0.6	5	0.3	3
2 y	10.6	(6.0–17.0)	3.5	(1.5–8.5)	33	6.3	(3.0–9.5)	59	0.5	5	0.3	3
4 y	9.1	(5.5–15.5)	3.8	(1.5–8.5)	42	4.5	(2.0–8.0)	50	0.5	5	0.3	3
6 y	8.5	(5.0–14.5)	4.3	(1.5–8.0)	51	3.5	(1.5–7.0)	42	0.4	5	0.2	3
8 y	8.3	(4.5–13.5)	4.4	(1.5–8.0)	53	3.3	(1.5–6.8)	39	0.4	4	0.2	2
10 y	8.1	(4.5–13.5)	4.4	(1.8–8.0)	54	3.1	(1.5–6.5)	38	0.4	4	0.2	2
16 y	7.8	(4.5–13.0)	4.4	(1.8–8.0)	57	2.8	(1.2–5.2)	35	0.4	5	0.2	3
21 y	7.4	(4.5–11.0)	4.4	(1.8–7.7)	59	2.5	(1.0–4.8)	34	0.3	4	0.2	3

[1]These data have been compiled from several sources. Emphasis is given to recent studies using electronic counters and to the selection of populations that are likely to exclude individuals with iron deficiency. The mean ± 2 SD can be expected to include 95% of the observations in a normal population. MCV = mean corpuscular volume, MCH = mean corpuscular hemoglobin, MCHC = mean corpuscular hemoglobin concentration. (Based on Cairo MS: In: *Pediatrics,* 20th ed. Rudolph AM [editor]. Appleton & Lange, 1996:1222. As modified in Lubin BH: Reference values in infancy and childhood. In: *Hematology of Infancy and Childhood,* 4th ed. Nathan DG, Oski FA [editors]. Saunders, 1993:Appendix iii.)

[2]Numbers of leukocytes are in thousands per cubic millimeter, ranges are estimates of 95% confidence limits, and percentages refer to differential counts. Neutrophils include band cells at all ages and a small number of metamyelocytes and myelocytes in the first few days of life. (From Cairo MS: In: *Pediatrics,* 20th ed. Rudolph AM [editor]. Appleton & Lange, 1996. As modified in Lubin BH: Reference values in infancy and childhood. In: *Hematology of Infancy and Childhood,* 4th ed. Nathan DG, Oski FA [editors]. Saunders, 1993:Appendix xi.)

Index

NOTE: Page numbers in bold face type indicate a major discussion. A *t* following a page number indicates tabular material and an *i* following a page number indicates an illustration. Drugs are listed under their generic names. When a drug trade name is listed, the reader is referred to the generic name.

A$_2$ component of second heart sound, 475
Aa$_D$O$_2$ (alveolar-arterial oxygen difference), in acute respiratory failure, 333, 333*i*, 334*t*
Aagenaes' syndrome, 574
Abdomen
    acute, **547**, 547*t*. *See also specific cause*
    assessment of
        in allergic disorders, 923
        in appendicitis, 547
        in cardiovascular disease, 478
        in newborn, 26
        in trauma patient, 296
        in intussusception, 548
Abdominal epilepsy, 560
Abdominal migraine, 560
Abdominal pain. *See also* Acute abdomen
    in celiac disease, 561
    in cholelithiasis, 589
    in pancreatitis, 600, 601
    in parasitic infections, 1062*t*
    recurrent, **560**
Abdominal surgical conditions. *See also* Acute abdomen
    in newborn, **59–62**
Abdominal wall defects, **61**
Abetalipoproteinemia, diarrhea in, 555*t*
ABO incompatibility, neonatal jaundice caused by, 49
ABO testing, 775
Abrasion, ocular, 379–380
Abrin, in Jequinty bean, poisoning due to, 324*t*
Abscesses, 365
    brain, **684–685**
        cerebrospinal fluid characteristics in, 634*t*
        mastoiditis complicated by, 412
    breast, 137*t*, 138
    liver, **592–593**, 1069, 1070
    lung, **461–462**
    nasal septum, **419**
    orbital, 389
        ethmoiditis and, 417
    peritonsillar, **421–422**
    retropharyngeal, **422**

subperiosteal, ethmoiditis and, 417
tubo-ovarian, in pelvic inflammatory disease, 1105
Absence seizures, 645*t*, 646*t*
    atypical, 645*t*, 646*t*
        electroencephalographic patterns in, 645*t*, 649
        laboratory studies in, 649*t*
    electroencephalographic patterns in, 645*t*, 649
    laboratory studies in, 649*t*
Abstinence, for contraception, 149–150
Abuse, child, **210–214**. *See also* Child abuse and neglect
    emotional, 210
        history in, 211–212
        management and reporting of, 213
        prevention of, 213
    physical, 210
        eye injuries and, 380–381
        fractures and, 716
        history in, 211, 211*t*
        management and reporting of, 213
        physical findings in, 212
        prevention of, 213
        radiologic and laboratory findings in, 212–213
        subluxation of radial head and, 715
    sexual, 210
        anal fissures and, 549
        forensic evaluation of, 213
        history in, 211, 211*t*
        management and reporting of, 213
        physical findings in, 212
        presentations of, 211, 211*t*
        prevention of, 213
    substance. *See also* Substance abuse
        by adolescent, **158–176**
        maternal
            breast-feeding and, 275
            infants affected by, **68–70**, 275
            neonatal seizures and, 68, 74*t*
ABVD regimen, for Hodgkin's disease, 790
Acanthamoeba
    encephalitis caused by, 1071
    keratitis in contact lens wearers caused by, 386, 1071

Accelerated idioventricular rhythm, 531
Acceleration-deceleration head and spinal injury, 659
Accidental injuries. *See* Trauma
Accommodative esotropia, 391
Accutane. *See* Isotretinoin
Acetaminophen
    for fever, 230
    for migraine, 658
    overdose/poisoning due to, **309**
    for pain control in critically ill child, 356
    therapeutic blood levels of, 1119*t*
    toxicity of, 309*i*
Acetate, nutritional requirements for, for intravenous nutrition, 281*i*
Acetazolamide, for seizures, 653*t*
Acetylcholine receptor protein, in myasthenia gravis, 694
Acetylcysteine, for acetaminophen overdose/poisoning, 309
Achalasia, esophageal, **537–538**
Achievement tests
    in developmental competence evaluation, 88–89, 95–96
    discrepancy with intelligence tests and, **97**
Achondroplasia, **709**
Achromatopsia, 391
Acid-base equilibrium, **1108**
Acid-base status
    in inborn errors of metabolism, 868*t*
    normal values for, 1126*t*
Acid load testing, in distal renal tubular acidosis, 625
Acid maltase deficiency, 870
Acid phosphatase, normal values for, 1126*t*
Acidemia
    arginosuccinic, 872–873
    glutaric
        type I, **879–880**
            clinical and laboratory features of, 878*t*
        type II, **880–881**
            clinical and laboratory features of, 878*t*

Myositis
  benign acute childhood, **694**
  ossificans, **714**
Myotomy, Heller, for esophageal achalasia, 538
Myotonias, 692–693*t*
  congenita (Thomsen), 692–693*t*
Myotonic dystrophy, 693–693*t*
Myringotomy, 409–410
Mysoline. *See* Primidone

Naegleria fowleri, **1065***t*, **1071**
Nafcillin, 947*t*, 954
  guidelines for use of, 949*t*
    in newborn, 951*t*
  for *Hameophilus influenzae* infection, 1042
  for staphylococcal infection, 1014
Nail polish remover, poisoning due to, 314
Nails, in psoriasis, 372
Nalidixic acid, 957
Naloxone, 356
  for diphenoxylate overdose/poisoning, 316
  emergency use of, 292*t*
Naltrexone
  for autism, 186, 208
  psychopharmacologic uses of, 208
Naphthalene, poisoning due to, **316**
Naprosyn. *See* Naproxen
Naproxen
  for dysmenorrhea, 146*t*
  for juvenile rheumatoid arthritis, 725
  for pain control in critically ill child, 356
  for spondyloarthropathy, 726
Naproxen sodium, for dysmenorrhea, 146*t*
Narcolepsy, 659
Narcotics. *See* Opioids
Nasal cannula, for oxygen therapy, 334*t*, 432
Nasal fracture, **419**
Nasal furuncle, **418**
Nasal polyps, mouth breathing and, 424
Nasal septum
  abscess of, **419**
  hematoma of, **419**
  subluxation of, **418–419**
Nasogastric intubation
  for distal intestinal obstruction, 60
  for high intestinal obstruction, 60
  for tracheoesophageal fistula and esophageal atresia, 59
  in trauma patient, 295
Nasolacrimal duct obstruction, 382
Nasolacrimal system
  disorders of, **382**
  obstruction of, 382
    tearing caused by, 375, 382
Nasopharyngeal airway, for resuscitation, 286, 290*i*
  in trauma patient, 294

Nasopharyngoscopy, fiberoptic, in adenoid assessment, 424
Nasopharynx, colonization of, in otitis media, 404–405
Natal teeth, 26, 393
National Childhood Vaccine Injury Act, 257
National Vaccine Injury Compensation Program, 257–258
National Vaccine Program, 257
Near drowning, prevention of, 225
Nearsightedness, 375
NEC. *See* Necrotizing enterocolitis
Necator americanus, 1077–1078
Neck, assessment of
  in newborn, 26
  at physical examination, 218*t*
Necrotizing enterocolitis, **61–62**
  intestinal perforation caused by, 62
Necrotizing fasciitis, 1004
Nedocromil, 927*t*, 928, 933
Needle cricothyroidotomy, for resuscitation, in trauma patient, 294
Negative nitrogen balance, management of, 283–284
Neglect. *See also* Child abuse and neglect
  emotional, 210
    history in, 212
    physical findings in, 212
    short stature and, 212, 821*t*, **823**
  physical, 210
    history in, 212
Neisseria
  gonorrhoeae (gonococcus), **1017–1020**, **1099–1100**. *See also* Gonorrhea
    antibiotic prophylaxis for exposure to, 952*t*
    antibiotics for infection caused by, 946*t*, 1097*t*
    conjunctivitis in newborn caused by, 57–58, 382–383
  meningitidis (meningococcus), **1015–1017**
    antibiotic prophylaxis for exposure to, 952*t*, 1016–1017
    antibiotics for infection caused by, 946*t*
    immunization against infection caused by, **255**, 1016
    meningitis caused by, 1016, 1017
      outcome of, 684*t*
Nematode infections, **1076–1080**. *See also specific type*
Neonatal acne, 359, 363
Neonatal Behavioral Assessment scale, 1
Neonatal circulation, **484–485**
Neonatal herpes, 56
Neonatal intensive care, **31–36**. *See also* Critical care
  general approach to, **31**
  perinatal resuscitation and, **32–35**
  transportation issues and, **32**
Neonatal jaundice. *See* Jaundice

Neonatal seizures, **74**, 646*t*
  differential diagnosis of, 74*t*
  in hypocalcemia, 67, 74*t*
  in hypoxic-ischemic encephalopathy, 71, 74*t*
  in intracranial hemorrhage, 72, 74*t*
Neonatal teeth, 393
Neoplastic disease, **781–803**. *See also specific type and* Cancer
  coma caused by, 642*t*
Neostigmine, for myasthenia gravis treatment, 695
Neostigmine test, for myasthenia gravis diagnosis, 695
Nephritis. *See also* Glomerulonephritis
  acute interstitial, **613**
Nephroblastoma (Wilms' tumor), **794–796**, 896*t*
Nephrogenic diabetes insipidus, **628**, 825
Nephrolithiasis, **627–628**
  in inflammatory bowel disease, 565*t*
Nephronophthisis, juvenile, 611, 612
Nephropathy
  IgA, 614*t*
  membranous, **616**
  mesangial, **616**
Nephrosis
  congenital, 611, **614**
  lipoid, **615**
Nephrotic syndrome. *See also* Nephropathy
  corticosteroid-resistant/relapsing focal glomerular sclerosis causing, **615–616**
  mesangial nephropathy causing, **616**
  idiopathic of childhood, **615**
Nerve deafness, mumps causing, 986
Nervous system. *See also* Central nervous system
  assessment of, **631–639**
  congenital malformations of, **668–670**
  disorders of, **639–689**. *See also* Neurologic disorders
  drug toxicity and, 1122*t*
  in leptospirosis, 1057
  in shock, 344, 344–345
Neural tube defects, **668**, **906–908**
Neuroaxonal degeneration (Seitelberger's disease), 676*t*
Neuroblastoma, **793–794**
  diarrhea associated with, 554*t*
  orbital, 390
Neurocutaneous dysplasia, **672–675**
Neurocysticercosis, 1080–1081
Neuroectodermal tumors, 664*t*, 787
Neurofibromatosis, **672–673**, **900–901**, 900*i*
  café au lait spots in, 360, 672, 901
Neurogenic (central) diabetes insipidus, **825–826**
Neurohypophysis (posterior pituitary gland), **825–826**
Neuroleptic malignant syndrome, 205

diagnostic tests for, 961*t*
immunization against, **244–245**. *See also* MMR vaccine
pharyngitis in, 420
Rufen. *See* Ibuprofen
Runyon classification, of mycobacteria, 1048–1049

S₁, 475
S₂, 475
   splitting of, 475
      in valvular aortic stenosis, 500
S₃, 475, 476
S₄, 475, 476
Saber shins, in syphilis, 1054
Sabin vaccine (OPV vaccine), 243–244
   adverse effects of, 244
   contraindications/precautions for, 236*t*
   schedule of administration for, 239*t*, 240*t*, 244
Sacral agenesis, 906–908
Sacral lipomas, 906–908
"Saddle" nose deformity, in syphilis, 1054
St. Louis encephalitis, 983*t*
Salicylates. *See also* Aspirin
   for juvenile rheumatoid arthritis, 725–726
   overdose/poisoning due to, **325–326**, 326*i*
   Reye's syndrome and, 598
Salivary gland disorders, **426**
   mumps, 985, 986
Salk vaccine (IPV), 243–244
   adverse effects of, 244
   contraindications/precautions for, 236*t*, 237*t*
   schedule of administration for, 244
Salmeterol, 926*t*
   for asthma, 933
Salmon patch, 361
Salmonella
   antibiotics for infection caused by, 946*t*, 1030–1031, 1032
   choleraesuis, 1029
   enteritidis, 1029
   gastroenteritis caused by, **1029–1031**
   hirschfeldii, 1031
   paratyphi A, 1031
   schottmülleri, 1031
   typhi, 1029, 1031
      immunization against, 254–255, 1032
Salpingitis, gonococcal, 1018, 1019
Salt, for Addison's disease, 849
Salt restriction, heart failure and, 487
Sandhoff disease, 676*t*, 884*t*
Sandpaper rash, in scarlet fever, 1003
Sanfilippo syndrome, 883*t*
Sani-Clor, poisoning due to, 313
Saquinavir, for HIV infection/AIDS, 998
Sarcoma
   Ewing's, **796–797**
   Kaposi's, in HIV infection/AIDS, 995

Scabies (*Sarcoptes scabei*), 369, 938, 1104
   treatment of, 1098*t*
Scald burns, in physically abused child, 212
Scalded skin syndrome, 365–366, 1012, 1013
   rash in, 968*t*, 1012
Scales of Independent Behavior, 94*t*, 96
Scales (skin), 357
Scapulohumeral muscular dystrophy (Erb's muscular dystrophy), 690–691*t*
Scar, 357
Scarf sign, in newborn, maturity evaluation and, 25*t*
Scarlet fever
   staphylococcal, rash in, 967*t*
   streptococcal
      differential diagnosis of, 1005
      rash in, 967*t*, 1003
Scheie syndrome, 883*t*
Schema, in Piaget's developmental theory, 2
Scheuemann's disease, 719*t*
Schistosoma (schistosomiasis), **1082–1083**
   haematobium, 1083
   japonicum, 1083
   mansoni, 1083
   mekongi, 1083
Schizophrenia, childhood, 185, **187**
   psychopharmacologic treatment of, 201*t*, 205–206
Schönlein-Henoch purpura. *See* Henoch-Schönlein purpura
School-age child
   anxiety sources and, 183*t*
   growth and development in
      in early childhood (ages 5 to 7), **15**, 16–17*t*
      in middle childhood (ages 7 to 11), **15**, 17*t*
   with HIV infection/AIDS, 1000
   parenthood issues and, 178
   percentile standards for weight and height in, 7–8*t*
   preventive health care services for, 219*t*
   psychosocial assessment of, interview for, 179–181
School avoidance/phobia, **135**, **190–192**
   differential diagnosis of, 191*t*
   recurrent abdominal pain and, 560
   recurrent pharyngitis and, 421
School failure, **135–137**, 136*t*
Schüffner's dots, in malaria, 1067*t*
Schwachman's syndrome, 602, 756
   diarrhea in, 554*t*
SCID. *See* Severe combined immunodeficiency disease
Sclera, laceration of, 379
Scleroderma, diffuse (progressive systemic sclerosis), **729**

Sclerosing cholangitis, primary, 590–591*t*
   in inflammatory bowel disease, 565*t*
Sclerotherapy, for esophageal varices, 560
Scoliosis, **466**, **709–710**
Scopolamine, overdose/poisoning due to, **312**
Scorpion stings, **326–327**
Scotochromogens (PPD-G), 1048–1049
Screening tests, **221–223**
   for adolescent substance abuse
      clinical instruments for, **166**
      context of, **160–161**
      medical assessment and, 166–167, 166*t*
      pharmacologic, 167–169
      physical and physiologic, **166–169**
      urine, 168–169
   for anemia, 222
   for bacteriuria, 222
   for bleeding disorders, 761
   for cystic fibrosis, 903
   for group B streptococcal infection, 1007–1008
   for hearing loss, 414–415
   for hypercholesterolemia/hyperlipidemia, 222
   for hypothyroidism, 221, 830
   for inborn errors of metabolism, **869**
   interpretation of, 1124–1125, 1125*i*
   for lead toxicity, 222
   in newborn, 27–28, 221–222
      for hearing, 414
   in pediatric historical database, 217*t*
   for phenylketonuria, 221, 873, 1125*i*
   for psychosocial problems and psychiatric disorders, **178–179**
   sensitivity and specificity of, 1124–1125, 1125*i*
   for sexually transmitted disorders, 223, **1096**
   for sickle cell disease, 748
   for syphilis, 1055, 1096
   for tuberculosis, 223, 1046, 1046*t*
      in HIV infection/AIDS, 999–1000
Scrotal tongue, 425
Seasonal allergic rhinitis (hay fever), 418, 935–936
   immunotherapy for, 925, 936
   mouth breathing and, 424, 936
Sebaceous follicles, obstruction of in acne, 364
Sebaceous gland hyperplasia, in newborn, 359
Sebaceous nevus of Judassohn, 362
Seborrheic dermatitis, 371, 937
Seckel's dwarfism, 823
Second-degree heart block, **532**, 533*i*
Second heart sound, 475
   split, 475
      in valvular aortic stenosis, 500
Second malignancies, cancer treatment and, 803

Basic Gynecology and Obstetrics
Gant & Cunningham
1993, ISBN 0-8385-9633-9, A9633-7

Review of General Psychiatry, 4/e
Goldman
1995, ISBN 0-8385-8421-7, A8421-8

Principles of Clinical Electrocardiography, 13/e
Goldschlager & Goldman
1990, ISBN 0-8385-7951-5, A7951-5

Medical Epidemiology, 2/e
Greenberg, Daniels, Flanders, Eley, & Boring
1995, ISBN 0-8385-6206-X, A6206-5

Basic and Clinical Endocrinology, 5/e
Greenspan & Strewler
1997, ISBN 0-8385-0588-0, A0588-2

Occupational Medicine
LaDou
1990, ISBN 0-8385-7207-3, A7207-2

Clinical Anesthesiology, 2/e
Morgan & Mikhail
1996, ISBN 0-8385-1381-6, A1381-1

Basic Surgery
Niederhuber
1997, ISBN 0-8385-0509-0, A0509-8

Dermatology
Orkin, Maibach, & Dahl
1991, ISBN 0-8385-1288-7, A1288-8

Rudolph's Fundamentals of Pediatrics
Rudolph & Kamei
1994, ISBN 0-8385-8233-8, A8233-7

Genetics in Primary Care & Clinical Medicine
Seashore
1995, ISBN 0-8385-3128-8, A3128-4

Clinical Thinking in Surgery
Sterns
1989, ISBN 0-8385-5686-8, A5686-9

The Principles and Practice of Medicine, 23/e
Stobo, Hellman, Ladenson, Petty, & Traill
1996, ISBN 0-8385-7963-9, A7963-0

Smith's General Urology, 14/e
Tanagho & McAninch
1995, ISBN 0-8385-8612-0, A8612-2

General Ophthalmology, 14/e
Vaughan, Asbury, & Riordan-Eva
1995, ISBN 0-8385-3127-X, A3127-6

Clinical Oncology
Weiss
1993, ISBN 0-8385-1325-5, A1325-8

CURRENT Clinical References

CURRENT Critical Care Diagnosis & Treatment, 2/e
Bongard & Sue
1997, ISBN 0-8385-1454-5, A1454-6

CURRENT Diagnosis & Treatment in Cardiology
Crawford
1995, ISBN 0-8385-1444-8, A1444-7

CURRENT Diagnosis & Treatment in Vascular Surgery
Dean, Yao, & Brewster
1995, ISBN 0-8385-1351-4, A1351-4

CURRENT Obstetric & Gynecologic Diagnosis & Treatment, 9/e
DeCherney
1997, ISBN 0-8385-1401-4, A1401-7

CURRENT Diagnosis & Treatment in Gastroenterology
Grendell, McQuaid, & Friedman
1996, ISBN 0-8385-1448-0, A1448-8

CURRENT Pediatric Diagnosis & Treatment, 13/e
Hay, Groothius, Hayward, & Levin
1997, ISBN 0-8385-1400-6, A1400-9

CURRENT Emergency Diagnosis & Treatment, 4/e
Saunders & Ho
1992, ISBN 0-8385-1347-6, A1347-2

CURRENT Diagnosis & Treatment in Orthopedics
Skinner
1995, ISBN 0-8385-1009-4, A1009-8

CURRENT Medical Diagnosis & Treatment 1997, 36/e
Tierney, McPhee, & Papadakis
1997, ISBN 0-8385-1489-8, A1489-2

CURRENT Surgical Diagnosis & Treatment, 11/e
Way
1997, ISBN 0-8385-1456-1, A1456-1

LANGE Clinical Manuals

Dermatology
Diagnosis and Therapy
Bondi, Jegasothy, & Lazarus
1991, ISBN 0-8385-1274-7, A1274-8

Practical Oncology
Cameron
1994, ISBN 0-8385-1326-3, A1326-6

Office & Bedside Procedures
Chesnutt, Dewar, & Locksley
1993, ISBN 0-8385-1095-7, A1095-7

Psychiatry
Diagnosis & Treatment, 2/e
Flaherty, Davis, & Janicak
1993, ISBN 0-8385-1267-4, A126 7-2

Practical Gynecology
Jacobs & Gast
1994, ISBN 0-8385-1336-0, A1336-5

Drug Therapy, 2/e
Katzung
1991, ISBN 0-8385-1312-3, A1312-6

Geriatrics
Lonergan
1996, ISBN 0-8385-1094-9, A1094-0

Ambulatory Medicine
The Primary Care of Families, 2/e
Mengel & Schwiebert
1996, ISBN 0-8385-1466-9, A1466-0

Practical Pain Management
Minzter
1997, ISBN 0-8385-8116-1, A8116-4

Poisoning & Drug Overdose, 2/e
Olson
1994, ISBN 0-8385-1108-2, A1108-8

Internal Medicine
Diagnosis and Therapy, 3/e
Stein
1993, ISBN 0-8385-1112-0, A1112-0

Surgery
Diagnosis and Therapy
Stillman
1989, ISBN 0-8385-1283-6, A1283-9

Medical Perioperative Management
Wolfsthal
1989, ISBN 0-8385-1298-4, A1298-7

LANGE Handbooks

Handbook of Gynecology & Obstetrics
Brown & Crombleholme
1993, ISBN 0-8385-3608-5, A3608-5

HIV/AIDS Primary Care Handbook
Carmichael, Carmichael, & Fischl
1995, ISBN 0-8385-3557-7, A3557-4

Handbook of Poisoning, 12/e
Prevention, Diagnosis, & Treatment
Dreisbach & Robertson
1987, ISBN 0-8385-3643-3, A3643-2

Handbook of Clinical Endocrinology
Fitzgerald
1992, ISBN 0-8385-3615-8, A3615-0

Clinician's Pocket Reference, 8/e
Gomella
1997, ISBN 0-8385-1476-6, A1476-9

Neonatology
Management, Procedures, On-Call Problems, Diseases, and Drugs, 3/e
Gomella
1994, ISBN 0-8385-1331-X, A1331-6

Surgery on Call, 2/e
Gomella & Lefor
1995, ISBN 0-8385-8746-1, A8746-8

Internal Medicine On Call, 2/e
Haist, Robbins, & Gomella
1997, ISBN 0-8385-4056-2, A4056-6

Obstetrics & Gynecology On Call
Horowitz & Gomella
1993, ISBN 0-8385-7174-3, A7174-4

Pocket Guide to Commonly Prescribed Drugs, 2/e
Levine
1996, ISBN 0-8385-8099-8, A8099-2

Handbook of Pediatrics, 18/e
Merenstein, Kaplan, & Rosenberg
1997, ISBN 0-8385-3625-5, A3625-9

Pocket Guide to Diagnostic Tests, 2/e
Nicoll, McPhee, Chou, & Detmer
1997, ISBN 0-8385-8100-5, A8100-8

Quick Medical Spanish
Rogers
1996, ISBN 0-8385-8258-3, A8258-4

Pocket Guide to the Essentials of Diagnosis & Treatment
Tierney
1997, ISBN 0-8385-3605-0, A3605-1

Appleton & Lange • P.O. Box 120041 • Stamford, CT • 06912-0041